PATHOLOGY OF THE GASTROINTESTINAL TRACT

SECOND EDITION

PATHOLOGY OF THE GASTROINTESTINAL TRACT

SECOND EDITION

EDITORS

SI-CHUN MING, M.D.
Professor Emeritus of Pathology
Department of Pathology and Laboratory Medicine
Temple University School of Medicine
Philadelphia, Pennsylvania

HARVEY GOLDMAN, M.D.
Professor of Pathology
Beth Israel Deaconess Medical Center
Harvard Medical School
Boston, Massachusetts

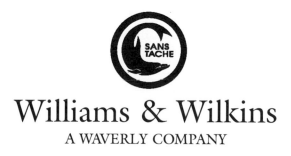

Williams & Wilkins
A WAVERLY COMPANY

BALTIMORE • PHILADELPHIA • LONDON • PARIS • BANGKOK
HONG KONG • MUNICH • SYDNEY • TOKYO • WROCLAW

Editor: Charles W. Mitchell
Managing Editor: Marjorie Kidd Keating
Marketing Manager: Lorraine A. Smith
Production Coordinator: Carol Eckhart
Copy Editor: Jeffrey S. Myers
Cover and Text Design: Shepherd, Inc.
Illustration Planner: Lorraine Wrzosek
Typesetter: Graphic World, Inc.
Printer/Binder: RR Donnelley & Sons Company

351 West Camden Street
Baltimore, Maryland 21201-2436 USA

Rose Tree Corporate Center
1400 North Providence Road
Building II, Suite 5025
Media, Pennsylvania 19063-2043 USA

Accurate indications, adverse reactions, and dosage schedules for drugs are provided in this book, but
it is possible that they may change. The reader is urged to review the package information data of the
manufacturers of the medications mentioned.

Printed in the United States of America

First Edition, 1992 by W.B. Saunders Company

Library of Congress Cataloging-in-Publication Data

Pathology of the gastrointestinal tract / editors, Si-Chun Ming,
    Harvey Goldman. — 2nd ed.
        p.   cm.
        Includes bibliographical references and index.
        ISBN 0-683-18007-X
        1. Gastrointestinal system—Diseases.   2. Gastrointestinal system—
    Histopathology.   I. Ming, Si-Chun.   II. Goldman, Harvey, 1932–   .
        [DNLM: 1. Gastrointestinal Diseases—pathology.
    2. Gastrointestinal Diseases—etiology.   3. Gastrointestinal
    Diseases—diagnosis.   4. Gastrointestinal System—physiology. WI
    140 P297 1998]
    RC802.9.P373   1998
    616.3′3—dc21
    DNLM/DLC
    for Library of Congress   97-22939
                                                                                   CIP

*The publishers have made every effort to trace the copyright holders for borrowed material. If they have
inadvertently overlooked any, they will be pleased to make the necessary arrangements at the first opportunity.*

To purchase additional copies of this book, call our customer service department at **(800) 638-0672**
or fax orders to **(800) 447-8438.** For other book services, including chapter reprints and large quantity
sales, ask for the Special Sales department.

Canadian customers should call **(800) 665-1148** or fax **(800) 665-0103.** For all other calls originating
outside the United States, please call **(410) 528-4223** or fax us at **(410) 528-8550.**

Visit Williams & Wilkins on the Internet: **http://www.wwilkins.com** or contact our customer
service department at **custserv@wwilkins.com**. Williams & Wilkins customer service representatives
are available from 8:30 am to 6:00 pm, EST, Monday through Friday, for telephone access.

                                                        98 99 00 01 02
                                                        1 2 3 4 5 6 7 8 9 10

With love
to
Pen-Ming, Carol, Ruby, Stephanie,
Jeffrey, Michael, and Eileen

and to
Eleonora, Palko, Sasha, and Vierku

PREFACE

This book is intended to provide a comprehensive analysis and presentation of the pathologic features of the disorders affecting the human gastrointestinal tract. Specific attention is directed to the etiology and evolution of these diseases, including basic biology and evolutional mechanisms of the disease processes. Differential diagnosis and clinicopathologic correlations are stressed. The text is organized in a logical format. The general principles and pathologic features shared by different organs are presented together to provide common bases of understanding and to eliminate redundancy and duplication in the presentation. This format also provides room for extended discussion of correlative topics.

The first edition fulfilled its purposes well. Since its publication, great advances have occurred in medicine and many of these achievements have been made in the basic science and pathology of gastrointestinal disorders. At the time of its release, the first edition was the only pathology book that presented and discussed cell biology and genetics affecting the digestive tract. In the second edition, we provide state-of-the-art information regarding newly developed knowledge and technology. In addition, the book is updated to include new materials and references in both pathologic and clinical aspects. The overall quality of the illustrations is improved and we added color illustrations, particularly in the new chapters, to enhance visual presentation.

To expand the coverage of the new knowledge, we added two chapters: Chapter 5 deals with advanced investigative and diagnostic techniques, such as immunohistochemistry and cytometry, and Chapter 8 presents the molecular biology of gastrointestinal diseases. These chapters cover the newly developed and rapidly advancing frontiers of basic medical research and investigation, include both theoretic and technologic aspects, and emphasize both diagnostic and investigative applications. Additional changes include expansion of the discussion of genetics and cytogenetics (Chapter 7) to include new concepts and clinical applications, as well as updating of material concerning cell proliferation and kinetics (Chapter 9) by new authors. Furthermore, these topics are supplemented and integrated with related observations in chapters dealing with specific disorders.

Some chapters were reorganized to accommodate new knowledge and to facilitate orderly presentation and discussion. The disorders of lymphoid system are now presented in two chapters by new authors, immunodeficiency disorders are addressed in Chapter 16 and lymphoproliferative disorders are the focus of Chapter 17. Chapters in the first edition concerning early and late stomach cancers are combined into a single chapter, with joint authorship (Chapter 27). The topics of squamous cell carcinoma of the esophagus (Chapter 21) and developmental disorders (Chapter 10) are addressed by new authors, and new coauthors have also been added to some other chapters. We are grateful to our returning authors who updated and expanded their already excellent contributions to the first edition of the book.

With the changes as outlined, we are confident that the book will continue to serve pathologists as well as our clinical colleagues in the special field of gastroenterology.

Si-Chun Ming, M.D.
Harvey Goldman, M.D.

Contributors

Gerald C. Abrams, M.D.
Professor of Pathology
Department of Pathology
The University of Michigan Hospital
Ann Arbor, Michigan

Charles W. Andrews, Jr., M.D.
Assistant Professor of Pathology
Department of Anatomic Pathology
Emory University Medical School
Atlanta, Georgia

Donald A. Antonioli, M.D.
Senior Pathologist
Department of Pathology
Beth Israel Deaconess Medical Center
Associate Professor of Pathology
Department of Pathology
Harvard Medical School
Boston, Massachusetts

Henry D. Appelman, M.D.
Professor of Pathology
Department of Pathology
The University of Michigan
Ann Arbor, Michigan

D. Bruce Baird, M.D.
Associate Professor of Pathology
Department of Pathology and Laboratory Medicine
East Carolina University School of Medicine
Greenville, North Carolina

Luigi Barbara, M.D.
Professor of Internal Medicine
Head, Department of Internal Medicine and Gastroenterology
University of Bologna and S. Orsola Hospital
Bologna, Italy

Guido Biasco, M.D.
Associate Professor of Clinical Oncology
"Giorgio Prodi" Center for Cancer Research
University of Bologna
Bologna, Italy

Mary P. Bronner, M.D.
Assistant Professor of Pathology
University of Washington
Attending Surgical Pathologist
University of Washington Medical Center
Seattle, Washington

Carlo Capella, M.D., Ph.D.
Professor of Pathology
Head, Surgical Pathology Service
Department of Pathology
II Faculty of Medicine
University of Pavia at Varese
Varese, Italy

Harry S. Cooper, M.D.
Senior Member and Director of Laboratory Services
    Department of Pathology
Fox Chase Cancer Center
Philadelphia, Pennsylvania

John D. Crissman, M.D.
Professor and Chairman
Department of Pathology
Wayne State University School of Medicine
Chief of Pathology
Harper Hospital
Detroit, Michigan

Roberto Fiocca, M.D.
Associate Professor of Pathology
Department of Human Pathology
University of Pavia
Pavia, Italy

Harvey Goldman, M.D.
Vice Chairman, Department of Pathology
Beth Israel Deaconess Medical Center
Professor of Pathology
Harvard Medical School
Boston, Massachusetts

Rodger C. Haggitt, M.D.
Professor of Pathology
Adjunct Professor of Medicine
University of Washington
Director of Hospital Pathology
University of Washington Medical Center
Seattle, Washington

Stanley R. Hamilton, M.D.
Department of Pathology
The Johns Hopkins University School of Medicine
Baltimore, Maryland

Jihad Hayek, M.D.
Department of Pathology
Beth Israel Deaconess Medical Center
Instructor of Pathology
Harvard Medical School
Boston, Massachusetts

Teruyuki Hirota, M.D.
Professor and Chief
Division of Pathology
Tokyo Medical College Hospital
Tokyo, Japan

Peter G. Isaacson, F.R.C.Path.
Professor and Head
Department of Histopathology
University College London Medical School
London, United Kingdom

David F. Keren, M.D.
Medical Director
Warde Medical Laboratory
Clinical Professor of Pathology
Department of Pathology
University of Michigan Medical School
Ann Arbor, Michigan

Harry B. W. Kozakewich, M.D.
Assistant Professor of Pathology
Harvard Medical School
Department of Pathology
The Children's Hospital
Boston, Massachusetts

Stefano La Rosa, M.D.
Department of Clinico-Biological Sciences
University of Pavia at Varese
Varese, Italy

Massimo Loda, M.D.
Director, Molecular Pathology and Immunohistochemistry
Beth Israel Deaconess Medical Center
Assistant Professor of Pathology
Department of Pathology
Harvard Medical School
Boston, Massachusetts

James L. Madara, M.D.
Professor and Chairman
Department of Pathology
Emory University School of Medicine
Atlanta, Georgia

Mario Miglioli, M.D.
Professor of Internal Medicine
Department of Internal Medicine and Gastroenterology
University of Bologna
Bologna, Italy

Jeffrey E. Ming, M.D., Ph.D.
Fellow, Division of Human Genetics and Molecular Biology
Department of Pediatrics
Children's Hospital of Philadelphia
University of Pennsylvania School of Medicine
Philadelphia, Pennsylvania

Si-Chun Ming, M.D.
Professor Emeritus of Pathology
Department of Pathology and Laboratory Medicine
Temple University School of Medicine
Philadelphia, Pennsylvania

Pen-Ming L. Ming, M.D.
Professor of Pathology and Laboratory Medicine
    and of Obstetrics and Gynecology
Temple University School of Medicine
Director of Cytogenetics Laboratory
Temple University Hospital
Philadelphia, Pennsylvania

Frank A. Mitros, M.D.
Professor of Pathology
Department of Pathology
University of Iowa
Iowa City, Iowa

H. Thomas Norris, M.D.
Professor and Chairman
Department of Pathology and Laboratory Medicine
East Carolina University School of Medicine
Chief of Pathology
Pitt County Memorial Hospital
Greenville, North Carolina

Robert D. Odze, M.D., F.R.C.Pc.
Assistant Professor of Pathology
Department of Surgical and Gastrointestinal Pathology
Brigham and Women's Hospital
Harvard Medical School
Boston, Massachusetts

Gian Maria Paganelli, M.D., Ph.D.
Assistant Professor
"Giorgio Prodi" Center for Cancer Research
University of Bologna
Bologna, Italy

Robert R. Rickert, M.D.
Co-Chairman, Department of Pathology
Saint Barnabas Medical Center
Livingston, New Jersey
Clinical Professor of Pathology
University of Medicine and Dentistry of New Jersey-
    New Jersey Medical School
Newark, New Jersey

Guido Rindi, M.D., Ph.D.
Lecturer of Pathology
Department of Human Pathology
University of Pavia
Pavia, Italy

Cyrus E. Rubin, M.D.
Emeritus Professor of Medicine and Professor of Pathology
University of Washington
Attending Physician
Division of Gastroenterology
University of Washington Medical Center
Seattle, Washington

Fausto Sessa, M.D.
Department of Pathology
University of Pavia at Varese
Varese, Italy

Daniel G. Sheahan, M.B., B.Ch., M.Sc.(Pathol.)
Chairman, Department of Pathology
Shadyside Hospital
Pittsburgh, Pennsylvania
Formerly Director of Anatomic Pathology
Harper Hospital and Professor of Pathology
Wayne State University
Detroit, Michigan

Lawrence K. Silbart, Ph.D.
Assistant Professor
The University of Connecticut
Center for Environmental Health
Department of Animal Science, CANR
Storrs, Connecticut

Enrico Solcia, M.D., Ph.D.
Professor of Pathology
Department of Human Pathology
University of Pavia
Pavia, Italy

Chik-Kwun Tang, M.D.
Professor of Pathology
Temple University School of Medicine
Director of Surgical Pathology
Temple University Hospital
Philadelphia, Pennsylvania

Jeffrey S. Warren, M.D.
Associate Professor and Director
Division of Clinical Pathology
Department of Pathology
University of Michigan Medical School
Ann Arbor, Michigan

Siegfried Witte, M.D.
Chief, Cytological Laboratories
Diakonissen Krankenhaus
Karlsruhe, Germany
Professor of Internal Medicine
University of Freiburg
Freiburg, Germany

John H. Yardley, M.D.
Professor of Pathology
Department of Pathology
The Johns Hopkins University School of Medicine
Baltimore, Maryland

CONTENTS

PART II: DISORDERS COMMON TO THE GASTROINTESTINAL TRACT

PART III: ESOPHAGUS

PART IV: STOMACH

COLOR PLATES

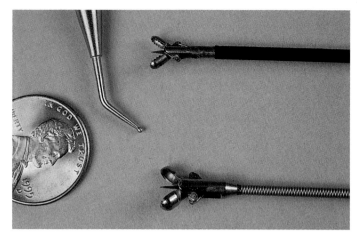

Figure 3.1

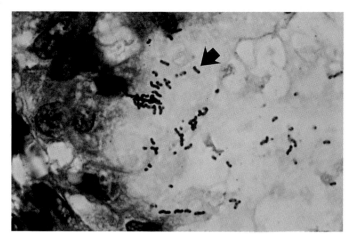

Figure 3.3

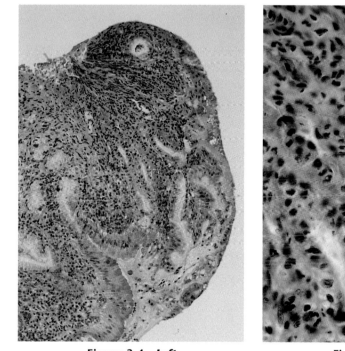

Figure 3.4 *Left*

Figure 3.4 *Right*

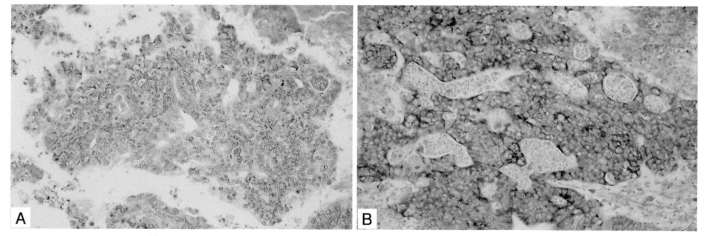

Figure 8.2 A

Figure 8.2 B

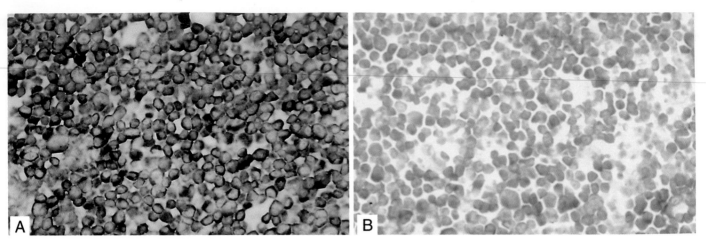

Figure 8.3 A

Figure 8.3 B

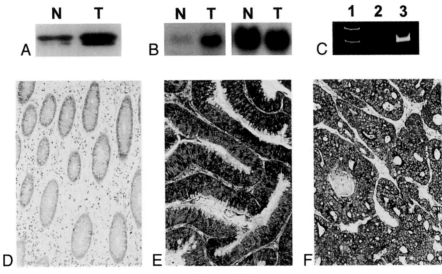

Figure 8.7

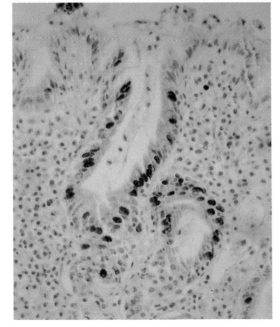

Figure 9.5

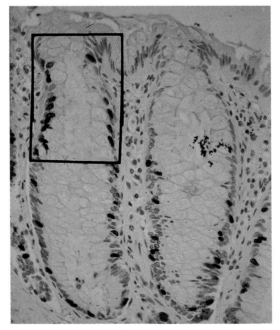

Figure 9.7

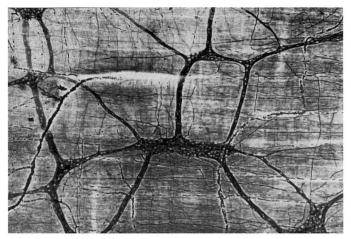

Figure 13.3

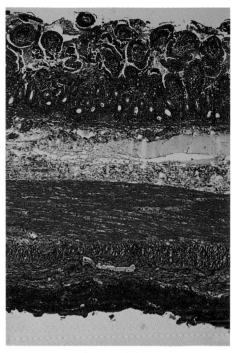

Figure 13.16 A

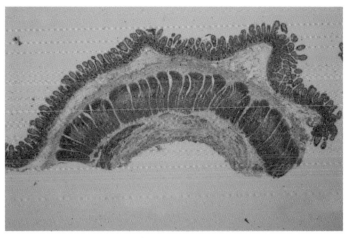

Figure 13.16 B

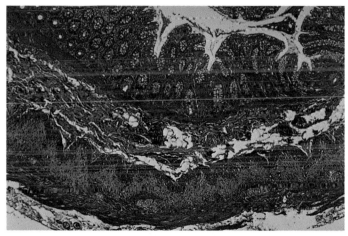

Figure 13.17

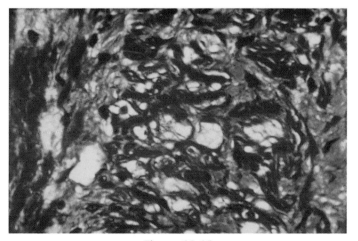

Figure 13.18

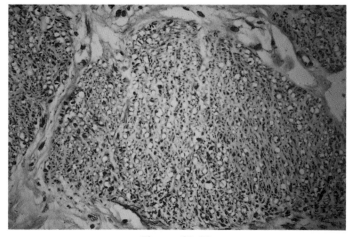

Figure 13.19

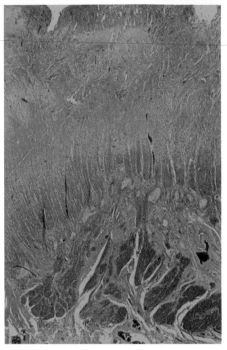

Figure 13.20

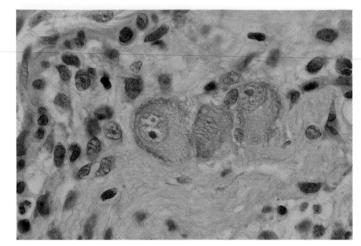

Figure 13.23

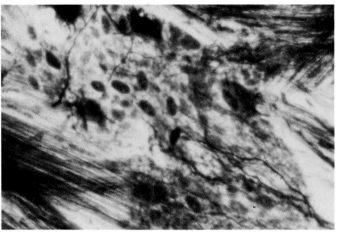

Figure 13.26

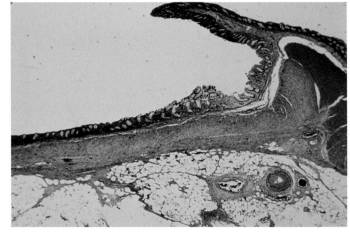

Figure 13.28

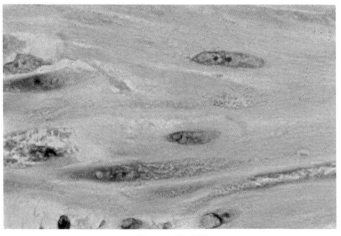

Figure 13.29

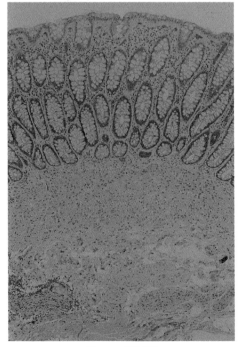

Figure 13.32

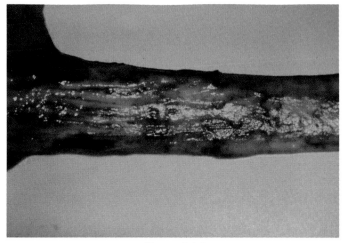

Figure 14.1

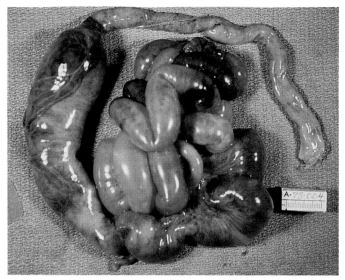

Figure 14.23

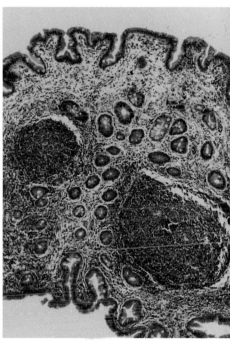

Figure 16.1

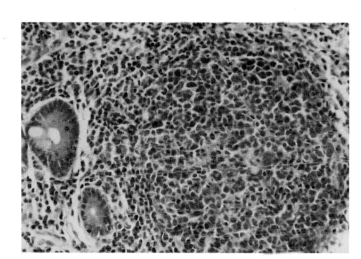

Figure 16.2

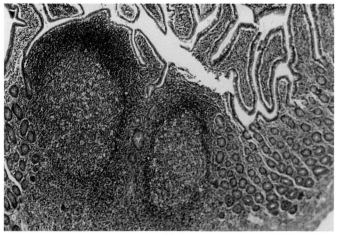

Figure 16.3

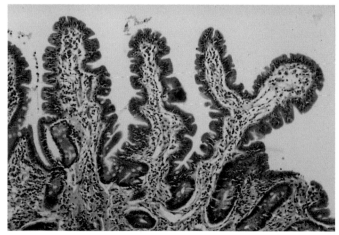

Figure 16.4

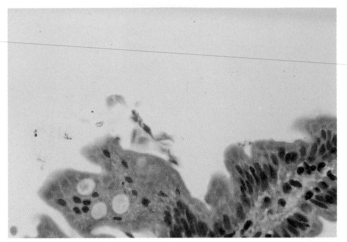

Figure 16.5

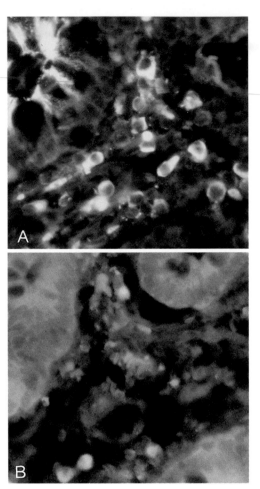

Figure 16.6 A&B

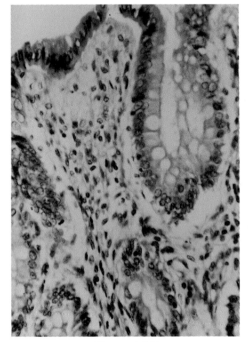

Figure 16.7

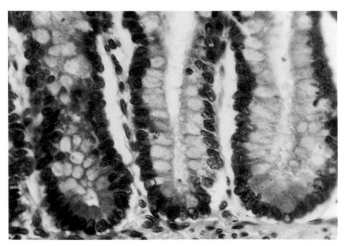

Figure 16.8

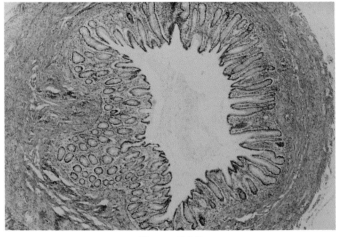

Figure 16.9

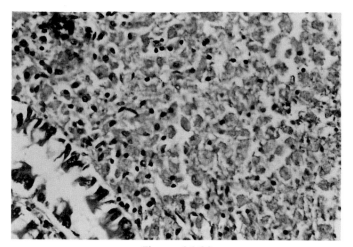

Figure 16.10

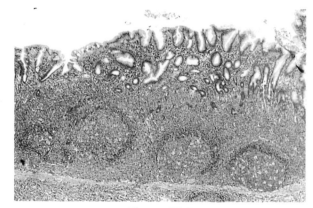

Figure 16.11

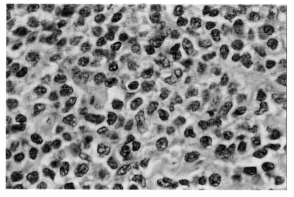

Figure 17.1

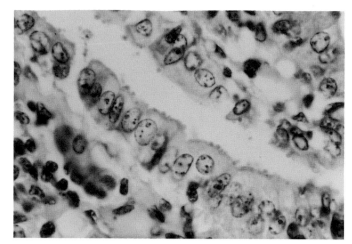

Figure 17.2

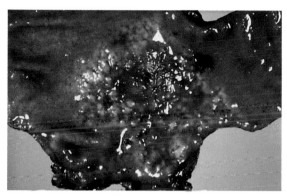

Figure 17.3

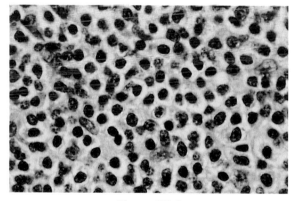

Figure 17.4

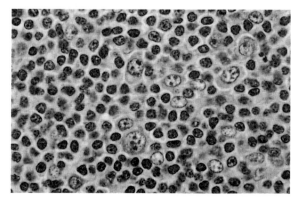

Figure 17.5

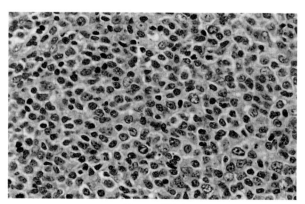

Figure 17.6

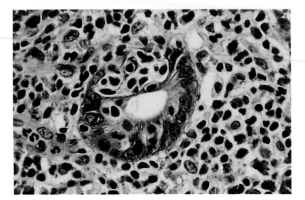

Figure 17.7

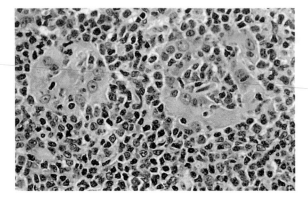

Figure 17.8

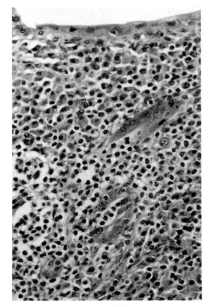

Figure 17.9

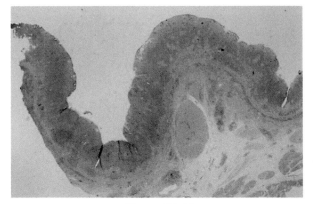

Figure 17.10

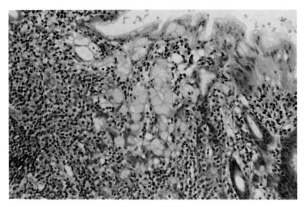

Figure 17.11

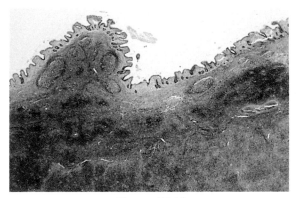

Figure 17.12

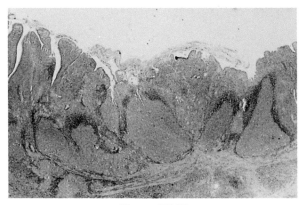

Figure 17.13

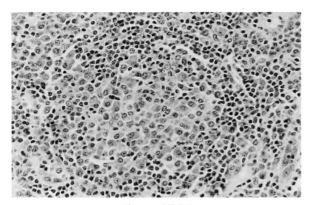

Figure 17.14

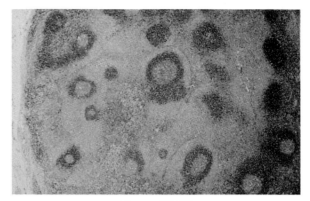

Figure 17.15

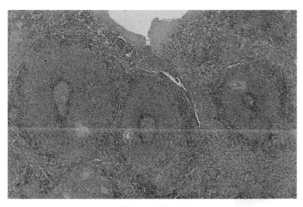

Figure 17.16

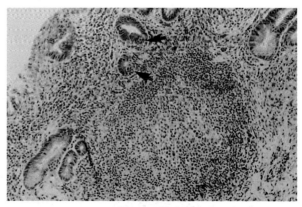

Figure 17.17

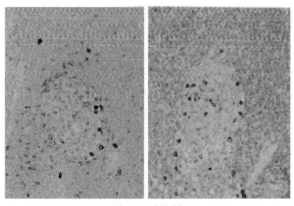

Figure 17.18

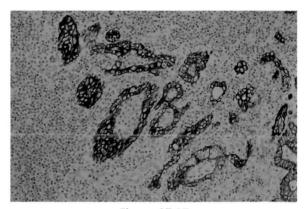

Figure 17.19

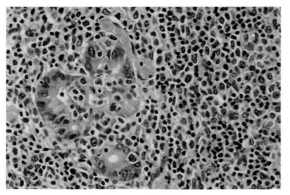

Figure 17.20

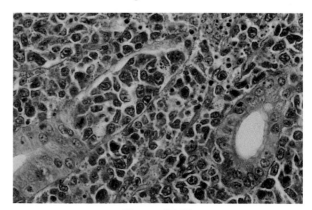

Figure 17.21

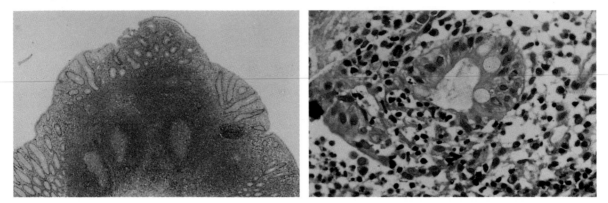

Figure 17.22 A

Figure 17.22 B

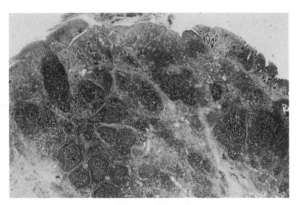

Figure 17.23

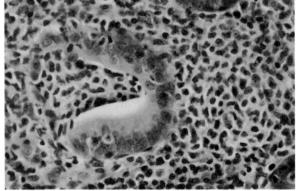

Figure 17.24

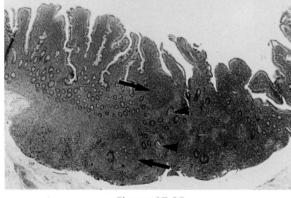

Figure 17.25

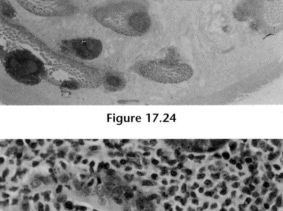

Figure 17.26

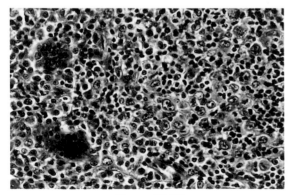

Figure 17.27

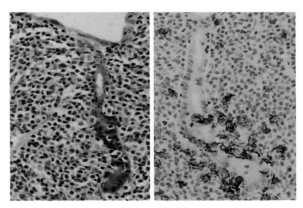

Figure 17.28

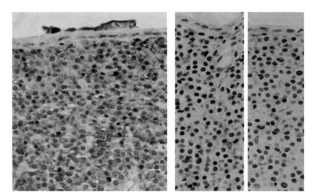

Figure 17.29

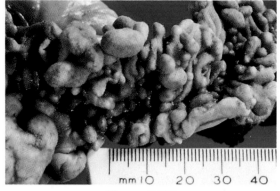

Figure 17.30

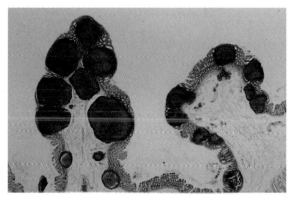

Figure 17.31

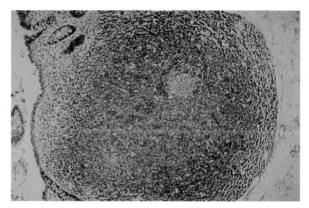

Figure 17.32

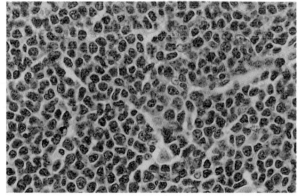

Figure 17.33

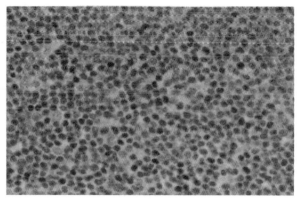

Figure 17.34

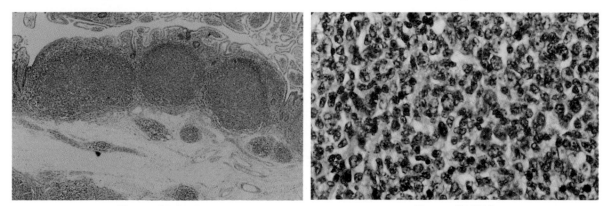

Figure 17.35 A
Figure 17.35 B

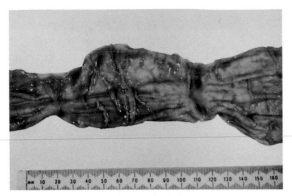

Figure 17.36

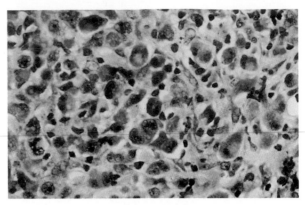

Figure 17.37

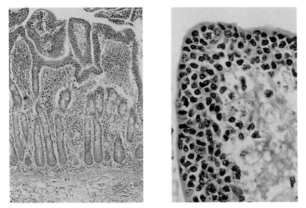

Figure 17.38

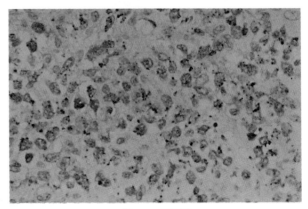

Figure 17.39

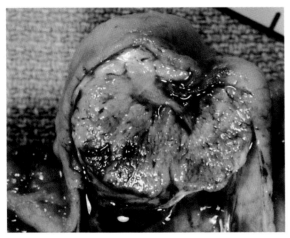

Figure 18.1

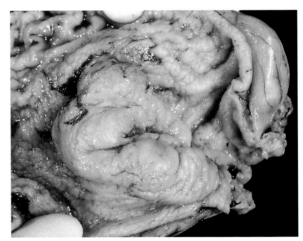

Figure 18.2

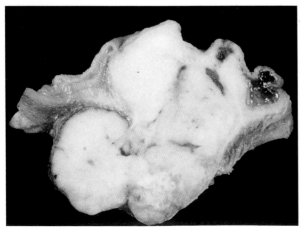

Figure 18.4

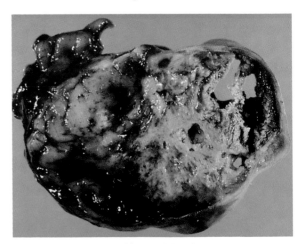

Figure 18.5

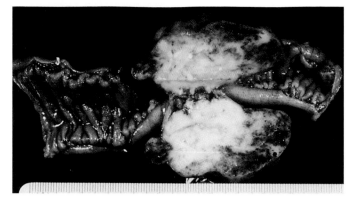

Figure 18.6

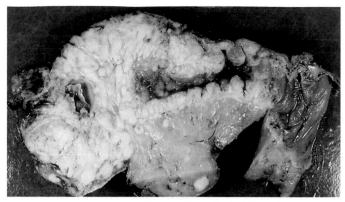

Figure 18.7

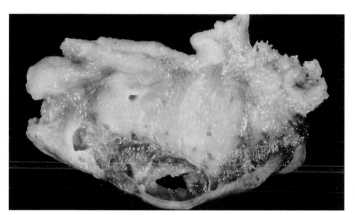

Figure 18.8

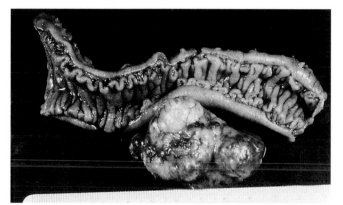

Figure 18.9

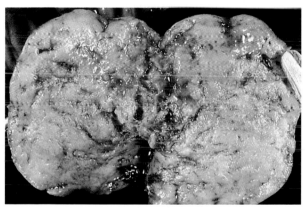

Figure 18.11

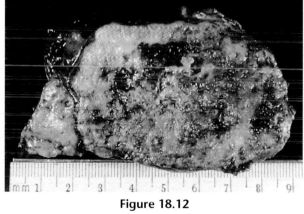

Figure 18.12

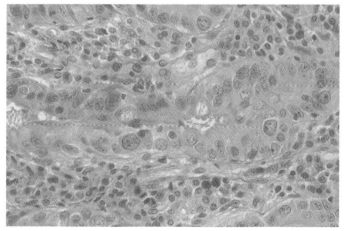

Figure 19.2

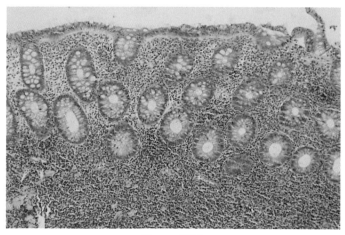

Figure 19.3

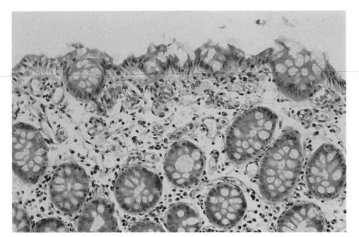

Figure 19.4

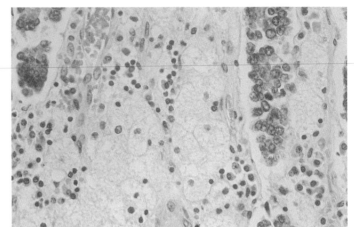

Figure 19.9

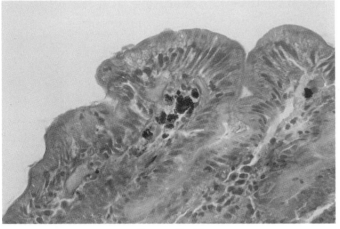

Figure 19.11

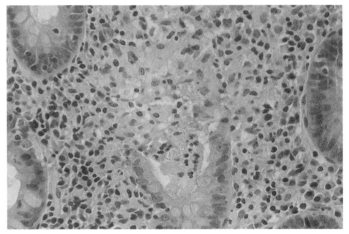

Figure 19.14

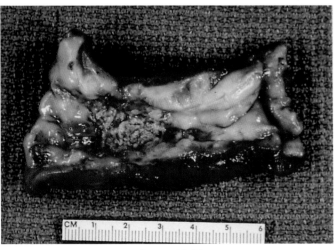

Figure 21.10

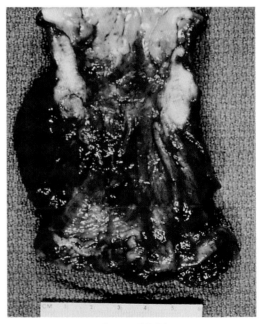

Figure 22.10

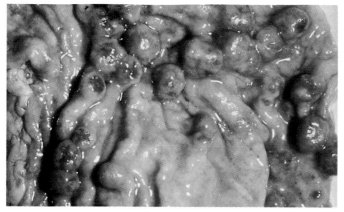

Figure 26.12

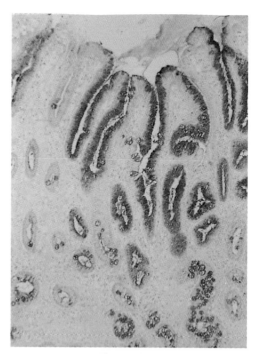

Figure 27.7

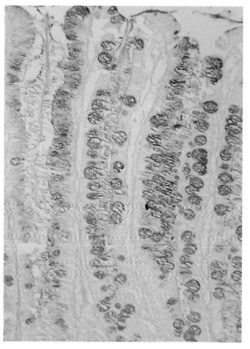

Figure 27.8

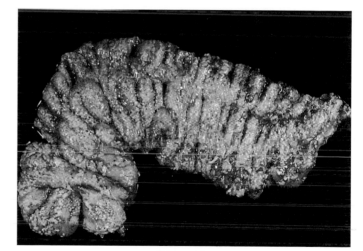

Figure 28.4

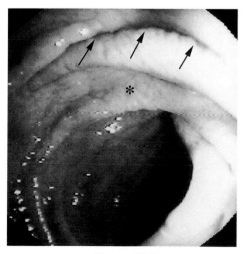

Figure 31.5

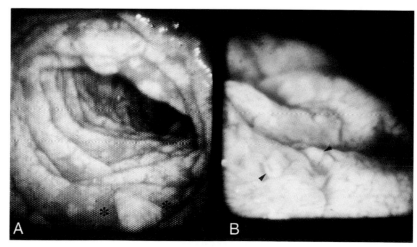

Figure 31.21 A&B

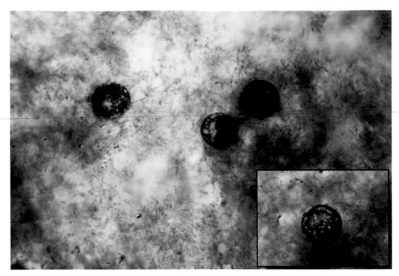

Figure 31.31

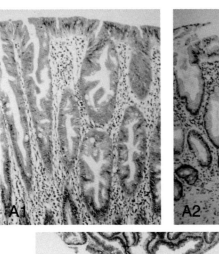

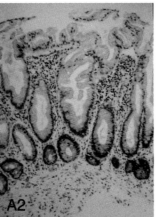

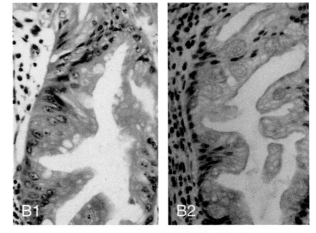

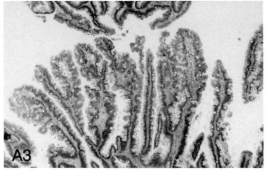

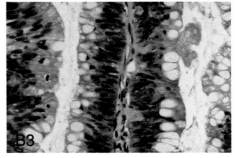

Figure 33.6 A

Figure 33.6 B

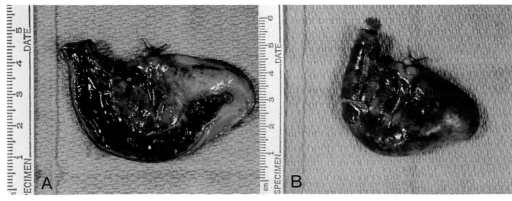

Figure 35.4 A&B

PART I

GENERAL PRINCIPLES

GENERAL CONCEPTS AND METHODS OF EXAMINATION

Harvey Goldman

This chapter presents the general nomenclature, classifications, and pathologic processes, as well as the methods of examination, used in the study of disorders of the various segments of the gastrointestinal tract. In subsequent chapters relating to specific organs and diseases, relevant and commonly used terms are repeated or introduced as needed to allow for the detailed presentation of a particular disorder.

GENERAL CONCEPTS OF GASTROINTESTINAL DISORDERS

A large array of terms are often used to describe a particular disorder of a single organ. In fact, the same disease affecting a different organ, including closely related organs, may be described using modified or sometimes strikingly different terms. Although this breadth of terminology serves as a testimony to the richness of the language, the basic concepts may be obscured. We therefore believe it is a worthwhile exercise to express the general tenets and foundations for the description of diseases.

CATEGORIES OF DISEASES

By common usage, it has proven convenient to separate disorders into broad categories of developmental anomalies, motor and mechanical disturbances (including dysfunctions of nerves and muscles), vascular disorders, endocrine and metabolic diseases, the many inflammatory lesions, and tumors (Table 1.1). Although all injuries ultimately evoke a standard and stereotyped inflammatory

reaction, the term "inflammatory disorders" has come to be used for those conditions that have a predominant, often primary, element of inflammatory reaction and its effects in their presentation. Within each of these broad categories of diseases, subgroups are formed to express particular etiologic factors, common pathogenetic or functional pathways, or anatomic divisions.

DEVELOPMENTAL DISORDERS

Considering the big volume of the gut and its embryologic complexity, it is not surprising to note a large array of congenital and developmental anomalies that affect all portions. The major effects are in the form of persistent masses from cysts, interference with luminal flow by stenoses and atresias or by extrinsic compression from hernias, and inflammation or bleeding from localized diverticula. The functional anatomy of the gut is detailed in Chapter 2 and the embryology and developmental anomalies is presented in Chapter 10.

MOTOR AND MECHANICAL DISORDERS

Food must pass through the gut at a steady and appropriate rate to permit optimal function by the gastrointestinal tract. A large assortment of congenital and acquired, primary and secondary conditions can interfere with this flow. Such conditions include mechanical disorders, which involve a discernable physical obstruction, such as an inflammatory stricture or tumor, and motor disturbances (pseudo-obstruction), in which no such obstructive element can be identified. The motor disorders may be attributed to local infiltrations (such as amyloid or tumor) or to specific diseases, either primary or secondary, of the bowel wall musculature or its nerve supply.

A mechanical disorder implies causation by a gross physical disturbance, such as the effects of trauma, foreign bodies, obstruction by any mass or other grossly visible lesion, and other alterations of anatomy that may interfere with normal flow or other function, such as diverticula and hernias. Such structural alterations may be congenital or acquired, and this information, together with the particular locations and pathogenetic data, form the basis for special classifications within each organ. A diverticulum represents a localized outpouching of the gut lumen and is divided into the true diverticula (with a wall containing all of the inherent structures, albeit often attenuated) and pseudodiverticula (with a wall at some point missing some of the intrinsic elements). More useful separations include designation as congenital versus acquired, or division into those resulting from the action of pressure, normal or elevated, applied to a weaker than normal portion of the wall (pulsion type) as opposed to those resulting from an extrinsic inflammatory process with subsequent retraction or pulling on the gut wall (inflammatory or traction type). Similarly, hernias are categorized in a variety of ways on the basis of anatomic location, etiology, nature of contents, and special morphologic forms.

Many other disorders start with a gross mechanical event, but this occurrence may be superseded by significant vascular obstruction or effects of inflammation. In such cases, we often discuss the condition under the heading with the greater amount of pathologic effect, i.e., as a vascular or inflammatory disorder. It is not surprising that the listing of causes of intestinal obstruction becomes part of the listing of causes of vascular insufficiency of the gut, which in turn is superseded by a designation of some of the disorders with a name that implies inflammation. (See Chapter 13 for a general presenta-

---

TABLE	
1.1	**Categories of Gastrointestinal Diseases**

Developmental disorders
Motor and mechanical disorders
    Muscular and nervous system diseases
    Obstruction, diverticula, hernias
Vascular disorders
    Varices and malformations
    Vasculitis
    Ischemic/hypoxic lesions
Endocrine and metabolic disorders
Inflammatory disorders
    Infections
    Physical and chemical injury
    Immunological disorders
    Idiopathic disorders
Tumors
    Heterotopias
    Polyps
    Neoplasms

TABLE	
1.2	**Causes and Effects of Ischemic/ Hypoxic Disease**

Causes
    Arterial occlusion by plaques, thrombi, and emboli
    Venous occlusion by thrombi
    Venous compression associated with adhesions, hernias,
        volvulus, etc.
    Low perfusion state
    Obstruction and distension of gut lumen
Promoting factors
    Anemia
    Cardiac and pulmonary diseases
Effects
    Functional effects of pain and diarrhea, without necrosis
    Mucosal infarct
    Mural infarct
    Transmural infarct

---

tion of motor and mechanical disorders, and Chapter 32 for a discussion of colonic diverticula.)

VASCULAR DISORDERS

This category can be separated into simple dilations or varices, other vascular malformations that are congenital or acquired, the vasculitides, and ischemic and anoxic disorders. The details of the pathologic findings and the designations of the various clinicopathologic entities of hypoxic damage of the gut are presented in Chapter 14. It is worthwhile here to consider the general principles underlying this damage, with particular reference to the need for greater clarity in nomenclature and classification.

Many classifications contain a generous admixture of terms dealing with particular location, causes, proposed pathogenetic mechanisms, standard pathologic effects, differences in morphologic forms usually due to various complicating factors, duration of events, clinical features, and subsequent outcome. It is more orderly and ultimately wiser to consider and critically analyze each of these factors separately (Table 1.2). Causes of hypoxic injury of the gut result from actual or mechanical obstruction of the blood vessels, including large or small arteries and veins, or other factors resulting in reduced blood flow (1). In an individual case, there may be a single factor, a dominant factor, or any combination. An important cause of increasing incidence is reduced perfusion in the absence of any mechanical vascular occlusion. Such decreased splanchnic perfusion may result from any type of shock (i.e., cardiogenic, hemorrhagic, etc.) and any major operative procedure.

Whatever the particular cause of hypoxia, it should be appreciated that the pathogenetic pathway, mechanism of injury, and ultimate effects on the gut are limited in expression. In simplest terms, with the evolution of a critical reduction in nutrients, particularly the supply of oxygen, the cells and tissues undergo hypoxic damage. The bowel injury may differ in speed of occurrence, incidence of complicating events, and therefore different functional and clinical effects, but the initial event of hypoxic damage is rigorously the same.

Hypoxia of short duration or of a mild degree may cause only a reversible functional derangement without structural damage, characterized by pain and altered absorption and/or secretion. With persistent and severe hypoxia, there ensues necrosis of the cells and tissues, termed an "infarct." Based on the severity and duration of the hypoxia, the infarction may be limited to the inner lining ("mucosal infarct") and be largely reversible without permanent damage; extend into the wall ("mural infarct") resulting in inflammatory and fibrous complications; or involve all layers ("transmural infarct") leading to the potential for perforation (2). Synonyms of historical interest but of uncertain utility include hemorrhagic necrosis, hemorrhagic enteropathy, reversible ischemia, and shock or low flow lesion for the mucosal infarct; chronic ischemia, ischemic enteritis or colitis, and ischemic stricture for the mural infarct; and strangulation, gangrene, or even the unqualified use of the word infarct for the transmural infarct.

In any analysis of ischemic disorders, it is best to list separately the particular location involved, the specific cause or combination of factors, the basic morphologic effects, and the clinical and functional sequelae (both acute and chronic). The bowel infarction may be further complicated by secondary events leading to a change in morphologic appearance, including prominent inflammation and inflammatory pseudopolyps, pseudomembrane formation, pneumatosis, and other effects of sepsis or perforation.

ENDOCRINE AND METABOLIC DISORDERS

Most hormonal and metabolic disturbances exhibit some effect on the gastrointestinal tract, ranging from altered motility to the presence of depositions or inflammatory lesions. These disturbances are described throughout the book, but principally in Chapters 15 and 19.

INFLAMMATORY DISORDERS

This category typically embraces conditions that manifest a prominent degree of tissue necrosis and inflammation, evident both structurally and clinically (3). As indicated previously, it is customary to exclude from this category those disorders that emanate from a primary mechanical, vascular, or tumorous event. Major causes of inflammatory lesions are infections, radiation, drugs and chemical agents, and allergic and other immunologic processes. Within the gut, several conditions lack definitive etiologic factors and so are referred to as primary or idiopathic inflammatory disorders. These common conditions include reflux esophagitis, chronic peptic ulcer disease, Crohn's disease, and ulcerative colitis. The inflammatory reactions in the idiopathic lesions are often of a nonspecific stereotyped nature, and precise diagnoses depend on history, location of disease, and exclusion of other specific disorders, such as infections.

The presentation concerning inflammatory lesions is extensive throughout the book. Concentrating on the etiology, this text offers information concerning disorders attributable to chemical and physical agents (see Chapter 11), allergic diseases (see Chapter 12), other immunologic conditions (see Chapters 6 and 16), and systemic disorders (see Chapter 19). In addition, diseases mainly affecting particular parts of the gut are covered as follows: the esophagus in Chapter 20, the stomach in Chapters 23 and 24, and the intestines in Chapters 28 to 31.

TUMORS

Tumors are common in the gastrointestinal tract and manifest as masses that protrude into the lumen or that infiltrate the gut wall. Included are heterotopic (ectopic) foci of gastric or pancreatic tissues; polyps, representing projections from the mucosal surface, that can be inflammatory, hamartomatous, hyperplastic, or neoplastic; and a wide variety of benign and malignant neoplasms originating from the many cellular and tissue elements present in the gut. It is essential to separate the epithelial polyps properly, because only the neoplastic type, the adenoma, is a proven precursor of carcinoma. Most important, because of their high prevalence and clinical significance, are the epithelial neoplasms, but tumors of the mesenchymal elements (see Chapter 18), of the lymphoid system (see Chapter 17), and of the endocrine cells (see Chapter 15) are also commonly observed.

Considerable heterogeneity exists in the structure and function of the epithelial cells of the different parts of the gastrointestinal tract, and the dissimilarity in their appearances is compounded by the frequent occurrence of metaplasia, as described in the following section. As a result of this mixture of normal and metaplastic elements, the composition of many of the epithelial tumors is complex, particularly in the stomach and lower esophagus. In response to increasing awareness of the existence and importance of precancerous conditions and lesions, particularly of dysplasia, in all parts of the gut, endoscopic surveillance programs have been developed that can detect cases of epithelial tumors at an early and potentially curative stage.

Other chapters include discussion of epithelial tumors in specific areas of the gastrointestinal tract, specifically the esophagus (see Chapters 21 and 22), the stomach (see Chapters 26 and 27), and the intestines (see Chapters 33 and 34). Considerable information related to the biology of the tumors and on their methods of identification is presented throughout part I.

RESPONSES TO INJURY: EFFECTS ON EPITHELIUM

The standard pathologic processes affecting epithelia include degeneration as a direct result of the injury, regeneration as part of the reparative response, metaplasia as a sign of chronicity, and dysplasia as a marker of neoplasia.

DEGENERATION AND REGENERATION

Signs of degeneration range from simple swelling of the cell (a reversible situation) to progressive autolysis and necrosis of the cell. Many conditions are associated with a programmed series of events leading to cell death, termed "apoptosis"(4). The nuclei show disintegration (karyorrhexis and karyolysis), either promptly or after a period of condensation (pyknosis). In some instances, special cytologic features help to indicate a particular etiologic process. A pronounced degree of nuclear enlargement and hyperchromasia suggests damage by radiation or certain drugs. Many immunologic disorders reveal a marked mononuclear cell infiltrate together with relatively slight light microscopic evidence of epithelial cell injury. In contrast, more extensive and prompt liquifaction of the cells is expected in those conditions with a prominent neutrophilic reaction, such as noted with many infections. It should be stressed that these special cellular features generally are quantitative and not always specific.

Regeneration is recognized by an expansion of the growing, immature, and less mature cells within given epithelia. Noted are an increase in the number of mitoses and an enlargement of the regenerative zone, located at the base of squamous epithelia, in the neck region at the bottom of the gastric foveolae (pits), and in the lower portion of the intestinal crypts. The regenerative cells are enlarged and have bigger and rounder nuclei with prominent nucleoli but a relatively faint chromatin pattern. The cytoplasm typically shows a decrease in mature products. It is essential to distinguish these cells, with their greater size and more prominent nuclei, from atypical growths (i.e., dysplasia and neoplasia). The latter typically reveal some combination of greater pleomorphism, hyperchromasia, loss of nuclear polarity, and reduced amount of cytoplasm.

METAPLASIA

This effect represents a change in cytoplasmic differentiation from the expected normal to an alternative but mature form. Metaplasia should be distinguished from heterotopia, which is an inborn or developmental misplacement of mature epithelium. This distinction can be accomplished in most instances, because the presence of heterotopic tissue is associated with some developmental anomaly and/or is not preceded by any inflammatory or degenerative condition. An example of heterotopia is the appearance of mature gastric corpus tissue within a Meckel's diverticulum and in other parts of the gut (see Chapter 19).

Acquired metaplasia is more common and appears to be a consequence of prior, usually chronic, inflammatory disease. After prolonged injury to any portion of the gut, all epithelial elements of the embryonic tract tend to appear as part of the regeneration. With time, probably in response to local but unknown stimuli, the native cells for that particular segment of the gut prevail and reconstitute the normal epithelial layer. With repeated episodes of injury, however, the tendency for metaplasia continues in concert with the regenerative signal.

The potential importance of metaplasia is that it is a marker of a chronic inflammatory condition, which in turn may be prone to the development of carcinoma. This feature is especially significant in Barrett's esophagus and in chronic gastritis with intestinal metaplasia (see Chapters 20, 22, 23, and 27).

In areas of metaplasia, one encounters and recognizes the elements from other portions of the gut, even within parts of the same organ (Table 1.3). After sustained esophagitis, the squamous epithelium of the esophagus may be replaced by glandular tissue, including elements of both the stomach and intestines as well as hybrid forms (5). Injury within the stomach is commonly associated with a proliferation of pyloric glandular tissue, resulting in replacement of the specialized glandular cells (including parietal and chief cells) within the fundus and corpus. The same process occurs within the antrum, but it is appreciated as a hyperplasia of pyloric glands, which is a native element to that area. Throughout the stomach, there may be metaplasia with intestinal-type epithelium, including the appearance of columnar absorptive cells, goblet mucous cells, Paneth cells, and uncommon full development of villi (6). The intestinal metaplasia structurally resembles small intestinal or co-lonic epithelium, and often a mixture.

TABLE 1.3	Types of Metaplasia in Gut Epithelium	
Location	Metaplasia	Condition
Esophagus	Glandular tissue	Barrett's esophagus
Stomach	Intestinal glands	Chronic gastritis
	Pyloric glands in corpus	
Duodenum	Gastric surface-type mucous cells	Chronic peptic duodenitis
Small intestine	Pyloric glands	Crohn's disease
Colon and rectum	Paneth cells	Ulcerative colitis

Injury to the small intestine is most often associated with pyloric glandular metaplasia, which on occasion is so pronounced as to produce gross nodules. This proliferation has been termed by others as pseudopyloric metaplasia, presumably to emphasize the change in location; however, no structural differences exist between the pyloric glandular cells that are noted in the native antrum and those in metaplastic sites. Commonly noted in cases of chronic duodenitis is a gastric surface-type mucous cell metaplasia replacing the intestinal epithelial cells on the villi (7). Finally, chronic colonic inflammation is invariably associated with Paneth cells (8), which are indigenous to the small intestine and proximal colon, and less often with pyloric glandular cells. It is rare to find more specialized gastric corpus and small intestinal absorptive cells within the colon, and squamous metaplasia is an unusual finding within any of the segments of the gut. Further details of metaplastic elements, together with information about their finer localization, are presented in organ-specific chapters, with particular reference to diagnosis and clinical significance.

DYSPLASIA AND NEOPLASIA

The term "neoplasia" should be reserved at all times for the growth of an abnormal cell line, which is cytologically distinct from the other simpler effects of injury (i.e., degeneration, regeneration, and metaplasia). Synonyms for the cellular features and process noted in neoplasia include atypical hyperplasia and dysplasia. These features can be further quantitated in degree of abnormality to denote a probability for a benign or malignant growth. Unfortunately, the full cellular alterations that may be encountered during simple degeneration or regeneration are not always appreciated, and use of the term "atypia" (atypism, atypical epithelium) or even "dysplasia" for such cellular changes has become common practice. At times, the terms "inflammatory atypia" or "inflammatory dysplasia" have been used to emphasize the probable inflammatory nature of such cellular changes. The liberal use of such terms, however, tends to obscure the real nature of the lesion and may lead to unnecessary concern on the part of the clinician about a true neoplastic process. Clearly, there are occasions when one cannot ascertain with certainty whether a cellular alteration is neoplastic; in such instances, some narrative statement or a less committed designation (e.g., cellular atypism—probably or possibly inflammatory, or of uncertain nature) could be provided. It is best, however, to reserve the term "dysplasia" for use when describing the cellular alterations that are clearly a part of neoplasia (9).

In the assessment of a neoplasm, the designation of benign or malignant is rendered in part by the degree of cellular alteration (i.e., dysplasia) and tissue organization. This designation is made more certain with the demonstration of invasion or metastasis. In some instances, it is possible to appreciate a full range—from microscopic dysplasia to grossly evident benign neoplasms and malignancy. Furthermore, the degree or staging of the malignancy can include a true in-situ state (i.e., malignant tumor that has not transgressed the basement membrane), infiltration of the other mucosal elements (i.e., lamina propria and muscularis mucosae), and invasion into deeper structures. This staging has been well established for carcinomas of the stomach and probably applies as well to carcinomas of other portions of the gut.

The term dysplasia has been used both as a descriptive microscopic term and to indicate a precancerous lesion, such as in patients with long-standing ulcerative colitis, chronic gastritis, and Barrett's esophagus. This double use of the term has led to some confusion in terminology. As indicated previously, this confusion should not be compounded by using the term to designate alterations that are thought to be the sequelae of inflammation alone. In disorders of the gut epithelia, there is an increased tendency to use the word dysplasia to signify a neoplastic lesion, to distinguish between microscopic foci and gross lesions, and to limit the rating of dysplasia to low-grade and high-grade degrees (9). This two-tier rating system is particularly helpful in the assessment of microscopic dysplastic lesions noted in patients with chronic inflammatory conditions, with the implication that low-grade lesions require further biopsy analysis and high-grade lesions deserve consideration of resection. Further details are provided elsewhere in this text regarding the dysplastic lesions of the esophagus (see Chapters 20 and 22), the stomach (see Chapter 27), and the colon (see Chapters 29 and 34).

RESPONSES TO INJURY: INFLAMMATORY EFFECTS

STANDARD REACTION

Inflammation is a stereotyped response to any injury and is characterized by a combination of the effects of acute inflammation, immunologic response, and repair. Whatever the cause of the disease, if there is destruction of tissue, there is a standard acute inflammatory reaction, consisting of vascular, fluid, and cellular components. Noteworthy is the presence of dilated vessels, edema, and an initial neutrophilic response; in most instances, the early reaction is followed in short order by a variable number of macrophages. The acute inflammatory reaction is enhanced by causative agents that promote chemotaxis (e.g., microorganisms that act at an extracellular level) or in any disorder with a large amount of necrosis. It should be stressed that this variation represents differences in degree and not in the quality of the acute inflammatory reaction. In those disorders that proceed to an immunologic response by the body, there are varying quantities of lymphocytes, plasma cells, and eosinophils; also, largely in response to the lymphokines, there are even greater quantities of macrophages. When the destruction of the tissue exceeds the capacity to provide prompt and orderly regeneration (e.g., when necrosis

extends beyond the mucosa into the submucosa), there is also the element of repair tissue, consisting essentially of the small vessels and fibroblasts of granulation tissue and their product of collagen. Although each of these processes (acute inflammation, immune response, and repair) may occur in any combination in association with a particular disorder, they each relate independently to a separate stimulus. One should avoid, in this regard, uniting any of these phenomena with the categorization of a disorder as acute or chronic; these latter labels more critically relate to the duration of the disorder.

SPECIAL FEATURES

In some disorders, largely determined by the particular etiologic agent or mechanism, a more restrictive or distinctive pattern of inflammation may be encountered. Examples include prominent cellular alterations without much acute inflammation, as may be seen in microorganisms that operate within the cells; granuloma formation in response to foreign bodies or various hypersensitivity reactions; and differences in the nature and quantity of necrosis. The demonstration of such types of inflammation and their particular subfeatures may assist in the determination of a particular etiology or at least in providing a more selective list. It should be emphasized that the only true specific features include the recognition of a particular microorganism, subject to confirmation by culture if possible; the identification of foreign material; or the unequivocal finding of neoplastic cells. In most instances, the particular features of the cellular injury and reactive inflammation are combined with other data (gross, radiographic, clinical) to provide a certain or presumptive diagnosis.

PATTERNS AND STAGES OF DISEASES

The terms "acute" and "chronic" injury are common descriptors, which in the strictest sense relate to the duration of the disorder. The pathologist, in this regard, attempts to relate the character of the inflammatory response to this estimate of acute or chronic disease, but this approach has its limitations. As noted previously, the standard inflammatory reactions (acute, immune, and repair) occur in response to specific stimuli that are independent of the duration of the disorder. More helpful in the gut are the changes noted in the epithelia, in the form of metaplasia or other disordered growth. Thus, chronic esophagitis is revealed by the finding of glandular metaplasia, chronic gastritis by the presence of intestinal metaplasia, and chronic colitis by the appearance of prominent budding of the crypts (10).

An acute injury is characterized by a relatively short and certain duration, followed by apparent complete recovery, although some injuries can recur. In contrast, a chronic injury may embrace multiple situations, including simple persistence of the acute disorder, the development of some complication of the acute injury, an uncontrolled tendency for repeated episodes of acute disease, a disorder that cannot be completely eliminated, and any combination. For those chronic disorders that wax and wane, corresponding to clinical relapses and remissions, the terms "active" and "inactive" disease are often used. In such instances, active disease corresponds to a situation with recurrent or enhanced destruction of tissue; as a consequence, such episodes are associated with increased acute inflammatory reaction. The inactive state usually differs from the completely normal tissue by showing some effects of the repeated injury, in the form of irregular healing of the glands (i.e., some degree of atrophy and metaplasia as well as regeneration) and increased fibrosis. These differences from normal tissue, in some instances, may help to discern between a complete recovery of an acute injury (e.g., an acute colitis) and an inactive state of a chronic disorder (e.g., chronic ulcerative colitis) (11).

Another term—"subacute inflammation or injury"—is used occasionally, but is of doubtful assistance. It appears to have been used in large part by clinicians to signify a duration or degree of a disorder that is more than expected in ordinary acute disease but not yet established as a chronic disorder. Some pathologists consider this term synonymous with situations of greater destruction or the appearance of some elements of the immune response, particularly large quantities of eosinophils or plasma cells. At best, subacute inflammation is a tentative term to denote a situation of greater destruction, and it is not clear in a particular case whether it relates to an acute, healing, or chronic disorder. It may be difficult to completely dismiss the term from our jargon, but it must be appreciated that it has a different meaning in different situations. Whenever and wherever it is applied, it must be defined specifically.

METHODS OF EXAMINATION

The pathologic features are usually not completely specific, and precision in diagnosis demands a combination of these features with the essential functional data. Furthermore, the information sought may not be just the diagnosis of the underlying condition, but rather the severity, activity or extent of disease, or the presence of complications. It is the responsibility of the clinician to provide the essential clinical data and also to indicate the special information that is sought in the examination. The pathologist, in turn, must attempt to respond to the specific questions.

NATURE OF SPECIMEN

The gastrointestinal specimens examined include a variety of mucosal biopsy samples obtained by blind aspiration or under direct vision at times of endoscopy, biopsy and resection specimens received at operations, and autopsy studies.

MUCOSAL BIOPSIES

With technologic advances involving flexible endoscopes has come an enormous increase in the number of mucosal biopsy samples obtained for examination (12–14). These tissue samples generally are small and require special consideration of the best methods for orientation, fixation, modes of examination, and interpretation (10, 15, 16). The pathologist must be prepared to consider this large volume of small and multiple biopsy samples in the recognition of the earlier stages of the many gastrointestinal disorders, in the greater appreciation of the evolution of the lesions, and in the expansion of the interpretations to include not only the diagnosis but also answers to the other questions posed. We endeavor throughout this book to include information dealing with mucosal biopsies in each organ-specific chapter. At present, such endoscopy-derived mucosal biopsy samples are regularly obtained from the esophagus, stomach, first and second portions of duodenum, all of the colon and rectum, and occasionally from the distal ileum.

In some of these sites, depending on the clinical circumstances, blind aspiration biopsies may be performed instead. This procedure provides a bigger specimen, including a larger portion of the submucosa, permitting better orientation and a larger sample for study. Such aspiration biopsies are more commonly performed to obtain tissue samples from areas beyond the reach of conventional endoscopes, such as in the distal duodenum and proximal jejunum.

A concern with all of these small mucosal biopsy samples is the necessity of appropriate orientation of the specimen. This need is greatest when judging nonneoplastic conditions of the small bowel, particularly in the determination of the relative and absolute heights of the villi and crypts (17). Optimal orientation can be readily accomplished by examining the gross specimen with a magnifying lens or dissecting microscope (see detailed description in Chapter 31). Although aesthetically desirable, perfect orientation is less important in evaluating mucosal biopsy samples from other segments of the gut; by the simple expediency of examining multiple sections of the biopsy, areas with reasonable orientation are obtained.

The subsequent fixation and processing of tissue from mucosal biopsies are also important considerations. Although standard formalin fixation proves sufficient in most cases, Bouin's and Hollende's solutions have been recommended to improve cytologic detail, particularly in the detection and typing of highly cellular tumors, such as lymphomas. The general subject of endoscopy and endoscopic biopsies is addressed in Chapter 3.

SURGICAL AND AUTOPSY SPECIMENS

In the examination of surgical biopsy and resection specimens, one must remember the tendency for the gut mucosa to undergo fairly rapid autolysis. The overlying epithelial cells are also extremely fragile and subject to excess shedding coincident with any manipulation of the mucosa in an unfixed state. For these reasons, it is important that the specimen is opened, examined grossly, and immersed in fixative without unnecessary delays. The same rules apply for examination of the gut at the time of autopsy. Although one has no control over the length of time before the autopsy is performed, once the tissue is removed from the body at room temperature, it should be rapidly examined and fixed.

GROSS PREPARATION AND EXAMINATION

As indicated previously, careful attention to orientation and fixation should be applied to small biopsy samples. Sections at multiple levels are recommended to provide areas of better orientation, to detect focal findings, and to provide the full range of abnormalities.

The need for prompt examination and fixation of larger specimens, including those obtained from surgery and autopsy, has been mentioned. In some instances, it is useful to distend the specimen of gut (prior to its opening) to achieve a more anatomic and functional state. This maneuver is particularly helpful in obtaining correlations with in vivo gross radiographic studies. Examples include specimens with any obstruction; with diverticular disease, particularly of the colon; and with sinuses or fistulous tracts. With such studies, the pathologist can better appreciate the luminal and muscular alterations and identify any openings in the bowel wall with greater precision. Specimen preparation involves gently washing out the luminal contents, clamping or tying off one end, and allowing fixative to flow in to completely fill the lumen of the specimen. The other end is then secured and the entire specimen is immersed in fixative, prior to its opening.

Vascular injection, mainly of the arterial segment, can be of use in the full delineation of vascular lesions and in determining the causation of ischemic bowel disease (18). In vascular lesions, such injection techniques may assist in correlation with in vivo angiographic studies, indicate the particular location of the lesion that is often small and difficult to appreciate by standard gross inspection, and appreciate the full scope and even pathogenesis of the lesion by providing a three-dimensional model. Vascular injections are particularly useful when defining vascular lesions that are especially small and do not have extensive communications with the mucosal aspect, for example, angiomatous malformations, acquired ectasias, and bleeding points in diverticula.

More specialized techniques, involving not only vascular injection but also subsequent clearing by xylol of the gross specimen and examination with the dissecting microscope, have been recommended and are probably essential for the full examination of tiny lesions, such as the vascular ectasias (also termed angiodysplasia) of the right side of the colon in elderly patients (19). This topic is discussed further in Chapter 14. Vascular injection may also assist in determining the particular cause of ischemic bowel disease by providing accurate delineation of the vascular anatomy, including any collaterals, and by noting any areas of narrowing or occlusion. Finally, alterations of the vascular system are being noted in some patients with acquired bowel disease not of an ischemic nature (e.g., some forms of enteritis and chronic colitis) (20), and it may prove useful to obtain correlative studies with the injected gross specimens.

Special techniques of preparation are also needed for accurate identification of the nervous tissue elements within the gut wall. This type of preparation involves the use of thick sections and silver impregnation, and such studies have provided useful information in many forms of pseudo-obstruction (21, 22). Details related to application of these techniques are provided in Chapter 13.

Regarding gross examination in general, the pathologists' attention is usually directed to the en face appearance of the mucosa. Noted in particular are any hemorrhages or other discolorations, loss or other alterations of the normal folds, ulcers, polyps, and other tumors. To better appreciate the events occurring in the rest of the bowel wall, these areas should be viewed on profile after appropriate cuts. In such a way, it is possible to discern depths of ulcers and of tumor invasion and the presence and extent of any diverticula, sinuses, or fistulae.

Microscopic Examination

There is often a need to obtain multiple sections at different levels of small biopsy samples. For the larger specimens, the best practice is to obtain sections from any grossly altered area to include representative lesions and any gross variations; i.e., the center and edges of tumors, and the different aspects of inflammatory disease to note the characters of active and inactive disease. Additional sections from uninvolved areas are often obtained to confirm normality or to verify particular anatomic regions.

In addition to the standard hematoxylin and eosin stain, a large variety of special stains are available for application in selected cases. Mucin stains are used to identify neutral, mildly, and strongly acidic types. They also may be helpful in determining areas and types of

metaplasia and in identifying the differentiation of a tumor. With such stains, transitional areas between the normal mucosa of the stomach and well-formed areas of intestinal metaplasia can be appreciated, and it is possible to discern the contribution of both gastric and intestinal types of epithelia in Barrett's esophagus. As required, additional stains are used to detect microorganisms; identify various stromal elements, particularly in tumors; define hormone-producing cells; and distinguish pigments.

Other Techniques

CYTOLOGY

Cytologic examination at the time of endoscopy has proven to be an important companion of mucosal biopsies (23, 24). As presently obtained by brushes, it covers a larger area of the mucosa than is possible in a single biopsy and can access strictured areas more readily. This technique is also associated with the potential for more rapid staining, examination, and interpretation. It should be noted, however, that false-negative cytologic preparations may be obtained from tumors with marked necrosis or infiltrative tumors that have minimal mucosal abnormality.

In the past, when fewer biopsy samples were obtained, cytologic examination was more often critical. At present, it is less so, as multiple mucosal biopsy samples may be readily obtained using flexible endoscopes. Nevertheless, it would be wrong to introduce an element of competition between the two examinations; rather, we emphasize that, with the same endoscopic examination, it is possible to obtain material for both cytologic and histologic examination, which provides the greatest yield with respect to diagnosis of tumors and their particular differentiation (25). Cytologic examination can also be performed on imprints of tumors from larger specimens, providing finer cellular detail and potentially accelerating the diagnostic process (26). Cytologic techniques and diagnosis are discussed in detail in Chapter 4.

IMMUNOCYTOCHEMISTRY

Immunologic techniques are used extensively at a tissue level, including both immunofluorescence and especially immunocytochemical methods (27). The stains help to establish monoclonality in lymphomatous cells, to distinguish carcinomas from lymphomas, and to separate the various mesenchymal and neurologic tumors (28, 29). They are also of value in specifically identifying particular hormone-producing cells, some microorganisms or their antigens, and oncofetal antigens (30). See Chapter 5 for further details.

ELECTRON MICROSCOPY

Ultrastructural examination by standard transmission electron microscopy is helpful in selected instances (10, 31, 32). To date, electron microscopy has proven to be of value in delineating some tumors (particularly stromal type, hormonal type, melanocytic, epithelial versus lymphoma), providing a general definition of hormonal cells, assessing the functional state of a particular cell (e.g., activity of parietal cells), recognizing early lesions (e.g., surface cell alterations in acute gastritis), identifying unusual microorganisms (e.g., bacterial rods in Whipple's disease, and uncommon protozoa such as microsporidia), and resolving the nature of storage deposits.

Examination by scanning electron microscopy can be helpful in the demonstration, often exquisite, of topographic markings and detailed microanatomy, but the technique has minimal use in standard diagnoses at the present time. It has been used to display the altered villous configurations in small bowel disorders and to help identify areas of epithelial dysplasia, including squamous cell lesions in the esophagus and glandular dysplasia in cases of long-standing ulcerative colitis (33).

SPECIAL TECHNIQUES

As needed, tissues are submitted for appropriate viral, bacterial, or fungal cultures. Recognition of the various parasitic infestations necessitates finding the organisms or their ova in the tissue sections. Histochemical techniques to identify enzymes were applied previously to help in determining the nature of epithelial and stromal populations, but their utility has proven limited and they have been largely supplanted by ultrastructural and immunocytochemical techniques. Biochemical analyses are used for the more precise identification of the various storage elements and to measure enzyme content in selected disorders.

Flow cytometric analyses are now routinely available for the subtyping of lymphomas and for the identification of the various immunodeficiency disorders. They are also being used with increasing frequency in the assessment of epithelial and stromal tumors (see Chapters 5 and 9). Aberrations in the chromosomal number and DNA content (such as aneuploidy) and in the cell cycle fractions can be identified and correlated with the nature of neoplastic tissue and behavior of malignant tumors (34, 35). We are also witnessing the rapid application of molecular techniques, including immunocytochemical stains, in-situ hybridization studies, and extraction of DNA and RNA (36–38). These techniques are being applied in an effort to define oncogenes, tumor suppressor genes, and other growth factors and their receptors to help in diagnosis and in correlations with tumor survival (see detailed discussion of this topic in Chapter 8).

PATHOLOGY REPORTS

Although the manner of reporting the pathologic analysis of a particular specimen cannot be made strictly uniform, we offer some suggestions about the type of information that should be included routinely in pathologic reports. First, list the particular diagnosis, accompanied as needed and desired by a list of the essential features that are supportive of this diagnosis. In the absence of completely specific features, you may offer some qualifying phase. Second, indicate the particular location and extent of the disorder, including both the longitudinal amount and the depth of bowel involved. Third, note explicitly the areas of the specimen, whether longitudinal or in depth, that are free of disease. This reiteration is of particular assistance to the clinician and surgeon in the evaluation of the disease-free gut. Fourth, record any complications of the basic disorder. Finally, list any other pathologic features of special interest and essential negative statements.

Much of the pathologic description can be readily contracted by using fairly precise collective pathologic terms, described previously in this chapter. For example, the designation of a chronic active colitis would embrace and make unnecessary the separate listing of acute and chronic inflammation, crypt abscesses, glandular regeneration, and metaplasia.

It is also necessary to answer any specific questions posed by the clinician, especially with respect to analyses of mucosal biopsy specimens, considering the multiple potential reasons for the procedure. Clinicians may seek a particular diagnosis, information concerning the extent or activity of the disease, or the presence of complications. They have an obligation to provide the particular reason for the procedure and biopsy, as does the pathologist to supply the best available answer.

REFERENCES

1. Williams LF. Vascular insufficiency of the intestine. Gastroenterology 1971;61:757–777.
2. Swerdlow SH, Antonioli DA, Goldman H. Intestinal infarctions: A new pathologic classification [letter]. Arch Pathol Lab Med 1981;10:218.
3. Owen DA, Kelly JK. Inflammatory diseases of the gastrointestinal tract. Modern Pathol 1995;8:97–108.
4. Que FG, Gores GJ. Viewpoints in digestive diseases. Cell death by apoptosis: Basic concepts and disease relevance for the gastroenterologist. Gastroenterology 1996;110:1238–1243.
5. Zwas F, Shields HM, Doos WG, et al. Scanning electron microscopy of Barrett's epithelium and its correlation with light microscopy and mucin stains. Gastroenterology 1986;90:1932–1941.
6. Stemmerman GN. Intestinal metaplasia of the stomach. A status report. Cancer 1994;74:556–564.
7. James AH. Gastric epithelium in the duodenum. Gut 1964;5:285.
8. Symonds DA. Paneth cell metaplasia in diseases of the colon and rectum. Arch Pathol Lab Med 1974;97:343.
9. Riddell RH, Goldman H, Ransohoff DF, et al. Dysplasia in inflammatory bowel disease: Standardized classification with provisional clinical applications. Hum Pathol 1983;14:931–968.
10. Goldman H. Gastrointestinal mucosal biopsy. New York: Churchill Livingstone, 1996.
11. Surawicz CM, Belic L. Rectal biopsy helps to distinguish acute self-limited colitis from idiopathic inflammatory bowel disease. Gastroenterology 1984;86:104–113.
12. Goldman H. Era of the mucosal biopsy. In: Goldman H, Appelman HD, Kaufman N, eds. Gastrointestinal pathology. Baltimore: Williams & Wilkins, 1990;1–10.
13. Morrissey JF, Reichelderfer M. Gastrointestinal endoscopy. N Engl J Med 1991;325:1142–1149,1214–1222.
14. Hirschowitz BI. Development and application of endoscopy. Gastroenterology 1993;104:337–342.
15. Rotterdam H, Sheahan DG, Sommers SC, eds. Biopsy diagnosis of the digestive tract. 2nd ed. New York: Raven Press, 1993.
16. Whitehead R. Mucosal biopsy of the gastrointestinal tract. 5th ed. Philadelphia: WB Saunders, 1996;1–25.
17. Perera DR, Weinstein WM, Rubin CE. Small intestinal biopsy. Hum Pathol 1975;6:157.
18. Ming SC, Bonakdarpour A. The evolution of lesions in intestinal ischemia. Arch Pathol Lab Med 1977;101:40.
19. Mitsudo SM, Boley SJ, Brandt LJ, et al. Vascular ectasias of the right colon in the elderly: A distinct pathologic entity. Hum Pathol 1979;10:585.
20. Wakefield AJ, Sawyer AM, Dhillan AP, et al. Pathogenesis of Crohn's disease: Multifocal gastrointestinal infarction. Lancet 1989;2:1057–1062.
21. Krisnamurthy S, Schuffler MD. Pathology of neuromuscular disorders of the small intestine and colon. Gastroenterology 1987;93:610–639.
22. Costa M, Brookes SJH. The enteric nervous system. Am J Gastroenterol 1994;89:5129–5137.
23. Qizilbash AH, Casteli M, Kowalski MA, et al. Endoscopic brush cytology and biopsy in the diagnosis of cancer of the upper gastrointestinal tract. Acta Cytol 1980;24:313.
24. Ehya H, O'Hara BJ. Brush cytology in the diagnosis of colonic neoplasms. Cancer 1990;66:1563–1567.
25. Marshall JB, Diaz-arias AA, Barthel JS, et al. Prospective evaluation of optimal number of biopsy specimens and brush cytology in the

diagnosis of cancer of the colorectum. Am J Gastroenterol 1993;88: 1352–1354.

26. Debongnie JC, Mairesse J, Donnay M, et al. Touch cytology. A quick, simple, sensitive screening test in the diagnosis of infections of the gastrointestinal mucosa. Arch Pathol Lab Med 1994;118:1115–1118.

27. Blackman E, Nash SV. Diagnosis of duodenal and ampullary epithelial neoplasms by endoscopic biopsy: A clinicopathologic and immuno-histochemical study. Hum Pathol 1985;16:901–910.

28. Mori M, Ambe K, Adachi Y, et al. Prognostic value of immunohis-tochemically identified CEA, SC, AFP, and S-100 protein-positive cells in gastric carcinoma. Cancer 1988;62:534–540.

29. Isaacson PG. Gastrointestinal lymphoma. Hum Pathol 1994;25: 1020–1029.

30. Lechago J. Gastrointestinal neuroendocrine cell proliferations. Hum Pathol 1994;25:1114–1122.

31. Frost AR, Orenstein JM, Abraham AA, et al. A comparison of the usefulness of electron microscopy and immunohistochemistry. One laboratory's experience. Arch Pathol Lab Med 1994;118:922–926.

32. Erlandson RA, Rosai J. A realistic approach to the use of electron microscopy and other ancillary diagnostic techniques in surgical pathology. Am J Surg Pathol 1995;19:247–250.

33. Shields HM, Best CJ, Goldman H. Distinction of dysplasia from inflammatory changes in ulcerative colitis. A scanning electron microscopy study with quantitative analyses. Surg Pathol 1988;1: 183–192.

34. Haggitt RC, Reid BJ, Rabinovitch PS, et al. Barrett's esophagus. Correlation between mucin histochemistry, flow cytometry, and histologic diagnosis for predicting increased cancer risk. Am J Pathol 1988;131:53–61.

35. Hood DL, Petras RE, Edinger M, et al. Deoxyribonucleic acid ploidy and cell cycle analysis of colorectal carcinoma by flow cytometry. Am J Clin Pathol 1990;93:615–620.

36. Grody WW, Gotti RA, Naeim F. Diagnostic molecular pathology. Modern Pathol 1990;2:553–568.

37. Stemmerman G, Heffelfinger SC, Noffsinger A, et al. The molecular biology of esophageal and gastric cancer and their precursors. Hum Pathol 1994;25:968–981.

38. Hamilton SR. The molecular genetics of colorectal neoplasia. Gastroenterology 1993;105:3–7.

FUNCTIONAL ANATOMY OF THE GASTROINTESTINAL TRACT

Donald A. Antonioli and James L. Madara

The objectives of this chapter are to review the organization of the gastrointestinal tract and to explore the gross and microscopic features of the various segments of that system. Excellent texts on the gross and microscopic anatomy of the gastrointestinal tract are readily available; in this chapter, we stress histologic features and structural-functional correlations of particular interest to pathologists.

GENERAL ORGANIZATION OF THE GASTROINTESTINAL TRACT

All segments of the gut are organized into four layers. The innermost layer is the mucosa, which is structurally and functionally the most complex area. The mucosa rests on the submucosa, beneath which is the muscularis propria. The outermost layer is termed the serosa or, if it lacks an outer limiting layer of mesothelial cells, the adventitia (Fig. 2.1).

The mucosa consists of three elements. The element facing the intestinal lumen is the epithelium, which varies in composition in different parts of the gut. The epithelium rests on and within a mesenchymal compartment termed the lamina propria; it contains connective tissue, smooth muscle fibers in some areas, a variety of vascular channels, nerve fibers, and inflammatory cells. The third and deepest layer of the mucosa is the muscularis mucosae, a double layer of smooth muscle, consisting of an inner circular and outer longitudinal band or spiral, that separates the lamina propria from the submucosa.

The submucosa is the branching and distribution zone for muscular arteries that have entered through the muscularis propria; in turn, small venous channels draining the mucosa converge to form larger veins that exit through the outer muscular layer. The submucosa is rich in lymphatics, a variety of inflammatory cells, autonomic neural fibers, and clusters of ganglion cells that form the submucosal plexus.

In most of the gastrointestinal tract, the muscularis propria consists of smooth muscle organized into a tightly coiled, inner circular layer and a more loosely helical, outer longitudinal layer. The smooth muscle cells are arranged in parallel arrays. Their cytoplasm is normally homogeneous and eosinophilic; however, formalin fixation often introduces an artifactual cytoplasmic vacuolar change that must be distinguished from true muscular vacuolar degeneration, as seen in association with certain types of myopathies. Specific topographic variations in the organization of the

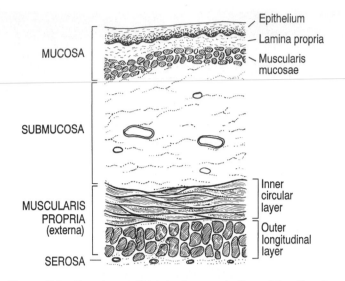

Figure 2.1   Four-layered histologic organization of the digestive tract.

muscularis propria are discussed in the appropriate subdivisions of this chapter.

Between the two layers of the muscularis propria are prominent autonomic neural fibers and clusters of ganglion cells forming the myenteric plexus. Both layers of the muscularis are additionally innervated by small neural twigs, which are not readily identified in routine hematoxylin and eosin preparations but are easily demonstrated by immunocytochemical techniques using antibodies to neuron-specific enolase or S-100 protein. Similarly, the vasculature of the muscular layer is inconspicuous, and inflammatory cells are not normally identified in this layer.

The function of the muscularis propria is to propel food through the gut by contractile peristaltic waves initiated and coordinated by neural and hormonal events. Flow is regulated by differing types of peristalsis and by sphincters located in the upper esophagus, in the distal portions of the esophagus, stomach, and ileum, and in the anus.

Most of the intestine is lined on its outer surface by a protective layer, the serosa. The serosa is formed of mesenchymal elements (fibroadipose tissue, vessels), lined externally by a single layer of mesothelial cells. In locations such as the esophagus, in which the mesothelial layer is absent, the outermost layer of the intestine is termed the adventitia. The serosa forms a natural barrier to the spread of inflammatory and malignant processes. A small number of mononuclear inflammatory cells normally may be identified in this layer (1).

Other chapters provide a more detailed discussion concerning inflammatory cells within the normal gut (see Chapter 5), cell renewal (see Chapter 7), and muscular and neural elements (see Chapter 11).

ESOPHAGUS

GROSS ANATOMY

The human esophagus is a hollow tube, with a smooth white mucosal surface, that is approximately 25 cm long. It extends from the cricopharyngeal muscle to its junction with the stomach at a point 2 to 3 cm below the diaphragm. Based on average endoscopic measurements in adults, the esophagus begins 15 cm distal to the central incisor teeth and ends 40 cm from that dental landmark. It lies behind the tracheobronchial tree, aortic arch, and heart, and in front of the vertebral column. At each end, it is demarcated by a sphincter. The upper sphincter is an anatomically definable structure composed of cricopharyngeal skeletal muscle fibers. In contrast, the lower esophageal sphincter, which is formed of smooth muscle, has no clearly defined gross or microscopic identity; rather, it is a zone of increased intraluminal pressure occupying the distal 5 cm of the esophagus (2, 3).

The arterial blood supply to the esophagus is complex, with anastomoses among the various components within the esophageal wall. The upper one third of the esophagus is supplied by the inferior thyroid arteries; the middle one third by intercostal arteries, the bronchial arteries, and branches directly from the aorta; and the lower one third by the left gastric and inferior phrenic arteries. The accompanying veins form mural complexes that connect the systemic and portal venous systems, thus permitting the possible development of esophageal varices in patients with portal hypertension.

The esophagus is well supplied with lymphatics that form a richly anastomosing network in the lamina propria and submucosa. Like the distribution of the arterial supply, lymphatic drainage is related to the three longitudinal segments of the esophagus. Drainage from the upper one third of the esophagus is to cervical and paratracheal lymph nodes, from the middle one third to bronchial and mediastinal lymph nodes, and from the lowest one third to mediastinal nodes and a variety of lymph nodes below the diaphragm. This extensive lymphatic drainage explains the wide dissemination sometimes noted in patients with primary esophageal malignancies (4).

FUNCTIONS

The primary functions of the normal esophagus are the propulsion of food from the mouth to the stomach and the prevention of significant reflux of gastric contents into the esophagus. The propulsive function is effected by involuntary peristalsis in the muscularis propria that, unlike the remainder of the digestive tract, is formed of two types of muscle fibers in humans. The upper one third consists of skeletal (striated) muscle fibers, the middle one third of mixed striated and smooth muscle, and the lowest one third of smooth muscle only (5). Nevertheless, innervation is similar throughout the esophagus, and peristalsis proceeds smoothly and uniformly throughout the organ. This variation in muscular composition accounts for the different types of neuromuscular disorders affecting the upper versus the lower esophagus. Normally closed to prevent reflux of gastric contents into the esophagus, the lower esophageal sphincter relaxes when the peristaltic wave reaches the distal esophagus, thus permitting entry of food into the stomach. Gravity also aids peristalsis in the movement of food to the stomach.

In the resting state, the esophagus is a collapsed tube, its lumen plicated by longitudinal folds. The elastic tissue in its walls accounts for its distensibility. Thus, during swallowing, the lumen dilates and the folds flatten so that the esophagus can normally accommodate the passage of even a large food bolus.

HISTOLOGIC FEATURES

The esophageal mucosa consists of squamous epithelium, lamina propria, and a thick muscularis mucosae. The inner lining of the esophageal mucosa is a multilayered, nonkeratinizing squamous epithelium that offers protection against injury from hard, jagged, or large food fragments (Fig. 2.2). The normal basal (regenerative) zone of the squamous epithelium, composed of cuboidal basophilic cells in an orderly arrangement along the basement lamina, occupies no more than 15 to 20% of the epithelial height, although it may be slightly thicker in the distal esophagus (6). Mitoses in this zone are usually difficult to identify, perhaps because cell turnover time is relatively long (more than 7 days) (7).

Above the basal zone, the postmitotic epithelial cells mature, a process characterized by accumulation of cytoplasmic glycogen, nuclear pyknosis, and a change in cell polarity from vertical to horizontal, the latter accompanied by conversion of the cell shape from round to elliptical. These changes in cell contour and polarity account for the characteristic "basket weave" appearance of the upper half of the esophageal epithelium. The ratio of the thickness of the basal zone to that of the mature epithelium is an important consideration in evaluating pathologic conditions of the esophagus. A simple method to determine the amount of mature epithelium is to perform the periodic acid-Schiff reaction to demonstrate cytoplasmic glycogen (8).

Ultrastructurally, the basal cells have large nuclei, relatively few cytoplasmic organelles, and no glycogen. In comparison, the maturing, postmitotic squamous cells are characterized by glycogen accumulation in the cytoplasm; increasing amounts of tonofilaments (keratins), especially beneath the cell membrane; and more numerous desmosomes. Cell degeneration occurs in the surface layers (5). Scanning electron microscopy reveals that the luminal surface of the most superficial squamous cells has a network of microridges. Their function is not known precisely, but they may offer protection by holding a thin layer of mucus for lubrication and cytoprotection (9) (Fig. 2.3).

Distally, the white esophageal squamous epithelium abruptly converts to the tan-pink gastric cardia glandular epithelium either at

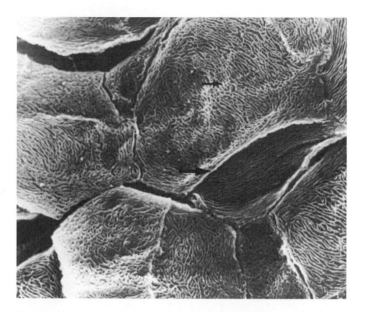

Figure 2.3 Luminal surface of normal esophageal squamous mucosa. Scanning electron micrograph demonstrates the complex pattern of surface microridges *(short arrow)*. Prominent intercellular ridges *(long arrow)* identify the junction of adjacent squamous cells (glutaraldehyde, ×2800). (Courtesy of Helen Shields, M.D., Beth Israel Hospital, Boston, MA.)

the gross anatomic gastroesophageal junction or at some point (1 to 3 cm) within the lowermost esophagus, in the high pressure zone of the lower esophageal sphincter. This sharply defined mucosal junction, called the Z-line, has a jagged appearance as it extends around the circumference of the esophagus (10).

The lowest layers of the squamous epithelium may contain scattered endocrine cells and melanocytes, whereas the lower and middle layers contain T lymphocytes and Langerhans' cells (Fig. 2.4)(11–13). The latter are antigen-presenting cells that characteristically have elongated, often angulated nuclei and inconspicuous cytoplasm in formalin-fixed and hematoxylin and eosin-stained sections. Their presence and their dendritic cytoplasmic processes can be highlighted immunocytochemically by staining the tissue with antibodies to S-100 protein. The presence of T lymphocytes and Langerhans' cells in the normal esophageal mucosa suggests an immunoregulatory function for this organ, but mechanisms of its action are as yet undefined (11, 14).

Glandular epithelium on the surface of the esophagus usually represents an acquired metaplastic change, known as Barrett's esophagus. In the upper 5 to 10 cm of the esophagus, however, in the area of the cricopharyngeal muscle, islands of corpus/fundic-type gastric mucosa of congenital origin (gastric heterotopia) have been identified in approximately 4% of patients at endoscopy (15); see Chapter 16 for further details. Indigenous mucous glands are also part of the normal esophagus and are of two types. Simple tubular mucous glands (termed "superficial" or "mucosal" mucous glands) are located in the lamina propria, but are confined to narrow zones at the two ends of the esophagus; i.e., adjacent to the cricopharyngeal muscle and next to the gastroesophageal junction. They produce neutral mucins and, because of their similarity to the glands of the gastric cardia, have also been called "cardiac glands."

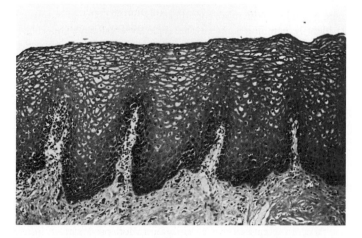

Figure 2.2 Normal squamous mucosa of the esophagus. The basal zone occupies less than 20% of the mucosal thickness, whereas the papillae of lamina propria extend approximately halfway through the height of the mucosa (×150).

In contrast, a more complex type of mucous gland (termed "deep" or "submucosal") is located in variable numbers in the submucosa along the length of the esophagus, with a tendency to a higher concentration in the proximal esophagus (Fig. 2.5). These glands, which produce acidic mucins, drain their secretions through the lamina propria and epithelium via ducts lined by columnar epithelium that is surrounded by myoepithelial cells (8, 16, 17). The glandular secretion is presumably to lubricate the luminal surface of the esophagus and perhaps to act as a barrier to damage caused by refluxed gastric acid and pepsin (18). The ducts of the submucosal glands are commonly surrounded by aggregates of mature lymphocytes in the lamina propria (19).

Projections of lamina propria, termed "papillae," extend into the squamous epithelium at regular intervals along the esophagus (see Fig. 2.2). The papillae and lamina propria contain fibrovascular tissue, lymphatics, elastic tissue, and occasional inflammatory cells. The papillae normally do not extend to more than 50 to 60% through the height of the epithelium (1, 6). The lamina propria otherwise lacks specific characteristics; it rests on a two-layered, but

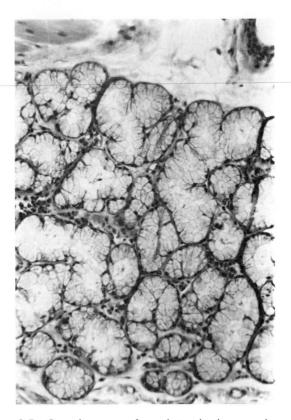

Figure 2.5 Complex array of esophageal submucosal mucous glands (×150).

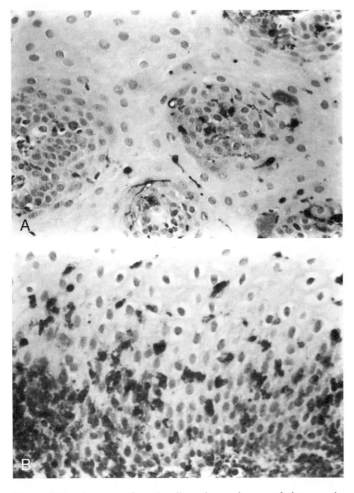

Figure 2.4 A. Langerhans' cells in lower layers of the esophageal epithelium. Note their elongated cytoplasmic processes extending between the squamous cells. (Staining for S-100 protein, PAP technique, ×300). **B.** Lymphocytes are identified within the lower portion of the esophageal epithelium. (Staining for leukocyte common antigen, PAP technique, ×300).

relatively thick, muscularis mucosae that, unlike the muscularis mucosae of the stomach and intestines, consists of longitudinal rather than spiraled fibers (17). The lamina propria may also contain ectopic sebaceous glands (20) or, in the lower esophagus-cardia region, foci of ectopic exocrine pancreas (21).

Vessels, lymphoid cells, and neural tissue occupy the wide submucosa. Unlike other parts of the gut, in which ganglion cells lie close to the muscularis mucosae, the ganglion cells of the esophageal submucosa are deep, adjacent to the muscularis propria; small nerve twigs extend into the more superficial zones (5). Thus, it is unusual to identify ganglion cells in the typically small and superficial, endoscopically derived grasp biopsy specimens of the esophagus.

STOMACH

GROSS ANATOMY

The stomach is variable in its gross configuration, but it is most often "J"-shaped. Normally located in the left upper quadrant of the abdomen, its upper portion lies beneath the dome of the left hemidiaphragm. Distally, it joins the duodenum in approximately the midline of the peritoneal cavity. As noted in the section on the esophagus, the junction of esophagus with stomach is normally several centimeters below the diaphragm. Because of defects in the diaphragm, however, the proximal stomach may extend into the thoracic cavity, a condition known as hiatal hernia (2, 22).

The stomach is divided grossly into four zones, each of which has a specific microscopic mucosal structure. The cardia is the narrow (approximately 1.0 cm long) portion of the stomach immediately distal to the gastroesophageal junction. The remainder of the stomach is divided into proximal and distal parts by an imaginary circumferential line drawn through the angle, or notch (incisura angularis), on the lesser curve of the stomach. The proximal portion is the body or corpus; the portion of the body that extends above the junction with the esophagus is the fundus. The distal part of the stomach, the pyloric antrum, is demarcated from the duodenum by the pyloric sphincter. The latter is closed in the resting state to prevent the reflux of intestinal contents into the stomach. Particularly in older patients (and perhaps as a consequence of chronic gastritis), the pyloric antral mucosa may extend proximal to the incisura along the lesser curvature, occasionally even reaching the cardia, a process termed "pseudopyloric metaplasia" (23, 24).

In the resting state, the gastric mucosa and submucosa form rugae, which are longitudinal folds, that lie parallel to, but are absent at, the lesser curvature. These rugae, which tend to be more prominent in the proximal than in the distal stomach, normally flatten during food ingestion to increase the capacity of the stomach. Retention of rugae in the distended stomach is seen occasionally in normal subjects, but this finding is usually secondary to inflammatory, hyperplastic, and neoplastic processes. In addition to rugae, the mucosa is divided into fixed mosaic-like areas, separated by furrows, that are termed areae gastricae. Unlike normal rugae, they are not changed by alterations in the configuration of the stomach (23).

The arterial blood supply to the stomach is complex and is subject to numerous congenital variations. In brief, the gastric blood supply is derived from three branches of the celiac artery: the splenic, common hepatic, and left gastric arteries. These vessels, in turn, give rise to the five major gastric arteries: the left and right gastric, left and right gastroepiploic, and short gastric arteries. Because of the rich anastomoses among the intramural gastric arteries, infarction of this organ is extremely rare. Venous drainage from the stomach is through the portal system to the liver. As in the esophagus, however, the potential for systemic-portal anastomoses (left gastric vein to azygous vein) exists in the stomach. Thus, gastric varices may develop in patients with portal hypertension. As discussed subsequently (see "Histology of the Gastric Mucosa"), lymphatics in the gastric mucosa are located only in the lowermost portion of the lamina propria and in the muscularis propria. Deeper in the wall is a rich lymphatic network that drains to regional perigastric lymph nodes and to nodes in the omentum, around the head of the pancreas, and in the splenic hilum (4).

Gastric Functions

In the stomach, solid food is fragmented and mixed by peristalsis. A semiliquid material (chyme) is formed that is released in small, regulated bursts into the duodenum by rhythmic openings of the pyloric sphincter. In humans, cells in the corpus and fundus of the stomach also produce hydrochloric acid and intrinsic factor; the latter is necessary for the absorption of Vitamin B_{12} in the terminal ileum. The physiologic roles of hydrochloric acid are not completely defined. It may aid the absorption of iron in the proximal duodenum by providing an acidic environment. Indirect evidence of a bacteriostatic function for hydrochloric acid is the fact that, compared with controls, enteric bacterial infections are more prevalent in

patients with atrophic gastritis. Also, an acid milieu is necessary for the activation of gastric proteolytic enzymes (25).

Although predominantly a small intestinal function, some digestion does occur in the stomach. Certain gastric mucosal cells produce pepsinogens, proteolytic enzymes that are secreted in an inactive form but are then activated by the acid environment of the gastric lumen during meals. In addition, lipase derived from gastric mucosal chief cells is active at a low gastric pH (26, 27).

Production of the hormone gastrin is another major gastric function. Produced by antropyloric endocrine cells, gastrin causes release of hydrochloric acid as one of its major physiologic effects. Gastric and intestinal endocrine cells are discussed fully in Chapter 13.

HISTOLOGY OF THE GASTRIC MUCOSA (SEE TABLE 2.1)

The mucosa is structurally and functionally the most complex layer of the gastric wall. The other layers do not contain special anatomic features except for the muscularis propria, which is organized into three (innermost oblique, inner circular, outer longitudinal) rather than two layers and forms a nodular pyloric sphincter at the distal end of the stomach (23).

The gastric mucosa varies in thickness; it is thinnest in the cardia and up to 1.5 mm thick in the corpus (17). It consists of the usual three components: epithelium, lamina propria, and muscularis mucosae. The epithelial cells vary in different parts of the stomach, and functionally are the most important elements in the mucosa. The lamina propria and muscularis mucosae are histologically similar to the analogous layers in the esophagus, although the gastric lamina propria does not contain lymphatics, except in its lowermost portion, adjacent to the muscularis mucosae (28, 29). In this regard, it is similar to the lamina propria of the colon but differs from that of the esophagus and small intestine, both of which are rich in lymphatics. The deep location of gastric mucosal lymphatics is an important factor in explaining the low frequency of nodal metastases in gastric carcinomas confined to the mucosa (28, 29).

The lamina propria contains elastic fibers and strands of smooth muscle, the latter derived from the muscularis mucosae and normally identified most prominently in the distal part of the stomach. A small number of inflammatory cells, chiefly mononuclear, are also present in the upper one third of the lamina propria in children and adults (23); however, they are typically absent in newborns and infants. Likewise, a few eosinophils may be identified in otherwise normal gastric mucosa (30). Other common findings noted in endoscopically derived biopsy specimens are edema and variable fresh hemorrhage in the lamina propria. If unaccompanied by epithelial cell necrosis and/or a polymorphonuclear leukocytic infiltrate, edema and hemorrhage in this location are best considered artifacts secondary to the trauma of the endoscopic procedure.

SURFACE-FOVEOLAR MUCOUS CELLS

The epithelium of the gastric mucosa forms glands that vary in density and cellular composition in different parts of the stomach. At their upper end, several glands connect with and drain their secretions into conical depressions of the mucosal surface known as gastric foveolae or pits. The foveolae and the mucosal surface between them are uniformly lined by surface-foveolar mucous cells,

TABLE

2.1   **Gastric Epithelial Cells: Ultrastructural Characteristics and Major Functions**

Cell Type	Distinctive Ultrastructural Features	Major Functions
Surface-foveolar mucous cells	Apical stippled granules up to 1 μm in diameter	Production of neutral glycoprotein and bicarbonate to form a gel on the gastric luminal surface; neutralization of HCl[a]
Mucous neck cell	Heterogeneous granules, 1-2 μm in diameter, dispersed throughout the cytoplasm	Progenitor cell for all other gastric epithelial cells Glycoprotein production Production of pepsinogens I and II
Oxyntic (parietal) cell	Surface membrane invaginations (canaliculi) Tubulovesicle structures Numerous mitochondria	Production of HCl Production of intrinsic factor Production of bicarbonate
Chief cell	Moderately dense apical granules up to 2 μm in diameter Prominent supranuclear Golgi apparatus Extensive basolateral granular endoplasmic reticulum	Production of pepsinogens I & II, and of lipase
Cardiopyloric mucous cell	Mixture of granules like those in mucous neck and chief cells Extensive basolateral granular endoplasmic reticulum	Production of glycoprotein Production of pepsinogen II
Endocrine cells	See Chapter 13	

[a]Bicarbonate is probably produced by other gastric epithelial cells in addition to surface-foveolar mucous cells.

which are columnar cells with a small basal nucleus, pale-staining apical cytoplasmic mucin, and a straight lateral border (Fig. 2.6). These cells produce predominantly neutral glycoproteins; thus, the apical cytoplasm stains positively in the periodic acid-Schiff (PAS) reaction (23). The deep foveolar mucous cells, however, also contain acidic mucins. In the corpus-fundic region, these mucins are nonsulfated (N-acylated sialomucins); in the pyloric antrum, sulfated mucins also may rarely be identified (Table 2.2) (31, 32). Ultrastructurally, the cells have sparse apical microvilli beneath

which the apical cytoplasm is filled with moderately dense, stippled secretory granules. The cells adhere to one another by circumferential tight junctions located in the upper one third of the lateral cell border (see Fig. 2.6) (33).

Surface mucous cells secrete their glycoprotein at a continuous baseline rate by exocytosis, but secretion is increased by vagal stimulation, irritants, prostaglandins, and various hormones. On the cell surface, the mucin forms a tightly adherent gel that contains bicarbonate; bicarbonate is also produced by the mucous cells via

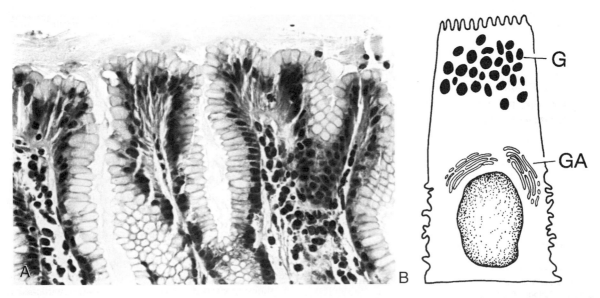

Figure 2.6   Gastric surface-foveolar mucous cells. **A.** In routine sections, they are columnar cells with pale granular apical cytoplasm (×300). **B.** Characteristic ultrastructural features are apical granules (G), prominent Golgi apparatus (GA), and complex basolateral cell membrane.

carbonic anhydrase activity. The gel with its trapped bicarbonate is important in neutralizing hydrochloric acid and in maintaining the pH at 7 at the mucosal cell surface. The mucin gel in association with the mucous cell tight junctions forms a mucosal barrier to the back-diffusion of acid (33–35). In humans, surface mucous cell turnover time is between 2 and 6 days (7).

MUCOUS NECK CELLS

The mucous neck cell is found throughout the stomach, predominantly in the upper portion (neck or isthmus) of each gland, immediately beneath the glandular junction with the foveolae, although a few neck cells may be scattered along the length of the glands (36). Light microscopy demonstrates that these cells are similar in appearance to the surface-foveolar mucous cells, but may be distinguished from them by their shorter size, more triangular shape, and slightly basophilic cytoplasm. Also, they stain less strongly than the surface mucous cells with the PAS reaction, but may stain with alcian blue at pH 2.5, because they contain some acidic mucins (see Table 2.2) (31, 36).

Neck cells have distinctive features when examined ultrastructurally: compared with surface-foveolar mucous cells, their secretory granules generally are larger and less dense, and they are dispersed more evenly throughout the cytoplasm (33).

Of critical importance, mucous neck cells are the gastric epithelial progenitor cells. In each gland, they form the zone of epithelial cell renewal, giving rise to new surface-foveolar mucous cells as well as to all the cell types within the glands. Despite the cellular renewal function of the neck zone, mitoses in adults are typically not observed in this area in sections of normal stomach. In fact, the presence of mitoses signifies regeneration, and is usually accompanied by other evidence of injury and repair.

EPITHELIAL CELLS OF THE GASTRIC GLANDS

The deeper portions of the gastric epithelial glands vary in their configuration and cellular content. In the corpus and fundus, the glands (gastric glands proper, or fundic glands) are long, straight, tightly packed, and associated with relatively short foveolae that

TABLE 2.2	Mucin Profiles of Gastric Epithelial Cells	
	Mucin Type	
Cell Type	Neutral	Acidic
Surface-foveolar mucous cells	Predominant	Trace[a] (in cells at base of foveoli)
Mucous neck cells	Predominant	Trace[a]
Cardiopyloric mucous cells	Predominant	Usually negative

Derived from Rotterdam H. The normal stomach and duodenum. In: Rotterdam H, Enterline HT, eds. Pathology of the stomach and duodenum. New York: Springer, 1989;1–12; Owen DA. Stomach. In: Sternberg SS, ed. Histology for pathologists. New York: Raven Press, 1992;533–545.

[a]Sialo- and sulfated mucins.

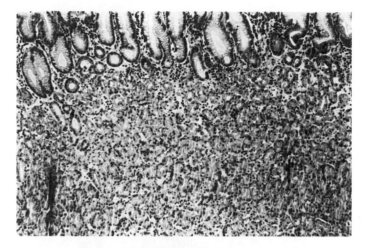

Figure 2.7 Architecture of the gastric glands proper. The glands are closely packed and the foveoli are relatively short (×75).

form no more than 25% of the mucosal thickness. These structures are the gastric glands proper; they contain mucous neck, oxyntic (parietal), zymogenic (chief) and endocrine cells (Fig. 2.7).

In the cardia and pyloric antrum, the glands (cardiopyloric glands) are shorter, coiled, more loosely arrayed, and associated with longer foveolae that may account for up to 50% of the mucosal height. These cardiopyloric glands are normally lined predominantly by mucous and endocrine cells, but they may contain variable numbers of oxyntic cells in many patients, a finding that signifies retention of the fetal pattern of oxyntic cell distribution (Fig. 2.8) (37). Large numbers of oxyntic cells in pyloric mucosa, however, should suggest the possibility of oxyntic cell hyperplasia secondary to hypergastrinemia. Zymogenic cells are not identified outside the corpus and fundus.

The border between the pyloric glands and the gastric glands proper is often not sharp. Rather, it is typically characterized by a transition zone of 1 to 2 cm width that may vary in location in the normal stomach and that contains an admixture of corpus-fundic and cardiopyloric glandular cell types (23). Awareness of the transition zone phenomenon prevents overinterpretation of corpus mucosa as showing pyloric metaplasia.

Oxyntic (Parietal) Cells

Most oxyntic cells occupy the midportion of the gastric glands, but they may be found in the neck region or at the base. They are pyramidal with a narrowed apex, a centrally placed nucleus, and deeply eosinophilic granular cytoplasm (23). Their ultrastructural appearance is distinctive. The cells have deep invaginations of the surface membrane, called canaliculi, that extend into the cytoplasm. The latter contains numerous cytoplasmic tubulovesicular structures in the resting state and many mitochondria that account for the deep cytoplasmic eosinophilia and granularity noted in hematoxylin and eosin-stained sections (Fig. 2.9) (33).

Production of hydrochloric acid by the oxyntic cells is effected by several mechanisms, chiefly through vagal stimulation and release of gastrin and histamine. These stimuli eventuate in intracellular energy production (cyclic AMP) and accumulation of calcium. Activation of the oxyntic cells sets into motion a specific hydrogen-

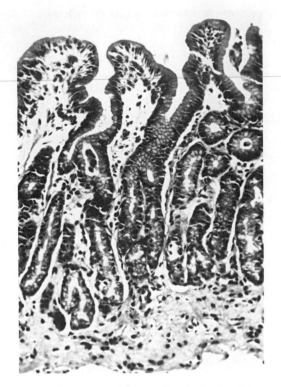

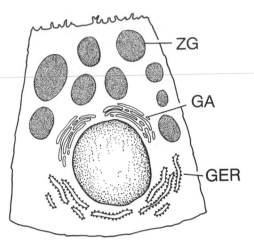

Figure 2.10 Major ultrastructural features of chief cells are basolateral granular endoplasmic reticulum (GER), supranuclear Golgi apparatus (GA), and apical zymogen granules (ZG).

Figure 2.8 Architecture of the cardiopyloric glands in a pediatric patient. Compared to the gastric glands proper, the glands are shorter, more irregular, and contain a different array of cells (see text for details). The foveoli may occupy up to 50% of the mucosal thickness (×50).

potassium-ATPase, located on the canalicular and tubulovesicular membranes, that acts as a proton pump to exchange hydrogen ions for potassium ions across the apical membrane (25). During acid production, the cytoplasmic tubulovesicles fuse with the canalicular

membrane, the latter becoming filled with microvilli, thus increasing the surface area for metabolic exchange. This process of fusion is reversed when acid production ceases (1, 25).

Oxyntic cells also contain carbonic anhydrase and produce bicarbonate (33). In fact, all of the major cell types of the gastric glands, except the endocrine cells, contain this enzyme (38). The release of bicarbonate into the gastric lumen and intercellular spaces presumably contributes to the protection against injury by acid (39).

In humans, oxyntic cells also produce intrinsic factor, necessary for the ileal absorption of Vitamin B_{12}. Intrinsic factor is widely distributed in the oxyntic cell, from the basal rough endoplasmic reticulum to the apical membrane (40).

Zymogenic (Chief) Cells

Zymogenic cells are concentrated at the base of the gastric glands proper. They are low columnar cells, with basal nuclei and deeply basophilic cytoplasm, that produce two immunologically distinct groups of proteolytic enzymes (pepsinogen I and II) in an inactive (proenzyme) form (41). Ultrastructurally, they are classic protein-synthesizing cells, having extensive subnuclear rough endoplasmic reticulum; a prominent supranuclear Golgi apparatus; and numerous apical, moderately dense secretory granules, the latter accounting for the cytoplasmic basophilia noted in hematoxylin and eosin-stained sections (Fig. 2.10). When the chief cells are stimulated, the pepsinogens contained in the granules are released from the cells by exocytosis and then activated by the low luminal pH during digestion (33, 42). As noted previously, lipase is also produced in reasonably large amounts in human chief cells (26, 27).

Cardiopyloric Mucous Cells

These cells, which line the cardiopyloric glands, produce predominantly neutral glycoproteins, presumably to aid in neutralizing gastric acid as it enters the duodenum (see Table 2.2). Although these cells superficially resemble surface-foveolar mucous cells at the light microscopic level, they differ from them ultrastructurally by

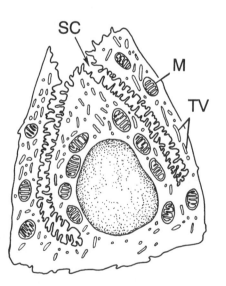

Figure 2.9 Major ultrastructural features of oxyntic cells are surface intracytoplasmic canaliculus (SC), cytoplasmic tubulovesicles (TV), and numerous mitochondria (M).

having mucin granules throughout the cytoplasm rather than confined to the cell apex. Also, the mucin granules are more irregular in size and shape and less dense than those in surface-foveolar mucous cells. Their secretory granules contain pepsinogen II and lysozyme as well as glycoprotein (33, 41, 42).

Endocrine Cells

The stomach is rich in endocrine cells that form part of the diffuse gastrointestinal endocrine system, which is analyzed in Chapter 13.

SMALL INTESTINE

Of all the segments of the alimentary tract, the small intestine is perhaps the most crucial because life may be sustained in the absence of the esophagus, stomach, or colon if direct access to the lumen of the small intestine is maintained. Thus, the fact that endoscopists routinely sample only the two extreme ends of the small intestine should not obviate the need to appreciate the structural detail of this vital organ. Here, we shall present an overview of the vast literature describing small intestinal structure and function. For more detailed reference, recent reviews may be useful (43, 44).

GROSS ANATOMY

The first portion of the small intestine, the duodenum, extends approximately 25 cm from the pyloric sphincter to a fibrous and muscular band, the ligament of Treitz. From its origin at the distal stomach, the duodenum enters the retroperitoneum, curves, then returns to the peritoneal cavity; thus, it has the contour of a C-shaped loop. Given this appearance, it is not surprising that the duodenum has descriptively (and arbitrarily) been divided into superior, descending, horizontal and ascending portions. The duodenal loop hugs the head of the pancreas and, focally, is in close apposition to the transverse colon. As a result, processes affecting these latter organs can distort the shape of the duodenal "C-loop" and be recognized by radiologists on upper gastrointestinal tract (upper GI) imaging studies.

One feature of duodenal gross anatomy has particular impact on the strategy used by clinicians in obtaining small intestinal mucosal biopsies. Because the entire duodenum is in a fixed position, the clinician can recognize by endoscopy the site at which an intraluminal biopsy capsule leaves the distal duodenum and enters the mobile proximal jejunum. This site, of course, corresponds to the ligament of Treitz. Recognition of this site permits the endoscopist to reproducibly and serially sample intestinal mucosa in a given patient at the same location.

Between the ligament of Treitz and the ileocecal sphincter lie the jejunum and ileum. Arbitrarily, the proximal one-third of this segment of the small intestine is referred to as jejunum and the remainder as the ileum. The structure and function of the jejunum and ileum are substantially different; however, these differences occur gradually, and clear anatomic or functional localization of a precise jejunal-ileal transition site is impossible. One gross alteration occurring along the jejunal-ileal axis that is important to radiologists (and to pathologists attempting to identify an unmarked segment of small intestine) is the presence of circumferential mucosal folds, or plicae circularis. They are densely distributed in the proximal jejunum and, by displacing luminal barium, impart a flocculent

appearance to this segment on upper GI series. In contrast, plicae are widely separated in the distal ileum. A second gross feature that permits identification of the ileum is the presence of Peyer's patches, which are dense collections of mucosal lymphoid nodules appearing as oval, 1- to 4-cm long mucosal distortions.

The duodenum is supplied chiefly by the pancreaticoduodenal artery off the celiac axis, with drainage primarily through superior and inferior pancreaticoduodenal veins to the portal system. Lymphatic drainage is to pyloric and lumbar preaortic lymph nodes. The jejunum and ileum are supplied by approximately a dozen branches of the superior mesenteric artery. These branches divide and anastomose several times in the mesentery, forming arcades, the last of which defines a marginal vessel along the small intestine (4). Because of this series of vascular anastomoses, the risk of small bowel infarction is greatly diminished if one portion of its proximal blood supply is compromised. The organization of the mucosal vasculature is discussed in the next section.

Venous drainage in the jejunum and ileum parallels the arterial supply, with the superior mesenteric vein joining the splenic vein to form the portal vein. The lymphatic system is highly developed in the small intestinal mucosa. Each villus contains one or more well-formed vertical lymphatic channels (lacteals) that drain into a complex submucosal lymphatic network. Unlike in the stomach, the lymphatics draining the small intestine are large (up to 1 mm in diameter). Drainage is to periaortic lymph nodes at the mesenteric root. Significant obstruction to the lymphatics may lead to intestinal mural edema and prominent intraluminal loss of protein and fluid (4).

ORGANIZATION OF THE MUCOSAL VASCULATURE

The general organization of the small intestinal wall is the same as described earlier in this chapter. More detail is provided here, however, because of the potentially major role that the architecture of the mucosal circulation plays in the function of the small intestine.

The mucosal lining is organized into villous projections, each of which is centrally penetrated by an arteriole. This arteriole splays at the villous tip into a network of capillaries that subsequently course down along the sides of the villus. Thus, the villous vasculature is endowed with a hairpin turn that could, in theory, permit countercurrent exchange of gases and solutes similar to that which occurs in the kidney. Evidence now exists that exchange between these ascending and descending vascular limbs occurs (45). Such exchange appears to play a crucial role in determining the distribution of lesions in pathologic disorders, such as ischemia.

EPITHELIAL STRUCTURE
GENERAL ASPECTS

The epithelial lining initiates and modulates the basic activities attributed to the small intestine: terminal digestion of nutrients and vectorial transport of nutrients, water, and ions. The epithelial surface is expanded not only by villous processes but also by the crypts present between villi (Fig. 2.11). The distance from the villous tips to the base of the crypts constitutes the mucosal thickness, because the crypts rest directly on the muscularis mucosae. Normally, the height of the villus, which is approximately 1 mm, exceeds that of the crypt by a factor of 4 to 5. The discrete anatomic nature of crypts and villi is substantiated by the fact that different cell populations reside in these two compartments: Paneth cells, undifferentiated crypt cells, endocrine cells, and goblet cells in the crypt and absorptive cells, goblet cells, and endocrine cells on the villus. Two additional, minor cell types of unknown function—tuft and cup cells—are present in both compartments.

The anatomic stratification of the epithelium into crypts and villi is paralleled by functional compartmentalization. Crypt cells secrete ions and water, synthesize secretory component, and transport IgA (synthesized by lamina propria plasma cells) into the lumen. In addition, the crypts are the site at which cell renewal occurs. Cell turnover time is approximately 5 to 6 days in the jejunum and 3 days in the ileum (see details in Chapter 7). In contrast, the villus is the site at which terminal digestion of nutrients and absorption of nutrients, ions, and water occur (43, 44).

Several expectations arise when considering the consequences of the stratification of epithelial function along the crypt-villus axis. Destruction of the crypt, the proliferative unit of this epithelium, should impair or destroy the ability of the small intestine to reconstitute its surface. Expansion of the crypt contribution to total epithelial surface (either by enlargement of this compartment, shrinkage of the villus compartment, or both) should result in

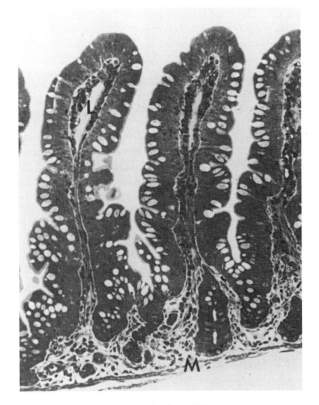

Figure 2.11   Light micrograph of small intestinal mucosa shows tall fingerlike villi and short crypts. Villi are predominantly lined by absorptive cells (cells with brush border) but also contain several goblet cells (clear goblet-shaped cells). A lymphatic (L) can be seen in a villus core, as can a fine wisp of the muscularis mucosae (M) (×250). (Reprinted with permission from Madara JL, Trier JS. Functional morphology of the mucosa of the small intestine. In: Johnson LR, ed. Physiology of the gastrointestinal tract. 3rd ed. New York: Raven Press, 1994;1577–1622.)

enhanced secretion of ions and water. Finally, diminution of the villous contribution to the epithelial surface should result in abnormal terminal digestion and malabsorption of nutrients, water, and ions. In general, these principles are realized in multiple small intestinal disease states (see Chapters 26–29).

Although crypts and villi constitute the majority of the surface area of the small intestine, a third compartment exists that, although small in area, may play an exceedingly important role in intestinal defense mechanisms. Throughout the small intestine, nodules of lymphoid cells distort the mucosal surface contour to produce broad domes rather than discrete villi. In the ileum, aggregates of such structures large enough to be visible macroscopically constitute the previously mentioned Peyer's patches. The so-called "follicular dome epithelium" overlying these lymphoid nodules (which contain "germinal" or "follicular" centers) consists predominantly of villous absorptive cells. Another minor and unique component of this epithelium is the "M," or membranous, epithelial cell (described in detail below) that is not found elsewhere (except, perhaps, in progenitor form). Moreover, it is this cell that imparts to the follicular dome epithelium the ability to absorb intact macromolecules and transport such antigenic "samples" to the underlying lymphoid tissue. Thus, the follicular dome epithelium and subjacent lymphoid tissue form the afferent limb of the intestinal immune response (43, 44).

A fourth epithelial compartment deserves brief mention. On the duodenal side of the pyloric sphincter are Brunner's glands, which are submucosal mucous glands lined by cells practically indistinguishable from pyloric gland mucous cells. Although present primarily in the duodenum, they may be identified in small numbers in the submucosa up to a foot distal to the ligament of Treitz; thus, their presence does not accurately define whether a biopsy comes from the duodenum or the proximal jejunum. These coiled glands focally penetrate the muscularis mucosae and are in continuity with crypt lumina into which they empty their secretory product. On the basis of ultrastructural, immunochemical, and histochemical evidence, these cells produce and secrete glycoproteins and pepsinogen II by simple exocytosis into their gland lumens. Although it had long been assumed that these cells were also the source of duodenal bicarbonate, which neutralizes gastric juice-derived acidity, results of recent studies indicate that duodenal villous cells are capable of bicarbonate secretion and call into question the contribution of Brunner's glands to duodenal neutralization (41, 46, 47).

INDIVIDUAL CELL TYPES (TABLE 2.3)

Absorptive Cells

Absorptive cells are the major cell type on the villus. In routine sections, they are characterized by a PAS-positive apical brush border, approximately 1.0 to 1.5 μ in height (see Fig. 2.11). These columnar cells display basal, oval nuclei and, in ideal 5-μ sections, a faint supranuclear lucency representing the Golgi apparatus. The remainder of the cytoplasm stains eosinophilic and is granular owing to the presence of organelles, such as lysosomes and mitochondria. The apical cytoplasmic area representing the terminal web, however, is devoid of organelles. The terminal bar, which contains the junctional zone (see below), can be identified as a faint basophilic structure just below the brush border at the interface of adjacent

TABLE	
2.3	**Small Intestine and Colonic and Epithelial Cells: Ultrastructural Characteristics and Major Functions**

Cell Type	Distinctive Ultrastructural Features	Major Functions

Absorptive cell (enterocyte)	Dense, tall apical microvilli, with external glycocalyx and internal microfilaments
	Apical terminal web
	Numerous intermediate filaments
	Microtubules
		Small intestine
		  Terminal digestion of nutrients
		  Absorption of nutrients
		  Intracellular lipid metabolism
		Colon
		  Electrolyte uptake; fluid reabsorption

Undifferentiated crypt cell	Short, sparse irregular microvilli Poorly developed terminal web Apical granules, 0.1 to 1.5 μm in diameter	Progenitor cell for all other intestinal cell types Synthesis of secretory component Release of IgA-receptor complex into crypt lumen "Secretion" of chloride and water
Goblet mucous cell	Sparse, irregular microvilli Apical granules that vary in size and density, depending on maturation of the cell (see text)	Production of acidic glycoproteins
Paneth cell	Large, dense apical granules Prominent supranuclear Golgi apparatus Extensive basolateral granular endoplasmic reticulum	Production of lysozyme
M cell	Smooth apical surface Central depression containing lymphoid cells; "inverted glass" appearance Numerous endocytotic vesicles	Uptake of luminal substances; role in intestinal immune response
Caveolated (tuft) cell	Long, wide microvilli containing microfilament bundles Membrane-bound spaces (caveoli) between microfilament bundles	Unknown
Cup cell	Concave brush border with short microvilli Poorly formed terminal web	Unknown
Endocrine cells	See Chapter 13	

cells by repeatedly focusing through the section. These cellular details are less apparent in formalin-fixed tissue than in tissue fixed in Bouin's or Hollende's solution.

The appearance of absorptive cells may change with differing physiologic states. During active absorption, the spaces between absorptive cells (paracellular spaces) may dilate (48), thus compressing the cells. In addition, because normal fat metabolism occurs in these cells (i.e., re-esterification of glycerol with absorbed fatty acids in the smooth endoplasmic reticulum, and subsequent combination of these lipids with newly synthesized apoproteins to form chylomicrons), transient intracellular lipid accumulation after a fatty meal may produce vacuoles in absorptive cells (43). Thus, moderate degrees of absorptive cell vacuolization in an otherwise normal villous epithelium must be interpreted with caution: such a finding may not indicate a disease state such as abetalipoproteinemia, but rather the residue of an ill-advised meal eaten shortly before the biopsy was performed.

Ultrastructurally, the apical plasma membrane of absorptive cells forms microvilli that regularly measure 0.1 μm in width and approximately 1 μm in height. Conversely, the basolateral membrane is relatively smooth and contains focal finger- and sheetlike processes that extend to interdigitate with those of adjacent cells. These two major domains of the plasma membrane

also differ strikingly in composition. The protein-lipid ratio of the apical membrane is exceedingly high (49). Thus, it is not surprising that, when visualized by the freeze-fracture technique, this domain exhibits densely distributed, P-face intramembrane particles (50), which probably represent integral membrane proteins (Fig. 2.12). At least 20 different protein bands can be identified in preparations derived from this membrane (51). This large number is not surprising, considering the array of hydrolases, transporters, and exchangers localized to this site. In contrast, the basolateral membrane exhibits protein and lipid profiles substantially different from those of the apical membrane. These chemical differences no doubt serve as the basis for physical differences between these two membranes, such as discrepant membrane fluidity (52).

A major basolateral membrane protein is the ATP-driven Na+/K+ exchanger (Na+/K+-ATPase). Na+/K+-ATPase-driven sodium extrusion from the cell results in an electrochemical gradient across the plasma membrane that favors sodium entry. This gradient provides the driving force for entry of many ions and nutrients into the cell (and is the reason that nutrient absorption, except lipids, is sodium dependent) (44). Absorption and transport of these substances is vectorial, from the apical membrane through the cell, with extrusion at the basolateral membrane. The highly polarized arrangement of pumps, transporters, and facilitated pathways on the apical and basolateral membranes permit this vectorial transport process to proceed.

Maintenance of the polarity of apical and basolateral membrane domains in absorptive cells is accomplished, in part, by the intercellular tight junction. The tight junction circumferentially belts the apical 0.5-μm portion of the lateral membrane (Fig. 2.13). It consists of a series of fusions between the outer membrane leaflets of adjacent cells that seal the lumen from the paracellular space and, thus, protect the subepithelial compartment from noxious luminal elements. These fusion sites actually are transmitted linearly in the plane of the lateral membrane. Hence, in freeze-fracture replicas, the tight junction appears as an array of anastomosing P-face strands and E-face grooves representing the fusion sites described above (Fig. 2.14). The tight junction may also represent a barrier that restricts movement of integral membrane proteins and plasma membrane outer leaflet lipids across it, thus helping to maintain the distinctive chemical profiles of the apical and basolateral membranes (43).

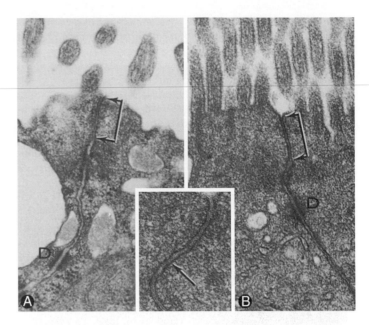

Figure 2.13   Thin sections of junctional complexes in the crypt *(left)* and on the villus *(right)*. The apical junctional complex includes tight junctions *(brackets)* and desmosomes (D). The organization and structure of tight junctions cannot be fully appreciated in thin sections (approximately ×52,700). **Inset:** Villus tight junction at higher magnification (approximately ×78,200). A point of fusion of the outer membrane leaflets of adjacent cells is indicated *(arrow)*. Fusion points correspond to P-face strands and E-face grooves revealed by freeze fracture. (Reprinted with permission from Madara JL, Trier JS. Functional morphology of the mucosa of the small intestine. In: Johnson LR, ed. Physiology of the gastrointestinal tract. 3rd ed. New York: Raven Press, 1994;1577–1622.)

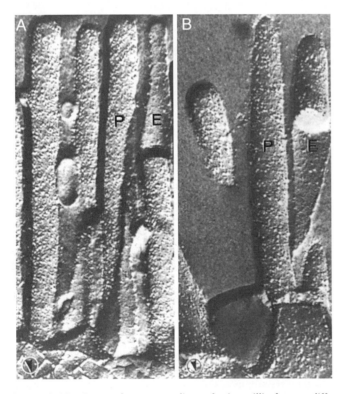

Figure 2.12   Freeze-fracture replicas of microvilli of an undifferentiated crypt cell *(left)* and a villus absorptive cell *(right)*. The majority of intramembrane particles are associated with the convex membrane half, which covers the microvillus core (protoplasmic or P face); fewer particles are associated with the concave membrane half, which abuts the extracellular space (extracellular or E face). P-face particles are more numerous in the microvillus membranes of villus cells than in those of crypt cells. E-face particle density is comparable in both sites (×135, 350). (Reprinted with permission from Madara JL, Trier JS, Neutra MR. Structural changes in the plasma membrane accompanying differentiation of epithelial cells in human and monkey small intestine. Gastroenterology 1980;78:963-975.)

Although this arrangement in part explains the maintenance of cell polarity, it does not explain the origin of cell polarity. Many constituents of the plasma membrane are replaced several times over the life span of the absorptive cells. For example, the half-life of sucrase-isomaltose may be as short as 4 to 6 hours (51). Newly synthesized replacement protein, however, is subsequently found only on the apical domain and is not equally intermixed in the basolateral membrane. This phenomenon, in which newly synthesized membrane components migrate to the appropriate domain, is termed membrane "addressing." The process is not well understood, but it clearly lies at the heart of how cells polarize themselves.

As noted previously, the tight junction not only assists in maintenance of polarity, but also impedes passive flow of molecules between cells. Whereas this barrier appears to be absolute for large molecules, it is relative for smaller ones. Indeed, at least 80% of passive ion permeation across ileal epithelium occurs via a transjunctional pathway. The distribution of this transjunction "leak" pathway, however, may not be uniform within the mucosa. Rather, in the baseline state, absorptive cells display tight junctions with relatively many strand barriers, while undifferentiated crypt cells have fewer strand barriers per junction (53) (see Fig. 2.14). The functional significance of less leaky villous epithelium was originally thought to be that the greatest barrier to passive flow of noxious luminal compounds occurs at the site closest to the lumen. The results of recent studies indicate, however, that tight junction structure and function may not be static and, thus, the view just described may be oversimplified (54). For example, brief osmotic loads, such as occur in the proximal jejunum during normal digestion, may elicit a reversible increase in the barrier function of the absorptive cell junction and be accompanied by an increase in the ability of the junction to exclude noxious cations, such as hydrogen ion (55). Conversely, contraction of components of the absorptive cell cytoskeleton may "pull" junctions apart and enhance permeability (56); such contractile events reversibly occur during physiologic glucose absorption (48). Thus, paracellular permeation may be transiently enhanced during meal-stimulated cytoskeletal contraction. In disease states, such processes may be magnified or

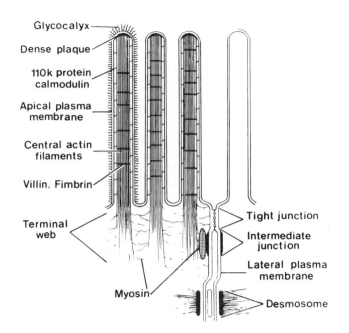

Figure 2.15 Schematic diagram of the structural features of the apical plasma membrane, the apical cytoplasm, and the junctional complexes of intestinal absorptive cells. (Reprinted with permission from Madara JL, Trier JS, Neutra MR. Structural changes in the plasma membrane accompanying differentiation of epithelial cells in human and monkey small intestine. Gastroenterology 1980;78:963-975.)

continuously expressed. For example, in active celiac sprue, discontinuities in absorptive cell junctions occur (57), like those seen with pharmacologically induced cytoskeletal contraction (56), and are paralleled by abnormalities in mucosal barrier function.

CYTOSKELETON Although all alimentary epithelial cells exhibit a complex cytoskeleton, the absorptive cell has served as a major model for studies of the molecular biology of nonmuscle cell cytoskeletal elements.

Each absorptive cell microvillus contains a central bundle of 20 to 30 actin microfilaments (58, 59) (Fig. 2.15). These microfilaments insert into a dense apical cap of unknown composition that lies directly under the plasma membrane at the microvillous tip. The ends of the microfilaments associated with this cap material may be viewed as equivalent to the Z bands of skeletal muscle; thus, associations with myosin would be expected at the opposite end. In fact, the distal ends of the parallel microfilaments project as "rootlets" into a "terminal web" of cytoskeletal elements beneath the microvilli (see Fig. 2.15), where they associate with myosin II and other proteins.

The actin microfilament bundle is cross-linked by proteins that presumably stabilize its structure (see Fig. 2.15). Two proteins—fimbrin and villin—are present at the cross-linking site (58, 59); the former appears to be the major "bundling" protein, and the latter is thought to regulate the physical state of the actin. Lastly, a 110,000-dalton unconventional form of myosin (myosin I), which associates with the calcium regulatory protein calmodulin, tethers the microvillous core bundle to the lateral microvillous membrane (60).

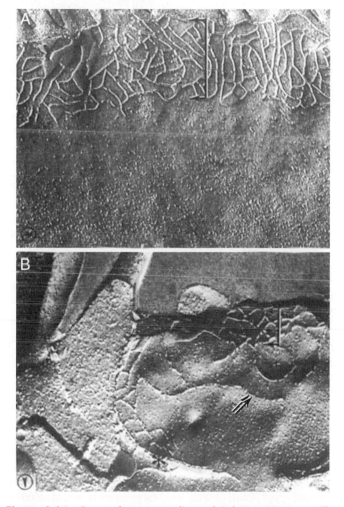

Figure 2.14 Freeze-fracture replicas of tight junctions on villus *(A)* and crypt cells *(B)*. Tight junctions of villus absorptive cells have greater depth (brackets) and are organized more uniformly than those of crypt cells. Unconnected lateral aberrant strands *(double arrow)* are common in the crypt, but rare on the villus. Cells in both crypts and villi show ladderlike specializations at three-cell junctions (*) (×80,000). (Reprinted with permission from Madara JL, Trier JS, Neutra MR. Structural changes in the plasma membrane accompanying differentiation of epithelial cells in human and monkey small intestine. Gastroenterology 1980;78:963-975.)

The terminal web itself is a distinctive cytoskeletal domain. Proteins identified in the microvillus may be present (villin) or absent in the terminal web, whereas other proteins are found here that are not in the microvillus (myosin II; spectrinlike TW 260/240 protein). Such proteins assist in tethering other cytoskeletal elements to each other and, probably, also to the plasma membrane.

One distinctive structure in the terminal web is the circumferential band of actin-myosin, known as the contractile ring. This ring not only can be stimulated to contract in isolated brush borders (61), but also can be induced experimentally to contract in epithelial sheets (56). Because the ring is tethered to the lateral membrane at the site of the intercellular junction, such contraction pulls tight junctions apart, thus disrupting the barrier function of this crucial structure. Surprisingly, ring contraction is the only clearly described function of brush border contractile proteins.

Cables of 10-nm intermediate filaments composed of keratin-like material course through the cell, loop through the terminal web (presumably stabilizing it), and anchor to desmosomes on the lateral plasma membrane. Also coursing through the cytoplasm, predominantly in the area between the nucleus and apical membrane, are 25-nm thick microtubules. They assist in routing intracellular movement, as evidenced by the fact that lipid movement through the cell is impeded when microtubular function is deranged (43), and membrane constituents are transported to inappropriate domains under these conditions (62).

OTHER ORGANELLES   The remaining organelles in the absorptive cells are similar to those in other cells (43), although sequential functional stratification of these organelles exists, as exemplified by intracellular lipid metabolism. After absorption of luminal free fatty acids and monoglycerides, re-esterification of these compounds to triglycerides occurs in the smooth endoplasmic reticulum; the results of this process are visualized as apical lipid droplets. The droplets are then transferred to the Golgi, during which time they are combined with apoproteins, cholesterol, and phospholipid to form chylomicrons. Next, chylomicrons are transported in vesicles to the lateral membrane and undergo exocytosis into the lateral intercellular space.

Derangement of one phase of a sequential cellular process during cell injury may result in a cascade of events. For example, in injured absorptive cells, lipid often accumulates in intracellular endoplasmic reticulumlike compartments, producing a vacuolated appearance to the apical cytoplasm when viewed by light microscopy. Lipid is passively absorbed, but energy is required for its subsequent intracellular metabolism (re-esterification, chylomicron formation). Thus, the morphologic finding of lipid vacuoles probably represents the "downstream" backup of internalized lipid in an energy-depleted cell.

Undifferentiated Crypt Cells

This cell is the major component of the crypt. It is termed "undifferentiated" because, in contrast to the absorptive cell, it has sparse, short, often irregular microvilli and a less well-developed terminal web (see Fig. 2.13), and it does not absorb lipid or floridly express functional integral membrane proteins necessary for terminal digestion and absorption of nutrients. This cell type is, however, capable of moving through the cell cycle and thus serves as the progenitor for other cell types in the intestinal epithelium (59). In addition,

these cells perform several unique and sophisticated functions. They synthesize a receptor for IgA, termed "secretory component," and, with precision, place this receptor on the lateral plasma membrane. After binding the ligand (IgA produced by lamina propria plasma cells), these cells immediately internalize the ligand-receptor complex, shuttle it to the apical membrane, and, by a process in which the receptor is chemically modified, extrude the ligand-receptor complex into the lumen. Thus, these cells are an integral part of the intestinal immune response (43). Also, in contrast to absorptive cells, these cells are structurally arranged to transport chloride actively into the lumen in response to secretogogues, such as cholera toxin or the heat-labile enterotoxin of *E. coli* (63).

Undifferentiated crypt cells have other structural modifications that facilitate secretory processes. For example, they have narrow apices (Fig. 2.16), resulting in large amounts of intercellular junction per unit crypt surface (1 cm^2 of crypt surface has 80 m of junction!) (56). Moreover, in comparison with absorptive cells, they have tight junctions that have fewer strand barriers (see Fig. 2.14) and are cation selective. These anatomic features facilitate the transjunctional movement of paracellular Na+ (driven by the favorable electrical gradient created by the active transcellular chloride secretory process) accompanied by H_2O "secretion," thus permitting what, in the extreme, we recognize as secretory diarrhea.

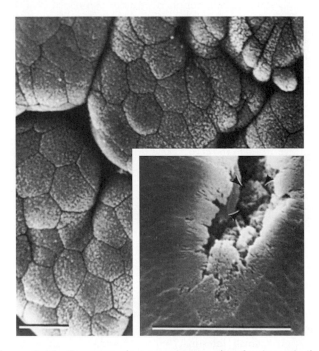

Figure 2.16   Scanning electron micrographs of guinea pig ileal villus and crypt *(inset)* epithelium. The villus surface is covered by polygonal absorptive cells that have estimated cell widths of 10 μm and produce a honeycomb appearance (×1,225). **Inset:** Crypt epithelial cells *(arrowheads)* are polygonal, but have apical cell widths of only 3.5 μm. Thus, the high linear junctional density in the crypt is not due to tortuous cell contours, but to diminished apical cell widths (×3,500). *Bars* represent 10 mm. (Reprinted with permission from Marcial MA, Carlson SL, Madara JL. Partitioning of paracellular conductance along the crypt-villus axis: A hypothesis based on structural analysis with detailed consideration of tight junction structure-function relationships. J Membr Biol 1994;80:59–70.)

Baseline secretion may cleanse the crypt lumen and wash other important crypt products, such as IgA, into the intestinal lumen proper. Enhanced secretion, as occurs in cholera, may clear the lumen of toxin-producing bacilli and thus shorten the clinical course of the disease. Because modulation of the rate of this normal Cl-secretory process occurs at the level of the chloride channel, it is not surprising that the intestinal mucosa may be structurally normal by light microscopy in some diarrheal diseases (e.g., cholera).

In general, the other architectural characteristics of undifferentiated crypt cells represent variations on the themes discussed in the absorptive cell section. In contrast to absorptive cells, however, undifferentiated crypt cells prominently display apical secretory vesicles of 0.1 to 1.5 nm diameter. These vesicles contain glycoprotein and exocytose their content when stimulated by cholinergic agonists, but have no known function (43).

Goblet Mucous Cells

Goblet cells are the second major cell population of both crypts and villi (43). They are more numerous in the ileum than in the jejunum and are relatively sparse on villous tips. They are identified easily in routine sections because of their brandy goblet shape and distended apical cytoplasm filled with pale-stained, 1- to 3-μ mucous granules. A densely staining, thin peripheral rim of compressed cytoplasm, termed the theca, surrounds this mucous granule mass. A brush border is absent.

Electron microscopy reveals only few, irregular, predominantly perijunctional microvilli, nearly devoid of intramembrane particles, on goblet cell apical membranes (Figs. 2.17 and 2.18). The mucous granules are membrane bound and originate from the well-developed supranuclear Golgi apparatus. Although both crypt and villus goblet cells generally share the same structural features, a subclass of less well-differentiated goblet cells, called "oligomucous cells," are found in the crypt. Their distinctive characteristic is that they are capable of cell division (43).

Goblet cells release the mucin contained in the secretory vesicles by simple and compound exocytosis (64). Although the rate of baseline secretion is imprecisely defined, newly synthesized mucin molecules appear to move from the Golgi apparatus, through the vesicle population, and onto the apical surface in approximately 4 hours (65). If stimulated with a goblet cell secretogogue, such as acetylcholine, massive mucin discharge occurs by a process in which multiple vesicles fuse in tandem (compound exocytosis) (64). It is now clear that "apocrine" secretion of goblet cell contents does not occur physiologically, but may be artifactually induced by inappropriate tissue handling before chemical fixation.

Human small intestinal mucin contains a high-molecular weight glycoprotein similar to that produced in the rat (66, 67) (2 x 10^6 daltons, 10% protein plus approximately 85% hexose consisting of at least six hexose species). Lectin labeling patterns are also well described. Lectins bind only the terminal sugars of the long carbohydrate chains and, thus, yield "superficial" (in a topographic sense, but some would also say in a real sense) information concerning mucin biochemistry. Thus, it should not be surprising if classes of mucins as defined biochemically bear no relationship to classes of mucins defined by lectin staining. Such lectin studies do demonstrate that goblet cells may be heterogeneous with respect to their secretory product, because goblet cell lectin stain patterns vary from jejunum to ileum. Of interest is the recent observation that goblet cells themselves may secrete lectinlike molecules (67). By

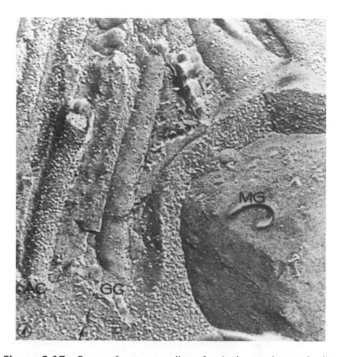

Figure 2.17 Freeze-fracture replica of apical cytoplasm of adjacent goblet and villus absorptive cells. *Arrow* indicates the position of the intercellular space separating the goblet (GC) and the absorptive cell (AC). The P-face of a microvillus from each cell is exposed. That of the goblet cell *(right)* is particle poor, whereas that of the absorptive cell *(left)* is particle rich. A mucin granule (MG) is visible in the goblet cell cytoplasm. (×146,000). (Reprinted with permission from Madara JL, Trier JS. Functional morphology of the mucosa of the small intestine. In: Johnson LR, ed. Physiology of the gastrointestinal tract. 3rd ed. New York: Raven Press, 1994;1577–1622.)

cross-linking terminal sugars, such molecules may stabilize or increase the rigidity of mucus in the intestinal lumen.

Goblet cell mucins are acidic and stain positively with alcian blue at pH 2.5. The mucins vary in composition and relative amounts in the small intestine and colon, with more sialomucin found in the small intestine and more sulfomucin in the colon. The sialomucins also vary in the two locations, with N-acylsialomucins common in the small intestine, but O-acylsialomucins predominating in the colon and most distal ileum (Table 2.4) (68, 69).

Mucins may assist intestinal function in a variety of ways. They act as surface lubricants, increase diffusion rates of threatening luminal molecules, and block the epithelial binding sites of bacteria. Of interest in this regard is the observation that exposure to certain bacterial products, particularly enterotoxins, results in massive mucin release (67).

A new class of peptides, termed "trefoil" peptides after the three-loop structure afforded by three disulfide bonds, is also produced and secreted by goblet cells. Trefoil peptides may assist in cross-linking mucin, thus providing a more viscous gel, and also may exert pro-repair influences on intestinal epithelia, perhaps by more direct effects on intestinal epithelial cells. Targeted disruption of the gene for one of these peptides has resulted in substantial impairment of the ability of mice to recover from intestinal injury (70).

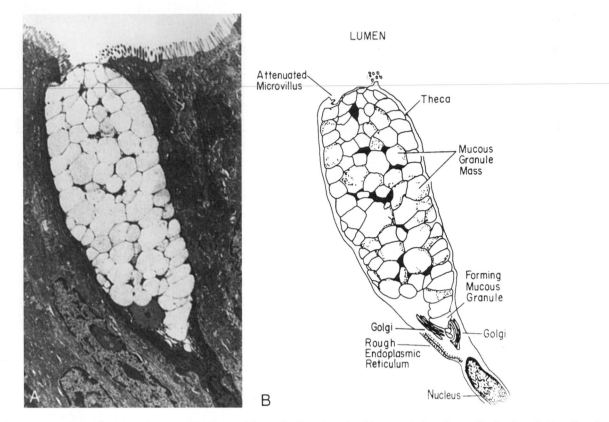

Figure 2.18   Electron micrograph *(A)* and trace *(B)* of a goblet cell. (Reprinted with permission from Shultz S, ed. Handbook of physiology, volume IV: The gastrointestinal system. Bethesda: American Physiological Association, 1991;84–120.)

Endocrine Cells (See Chapter 13)

Paneth Cells

Located at the base of the crypts, Paneth cells by light microscopic analysis have intensely eosinophilic apical secretory granules. Unlike most other small intestinal epithelial cells, Paneth cells are renewed only after approximately 20 days (43). Like other cell types, however, these cells appear to originate from undifferentiated crypt cells. Although the ultrastructural appearance of this cell resembles that of the goblet cell, Paneth cells have broader bases and their granules contain a dark, homogeneously staining protein product, with an appearance similar to that in zymogen-producing cells.

Paneth cells also exhibit not only baseline secretion, but also secretion stimulated by cholinergic agents and inhibited by atropine (71).

The precise secretory product(s) and function(s) of Paneth cells are unclear. Lysozyme may be one Paneth cell product, and Paneth cells can internalize extracellular matter, such as bacteria and immunoglobulin (43). Such observations have led to the speculation that these cells help to regulate the bacterial microenvironment of the crypt. Many species (such as cats and dogs) do not have Paneth cells, however, and these animals do not have any detectable deficiencies in bacteriologic surveillance.

Newly discovered Paneth cell products, termed "cryptdins" (72), are related to neutrophil defensins and appear to be secreted

TABLE	
2.4	**Mucin Profiles of Intestinal Goblet Cells**

| | | Mucin Type[a] | | |
| | | Sialomucin | Sialomucin | |
Location	Neutral	(N-acetyl)	(O-acetyl)	Sulfomucin
Small intestine	+	+ (predominant)	+ (minor)	−
Colon	+	+	+	+ (predominant)

[a]Mucin types also vary along the length of the crypt and/or villus, and in different parts of the small or large intestine.

antimicrobial agents. Differing species of cryptdin peptides, altered in single amino acids, can show distinctive specificities toward target microorganisms. It is possible that secretion of such antimicrobial agents into the crypt lumen, along with fluid secretion at this site, creates a relatively sterile microenvironment within the crypt compartment.

Membranous (M) Cells

Membranous, or "M," cells are present only on the epithelium above sites where lymphoid follicles protrude from the lamina propria and distort the overlying epithelium into a dome-like contour, hence the name "follicular dome epithelium" (73, 74). Although this epithelium represents only a tiny fraction of the total intestinal surface, and M cells are a numerically minor constituent even in this epithelium, the M cells play a vital role in intestinal immune responses (see previous discussion).

M cells are difficult to appreciate by light microscopy, but this observation is not surprising in view of their ultrastructural appearance. By electron microscopy (Fig. 2.19), M cells have the appearance of an inverted glass: they have thin walls that connect with a confluent surface and exhibit a central depression. They also have thin cytoplasmic processes that extend laterally over the basal

lamina. Their apical surfaces display small folds or notably attenuated microvilli (see Fig. 2.19), whereas lymphoid cells, which may be either macrophages or mark as B or T cells, reside within the aforementioned hollow.

In addition to the usual allotment of cellular organelles, M cells contain numerous endocytotic vesicles that are crucial to their function. These vesicles internalize luminal matter ranging from macromolecules to virions, bacteria, and parasites, and are capable of shuttling such material across the M cell and depositing it in the centered hollow, to be engulfed and processed by lymphoid cells (74). Hence, uptake of luminal substances by M cells appears to be the initial event in the afferent limb of the intestinal immune response.

Although nonselective to some degree, transport of some luminal agents across M cells may be receptor mediated and, therefore, selective. This biologic strategy, of value, for example, in initiating a specific IgA response to a luminal organism, is not always beneficial. For instance, neurotropic virions may gain entrance to the individual through this same pathway. Of interest, the initial lesions of salmonella infection and of Crohn's disease localize to the region of the follicular dome (see appropriate chapters). Such observations may represent important clues about the initial steps of intestinal injury in these disorders.

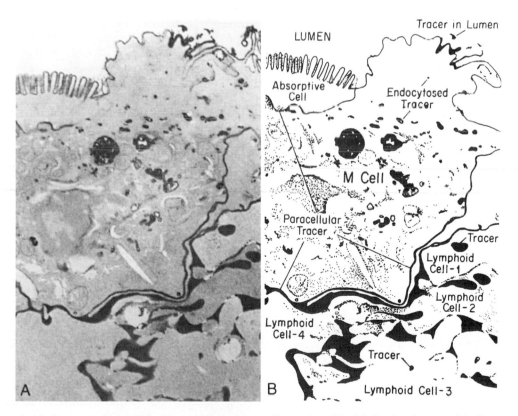

Figure 2.19 Unstained electron micrograph (A) and labeled trace illustration (B) of follicular dome epithelium exposed on luminal surface to macromolecule horseradish peroxidase. Dark reaction product indicating presence of this molecule can be seen within vesicles in M cell, within spaces surrounding M cell, and within vesicles of lymphoid cells under M cells. Comparable transport of this macromolecule across other types of epithelial cells is not known to occur in adult small intestine (×9,000). (Reprinted with permission from Shultz S, ed. Handbook of physiology, volume IV: The gastrointestinal system. Bethesda: American Physiological Association, 1991;84–120.)

Caveolated Cells

Caveolated, or tuft, cells are of necessity defined by their unique structural characteristics, because their function is completely unknown (43). They occur in the stomach and throughout the small intestine and colon, and are present in crypts and on villi. Although somewhat difficult to identify by light microscopy, they can be recognized in 1-µ sections by the tuftlike brush border that projects above those of adjacent absorptive cells. Ultrastructurally, the microvilli are longer and wider than those of adjacent cells, and by freeze fracture, relatively few intramembrane particles are present at this site. Each microvillus contains a microfilament bundle that projects deeply into the underlying cytoplasm. Round and tubular membrane-bound spaces, termed "caveoli," are located between the microfilament bundles. These spaces may be in continuity with the lumen to some degree, but their significance is unknown (43, 44).

Cells with "long rootlets" are often recognized in carcinomas arising from the intestine and have been touted as useful in identifying the origin of a metastatic lesion. Such cells are likely to represent differentiation toward caveolated phenotypes. Further verification of their uniqueness to intestinal carcinomas is needed, because this cell phenotype is also a constituent of other normal epithelia, such as those lining the biliary and respiratory trees.

Cup Cells

A numerically minor class of small intestinal epithelial cells, cup cells occur in many species, including monkeys, but it is not specifically known if they are present in humans. Often, they are more densely distributed in the ileum than in the jejunum (43).

In 1-µ sections, they generally display lighter cytoplasmic staining than neighboring absorptive cells. More readily appreciated, however, is the short, concave ("cupped") brush border. By electron microscopy, cup cell microvilli are short but regular, and by freeze fracture, they have linear P-face particle arrays with complementary E-face grooves. Cup cells also often exhibit thick, poorly defined terminal webs and small mitochondria with dense inner matrices. They do not vigorously absorb lipid nor do they express significant surface alkaline phosphatase activity. Their function is unknown. In guinea pigs, however, they have been reported to serve as a site for selective attachment of an unidentified species of bacteria.

COLON

The purpose of the colon is to reclaim luminal water and ions. In most instances, this function translates into the absorption of 250 to 270 ml of isotonic fluid per day, a small amount relative to the quantity of fluid and salt absorbed by the small intestine.

The structure of the colon in many respects overlaps that of the small intestine. Thus, for some topics, the reader is referred to the immediately preceding section as well as to other discussions of the appendix (see Chapter 33) and the anal canal (see Chapter 34).

GROSS ANATOMY

In adults, the colon is approximately 1.5 m in length. Anatomic divisions, from proximal to distal, include the cecum (that portion between the ileocecal valve and the appendix), ascending colon, hepatic flexure, transverse colon, splenic flexure, descending colon, sigmoid colon, rectum, and anus. The posterolateral wall of the ascending colon, sigmoid colon, and rectum are not covered with a serosa, and thus have immediate access to the retroperitoneum. It is, therefore, no surprise that disease processes can penetrate the intestinal wall at these sites and involve retroperitoneal structures or even the joints of the pelvis.

The outer longitudinal layer of the muscularis propria is divided into three equidistant visible cables, or taeniae, that begin at the cecum, extend along most of the colon, then become one confluent sheet as the colon leaves the peritoneal cavity at the distal sigmoid. Presumably because of tension within the taeniae, the colonic wall displays many prominent pouches, or haustra. At the center of such haustra, the colonic lumen is widest; at the periphery of the haustra, the lumen is most narrow. These features produce the impression of luminal arclike constrictions or plicae semilunares.

The ascending and transverse colon are supplied by three branches of the superior mesenteric artery (ileocolic, and right and middle colic arteries), whereas the splenic flexure, descending colon, and sigmoid are nourished by branches of the inferior mesenteric artery (left colic and sigmoid arteries). These vessels form arcades that are less numerous and complex than those in the small intestinal vasculature. The rectum has a richly anastomosing arterial system derived from the inferior mesenteric and internal iliac arteries (4).

In general, the venous drainage of the colon parallels its arteries, with the right and transverse colonic flow directed into the superior mesenteric vein and the left colonic drainage into the inferior mesenteric vein. As in the esophagus and stomach, the rectum has systemic-portal anastomoses, offering the potential for development of varices in patients with portal hypertension. Also like the stomach, lymphatic channels in the colonic mucosa are confined to the lowermost portion of the lamina propria and within the muscularis mucosae. For this reason, carcinomas confined to the colonic mucosa have essentially no metastatic potential. Lymph nodes are located adjacent to the colonic wall and along the course of the major arteries. These nodes drain to the superior and inferior mesenteric nodes. The lymphatic drainage from the rectum is complex, with flow to inferior mesenteric and internal iliac nodes (4).

ORGANIZATION OF THE COLONIC WALL

As in the small intestine, the mucosa is structurally and functionally the most important layer of the colon. The colonic mucosal surface is flat and peppered with well-like orifices that represent the mouths of the tubular crypts (Fig. 2.20). The crypts are straight in normal biopsy-derived tissue and are unbranched, except during embryologic development, when the colonic surface expands by a process in which crypts bifurcate and subsequently "divide" into two crypts.

Occasionally, light microscopic sections show a vaguely nodular pattern to the mucosa produced by the periodic appearance of pairs of crypts that are shorter than their neighbors. At such sites, the colonic surface is gently indented. This normal mucosal structural variant is called the anthemea or anthemean folds. These anthemea are analogous to the areae gastrica in the stomach.

As in the small intestine, lymphoid nodules that distort the normal mucosal architecture are present in the colon. Unlike the small intestine, however, such lymphoid nodules usually are not

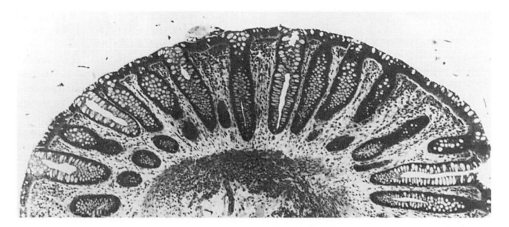

Figure 2.20   Sections of colonic mucosa obtained by endoscopic biopsy. The specimen is curved owing to postbiopsy contraction of the muscularis mucosae. The surface is flat and lined by columnar absorptive and goblet cells. Straight well-like crypts occupy the depth of the lamina propria (×125). (Courtesy of Marian Neutra, M.D., Department of Pediatrics, Harvard Medical School and Children's Hospital, Boston, MA.)

densely clustered enough to become grossly obvious. Like the small intestine, the colonic epithelium renews itself almost weekly, and the undifferentiated crypt cell appears to be the progenitor for all cell types.

EPITHELIAL STRUCTURE

GENERAL FEATURES

The colonic mucosa may be divided into three compartments that are anatomically and functionally distinct. The surface, which contains columnar absorptive cells and goblet cells, is the site of water and electrolyte resorption and mucin production (see Fig. 2.20). The crypt contains undifferentiated columnar cells, goblet cells, endocrine cells, and the cecum and ascending colon contain scattered, basally located Paneth cells. The crypt is the site of colonic water and electrolyte secretion, mucus secretion, and secretion of poorly characterized non-goblet cell glycoprotein(s). Lastly, the epithelium overlying the lymphoid nodules contains M cells and is presumably the site at which luminal antigens can be sampled by the underlying lymphoid stroma.

COLONIC MUCOSAL EPITHELIAL CELLS (SEE TABLE 2.3)

Absorptive Cells

In the colon, absorptive cells are tall, columnar structures (see Fig. 2.20) with microvilli that are the same diameter as, but shorter and less abundant than, those of small intestine absorptive cells. Thus, by light microscopy, it is difficult to identify the colonic microvillous surface as a "brush border." The fine structure of the colonic absorptive cell is otherwise similar to that of its small intestinal equivalent, but with one subtle variation: colonic cells have tight junctions with more strands than those of small intestinal absorptive cells. This difference may, in part, determine the higher resistance to passive transepithelial ion flow exhibited by the colon. In some animals, a subset of colonic absorptive cells exhibits linear P-face microvillous particle arrays reminiscent of those noted in small intestinal cup cells. Whether these cells represent the colonic cup cell equivalent is unclear.

The colonic absorptive cell exhibits functional differences from its counterpart in the small intestine. The apical membrane proteins involved in terminal digestion and nutrient uptake are depleted or absent in colonic absorptive cells. Rather, the apical membranes primarily contain transport proteins responsible for electrolyte uptake; specifically, an amiloride-inhibited, aldosterone-stimulated, electrogenic sodium uptake mechanism may dominate the surface of this cell (75). The importance of this mechanism for pathologists is that, on cellular injury and consequent energy depletion, Na+/K+-ATPase is inhibited, but a gradient for sodium entry into colonic absorptive cells still transiently exists. This gradient would be diminished as sodium enters the cell through the selective apical membrane pathway. The result might well be sodium accumulation until the gradient favoring sodium entry is dispersed, with a resulting increase in cell volume, i.e., the cells swell.

Other transport-related molecules present on the apical membrane include a bicarbonate-chloride exchanger that may be of importance in disease states (75). As previously discussed, secretory diarrheas originating in the small intestine (and in the colon) result from chloride secretion by undifferentiated crypt cells. As this chloride-loaded solution moves into the colon, bicarbonate-chloride exchange at the apical membrane occurs and the luminal content becomes bicarbonate enriched. This mechanism may well serve as the basis for the bicarbonate loss seen in patients with secretory diarrhea.

Goblet Mucous Cells

Colonic goblet cells are structurally comparable to those of the small intestine. Cholinergic stimulation results in massive exocytosis of mucin secretory granules of crypt, but not of surface, goblet cells (67). Thus, just as goblet cells vary from region to region and from crypt to surface in the type of mucin they synthesize, so too do they vary in expression of basolateral receptors for secretogogues and/or basolateral innervation. As noted previously, colonic goblet cell mucin is enriched in sulfomucins, whereas that in the small intestine is enriched in sialomucin (see Table 2.4) (76). Colonic goblet cells, like those in the small intestine, also produce trefoil peptides.

Undifferentiated Columnar Crypt Cells

These cells are interposed between crypt goblet cells and are similar in structure to their counterparts in the small intestine, with one major exception: they contain numerous membrane-bound vesicles containing flocculent material that presumptively represents a nonmucin glycoprotein. As in the small intestine, these cells are the site of electrogenic chloride secretion.

Other Cells

Caveolated cells, Paneth cells, and M cells are also present in the colonic mucosa and are identical to those described in the small intestine. Endocrine cells are discussed in Chapter 13.

REFERENCES

1. Fawcett DW. Bloom & Fawcett — A textbook of histology. 11th ed. Philadelphia: WB Saunders, 1986;619–640.
2. Pick TP, Howden R, eds. Gray's anatomy. New York: Bounty Books, 1977.
3. Enterline H, Thompson J. Pathology of the esophagus. New York: Springer, 1984;1–22.
4. Gannon B. The vasculature and lymphatic drainage. In: Whitehead R, ed. Gastrointestinal and oesophageal pathology. 2nd ed. Edinburgh: Churchill Livingstone, 1995;129–199.
5. Geboes K, Mebis J, Desmet V. The esophagus: Normal ultrastructure and pathological patterns. In: Motta PM, Fujita H, eds. Ultrastructure of the digestive tract. Boston: Martinus Nijhoff, 1988;17–34.
6. Weinstein WM, Bogoch ER, Bowes KL. The normal human esophageal mucosa: A histological reappraisal. Gastroenterology 1975;68:40–44.
7. Eastwood GL. Gastrointestinal epithelial renewal. Gastroenterology 1977;72:962–975.
8. DeNardi FG, Riddell RH. Esophagus. In: Sternberg SS, ed. Histology for pathologists. New York: Raven Press, 1992;515–532.
9. Andrews PM. Microplicae: Characteristic ridgelike folds of the plasmalemma. J Cell Biol 1976;68:420–429.
10. Spechler SJ, Zeroogian JM, Antonioli DA, et al. Short-segment Barrett's esophagus. Lancet 1994;344:1533–1536.
11. Geboes K, DeWolf-Peeters C, Rutgeerts P, et al. Lymphocytes and Langerhans' cells in the human oesophageal epithelium. Virchows Arch [A] 1983;401:45–55.
12. Tateishi R, Taniguchi H, Wada A, et al. Argyrophil cells and melanocytes in esophageal mucosa. Arch Pathol Lab Med 1974;98:87–89.
13. Mangano MM, Antonioli DA, Schnitt SJ, et al. Nature and significance of cells with irregular nuclear contours in esophageal mucosal biopsies. Mod Pathol 1992;5:191–196.
14. Hammar S. Langerhans' cells. In: Rosen PP, Fechner RE, eds. Pathology annual: 1988, Part 2. Norwalk: Appleton & Lange, 1988;293–328.
15. Jabbari M, Goresky CA, Lough J, et al. The inlet patch: Heterotopic gastric mucosa in the upper esophagus. Gastroenterology 1985;89:352–356.
16. Hopwood D, Coghill G, Sanders DSA. Human oesophageal submucosal glands: Their detection, mucin, enzyme and secretory protein content. Histochemistry 1986;86:107–112.
17. Neutra MR, Padykula HA. The gastrointestinal tract. In: Weiss L, ed. Modern concepts of gastrointestinal histology. New York: Elsevier, 1984;659–706.
18. Namiot Z, Sarosiek J, Rourk M, et al. Human esophageal secretion: Mucosal response to luminal acid and pepsin. Gastroenterology 1994;106:973–981.
19. McClave SA, Boyce Jr HW, Gottfried MR. Early diagnosis of columnar-lined esophagus: A new endoscopic diagnostic criterion. Gastrointest Endosc 1987;33:413–416.
20. Bertoni G, Sassatelli R, Nigrisoli E, et al. Ectopic sebaceous glands in the esophagus: Report of three new cases and review of the literature. Am J Gastroenterol 1994;89:1884–1887.
21. Wang HH, Zeroogian JM, Spechler SJ, et al. Prevalence and significance of pancreatic acinar metaplasia at the gastroesophageal junction. Am J Surg Pathol 1996;20:1507–1510.
22. Rotterdam H. The normal stomach and duodenum. In: Rotterdam H, Enterline HT, eds. Pathology of the stomach and duodenum. New York: Springer, 1989;1–12.
23. Owen DA. Stomach. In: Sternberg SS, ed. Histology for pathologists. New York: Raven Press, 1992;533–545.
24. Kimura K. Chronological transition of the fundic-pyloric border determined by stepwise biopsy of the lesser and greater curvatures of the stomach. Gastroenterology 1972;63:584–592.
25. Wolfe MM, Soll AH. The physiology of gastric acid secretion. N Engl J Med 1988;319:1707–1715.
26. Moreau H, Laugier R, Gargouri Y, et al. Human preduodenal lipase is entirely of gastric fundic origin. Gastroenterology 1988;95:122–126.
27. Ménard D, Monfils S, Tremblay E. Ontogeny of human gastric lipase and pepsin activities. Gastroenterology 1995;108:1650–1656.
28. Lehnert T, Erlandson RA, Decosse JJ. Lymph and blood capillaries of the human gastric mucosa: A morphologic basis for metastasis in early gastric carcinoma. Gastroenterology 1985;89:939–950.
29. Listrom MB, Fenoglio-Preiser CM. Lymphatic distribution of the stomach in normal, inflammatory, hyperplastic, and neoplastic tissue. Gastroenterology 1987;93:506–514.
30. Lowichik A, Weinberg AG. A quantitative evaluation of mucosal eosinophils in the pediatric gastrointestinal tract. Mod Pathol 1996;9:110–114.
31. Goldman H, Ming S-C. Mucins in normal and neoplastic gastrointestinal epithelium. Arch Pathol Lab Med 1968;85:580–586.
32. Jass JR, Filipe MI. The mucin profile of normal gastric mucosa, intestinal metaplasia and its variants and gastric carcinoma. Histochem J 1981;13:931–939.
33. Helander HF. Fine structure of gastric glands. In: Motta PM, Fujita H, eds. Ultrastructure of the digestive tract. Boston: Martinus-Nijhoff, 1988;35–51.
34. LaMont JT. Structure and function of gastrointestinal mucus. Viewpoints Dig Dis 1985;17:1–4.
35. Goldman H, Antonioli DA. Mucosal biopsy of the esophagus, stomach, and proximal duodenum. Hum Pathol 1982;13:423–448.
36. Toner PG, Watt PCH, Boyd SM. The gastric mucosa. In: Whitehead R, ed. Gastrointestinal and oesophageal pathology. 2nd ed. Edinburgh: Churchill Livingstone, 1995;15–32.
37. Kelly EJ, Lagopoulos M, Primrose JN. Immunocytochemical localisation of parietal cells and G cells in the developing human stomach. Gut 1993;34:1057–1059.
38. O'Brien P, Rosen S, Trencis-Buck L, et al. Distribution of carbonic anhydrase within the gastric mucosa. Gastroenterology 1977;72:870–874.
39. Parkkila S, Parkkila A-K, Rajaniemi H. Distribution of the carbonic anhydrase isoenzymes I, II, and VI in the human alimentary tract. Gut 1994;35:646–650.
40. Levine JS, Nakane PK, Allen RH. Immunocytochemical localization of human intrinsic factor: The nonstimulated stomach. Gastroenterology 1980;79:493–502.
41. Samloff IM. Pepsinogens I & II: Purification from gastric mucosa and radioimmunoassay in serum. Gastroenterology 1982;82:26–33.
42. Basson MD, Modlin IM. Pepsinogen: Prolate ellipsoid or unrecognized pathogen? J Clin Gastroenterol 1987;9:475–479.
43. Madara JL, Trier JS. Functional morphology of the mucosa of the small intestine. In: Johnson LR, ed. Physiology of the gastrointestinal tract. 3rd ed. New York: Raven Press, 1994;1577–1622.
44. Madara JL. Functional morphology of the epithelium of the small intestine. In: Shultz S, ed. Handbook of physiology, volume IV: The gastrointestinal system. Bethesda: American Physiological Association, 1991;84–120.
45. Lundgren O, Haglund U. The pathophysiology of the intestinal countercurrent exchanger. Life Sci 1978;23:1411–1422.
46. Harmon JW, Woods M, Gurll NJ. Different mechanisms of hydrogen ion removal in stomach and duodenum. Am J Physiol 1978;235 (Endocrinol Metab Gastrointest Physiol 4):E692–E698.
47. Simson JNL, Merhav A, Silen W. Alkaline secretion by amphibian

duodenum. I. General characteristics. Am J Physiol 1981;240 (Gastrointest Liver Physiol 3):G401–G408.

48. Madara JL, Pappenheimer JR. The structural basis for physiological regulation of paracellular pathways in intestinal epithelia. J Membr Biol 1987;100:149–164.

49. Eichholz A. Structural and functional organization of the brush border of intestinal epithelial cells. III. Enzymic activities and chemical composition of various fractions of Tris-disrupted brush borders. Biochem Biophys Acta 1967;135:475–482.

50. Madara JL, Trier JS, Neutra MR. Structural changes in the plasma membrane accompanying differentiation of epithelial cells in human and monkey small intestine. Gastroenterology 1980;78:963–975.

51. Alpers DH. The relation of size to the relative rates of degradation of intestinal brush border proteins. J Clin Invest 1972;51:2621–2630.

52. Brasitus TA, Schachter D. Lipid dynamics and lipid-protein interactions in rat enterocyte basolateral and microvillus membranes. Biochemistry 1980;19:2763–2769.

53. Marcial MA, Carlson SL, Madara JL. Partitioning of paracellular conductance along the crypt-villus axis: A hypothesis based on structural analysis with detailed consideration of tight junction structure-function relationships. J Membr Biol 1984;80:59–70.

54. Madara JL. Loosening tight junctions: Lessons from the intestine. J Clin Invest 1989;83:1089–1094.

55. Madara JL. Increases in guinea pig small intestinal transepithelial resistance induced by osmotic loads are accompanied by rapid alterations in absorptive-cell tight-junction structure. J Cell Biol 1983;97:125–136.

56. Madara JL, Moore R, Carlson S. Alteration of intestinal tight junction structure and permeability by cytoskeletal contraction. Am J Physiol 1987;253 (Cell Physiol 22):C854–C861.

57. Madara JL, Trier JS. Structural abnormalities of jejunal epithelial cell membranes in celiac sprue. Lab Invest 1980;43:254–261.

58. Mooseker MS. Actin binding proteins of the brush border. Cell 1983;35:11–13.

59. Louvard D, Kedinger M, Hauri HP. The differentiating intestinal epithelial cell. Annu Rev Cell Biol 1992,8.157.

60. Pollard TD, Doberstein SK, Zot HG. Myosin I. Annu Rev Physiol 1991;53:653–681.

61. Rodewald R, Newman SB, Karnovsky MJ. Contraction of isolated brush borders from intestinal epithelia. J Cell Biol 1976;70:541–554.

62. Pavelka M, Ellinger A, Gangl A. Effect of colchicine on rat small intestinal absorptive cells. I. Formation of basolateral microvillus borders. J Ultrastruct Res 1981;85:249–259.

63. Kaunitz JD, Barrett KE, McRoberts JA. Electrolyte secretion and absorption: Small intestine and colon. In: Yamada T, ed. Textbook of gastroenterology. Philadelphia: Lippincott, 1995;326–360.

64. Specian RD, Neutra MR. Acceleration of secretion in colonic goblet cells by acetylcholine. J Cell Biol 1980;85:626–640.

65. Neutra MR, Leblond CP. Radioautographic comparison of the uptake of galactose-H^3 and glucose-H^3 in the Golgi region of various cells secreting glycoproteins or mucopolysaccharides. J Cell Biol 1966;30:137–150.

66. Forstner JF, Jabbal I, Forstner GG. Goblet cell mucin of the rat small intestine. Chemical and physical characterization. Can J Biochem 1973;51:1154–1166.

67. Neutra MR, Forstner JF. Gastrointestinal mucus. In: Johnson LR, ed. Physiology of the gastrointestinal tract. 2nd ed. New York: Raven Press, 1987;975–1010.

68. Culling CFA, Reid PE, Burton JD, et al. A histochemical method of differentiating lower gastrointestinal tract mucin from other mucins in primary or metastatic tumors. J Clin Pathol 1975;28:656–658.

69. Filipe MI, Fenger C. Histochemical characteristics of mucins in the small intestine. A comparative study of normal mucosa, benign epithelial tumours and carcinoma. Histochem J 1979;11:277–287.

70. Mashimo H, Wu D, Podolsky DK, et al. Impaired defense of intestinal mucosa in mice lacking intestinal trefoil factor. Science 1996; 262–265.

71. Toner PG, Carr KE, Al-Yassin TM. The gastrointestinal tract. In: Johanessen JV, ed. Electron microscopy in human medicine, volume 7: Digestive system. New York: McGraw-Hill, 1980;87–185.

72. Ouellette AJ, Selsted ME. Paneth cell defensins: Endogenous peptide components of intestinal host defense. FASEB J 1996;10:1280–1289.

73. Owen RL, Jones AL. Epithelial cell specialization within human Peyer's patches: An ultrastructural study of intestinal lymphoid follicles. Gastroenterology 1974;66:189–203.

74. Owen RL. Sequential uptake of horseradish peroxidase by lymphoid follicle epithelium of Peyer's patches in the normal unobstructed mouse intestine: An ultrastructural study. Gastroenterology 1977;72:440–451.

75. Binder HJ, Sandle GI. Electrolyte absorption and secretion in the mammalian colon. In: Johnson LK, ed. Physiology of the gastrointestinal tract. 2nd ed. New York: Raven Press, 1987;1389–1418.

76. Filipe MI, Branfoot AC. Mucin histochemistry of the colon. In: Morson BC, ed. Current topics in pathology, volume 63: Pathology of the gastro-intestinal tract. Berlin: Springer, 1976;143–178.

ENDOSCOPY AND ENDOSCOPIC BIOPSY

Mary P. Bronner, Rodger C. Haggitt, and Cyrus E. Rubin

HISTORY OF GASTROINTESTINAL ENDOSCOPY

Attempts to visualize the interior of the esophagus and stomach using a rigid tube passed perorally began more than a century ago in Germany. Whereas visualization of the esophagus was adequate if magnifying lenses were used, and safe if the operator was expert, this was not the case in the stomach. Even in the hands of an expert endoscopist such as the pioneer Rudolph Schindler, a stiff tube occasionally caused perforations while negotiating the esophagogastric junction. Furthermore, the area of the stomach visualized was extremely limited. Schindler therefore abandoned the rigid gastroscope in 1928 and in collaboration with George Wolf, an instrument maker, designed a new "flexirigid" gastroscope (1). It was first demonstrated in 1932 and incorporated a flexible optical axis made possible by multiple short focal-length lenses. This instrument was slightly flexible distally and rigid proximally. Its tip was made of a flexible rubber introducer, and the viewing lens faced laterally just proximal to the flexible rubber tip. The instrument could be passed without causing perforation. The area of stomach visualized was greater than with the rigid tube but was still very limited; the duodenum and some parts of the stomach could not be visualized at all. There was no channel by which to pass a biopsy forceps for direct sampling of lesions.

The modern era of gastrointestinal endoscopy began in 1957 when Basil Hirschowitz and Lawrence Curtis at the University of Michigan developed the first fiberoptic gastroscope (2). The technical advances that made the fiberoptic instrument possible began in 1927 when Baird proposed the idea of transmitting light along the axis of a flexible glass fiber (3). Hopkins and Kapany constructed a 9-inch long coherent fiberglass bundle capable of transmitting an image, and described their invention in an article that appeared in

Nature in 1954 (2). Hirschowitz's attention was directed to this invention, and he traveled to London to examine the device first hand. The image transmitted by the fiber bundle had sufficient definition to make large print readable, but the color was green and the light loss was so great that a long fiber bundle would be impractical. Hirschowitz returned to Ann Arbor and was able to interest his colleagues in the physics department at the University of Michigan in the problem. Lawrence Curtis, a physics student, solved the problem of cross-talk (light loss caused by leakage of light from one fiber into the adjacent one) by inventing a technique for coating the glass fibers with glass of a lower refractive index (2). This development in 1956 turned out to be the breakthrough that permitted steady improvement in the quality of fiberoptic instruments. A usable prototype fiberscope was soon developed, and the first endoscopy was carried out by Hirschowitz on himself: "I took the instrument and my courage in both hands, and swallowed it over the protest of my unanesthetized pharynx and my vomiting center (2)." Some endoscopists to this day retain this penchant for autoendoscopy (4).

The first fiberoptic endoscopes became available in the United States in 1960. With the stimulus of the American gastroenterologist John Morrissey, an endoscope was developed in Japan that could be passed into the proximal duodenum, making the diagnosis of duodenal ulcer practical (5). The ability to control the endoscope tip and the resolution of the image improved substantially with time. A channel for passage of diagnostic biopsy forceps and therapeutic instruments for the control of bleeding assumed increasing importance. Development of fiberoptic colonoscopes followed in 1961, and by 1969, Wolf and Shinya had introduced flexible endoscopic polypectomy for colonic adenomas located beyond the reach of the rigid sigmoidoscope (6).

A more recent development in endoscopy has been the introduction of the video endoscope, which has largely replaced the use of the older fiberoptic endoscopes. By placing a television chip on the tip of the endoscope, video images can be projected onto a television screen, recorded photographically, or videotaped. By using video endoscopy, the endoscopist, assistant, and even pathologist can review the endoscopic findings. This capability has improved coordination of endoscopic therapy and has made teaching endoscopy much easier.

Since its introduction nearly 30 years ago, endoscopy has become the most important part of the gastroenterologist's diagnostic methodology.

MODERN ENDOSCOPY

CLINICAL APPLICATION

Esophagogastroduodenoscopy is the primary method for the diagnosis of upper gastrointestinal bleeding. In an increasing number of centers in the Western world, endoscopy has replaced upper gastrointestinal radiography as the primary method of diagnosing upper gastrointestinal illness.

Endoscopy plays a large role in the management of peptic ulcer and gastroesophageal regurgitant disease, and it is being used increasingly for surveillance of premalignant conditions of the upper gastrointestinal tract. Flexible sigmoidoscopy is now recommended as a routine screening procedure in patients over 50 to detect colorectal adenomas and unsuspected carcinomas. Colonoscopy has become the primary method of investigation of lower gastrointestinal bleeding of unknown origin.

THERAPEUTIC ENDOSCOPY

The ability to pass various instruments via a channel in the endoscope has made therapeutic endoscopy a reality. Endoscopic techniques have replaced some invasive surgical techniques, e.g., polypectomy via the colonoscope, and less frequently via the gastroscope. In the esophagus, the channel is used to extract foreign bodies, to dilate strictures, and to treat varices. It is also used to palliate esophageal malignancy under direct vision by insertion of an inlying stent after mechanical dilatation or by the opening of a channel through occluding cancer with a laser. More recently, other endoscopic photoablation techniques for esophageal neoplasia have been developed. A variety of methods have been developed for the control of bleeding in the stomach, duodenum, and colon, such as electrocoagulation devices, heater probes, and various types of laser. Gastrostomy can be accomplished percutaneously with the aid of gastroscopy. Tubes can be introduced through the papilla of Vater to visualize the pancreatic and biliary ducts. The papilla of Vater can be incised to release a common duct stone, and balloons can be passed to dilate strictured biliary ducts, which are then kept open with stents inserted via the endoscope.

IMPORTANCE OF BIOPSY

The importance of being able to obtain biopsy samples from lesions under direct vision cannot be overemphasized. There are limitations to this technique, however; for example, submucosal lesions may not be reached by the biopsy forceps, especially if the lesion is not raised and cannot be excised with a snare. The possibility of follow-up of an unhealed gastric ulcer makes prompt diagnosis of early-stage cancer more feasible. Endoscopy is useful clinically in patients with inflammatory conditions of the colon to differentiate between idiopathic inflammatory bowel disease and other inflammatory disorders, and to carry out endoscopic surveillance for neoplasia.

Screening for cancer is performed most often in the colon in patients with a history of colonic cancer, a family history of colonic cancer, or ulcerative colitis of more than 8 years' duration. Screening of patients with Barrett's esophagus for dysplasia or early, curable cancer is widely performed.

Esophagoscopy, often with biopsy or brush cytology, is essential to the modern diagnosis of esophageal disease. Endoscopy is used in the diagnosis of regurgitant esophagitis, peptic stricture, esophageal ulcer, squamous carcinoma, adenocarcinoma, Mallory-Weiss tear, varices, Barrett's esophagus, hiatal hernia, and a variety of opportunistic infections in the immunocompromised patient. Gastroscopy within the first 24 hours of bleeding is the best method of finding a bleeding gastric or duodenal source. Gastroscopy with biopsy is also essential for the diagnosis of gastritis, for differentiating a malignant from a benign gastric ulcer, and for the diagnosis of polypoid lesions and various postgastrectomy problems.

Intramural, extramucosal lesions may have a characteristic endoscopic appearance, with bridging folds from the mass to the surrounding mucosa. Biopsy diagnosis usually fails because the overlying mucosa is uninvolved and the lesion is too deep to reach. The addition of an ultrasound transducer to the tip of an endoscope, however, has allowed imaging of the gastrointestinal wall and immediately surrounding structures (7). This technique has been applied predominantly for the staging of gastrointestinal and pancreatic cancer but has also permitted a more precise diagnosis of submucosal masses (8). The depth of invasion of a gastrointestinal malignancy and the presence of enlarged, suspicious lymph nodes can be readily detected. Intramural masses that are not accessible to endoscopic biopsy can be defined according to their echo character, as well as by their precise location within the gastrointestinal wall. Lymphoma, stromal tumors, cysts, and other mural lesions may be defined by using endoscopic ultrasound. Sonography does not supplant histology; however, a tissue diagnosis can often be obtained with endoscopic, ultrasound-guided fine-needle aspiration through the gastrointestinal wall (9).

Biopsy of the gastric mucosa frequently determines the diagnosis of specific types of gastritis. Now that *Helicobacter pylori* is a proven etiologic agent in gastritis and duodenal ulcer, gastroscopy with biopsy has become increasingly important diagnostically. Diagnoses of the reactive gastropathies, opportunistic infections of the stomach with cytomegalovirus and other herpes viruses, or systemic diseases such as Crohn's disease and sarcoidosis may also be rendered. In the duodenum, duodenoscopy is primarily useful for the diagnosis of duodenal ulcer and associated diffuse antral predominant gastritis with *H. pylori*. Occasionally, periampullary adenoma or carcinoma and other disorders such as celiac sprue, immunodeficiency disorders, and infections, especially in immunodeficient patients, can also be diagnosed on the basis of biopsy findings.

CONTRAINDICATIONS

All types of fiberoptic endoscopy are contraindicated without informed consent and should never be performed in the uncooperative or combative patient. Medical contraindications may be present, and the endoscopy procedure can usually be postponed until the patient is stable. Acute perforation anywhere in the gastrointestinal tract is also a contraindication.

COMPLICATIONS

Complications of endoscopy are rare, except when it is performed by the inexperienced (10). Nevertheless, aspiration may occur during upper endoscopy and may be catastrophic in patients with underlying pulmonary compromise. Perforations of the colon occur occasionally during colonoscopy. Reported results from a prospective study involving almost 13,000 patients included a perforation rate of 0.6% for diagnostic colonoscopy and 0.8% for polypectomies (11). The more "invasive" therapeutic procedures, such as creating a channel with a laser through a malignant stenosis of the esophagus or endoscopic sclerosis of esophageal varices, are associated with a somewhat higher complication rate.

ENDOSCOPIC EQUIPMENT

A variety of endoscopes have been designed for specific applications in different organs. The endoscope most commonly used is a forward-looking instrument that can be used for examining the esophagus, stomach, and duodenum at a single sitting. The side-viewing upper endoscope is used primarily for cannulating the papilla of Vater to visualize the biliary tract and pancreatic tree. The colonoscope is longer and has different flexibility characteristics, which enable it to be passed all the way from the anus to the cecum and even into the terminal ileum. The larger endoscopes are used primarily for therapy because they contain a larger channel. They also are of great use for obtaining biopsy specimens of adequate size with jumbo forceps to facilitate diagnosis.

ENDOSCOPIC CHANNEL SIZE

Contemporary endoscopes contain biopsy channels that vary from 2.0 to 3.7 mm in diameter, depending on the size of the specimen desired and whether a larger channel is needed for therapy. We believe that an endoscope with the largest channel should be used for obtaining diagnostic biopsy specimens with the largest forceps, if at all possible. All endoscopic biopsy forceps have two cup-shaped jaws that may be either round or elliptical (Fig. 3.1). It is best to use a forceps with a central spike (see Fig. 3.1) to fix the instrument on the mucosa, thus assuring retrieval of a biopsy specimen of adequate size.

OPTIMAL BIOPSY TECHNIQUE

To take a biopsy specimen, the forceps' jaws are opened and pressed against the mucosa. The forceps' jaws are then closed, and the specimen is pulled off. Typical endoscopic biopsies are about 1 mm in depth and 2 to 5 mm in diameter, depending on the size of the forceps. The specimens usually include only mucosa and a variable amount of the muscularis mucosae; occasionally, they include small slivers of submucosa. Thus, the vascular submucosa is mostly avoided, and bleeding is minimal if the patient's coagulation is normal.

The size of the forceps is the most important factor in determining the size and quality of the biopsy specimen. The smallest forceps is 1.8 mm in diameter and obtains biopsy specimens

that average 3.3 mg (12). Such small biopsy specimens are often inadequate for diagnosis. The standard biopsy forceps is 2.4 mm in diameter and obtains specimens averaging 5.9 mg, a size more likely to be diagnostic. The 3.4-mm jumbo forceps obtains specimens averaging 15.5 mg; these large specimens are the best for diagnostic purposes (see Fig. 3.1) (12). Elliptical forceps cups and those with serrated edges consistently obtain larger specimens than round or nonserrated ones. Muscularis mucosae was obtained in only one third of biopsies with the smallest forceps but in two thirds of biopsies with the standard forceps and in almost all biopsies with the largest forceps in the study reported by Danesh and colleagues (12). Use of the large forceps is not associated with a higher risk of complications (13). In our own experience with thousands of jumbo biopsies, the complication rate has been just as low as that obtained using smaller forceps.

Some endoscopists obtain biopsy specimens by simply opening the forceps and approximating it to the mucosa, rather than pressing it into the mucosa. The use of pressure on the forceps sufficient to put a slight bend in the cable produces significantly larger specimens with no increase in the risk of complications. Obtaining larger biopsy specimens is critical for making more accurate diagnoses, because larger samples contain more tissue, have proportionately less crush artifact, are less liable to fragment, and are easier to orient.

Endoscopic biopsies rarely contain much submucosa and are therefore generally most useful only for evaluating conditions that affect the mucosa. Various techniques that overcome this difficulty in sampling the submucosa and in obtaining full-thickness biopsy specimens of the mucosa include fine-needle aspiration biopsy performed under direct vision through the endoscope (9, 14); the snare biopsy technique, in which an electrosurgical snare is used to obtain a larger specimen (15); and saline assisted polypectomy (16).

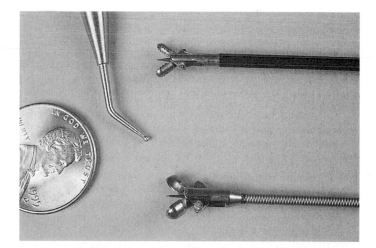

Figure 3.1   *Left:* Penny for size reference; *Above vertically:* End of specimen-orienting tool (Dycal-dental instrument); *Right horizontally at top:* Small biopsy forceps with elliptical, serrated cup edge and impaling spike; *Right horizontally at bottom:* Large "jumbo" biopsy forceps with impaling spike. The specimen size obtained with smaller forceps may be enhanced through the use of elliptical cups and serrated edges; however, jumbo forceps obtain the largest and best specimens without increased complications. (See color plate.)

Snare excision of a fold pulled into the snare is more likely to cause bleeding or, on occasion, perforation (15). Submucosal lesions are, in general, difficult to sample.

Another technique applied in the colon is use of an insulated monopolar forceps to obtain a biopsy by electrocoagulation, the so-called hot biopsy (17). For this procedure, a standard forceps is coated with plastic insulation on its external surface. The mucosa is grasped and tented into the lumen and heated for 1 to 2 seconds by the application of an electrosurgical current before the biopsy is pulled away from the mucosa (17). This technique is used to obliterate small colonic polyps and yet provide some tissue for histologic examination. The tissue provided is barely adequate, and the technique has been associated with bleeding and perforation, especially in the ascending colon.

TECHNICAL FACTORS AND METHODS FOR HANDLING ENDOSCOPIC BIOPSY SPECIMENS

ORIENTATION

Correctly oriented biopsy specimens, which permit taking histologic sections perpendicular to the mucosal surface, are critical for the diagnosis of reflux esophagitis, for the evaluation of small intestinal villi, and for the diagnosis of dysplasia in all sites. Although some diagnoses can be made confidently with inadequately oriented biopsy specimens, diagnosis is easier and more accurate when specimens are well oriented. Endoscopic biopsy specimens of the small bowel are only adequate if they are properly handled and taken with the largest biopsy forceps (18, 19).

We prefer to orient endoscopic biopsy specimens before fixation immediately after they are removed from the patient. In our endoscopy unit, this task is accomplished by a trained endoscopy assistant. The specimen should be handled gently at all times, preferably with the side, rather than the point, of a dissecting needle. To avoid damaging the specimen with a dissecting needle, we routinely use a blunt-ended generic dental tool called a "Dycal" (see Fig. 3.1) that is available through dental supply houses throughout the United States. The specimen is gently teased out of the biopsy forceps onto the tip of the index finger. It is placed lumen-side down on the finger and then unrolled with the aid of the side of the dissecting needle or the Dycal tool just mentioned (see Fig. 3.1), so that the cut, submucosal side faces up. The cut side of the biopsy is then gently placed onto a adherent surface that can be dropped into the fixative. The inside of the lid of a standard plastic cassette used for histologic tissue processing is adequate for this purpose and saves technician time. The need for other mounting substrates, such as plastic mesh, cucumber slices (20), ™Gelfoam, ™Millipore filters, and thin plastic cards is also made unnecessary by this technique. These other substrates can be used for mounting, but we find the cassette top is the simplest approach. In all cases, it is important to mount the biopsy so that the mucosal surface faces away from the orienting substrate. The specimen should be dropped into the fixative as quickly as possible and never allowed to dry (21). Orientation may be facilitated by using magnifying aids, such as a fluorescent ring light with a magnifying lens or a jeweler's loupe worn with a headband.

This orientation operation must be performed rapidly and carefully to avoid damaging the mucosa through rough handling. For most biopsy specimens, it is less desirable to drop the biopsy specimen into fixative directly from the forceps and then perform orientation later during embedding. In certain select situations, however, it is best to drop the specimen directly into the fixative using as little manipulation as possible, i.e., when trying to preserve adherent membranes to diagnose pseudomembranous colitis or amebiasis.

FIXATION

The ideal fixative for endoscopic biopsies should be reliable and inexpensive; preserve all tissue structures; be compatible with most histochemical, immunohistochemical, and molecular methods; and not require mixing immediately before use. It should have a long shelf life, be relatively safe, and penetrate the tissue deeply and rapidly.

FORMALIN

Because formalin satisfies many of these requirements, it has been widely adopted as a routine fixative in pathology laboratories. The formaldehyde gas in aqueous solution (formalin) is 99.9% hydrated to methylene glycol; only 0.1% exists as the active form, carbonyl formaldehyde (22). For this reason, formalin fixes slowly, and requires a minimum of 20 hours for complete fixation. Unfortunately, biopsy specimens in most laboratories receive no more than 3 to 4 hours of fixation in formalin, and therefore are fixed in alcohol on the tissue processor. Formalin has a relatively delicate chemical action on proteins, forming methylene bridges between adjacent reactive groups in the protein molecules (23). Because of the delicate nature of formalin fixation, the tissue is not protected from the disruptive effects of tissue processing, sectioning, deparaffinization, and staining. In contrast, protein precipitant fixatives, such as solutions containing various metallic cations (mercury, copper, or zinc) and acids (picric and acetic) produce a more profound denaturation of cellular proteins and in doing so render the tissue resistant to the harmful effects of processing, sectioning, deparaffinization, and staining (23). As a result, the sections have much better preservation of tissue detail. In addition, formalin is not a good preservative for nucleoproteins (24) and consequently gives poor nuclear definition, especially in very cellular tissues (25). Pierre Masson's objection to formalin as a fixative for gastrointestinal tissues is just as valid today as it was when he expressed it in 1928: "Formol itself fixes the granules well but fixes the tissues very badly (I am perhaps alone in this opinion but the greater my experience the more I am convinced of its truth.)" (26).

OTHER FIXATIVES

Many gastrointestinal pathologists prefer Bouin's fluid, Hollande's modification of Bouin's fluid (Table 3.1), B-5, or others. Alcohol-based fixatives and those containing heavy metals do not preserve Paneth cell and eosinophil granules, and acidic fixatives lake red cells. We prefer the Hollande's modification of Bouin's fluid for routine fixation of gastrointestinal biopsy specimens because it produces excellent nuclear detail, is associated with minimal tissue shrinkage, and preserves red cells and Paneth cell granules (27, 28). The cupric acetate and picric acid in Hollande's probably explain the

TABLE	
3.1	**Formula for Hollande's Solution**

Formalin (40% formaldehyde)	100 mL
Glacial acetic acid	15 mL
Picric acid	40 g
Cupric acetate	25 g
Water	1000 mL

Dissolve cupric acetate in water without heat, add picric acid slowly with stirring. When dissolved, filter and add formalin and acetic acid. Hollande's solution has a shelf life of at least 1 year. To avoid storing dry picric acid in the laboratory, substitute 1000 mL saturated picric acid solution for the picric acid and water.

excellent mordanting (dye fixation of colors) characteristic of Hollande's solution. Picric acid tends to cause tissue shrinkage, and this effect is counteracted by the swelling action of acetic acid in Bouin's and Hollande's. Formalin-fixed tissues from remote sites can be postfixed in Hollande's, B-5, and so on for 2 hours with some improvement in histologic appearance (see subsequent discussion for details regarding histologic tissue processing if placing Hollande's fixed tissue in a processor also using formalin).

The shelf life of Hollande's solution is at least 1 year. Specimens should remain in Hollande's solution for a minimum of 2 hours, but not longer than 3 days, because they become brittle. Specimens that need to be held for more than 3 days should be transferred to 70% ethanol. Tissues fixed in Hollande's solution should be washed in running tap water until the water becomes clear before they are placed in a tissue processor containing formalin, unless a tissue processor without a formalin step is used. If tissues fixed in Hollande's solution are placed in phosphate-buffered formalin, a precipitate of small, round, basophilic granules develops, usually in association with mucus, and can be mistaken for fungi or parasites. To obviate this precipitate, unbuffered formalin should be used in the tissue processor. The lack of a buffer in the processor does not cause problems because the solution is changed often.

The pathologist accustomed to formalin fixation may find that the superior nuclear detail achieved by the various special fixatives requires some initial adjustment of diagnostic criteria, particularly regarding the improved nuclear detail that may lead to the overdiagnosis of dysplasia.

MOLECULAR ASSAY FIXATIVES

The major disadvantage associated with the use of Hollande's, Bouin's, or similar fixatives is that DNA and RNA are degraded to small fragments by these fixatives. This degradation precludes many molecular analyses, except those for which very short nucleic acid sequences suffice. In general, these fixatives make most polymerase chain reaction-based assays, as well as Northern, Southern, and other blotting assays difficult or impossible (29–32). If such assays are anticipated, especially for clinical molecular diagnostic purposes or for research, aldehyde-based cross-linking fixatives such as formalin or alcohol-based fixatives are recommended. These latter fixatives do not produce as much nucleic acid degradation. Fresh or fresh frozen tissues are preferable for many molecular studies, but aldehyde or alcohol-based fixatives usually provide adequate nucleic acid preservation for many molecular applications. In the current

clinical molecular diagnostic field, this issue is most important for confirming the diagnosis of lymphoma by gene rearrangement assays. Finally, for in situ hybridization, aldehyde-based cross-linking fixatives are also preferred (29, 30, 33).

PROCESSING

Endoscopic biopsy specimens are small enough that most fixatives penetrate them completely within 2 to 3 hours. After fixation, it is best to leave them on mesh and place them in biopsy cassettes with small openings, or wrap them in lens paper or place them in embedding bags to ensure that they are not lost during further processing. ™Polyfoam pads are not used because they produce triangular holes in the tissue sections (34). If the cassette top is used as the mounting surface before fixation, as mentioned previously, this transfer step is avoided.

Most of the standard processing schedules in use on automatic tissue processors should provide satisfactory results with endoscopic biopsy specimens. If the volume of biopsies is large enough that the use of an individual tissue processor for them is possible, the processing cycle usually can be shortened by decreasing the amount of time in each solution.

EMBEDDING

If the specimen is oriented on plastic mesh or some other substrate that cannot be sectioned in the microtome, the biopsy specimen must be carefully removed from the substrate. When the biopsy specimen is brought to paraffin, it is turned on edge and embedded in the paraffin block by means of a heated forceps. The long axis of the specimen should be oriented in such a way that in subsequent microtome sectioning, the specimen is cut through its longest axis. If two or more biopsy samples are to be embedded in the same block, they are easier to cut if they are placed fairly close together, with their long axes and cut surfaces oriented in the same direction. We do not recommend placing more than four biopsy specimens in a block, because step-serial sections are then hard to obtain.

If the specimen is oriented on a cucumber slice or Gelfoam, it may not be necessary to remove it before embedding, because these materials can be sectioned like tissue; the histotechnologist simply trims the excess substrate, turns the mount on edge, and embeds it intact. Should the Gelfoam or cucumber cause difficulty in ribboning the paraffin sections, the specimen can be removed from the substrate before embedding.

Biopsy specimens not mounted onto a substrate should be oriented during the embedding procedure with the aid of a ring light encompassing a central magnifying lens, a jeweler's loupe, or some other aid. Although it is far more desirable to perform orientation in the endoscopy unit, this procedure can deliver acceptable results provided the histotechnologist understands what is required and has the skill, patience, and interest necessary for carrying it out.

In most laboratories, better results can be achieved if only one or two individuals are assigned to handle gastrointestinal mucosal biopsy specimens.

SECTIONING

Before sectioning, the blocks are trimmed close to the specimen itself, and the upper and lower edges of the block are kept as parallel as possible; a rectangle is the desired shape. Trimming the blocks close to the specimen permits many more sections to be included in a given length of a paraffin ribbon and consequently on the glass slide. The cuts made to trim the block should be as shallow as possible, because if the tissue protrudes too far from the underlying paraffin block, it is not stable during sectioning and may fracture.

The biopsy specimens are step-serial sectioned after entering the initial portion of the well-oriented area of the biopsy sample (35). Histologic sections are better if the submucosal surface, rather than the luminal surface, meets the knife first during sectioning.

The sections are floated on a 45° to 50° C waterbath. The water in the bath should be changed daily, and its surface should be cleaned repeatedly during cutting by drawing a tissue across its surface. The slides are allowed to drain dry. After floating the sections onto the slides, the technician must check them to see whether they are in the central, oriented core by using a microscope with the condenser diaphragm partially closed. The slides are then placed in a 62° C oven or into a slide dryer on high temperature for a minimum of 30 minutes (2 hours is preferable) before staining. We prefer leaving esophageal sections and those containing much blood in the oven overnight to keep them from falling off during subsequent staining. We place two ribbons on each slide, leaving an ample margin on each edge of the slide, to avoid the fading from oxidation that occurs near the edge of the coverslip (Fig. 3.2). Each ribbon should contain 12 or more sections. We cut five slides, of which three are stained and two are saved for special stains should they be required (see Fig. 3.2) (35). For routine work, three stained slides may be sufficient, provided they were taken from the central, properly oriented core of the biopsy.

Our practice of step-serial sectioning of gastrointestinal biopsy specimens is practical not only for academic institutions but also for the community hospital laboratory. Once the blocks are trimmed, it takes no longer to cut a ribbon or two of serial sections than it does to cut individual step sections. As an absolute minimum, three levels of each block, each containing a ribbon of sections, should be made; additional levels should be obtained liberally in certain situations.

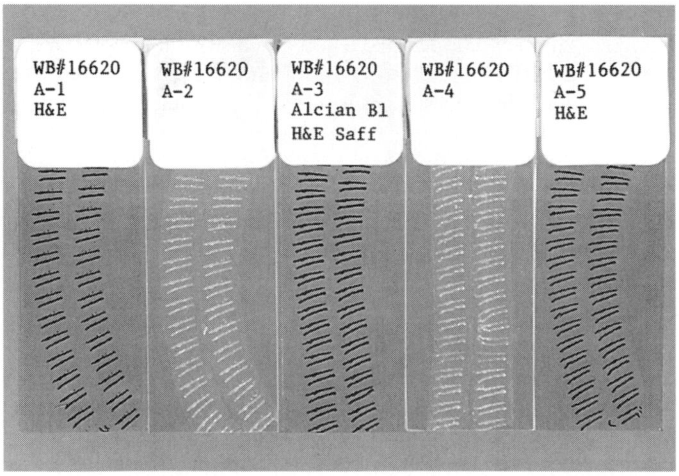

Figure 3.2 Step-serial sections of a gastrointestinal mucosal biopsy. Note that two ribbons of sections have been placed on each slide. Five slides were made, the first, third, and fifth of which were stained; the second and fourth were retained unstained for later use if necessary.

Indications for additional levels include: incorrect orientation on initial sections, a search for granulomas when clinical or biopsy findings are suggestive of Crohn's disease, surveillance biopsies for dysplasia, biopsy specimens that show no evidence of malignant tumor that is thought to be present clinically, findings on initial sections that are equivocal, and any other circumstance in which the pathologist judges that levels might be helpful.

STAINING

We routinely stain all gastrointestinal biopsy samples on one of three stained levels with a combination of hematoxylin and eosin (H & E), Alcian blue, and saffron (Table 3.2). The rationale for this routine stain is that acid mucins are demonstrated by the Alcian blue at pH 2.5, and collagen can be differentiated from smooth muscle by the saffron. When used as a routine stain on gastrointestinal material, this combination results in more timely diagnosis because it eliminates the need for separate special stains for mucin and collagen. Alcian blue has repeatedly proved useful in diagnosing specialized metaplastic columnar epithelium in Barrett's esophagus, in determining the presence of intestinal metaplasia in the stomach, in identifying signet-ring cell carcinoma infiltrating the gastric mucosa, and in determining that giant cells and granulomas in the lamina propria are foreign-body reactions to mucus. Saffron is useful in diagnosing collagenous sprue in small bowel biopsies; in identifying the diagnostic fibromuscular obliteration of the lamina propria in solitary rectal ulcer syndrome; and in diagnosing ischemic colitis, collagenous colitis, healed erosions, and ulcers.

We also routinely apply the special stain developed by Genta (Table 3.3, Fig. 3.3) on all gastric biopsy tissues (36). This stain contains H & E, Alcian blue at pH 2.5, and a modified Warthin-Starry silver impregnation technique. As just mentioned, the Alcian blue aids in the identification of intestinal metaplasia, which assists in the classification of gastritis into atrophic versus nonatrophic categories. The silver component of Genta stain is extremely valuable for the detection of H. pylori. Some form of special stain is now mandatory for all gastric biopsies in which Helicobacter cannot be identified with certainty on an H & E-stained section, because H. pylori is a proven and treatable cause of gastritis and its associated duodenal and gastric ulcers. The organisms can be difficult or impossible to identify with any degree of certainty when using H & E alone, particularly if they are few in number, and thus H. pylori cannot be excluded without benefit of a special stain.

The Genta stain may be specific for H. pylori, as it produces a black dot at both poles of an orange organism (see Fig. 3.3). Because of the silver impregnation, the stain also makes the organism larger and easier to identify, even at lower power screening magnification. In practice, this improved detection and enhanced specificity have served to dramatically decrease professional screening time. For these reasons, we routinely perform the Genta stain on one of the three step-serial sections on all gastric biopsies processed in our histology laboratory, even though it is difficult to perform and requires dedicated, knowledgeable histotechnologists in order to obtain uniform results.

The use of a routine periodic acid-Schiff (PAS) stain in screening for Whipple's disease is not cost effective because the foamy macrophages of this rare condition are easily recognized in H & E sections; when they are identified, appropriate special studies can then be undertaken to confirm the diagnosis.

TABLE 3.2 | Method for Hematoxylin and Eosin (H & E), Alcian Blue, and Saffron Stain

Rationale

Alcian blue and saffron used in combination with the routine H & E stain have the added benefits of demonstrating acidic mucins (Alcian blue) and staining collagen yellow (saffron). When used as a routine stain on gastrointestinal material, it results in earlier diagnosis, as it eliminates the need to use separate special stains for mucin and collagen.

Precautions

Care must be taken not to overstain in saffron. If sections are overstained, decolorize slides in ammonia water, wash well, and restain, starting with eosin.

Results

Nuclei	Blue
Cytoplasm	Pink to red
Goblet mucin	Aqua blue
Collagen	Yellow
Smooth muscle	Salmon pink
Other elements	Shades of pink and blue

Fixation

Any good fixative; excellent results with Hollande's fixed tissues.

Technique

Paraffin sections 4–6 m.

Solutions

Routine H & E
1% Alcian Blue (pH 2.5)

Alcian blue 8 GS (C.I. 74240)	2.0 g
Acetic acid	6.0 mL
Distilled H₂O	194.0 ml

Mix until dissolved and add two or three crystals of thymol as a preservative.

Alcian blue has a normal shelf life of about 3 months, but one must be aware of the more rapid deterioration of solutions when large numbers of slides are stained and change accordingly.

Alcoholic Saffron

Saffron (ground pure Mancha)	7.5 g
Absolute alcohol	400.0 mL

Mix, heat for 6 hours in 60° C dry oven, cool, and filter.
Keeps well, but change once a week for consistent staining.

0.5% Lithium Carbonate

Lithium carbonate	5.0 g
Distilled water	1000.0 mL

Mix well.

Procedure

1. Deparaffinize and bring to water; remove pigment when necessary	
2. Alcian blue	4 min
3. Water	Wash
4. Lithium carbonate	1 min
5. Water	Wash
6. Hematoxylin (Harris)	10 min
7. Water	Wash
8. Acid alcohol (to differentiate)	Dip as needed
9. Water	Wash
10. Lithium carbonate	1 min
11. Water	Wash
12. Check microscopically for nuclear detail	
13. 95% Alcohol	10 dips
14. Eosin	25 dips
15. 70% Alcohol	15 dips
16. 95% Alcohol	15 dips
17. Absolute alcohol	15 dips
18. Absolute alcohol	15 dips
19. Saffron	1 min
20. Absolute alcohol	10 dips
21. Absolute alcohol	10 dips
22. Xylene	10 dips
23. Xylene	2 min
24. Xylene	2 min
25. Coverslip	

Notes: Metanil yellow (C.I. 13065) can be substituted for saffron for purposes of economy.

Staining time in saffron is variable; 1 minute seems to work well with freshly made batches. The solution should be discarded weekly because it gets stronger with age.

Any of the special histochemical stains in common use can be applied to gastrointestinal biopsy specimens as needed. Special stains are particularly useful for identifying infectious organisms, such as mycobacteria or fungi. If unstained slides are saved, these stains can be performed more readily on an ad hoc basis, as the need arises.

SPECIAL PROCEDURES

The use of Giemsa-stained smears made from mucus teased from the fresh biopsy specimen before fixation can be valuable in diagnosing *Giardia lamblia.* Young, Hughes, and Lee advocate touch preparations of biopsy specimens for the diagnosis of gastrointestinal

malignancies (37), citing a sensitivity of 100% for carcinoma of the esophagogastric junction. We have not had personal experience with this technique.

Immunohistochemical localization of various antigens is readily performed on gastrointestinal biopsy specimens. Its principal diagnostic value is in the classification of poorly differentiated malignant tumors, but many other questions can be addressed by the appropriate use of immunohistochemistry. The majority of questions in this regard can be addressed in the context of deparaffinized sections of standard formalin-fixed tissues, including studies requiring antibodies to cell- and tissue-specific markers and hormones, as well as lymphoid cell surface antigens. Fixatives such as Bouin's or B-5 do not offer any significant advantages over

TABLE 3.3 | Genta Stain Method for *Helicobacter pylori* (Revised for Hollande's Fixative)

Rationale

Using a modified Warthin-Starry silver technique, this stain provides excellent diagnostic accuracy for *Helicobacter pylori* and reduces professional screening time. The combined H & E and Alcian blue stains allow simultaneous diagnostic analysis of the gastric tissue with identification of acidic mucins.

Precautions

Take care not to overstain the organisms with silver in the reducing step, so that the characteristic morphology (two black dots at either pole of the bacterium with an orange center) is not obscured. Do not use metal spoons to weigh any of the reagents.

Results (Fig. 3.3)

Nuclei	Blue and black
Cytoplasm	Pink to orange
Goblet mucin	Aqua blue
Collagen	Pink
Smooth muscle	Pink
Helicobacter pylori	Black poles with orange center

Fixation

Hollande's (modified from formalin protocol by Genta et al.[36])

Technical

Paraffin sections 4–6 μm

Solutions

1% Aqueous Uranyl Nitrate

Prepared solution keeps for 2 months. Keep dates current.

1% Silver Nitrate

Silver nitrate	0.5 g
Distilled water	50.0 mL

Mix in coplin jar/staining boat when staining >5 slides. Solution is prepared fresh every time.

2.5% Gum Mastic

Prepared solution is kept refrigerated for up to 2 months.

2% Hydroquinone

Hydroquinone	1.0 g
Distilled water	50.0 mL

Mix in coplin jar/staining boat when staining >5 slides. Solution is prepared fresh every time.

0.4% Silver Nitrate

Prepared solution is kept refrigerated for up to 3 months.

Reducing Solution

Into an acid-washed graduated glass cylinder or plastic cylinder, add the following in order:

2.5% Gum mastic	10.0 mL
2% Hydroquinone	25.0 mL
Absolute alcohol	5.0 mL
0.4% Silver nitrate	2.5 mL

Reducing solution is prepared a few minutes before the reduction process each day. Place milky solution in coplin jar and put in water bath about 1 minute before reduction process.

1% Alcian Blue (pH 2.5)

Alcian blue 8 G5 (C.I. 74240)	2.0 g
Acetic acid	6.0 mL
Distilled H$_2$O	194.0 mL

Mix until dissolved; add two or three crystals of thymol as a preservative. Alcian blue has a normal shelf life of ~3 months, but one must note the more rapid deterioration of solutions when large numbers of slides are stained and change accordingly.

Procedure

1. Place coplin jar in 45° C H$_2$O bath	
2. Deparaffinize and bring to distilled water	
3. 1% uranyl nitrate at RT (to sensitize)	3 min
4. Distilled water (to prevent cross contamination)	Wash
5. 1% Silver nitrate at RT	2 min
6. 1% Silver nitrate, microwave to just below boiling point—do not boil	Time varies by microwave
7. Remove from microwave, and let stain in hot silver nitrate solution	2 min
8. Distilled water, 3 changes	Wash
9. 95% Alcohol, 2 changes	Wash
10. Absolute alcohol, 2 changes	Wash
11. 2.5% Gum mastic	5 min
12. Air dry slides	1 min
13. Distilled water, 2 changes	Wash
14. Reducing solution in 45° C H$_2$O bath; check microscopically at 10 min, 11 min, etc. for development of dark brown or black *Helicobacter pylori* and light yellow background	10–15 min
15. Distilled water	Wash
16. 95% Alcohol, quickly (2 changes)	2 dips each
17. Absolute alcohol, quickly (2 changes)	2 dips each
18. Distilled water	Wash
19. Alcian blue pH 2.5	10 min
20. Running water	Wash
21. Harris hematoxylin	7 min
22. Running water	Wash
23. Acid alcohol to differentiate	Dip as needed
24. Running water	Wash
25. Lithium carbonate	1 min
26. Running water	Wash
27. 95% alcohol, quickly	1–2 dips
28. Eosin	90 sec
29. Tap water, quickly	1–2 dips
30. 95% alcohol, 2 changes	Dehydrate
31. Absolute alcohol, 3 changes	Dehydrate
32. Xylene, 3 changes	
33. Coverslip and check positive control	

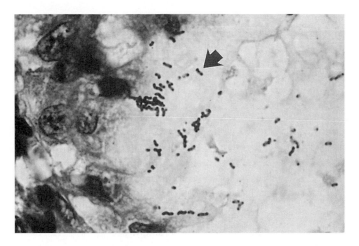

Figure 3.3 Gastric biopsy stained with the Genta stain. This combination stain includes hematoxylin & eosin (H & E), Alcian blue at pH 2.5, and a modified Warthin-Starry silver technique. This stain may be specific for *Helicobacter pylori,* based on the black dot it produces at both poles with an intervening orange-center (*arrow*) (Genta stain). (See color plate.)

formalin-fixed tissues, particularly with the use of new "heat-induced epitope retrieval" techniques that greatly enhance and enlarge the number and range of antibodies that can be applied to deparaffinized, formalin-fixed tissues (38).

Electron microscopy likewise requires advance planning so that the specimen can be properly prepared. The indications for electron microscopy have diminished since immunohistochemistry became widely available. The activity of Whipple's disease can be assessed by demonstrating Whipple's bacilli by light microscopy of sections of jejunum fixed in osmic acid and embedded in plastic.

Other techniques that we have used successfully on endoscopic biopsies include flow cytometry for analysis of nuclear DNA content and cell cycle parameters (39).

INTERPRETATION OF BIOPSY FINDINGS

Optimal interpretation of endoscopic biopsy findings requires close communication between the endoscopist and the pathologist. Endoscopic biopsy specimens challenge the pathologist not only because they are small, but also because they pose questions that require more than a diagnosis of "benign" or "malignant"; they require that the pathologist know and recognize diagnostic criteria for a broad spectrum of medical and surgical conditions. In each case, the pathologist must know the pertinent clinical history and physical findings, the results of radiographic and laboratory studies, indications for endoscopy, endoscopic findings, and detailed information concerning the sites of biopsy. Because a complete endoscopy report should contain most of these data, the practice of sending a copy to the laboratory along with each biopsy specimen provides a convenient method of transmitting the necessary information.

The endoscopist should avoid the tendency to group specimens from different locations and place them in the same bottle of fixative. If one biopsy then shows equivocal findings that need to be investigated, one does not know which site to target for additional biopsies. In addition, certain diagnoses require information concerning the distribution of pathologic changes in the tissues. A good example is idiopathic inflammatory bowel disease. Crohn's disease tends to be segmental and to spare the rectum, whereas ulcerative colitis usually involves the rectum and a variable length of contiguous proximal colon diffusely and circumferentially. Well-placed biopsies can detect these distributional phenomena and facilitate the differentiation of ulcerative colitis and Crohn's disease.

On the other hand, as many as four biopsies from the same level within the esophagus or colon or the same lesion can be placed in one block and still be serially sectioned. This step increases information and reduces costs. For example, in screening for Helicobacter-associated gastritis, we routinely place three biopsies, two from the lesser curvature of the antrum near the pyloris and one from the middle of the greater curvature of the body of the stomach, into one block and charge for a single biopsy. The anatomic biopsy site information is maintained by having the clinicians place the biopsies in separate fixative containers. The histotechnologists then embed all three biopsies in one paraffin block, placing the fundal site in the center.

ARTIFACTS

Endoscopic biopsy forceps are designed to tear, rather than cut, tissue fragments from the mucosa. Thus, mechanical artifacts are unavoidable. Crush artifacts occur consistently because of the squeezing of the tissue at the point of closure of the biopsy forceps (Fig. 3.4). Glandular tissue distorted in this manner can be mistaken for carcinoma (see Fig. 3.4). Crush artifact may also compress the component of normal mononuclear cells present at the edges of the biopsy specimens in the small bowel and colon, causing them to appear increased and thus suggestive of inflammation. A similar effect on normal fibrous tissue may simulate fibrosis. In biopsy specimens oriented onto a substrate, some crush artifact is evident at either end of the specimen. In these specimens, the two or three glands at either edge may not be grossly distorted, but the nuclei may be damaged, so that their shape is altered: from round (normal) to oval to angulated. Such nuclei may also become artifactually hyperchromatic, opaque, and distorted, which can mistakenly lead to a diagnosis of dysplasia or carcinoma.

Hemorrhages in biopsy specimens are difficult to interpret because the trauma from the biopsy forceps may cause extravasation of blood. Unless associated necrosis, fibrin, or hemosiderin deposition is present, it is difficult to be certain that such extravasates represent true hemorrhage. In the face of uncertainty about the significance of extravasated red cells, the pathologist should note their presence and add a comment to the effect that they may represent biopsy artifact.

Enemas and/or laxatives used before proctosigmoidoscopy and colonoscopy may produce changes in the normal mucosa that can be seen both at endoscopy and in biopsy samples (40–43). Endoscopic changes induced by a hypertonic sodium phosphate enema ™(Fleet Phospho-Soda) include hyperemia, loss of the normal vascular pattern, production of petechiae, and occasionally production of increased mucosal fragility. Histologically, bisacodyl

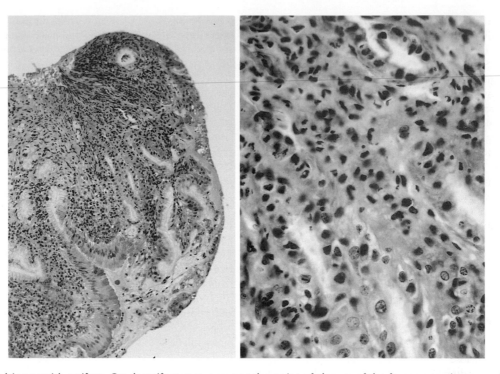

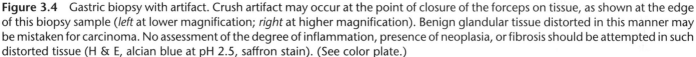

Figure 3.4   Gastric biopsy with artifact. Crush artifact may occur at the point of closure of the forceps on tissue, as shown at the edge of this biopsy sample (*left* at lower magnification; *right* at higher magnification). Benign glandular tissue distorted in this manner may be mistaken for carcinoma. No assessment of the degree of inflammation, presence of neoplasia, or fibrosis should be attempted in such distorted tissue (H & E, alcian blue at pH 2.5, saffron stain). (See color plate.)

(Dulcolax™) can cause a specific "erased" appearance of the superficial half of the mucosa (40). All of these bowel preparations, as well as magnesium citrate and senna derivatives (Senna X-Prep™), can produce lamina propria edema, subnuclear vacuoles and nuclear apoptotic debris in the surface epithelium, separation of the surface epithelium from the basal lamina, and depletion or diminution of goblet cell mucin. Mild hyperplasia of crypt epithelium, with crowding of nuclei and mitotic figures in the upper region of the crypt, and hemorrhages in the lamina propria may also be seen. Mucosa from patients prepared for colonoscopy with Golytely™, an electrolyte solution, does not show these artifacts (43, 44). Thus, the pathologist must consider the effects of preparation to avoid overinterpretation of the biopsy.

FACTORS AFFECTING THE ACCURACY OF ENDOSCOPIC BIOPSY

Provided that the pathologist knows and is able to identify the diagnostic criteria for each condition being evaluated, the accuracy of endoscopic biopsy depends on several other factors, foremost among which is the adequacy of tissue sampling. Some disease processes, such as ulcerative colitis, affect the target organ diffusely, and the site and number of biopsy samples are less critical than when a discrete lesion is sampled. In focal or discrete lesions, the number of biopsy specimens required to establish or to confidently exclude a diagnosis is important; this number depends on whether a layer of necrotic debris covers the lesion, whether residual benign tissue surrounds the malignant tumor, the size of the lesion (e.g., gastric ulcer), and so forth. Multiple biopsies increase the tissue

sample and reduce the incidence of false-negative results. Sancho-Poch and colleagues showed that the positive yield of biopsies for gastric cancers rose from 45% when a single biopsy specimen was taken to 99% for eight or more specimens (45). Other studies confirm this high positive yield with multiple specimens of gastric cancer (46) and show that the best results are achieved with biopsy specimens taken from the rim or edge of an ulcerated carcinoma (47). Although the rate varies somewhat from organ to organ, increasing the number of biopsy specimens consistently increases the number of positive cancer diagnoses for all sites. Graham and colleagues showed that a minimum of four biopsy specimens, combined with brush cytology, produced a high diagnostic yield (48).

The endoscopist must be aware that these comments apply equally to lesions that have been interpreted as benign on the basis of their endoscopic and radiographic features. Because submucosal lesions such as lipomas and leiomyomas are covered by normal mucosa, the biopsy forceps does not reach them. In these cases, needle aspiration via the endoscope may permit a cytologic diagnosis (9, 14). The same is true of carcinomas that undermine mucosa at their edges or that have benign neoplasia at the edges, as frequently occurs in the colon. In both situations, a snare biopsy may be necessary to confirm the clinical impression of carcinoma (15); better yet, the whole lesion should be removed with a snare, if possible. In certain situations, biopsy cannot confidently exclude a diagnosis; for example, to rule out a focus of invasive carcinoma in a colonic adenoma, the entire lesion must be removed and evaluated (49). The diagnosis of well-differentiated lymphoproliferative disorders may be difficult or impossible with biopsies.

In the hands of a skilled, conservative pathologist, the incidence of false-positive results should be nil. Negative (benign) biopsy results in specimens of clinically suspicious lesions do not exclude malignancy. Several studies have shown that a combination of brush cytology and biopsy provides more positive diagnoses of cancer than biopsy alone (50); however, if multiple biopsy specimens are obtained, brush cytology adds little to the diagnostic yield (46). One study found that brush cytology was poor at establishing the diagnosis of early gastric cancer (51). Brush cytology generally has a false-positive rate of 4 to 5% (50). Brush cytology may be useful when biopy findings of a clinically malignant lesion are negative or when there is a stricture proximal to the lesion that does not permit passage of the endoscope for biopsy but does allow use of the cytology brush (46). Cytology may be more accurate in the diagnosis of lymphoma (50). Touch smears made from the endoscopic biopsy were shown in one study to have a high sensitivity in diagnosing carcinoma (37).

VALUE TO THE PATIENT OF GOOD TECHNIQUE AND OPTIMUM INTERPRETATION

The approach to endoscopic biopsy may seem complicated and not worth the effort to those who are not accustomed to such procedures. In fact, the additional effort required to obtain biopsy specimens of optimum technical quality is relatively small and amply rewarded by the improvement in patient care. The main advantage of this additional effort is more accurate diagnosis. We frequently see biopsy specimens of the esophagus, stomach, or colon for a second opinion in which the original pathologist was concerned about the possibility of a malignant neoplasm, that, when evaluated with the use of the methods described here, were found to indicate reactive changes caused by inflammation or some other benign condition. Thus, some of the errors in interpretation are attributable to the inadequacy of the material provided to the pathologist or to the inadequacy of its processing in the histology laboratory. Properly obtained, processed, and interpreted biopsy specimens avoid unnecessary operations and foster earlier operative intervention when cancers are potentially curable.

In some clinical situations, it is difficult to differentiate between two related diseases. For example, a patient who has had bloody diarrhea for 1 month may have chronic idiopathic inflammatory bowel disease or may still have an acute self-limited process, presumably of infectious origin. Histologic criteria that can be identified in well-processed rectal biopsies differentiate these two distinct conditions with a high degree of accuracy (52, 53). Similarly, the clinician cannot always differentiate Crohn's colitis from ulcerative colitis. The prognosis and surgical treatment are quite different, and it is therefore helpful to be able to identify Crohn's disease with certainty by finding typical epithelioid granulomas in endoscopic colonic biopsy specimens. Granulomas can be quite small and missed when the biopsy is not step-serial sectioned or when only a single biopsy has been taken (54).

Assessment of villous architecture is the main basis of classifying small bowel biopsy pathology (21, 55). Similarly, crypt architecture is a prime diagnostic feature in differentiating idiopathic inflammatory bowel disease from acute self-limited and infectious colitis. Thus, step-serial sections taken through the central, properly oriented core of the biopsy are essential because it may be impossible to identify anything but gross changes in villous or crypt architecture in biopsies not properly oriented or in occasional step sections. Finally, the diagnosis of dysplasia throughout the gastrointestinal tract requires observing how the nuclear changes persist or mature from the base to the surface—a critical aspect that can only be achieved in oriented material. Patients, clinicians, and pathologists all benefit from better processing of endoscopic biopsies.

SUMMARY

Over the past decade, practicing pathologists have seen a dramatic increase in the number of endoscopic biopsies of the gastrointestinal tract. Because these biopsies permit earlier diagnosis and aid in the clinical evaluation of many different lesions, this increase can be expected to continue. Accurate interpretation of endoscopic biopsy findings requires close communication with the clinician, technically optimal histologic sections, and the knowledge of and ability to recognize diagnostic criteria for a broad spectrum of medical and surgical conditions. This chapter includes technical pointers and information that are helpful in dealing with an ever-increasing volume of biopsy specimens.

ACKNOWLEDGMENTS

The authors thank Dr. Michael Kimmey for helpful suggestions concerning this chapter revision.

REFERENCES

1. Gordon ME, Kirsner JB. Rudolf Schindler, pioneer endoscopist: Glimpses of the man and his work. Gastroenterology 1979;77: 354–361.
2. Hirschowitz BI. A personal history of the fiberscope. Gastroenterology 1979;76.864–869.
3. Hirschowitz BI. History of fiberoptic endoscopy (letter to the editor). Gastroenterology 1980;78:1123.
4. Jackson FW. Autoendoscopy (letter to the editor). Gastrointest Endosc 1981;77:111.
5. Morrissey JF. The 1982 ASGE Distinguished Lecture. Gastrointestinal endoscopy—20 years of progress. Gastrointest Endosc 1983; 29:53–56.
6. Wolf WI, Shinya H. Polypectomy via the fiberoptic colonoscope: Removal of lesions beyond reach of the sigmoidoscope. N Engl J Med 1973;288:329–332.
7. Kimmey MB, Martin RW, Haggitt RC, et al. Histologic correlates of gastrointestinal ultrasound images. Gastroenterology 1989; 96:433.
8. Botet JF, Lightdale CJ, Zauber AG, et al. Preoperative staging of esophageal cancer: Comparison of endoscopic US and dynamic CT. Radiology 1991;181:419.
9. Vilmann P, Jacobsen GK, Henriksen FW, et al. Endoscopic ultrasonography with guided fine needle aspiration biopsy in pancreatic disease. Gastrointest Endosc 1992;38:172.
10. Shahmir M, Schuman BM. Complications of fiberoptic endoscopy. Gastrointest Endosc 1980;26:86–91.
11. Jentshura D, Raute M, Winter J, et al. Complications in endoscopy of the lower gastrointestinal tract. Surg Endosc 1994;8:672–676.
12. Danesh BJZ, Burke M, Newman J, et al. Comparison of weight, depth, and diagnostic adequacy of specimens obtained with 16 different biopsy forceps designed for upper gastrointestinal endoscopy. Gut 1985;26:227–231.
13. Siegel M, Barkin JS, Rogers AL, et al. Gastric biopsy: A comparison of biopsy forceps. Gastrointest Endosc 1983;29:35–36.

14. Iishi H, Yamamoto R, Tatsuta M, et al. Evaluation of fine needle aspiration biopsy under direct vision gastrofiberscopy in diagnosis of diffusely infiltrative carcinoma of the stomach. Cancer 1986;57:1365–1369.

15. Komorowski RA, Caya JG, Geenen JE. The morphologic spectrum of large gastric folds: Utility of the snare biopsy. Gastrointest Endosc 1986;32:190–192.

16. Waye JD. Saline injection colonoscopic polypectomy: Editorial. Am J Gastroenterol 1994;89:305–306.

17. Williams CB. Diathermy-biopsy: A technique for the endoscopic management of small polyps. Endoscopy 1973;5:215–218.

18. Achkar E, Carey WD, Petras R, et al. Comparison of suction capsule and endoscopic biopsy of small bowel mucosa. Gastrointest Endosc 1986;32:278–281.

19. Scott BB, Jenkins D. Endoscopic small intestinal biopsy. Gastrointest Endosc 1981;27:162–167.

20. Allen TV, Achord JL. The pickle of proper bowel biopsy orientation. Gastroenterology 1977;72:774–775.

21. Perera DR, Weinstein WM, Rubin CE. Small intestinal biopsy. Hum Pathol 1975;6:157–217.

22. Fox CH, Johnson FB, Whiting J, et al. Formaldehyde fixation. J Histochem Cytochem 1985;33:845–853.

23. Banks PM. Technical aspects of specimen preparation and special studies. In: Jaffe ES, ed. Surgical pathology of the lymph nodes and related organs. Philadelphia: WB Saunders, 1985;7.

24. Hopwood D. General principles of fixation. In: Filipe MI, Lake BD. Histochemistry in pathology. New York: Churchill Livingstone, 1983;3–4.

25. Pearse AGE. Histochemistry theoretical and applied, vol 1. New York: Churchill Livingstone, 1980;97.

26. Masson P. Carcinoids (argentaffin–cell tumors) and nerve hyperplasia of the appendicular mucosa. Am J Pathol 1928;4:181–211.

27. Hartz PH. Simultaneous histologic fixation and gross demonstration of calcification. Am J Clin Pathol 1947;17:750.

28. Haggitt RC. Handling of gastrointestinal biopsies in the surgical pathology laboratory. Lab Med 1982;13:272–278.

29. Tyrrell L, Elias J, Longley J. Detection of specific mRNAs in routinely processed dermatopathology specimens. Am J Dermatopathol 1995;17:476–483.

30. O'Leary JJ, Browne G, Landers RJ, et al. The importance of fixation procedures on DNA template and its suitability for solution–phase polymerase chain reaction and PCR in situ hybridization. Histochem J 1994;26:337–346.

31. Greer CE, Peterson SL, Kiviat NB, et al. PCR amplification from paraffin-embedded tissues. Effects of fixative and fixation time (see comments). Am J Clin Pathol 1991;95:117–124.

32. Ben-Ezra J, Johnson DA, Rossi J, et al. Effect of fixation on the amplification of nucleic acids from paraffin-embedded material by the polymerase chain reaction. J Histochem Cytochem 1991;39:351–354.

33. Weiss LM, Chen YY. Effects of different fixatives on detection of nucleic acids from paraffin-embedded tissues by in situ hybridization using oligonucleotide probes. J Histochem Cytochem 1991;39:1237–1242.

34. Carson FL. Polyfoam pads—a source of artifact. J Histotechnology 1981;4:33–34.

35. Surawicz CM. Serial sectioning of a portion of a rectal biopsy detects more focal abnormalities. Dig Dis Sci 1982;27:434–436.

36. Genta RM, Robason GO, Graham DY. Inflammatory responses and intensity of Helicobacter pylori infection in patients with duodenal and gastric ulcer: Histopathologic analysis with a new stain. Acta Histochem 1995;28:67–72.

37. Young JA, Hughes HE, Lee FD. Evaluation of endoscopic brush and biopsy touch smear cytology and biopsy histology in the diagnosis of carcinoma of the lower esophagus and cardia. J Clin Pathol 1980;33:811–814.

38. Gown AM, deWever N, Battifora H. Microwave-based antigenic unmasking: A revolutionary new technique for routine immunohistochemistry. Appl Immunohistochemistry 1993; 1:256–266.

39. Rubin CE, Haggitt RC, Burmer GC, et al. DNA aneuploidy in colonic biopsies predicts future development of dysplasia in ulcerative colitis. Gastroenterology 1992;103:1611–1620.

40. Saunders DR, Haggitt RC, Kimmey MB, et al. Morphological consequences of bisacodyl on normal human rectal mucosa: Effects of a prostaglandin El analog on mucosal injury. Gastrointest Endosc 1990;36:101–104.

41. Meisel JL, Bergman D, Graney D, et al. Human rectal mucosa. Proctoscopic and morphological changes caused by laxatives. Gastroenterology 1977;72:1274–1279.

42. Leriche M, Devroede G, Sanchez G, et al. Changes in the rectal mucosa induced by hypertonic enemas. Dis Colon Rectum 1978;21:227–236.

43. Pockros PJ, Foroozan P. Golytely lavage versus a standard colonoscopy preparation. Gastroenterology 1985;88;545–548.

44. David GR, Santa Ana CA, Morawski SG, et al. Development of a lavage solution associated with minimal water and electrolyte absorption or secretion. Gastroenterology 1980;78:991–995.

45. Sancho-Pocb FJ, Balanzo J, Ocana J, et al. An evaluation of gastric biopsy in the diagnosis of gastric cancer. Gastrointest Endosc 1978;24:281–282.

46. Kobayashi S, Yoshii Y, Kasugai T. Biopsy and cytology in the diagnosis of early gastric cancer. Endoscopy 1976;8:53–58.

47. Hatfield ARW, Slavin C, Segal AW, et al. Importance of the site of endoscopic gastric biopsy in ulcerating lesions of the stomach. Gut 1975;16:884–886.

48. Graham DY, Schwartz JT, Cain GD, et al. Prospective evaluation of biopsy number in the diagnosis of esophageal and gastric carcinoma. Gastroenterology 1982;82:228–231.

49. Livstone EM, Troncale FJ, Sheahan DG. Value of a single forceps biopsy of colonic polyps. Gastroenterology 1977;73:1296–1298.

50. Bemvenuti GA, Hattori K, Levin B, et al. Endoscopic sampling for tissue diagnosis in gastrointestinal malignancy. Gastrointest Endosc 1975;21:159–161.

51. Ito Y, Blackstone MO, Riddell RH, et al. The endoscopic diagnosis of early gastric cancer. Gastrointest Endosc 1979;25:96–101.

52. Surawicz CM, Belic L. Rectal biopsy helps to distinguish acute self-limited colitis from idiopathic inflammatory bowel disease. Gastroenterology 1984;86:104–113.

53. Surawicz CM, Haggitt RC, Husseman M, et al. Mucosal biopsy diagnosis of colitis: Acute self–limited colitis and idiopathic inflammatory bowel disease. Gastroenterology 1994;107:755–763.

54. Surawicz CM, Meisel JL, Ylvisaker T, et al. Rectal biopsy in the diagnosis of Crohn's disease: Value of multiple biopsies and serial sectioning. Gastroenterology 1981;81:66–71.

55. Dobbins WO. Small bowel biopsy in malabsorptive states. Contemp Issues Surg Pathol 1983;4:121–165.

CYTOLOGIC TECHNIQUES AND DIAGNOSIS

Siegfried Witte

COLLECTION OF MATERIAL
ESOPHAGUS
STOMACH
DUODENUM
COLON AND RECTUM
    ACCESSIBLE TISSUES
    DEEP-SEATED LESIONS
METHODS OF MICROSCOPIC EXAMINATION
FRESH UNFIXED PREPARATIONS
    PHASE CONTRAST MICROSCOPY
    NOMARSKI DIFFERENTIAL INTERFERENCE CONTRAST
        MICROSCOPY
    ULTRAVIOLET-LIGHT MICROSCOPY
    FLUORESCENCE MICROSCOPY
STAINING TECHNIQUES
QUANTITATIVE METHODS
    MICROMORPHOMETRY

FLUORESCENCE CYTOPHOTOMETRY
HIGH-RESOLUTION IMAGE ANALYSIS
TELEMICROSCOPY
CYTOMORPHOLOGY AND CYTODIAGNOSIS
ESOPHAGUS
STOMACH
DUODENUM
COLON AND RECTUM
STATISTICAL EVALUATION OF CYTODIAGNOSES
ESOPHAGUS
STOMACH
    QUALITATIVE STUDIES
    QUANTITATIVE STUDIES
DUODENUM
COLON AND RECTUM

Gastroenterologic cytodiagnosis is based on the desquamation of superficial cells from the mucosa of the gastrointestinal tract. Under pathologic conditions, such desquamation can increase substantially. The foremost role of cytology is the identification of malignant tumors. The criteria for recognition of tumor cells by microscopy have been defined in the practice of clinical cytology. These criteria in principle hold for all organs, but differences exist with respect to various tumors. In practice, diagnosis must also take into account organ-specific changes in cells, generally of inflammatory origin, which must be recognized and distinguished from tumor cells.

The yield of cells that can contribute to making a diagnosis is increased when the desquamation of cells is promoted by appropriate technical methods and when cellular material is obtained as specifically as possible. Cytologic samples should be taken only from the suspected regions of the mucosa of only the desired organ, without contamination from other areas. Furthermore, assessment by microscopy requires cells in well-preserved condition and appropriate methods of preparing the cells and of microscopic examination.

Finally, the level of experience of the cytologist plays an important part, although even the best cytologist obtains good results only when he or she receives appropriate cellular material from a good endoscopist. At present, the yield of cells usually depends on endoscopic technique. The cells must be sampled specifically; that is, macroscopically suspected findings must be identified for localization. When indicators of this sort are absent, or when endoscopic investigation cannot be performed, the material must be sampled "blind." In such instances, it is necessary to sample as much as possible of the entire mucosal surface of the organ being investigated, as in screening of populations in which certain malignant tumors occur at high rates. Additionally, the cytologist can collect material by fine-needle aspiration of deep-seated lesions.

COLLECTION OF MATERIAL

ESOPHAGUS

Nonselective esophageal sampling techniques for screening are justified in regions in which esophageal carcinoma is frequent. In China, an abrasive balloon is used (1), a technique whose development is traced back to Panico and Papanicolaou (2). A gauze sheath is tied in place over an inflatable balloon attached to tubing. After the balloon has been advanced to the chosen level, generally that of the cardia, the balloon is inflated using a syringe attached to the oral end of the tubing. The tube is then pulled back to the level of the proximal esophagus, and the balloon is deflated. The procedure can be repeated.

The best yield of cellular material is given by rinsing the balloon in a few milliliters of physiologic saline solution. The sediment obtained by centrifugation can be microscopically examined.

Another technique involves the use of a nonendoscopic abrasive cytology tube containing four brushes. This method has been used for screening dysphagic patients (3).

Our own experience includes collection using the cell-swab method described by Henning (4). A foam-rubber swab is fastened to a wire. The wire slides freely within a thin and flexible tube that widens at one end to form a rubber sheath. The swab is introduced while covered by this sheath. At a chosen level, the head of the swab is advanced by means of a handle at the oral end of the tube, and the tube is moved backward and forward a few times. By these movements, the swab abrades the suspected area and is then drawn back into the protective rubber sheath. The tube is then removed. Cellular material is collected from the foam rubber by rinsing in physiologic saline solution and centrifugation, as just described for the abrasive balloon technique.

The advantage of the abrasive balloon is that it abrades the entire superficial mucosal surface; the disadvantages are that patients find it unpleasant and that it also yields cells from the pharynx and oral cavity. The advantages of the cell-swab method are that the level of sampling is relatively specific, that undesirable contamination is avoided, and that the procedure is rapid.

The high level to which flexible endoscopy has been developed makes endoscopically guided sampling the optimal and clinically preferred technique for obtaining material. An abrasive brush is fastened to a sound that is introduced through the instrument channel of the endoscope. Under direct endoscopic observation, the brush is advanced to the chosen site. By working the guidance lever of the endoscope, one scrapes the brush gently, several times and as tangentially as possible, across the surface of the lesion. The brush is then retracted into the protective opening of the instrument channel, and endoscopy is concluded. Any necessary forceps biopsy specimens are taken before brush abrasion. After removal of the endoscope from the patient, the brush is again advanced out of the opening of the instrument channel and rinsed in a few milliliters of physiologic saline solution. The cellular sediment is collected by centrifugation.

It is important to perform biopsies before cell-brush abrasion during endoscopy, because the tissues are slightly disrupted by the biopsy and the yield of cells on brush abrasion is increased. Additionally, a superficial film of blood affects brush sampling less than it does biopsy.

STOMACH

Gastric cell sampling currently is performed only under endoscopic observation (5, 6). When attempting cytologically to identify a malignant tumor in the stomach, one must also determine the location of the tumor. Only in this way is diagnosis of practical value, leading as it must to surgical treatment to extirpate the tumor. It is generally recognized that, even in its early stages, gastric carcinoma manifests as an endoscopically recognizable lesion of the gastric mucosa. The endoscopist, however, generally cannot confirm that a lesion seen at endoscopy is malignant.

The technical conditions under which material is sampled are accordingly of decisive importance for successful diagnosis. They depend on the endoscopist's ability to inspect the entire stomach, to recognize suspicious areas, and to obtain and retrieve material from precisely those areas.

The technique of brush abrasion is in principle the same as that used in the esophagus. Tangential contact with the entire surface of the lesion is necessary, with exertion of light pressure. We avoid pushing the brush away from the instrument; instead, we draw it toward the endoscope. Strong pressure can cause linear superficial erosions.

If cytologic investigation of more than one gastric lesion during a single session is desired, covered abrasion brushes must be used to allow repeated sampling. They are introduced in plastic tubes that fit within the instrument channel of the gastroscope. The brush is advanced out of the protective tube only in the stomach. After abrasion, it is retracted into the tube, and tube and brush are removed together. Covered brushes are smaller than the normal brushes that are used without a cover, and accordingly the yield of cellular material is less. We therefore recommend sampling the most important lesion with an uncovered brush at the end of endoscopic investigation.

Zargar et al. (7) compared the value of brushing before or after biopsy in the endoscopic diagnosis of gastroesophageal malignancy and found a significantly higher diagnostic yield when the brushing was performed first.

Needle aspiration can be used for obtaining cells from endoscopically identifiable foci of disease in the submucosa. The injection cannulas used for sclerotherapy of esophageal varices are particularly well suited to this purpose. While exerting negative pressure using a 20-ml syringe at the oral end, it is important to move the cannula slightly backward and forward in the tissues several times. Before the tip of the needle is withdrawn from the mucosa, however, the vacuum must be released. After the cannula is withdrawn, the syringe is removed, its plunger is drawn back, and the syringe is attached again, for squirting the aspirated cellular material within the tip of the cannula carefully out onto a slide, where it can be smeared as a blood film is smeared.

Layfield et al. (8) described a similar technique with a Stifcor™ transbronchial aspiration needle.

DUODENUM

From a cytologic standpoint, the papilla of Vater is the most important region of the duodenum. We use abrasion brushes in conjunction with duodenoscopy to sample tangentially the papilla or other suspected regions in the proximal horizontal portion, the descending portion, or the distal horizontal portion of the duodenum. The technique is the same as that used in the stomach. With the covered brushes described previously, it is possible to enter the lumen of the papilla to obtain cellular material.

Although the techniques for sampling the excretory ducts of the pancreas and the biliary tree are not discussed here, it should be mentioned that using a probe to aspirate secretions from the immediate vicinity of the papilla (prepapillary aspiration, with or without stimulation using intravenous secretin) is a routine procedure for cytologic studies of those regions (9).

COLON AND RECTUM

ACCESSIBLE TISSUES

In these regions, we favor endoscopically directed abrasion techniques, using either the sigmoidoscope or the colonoscope for localization. If polypoid lesions can be removed endoscopically using an electrical snare, that maneuver has diagnostic priority. In such instances, the cytologist must be content with blotting the resected polyp on several microscope slides.

In the presence of diffuse inflammatory changes, ulcerative lesions, or polypoid tumors that cannot be endoscopically resected in toto, we use brush abrasion. Multiple sampling is possible with the use of covered brushes. We never draw an uncovered brush through the instrument channel of the colonoscope after abrasion; this maneuver decreases the cellular yield and soils the instrument channel. Forceps biopsy specimens are always taken before brush abrasion. Some authors (10, 11) use endoscopic fine-needle aspiration cytology, particularly in submucosal processes.

We obtain cytologic material from the anal canal by means of a firm, dry cotton swab on a wooden stick, introduced through an open proctoscope. The swab is then rolled and blotted on dry microscope slides.

DEEP-SEATED LESIONS

Cellular material from deep-seated lesions that cannot be reached by endoscopic techniques is collected by ultrasound-guided or ultrasound-assisted needle aspiration with relatively moderate means and a minimum invasive manner. These interventions are most useful for the assessment of focal lesions of parenchymatous organs. In our institution, this technique is indicated in 20 to 40 cases per year (unpublished results).

In contrast to CT-guided puncture, sonographic intervention involves continuous observation of the biopsy needle on the screen, made possible by special biopsy scanners with integrated or laterally fixed needles. The puncture tract thus predefined is shown on the screen as an electrical guideline; the needle is observed from the time it pierces the skin until its penetration into the target object. Because this technique is performed under real-time conditions and not with a static, frozen picture, the accuracy is high.

Depending on the location of the process, the quality of the picture, patient compliance, and the experience of the investigator, biopsies of objects less than 1 cm in diameter are possible using either fine needles (up to 1 mm in diameter) or thick needles (more than 1 mm in diameter), according to the investigational problem. Cytologic fine-needle biopsies are carried out by aspiration; histologic biopsies are performed with cutting needles of larger caliber.

With a sufficiently experienced investigator and respecting the contraindications, the rate of complications is low. Bleeding represents the main risk; local infections or subsequent needle tract seeding occur less frequently.

METHODS OF MICROSCOPIC EXAMINATION

FRESH UNFIXED PREPARATIONS

The cytology laboratory should be in close proximity to the endoscopy suite to make the best use of cytologic diagnosis of unfixed material. In our hospital, they open off the same corridor.

The centrifuge tubes containing either the physiologic saline solution, in which the abrasion brushes were rinsed, or the aspirated secretions are sealed and brought to the cytology labo-

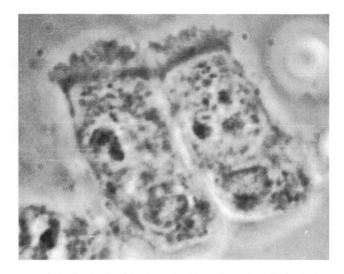

Figure 4.1 Jejunal epithelial cells. Note the cylindrical cell shape and brush border (unfixed wet preparation, phase contrast, ×1250).

ratory, where they are processed within 1 hour of being obtained by endoscopy.

The tubes are centrifuged for 5 minutes in a normal laboratory centrifuge at a moderate number of revolutions per minute. All of the supernatant is decanted. With a glass rod, the sediment is distributed among three or four dry microscope slides to which coverslips are applied. Careful pressure should produce equal distribution of the material to the rim of the coverslip. Processing these samples quickly avoids osmotic changes related to drying. These preparations are then immediately examined under the microscope. They can also be stored for up to 2 hours in a high-humidity container.

PHASE CONTRAST MICROSCOPY

This method is used most frequently for microscopic examination of unfixed wet smear preparations. We use it routinely to scan all preparations (12). Cell-free preparations can be scanned quickly in this manner. An assessment of cellular content is essential to permit the endoscopist to develop his or her sampling technique as highly as possible. Protozoa, such as *Giardia lamblia*, trichomonads, and amoebae, are immediately recognizable in unfixed preparations because they are motile.

The optical characteristics of phase contrast microscopy (Figs. 4.1 and 4.2) permit identification of the following cytologic details: *(a)* nuclear size (anisokaryosis, alterations in nuclear/cytoplasmic ratio), nuclear shape, nuclear membrane (irregular thickening, double contouring), nucleoli (number, size, shape, definition with regard to the remainder of the optically homogeneous nucleoplasm); *(b)* cytoplasmic and cellular shape, definition by cellular organelles (such as the brush border), fine structure of the cytoplasm (granularity, vacuolation); and *(c)* *Campylobacter* (*Helicobacter*) *pylori* (13) or protozoa. Thin preparations are optimal for phase contrast illumination. If several cells overlie one another, disturbing halation effects appear in thicker regions. Such instances provide an indication for examination by Nomarski contrast microscopy.

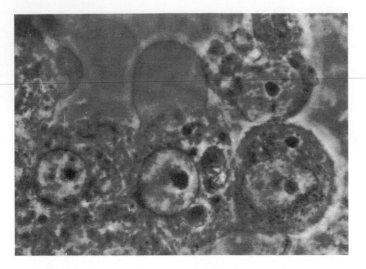

Figure 4.2 Tumor cell cluster, gastric adenocarcinoma (unfixed wet preparation, phase contrast, ×1250).

NOMARSKI DIFFERENTIAL INTERFERENCE CONTRAST MICROSCOPY (14)

Preparations are made in the same manner as just described. The technique, however, is somewhat more painstaking than that used for phase contrast microscopy. Its advantage is good resolution even in thick clumps of cells, provided by a narrow depth of focus (Fig. 4.3).

ULTRAVIOLET-LIGHT MICROSCOPY (14, 15)

Neither phase contrast nor Nomarski contrast microscopy adequately details nuclear internal structure. This disadvantage is

compensated for by ultraviolet-light microscopy, which takes advantage of specific absorbance by nucleic acids and nonhistone proteins on illumination with short-wavelength ultraviolet light. We have demonstrated that the nuclei of unfixed cells display an internal structure that resembles the chromatin structure of fixed and stained cells and that provides information of substantial value in cytodiagnosis (16). Special equipment (quartz optics, monochromatization, image transformers) is required (Fig. 4.4). A new developed ultraviolet microscope is now available commercially (17).

FLUORESCENCE MICROSCOPY

Staining of unfixed cells with fluorescent dyes, such as acridine orange, also permits chemical differentiation among nucleic acids, in particular distinction of desoxyribonucleic acids within the nucleus from ribonucleic acids within nucleoli and the cytoplasm (18). This differentiation facilitates the recognition of cellular atypia and of tumor cells.

Staining Techniques

After the investigations of unfixed preparations are completed, the same preparations are processed for fixation. To this end, the coverslips are pushed sideways across the microscope slides, smearing out the cellular material. The coverslips are removed and the smears are fixed on the microscope slides. We use a fixative spray. Even when microscopic scanning of wet unfixed preparations is not performed, we use the same technique for smearing and fixation. After fixation the preparations are suitable for mailing to a cytologic laboratory.

Routine staining of fixed preparations is performed according to the methods described by Papanicolaou (19). These methods do not specifically identify tumor cells. They have the advantage,

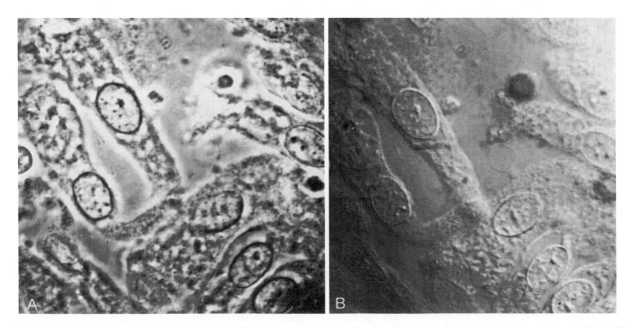

Figure 4.3 Normal columnar cells of gastric epithelium (unfixed wet preparation, ×800). **A.** Phase contrast. **B.** Differential interference contrast.

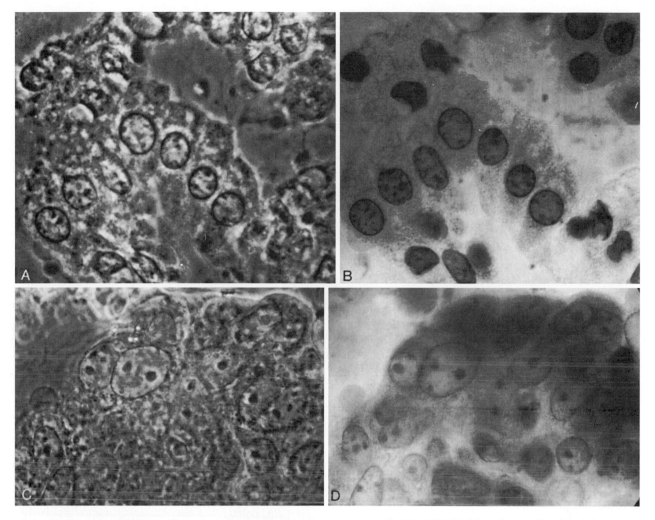

Figure 4.4 A. Gastric epithelial cells in superficial gastritis. Phase contrast. **B.** Same field, monochromatic ultraviolet microscope. Specific absorbance of nucleic acids, $\lambda = 263$ nm. **C.** Tumor cell cluster, adenocarcinoma of the rectum. Phase contrast. **D.** Same field, monochromatic ultraviolet microscope. Specific absorbance of nucleic acids, $\lambda = 263$ nm. (Unfixed wet preparations, ×800.)

however, of adequately detailing the nuclear features that are particularly important for diagnosis, such as chromatin structure, nucleoli, and the nuclear membrane, even in regions of dense cellularity and in clumps of cells. In addition, distraction due to epithelial mucus staining is only slight.

If the material contains little mucus, hematologic stains such as the May-Grünwald-Giemsa stain also can be used. They provide optimal cytoplasmic differentiation. If the preparations contain abundant mucus or proteinaceous material in the background, they are generally so overstained by this technique that evaluation is not possible. A detailed and precise description about the preparation of a smear for cytologic medicine and the most important color processes is available elsewhere (20).

QUANTITATIVE METHODS

Cytologic methods are suited for quantitative studies, a significant advantage over biopsy-histology methods. Even automated techniques for quantitative cytology are now available. The results

mentioned subsequently are based only on cell material collected by the endoscopic cytologic techniques.

MICROMORPHOMETRY

Individual cells were once measured subjectively by means of a microscope equipped with an ocular on which a micrometer was engraved. At present, micromorphometry is generally performed in combination with projection equipment and a graphics tablet or with a system coupling a video camera and a computer.

Determination of nuclear diameter is the oldest quantitative approach, permitting calculation of nuclear area. This method was used to identify significant increases in the dimensions of esophageal and gastric epithelial nuclei in pernicious anemia (21) and tropical sprue (22). Squamous but not gastric epithelial nuclear measurements returned to normal after therapy with Vitamin B_{12}. The area of esophageal squamous epithelial nuclei increases significantly from normal intermediate cells through mild hyperplasia, moderate dysplasia and severe dysplasia, to malignant change (23).

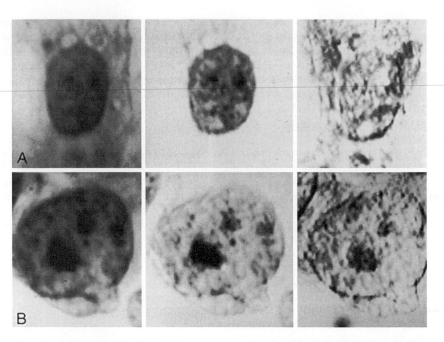

Figure 4.5   From left to right, original absorbance, $\lambda = 263$ nm; pure nucleic acid picture, $\lambda = 280$ nm pure nonhistone protein picture. **A.** Atypical colonic epithelial cell in a case of ulcerative colitis. **B.** Tumor cell in a case of adenocarcinoma of the colon. (Monochromatic ultraviolet absorbance of unfixed wet cells, ×800, processed by means of image analysis computer technique.)

Among many additional morphometric parameters, one of the most important is standard deviation in nuclear area, which quantitatively describes anisokaryosis. In gastric carcinoma, the standard deviation in nuclear area is significantly greater than that in the nuclear area of normal cells. A similar parameter is the nuclear-cytoplasmic ratio, which is smaller for normal gastric epithelium than for malignant cells (24).

FLUORESCENCE CYTOPHOTOMETRY

Stoichiometric cytochemical demonstration of desoxyribonucleic acid using the Feulgen reaction is the oldest, and to date the most important, method. It is now generally used for individual-cell fluorometry, with a fluorescent dye as an indicator. Measurement of intensity of nuclear fluorescence (25) in individual cells, using a fluorescence microscope equipped for photometry, yields a histogram of fluorescence intensities integrated over nuclear areas. With normal diploid cells used as standards for comparison, the DNA content of a cytologic smear can be measured, enabling a determination of whether DNA complements are diploid, polyploid, or aneuploid. Statistical evaluation of measured values is necessary for arriving at results of value in diagnosis. The technique is still evolving.

At present, it is not possible to make the diagnosis of cytologic malignancy from DNA histograms alone (26). Still, quantitative measurement of DNA remains the cornerstone of cytophotometric techniques. Photometry of individual cells is a time-consuming technique. The advantage of being able to assay cells subjectively identified as suspicious is countered by the disadvantage that only a limited number of cells can be evaluated in a reasonable amount of time.

FLOW CYTOPHOTOMETRY

Large numbers of suspensions of individual cells can be assayed in short periods of time by commercially available flow-through systems. A fine stream of liquid transports the cells past one or more ports where fluorescence or light-beam diffraction is measured. Although determination of fluorescence-stained DNA content is important, systems that assay multiple parameters also exist. Flow techniques have definite disadvantages: they have no microscopic optical resolution, microscopic images are not obtained, and permanent preparations for microscopic documentation are not generated. Suspensions of abraded cellular material from clinical sources generally consist of a mixed population of a wide variety of cells, of which only a small proportion can be atypical cells or cells suspected of malignancy. In many instances, therefore, the number of tumor cells is insignificant by comparison with the number of nonmalignant cells. Interpretation of histographic findings is then difficult or inconclusive (27). The development of cell-sorting methods that deposit enriched populations of atypical cells on permanent substrates would significantly increase the value of flow techniques for our specialty. A new approach is provided by staining with fluorescence-labeled monoclonal antibodies.

HIGH-RESOLUTION IMAGE ANALYSIS

High-power magnification permits quantitative description of cells and, in particular, nuclear structure using digital video image generation and computer-directed image processing. These methods are suitable for automation and rapid image analysis. Their goal is completely automated evaluation of smear preparations for tumor identification (28). Preparations can be stained conventionally, with the Papanicolaou stain, or by using fluorescence techniques.

My colleagues and I have gained experience using absorption of monochromatic ultraviolet light by unfixed and unstained cell smears to analyze nucleic acid and nonhistone-protein configurations of nuclei in preparations of gastroenterologic material. Distinction between these nuclear components on high-magnification microscopy is possible with computer-directed image analysis (29). We found epithelial cell nuclei that are normal or show inflammatory changes are readily separable from atypical, neoplastic cell nuclei (30) (Fig. 4.5; Table 4.1).

It is necessary to combine quantitative assessments of various characteristics of cells—DNA content, nuclear size, variation in nuclear size—with high-resolution analysis of nuclear texture to identify tumors in cytologic material objectively, independent of subjective assessments. Investigators in many laboratories are working toward this goal.

TELEMICROSCOPY

A new development to improve cytodiagnostic efficiency is telemicroscopy as a means to share expensive equipment and human expertise. A remote controllable microscope system is connected by online TV transmission of the fields of view to a cytodiagnostic expert. Various concepts and systems have been realized (31).

CYTOMORPHOLOGY AND CYTODIAGNOSIS

ESOPHAGUS

A cytologic abrasion smear prepared from the normal esophagus shows a uniform pattern of cells, consisting of squamous epithelial cells of the intermediate type. Superficial cells are rare, and no keratinization is present. Hyperplasia is manifested by intermediate cells containing enlarged nuclei with normal finely granular chromatin. Patients with pernicious anemia tend to have enlarged, multiple nuclei that regress with institution of Vitamin B_{12} therapy. In esophagitis, epithelial cells from deeper layers, the parabasal cells, appear. The nuclei of these cells are larger and their cytoplasm more basophilic and less extensive than that of intermediate cells. In acute esophagitis, intraepithelial leukocytes are found. When severely necrotizing inflammation is present, large numbers of bacteria and/or fungal hyphae and yeasts are seen. Oxyphilic staining of the cytoplasm reveals a tendency to keratinization, which may occur in normal squamous epithelium and also as a sign of atypia in dysplastic cells. Small squamous-type cells with small, round nuclei and bright oxyphilic cytoplasm are termed ductal cells. These cells occur in small groups and are shed from the ducts of mucous glands in the squamous epithelial layer.

Displaced cell types that may be found include gastric columnar cells or even cells from the duodenal mucosa. They demonstrate heterotopy of the corresponding gastric or duodenal mucosa in the esophagus.

Of particular importance are dysplastic squamous cells (32) (Fig. 4.6). This term implies a dissociation between the maturation of the nuclei and that of the cytoplasm. Nuclei are enlarged, particularly in relation to the more mature cytoplasm. The nuclei are also hyperchromatic, and the nuclear membrane is emphasized. In moderate dysplasia, the nuclear enlargement is found in the intermediate cells; in more severe dysplasia, it also affects the parabasal cells. Hyperchromasia and nuclear enlargement are most pronounced in such cases. Malignancy is suspected when the smear contains numerous, highly dysplastic, polymorphic parabasal cells.

Tumor cells of the squamous epithelium are enlarged and show anisokaryosis and hyperchromia of the nucleus, a thickened nuclear membrane, and a significant shift in the nuclear-cytoplasmic ratio in favor of the nucleus. Enlarged nucleoli are seen in increased numbers. Tumor cells may occur singly or, particularly characteristically, in three-dimensional clumps of cells ("clusters") (Fig. 4.7). The smears may be assessed in accordance with criteria presented in Table 4.2. Rarely, small cell carcinoma arising from the esophagus can be found (33). As a rare variety, the polypoid esophageal carcinoma is characterized cytologically by an association of spindle-shaped cells with malignant squamous cells (34). The diagnostic cytologic features of primary esophageal adenocarcinoma were analyzed by Shurbaji and Erozan (35) in 18 consecutive cases obtained by brushing.

STOMACH

The mucosal cells of the stomach are columnar cells. They are rather tall, with oval nuclei situated in the basal one third of the cells, which often come to a point. The cytoplasm becomes less dense toward the gastric lumen. This secretory area of the gastric mucosa can be seen with particular clarity under phase contrast microscopy. Only a few columnar cells, often lying singly or altered by cytolytic processes, or even free cell nuclei are found in the normal stomach. Columnar

| TABLE 4.1 | Comparison of Cytologic Classification by Light Microscopy and Reclassification by Automated Image Analysis[a] | | |

Light Microscopy		Automated Analysis	
Cell Class	Cases	Normal	Pathologic
1	137	129(131)	8(6)
2	51	43(44)	8(7)
3	62	55(57)	7(5)
4	150	67(–)	83(–)
5	174	26(34)	148(140)
6	137	11(5)	126(132)
Total cases	711	331(271)	380(290)

Automated, high-resolution image analysis is performed on unfixed, unstained cells, with monochromatic ultraviolet microscopy; wavelength, 263 nm.

Six cell classes: 1, normal cylindrical cell; 2, rounded epithelial cell; 3, epithelial cell with nuclear swelling; 4, epithelial cell with slight to moderate nuclear atypia, solitary enlarged nucleolus ("ulcer cells"); 5, cell with severe nuclear atypia; 6, malignant cell.

In automated analysis, normal cells include cells in classes 1 to 3 and pathologic cells include cells in classes 4 to 6. Classification after omission of class 4 is given in parentheses.

[a]Misclassified cases by automated analysis: 17% (10%)

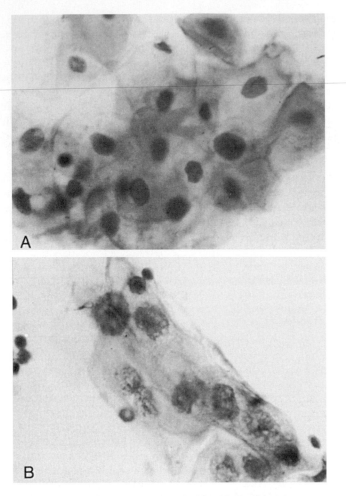

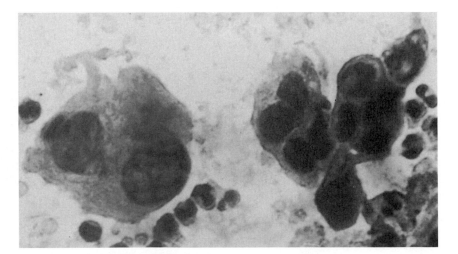

cells found in large numbers and in clusters are taken as a sign of shedding of the epithelium from the basement membrane as a result of inflammation. The columnar cells can be recognized in these clusters by elicitation of the so-called honeycomb phenomenon. It is possible to focus the microscope down onto a deep plane, in which the cell nuclei appear sharp and round, and onto a plane lying above these that passes through the foamy cytoplasm and gives a honeycomb-like pattern as the result of the network of interepithelial boundaries (Fig. 4.8).

The second variety of epithelial cells is the goblet cells. Their cytoplasm is transformed into a vast homogeneous mucous vacuole with a basal nucleus that is distorted into a semilunar shape. Goblet cells are not found in the normal stomach. They are an accompaniment of chronic gastritis, particularly the atrophic form.

Columnar cells whose short ends do not show the loose density of a vacuole but have a sharply delineated edge with a thick border of short bristles (cuticular fringe) are usually found only in the small intestine. Their occurrence in the stomach is a sign of intestinal metaplasia. Together with other signs of chronic gastritis, they are a sign of metaplastic gastritis. When these intestinal cells are found in the stomach, they are always of a mature type, with regular round to oval nuclei and no signs of cellular atypia (Fig. 4.9).

The characteristic representative cells of the glands in the fundus are the parietal cells. They are definitely smaller than the intermediate squamous cells with which they are sometimes confused. They have a relatively extensive cytoplasm and one or more small, round chromatin-rich nuclei. The cell is pyramidal, and its main feature is dense, fine-grained, eosinophilic granulation that fills the cytoplasm evenly with the exception of indistinct "roads." The cells mostly occur in groups, sometimes as cell casts, together with small, heavily vacuolated columnar cells with relatively large nuclei, the mucous neck cells. Parietal cells and mucous neck cells in clusters (Fig. 4.10), suggestive of the tubular structure of glands, indicate increased desquamation of glandular cells as the morphologic expression of an increase in the functional activity of the gastric glands, as has been confirmed by bioptic histology (36). This finding

Figure 4.6   Dysplastic squamous cells of the esophagus. **A.** Slight to moderate dysplasia. **B.** Severe dysplasia in a case of pernicious anemia (Papanicolaou, ×500).

Figure 4.7   Tumor cells in squamous carcinoma of the esophagus. Note also degenerative cell changes after irradiation therapy (Papanicolaou, ×325).

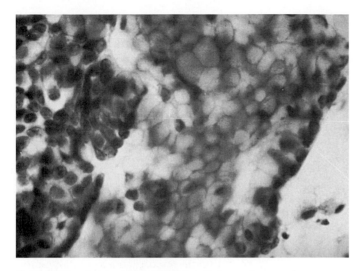

Figure 4.8 Columnar epithelial cells from the gastric mucosa. Note monolayer sheet with honeycomb pattern. Case of superficial gastritis (Papanicolaou, ×108).

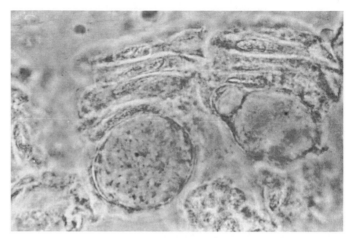

Figure 4.9 Goblet cells and elongated cylindrical cells in chronic atrophic gastritis (wet unfixed preparation, phase contrast, ×800).

is not present when there is mucosal atrophy of the body of the stomach, but it is noted in cases of basal hypersecretion of the stomach and also in cases of duodenal ulcer.

The cells of the mucosal surface are altered in all forms of severe gastritis, and so it is not surprising that this alteration constitutes the most frequent cytopathologic finding in the stomach. Systematically, we must make the following distinction: changes in the cell shape, changes in the cytoplasm, and changes in the nucleus. The

cell shape ranges from tall columnar to plump, short columnar, to pyramidal, cuboidal, and round. Therefore, anisocytosis is significant. The cell content is generally high, and the cells lie in clusters. On the other hand, it is characteristic that they are separated from one another, which indicates a loss of cellular adherence. A further characteristic finding in the cytoplasm is the presence of perinuclear vacuoles that indent the pyknotic nucleus from one or both sides. The cytoplasmic changes are indicative of chronic gastritis and the perinuclear vacuoles are a sign of hypoxic cell damage (Fig. 4.11).

Nuclear changes are of even greater diagnostic significance than changes in cell shape. The normal oval nuclei may be rounded, often dense, and pyknotic, a sign of aged, damaged cells. Swollen nuclei with loose chromatin structure may also be found, leading to anisokaryosis. When the nuclei are enlarged as the result of swelling

TABLE	
4.2	**Cytologic Assessment Criteria for Esophageal Preparations**

Cell content
Squamous cells
  Superficial
  Intermediate
  Parabasal
Keratinization
  Parakeratosis
  Dyskeratosis
  Hyperkeratosis
Characteristics of the nucleus
  Size
  Hyperchromasia
  Thickened nuclear membrane
  Chromatin structure
  Number of nucleoli
  Size of nucleoli
Inflammatory cells
  Count
  Intraepithelial collections
  Bacterial clusters
  Fungi/yeasts

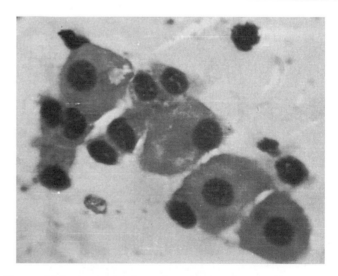

Figure 4.10 Parietal cells and mucous neck cells, obtained by gastric brushing, in a case of hyperchlorhydria (Papanicolaou, ×500).

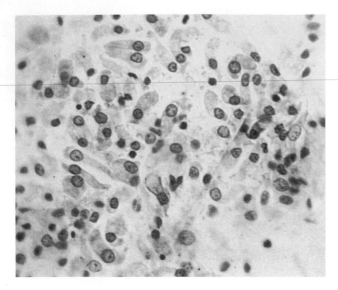

Figure 4.11 Anisokaryosis and anisocytosis of gastric epithelial cells and some perinuclear vacuoles in a case of chronic superficial gastritis (Papanicolaou, ×108).

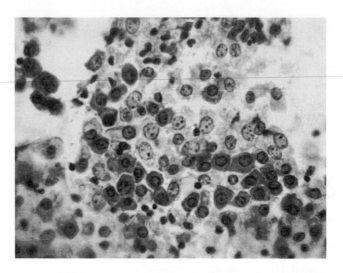

Figure 4.12 Gastric epithelial cells with enlarged nuclei, anisokaryosis, enlarged nucleoli, basophilic cytoplasm, cuboid shaped, in a case of chronic gastric erosions (Papanicolaou, ×325).

(edema of the nucleus), the chromatin structure is pale, which indicates a higher level of functional activity associated with increased regeneration. The nucleoli, which are usually not visible or appear only as dots, are often enlarged and have their own staining characteristics, e.g., being copper colored in Papanicolaou stains. Condensations of chromatin, centromeres, have the violet color of nuclear chromatin (Fig. 4.12). These cell changes bring about a shift in the normal nuclear-cytoplasmic ratio in favor of the nucleus. Anisokaryosis and anisocytosis occur simultaneously. In cell clusters, the cell boundaries are often no longer visible when the cell changes are advanced (Fig. 4.13).

All these variations in the surface epithelium are signs of a maturational disturbance. The normal process of differentiation of the surface epithelium from the less differentiated cells of the regeneration zones in the lacunar region is disturbed or completely abolished. The severity of this maturation disturbance parallels the severity of the gastritis. In superficial gastritis, the cytologic findings are more or less those of normal columnar epithelium. In severe chronic gastritis, generally reported as "atrophic" on histologic

examination if the normal glands of the body of the stomach are destroyed, the preponderant cytologic finding is the presence of round cells with significant anisokaryosis. The most severe changes are seen in the surface epithelium of patients with pernicious anemia and include anisomacrokaryosis and enlarged nucleoli. The epithelial changes found in gastritis are irreversible and can be demonstrated constantly over a number of years.

The correlation between the degree of cytologic changes in the epithelial cells and the histologic diagnosis of gastritis has been documented impressively by Bigotti and Crespi (37) (Table 4.3).

In peptic ulcer and complete erosions, so-called ulcer cells at the edge of these lesions are the characteristic cell type of a regenerating surface epithelium. These large columnar cells have enlarged nuclei and pronounced anisokaryosis. The chromatin structure is delicate, and the nuclei generally have single, enlarged, sharply demarcated nucleoli. It is striking that these changes can be demonstrated continuously over a number of months in the case of erosions (Fig. 4.13).

| TABLE 4.3 | Comparison of Cytologic Changes and Histologic Diagnosis of Gastritis |

Severity of the Predominant Cell Changes	Number of Cases	Histologic Diagnosis				
		Normal	Superficial Gastritis	Atrophic Gastritis		Gastric Atrophy
				Moderate	Severe	
0 (normal)	29	29	—	—	—	—
I	56	51	5	—	—	—
II	125	4	78	32	11	—
III	129	—	21	45	60	3
IV	45	—	2	2	9	32

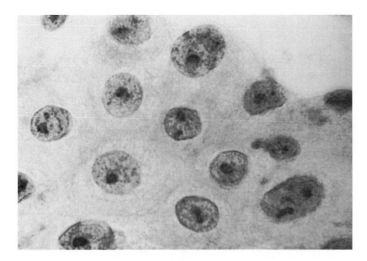

Figure 4.13 Gastric epithelial cells with enlarged nuclei, very prominent nucleoli, anisokaryosis, cell borders not visible, in a case of gastric ulcer (Papanicolaou, ×800).

In all slides obtained by gastroscopic brushings, it is important to look for *Helicobacter pylori*. These organisms can be identified readily in Papanicolaou-stained smears by their characteristic spiral form arranged in groups, running parallel to each other, mostly in gastric mucus or on the surface of gastric epithelial cells (Fig. 4.14) (38).

A knowledge of the cell changes just described is a basis for the recognition of tumor cells in cancer of the stomach, because such changes often accompany or even mask malignant cells in cytologic preparations. Recognizing tumor cells in gastric abrasion smears under the microscope requires taking into account many features that can only be assessed in combination (Table 4.4; Fig. 4.15).

In contrast, greater difficulties are presented by signet-ring cell carcinoma, in which tumor cells occur singly, as a rule, sometimes being scattered and present only in scanty numbers in the preparation. The characteristic feature is the large mucous vacuole

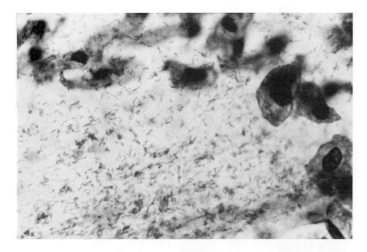

Figure 4.14 Gastric mucus, obtained by endoscopic brushing of the antrum with groups of Helicobacter pylori (Papanicolaou, ×504).

TABLE	
4.4	**Cytologic Characteristics of Gastric Carcinoma Cells**

Nuclei
  Anisokaryosis
  Tendency to nuclear enlargement
  Hyperchromasia
  Irregular, coarse-grained or lumpy chromatin
  Nuclear membrane thickened irregularly
  Pathologic mitoses
Cytoplasm
  Deviation from the normal shape of epithelial cells ("foreign" cells)
  Anisocytosis
  Increased basophilia
  Shift of nuclear/cytoplasmic ratio in favor of the nucleus
In fixed preparations stained with Papanicolaou stains
  Hyperchromia with coarsened chromatin structure in the nucleus
  Irregular thickening of the nuclear membrane
  Multiplication, enlargement, distortion of the nucleoli
  Shift of the nuclear-cytoplasmic ratio with nuclear enlargement and anisokaryosis
  Three-dimensional arrangement of cells into clusters
  Cell boundaries in the cluster not clearly visible
In unfixed, unstained, phase contrast preparations
  Double contouring of the nuclear membrane with irregular thickening
  Atypical nuclei
  Shift of the nuclear-cytoplasmic ratio with nuclear enlargement and anisokaryosis, granular and vacuolar structures in the cytoplasm
  Honeycomb effect never present in clusters of cells

that fills the entire cell, with the result that the cell becomes rounded and the hyperchromic nucleus is distorted and displaced to the edge of the cell (Fig. 4.16). Highly atypical malignant cells with bizarre nuclei and prominent nucleoli have been found in a case of primary gastric choriocarcinoma by endoscopic brushing (39). So-called premalignant glandular lesions (40) cannot be defined by cytologic technique only. Signs of secretory vesicles are seen with particular clarity by phase contrast microscopy. Squamous cell carcinomas in the region of the cardia have the following features already noted for the esophagus: relatively extensive cytoplasm and significant anisokaryosis of the hyperchromatic central, round to oval nucleus. Single cell deposits are more frequent than in adenocarcinoma.

The rare mesenchymal tumors of the stomach also furnish typical cytologic findings. Malignant, non-Hodgkin's lymphomas yield single, pathologic lymphatic round cells mostly with a small to moderate amount of homogeneous basophilic cytoplasm. The nuclei have a condensed, coarse-grained chromatin structure and an enlarged, round, solitary nucleolus (Fig. 4.17). In highly malignant types of lymphoma, the enlargement and irregularity of the nuclei is pronounced, as is the cytoplasmic basophilia (41). The rare Hodgkin's lymphoma can be recognized by the characteristic basophilic cells with giant nuclei and the multinucleated giant cells of the Sternberg type, with pale chromatin and enlargement of the

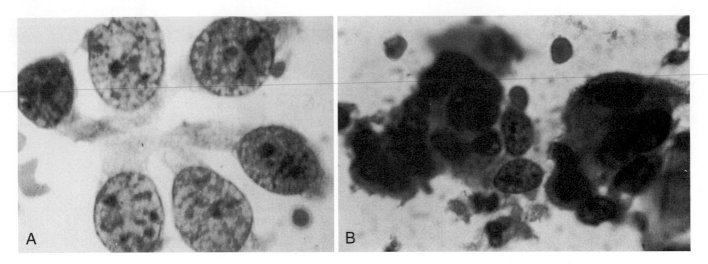

Figure 4.15   A. Tumor cells, cylindrical cell type, in a case of early gastric cancer (Papanicolaou, ×800). **B.** Tumor cell cluster obtained by gastroscopic brushing in a case of adenocarcinoma (Papanicolaou, ×504).

multiple nucleoli. Leiomyosarcoma is characterized by spindle-shaped or long, drawn-out cells with elliptical nuclei adjacent to basophilic cells with round nuclei (42).

Tumor cell-containing smears show secondary cell changes of a regressive type, as the result of necrotic phenomena at the tumor surface. The cells take up stain poorly, and the nuclei are reduced to nuclear ghosts. In such cases, there are also many leukocytes, mixed bacterial flora, fungal mycelia, and occasional protozoa (usually trichomonads), which are easy to identify in unstained preparations because of their motility but are more or less impossible to detect in stained preparations. Microfilariae were found as an exceptional experience (43). Campylobacter (Helicobacter) pylori can be detected with high specificity (44–48). When tumor growth has produced stenosis, food remnants may be the predominant finding in cytologic preparations.

As a rule, large, necrotic tumors are substantially more difficult to identify cytologically because of the secondary changes just described. Small tumors produce "clean" preparations with well-preserved tumor cells, and therefore are easier to diagnose by cytologic examination. This fact is of relevance to the clinical significance of cytodiagnosis (49, 50).

DUODENUM

The characteristic cell type of the duodenum is the intestinal epithelial cell, a narrow columnar cell with a round or slightly oval, chromatin-rich nucleus situated in the basal one third of the cell. The cell surface facing the lumen is marked sharply by a border-like area of condensation on which sits a dense, short cuticular fringe.

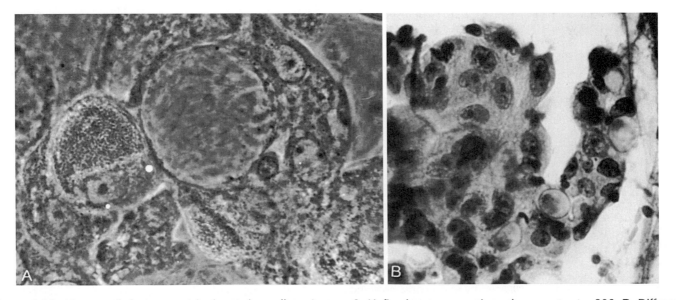

Figure 4.16   Tumor cell clusters, gastric signet-ring cell carcinoma. A. Unfixed wet preparation, phase contrast, ×800. **B.** Different case, Papanicolaou, ×400.

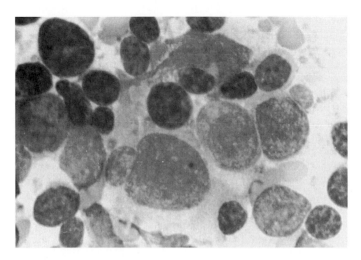

Figure 4.17 Malignant non-Hodgkin's lymphoma, high grade, of the gastrointestinal tract (May-Grünwald-Giemsa, ×800).

In duodenal ulcer, the intestinal cell type disappears. From the edge of the ulcer, regeneration cells are obtained, similar to those described for gastric ulcer, with swollen nuclei and an enlarged, solitary nucleolus. These cells show clear anisokaryosis, in contrast to the intestinal cells with their monomorphic nuclei. Heterotopic gastric mucosa in the duodenum can be recognized easily by the occurrence of parietal cells.

In duodenitis, lymphocytes are mixed with the intestinal cells in greater or lesser numbers (51). This intermixing is particularly the case in Crohn's disease of the duodenum, in which findings include undifferentiated cells with large nuclei and extensive cytoplasm.

Cytologic examination of the unfixed duodenal mucosa by phase contrast microscopy may reveal the presence of *Giardia lamblia*, now present in large numbers, as the cause of long-standing undiagnosed symptoms in the upper abdomen. They manifest a lively motility as a result of the pair of flagella at the hind end and the cilia attached to the pear-shaped, flattened cytoplasm. Motility remains for several hours after sampling if the specimen is kept in a moist chamber. On Papanicolaou staining, these protozoa can also be recognized, although with greater difficulty, by the pear shape and the two typical eyelike nuclei.

Tumor cells in the duodenum, other than those from the papilla, are a rare finding. These cases are generally the result of a pancreatic adenocarcinoma invading the duodenal wall. The major papilla has a short, plump columnar epithelium without a cuticular fringe, which distinguishes it from the duodenal epithelium. Within the pore of the papilla is a border zone in which the surface epithelium of the papilla meets the ductal epithelium of the choledochus and pancreatic ducts. Such border zones are the most common sites for cell transformation, and they can be investigated satisfactorily by obtaining brush abrasions under endoscopic guidance or by endopapillary aspiration. Most important is the recognition of carcinoma of the papilla, which is susceptible to early cytologic diagnosis and which is more difficult to reach with biopsy forceps. The tumor cells are of the adenocarcinoma type, or there may also be clusters of papillary tumor cells, which are characterized by a drawn out cytoplasm and an elliptical nucleus with the cytologic criteria of malignancy (Fig. 4.18). Atypical columnar cells arranged in a papillary pattern associated with villous papillary adenoma must

be differentiated from these cells because they also have elliptical nuclei. Anisokaryosis is rare, however, and there is no shift in the nuclear-cytoplasmic ratio (52). Findings from a retrospective study provided strong evidence that most ampullary and duodenal carcinomas develop in preexisting adenomas (53), confirming former studies on step-wise sections of the ampulla (54). My colleagues and I were able to make an early diagnosis of the recurrence of a villous papillary carcinoma, excised at operation, by constantly demonstrating tumor cells in the brush smear of the papilla.

Only brief mention can be made here of the cytologic diagnosis of the biliary tract and pancreatic juice (55–57). This topic is clinically important because bioptic methods are not available and tumors in these areas are becoming more frequent both in our practice and in other countries.

COLON AND RECTUM

The colon is lined with a single layer of tall, blunted columnar cells. The nuclei are large and elliptical and lie within the basal one third of the cell. The cytoplasm loses density toward the lumen. These cells have no cuticular fringe. Only sparse scrapings can be obtained from healthy mucosa. Larger numbers and clusters of single-layered cells obtained by brush abrasion are indicative of increased desquamation and friability of the mucosa. This finding is regarded as cytologic evidence of simple colitis.

The cells termed "colic cells" are a singular cytologic finding. They are degenerative forms of intestinal epithelial cells, rounded cells with karyorrhexis, a fragmentation of the pyknotic nucleus into numerous, homogeneous particles of varying size, together with hyaline inclusions in the cytoplasm. These colic cells are the only highly characteristic microscopic feature of the colitic mucosa (Fig. 4.19).

In the acute stage of ulcerative colitis, neutrophilic granulocytes dominate the cytologic picture. In the chronic stages, the surface epithelium shows more or less clear signs of atypia. The nuclei may be enlarged and may show significant anisokaryosis. Confusion with tumor cells is prevented by the absence of hyper-

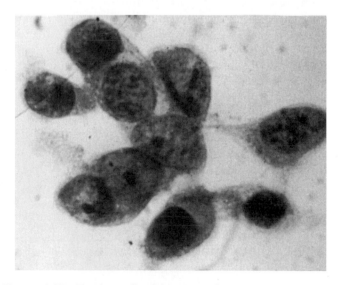

Figure 4.18 Tumor cells from an adenocarcinoma of the duodenal papilla (Papanicolaou, ×800).

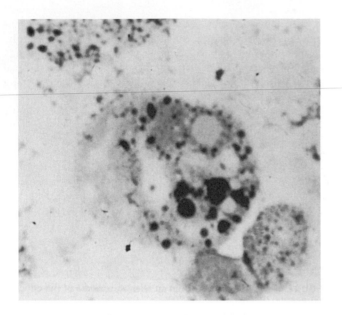

Figure 4.19 So-called colic cells, degenerated colonic epithelia, in a case of colitic mucosa (May-Grünwald-Giemsa, ×800).

chromatic nuclear chromatin and the absence of nuclear atypia (58). Nuclear atypia may be present for months; therefore, careful examination is necessary. Such examination may be a difficult undertaking in patients with long-standing active ulcerative colitis. Brush cytology is most helpful in patients who have developed strictures (59). The value of segmental colonic lavage in areas of stricture have been discussed by Katz et al. (60).

Crohn's disease is, by way of contrast, more difficult to diagnose cytologically than ulcerative colitis. One feature is the predominance of lymphatic cells. The occurrence of epithelioid cells; pale cells with extensive cytoplasm; large, oval nuclei; and a

fine network of chromatin is characteristic, although rare. The presence of multinucleated giant cells helps to establish the diagnosis (Fig. 4.20).

In cancer of the large bowel, tumor cells of the adenocarcinoma type are delivered regularly, singly and in clusters, generally with accompanying signs of necrosis and collections of leukocytes. Cytodiagnosis is reliable in these circumstances (61), particularly in regard to stenosing tumors. Obtaining biopsy specimens from such tumors with forceps under endoscopic control is difficult. In such cases, histologic diagnosis of the tumor is secondary to cytologic diagnosis by abrasion. In polypoid tumors, on the other hand, histologic examination of the polyp removed in its entirety by endoscopic snare is preferable for two reasons. First, only histologic examination can determine whether the stalk of a polyp has been invaded by tumor, which is an important piece of information in terms of further treatment. Second, the demonstration of a focal malignant transformation in an otherwise nonmalignant polyp is not of particular clinical importance if the polyp has been fully excised.

A cytologic swab preparation made from a fully excised polyp provides interesting material for the cytologist nonetheless. It shows clusters of colonic epithelial cells that are characteristic of the various histologic types of polyp. The predominant type in hyperplastic polyp is the normal columnar cell, changed only by a slight nuclear enlargement and anisokaryosis and found in large cell clusters. Adenomatous polyps predominantly produce cuboid cells with large, round nuclei that are arranged in formations suggestive of tubules. Anisokaryosis and enlargement of the solitary nucleolus are variable findings that are regarded as examples of cellular atypia. The more a polyp of the tubular adenomatous variety shows signs of a villous component, the more predominant is cellular atypia. The nuclei show hyperchromasia, irregular condensation of the chromatin. The elliptical nucleus is a general cytologic feature of villous polyps and must be distinguished from the atypical features of the nuclear chromatin that have been mentioned. Polypoid carcinomas,

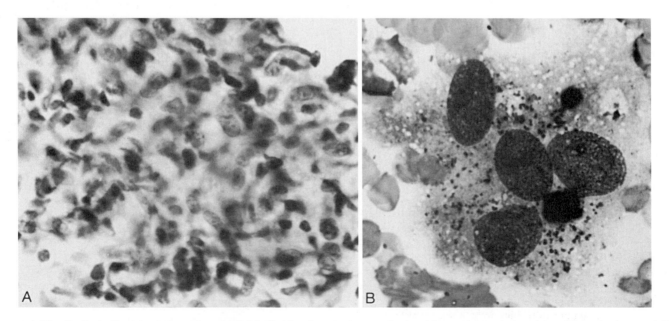

Figure 4.20 Crohn's disease of the colon. **A.** Epithelioid cell granuloma, obtained by endoscopic brushing (Papanicolaou, ×160). **B.** Multinucleated giant cell (May-Grünwald-Giemsa, ×800).

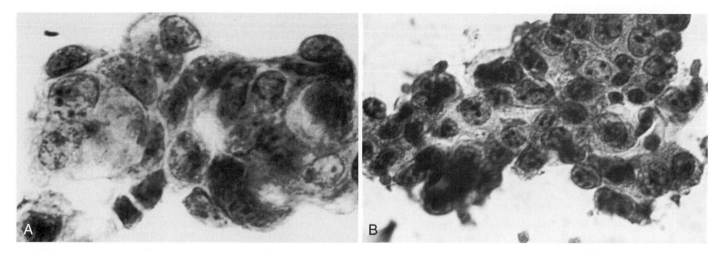

Figure 4.21   A. Tubular adenoma of the colon with severe cellular atypia (Papanicolaou, ×1000). **B.** Tumor cells in adenocarcinoma of Barrett's esophagus (Papanicolaou, ×504).

then, show all the nuclear features of malignancy in addition to the lengthening of the cell and the nucleus (Fig. 4.21A). Thus, it is possible to devise a cytologic spectrum of increasing cellular atypia, embracing hyperplastic polyps; adenomas of the tubular, tubulo-villous, and villous types; and polypoid carcinoma.

In patients with a malignancy of the rectum, a transprocto-scopic, fine-needle aspiration cytology can be most helpful (62). It is also possible to cytologically diagnose mesenchymal malignancies, in particular, lymphosarcomas, the differentiation of which requires techniques of microscopy adapted from hematology.

The rare, and unfortunately often misdiagnosed, carcinoma of the anus warrants some mention. This squamous cell carcinoma with some signs of keratinization can be diagnosed easily and correctly by the cytologic examination of a smear prepared by means of a cotton wool swab, with or without the aid of a proc-toscope.

STATISTICAL EVALUATION OF CYTODIAGNOSES

ESOPHAGUS

Experimental evidence from China concerning the nuclear area in the surface epithelium (23) is presented in Table 4.5. In our own investigations (23), we examined cytologic abrasion smears from the esophagus in a series of patients from two Chinese counties with different incidences of carcinoma of the esophagus (Table 4.6). The incidence of cancer of the esophagus is also high in South Africa (63). Among 500 smears from patients without symptoms were 26 showing dysplasia and 15 showing carcinoma. Mass screening in 1000 residents of low-, intermediate-, and high-risk areas for esophageal cancer in Transkei by brush biopsy capsules revealed dysplastic changes in 9% and carcinoma in 2% of the high-risk population (64). A prospective cytologic study in a high-risk area in China showed that the incidence of esoph-ageal cancer was significantly higher in subjects with notable cytologic atypia than in the control group with normal cytologic findings (65).

In the personal experience of the author, 16 cases of cancer of the esophagus occurred in the period from 1981 to 1986. Endos-copy led to a correct diagnosis in 15 of the 16 cases. Both histologic and abrasion cytologic examinations were positive for tumor in each of 14 cases. In one case, cytologic analysis yielded tumor cells when biopsy results were falsely negative. In another case, the result of histologic examination was positive and that of cytologic examina-tion was negative.

In an Italian study involving the combined endoscopic inves-tigation of 173 cases of cancer of the esophagus over a 5-year period, investigators used toluidine blue staining of the mucosa for better identification of the lesions (66). Cytologic findings were positive in 89%; histologic findings were positive in 84%. Both microscopic examinations had a 3% false-negative rate. In 31 proven cases of esophageal carcinoma, tumor cells were found definitely in 25 cases and probably in 6 over a 5-year period in Australia (67).

In a Spanish study, 858 endoscopic examinations of the esophagus and the cardia were performed over a 6-year period, including 309 cases with confirmed malignancies (68). Cytologic findings were positive for cancer in 93.5%, and no false-positive

TABLE	
4.5	**Nuclear Area of Squamous Cells in Esophageal Mucosa**

	Nuclear Area	
Cell Type	µm²	RV[a]
Normal	49.1	1.0
Mild hyperplasia	135.8	2.8
Moderate dysplasia	181.9	3.7
Severe dysplasia	231.9	4.7
"Near carcinoma"	291.2	5.9
Carcinoma	312.8	6.4

[a]Relative value of nuclear area size as compared with that of the normal cell.

TABLE 4.6 | Cytodiagnosis of Esophagus in Patients From Two Chinese Counties

| | | | | | Cytodiagnosis (%) | | | |
| | | | | | | Dysplasia | | | |
County	Rate of Carcinoma	No. of Cases	Normal	Mild Hyperplasia	Moderate	Severe	Near Carcinoma	Carcinoma
Linxian	High	492	52.4	27.3	13.6	2.0	1.2	2.3
Jaoxian	Low	240	74.7	22.5	1.8	0	0	0

diagnosis was made in the patients with benign conditions. Biopsy specimens were obtained in only 269 of the tumor cases because of obstructing lesions in 40 patients in whom no satisfactory biopsies could be made, with overall positivity of 77.02%. Cytologic analysis increased the yield of biopsy by 20.8%.

Findings of a Swiss study (69) involving 100 cases, including 20 cancers, showed 70% sensitivity of cytologic diagnosis, 80% for histologic biopsy, and 95% for both, with no false-positive results.

In an Irish study, the role of cytology in the differentiation of benign from malignant mucosal lesions in 2183 consecutive patients by esophagogastroduodenoscopy was examined (70). From 58 cases of esophageal cancer, cytologic and biopsy findings were both positive in 71%, biopsy alone in 17%, and cytology alone in 12%. All cases could be diagnosed correctly.

A prognostically relevant classification of 37 cases of esophageal carcinoma was undertaken with Feulgen-DNA measurement (71). In this study, the most favorable prognosis was associated with a predominant hypotriploidy, the least favorable with a hypertetraploidal polyploidy. The problems of standardized diagnostic image cytometry are not discussed here in detail because the material is mostly not obtained by cytologic methods (72).

Special mention should be made about the cytology of Barrett esophagus. As a consequence of the chronic gastroesophageal reflux, columnar epithelia dysplasia develops with the presence of goblet cells. Barrett-associated carcinomas show regularly cytologic flagrant malignant features (73, 74). A significant increase during the last 5 to 8 years of esophageal cancer, including the cardia region, detected by endoscope-guided cell brushing technique, points to the disputed role of Barrett esophagus in our gastroenterologic patients. This increase is in contrast to the number of gastric cancers, which remained rather stationary.

The differential diagnosis between moderate or severe cellular atypias and tumor cells is often difficult. Such features of the nucleoli as their increase in size and number and especially their deviation from the round shape with deformations and irregularities are best suited for a tumor cell diagnosis (Fig. 4.21B).

Koga et al. (75) found a good correlation of the proliferating cell nuclear antigen (PCNA) with the severity of esophageal epithelial dysplasia, suggesting that a high grade of dysplasia may be as serious a lesion as esophageal carcinoma.

Zhuang et al. (76), applying a microdissection technique for genetic evaluation using polymorphic markers flanking the APC gene locus, found identical HPC gene alterations in all 12 esophagectomy specimens of Barrett esophagus patients and the same APC alterations in dysplastic and adenocarcinoma cases, even in some metaplastic foci adjacent to dysplasia.

The DNA ploidy of tumor cells did not correlate significantly with the TNM-stage or histologic differentiation grade of the tumor in 40 patients with an adenocarcinoma in Barrett's esophagus and is, therefore, an independent prognostic factor for survival (77).

Superficial esophageal squamous cell carcinoma without invasion beyond the muscularis mucosae showed a lesser p53 protein expression and lower [67]Ki-labeling index than cases with a deeper tumor invasion (78).

STOMACH

QUALITATIVE STUDIES

Five years ago, my colleagues and I investigated 145 cases of proven carcinoma of the stomach, comparing material obtained endoscopically for cytologic and histologic analysis. The endoscopic findings were judged to be neoplastic in 74.5%. Tumor cells were demonstrated cytologically in 70% and histologically confirmed in 89.4% of the tumors. In 17 cases (10.8%), histologic results were positive for tumor, whereas tumor cells were not found cytologically. On the other hand, we had 9 cases (6.2%) with cytologic evidence of tumor in whom no tumor was detectable on histologic biopsy. Tumor cells

TABLE 4.7 | Review of Recent Reports on Endoscopically Diagnosed Gastric Carcinoma

Reference	Number of Cases	Cytologically Positive	Histologically Positive
Rachail-Amoux et al. (81)	114	98	104
Simon et al. (82)	72	57	61
Debongnie et al. (83)	96	79	84
Chambers and Clark (84)	163	134	157
Moreno-Otero et al. (85)	194	176	153
Qizilbash et al. (86)	37	33	35
Marbet et al. (69)	49	30	40
O'Donoghue et al. (70)	332	260	294
Total	1057	867 (82.0%)	928 (87.8%)

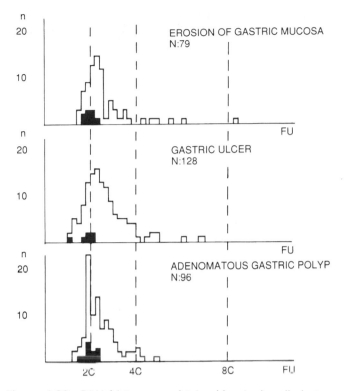

Figure 4.22   DNA histograms obtained by single-cell photometry of gastric cell samples from cases of benign gastric lesions. FU, fluorescence units (relative amounts of DNA); n, number of nuclei; 2c, 4c DNA content, which corresponds to diploid, tetraploid chromosomal set; N, total number of nuclei measured; black columns, white blood cells within the smear as internal standard. (Redrawn with permission from Sprenger F, Witte S: Der diagnostische Wert der Zellkern-DNS-Bestimmung an zytologischen Ausstrichen von gutartigen und bösartigen Veränderungen des Magens. Pathol Res Pract 1978;163:148.)

permit material suitable for microscopy to be obtained because of advanced necrosis. The diagnoses were, however, readily established visually at endoscopy.

QUANTITATIVE STUDIES

Among the quantitative methods of gastric cytology, a distinction should be made between cytophotometric methods and flow methods. Both are concerned, above all, with measurement of DNA, but micromorphology plays no part in flow methods.

In association with Sprenger (26), the author performed investigations with the use of single-cell fluorophotometry. We first stained the abrasion preparations by Papanicolaou's method before examination. The same preparations were then decolorized, and DNA was measured with Feulgen-acriflavine staining. Histograms were prepared for each case, together with data on the frequency distribution of DNA values characterized by the following two variables:

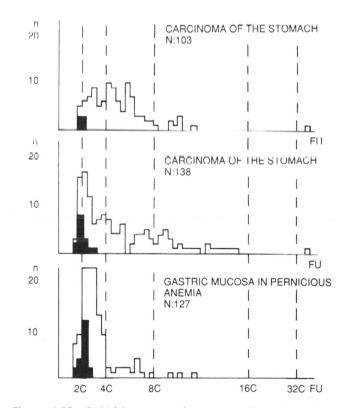

Figure 4.23   DNA histograms of two cases of gastric carcinoma and a case of pernicious anemia. FU, fluorescence units (relative amounts of DNA); n, number of nuclei; 2c, 4c DNA content, which corresponds to diploid, tetraploid chromosomal set; N, total number of nuclei measured; black columns, white blood cells within the smear as internal standard. (Redrawn with permission from Sprenger E, Witte S: Der diagnostische Wert der Zellkern-DNS-Bestimmung an zytologischen Ausstrichen von gutartigen und bösartigen Veränderungen des Magens. Pathol Res Pract 1978;163:148.)

were described in 3 of 1524 gastroscopic investigations in which no tumor was demonstrable clinically (false-positive rate of cytodiagnosis, 0.2%).

From the literature, we had collected 924 cases of proven carcinoma of the stomach. Cytologic examination yielded tumor cells in 92.6% and biopsy showed tumor in 85.1%. In 296 cases of early cancer, the corresponding figures for cytologic study and biopsy are 91.6% and 88.9%, respectively (79, 80).

From recent literature, we collected a further 676 cases of endoscopically demonstrated carcinoma of the stomach (Table 4.7). In this series, cytology yielded tumor cells in 83.6%; biopsy, with diagnosis of tumor in 85.9%, showed a comparable success rate. We found a false-positive cytologic diagnosis of tumor in 1.8% of 4941 cases in the literature (80).

In summary, all investigations show agreement that the certainty of making a correct diagnosis of tumor is increased if both cytologic and histologic examination is carried out in the same patient. In our experience, we have had a false-negative rate for both microscopic methods of between 1 and 2%. In reality, however, there were no true diagnostic failures because the 1 to 2% represented cases of advanced carcinoma of the stomach that did not

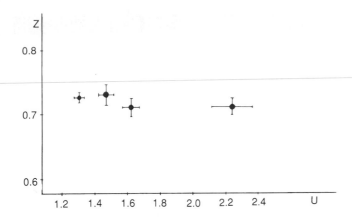

Figure 4.24 Mean ploidy DNA values (U) and relative frequency of euploid and polyploid DNA values (Z). Standard deviations of the mean, 126 cases of single-cell DNA measurements in gastric smears. From left to right, cases with normal gastric mucosa, gastric erosions, gastric ulcers, gastric carcinomas. (Reprinted with permission from Sprenger E, Witte S: Der diagnostische Wert der Zellkern-DNS-Bestimmung an zytologischen Ausstrichen von gutartigen und bösartigen Veränderungen des Magens. Pathol Res Pract 1978;163:148.)

1. The relative mean ploidy (U):

$$U = \frac{x \text{ FU in sample population}}{x \text{ FU in reference population}}$$

in which x = mean of the measured counts; FU = fluorescent units; reference population = number of leukocytes, normal intermediate squamous cells, or columnar cells in the preparation; and sample population = number of pathologic cells found in the preparation.

2. The relative frequency of euploid and polyploid DNA values in the sample population (Z):

$$Z = \frac{Nx}{Nx + Ny}$$

in which N = total number of cells measured; x = all euploid and polyploid cells (mean of the diploid standard population ± 25% or of its multiples + 25%); y = all cells not included in x (aneuploid).

We investigated 126 patients with various findings in the gastric mucosa. Histograms of the normal gastric mucosa, of superficial gastritis, and of atrophic gastritis show a peak frequency of diploid cells (stem line). In gastritis, the histogram is expanded as a result of increased cell proliferation to include tetraploid values and, in atrophic gastritis, to include octoploid values (Fig. 4.22). Two cases of carcinoma of the stomach (Fig. 4.23) show a varying histogram. In the first example is an aneuploid stem line at 3c with doubling peaks at 6c and 12c, together with a stem line at 4c. In the second case, a stem line is at 2c with doubling peaks at 4c and 8c. Both histograms demonstrate wide polyploidal scatter up to 32c.

Statistical evaluation of the variables U and Z allows separating the various groups of cytologic findings and the endoscopic diagnostic categories (Fig. 4.24) into significantly different groups. This organization shows that the relative mean ploidy value (U) is a suitable criterion for differentiating tumor cells from normal cells and from gastric cells that show reactive change. In 20 cases of early gastric cancer, Czernak and associates (87) found two DNA histogram patterns: a diploid type in 6 of 7 signet-ring cell carcinomas (diffuse type), and an aneuploid type in 11 of 13 adenocarcinomas of the intestinal type.

Using flow DNA cytometry, we collected results from 161 examples of gastric abrasion cytology smears (27). In normal gastric mucosa, most cells are found in the diploid region; only a few are in the area between 2c and 4c. Below 2c is a fraction representing cell debris. In gastric cancer, the DNA flow histogram is also characterized by a main peak in the diploid region owing to the preponder-

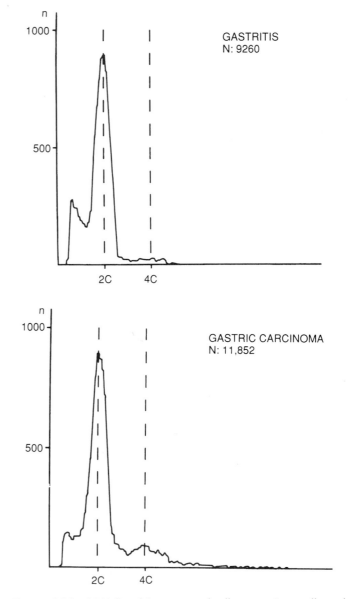

Figure 4.25 DNA flow histograms of cell suspensions collected by gastroscopic brushing from a patient with superficial gastritis and a patient with gastric carcinoma. n, number of nuclei; 2c, 4c, DNA content, which corresponds to diploid, tetraploid chromosomal set; N, total number of nuclei measured. (Reprinted with permission from Sprenger E, Witte S: The diagnostic significance of flow cytometric nuclear DNA measurement in gastroscopic diagnosis of the stomach. Pathol Res Pract 1980;169:269.)

TABLE 4.8	Results of Conventional Smear Cytologic Study Compared with DNA Flow Cytometry On Cell Samples Obtained By Routine Gastroscopic Brushing				
	Cytologic Diagnosis				
Flow Cytometric Diagnosis	Benign	Suspicious	Malignant	Unsatisfactory	Total
Negative	68	6	1	2	77
Positive	47	12	17	0	76
Unsatisfactory	7	1	0	0	8
Total	122	19	18	2	161

Reprinted with permission from Sprenger E, Witte S: The diagnostic significance of flow cytometric nuclear DNA measurement in gastroscopic diagnosis of the stomach. Pathol Res Pract 1980;169:269.

Values are calculated by discriminate analysis (27).

ance of nonmalignant gastric cells in the sample. A second peak at 4c represents a second stem line with scatter to 8c, which is attributed to tumor cells (Fig. 4.25).

We have undertaken a classification of these DNA flow histograms, using discriminance analysis in benign and malignant and "unsatisfactory" samples, and compared this classification with results from conventional cytodiagnosis of the same abrasion smear material (Table 4.8). Of the 37 cases diagnosed as possibly or definitely malignant by conventional techniques, 7 (19%) were not recognized by the DNA flow histogram. Of 122 cases judged to be benign cytologically, 47 (38%) were falsely judged to be positive by the flow method. From these findings, it appears that this method on its own is not capable of achieving a discrimination of practical usefulness between gastric cytograms

DUODENUM

From 57 cases of carcinoma of Papilla major we were able to diagnose 18 from brush abrasion under endoscopic control by cytologic methods. In 51 instances, we were able to obtain

histologic material by forceps biopsies; a tumor diagnosis could be rendered in 28 of the 51. The false-negative rate by cytologic examination was 9 of 57 cases (15.8%). The false-negative rate of the histologic biopsy material was 20 out of 51 cases (39.2%). In 13 cases only, the cytologic diagnosis reflected tumor cell involvement, whereas the histologic biopsy missed the tumor. In 8 cases, both methods gave false-negative results. The false negative rate was, therefore, only 4.8%. In 2 cases, cytologic examination led to an early diagnosis, although on endoscopic examination, a tumor lesion was not seen.

The reason for the discrepancy between the cytologic and the bioptic histologic results may be seen in technical details of the sampling procedures. It seems to be easier to brush the papillary region completely than to obtain representative material by forceps biopsy.

COLON AND RECTUM

In 182 cases of adenocarcinoma in this anatomic region in which biopsy using both brush abrasion and forceps was indicated (in

TABLE 4.9	Comparison of Results of Investigation at Endoscopy in 545 Cases of Proven Colon and Rectal Carcinoma			
Reference	Number of Cases	Cytologically Positive	Histologically Positive	Either Positive
Halter (88)	77	70	46	74
Debongnie et al. (89)	60	42	51	56
Watanabe (61)	44	42	38	?
Rachail-Arnoux et al. (81)	86	74	82	83
Miczban and Feher (90)	11	1.1	1.1	11
Marbet et al. (69)	62	5.1	42	59
Dinkov et al. (91)	123	117	116	122
Ehya and O'Hara (92)	82	67	60	74
Total	545	474 (87%)	446 (82%)	479[a] (95.6%)

[a]Numbers do not include Watanabe's cases.

other words, in those cases in which complete polypectomy was not undertaken), tumor cells were found on cytologic examination in 136 cases (75%). The histologic examination resulted in finding malignant tumor in 141 (77%). In 3 of these 182 cases, cytologic results were negative and histologic results were positive; in 8 cases, the cytologic results were positive and the histologic results were negative. In 3 cases, the preparation for cytologic and histologic examinations contained only necrotic cells. There were no examples of false-positive cytodiagnosis in material obtained from 287 endoscopies performed in patients with nonmalignant disease of the colon.

A literature search led to the collection of 545 cases of colorectal carcinoma in which cytologic and histologic investigations were undertaken (Table 4.9). The results show that biopsy and cytologic analysis have fairly similar diagnostic success, which was improved by cytologic examination in 5% of cases.

Winawer et al. (93) confirmed that the use of brush cytology improved the yield of tissue diagnosis considerably when added to the biopsy technique (from 60 to 89%), whereas lavage cytology did not seem to increase the diagnostic yield significantly. The diagnosis of exophytic cancer was easier to obtain than that of infiltrative cancer for all techniques. Rectal cancer was diagnosed in 30 patients on the basis of findings from transproctoscopic fine-needle aspiration, brush cytology, and biopsy (62). Biopsy results were positive in 27, brush cytology showed positive findings in 25, and fine-needle aspiration yielded positive results in 29.

Quantitative investigations of the DNA in cell material from the colon or rectum are only available from the flow analysis of DNA in tissue samples excised or resected for histologic examination, mainly from polyps. Preparations made especially for cytologic study were not evaluated.

In a morphometric study (94) of 35 cases with cytologic smears prepared by rectal scraping, including 12 benign adenomas, 14 carcinomas, and 9 irradiated carcinomas free of disease at the time of sampling, a nuclear area of $30\,\mu m^2$ was found in 21% of tumor cells but in only 5% of adenoma cells. The nuclear-cytoplasmic ratio of more than 0.5 showed significant differences between malignant and benign cases and between malignant and treated nonrecurrent cases.

Analysis of chromosomes in abrasion smears taken from the rectum by Xavier and associates (95) showed a normal karyotype in all examples of normal mucosa and from mucosa from patients with Crohn's disease. Hypotetraploid cells were found in some cases of ulcerative colitis. In patients with carcinoma, aneuploidy with breakage of chromosomes and marker chromosomes were always present.

REFERENCES

1. Shu YJ. Cytopathology of the esophagus. Acta Cytol 1983;27:7–16.
2. Panico FG, Papanicolaou GN, Cooper WA. Abrasive balloon for exfoliation of gastric cancer cells. JAMA 1950;143:1308–1311.
3. Aste H, Saccomanno S, Munizzi F. Blind pan-esophageal brush cytology. Diagnostic accuracy. Endoscopy 1984;16:165–167.
4. Henning N. Zytodiagnostik von Tumoren. Folia Haematol 1950;70:198–202.
5. Fukuda T, Shida S, Takita T, et al. Cytologic diagnosis of early gastric cancer by the endoscopic method with gastrofiberscope. Acta Cytol 1967;11:456–459.
6. Witte S. Gastroscopic cytology. Endoscopy 1970;2:88–93.
7. Zargar SA, Khuroo MS, Jan GM, et al. Prospective comparison of the value of brushing before and after biopsy in the endoscopic diagnosis of gastroesophageal malignancy. Acta Cytol 1991;35:549–552.
8. Layfield LJ, Reichman A, Weinstein WM. Endoscopically directed fine needle aspiration biopsy of gastric and esophageal lesions. Acta Cytol 1992;36:69–74.
9. Witte S: Die endoskopische Tumorzelldiagnostik im Bereich des Duodenums. Z Gastroenterol 1976;14:508–514.
10. Kochhar R, Rajwanski A, Goenka MK, et al. Colonoscopic fine needle aspiration cytology in the diagnosis of ileocecal tuberculosis. Am J Gastroenterol 1991;86:102–104.
11. Zargar SA, Khuroo MS, Mahajan R, et al. Endoscopic fine needle aspiration cytology in the diagnosis of gastro-oesophageal and colorectal malignancies. Gut 1991;32:745–748.
12. Henning N, Witte S. Atlas of gastrointestinal cytodiagnosis. 2nd ed. Stuttgart: Georg Thieme, 1970;132.
13. Pinkard KI, Harrison B, Capstick JA, et al. Detection of Campylobacter pyloridis in gastric mucosa by phase contrast micoscopy. J Clin Pathol 1986;39:112–113.
14. Witte S, Ruch F: Moderne Untersuchungsmethoden in der Zytologie. 2. Aufl. Baden-Baden: Gerhard Witzstrock, 1979;155.
15. Witte S. Innovations of ultraviolet microscopy in clinical diagnosis. GBK Fortbld Aktuelle 1994;22:Suppl. 10–11.
16. Witte S, Bloss WH, Schwarzmann P, et al. Quantitative ultraviolet microscopy. In: Goerttler K, Feichter GE, Witte S, eds. New frontiers in cytology. Berlin: Springer, 1988;140–148.
17. Zeiss C. MPM 400/800, Mikroskop-Photometer, Oberkochen, Germany, 1990.
18. Schümmelfeder N, Ebscher KJ, Krogh E. Acridine orange fluorescence staining. Naturwissensch 1957;44:467.
19. Papanicolaou GN. Atlas of Exfoliative Cytology. Cambridge: Harvard University Press, 1954;5.
20. Takahashi M. Color atlas of cancer cytology. 2nd ed. Tokyo: Igaktu-Shoin Ltd. 1981.
21. Farrant PC. Oral epithelial cells in pernicous anemia. Br Med J 1964;1:1694–1697.
22. Gardner FH. Cell changes in tropical sprue. J Lab Clin Med 1956;47:529–539.
23. Witte S. Zytologische Diagnostik des oberen Gastrointestinaltraktes. Leber Magen Darm 1984;14:8–17.
24. Boon ME, Kurver PHJ, Baak JPA, et al. The application of morphometry in gastric cytological diagnosis. Virchows Arch [A] 1981;393:159–164.
25. Böhm N, Sprenger E. Fluorescence cytophotometry, a valuable method for the quantitative determination of nuclear Feulgen-DNA. Histochemie 1968;16:100–118.
26. Sprenger E, Witte S. Der diagnostische Wert der Zellkern-DNS-Bestimmung an zytologischen Ausstrichen von gutartigen und bösartigen Veränderungen des Magens. Pathol Res Pract 1978;163:148–157.
27. Sprenger E, Witte S. The diagnostic significance of flow cytometric nuclear DNA measurement in gastroscopic diagnosis of the stomach. Pathol Res Pract 1980;169:269–275.
28. Erhardt R, Reinhardt ER, Schlipf W, et al. FAZYTAN, a system for fast automated cell segmentation, cell image analyses and feature extraction based on TV-image pickup and parallel processing. Anal Quant Cytol Histol 1980;2:25–40.
29. Witte S, Bloss WH, Reinhardt ER. Differential texture analysis of short wavelength absorbances in unfixed cells. Presented at the International Conference on High Resolution Cell Image Analysis, North Hollywood, CA, 1982.
30. Witte S, Sträßle G. Quantitative UV microscopy: Analysis of DNA and nuclear protein textures including 3D-techniques. GBK Fortbld Aktuell 1992;62:44–47.
31. Schwarzmann P, Schmid J, Schnoerr C, et al. Two telemicroscopic systems for telepathology based on ISDN or video band (VBN) networks. GBK Fortbld Aktuelle 1994;22(Suppl):26.
32. Shen Q. Diagnostic cytology and early detection. In: Huang GJ, Kai WY, eds. Carcinoma of the esophagus and gastric cardia. Berlin: Springer, 1984;155–190.
33. Horai T, Kobayashi A, Tateishi R, et al. A cytologic study on small cell carcinoma of the esophagus. Cancer 1978;41:1890–1896.

34. Selvaggi SM. Polypoid carcinoma of the esophagus on brush cytology. Acta Cytol 1992;36:650–651.

35. Shurbaji MS, Erozan YS: The cytopathologic diagnosis of esophageal adenocarcinoma. Acta Cytol 1991;35:189–194.

36. Elster K, Heinkel K, Henning N: Glandular cells in gastric biopsy. Zentralbl Pathol 1957;67:170–176.

37. Bigotti A, Crespi M: Citopatologia e citodiagnostica apparato digerente. In: Cavallero M, ed. Trattato di citopatologia e citodiagnostica. Roma: Marrapesa, 1976;387–441.

38. Pinto MM, Mersiano FV, Afridi S, et al. Cytodiagnosis of campylobacter pylori in Papanicolaou-stained imprints of gastric biopsy specimens. Acta Cytol 1991;35:204–206.

39. Gorczyca W, Woyke S: Endoscopic brushing cytology of primary gastric choriocarcinoma. Acta Cytol 1992;36:551–554.

40. Wang HH, Ducatman BS, Thinbault S. Cytologic features of premalignant glandular lesions in the upper gastrointestinal tract. Acta Cytol 1991;35:199–203.

41. Cabré-Fiol V, Vilardell F. Progress in the cytological diagnosis of gastric lymphoma. Cancer 1978;41:1456–1461.

42. Sato A, Ishioka K, Kobiyama M, et al. Cytological diagnosis of leiomyogenic tumors of the stomach. Tohoku J Exp Med 1980;132:213–223.

43. Whitaker D, Reed WD, Shilkin KB: A case of filariasis diagnosed on gastric cytology. Pathology 1980;12:438–448.

44. Gad A: Rapid diagnosis of Campylobacter pylori by brush cytology. Scand J Gastroenterol 1989;24 (Suppl 167):101–103.

45. Estrin HM, Hansan MO, Carr HS, et al. Antral brushing and biopsies for gastric campylobacter pylori: A comparative study of a rapid urease test, culture and histology. Can J Gastroenterol 1989;3:91–94.

46. Faverly D, Famerée D, Lamy V, et al. Identification of Campylobacter pylori in gastric biopsy smears. Acta Cytol 1990;34:205–210.

47. Davenport RD: Cytologic diagnosis of Campylobacter pylori-associated gastritis. Acta Cytol 1990;34:211–213.

48. Debougnie JC, Delmee M, Mainguet P, et al. Cytology: A simple, rapid sensitive method in the diagnosis of helicobacter pylori. Am J Gastroenterol 1992;87:20–23.

49. Au FC, Koprowska I, Berger A, et al. The role of cytology in the diagnosis of carcinoma of the stomach. Surg Gynecol Obstet 1980;151:601–603.

50. Takeda T, Yamada S, Amakasu H, et al. Histologic studies of atypical epithelial growth of the stomach. Nippon Shokakibyo Gakkai Zasshi 1981;16:232–235.

51. Cheli R, Aste H, Nicoló G, et al. Cytological findings in chronic non-specific duodenitis. Endoscopy 1974;6:110–115.

52. Baczako K, Büchler M, Beger HG, et al: Morphogenesis and possible precursor lesions of invasive carcinoma of the papilla of Vater: Epithelial dysplasia and adenoma. Hum Pathol 1985;16:305–310.

53. Seifert E, Schulte F, Stolte M: Adenoma and carcinoma of the duodenum and papilla of Vater: A clinicopathologic study. Am J Gastroenterol 1992;87:37–42.

54. Yamaguchi K, Enjoji M: Carcinoma of the ampulla of Vater. Cancer 1987;59:506–515.

55. Witte S: Die endoskopische Tumorzelldiagnostik im Bereich des Duodenums. Zentralbl Gastroenterol 1976;14:508–514.

56. Rupp M, Hawthorne CM, Ehya H: Brushing cytology in biliary tract obstruction. Acta Cytol 1990;34:221–226.

57. Witte S, Langer J: Die endoskopische Zytodiagnostik des Pankreas und der Gallengänge. Med Klin 1991;86:449–453.

58. Witte S, Göbel D: Zytodiagnostik der Colitis ulcerosa. Leber Magen Darm 1973;3:131–134.

59. Melville DM, Richman PI, Shepherd NA, et al. Brush cytology of the colon and rectum in ulcerative colitis: An aid to cancer diagnosis. J Clin Pathol 1988;41:1180–1186.

60. Katz S, Katz I, Platt N, et al. Cancer in chronic ulcerative colitis. Diagnostic role of segmental colonic lavage. Dig Dis Sci 1977;22:355–364.

61. Watanabe H: Cytological diagnosis of cancer of the colon and rectum. Tohoku J Exp Med 1987;154:169–176.

62. Kochhar R, Rajwanshi A, Wig JD, et al. Fine needle aspiration cytology of rectal masses. Gut 1990;31:334–336.

63. Berry AV, Baskind AF, Handlton DC. Cytologic screening for esophageal cancer. Acta Cytol 1981;25:135–147.

64. Jaskiewicz K, Venter FS, Marasas WF. Cytopathology of the esophagus in Transkei. J Natl Cancer Inst 1987;79:961–967.

65. Lu J-B, Yang WX, Dong W-Z, et al. A prospective study of esophageal cytological atypia in linxian county. Int J Cancer 1988;41:805–808.

66. Norberto L, Cusumano A, Martella B, et al. Evaluation critique des prélèvements cyto-histologiques perendoscopiques après coloration vitale au bleu de Toluidine dans le cancer de l'oesophage. Acta Endosc 1985;15:327–329.

67. Drake M: Gastro-esophageal cytology. Basel: S. Karger, 1985;267.

68. Cussó X, Monés-Xiol J, Vilardell F: Endoscopic cytology of cancer of the esophagus and cardia: A long-term evaluation. Gastrointest Endosc 1989;35:321–323.

69. Marbet UA, Dalquen P, Stalder GA, et al. Wertigkeit von Biopsie und gezielter Bürstenzytologie bei der gastrointestinalen Karzinomdiagnostik aufgrund der Endoskopien von 1979–1984. Schweiz Med Wochenschr 1985;115:1007–1009.

70. O'Donoghue JM, Horgan PF, O'Donohoe MK, et al. Adjunctive endoscopic brush cytology in the detection of upper gastrointestinal malignancy. Acta Cytol 1995;39:28–34.

71. Hiratsuka R: Clinicopathological studies of DNA content in nuclei of cells isolated from patients with esophageal carcinoma. Fukuoka Acta Med 1981;72:556.

72. Böcking H, Giroud F, Reith A: Consensus report of the european society for analytical cellular pathology task force on standardization of diagnostic DNA image cytometry. Anal Quant Cytol Histol 1995;17:1–7.

73. Robey SS, Hamilton SR, Gupta PK, et al. Diagnostic value of cytopathology in Barrett esophagus and associated carcinoma. Am J Clin Pathol 1988;89:493–498.

74. Wang HH, Doria Jr WI, Purohit-Buch S, et al. Barrett's esophagus. The cytology of dysplasia in comparison to benign and malignant lesions. Acta Cytol 1992;36:60–64.

75. Koga Y: Biologic characteristics of esophageal epithelial dysplasia assessed by proliferating cell nuclear antigen. Cancer 1996;77:237–244.

76. Zhuang ZH, Vortmeyer AO, Mark EJ, et al. Barrett's esophagus: Metaplastic cells with loss of heterozygosity at the APC gene locus are clonal precursors to invasive adenocarcinoma. Cancer Res 1996;56:1961–1964.

77. Menke-Pluymers MBE, Hop WCJ, Mulder AH, et al. DNA ploidy as a prognostic factor for patients with an adenocarcinoma in Barrett's esophagus. Hepatogastroenterology 1995;42:786–788.

78. Kawamura T, Goseki N, Koike M, et al. Acceleration of proliferative activity of esophageal squamous cell carcinoma with invasion beyond the mucosa. Cancer 1996;77:843–849.

79. Witte S: Cytologie des Magens. In: Demling L, ed. Handbuch der inneren Medizin. 5. Aufl. Berlin: Springer, 1974;355–380.

80. Witte S: Magenzytologie. Baden-Baden: Gerhard Witzstrock, 1987,80.

81. Rachail-Amoux M, Aubert H, Zarski J-P, et al. Résultats du cytodiagnostic dirigé sous contrôle endoscopique dans 248 cas de cancers digestifs. Gastroenterol Clin Biol 1983;7:158–163.

82. Simon L, Bajtai A, Figus I, et al. Clinical value of exfoliative and abrasive cytology in the diagnostics of gastric cancer and precanceroses. Arch Geschwulstforsch 1977;47:719–727.

83. Debongnie I-C, Legros G, Beyaert C. Apport de la cytologie du tractus digestif supérieur dans un hôpital général. Acta Endosc 1985;15:337–342.

84. Chambers LA, Clark II WE. The endoscopic diagnosis of gastroesophageal malignancy: A cytologic review. Acta Cytol 1986;30:110–114.

85. Moreno-Otero R, Martinez-Raposo A, Cantero J, et al. Exfoliative cytodiagnosis of gastric adenocarcinoma. Comparison with biopsy and endoscopy. Acta Cytol 1983;27:485–488.

86. Qizilbash AH, Castelli M, Kowalski MA, et al. Endoscopic brush cytology and biopsy in the diagnosis of cancer of the upper gastrointestinal tract. Acta Cytol 1980;24:313–318.

87. Czernak B, Herz F, Koss LG. DNA distribution patterns in early gastric carcinomas. Cancer 1987;59:113–117.

88. Halter F. Brush cytology in colonic malignancies. Hepatogastroenterology 1981;28:178.

89. Debongnie I-C, Legros G, Beyaert C. Cytologie des lésions inflammatoires et néoplasiques du colon. Acta Endosc 1985;15:331–336.

90. Miczban I, Feher M. Die Bedeutung der zytologischen Untersuchungen in der Erkennung der neoplastischen Veränderungen des Rectosigmoideums. Tijdschr Gastroenterol 1977;20(4):237–249.

91. Dinkov L, Bakalov W, Donov M. Zytodiagnostik kolorektaler Präkanzerosen und Karzinome. Arch Geschwulstforsch 1982;52:649–655.

92. Ehya H, O'Hara BJ. Brush cytology in the diagnosis of colonic neoplasms. Cancer 1990;66:1563–1567.

93. Winawer SJ, Leidner SD, Hajdu SI, et al. Colonoscopic biopsy and cytology in the diagnosis of colon cancer. Cancer 1978;42:2849–2853.

94. Gérard F, Guerret S, Gérard J-P, et al. Usefulness of morphometry in the cytologic assessment of rectal tumors. Anal Quant Cytol Histol 1990;12:181.

95. Xavier RG, Prolla JC, Benvenuti GA, et al. Tissue cytogenetic studies in chronic ulcerative colitis and carcinoma of the colon. Cancer 1974;34:684–695.

5

IMMUNOHISTOLOGY AND CYTOMETRY OF THE GASTROINTESTINAL TRACT

Daniel G. Sheahan and John D. Crissman

Because the immunohistology and cytometry of the gastrointestinal (GI) tract is complex and the depth of material available on the subject is extensive, this chapter is intended to be an overview. The authors present a broad spectrum of diseases and include an extensive, representative bibliography that may be the starting point for in-depth study.

DNA quantitation is the focus of the section on cytometry,

recognizing that any immunologic stain could be measured using these techniques. Because of current interests in DNA quantitation, we provide background information to help the reader interpret this literature. DNA quantitation data are available for a number of gastrointestinal neoplasms; because the greatest amount of data available is for colon cancer, these data are reviewed in detail.

IMMUNOHISTOLOGY

Thirty years after the inception of immunofluorescent studies (1) on frozen tissue, immunohistochemical localization of antigens in fixed tissues became a reality with the demonstration of immuno-globulin-containing cells in formalin-fixed, paraffin-embedded tissues using an enzyme-labeled antibody (2). With recognition of the value of this application to "routine" histologically prepared tissues came a dramatic increase in the number of antibodies, initially polyclonal and subsequently monoclonal, that became available. Immunohistochemistry rapidly became commonplace in practice and immunohistochemical studies assumed the mantle of sophisticated special stains.

The true and ever increasing value of immunohistochemistry as an adjunct to traditional histologic evaluation of normal and pathologically altered tissues is a function of a number of diverse factors, including: *(a)* various aspects of tissue procurement, preparation, fixation, and processing that impinge on antigenic molecular structural preservation; *(b)* variations in the technical reproducibility of results between different laboratories; *(c)* variations in the professional skills in the interpretation of immunohistochemically stained tissue preparations; and *(d)* the availability of antibodies prepared against specific antigens that are of reliable standards.

METHODOLOGY

As is true for routine histology, a variety of factors, the most important of which are tissue fixation and paraffin embedding, influence immunohistochemical results. Of utmost importance in immunohistochemistry is preservation of tissue morphology to allow accurate localization of antigens to specific tissue cells or cell components. In addition, the antigens in the tissue cannot be allowed to lose their immunoreactivity.

The most satisfactory fixatives in routine use—formaldehyde, Bouin's, and especially those with a mercuric base such as B5—permit good to excellent antigenic preservation with consequent optimal immunohistochemical detection and localization in tissues. Surface and nuclear antigens are well preserved in frozen tissue samples, and with the increasing availability of frozen tissue bank repositories, the immunohistochemical study of frozen-section tissue samples can be used more often.

AUTOMATED IMMUNOHISTOCHEMISTRY

Automation was introduced to immunohistochemistry by Dr. David Brigati. Today, a number of automated "immunostainers" are commercially available. The authors have experience with one of these types of instruments and have found it to be reliable, superior to manual procedural methods, and capable of handling large volumes of slides, producing results that are of constant high quality in a rapid time frame, usually within 2 hours. This efficiency permits same-day response. On occasion, the immunostains are ready before some routine special stains, with consequent improvement in turnaround time in surgical pathologic assessment, release of technical personnel for other duties, and reduction in the overall cost of performance of immunohistochemical stains. Because these instruments are programmable using computerized control, more

than one daily and an overnight run can be performed, which is of enormous benefit to both service and research activities.

ENZYME DIGESTION

The unmasking of antigens for immunohistochemical detection by exposure of the tissue sections to specific protease enzymes has been in existence for more than 20 years (3). For optimal results, the glass slides should be coated with adhesive compounds or electrostatically charged to ensure tissue section adhesion to the slides, and the duration of enzyme digestion should be sufficient to maximize antigenic exposure without incurring morphologic tissue damage. There is no magic formula for enzyme digestion methods and they must be individualized in each laboratory for the improved detection of each individual antigen. In gastrointestinal pathology practice, the antigens that routinely require enzyme digestion include cytomegalovirus (CMV) and human immunodeficiency virus (HIV) when using monoclonal antibody detection, *Pneumocystis carinii,* cytokeratin, and desmin.

ANTIGEN RETRIEVAL

Formalin fixation-induced protein cross-linking, which may mask the presence of antigenic sites, can be altered by exposure to intense heat or to strong alkali (4). It is also known that refixing deparaffinized tissue sections in zinc formalin improves the results of immunohistochemical staining (5). Incorporation of the principles of these two observations into immunohistochemical methodology has led to the development of antigen retrieval methods, the most common of which is exposure of tissue sections in a microwave oven to high heat (~100° C) for varying times that depend on the antigen type in the presence of lead thiocyanate, zinc sulfate, or, especially for nuclear antigens, glycine HCl or citrate buffer (6, 7).

OTHER TECHNIQUES

Other types of tissue evaluation that parallel the immunohistochemical technique have been developed. In situ hybridization is a technique whereby a labeled oligonucleotide probe binds reciprocally with a complementary DNA or RNA nucleotide sequence in tissue, producing identifiable and specific stable base pairs. Biotinylated probes incorporating enzymatic labeling are currently the most frequently used types, which further enhances their similarity to immunohistochemical methods.

In situ hybridization has advantages over immunohistochemistry because of its high specificity and the fact that nucleotides are more resistant than proteins to formalin fixation, producing a more selectively sensitive test. This technique, however, is slower and more expensive than immunohistochemical methods.

CONTROLS

The use of antibody controls, both positive and negative, is intrinsic to the appropriate interpretation of immunohistochemical stains and as a corollary to the quality assurance of the materials and methods used.

The three types of controls, which are important in the use of immunohistochemistry, are those that pertain to primary antibody specificity, method of localization of the primary antibody, and integrity of the tissue being studied. Positive controls are represented by detectable staining of specific antigens by their appropriately labeled specific antibodies in a tissue section known to harbor such antigens. This result validates both the active antigenicity within the tissue sections and the specificity of the applied antibody. Positive control sections must accompany each run of test tissue sections within which the specific antigen is sought.

Many types of negative controls are used to test the efficacy and accuracy of the immunohistochemical methods. Each individual test slide of each run must have its own individual negative control to ensure the tissue specificity of the primary antibody. In routine laboratory practice, saline or normal serum are used as negative controls in place of the specific primary antibody. Absence of staining supports the specificity of the primary antibody used, and any staining reaction elicited is considered attributable to components of the staining reaction other than the specific antibody. Usage of preimmune serum, absorbed antibody, or blocking antibody as negative controls has no application in routine practice. When a panel of antibodies is applied to serial tissue sections, those that do not show immunoreactivity may be considered irrelevant antibodies and, in this circumstance, serve inadvertently as negative antibody controls.

Tissue controls are also of positive and negative varieties. A positive tissue control is one that is known to harbor a specific antigen; reciprocally, a negative tissue control does not contain the specific antigen in question. The assurance that the tissue submitted to immunohistochemical analysis has sufficient integrity and retention of antigenic structure is best served by the degree of expression of the labile but ubiquitous antigen vimentin in the tissue (8) (Fig. 5.1).

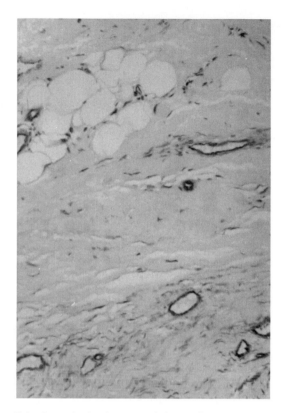

Figure 5.1 Intestinal submucosal tissue shows positive immunohistochemical staining in vascular structures and stromal fibroblasts indicating retained integrity of tissue antigenic structure.

IDENTIFICATION OF NORMAL STRUCTURES

In addition to the normal cytokeratin immunopositivity of the gastrointestinal surface epithelium, some specific epithelial cell types and the different stromal cells of the gastrointestinal wall manifest different specific cell markers that are detectable by immunohistochemical methods. Neoplasms derived from these cell types may show immunohistochemical expression of these same cell markers, which facilitates their specific diagnostic identification.

In the basal layer of the esophageal and the anal squamous mucosae, occasional melanocytes may be identified both by routine special and immunohistochemical stains. As elsewhere in the body, melanocytes manifest S-100 protein but not the "melanoma" associated antigen (HMB 45) that is expressed in most malignant melanomas. Rarely, benign proliferation of melanocytes is seen throughout the central esophageal squamous mucosa, and melanin-containing cells are detected on occasion in the rectal mucosa (9). It is important to recognize that with routine hematoxylin and eosin (H & E) staining, certain cells, especially lamina propria macrophages, may show brown pigmentation that is not melanin. Such conditions include vitamin E deficiency-induced intestinal lipofuscinosis (10) and ceroidosis (11). Siderophages, which contain hemosiderin, can be confirmed by iron stains. Melanosis coli and pseudomelanosis of the duodenum and small intestine, despite their appellation, are entities in which the lamina propria macrophages contain pigmented material other than melanin (12–15). None of these conditions show S-100 protein immunoreactivity.

It is important to avoid misinterpreting these pigments as labeled sites of antigen localization. Malignant melanoma, whether well differentiated or anaplastic, primary or metastatic in the GI tract, immunostains positively with S-100 protein and the premelanosome glycoprotein monoclonal antibody HMB-45.

The gastric mucosa contains a multiplicity of epithelial cell types possessing a variety of interrelated functions. All regions of the stomach, cardia, fundus, and antrum have a surface layer of neutral mucus-secreting columnar epithelium extending into the foveolar pits with subjacent tubular or branching glands lined by specialized epithelium. Within these glands is a diffusely distributed neuroendocrine cell population with different cell types predominating in various regions of the mucosa.

In the middle one third of the antral mucosa are endocrine cells with vesicular nuclei and clear perinuclear cytoplasm. These cells produce somatostatin and the hormones gastrin and adrenocorticotropic hormone (ACTH), both of which are easily demonstrated immunohistochemically in normal (Fig. 5.2), hyperplastic, or neoplastic conditions.

In the fundic mucosa is a population of argyrophilic neuroendocrine cells that have not yet been shown to contain an immunohistochemically detectable hormone product. These cells are called ECL cells because of their resemblance to enterochromaffin cells. ECL cells are under the trophic influence of antral G cells and proliferate in conditions characterized by G-cell hyperplasia.

Throughout the intestines is a wide variety of immunohistochemically detectable mucosal endocrine cells, the most common of which is the serotonin-producing enterochromaffin EC cell.

The lamina propria contains a range of inflammatory cells that normally immunoexpress the various immunoglobulins in plasma cells, T- and B-cell markers on lymphocytes, endothelial cell markers on vascular lining cells, actin and desmin on muscle, and S-100 on nerve structures. The pervasive presence of vimentin throughout all stromal tissue is also easily confirmed immunohistochemically (see Fig. 5.1).

INFECTIOUS DISEASE

GENERAL PRINCIPLES

The application of immunohistochemistry to the diagnosis of infectious disease has provided many advantages to clinician, pathologist, and patient alike. As a diagnostic adjunct to routine histology, it provides faster results than culture methods, reduces hazardous exposure of laboratory personnel, allows specific identification of pathogens with a high level of sensitivity, and their localization in tissue sometimes even before traditional histologic changes, e.g. viral inclusions, are manifest. It also permits recognition of pathogens that are difficult if not impossible to grow on culture media.

With ever increasing methodologic advances, newer molecular based techniques, which incorporate increased sensitivity and specificity, have been introduced into the diagnostic laboratory. These techniques include in situ hybridization and polymerase chain reaction (PCR) applied to Southern blot analysis. Despite their advantages, these techniques have limitations. This methodology is slow, time consuming, and expensive; at present, in the stringent financial arena emanating from managed care, it is not optimally reimbursable. These pure molecular techniques do not provide tissue localization of putative pathogens, and even though they detect a specific antigen within a test sample, it may not necessarily imply that the identified pathogen is viable or necessarily causative of the clinical infectious disease at that tissue site.

The diagnosis of infectious disease embraces the recognition of bacterial, viral, fungal, and protozoal pathogenic organisms. The following section includes a discussion of the impact of precise identification using immunohistochemical methods.

BACTERIAL DISEASES

In routine diagnostic practice, the need for immunohistochemical detection of bacterial infection is minimal and is even less for confirmation of its presence. Antibodies have been produced against a wide variety of bacteria, but extensive cross-reactivity among different bacterial strains imposes limitations on the applicability of immunohistochemistry to the diagnosis of infectious disease.

Identification of specific gastrointestinal infectious pathogens, however, is readily feasible by immunohistochemical means. Gastrointestinal syphilitic disease, most frequently anorectal, is usually histologically indistinguishable in routine H & E-stained sections from other anoproctitides and requires specific immunohistochemical identification of the *Treponema pallidum* organism to verify the cause of the proctitis. Dark-field illumination may be considered specifically diagnostic of syphilis in lesions involving the perianal mucosa or skin, but because of the existence of nontreponemal intestinal spirochetosis in the distal colon and rectum, immunohistochemical studies are required for the specific diagnosis of syphilis (16) in this location, especially in populations that participate in anal sexual practices.

In the appropriate clinical context, mycobacterial disease is easily recognized histologically. The most common mycobacterial disease affecting the GI tract is due to *Mycobacterium avium intracellulare* (MAI), with rarer instances of *Mycobacterium gordona* infection noted in recent years in AIDS patients. In these variants of mycobacterial disease, a characteristic histologic feature is macrophages packed with numerous acid-fast bacilli in the gastroenteric mucosa, with lesser degrees of involvement of the enteric wall. Occasionally, only rare acid-fast organisms are recognized. Although rarely required, immunohistochemical methods can demonstrate mycobacteria, both tuberculous as well as atypical, in tissue specimens (17).

CHLAMYDIA TRACHOMATIS

This obligate intracellular bacterium-like organism is responsible for lymphogranuloma venereum (LGV), a sexually transmitted disease, and for chlamydial proctitis. Multiple C. trachomatis serotypes are causative of LGV, whereas fewer numbers of such serotypes and some non-LGV stains are associated with chlamydial proctitis.

The endoscopic and histologic appearances of chlamydial proctitis are not specific and its distinction from other causes can be established by identification of the organism from cultures of rectal swabs. An additional complicating factor is the occasional coexistence of more than one colorectal infectious disease in immunocompetent, but especially in immunocompromised, patients who practice anal intercourse. Applications of immunohistochemical

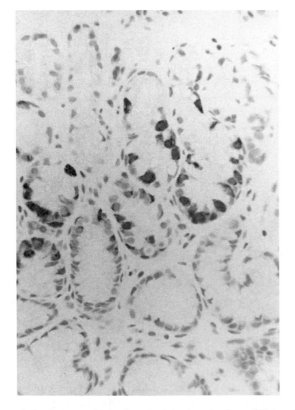

Figure 5.2   Immunohistochemical demonstration of G (gastrin) cells in normal gastric antral mucosa.

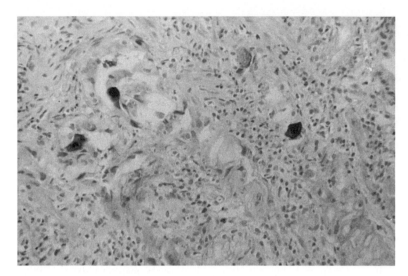

Figure 5.3 Immunohistochemical demonstration of cytomegalovirus in both epithelial and stromal cells of stomach. The nuclear staining is more intense than that seen in the cytoplasm.

methods to the localization of chlamydia species in rectal biopsy is now feasible with the use of monoclonal antibodies directed against chlamydia antigens (18). This diagnostic approach permits specific identification of chlamydia organisms as a causative agent of the inflammatory process at the site of mucosal disease.

Yersinia enterocolitis is a diarrheal disease of abrupt onset that results from food contamination by the coccobacillary forms of *Yersinia pseudotuberculosis* organisms. Although difficult to recognize in the mucosal inflammatory exudate on routine gram stains, the organisms can be detected immunohistochemically (19), which permits the distinction of Yersiniosis from Crohn's disease, tuberculosis, and lymphoma, particularly in the ileocolic region.

VIRAL GASTROENTERITIS

The two most common viruses that affect the GI tract are herpes virus and CMV, each of which has an easily recognizable routine histologic appearance with characteristic cellular viral inclusions. Routine immunohistochemical staining of formalin or Bouin's fixed tissue can demonstrate with ease the presence of the appropriate viral antigen in infected tissues (Fig. 5.3), reducing the need to apply more sensitive and more expensive molecular techniques, such as in situ hybridization or PCR.

Immunoelectronmicroscopy has limited application to the diagnosis of enteric viral infectious disease. It can be used to detect the presence in stool of small RNA and DNA diarrheagenic viruses such as rotavirus, Norwalk agent, and enteric adenovirus (20).

Most cases of infant diarrhea attributed to adenoviral infection are considered to be attributable to serotypes Ad40 and Ad41. Corroborative evidence of enteric adenoviral infection is provided by the presence of intraepithelial intranuclear inclusions and its demonstration ultrastructurally (21).

HERPES VIRUS INFECTION

Herpetic infection of the GI tract is most common in the esophagus and in the anorectum, particularly among male homosexual patients. This ulcerative infection causes epithelial cell multinucleation and ground glass intranuclear Cowdry type A inclusions, with scattered granular cytoplasmic Cowdry type B inclusions. Because the infected epithelial cells become immersed in the inflammatory exudate, immunohistochemical identification of herpes virus types I or II antigen may be required to establish the diagnosis in such situations. In immunocompromised hosts, we routinely order both fungal and viral immunostains for Herpes and CMV on biopsy samples from the esophagus or anal canal that manifest severe ulcerative inflammation.

Herpetic infection of the stomach is uncommon and has been detected immunohistochemically (22). Herpetic enterocolitis is extremely rare (23), but herpes proctitis, a severely painful condition, is a common sexually transmitted disease. This ulcerative disease is associated with a prominent mucosal mixed inflammatory cell infiltrate, but the characteristic epithelial cell inclusions or multinucleated cells may not be seen. In these circumstances, immunohistochemistry is useful for identifying herpes virus antigen. As in all such squamous mucosal ulcerated inflammatory conditions in immunocompromised hosts, diligent search for other pathogens—viral, fungal, and bacterial—is warranted.

CYTOMEGALOVIRUS INFECTION (CMV)

The prevalence of CMV infection increased dramatically with the onset of enlarging populations of immunosuppressed patients, especially AIDS patients and transplant recipients. Cytomegalovirus infection affects all levels of the GI tract and shows a spectrum of morphologic change, from isolated viral cellular inclusions unassociated with inflammation to extensive ulceration with or without ischemic compromise. When the typical viral inclusion is seen, additional histochemical confirmation is not necessary. When immunocompromised individuals show mucosal inflammation without obvious presence of a pathogen, however, it is advisable to attempt immunohistochemical identification of CMV antigen in the cytoplasm and nucleus of both epithelial and stromal cells (see Fig. 5.3) as well as other coexistent pathogens to establish the appropriate diagnosis with resultant appropriate therapy. In an endoscopic study involving 66 liver transplant recipients (24), gastroduodenal CMV infection was found in 31.8%, mostly during the second month after transplantation. The most sensitive method of detection was viral culture and the least sensitive but most rapid was histomorphology.

In this study, immunohistology was not used. Personal experience indicates that the yield of CMV infection, as determined from the study of routine H & E-stained sections of gastrointestinal biopsy samples, is minimally, if at all, enhanced by the addition of immunohistochemical studies. In biopsy specimens that show positive CMV immunoreactivity but the initial evaluation of the H & E stained sections failed to reveal CMV inclusions, careful review of the initial H & E sections frequently disclosed histologic evidence of CMV infection.

HUMAN PAPILLOMAVIRUS (HPV)

Human papillomavirus (HPV) infection of the GI tract is limited to involvement of the esophagus and the anorectal region in two distinctly different patterns.

Esophageal involvement is rare (25, 26) and usually manifests as single or multiple squamous papillomas, commonly in infants. Viral types 6 and 11 can be detected immunohistochemically in some lesions (27, 28) (Fig. 5.4), which allows their differentiation from esophageal inflammatory or fibrovascular polyps, especially when the characteristic koilocytotic epithelial cell changes or papillary formation of HPV-related squamous papillomas are not identifiable. Malignant sequelae from esophageal HPV infection have not been recognized (26).

The association of HPV with both papillomas and carcinomas of the anal canal is now recognized. Of the more than 60 subtypes of HPV so far identified, types 6 and 11 are recognized in the benign condylomatous lesions, and types 16 and 18 are more frequent in anal dysplasia and carcinoma (29–34). HPV can be demonstrated in

anal canal lesions of squamous but not cloacogenic or rectal origins by in situ hybridization (32, 35) and the more sensitive PCR (36). Vincent-Salomon and colleagues (33), using PCR and Southern blot hybridization, showed that 66% of squamous and 90% of basaloid anal carcinomas had HPV infection, with subtype HPV 16 encountered most commonly. Of significant importance is the capability of these techniques to identify HPV infection in populations at increased risk for anal cancer. In more than 50% of symptomatic, HIV-positive homosexual males, without evidence of AIDS, HPV 6, 11, 16, and 18 were detected, indicating that HPV infection in immunocompromised individuals may represent a risk factor in the development of anal carcinoma.

MEASLES

The classic histopathologic feature of measles infection is the Warthin-Finkeldy giant cell (37). The measles viral antigen can be demonstrated immunohistochemically by means of polyclonal and monoclonal antibodies. Its detection is not usually required in gastrointestinal disease, in contrast to more symptomatic measles infection of the respiratory and central nervous systems (38, 39).

HUMAN IMMUNODEFICIENCY VIRUS (HIV)

Human immunodeficiency virus (HIV) appears capable of causing malabsorption with small intestinal partial mucosal atrophy in the absence of associated opportunistic enteric infection—so-called AIDS enteropathy (40, 41). The HIV p24 antigen has been identified immunohistochemically in the mononuclear cells of the lamina propria (42) and by in situ hybridization in both crypt epithelial and lamina propria inflammatory cells (43).

FUNGAL LESIONS

Although routine diagnostic confirmation of the presence of fungal organisms in tissue sections can be established relatively easily using silver and other special stains, specific individual fungal species can be identified, when necessary, by immunohistochemical means. Polyclonal and monoclonal antibodies are available for the detection of *Cryptococcus neoformans* (44), *Aspergillus* (45), *Candida*, and *Histoplasma capsulatum* (46, 47).

PROTOZOAL INFESTATIONS

Cryptosporidiosis, which most often affects the upper small bowel but may be seen anywhere from esophagus to anorectum, is a common infectious complication of immunosuppressed patients, especially those with AIDS. *Cryptosporidia* is usually detectable in routine H & E-stained sections. If required, specific immunohistochemical identification of cryptosporidial species can be established (48). Other protozoal infections in which the etiologic agent can be identified by immunohistochemical means include toxoplasmosis (Fig. 5.5), a disease that can be seen throughout the full length of the GI tract in immunocompromised hosts (49), and Pneumocystis carinii infection (50, 51), although some authors consider this infection to be more fungal than protozoal (52, 53). Other coccidial protozoal infestations of the GI tract attributable to minute intracellular organisms, such as *Isospora belli* and microsporidia, are not yet detectable by immunohistochemical means.

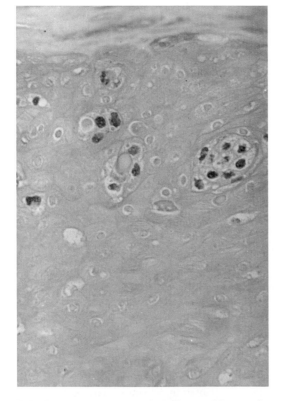

Figure 5.4 Squamous mucosa showing positive nuclear staining for human papillomavirus in nests of koilocytotic cells.

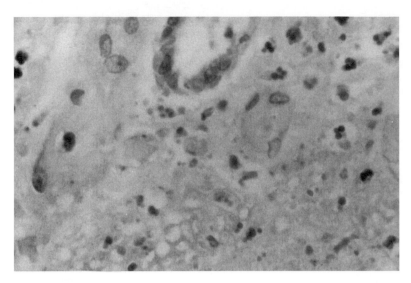

Figure 5.5 Immunohistochemical demonstration of Toxoplasma gondii organisms in small bowel. The organisms present diffusely stain with varying intensity.

AMEBIC COLITIS

The presence of an acute inflammatory exudate in ulcerated colonic mucosal specimens induces efforts to identify the possible causative pathogen. *Entamoeba histolytica* causes amebic colitis, a disease of varying prevalence throughout the world. This pathogenic trophozoite is of similar size and shares some mucin histochemical features with lamina propria macrophages, which can lead to diagnostic difficulty. Their distinction from one another is aided considerably by immunohistochemical application of the histiocytic cell markers α_1-antitrypsin and α_1-chymotrypsin, with which the amebic trophozoite is negative but macrophages are positive.

Specific antibodies that permit the immunohistochemical identification of the E. histolytica organism are available (54).

RICKETTSIAL DISEASE

The tick-borne rickettsial disease Rocky Mountain spotted fever is characterized by systemic febrile symptoms and a skin rash involving wrists and ankles secondary to endothelial cell involvement by the organism. GI tract infection results in ischemia with ulceration and even massive bleeding. The organisms can be detected immunohistochemically in the endothelial cells (55) of the gastrointestinal vasculature.

PRIMARY CARCINOMA

Because of a common embryologic origin, most gastrointestinal carcinomas are of glandular origin, the esophagus and anal canal being the primary sources of the less frequently seen squamous malignancy. They each have their own specific and distinct immunohistochemical profile, but for routine diagnostic work, application of such profiles is not usually required.

Specific variants of carcinoma can manifest particular patterns of immunohistochemical characteristics. For example, small cell carcinoma of the esophagus may show positive staining for ACTH and calcitonin (56–58).

Spindle cell carcinomas (carcinosarcomas) are now considered

purely epithelial in origin, based on immunohistochemical (59, 60) as well as other observations. Vimentin (61), α_1-antitrypsin, and α_1-antichymotrypsin expression (62) may also be seen in some tumors.

Many genes show alterations in gastrointestinal neoplasia that do not, as yet, have an immunohistochemically detectable protein product. These genes include the APC (adenomatous polyposis coli) and the MCC (mutated in colon cancer) genes.

It is important to remember that immunohistochemistry can be relied on only to detect increased expression of tumor marker proteins, such as p53, and that gene deletions or binding of the protein by other agents prevent its immunodetection. As a result, immunohistochemical analysis does not detect all genetic alterations.

Growth factors and their receptors are coded by oncogenes. When overexpressed, these factors and receptors promote angiogenesis and induce altered cell growth as a result of activation of signal transduction pathways (63). The most frequently encountered growth factors and growth factor receptors in the GI tract are epidermal growth factor (EGF) and its receptor EGFR, transforming growth factor (TGF)-α and erb B2.

ESOPHAGEAL CARCINOMA

Both EGF and TGF-α are overexpressed in EGFR-overexpressing squamous cell carcinoma cell lines (64, 65). EGF expression correlates with depth of tumor invasion and prognosis (64). TGF-α immunoreactivity has been reported in 42% (66) and 35% (67) of squamous carcinomas. The latter group noted poorer survival rates in TGF-α-positive than in TGF-α-negative tumors.

EGFR abnormalities are more common in association with esophageal squamous carcinoma than with other cancers (68), and are 10 fold more common in esophageal than in gastric carcinoma (69). Overexpression of EGFR can be detected immunohistochemically in up to 50% of squamous esophageal carcinomas and is associated with grade of dysplasia, frequency of lymph node metastasis, and shortest survival, especially in tumors that also coexpress TGF-α (70–73). Immunohistochemical staining of EGFR is located in the cell membranes of the basal zone of the normal squamous mucosa; stronger staining occurs in dysplasia and in situ carcinoma and is seen with varying degrees of intensity in most invasive carcinomas.

In esophageal glandular neoplasia, the expression of both EGFR and TGF-α shows a progressive increase from normal to metaplasia to dysplasia to invasive adenocarcinoma (74). EGFR expression correlates with the grade of dysplasia and the frequency of lymph node metastasis (67), as well as with poorer prognosis when both EGFR and TGF-α are overexpressed in the same tumor (68).

Mutations or deletions of the tumor suppressor gene p53 produce functional derangements that appear to play a role in carcinogenesis, including that of the esophagus (75), stomach (76), and colon (77). It regulates DNA replication and initiates apoptosis in response to DNA damage (78). When the p53 gene becomes mutated, abnormal cell growth may result (79).

Immunohistochemically, p53 alterations are noted in from one third to one half of esophageal carcinomas, squamous and glandular (80, 81), as well as in the histologically normal contiguous squamous or Barrett's metaplastic mucosa (82, 83). It has also been shown that the immunohistochemical expression of p53 increases with increasing grades of dysplasia (84). These observations indicate that p53 alterations exist throughout the full spectrum of esophageal carcinogenesis, from the precursor stages to fully established invasive carcinoma.

Ras oncogenes participate in cell growth and differentiation and the p21 protein product is involved in membrane signal transduction pathways. Numerous studies worldwide (85–87) have failed to show an association between Ras mutations and squamous carcinoma of the esophagus, including those tumors that occur in populations of high prevalence in association with potentially carcinogenic environmental exposure. Overexpression of h-Ras, however, has been reported in adenocarcinoma and in high- but not low-grade dysplasia arising in Barrett's metaplastic mucosa (88), and has been suggested as a possible marker for high-grade glandular dysplasia occurring in a background of Barrett's esophageal mucosa.

The erb B2 (Her 2/neu) protooncogene, which encodes a transmembrane tyrosine kinase, is amplified (89) and overexpressed (71) in approximately one sixth of esophageal adenocarcinomas (Fig. 5.6).

Immunohistochemical studies using PCNA antibodies have demonstrated an expanded proliferative zone in Barrett's mucosa. Gray et al. and Ramel et al. showed overexpression of the tumor suppressor gene p53 protein product (81, 90), ranging from 5% in Barrett's nondysplastic metaplastic mucosa to 15% in low-grade dysplasia to 45% in high-grade dysplasia to 53% in adenocarcinoma arising in Barrett's epithelium. Younes et al. noted similar findings (84). These observations indicate that the overexpression of p53 may play a significant role in the development of adenocarcinoma arising in Barrett's mucosa. Oncogene and growth factors are also overexpressed in Barrett's mucosa and in the adenocarcinoma that arises from it (88, 91, 92).

GASTRIC CARCINOMA

The usual immunohistochemical profile of gastric adenocarcinoma is cytokeratin, epithelial membrane antigen, and carcinoembryonic antigen positivity, with the latter detectable in up to 90% of cases (93). Other markers include (a) CA19-9, which is more frequent in rapidly compared to slowly progressive poorly differentiated carcinomas (94), (b) epidermal growth factor (EPG) and its receptor (EPGR), both of which correlate with poor differentiation and aggressive behavior (95), and (c) the protease inhibitors α1-antitrypsin, α1-antichymotrypsin, and α2-macroglobulin, all of which show increased expression in advanced compared to early gastric carcinoma (96).

The immunodetectable antigens just described are not sufficiently specific or sensitive to be of selective value in establishing the diagnosis of gastric carcinoma. Immunohistochemistry is, however, of value in the diagnostic evaluation of gastric carcinoma, especially in biopsy specimens, by (a) identifying specific types of gastric carcinoma; (b) distinguishing poorly differentiated primary gastric carcinoma from lymphoma, malignant melanoma, and sarcoma; and (c) providing some prognostic information.

Specific, although rare, subtypes of gastric adenocarcinoma can be distinguished immunohistochemically. The hepatoid pattern, which is composed of large eosinophilic hepatocyte-like cells, shows immunodetectable albumin, α1-antitrypsin, and intracytoplasmic hyaline PAS-positive globules that are immunopositive for

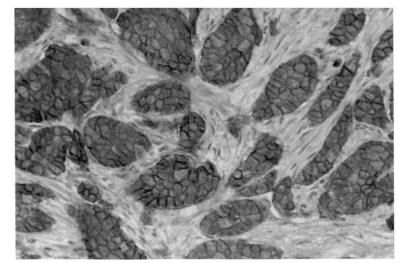

Figure 5.6   Poorly differentiated adenocarcinoma showing the typical pattern of cell membrane staining with c-erb-2 proto-oncogene.

α-fetoprotein (97). The rare primary gastric endodermal sinus tumor also manifests α-fetoprotein immunohistochemically (98).

The stomach is the most common gastrointestinal site of choriocarcinoma, either as an exclusive tumor or as partial differentiation within an adenocarcinoma. Immunohistochemically, the β-subunit of human chorionic gonadotropin (HCG) is demonstrable in the syncytiotrophoblast, and placental lactogen is noted in the cytotrophoblast (99). These findings are nonspecific, however; other tumors, including gastric adenocarcinoma, may also produce these factors (100). Thrombomodulin, an anticoagulant found in normal placental trophoblast, is demonstrable in the trophoblast of gonadal but not of primary gastric choriocarcinoma (101), a feature that may be helpful in distinguishing the two processes (99).

Various immunohistochemically identifiable endocrine cells, including chromogranin, neurone-specific enolase, and polypeptide hormone-containing cells, may be seen in close to 20% of gastric carcinomas (102), without them being considered as adenoendocrine carcinomas (103). Neuroendocrine, including small (oat cell), carcinomas are composed predominantly of argyrophil endocrine cells, have ultrastructural evidence of dense core granules, and show neuroendocrine marker expression ranging from total nonreactivity to diffuse positive reactivity. Gastric lymphoepithelial-like carcinoma, similar to that seen in the nasopharynx, consists of undifferentiated, non-small cell carcinoma cells separated by a dense lymphoplasmacytic infiltrate. Its prognosis is considered better than that of the usual gastric cancer. Distinction of this neoplasm from lymphoma is revealed by its carcinoembryonic antigen (CEA) and keratin immunopositivity, and the recent demonstration of Epstein-Barr virus (EBV) in the tumor cells, by both in situ hybridization (104) and immunohistochemistry (105). EBV has also been detected in a small percentage of the more usual variants of gastric adenocarcinoma, but it does not appear to correlate with either bcl-2 expression or p53 accumulation (106). The rare gastric carcinosarcoma (107, 108) can be distinguished from spindle cell carcinoma by the immunohistochemical demonstration of smooth muscle tissue markers in the former.

The identification and study of prognostic markers has provided controversial results, in part because of the different techniques and various types of antibodies used and the different populations studied. Nevertheless, it appears that differences exist in the expression of molecular "markers" between the different morphologic phenotypes of gastric carcinoma (109). Specific dominant oncogenes, when mutated, lead to an increased protein product that causes augmented function.

The Ras gene family is rarely mutated in gastric cancer (110) and produces the Ras p21 protein that is considered to be involved in differentiation and proliferation. Ras immunostaining has been noted more frequently in advanced compared to early gastric cancer (111), in the intestinal compared to the diffuse type (112, 113), and has been correlated with depth of invasion, metastases, and poor prognosis (111). Immunohistochemical evidence of Ras overexpression in normal intestinal metaplastic and dysplastic epithelium has been documented (112), suggesting that Ras overexpression may result from the trophic effect of the tumor or play a continuous role throughout gastric carcinogenesis. These observations are best confirmed with the use of more sensitive detection methods (114).

The p62 nuclear protein, which is encoded by the myc genes, is considered to play a role in transcription, proliferation, and cell cycle control. C-myc overexpression has been noted immunohistochemically in advanced but not in early gastric carcinoma (115),

as well as in a wide range of inflammatory, metaplastic, and dysplastic conditions of the stomach (116). It is possible, therefore, that c-myc is a marker of proliferation rather than a specific marker of malignant transformation.

In contrast, tumor suppressor genes, when mutated, lead to a loss of function. The p53 gene plays a role in the control of DNA replication and in the initiation of programmed cell death after DNA damage. Its protein product is immunohistochemically detectable. Mutations of this gene have been reported in intestinal metaplasia, dysplasia and the intestinal but not the diffuse type of carcinoma of the stomach (117), and in aneuploid but not diploid tumors (118), and correlate with depth of invasion, stage, and poor prognosis (119, 120). Immunohistochemical studies, however, which have shown p53 expression in 28% of early and 46% of advanced carcinoma (119, 121), have not demonstrated that p53 expression is able to predict survival or show an association with established prognostic factors. Consequently, it appears that detection of p53 immunohistochemical expression is not as sensitive as p53 gene mutation by molecular analysis.

Growth factors are regulatory polypeptides that stimulate cell proliferation and promote cell differentiation through specific cell membrane receptors. Overexpression of epidermal growth factor receptor (EGFR) has been detected immunohistochemically in gastric cancer (122, 123) but also in normal and inflamed atrophic gastric mucosa, indicating its poor prognostic value. Similarly, immunohistochemical expression of the related c-erb-B2 gene has been described more frequently in intestinal than in diffuse gastric cancer (124), but its prognostic significance remains unclear.

Immunohistochemical studies of epithelial cell proliferation in gastric inflammatory (Fig. 5.7) and neoplastic conditions (Fig. 5.8) using proliferating cell nuclear antigens (125) and Ki-67 (126) may provide valuable prognostic information, but overexpression of growth factors such as EGF and TGF-α has been noted in both of these conditions, limiting their applicability as prognostic factors in gastric carcinoma.

Immunohistochemical expression of cathepsins has been demonstrated in gastric adenocarcinoma (127). The greatest concentration of positively stained carcinoma cells was at the advancing edge of the tumor and correlated with the incidence of lymph node metastasis (128). Because of the capacity of cathepsins to degrade extracellular matrices (129), their expression, especially that of cathepsin D, at the periphery of malignant tumors may be related to the tumor's invasive and metastatic capability.

COLONIC CARCINOMA

The first recognized immunohistochemical tumor marker that is best related to colonic carcinoma is carcinoembryonic antigen (CEA) (130). Although present immunohistochemically in up to 100% of colon cancers, CEA has also been noticed in a wide variety of other carcinomas, including those at other major gastrointestinal sites such as the stomach, pancreas, and small intestine, as well as those arising in extraintestinal sites, such as lung, breast, ovary, cervix, and endometrium. As a result, CEA has remarkable sensitivity but little specificity as a tumor marker for any one specific site with resultant limited diagnostic applicability. CEA can be detected immunohistochemically in normal appearing but proliferating colonocytes at the edge of colon cancers and also in colonic adenomas, thus further limiting the diagnostic capabilities of this antigen (131).

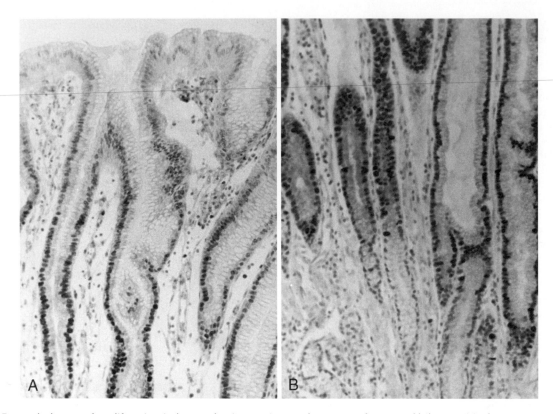

Figure 5.7   Expanded zone of proliferation in hyperplastic gastric antral mucosa of a case of bile gastritis demonstrated by increased proliferating cell nuclear antigen (PCNA) staining extending toward the surface of mucosa **(A)** and into the deep antral gland region of mucosa **(B)**.

Nevertheless, positive CEA immunostaining may help in certain specific circumstances. It can indicate the possible primary site of a CEA-positive metastatic tumor, and it virtually excludes other sites such as prostate, melanoma, lymphoma, or sarcoma. Immunohistochemical identification of micrometastases using cytokeratin with (132) or without CEA (133) antibodies or with TAG-72 (CC49) antibodies in lymph nodes of patients with Dukes

B carcinoma as established by examination of H & E-stained slides only enables tumor reclassification, which reflects survival rates that are more accurate (134).

Antibodies have been created against various CEA epitopes with partial success in so far as some such antigens can separate tumors of primary gastrointestinal origin from extraintestinal primary carcinomas, such as breast (135). In similar fashion, a

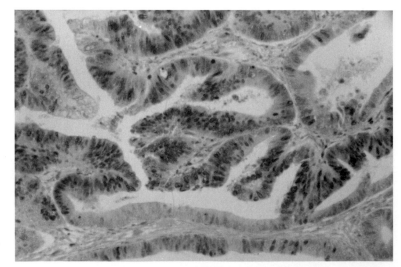

Figure 5.8   Well-differentiated adenocarcinoma showing strong PCNA staining.

monosialoganglioside marker known as the gastrointestinal carcinoma antigen (GICA), which is distinct from CEA, has been shown to react positively with colon, stomach, and pancreas but not with primary extraintestinal carcinoma (136, 137). Other putative tumor markers, including small and large intestine mucosubstance antigens (SIMA, LIMA), have been studied in cases of colorectal cancer, but they are not specific markers of malignancy nor can they indicate sole colonic origin of these tumors (138).

Molecular pathologic analysis of the pathogenesis of colorectal neoplasia has provided evidence that a progressive accumulation of genotypic changes (139) complements the phenotypic alterations already recognized as supporting the colonic adenomacarcinoma sequence. Most of the gene changes have been established by use of molecular techniques, whereas immunohistochemistry is only applicable to the protein product attributable to such gene changes. This newly acquired information has provided a better understanding of colorectal neoplasia. In routine practice, however, definitive and affordable application of these new observations to diagnostic and prognostic evaluation is not yet at hand. The immunohistochemical expression of the known antigens is limited, which compromises the value of what is currently applicable to diagnosis or prognosis of colorectal cancer. It appears also that immunohistochemical methods are less sensitive than in situ hybridization for the localization of antigenic proteins in tissue. Combining more sensitive techniques, such as PCR, with in situ hybridization or with immunohistochemistry may enable the application of more specific and sensitive methods to tumor marker identification and tissue localization (140, 141).

Molecular genetic alterations that occur during the development of colorectal neoplasia include changes in oncogenes (K-Ras, cyclins, myc, neu/HER2) and tumor suppressor genes (APC, DCC, p53) (142). In addition, a variety of the same factors related to cellular proliferation, such as PCNA and Ki-67 antigen, as well as those of stromal origin, such as collagen IV and laminin, have shown changes.

The immunohistochemical expression of the protein product of many of the oncogene and tumor suppressor gene changes has been described. The reported patterns are not uniform in the different investigations and presumably reflect the different antibody sources and preparations used, fixation differences, and the many other variables that are common to immunohistochemical procedures.

The Ras oncogene encodes the Ras p21 protein, which is expressed in 26% of colonic adenomas and in 61% of carcinomas, an observation that was interpreted as the oncogene having a role in the progression of colonic neoplasia (143). Other authors noted relatively similar incidences of Ras protein expression in colorectal carcinoma and related them to short recurrence-free intervals when compared to those tumors that did not express Ras protein (144, 145). Nuclear immunohistochemical myc-oncogene expression has been described in 100% of colonic adenocarcinomas and lesser numbers of colonic adenomas (146). This expression has been noted also in increasing amounts with increasing grades of dysplasia, with the greatest occurring in invasive adenocarcinoma (147). These observations may indicate that c-myc is related to the progression of colorectal neoplasia. Immunoexpression of Ras protein was associated with a poorer 5-year survival rate compared to Ras-negative tumors, but no similar prognostic pattern was established for the c-myc protein (148).

More prevalent than oncogene alterations are those that occur in tumor suppressor genes, especially in familial colonic carcinoma (142). Immunohistochemical expression of the p53 gene protein product is demonstrated most frequently, with varying incidences in colon carcinoma ranging from 76% (149) to 70% (150, 151) to other studies in which the incidence was related to the presence (62%) or absence (36%) of metastases. Sun and colleagues (152) noted that p53 expression in colorectal carcinoma was more frequent in nondiploid than in diploid tumors and was more significantly associated with a poor prognosis. These observations were subsequently confirmed by Lanza et al. (153). Yamaguchi et al. (154) provided evidence to suggest that p53 expression in colorectal cancers is of prognostic significance, based on their observations that p53-positive tumors recurred more frequently and had shorter survival rates than p53-negative tumors. The observation that mucinous carcinomas of the colon show less expression of p53 than nonmucinous carcinomas (149, 153) provides additional evidence that mucinous adenocarcinoma of the colon may be a distinctly different and possibly specific type of colonic carcinoma.

In another study, although no correlation was established in either colonic adenomas or carcinomas between bcl-2 protein expression and proliferative activity as determined by MIB-1 antigen expression, bcl-2 protein expression in adenomas (90%) was markedly different compared to that in carcinomas (20%) (155). These results may indicate that decreased apoptosis is not a significant factor in the genesis of colorectal neoplasia.

The p53 and bcl-2 genes are involved in cell proliferation and inhibition of apoptosis, respectively. Immunohistochemical expression of bcl-2 was 98% in adenomas and 56% in carcinomas of the colon, whereas that of p53 was 38% in adenomas and 74% in carcinomas (156). These results suggest that the increased expression of bcl-2 is early and that of p53 is late in the evolution of the colonic adenoma-carcinoma sequence.

Immunoexpression of nucleophosmin B23, a phosphoprotein involved in ribosomal assembly and transport, is increased in colorectal neoplasia compared to normal colonic mucosa and shifts from a nuclear to a nucleolar location early in the adenoma carcinoma sequence (157). Its role in colorectal neoplasia is otherwise unknown.

The metastasis suppressor gene nm23 is expressed at a higher degree in colonic carcinomas with poorer survival and in hepatic metastases compared to those with better survival. These data, however, are not consistent with the idea that nm23 operates as a metastasis suppressor gene (158).

The immunohistochemically detectable markers of tumor cell proliferation include proliferating cell nuclear antigen (PCNA) (159) and Ki-67, a nuclear antigen, both of which are present during the synthetic and mitotic phases of the cell cycle (G1,S,G2,M). The Ki-67 antigen originally was detectable only in frozen tissue, but now MIB-1, created against recombinant KI-67, can be used on paraffin sections with equally good results (160) (Fig. 5.9). The degree of positivity of these two cell proliferation-related antigens correlates well with both thymidine-labeled and mitotic indices. It should be recognized, however, that cell proliferation may not be a major risk factor for carcinoma (161). It is known that no relationship exists between proliferation markers and p53 expression (153, 162).

A critical component of colorectal carcinoma, as it affects patient outcome, is its capacity to invade stromal tissue and to produce metastases. The ability of tumor cells to modify the

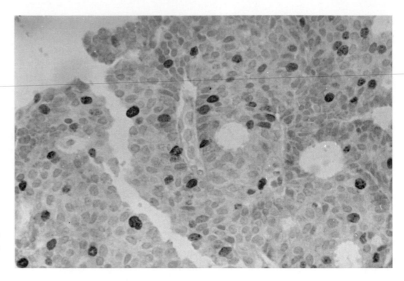

Figure 5.9 Ki-67 expressed immunohistochemically using M1B-1 antibody in paraffin sections of moderately differentiated adenocarcinoma of colon.

surrounding stromal tissue is mediated largely through the metalloproteinases (163), which include the interstitial collagenases, type IV collagenases, and stromelysins (164). These proteinases are under the inhibitory control of their tissue specific inhibitors (TIMPS) (165), which also have cell growth promotion properties (166).

Carcinomas, including gastrointestinal neoplasms, express greater amounts of metalloproteinases than normal tissue (167). Different tumor cells and stromal cells produce different metalloproteinase enzymes and tissue-specific inhibitors. Urbanski and colleagues (168) provided evidence that certain metalloproteinases are expressed more often in adenocarcinomas than in benign adenomas of the colon. These observations, coupled with observations from study of pulmonary neoplasia (168), suggest that the expression of specific metalloproteinases may antedate the occurrence of tumor cell invasion and that the detection of such enzymes within benign adenomas may be predictive of malignant change.

Certain metalloproteinases (e.g., MMP-9) are immunohistochemically detectable in carcinomas and in adenomas with high-grade dysplasia. Other proteinases that possess elastolytic activity, such as the cysteine proteinases (cathepsins), are also detectable immunohistochemically. Despite the potential for increased understanding of tumor invasion and metastasis from study of these enzymes, their applicability to diagnostic or prognostic usage is not established at this time.

ULCERATIVE COLITIS

As elsewhere, application of immunohistochemistry to detect early neoplastic change in chronic ulcerative colitis has not been sufficiently sensitive or specific to be of diagnostic value. The multiplicity of gene alterations in colorectal neoplasia is well established. Many tumor-related markers, including P-glycoprotein and CEA, that are expressed in neoplastic cells may also be identified in colitic regenerative epithelium (169, 170). The association of aneuploidy and p53 deletion has been suggested as a possible marker for dysplasia in chronic ulcerative colitis (171). Ras mutations have been detected in dysplasia and in carcinomas associated with ulcerative colitis (172, 173).

ANAL CANAL NEOPLASIA

Anal condylomas and carcinomas are associated with HPV infection. Of the more than 60 HPV subtypes, subtypes 2, 6, 10, and 11 are associated with condylomas and subtypes 6, 11, 16, and 18 and less frequently 31 and 33 are seen in anal squamous (174) but not cloacogenic or rectal carcinoma (175, 176). The role of HPV is related to the formation of a complex between the virally encoded protein E6 forms and the wild type p53 protein (177) producing rapid proteolytic degradation of p53 (178). The viral capsid antigens are detectable in the nuclei of the koilocytotic cells of the condylomatous epithelium by immunohistochemical (see Fig. 5.4) (179) and by in situ hybridization using HPV DNA probes (180). The recognition that HPV infection may be seen in up to 50% of HIV positive homosexual men without AIDS or anal carcinoma indicates that HPV infection may be a risk factor for anal carcinoma (34, 181). The prognosis of anal cancer may be better in patients with, than in those without, prior HPV infection.

MALIGNANT MELANOMA

Malignant melanoma, whether a primary lesion in the esophagus or anal region or a metastasis to any region of the gastrointestinal tract, is immunopositive with vimentin, S-100 protein, and melanosome-based malignant melanoma antigen (HMB-45) (182) and negative with keratin and leukocyte common antigen. The positive immunoreactive antibodies are individually sensitive but not highly specific (183–185). Therefore, application of all three antibodies is strongly recommended, and positive reactions with all three provide the greatest likelihood of correctly identifying the tumor as malignant melanoma.

THE UNKNOWN PRIMARY NEOPLASM

The gastrointestinal tract has its complement of metastatic lesions and a wide spectrum of such tumors has been recognized. In many instances, these lesions are incidental findings. On occasion, however, the first clinical presence of a malignancy may be recognized by metastatic spread to the GI tract. Secondary tumor involvement of the gut may be attributable to direct extension from neighboring organs or to true lymphatic or hematogenous spread.

In many instances, the traditional histologic picture is sufficient to suggest the primary source of the tumor. When the tumor is too anaplastic to permit histologic identification, immunohistochemistry can be of value. Initial use of a simple panel of antibodies can help to identify the tumor type. Positive staining with cytokeratin indicates carcinoma; with S-100, protein malignant melanoma; with leukocyte common antigen, lymphoma; and with vimentin, soft tissue tumors (Table 5.1). Additional antibodies can further define specific tumor types within these groups. Which antibodies are chosen reflects the clinical and laboratory findings, the location and morphologic appearances of the tumor, and the experience and bias of the pathologist. This sequential selective approach, though slower, is economically preferable to the initial application of a "broad battery" of antibodies to the immunohistochemical identification of the tumor.

Positive results support specific tumor diagnoses. False-positive reactions may occur in areas of necrosis owing to nonspecific spread of antigen from necrotic cells or from tissue crush injury into contiguous tissue. The exact location of the antigen—membranous, cytoplasmic, or nuclear—is imperative to proper interpretation of positive immunohistochemical reactions. Reciprocally, although negative results may correctly reflect absence of a specific antigen in tissue, false-negative results may also occur. Methodologic error or antigenic mutational change can contribute to a negative immunohistologic result.

Keratin staining is of limited value in distinguishing between primary and metastatic carcinoma involving the GI tract. Specific organ derivation of carcinoma metastatic to the alimentary tract by immunohistochemical means is also limited. Breast metastases may be suggested by the detection of estrogen and progesterone receptors and further emphasized if other "breast-specific" antibodies, such as lactalbumin, are used (186).

Direct spread from extraintestinal carcinomas can be a source of diagnostic confusion. Prostatic adenocarcinoma, whether truly metastatic or directly infiltrating into rectal mucosa, particularly when poorly differentiated, can be mistaken for other tumors. The immunohistochemical expression of both prostatic acid phosphatase (PAP) and prostate specific antigen (PSA) can be considered strongly supportive of the diagnosis of prostate cancer. It should be noted that a high percentage of rectal carcinoid tumors, some variants of which may resemble prostatic adenocarcinoma, show PAP but not PSA activity (187).

TABLE 5.2	Pan Neuroendocrine Markers	
Common Usage	Rare Usage
Synaptophysin	Leu 7
Chromogranin	PGP 9.5
Neurone-specific enolase	HISL-19
	7B2
	Bombesin
	Histaminase

NEUROENDOCRINE CELLS

The other extensive epithelial cell component of the GI mucosa is the neuroendocrine cell population. The evolution of the diagnostic usage of immunohistochemistry has identified two types of tissue markers in neuroendocrine cells: one generalized and known as pan-neurendocrine and the other specific for hormonal or peptide components of individual cells. The former group, which includes chromogranin, synaptophysin, and the relatively nonspecific neurone specific enolase, is used as a screening mechanism to identify the neuroendocrine nature of tumors, including those that do not manifest specific hormonal or peptide products (Table 5.2). The individual cell types and the specific neuroendocrine hyperplasias, as well as neoplasias derived from them, can be identified immunohistochemically by their specific hormonal or peptide product (Table 5.3).

NEUROENDOCRINE CELL PROLIFERATIVE DISORDERS

Neuroendocrine proliferations, both hyperplastic and neoplastic, occur throughout the entire GI tract, the most frequently encountered of which are listed in Table 5.4.

The enterochromaffin cell, which is the most ubiquitous gastrointestinal mucosal endocrine cell, is increased in number nonspecifically in the small intestinal mucosa of untreated celiac disease (188, 189), in chronic active gastritis, and in appendicitis (190). These cells are argentaffin and argyrophilic and are specifically identified by the immunohistochemical demonstration of serotonin, secretin, or substance P (191). They are also increased in Barrett's and intestinal metaplastic mucosae (192) and in the colonic mucosa of patients with ulcerative colitis, the significance of which is not clear (193).

Enterochromaffin-like (ECL) cell hyperplasia occurs in the atrophic fundic mucosa of patients with pernicious anemia (194) and to a lesser extent in the otherwise normal fundic mucosa of individuals with the Zollinger-Ellison syndrome or primary G-cell hyperplasia secondary to the trophic effect of gastrin (195). These cells are argyrophilic but do not manifest any immunohistochemically demonstrable peptide or endocrine product.

Hyperplasia of G cells may occur as a result of a variety of conditions, some of which are associated with hypochlorhydria such as fundic atrophic gastritis, antral exclusion, truncal vagotomy, and H-2 blocker or proton pump inhibitor therapy (190). The persistent

TABLE 5.1	Immunohistochemical Detection of Cellular Origin of Undifferentiated Neoplasms	
Antigen	Tumor Type
Cytokeratin (CK)	Carcinoma
Leukocyte common antigen (LCA)	Lymphoma
S-100 protein (S-100)	Neural/melanoma
Vimentin (VIM)	Soft tissue

TABLE

5.3   Gastrointestinal Tract Neuroendocrine Cells: Product and Location

Endocrine Cell Type	Product	Fundus	Antrum	Duodenum	Intestines
G	Gastrin	−	+	+	−
D	Somatostatin	+	+	+	+
EC	Substance P	−	−	+	+
EC	5-HT	−	−	+	+
ECL	Unknown	+	−	−	−
Unknown	VIP	+	+	+	+
I	Cholecystokinin	−	−	+	+
L	Enteroglucagon	−	−	+	+
K	GIP	−	−	+	+
Unknown	Bombesin	−	+	+	−
S	Secretin	−	−	+	+
PP	Pancreatic polypeptide	−	−	+	+

lack of intraluminal gastric acid leads to a continuous gastrin mediated stimulus to G-cell proliferation. In rare instances, the number of G cells increases in the absence of associated predisposing conditions, a condition known as primary G-cell hyperplasia (196). Greater numbers of antral G cells are seen in the middle one third of the mucosa and are identifiable immunohistochemically by the presence of intracellular gastrin (Fig. 5.10). Increased numbers of fundic mucosal endocrine cells, which are immunoreactive for the α-subunit of HCG, have also been reported in patients with hypergastrinemia owing to any cause (197).

A rare instance of somatostatin cell hyperplasia has been recognized by the immunohistochemical demonstration of increased numbers of somatostatin-containing cells in the mucosa of the stomach and duodenum (198).

CARCINOID TUMORS

Carcinoid tumors are classified into foregut, midgut, and hindgut types based on their embryonic origin (199). Notably, the immunohistochemical profile of gastrointestinal carcinoid tumors is extremely variable. In some situations, the tumor is composed of cells showing *(a)* a single hormone or peptide, such as a gastrinoma; *(b)* a multihormonal or peptide pattern within the tumor cells; or *(c)*

TABLE

5.4   Gastrointestinal Neuroendocrine Proliferations

Hyperplasia	Neoplasia
Gastrin (G) cell	Carcinoid tumors
Enterochromaffin-like (ECL) cell	Neuroendocrine
Enterochromaffin (EC) cell	Carcinoma
Somatostatin (D) cell	Mixed endocrine/exocrine tumors

a completely negative immunohistochemical pattern (200). In addition, the tumor may demonstrate the following: immunohistochemical markers similar to those seen in the normal mucosa overlying the tumor (201), markers not normally encountered at that mucosal site (200), or immunodetectable peptides, such as vasoactive intestinal peptide (VIP), which are not normally identified within gastrointestinal endocrine cells (202).

In general, specific hormonal peptides such as gastrin are encountered in foregut carcinoids, serotonin and substance P are found in midgut carcinoids, and enteroglucagon and pancreatic polypeptide are noted in hindgut carcinoids (200, 203). Immunohistochemical demonstration of specific hormones or peptides in tumors may correlate well with the clinical presentation and behavior, such as occurs with serotonin- or gastrin-containing tumors, but frequently, no clinical manifestations are attributable to the immunohistochemically detected hormonal or peptide factors in the tumor. It is emphasized that immunohistochemical findings in carcinoid tumors do not distinguish between benign and malignant tumors and have no prognostic significance.

Although relatively uniform in their histologic appearance, foregut carcinoids, other than those in the esophagus (most of which are neuroendocrine [oat cell] carcinomas), are heterogeneous in terms of histochemical, immunohistochemical, and ultrastructural features (204). Gastric carcinoids may be the result of ECL cell hyperplasia and fundic atrophy (194) or they may occur spontaneously (205) with or without the atypical carcinoid syndrome (206). They usually show 5-hydroxytryptophan rather than serotonin and, immunohistochemically, may manifest gastrin or ACTH (207). Their distinction from glomus tumors is facilitated by the smooth muscle actin and factor VIII-related antigen immunoreactivity seen in these tumors (208).

In the duodenum, the most frequently encountered carcinoid tumors are the small gastrinomas, which cause 13% of the cases of Zollinger-Ellison syndrome (209), and the larger, histologically unique psammomatous somatostatinomas, which do not manifest clinical hormonal expression but may be associated with multiple endocrine neoplasia (MEN) and von Recklinghausen's syndromes (210).

The cytologically more homogeneous midgut carcinoids are most common in the ileum and appendix, are associated with the carcinoid syndrome in 20% of cases, and show the typical ultrastructural features of EC cells (211). Immunohistochemically, these tumors characteristically express serotonin and substance P (212). Less commonly, immunodetection reveals other secretory products, including calcitonin, somatostatin, gastrin, ACTH, enteroglucagon, and VIP (200, 213).

Hindgut carcinoids are most frequent in the rectosigmoid region (214), may be histologically atypical, with increased mitoses, and are aggressive. They usually are nonreactive with silver stains and do not show uniform ultrastructural features, reflected in the diverse immunohistochemical expression of multiple peptides, including enteroglucagon, pancreatic polypeptide, substance P, and somatostatin, although their presence usually remains clinically silent (215).

MIXED ENDOCRINE/EXOCRINE TUMORS

Small numbers of endocrine cells are commonly seen in gastrointestinal carcinomas and may be associated with a poorer prognosis (216, 217). Reciprocally, endocrine tumors may show focal areas of squamous or glandular differentiation (218, 219). From this background, recognition of tumors composed of mixed endocrine and exocrine cell populations has become established (220, 221). The term mixed/composite tumors is reserved for those lesions of which at least one third is composed of endocrine cells.

One variant, known as goblet cell carcinoid (adenocarcinoid), is seen most often in the appendix, although it can occur elsewhere in the GI tract. These lesions are composed of mucin-secreting and endocrine cells that are immunoreactive for serotonin. They are intermediate between the usual carcinoid tumor and adenocarcinoma in terms of aggressive behavior (222).

The other variant, the adenoendocrine carcinoma, also occurs throughout the GI tract (220) and histologically resembles ordinary adenocarcinoma. At least one third of the tumor cells are of neuroendocrine type and are either scattered or found in discrete areas within the tumor (223); occasionally, they are associated with a significant desmoplastic reaction (224). The presence of immunoreactive gastrin, serotonin, somatostatin, and calcitonin has been

reported (221, 223). The behavior of these tumors, however, is similar to that of ordinary adenocarcinoma from the same region of the alimentary tract, and so the immunohistochemical findings in these tumors have no prognostic significance.

PARAGANGLIOMA

Paragangliomas are rare primary tumors of the GI tract, but they may infiltrate from extraintestinal sites. These tumors express synaptophysin, chromogranin, neuron-specific enolase, and neurofilament but do not manifest cytokeratins, which distinguishes them from the keratin-positive carcinoid tumors and neuroendocrine carcinomas. It has been suggested that benign paragangliomas are frequently positive for S-100 protein and glial fibrillary acidic protein in contrast to the malignant variant, which usually fails to express these two proteins (225). The rare duodenal gangliocytic paraganglioma may express immunohistochemically a large number of hormonal polypeptides without clinical evidence of their production (226).

NEUROENDOCRINE CARCINOMAS

Neuroendocrine (small cell, oat cell) carcinomas have been recorded in the stomach (227), duodenum (228), small bowel (229), colon (230, 231), and most frequently in the esophagus (218). The characteristic histologic appearance seen in pulmonary tumors is replicated in gastrointestinal neoplasms. In addition to focal argyrophilia, at least some tumor cells manifest multiple peptide hormones, including vasoactive intestinal peptide, calcitonin, and adrenocorticotropic hormone (228). Diagnostic application of these immunohistochemical markers is rarely required because the histologic appearance is characteristic and the tumor peptide hormone content invariably remains clinically inapparent. Nevertheless, in the colon, distinction between neuroendocrine carcinomas and poorly or undifferentiated carcinomas, which show lesser degrees of immunohistochemically detectable endocrine markers, is important because of the more dismal prognosis of colonic neuroendocrine carcinomas (231).

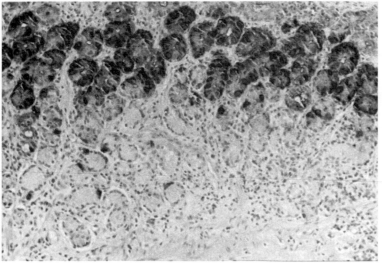

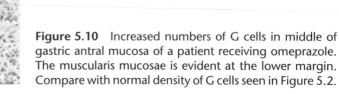

Figure 5.10 Increased numbers of G cells in middle of gastric antral mucosa of a patient receiving omeprazole. The muscularis mucosae is evident at the lower margin. Compare with normal density of G cells seen in Figure 5.2.

TABLE 5.5 | Gastrointestinal B-Cell Lymphoma Immunohistochemical Profile

	Low-Grade MALToma	High-Grade MALToma	Burkitt's Lymphoma	Lymphomatous Polyposis	Follicular Center Cell Lymphoma	Chronic Lymphocytic Leukemia
Pan B	+	+	+	+	+	+
Surface IG	+ (M)	+	+ (M)	+ (M)	+	± (M)
Cytoplasmic Ig	±	+	–	–	–	(M)
CD45	+	+	+	+	+	+
CD23	+	–			±	+
CD35	+			+	–	
CD5	–	–	–	+	–	+
CD10	–	±	+	±	±	–
bcl-2	+	–			±	

LYMPHOPROLIFERATIVE DISORDERS

Gastrointestinal lymphoproliferative disorders are fairly common and are derived from the extensive lymphoid tissue in the normal or chronically inflamed alimentary tract. Recent developments in the genotypic and immunophenotypic expression of the lymphoproliferative disorders have greatly facilitated the distinction between lymphoid hyperplasia and malignant lymphoma and the development of an improved classification of gastrointestinal lymphomas (Table 5.5) (232).

Lymphoid hyperplasias occur as focal or diffuse lesions from the esophagus (233) to the rectum (234) and include the increase in gastric lymphoid follicles associated with *Helicobacter pylori*-associated chronic active gastritis and with gastric peptic ulcer, or with the adult form of focal lymphoid hyperplasia of the small intestine, which may resemble MALT lymphoma histologically. The polytypic immunoexpression of immunoglobulin light chains by the lymphoplasmacytic infiltrate separates these hyperplastic lesions from the monotypic pattern seen in malignant lymphomas.

A variety of primary extranodal lymphomas involve the GI tract (Table 5.6). Involvement of the gut by other lymphomas is also recognized as a rare occurrence.

LOW-GRADE MALTOMA

Low-grade MALTomas occur most frequently in the stomach, with rare examples in the intestines. They consist of polymorphous infiltrates of mature, monocytoid B, small cleaved lymphocytes; plasma cells; blast forms; and lymphoplasmacytoid cells. The characteristic lymphoepithelial lesions and reactive lymphoid follicles are occasionally colonized by the malignant cell infiltrate (235). Immunohistochemically, surface and cytoplasmic immunoglobulin, mostly IgM, with light chain restriction, pan B-cell markers, and Bcl-2 protein are expressed; neither CD5 nor CD10 are expressed. The complete or residual component of the follicular centers can be detected by CD23 and CD35, which identify the dendritic cell population of these centers.

HIGH-GRADE T- OR B-CELL LYMPHOMA

These aggressive tumors account for more than one half of adult gastrointestinal lymphomas. In the Western world, most are considered to derive from low-grade MALTomas, whereas in the Middle East, many are derived from immunoproliferative small intestinal disease (IPSID).

Histologically, it may be difficult if not impossible to distinguish primary gastrointestinal from primary nodal high-grade lymphoma, which secondarily involves the GI tract. The presence of lymphoepithelial lesions and residual follicles suggest the former origin. They are composed of large noncleaved cells and numerous multinucleated forms with large round vesicular nuclei showing numerous nucleoli. Immunohistochemically, they may show T-cell or B-cell lineage. The latter manifest cytoplasmic immunoglobulin in some cases and may express lymphocyte homing receptor CD44 and other adhesion molecules. The bcl-2 protein, which is usually expressed in follicular center cell lymphomas, is not seen in high-grade MALTomas (236).

The different histologic appearances for diffuse mixed, diffuse large-cell, or immunoblastic lymphomas confer no prognostic significance to this group of tumors. The immunophenotypically

TABLE 5.6 | Primary Gastrointestinal Non-Hodgkin's Lymphoma

B Cell	T Cell
Low-grade MALToma	Enteropathy-associated lymphoma
High-grade MALToma	Other
Immunoproliferative small intestinal disease (IPSID) (α-heavy chain disease)	
Lymphomatous polyposis (Mantle cell zone lymphoma)	
Burkitt's-(like)	
Other	

identified diffuse large T-cell lymphoma has the worst prognosis. Variable immunohistochemical expression of CD30, p53, and HLA-DR proteins is noted in all the various histologic subtypes, the prognostic significance of which is not yet established. Discordance between genotypic and immunophenotypic p53 expression and lack of understanding of the role that drug resistance mechanisms play in these tumors further limits the identification of valuable prognostic factors in diffuse large-cell lymphoma (237).

IMMUNOPROLIFERATIVE SMALL INTESTINAL DISEASE (IPSID)

Now recognized for 30 years (238), this variant of MALT lymphoma, which is associated with malabsorption in young adults, occurs predominantly in Middle Eastern populations. It is composed of a lymphoplasmacytic and centrocytic-like infiltrate of the small intestinal mucosa with lymphoepithelial lesions, colonization of follicles, and plasma cell differentiation. In contrast to light chain synthesis by other lymphomas, immunoglobulin A α-heavy chains are synthesized by and immunohistochemically detectable in plasma cells, centrocyte-like cells, and transformed blast forms (239).

BURKITT'S LYMPHOMA

Gastrointestinal Burkitt's lymphoma, common in children in Africa, is an aggressive small, noncleaved cell lymphoma that involves the ileocecal region. The tumor is composed of cells with round to oval nuclei, showing clumped nuclear chromatin, multiple (two to five) nucleoli, and scant basophilic cytoplasm containing multiple cytoplasmic lipid vacuoles best appreciated on cell smears. Interspersed are multiple tingible body macrophages, which provide the "starry-sky" pattern. Immunohistochemically, the tumor cells show pan-B-cell markers, surface immunoglobulins (predominantly IgM), and κ- or λ-light chain restriction. They are positive for the common ALL antigen (CD10) and negative for CD5, which helps to distinguish them from mantle zone B cell lymphoma cells. They are also negative for TdT, a marker of lymphoid precursor cells, which distinguishes them from TdT positive lymphoblastic lymphoma cells.

LYMPHOMATOUS POLYPOSIS

This uncommon disease of Western adults manifests as multiple small, grey-white polyps throughout the GI tract. The polyps are composed of nodules of lymphoma cells that replace the mantle zones and occasionally entrap reactive follicle centers within them. The nodules consist of a uniform population of small/medium-sized lymphocytes that show irregular nuclei devoid of prominent nucleoli and minimal cytoplasm (centrocytes) (240) identical to that seen in systemic mantle zone lymphoma (241). Usual findings include positive immunohistochemical expression of pan-B cell markers, surface immunoglobulin showing light chain restriction, and CD5 with negative CD10 and CD23. Strong expression of CD35 and CD43 has been noted also.

In 1992, bcl-1 gene rearrangement, the characteristic molecular lesion of mantle cell lymphoma (242), was detected in approximately one third of multiple lymphomatous polyposis cases studied (243). These authors also noted overexpression of the cyclin D1 protein, also characteristic of mantle cell lymphoma (244), in more than 75% of the multiple lymphomatous polyposis cases. In contrast,

none of the MALT lymphomas studied showed any of these changes. These observations, in addition to further supporting the centrocytic (mantle cell) nature of multiple lymphomatous polyposis, provide further diagnostic means by which to distinguish these different primary gastrointestinal lymphomas with significantly different prognoses.

FOLLICULAR (CENTER CELL) LYMPHOMA

Secondary involvement of the GI tract by nodal lymphoma has been reported (245, 246). Primary gastrointestinal follicular center (nodal type) lymphoma is rare and shows a follicular, diffuse, or mixed histologic pattern with an immunophenotypic profile similar to that seen in peripheral lymph node follicular lymphomas. When MALTomas colonize hyperplastic lymphoid follicles, distinction between them and follicular lymphomas may be difficult. In such circumstances, immunohistochemical profiles, which include bcl-2, CD5, and CD10 markers, are helpful.

AIDS-ASSOCIATED LYMPHOMA

The GI tract, in particular the small bowel and anorectum, is the commonest site of AIDS-related lymphomas. They are B-cell, large, immunoblastic, or Burkitt's-like lymphomas with a dismal prognosis. The immunophenotype in the Burkitt's-like variant is composed of the monotypic expression of surface immunoglobulin (IgM) and CD10 positivity without EBV receptor expression. In the more immature variants, the CD10 and EBV receptor expression is reversed and, on occasion, they may be immunophenotypically unidentifiable as B-cell lymphomas.

POSTTRANSPLANT LYMPHOPROLIFERATIVE DISORDER (PTLD)

The GI tract is one of the common sites of extranodal PTLD, the lesions of which are of B-cell origin. They may be monomorphous, composed of atypical lymphocytes, or polymorphous, consisting of a mixture of small and large lymphocytes, lymphoplasmacytoid cells, and immunoblasts. Because these lymphomas may be monoclonal, polyclonal, or of mixed clonality, this feature cannot be used to accurately predict outcome.

Immunohistochemically, they may express either polyclonal or monoclonal surface and cytoplasmic immunoglobulins or they may not express any immunoglobulins. In addition to HLA-DR expression, the B-cells express EBV gene products (EBNA-2,3) (247) and cell adhesion molecules, including lymphocyte function antigens (LFA-1), intercellular adhesion molecule-1 (1CAM-1), and activation markers (CD23).

ENTEROPATHY-ASSOCIATED T-CELL LYMPHOMA (EATCL)

This tumor is usually, but not always, associated with celiac disease (248). It has a poor prognosis and usually occurs as ulcerative lesions in the jejunum. These polymorphous, high-grade T-cell lesions are composed of atypical lymphocytes, histiocytes, and eosinophils. Immunophenotypic expression comprises CD3, CD7, and variable CD8 positivity, with CD4 and TdT negativity. Immunohistochemical expression of human mucosal lymphocyte-1 (HML-1) in these tumors reflects their origin from intraepithelial T lymphyocytes (249). CD30 expression may be seen in cases manifesting large multinucleated and immunoblast type cells.

NATURAL KILLER CELL LYMPHOMA

The natural killer subset of T cells has been identified immunohistochemically in fresh-frozen tissue sections using the CD56 neural cell adhesion molecule, and also as the characteristic cells of the rare extranodal T/NK-cell lymphomas, including those in the GI tract (250, 251). With the use of antigen retrieval techniques, a CD56 antibody (123C3) can be demonstrated immunohistochemically in paraffin-embedded tissue (252, 253), thereby expanding the tumor's immunophenotype to CD2+, CD3-, and CD56+ with a strong EBV association.

GRANULOCYTIC SARCOMA

Gastrointestinal granulocytic sarcoma develops in 13% of myeloproliferative disorders (254). These lesions are distinguished from lymphomas by the characteristic sheets of atypical mononuclear cells of the myeloid series that are lysozyme and chloroacetate esterase positive (255) and immunoreactive for myeloperoxidase (256).

SOFT TISSUE TUMORS

Benign mesodermal tumors may be found throughout the gastrointestinal tract. The most common are of vascular, smooth muscle, adipose, and neural tissue origin, with some others of indeterminate origin and behavior, termed "gastrointestinal stromal tumors." Sarcomas are rare primary gastrointestinal lesions. Those of extraintestinal origin usually have spread directly from contiguous organs or from the retroperitoneum to involve the intestine.

Among the stromal cells and the tumors that are derived from them, vascular endothelium is factor VIII-related antigen, actin, and CD34 (257) positive; ganglion cell and nerve tissue is neurofilament and S-100 protein positive; and the smooth muscle of vascular walls and the muscularis is desmin and smooth muscle actin positive. In addition, vimentin can be detected in most mesenchymal cell types of the GI tract, including fibroblasts and smooth muscle, nerve, and endothelial cells (see Fig. 5.1). In fact, because of its pervasive presence in soft tissues and its sensitivity to formalin exposure, vimentin has been proposed as the universal positive tissue control (258).

There are exceptions to these general patterns of stromal cell immunoreactivity. Keratin positivity may be seen in mesodermal tumors (259, 260), and vimentin has been demonstrated in lymphoma, malignant melanoma (261), and some poorly differentiated carcinomas (262). In addition, CD34 (human progenitor cell antigen) has been reported in benign nerve sheath and gastrointestinal epithelioid smooth muscle tumors (263).

MESENCHYMAL TUMORS

Mesenchymal stromal tumors, both benign and malignant, may possess (a) clearly defined morphologic features that characterize them as being of adipose, smooth muscle, neural, or vascular origin; (b) specific histologic patterns, such as granular cell or glomus tumors; or (c) gross appearances that differ from those of the typical leiomyoma or neurofibroma, with nondefined histologic or cellular differentiation and indeterminate biologic behavior (264). In this discussion, the more usual immunophenotypic patterns are emphasized while recognizing that many of these lesions may show aberrant antigenic expression.

ADIPOSE TUMORS

Both lipomas, which do not usually present diagnostic problems, and liposarcomas may show S-100 immunoreactivity (265).

MUSCLE TUMORS

The immunohistochemical markers indicating the myogenic nature of tumors are the contractile proteins known as actins, especially muscle specific actin (HHF35); an intermediate filament known as desmin; and myoglobin. Desmin detection is better in frozen than in formalin-fixed paraffin-embedded tissues, the latter often requiring enzyme digestion to optimize results. Myoglobin, produced by mature skeletal muscle, is not frequently demonstrable in anaplastic skeletal muscle tumors. As a result, actin antibody is more appropriate for the identification of muscle tumors, especially when poorly differentiated or undifferentiated. The classic leiomyoma is frequently immunoreactive for desmin and smooth muscle actin (HHF35) (260, 266). Desmin, when diffuse, is characteristic of all

TABLE								
5.7	**Comparative Immunohistochemistry of Tumors of Neural Origin**							
	S-100	Vimentin	Leu 7	Myelin Basic Protein	Type IV Collagen	Epithelial Markers	Histiocytic Markers	Neurone-specific Enolase
Neurilemmoma	+	+	+	+	+	−	−	+
Neurofibroma	+foc	+	+	+	−	−	−	+
Granular cell tumor	+	+	−	−	−	−	+	+
Malignant schwannoma	±	+	+	+	−	−	−	−
Chordoma	+	+				+		−
Malignant melanoma	+	+				−		

benign smooth muscle tumors, but it is seen in less than one half of leiomyosarcomas (267). When desmin is present focally, myofibroblastic proliferations should be considered.

Monoclonal antibodies to muscle actin epitopes, the most common of which is HHF35, are detectable in all types of muscle (266) as well as in myofibroblasts, pericytes, and myoepithelial cells. Their presence indicates a less than complete specificity for smooth muscle fibers, although they are usually helpful in distinguishing between smooth muscle and neural tumors of the gut.

The primitive stromal cell tumors, in addition to having ultrastructural features that do not permit identification of their cell of origin, have controversial immunohistochemical findings. In several investigations, most tumors were vimentin positive but showed no uniform expression of either desmin or S-100 protein (268–270). Ma et al. (271) noted smooth muscle actin in as many as 60% of cases, but almost no desmin reactivity in the tumors they studied. The immunohistochemical profile of this primitive stromal cell tumor group appears to be heterogeneous, provides little histogenetic information, and is of no value in distinguishing benign from malignant variants.

NEURAL TUMORS

Most neural tumors that affect the GI tract are benign and consist of neurilemmomas and neurofibromas. Both of these lesions show no immunohistochemical evidence of epithelial antigens, but do manifest vimentin, Leu 7, myelin basic protein (272, 273), and focal glial fibrillary acidic protein immunohistochemical positivity. In addition, some neurofibromas and virtually all neurilemmomas are S-100 protein positive, showing nuclear and cytoplasmic reactivity (265). Type IV collagen antibody can be used to demonstrate the prominent basement membrane, a characteristic feature of neurilemmomas. Malignant schwannomas rarely show desmin positivity and are S-100 positive in less than 50% of cases (265). Granular cell tumor, which is rarely seen in the GI tract, is S-100 positive (274), indicating its probable neural origin. This tumor also expresses neurone-specific enolase, vimentin, and α_1-antitrypsin (Table 5.7).

Whereas S-100 protein immunoreactivity is well recognized in malignant melanoma (275), a tumor that is also of putative neural origin, this protein is also immunoreactive in non-neural tumors, including lipoma, liposarcoma, chondroma, chondrosarcoma (265), and some carcinomas (184). This broad spectrum of S-100 protein immunoreactivity emphasizes yet again the value of applying a battery of immunohistochemical stains to the study of diagnostically difficult lesions. Awareness of this aberrant antigen expression, coupled with the technical and artifactual tissue-related changes, is of great value in the proper interpretation of immunohistochemical findings in the mesenchymal tumors involving the GI tract.

Other immunohistochemical neural tissue markers that show considerably less specificity include the γ-subunit of neuron-specific enolase and Leu 7, the natural killer lymphocyte antigen (273), neither of which are superior to S-100 protein in the immunohistochemical evaluation of neural tumors.

GRANULAR CELL TUMOR

Granular cell tumor occurs throughout the GI tract (276) and can present diagnostic difficulty. Taking advantage of their presumed

Schwann cell origin, the diagnosis of granular cell tumors can be established by demonstrating S-100 protein (277); myelin-associated glycoprotein (CD57) using monoclonal antibody HNK-1 (278); vimentin (279); and the lysosome-associated glycoprotein (CD68) (280) that has been reported to occur in schwannomas (281, 282).

VASCULAR TUMORS

Benign vasoformative tumors, including hemangioma, lymphangioma, and arteriovenous malformations, are rarely if ever a histopathologic diagnostic problem in gastrointestinal pathology. On the other hand, both angiosarcoma and Kaposi's sarcoma are often included in the differential diagnosis of undifferentiated or spindle cell tumors. Immunohistochemical markers that are useful and sensitive if not completely specific for vascular tumors are factor VIII-related antigen, the lectin *Ulex europaeus* (283, 284), and the human hematopoietic progenitor cell antigen (CD34) (285). Positive immunostaining pattern with these antigens coupled with the ultrastructural finding of Weibel-Palade bodies in an undifferentiated tumor is strong evidence of its vascular nature.

Most benign vascular tumors express factor VIII-related antigen after enzymatic digestion (286). Recognition that granulation tissue normally expresses factor VIII Rag is always a consideration in the interpretation of ulcerated lesions.

Gastrointestinal involvement by Kaposi's sarcoma occurs in transplant recipients and in approximately 40% of AIDS patients with skin or lymph nodal Kaposi's sarcoma (287). Expression of this antigen in malignant vascular tumors of the GI tract is variable, ranging from negative immunoreactivity in the spindle cell population but positive immunoreactivity in the normal appearing constitutive vascular channels of the submucosal Kaposi's sarcoma lesions (288) to sparse, focal, or complete absence of immunoreactivity in the rarely encountered angiosarcoma.

Other antigens that are immunohistochemically demonstrable in endothelial cell tumors include CD34, CD31, and the blood group isoantigens. CD34, the human progenitor cell antigen, is present in all benign lesions and more than 80% of angiosarcoma and Kaposi's sarcoma (257). It is not specific, however, because it has been noted in a variety of other tumors, including smooth muscle and peripheral nerve sheath tumors (263). CD31 (PECAM-1) has a similar distribution in vascular tumors to that of CD34, but it is more specific, being noted only rarely in other tumors, such as leiomyosarcoma or carcinoma (289). The lectin U. europaeus, which identifies the H antigen of the ABO blood group system, is immunohistochemically more sensitive but significantly less specific than factor VIII-related antigen in the recognition of angiosarcomas (290), which limits its diagnostic applicability.

SARCOMAS

Primary gastrointestinal sarcomas are rare and most commonly are of smooth muscle origin. Even more rare is direct invasion of the GI tract by extraintestinal retroperitoneal sarcomas, such as liposarcoma, chondrosarcoma, malignant fibrous histiocytoma, and rhabdomyosarcoma. Of these four lesions, all are vimentin positive; in addition, the former three are S-100 positive and the latter is myoglobin, actin, and desmin positive. Sacral chordoma, which has the potential to infiltrate the rectum, shows keratin in addition to vimentin and S-100 protein positivity. This tumor is negative for

CEA, however, which helps to distinguish it from mucinous carcinomas and from keratin-negative chondrosarcomas (291).

MISCELLANEOUS GASTROINTESTINAL DISEASES

ESOPHAGEAL BULLOUS DISEASE

The esophagus is rarely involved by bullous dermatologic disease. Pemphigus vulgaris, an acantholytic disease associated with formation of suprabasal bullae, is characterized immunohistochemically by the intercellular deposition of IgG in the squamous epithelium (292). In contrast, the bullae in pemphigoid commence at the subepithelial level and the immunohistochemical expression of IgG is limited to the mucosal basement membrane in linear fashion. Easier biopsy access to skin or oral mucosal tissue usually precludes such study of the esophageal mucosa.

HIRSCHSPRUNG'S DISEASE

This congenital disease of early life is characterized by submucosal neural hypertrophy and, most specifically, the absence of ganglion cells in the affected region of the colorectum. Recognition of the neuron-specific enolase staining of neural elements and S-100 protein staining of Schwann cell elements, which identify the immature ganglioneuronal plexus in these young patients, prevents the erroneous diagnosis of Hirschsprung's disease (293). Loss of immunoreactive VIP, together with acetylcholinesterase and PGP 9.5 staining of the expanded cholinergic nerve fiber network (294, 295), has been documented in the aganglionic segment of Hirschsprung's disease (296). In contrast, the expression of VIP in the neural fibers and in the ganglia of patients with chronic idiopathic pseudoobstruction is increased, but this marker is not sufficiently sensitive or specific to distinguish between these disorders (297).

LANGERHANS' CELL HISTIOCYTOSIS

This disease of pediatric age groups is usually disseminated and rarely involves the GI tract as a primary manifestation (298, 299). The small or large intestine may be involved by a severe diffuse lamina propria infiltrate of histiocytes that express S-100 protein and CD1 immunohistochemically in addition to electronmicroscopic evidence of Birbeck granules. The infiltrate may invade and destroy glands with formation of mucosal ulcers.

DNA CONTENT AND CELL CYCLE ANALYSIS BY FLOW CYTOMETRY

Clinical application for the measurement of nuclear DNA quantity and cell cycle compartments has developed with the advent of practical flow cytometry instrumentation (FCM) (300–302). DNA analysis involves the use of a number of fluorescent dyes that bind stoichiometrically with nuclear DNA in nuclei of individual cells. The principle of DNA analysis is the measurement of the DNA content in numerous (10^4 to 10^5) single cells harvested from solid tumors and the construction of a histogram reflecting the distribution of individual cell DNA content within the study cell population.

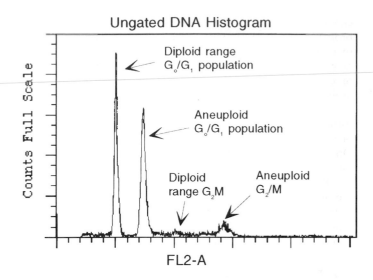

Figure 5.11 Complex histogram comprises an admixture of diploid range and aneuploid cells. The diploid subset may represent normal/non-neoplastic cells or may be mixed with neoplastic diploid range cells. The overlapping cell populations complicate measurement of SPF.

CELL CYCLE ANALYSIS

The distribution of DNA content is primarily in the G0 and G1 phases of the cell cycle, which both contain a normal complement of DNA, representing 46 chromosomes (303, 304) (Figs. 5.11 and 5.12). G0 is the resting phase and G1 is the preliminary phase before the sequence of events leading to cell division. G0 and G1 have the same nuclear DNA content and cannot be separated, although immunostaining identifies a number of gene products separating G0 and G1 phases. In contrast, cells in the G2 and M or mitotic phase contain twice the normal DNA cell content, i.e., 92 chromosomes, which represent the duplication of genetic information required before cell division. The distribution of DNA content of cells in normal tissues consists primarily of cells in G0 and G1 phase with 46 chromosome DNA content (defined as 2N). The second and smaller peak (usually 5 to 15% of the cell population) comprises the second DNA content peak of 92 chromosomes (defined as 4N) and contains cells in G2/M phase. The cells between 2N and 4N peaks are in the process of synthesizing DNA to double the cellular content before cell division; the cells within this compartment are synthesis phase or SPF.

It would be convenient if quantitation of the proportion of the cell population in the G2/M component represented the replicating cell fraction. Although the G2/M component is relatively easy to measure, the cells in this compartment of the cell cycle do not necessarily enter and exit this fraction in a uniform manner that accurately reflects the proliferation of a cell population. As a result, the G2/M component provides a rough estimate but an inaccurate parameter for calculating cell division or proliferation.

CELL PROLIFERATION ANALYSIS

Measurement of cell proliferation is particularly difficult in solid tumors for a variety of reasons. The most accurate method of determining cell proliferation is by incorporating identifiable precursors into the genomic DNA, such as with tritiated thymidine and bromodeoxyuridine (BUdR) (305). The radioisotope, tritiated thymidine, is measured by autoradiographs and BUdR can be detected by immunostaining techniques. Dual labeling at specific time intervals is the most accurate method of measuring cell proliferation, with single labels the next best approach.

Mitotic figures have been incorporated into traditional histo-pathology as an indicator of cell proliferation, but they represent only a rough estimate of the proliferative fraction of solid tumors. Other cytologic indicators include AgNOR and immunostaining for features involved in DNA replication, such as Ki-67. AgNOR and Ki-67 staining have proven to have some predictive value for tumor prognosis, but measurement is tedious, especially in tissue sections. As a result, there have been numerous evaluations of similar approaches but none have received widespread acceptance as an adjunct to routine tumor classification.

HISTOGRAM INTERPRETATION

The two major observations that result from flow cytometric DNA analysis are the presence (or absence) of G0/G1 populations with abnormal DNA content and the quantitation of the SPF compartment (or rarely the SPF and G2/M populations). The former is a measurement of cells in G0/G1 containing abnormal amounts of DNA (aneuploidy). Aneuploidy is a cytogenetic term defined as abnormal chromosomal content—usually increased numbers of complete or portions of chromosomes. The term often appears (erroneously) in the flow cytometry (and image analysis) literature as synonymous with increased cellular DNA content. Measurement of DNA content requires a reference population, usually normal diploid cell populations, such as lymphocytes for comparison, allowing confirmation that an abnormal cell population is present. Most disaggregated solid tumor cell (or nuclear) preparations contain non-neoplastic cells, however, including stroma, inflammatory, and, in many instances, non-neoplastic epithelial cells. The presence of these diploid range cells overlaps the diploid or

"near-diploid" neoplastic cell populations, often obscuring the latter neoplastic cell population (see Fig. 5.11). In addition, measurement of SPF in these overlapping cell populations is potentially misleading. Occasionally cells from chicken or trout are used as they contain less DNA than a human normal diploid cell population, eliminating the problem of overlapping cell populations (306).

The overlapping cell populations remain one of the major problems in interpreting tumor cell DNA content as well as measuring the SPF population. The ratio of DNA cell content in the tumor cell population is compared to normal diploid cells, and this ratio is defined as the DNA index (DI). The DI is calculated as the ratio of the mean channel of the abnormal FCM aneuploid peak divided by the mean channel of the control normal (diploid) G0/G1 peak. The denominator is determined by the use of appropriate control cells known to have a diploid DNA content. To identify the normal peak, the control cell system must be carefully calibrated, because slight shifts in DNA staining occur with different methods of solid tumor disaggregation. We have found that diploid cells in the tumor provide a reliable basis on which to establish the diploid channel.

Minor chromosomal abnormalities involving single chromosomes, such as deletions, translocations, point mutations, and other changes common in neoplasms, may not appreciably change the total cell DNA content (307). In tumors with minor chromosomal abnormalities, identification of DNA content changes depends on the sensitivity and resolution of the histogram. Optimum sample preparation to provide a narrow peak width (low coefficient of variation or CV) for diploid control and tumor cells allows better resolution of peridiploid tumor populations. We define abnormal or aneuploid DNA peaks as second peaks that can be resolved from the known diploid DNA peak. Other investigators use arbitrary definitions such as a 10% difference. The limits of resolution depend on the quality of the sample preparation as reflected by the CV of the normal and abnormal peaks.

CELL SAMPLE PREPARATION

Dissociation and fixation artifacts may alter DNA staining, which mandates careful control of cell populations and preparation by the same procedure as the tumor cell population (308). In many studies, human lymphocytes prepared and stored differently from the cells dissociated from solid tumors are used as controls and they may or may not correspond with diploid non-neoplastic cells from the tumor. The process of dissociation of human tumors has the potential to alter DNA staining characteristics, especially if enzymes are used (309). We strongly recommend handling exogenous diploid control cells and the dissociated tumor cells in similar fashion. In addition, we have found that the number of diploid cells present in human colon cancer is sufficient to determine the diploid standard channel. Ideally, normal diploid non-neoplastic cells within the dissociated tumor serve as the optimum internal diploid standard. When a question arises as to which peak represents the non-neoplastic cells, we can document their location by dual labeling for cytoplasmic keratin or LCA antigens.

Two general approaches have evolved to produce single cell samples suitable for FCM DNA analysis. The most common method is the use of bare nuclei extracted from solid tumors by a combination of detergents and enzymes. This approach was pioneered by Vindelov and is used in many laboratories (310). Similar

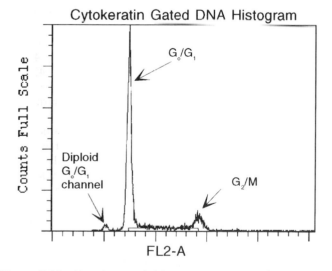

Figure 5.12 Keratin-gated histogram restricts the measurement to epithelial cells. In this example, the host stromal and inflammatory cells are "gated out." The resulting histogram is "cleaner" and allows more accurate SPF determination.

TABLE

5.8   Prospective Flow Cytometry Analysis of Colonic Adenocarcinoma

Authors	Number of Tumors	Colon/Rectum	Diploid Number	(%)	Aneuploid Number	(%)
Wolley et al.[317]	33	33/0	20	(61)	13	(39)
Rognum et al.[318]	85	NS	28	(33)	57	(67)
Banner et al.[319]	56	51/5	14	(25)	42	(75)
Teodori et al.[320]	24	19/5	10	(37)	14	(63)
Melamed et al.[321]	33	20/13	15	(45)	18	(55)
Durrant et al.[322]	31	18/13	20	(65)	11	(35)
Hiddemann et al.[323]	88	45/45[a]	16	(18)	72	(82)
Scott et al.[324]	30	Ns[b]	12	(40)	18	(60)
Emdin et al.[325]	37	22/15	14	(38)	23	(62)
Visscher et al.[313]	74	64/10	26	(35)	48	(65)
Lanza et al.[326]	123	123/0	33	(27)	90	(73)
Armitage et al.[327]	320	209/111	129	(40)	191	(60)
Tang et al.[328]	653	285/368	272	(42)	381	(58)
Chapman et al.[329]	351	234/117	139	(40)	212	(60)
Witzig et al.[330]	694	515/179	353	(51)	341	(49)
TOTAL	2632	1638/881	1101	(42)	1531	(58)

[a] Two squamous carcinomas.

[b] Not specified.

techniques have been suggested for extracting nuclei from paraffin tissue blocks for DNA analysis and include the use of different proteases with varying digestion times. At present, the most popular protocol is one proposed by Hedley et al. (311).

A second method for preparation of samples for FCM analysis is to produce suspensions of intact cells by either enzymatic digestion or mechanical dissociation. This approach is more difficult because the disruption of desmosomes or other cell-cell attachments requires great care. In many instances, only portions of the cytoplasm remain and the injured cells are not viable.

TABLE

5.9   Patient Outcome Related to DNA Content

Authors	Number of Cases	Colon/Rectum	Survivor Total (%) Diploid	Aneuploid	Follow Up
Wolley et al.[317]	33	33/0	14/20 (70)	0/13 (0)	2–3 years survival
Melamed et al.[321]	33	20/13	8/15 (53)	12/18 (67)	2–3 years survival
Emdin et al.[325]	37	22/15	12/14 (86)[a]	10/20 (60)	Mean follow up, 30.4 months
Armitage et al.[327]	134	NA	27/62 (44)	14/72 (19)	Survival minimum 5 years
Kokal et al.[331]	77	47/30	24/24 (100)	34/53 (64)	Disease-free minimum survival 5 years
Scott et al.[324]	121	0/121	38/61 (62)	24/51 (47)	Survival minimum 15 years
Schutte et al.[332b]	279	NA	79/105 (75)	85/174 (49)	Survival minimum 5 years
Visscher et al.[313]	95	95/0[c]	34/56 (61)	20/39 (51)	Survival minimum 5 years
Armitage et al.[327]	236	152/84	71/94 (76)	90/142 (63)	Disease-free survival minimum 2 years
Tang et al.[328]	653	285/368	180/272 (66)	225/381 (59)	Survival 10 years
Chapman et al.[329]	258		79/104 (76)	98/154 (64)	5 years
Witzig et al.[330]	694	515/179	229/353 (65)	181/341 (53)	5 years
TOTAL	2650	1188/988	761/1131 (67)	762/1404 (54)	

[a] Two patients progressing; both have wound recurrences.

[b] Calculated from survival curves.

[c] Confined to right colon, stages A and B.

One critical issue in any dissociation technique is whether the resulting nuclear or cellular suspension is truly representative of the tumor population. As obvious as this statement appears, few investigators have performed appropriate studies to define the efficiency of extraction and to determine if the recovered cells are representative of the cell components comprising the tumor. Nuclear suspensions are technically less difficult and time consuming to prepare, but discrimination of diploid tumor from contaminating inflammatory and stromal nuclei is difficult or impossible to achieve. In addition, the possibility of applying multiparameter analyses using cytoplasmic or cell membrane markers is lost.

Mechanical disaggregation of most adenocarcinomas, including colonic adenocarcinomas, to produce intact cells is a relatively simple procedure that is an attractive alternative to enucleation procedures. We recommend quality control procedures for this method in each laboratory, however, to ensure that the dissociated cells are representative of the tumor (309).

MULTIPLE MARKERS

The ability of the flow cytometer to quantitate multiple markers has prompted the use of secondary tissue-specific markers for solid tumors to allow electronic gating to select defined cell populations. In suspensions of intact cells, it is possible to use a variety of dual labeling techniques to cytoplasmic antigens for better definition of tumor cell populations and, by electronic gating, to restrict the DNA analysis to tumor cells (303, 310, 313).

The ultimate goal of observing multiple parameters is to identify tumor cells subsets, to restrict the DNA analysis to tumor cells, and to exclude contaminating host cell components. This effort results in "clean" nonoverlapping histogram peaks of defined cell populations with better resolution of tumor DNA content and more accurate SPF calculations by excluding the dilutional effect of non-neoplastic cells and the overlap of diploid and aneuploid DNA histograms (see Fig. 5.12).

No true tumor-specific markers for epithelial-derived neoplasms are currently available. In our laboratory, we use antibodies directed to keratin intermediate filaments to discriminate epithelial cells. Although discrimination between normal and neoplastic epithelial cells is not possible on this basis, normal host stroma and inflammatory cells can be excluded from the DNA analysis. In colon carcinomas, the inflammatory component can be significant, diluting malignant diploid populations. This effect becomes of increasing importance if SPF measurements are planned. Even when the tissue is selected by a pathologist, the disaggregated cells represent a combination of normal and neoplastic epithelial cells and substantial numbers of host stromal and inflammatory cells. The latter do not stain with antibodies to keratin but can be identified by antibodies directed to the leukocyte common antigen epitope.

We recently compared the disaggregation of fresh surgical specimens and formalin-fixed paraffin-embedded colon carcinomas (309). We examined mechanical versus enzymatic disaggregation methods, cell fixation parameters, nuclear extraction from paraffin blocks, and keratin gating of intact epithelial cells to exclude the abundant inflammatory and stromal cells associated with colon adenocarcinomas. These parameters were initially evaluated using established diploid and aneuploid murine colon adenocarcinoma lines grown in syngeneic mice. This use of established lines permitted the comparison of results in sequential studies, including

comparing cell yields and efficiency of dissociation techniques. Once optimum conditions were identified for the animal models, we studied a series of 30 human colon carcinomas for comparison of fresh and formalin-fixed, paraffin-embedded disaggregation techniques. The aneuploid murine colon adenocarcinoma line (#36-A) was best dissociated by mechanical means, with approximately 40% of the recovered cells being aneuploid. The remaining cells presumably represented stromal and inflammatory (diploid) populations. Enzyme (collagenase, class III) dissociation resulted in tumor cell yields that were approximately one half those achieved by mechanical methods. This observation is important because mechanical disaggregation is simpler and requires less time to prepare.

Comparison of 30 fresh, mechanically disaggregated human colon adenocarcinomas with formalin-fixed and paraffin-embedded tissues from the same tumors revealed a decreased detection of aneuploid cells in the latter group. Twenty-two aneuploid human colonic adenocarcinomas were detected by analysis of fresh intact cells, but only 17 were reportedly aneuploid by the standard Hedley analysis of corresponding paraffin-embedded tumor. The analysis of nuclei retrieved from paraffin often resulted in poor quality histograms (wide CV) with less sensitivity in the detection of peridiploid DNA peaks. Small populations of aneuploid cells can also be masked by debris, especially when the number of aneuploid cells is low.

PROGNOSIS AND CELL DNA MEASUREMENT

Initial reports concluded that the clinical prognostic value of DNA measurements in colorectal cancer was promising. Consensus on the clinical utility of DNA measurements in colorectal neoplasia, however, has not been demonstrated (313, 314). Although aneuploidy is correlated with clinical parameters, such as Dukes' stages, careful statistical analysis of follow up is lacking from much of the published data (314, 315). Tumors arising from the distal bowel and rectum are clinically, epidemiologically, and possibly biologically different from right-sided bowel tumors, with the former having a higher incidence of DNA aneuploidy (316). Individual studies are extremely difficult to compare because of variations in selection of cases, particularly by stage, in follow-up intervals, and in flow cytometric techniques. In 1989, we published an extensive review of the literature on DNA measurements in colorectal carcinomas, concluding the following. First, many series were missing critical data, not allowing comparisons to other series. Second, in the 491 patients we thought were carefully studied, 64.4% of the cases were aneuploid. Third, the frequency of aneuploidy was higher in advanced stage tumors. Finally, patients with diploid range tumors had a better survival but the data were variable and, as a result, not conclusive.

Numerous studies since our review have not changed our initial impressions. An extensive review of the clinical relevance of prognostic markers in colorectal cancer reported by the College of American Pathologists in 1995 has similar conclusions (315), among which is that DNA ploidy is a weak independent prognostic marker. They likewise concluded that sampling and technical issues clouded many of the studies, not allowing valid comparisons.

Interestingly, this retrospective analysis was more positive about the potential for cell proliferation measurements, concluding that they had the potential to be a powerful predictor of outcome (315). Both studies provide extensive bibliographies for further study (314, 315) (Tables 5.8 and 5.9).

REFERENCES

1. Coons AH, Creech HJ, Jones RN. Immunological properties of an antibody containing a fluorescent group. Proc Soc Exp Biol Med 1941;47:200–202.
2. Taylor CR, Burns J. The demonstration of plasma cells and other immunoglobulin containing cells in formalin-fixed, paraffin-embedded tissues using peroxidase-labelled antibody. J Clin Pathol 1974;27:14–20.
3. Huang S-N. Immunohistochemical demonstration of hepatitis B core and surface antigens in paraffin section. Lab Invest 1975; 33:88–95.
4. Fraenkel-Conrat H, Olcott HS. Reaction of formaldehyde with proteins. VI. Crosslinking of amino groups with phenol, imidazole or indole groups. J Biol Chem 1948;174:827–834.
5. Banks PM. Diagnostic applications of an immunoperoxidase method in hematopathology. J Histochem Cytochem 1979;27: 1192–1194.
6. Taylor CR, Shi S-R, Chaiwun B, et al. Strategies for improving the immunohistochemical staining of various intranuclear prognostic markers in formalin paraffin sections. Hum Pathol 1994;25: 263–270.
7. Taylor CR, Shi S-R, Tandon A, et al. Antigen retrieval technique used for immunohistochemistry. Hypothesis principle and application. Mod Pathol 1992;5:121A.
8. Azumi N, Battifora H. The distribution of vimentin and keratin in epithelial and non-epithelial neoplasms. A comprehensive immunohistochemical study on formalin and alcohol fixed tumors. Am J Clin Pathol 1987;88:286–296.
9. Werdin C, Limas C, Knodell RG. Primary malignant melanoma of the rectum. Evidence for origination from rectal mucosal melanocytes. Cancer 1988;61:1364–1371.
10. Kaiserling E, Schaffer R, Weckermann J. Brown bowel syndrome with manifestations in the gastrointestinal tract and thyroid gland. Pathol Res Pract 1988;183:65–74.
11. Hitzman JL, Weiland LH, Oftedahl GL, et al. Ceroidosis in the "brown bowel syndrome." Mayo Clin Proc 1979;54:251–257.
12. West B. Pseudomelanosis duodeni. J Clin Gastroenterol 1988;10: 127–129.
13. Won KH, Ramchaud S. Melanosis of the ileum. Dig Dis Sci 1970;15:57–64.
14. Balasz M. Melanosis coli. Dis Colon Rectum 1986;29:839–844.
15. Walker NI, Bennett RE, Axelsen RA. Melanosis. Am J Pathol 1988;131:465–476.
16. Beckett JH, Bigbee JW. Immunoperoxidase localization of Treponema pallidum. Arch Pathol Lab Med 1979;103:135–138.
17. Wiley EL, Mulhollan TJ, Beck B, et al. Polyclonal antibodies raised against bacillus Calmette-Guerin, Mycobacterium duvalii and Mycobacterium paratuberculosis used to detect mycobacteria in tissue with the use of immunohistochemical techniques. Am J Clin Pathol 1990;94:307–312.
18. Shurbaji MS, Dumler JS, Gage WR, et al. Immunohistochemical detection of chlamydial antigens in association with cystitis. Am J Clin Pathol 1990;93:363–366.
19. Rotterdam H, Sheahan DG, Sommers S. In: Biopsy diagnosis of the digestive tract. 2nd ed. New York: Raven Press, 1993;2: 381–382.
20. Wadell G, Allard A, Svensson L, et al. Enteric adenoviruses. In: Farthing MJG, ed. Viruses and the gut. Proceedings of the 9th British Society of Gastroenterology—International Workshop. London: Smith Kline & French, 1989;70–78.
21. Yunis EJ, Hashida Y. Electron microscopic demonstration of adenovirus in appendix vermiformis in a case of ileocecal intussusception. Pediatrics 1973;51:566–570.
22. Lohr JM, Nelson JA, Oldstone MB. Is herpes simplex virus associated with peptic ulcer disease? J Virol 1990;64:2168–2174.
23. Boulton AJM, Slater DN, Hancock BW. Herpes virus colitis. A new cause of diarrhoea in a patient with Hodgkin's disease. Gut 1982;23: 247–249.
24. Hassanein TI, Shetty B, Gavaler JS, et al. The timing, location and histologic characterization of upper gastrointestinal cytomegalovirus infection occurring in a liver transplant population. Eur J Gastroenterol Hepatol 1993;5:1021–1027.
25. Colina F, Solis JA, Munoz MT. Squamous papilloma of the esophagus. Am J Gastroenterol 1980;74:410–414.
26. Fernandez-Rodriguez CM, Badia-Figuerola N, Ruiz del Arbol L, et al. Squamous papilloma of the esophagus: Report of 6 cases with long-term follow up in four patients. Am J Gastroenterol 1986;81: 1059–1062.
27. Winkler B, Capo V, Reumann W, et al. Human papillomavirus of the esophagus. A clinicopathologic study with demonstration of papillomavirus antigen by the immunoperoxidase technique. Cancer 1985; 55:149–155.
28. Odze R, Upton M, Shocket D, et al. Esophageal squamous papillomas: Clinical-pathologic evaluation and analysis for humanpapillomavirus (HPV) by immunoperoxidase (IP) DNA in situ hybridization (ISH) and polymerase chain reaction (PCR) techniques. Mod Pathol 1992;5:46A.
29. Noffsinger A, Witte D, Fenoglio-Preiser CM. The relationship of human papillomaviruses to anorectal neoplasia. Cancer 1992;70: 1276–1287.
30. Palefsky JM, Holly EA, Gonzales J, et al. Detection of human papillomavirus DNA in anal intraepithelial neoplasia and in anal cancer. Cancer Res 1991;51:1014–1019.
31. Palmer JG, Scholefield JH, Coates PJ, et al. Anal cancer and human papillomaviruses. Dis Colon Rectum 1989;32:1016–1022.
32. Beckmann AM, Daling JR, Sherman KJ, et al. Human papillomavirus infection and anal cancer. Int J Cancer 1989;43:1042–1049.
33. Vincent-Salomon A, de la Rochfordiere A, Salmon R, et al. Frequent association of human papillomavirus 16 and 18 DNA with anal squamous cell and basaloid carcinoma. Mod Pathol 1996;9:614–620.
34. Palefsky JM, Gonzales J, Greenblatt RM, et al. Anal intra-epithelial neoplasia and anal papillomavirus infection among homosexual males with group IV HIV disease. JAMA 1990;263:2911–2916.
35. Wolber R, Dupuis B, Thiyagaratnam P, et al. Anal cloacogenic and squamous carcinomas: Comparative histologic analysis using in situ hybridization for humanpapillomavirus DNA. Am J Surg Pathol 1990;14:176–182.
36. Zaki SR, Judd R, Coffield LM, et al. Human papillomavirus infection and anal carcinoma. Retrospective analysis by in situ hybridization and the polymerase chain reaction. Am J Pathol 1992;140: 1345–1355.
37. Watson AJ, Parkin JM. Jejunal biopsy findings during prodromal stage of measles in a child with coeliac disease. Lancet 1970;2:1134–1135.
38. Sata T, Kurata T, Aoyama Y, et al. Analysis of viral antigens in giant cells of measles pneumonia by immunoperoxidase method. Virchows Arch [A] 1986;410:133–138.
39. McQuaid S, Isserte S, Allan GM, et al. Use of immunocytochemistry and biotinylated in situ hybridization for detecting measles virus in central nervous system tissue. J Clin Pathol 1990;43:329–333.
40. Kotler DP, Gaetz HP, Lange M, et al. Enteropathy associated with the acquired immunodeficiency syndrome. Ann Intern Med 1984;101: 421–428.
41. Gillin JS, Shike M, Alcock N, et al. Malabsorption and mucosal abnormalities of the small intestine in the acquired immunodeficiency syndrome. Ann Intern Med 1985;102:619–622.
42. Ullrich R, Zieitz M, Heise N, et al. Small intestinal structure and function in patients infected with human immunodeficiency virus (HIV): Evidence for HIV-induced enteropathy. Ann Intern Med 1989;111:15–21.
43. Nelson JA, Reynolds-Kohler C, Margaretten W, et al. Human immunodeficiency virus detected in bowel epithelium from patients with gastrointestinal symptoms. Lancet 1988;ii:259–262.
44. Russel B, Beckett JH, Jacobs PH. Immunoperoxidase localization of Sporothrix schenckii and Cryptococcus neoformans. Arch Dermatol 1979;115:433–435.
45. Philips P, Weiner MH. Invasive aspergillosis diagnosed by immunohistochemistry with monoclonal and polyclonal reagents. Hum Pathol 1987;18:1015–1024.
46. Moskowitz LB, Ganjei P, Ziegels-Weissman J, et al. Immunohistological identification of fungi in systemic and cutaneous mycosis. Arch Pathol Lab Med 1986;110:433–436.
47. Klatt EC, Cosgrove M, Meyer PR. Rapid diagnosis of disseminated histoplasmosis in tissues. Arch Pathol Lab Med 1986;110: 1173–1175.

48. Bonnin A, Petrella T, Dubremetz JF, et al. Histopathologic method for diagnosis of cryptosporidiosis using monoclonal antibodies. Eur J Clin Microbiol Infect Dis 1990;9:664–666.
49. Pauwels A, Meyohas MC, Eliaszewicz M, et al. Toxoplasma colitis in the acquired immunodeficiency syndrome. Am J Gastroenterol 1992;87:518–519.
50. Carter TR, Cooper PH, Petri WA, et al. Pneumocystis carinii infection of the small intestine in a patient with acquired immunodeficiency syndrome. Am J Clin Pathol 1988;89:679–683.
51. Cote RJ, Rosenblum M, Telzak EE, et al. Disseminated Pneumocystis carinii infection causing extrapulmonary organ failure. Clinical, pathological and immunohistochemical analysis. Mod Pathol 1990; 3:25–30.
52. Stringer SI, Hudson K, Blase MA, et al. Sequence from ribosomal RNA of Pneumocystis carinii compared to those of four fungi suggests an ascomycetous affinity. J Protozool 1989;36:14S–16S.
53. Edman JC, Kovacs JA, Masur H, et al. Ribosomal RNA sequence shows Pneumocystis carinii to be a member of the fungi. Nature 1988;334:519–522.
54. Perez de Suarez E, Perez-Schael I, Perozo-Ruggeri G, et al. Immunocytochemical detection of Entamoeba histolytica. Trans R Soc Trop Med Hyg 1987;81:624–626.
55. Randall MB, Walker DH. Rocky Mountain spotted fever. Gastrointestinal and pancreatic lesions and rickettsial disease. Arch Pathol Lab Med 1984;108:963–967.
56. Mori M, Matsukuma A, Adachi Y, et al. Small cell carcinoma of the esophagus. Cancer 1989;63:564–573.
57. Johnson FE, Clawson MC, Bashiti HM, et al. Small cell undifferentiated carcinoma of the esophagus. Cancer 1984;53:1746–1751.
58. Chejfec G, Falkmer S, Askensten U, et al. Neuroendocrine tumors of the gastrointestinal tract. Pathol Res Pract 1988;183:143–154.
59. Ellis GL, Langloss JM, Heffner DK, et al. Spindle cell carcinoma of the aerodigestive tract. An immunohistochemical analysis of 21 cases. Am J Surg Pathol 1987;11:335–342.
60. Zarbo RJ, Crissman JD, Venkat H, et al. Spindle cell carcinoma of the upper aerodigestive tract mucosa. An immunologic and ultrastructural study of 18 biphasic tumors and comparison with seven monophasic tumors. Am J Surg Pathol 1986;10.741–753.
61. Gal AA, Martin SE, Kernen JA, et al. Esophageal carcinoma with prominent spindle cells. Cancer 1987;60:2244–2250.
62. Linder J, Stein RB, Roggli VL, et al. Polypoid tumor of the esophagus. Hum Pathol 1987;18:692–700.
63. Cross M, Dexter TM. Growth factors in development, transformation and tumorigenesis. Cell 1991;64:271–280.
64. Tahara E. Growth factors and oncogenes in human gastrointestinal carcinomas. J Cancer Res Clin Oncol 1990;116:121–131.
65. Yoshida K, Kyo E, Tsuda T, et al. EGF and TGF-alpha, the ligands of hyperproduced EGFR in human esophageal carcinoma cells, act as autocrine growth factors. Int J Cancer 1990;45:131–135.
66. Stemmerman G, Heffelfinger SC, Noffsinger A, et al. The molecular biology of esophageal and gastric cancer and their precursors. Hum Pathol 1994;25:968–981.
67. Iihara K, Shiozaki H, Tahara H, et al. Prognostic significance of transforming growth factor-alpha in human esophageal carcinoma. Implication for the autocrine proliferation. Cancer 1993;71:2902–2909.
68. Mukaida H, Toi M, Hirai T, et al. Clinical significance of the expression of epidermal growth factor and its receptor in esophageal cancer. Cancer 1991;68:142–148.
69. Ochiai A, Takanashi A, Takekura M, et al. Effect of human epidermal growth factor on cell growth and its receptor in human gastric carcinoma cell lines. Jpn J Clin Oncol 1988;18:15–25.
70. Yano H, Shiozaki H, Kobayashi K, et al. Immunohistochemical detection of the epidermal growth factor receptor in human esophageal squamous cell carcinoma. Cancer 1991;67:91–98.
71. Al-Kasspooles M, Moore JH, Ottinger MB, et al. Amplification and overexpression of EGFR and erb B-2 genes in human esophageal adenocarcinoma. Int J Cancer 1993;54:213–219.
72. Hollstein MC, Smits AM, Galiana C, et al. Amplification of epidermal growth factor receptor gene but no evidence of Ras mutations in primary human esophageal cancers. Cancer Res 1988;48:5119–5123.
73. Ozawa S, Ueda M, Ando N, et al. High incidence of EGF receptor hyperproduction in esophageal squamous cell carcinoma. Int J Cancer 1987;39:333–337.
74. Filipe MI, Jankowski J. Growth factors and oncogenes in Barrett's esophagus and gastric metaplasia. Endoscopy 1993;25:637–641.
75. Jankowski J, Coghill G, Hopwood D, et al. Oncogenes and oncosuppressor gene in adenocarcinoma of the esophagus. Gut 1992;33:1033–1038.
76. Martin HM, Filipe MI, Morris RW, et al. p53 expression and prognosis in gastric carcinoma. Int J Cancer 1992;50:859–862.
77. Baker SJ, Fearson ER, Nigro JM, et al. Chromosome 17 deletions and p53 gene mutations in colorectal carcinomas. Science 1989;244:217–221.
78. Lane DP. Worrying about p53. Curr Biol 1992;2:581–583.
79. Vogelstein B, Kinzler KW. p53 function and dysfunction. Cell 1992;70:523–526.
80. Bennett WP, Hollstein MC, He A, et al. Archival analysis of p53 genetic and protein alterations in Chinese esophageal cancer. Oncogene 1991;6:1779–1784.
81. Ramel S, Reid BJ, Sanchez CA, et al. Evaluation of p53 protein expression in Barrett's esophagus by two parameter flow cytometry. Gastroenterology 1992;102:1220–1228.
82. Wang LD, Hong JY, Qiu SL, et al. Accumulation of p53 protein in human esophageal precancerous lesions: A possible early biomarker of carcinogenesis. Cancer Res 1993;53:1783–1787.
83. Sasano H, Miyazaki A, Gooukon Y, et al. Expression of p53 in human esophageal cancer: An immunohistochemical study with correlation to proliferating cell nuclear antigen expression. Hum Pathol 1992;23:1238–1243.
84. Younes M, Lebovitz RM, Lechago LV, et al. p53 protein accumulation in Barrett's metaplasia, dysplasia and carcinoma. A follow-up study. Gastroenterology 1993;105:1637–1642.
85. Galiana C, Fusco A, Martel N, et al. Possible role of activated Ras genes in human esophageal carcinogenesis. Int J Cancer 1993;54:978–982.
86. Hollstein MC, Peri L, Mandard AM, et al. Genetic analysis of human esophageal tumors from two high incidence geographic areas: Frequent p53 base substitutions and absence of Ras mutations. Cancer Res 1991;51:4102–4106.
87. Shiga C, Shiga K, Sasano H, et al. A point mutation of c-ki-Ras gene was found in human esophageal carcinoma cell lines but not in primary esophageal carcinomas. Biochem Biophys Res Commun 1992;187:515–521.
88. Abdelatif OMA, Chandler FW, Mills LR, et al. Differential expression of c-myc and H-Ras oncogenes in Barrett's epithelium: A study using colorimetric in situ hybridization. Arch Pathol Lab Med 1991;115:880–885.
89. Houldsworth J, Gordon-Cardo C, Ladanyi M, et al. Gene amplification in gastric and esophageal adenocarcinomas. Cancer Res 1990;50:6417–6422.
90. Gray MR, Hall PA, Nash J, et al. Epithelial proliferation in Barrett's esophagus by proliferating cell nuclear antigen immunolocalization. Gastroenterology 1992;103:1769–1776.
91. Jankowski J, McMenamin R, Hopwood D, et al. Abnormal expression of growth regulatory factors in Barrett's oesophagus. Clin Sci 1991;81:663–668.
92. Poller DN, Steele RJC, Morrell K. Epidermal growth factor receptor expression in Barrett's esophagus. Arch Pathol Lab Med 1992;116:1226–1227.
93. Mori M, Ambe K, Adachi Y, et al. Prognostic value of immunohistochemically identified CEA, SC, AFP and S-100 protein positive cells in gastric carcinoma. Cancer 1988;62:534–540.
94. Ikeda Y, Mori M, Kido A, et al. Immunohistochemical expression of carbohydrate antigen 19-9 in gastric carcinoma. Am J Gastroenterol 1991;86:1163–1166.
95. Sugiyama K, Yonemura Y, Miyazaki I. Immunohistochemical study of epidermal growth factor and epidermal growth factor receptor in gastric carcinoma. Cancer 1985;33:1557–1561.
96. Tahara E, Ito H, Taniyama K, et al. α1-Antitrypsin, α1-antichymotrypsin and α1-macroglobulin in human gastric carcinomas. Hum Pathol 1984;15:957–964.
97. Ishikura H, Fukasawa T, Ogasawara K, et al. An AFP producing gastric carcinoma with features of hepatic differentiation. Cancer 1985;56:840–848.

98. Motoyama T, Saito K, Iwafuchi M. Endodermal sinus tumor of the stomach. Acta Pathol Jpn 1985;39:497.

99. Ramponi A, Angeri G, Arceci F, et al. Gastric choriocarcinoma: An immunohistochemical study. Pathol Res Pract 1986;181:390–396.

100. Wurzel J, Brooks JJ. Primary gastric choriocarcinoma. Cancer 1981; 48:2756–2761.

101. Yonezawa S, Maruyama I, Tanaka S, et al. Immunohistochemical localization of thrombomodulin in chronic diseases of the uterus and choriocarcinoma of the stomach. Cancer 1988;62:569–576.

102. Ooi A, Mai M, Ogino T, et al. Endocrine differentiation of gastric adenocarcinoma. Cancer 1988;62:1090–1104.

103. Yang GCH, Rotterdam H. Mixed (composite) glandular-endocrine cell carcinoma of the stomach. Am J Surg Pathol 1991;15:592–598.

104. Shibata D, Tokunaga M, Uemura T, et al. Association of the Epstein-Barr virus with undifferentiated gastric carcinomas with intense lymphoid infiltration. Lymphoepithelioma-like carcinoma. Am J Pathol 1991;139:469–476.

105. Shin WS, Kang MW, Kang JH, et al. Epstein-Barr virus-associated gastric adenocarcinomas among Koreans. Am J Clin Pathol 1996; 105:174–181.

106. Gulley ML, Pulitzer DR, Eagan PA, et al. Epstein-Barr virus infection is an early event in gastric carcinogenesis and is independent of bcl-2 expression and p53 accumulation. Hum Pathol 1996;27:20–27.

107. Siegal A, Freund U, Gal R. Carcinosarcoma of the stomach. Histopathology 1988;13:350–353.

108. Aiba M, Hirayama A, Suzuki T, et al. Carcinosarcoma of the stomach: Report of a case with review of the literature of gastrectomized patients. Surg Pathol 1991;4:75–83.

109. Wright PA, Quirke P, Attanoos R, et al. Molecular pathology of gastric carcinoma. Hum Pathol 1992;23:848–859.

110. Koshiba M, Ogawa O, Habuchi T, et al. Infrequent Ras mutation in human stomach cancers. Jpn J Cancer Res 1993;84:163–167.

111. Tahara E, Yasui W, Taniyama K, et al. Ha-Ras oncogene product in human gastric carcinoma: Correlation with invasiveness, metastasis or prognosis. Jpn J Cancer Res 1986;77:517–522.

112. Yoshida K, Hamatani K, Koide H, et al. Analysis of Ras gene expression in stomach cancer by anti-Ras p21 monoclonal antibodies. Cancer Detect Prev 1988;12:369–376.

113. Czerniak B, Herz F, Gorczyca W, et al. Expression of Ras oncogene p21 protein in early gastric carcinoma and adjacent gastric epithelia. Cancer 1989;64:1467–1473.

114. Gulbis B, Galand P. Immunodetection of the p21 Ras products in human normal and preneoplastic tissues and solid tumors. Hum Pathol 1993;24:1271–1285.

115. Yamamoto T, Yasui W, Ochiai A, et al. Immunohistochemical detection of c-myc oncogene product in human gastric carcinomas: Expression in tumor cells and stromal cells. Jpn J Cancer Res 1987;78:1169–1174.

116. Ciclitira PJ, Macartney JC, Evan G. Expression of c-myc in non-malignant and premalignant gastrointestinal disorders. J Pathol 1987;151:293–296.

117. Matozaki T, Sakamoto C, Matsuda K, et al. Missense mutations and a deletion of the p53 gene in human gastric cancer. Biochem Biophys Res Commun 1992;182:215–223.

118. Tamura G, Kihana T, Nomura K, et al. Detection of frequent p53 gene mutations in primary gastric cancer by cell sorting and polymerase chain reaction single-strand conformation polymorphism analysis. Cancer Res 1991;51:3056–3058.

119. Starzynska T, Bromley M, Ghosh A, et al. Prognostic significance of p53 overexpression in gastric and colorectal carcinoma. Br J Cancer 1992;66:558–562.

120. Kakeji Y, Maehara Y, Adachi Y, et al. Proliferative activity as a prognostic factor in Borrmann type 4 gastric carcinoma. Br J Cancer 1994;69:749–753.

121. Muller W, Borchard F. Prognostic influence of p53 expression in gastric cancer. J Pathol 1996;178:255–258.

122. Lemoine NR, Jain S, Silvestre F, et al. Amplification and overexpression of the EGF receptor and c-erb-B2 protooncogenes in human stomach cancer. Br J Cancer 1991;64:79–83.

123. Bennett C, Paterson IM, Corbishley CM, et al. Expression of growth factor and epidermal growth factor receptor-encoded transcripts in human gastric tissues. Cancer Res 1989;49:2104–2111.

124. Falck VG, Gullick WJ. c-erb-B2 oncogene product staining in gastric adenocarcinoma. An immunohistochemical study. J Pathol 1989; 159:107–111.

125. Jain S, Filipe MI, Hall PA, et al. Prognostic value of proliferating cell nuclear antigen in gastric carcinoma. J Clin Pathol 1990;44: 655–659.

126. Yonemura Y, Ooyama S, Sugiyama K, et al. Growth fractions in gastric carcinomas determined with monoclonal antibody Ki-67. Cancer 1990;65:1130–1134.

127. Saku T, Sakai H, Tsuda M, et al. Cathepsins D and E in normal, metaplastic, dysplastic and carcinomatous gastric tissue. An immunohistochemical study. Gut 1990;31:1250–1255.

128. Matsuo K, Ieyoshi K, Tsukuba T, et al. Immunohistochemical localization of cathepsins D and E in human gastric cancer. Hum Pathol 1996;27:184–190.

129. Montcourrier P, Mangeat PH, Salazar G, et al. Cathepsin D in breast cancer cell can digest extracellular matrix in large acidic vesicles. Cancer Res 1990;50:6045–6054.

130. Wiggers T, Arends JW, Verstijnen C, et al. Prognostic significance of CEA immunoreactivity patterns in large bowel carcinoma tissue. Br J Cancer 1986;54:409–414.

131. Zamcheck N, Liu P, Thomas P., et al. Search for useful biomarkers of pre or early malignant colonic tumors. Prog Clin Biol Res 1988;279: 251–275.

132. Cutait R, Alves VAF, Lopes LC, et al. Restaging of colorectal cancer based on the identification of lymph node micrometastases through immunoperoxidase staining of CEA and cytokeratins. Dis Colon Rectum 1991;34:917–922.

133. Haboubi NY, Clark P, Kaftan SM, et al. The importance of combining xylene clearance and immunohistochemistry in the accurate staging of colorectal carcinoma. J R Soc Med 1992;85:386–388.

134. Greenson JK, Isenhart CE, Rice R, et al. Identification of occult micrometastases in pericolic lymph nodes of Dukes' colorectal cancer patients using monoclonal antibodies against cytokeratin and CC49. Cancer 1994;73:563–569.

135. Kahn HJ, Yeger H, Loftus R, et al. Monoclonal antibodies to human pancreatic carcinoma cell line recognizes gastrointestinal neoplasms. Am J Pathol 1989;134:641–649.

136. Arends JW, Wiggers T, Verstijnen C, et al. Gastrointestinal cancer-associated antigen (GICA) immunoreactivity in colorectal carcinoma in relationship to patient survival. Int J Cancer 1984;34:193–196.

137. Atkinson BF, Erst CS, Herilyn M, et al. Gastrointestinal cancer associated antigen immunoperoxidase assay. Cancer Res 1982;42: 4820–4823.

138. Hertzog PJ, Pilbrow SJ, Pederson J, et al. Aberrant expression of intestinal mucin antigens associated with colorectal carcinoma defined by a panel of monoclonal antibodies. Br J Cancer 1991;64: 799–808.

139. Vogelstein B, Fearon ER, Hamilton SR, et al. Genetic alterations during colo-rectal tumor development. N Engl J Med 1988;319: 525–532.

140. Teo A, Shaunak S. Polymerase chain reaction in situ: An appraisal of an emerging technique. Histochem J 1995;27:647–659.

141. Bagasara O, Seshamma T, Pomerantz RJ. Polymerase chain reaction in situ: Intracellular amplification and detection of HIV-1 proviral DNA and other specific genes. J Immunol Methods 1993; 158:131–145.

142. Marx J. New colon cancer gene discovered. Science 1993;260: 751–752.

143. Hayashi Y, Widjono YW, Ohta K, et al. Expression of EGF, ECF-receptor, p53, v-erb B and Ras p21 in colorectal neoplasms by immunostaining paraffin-embedded tissues. Pathol Int 1994;44: 124–130.

144. Sun X-F, Hatschek T, Wingren S, et al. Ras p21 expression in relation to histopathological variables and prognosis in colorectal adenocarcinoma. Acta Oncol 1991;30:933–939.

145. Sun X-F, Wingren S, Carstensen JM, et al. Ras p21 expression in relation to DNA ploidy, S-phase fraction and prognosis in colorectal adenocarcinoma. Eur J Cancer 1991;27:1646–1649.

146. Melhem MF, Meisler AI, Finley GG, et al. Distribution of cells expressing myc proteins in human colorectal epithelium, polyps, and malignant tumors. Cancer Res 1992;52:5853–5864.

147. Tulchin N, Ornstein L, Harpaz N, et al. C-myc protein distribution. Am J Pathol 1992;140:719–729.

148. Miller F, Heimann TM, Quish A, et al. Ras and c-myc protein expression in colorectal carcinoma. Dis Colon Rectum 1992;35: 430–435.

149. Hanski C, Bornhoeft G, Shimoda T, et al. Expression of p53 protein in invasive colorectal carcinomas of different histologic types. Cancer 1992;70:2272–2277.

150. Cunningham J, Lust JA, Shaid DJ, et al. Expression of p53 and 17p allelic loss in colorectal carcinoma. Cancer Res 1992;52:1974–1980.

151. Kaklamanis L, Gatter KC, Mortensen N, et al. p53 expression in colorectal adenomas. Am J Pathol 1993;142:87–93.

152. Sun X-F, Carstensen JM, Stal O, et al. Prognostic significance of p53 expression in relation to DNA ploidy in colorectal adenocarcinoma. Virchows Arch [A] 1993;423:443–448.

153. Lanza G, Maestri I, Dubini A, et al. p53 expression in colorectal cancer. Am J Clin Pathol 1996;105:604–612.

154. Yamaguchi A, Kurosaka Y, Fushida S, et al. Expression of p53 protein in colorectal cancer and its relationship to short-term prognosis. Cancer 1992;70:2778–2784.

155. Flohil CC, Janssen PA, Bosman FT. Expression of bcl-2 protein in hyperplastic polyps, adenomas and carcinomas of the colon. J Pathol 1996;178:393–397.

156. Hao X, Talbot IC, Ilyas M. Overexpression of bcl-2 and p53 oncoprotein in the adenoma-carcinoma sequence (abstract). J Pathol 1996;179:3A.

157. Nozawa Y, van Belzen N, van der Made ACJ, et al. Expression of nucleophosmin/B23 in normal and neoplastic colorectal mucosa. J Pathol 1996;178:48–52.

158. Smith C, Lamb RF, Birnie GD, et al. Increased expression of nm23 protein is associated with decreased survival in colorectal carcinoma. J Pathol 1996;179:36A.

159. Galand P, Degraef C. Cyclin/PCNA immunostaining as an alternative to tritiated thymidine pulse labelling for marking S-phase cells in paraffin sections from animal and human tissues. Cell Tissue Kinet 1989;22:383 392.

160. Gerdes J, Becker MH, Key G, et al. Immunohistologic detection of tumor growth fraction (Ki-67) in formalin fixed and routinely processed tissue. J Pathol 1992;168:85–86.

161. Farber E. Cell proliferation is not a major risk factor for cancer. Mod Pathol 1996;9:606.

162. Campo E, de la Calle-Martin O, Miquel R, et al. Loss of heterozygosity of p53 gene and p53 protein expression in human colorectal carcinomas. Cancer Res 1991;51:4436–4442.

163. Matrisian LM. The matrix-degrading metalloproteinases. Bioessays 1992;14:455–463.

164. Birkedal Hansen H, Moor WGI, Bodden MK, et al. Matrix metalloproteinases: A review. Oral Biol Med 1993;4:197-250.

165. Denhardt DT, Feng B, Edwards DR, et al. Tissue inhibitor of metalloproteinases (TIMP, aka EPA): Structure, control of expression and biological functions. J Pharmacol Exp Ther 1993;59: 329–341.

166. Hayakawa T, Yamashita K, Tanzawa K, et al. Growth promoting activity of tissue inhibitor of metalloproteinases-1 (TIMP-1) for a wide range of cells: A possible new growth factor in serum. FEBS Lett 1992;298:29–32.

167. Shima I, Sasguri Y, Kusukawa J, et al. Production of matrix metalloproteinase-2 and metalloproteinase-3 related to malignant behavior of esophageal carcinoma: A clinicopathologic study. Cancer 1992;70:2747–2753.

168. Urbanski SJ, Edwards DR, Maitland A, et al. Expression of metalloproteinases and their tissue inhibitors in primary pulmonary carcinomas. Br J Cancer 1992;66:1184–1188.

169. Saclarides TJ, Jakate SM, Coon JS, et al. Variable expression of P-glycoprotein in normal, inflamed, and dysplastic areas in ulcerative colitis. Dis Colon Rectum 1992;35:747–752.

170. Fischbach W, Mossner J, Seyschab H, et al. Tissue carcinoembryonic antigen and DNA aneuploidy in precancerous and cancerous colorectal lesions. Cancer 1990;65:1820–1824.

171. Burmer GC, Rabinovitch PS, Haggitt RC, et al. Neoplastic progression in ulcerative colitis: Histology, DNA content and loss of a p53 allele. Gastroenterology 1992;103:1602–1610.

172. Chen J, Compton C, Cheng E, et al. c-Ki-Ras mutations in dysplastic fields and cancers in ulcerative colitis. Gastroenterology 1992;102: 1983–1987.

173. Burmer GC, Crispin DA, Kolli VR, et al. Frequent loss of a p53 allele in carcinomas and their precursors in ulcerative colitis. Cancer Commun 1991;3:167–172.

174. Zaki SR, Judd R, Coffield LM, et al. Human papillomavirus infection and anal carcinoma. Am J Pathol 1992;140:1345–1355.

175. Beckman AM, Daling JR, Sherman KJ, et al. Human papillomavirus infection and anal cancer. Int J Cancer 1989;43:1042–1049.

176. Wolber R, Dupuis B, Thiyagatatnam P, et al. Anal cloacogenic and squamous carcinomas: Comparative histogenic analysis using in situ hybridization for human papillomavirus DNA. Am J Surg Pathol 1990;14:176–182.

177. Werness BA, Levine AJ, Howley PM. Association of human papillomavirus types 16 and 18 E6 proteins with p53. Science 1990;248: 76–79.

178. Scheffner M, Werness BA, Huibregtse JM, et al. The E6 oncoprotein encoded by human papillomavirus types 16 and 18 promotes the degradation of p53. Cell 1990;63:1129–1136.

179. Gal AA, Meyer PR, Taylor CR. Papillomavirus antigens in anorectal condyloma and carcinoma in homosexual men. JAMA 1987;257: 337–340.

180. Beckmann AM, Myerson D, Daling JR, et al. Detection of human papillomavirus DNA in carcinoma by in situ hybridization with biotinylated probes. J Med Virol 1985;16:265–273.

181. Holly EA, Whittemore AS, Aston DA, et al. Anal cancer incidence: Genital warts, anal fissure or fistula, hemorrhoids, and smoking. J Natl Cancer Inst 1989;81:1726–1731.

182. Duray PH, Palazzo J, Gown AM, et al. Melanoma cell heterogeneity. A study of two monoclonal antibodies compared with S-100 protein in paraffin sections. Cancer 1988; 61:2460–2468.

183. Bonetti F, Colombari R, Manfrin E, et al. Breast carcinoma with positive results for melanoma marker (HMB-45). HMB-45 immunoreactivity in normal and neoplastic breast. Am J Clin Pathol 1989;92:491–495.

184. Dwarakanath S, Lee AKC, DeLellis RA, et al. S-100 protein positivity in breast carcinoma. A potential pitfall in diagnostic immunohistochemistry. Hum Pathol 1987;18:1144–1148.

185. Drier JK, Swanson DI, Cherwitz DI, et al. S-100 protein immunoreactivity in poorly differentiated carcinomas. Immunohistochemical comparison with malignant melanoma. Arch Pathol Lab Med 1987; 111:447–452.

186. Lee AK, DeLellis RA, Rosen PP, et al. Alpha lactalbumin as an immunohistochemical marker for metastatic breast carcinomas. Am J Surg Pathol 1984;8:93–100.

187. Azumi N, Traweek ST, Battifora H. Prostatic acid phosphatase in carcinoid tumors. Immunohistochemical and immunoblot studies. Am J Surg Pathol 1991;15:785–790.

188. Pietroletti R, Bishop AE, Carlei F, et al. Gut endocrine cell population in coeliac disease estimated by immunohistochemistry using a monoclonal antibody to chromogranin. Gut 1986,27:838 843.

189. Sjolund K, Alumets J, Berg NO, et al. Enteropathy of coeliac disease in adults: Increase number of enterochromaffin cells in the duodenal mucosa. Gut 1982;23:42–48.

190. Dayal Y, DeLellis RA, Wolfe HJ. Hyperplastic lesions of the gastrointestinal endocrine cells. Am J Surg Pathol 1987;11(Suppl 1):87–101.

191. Polak JM, Pearse AGE, Van Noorden S, et al. Secretin cells in coeliac disease. Gut 1973;14:870–874.

192. Rindi G, Bishop AE, Daly MJ, et al. A mixed pattern of endocrine cells in metaplastic Barrett's oesophagus. Evidence that the epithelium derives from a pluripotential stem cell. Histochemistry 1987;87:377–383.

193. Gledhill A, Hall PA, Cruse JP, et al. Enteroendocrine cell hyperplasia, carcinoid tumors and adenocarcinoma in long standing ulcerative colitis. Histopatholoy 1986;10:501–508.

194. Hodges JR, Isaacson P, Wright R. Diffuse enterochromaffin-like (ECL) cell hyperplasia and multiple gastric carcinoids. A complication of pernicious anemia. Gut 1981;22:237–241.

195. Lehy T, Mignon M, Cadiot G, et al. Gastric endocrine cell behavior in Zollinger-Ellison patients upon long-term potent antisecretory treatment. Gastroenterology 1989;96:1029–1040.

196. Lewin KJ, Yang K, Ulich T, et al. Primary gastrin cell hyperplasia. Report of 5 cases with a review of the literature. Am J Surg Pathol 1984;8:821–832.

197. Bordi C, Pilato FP, Bartele A, et al. Expression of glycoprotein hormone α-subunit by endocrine cells of the oxyntic mucosa is associated with hypergastrinemia. Hum Pathol 1988;19:580–585.

198. Hakanson R, Bottcher G, Sundler F, et al. Activation and hyperplasia of gastrin and enterochromaffin-like cells in the stomach. Digestion 1986;35(Suppl 1):23–41.

199. Williams ED, Sandler M. The classification of carcinoid tumours. Lancet 1963;1:238–243.

200. Yang K, Ulich T, Cheng L, et al. The neuroendocrine products of intestinal carcinoids. An immunoperoxidase study of 35 carcinoid tumors stained for serotonin and eight polypeptide hormones. Cancer 1983;51:1918–1926.

201. Alumets J, Alm P, Falkmer S, et al. Immunohistochemical evidence of peptide hormones in endocrine tumors of the rectum. Cancer 1981;48:2409–2415.

202. Capella C, Polak JM, Buffa R, et al. Morphologic patterns and diagnostic criteria of VIP producing endocrine tumors. Cancer 1983;52:1860–1874.

203. Alumets J, Sundler F, Falkmer S, et al. Neurohormonal peptides in endocrine tumors of the pancreas, stomach and upper small intestine. I. Immunohistochemical study of 27 cases. Ultrastruct Pathol 1983; 5:55–72.

204. Lechago J. Gastrointestinal neuroendocrine cell proliferations. Hum Pathol 1994;25:1114–1122.

205. Rindi G, Luinetti O, Cornaggia M, et al. Three subtypes of gastric argyrophil carcinoid and the gastric neuroendocrine carcinoma; a clinicopathologic study. Gastroenterology 1993;104:994–1006.

206. Oates JA, Sjoerdsma A. A unique syndrome associated with secretion of 5-hydroxytryptophan by metastatic gastric carcinoids. Am J Med 1962;32:333–342.

207. Hirata Y, Sakamoto N, Yamamoto H, et al. Gastric carcinoid with ectopic production of ACTH and B-MSH. Cancer 1976;37: 377–385.

208. Caccano D, Kaneko M, Gordon RE. Glomus tumor of the stomach. Mt Sinai J Med 1987;54:344–347.

209. Hoffman JW, Fox PS, Wilson SD. Duodenal wall tumors and the Zollinger-Ellison syndrome: Surgical management. Arch Surg 1973; 107:334–339.

210. Dayal Y, Tallberg KA, Nunnemacher G, et al. Duodenal carcinoids in patients with and without neurofibromatosis. A comparative study. Am J Surg Pathol 1986;10:348–357.

211. Chejfec G, Falkmer S, Askensten U, et al. Neuroendocrine tumors of the gastrointestinal tract. Pathol Res Pract 1988;183:143–154.

212. Lechago J, Shah IA. Gastro-entero-pancreatic hormones. In: True L, ed. Atlas of diagnostic immunohistochemistry. New York: Grover Medical, 1990;1–20.

213. Imura H, Matasukura S, Yamamoto H, et al. Studies on ectopic ACTH-producing tumors. II. Clinical and biochemical features of 30 cases. Cancer 1975;35:1430–1437.

214. Ballantyne GH, Savoca PE, Flannery JT, et al. Incidence and mortality of carcinoids of the colon. Data from the Connecticut Tumor Registry. Cancer 1992;69:2400–2405.

215. Kanter M, Lechago J. Multiple malignant rectal carcinoid tumors with immunocytochemical demonstration of multiple hormonal substances. Cancer 1987;60:1782–1786.

216. deBruine AP, Wiggers T, Beek C, et al. Endocrine cells in colorectal adenocarcinomas: Incidence, hormone profile and prognostic relevance. Int J Cancer 1993;54:765–771.

217. Banner BF, Memoli VA, Warren WH, et al. Carcinoma with multidirectional differentiation arising in Barrett's esophagus. Ultrastruct Pathol 1983;4:205–214.

218. Reyes CV, Chejfec G, Jao W, et al. Neuroendocrine carcinoma of the esophagus. Ultrastruct Pathol 1980;1:367–376.

219. Petrelli M, Tetancro E, Reid JD. Carcinoma of the colon with undifferentiated, carcinoid and squamous cell features. Am J Clin Pathol 1981;75:581–584.

220. Klappenbach RS, Kurman RJ, Sinclair CF, et al. Composite carcinoma—carcinoid tumors of the gastrointestinal tract. Am J Clin Pathol 1985;84:137–143.

221. Ulich TR, Kellin M, Lewin KJ. Composite gastric carcinoma. Report of a tumor of the carcinoma-carcinoid spectrum. Arch Pathol Lab Med 1988;112:91–93.

222. Warkel RI, Cooper PH, Helwig EB. Adenocarcinoid: A mucin-

223. Ali MH, Davidson A, Azzopardi JG. Composite gastric carcinoid and adenocarcinoma. Histopathology 1984;8:529–536.

224. Soga J, Tazawa K, Wada K, et al. Argyrophil cell carcinoid of the stomach-A light and electron-microscopic observation. Acta Pathol Jpn 1972;22:541–553.

225. Achilles E, Padberg B-C, Holl K, et al. Immunocytochemistry of paragangliomas. Value of staining for S-100 protein and glial fibrillary acidic protein in diagnosis and prognosis. Histopathology 1991;18: 453–458.

226. Hamid QA, Bishop AE, Rode J, et al. Duodenal gangliocytic paragangliomas. A study of 10 cases with immunocytochemical neuroendocrine markers. Hum Pathol 1986;17:1151–1157.

227. Matsusaka T, Watanabe H, Enjoji M. Oat cell carcinoma of the stomach. Fukuoka Igaku Zasshi 1976;67:65–73.

228. Swanson PE, Dykoski D, Wick MR, et al. Primary duodenal small-cell neuroendocrine carcinoma with production of vasoactive intestinal polypeptide. Arch Pathol Lab Med 1986;110:317–320.

229. Toker C. Oat cell tumor of the small bowel. Am J Gastroenterol 1974;61:481–483.

230. Mills ES, Allen MS, Cohen AR. Small cell undifferentiated carcinoma of the colon. A clinicopathologic study of five cases and their association with adenomas. Am J Surg Pathol 1983;7:643–651.

231. Burke AB, Shekitka KM, Sobin LH. Small cell carcinomas of the large intestine. Am J Clin Pathol 1991;95:315–321.

232. Isaacson PG. Gastrointestinal lymphoma. Hum Pathol 1994;25: 1020–1029.

233. Sheahan DG, West AB. Focal lymphoid hyperplasia (pseudolymphoma) of the esophagus. Am J Surg Pathol 1985;9:141–147.

234. Ranchod M, Lewin KL, Dorfman RF. Lymphoid hyperplasia of the gastrointestinal tract; a study of 26 cases and review of the literature. Am J Surg Pathol 1978;2:383–400.

235. Isaacson PG, Wotherspoon AC, Diss T, et al. Follicular colonization in B-cell lymphoma of mucosa Pan LX-associated lymphoid tissue. Am J Surg Pathol 1991;15:819–828.

236. Villuendas R, Piris MA, Orradre JL, et al. Different bcl-2 protein expression in high grade B-cell lymphomas derived from lymph node or mucosa-associated lymphoid tissue. Am J Pathol 1991;139: 989–993.

237. Gascoyne RD. Prognostic factors in non-Hodgkins lymphoma. A single institution perspective: The Vancouver experience with identification of prognostic factors. Am J Surg Pathol 1996;20: 373–375.

238. Ramot B, Shahin M, Bubis JJ. Malabsorption syndrome in lymphoma of small intestine. A study of 13 cases. Isr J Med Sci 1965;1:221–226.

239. Isaacson PG, Dogan A, Price SK, et al. Immunoproliferative small intestinal disease: An immunohistochemical study. Am J Surg Pathol 1989;13:1023–1033.

240. O'Brian DS, Kennedy MJ, Daly PA, et al. Multiple lymphomatous polyposis of the gastrointestinal tract. A clinicopathologically distinctive form of non-Hodgkin's lymphoma of B-cell centrocytic type. Am J Surg Pathol 1989;13:691–699.

241. Banks PM, Chan J, Cleary ML, et al. Mantle cell lymphoma. A proposal for unification of morphologic, immunologic, and molecular data. Am J Surg Pathol 1992;16:637–640.

242. Williams ME, Swerdlow SH, Rosenberg CL, et al. Characterization of chromosome 11 translocation breakpoints in the bcl-1 and PRAD1 loci in centrocytic lymphoma. Cancer Res 1992;52:5541S–5544S.

243. Kumar S, Krenacs L, Otsuki T, et al. bcl-1 rearrangement and cyclin D-1 protein expression in multiple lymphomatous polyposis. Am J Clin Pathol 1996;105:737–743.

244. Swerdlow SH, Yang WI, Zuckerberg LR, et al. Expression of cyclin D1 protein in centrocytic/mantle cell lymphoma with and without rearrangement of the bcl-1/cyclin D1 gene. Hum Pathol 1995;26: 999–1004.

245. Berger F, Coiffier B, Bonneville C, et al. Gastrointestinal lymphomas: Immunohistochemical study of 23 cases. Am J Clin Pathol 1987;88: 707–712.

246. Fischbach W, Kestel W, Kirchner T, et al. Malignant lymphoma of the upper gastrointestinal tract. Results of a prospective study in 103 patients. Cancer 1992;70:1075–1080.

247. Thomas JA, Hotchin MA, Allday MJ, et al. Immunohistology of

Epstein-Barr virus-associated antigens in B-cell disorders from immunocompromised individuals. Transplantation 1990;49:944–953.

248. O'Farrelly C, Feighery C, O'Briain DS, et al. Humoral response to wheat protein in patients with coeliac disease and enteropathy-associated T cell lymphoma. Br Med J 1986;292:908–910.

249. Spencer J, Cerf-Bensussan N, Jarry A, et al. Enteropathy-associated T-cell lymphoma (malignant histiocytosis of the intestine) is recognized by a monoclonal antibody (HML-1) that defines a membrane molecule on human mucosal lymphocytes. Am J Pathol 1988;132:1–5.

250. Wong KF, Chan JKC, Ng CS. CD 56 (NCAM)-positive malignant lymphoma. Leuk Lymphoma 1994;14:29–36.

251. Wong KF, Chan JKC, Ng CS, et al. CD 56 (NKHI)-positive hematolymphoid malignancies: An aggressive neoplasm featuring frequent cutaneous/mucosal involvement, cytoplasmic azurophilic granules and angiocentricity. Hum Pathol 1992;23:798–804.

252. Van Gorp J, Weiping L, Jacobse K, et al. Epstein-Barr virus in nasal T-cell lymphomas (polymorphic reticulosis/midline malignant reticulosis) in Western China. J Pathol 1994;173:81–87.

253. Tsang WYW, Chan JKC, Ng CS, et al. Utility of a paraffin section-reactive CD 56 antibody (123C3) for characterization and diagnosis of lymphomas. Am J Surg Pathol 1996;20:202–210.

254. Meis JM, Butler JJ, Osborn BM, et al. Granulocytic sarcoma in nonleukemic patients. Cancer 1986;58:2697–2709.

255. Neiman RS, Barcos M, Berard C, et al. Granulocytic sarcoma: A clinicopathologic study of 61 biopsied cases. Cancer 1981;48:1426–1437.

256. Pinkus GS, Pinkus JL. Myeloperoxidase: A specific marker for myeloid cells in paraffin sections. Mod Pathol 1991;4:733–741.

257. Nickoloff BJ. The human progenitor cell antigen (CD-34) is localized on endothelial cells, dermal dendritic cells, and perifollicular cells in formalin-fixed normal skin, and on proliferating endothelial cells and stromal spindle-shaped cells in Kaposi's sarcoma. Arch Dermatol 1991;127:523–529.

258. Battifora H. Assessment of antigen damage in immunohistochemistry. The vimentin internal control. Am J Clin Pathol 1991;96:669–671.

259. Swanson PE. Hedffalumps, jagulars and cheshire cats: A commentary on cytokeratins and soft tissue sarcomas. Am J Clin Pathol 1991;95(Suppl 1):S2–S7.

260. Miettinen M. Immunoreactivity for cytokeratin and epithelial membrane antigen in leiomyosarcoma. Arch Pathol Lab Med 1988;112:637–640

261. Miettinen M. Gastrointestinal stromal tumors. Am J Clin Pathol 1983;89:601–610.

262. Azumi N, Battifora H. The distribution of vimentin and keratin in epithelial and non-epithelial neoplasms, a comprehensive immunohistochemical study on formalin and alcohol-fixed tissues. Am J Clin Pathol 1987;88:286–296.

263. Weiss SW, Nickoloff BJ. CD 34 is expressed by a distinctive cell population in peripheral nerve, nerve sheath tumors, and related lesions. Am J Surg Pathol 1993;17:1039–1045.

264. Appelman HD. Mesenchymal tumors of the gut: Historical perspectives, new approaches, new results and does it make any difference? In: Goldman H, Appelman HD, Kaufman N. eds. Gastrointestinal pathology. International Academy of Pathology monograph. Baltimore: Williams & Wilkins 1990;220–246.

265. Weiss SW, Langloss JM, Enzinger FM. Value of S-100 protein in the diagnosis of soft tissue tumors with particular reference to benign and malignant Schwann cell tumors. Lab Invest 1983;49:299–308.

266. Tsukada T, Tippens D, Gordon D, et al. HHF35, a muscle-actin-specific monoclonal antibody. I. Immunocytochemical and biochemical characterization. Am J Pathol 1987;126:51–60.

267. Azumi N, Ben-Ezra J, Battifora H. Immunophenotypic diagnosis of leiomyosarcomas and rhabdomyosarcomas with monoclonal antibodies to muscle-specific actin and desmin in formalin-fixed tissues. Mod Pathol 1988;1:469–474.

268. Hjermstad BM, Sobin LH, Helwig EB. Stromal tumors of the gastrointestinal tract: Myogenic or neurogenic? Am J Surg Pathol 1987;11:383–386.

269. Pike AM, Appelman HD, Lloyd RV. Cell markers in gastrointestinal stromal tumors. Hum Pathol 1988;19:830–834.

270. Saul SH, Rast ML, Brooks JJ. The immunohistochemistry of gas-

trointestinal stromal tumors. Am J Surg Pathol 1987;11:464–473.

271. Ma CK, Amin MB, Kintaner E, et al. Immunohistologic characterization of gastrointestinal stromal tumors. Mod Pathol 1992;5:45A.

272. Gould VE, Moll R, Lee I, et al. The intermediate filament complement of the spectrum of nerve sheath neoplasms. Lab Invest 1986;55:463–474.

273. Wick MR, Swanson PE, Scheithauer BW, et al. Malignant peripheral nerve sheath tumor: An immunohistochemical study of 62 cases. Am J Clin Pathol 1987;87:425–433.

274. Mukai M. Immunohistochemical localization of S-100 protein and peripheral nerve myelin proteins (P2 protein, P0 protein) in granular cell tumors. Am J Pathol 1983;112:139–146.

275. Nakajima T, Watanabe S, Sato Y, et al. An immunoperoxidase study of S-100 protein distribution in normal and neoplastic tissues. Am J Surg Pathol 1982;6:715–727.

276. Johnston J, Helwig EB. Granular cell tumors of the gastrointestinal tract and perianal region. A study of 74 cases. Dig Dis Sci 1981;26:807–816.

277. Buley ID, Gattler KC, Kelly PM, et al. Granular cell tumours revisited. An immunohistological and ultrastructural study. Histopathology 1988;12:263–274.

278. Smolle J, Konrad K, Kerl H. Granular cell tumors contain myelin associated glycoprotein. An immunohistochemical study using Leu-7 monoclonal antibody. Virchow Arch [A] 1985;406:1–5.

279. Mazur MT, Shultz JJ, Myers JL. Granular cell tumor. Immunohistochemical analysis of 21 benign tumors and one malignant tumor. Arch Pathol Lab Med 1990;114:692–696.

280. Kurtin PJ, Bonin DM. Immunohistochemical demonstration of the lysosome-associated glycoprotien CD68 (KP-1) in granular cell tumors and schwannomas. Hum Pathol 1994;25:1172–1178.

281. Dei Tos AP, Doglioni C, Laurino L, et al. KPI (CD 68) expression in benign neural tumors further evidence of its low specificity as a histiocyte/myeloid marker. Histopathology 1993;22:185–187.

282. Kaiserling E, Xaio J-C, Ruck P, et al. Aberrant expression of macrophase-associated antigens (DC68 and Ki-MIP) by Schwann cells in reactive and neoplastic neural tissue. Light and electron microscopic findings. Mod Pathol 1993;6:463–468.

283. Alles JU, Bosslet K. Immunocytochemistry of angiosarcomas. A study of 19 cases with special emphasis on the applicability of endothelial cell specific markers to routinely prepared tissues. Am J Clin Pathol 1988;89:463–471.

284. Ordonez NG. Comparison of Ulex europaeus I lectin and factor VIII-related antigen in vascular lesions. Arch Pathol Lab Med 1984;120.129–132.

285. Traweek ST, Kandalaft PI, Mehta P, et al. The human hematopoietic progenitor cell antigen (CD 34) in vascular neoplasia. Am J Clin Pathol 1991;96:25–31.

286. Sehested M, Hou-Jensen K. Factor VIII-related antigen as an endothelial cell marker in benign and malignant diseases. Virchows Arch [A] 1981;391:217–225.

287. Friedman SL, Wright TL, Altman DF. Gastrointestinal Kaposi's sarcoma in patients with acquired immunodeficiency syndrome. Endoscopic and autopsy findings. Gastroenterology 1985;89:102–108.

288. Millard PR, Heryet AR. An immunohistochemical study of Factor VIII-related antigen and Kaposi's sarcoma using polyclonal and monoclonal antibodies. J Pathol 1985;146:31–38.

289. Miettinen M, Lindenmayer AE, Chaubal A. Endothelial cell markers CD31, CD 34, and BNH 9 antibody to H-and Y-antigens: Evaluation of their specificity and sensitivity in the diagnosis of vascular tumors and comparison with von Willebrand factor. Mod Pathol 1994;7:82–90.

290. Ordonez NG, Batsakis JG. Comparison of Ulex europaeus lectin and factor VIII-related antigen in vascular lesions. Arch Pathol Lab Med 1984;108:129–132.

291. Meis JM, Giraldo AA. Chordoma: An immunohistochemical study of 20 cases. Arch Pathol Lab Med 1988;112:553–556.

292. Meurer M, Millus JL, Rogers III RS, et al. Oral pemphigus vulgaris. Arch Dermatol 1977;113:1520–1524.

293. Robey SS, Kuhajda FP, Yardley JH. Immunoperoxidase stains of ganglion cells and abnormal mucosal nerve proliferations in Hirschsprung's disease. Hum Pathol 1988;19:432–437.

294. Sams VR, Bobrow L, Keeling J, et al. The evaluation of PGP9.5 in the

diagnosis of Hirschsprung's disease. J Pathol 1987;151:78A.

295. Wakely Jr PE, McAdams JA. Acetylcholinesterase histochemistry and the diagnosis of Hirschsprung's disease. Pediatr Pathol 1984;2:35–46.

296. Larsson LT, Malmfors G, Sundler F. Defects in peptidergic innervations in Hirschsprung's disease. Pediatr Surg Int 1988;3:147–155.

297. Qualman SJ, Murray R. Aganglionosis and related disorders. Hum Pathol 1994;25:1141–1149.

298. Jaffe R, Wollman MR, Kocoskis S, et al. Langerhans' cell histiocytosis with gastrointestinal involvement. Am J Dis Child 1993;147:79–80.

299. Hage C, Willman CL, Favara BE, et al. Langerhans's cell histiocytosis (Histiocytosis X): Immunophenotype and growth fraction. Hum Pathol 1993;24:840–845.

300. Koss LG, Czerniak B, Herz F, et al. Flow cytometric measurements of DNA and other cell components in human tumors: A critical appraisal. Hum Pathol 1989;20:528–548.

301. Lovett EJ, Schnitzer B, Keren DF, et al. Application of flow cytometry to diagnostic pathology. Lab Invest 1984;50:115.

302. Braylan RC. Flow cytometry. Arch Pathol Lab Med 1983;107:1–3.

303. Quinn CM, Wright NA. The clinical assessment of proliferation and growth in human tumours: Evaluation of methods and applications as prognostic variables. J Pathol 1990;160:93–102.

304. Woosley JT. Measuring cell proliferation. Arch Pathol Lab Med 1991;115:555–557.

305. Feichter G, Czech W, Haag D, et al. Comparison of S-phase fractions measured by flow cytometry and autoradiography in human transplant tumors. Cytometry 1988;9:605–611.

306. Vindelov LL, Christensen IJ, Nissen NI. Standardization of high resolution flow cytometric DNA analysis by the simultaneous use of chicken and trout red blood cells as internal reference standards. Cytometry 1983;5:328–331.

307. Tribukait B. Clinical DNA flow cytometry. Med Oncol 1984;1:211–218.

308. Danque POV, Chen HB, Patil J, et al. Image analysis versus flow cytometry for DNA ploidy quantitation of solid tumors: A comparison of six methods of sample preparation. Mod Pathol 1993;6:270–275.

309. Crissman JD, Zarbo RJ, Niebylski CD, et al. Flow cytometric DNA analysis of colon adenocarcinomas: A comparative study of preparatory techniques. Mod Pathol 1988;1:198–204.

310. Vindelov LL. Flow microfluorometric analysis of nuclear DNA in cells from solid tumors and cell suspensions. A new method for rapid isolation and staining of nuclei. Virchows Archiv [B] 1977;24:227–242.

311. Hedley DW, Friedlander ML, Taylor IW, et al. Method for analysis of cellular DNA content of paraffin-embedded pathological material using flow cytometry. J Histochem Cytochem 1983;31:1333–1335.

312. Zarbo RJ, Visscher DW, Crissman JD. Two-color multiparametric method for flow cytometric DNA analysis of carcinomas using staining for cytokeratin and leukocyte-common antigen. Anal Quant Cytol Histol 1989;11:391–402.

313. Visscher DW, Zarbo RJ, Ma CK, et al. Flow cytometric DNA and clinicopathologic analysis of Dukes' A&B colonic adenocarcinomas: A retrospective study. Mod Pathol 1990;3:709–712.

314. Crissman JD, Zarbo RJ, Ma CK, et al. Histopathologic parameters and DNA analysis in colorectal adenocarcinomas. In: Rosen PP, Fechner RE, eds. Pathology annual. East Norwalk: Appleton and Lange, 1989;103–147.

315. Fielding LP, Pettigrew N. College of American Pathologists Conference XXVI on clinical relevance of prognostic markers in solid tumors. Report of the colorectal cancer working group. Arch Pathol Lab Med 1995;119:1115–1121.

316. Wolman SR, Visscher DW. Cellular genetics alterations: Models of breast and colon cancer. Mol Cell Biol 1993;7:1–34.

317. Wolley RC, Schreiber K, Loss LG, et al. DNA distribution in human colon carcinomas and its relationship to clinical behavior. J Natl Cancer Inst 1982;69:15–22.

318. Rognum TO, Thorud E, Elgjo K, et al. Large bowel carcinomas with different ploidy, related to secretory component, IgA, and CEA in epithelium and plasma. Br J Cancer 1982;45:921–934.

319. Banner BF, Tomas-De La Vega JE, Roseman DL, et al. Should flow cytometric DNA analysis precede definitive surgery for colon carcinoma? Ann Surg 1985;202:740–744.

320. Teodori L, Tirindelli-Danesi D, Cordelli E, et al. Potential prognostic significance of cytometrically determined DNA abnormality in GI tract human tumors. Ann NY Acad Sci 1986;468:291–301.

321. Melamed MR, Enker WE, Banner P, et al. Flow cytometry of colorectal carcinoma with three-year follow-up. Dis Colon Rectum 1986;29:184–186.

322. Durrant LG, Robins RA, Armitage NC, et al. Association of antigen expression and DNA ploidy in human colorectal tumors. Cancer Res 1986;46:3543–3549.

323. Hiddemann W, Von Bassewitz DB, Kleinemeier H-J, et al. DNA stemline heterogeneity in colorectal cancer. Cancer 1986;58:258–263.

324. Scott NA, Grande JP, Weiland LH, et al. Flow cytometric DNA patterns from colorectal cancers—how reproducible are they? Mayo Clin Proc 1987;62:331–337.

325. Emdin SO, Stenling R, Roos G. Prognostic value of DNA content in colorectal carcinoma. A flow cytometric study with some methodologic aspects. Cancer 1987;60:1282–1287.

326. Lanza G, Muestri I, Bullotta MR, et al. Relationship of nuclear DNA content to clinicopathologic features in colorectal cancer. Mod Pathol 1994;7:161–165.

327. Armitage NCM, Ballantyne KC, Sheffield JP, et al. A prospective evaluation of the effect of tumor cell DNA content on recurrence in colorectal cancer. Cancer 1991;67:2599–2604.

328. Tang R, Ho Y-S, You YT, et al. Prognostic evaluation of DNA flow cytometric and histopathologic parameters of colorectal cancer. Cancer 1995;76:1724–1730.

329. Chapman MAS, Hardcastle JD, Armitage NCM. Five-year prospective study of DNA tumor ploidy and colorectal cancer survival. Cancer 1995;76:383–387.

330. Witzig TE, Loprinzi CL, Gonchoroff NJ, et al. DNA ploidy and cell kinetic measurements as predictors of recurrence and survival in stages B2 and C colorectal adenocarcioma. Cancer 1991;68:879–888.

331. Kokal W, Sheibani K, Terz J, et al. Tumor DNA content in the prognosis of colorectal carcinoma. JAMA 1986;255:3123–3127.

332. Schutte B, Reynders MMJ, Wiggers T, et al. Retrospective analysis of the prognostic significance of DNA content and proliferative activity in large bowel carcinoma. Cancer Res 1987;47:5494–5496.

STRUCTURE AND FUNCTION OF THE GASTROINTESTINAL IMMUNE SYSTEM

Lawrence K. Silbart and David F. Keren

The mucosa-associated lymphoid tissues (MALT) provide immunologic defense at all mucosal surfaces. The gut-associated lymphoid tissues (GALT), a subset of MALT, provide protection to the entire gastrointestinal tract and recently has come under intense scrutiny with increased awareness of the following facts: (*a*) nearly two thirds of the lymphocytes in the body are located in the GALT; (*b*) the majority of antigen exposure occurs at mucosal surfaces; and (*c*) many vaccines applied to mucosal surfaces elicit both mucosal and systemic (humoral) immunity.

The immense commitment of lymphocytes to GALT is common throughout vertebrate evolution. The lowest vertebrate order, agnatha, has only GALT, whereas higher order vertebrates have evolved additional lymphoid tissues, including the thymus, spleen, bone marrow, and lymph nodes (1). In humans, it is estimated that a single meter of intestine contains as many as 10^{10} lymphocytes (2), or nearly the equivalent of an entire spleen. The plasma cells contained in GALT produce more than 70% of the total amount of immunoglobulin synthesized on a daily basis (2).

Although cross-regulation of MALT and the systemic immune system is significant, there is a clear compartmentalization in terms of their respective anatomy, antigenic stimulation, lymphocyte trafficking, duration of responsiveness, and effector mechanisms. By studying the similarities, differences, and interactions between the systemic and mucosal immune systems, complex phenomena such as oral tolerance, mucosal responsiveness, and certain allergic and autoimmune conditions can be better understood.

PROTECTION OF GASTROINTESTINAL TRACT MUCOSA

NONSPECIFIC FACTORS

A delicate balance must be maintained across the gastrointestinal mucosa, allowing the absorption of fluids, electrolytes, and micro- and macro-nutrients while excluding potentially pathogenic microorganisms and their associated toxins. To maintain this balance, an elaborate system of specific and nonspecific defense strategies has evolved that comprises chemical, physical, and immunologic barriers to such organisms and toxins. The entire lumen of the gastrointestinal tract is nonsterile, with large numbers of organisms present in the mouth, ileum, colon, and rectum. Relatively low numbers of organisms are found in the stomach and proximal small intestine, principally because of destruction of many microorganisms by the extremely low pH of the stomach, and the rapid transit time of chyme passing through the duodenum and jejunum. Nonspecific factors such as mucus secretion, peristalsis, gastric acidity, digestive enzymes, bile salts, and the presence of commensal bacteria all play important roles in minimizing the colonization of the gut by pathogenic microorganisms.

SPECIFIC IMMUNOLOGIC FACTORS

The hallmark of mucosal immunity is the secretion of antigen-specific secretory IgA (S-IgA) into the gut lumen. The dissemination of antigen-specific, IgA-committed plasma cells to a wide variety of mucosal and glandular tissues has led to its designation as "the common mucosal immune system." Mucosal immunity is passively transferred to infants via colostrum and breast milk, both of which contain high titer antibodies and numerous lymphocytes (reviewed by Kleinman and Walker [3]). Antibodies of the IgG isotype are actively transported from the gut to the circulation to confer passive humoral immunity; those of the IgA and IgM isotype remain in the gut lumen.

In the adult, gastrointestinal immunity actually begins in the oral cavity, with high concentrations of secretory immunoglobulins present in saliva. These antibodies are produced by plasma cells lining the parotid, sublingual, submaxillary, and minor salivary glands (4, 5). Although the lumen of the stomach is primarily protected by gastric acid, its lining contains IgA-secreting plasma cells that have been shown to protect mice from *Helicobacter felis*-induced gastritis (6). This finding raises the intriguing possibility that mucosal vaccination may lead to protection against *H. pylori* in humans.

The small intestine contains a large population of lymphocytes and antigen-presenting cells for both the induction of mucosal immune responses and the secretion of S-IgA. Pathogenic organisms and their associated toxins (i.e., endo- and exotoxins such as lipopolysaccharide and cholera toxin, respectively) can be prevented from interacting with or colonizing the epithelium via "immune exclusion." The focus of this chapter is on the anatomic structures and cell populations responsible for eliciting and maintaining these responses.

HISTORICAL PERSPECTIVE

In 1880, Louis Pasteur reported that chickens became immune to "chicken cholera" (later classified as *Pasteurella*) after being given food supplemented with an attenuated form of the organism (7). Unfortunately, he obtained inconsistent results when using the oral route to protect sheep from anthrax and he discontinued the work. Soon thereafter, Ferran demonstrated that humans and animals could be protected from cholera after ingestion of an oral dose of attenuated *Vibrio cholerae* (8).

In 1891, Paul Ehrlich found that antibodies to vegetable poisons could be found in both serum and milk after feeding these toxins to mice (9). Furthermore, these mammary secretions were capable of protecting suckling mice from the poisons for several weeks. This finding was the first scientific evidence that stimulation of one mucosal surface (the intestine) could elicit protection at other mucosal surfaces (lactating mammary gland).

Metchnikoff first described the dichotomy between the systemic and mucosal immune system in 1894 when he observed that subcutaneous immunization of young rabbits with *V. cholerae* conferred protection against intraperitoneal challenge, but not oral challenge, with the organism (10).

Besredka further developed the concept of mucosal immunity while studying the immune response to paratyphoid in mice. Finding himself short one mouse, he used an animal that had received an oral dose of paratyphoid 1 month earlier. Much to his surprise, this mouse survived inoculation with what normally would have been a lethal dose of paratyphoid (11). After World War I, Besredka vigorously pursued the study of local immunity and was successful in using oral immunization to protect against dysentery,

cholera, and typhoid in both laboratory and clinical trials (12). He also observed a close concordance between the presence of agglutinating antibodies in stool specimens and recovery from illness; however, serum antibody levels were unrelated to recovery (13). As a result, Besredka hypothesized that stimulation of mucosal immunity was largely independent from that of systemic immunity.

The modern era of mucosal immunology began with the discovery by Tomasi and colleagues that IgA is the predominant antibody isotype in mucosal secretions (14). Whereas surfaces other than the gastrointestinal tract are involved in mucosal immunity (i.e. bronchial mucosa, mammary glands, conjunctiva, genitourinary tract, etc.), the gastrointestinal tract is unique in that it is constantly exposed to large quantities of foreign antigens (15), the majority of which are nonpathogenic dietary molecules or commensal bacteria. Thus regulating gastrointestinal immune responses to the complex milieu of material present in the gut is imperative to host survival.

ANATOMY OF GUT-ASSOCIATED LYMPHOID TISSUES (GALT)

GALT comprises discrete organs and diffuse tissues, including Peyer patches, isolated lymphoid follicles dispersed throughout the small and large intestine, the appendix, mesenteric lymph nodes, and the lamina propria. These structures have in common the presence of lymphocytes with functional capabilities that differ from lymphocytes in peripheral lymph nodes, including regulator T lymphocytes, CD8+ effector cytotoxic T lymphocytes, IgA-committed precursor B cells, and plasma cells.

PEYER PATCHES

Peyer patches were first described by butchers as areas of weakness in the intestine that often ruptured during sausage making (16). Johann Conrad Peyer later described these structures as aggregates of glands resembling "small grapes" (16). Peyer patches are grossly identifiable aggregates of five or more lymphoid follicles that are present throughout the small intestine but are larger and more numerous in the distal 2 m of small bowel; a prominent patch frequently encircles the area just proximal to the ileocecal valve (17). In many species, Peyer patches can be identified on gross physical examination as outcroppings on the serosal, antimesenteric side of the intestine. Any given patch may be barely visible or as large as 30 cm, and may contain as many as 100 follicles. Cornes demonstrated that Peyer patches are dynamic structures, with the size of an individual patch related to its current state of antigenic stimulation (17). In support of this concept, germ-free animals have exceedingly low numbers of Peyer patches, most of which are quite small. When these animal are moved to conventional housing and dietary conditions, both the number and size of the patches increases with exposure to microorganisms (18). The appearance of Peyer patches is more subtle in humans and nonhuman primates, and often requires the use of special fixatives (2% acetic acid) and stains (17, 19).

The Peyer patch also impinges on the lumen of the intestine, and is lined with a specialized "follicle-associated epithelia" (FAE) containing numerous "M" (or "microfold") cells. These cells function as antigen sampling cells that regularly pinocytose soluble, particulate, and adherent material, including bacteria (20), viruses (21), parasites, and macromolecules (22) from the apical membrane. They deliver these antigens to an intraepithelial pocket

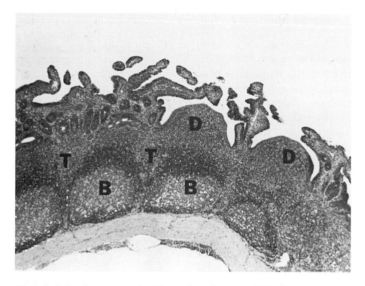

Figure 6.1 Peyer patch. Note the characteristic dome-corona area (D) where antigen is first processed, the B cell follicular areas (B), and the T cell interfollicular regions (T).

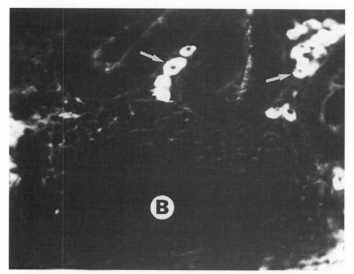

Figure 6.2 Peyer patch stained with fluorescein-conjugated anti-IgA. Note that the lymphoid nodule that contains precursor B lymphocytes (B) is negative, while IgA-containing plasma cells in adjacent villi are clearly evident *(arrows)*. (Reprinted with permission from Keren DF. Immunology and immunopathology of the gastrointestinal tract. Chicago: American Society of Clinical Pathologists, 1980.)

wherein reside lymphocytes and macrophages (22). M cells are flatter than normal absorptive villus epithelial cells and have fewer and shorter microvilli. The absence of goblet cells in the FAE explains the paucity of mucus overlying the patch, facilitating antigen sampling without interference from the glycocalyx (23).

Several species of bacteria and viruses have exploited the properties of Peyer patches to gain access across the epithelium. For example, *V. cholerae* (24), *E. coli* (25), *Shigella dysenteria* (26), *Listeria monocytogenes* (27), *Salmonella typhimurium* (20), *Mycobacterium paratuberculosis* (28), *Campylobacter jejuni* (29), *Yersinia enterocolitica* (30), bacillus Calmette-Guérin (31), poliovirus (32), reovirus (21) and possibly human immunodeficiency virus (HIV) (33) appear to be taken up selectively across Peyer patches after adhering to the M cell surface.

Immediately beneath the Peyer patch FAE is the dome-corona region (Fig. 6.1). This area is populated by a mixture of cells, many of which are major histocompatibility complex (MHC) II positive (B lymphocytes, dendritic cells, and macrophages). These cells process and present antigen, in the context of the MHC II binding groove (34), to T cells. Macrophages filled with cell debris, lipofuscin-like material, and bacterial remnants are frequently seen in this region. Suppressor T cells, also present in MALT, inhibit production of systemic immunity to orally administered antigens, as discussed subsequently. Few plasma cells are found within the Peyer patch, although they are abundant in the surrounding lamina propria (Fig. 6.2).

The average number of Peyer patches in humans increases from about 50 at 24 to 29 weeks of gestation to almost 250 by adolescence (Table 6.1) (17). The number of these structures gradually declines during adulthood, with fewer than 100 observed in individuals older than age 70 years. This attrition in the number of Peyer patches is generally accompanied by a thickening in the villi, attributable in part to the accumulation of plasma cells and memory B and T cells in the lamina propria. The variation in numbers of Peyer patches at different ages indicates that this lymphoid tissue is actively involved in interactions with luminal antigens.

TABLE 6 . 1	Peyer's Patches in Humans		
	Average Number of Peyer's Patches		
Age	(N)	Mean	Standard Deviation
Gestation 24–29 weeks	6	59	8.4
Gestation 30–37 weeks	8	77	18.1
Newborn	7	102	15.6
>Newborn to 6 months	5	96	24.9
>6 months to 6 years	7	159	39.7
>6 years to 12 years	5	239	68.9

Data summarized from Cornes JS. Number, size, and distribution of Peyer's patches in the human small intestine. Gut 1965; 6:225–238.

In some animals and humans, primordial Peyer patches can be detected along the intestine about halfway through gestation (19, 35). Within a few days after their appearance, a striking proliferation of the follicular areas occurs. At birth, Peyer patches have the greatest density of proliferating lymphoid cells in the body (19). The increase in the numbers of Peyer patches after birth likely reflects the initial response of the host immune system to the wide variety of environmental antigens that pass through the gastrointestinal tract.

ISOLATED LYMPHOID FOLLICLES

Isolated lymphoid follicles are present throughout the gastrointestinal tract and represent the most abundant discrete lymphoid structure of MALT. Random sections of small intestine or colon

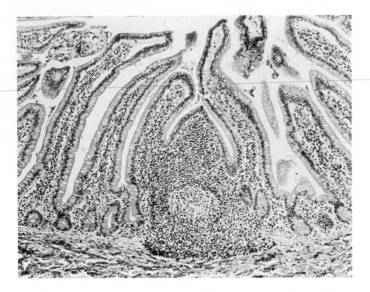

Figure 6.3   Isolated lymphoid follicles, which occur throughout the gastrointestinal tract. They have specialized surface epithelium for antigen uptake, as do Peyer patches. (Reprinted with permission from Keren DF. Immunology and immunopathology of the gastrointestinal tract. Chicago: American Society of Clinical Pathologists, 1980.)

frequently contain one or more isolated follicles. Indeed, in many instances of colonic biopsy, the "small polyps" identified by the gastroenterologist are actually isolated lymphoid follicles. In the colon, an average of three such nodules may be present per square centimeter (37). Although they look like small Peyer patches histologically (Fig. 6.3), their size (1 to 3 mm) has precluded their isolation for functional studies in vitro. Some evidence exists, however, that their function is similar to that of Peyer patches. For example, an M cell epithelium is associated with these follicles (38), and ileal loops isolated from regions of the rabbit intestine not containing Peyer patches were capable of initiating a secretory immune response when stimulated with luminal antigen (39).

APPENDIX

In humans, the appendix is a relatively small, blind tubular process of the cecum with no digestive function. Although its role in generating mucosal immunity is unclear, the large commitment of lymphocytes and M cell epithelium suggest it may be an important structure for the induction of such responses (40).

MESENTERIC LYMPH NODES

These structures receive lymphatic drainage from the villous epithelium as well as from Peyer patches, and contain large numbers of IgA+ B lymphocytes (41). Their presence allows a second interaction of lymphocytes with antigen draining from either area, and is thought to play an important role in the activation and maturation of lymphocytes emigrating from the Peyer patches. Despite their unique immunologic composition, the mesenteric lymph nodes cannot be distinguished histologically from peripheral lymph nodes.

LAMINA PROPRIA

The lamina propria is the principle effector tissue of the GALT by virtue of its capacity to house an immense number of lymphocytes. It contains a dense layer of connective tissue that is sandwiched between the epithelium of the gastrointestinal tract and the submucosal muscle layers. Among the lymphocytes that lodge in this tissue are memory B and T cells, CD4+ T-helper cells (Th1 and Th2), CD8+ cytotoxic/suppressor T cells, and IgA+ B cells. Approximately 40% of lymphocytes found in this tissue are B cells, which lodge and proliferate in the presence of antigen and then terminally differentiate into IgA-secreting plasma cells (42).

MUCOSAL LYMPHOID CELLS AND THEIR INTERACTIONS

The intestinal mucosa contains the largest collection of cells actively engaged in immune responses in the body. Included among these cells are plasma cells, lymphocytes, macrophages, granulocytes, and mast cells. Most of these cells are located in the lamina propria, although some important subpopulations of cells are found between epithelial cells (interepithelial lymphocytes [IEL]), and other important populations are present within the submucosa. To maintain the delicate balance between immunologic responsiveness, tolerance, and memory, a highly coordinated system of communication must exist between these cells. These interactions are governed primarily by direct interaction between cells and through the secretion of soluble cytokines that interact with membrane-bound receptors in an autocrine and paracrine fashion.

Plasma cells are abundant in the lamina propria throughout the gastrointestinal tract. Human infants usually lack immunoglobulin-containing cells for the first week of life (43), but by the second week, predominantly IgM-containing cells, and some IgA-containing plasma cells, are present. After 1 month of age, IgA assumes its role as the main immunoglobulin of lamina propria plasma cells (Table 6.2), with adult numbers of plasma cells attained by 1 year of age. Relatively few (about 10%) IgG-containing plasma cells are normally present in the gut. In adults, lamina propria plasma cells are continually replaced (with a half-life of about 6 days) depending on the level of local antigen stimulation in the gut (44). The inflammation associated with active ulcerative colitis frequently results in an increase in all three isotypes of plasma cells (45). In

TABLE 6.2	Development of Gut Plasma Cells		
Age	IgA Plasma Cells[a]	IgM Plasma Cells	IgG Plasma Cells
0–1 mo	14	26	5
1–3 mo	112	53	4
3–6 mo	163	59	6
6 mo–2 yr	408	137	54

Data from Perkkio M, Savilahti E. Time of appearance of immunoglobulin-containing cells in the mucosa of the neonatal intestine. Pediatr Res 1980; 14:953–995.

[a]Cells per high-power field.

TABLE 6.3	Phenotypes of Mucosal Lymphocytes		
Location	CD8	CD4	CD4/CD8
Intraepithelial (IEL)[a]			
Ileum	13.1 + 6.9	2.0 + 2.1	0.13 + 0.1
Colon	4.8 + 2.3	0.69 + 1.1	0.20 + 0.1
Lamina propria (LPL)[b]			
Ileum	13.0 + 3.5	24.8 + 3.7	2.0 + 0.6
Colon	10.8 + 4.1	19.0 + 5.9	1.9 + 0.6

Reprinted with permission from Hirata I, Berrebi G, Austin LL, et al. Immunohistological characterization of intraepithelial and lamina propria lymphocytes in control ileum and colon and in inflammatory bowel disease. Dig Dis Sci 1986; 31:593–603.

[a]IEL data expressed as positive lymphoid cells per 100 epithelial cell nuclei.

[b]LEL data expressed as positive lymphoid cells per 100 mononuclear cells.

patients with IgA deficiency (1 in 700 individuals), a compensatory increase in IgM-containing plasma cells is usually seen.

Normal adults have about 350,000 IgA-, 50,000 IgM , and 10,000 IgG-containing plasma cells per cubic millimeter along the lamina propria (46). IgE- and IgD-containing plasma cells are also present, but in lower numbers (47, 48). In some studies, investigators have detected considerably more IgE-containing plasma cells in the upper small intestine (49), possibly as a result of mild gut allergies (50).

INTRAEPITHELIAL LYMPHOCYTES (IEL)

These lymphocytes are interspersed between normal villous epithelial cells, and are estimated to make up about one sixth of the cells lining the epithelium. Near the turn of the century, anatomists thought that these lymphocytes were merely senescent cells ready to be sloughed along with the villous epithelial cells. Immunohistochemical and in vitro studies have shown that IEL are actually an important population of lymphocytes, the majority of which are in an activated state (51) and express the CD8 surface antigen associated with suppressor/cytotoxic T cells (Table 6.3) (53, 54). Many of these medium-sized lymphocytes contain lysosomal granules (55) and exist between, not within, epithelial cells (Fig. 6.4). IEL form intimate contacts with the adjacent epithelial cells, and often extend pseudopodia into neighboring cells (51). Different subpopulations of IEL are thought to provide a surveillance function similar to that of natural killer (NK) cells for damaged or virally infected cells, whereas others are responsible for responding to luminal antigens (51, 56).

It is possible to segregate IEL into two distinct lineages of T cells, each derived from a common progenitor cell. The difference between these cell populations lies in their usage of T cell receptor (TCR) genes, with about 50% using the αβ-TCR, and 50% using γδ-TCR genes (57). The γδ-TCR+ IEL are unusual in a number of respects. They appear to mature extrathymically and bear an unusual phenotype in which CD8 is expressed on their surface as an αα-homodimer (rather than the traditional αβ-heterodimer) (58). In addition, their T cell receptor is more immunoglobulin-like in its

binding characteristics than that of αβ-T cells. These T cells can bind unprocessed antigens, antigens expressed in nonclassical MHC molecules (59), and certain nonpeptide structures. For example, γδ-T cells have been found to recognize the isopentenyl pyrophosphate mycobacterial antigen (60).

IEL do not appear to originate or reside in the Peyer patches (61), but traffic directly to the intestinal epithelium, relying at least in part on the interaction of the $\alpha_{IEL}\beta_7$ integrin:E-cadherin interaction (62). Several studies have shown that γδ-TCR+ IEL can mediate protective responses to enteric organisms, most notably *L. monocytogenes* (63). Activation of these cells occurs through ligation of their T cell receptor, and can be assessed through the expression of CD11c (a β2-integrin) on the cell membrane (64). The fact that the number of IELs is greatly reduced in germfree mice suggests that they play an active role in responding to environmental antigens in the normal gut flora (65). In addition, IEL have been associated with the pathogenesis of some inflammatory conditions of the gut, including gluten-sensitive enteropathy (66) and reflux esophagitis (66), but not in inflammatory bowel disease (66).

LAMINA PROPRIA LYMPHOCYTES (LPL)

LPL have the same 2:1 CD4:CD8 phenotype ratio as do lymphocytes in the peripheral blood (42, 52, 67, 68), which strongly favors the induction of antibody responses. Under the influence of interleukin (IL)-6 and other type II cytokines, immigrating IgA-committed B cells are induced to terminally differentiate into

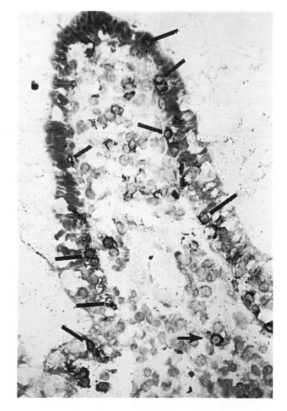

Figure 6.4 Interepithelial lymphocytes (IEL) have been identified by anti-CD8 (formerly T8), indicating their suppressor/cytotoxic phenotype. Note the occasional positive cell in the lamina propria *(arrow)*. (Courtesy of Dr. William O. Dobbins.)

plasma cells. At any point in time, a high proportion of LPL T cells are active, suggesting that this tissue is constantly reacting to gut antigens (42, 65).

Natural killer (NK) cells are large granular lymphocytes that do not express any known T cell receptor on their surface. They have the intrinsic ability to kill target cells without prior sensitization, in an MHC-unrestricted manner. In fact, binding to certain MHC I allelic forms actually provides a negative signal for lysis (69, 70). NK cells are thus considered part of the innate immune system, and play an important role in lysing cells infected with certain intracellular bacteria, viruses, and cancer cells. They can be identified or sorted based on the surface expression of CD16 (FCγRIIIA) or CD56 (N-CAM), and are capable of secreting a variety of important cytokines. NK cells are stimulated and activated by IL-1, IL-2, IL-12, and IFN-α, after which they are sometimes referred to as "lymphokine-activated killer" cells (LAK). Early in infection, NK cells may play a pivotal role in influencing responsiveness via cell-mediated immunity by secreting primarily Th1 (type 1) cytokines (IL-3, IL-8, GM-CSF, M-CSF, TNF-α, and IFN-γ) (71). As described in a review by Scott and Trinchieri (71), NK cells also confer protection to a wide variety of infectious organisms, including *Cryptococcus neoformans, Mycobacterium tuberculosis, L. monocytogenes, Toxoplasma,* and others.

B1 B cells/Plasma Cells

B1 B cells are derived from self-renewing stem cells in the peritoneal and pleural cavities (72). These cells have come under intense scrutiny because of their capacity to secrete relatively low affinity antibodies that exhibit cross-reactivity with a wide variety of antigens, sometimes resulting in autoimmunity (73, 74). These polyspecific or "plastic" antibodies are frequently IgM+, and only rarely exhibit isotype switch or affinity maturation. They bear an unusual surface marker, CD5 (formerly known as Ly-1), which originally was thought to be unique to T cells (72). These B cells proliferate in response to a number of bacterial polysaccharide antigens in a T cell-independent fashion. In mice, they have been shown to home selectively to the lamina propria and secrete S-IgA under the influence of IL-5 (75, 76). Much remains to be learned about this potentially important cell population in the human intestine.

Villous Epithelial Cells

The primary role of villous epithelial cells in host defense is to maintain a barrier to pathogenic organisms via tight junctions and a dense brush border coated with mucins and secretory immunoglobulins. Nonetheless, these epithelial cells are capable of endocytosing luminal antigen and, under the appropriate cytokine signalling, can express MHC II for presentation of processed exogenous antigens (77). This activity may be more important for generating "oral tolerance," as these epithelial cells are relatively inefficient at processing and presenting antigen on their surface (78) and lack essential costimulatory molecules necessary for inducing mucosal responsiveness, resulting in T cell anergy (79). Expression of MHC II on epithelial cells can be induced by IFN-γ, which may play a role in several inflammatory processes in the gut (78).

Another important role of villous epithelial cells in mucosal immunity is as a conduit for polymeric immunoglobulins (S-IgA and IgM) secreted by lamina propria plasma cells. Polymeric immunoglobulin receptor (pIgR) on the basal and lateral sides of the epithelial cells binds with high affinity to polymeric immunoglobulins and shuttles them to the apical membrane within transcytotic vesicles (15). This process allows the excretion of the $(IgA)_2$-J chain-secretory component ternary complex known as S-IgA.

Paneth Cells

Paneth cells reside in the crypts of the small intestine, and to a lesser extent in the appendix and ascending colon. Paneth cell metaplasia is frequently observed in chronic gastritis and ulcerative colitis (80). Although their location in the bottom of the crypts does not suggest an important role in sampling luminal antigens, these cells have phagocytic capabilities in vivo and in vitro and respond to microorganisms in the gut lumen by secreting lysozyme and defensins (81–84).

Moller et al. noted that Paneth cells express high levels of CD95 ligand, which is known to mediate apoptosis of cells expressing CD95 (APO-1/fas) (84). Thus, Paneth cells may aid in the maintenance of mucosal integrity by inducing apoptosis of self-reactive B and T cells, as well as transformed epithelial cell (80).

Other Cellular Cytotoxic Mechanisms in MALT

A complex type of cytotoxic activity involving a collaboration between killer cells (which may be lymphocytes, monocytes, or granulocytes) and antibody has been described in the gastrointestinal tract. This antibody-dependent cell-mediated cytotoxicity (ADCC) has been demonstrated in vitro with S-IgA directed against specific bacterial pathogens such as *Shigella flexneri* and *Salmonella typhi* (85, 86), although its role in vivo is not yet clear. Capron et al. found that eosinophils could destroy schistosomes that were coated with a reagenic form of mouse IgG (87). Such a role for eosinophils in host defense against parasites provides a logical explanation for the eosinophilia commonly observed in patients with parasitic infestations. The demonstration of a receptor for secretory component on human eosinophil cytoplasmic membranes by the same group suggests that this mechanism may be relevant to human mucosal defense (88).

Activated macrophages are present both in the lamina propria and within the organized GALT (Table 6.4) (89). The activated state may be due to upregulation of Fcα receptors on monocytes by

TABLE 6.4	Characteristics of Mucosal Macrophages	
	Macrophage Source	
Characteristic	Intestinal	Peripheral Blood
Granularity	4+	1+
Phagocytosis	4+	1-2+
Pseudopod	Present	Usually absent

Data from Bull DM, Bookman MA. Isolation and functional characterization of human intestinal mucosal lymphoid cells. J Clin Invest 1977; 59:966.

endotoxin and cytokines, such as tumor necrosis factor and IL-1, that are produced locally in response to lipopolysaccharide (90). Despite early questions concerning the existence of functional macrophages within Peyer patches, it is now clear that macrophages are present in these and other MALT structures (91) and play a major role in processing luminal antigens (92).

A large number of granulocytes are also found in normal human intestine, with eosinophils representing as many as 3% of cells isolated from human colonic mucosa (88). Neutrophils are associated with acute inflammation and are present in relatively small numbers in histologic sections of noninflamed human bowel. Mast cells are a heterogeneous group of cells that respond to parasitic infestations and also play a role in allergic reactions (93). They arise from the bone marrow (94), are influenced by the microflora of the gut (95), and are attracted by the production of IL-3 by T cells in the mucosa (96). Mast cells are active in the expulsion of a variety of intestinal parasites (97, 98). Befus et al. found that these cells could be stained readily when the tissues were fixed in Carnoy's fixative, but not when routine formalin fixation was used (99). This result implies that most tissues examined by pathologists do not show the mast cell content to advantage.

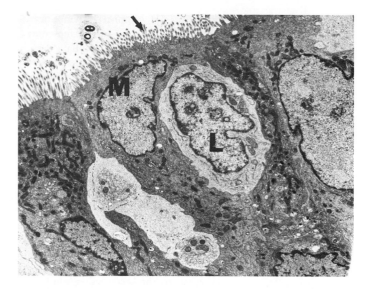

Figure 6.5 "M" cell (M) between two absorptive epithelial cells. Note the irregular microvilli *(arrow)* and lymphocyte (L) associated with the "M" cell. (Reprinted with permission from Keren DF. Immunology and immunopathology of the gastrointestinal tract. Chicago: American Society of Clinical Pathologists, 1980.)

ANTIGEN PROCESSING IN THE GUT

FUNCTION AND INTERACTION OF CELL POPULATIONS

Bookman and Cooper demonstrated that the epithelium overlying lymphoid follicles in Peyer patches, appendix, or Bursa of Fabricius (in the chicken) could imbibe intraluminal antigens (40). The specific nature of these cells was determined by Owen, who observed uptake of macromolecules by this specialized follicle-associated epithelial cells that he termed "M-cells" (22). These cells have also been identified overlying isolated lymphoid follicles in the gut, implying a similar function for these structures (38).

M cells have shorter, more irregular microvilli than adjacent absorptive columnar epithelial cells. They originate from the adjacent crypt epithelium (100) and have more intense esterase, but weaker alkaline phosphatase activity than surrounding epithelial cells (101). They are a dynamic population, showing increased numbers in inflamed mucosa (102). In an attempt to explain the unique functions of these cells, Madara et al. found that M cell membranes have a low protein-to-lipid ratio, compared to absorptive epithelium, and contain abundant morphologically detectable cholesterol, except in areas involved in endocytosis (103). Adhesion of virus, parasites, and bacteria to these cells is the first step in processing of luminal antigens by the MALT (104). The adhesion of these microorganisms may, however, provide an important route for invasion of host cells (26, 105, 106) (Fig. 6.5). In addition to passage of antigen into MALT, M cells represent a prominent site by which lymphocytes traffic from the mucosa into the gut lumen in rabbit (107).

During the inductive phase of the mucosal immune response, antigen is taken up from the gut lumen by M cells and passed to the underlying lymphoid tissues in MALT, where it can be processed by macrophages and dendritic cells and may contact antigen-specific precursors for IgA-secreting plasma cells (108). Elaborate capillary

flow in these follicles may facilitate distribution of antigen to numerous lymphocytes, especially T-helper cells (109). Resting B cells in the dome-corona region are generally surface IgM+, whereas germinal center B cells have undergone heavy chain switch to a surface IgA+ phenotype under the local influence of cytokines, including IL-4, IL-5, and transforming growth factor beta (TGF-β) (110–112). Activated B cells clonally expand in these germinal centers, and undergo affinity maturation via somatic hypermutation.

T cells found within the follicles are frequently CD4+ Th2 (type 2 helper cells) that support B cell activation and isotype switching through cognate B cell-T cell interactions and by the secretion of a "type 2" cytokine profile (IL-4, 5, 6, 10, 13). Coactivation of these cells occurs on ligation of gp39 (or CD40 ligand) expressed on the T cell surface, and CD40 on the surface of the B lymphocyte (113, 114). In mice, the type II cytokines released by TL2 cells play important roles in proliferation and maturation of the precursor B lymphocytes within the Peyer patches (115).

Th2 cells can be stimulated by microbial toxins such as cholera toxin and the heat-labile enterotoxin from *E coli*. These toxins, and their associated subunits, are frequently used as adjuvants for augmenting the secretory IgA response in experimental animals (116–120) and humans (121, 122). The precursor B lymphocytes must first be stimulated by antigen, and then TGF-β and IL-5 promote a recombinatorial switch of the immunoglobulin isotype expressed by these cells from IgM to IgA. Cell populations capable of mediating this switch exist among MALT T cell populations, but not among spleen T cells (123), and have been detected in some human T cell neoplasms (124). Prominent high-endothelial venules (HEV) are also found in the interfollicular region, and serve an important role in lymphocytes trafficking to and from the Peyer patch (125).

Soon after antigen stimulation, IgA-committed B lymphocytes leave MALT and travel through lymphatic vessels to mesenteric lymph nodes (41). These cells then enter afferent lymphatic vessels that flow into the thoracic duct. By this time, most of the lymphocytes are large, rapidly dividing lymphoblasts. After 4 to 6 days, these cells return via the HEV to effector sites in the gut mucosa, but also to other mucosal surfaces, including the bronchial mucosa, salivary glands, mammary glands, conjunctiva, and genitourinary tract. At these sites, they come under the influence of cytokines, including IL-5 and IL-6, that complete the maturation of the IgA-committed, antigen-specific B lymphocytes to plasma cells (109, 115). Vasoactive intestinal peptide is a major factor in the amount of IgA produced in human mucosa (126). A mucosal memory response can be elicited by multiple oral challenges with live microorganisms (127, 128).

The circuitous route for B lymphocyte migration is hypothesized to arm all mucosal surfaces to an antigen present in the environment (129). The survival advantage of this mechanism may be to aid the paltry defenses of neonates by the secretory IgA in breast milk. Studies in newborn nurseries demonstrate that babies fed breast milk have a significantly lower rate of enterotoxigenic E. coli diarrhea compared to formula-fed infants. IgA in maternal secretions principally reacts with specific microorganisms present in their own gastrointestinal tract (130). Some authors have suggested that development of vaccines for diseases such as acquired immunodeficiency syndrome (AIDS) could take advantage of this circuitous B cell migration to provide protection at genitourinary sites (131).

In studies involving the use of isolated ileal (Thiry-Vella) loops in rabbits, mucosal immunity was detected in loop secretions even when no antigen was directly applied to the loops (128, 132). Therefore, oral antigen stimulation arms a wide variety of mucosal surfaces, especially the gut, to antigens sampled from the environment. Other work, however, indicates that whereas all areas of the mucosal immune system contain secretory IgA, the immune response is stronger in areas exposed to antigen (130).

ORAL TOLERANCE

Oral tolerance is generally defined as systemic hyporesponsiveness to parenteral antigen challenge after oral exposure to the same antigen. Tolerance has been adoptively transfered by injecting lymphocytes from orally immunized animals into previously unchallenged animals (134). The cells responsible for transfering antigen-induced systemic tolerance in experimental systems are mainly T lymphocytes (134). As with the switch process, cytokines such as TGF-β and IL-2 potentiate induction of oral tolerance (133, 135, 136). These antigen-specific suppressor T cells are found in MALT within 2 days after feeding protein antigen (137). Soon after, however, these cells leave MALT such that by 4 days after feeding, the suppressor T cells are absent from Peyer patches but are present in systemic lymphoid tissues. T cells responsible for suppressing IgG responses and other T cells that enhance the IgA response are present in MALT, whereas the converse is true in the spleen (138). In older animals, functional defects in the suppressor T cells may explain the increased incidence of both infection and neoplasia with aging (139).

Oral tolerance in adults results in a reduction in cell-mediated immunity and T cell-dependent proliferation, but not B cell tolerance (140). Thus, oral tolerance could be exploited to treat certain types of immunologic conditions that are largely T-cell based, including allergies and autoimmune diseases (141). In MALT, oral antigen administration induces precursor T cells to become suppressor T cells that inhibit the production of systemic IgG or IgM responses to that antigen (142). Suppressor T cells leave MALT and travel to the spleen and other sites, where they may act on cells stimulated by mucosal antigens (137). In humans, suppressor cells for the IgA response bear surface receptors for IgA (143).

CHARACTERISTICS OF SECRETORY IgA

The end result of the cellular interactions just described is the synthesis and secretion of an antigen-specific secretory IgA (S-IgA) by plasma cells lodged in the lamina propria. IgA is synthesized as a 7S monomer consisting of two α-heavy chains and two light chains linked in a dimeric, "tail-to-tail" arrangement by a 15.6-kDa polypeptide called the J (for joining) chain (144–146). In humans, there are two subclasses of IgA: IgA1 and IgA2. Whereas IgA1 predominates in the serum, a disproportionately large number of IgA2-secreting plasma cells are present along the lamina propria of the gastrointestinal tract (147). The IgA2 subclass is divided into two allotypes, namely A2m(1) and A2m(2). The IgA2m(1) allotype is unique among immunoglobulins because the two light chains are covalently bound to each other and are linked to the α-heavy chains by relatively weak noncovalent forces (148).

Transport of polymeric IgA across epithelial cells is mediated by an 86-kDa membrane-bound glycoprotein expressed on the basal and lateral surfaces of the epithelial cells known as the polymeric immunoglobulin receptor (pIgR) (Fig. 6.6) (149–152). Polymeric IgA molecules bind to pIgR and are "transcytosed" across the epithelial cell in vesicles (153, 154). Before their release into the intestinal lumen, pIgR becomes covalently bound to the immunoglobulin, and is cleaved from its membrane attachment. The majority of the pIgR molecule remains covalently associated with the IgA dimer, and is then called secretory component (SC). The pIgR receptors can be upregulated by cytokines such as TGF-β (155) and IFN-γ during inflammation (156), an effect that may influence the amount of IgA transported into the gut lumen. SC helps to prevent degradation of IgA in the proteolytic environment of the gut lumen. The form released into the lumen, then, is the 11S, 385-kD complex of dimeric IgA2-J chain and SC known as S-IgA (157). pIgR is also able to combine with IgM and provides a similar mechanism of secretion into the gut lumen (157). Although the SC is able to prevent digestion of the dimeric IgA by most human proteases, some bacteria produce proteases that are able to cleave IgA1 in its hinge region (158). IgA2 is more resistant to microbial proteases than IgA1; a fact that may explain the increased proportion of IgA2 in the intestine relative to the systemic circulation.

The stimulus responsible for release of IgA-J chain SC into the gut lumen is still unclear, although results of some studies suggest that biologically active molecules such as cholera toxin can promote this secretion (159). Once released into the bowel lumen, S-IgA mediates protection against microorganisms and their toxic products (160) by interfering with the uptake of microorganisms and their products. This process, termed immune exclusion, requires S-IgA to coat the surface of luminal antigens, thereby preventing the adherence of the antigen to the glycocalyx of the surface epithelium. Clearly, microorganisms and toxins rendered incapable of binding

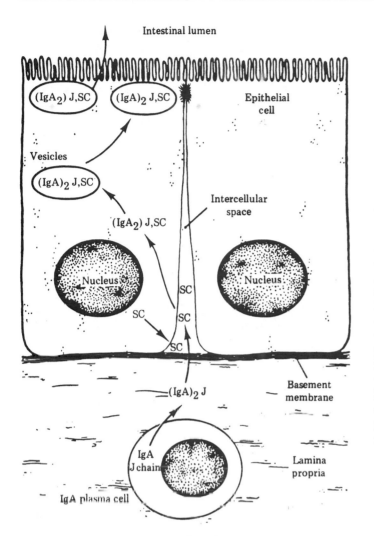

Intestinal lumen

Figure 6.6   IgA is synthesized by plasma cells in the lamina propria mainly as a dimer combined with J chain (also made by the plasma cell). IgA is attracted to the surface epithelial cells, which synthesize secretory component and express it on their basal and lateral borders. The IgA attaches to the secretory component and is taken up by the epithelial cell. This complex is packaged into vesicles that concentrate near the surface epithelium and is eventually secreted into the gut lumen. IgM is transported into the lumen by the same mechanism. IgG, IgE, and IgD do not combine with secretory component and do not share this secretory pathway.

to the surface epithelium are not able to damage tissues. This mechanism has been shown to protect against *V. cholerae, Streptococcus sanguis, S. mutans, E. histolytica,* and *H. influenza* (161–164). Some microbial products, such as cholera toxin, and microorganisms, such as *Bifidobacterium breve* have been proposed as adjuvants for stimulating mucosal immunity against mucosal pathogens and carcinogens (165, 166).

In addition to antigen-specific activity, S-IgA carbohydrates have a lectin-like affinity for enterobacteria that may facilitate aggregation in the lumen and prevent their attachment to the surface epithelium (167). A similar mechanism has been hypoth-

esized to result in neutralization of viruses within epithelial cells (168). In this model, however, the dimeric IgA attached to a virus that was already residing within the cell, before the destruction of the cell. Combination of S-IgA with the virus facilitated removal of the virus from the cell, following the normal transcellular transport pathways described previously.

Some additional evidence shows that antigen-specific S-IgA can collaborate with killer cells and damage microorganisms by means of ADCC (85, 86). IgA is a poor activator of complement, and does not effectively opsonize antigens for phagocytosis by neutrophils or macrophages (169–173).

Overall, the GALT handles the complex array of antigens present in the gut lumen with extraordinary efficiency, allowing the maintenance of homeostasis on both sides of the mucosa. Loss of homeostasis is manifest in a number of immunodeficiency or hyperreactivity states, as exemplified by infection with unusual pathogens such as *Mycobacterium avium-intracellulare* in AIDS patients. Much remains to be learned about the etiology of the apparent immune dysregulation that leads to the infiltration of the mucosa by lymphocytes, plasma cells, eosinophils, and mast cells in poorly understood conditions such as inflammatory bowel diseases. It remains unclear whether or not these conditions represent primary immunopathologic reactions or are secondary to provocation by as yet unrecognized pathogens. The goal of future studies will be to influence mucosal responses so that such dread diseases as autoimmunity, hypersensitivity, and gastrointestinal cancers can be reduced or eliminated. In addition, the collective MALT has an almost limitless potential for stimulation through use of oral and nasal vaccines, many of which may replace parenteral vaccination protocols.

REFERENCES

1. Du Pasquier L. Evolution of the immune system. In Paul WE, ed. Fundamental immunology. New York: Raven 1993;199–233.
2. Brandtzaeg P. Overview of the mucosal immune system. Curr Top Microbiol Immunol 1989;146:13–25.
3. Kleinman RE, Walker WA. The enteromammary immune system: An important new concept in breast milk host defense. Dig Dis Sci 1979;24:876–882.
4. Archibald DW, Barr CE, Torosian JP, et al. Secretory IgA antibodies to human immunodeficiency virus in the parotid saliva of patients with AIDS and AIDS-related complex. J Infect Dis 1987;155: 793–796.
5. Vigneswaran N, Haneke E, Hornstein OP, et al. Localization of epithelial markers and defense proteins in minor and major salivary glands. Acta Histochem 1989;37:S235–S239.
6. Lee CK, Weltzin R, Thomas WD, et al. Oral immunization with recombinant *Helicobacter pylori* urease induces secretory IgA antibodies and protects mice from challenge with *Helicobacter felis.* J Infect Dis 1995;172:161–172.
7. Pasteur L (1880), cited by Calmette A: Les vaccinations microbiennes par voie buccale. Ann Inst Pasteur 1923;37:900–920.
8. Ferran J. Nota sobre la profilaxis del colera por medio de infecciones hipodermicas de cultivo puro del bacilo virgula. Siglo Med 1885; 37:480.
9. Ehrlich P. Experimentelle Untersuchungen uber Immunitat. II. Ueber Arbin. Dtsch Med Wochenschr 1891;17:1218–1249.
10. Metchnikoff E. (1894), cited by Cantacuzene J. La pathognie du cholera et la vaccination anticholerigene. Ann Inst Pasteur 1920;34: 57–87.
11. Besredka A. De la vaccination contre les etats typhoides par la voie buccale. Ann Inst Pasteur 1919;33:882–903.
12. Besredka A. De la vaccination par voie buccale contre la dysenterie, la fievre typhoide et le cholera. Oral vaccination against dysentery, Typhoid and cholera. Rev Hyg Med Prev 1927;49:445–463.

13. Davies A. An investigation into the serological properties of dysentery stools. Lancet 1922;2:1009–1012.

14. Tomasi Jr TB, Tan EM, Solomon A, et al. Characteristics of an immune system common to certain external secretions. J Exp Med 1965;121:101–125.

15. Brandtzaeg P. Research in gastrointestinal immunology: State of the art. Scand J Gastroenterol 1985;20(S114):137–156.

16. Griebel PJ, Hein WR. Expanding the role of Peyer's patches in B-cell ontogeny. Immunol Today 1996;17:30–39.

17. Cornes JS. Number, size, and distribution of Peyer's patches in the human small intestine. Gut 1965;6:225–238.

18. Crabbe PA, Nash DR, Bazin H, et al. Immunohistochemical observations on lymphoid tissues from conventional and germ-free mice. Lab Invest 1970;22:448.

19. Reynolds JD, Morris B. The evolution and involution of Peyer's patches in fetal and postnatal sheep. Eur J Immunol 1983;13:627–631.

20. Jones BD, Ghori N, Falkow S. *Salmonella typhimurium* initiates murine infection by penetrating and destroying the specialized epithelial M-cell of the Peyer's patches. J Exp Med 1994;180:15–23.

21. Wolf JL, Rubin DH, Finberg R, et al. Intestinal M-cells: A pathway for entry of reovirus into the host. Science 1981;212:471–472.

22. Owen RL. Sequential uptake of horseradish peroxidase by lymphoid follicle epithelium of Peyer's patches in the normal unobstructed mouse intestine: An ultrastructural study. Gastroenterology 1977;72:440–451.

23. Wolf JL, Bye WA. The membranous epithelial (M) cell and the mucosal immune system. Annu Rev Med 1984;35:95–112.

24. Owen RL, Pierce NF, Apple RT, et al. M cell transport of Vibrio cholerae from the intestinal lumen into Peyer's patches: A mechanism for antigen sampling and for microbial transepithelial migration. J Infect Dis 1986;153:1108–1118.

25. Inman LR, Cantey JR. Specific adherence of *Escherichia coli* (strain RDEC-1) to membranous (M) cells of the Peyer's patch in Escherichia coli diarrhea in the rabbit. J Clin Invest 1983;71:1–8.

26. Wassef JS, Keren DF, Mailloux JL. Role of M cells in initial antigen uptake and in ulcer formation in the rabbit intestinal loop model of shigellosis. Infect Immun 1989;57:858–863.

27. MacDonald TT, Carter PB. Cell mediated immunity to intestinal infection. Infect Immun 1980;28:516–523.

28. Momotani E, Whipple DL, Thiermann AB, et al. Role of M-cells and macrophages in the entrance of Mycobacterium paratuberculosis into domes of ileal Peyer's patches in calves. Vet Pathol 1988;25:131–137.

29. Walker RI, Schmauder-Chock EA, Parker JL, et al. Selective association and transport of *Campylobacter jejuni* through M-cells of rabbit Peyer's patches. Can J Microbiol 1988;34:1142–1147.

30. Grutzkau A, Hanski C, Naumann M. Comparative study of histopathological alterations during intestinal infection of mice with pathogenic and non-pathogenic strains of *Yersinia enterocolitica* serotype O:8. Virchows Arch (A) 1993;423:97–103.

31. Fujimura Y. Functional morphology of microfold cells (M cells) in Peyer's patches—phagocytosis and transport of BCG by M cells into rabbit Peyer's patches. Gastroenterologia Japonica 1986;21:325–335.

32. Sicinski P, Rowinski J, Warchol JB, et al. Poliovirus type I enters the human host through intestinal M cells. Gastroenterology 1990;98:56–58.

33. Amerongen HM, Weltzin R, Farnet CM, et al. Transepithelial transport of HIV-1 by intestinal M cells: A mechanism for transmission of AIDS. J Acquir Immune Defic Syndr Hum Retrovirol 1991;4:760–765.

34. Cebra JJ, Cebra ER, Clough ER, et al. IgA commitment: Models for B-cell differentiation and possible roles for T-cells in regulating B-cell development. Ann NY Acad Sci 1983;409:25–38.

35. Keren D. Immunology and immunopathology of the gastrointestinal tract. Chicago: American Society of Clinical Pathologists, 1980.

36. Spencer J, MacDonald TT, Finn T, et al. The development of gut associated lymphoid tissue in the terminal ileum of fetal human intestine. Clin Exp Immunol 1986;64:536–543.

37. Dukes C, Bussey HJR. The number of lymphoid follicles of the human large intestine. J Pathol 1926;29:111–118.

38. Rosner AJ, Keren DF. Demonstration of M cells in the specialized follicle-associated epithelium overlying isolated lymphoid follicles in the gut. J Leukoc Biol 1984;35:397–404.

39. Keren DF, Holt PS, Collins HH, et al. The role of Peyer's patches in the local immune response of rabbit ileum to live bacteria. J Immunol 1978;120:1892–1896.

40. Bockman DE, Cooper MD. Early lymphoepithelial relationships in human appendix. A combined light and electron-microscopic study. Gastroenterology 1975;68:1160.

41. McWilliams M, Phillips-Quagliata JM, Lamm ME. Mesenteric lymph node B lymphoblasts which to the small intestine are precommitted to IgA synthesis. J Exp Med 1977;145:866–875.

42. Selby WS, Janossy G, Bofill M, et al. Lymphocyte subpopulations in the human small intestine. The findings in normal mucosa and in the mucosa of patients with adult coeliac disease. Clin Exp Immunol 1983;52:219–224.

43. Perkkio M, Savilahti E. Time of appearance of immunoglobulin-containing cells in the mucosa of the neonatal intestine. Pediatr Res 1980;14:953–995.

44. Iscaki S, Bouvert JP. Human secretory immunoglobulin A and its role in mucosal defence. Bull Inst Pasteur 1993;91:203–224.

45. Keren DF, Appelman HD, Dobbins III WO, et al. Correlation of histopathologic evidence of disease activity with the immunoglobulin-containing cells in the colon of patients with inflammatory bowel disease. Hum Pathol 1984;15:757–763.

46. Carbbe PA, Heremans JF. The distribution of immunoglobulin-containing cells along the human gastrointestinal tract. Gastroenterology 1966;51:305–316.

47. Patterson S, Roebuck P, Mills TAE, et al. IgE plasma cells in human jejunum demonstrated by immune electron microscopy. Clin Exp Immunol 1981;46:301–310.

48. Slaoui H, Andre C, Dechavanne M, et al. Immunofluorescence study of mucosal B lymphocytes in bile reflux gastritis. Digestion 1979;19:131–133.

49. Scott BB, Goodall A, Stephenson P, et al. Duodenal bulb plasma cells in duodenitis and duodenal ulceration. Gut 1985;26:1032–1037.

50. Rosekrans PCM, Meijer CJLM, Cornelisse CJ, et al. Use of morphometry and immunohistochemistry of small intestinal biopsy specimens in the diagnosis of food allergy. J Clin Pathol 1980;33:125–130.

51. Lundqvist C, Hammarstrom BS, Athlin L, et al. Intra-epithelial lyphocytes. Evidence for regional specialization and extrathymic T cell maturation in the human gut epithelium. Int Immunol 1995;7:1473–1487.

52. Hirata I, Berrebi G, Austin LL, et al. Immunohistological characterization of intraepithellial and lamina propria lymphocytes in control ileum and colon and in inflammatory bowel disease. Dig Dis Sci 1986;31:593–603.

53. Meuwissen SGM, Feltkamp-Vroom TM, der la Reviere AB, et al. Analysis of the lympho-plasmacytic infiltrate in Crohn's disease with special reference to identification of lymphocyte-subpopulations. Gut 1976;17:770–780.

54. Janossy G, Tidman N, Selby WS, et al. Human T lymphocytes of inducer and suppressor type occupy different microenvironments. Nature 1980;288:81–84.

55. Dobbins III WO. Human intestinal intraepithelial lymphocytes progress report. Gut 1986;27:972–985.

56. Ellison CA, MacDonald GC, Rector ES, et al. Gamma delta T cells in the pathobiology of murine acute graft-versus-host disease. Evidence that gamma delta T cells mediate natural killer-like cytotoxicity in the host and that elimination of these cells from donors significantly reduces mortality. J Immunol 1995;155:4189–4198.

57. Goodman T, Lefrancois L. Intraepithelial lymphocytes: Anatomical site, not T cell receptor form, dictates phenotype and function. J Exp Med 1989;170:1569.

58. Rocha B, von Boehmer H, Guy-Grand D. Selection of intraepithelial lymphocytes with CD8 alpha/alpha co-receptors by self-antigen in the murine gut. Proc Natl Acad Sci USA 1992;89:5336–5340.

59. Chien YH, Jores R, Crowley MP. Recognition by gamma delta T cells. Annu Rev Immunol 1996;14:511–532.

60. Tanaka Y, Morita C, Nieves E, et al. Natural and synthetic non-peptide antigens recognized by human gamma delta T cells. Nature 1995;375:155–158.

61. Nanno M, Matsumoto S, Koike R, et al. Development of intestinal intraepithelial T lymphocytes is independent of Peyer's patches and lymph nodes in aly mutant mice. J Immunol 1994;153:2014–2020.

62. Cepek KL, Parker CM, Madara JL, et al. Integrin alpha E beta 7 mediates adhesion of T lymphocytes to epithelial cells. J Immunol 1993;150:3459–3470.

63. Hiromatsu K, Yoshikai Y, Matsuzaki G, et al. A protective role of gamma delta T cells in primary infection with *Listeria monocytogenes* in mice. J Exp Med 1992;175:49–56.

64. Huleatt JW, Lefrancois L. Antigen-driven induction of CD11c on intestinal intraepithelial lymphocytes and CD8+ T cells in vivo. J Immunol 1995;154:5684–5693.

65. Guy-Grand D, Griscelli C, Vassalli P. The mouse gut T lymphocytes, a novel type of T cell. Nature, origin, and traffic in mice in normal and graft-versus-host conditions. J Exp Med 1978;148:1661–1677.

66. Wang HH, Mangano MM, Antonioli DA. Evaluation of T-lymphocytes in esophageal mucosal biopsies. Mod Pathol 1994;7:55–58.

67. Cerf-Benussan N, Guy-Grand D, Griscelli C. Intraepithelial lymphocytes of human gut: Isolation, characterization and study of natural killer activity. Gut 1985;26:81–88.

68. Selby WS, Janossy G, Bofill M, et al. Intestinal lymphocyte subpopulations in inflammatory bowel disease; an analysis by immunohistological and cell isolation techniques. Gut 1984;25:32–40.

69. Moretta L, Ciccone E, Mingari MC, et al. Human natural killer cells: Origin, clonality, specificity, and receptors. Adv Immunol 1994;55:341–380.

70. Trinchieri G. Recognition of class I major histocompatibility complex antigens by natural killer cells. J Exp Med 1994;180:417–421.

71. Scott P, Trinchieri G. The role of natural killer cells in host-parasite interactions. Curr Opin Immunol 1995;7:34–40.

72. Buskila D, MacKenzie LE, Shoenfeld Y, et al. The biology of CD5+ B cells. In: Shoenfeld Y, Isenberg DA, eds. Natural autoantibodies: Their physiological role and regulatory significance. Boca Raton: CRC Press, 1993;125–142.

73. Youinou P, Buskila D, MacKenzie LE, et al. CD5+ B cells and disease. In: Shoenfeld Y, Isenberg DA, eds. Natural autoantibodies: Their physiological role and regulatory significance. Boca Raton: CRC Press, 1993;143–165.

74. Murakami M, Tsubata T, Okamoto M, et al. Antigen induced apoptotic death of Ly-1 B cells responsible for autoimmune disease in transgenic mice. Nature 1992;357:77–80.

75. Beagley KW, Murray AM, McGhee JR, et al. Peritoneal cavity CD5 (B1a) B cells: Cytokine-induced IgA secretion and homing to intestinal lamina propria in SCID mice. Immunol Cell Biol 1995;73:425–432.

76. Beagley KW, Bao S, Ramsay AJ, et al. IgA production by peritoneal cavity B cells is IL-6 independent: Implications for intestinal IgA responses. Eur J Immunol 1995;25:2123–2126.

77. Mayer L, Shlien R. Evidence for function of Ia molecules on gut epithelial cells in man. J Exp Med 1987;166:1471–1483.

78. Mayer L. Interferon-gamma and class II antigen expression on enterocytes. In: Walker WA, Harmatz PR, Wershil BK, eds. Immunophysiology of the gut. San Diego: Academic Press, 1993;111–118.

79. Brandtzaeg P, Halstensen TS, Huitfeldt HS, et al. Epithelial expression of HLA, secretory component (poly-Ig receptor), and adhesion molecules in the human alimentary tract. Ann NY Acad Sci 1992;664:157–179.

80. Sandow JF, Whitehead R. The paneth cell. Gut 1979;20:420–431.

81. Kagan BL, Ganz T, Lehrer RI. Defensins: A family of antimicrobial and cytotoxic peptides. Toxicology 1994;87:131–149.

82. Kern SE, Keren DF, Beals TF, et al. A model for Paneth cell study: Tissue culture of the hyperplastic Paneth cell population of rabbit Thiry-Vella ileal loops. Adv Exp Med Biol 1987;216:419–426.

83. Yardley JH, Keren DF. "Precancer" lesions in ulcerative colitis. A retrospective study of rectal biopsy and colectomy specimens. Cancer 1974;34:835.

84. Moller P, Walczak H, Riedl S, et al. Paneth cells express high levels of CD95 ligand transcripts. Am J Pathol 1996;149:9–13.

85. Tagliabue A, Nencioni L, Villa L, et al. Antibody-dependent cell-mediated antibacterial activity of intestinal lymphocytes with secretory IgA. Nature 1983;306:184–186.

86. Taliabue A, Villa L, Boraschi D, et al. Natural anti-bacterial activity against *Salmonella typhi* by human T4+ lymphocytes armed with IgA antibodies. J Immunol 1985;135:4178–4181.

87. Capron M, Capron A, Torpier G, et al. Eosinophil-dependent cytotoxicity in rat schistosomiasis. Involvement of IgG2a antibody and role of mast cells. Eur J Immunol 1978;8:127–133.

88. Lamkhioued B, Gounni AS, Gruart V, et al. Human eosinophils express a receptor for secretory component. Role in secretory IgA-dependent activation. Eur J Immunol 1995;25:117–125.

89. Bull DM, Bookman MA. Isolation and functional characterization of human intestinal mucosal lymphoid cells. J Clin Invest 1977;59:966.

90. Shen L, Collins JE, Schoenborn MA, et al. Lipopolysaccharide and cytokine augmentation of human monocyte IgA receptor expression and function. J Immunol 1994;152:4080–4086.

91. LeFevre ME, Vanderhoff JW, Laisue JA, et al. Accumulation of 2-μ latex particles in mouse Peyer's patches during chronic latex feeding. Experientia 1978;15:120–123.

92. Owen RL, Allen CL, Stevens DP. Phagocytosis of *Giardia muris* by macrophages in Peyer's patch epithelium in mice. Infect Immun 1981;33:591–601.

93. Guy-Grand D, Dy M, Luffau G, et al. Gut mucosal mast cells. Origin, traffic and differentiation. J Exp Med 1984;160:12–28.

94. Crowle PK, Reed ND. Bone marrow origin of mucosal mast cells. Int Arch Allergy Appl Immunol 1984;73:242–247.

95. Wal JM, Meslin JC, Weyer A, et al. Histamine and mast cell distribution in the gastrointestinal wall of the rat: Comparison between germ-free and conventional rats. Int Arch Allergy Appl Immunol 1985;77:308–313.

96. Kawanishi H. Role of IgE as a mast cell development co-factor in the differentiation of murine gut associated mast cells in vitro. Eur J Immunol 1986;16:689–692.

97. Woodbury RG, Miller HRP, Huntley JF, et al. Mucosal mast cells are functionally active during spontaneous expulsion of intestinal nematode infections in rat. Nature 1984;312:450.

98. Handlinger JH, Rothwell TLW. Intestinal mast cell changes in guinea pigs infected with the nematode Trichostrongylus colubriformis. Int Arch Allergy Appl Immunol 1984;74:165–171.

99. Befus D, Goodacre R, Dyck N, et al. The mast cell populations of the human intestine. Selected summaries. Gastroenterology 1985;89:1437–1438.

100. Smith MW, Jarvis LG, King IS. Cell proliferation in follicle-associated epithelium of mouse Peyer's patch. Am J Anat 1980;159:157–166.

101. Bhalla DK, Owen RL. Migration of B and T lymphocytes to M cells in Peyer's patch follicle epithelium: An autoradiographic and immunocytochemical study in mice. Cell Immunol 1983;81:105–117.

102. Cuvelier CA, Quatacker J, Mielants H, et al. M-cells are damaged and increased in number in inflamed human ileal mucosa. Histopathology 1994;24:417–426.

103. Madara JL, Bye WA, Trier JS. Structural features of and cholesterol distribution in M-cell membranes in guinea pig, rat, and mouse Peyer's patches. Gastroenterology 1984;87:1091–1103.

104. Neutra MR, Kraehenbuhl FP. The role of transepithelial transport by M cells in microbial invasion and host defense. J Cell Science Suppl 1993;17:209–215.

105. Kauffman RS, Finberg R, Dambrauskas R, et al. Determinants of reovirus interaction with the intestinal M cells and absorptive cells of murine intestine. Gastroenterology 1983;85:291–300.

106. Dhar R, Ogra PL. Local immune responses. Br Med Bull 1985;41:28–33.

107. Regoli M, Borghesi C, Bertelli E, et al. A morphological study of the lymphocyte traffic in Peyer's patches after an in vivo antigenic stimulation. Anat Rec 1994;239:47–54.

108. Cebra JJ, Kamat R, Gearhart P, et al. The secretory IgA system of the gut. Ciba Found Symp 1977;5–28.

109. Bhalla DK, Murakami T, Owen RL. Microcirculation of intestinal lymphoid follicles in rat Peyer's patches. Gastroenterology 1981;81:481–491.

110. Ehrhardt RO, Strober W, Harriman GR. Effect of transforming growth factor (TGF)-B1 on IgA isotype expression: TGF-B1 induces a small increase in sIgA+ B cells regardless of the method of B cell activation. J Immunol 1992;148:3830–3836.

111. Kunimoto DY, Ritzel M, Tsang M. The roles of IL-4, TGF-beta and LPS in IgA switching. Eur Cytokine Netw 1992;3:407–415.

112. Islam KB, Nilsson L, Sideras P, et al. TGF-beta 1 induces germ-line transcripts of both IgA subclasses in human B lymphocytes. Int Immunol 1991;3:1099–1106.

113. Defrance T, Vanbervliet B, Briere F, et al. Interleukin 10 and transforming growth factor beta cooperate to induce anti-CD40-activated naive human B cells to secrete immunoglobulin A. J Exp Med 1992;175:671–682.

114. Geha RS, Rosen FS. The genetic basis of immunoglobulin-class switching (editorial). N Engl J Med 1994;330:1008–1009.

115. McGhee JR, Mestecky J, Dertzbaugh MT, et al. The mucosal immune system: From fundamental concepts to vaccine development. Vaccine 1992;10:75–88.

116. Xu-Amano J, Kiyono H, Jackson RJ, et al. Helper T cell subsets for immunoglobulin A responses: Oral immunization with tetanus toxoid and cholera toxin as adjuvant selectively induces Th2 cells in mucosa associated tissues. J Exp Med 1993;178:1309–1320.

117. Dertzbaugh MT, Elson CO. Comparative effectiveness of the cholera toxin B subunit and alkaline phosphatase as carriers for oral vaccines. Infect Immun 1993;61:48–55.

118. Jackson RJ, Fujihashi K, Xu-Amano J, et al. Optimizing oral vaccines: Induction of systemic and mucosal B-cell and antibody responses to tetanus toxoid by use of cholera toxin as an adjuvant. Infect Immun 1993;61.

119. Clements JD, Lyon FL, Lowe KL, et al. Oral immunization of mice with attenuated *Salmonella enteritidis* containing a recombinant plasmid which codes for production of the subunit of heat-labile *Escherichia coli* enterotoxin. Infect Immun 1986;53:685–692.

120. Clements JD, Hartzog NM, Lyon FL. Adjuvant activity of Escherichia coli heat-labile enterotoxin and effect on the induction of oral tolerance in mice to unrelated protein antigens. Vaccine 1988;6: 269–277.

121. Holmgren J, Svennerholm A-M. Development of oral vaccines against cholera and enterotoxinogenic *Escherichia coli* diarrhea. Scand J Infect Dis 1990;23 (Suppl 76):47–53.

122. Levine MM, Kaper JB. Live oral vaccines against cholera: An update. Vaccine 1993;11:207–212.

123. Pierce NF. The role of antigen form and function in the primary and secondary intestinal immune responses to cholera toxin and toxoid in rats. J Exp Med 1978;148:195–206.

124. Kawanishi H, Saltzman LE, Strober W. New understanding of regulatory mechanisms of immunoglobulin A secretion by intestinal cells. Selected summaries. Gastroenterology 1983;85:1219.

125. Berlin C, Berg EL, Briskin MJ, et al. Alpha4-beta7 integrin mediates lymphocyte binding to the mucosal vascular addressin MAdCAM-1. Cell 1993;74:185–195.

126. Boirivant M, Fais S, Annibale B, et al. Vasoactive intestinal polypeptide modulates the in vitro immunoglobulin A production by intestinal lamina propria lymphocytes. Gastroenterology 1994;106: 576–582.

127. Tseng J. Expression of immunoglobulin heavy chain isotypes by Peyer's patch lymphocytes stimulated with mitogens in culture. J Immunol 1982;128:2719–2725.

128. Keren DF, Kern SE, Bauer DH, et al. Direct demonstration in intestinal secretions of an IgA memory response to orally administered *Shigella flexneri* antigens. J Immunol 1982;128:475–479.

129. Ruedl C, Fruhwirth M, Wick G, et al. Immune response in the lungs following oral immunization with bacterial lysates of respiratory pathogens. Clin Diag Lab Immunol 1985;47:123–128.

130. Goldblum RM, Ahlstedt S, Carlson B, et al. Antibody-forming cells in human colostrum after oral immunization. Nature 1975;257: 797–798.

131. Mestecky J, Kutteh WH, Jackson S. Mucosal immunity in the female genital tract: Relevance to vaccination efforts against the human immunodeficiency virus. AIDS Res Hum Retroviruses 1994;10: S11–S20.

132. Keren DF, McDonald RA, Scott PJ, et al. Effect of antigen form on local immunoglobulin A memory response of intestinal secretions to *Shigella flexneri*. Infect Immun 1985;47:123–128.

133. Mayer L, Posnett DN, Kunkel HG. Human malignant T cells capable of inducing an immunoglobulin class switch. J Exp Med 1985;161: 134–144.

134. Mowat AM. The regulation of immune responses to dietary protein antigens. Immunol Today 1987;8:93–98.

135. Santos LM, Al-Sabbagh A, Londono A, et al. Oral tolerance to myelin basic protein induces regulatory TGF-beta secreting T cells in Peyer's patches of SJL mice. Cell Immunol 1994;157:439–447.

136. Rizzo L, Miller-Rivero NE, Chan C, et al. Interleukin-2 treatment potentiates induction of oral tolerance in a murine model of autoimmunity. J Clin Invest 1994;94:1668–1672.

137. Richman LK, Chiller JM, Brown WR, et al. Enterically induced immunologic tolerance. I. Induction of suppressor T lymphocytes by intragastric administration of soluble proteins. J Immunol 1978;121: 2429–2434.

138. Mattingly JA, Waksman BH. I. Specific suppressor cells formed in rat Peyer's patches after oral administration of sheep erythrocytes and their systemic migration. J Immunol 1978;121:1878–1883.

139. Kawanishi H: Recent progress in senescence-associated gut mucosal immunity. Dig Dis Sci 1993;11:157–172.

140. Husby S, Mestecky J, Moldoveanu Z, et al. Oral tolerance in humans T cell but not B cell tolerance after antigen feeding. J Immunol 1994;152:4663–4670.

141. Weiner HL. Treatment of autoimmune diseases by oral tolerance. Mucosal Immunol Update 1993;1:1–3.

142. Elson CO, Heck JA, Strober W. T-cell regulation of murine IgA synthesis. J Exp Med 1979;149:632–643.

143. Elson CO. Induction and control of the gastrointestinal immune system. Scand J Gastroenterol (Suppl) 1985;114:1–15.

144. Niedermeier W, Tomana M, Mestecky J. The carbohydrate composition of J chain from human serum and secretory IgA. Biochim Biophys Acta 1972;257:527–530.

145. Mestecky J, Schrohenloher RE, Kulhavy R, et al. Site of J chain attachment to human polymeric IgA. Proc Natl Acad Sci USA 1974;71:544–548.

146. Bastian A, Kratzin H, Eckart K, et al. Intra- and interchain disulfide bridges of the human J chain in secretory immunoglobulin A. Biol Chem 1992;373:1255–1263.

147. Crago SS, Kutteh WH, Moro I, et al. Distribution of IgA1-, IgA2-, and J chain-containing cells in human tissues. J Immunol 1984;132: 16–18.

148. Tsuzukida Y, Wang CC, Putnam FW. Structure of the A2m(1) allotype of human IgA—a recombinant molecule. Proc Natl Acad Sci USA 1979;76:1104–1108.

149. Huling S, Fournier GR, Feren A, et al. Ontogeny of the secretory immune system: Maturation of a functional polymeric immunoglobulin receptor regulated by gene expression. Proc Natl Acad Sci USA 1992;89:4260–4264.

150. Chintalacharuvu KR, Piskurich JF, Lamm ME, et al. Cell polarity regulates the release of secretory component, the epithelial receptor for polymeric immunoglobulins, from the surface of HT-29 colon carcinoma cells. J Cell Physiol 1991;148:35–47.

151. Delacroix DL, Malburny GN, Vaerman JP. Hepatobiliary transport of plasma IgA in the mouse: Contribution to clearance of intravascular IgA. Eur J Immunol 1985;15:893–899.

152. Brown WR, Isobe Y, Nakane PK. Studies on the translocation of immunoglobulins across intestinal epithelium. II. Immunoelectron microscopic localization of immunoglobulins and secretory component in human intestinal mucosa. Gastroenterology 1976;71: 985–995.

153. Mostov KE, Kraehenbuhl JP, Blobel G. Receptor-mediated transcellular transport of immunoglobulin: Synthesis of secretory component as multiple and larger transmembrane forms. Proc Natl Acad Sci USA 1980;77:7257–7261.

154. Song W, Vaerman JP, Mostov K. Dimeric and tetrameric IgA are transcytosed equally by the polymeric Ig receptor. J Immunol 1995;155:715–721.

155. McGee DW, Aicher WK, Eldridge JH, et al. Transforming growth factor-beta enhances secretory component and major histocompatability complex class-1 antigen expression on rat IEC-6 intestinal epithelial cells. Cyotkine 1991;3:543–550.

156. Youngman KR, Fiocchi C, Kaetzel CS. Inhibition of IFN-γ in supernatants from stimulated human intestinal mononuclear cells prevents up-regulation of the polymeric Ig receptor in an intestinal epithelial cell line. J Immunol 1994;153: 675–681.

157. Brown WR, Isobe Y, Nakane PK, et al. Studies on translocation of immunoglobulins across intestinal epithelium. IV. Evidence for

binding of IgA and IgM to secretory component in intestinal epithelium. Gastroenterology 1977;73:1333–1339.

158. Kerr MA. The structure and function of human IgA. Biochem J 1990;271:285–296.

159. Ahnen DJ, Brown WR, Kloppel TM. Secretory component: The polymeric immunoglobulin receptor. What is in it for the gastroenterologist and hepatologist? Gastroenterology 1985;89: 667–682.

160. Hamilton SR, Keren DF, Boitnott JK, et al. IgA content of intestinal epithelium and secreted fluid in experimental cholera: Comparison with net fluid production and goblet cell mucin content. Gut 1980;21:365–369.

161. Yardley JH, Keren DF, Hamilton SR, et al. Local (immunoglobulin A) immune response by the intestine to cholera toxin and its partial suppression with combined systemic and intra-intestinal immunization. Infect Immun 1978;19:589–597.

162. Fubara ES, Freter R. Source and protective function of coproantibodies in intestinal disease. Am J Clin Nutr 1972;25:1357–1362.

163. Carrero JC, Diaz MY, Viveros M, et al. Human secretory immunoglobulin A anti-*Entamoeba histolytica* antibodies inhibit adherence of amebae to MDCK cells. Infect Immun 1994; 62:764–767.

164. Harabuchi Y, Faden H, Yamanaka N, et al. Human milk secretory IgA antibody to nontypeable *Haemophilius influenzae*; possible protective effects against nasopharyngeal colonization. J Pediatr 1994;124: 193–198.

165. Silbart LK, Keren DF. Reduction of intestinal carcinogen absorption by carcinogen-specific secretory immunity. Science 1989;243: 1462–1464.

166. Yasui H, Nagaoka N, Hayakawa K. Augmentation of anti-influenza virus hemagglutinin antibody production by Peyer's patch cells with *Bifidobacterium breve* YIT4064. Clin Diag Lab Immunol 1994;1: 244–246.

167. Wold AE, Mestecky J, Tomana M, et al. Secretory immunoglobulin A carries oligosaccharide receptors for *Escherichia coli* type 1 fimbrial lectin. Infect Immun 1990;58:3073–3077.

168. Mazanec MB, Kaetzel CS, Lamm ME, et al. Intracellular neutralization of virus by immunoglobulin A antibodies. Proc Natl Acad Sci USA 1992;89:6901–6905.

169. Williams RC, Gibbons RJ. Inhibition of bacterial adherence by secretory immunoglobulin A: A mechanism of antigen disposal. Science 1972;177:697–699.

170. Zipursky A, Brown EJ, Bienenstock J. Lack of opsonization potential of 11S human secretory IgA. Proc Soc Exp Biol Med 1973;142: 181–184.

171. Adinolfi M, Glynn AA, Lindsay M, et al. Serological properties of IgA antibodies to *Escherichia coli* present in human colostrum. Immunology 1966;10:517–526.

172. Ishizaka T, Ishizaka K, Borsos T, et al. C'-1 fixation by human isoagglutinins: Fixation of C'-1 by gamma-G and gamma-M but not by gamma-A antibody. J Immunol 1966;97:716–726.

173. Iida K, Fujita T, Inai S, et al. Complement fixing abilities of IgA myeloma proteins and their fragments: The activation of complement through the classical pathway. Immunochemistry 1976;13: 747–752.

GENETICS AND CYTOGENETICS OF GASTROINTESTINAL DISORDERS

Jeffrey E. Ming and Pen-Ming L. Ming

Genetic factors play an important role in many gastrointestinal diseases. Some conditions are hereditary and may be transmitted in a Mendelian or multifactorial fashion. Detailed family pedigree analysis is essential for differentiating familial forms of a disease from sporadic, noninherited forms. The hereditary diseases should also be distinguished from conditions that occur more frequently within a family than in the general population, but are attributable to environmental influences. Environmental factors shared by family members because of their lifestyle or dietary habits may cause a disease to "run in the family." Similarly, the racial and geographic differences in the incidence of many diseases, such as esophageal cancer, can be explained on an environmental rather than a genetic basis.

Recent advances in molecular biology have resulted in the identification of the genes responsible for a number of diseases. This technology has also been instrumental in elucidating a sequence of cytogenetic and genetic alterations in the evolution of malignant changes. In addition, mutations, gene amplification, or changes in gene expression have been found in many types of neoplastic cells. It should be emphasized, however, that such alterations in tumor cells may also be affected by environmental factors and not solely by inherited genetic defects.

Cytogenetic studies of a variety of tumor types have revealed various numeric or structural chromosomal aberrations. The pattern of abnormality can form the basis for identification and localization of the specific gene(s) involved in a certain disease. Thus, the combination of cytogenetic and molecular techniques provides a powerful tool for understanding cellular as well as genetic changes in many diseases. These advances in the molecular basis of disease improve the accuracy of diagnosis, genetic counseling, and disease risk for family members.

PATTERN OF INHERITANCE

Inheritance patterns are traditionally divided into two major categories: Mendelian and multifactorial inheritance. Mendelian inheritance involves the transmission of a single mutant gene (monogenic) and can be classified into autosomal dominant, autosomal recessive, and X-linked types. Multifactorial inheritance results from the interaction of multiple genes (polygenic) and multiple environmental factors. Risks to relatives of affected individuals are generally lower than those for Mendelian disorders, except when multiple family members are affected. Certain inheritance patterns do not fit into either category. These "nontraditional" modes of inheritance are discussed in a subsequent section.

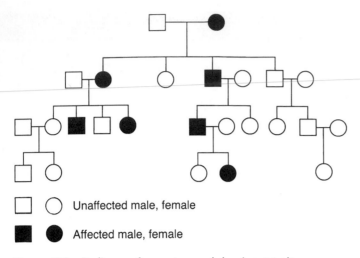

Unaffected male, female

Affected male, female

Figure 7.1   Pedigree of an autosomal dominant trait.

Genetic heterogeneity is a common phenomenon in inherited diseases. It occurs when mutations in two or more different genes produce a similar clinical condition. For instance, congenital deafness can be inherited as an autosomal dominant trait in some families, as an autosomal recessive trait in others, and as an X-linked trait in still others. On the other hand, a syndrome due to a single gene alteration may exhibit multiple clinical manifestations involving several organ systems. This phenomenon is known as pleiotropy. For example, in Peutz-Jeghers syndrome, the clinical manifestations can be as varied as polyposis of the intestine and pigmentation of the oral mucosa.

Mendelian Inheritance

AUTOSOMAL DOMINANT INHERITANCE

Dominant disorders manifest in individuals who carry one abnormal gene and one normal gene (heterozygotes). Autosomal dominant inheritance is characterized by the following: *(a)* Affected individuals often have an affected parent. Examination of the parents may be required to detect subtle signs of the condition. *(b)* A child of an affected and a normal parent has a 50% chance of being affected. *(c)* Males and females are affected in equal proportions. *(d)* Affected males and females can transmit the condition to either a son or a daughter.

Figure 7.1 shows a typical pedigree of autosomal dominant inheritance. Note the vertical transmission pattern from generation to generation. Two common clinical features of diseases associated with autosomal dominant inheritance are: delayed age of onset (although the mutant gene is present from the time of conception, the disease may not be diagnosed until adulthood) and variability in expression; the severity and extent of disease and the clinical manifestations may vary greatly among affected individuals, even within a family.

Some individuals who carry a defective gene for an autosomal dominant condition do not have any clinical signs. This phenomenon is known as lack of penetrance. If only 50% of individuals who carry the defective gene are clinically affected, the gene has 50% penetrance. Some gastrointestinal diseases with autosomal dominant inheritance are summarized in Table 7.1.

AUTOSOMAL RECESSIVE INHERITANCE

Unlike autosomal dominant inheritance, the autosomal recessive disorders manifest in an individual only when both alleles at a particular genetic locus are mutant (homozygotes). Features of autosomal recessive inheritance include: *(a)* The parents are usually clinically normal, but each parent carries one copy of the abnormal gene, while the other copy is normal (heterozygotes); i.e., they are asymptomatic carriers. *(b)* If both parents are carriers, each child has a 25% chance of being affected, a 50% chance of being a heterozygote carrier, and a 25% chance of inheriting neither mutant gene. *(c)* Males and females are affected in equal proportions.

Figure 7.2 shows a pedigree with autosomal recessive inheritance. Note the horizontal distribution of affected siblings and cousins of the same generation. Several characteristic clinical features of diseases showing autosomal recessive inheritance follow: *(a)* The disease is usually diagnosed early in life. *(b)* The clinical manifestations tend to be more uniform than those in dominant diseases. *(c)* The frequency of affected offspring is higher in consanguineous matings. *(d)* Unless the carrier state is clinically

TABLE 7.1	Gastrointestinal Disease With Autosomal Dominant Inheritance

Inheritance proved
  Cowden disease
  Duodenal peptic ulcer with hyperpepsinogenemia I
  Duodenal peptic ulcer with tremor and nystagmus
  Familial adenomatous polyposis
  Familial intestinal neurofibromatosis
  Familial juvenile polyposis
  Familial megaduodenum and/or megacystitis
  Familial midgut volvulus
  Familial tylosis (keratosis plamaris et plantaris) with esophageal
    cancer
  Gardner syndrome
  Hereditary nonpolyposis colon cancer
  Hirschsprung's disease (RET gene mutation)
  Monosaccharide malabsorption owing to sodium-glucose transport
    deficiency
  Mucosal neuroma syndromes with endocrine tumors
  Muir-Torre syndrome
  Osler-Weber-Rendu disease
  Peutz-Jeghers syndrome
Inheritance suspected
  Anorectal anomalies (anorectal stenosis or imperforate anus)
  Barrett esophagus
  Congenital hypertrophic pyloric stenosis
  Duodenal ulcer owing to antral G cell hyperfunction
  Enteropathy with villous edema and IgG2 deficiency
  Gastric peptic ulcer with hyperpigmentation and myopia
  Neuronal intestinal dysplasia, type B
  Omphalocele

Data from McKusick VA. Mendelian inheritance in man—Catalogs of autosomal dominant, autosomal recessive, and X-linked phenotypes. 11th ed. Baltimore: Johns Hopkins University Press, 1994.

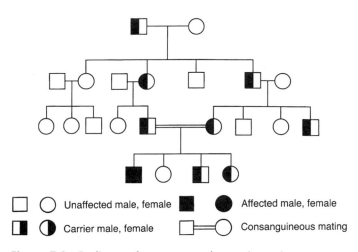

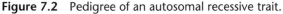

Figure 7.2   Pedigree of an autosomal recessive trait.

detectable, the parents frequently do not know that they are at risk of having affected offspring until a child with the recessive disease is born into the family. Some gastrointestinal diseases with autosomal recessive inheritance are listed in Table 7.2.

X-LINKED INHERITANCE

By definition, the genes responsible for X-linked disorders are located on the X chromosome. Therefore, the risk and clinical expression of the disease are different in the two sexes. Characteristics of X-linked inheritance include the following: (*a*) Males show clinical effects more frequently and with greater severity than females. (*b*) Fifty percent of the sons of a female carrier are clinically affected. Daughters typically do not show clinical signs, but 50% of the daughters of a carrier mother are carriers. (*c*) All female offspring of affected males are carriers. (*d*) Affected males do not transmit the mutant gene to their sons.

Figure 7.3 illustrates a typical pedigree of X-linked recessive inheritance. Note that males are clinically affected, and there is no father-to-son transmission. To date, no commonly occurring gastrointestinal disease clearly shows X-linked inheritance. Some malformations, however, such as anal atresia, have shown familial aggregation suggestive of X-linked inheritance (1, 2). One form of neuronal intestinal pseudo-obstruction has been linked to Xq28 (3).

MULTIFACTORIAL INHERITANCE

A variety of common diseases (such as hypertension) and congenital malformations (such as cleft palate) have been known to "run in families" but do not follow a pattern of Mendelian inheritance. They are usually the result of a number of interacting genetic and environmental factors. Many gastrointestinal diseases fit best into this category. In multifactorial inheritance, the interacting genetic and environmental factors often must pass beyond a "threshold" to produce clinically overt disease. In addition, the recurrence risk is influenced by the number of affected persons in the family and the severity of the disorder in the affected individuals. In general, the greater the number of affected relatives and the more severe their disease, the greater the risk to other family members.

NONTRADITIONAL INHERITANCE

MITOCHONDRIAL INHERITANCE

Hereditary diseases can be attributed to defects in mitochondrial DNA. Because the cytoplasm of the zygote is almost completely contributed by the ovum, and not by the spermatozoa, the mode of inheritance is exclusively maternal. Although mitochondrial mutations can be passed down to both males and females, only females

TABLE 7.2	Gastrointestinal Diseases With Autosomal Recessive Inheritance

Inheritance proved
  Achalasia and glucocorticoid deficiency
  Acrodermatitis enteropathica
  Congenital chloridorrhea (familial chloride diarrhea)
  Disaccharide intolerance, type I (congenital sucrase isomaltase deficiency)
  Disaccharide intolerance, type II (congenital lactase deficiency)
  Disaccharide intolerance, type III (adult lactase deficiency)
  Enterokinase deficiency
  Familial esophageal achalasia
  Familial intestinal polyatresia syndrome
  Familial intestinal pseudoobstruction with ophthalmoplegia
  Hirschsprung's disease (endothelin-B receptor mutation)
  Jejunal atresia
  Lipid transport defect of intestine with hypobetalipoproteinemia
  Megacystitis-microcolon-intestinal hypoperistalsis syndrome
  Microvillus inclusion disease
  Neuronal intestinal dysplasia, type A (intestinal pseudoobstruction)
  Turcot syndrome
Inheritance suspected
  Celiac disease
  Groll-Hirschowitz syndrome (familial nerve-type deafness, mesenteric diverticula of small bowel and progressive neuropathy)

Data from McKusick VA. Mendelian inheritance in man—Catalogs of autosomal dominant, autosomal recessive, and X-linked phenotypes. 11th ed. Baltimore: Johns Hopkins University Press, 1994.

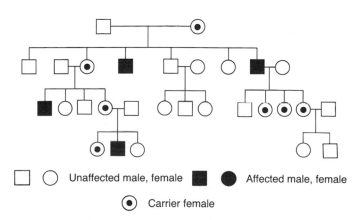

Figure 7.3   Pedigree of an X-linked recessive trait.

can transmit the disease. Because each ovum likely contains some abnormal mitochondria, all children of an affected mother will theoretically inherit the condition. Complex III deficiency owing to mitochondrial DNA deletion led to chronic diarrhea with villous atrophy (4). Multiple deletions of mitochondrial DNA were detected in the mitochondrial neurogastrointestinal encephalomyopathy syndrome, although the defective gene may be nuclear (5).

IMPRINTING AND UNIPARENTAL DISOMY

Classically, a given gene in either sex has a similar expression pattern. Although this statement is true for most genes, some genes are expressed only on the maternally derived chromosome, and other genes only on the paternally derived chromosome. A gene that has a different expression pattern depending on the parent of origin is said to be "imprinted." In effect, only one copy of an imprinted gene is functional in a given individual. Loss of the functional allele can occur by a deletion or by uniparental disomy. In uniparental disomy, both homologues of a chromosome pair are derived from the same parent. Webb and colleagues described a case in which a fetus with paternal uniparental disomy for chromosome 11 had intestinal malrotation and hypospadias (6).

GERMLINE MOSAICISM

Mosaicism refers to two or more cell lines with different genotypes derived from a single zygote. Germline mosaicism occurs when a gene mutation occurs in some, but not all, of the germ cells in an individual. This person may not have any clinical manifestations because the mutation is not present in all the cells. This state must be considered when two parents who have a normal phenotype and genotype by all known tests have more than one child with the same autosomal dominant condition. Germline mosaicism was demonstrated for osteogenesis imperfecta when approximately 12% of sperms in a clinically normal man were found to carry the abnormal gene (7).

CHROMOSOMAL SYNDROMES AFFECTING THE GASTROINTESTINAL TRACT

Chromosome imbalance may either be inherited or occur de novo. With the exception of balanced translocation, chromosomal rearrangements usually lead to an abnormal phenotype, which may include mental and growth retardation and malformations of multiple organ systems. Although a balanced translocation can be transmitted from generation to generation without producing deleterious clinical effects, the carrier of such a translocation has a greatly increased risk of genetically imbalanced offspring.

DOWN SYNDROME

Down syndrome is most frequently caused by trisomy 21. Duodenal atresia occurs in 8% of affected patients (8). Conversely, about one third of all patients with duodenal atresia have Down syndrome (8). Hirschsprung's disease occurs in approximately 2 to 6% of patients with Down syndrome (9, 10). Of 697 infants studied with anorectal malformation, 10 patients had Down syndrome (10). Anorectal malformations, including imperforate anus, occur in 0.36 to 2.2% of affected infants (11, 12). This rate is 10 to 60 times greater than that of the general population (0.035%) (13). Tracheoesophageal fistula or esophageal atresia occurs in approximately 0.5%, which is 17 times higher than the rate of the general population (13). Other associated gastrointestinal malformations include malrotation of the colon and Meckel's diverticulum.

TRISOMY 18 SYNDROME

Trisomy 18 is less common than Down syndrome but is associated with more severe malformations. In one series of 84 patients, 64 (85%) had malformations of the gastrointestinal tract (10). Other gastrointestinal abnormalities include esophageal atresia, Meckel's diverticulum, intestinal malrotation, tracheoesophageal fistula, omphalocele, imperforate anus, and pyloric stenosis (10, 14).

TRISOMY 13 SYNDROME

Among the autosomal trisomy syndromes, trisomy 13 has the most severe congenital anomalies, particularly involving the central nervous system. Associated gastrointestinal malformations are found in approximately 60% of infants (10). In decreasing order of frequency, these anomalies include malrotation, unattached mesentery, Meckel's diverticulum, omphalocele, true diverticula of the appendix, and mesenteric cyst.

OTHER CHROMOSOMAL SYNDROMES

Gastrointestinal manifestations are a part of many chromosomal syndromes. These anomalies are summarized in Table 7.3. In a study of 235 fetuses with an abdominal wall or gastrointestinal defect, Nicolaides and coworkers (20) reported chromosome abnormalities in 29%. Abnormal chromosomal changes were present in 36% of fetuses with exomphalos, 43% of those with duodenal atresia, and 75% of those with gastric agenesis, but in none of 26 fetuses with gastroschisis. The chromosomal aberrations included trisomy 18, trisomy 21, trisomy 13, 5q-, t(4;15), triploidy, XXY, and dup(11)(p15). In a cohort of 597 women with Turner syndrome, colon cancer was detected in five individuals, yielding a relative risk of 6.9 (21).

GENETICS OF NONNEOPLASTIC DISEASES OF THE GASTROINTESTINAL TRACT

As our knowledge and understanding in human genetics have dramatically increased during the last 20 years, more and more clinical disorders have been found to be genetically influenced, if not genetically controlled. Gastrointestinal diseases are no exception. This section is a discussion of only a few relatively common diseases with a strong genetic basis.

PEPTIC ULCER

Studies have shown that both gastric and duodenal ulcers are more common in the siblings of affected patients than in the general population (22), and that first-degree relatives of gastric ulcer patients tend to have gastric ulcers whereas relatives of duodenal

TABLE 7.3	Chromosomal Syndromes Affecting the Gastrointestinal Tract

Chromosome Abnormality	Gastrointestinal Manifestations
Trisomy 1q	Intestinal stenosis and atresia, pyloric stenosis
Deletion of 4p	Malrotation of the intestine
Deletion of 5p (Cri-du-chat syndrome)	Inguinal hernia
Trisomy 9 mosaic	Diaphragmatic hernia
Deletion of 9p	Diaphragmatic hernia
Partial trisomy 10q	Malrotation of intestine
Deletion of 11p (Aniridia-Wilms tumor syndrome)	Inguinal hernia
Deletion of 11q	Pyloric stenosis
Tetrasomy 12p	Diaphragmatic hernia, inguinal hernia, malrotation of intestine
Trisomy 12q	Malrotation of intestine
Trisomy 13 (Patau syndrome)	Malrotation of the colon, omphalocele, Meckel's diverticulum, unattached mesentery
Deletion of 13q	Imperforate anus, Hirschsprung's disease
Trisomy 16q	Malrotation of the colon
Trisomy 18 (Edwards syndrome)	Malrotation of intestine, omphalocele, diaphragmatic or inguinal hernia, pyloric stenosis, Meckel's diverticulum, tracheoesophageal fistula, imperforate anus
Deletion of 18p	Inguinal hernia
Trisomy 19q	Malrotation of intestine
Trisomy 21 (Down syndrome)	Hirschsprung's disease, duodenal atresia, anal atresia, rectal prolapse, malrotation of colon, Meckel's diverticulum, tracheoesophageal fistula, esophageal atresia
Ring chromosome 21	Pyloric stenosis, inguinal hernia
Partial duplication 22 (Cat eye syndrome)	Malrotation of intestine, anal atresia, Hirschsprung's disease
Monosomy X (Turner syndrome)	Pyloric stenosis
Triploidy	Malrotation of intestine

Data from Warkany J, Passarge E, Smith LB. Congenital malformations in autosomal trisomy syndromes. Am J Dis Child 1966; 112:502–517; Thompson JS. The genetics of multiple congenital anomalies. In: Shafie ME, Klipple CH, eds. Associated congenital anomalies. Baltimore: Williams & Wilkins, 1981:9–15; DeGrouchy J, Turleau C. Clinical atlas of human chromosomes. 2nd ed. New York: John Wiley and Sons, 1984; Jones KL. Smith's recognizable patterns of human malformation. 5th ed. Philadelphia: WB Saunders, 1996; Beedgen B, Nutzendel W, Querfeld V, et al. Partial trisomy 22 and 11 due to a paternal 11;22 translocation associated with Hirschsprung's disease. Eur J Pediatr 1986; 145:229–232; Lamont MA, Fitchett M, Dennis NR. Interstitial deletion of distal 13q associated with Hirschsprung's disease. J Med Genet 1989; 26:100–104.

Note: p = short arm of chromosome, q = long arm of chromosome.

ulcer patients tend to have duodenal ulcers (23). These findings suggest that gastric and duodenal ulcers are two distinct entities with independent segregation. This concept was supported by the discovery of a strong association of blood group O and nonsecretor status with duodenal ulcer, but not with gastric ulcer (24). Individuals of blood group O are about 30 to 40% more likely to develop duodenal ulcer than people of the other blood groups (25, 26). In addition, the nonsecretors are 50% more likely to develop duodenal ulcer than secretors (27, 28). Individuals with both blood group O and nonsecretor status have a 150% increased risk of developing duodenal ulcers. The association between blood group antigens and gastric ulcer however, is not clear.

Concordance of peptic ulcer in monozygotic twins is less than 100%, but consistently exceeds that of dizygotic twins (26, 29). The twins shared either gastric or duodenal ulcer, further supporting separate genetic transmission of these two types of peptic ulcers (29). On the other hand, the less than 100% concordance for duodenal ulcer in monozygotic twins indicates that other factors must be involved in the pathogenesis of peptic ulcers. One possi-

bility is a polygenic background on which the major predisposing genes act. It has been estimated that 20% of first-degree relatives of an ulcer patient will develop peptic ulcer disease during their lifetime (29).

An association between HLA antigens and duodenal ulcers has been identified in some, but not all, patients (29–33), although the associations are not consistently present among studies. Each HLA association may represent a selected subgroup of patients (32). Studies with biochemical and physiologic markers have in fact shown that there are genetic subtypes of duodenal ulcer. Among these subtypes, only duodenal ulcer with hyperpepsinogenemia I is generally an inherited (autosomal dominant) trait (34, 35). Duodenal ulcer with hypergastrinemia owing to increased antral G-cell activity showed autosomal dominant inheritance in one kindred (36).

Peptic ulcer disease can be inherited as part of a syndrome. Multiple endocrine neoplasia type 1 is associated with pancreatic islet cell tumors, pituitary adenomas, and hyperparathyroidism. The increased risk for peptic ulcer is associated with the Zollinger-Ellison syndrome, or excessive gastrin production related to a gastrinoma. Two other rare autosomal dominant conditions feature peptic ulcers. In one kindred, duodenal ulcer occurred with tremor and nystagmus (37). Another family had gastric ulcers, hyperpigmentation, and early onset of myopia (38).

CELIAC DISEASE (NONTROPICAL SPRUE)

Celiac disease, or gluten-sensitive enteropathy, is characterized by generalized malabsorption and abnormal small intestinal mucosa. The ingestion of wheat gluten and similar alcohol-soluble proteins (prolamins) in rye, barley, and oats damages the mucosa of the small intestine, resulting in atrophy of the villi and elongation of the crypts. The pathogenesis of celiac disease may involve the interplay of multiple genetic factors and an abnormal immunologic response to ingested gluten-related proteins.

The tendency for celiac disease to recur in families is well recognized. The incidence of celiac disease varies from 8.2 to 18.3% in first-degree relatives (39). Celiac disease was concordant in 70% of monozygotic twins and in about 30% of serologically HLA-identical siblings (40). About 80 to 90% of patients with celiac disease carry the histocompatibility antigens HLA-DR3 and HLA-DQw2 as compared with 20 to 30% of normal adults. Individuals with DR3 antigens have an 11.6 times higher risk of developing celiac disease (41). Nonetheless, only 1% of individuals with those antigens develop celiac disease (40). Further studies showed that a particular polymorphism of the DQ β-chain confers an additional risk of celiac disease beyond that of having HLA-DR3 and HLA-DQw2 (42, 43). Western Ireland has a high prevalence of celiac disease, and 50% of the patients studied from this region had a single extended MHC haplotype, compared to 27% of nontransmitting parents (44). A non-MHC locus that may contribute to celiac disease susceptibility has been linked to 6p (45).

INFLAMMATORY BOWEL DISEASE

Inflammatory bowel disease (IBD) includes ulcerative colitis and Crohn disease. Although these two entities can be distinguished clinically and pathologically, they share a number of features. Family studies of IBD show a strong genetic influence in at least 15 to 20% of patients (46). It is estimated that 2 to 8% of all patients with IBD will have one or more relatives affected, usually a first-degree relative (47).

The prevalence of ulcerative colitis in first-degree relatives was 15 times higher than that in nonrelatives. The age of onset was significantly lower among patients with a family history of ulcerative colitis. It is interesting to note that ulcerative colitis is more likely than Crohn's disease to occur among the families of probands with ulcerative colitis, and the same relationship holds true for Crohn disease; however, an intermingling of these two disorders is found in some families (46).

In a study of 204 individuals with Crohn disease who had a relative with IBD, concordance for Crohn's disease was found in 75% of parent-child pairs and in 82% of sibling pairs, with the remainder of the affected individuals having ulcerative colitis (48). Case reports have documented concordance in five of eight pairs of monozygotic twins with ulcerative colitis and in seven of eight pairs of monozygotic twins with Crohn disease (46).

A genome-wide linkage study of Crohn disease families yielded a potential locus at 16p12-p13 (49). Another screen showed strong linkage for a susceptibility gene for both Crohn disease and ulcerative colitis to chromosome 12 (50). Linkage to chromosomes 7q22 and 3p21 were also noted. Region 3p21 includes the G protein subunit α-i2. Transgenic mice lacking this protein developed severe colitis resembling human ulcerative colitis, and some mice developed adenocarcinoma of the colon (51). The accumulated evidence supports a strong genetic influence in the development of IBD, but the exact genetic mechanism has not been identified. It is most likely that both genetic and environmental factors are important in its development.

HIRSCHSPRUNG'S DISEASE (CONGENITAL AGANGLIONIC MEGACOLON)

Hirschsprung's disease is associated with absence of intramural ganglion cells in the intestine. In short-segment involvement (present in about 90% of patients), aganglionosis extends from the rectum to the splenic flexure of the colon. In long-segment involvement, aganglionosis extends into the transverse colon or even through the entire colon into the small intestine.

Approximately 4% of the cases are familial (2). The risk of recurrence in siblings depends on the length of the aganglionic segment. In general, the longer the involved segment, the higher the recurrence risk. The sex ratio also varies with the extent of aganglionosis. In long-segment cases, the male-to-female ratio is 1.86:1; in short-segment cases, the sex ratio is 5.2:1 (2). In short-segment disease, the recurrence risk for siblings of an affected male is about 1% for sisters and 6% for brothers, whereas that of an affected female is 3% for sisters and 8% for brothers. In long-segment disease, the risk for siblings of an affected male is about 10% for sisters and 7% for brothers, whereas that of an affected female is 9% for sisters and 18% for brothers (2). Both short- and long-segment disease, however, may be present in the same kindred (52, 53). In a study of 487 probands and their families, Badner et al. (54) observed a risk to siblings of 4%, as compared with 0.02% in the general population.

Molecular genetic studies have demonstrated that Hirschsprung's disease is etiologically heterogeneous, as several genes play a role in the pathogenesis of this condition. Although the gene defect has been identified in many cases, the genetic cause remains unknown in others. Analysis of families with long-segment disease and those with short-segment disease showed a mutation in the RET proto-oncogene on chromosome 10q11.2 (55, 56). The gene codes for a receptor tyrosine kinase. Results showed that both long- and short-segment disease can arise from mutations in the RET gene, and, in fact, the same mutation has been found to cause both short- and long-segment disease (55).

The form of Hirschsprung's disease attributable to RET gene mutations is autosomal dominant. The RET gene may play a role in ganglion cell migration or differentiation (57). Mutations in the RET gene may also cause medullary thyroid carcinoma and multiple endocrine neoplasia types 2A and 2B.

In a large inbred Mennonite kindred, another locus for Hirschsprung's disease was detected on 13q22 (58). The fraction of affected individuals in this kindred was most consistent with an autosomal recessive mode of inheritance. Mutations in the gene encoding the endothelin-B receptor (EDNRB), a receptor for vasoactive peptides, were subsequently identified (59). This allele was not completely penetrant, because 74% of individuals homozygous for the mutation were affected compared to 21% of heterozygotes. Penetrance was higher in males than in females. Homozygotes were more likely to have deafness or pigment abnormalities of the skin, hair, or iris. Both epidermal melanocytes and intestinal ganglion cells are derived from neural crest cells. Of interest, Hirschsprung's disease can occur in association with Waardenburg syndrome (60), which is characterized by pigment abnormalities and deafness.

Mutations have been identified in both the EDNRB gene (59) and the endothelin-3 gene (61), which is a ligand for the endothelin-B receptor. Other genes are involved in the pathogenesis of Hirschsprung's disease, because even within the Mennonite kindred, five individuals with congenital megacolon did not have the specific mutation present in other family members. Preliminary evidence for an additional locus at 21q22 was obtained in this kindred (58).

Mutations in the RET gene may account for 50% of familial Hirschsprung's disease and 15 to 20% of sporadic cases (62, 63). Mutations in EDNRB account for 5% of cases. Long-segment disease occurs in 75% of individuals with a RET mutation, but in less than 5% of those with an EDNRB mutation (63).

Hirschsprung's disease may be associated with several other disorders, most notably Down syndrome. About 2 to 6% of Down syndrome patients have Hirschsprung's disease (9, 10). Other associated conditions include chromosomal syndromes (see Table 7.3), cleft palate, cartilage-hair hypoplasia, deafness, multiple endocrine neoplasia type 2A (64) or 2B (65), congenital central hypoventilation syndrome (66), neuroblastoma (67), pheochromocytoma, rubella embryopathy, colonic atresia, Smith-Lemli-Opitz syndrome, and Aarskog syndrome (68). The association of Hirschsprung's disease with such a wide range of disorders further underlines the genetic heterogeneity of this condition.

CONGENITAL HYPERTROPHIC PYLORIC STENOSIS

Siblings of children with congenital hypertrophic pyloric stenosis (CHPS) have a 12-fold increased risk for CHPS compared to the general population (69). The inheritance pattern is most consistent with multifactorial inheritance or the effects of multiple interacting loci (70). The incidence of CHPS has been decreasing in recent years to approximately 1.5 to 3/1000 live births (2). The distribution of the disease in the two sexes is remarkably different: the incidence in females is 1/1000 and that in males is 1/200. When a female develops CHPS, her children have a higher risk of the disease than do the offspring of an affected male. Sons of affected females are affected 18.9% of the time, and daughters are affected 7.0% of the time. Sons of affected males are affected only 5.5% of the time, and 2.4% of the daughters are affected (69).

Patients with Turner syndrome (monosomy X) have an increased incidence of CHPS, suggesting that the presence of a second X chromosome may have a mitigating effect (71). It is postulated that females carry a higher concentration of the genes determining susceptibility, so a woman's chances of transmitting these genes to her offspring is greater than that for an affected male. CHPS was the first multifactorial condition identified in which the risk of transmission depended on the sex of the affected parent.

Twin studies showed higher concordance for monozygotic twins than for dizygotic twins, but the concordance is only about 50% (2), suggesting that the overall influence of genetic factors may be limited. In an analysis of biopsy specimens from the hypertrophied pylorus, neurons innervating the circular muscle of the pylorus did not stain with NADPH-diaphorase, reflecting a lack of activity of neuronal nitric oxide synthase (NOS) (72). Targeted disruption of the neuronal NOS gene in mice results in an enlarged stomach with hypertrophy of the sphincter and circular muscle layer of the pylorus (73). Examination of two alleles of NOS was performed in 27 families, and inheritance of a specific allele was found to correlate with CHPS (74). Thus, NOS may be a susceptibility locus for CHPS. The heterogeneous nature of CHPS is manifest by its association with a number of other disorders, including chromosomal syndromes (see Table 7.3), phenylketonuria, esophageal atresia, hiatal hernia, peptic ulcer, Smith-Lemli-Opitz syndrome, rubella embryopathy, and Cornelia de Lange syndrome.

ESOPHAGEAL ACHALASIA

The majority of cases of esophageal achalasia are not familial, although several reports describe recurrences in a kindred. Most familial cases involve affected siblings with normal parents, suggesting autosomal recessive inheritance (75–78). Onset of familial achalasia is often in the first decade and sometimes in adolescence. Achalasia can also appear in association with adrenal glucocorticoid insufficiency, an autosomal recessive disorder (79). One Mexican kindred with achalasia and microcephaly has been described (80).

GENETICS OF NEOPLASTIC DISEASES OF THE GASTROINTESTINAL TRACT

ESOPHAGEAL NEOPLASMS

Among the malignant esophageal tumors, 70% are squamous cell carcinomas and 30% are adenocarcinomas. Focal palmoplantar keratosis, or tylosis, is the only hereditary disease associated with esophageal squamous cell carcinoma. Patients with tylosis have a 90% risk of developing carcinoma of the esophagus by age 65 (81). The condition shows autosomal dominant inheritance with complete penetrance, and it has been mapped to 17q23-qter, telomeric to the keratin gene cluster (82, 83).

A strong family history of esophageal carcinoma has been reported in some high-risk areas, such as the Northern Caspian Littoral of Iran. Ghadirian (84) studied family histories among Turkoman (a high-risk population) and non-Turkoman (a low-risk population) people in that region. A positive family history was obtained in 47% of the former, of whom 82% were blood relatives and 18% by marriage. In contrast, only 2% of the non-Turkoman group had a positive family history. Thus, a genetic factor apparently is involved in the development of esophageal cancer in the high-risk population.

Adenocarcinoma is primarily a complication of Barrett's esophagus secondary to reflux esophagitis. Familial recurrences of Barrett's esophagus and adenocarcinoma have been reported (85–87).

Cytogenetic studies of esophageal carcinoma revealed extensive numeric and structural abnormalities involving almost every chromosome. Chromosome numbers varied from 45 to 100 per cell (88). The only consistent finding was loss of the Y chromosome

(89, 90). Using in situ hybridization of formalin-fixed tissue sections, Hunter et al. (91) demonstrated absence of the Y chromosome in 13 of the 14 adenocarcinomas (93%) and 8 of the 13 squamous cell carcinomas (62%). The structural changes were also extremely diverse, including deletion, duplication, inversion, insertion, and translocation. The chromosomes frequently involved in rearrangements included 1, 2, 3, 4, 6, 7, 9, 10, and 11 (88, 89, 92). Deletion of chromosome 3p14.2-p21.3 and chromosome 9q31-q32 was most common in squamous cell carcinomas (93–95), whereas deletion of chromosome 3q13.2-q23 was often seen in adenocarcinomas (92). Rodriguez and coworkers reported rearrangement of chromosome 11p13-p15 in three adenocarcinomas associated with Barrett's esophagus (96). Cytogenetic studies of short-term cultures of epithelium from Barrett's esophagus demonstrated chromosome abnormalities in 9 of 10 cases, including a t(3;6) in 1 patient, trisomy 5 and trisomy 7 in one other patient, and loss of the Y chromosome in the remaining 7 patients (97).

Allelotype analysis of esophageal carcinoma showed loss of heterozygosity (LOH) at frequencies of at least 30% at chromosomes 3p, 3q, 5q, 6p, 8p, 9p, 9q, 10p, 11p, 13q, 17p, 17q, 18q, 19q, and 21q (98, 99). These chromosome regions could contain tumor suppressor genes that may be associated with development and/or progression of esophageal cancer. Loss of heterozygosity of 9p22 and 17p13 (the p53 site) was noted in high-grade dysplasias and carcinomas (95). Abnormalities of p53 were found in adenocarcinomas and were associated with 17p deletions (100). Mutations in p53 (101) and MTS1 (95) have been detected in squamous tumors. Squamous cell carcinoma of the esophagus has shown amplification of c-myc and c-erb B genes (102, 103). Amplification of a region of chromosome 11q13, which includes the hst-1 and int-2 oncogenes, was found in 47% of primary esophageal carcinomas and 100% of metastatic lesions (104). Another amplified gene in the region, cyclin D, plays a role in the regulation of cell proliferation (105). DNA instability is frequently found in adenocarcinomas, but is rare in squamous tumors (106). LOH of the retinoblastoma gene (107) and the APC and MCC genes (108) have been found in the majority of esophageal cancers.

Although 35 of the 61 esophageal carcinomas studied by Ogasawara et al. (109) showed LOH on 5q, none of them had mutation of the remaining APC gene allele. Similarly, in a deletion analysis of chromosome 18q, Shibagaki and colleagues (99) found that the region on 18q commonly lost in esophageal carcinoma did not include the DCC locus. These findings suggest that tumor suppressor genes on 5q and 18q other than APC and DCC were involved in esophageal carcinogenesis.

Twenty percent of esophageal tumors are benign, mostly leiomyomas. Diffuse esophageal leiomyomatosis can occur in association with Alport's syndrome (glomerulonephritis, deafness, and congenital cataracts) (110). Alport's syndrome is associated with a mutation in the gene COL4A5, which encodes the α-5 chain of type IV collagen (111) and is located on Xq22 (112). Patients with esophageal leiomyomatosis have a contiguous gene deletion, which not only includes COL4A5, but also affects the α-6 chain of type IV collagen, the COL4A6 gene (113).

Gastric Neoplasms

Greater than 90% of the neoplasms in the stomach are malignant, mainly adenocarcinomas. Adenomas have a high incidence of malignant transformation but are not the main precursor of carcinoma, as in the colon. Other precursors include chronic atrophic gastritis with or without intestinal metaplasia; chronic gastric ulcer; mucosal hyperplasia, including Ménétrier's disease; postgastrectomy remnants; and, occasionally, nonneoplastic polyps. Detailed information about these conditions is presented in Chapters 26 and 27.

The most important precursor is chronic atrophic gastritis (CAG). Type A involves the fundic mucosa and is related to pernicious anemia. Type B involves the central mucosa and is the most important precancerous condition for gastric cancer. Study of Colombian families revealed that CAG may be transmitted as an autosomal recessive trait with penetrance dependent on the age of the patient and the CAG status of the mother (114). Homozygous recessives had a penetrance of 73 or 41% at age 30 years, depending on whether or not the mother was affected.

Gastric carcinoma itself may be affected by genetic factors. Individuals with blood group A have a 20% increased risk of gastric carcinoma compared to those with the other blood groups (115). No such association has been found, however, in patients with intestinal metaplasia, which is considered a precursor of gastric cancer. The incidence of gastric carcinoma is significantly lower in blood group O women and the survival time is longer in group O individuals than in patients with other blood groups (111). These findings suggest that gastric cancer cells produce an antigen immunologically related to blood group A, so that group O individuals may not be as susceptible to tumor growth as individuals of other blood groups.

Familial cases of gastric carcinoma are not unusual. The best known example is that of Napoleon Bonaparte: Napoleon, his grandfather, his father, and five siblings were said to be affected with gastric carcinoma (117). There appears to be a threefold increased risk among relatives of patients with gastric cancer (118). Gastric carcinoma also occurs in patients with genetically transmitted intestinal diseases, such as familial adenomatous polyposis and cancer family syndrome.

Cytogenetic studies with G banding on gastric carcinomas revealed many aberrations. Ochi et al. (119) studied 5 primary, stage IV carcinomas and found 67 numeric and 83 structural chromosome abnormalities. The most consistent numeric alteration was loss of the Y chromosome in three of the four male patients. No recurring structural changes were recorded, although breakpoints at 1p22, 3p21, and 19p13 were frequent. In another study involving two primary gastric carcinomas and three metastatic effusions, karyotypic abnormalities were noted on chromosomes 1, 7, 8, and 9. The most common aberrations included trisomy 9, i(9q), 9p+, trisomy 8, and i(8q) (120). In a study on the effusion of six gastric carcinomas, Misawa et al. (121) reported nonrecurrent changes in chromosomes 3, 5, 13, and 17. Using fluorescence in situ hybridization (FISH) with centromere-specific α-satellite DNA probes on interphase nuclei of six gastric adenocarcinomas, Rao et al. demonstrated that the most common numeric changes were loss of the Y chromosome, monosomy 10, and trisomy of chromosomes 7, 8, 11, and 17 (122). Seruca and colleagues performed cytogenetic studies on 11 gastric carcinomas by direct harvesting or short-term in vitro culture (123). They reported that polysomy of chromosomes 2 and 20 were the most common numeric changes whereas chromosomes 1, 3, 7, and 13 were most frequently involved in structural rearrangements. Partial deletion of 6q, i(8q), and i(17q) were among the recurrent changes in several tumors. Homogeneously staining regions and double minutes were also seen repeatedly.

Chromosome aberrations are different in the two types of gastric carcinoma: the expanding (intestinal) type and the infiltrative (diffuse) type. Ming et al. (124) reported cytogenetic and molecular changes in two such tumor cell lines: (a) MGc80-3 derived from an expanding poorly differentiated adenocarcinoma in a 53-year-old man (125), and (b) KATO II established from pleural effusion in a 55-year-old man with an infiltrative signet ring cell carcinoma (126). Both cell lines showed multiple nonrandom chromosome aberrations but with considerable differences between them.

MGc80-3 cells had a modal number of 63 to 70 chromosomes with many different types of structural rearrangements and 3 to 5 marker chromosomes (Fig. 7.4), whereas KATO II cells had a modal number of 69 to 84 chromosomes with only two types of structural changes, i(5q) and i(15q) (Fig. 7.5). Loss of the Y chromosome was the only finding shared by both cell lines. By Southern blot hybridization techniques, ets-1 expression was negative in MGc80-3 cells but positive in KATO II cells. In contrast, c-myc expression was positive in MGc80-3 cells but negative in KATO II cells. Cytogenetic differences between these two types of gastric cancer were also observed by Saal et al. (127).

In carcinomas of the infiltrative type, the only numeric changes were loss of the Y chromosome in four of the seven male patients and occasional structural changes involving chromosomes 1 and 18. In contrast, expanding type tumors were exclusively aneuploid, with many structural alterations involving chromosomes 1, 6, 12, and 13. It is surprising that the clinically less aggressive tumor (expanding type) shows more chromosome abnormalities than the infiltrative

type, which is usually associated with a less favorable prognosis. These studies suggest that the morphologic and biologic differences between these two types of gastric cancer may be related, in part, to the different cytogenetic and molecular changes in their constitutional cells.

Molecular studies of gastric carcinoma revealed frequent LOH at 3p (128), 6q (129), 7q (130), 9p (131), 11q (132), 2p, 5q and 13q (133), 12q, 17p, and 17q (128). It is possible that these sites are those that contain loci of tumor suppressor genes.

Several genes have been identified that may play a role in gastric carcinogenesis. Amplification, loss of heterozygosity, and/or mutations in these genes may be responsible for the multistep pathway that eventually leads to gastric cancer. Ras oncogenes have been studied by many investigators with varying results, but the overall prevalence of mutations of these genes in gastric cancers is low (134–137).

Several oncogenes are amplified in some gastric tumors. Amplification of the c-myc and c-erb B2 (138, 139) proto-oncogenes have been reported. The proto-oncogene c-met, the receptor for hepatocyte growth factor, is amplified in advanced gastric cancer (140). K-sam, which encodes the receptor for keratinocyte growth factor, can also be amplified (141). c-met and K-sam are rarely amplified in esophageal or colorectal cancers.

Allelic loss and mutation of p53 have been noted in the majority of cases of both early and advanced gastric cancer (142–145). Abnormalities of this gene are also present in 30% of gastric adenomas (146).

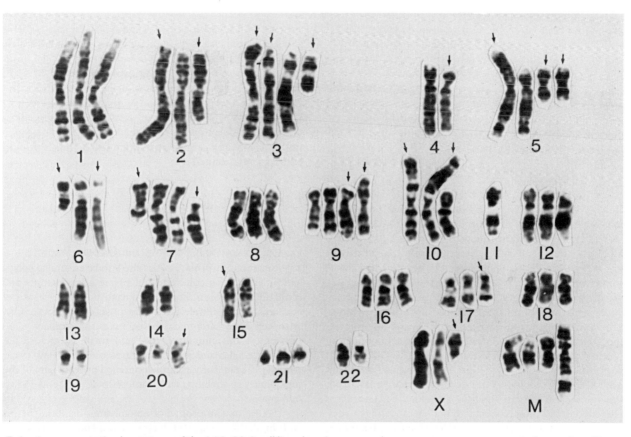

Figure 7.4 A representative karyotype of the MGc80-3 cell line showing many chromosome rearrangements (arrows) and four marker chromosomes (M).

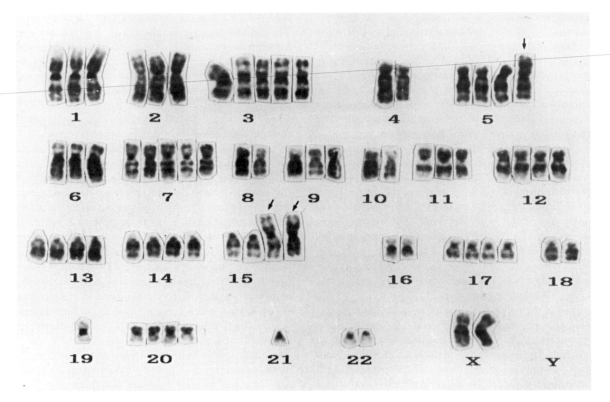

Figure 7.5   A representative karyotype of the KATO II cell line with i(5q) and i(15q) as the only structural abnormalities *(arrows)*.

LOH and mutation of the APC gene occur in gastric cancers (147–149). The APC gene may also be mutated in adenomas (150). Mutations in the E-cadherin gene (151) have been noted, and expression of E-cadherin and α-catenin may be decreased in some gastric cancers (152). The APC gene product binds to catenins. LOH of the DCC gene on chromosome 18q has also been reported (153). Instability of microsatellite regions, probably reflecting errors in DNA mismatch repair, has been noted in approximately 30% of primary gastric cancers (154, 155).

INTESTINAL NEOPLASMS

In contrast to the esophagus and stomach, benign tumors are common in the intestine, particularly the colorectum. Mesenchymal tumors are common in the small intestine, but rare in the large intestine. In the latter, most of the primary tumors are epithelial in origin—about two-thirds are adenomas and one-third are adenocarcinomas. Even though the small intestine is longer than the colon, carcinomas occur almost 60 times more often in the colorectum than in the small intestine. Detailed information of tumor types in the intestines is provided in Chapters 33 and 34.

Genetic factors play an important role in the development of intestinal adenomas and carcinomas. Results of studies suggest that 15% of colorectal cancers may be related to autosomal dominant conditions (156, 157). Multiple intestinal polyps represent a major manifestation in several genetic conditions (Table 7.4). The polyps are heterogeneous and their tendency to malignant change varies. The pathologic features of the polyps are described in Chapter 33.

Genetic factors are also important in the development of intestinal cancers in patients without polyposis, including many patients with sporadic tumors (158, 159). In such patients, colorectal carcinoma is the main presentation. Adenomas are also often present, even though they are not numerically or symptomatically significant. Adenomas are nevertheless important components of these cases and may be the seat of malignant transformation.

Polyposis of the intestine is not always hereditary. In the Cronkhite-Canada syndrome, all cases have been sporadic, and the condition is not considered a genetic disease. These polyps are inflammatory, not premalignant, and are present throughout the entire gastrointestinal tract.

CLINICAL SYNDROMES

Familial Polyposis Syndromes

FAMILIAL ADENOMATOUS POLYPOSIS AND GARDNER SYNDROME   Familial adenomatous polyposis (FAP) is also known as familial polyposis coli and adenomatosis coli. The polyps are adenomatous and occur primarily in the colon. The carcinomas occur mostly in the left colon and are often multiple. It is also possible, however, for polyps, adenomas, and carcinomas to occur in the stomach (160–162), duodenum and ampulla (163), and small intestine (163, 164). Extraintestinal manifestations include osteomas, jaw cysts, dental anomalies, brain tumors, and congenital hypertrophy of the retinal pigmentary epithelium (see Chapters 26, 27, 33, and 34 for further information).

FAP shows autosomal dominant transmission. The frequency is 1 in 8300 to 13,500 births (165, 166). In Denmark, new mutations account for 25% of cases (166). The average age at the time of diagnosis of polyps is 35 years (167); the average age of cancer diagnosis is 39 years (168). About 50% of symptomatic and 6 to 12% of asymptomatic patients have carcinoma of the colon at the time of diagnosis (169, 170). Carcinoma may be present in all cases by the age of 50 years. Penetrance is nearly complete by age 40 years. Expressivity can be variable both within and between families (166).

The altered gene in FAP, termed APC, was mapped to 5q21 (171). Loss of heterozygosity of chromosome 5 is often noted in both familial and sporadic colon cancers, and the APC locus is lost in these cases (172–174). Mutations in APC lead to FAP (175–178). The APC gene product associates with α-catenin and β-catenin (179, 180). These proteins bind to the cell adhesion molecule E-cadherin. Thus, the APC product may play a role in cell adhesion and/or cell-to-cell communication.

Greater than 98% of the identified mutations in FAP result in premature termination of the protein, owing to either nonsense or frameshift mutations (181, 182). The majority of mutations occur in the proximal half of the gene (182), and many are in the 5′ portion of exon 15, the mutation cluster region (182). Because so many of the mutations result in premature protein termination, an assay to identify truncated forms of the protein has been developed for mutation screening (183, 184).

Studies that show some genotype-phenotype relationships are emerging. Mutations between codons 1250 and 1464 were associated with an increased number of polyps (185). Patients with mutations proximal to exon 10 had fewer polyps, and the average age of diagnosis was 39 years (186). Those with mutations distal to exon 9 generally had many more polyps and were diagnosed at an average age of 25 years. Desmoid tumors and mandibular lesions were more frequent in patients with truncating mutations between codons 1403 and 1528 (187). Four families with "attenuated" FAP and relatively few colonic polyps (often less than 100) had mutations in the APC gene more proximal than in other described cases (188). The presence of congenital hypertrophy of the retinal pigmentary epithelium correlated with mutations occurring after exon 9 (189).

In one study of both familial and sporadic adenomas and carcinomas, more than 80% of tumors had at least one mutation in the APC gene, and of these, 60% had two mutations (174). Another group of investigators found that at least 60% of colorectal carcinomas and adenomas had a mutation in the APC gene, including adenomas as small as 0.5 cm in diameter (190). The frequency of mutation did not increase as the tumors progressed from benign to malignant, implying that APC mutation is an early event and that mutations in other genes occur during later stages of carcinogenesis.

Gardner syndrome was originally described in individuals with FAP-like polyps who had additional findings outside of the gastrointestinal tract, including epidermal cysts and subcutaneous fibromas of the skin, desmoids of the skin and abdomen, osteomas, dental abnormalities, pigmented patches in the retina, and tumors of other organs (191, 192). The distinction between Gardner syndrome and FAP was unclear, however, because some individuals diagnosed with FAP also had extraintestinal signs. Clinical Gardner syndrome and FAP can occur in the same kindred. It was subsequently found that both conditions can result from the same mutation in the APC gene (173). Thus, Gardner syndrome and FAP are allelic and both are attributable to mutations in the APC gene.

A mutation in the APC gene can also cause the form of Turcot syndrome associated with medulloblastoma (193) (see next section).

TURCOT SYNDROME   Turcot syndrome is characterized by the presence of malignant brain tumor in patients with colonic adenomatous polyps (194). Recent advances have clarified the relationship between Turcot syndrome and Gardner's syndrome, which may also be associated with brain tumors. The gene mutation causing Turcot syndrome was identified in 13 families (193). In 10 families, the most frequent brain tumor was medulloblastoma. These families had mutations in APC, the gene responsible for familial adenomatous polyposis and Gardner's syndrome. In three other families, glioblastomas were present. The glioblastomas and colorectal tumors had DNA replication errors similar to those found in hereditary nonpolyposis colorectal cancer. Mutations in the mismatch repair genes MLH1 or PMS2 were identified in two of the kindreds. Thus, brain tumors occur in association with

---

TABLE 7.4	Hereditary Syndromes of Gastrointestinal Tumors	

Syndrome	Initial Tumor Type	Other Major Manifestations
Familial polyposis		
Familial adenomatous polyposis	Adenoma	Upper gastrointestinal lesions
Gardner syndrome	Adenoma	Osteoma, skin and soft tissue tumors
Turcot syndrome	Adenoma	Brain tumor
Peutz-Jeghers syndrome	Hamartoma	Mucocutaneous melanin spots
Famillal juvenile polyposis	Hamartoma	None
Muir-Torre syndrome	Adenoma or carcinoma	Skin tumors
Hereditary nonpolyposis colorectal cancer		
Lynch syndrome I (HSSCC)	Carcinoma	None
Lynch syndrome II (CFS)	Carcinoma	Other cancers in family
Discrete colorectal tumors	Adenoma or carcinoma	None
Cowden disease	Hamartoma	Hamartomas of skin, mucous membranes, breast, and thyroid

CFS, cancer family syndrome; GI, gastrointestinal; HSSCC, hereditary site-specific colorectal cancer.

colonic tumors in at least two different clinical conditions. In the autosomal dominant FAP/Gardner syndrome, mutations occur in the APC gene, and the brain tumor is generally a medulloblastoma. In the autosomal recessive Turcot syndrome, the tumor type is glioblastoma, and the mutations occur in mismatch repair genes.

HAMARTOMATOUS POLYPOSIS The polyps in both Peutz-Jeghers syndrome and familial juvenile polyposis are hamartomatous, but the major tissue components are different. The Peutz-Jeghers polyp is composed of intestinal crypts and villi and smooth muscle bundles in a disorganized fashion. Inflammatory cells are absent or scanty and the glandular structures are not excessively dilated. The juvenile polyp is composed of dilated intestinal glands and abundant connective tissue of the lamina propria. Smooth muscle elements are usually absent, and lymphoid cells are common. These features closely resemble those of inflammatory retention polyps in children, also known as juvenile polyps, as well as inflammatory polyps of Cronkhite-Canada syndrome, which occur among the elderly.

Peutz-Jeghers syndrome is characterized by the presence of Peutz-Jeghers polyps throughout the entire gastrointestinal tract and melanin spots on the lip (96%), buccal mucosa (83%), face (36%), and extremities (32%) (195, 196). Small bowel is the favored site of the polyposis, and the number of polyps is small. Other associated abnormalities include polyps in the urinary bladder and nasal cavity, bone deformities, congenital heart disease, and retarded development (197).

The symptoms of Peutz-Jeghers syndrome develop before the age of 20 year in two-thirds of cases, with an average age at time of diagnosis of 22.5 years (168). Symptoms of Peutz-Jeghers syndrome are noted at a younger age than those associated with FAP. Peutz-Jeghers polyps are generally not prone to malignant change; however, carcinomas of the gastrointestinal tract have been reported in about 2 to 3% of cases, most commonly in the proximal small intestine (198, 199). In many reports, the relationship between polyp and carcinoma is unclear. When the origin of malignancy was carefully studied, the carcinoma was usually found to arise in the adenomatous or dysplastic epithelium in the polyp (200). Malignancy can also occur outside of the gastrointestinal tract (201). The condition is linked to 19p in at least some families (202).

Isolated juvenile polyps may occur in the colon and rectum of children. In 1966, Veale et al. (203) reported 11 cases in 8 families. The principal symptoms were bleeding and prolapse of the polyp from the rectum; the average age at onset of symptoms was 6 years. The polyps in these patients were mostly in the rectum, and thereby the term of juvenile polyposis coli was given. Subsequently, polyps have been reported in other parts of the gastrointestinal tract (204, 205). Sachatello and coworkers (206) reported generalized juvenile polyposis involving the entire gastrointestinal tract in infants. The age of diagnosis shows a wide range (207, 208). Although many patients lack a family history (167, 209), the familial cases were transmitted as an autosomal dominant trait (168). The incidence of juvenile polyposis coli was estimated to be 1 in 24,000 births (209).

Dysplasia and adenomatous changes have been found in the polyps (204, 210), and carcinomas may have developed in them (207, 211). The average age at cancer diagnosis is about 40 years (204). Individuals with juvenile polyposis of the stomach, which may be the same entity as juvenile polyposis, may develop gastric cancer (212, 213).

Hereditary Nonpolyposis Colorectal Cancer (HNPCC)

It is estimated that familial polyposis accounts for only 0.2% of all colorectal carcinomas, whereas hereditary nonpolyposis colorectal cancer accounts for 1 to 5% of such cases (159, 214–216). The HNPCC syndrome is heterogenous and includes two major entities: cancer family syndrome (Lynch syndrome II) and hereditary site-specific colorectal cancer (Lynch syndrome I) (118, 158, 217).

Characteristics of the Lynch syndromes include: (a) a relatively young mean age at the time of diagnosis, 44.6 years; (b) the first cancer is usually in the proximal colon (72.3%) and only 25% are in the sigmoid or rectum; (c) a high incidence of multiple colon cancers, synchronous in 18.1% of cases and metachronous in 24.2%. The risk for developing metachronous cancers within 10 years is 40%. Because of the prevalence of cancer in the right colon, these cases have been termed hereditary site-specific colon cancer (118). When family members also exhibit cancers of other organs, the term cancer family syndrome, or Lynch syndrome II, is applied. When there is no other cancer in the family, it is referred to as Lynch syndrome I. The HNPCC syndromes show autosomal dominant transmission (118).

The broad spectrum of organs that may be affected by cancer in Lynch syndrome II includes endometrium, ovary, pancreas, and less commonly brain, bile duct, stomach, small intestine, breast, urinary system, and leukemia and lymphoma (217). The frequency of cancers in cancer family syndromes was studied in 196 individuals from 22 Finnish kindreds (214). Cancers included colorectal cancer in 61%, undefined intraabdominal cancer 15%, endometrial cancer 10%, gastric cancer 7%, biliary tract cancer 3%, and other cancers 7%. An autosomal dominant pattern of inheritance was shown by the colorectal and uterine cancers. The cumulative risk in the descendants increased to 50% by the age of 69 years.

The carcinomas in cancer family patients are more likely mucinous and poorly differentiated than are the sporadic colon cancers (218). Although HNPCC patients do not have polyposis, adenomas do occur in the colon. The incidence of adenoma is not increased, although some adenomas demonstrate a high grade of dysplasia (218) and are precursors of invasive carcinoma (219). No other lesions have been found to account for the high incidence of colon cancer in these patients.

Approximately 75 to 80% of HNPCC families (220) show linkage to chromosome 2p (221) or 3p (222). Some of the tumors in these HNPCC kindreds show a wide variation in short repeated dinucleotide segments. This finding is consistent with replication errors during development of the tumor that could be associated with mutations in a gene needed for maintaining stability of the DNA (221, 223). Evidence for DNA instability was subsequently found in 92% of HNPCC families (224). In other investigations, both sporadic and familial HNPCC colon tumors were found to have mutations in the MSH2 gene, which is involved in DNA mismatch repair (225–227). This gene maps to 2p22-p21.

On the basis of the finding that mutations in the MSH2 gene correlate with HNPCC, another mismatch repair gene, MLH1, which maps to 3p21, was examined for mutations in other HNPCC families (228). A variety of mutations were found in the MLH1 gene in tumors (228–230). There is no functional effect of mutations of the MSH2 and MLH1 genes in heterozygotes, and loss of heterozygosity with loss of the normal allele was demonstrated in several affected families (231). Mutations have now been reported in the following DNA mismatch repair genes: MSH2, MLH1, PMS1, and PMS2 (224, 232). Approximately 40% of HNPCC cases may be associated with mutations in MSH2 (233). Up to 13% of sporadic tumors show DNA instability, although the proportion that correlate to one of the identified DNA repair genes is unknown (234) (see Chapter 8 for more details).

The Muir-Torre syndrome was noted in some members of a cancer family (235). This syndrome is characterized by multiple intestinal cancers associated with genitourinary and skin tumors, particularly of the sebaceous gland. Mutations in both MLH1 and MSH2 have been identified in patients with the Muir-Torre syndrome (236, 237).

Discrete Adenomas and Carcinomas of the Colon

Whereas polyposis syndromes are rare, discrete adenomas in small numbers occur in from 10 to 50% of the general population. Overall, colorectal cancer may affect 3% of the population (204). The inheritance pattern of these cases is largely unknown. Recently, Burt et al. (238) studied a large Utah kindred with clusters of colorectal cancer. Extensive screening with flexible proctosigmoidoscopy revealed adenomas in 21% of the 191 pedigree members in contrast to 9% in the controls. The excess of adenomas showed autosomal dominant inheritance. A subsequent expanded study of 670 persons in 34 kindreds revealed the estimated prevalence of adenoma at age 60 years in related family members was 24%, whereas that in unrelated spouses was 12% (156). Such studies emphasize the importance of screening for colorectal tumors in first-degree relatives of patients with these lesions.

CYTOGENETIC AND MOLECULAR CHANGES

The use of new techniques in molecular cytogenetics has enhanced our understanding of colorectal carcinogenesis. It is well known that adenomatous polyps and adenomas are precursors of carcinomas. Now, cytogenetic and molecular data have substantiated this observation. Indeed, the sequential involvement of oncogenes, tumor suppressor genes and related chromosomic changes in colorectal tumorigenesis has been elegantly delineated by Vogelstein and coworkers (234, 239, 240). (For additional details, see Chapter 8.)

As noted previously in this chapter, mutations in APC and DNA mismatch repair genes are associated with familial colorectal cancer syndromes. Mutations in the APC gene, a tumor suppressor, have also been noted in more than two thirds of sporadic tumors (174, 190). These mutations occur early in tumorigenesis because the majority of adenomas also contain an APC mutation. Approximately 15 to 20% of sporadic colorectal cancers seem to have phenotypic defects in mismatch repair (241), although the genetic basis for this finding is not delineated at present.

Mutations in other genes have also been identified in colorectal cancers. A Ras gene mutation occurs in more than one third of colorectal cancers (242). Located on chromosome 12p, this gene has GTPase activity. Point mutations occur most frequently at codon 12 or 13 in K-ras (239). Mutations in codon 12 may be associated with more aggressive tumors (243). K-ras mutations have also been detected in adenomatous polyps (244).

The tumor suppressor gene p53, located on chromosome 17p, undergoes allelic loss in more than 75% of colorectal cancers (245).

The retained allele is generally mutated (246, 247), although allele loss or mutation of p53 is uncommon in adenomas (248). Thus, changes in p53 are associated with later stages of tumorigenesis.

The chromosomal region 18q21 is often deleted in colorectal carcinomas and advanced adenomas (249). A gene in this region that may be a tumor suppressor gene was named DCC (*d*eleted in *c*olorectal *c*ancer) (249). Studies show that the expression of the DCC gene is decreased in most colorectal carcinomas, and many primary colorectal tumors have a deletion of the DCC gene (250). The gene's product is a transmembrane protein with similarity to neural cell adhesion molecules. The protein likely plays a role in cell-to-cell or cell-to-matrix interactions in the development of colon carcinoma, and loss of the gene is found more frequently in metastatic colorectal cancers compared to nonmetastatic cancers (251). Nearly all hepatic metastases of primary colorectal cancers have LOH of 18q (252).

The MCC gene (*m*utated in *c*olon *c*ancer) also maps to 5q21 (253). Mutations in MCC have been found in some colon cancers (254). However, the remaining allele of MCC in tumors with LOH of 5q21 generally do not show a mutation, which is an unexpected finding for a tumor suppressor gene (255).

Amplification and overexpression of c-myc have been found in some colorectal cancers (256–260). c-erb-B is amplified in a small number of colon cancers (261).

Cytogenetic changes in the colonic tumors may be numeric and/or structural. The study of 38 colonic adenomas by Reichman et al. (262) revealed analyzable karyotypes in 18 tumors. These adenomas showed normal diploid karyotype in 5, numeric abnormalities in 6, and both numeric and structural abnormalities in 7 of the 18. The latter included extra chromosomes 7, 8, or 13 and marker chromosomes. In one villous adenoma, there was an extra chromosome 8, loss of a Y chromosome, and an abnormal chromosome 1 with duplication of the long arm (263). Griffin and colleagues studied 27 adenomatous polyps from patients with FAP, 2 polyps from the small intestine in Peutz-Jeghers syndrome, and 4 polyps from juvenile polyposis syndrome (264). Chromosome abnormalities were found in 5 of 27 polyps from FAP, compared to 14 of 32 sporadic colorectal adenomas. Trisomy 7 and trisomy 13 were the most common numeric aberrations; structural changes were present only in sporadic polyps. The most common changes were deletion of 1p with various breakpoints, del(8p), and i(13q). Longy et al. (265) reported chromosome abnormalities in 22 of 42 adenomatous polyps of the colon: trisomy 7 in 13, trisomy 13 in 9, and monosomy 18 in 2 polyps. One of the two polyps with monosomy 18 showed areas of intramucosal carcinoma and also had a deletion of 17p. It is interesting to note that these two types of aberration, trisomy 7 versus monosomy 18 and del(17p), were not found in the same lesion, suggesting that they were involved in different stages of tumorigenesis.

On the basis of these cytogenetic studies and other reports (266, 267), colorectal adenomas may be classified into two groups: those with only numeric changes, and those with both numeric and structural aberrations. All tubulovillous and villous adenomas showed structural abnormalities. In general, adenomas with structural aberrations were usually larger and had a higher degree of dysplasia than those with only numeric changes or a normal karyotype. It seems that the more complex the chromosome changes, the higher the malignant potential of the adenomas. No single aberration, however, could be identified as the prerequisite marker for malignant transformation.

Cytogenetic studies of colorectal carcinomas have been more extensive than those of adenomas. Levin and Reichman (268) studied 49 colonic adenocarcinomas. They reported that only 8% of the tumors had normal karyotypes. Hypodiploidy or hypotriploidy were observed in 50%. Thirty-eight tumors had a total of 257 abnormal chromosomes, of which 44% had recognizable patterns, most frequently involving chromosomes 1, 5, 8, 9, 13, and 17. Trisomies were common. Homogeneously staining regions and double minutes were also observed. Tumors with significant chromosomal aberrations were often located in the left colon, whereas tumors with normal karyotypes or few abnormalities were more common in the right colon.

Muleris et al. (269) performed cytogenetic studies on 100 colorectal carcinomas. Seven tumors had normal karyotypes (NT). On the basis of chromosomal abnormalities, the tumors were classified into three types: (a) monosomic-type near diploid (MD) tumors in 28 cases, characterized by a monosomy of both chromosomes 17p and 18; (b) monosomic-type polyploid (MP) tumors in 42 cases, derived from the MD tumors by endoreduplication; and (c) trisomic-type (TT) tumors in 22 cases, with or without loss of 17p or 18. One tumor could not be classified. The MD and MP tumors were predominantly located in the distal colon and rectum, whereas TT and NT tumors were found mainly in the proximal colon. Structural rearrangements of the chromosomes per tumor in MD and MP tumors were two to three times higher than those in the TT tumors. Sixty percent of the rearrangements were unbalanced and 5% were balanced. Deletions occurred in 20% and isochromosomes in 10 to 20%.

Dutrillaux (270) noted that the monosomic-type tumors had losses or deletions involving, in order of decreasing frequency, chromosomes 18, 17, 1p, 4, 14, 5, and 21. Trisomy frequently involved chromosomes 7, 12, X, 5, and 8. The study concerning near-diploid tumors showed monosomies 17p, 18, and 1p and trisomies 20q, 13, X, and 8q (271).

The largest series of cytogenetic studies of primary colorectal carcinoma was carried out by Bardi et al. (272–274). A total of 153 primary adenocarcinomas were analyzed by short-term culture techniques; 116 of them showed chromosome abnormalities. The most common numeric changes were, in order of decreasing frequency, gains of chromosomes 7, 13, 20, and Y and losses of chromosomes 18, Y, 14, 21, 4, 8, and 15. The structural rearrangements most commonly involved chromosomes 13q, 17p, 17q, 1p, 8q, 11q, 10p, 7p, 7q, 12q, 16p, and 19p. Frequently recurring aberrations included del(1p), i(8q), i(13q), and del(17p).

The results of these cytogenetic studies and those by other investigators (275–278) generally agree that nonrandom rearrangements most frequently involve chromosomes 1, 7, 8, 13, 14, 17, and 18 either numerically or structurally and eventually lead to genetic imbalances. The diagnostic significance of chromosomal aberrations was evaluated by multivariate analysis in relation to the stage of carcinoma (279). Distant metastasis was associated with allele loss and deletions of 17p and 18q, but not with the ras gene and deletion of 5q. The clonal origin of colorectal tumors was investigated by means of X-linked restriction fragment length polymorphisms (280). All tumors examined, including both adenomas and carcinomas, showed a monoclonal pattern of X chromosome inactivation.

Based on the correlation analysis between the karyotypes and clinicopathologic features of the tumors, Bardi et al. found a statistically significant association between the chromosome changes and tumor grade and site (272, 274). Poorly differentiated carcinomas usually show structural rearrangements, whereas well- or moderately differentiated tumors often have only numeric aberrations or normal karyotypes. The cytogenetic changes also varied with the location of the tumor. Carcinomas in the proximal colon and rectum were usually quasidiploid with simple chromosome changes, whereas the tumors of the distal colon often had complex triploid-tetraploid karyotypes. Furthermore, the patients who had tumors with multiple chromosomal abnormalities had a shorter survival time than those who had tumors with simple changes or normal karyotype (274, 281). Therefore, karyotypes could be used as one of the prognostic parameters in patients with colorectal carcinoma. The feasibility of the application of karyotypic study to clinical diagnosis is exemplified by the report of a rectosigmoid tumor in a 74-year-old man (282). Interpretation of the results of tissue biopsy was that the lesion was histologically benign. The karyotype of the same biopsy specimen showed several chromosomal changes, including trisomy 7, t(3;12), t(1;17), interstitial deletion of 5p, loss of the Y chromosome, and an extra X chromosome. These changes strongly suggested malignancy. A 5-cm, well to moderately differentiated adenocarcinoma in Dukes' stage B1 was subsequently excised.

Finally, the cytogenetic studies of squamous cell carcinoma of the anal canal should be mentioned. Muleris et al. (283) examined seven such tumors and found that deletions of chromosomes 11q and 3p were the most common recurring aberrations.

References

1. McKusick VA. Mendelian inheritance in man—Catalogs of autosomal dominant, autosomal recessive and X-linked phenotypes. 11th ed. Baltimore: Johns Hopkins University Press, 1994.
2. Passarge E. Developmental defects of the gastrointestinal tract. In: Rimoin DL, Connor JM, Pyeritz RE, eds. Principles and practice of medical genetics. 3rd ed. New York: Churchill Livingstone, 1997: 1525–1532.
3. Auricchio A, Brancolini V, Casari G, et al. The locus for a novel syndromic form of neuronal intestinal pseudo-obstruction maps to Xq28. Am J Hum Genet 1996;58:743–748.
4. Cormier-Daire V, Bonnefont J-P, Rustin P, et al. Mitochondrial DNA rearrangements with onset as chronic diarrhea with villous atrophy. J Pediatr 1994;124:63–70.
5. Hirano M, Silvestri G, Blake DM, et al. Mitochondrial neurogastrointestinal encephalomyopathy (MNGIE): Clinical, biochemical, and genetic features of an autosomal recessive mitochondrial disorder. Neurology 1994;44:721–727.
6. Webb A, Beard J, Wright C, et al. A case of paternal uniparental disomy for chromosome 11. Prenat Diagn 1995;15:773–777.
7. Cohn DH, Starman BJ, Blumberg B, et al. Recurrence of lethal osteogenesis imperfecta due to parental mosaicism for a dominant mutation in a human type I collagen gene (COL1A1). Am J Hum Genet 1990;46:591–601.
8. Warkany J. Uses and misuses of syndromes. In: Shafie ME, Kippel CH Jr, eds. Associated congenital anomalies. Baltimore: Williams & Wilkins, 1981:21–23.
9. Garver KL, Law JC, Garver B. Hirschsprung's disease: A genetic study. Clin Genet 1985;28:503–508.
10. Warkany J, Passarge E, Smith LB. Congenital malformations in autosomal trisomy syndromes. Am J Dis Child 1966;112:502–517.
11. Zlotogora J, Abu-Dalu K, Lernau O, et al. Anorectal malformations and Down's syndrome. Am J Med Genet 1989;34:330–331.
12. Urioste M, Martinez-Frias ML. Anorectal anomalies and Down's syndrome [letter]. Am J Med Genet 1991;39:493.
13. Torfs CP, Bateson TF, Curry CJR. Anorectal and esophageal anomalies with Down's syndrome [letter]. Am J Med Genet 1992; 44:847.

14. Baty BJ, Blackburn BL, Carey JC: Natural history of trisomy 18 and trisomy 13. I. Growth, physical assessment, medical histories, survival, and recurrence risk. Am J Med Genet 1994;49: 175–188.
15. Thompson JS. The genetics of multiple congenital anomalies. In: Shafie ME, Klipple CH, eds. Associated congenital anomalies. Baltimore: Williams & Wilkins, 1981:9–15.
16. DeGrouchy J, Turleau C. Clinical atlas of human chromosomes. 2nd ed. New York: John Wiley and Sons, 1984.
17. Jones KL. Smith's recognizable patterns of human malformation. 5th ed. Philadelphia: WB Saunders, 1996.
18. Beedgen B, Nutzendel W, Querfeld V, et al. Partial trisomy 22 and 11 due to a paternal 11;22 translocation associated with Hirschsprung's disease. Eur J Pediatr 1986;145:229–232.
19. Lamont MA, Fitchett M, Dennis NR. Interstitial deletion of distal 13q associated with Hirschsprung's disease. J Med Genet 1989;26: 100–104.
20. Nicolaides KH, Snijders RJ, Cheng HH, et al. Fetal gastro-intestinal and abdominal wall defects: Associated malformations and chromosomal abnormalities. Fetal Diagn Ther 1992;7:102–115.
21. Hasle H, Olsen JH, Nielsen J, et al. Occurrence of cancer in women with Turner syndrome. Br J Cancer 1996;73:1156–1159.
22. Doll R, Buch J. Hereditary factors in peptic ulcer. Ann Eugenics 1950;15:135–146.
23. Doll R, Kellock TD. The separate inheritance of gastric and duodenal ulcers. Ann Eugenics 1951;16:231–240.
24. Aird I, Bentall HH, Mehigan JA, et al. The blood groups in relation to peptic ulceration and carcinoma of colon, rectum, breast and bronchus. Br Med J 1954;2:315–321.
25. McConnell RB. The genetics of gastrointestinal disorders. London: Oxford University Press, 1966.
26. McConnell RB. Peptic ulcer, early genetic evidence families twins and markers. In: Rotter JI, Samloff IM, Rimoin DL, eds. The genetics and heterogeneity of common gastrointestinal disorders. New York: Academic Press, 1980: 31–41.
27. Cowan WK Genetics of duodenal and gastric ulcer. Clin Gastroenterol 1973;2:539–546.
28. Mourant AE, Kopec AC, Domaniewska-Sobczak K. Blood groups and disease: A study of associations of disease with blood groups and other polymorphisms. London. Oxford University Press, 1978.
29. Rotter JI, Shohat T. Peptic ulcer. In: Emery AEH, Rimoin DL, eds. Principles and practice of medical genetics. 2nd ed. New York: Churchill Livingstone, 1990:1097–1115.
30. Ellis A, Woodrow JC. HLA and duodenal ulcer. Gut 1979;20: 760–762.
31. Goldhard JG, Biemond I, Pena AS, et al. HLA and duodenal ulcer in Netherlands. Tissue Antigens 1983;22:213–218.
32. Soll AH. Duodenal ulcer and drug therapy. In: Sleisenger MH, Fordtran JS, eds. Gastrointestinal disease. 4th ed. Philadelphia: WB Saunders, 1989:814–879.
33. Ellis A. The genetics of peptic ulcer. Scand J Gastroenterol 1985; 110(Suppl):25–27.
34. Rotter JI, Petersen G, Samloff IM, et al. Genetic heterogeneity of hyperpepsinogenemic I and normopepsinogenemic I duodenal ulcer disease. Ann Intern Med 1979;91:372–377.
35. Habibullah CM, Ali MM, Ishaq M, et al. Study of duodenal ulcer disease in 100 families using total serum pepsinogen as a genetic marker. Gut 1984;25:1380–1383.
36. Taylor IL, Calam J, Rotter JI, et al. Family studies of hypergastrinemic, hyperpepsinogenemic I duodenal ulcer. Ann Intern Med 1981; 95:421–425.
37. Neuhauser G, Daly RR, Magnelli NC, et al. Essential tremors, nystagmus and duodenal ulceration: A "new" dominantly inherited condition. Clin Genet 1976;9:81–91.
38. Halal F, Gervais M-H, Baillargeon J, et al. Gastro-cutaneous syndrome: Peptic ulcer-hiatal hernia, multiple lentigenes-cafe-au-lait spots, hypertelorism, and myopia. Am J Med Genet 1982;11: 161–176.
39. Stokes PL, Asquith P, Cooke WT. Genetics of celiac disease. Clin Gastroenterol 1973;2:547–556.
40. Cole SG, Kagnoff MF. Celiac disease. Annu Rev Nutr 1983: 241.
41. Carpenter CB. The major histocompatibility gene complex. In: Isselbacher KJ, Braunwald E, Wilson J, et al., eds. Harrison's

42. principles of internal medicine. 13th ed. New York: McGraw-Hill, 1994:380–386.
43. Howell MD, Austin RK, Kelleher D, et al. An HLA-D region restriction fragment length polymorphism associated with celiac disease. J Exp Med 1986;164:333–338.
44. Howell MD, Resner J, Austin RK, et al. Rapid identification of hybridization probes for chromosomal walking. Gene 1987;55: 41–45.
45. Mannion A, Stevens FM, McCarthy CF, et al. Extended major histocompatibility complex haplotypes in celiac patients in the west of Ireland. Am J Med Genet 1993;45:373–377.
46. Zhong F, McCombs CC, Oslon JM, et al. An autosomal screen for genes that predispose to celiac disease in the western counties of Ireland. Nature Genet 1996;14:329–333.
47. Kirsner JB. Genetic aspects of inflammatory bowel disease. Clin Gastroenterol 1973;2:556–575.
48. Monsen U, Brostrom O, Nordenvall B. Prevalence of inflammatory bowel disease among relatives of patients with ulcerative colitis. Scand J Gastroenterol 1987;22:214–218.
49. Satsangi J, Grootscholten C, Holt H, et al. Clinical patterns of familial inflammatory bowel disease. Gut 1996;38:738–741.
50. Hugot J-P, Laurent-Puig P, Gower-Rousseau C, et al. Mapping of a susceptibility locus for Crohn's disease on chromosome 16. Nature Genet 1996;379:821–823.
51. Satsangi J, Parkes M, Louis E, et al. Two stage genome-wide search in inflammatory bowel disease provides evidence for susceptibility loci on chromosome 3, 7 and 12. Nature Genet 1996;14:199–202.
52. Rudolph U, Finegold MJ, Rich SS, et al. Ulcerative colitis and adenocarcinoma of the colon in G-alpha-i2-deficient mice. Nature Genet 1995,10:143–150.
53. Carter CO, Evans K, Hickman V. Children of those treated surgically for Hirschsprung's disease. J Med Genet 1981;18:87–90.
54. Lipson AH, Harvey J. Three-generation transmission of Hirschsprung's disease. Clin Genet 1987;32:175–178.
55. Badner JA, Sieber WK, Garver KL. A genetic study of Hirschsprung's disease. Am J Hum Genet 1990;45:568–580.
56. Edery P, Pelet A, Mulligan LM, et al. Long segment and short segment familial Hirschsprung's disease: Variable clinical expression at the RET locus. J Med Genet 1994;31:6023–6026.
57. Edery P, Lyonnet S, Mulligan L, et al. Mutations of the RET proto-oncogene in Hirschsprung's disease. Nature 1994;367: 378–380.
58. Iwashita T, Murakami H, Asai N, et al. Mechanism of RET dysfunction by Hirschsprung's mutations affecting its extracellular domain. Hum Mol Genet 1996;5:1577–1580.
59. Puffenberger EG, Kauffman ER, Bolk S, et al. Identity-by-descent and association mapping of a recessive gene for Hirschsprung's disease on human chromosome 13q22. Hum Mol Genet 1994;3: 1217–1225.
60. Puffenberger EG, Hosoda K, Washington SS, et al. A missense mutation of the endothelin-B receptor gene in multigenic Hirschsprung's disease. Cell 1994;79:1257–1266.
61. Shah KN, Dalal SJ, Desai MP, et al. White forelock, pigmentary disorder of irides, and long segment Hirschsprung's disease: Possible variant of Waardenburg syndrome. J Pediatr 1981;99: 432–435.
62. Edery P, Attié T, Amiel J, et al. Mutation of the endothelin-3 gene in the Waardenburg-Hirschsprung's disease (Shah-Waardenburg syndrome). Nature Genet 1996;12:442–444.
63. Attié T, Pelet A, Edery P, et al. Diversity of RET proto-oncogene mutations in familial and sporadic Hirschsprung's disease. Hum Mol Genet 1995;4:1381–1386.
64. Chakravarti A. Endothelin receptor-mediated signaling in Hirschsprung's disease. Hum Mol Genet 1996;5:303–307.
65. Verdy M, Weber AM, Roy CC, et al. Hirschsprung's disease in a family with multiple endocrine neoplasia type 2. J Pediatr Gastroenterol Nutr 1982;1:603–607.
66. Mahaffey SM, Martin LW, McAdams AJ, et al. Multiple endocrine neoplasia type IIB with symptoms suggesting Hirschsprung's disease: A case report. J Pediatr Surg 1990;25:101–103.
67. O'Dell K, Staren E, Bassuk A. Total colonic aganglionosis (Zuelzer-Wilson syndrome) and congenital failure of automatic control of ventilation (Ondine's curse). J Pediatr Surg 1987;22:1019–1020.

67. Clausen N, Anderson P, Tommerup N. Familial occurrence of neuroblastoma, Von Recklinghausen's neurofibromatosis, Hirschsprung's aganglionosis and jaw-winking syndrome. Acta Pediatr Scand 1989;78:736–741.
68. Hassinger DD, Mulvihill JJ, Chandler JB. Aarskog's syndrome with Hirschsprung's disease, midgut malrotation and dental anomalies. J Med Genet 1989;17:235–238.
69. Carter CO, Evans KA. Inheritance of congenital pyloric stenosis. J Med Genet 1969;6:233–254.
70. Mitchell LE, Risch N. The genetics of infantile hypertrophic pyloric stenosis: A reanalysis. Am J Dis Child 1993;147:1203–1211.
71. Benson PF, King MMR. An increased incidence of congenital pyloric stenosis in patients with ovarian dysgenesis. Guy's Hosp Reports 1964;113:254–258.
72. Vanderwinden J-M, Mailleux P, Schiffmann SN, et al. Nitric oxide synthase activity in infantile hypertrophic pyloric stenosis. N Engl J Med 1992;327:511–515.
73. Huang PL, Dawson TM, Bredt DS, et al. Targeted disruption of the neuronal nitric oxide synthase gene. Cell 1993;75:1273–1286.
74. Chung E, Curtis D, Chen G, et al. Genetic evidence for the neuronal nitric oxide synthase gene (NOS1) as a susceptibility locus for infantile pyloric stenosis. Am J Hum Genet 1996;58:363–370.
75. Dayalan N, Chettur L, Ramakrishnan MS. Achalasia of the cardia in sibs. Arch Dis Child 1972;47:115–118.
76. Westley CR, Herbst JJ, Goldman S, et al. Infantile achalasia: Inherited as an autosomal recessive disorder. J Pediatr 1975;87:243–246.
77. Frieling T, Berges W, Borchard F, et al. Family occurrence of achalasia and diffuse spasm of the oesophagus. Gut 1988;29:1595–1602.
78. O'Brien CJ, Smart HL. Familial coexistence of achalasia and non-achalasia oesophageal dysmotility: Evidence for a common pathogenesis. Gut 1992;33:1421–1423.
79. Allgrove J, Clayden GS, Grant DB, et al. Familial glucocorticoid deficiency with achalasia of the cardia and deficient tear production. Lancet 1978;I:1284–1286.
80. Polonsky L, Guth PH. Familial achalasia. Dig Dis Sci 1970;15:291–295.
81. Marger RS, Marger D. Carcinoma of the esophagus and tylosis: A lethal genetic combination. Cancer 1993;372:17–19.
82. Hennies H-C, Hagedorn M, Reis A. Palmoplantar keratoderma in association with carcinoma of the esophagus maps to chromosome 17q distal to the keratin gene cluster. Genomics 1995;29:537–540.
83. Stevens HP, Kelsell DP, Bryant SP, et al. Linkage of an American pedigree with palmoplantar keratoderma and malignancy (palmoplantar ectodermal dysplasia type III) to 17q24: Literature survey and proposed updated classification of the keratodermas. Arch Dermatol 1996;132:640–651.
84. Ghadirian P. Familial history of esophageal cancer. Cancer 1985;56:2112–2116.
85. Jochem VJ, Fuerst PA, Fromkes JJ. Familial Barrett's esophagus associated with adenocarcinoma. Gastroenterology 1992;102:1400–1402.
86. Eng C, Spechler SJ, Ruben R, et al. Familial Barrett esophagus and adenocarcinoma of the gastroesophageal junction. Cancer Epidemiol Biomarkers Prev 1993;2:397–399.
87. Crabb DW, Berk MA, Hall TR, et al. Familial gastroesophageal reflux and development of Barrett's esophagus. Ann Intern Med 1995;103:52–54.
88. Wuu KD, Wang-Wuu S. Karyotypic analysis of seven established human esophageal carcinoma cell lines. J Formos Med Assoc 1994;93:5–10.
89. Rao PH, Mathew S, Lauwers G, et al. Interphase cytogenetics of gastric and esophageal adenocarcinomas. Diagn Mol Pathol 1993;2:264–268.
90. Rosenblum-Vos LS, Meltzer S, Leana-Cox J, et al. Cytogenetics studies of primary cultures of esophageal squamous cell carcinoma. Cancer Genet Cytogenet 1993;70:127–131.
91. Hunter S, Gramlich T, Abbott K, et al. Y chromosome loss in esophageal carcinoma: An in situ hybridization study. Genes Chromosom Cancer 1993;8:172–177.
92. Rao PH, Mathew S, Kelsen DP, et al. Cytogenetics of gastric and esophageal adenocarcinomas. 3q deletion as a possible primary chromosomal change. Cancer Genet Cytogenet 1995;81:139–143.
93. Wang L, Li W, Wang X, et al. Genetic alterations on chromosomes 3 and 9 of esophageal cancer tissues from China. Oncogene 1996;12:699–703.
94. Miura K, Suzuki K, Tokino T, et al. Detailed deletion mapping in squamous cell carcinomas of the esophagus narrows a region containing a putative tumor suppressor gene to about 200 kilobases on distal chromosome 9q. Cancer Res 1996;56:1629–1634.
95. Mori T, Yanagisawa A, Kato Y, et al: Accumulation of genetic alterations during esophageal carcinogenesis. Hum Molec Genet 1994;3:1969–1971.
96. Rodriguez E, Rao PH, Ladanyi M, et al. 11p13-15 is a specific region of chromosomal rearrangement in gastric and esophageal adenocarcinomas. Cancer Res 1990;50:6410–6416.
97. Garewal HS, Sampliner R, Liu Y, et al. Chromosomal rearrangements in Barrett's esophagus: A premalignant lesion of esophageal carcinoma. Cancer Genet Cytogenet 1989;42:281–296.
98. Aoki T, Mori T, Du X, et al. Allelotype study of esophageal carcinoma. Genes Chromosomes Cancer 1994;10:177–182.
99. Shibagaki I, Shimada Y, Wagata T, et al. Allelotype analysis of esophageal squamous cell carcinoma. Cancer Res 1994;54:2996–3000.
100. Blount PL, Ramel S, Raskind WH, et al. 17p allelic deletions and p53 protein overexpression in Barrett's adenocarcinoma. Cancer Res 1991;51:5482–5486.
101. Hollstein MC, Metcalf RA, Welsh JA, et al. Frequent mutations of the p53 gene in human esophageal cancer. Proc Natl Acad Sci USA 1990;87:9958–9961.
102. Lu SH, Hsieh LL, Luo FC, et al. Amplification of the EGF receptor and c-myc genes in human esophageal cancers. Int J Cancer 1988;42:502–505.
103. Hollstein MC, Smits AM, Galiana C, et al. Amplification of epidermal growth factor receptor gene but no evidence of Ras mutations in primary human esophageal cancers. Cancer Res 1988;48:5119–5123.
104. Tsuda T, Tahara E, Kajiyama G, et al. High incidence of coamplification of hst-1 and int-2 genes in human esophageal carcinomas. Cancer Res 1989;49:5505–5508.
105. Jiang W, Kahan N, Tomira N, et al. Amplification and expression of the human cyclin D gene in esophageal cancer. Cancer Res 1992;52:2980–2983.
106. Meltzer SJ, Yin J, Manin B, et al. Microsatellite instability occurs frequently in both diploid and aneuploid cell populations of Barrett's-associated esophageal adenocarcinoma. Cancer Res 1994;54:3379–3382.
107. Boynton RF, Huang Y, Blount PL, et al. Frequent loss of heterozygosity at the retinoblastoma locus in human esophageal cancers. Cancer Res 1991;51:5766–5769.
108. Boynton RF, Blount PL, Yin J, et al. Loss of heterozygosity involving the APC and MCC genetic loci occurs in the majority of human esophageal cancers. Proc Natl Acad Sci USA 1992;89:3385–3388.
109. Ogasawara S, Tamura G, Maesawa G, et al. Common deleted region on the long arm of chromosome 5 in esophageal carcinoma. Gastroenterology 1996;110:52–57.
110. Cochat P, Guibaud P, Garcia-Torres R, et al. Diffuse leiomyomatosis in Alport syndrome. J Pediatr 1988;113:339–343.
111. Barker DF, Hostikka SL, Zhou J, et al. Identification of mutations in the COL4A5 collagen gene in Alport syndrome. Science 1990;248:1224–1227.
112. Hostikka SL, Eddy RL, Byers MG, et al. Identification of a distinct type IV collagen alpha chain with restricted kidney distribution and assignment of its gene to the locus of X chromosome-linked Alport syndrome. Proc Natl Acad Sci USA 1990;87:1606–1610.
113. Heidet L, Dahan K, Zhou J, et al. Deletions of both alpha-5(IV) and alpha-6(IV) collagen genes in Alport syndrome and in Alport syndrome associated with smooth muscle tumours. Hum Mol Genet 1995;4:99–108.
114. Bonney GE, Elston EC, Correa P, et al. Genetic etiology of gastric carcinoma. I. Chronic atrophic gastritis. Genet Epidemiol 1986;3:213–224.
115. McConnel RB. The genetics of carcinoma of the stomach. In: Shivas AM, ed. Racial and geographical factors in tumour incidence. Edinburgh: University Press, 1967:107–113.

116. Beckman L, Angqvist KA. On the mechanism behind the association between ABO blood groups and gastric carcinoma. Hum Hered 1987;37:410–413.

117. Sokoloff B. Predisposition to cancer in the Bonaparte Family. Am J Surg 1938;40:673–678.

118. Lynch HT, Lynch PM. Heredity and gastrointestinal tract cancer. In: Lipkin M, Good RA eds. Gastrointestinal tract cancer. New York: Plenum, 1978:241–274.

119. Ochi H, Douglass Jr HO, Sandberg AA. Cytogenetic studies in primary gastric cancer. Cancer Genet Cytogenet 1986;22:295–307.

120. Ferti-Passantonopoulou AD, Panani AD, Vlachos JD, et al. Common cytogenetic findings in gastric cancer. Cancer Genet Cytogenet 1987;24:63–73.

121. Misawa S, Horiike S, Taniwaki M, et al. Chromosome abnormalities of gastric cancer detected in cancerous effusions. Jpn J Cancer Res 1990;81:148–152.

122. Rao PH, Mathew S, Lauwers G, et al. Interphase cytogenetics of gastric and esophageal adenocarcinomas. Diagn Mol Pathol 1993;2:264–268.

123. Seruca R, Castedo S, Correia C, et al. Cytogenetic findings in eleven gastric carcinomas. Cancer Genet Cytogenet 1993;68:42–48.

124. Ming PL, Yuan ZA, Baffa R, et al. Molecular and cytogenetic characteristics of two cell lines derived from biologically distinct gastric carcinomas. Am J Hum Genet 1992;51:A278.

125. Wang KH. Establishment of a cell line from a poorly differentiated mucoid adenocarcinoma of human stomach. Acta Biol Exp Sinica 1983;16:257–262.

126. Sekiguchi M, Sakakibara K, Fujii G. Establishment of cultured cell lines derived from a human gastric carcinoma. Jpn J Exp Med 1978;48:61–68.

127. Saal K, Vollmers HP, Muller J, et al. Cytogenetic differences between intestinal and diffuse types of human gastric carcinoma. Virchows Arch [B] 1993;64:145–150.

128. Schneider BG, Pulitzer DR, Brown RD, et al. Allelic imbalance in gastric cancer: An affected site on chromosome arm 3p. Genes Chromosom Cancer 1995;13:263–271.

129. Queimado L, Seruca R, Costa-Pereira A, et al. Identification of two distinct regions of deletion at 6q in gastric carcinoma. Genes Chromosom Cancer 1995;14:28–34.

130. Kuniyasu H, Yasui W, Yokozaki H, et al. Frequent loss of heterozygosity of the long arm of chromosome 7 is closely associated with progression of human gastric carcinomas. Int J Cancer 1994;59:597–600.

131. Sakata K, Tamura G, Maesawa C, et al. Loss of heterozygosity on the short arm of chromosome 9 without p16 gene mutation in gastric carcinomas. Jpn J Cancer Res 1995;86:333–335.

132. Baffa R, Negrini M, Mandes B, et al. Loss of heterozygosity for chromosome 11 in adenocarcinoma of the stomach. Cancer Res 1996;56:268–272.

133. Tamura G, Sakata K, Maesawa C, et al. Microsatellite alterations in adenoma and differentiated adenocarcinoma of the stomach. Cancer Res 1995;55:1933–1936.

134. Lee KH, Lee JS, Suh C, et al. Clinicopathologic significance of the K-ras gene codon 12 point mutation in stomach cancer. An analysis of 140 cases. Cancer 1995;75:2794–2801.

135. Deng GR. A sensitive nonradioactive PCR-RFLP analysis for detecting point mutations at 12th codon on oncogene c-Ha-ras in DNAs of gastric cancer. Nucleic Acids Res 1988;16:6231.

136. Bos JL, Verlaan de Vries M, Marshall CJ, et al. A human gastric carcinoma contains a single mutated and an amplified normal allele of the Ki-ras oncogene. Nucleic Acids Res 1986;14:1209–1217.

137. Nishida J, Kobayashi Y, Hirai H, et al. A point mutation at codon 13 in the N-ras oncogene in a human stomach cancer. Biochem Biophys Res Commun 1987;146:247–252.

138. Gutman M, Ravia Y, Assaf D, et al. Amplification of c-myc and c-erb-B-2 proto-oncogenes in human solid tumors: Frequency and clinical significance. Int J Cancer 1989;44:802–805.

139. Tsuchiya T, Ueyama Y, Tamaoki N, et al. Co-amplification of c-myc and c-erbB-2 oncogenes in a poorly differentiated human gastric cancer. Jpn J Cancer Res 1989;80:920–923.

140. Kuniyasu H, Yasui W, Kitadai Y, et al. Frequent amplification of c-met gene in the scirrhous type stomach cancer. Biochem Biophys Res Commun 1992;189:227–232.

141. Katoh M, Hattori Y, Sasaki H, et al. K-sam gene encodes secreted as well as transmembrane receptor tyrosine kinase. Proc Natl Acad Sci USA 1992;89:2960–2964.

142. Sano T, Tsugino T, Yoshida K, et al. Frequent loss of heterozygosity of chromosomes 1q, 5q, and 17p in human gastric carcinomas. Cancer Res 1991;51:1926–1931.

143. Kim JH, Takahashi T, Chiba I, et al. Occurrence of p53 gene abnormalities in gastric carcinoma tumors and cell lines. J Natl Cancer Inst 1991;83:938–943.

144. Tamura G, Kihana T, Nomura K, et al. Detection of frequent p53 gene mutations in primary gastric cancer by cell sorting and polymerase chain reaction single-strand conformation polymorphism analysis. Cancer Res 1991;51:3056–3058.

145. Yamada Y, Yoshida T, Hayashi K, et al. p53 gene mutations in gastric cancer metastases and in gastric cancer cell lines derived from metastases. Cancer Res 1991;51:5800–5805.

146. Tohdo H, Yokozaki H, Haruma K, et al. p53 gene mutations in gastric adenomas. Virchows Arch [B] 1993;63:191–195.

147. Horii A, Nakatsuru S, Miyoshi Y, et al. The APC gene, responsible for familial adenomatous polyposis, is mutated in human gastric cancer. Cancer Res 1992;52:3231–3233.

148. Nakatsuru S, Yanagisawa A, Ichii S, et al. Somatic mutation of the APC gene in gastric cancer: Frequent mutations in very well differentiated adenocarcinoma and signet-ring cell carcinoma. Hum Molec Genet 1992;1:559–563.

149. McKie AB, Filipe MI, Lemoine NR. Abnormalities affecting the APC and MCC tumour suppressor gene loci on chromosome 5q occur frequently in gastric cancer but not in pancreatic cancer. Int J Cancer 1993;55:598–603.

150. Nishimura K, Yokozaki H, Haruma K, et al. Alterations of the APC gene in carcinoma cell lines and precancerous lesions of the stomach. Int J Oncol 1995;7:587–592.

151. Oda T, Kanai T, Oyama T, et al. E-cadherin gene mutations in human carcinoma cell lines. Proc Natl Acad Sci USA 1994;91:1858–1862.

152. Becker K-F, Atkinson MJ, Reich U, et al. E-cadherin gene mutations provide clues to diffuse type gastric carcinomas. Cancer Res 1994;54:3845–3852.

153. Uchino S, Tsuda H, Noguchi M, et al. Frequent loss of heterozygosity at the DCC locus in gastric cancer. Cancer Res 1992;52:3099–3102.

154. Han H-J, Yanagisawa A, Kato Y, et al. Genetic instability in pancreatic cancer and poorly differentiated type of gastric cancer. Cancer Res 1993;53:5087–5089.

155. Rhyu M-G, Park W S, Meltzer SJ. Microsatellite instability occurs frequently in human gastric carcinoma. Oncogene 1994;9:29–32.

156. Cannon-Albright LA, Skolnick MH, Bishop DT, et al. Common inheritance of susceptibility to colonic adenomatous polyps and associated colorectal cancers. N Engl J Med 1988;319:533–537.

157. Houlston RS, Collins A, Slack J, et al. Dominant genes for colorectal cancer are not rare. Ann Hum Genet 1992;56:99–103.

158. Lynch HT, Watson P, Lanspa SJ, et al. Natural history of colorectal cancer in hereditary nonpolyposis colorectal cancer (Lynch syndrome I and II). Dis Colon Rectum 1988;32:439–444.

159. Mecklin JP. Frequency of hereditary colorectal carcinoma. Gastroenterology 1987;93:1021–1025.

160. Utsunomiya J, Maki T, Iwama T, et al. Gastric lesion of familial polyposis coli. Cancer 1974;34:745–754.

161. Watanabe H, Munetomo E, Yao T, et al. Gastric lesions in familial adenomatosis coli. Hum Pathol 1978;9:269–283.

162. Offerhaus GJA, Giardiello FM, Krush AJ, et al. The risk of upper gastrointestinal cancer in familial adenomatous polyposis. Gastroenterology 1992;102:1980–1982.

163. Phillips LG. Polyposis and carcinoma of the small bowel and familial colonic polyposis. Dis Colon Rectum 1981;24:478–481.

164. Ross JE, Mara JE. Small bowel polyps and carcinoma in multiple intestinal polyposis. Arch Surg 1974;208:736–738.

165. Weenstrom J, Pierce ER, McKusick VA. Hereditary benign and malignant lesions of the large bowel. Cancer 1974;34:850–857.

166. Bisgaard ML, Fenger K, Bulow S, et al. Familial adenomatous polyposis (FAP): Frequency, penetrance, and mutation rate. Hum Mutat 1994;3:121–125.

167. Veale AMO. The polyposes. In: Emery AEH, Rimoin DL, eds. Principles and practice of medical genetics. New York: Churchill Livingstone, 1990:1125–1133.

168. Burt RW, Samowitz WS. The adenomatous polyp and the hereditary polyposis syndromes. Gastroenterol Clin North Am 1988;17:657–678.

169. Veale AMO. Intestinal polyposis. Eugenics Laboratory Memoirs. London: Cambridge University Press, 1965.

170. Asman HB, Pierce ER. Familial multiple polyposis—A statistical study of a large Kentucky kindred. Cancer 1970;25:972–981.

171. Nakamura Y, Lathrop M, Leppert M, et al. Localization of the genetic defect in familial adenomatous polyposis within a small region of chromosome 5. Am J Hum Genet 1988;43:638–644.

172. Ashton-Rickardt PG, Dunlop MG, Nakamura Y, et al. High frequency of APC loss in sporadic colorectal carcinoma due to breaks clustered in 5q21-q22. Oncogene 1989;4:1169–1174.

173. Okamoto M, Sato C, Kohno Y, et al. Molecular nature of chromosome 5q loss in colorectal trumors and desmoids from patients with familial adenomatous polyposis. Hum Genet 1990;85:595–599.

174. Miyoshi Y, Nagase H, Ando H, et al. Somatic mutations of the APC gene in colorectal tumors: Mutation cluster region in the APC gene. Hum Mol Genet 1992;1:229–233.

175. Groden J, Thliveris A, Samowitz W, et al. Identification and characterization of the familial adenomatous polyposis coli gene. Cell 1991;66:589–600.

176. Joslyn G, Carlson M, Thliveris A, et al. Identification of deletion mutations and three new genes at the familial polyposis locus. Cell 1991;66:601–613.

177. Kinzler KW, Nilbert MC, Su L-K, et al. Identification of FAP locus genes from chromosome 5q21. Science 1991;253:661–665.

178. Nishisho I, Nakamura Y, Miyoshi Y, et al. Mutations of chromosome 5q21 genes in FAP and colorectal cancer patients. Science 1991;253:665–669.

179. Rubinfeld B, Souza B, Albert I, et al. Association of the APC gene product with beta-catenin. Science 1993;262:1731–1734.

180. Su L-K, Vogelstein B, Kinzler KW. Association of the APC tumor suppressor protein with catenins. Science 1993;262:1734–1737.

181. Miyoshi Y, Ando H, Nagase H, et al. Germ-line mutations of the APC gene in 53 familial adenomatous polyposis patients. Proc Natl Acad Sci USA 1992;89:4452–4456.

182. Beroud C, Soussi T. APC gene: Database of germline and somatic mutations in human tumors and cell lines. Nucleic Acids Res 1996;24:121–124.

183. Powell SM, Petersen GM, Krush AJ, et al. Molecular diagnosis of familial adenomatous polyposis. N Engl J Med 1987;329:1982–1987.

184. van der Lujit R, Meera Khan P, Vasen H, et al. Rapid detection of translation-terminating mutations at the adenomatous polyposis coli (APC) gene by direct protein truncation test. Genomics 1994;20:1–4.

185. Nagase H, Miyoshi Y, Horii A, et al. Correlation between the location of germ-line mutations in the APC gene and the number of colorectal polyps in familial adenomatous polyposis patients. Cancer Res 1992;52:4055–4057.

186. Bunyan DJ, Shea-Simonds J, Reck AC, et al. Genotype-phenotype correlations of new causative APC gene mutations in patients with familial adenomatous polyposis. J Med Genet 1995;32:728–731.

187. Davies D, Armstrong J, Thakker N, et al. Severe Gardner's syndrome in families with mutations restricted to a specific region of the APC gene. Am J Hum Genet 1995;57:1151–1158.

188. Spirio L, Olschwang S, Groden J, et al. Alleles of the APC gene: An attenuated form of familial polyposis. Cell 1993;75:951–957.

189. Olschwang S, Tiret A, Laurent-Puig P, et al. Restriction of ocular fundus lesions to a specific subgroup of APC mutations in adenomatous polyposis coli patients. Cell 1993;75:959–968.

190. Powell SM, Zilz N, Beazer-Barclay Y, et al. APC mutations occur early during colorectal tumorigenesis. Nature 1992;359:235–237.

191. Gardner EJ, Plenk HP. Hereditary pattern for multiple osteomas in a family group. Am J Hum Genet 1952;5:139–147.

192. Gardner EJ, Richards RC. Multiple cutaneous and subcutaneous lesions occurring simultaneously with hereditary polyposis and carcinomatosis. Am J Hum Genet 1953;5:139–147.

193. Hamilton SR, Liu B, Parsons RE, et al. The molecular basis of Turcot's syndrome. N Engl J Med 1995;332:839–847.

194. Turcot J, Depres JP, St Pierre F. Malignant tumours of the central nervous system associated with familial polyposis of the colon. Dis Colon Rectum 1959;2:465–468.

195. Bartholomew LG, Moore CE, Dahlin DC, et al. Intestinal polyposis associated with mucocutaneous pigmentation. Surg Gynecol Obstet 1962;115:1–11.

196. Staley CJ, Schwarz H: Gastrointestinal polyposis and pigmentation of the oral mucosa (Peutz-Jeghers syndrome). Int Abstract Surg 1957;205:1–15.

197. Normandy TL. Gastrointestinal polyposis with mucocutaneous pigmentation (Peutz-Jeghers syndrome). N Engl J Med 1957;256:1093–1190.

198. Dodds WJ, Schulte WJ, Hensley Gt, et al. Peutz-Jeghers syndrome and gastrointestinal malignancy. AJR Am J Roentgenol 1972;115:374–377.

199. Reid JD. Intestinal carcinoma in the Peutz-Jeghers syndrome. JAMA 1974;229:833–834.

200. Perzin KH, Ridge MF. Adenomatous and carcinomatous changes in hamartomatous polyps of the small intestine (Peutz-Jeghers syndrome): Report of a case and review of the literature. Cancer 1982;49:971–983.

201. Giardiello FM, Welsh SB, Hamilton SR, et al. Increased risk of cancer in the Peutz-Jeghers syndrome. N Engl J Med 1987;316:1511–1514.

202. Hemminki A, Tomlinson I, Markie D, et al. Localization of a susceptibility locus for Peutz-Jeghers syndrome to 19p using comparative genomic hybridization and targeted linkage analysis. Nat Genet 1997;15:87–90.

203. Veale AMO, McCall I, Bussey HJR, et al. Juvenile polyposis coli. J Med Genet 1966;3:5–16.

204. Bussey HJR. Polyposis syndromes of the gastrointestinal tract. New York: Raven Press, 1983:43–51.

205. Desai DC, Neal KF, Talbot IC, et al. Juvenile polyposis. Br J Surg 1995;82:14–17.

206. Sachatello CR, Pickren JW, Grace Jr JT. Generalized juvenile gastrointestinal polyposis. A hereditary syndrome. Gastroenterology 1979;58:699–708.

207. Stemper TJ, Kent TH, Summers RW. Juvenile polyposis and gastrointestinal carcinoma. A study of a kindred. Ann Intern Med 1975;83:639–646.

208. Goodman ZD, Yardley JH, Milligan FD. Pathogenesis of colonic polyps in multiple juvenile polyposis: Report of a case associated with gastric polyps and carcinoma of the rectum. Cancer 1979;43:1906–1913.

209. Bussey HJR. Gastrointestinal polyposis. Gut 1970;11:970–978.

210. Rozen P, Baratz M. Familial juvenile colonic polyposis with associated colon cancer. Cancer 1982;49:1500–1503.

211. Sharma AK, Sharma SS, Mathur P. Familial juvenile polyposis with adenomatous-carcinomatous change. J Gastroenterol Hepatol 1995;10:131–134.

212. Watanabe A, Nagashima H, Motoi M, et al. Familial juvenile polyposis of the stomach. Gastroenterology 1979;77:148–151.

213. Sassatelli R, Betoni G, Serra L, et al. Generalized juvenile polyposis with mixed pattern and gastric cancer. Gastroenterology 1993;104:910–915.

214. Mecklin J-P, Jarvinen HJ, Peltokallio P. Cancer family syndrome: Genetic analysis of 22 Finnish kindreds. Gastroenterology 1986;90:328–333.

215. Ponz de Leon M. Prevalence of hereditary nonpolyposis colorectal cancer (HNPCC). Ann Med 1994:26:209–214.

216. Lynch HT, Smyrk T, Lynch JF. Overview of natural history, pathology, molecular genetics and management of HNPCC (Lynch syndrome). Int J Cancer 1996;69:38–43.

217. Lynch HT, Lanspa SJ, Bowman BM. Hereditary nonpolyposis colorectal cancer—Lynch syndromes I and II. Gastroenterol Clin North Am 1988;17:679–713.

218. Mecklin J-P, Sipponene P, Jarvinen HJ. Histopathology of colorectal carcinomas and adenomas in cancer family syndrome. Dis Colon Rectum 1986;29:849.

219. Love RR. Adenomas are precursor lesions for malignant growth in nonpolyposis hereditary carcinoma of the colon and rectum. Surg Gynecol Obstet 1986;162:8–12.

220. Nystrom-Lahti M, Parsons R, Sistonen P, et al. Mismatch repair genes on chromosomes 2p and 3p account for a major share of hereditary nonpolyposis colorectal cancer families evaluable by linkage. Am J Hum Genet 1994;55:659–665.

221. Aaltonen LA, Peltomaki P, Leach FS, et al. Clues to the pathogenesis of familial colorectal cancer. Science 1993;260:812–816.

222. Lindblom A, Tannergard P, Werelius B, et al. Genetic mapping of a second locus predisposing to hereditary non-polyposis colon cancer. Nat Genet 1993;5:279–282.

223. Parsons R, Li G-M, Longley MJ, et al. Hypermutability and mismatch repair deficiency in RER(+) tumor cells. Cell 1993;75:1227–1236.

224. Liu B, Parsons R, Papadopoulos N, et al. Analysis of mismatch repair genes in hereditary non-polyposis colorectal cancer patients. Nature Med 1996;72:169–174.

225. Fishel R, Lescoe MK, Rao MRS, et al. The human mutator gene homolog MSH2 and its association with hereditary nonpolyposis colon cancer. Cell 1993;75:1027–1038.

226. Leach FS, Nicolaides NC, Papadopoulos N, et al. Mutations of a MutS homolog in hereditary non-polyposis colorectal cancer. Cell 1993;75:1215–1225.

227. Kolodner RD, Hall NR, Lipford J, et al. Structure of the human MSH2 locus and analysis of two Muir-Torre kindreds for MSH2 mutations. Genomics 1994;24:516–526.

228. Papadopoulos N, Nicolaides NC, Wei Y-F, et al. Mutation of a mutL homolog in hereditary colon cancer. Science 1994;263:1625–1629.

229. Bronner CE, Baker SM, Morrison PT, et al. Mutation in the DNA mismatch repair gene homologue hMLH1 is associated with hereditary non-polyposis colon cancer. Nature 1994;368:258–261.

230. Han H-J, Maruyama M, Baba S, et al. Genomic structure of human mismatch repair gene, hMLH1, and its mutation analysis in patients with hereditary non-polyposis colorectal cancer (HNPCC). Hum Mol Genet 1995;4:237–242.

231. Hemminki A, Peltomaki P, Mecklin J-P, et al. Loss of the wild type MLH1 gene is a feature of hereditary nonpolyposis colorectal cancer. Nat Genet 1994;8:405–410.

232. Nicolaides NC, Papadopoulos N, Liu B, et al. Mutations of two PMS homologues in hereditary nonpolyposis colon cancer. Nature 1994; 371:75–80.

233. Bellacosa A, Genuardi M, Anti M, et al. Hereditary nonpolyposis colorectal cancer: Review of clinical, molecular genetics, and counseling aspects. Am J Med Genet 1996;62:353–364.

234. Kinzler KW, Vogelstein B. Lessons from hereditary colorectal cancer. Cell 1996;87:159–170.

235. Lynch HT, Fusaro RM, Roberts L, et al. Muir-Torre syndrome in several members of a family with a variant of the cancer family syndrome. Br J Dermatol 1985;113:295–301.

236. Bapat B, Xia L, Madlensky L, et al. The genetic basis of Muir-Torre syndrome includes the hMLH1 locus [letter]. Am J Hum Genet 1996;59:736–739.

237. Kruse R, Lamberti C, Wang Y, et al. Is the mismatch repair deficient type of Muir-Torre syndrome confined to mutations in the MSH2 gene? Hum Genet 1996;98:747–750.

238. Burt RW, Bishop OT, Cannon ML, et al. Dominant inheritance of adenomatous colonic polyps and colorectal cancer. N Engl J Med 1985;312:1540–1544.

239. Vogelstein B, Fearon ER, Hamilton SR, et al. Genetic alterations during colorectal tumor development. N Engl J Med 1988;319: 525–532.

240. Fearon ER. Molecular genetic studies of the adenoma-carcinoma sequence. Adv Intern Med 1994;39:123–147.

241. Thibodeau SN, Bren G, Schaid D. Microsatellite instability in cancer of the proximal colon. Science 1993;260:816–819.

242. Bos JL, Fearon ER, Hamilton SR, et al. Prevalence of Ras gene mutations in human colorectal cancers. Nature 1987;327:293–297.

243. Finkelstein SD, Sayegh R, Bakker A, et al. Determination of tumor aggressiveness in colorectal cancer by K-ras-2 analysis. Arch Surg 1993;128:526–532.

244. Burmer GC, Loeb LA. Mutations in the KRAS2 oncogene during progressive stages of human colon carcinoma. Proc Natl Acad Sci USA 1989;86:2403–2407.

245. Baker SJ, Fearon EJ, Nigro JM, et al. Chromosome 17 deletions and p53 gene mutations in colorectal carcinomas. Science 1989;244: 217–221.

246. Nigro JM, Baker SJ, Preisinger AC, et al. Mutations in the p53 gene occur in diverse human tumour types. Nature 1989;342: 705–708.

247. Baker SJ, Preisinger AC, Jessup JM, et al. p53 gene mutations occur in combination with 17p allelic deletions as late events in colorectal tumorigenesis. Cancer Res 1990;50:7717–7722.

248. Kikuchi-Yanoshita R, Konishi M, Ito S, et al. Genetic changes of both p53 alleles associated with the conversion from colorectal adenoma to early carcinoma in familial adenomatous polyposis and non-familial adenomatous polyposis patients. Cancer Res 1992; 52:3965–3971.

249. Fearon ER, Cho KR, Nigro JM, et al. Identification of a chromosome 18q gene that is altered in colorectal cancers. Science 1990; 247:49–56.

250. Cho KR, Oliner JD, Simons JW, et al. The DCC gene: Structural analysis and mutations in colorectal carcinomas. Genomics 1994;19: 525–531.

251. Zetter BR. Adhesion molecules in tumor metastasis. Semin Cancer Biol 1993;4:219–229.

252. Ookawa K, Sakamoto M, Hirohashi S, et al. Concordant p53 and DCC alterations and allelic losses on chromosomes 13q and 14q associated with liver metastases of colorectal carcinoma. Int J Cancer 1993;53:382–387.

253. Lindgren V, Bryke CR, Ozcelik T, et al. Phenotypic, cytogenetic, and molecular studies of three patients with constitutional deletions of chromosome 5 in the region of the gene for familial adenomatous polyposis. Am J Hum Genet 1992;50:988–997.

254. Kinzler KW, Nilbert MC, Vogelstein B, et al. Identification of a gene located at chromosome 5q21 that is mutated in colorectal cancers. Science 1991;251:1366–1370.

255. Curtis LJ, Bubb VJ, Gledhill S, et al. Loss of heterozygosity of MCC is not associated with mutation of the retained allele in sporadic colorectal cancer. Hum Mol Genet 1994;3:443–446.

256. Sugio K, Kurata S, Sasaki M, et al. Differential expression of c-myc and c-fos genes in premalignant and malignant tissues from patients with familial polyposis coli. Cancer Res 1988;48:4855–4861.

257. Calabretta B, Kaczmarek L, Ming P-ML, et al. Expression of c-myc and other cell cycle-dependent genes in human colon neoplasia. Cancer Res 1985;45:6000–6004.

258. Mariani-Costantini R, Theillet C, Hutzell P, et al. In situ detection of c-myc mRNA in adenocarcinomas, adenomas, and mucosa of human colon. J Histochem Cytochem 1989;37:293–298.

259. Royds JA, Sharrard M, Wagner B, et al. Cellular localisation of c-myc product in human colorectal epithelial neoplasia. J Pathol 1992;166: 225–233.

260. Stewart J, Evan G, Watson J, et al. Detection of the c-myc oncogene product in colonic polyps and carcinomas. Br J Cancer 1986; 53:1–6.

261. Meltzer SJ, Ahnen DJ, Battifora H, et al. Protooncogene abnormalities in colon cancers and adenomatous polyps. Gastroenterology 1987;92:1174–1180.

262. Reichmann A, Martin P, Levin B. Chromosomal banding patterns in human large bowel adenomas. Hum Genet 1985;70:28–31.

263. Reichmann A, Martin P, Levin B. Karyotypic findings in a colonic villous adenoma. Cancer Genet Cytogenet 1982;7:51–57.

264. Griffin CA, Lazar S, Hamilton SR, et al. Cytogenetic analysis of intestinal polyps in polyposis syndromes: Comparison with sporadic colorectal adenomas. Cancer Genet Cytogenet 1993;67:14–20.

265. Longy M, Saura R, Dumas F, et al. Chromosome analysis of adenomatous polyps of the colon: Possible existence of two differently evolving cytogenetic groups. Cancer Genet Cytogenet 1993; 67:7–13.

266. Bomme L, Bardi G, Pandis N, et al. Clonal karyotypic abnormalities in colorectal adenomas: Clues to the early genetic events in the adenoma-carcinoma sequence. Genes Chromosom Cancer 1994;10: 190–196.

267. Muleris M, Zafrani B, Validire P, et al. Cytogenetic study of 30 colorectal adenomas. Cancer Genet Cytogenet 1994;74:104–108.

268. Levin B, Reichmann A. Chromosomes and large bowel tumors. Cancer Genet Cytogenet 1986;19:159–162.

269. Muleris M, Salmon RJ, Dutrillaux B. Cytogenetics of colorectal adenocarcinomas. Cancer Genet Cytogenet 1980;46:143–156.

270. Dutrillaux B. Recent data on the cytogenetics of colorectal adenocarcinoma. Bull Cancer (Paris) 1988;75:509–516.

271. Muleris M, Salmon RJ, Dutrillaux AM, et al. Characteristic chromosomal imbalances in 18 near-diploid colorectal tumors. Cancer Genet Cytogenet 1987;29:289–301.

272. Bardi G, Johansson B, Pandis N, et al. Cytogenetic aberrations in colorectal adenocarcinomas and their correlation with clinicopathologic features. Cancer 1993;71:306–314.

273. Bardi G, Johansson B, Pandis N, et al. Cytogenetic analysis of 52 colorectal carcinomas—non-random aberration pattern and correlation with pathologic parameters. Int J Cancer 1993;55:422–428.

274. Bardi G, Sukhikh T, Pandis N, et al. Karyotypic characterization of colorectal adenocarcinomas. Genes Chromosom Cancer 1995;12:97–109.

275. Herbergs J, de Bruine AP, Marx PT, et al. Chromosome aberrations in adenomas of the colon. Proof of trisomy 7 in tumor cells by combined interphase cytogenetics and immunocytochemistry. Int J Cancer 1994;57:781–785.

276. Keldysh PL, Dragani TA, Fleischman EW, et al. 11q deletions in human colorectal carcinomas: Cytogenetics and restriction fragment length polymorphism analysis. Genes Chromosom Cancer 1993;6:45–50.

277. Bardi G, Pandis N, Fenger C, et al. Deletion of 1p36 as a primary chromosomal aberration in intestinal tumorigenesis. Cancer Res 1993;53:1895–1898.

278. Dutrillaux B, Gerbault-Seureau M, Saint-Ruf C, et al. Cytogenetic characterization of colorectal and breast carcinomas. In: Kirsch IR, ed. The causes and consequences of chromosomal aberrations. Boca Raton: CRC Press, 1993:447–467.

279. Kern SE, Fearon ER, Tersmette KWF, et al. Allelic loss in colorectal carcinoma. JAMA 1989;261:3099–3103.

280. Fearon ER, Hamilton SR, Vogelstein B. Clonal analysis of human colorectal tumors. Science 1987;238:1193–1197.

281. Laurent-Puig P, Olschwang S, Delattre O, et al. Survival and acquired genetic alterations in colorectal cancer. Gastroenterology 1992;102;1136–1141.

282. Ferti-Passantonopoulou A, Panani A, Avgerinos A, et al. Cytogenetic findings in a large bowel adenocarcinoma. Cancer Genet Cytogenet 1986;21:361–364.

283. Muleris M, Salmon R-J, Girodet J, et al. Recurrent deletions of chromosomes 11q and 3p in anal canal carcinoma. Int J Cancer 1987;39:595–598.

MOLECULAR BIOLOGY OF GASTROINTESTINAL DISORDERS

Massimo Loda

Molecular medicine is the newest and most advanced branch of medical science. Diagnostic methods and therapeutic interventions made possible by recombinant DNA technology are being used for patient care. Because treatment is based increasingly on new information concerning the mechanisms of action of genes that are involved in diseases, pathologists must be in the position to analyze specimens using recombinant DNA technology. Considerable effort has thus far been directed toward the assessment of the molecular mechanisms by which cancers develop and progress.

Adenocarcinoma of the colon and rectum is the second most prevalent cancer in the United States (1, 2); gastric and esophageal cancers are among the most common malignant neoplasms worldwide (3). Survival of patients with these diseases, however, has shown little change (1). Using the basic principles of molecular genetics, our understanding of these neoplasms has improved, and this knowledge is being applied to elucidate the various steps of tumor initiation, progression, and metastasis. In addition, technical advances in recombinant DNA technology have allowed the identification of prognostic tumor markers that have led to early diag-

nosis. Understanding the molecular events underlying neoplastic transformation will hopefully translate to improved survival as well as prevention of cancer.

GENE EXPRESSION AND REGULATION

Three molecules designed to store, keep, and eventually express genetic information are DNA, RNA, and proteins. Deoxyribonucleic acid (DNA) is the molecule that permanently encodes the data for all cellular functions. DNA consists of two antiparallel strands of nucleotide bases aligned on a phosphate/sugar backbone. The bases attached to one-strand hydrogen bond to the bases on the other in a complementary fashion such that adenine (A) bonds with thymine (T) and guanine (G) bonds with cytosine (C). This complementarity is the cornerstone of the ability to manipulate nucleic acids in vitro.

Ribonucleic acid (RNA) differs from DNA in that it is single stranded and contains uracil (U) in place of thymine bases. It is messenger RNA (mRNA) that is finally translated into functional protein products made up of the 20 amino acids.

The flow of information from DNA to protein begins with the process of transcription, which is the synthesis of a complementary single-stranded mRNA polymer from the 5′-3′ DNA strand of the double helix. Genomic coding DNA sequence information is amplified by this process. mRNA is then transported from the nucleus to the cytoplasm where its linear sequence of triplet codons is translated on the ribosomes to a linear sequence of amino acids. Control of the process of gene expression (Fig. 8.1) ultimately influences the activity or amount of protein gene product.

Although a given gene can be regulated at the transcriptional, translational, and posttranslational (degradative pathways) levels, control over gene expression takes place predominantly at the transcriptional level. The RNA polymerase, which stitches together the nascent mRNA polymer, must latch on to the DNA initially at a sequence termed the "promoter" before the transcription process may begin. Certain genes, called transcription factors, can influence mRNA production of other genes because they enable the polymerase to recognize this site. Transcription factors are regulated by other upstream proteins or by phosphorylation. Protein binding sites called "enhancer regions" up or downstream from the promoter can upregulate transcription. Repressors have the opposite action.

NONCODING DNA

Sequences that are ultimately translated into proteins (coding regions) are separated by noncoding regions of DNA. Most of the variability ("genetic polymorphism") among individuals' DNA occurs in noncoding regions. Simple sequences are present in tandem arrays called satellites, minisatellites, or microsatellites, depending on their length. The length of a set of satellites is unique to each individual. Modifications in length of these untranslated repetitive sequences present in multiple copies throughout the genome are used in the assessment of Mendelian inheritance of alleles, forensic testing, and genetic instability. Several tumor types display alterations in microsatellite sequences ("microsatellite instability") that is often the result of malfunctioning DNA repair enzymes involved in some forms of hereditary colon cancer syndromes.

RECOMBINANT DNA TECHNOLOGY: PRINCIPLES AND TECHNIQUES

Recombinant DNA technology allows the isolation of a single gene from a background of "contaminating" DNA and its subsequent amplification and manipulation. The use of enzymes that modify nucleic acids by cutting DNA at predetermined loci (restriction endonucleases), reattach loose ends (ligases), or synthesize identical copies of template nucleic acids (polymerases) are essential to their manipulation in vitro.

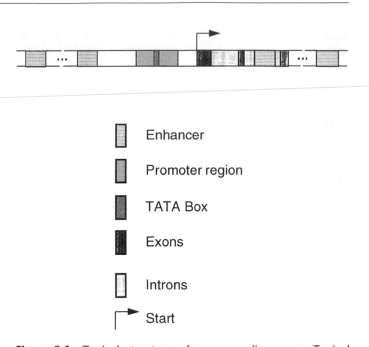

Enhancer

Promoter region

TATA Box

Exons

Introns

Start

Figure 8.1 Typical structure of a mammalian gene. Typical mammalian genes are flanked by regulatory elements, such as enhancers and repressors; by a promoter region, which includes the TATA box where transcription factors bind. The gene itself is made up of coding exons separated by intervening noncoding introns. *Arrow,* start of transcription. (Adapted from Lodish H, Baltimore D, Berk A, et al., eds: Molecular cell biology. 3rd ed. New York: Scientific American Books, 1995.)

MOLECULAR HYBRIDIZATION

Hybridization is the duplex molecule formation caused by the complementary base pairing between two nucleic acid strands. Molecular techniques use nucleic acid "probes" that are complementary to DNA or RNA molecules of interest, which represent the "target." Hybridization can occur in solution, on solid support, or at the cellular and subcellular levels.

PROBES

Nucleic acid probes are segments of DNA or RNA of variable length that may be labeled either radioisotopically or with a variety of nonisotopic reporter molecules, and revealed with a color reaction. In routine molecular diagnostics, nonisotopic probes are rapidly replacing costly and hazardous radiolabeled probes.

Probes range from short (up to 50 base pairs [bp]) single-stranded, synthetic oligonucleotides to complementary RNA probes of intermediate size (up to 1000 bp in length) to long (one to several thousand of bases in length), double-stranded DNA probes. The longer the probe, the more reporter molecules can be incorporated in the labeling reaction.

Single-stranded DNA oligonucleotide probes are used primarily in polymerase chain reactions (PCR), in allele-specific filter hybridization assays for the detection of point mutations (4), and in in situ hybridization when the target is a high copy number gene. Oligonucleotides can be custom synthesized if the target sequence is known. If appropriately stringent conditions are used, oligonucleotides can detect even single base pair mismatches, either by PCR (see subsequent section) (5, 6) or in filter hybridization (7), making these probes ideal for screening assays.

RNA polymerases drive the synthesis of RNA probes (riboprobes) in vitro. Cloned DNA, inserted in transcription-efficient plasmids with promoter sequences recognized by these polymerases, is used as template. Riboprobes are particularly suited for use in in situ hybridization. When riboprobes are compared to oligonucleotide probes in in situ detection, their intermediate length affords greater likelihood and more stable hybridization to stretches of RNA that remain available for binding after tissue processing. The use of riboprobes in in situ hybridization results in better sensitivity compared to oligonucleotide probes. Riboprobes are, however, more unstable and thus more difficult to manipulate.

Longer DNA probes are particularly suitable for use in solid support hybridization assays as well as in fluorescent in situ hybridization (FISH) for the identification of single copy genes.

FILTER HYBRIDIZATION

Filter hybridization entails the detection by a specific probe of target DNA or RNA sequences irreversibly bound to a solid substrate such as nylon or nitrocellulose. After endonuclease restriction, DNA run on a gel is transferred to filters that are hybridized with a labeled probe directed toward the gene of interest. Such a technique, known as Southern hybridization, requires intact (fresh or snap-frozen) genomic DNA. In addition to gene quantitation, this assay permits the determination of the size of the restriction fragment to which the probe hybridizes.

When RNA is the target, the technique is known as Northern hybridization. Contrary to DNA, RNA is not enzymatically modified before gel electrophoresis. Northern analysis allows quantitation of gene expression as well as size determination (i.e., specificity) of the mRNA species that is targeted. It requires large quantities (10 to 15 μg) of intact total RNA, which must also be extracted from fresh or snap-frozen material.

POLYMERASE CHAIN REACTION

Using repetitive cycles of heat denaturation of DNA, annealing of the oligonucleotide primers flanking the DNA fragment of interest, and extension of the annealed primers by temperature-stable DNA polymerases, it is possible to synthesize exponentially virtually unlimited amounts of identical molecules to the target of interest (8). This process is known as PCR. The scant availability of starting material is thus less of an obstacle when this technique is used for diagnostic purposes. Furthermore, it is possible to amplify short segments of DNA extracted from archival material.

Techniques to quantitate gene expression from small tissue samples use PCR amplification of target RNA previously converted to complementary DNA (cDNA) by the enzyme reverse transcriptase (RT)(9). Reverse transcriptase-PCR (RT-PCR) can also be applied to paraffin-embedded tissue (10, 11).

Because short stretches of DNA can be amplified in such large numbers, extreme care must be taken, when performing PCR reactions, to avoid contaminations that can result in false-positive results. These protective measures include interspersed negative control samples, frequent change of gloves, use of positive displace-

ment pipettes, decontamination of instrumentation by ultraviolet irradiation, use of separately ventilated rooms, as well as utilization of interfering synthetic nucleotides (12).

Other techniques such as the ligase chain reaction (13), the strand displacement assay (14) and the self-sustained sequence replication or 3SR (15) are also used, albeit more infrequently, to amplify nucleic acids.

IN SITU HYBRIDIZATION

In situ hybridization (ISH) involves the localization on tissue sections or cytologic preparations of labeled RNA or DNA molecules that hybridize with complementary target DNA or RNA sequences in the cell (16). ISH techniques have been used successfully to localize oncogenes in tumor cells (17). In addition, messenger RNAs for hormones have been localized in endocrine tumor cells in the absence of the protein product of the same gene as assessed by immunohistochemistry. ISH also effectively demonstrates receptors to gastrointestinal hormones (Fig. 8.2).

One of the more recent developments of in situ hybridization is known as fluorescent in situ hybridization (FISH). The FISH technique allows localization of chromosomal sequences, including genes, as well as identification of translocations, deletions, loss of heterozygosities (LOH), assessment of gene amplification, and assignment of genetic loci to newly cloned genes (18–21). Probe types available for FISH analyses include tandem repeat (centromeric or satellite) probes, which are useful for assessing chromosome copy number; regional or locus-specific probes, which are useful for identification of translocations, amplifications, and deletions; and whole chromosome probes (painting probes), which are useful for identifying structural rearrangements.

In recent years, strategies to improve the threshold of detectable copy number per cell has resulted in the development of a technique known as in situ-PCR, which entails amplification via PCR of target sequences (DNA or RNA) at the cellular level prior to in situ hybridization (indirect in situ PCR) (22). Optimization of such techniques, however, is still in the developmental stage (23).

Finally, one of the most recent developments of molecular hybridization makes use of several thousand oligonucleotides bound to silicone chips, which can be rapidly localized with complementary fluorescent probes and subsequently analyzed by computer (24).

TISSUES

Large fragments of nucleic acids used as targets in Northern and Southern blots are extracted from fresh or snap-frozen tissue specimens. Archival tissue, however, can also be used for molecular analyses. DNA and RNA can be successfully extracted from paraffin-embedded tissue and then hybridized (10, 25–27). It is important to remember, however, that nucleic acids are fragmented during routine tissue processing. As a result, methods applied for their detection or amplification need to be modified from those directed to the same target nucleic acid extracted from fresh tissue (5). RNA obtained from archival material is also amenable to reverse transcription to generate cDNA (11).

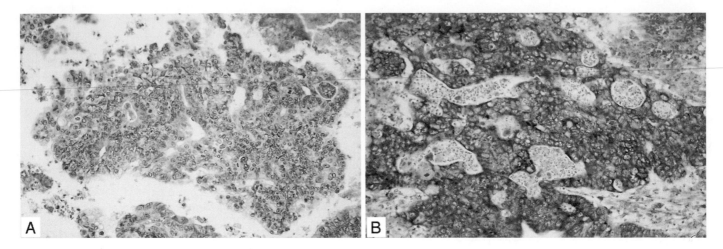

Figure 8.2 Colorectal carcinoma (**A**, hematoxylin & eosin) hybridized with digoxigenin-labeled riboprobe complementary to somatostatin receptor I (SSR I) mRNA (**B**). BCIP-NBT cytoplasmic blue reaction, methyl green counterstain. (See color plate.)

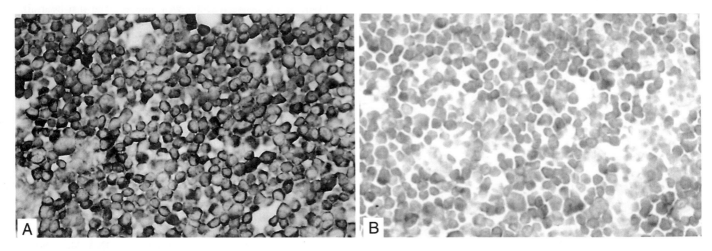

Figure 8.3 Stable transfection of Chinese hamster ovary (CHO) K1 cells with SSR I. Cells were formalin-fixed, paraffin-embedded, and probed with specific antisense riboprobe (**A**) or its sense control (**B**). BCIP-NBT cytoplasmic blue reaction, methyl green counterstain. (See color plate.)

EXPERIMENTAL MODELS

IN VITRO SYSTEMS

To study regulatory elements, specific genes can be transfected in replicating mammalian cells. DNA can be introduced into cells by such methods as calcium phosphate precipitation, electroporation, or liposome-mediated transfection (28). Expression of the gene can be transient, with short-lived extrachromosomal replication. To achieve long-term expression, a selection gene, usually encoding antibiotic resistance, and prolonged subculture, are used. DNA will then become permanently incorporated into host chromosomes, replicate with each cell division, and be transcribed and translated (Fig. 8.3). Another approach to determine regulation of gene expression is the construction and subsequent transfection of chimeric genes, in which the regulatory region of the gene is juxtaposed to the coding region of a reporter gene.

ANIMAL MODELS

Animal models of human disease form the basis of experimental pathology and provide the best paradigm for the assessment of molecular findings in routine pathology practice. Two models used widely for the study of gene function as it relates to human diseases are transgenic and knockout animals.

Transgenic animals are those in which foreign DNA (usually a human gene) is introduced into fertilized cells and is subsequently inherited in the progeny of the host (Fig. 8.4). The inserted gene can become integrated in the host genome at several chromosomal sites. By virtue of the way in which the construct is designed, it can be overexpressed in all tissues when transcription is driven by a strong constitutive promoter (e.g., CMV promoter), or its expression can be restricted by tissue-specific or developmentally regulated promoters (29–31). Transgenic animals provide the means to explore complex biologic functions of a given gene in vivo (32).

When it is important to assess the consequences of loss of function of a gene, knockout mice provide the ideal experimental setting (33). Standard knockout mice are made by specifically inactivating the gene of choice in embryonic stem cells. These cells are then injected into the mouse embryo in which they have the potential to develop into the different cell types. As in transgenic mice, the inactivated gene is carried in the germ line and passed to the progeny. A major problem is death in utero when, as is often the case, the gene turns out to be essential for normal development. To overcome this problem, genes may be knocked out selectively using cell type-specific gene targeting (34). Recently, models mimicking inflammatory bowel disease (IBD) have been described (35, 36).

Athymic (nude) mice are often used to assess tumorigenicity of carcinogens or to assess behavior of tumor cell lines in vivo. For instance, induction of gastrointestinal tumors may be accomplished by a variety of carcinogens such as azoxymethane (37). Interestingly,

it has been shown that mimicking human colorectal carcinoma growth, invasiveness, and metastatic events in nude mice requires orthotopic implantation of tumor tissue (38). The use of this model is particularly suited to test genes that are thought to either suppress or enhance the metastatic process (39, 40).

Throughout this chapter, relevant animal models are discussed in the context of the various entities.

MOLECULAR BIOLOGY OF DEVELOPMENT OF THE GASTROINTESTINAL TRACT

NORMAL DEVELOPMENT

The embryonic gut ultimately develops into various organs involved in digestion and respiration. Functionally differentiated organs, such as lung or liver, develop along the anteroposterior axis from simple endoderm surrounded by splanchnic mesoderm. Three subsequent phases of development are characterized by midline fusion of the splanchnopleure, protrusion of simple ducts and buds, and finally differentiation of the endoderm into histologically and biochemically specialized epithelium of the various organs.

DNA holds all the information necessary for the normal development of tissues and organs in its sequences, but developmental events require a coordinated spacial and temporal pattern of expression of the structural genes. Developmental genes known as "homeotic genes" were first identified in *Drosophila* and subsequently in other organisms, including humans. In *Drosophila*, mutations in these genes resulted in the development of entire body segments that were either temporally or spacially inappropriate. In other words, these genes appear to act as "switches" that specify the identity and spacial arrangement of body segments. Homeotic genes contain a conserved, roughly 180 bp DNA motif near the carboxyl terminus named the "homeobox," which is translated into the homeodomain of a protein that binds to DNA. Many homeodomains have DNA-binding motifs, such as the helix-turn-helix structure, which fits into the major groove of DNA. The homeobox domain is most likely a controlling element within major developmental "switch" genes. Thus, proteins encoded by homeotic genes are transcription factors that regulate pattern formation and confer cell fates in animals by coordinating transcription of downstream target genes. The observed level of conservation within these domains throughout evolution suggests how critical these proteins are to development.

In vertebrates, many lines of evidence suggest that a cluster of genes known as "Hox" (for homeobox) are the homologues of homeotic genes studied in lower organisms (41). For example, the human HOXA7 homeodomain differs from the one from *Drosophila* by only 1 of 60 amino acids (42). This high degree of conservation between species also allows the identification of homeotic sequences in an organism using a known probe from a different organism. Hox genes are organized in four clusters on different chromosomes (43). Gene order within each cluster is highly conserved and probably in direct relationship with expression. These genes have been implicated in regional specification of the digestive tract along the anteroposterior axis in vertebrates (41). In early stages of development before hindgut closure, hox genes are

Transgenic Model

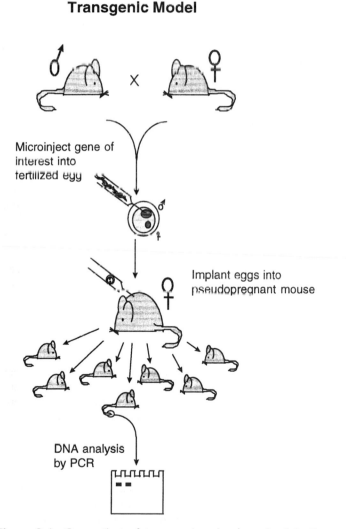

Microinject gene of interest into fertilized egg

Implant eggs into pseudopregnant mouse

DNA analysis by PCR

Figure 8.4 Generation of transgenic mice by microinjection of fertilized eggs. Microinjected eggs are transferred to a pseudopregnant female. Finally, offspring are checked for the presence of the transgene by PCR of DNA extracted from the tail.

expressed in a "Russian doll pattern" with the most 5′ gene on the cluster showing the most posteriorly restricted expression.

Another specific group of conserved homeotic genes in vertebrates is that of the caudal family. Studies have suggested a dual role for caudal genes in development. They are thought to determine anterior-posterior axis during gastrulation and may be involved in intestinal morphogenesis during late embryogenesis and adulthood in that they determine terminal differentiation of intestinal epithelial cells (42, 44). Homeobox genes of the caudal type have also been shown to be involved in gut closure (44). The serpent gene (srp) suppresses foregut-specific genes in order to mediate midgut-specific differentiation and morphogenesis (45). The putative transcription factor fork head (fkh), normally expressed in the stomodeum, developing esophagus, and proctodeum is thought to promote terminal rather than segmental development in the ectodermal portions of the developing gut (45). LOX-3C genes, segmentally expressed in the leech midgut, are related to vertebrate transcription factors involved in gut regionalization and in the differentiation of insulin and somatostatin-producing cells (46).

In summary, normal developmental functions of growth factors include the induction of gene expression across germ layers, the formation of concentration or activity gradients of morphogenetic activity, and coordination of cell fate decisions in groups of cells (47).

ABNORMAL DEVELOPMENT

Classically, gain-of-function (with or without overexpression) or inactivation of a gene have been used to establish whether a gene product plays a role in specifying cell fate. Intestinal epithelial cells prove to be a good environment for the study of cell commitment and differentiation as these cells undergo continuous renewal and there is sufficient phenotypic diversity among them. Sebastio et al. determined that the Caco-2 cell line, which is derived from human colon carcinoma and exhibits spontaneous enterocyte differentiation at cellular confluency in vitro, showed a pattern of homeobox gene expression that paralleled that observed in the adult small intestine (48). Even in vitro systems can thus provide a useful model for the analysis of cellular factors controlling homeobox gene expression.

Embryos that lack srp are missing the entire midgut and do not show endodermal differentiation. The anterior midgut and the posterior midgut become, respectively, ectodermal foregut and an additional hindgut in series with the normal hindgut.

Using a transgenic model, Wolgemuth and coworkers induced overexpression of the Hox 1.4 transgene in the embryonic gut (49). The transgenic offspring were dying between birth and young adulthood from megacolon. Hirschsprung's disease, which results in megacolon, is associated with a deficiency of myenteric ganglion cells in the colon. These ganglion cells are neural crest cell derivatives that migrate into the developing gut to innervate the bowel. The defect resulting in megacolon may thus occur in cells in the various layers of the developing gut that provide cues to migrating neural crest cells (49). Overexpression of another member of the hox family in transgenic mice resulted in hamartomatous lesions of the gut (50).

Homeotic genes are thought to play a role in neoplastic transformation as well. Differential expression of some of the hox genes in primary and metastatic colon cancer suggests an association between hox genes and colon cancer progression (43).

The process of differentiation of intestinal epithelial cells from putative stem cells located in the crypts is still poorly understood. The discovery and analysis of homeobox genes have begun to shed light on this process. Knowledge of the regulation of proliferation and differentiation may help us to understand the intricate mechanisms of neoplastic transformation in which such processes are no longer regulated. The specific function of homeotic genes in gastrointestinal development, however, is still in its early phases. Thus, their potential involvement in human gastrointestinal disease can only be inferred.

MOLECULAR BIOLOGY OF THE GASTROINTESTINAL NEUROENDOCRINE SYSTEM

The digestive tract is regarded as the largest "endocrine" organ system in the body (51). Gastrointestinal hormones, including hormonal peptides and neuropeptides, act on a variety of target tissues by binding receptors eliciting signals that lead to diverse biologic responses. The endocrine cell of the digestive system is thought to be of endodermal origin (51). These cells display classic endocrine, paracrine, and autocrine regulation by gastrointestinal hormones (52). In addition, tumor cells can express functional receptors to gastrointestinal hormones and may themselves produce molecules that may act in an autocrine manner (53, 54). Elucidation of the molecular mechanisms of action of one particular gastrointestinal hormone, gastrin, can serve as a paradigm for the role of neuroendocrine peptides and hormones in gastrointestinal pathophysiology.

Gastrin is a polypeptide hormone, the functions of which include stimulation of gastric secretion of gastric acid, pepsin, pancreatic enzyme, and intrinsic factor (51). Gastrin shares with cholecystokinin a common carboxy terminal, which is required for full biologic activity. Gastrin is secreted by the G cell, mainly in the antropyloric mucosa and has a well-documented trophic effect on the gastrointestinal tract mucosa (55). Some tumors secrete gastrin, whereas chronic hypergastrinemia produces hyperplasia of the enterochromaffin-like cell and the development of gastric carcinoids in rats and humans (56, 57).

Radioimmunoassays are used to measure gastrin secretion in an effort to detect and localize gastrinomas (58, 59), and antibodies directed against different intermediate forms of gastrin have been used to detect incomplete processing of gastrin in G cells of patients with duodenal ulcers, varied tumor types, and in aging (60–62).

Molecular cloning of the gene encoding the gastrin receptor (GR) has been difficult (63–65). Localization, size determination, affinity, and specificity of the gastrin receptor (GR) was initially accomplished with the use of radioligands (66–68). Determining the specificity of the receptor has been difficult, however, owing to the significant homology of gastrin and cholecystokinin (65). There is more than one gastrin/cholecystokinin receptor with different tissue distribution and affinities for the two peptides (63). The molecular structure of GR indicates that it may be linked to G proteins as second messengers. G protein-linked pathways, such as cAMP, play an important role in endocrine cells (69). In fact, an important target in the signal transduction pathway of most neuroendocrine hormones is the *c*AMP *r*esponse *e*lement *b*inding protein CREB, a transcription factor (70, 71). Knowledge of properties such as affinity and location of specific regions necessary for ligand binding allows for the development of specific receptor antagonists that may have therapeutic value. For example, different GR antagonists can block gastrin-mediated proliferation in a variety of gastric and colonic tumor cells (72–75).

Gastrointestinal neurons, which collectively constitute the enteric nervous system (76), are also important regulators of endocrine secretions in the gut. Receptors with tyrosine kinase activity are important to the normal migration and development of neuroblasts in the gut, and several of these receptors have been implicated in various gastrointestinal abnormalities. For example, the RET proto-oncogene was involved in the development of ganglia from vagal-neural crest cells in knockout mice (77). As a result, mutations of the RET gene are associated not only with multiple endocrine neoplasia type 2B (MEN-2B) but also with megacolon (78, 79). In addition, the receptor tyrosine kinase KIT has been implicated in the development of interstitial cells of Cajal, which are noneuronal pacemaker cells. Mice with mutated KIT genes have no interstitial cells and abnormal intestinal motility. Defects in interstitial cells owing to KIT mutations may explain the functional gut abnormalities reported in some patients with piebaldism, a disorder of hypopigmentation (80). Finally, mutations in both the endothelin-3 and endothelin-B receptors have been noted to cause megacolon and pigmentary disorders in mice and humans (81, 82). Interestingly, mutations in the endothelin-B receptor have been reported in patients with Hirschsprung's disease (83).

Another important gastrointestinal hormone is somatostatin, which inhibits a wide range of biologic actions, including cell growth and hormone secretion. Its antiproliferative actions account for some of the therapeutic effects of nonhydrolizable analogs of somatostatin, including sandostatin and RC-160. Colon carcinoma cells are sensitive to this growth-inhibitory effect both in vitro and in vivo (nude mice). The growth-inhibitory action of this hormone is mediated by highly specific receptors via stimulation of phosphotyrosine phosphatase activity (84). Radioligand assays have shown that approximately 10% of colorectal neoplasms express somatostatin receptors. The cloning and characterization of five subtypes of somatostatin receptors prompted an evaluation of their expression in normal and neoplastic colon tissues. Results showed no expression in the normal mucosa, and increasing expression of somatostatin receptor II with advancing stage of disease (Brook DL, Magi-Galluzzi C, Loda M, unpublished observations) (see Fig. 8.2). It may be possible to identify subgroups of cancer patients who express receptor subtypes responsible for growth inhibitory functions, with obvious therapeutic implications. (See Chapter 15 for details concerning the pathology of endocrine disorders.)

MOLECULAR BIOLOGY OF PREMALIGNANT DISORDERS

GENERAL PRINCIPLES

Permanent variations in DNA involving a change in either the sequence (mutation) or location of a gene (rearrangement) cause genetic alterations that form the basis of neoplastic transformation. Such genetic alterations can be caused by exogenous agents or errors during replication, and result in altered expression of the protein products of the gene involved.

Tumors are believed to be acquired through a multistep process (85) involving many genetic alterations. These changes result in the loss of function of genes that encode products that normally hold cell growth in check (tumor suppressor genes) or the activation of dominant genes that stimulate cell proliferation (proto-oncogenes) (Fig. 8.5). Rearrangement of chromosomes, resulting in translocations, insertions, or deletions, may result in oncogene activation or inactivation of suppressor genes. Microinsertion/deletions of DNA, or single base-pair changes (point mutations), may also cause oncogene activation or render a suppressor gene inoperative. Point mutations may cause amino acid substitution (missense mutations),

Genetic Alterations in Colon Tumorigenesis

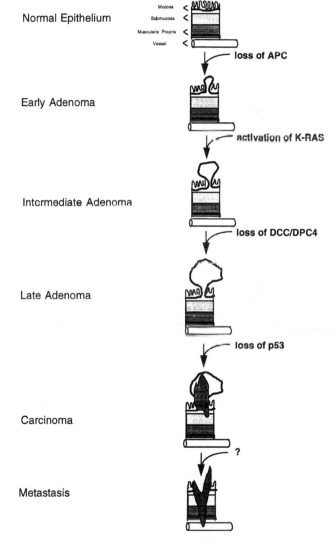

Figure 8.5 Genetic alterations in colorectal tumorigenesis. Genetic alterations are thought to occur sequentially in the initiation, progression, and metastasis of colorectal carcinomas. One of the earliest events is the genetic alteration of the APC gene. In addition, defective RER+ enhances genetic instability and mutations in several genes (211). Adhesion molecules likely play a significant role in the process of invasion (250). See text for abbreviations of genes.

premature truncation of message and protein (nonsense mutations), frameshift mutations with altered amino acid sequence downstream of the mutation, or aberrantly spliced RNA resulting from mutations in sequences at intron-exon junctions important for RNA splicing. As a result of these events, the biologic properties of the gene product may be altered.

Molecular techniques in cancer diagnosis help to determine overexpression or mutations of oncogenes or loss of function for suppressor genes. In addition, it is possible to assess clonality of tumors and to trace susceptibility to cancer in families with genetic linkage analysis.

Proto-oncogenes are highly conserved and are important in cellular pathways involved in growth and differentiation. Only one of the two alleles needs to be mutated to confer (dominant) oncogenic properties to that gene. The majority of oncogenes identified to date are part of the cell's growth regulatory pathways and range from growth factors to their receptors, intracellular signal transducers, cell cycle regulators, and transcription factors. The activation of oncogenes is usually associated with increased expression of their protein product. The assessment of oncogene mutations or overexpression may have both diagnostic and prognostic utility.

Tumor suppressor genes code for proteins the loss of function of which results in transformation. For this loss of function to occur, both alleles must be inactivated. When one allele is inactivated in the germline, such a genotype is transmitted to all somatic cells, rendering them more susceptible to a second mutational event on the remaining functional allele. The result is a greater predisposition to cancers in families carrying such germline mutations (86–91). Because germline mutations are present in all cells, comparison with DNA extracted from normal tissue is important in the assessment of the inactivation of the second allele in tumor DNA. Germline inactivation of a tumor suppressor gene is often the result of gross rearrangements in the region in which the gene is located. Studies determining LOH play an important role in the discovery of such genes as well as in genetic linkage analysis (92). Two tumor suppressor genes studied most intensely are the retinoblastoma (Rb) and the p53 genes. Hereditary retinoblastoma is a prototype of hereditary human cancer (87). Retinoblastoma develops in about 90% of individuals who harbor an inactivating mutation at this locus. In addition, Rb hereditary inactivating mutations have been implicated in the development of other types of tumors, including osteosarcomas, soft tissue tumors, small cell carcinoma of the lung, breast, and bladder cancers (93).

The p53 protein, the product of a tumor suppressor gene on chromosome 17p, has been implicated as a gatekeeper at the G1/S checkpoint in the cell cycle. Its role is to block progression of genetically damaged cells into S phase. Somatic mutations affecting the p53 gene are extremely common in human tumors, whereas germline allelic inactivations confer predisposition to cancer. As a result, malfunctioning of p53 has been associated with various cancers (94).

BARRETT'S ESOPHAGUS

In Barrett's esophagus, the stratified squamous epithelium of the distal esophagus is replaced by abnormal columnar epithelium. Patients with this condition have a 30-to 125-fold excess risk of developing adenocarcinoma (95), preceded by the progression of simple metaplasia into epithelial dysplasia of various severity. Grad-

ing of dysplasia may thus be of significant clinical importance in identifying patients with Barrett's esophagus who are most at risk for developing this complication.

Investigators have identified markers that correlate with the progression of Barrett's esophagus from metaplasia to carcinoma, including proliferation markers, such as PCNA (96) and Ki-67 (97); mutated tumor suppressor gene products, such as p53 (3); sucrase isomaltase (SI), a membrane disaccharidase (98); and growth factors (TGF-α) (99) and their receptors (EGFR) (100).

Increased proliferative activity is a hallmark of dysplastic lesions of the esophagus. The number of Ki-67-positive nuclei was shown to increase relative to changes from normal gastric mucosa to Barrett's metaplasia to high-grade dysplasia (97). Lapertosa et al. also found increased numbers of PCNA-positive cells in high-grade dysplasia, although they reported an overlap in the number of proliferating cells in the tissues determined to be positive, indefinite, and negative for dysplasia (101).

SI is a brush border enzyme normally expressed in the small intestine in adults or in fetal colon, but not usually detected in the normal adult colon. SI has been found in 76% of patients with Barrett's esophagus and in 82% of those with adenocarcinomas. Immunohistochemistry studies show that SI is localized in the apical membrane in Barrett's esophagus in contrast to the more diffuse cytoplasmic staining seen in esophageal dysplasia and carcinoma (98, 102).

Stepwise alteration of TGF-α, a ligand for the EGFR proto-oncogene, from low levels of expression in cardiac type metaplasia to higher levels in intestinal type metaplasia and adenocarcinoma, has been reported (100, 103).

Tumor suppressor genes are also involved in the early phases of esophageal carcinogenesis. Mutations in p53 that appear in Barrett's esophagus occur predominantly in exons 5 to 9, and evidence supports a tendency toward GC to AT transitions (3, 104). Overexpression of p53 can be assessed immunohistochemically (Fig. 8.6). This analysis usually reflects genetic missense mutations, which confer a longer half-life to the protein. Mutations of the adenomatous polyposis coli (APC) gene have been found in dysplastic and adenocarcinoma foci as well as some in metaplastic foci adjacent to dysplasia. In contrast, no APC gene alterations were found in the normal epithelium and metaplasia distant from dysplasia (105). Clonality analysis determined by X-chromosome inactivation revealed the same pattern in carcinoma, dysplasia, and metaplasia adjacent to dysplasia. Finally, the cyclin-dependent kinase inhibitor and putative tumor suppressor p27 is overexpressed in dysplastic Barrett's mucosa, and its sustained expression in a subset of invasive cancers is indicative of a favorable prognosis (Singh SP, Goldman H, Loda M, et al., unpublished results).

H. PYLORI/CHRONIC GASTRITIS

Helicobacter pylori infection of the stomach has been implicated in the pathogenesis of gastric cancer (106–108). Hansson and colleagues reported that patients with duodenal ulcer have a decreased risk of developing gastric cancer, whereas those with gastric ulcers are at higher risk (109). Because both conditions are associated with *H. pylori* infection, the timing of infection has been advocated as critical. Infection in childhood frequently results in atrophic gastritis, a premalignant condition, by early childhood. Multifocal atrophic gastritis, however, is uncommon when infection occurs after childhood. In young adults, acid-secreting capacity is maintained in

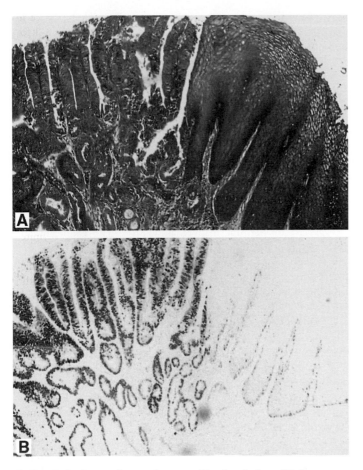

Figure 8.6 Barrett's esophagus with dysplasia: p53 immunostaining. **A**, Gastroesophageal junction with dysplastic Barrett's esophagus (H & E). Immunohistochemistry for p53 (**B**) reveals intense nuclear staining in the majority of dysplastic cells.

the face of mucosal damage caused by *H. pylori*, with a resulting endemic duodenal ulcer disease. These findings explain the epidemiology of gastric cancer, still prevalent in developing countries, where *H. pylori* childhood infection is the rule, and diminishing in developed countries in which improved hygienic conditions result in infections in adults (110).

Neither a definite causative link between the bacteria and cancer nor an underlying mechanism has been confirmed. Recent studies indicate that *H. pylori* infection is associated with increased proliferation (111–113). Because *H. pylori* induces a chronic inflammatory response that results in a greater rate of mucosal proliferation (114, 115), it has been proposed that mutagenic events may occur more frequently with a resultant increased risk of malignant transformation (see review by Goldstone et al. [116]). In laboratory animals (mice), *H. felis,* a spiral organism originally isolated from feline gastric tissue, causes gastritis that closely mimics many of the pathologic features noted in human *H. pylori* infection (117). Mice with a LOH at the p53 locus were inoculated with *H. felis,* followed for 1 year, and compared with uninfected controls of the same genotype. p53 heterozygous mice showed severe adenomatous and cystic hyperplasia of the surface foveolar epithelium. Whereas the wild-type infected mice showed the same pathologic change as the infected heterozygous mice, the latter group had

significantly higher proliferative indices. It may be that loss of p53 offers a genetic advantage in *H. pylori*-induced gastric carcinogenesis (118).

INFLAMMATORY BOWEL DISEASE (IBD)

Ulcerative colitis (UC) and Crohn's disease have a high morbidity and are associated with an increased risk of cancer development. This risk correlates with the extent and duration of the disease. The cumulative risk for cancer is 0.5 to 1% per year after the first 10 years, and the relative risk is 15-fold higher than expected in age-matched populations without colitis (119–121). Both genetic and environmental factors, such as repeated episodes of inflammation and repair, may have a role in the pathogenesis of IBD. Epithelial cells in ulcerative colitis and Crohn's colitis in relapse show increased proliferation indices compared to quiescent disease or control patients (122). Akin to sporadic tumors arising in normal colon, adenocarcinomas in the context of IBD are preceded by dysplastic lesions that progress from indefinite to low grade to high grade before transformation (123).

Although point mutations in proto-oncogenes such as ras appear to be important players in sporadic cancers of the colon, tumor suppressor genes such as p53 may play a more significant role in colon cancers arising from inflammatory dysplastic lesions. A higher percentage of c-Ki-ras mutations have been noted in sporadic colon cancers than in ulcerative colitis-associated cancers (122, 124–127). Although 75% of sporadic colon cancers show allelic loss of the p53 gene and greater than 90% of these tumors have mutations in the remaining allele (128), p53 inactivation seems to be a relatively late event in tumor progression (129)(see Fig. 8.5). In contrast to sporadic colon cancers, p53 mutation in ulcerative colitis-arising tumors appears to be a relatively early event in tumorigenesis (124). Although about two-thirds of patients with dysplasia have p53 mutations, not all of these patients have a loss of the remaining allele.

Other markers found to correlate with degree of dysplasia in IBD include SI, a mucosal disaccharidase that has been detected in colon cancer (130), and c-src, an oncogene previously observed to have elevated activity in both adenomas and colon cancers (131). Fetal rat colon infected with src containing retroviruses developed significant dysplasia throughout the colonic epithelium. In addition, the oncogenes myc and src appear to act synergistically to induce dysplasia and invasive cancer (132).

The availability of animal models in which the manipulation of both genetic and environmental factors can occur is essential to the assessment of the pathogenetic mechanisms involved in IBD. Recent advances in embryonic stem (ES) cell technology have made it possible to develop mutant mice that are specifically deficient for a given cytokine or cytokine receptor by using gene targeting. Aberrant regulation of the immune system coupled with environmental factors act synergistically in the pathogenesis of IBD (35, 36, 133). The interleukin-2 knockout mouse (IL-2-/-) is one of the closest animal models to human ulcerative colitis. IL-2 is a cytokine that promotes T-cell proliferation and differentiation of B cells in vitro. IL-2-/- mice become severely immunocompromised after the first 3 to 4 weeks of life. Fifty percent of these animals die, and those who survive develop human UC-like IBD. Histologic analysis of the mutant mice that develop IBD is not indicative of any known infectious process or pathogen. In a germfree environment, however, IL-2-/- mice showed no evidence of IBD; only the beginnings of an inflammatory process were seen at 17 to 20 weeks. IL-2-/- mice display immune system alterations, such as increased number of activated T and B cells, increased immunoglobulin secretion, anticolon antibodies, and aberrant MHC class II expression, all of which are also found in UC patients (36).

T cell receptor (TCR) mutant mice may also provide a useful animal model because of the similarity between IBD in these mutant mice and human UC, with selective involvement of the large intestine. One study of TCR and MHC class II mutants suggests that the disease requires the presence of B cells and the absence of class II MHC-restricted CD4-positive αβ T cells, which are the cells that produce IL-2. These mutant mice, when kept in a specific pathogen-free (SPF) environment, develop IBD, whereas nude mice and RAG-1 mutants (mice mutated in the recombination activating gene that renders them totally deficient in mature B and T cells) kept in the same SPF facility do not. Because all mice that developed IBD had B cells but lacked αβ-T cells, it is possible that underlying the pathogenesis of some types of IBD is a lack of αβ-T cell-mediated suppression of B cells. These findings further support the concept that diminished IL-2 levels are necessary, albeit not sufficient, to induce IBD.

To further underscore the role of cytokine-mediated immunity in the pathogenesis of IBD, the role of IL-10 has been partially elucidated. IL-10 is a potent cytokine-synthesis suppressor. IL-10 mutant mice kept in a noncontrolled environment develop chronic enterocolitis (35), whereas IL-10 mutants kept under SPF conditions suffer only from inflammation limited to the proximal colon.

A dysfunction in the mucosal immune system may lead to autoimmunity, possibly via formation of autoantibodies directed against an antigen derived from food and/or intestinal microorganisms. The selective involvement of the large intestine might be a result of the high concentration of microorganisms in this region (133).

MOLECULAR BIOLOGY OF GASTROINTESTINAL NEOPLASMS

ESOPHAGEAL CARCINOMA

Approximately 12,000 cases of esophageal cancer occur annually in the United States, with a male-to-female ratio of 3:1. Squamous cell carcinoma (SCC) represents the most common esophageal malignancy, although the incidence of adenocarcinoma is steadily increasing, particularly in white males (134). Both oncogenes and tumor suppressor genes are altered in SCC and adenocarcinoma of the esophagus (see review by Stemmermann G et al. [135]). Loss of heterozygosity (LOH) of the tumor suppressor genes p53, pRb, APC, mutated in colorectal cancer (MCC), and deleted in colorectal cancer (DCC) have been found alone or in combination in SCC (136). The p53 gene is altered in 50% of esophageal cancers, inclusive of both SCC and adenocarcinoma. Alterations include both missense mutations and loss of LOH. Inactivation of the cell cycle inhibitors p16 and p27 occur in esophageal cancers (137). Akin to mantle cell lymphomas, parathyroid adenomas, and breast carcinomas, overexpression of the oncogene cyclin D1 is also

associated with esophageal tumorigenesis (138). Human papillomavirus (HPV) DNA has been demonstrated by in situ hybridization in about 25% of patients with esophageal SCC (139).

GASTRIC CARCINOMA

Although the incidence of gastric cancer is declining worldwide, more than 20,000 cases per year are diagnosed in the United States, with a dismal 10% probability of survival at 5 years (140). A relationship between gastric cancer and *H. pylori* infection together with atrophic achlorhydric gastritis (see above) has been established (106–109, 141). Tumor suppressor genes (i.e., p53, DCC, APC) as well as oncogenes (i.e., EGF, EGFR, TGF-α, and erb-B2) have been implicated in the pathogenesis of gastric cancer (see review by Stemmerman et al. [135]). The cadherins and associated proteins have been shown experimentally to modulate cell migration, proliferation, and programmed cell death (29). Interestingly, decreased expression of the adhesion molecule E-cadherin has been shown to correlate with increasing histologic grade, metastatic potential, and survival in patients with gastric carcinomas (142). Expression of another cell adhesion molecule, CD44, a transmembrane glycoprotein associated with metastatic potential in experimental animals and unfavorable outcome in human colon carcinomas (143), is associated with poor prognosis in gastric adenocarcinoma as well (144).

COLON CARCINOMAS

Despite considerable progress in the elucidation of the molecular mechanisms responsible for colonic malignancies, colorectal cancer remains one of three most common causes of cancer death in the United States (145, 146). The prognosis of colorectal cancer after curative resection depends on pathologic and clinical staging. This staging system creates categories in which survival can range by as much as 40% for stage II and stage III disease. Better definition of the risk of recurrence by molecular methods will ensure that adjuvant therapy is given to those patients who are most likely to benefit from it.

RAS/MITOGEN ACTIVATED PROTEIN (MAP) KINASE PATHWAY

Because many proto-oncogenes are tyrosine kinases, it follows that the function of such proteins involved in pathways of growth and differentiation can be modulated by reversible phosphorylation (147).

Several oncogenes transmit signals through the proto-oncogene ras, which is mutated in about 30% of human cancers (148) and is one of the early events in colon carcinogenesis (127) leading to the activation by phosphorylation of mitogen activated protein (MAP) kinases. MAP kinase activation is thus a central step in tumor growth stimulation. MAP kinases ultimately relay the information (proliferation, differentiation, or programmed cell death) to the nucleus (149).

A novel family of phosphatases inactivates MAP kinase by dephosphorylating both threonine and tyrosine residues (150). These enzymes, which have a similarity to cdc 25 (a putative oncogene that controls cell entry into mitosis) (151, 152), are called MAP kinase phosphatases or MKP. Such dual-specific phosphatases are highly conserved through evolution (153–155). The human prototype of MKP, MKP-1 (156), regulates MAP kinase activity. Using in situ hybridization, MKP-1 was found to be overexpressed early in the carcinogenic pathway in colon as well as other epithelial tumors, with progressive loss of expression in higher grade and late stages in the absence of inactivating mutations or chromosomal loss (Fig. 8.7) (157). Aggressive tumors with poor prognosis (hepatocellular and pancreatic) express little or none of this phosphatase. MKP-1 may thus be a regulatory checkpoint in cancers that are activated by oncogenes encoding upstream components along the MAP kinase cascade, such as ras, as is the case in colorectal carcinomas.

p53 TUMOR SUPPRESSOR GENE

Sporadic mutations in the p53 tumor suppressor gene are the single most common genetic alteration observed in human cancer (158, 159). In addition, germline p53 mutations confer predisposition to cancer (89–91). Genomic DNA damage, hypoxia, oncogene activation, and certain viral infections result in a block of the cell cycle mediated by p53 and its effector p21. Whereas most research has centered on p53's control of the G1/S checkpoint, recent evidence points to a possible control by p53/p21 of the G2/M checkpoint as well, further underscoring the central role of p53 in cancer (160). A colon carcinoma cell line with mutant p53 and p21-/- was shown to undergo active cell division in spite of DNA damage induced by treatment with radiation or Adriamycin. These cells then acquired deformed polyploid nuclei and died through apoptosis. In contrast, p21+/+ colon cancer cells appeared unaltered after the same treatment because they growth arrested after DNA damage (160). p21 status of colorectal cancers may thus have important therapeutic implications.

In the gastrointestinal tract, p53 mutations have been studied extensively (see review by Bosari and Viale [161]). As just outlined, studies published to date have shown unfavorable prognostic

significance of p53 accumulation in esophageal cancer. Multivariate analysis, however, was not used to confirm these results. In contrast, two groups of investigators reported that p53 accumulation is associated with decreased survival in gastric cancer by multivariate analysis. p53 mutations are the most common genetic alteration found in colorectal cancer (162, 163). Deletions of chromosome 17p, which contains the gene for p53, are found in 75% of colorectal cancers and are often associated with mutation of the remaining p53 gene (164). Most immunohistochemical investigations of p53 in colorectal cancers have yielded conflicting results as to the role of this gene in predicting outcome, perhaps because of the late occurrence of p53 mutations in colorectal tumor progression (127, 129, 165).

Cancers tend to develop over 3- to 6-month periods in p53 knockout mice (166–168). Although several murine models of neoplasia in which p53 is constitutively inactivated exist (166, 169), these mice predominantly succumb to tumors of the lymphoid lineages (169).

DELETED IN COLORECTAL CANCER (DCC) GENE

Chromosome 18 is frequently deleted in colon carcinoma and its loss is associated with poor prognosis (170). The candidate suppressor gene located on chromosome 18q21.2 is the gene deleted in colorectal cancer, or DCC. DCC encodes an adhesion molecule belonging to the immunoglobulin superfamily and encodes the receptor for netrin, a conserved family of genes related to laminins (171). DCC may thus be involved in the regulation of cell-to-cell or cell-to-interstitium interactions. In addition, it likely plays an important role in the control of tumor growth and metastatic process because its inactivation appears to be a late event in the neoplastic progression of several human tumors, including a substantial number (70%) of colorectal neoplasms. The 18q chromosomal deletion was previously assessed by LOH assays, although these studies did not rule out that another candidate tumor suppressor gene, named deleted in pancreatic cancer locus 4, or

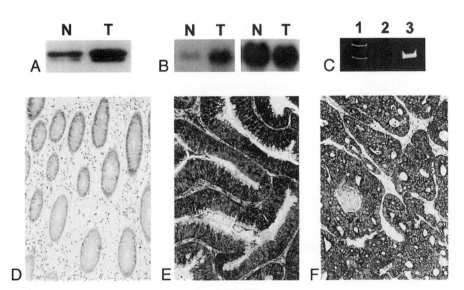

Figure 8.7 MKP-1 expression in colon carcinomas. **A,** Western blot of normal (N) and tumor (T) tissue; **B,** Northern blot of MKP-1 (first two lanes) and control housekeeping gene G3PDH (third and fourth lanes); **C,** RT-PCR with specific primers to MKP-1: lane 1, molecular weight marker; lane 2: no reverse transcriptase negative control; lane 3: specific 435 bp MKP-1 band; in situ hybridization of normal mucosa (**D**), adenoma (**E**), and carcinoma (**F**) with MKP-1 antisense riboprobe. (See color plate.)

DPC4, localized to 18q21.1 was responsible for the phenotype (172). Using immunohistochemical techniques, however, it was confirmed that specific loss of DCC protein product, akin to 18q LOH, was a powerful indicator of poor prognosis, particularly in stage II cancers (173). DCC likely plays an important role in colorectal carcinogenesis and assessment of its status may help to identify subsets of patients who may benefit from adjuvant therapy.

CELL DIVISION CYCLE AND CANCER

Progression through the eukaryotic cell division cycle is regulated by a number of cyclin-dependent kinases (Cdk) consisting of a regulatory cyclin subunit and a catalytic serine/threonine kinase subunit (see review by Lee [174]). Several distinct cyclin-Cdk complexes are active and required at various stages of the cell cycle. The activity of Cdk is tightly regulated by both activating and inactivating phosphorylation events (see review by Coleman and Dunphy [175]). A third class of subunits has been identified and shown to inhibit the activity of Cdk. For this reason, these proteins have been named *cyclin-dependent kinase inhibitors* (Cki) (see Sherr and Roberts [176]). Most known Cki promote cell cycle arrest in response to antimitogenic extracellular signals. Other Cki might function as intrinsic checkpoints of the cell cycle, ensuring that cells pass the G1 restriction point and replicate their genomes only under appropriate conditions.

In mammalian cells, two families of inhibitors have been cloned and characterized based on sequence homology and specificity of interaction with Cdk (Table 8.1) (177–193). Cki have been suggested as the products of potential antioncogenes because their function is often missing in transformed cells. For instance, p15 and p16 genes have been found mutated, deleted, or inactivated by methylation in a large number of human malignancies (194). p21 is transcriptionally induced by the tumor suppressor p53 (179, 195), which lacks function in about 50% of human tumors, including some gastrointestinal cancers (129, 159). Whereas p21 is expressed in normal nonproliferating cells in colonic crypts, compartmentalization of p21 with regard to proliferation was abrogated in colorectal neoplasms (196). The p27 gene analyzed by Southern

blot and PCR-SSCP in a large number of human cancers and human cell lines showed no structural alterations or point mutations (197–199).

Unlike p21, which is primarily regulated at the level of transcription, the down-regulation of p27 protein levels during G1 is the result of ubiquitin-mediated degradation (200). In a series of patients with colon cancer who had long-term follow up, p27 was found to be an independent prognostic variable by multivariate analysis. When compared to individuals with tumors that have high p27 expression, patients with tumors that lacked p27 had a 3.2 increased risk of death from the disease. More importantly, in stage II carcinomas, p27 absence increased the risk of death 32.3-fold, compared to tumors with high expression. Patients in stage II who had greater than 50% p27 staining had a median survival in excess of 219 months, whereas patients who had less than 50% p27 expression or no p27 expression had median survivals of 140 months and 69 months, respectively. Carcinomas with low or absent protein and high mRNA for p27 displayed enhanced proteolytic activity specific for p27, suggesting that loss of p27 expression appears to result from tumor-mediated degradation rather than from altered gene transcription (201). Hopefully, modulation of the degradation process will lead to improved therapeutic control of colon cancer.

TRANSFORMING GROWTH FACTOR β-GENE FAMILY

TGF-β are potent autocrine and paracrine negative regulators of growth in normal epithelial and neuroectodermal cells (202). The three mammalian forms (TGF-β1, 2, and 3), located on different chromosomes, share significant sequence homology and are highly conserved in mammalian species (202, 203). They are differentially expressed during embryogenesis and carcinogenesis, inhibit growth of cells of intestinal origin in vitro, and suppress genomic instability independently of G1 arrest (204). Akin to p27, TGF-β is expressed in the upper one third of intestinal villi and colonic crypts (205). In addition, TGF-β exerts a growth-inhibitory effect on well-differentiated, but not on poorly differentiated, colon carcinoma cell lines. TGF-β expression has been correlated with disease progression and metastases in colon cancer. Recently, an important component of the signaling pathway for TGF-β was shown to be a target for inactivating mutations in colorectal carcinomas (206). This finding, together with the chromosomal location of this protein, 18q21 (the site of DCC and DPC4, as just described), argue for a role of disrupted TGF-β signaling in colorectal tumorigenesis. Finally, loss of the functional receptor for TGF-β appears to be associated with adenocarcinomas and squamous cell carcinomas of the esophagus (207).

Other genes, such as DF3, a breast cancer-derived glycoprotein, and SI, have also been used as prognostic markers in colorectal carcinomas (208, 209).

INHERITED COLON CANCER SYNDROMES

HEREDITARY NONPOLYPOSIS COLON CANCER (HNPCC) SYNDROME — MISMATCH REPAIR

Because mutations play such an important role in cancer and inherited genetic diseases, it follows that highly conserved mechanisms that maintain genetic integrity should be in place in normal cells. The enzymes responsible for the maintenance of genetic

TABLE 8.1   Cyclin-Dependent Kinase Inhibitors Subdivided According to Sequence Homology and Specificity of Interaction

Group 1	
p21	Cip1, Pic1, Sdi1, Waf1
p27	Ick, Kip1, Pic2
p57	Kip2
Group2	
p16	Ink4A, Mys1, Cdkn2, Cdk4i
p15	Ink4B, Mts2
p18	Ink4C, Ink6A
p19/p20	Ink4D, Ink6B

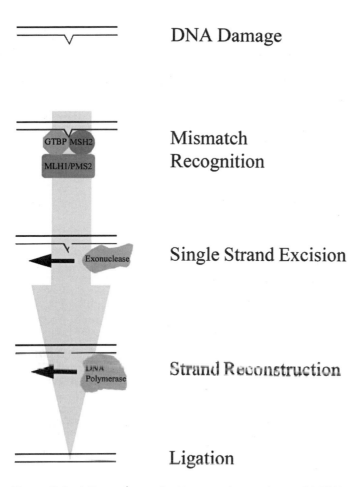

DNA Damage

Mismatch
Recognition

Single Strand Excision

Strand Reconstruction

Ligation

Figure 8.8 Mismatch repair. The protein products of MSH2, GTBP, MLH1, and PMS2 form a complex that binds to under-methylated DNA. Single-strand cleavage and repair then occur by the action of exonucleases and DNA polymerases.

integrity were discovered in bacteria (210). This mismatch repair system consists of five enzymes that work in concert to correct violations of G-C and A-T base-pair matching (Fig. 8.8). Yeast and human homologues have been demonstrated (211, 212). The importance of mismatch repair in human cancer is underscored by the fact that microsatellite instability reflecting defective genetic repair, also known as *r*eplication *e*rror (or RER) phenotype, is present in several human cancers of diverse tissue origin (213). In addition, inherited cancer syndromes, such as the autosomal dominant hereditary nonpolyposis colon cancer (HNPCC), have been found to harbor defects in mismatch repair genes (211, 212, 214). These genes—MLH1, MSH2, MSH3, PMS2 (called PMS1 in *Saccaromyces cerevisiae*) and GTBP or MSH6 seem to be inherited as recessive genes in that normal cells in patients who inherit an altered allele show low mutability, whereas when both copies are inactivated in tumors, the result is hypermutability (211, 214). Murine models with targeted disruption of the MSH2 gene display an increased predisposition to cancer, particularly lymphomas (215).

The HNPCC syndrome is associated with the autosomal dominant inheritance of defective mismatch repair genes and is estimated to account for 4 to 13% of colon cancers (216). Muta-

tions in hMLH1 and hMSH2 are present in up to 80% of HNPCC kindreds (213, 217, 218). Mismatch repair defects have also been implicated in at least 10% of sporadic colorectal carcinomas (214, 219, 220). Monoclonal antibodies to the hMLH1 and hMSH2 gene products have been used to screen for mismatch repair defects in routinely processed (formalin-fixed, paraffin-embedded) colorectal cancer tissues. Positive nuclear staining of normal colonic epithelium was observed in all cases in which normal mucosa was present. An intensity gradient was observed, with heavier staining in the crypts and decreasing signal toward the surface epithelium. Positive nuclear staining was present in 62 of 66 evaluated colorectal carcinomas. Lack of staining in three cases and partial staining in another was attributable to promoter methylation (221).

MSH2-deficient mice develop lymphomas (80%) and 70% of older mice develop intestinal neoplasms associated with APC inactivation (222). This phenotype is strikingly similar to that of humans with HNPCC and represents an extremely useful animal model to study the relationship between mismatch repair defects and mutations in the other genes implicated in colorectal tumorigenesis.

FAMILIAL ADENOMATOUS POLYPOSIS SYNDROMES— APC GENE

Familial adenomatous polyposis (FAP), a genetic syndrome that predisposes to colon cancer, affects 1 in 5000 Americans (1). Inheritance of the adenomatous polyposis coli (APC) gene located on 5q21-22 is autosomal dominant. Mutations in the APC gene are associated with the earliest stages of sporadic colorectal tumorigenesis (223). The phenotype of the inherited syndrome consists of multiple adenomatous polyps that progress to cancer unless removed. Molecular techniques have allowed the detection of at least 99 different mutations in the APC locus resulting in FAP in 173 unrelated patients (224). The mechanism of action of APC has been elucidated and described elsewhere (223). Using a novel inducible expression system in a colorectal cell line that does not contain APC protein, Morin et al. demonstrated a substantial diminution of cell growth by induction of apoptosis by the exogenous APC (225). Presymptomatic molecular diagnosis among at-risk family members is now possible by screening for germline mutations in the APC gene (224, 226–231).

A dominantly transmitted mutation in mice, named min for *m*ultiple *i*ntestinal *n*eoplasia, causes a phenotype resembling human FAP (232). Subsequent studies have shown that the min mutation is recombinationally inseparable from the exon 15 mutation of the APC gene in this animal model (233). Min mice provide an ideal environment in which to study the effects of both environmental and genetic factors on adenomatous polyposis syndromes. Dietrich et al. used this model to demonstrate the presence of another inherited gene (named *m*odifier *o*f *m*in, or mom) that modifies the phenotype of min mice by significantly reducing tumor numbers (234). Kennedy et al. used min mice to demonstrate that a soybean-derived protease inhibitor as a dietary supplement can suppress tumorigenesis significantly in those situations in which there is a genetic predisposition to the development of intestinal tumors (235). Such studies provide evidence of how genetic and environmental factors can influence the penetrance of a gene.

LYMPHOMAS

GENERAL ASPECTS

The application of molecular techniques is particularly important in leukemias and lymphomas. Southern blotting allows molecular analysis of rearranged immunoglobulin and T-cell receptor genes for the measurement of both clonality and lineage (236–238). Polymerase chain reaction (PCR) or RT-PCR also achieves these goals but does not require ample amounts of tissue and is more sensitive than Southern blotting. Great care, however, must be taken to avoid artifactual results (239–241).

Certain chromosomal translocations can be identified by FISH, and ISH is ideally suited to detect integrated viral DNA, such as that of the Epstein-Barr virus, commonly associated with certain lymphomas, (e.g., posttransplant lymphoproliferative disorders) (239).

MALT-ASSOCIATED LYMPHOMAS

The gastrointestinal tract is the most common site of primary extranodal non-Hodgkin's lymphoma (242). In 1984, Isaacson and Wright (243) proposed that B-cell lymphomas arising in mucosa-associated lymphoid tissue (MALT) in various sites, such as the gastrointestinal tract, lung, and thyroid, were a single pathologic entity. Until then, these lymphoproliferative lesions were somewhat of an enigma (239), but refined immunocytochemistry methods combined with molecular biology techniques have helped to define MALT lesions as a specific biologic entity (243–246).

Some evidence indicates that, like other tumors, MALT lymphomas may be a multistage tumorigenic process characterized by the progressive accumulation of genetic defects. The relationship between low-grade MALT lymphomas and high-grade B-cell lymphomas arising in mucosal sites, however, is uncertain. Chronic inflammation is thought to be associated with genetic instability. Low-grade MALT lymphomas commonly arise in the background of chronic inflammatory processes and can transform into high grade at a late stage (247). Although some investigators found no rearrangement of bcl-1, bcl-2, or the c-myc loci in any lymphoma of MALT type (248), other authors reported rearrangement involving the c-myc gene in 50% of high-grade MALT lymphomas (249). A difference in the extent of p53 mutations in low-grade versus high-grade MALT lymphomas has also been documented (250). These findings, along with data indicating an association between the RER-positive phenotype, a display of alterations in microsatellite sequences, and p53 mutations in MALT lesions (251), suggest that genetic events may play a pivotal role in the development of MALT lymphomas, particularly in high-grade transformation. To corroborate these findings, high-grade transformation of B-cell lymphomas, such as follicular lymphoma (252), and of chronic lymphocytic leukemia (253) are also associated with an increase in p53 mutations. A high frequency of p53 mutations was reported in the marginal zone of splenic B-cell lymphoma (254), which is analogous to MALT lymphoma in its origin of cell lineage, immunophenotype, histology, and molecular genetics (absence of bcl-2 and bcl-1 gene rearrangement) (255).

METASTASIS

Metastasis of tumor cells is a multistep process involving tumor cell entry and exit from the bloodstream and subsequent growth into new tissue (see review elsewhere [256, 257]). Such a process requires that the tissue provides a fertile "soil" for the tumor cell, that the organ in which the metastasis occurs is on the blood flow route draining the organ in which the tumor originated, or more likely, a combination of the two mechanisms. Factors responsible for metastasis include recruitment of new blood vessels to the primary tumor (angiogenesis), matrix degradation and stromal invasion by tumor cells, entry of tumor cells in the vasculature, adherence to the endothelium at the metastatic site, extravasation, and invasion of the organ parenchyma. Degradative enzymes secreted by tumor cells; enhanced motility of the tumor cell; altered expression of molecules responsible for cell-cell adhesion, such as E-cadherin, or cell-matrix adhesion, such as integrins; and growth factor secretion by a tissue may all favor the metastatic process (258–263).

In melanomas, breast carcinomas, and hepatocellular carcinomas, expression of the nm23 gene is inversely proportional to tumor metastatic potential. Murine melanoma cells and human breast carcinomas that are stably transfected with this gene lose their ability to migrate in response to a variety of chemoattractants, such as whole serum, platelet-derived growth factor (PDGF), and insulin-like growth factor (IGF-1). The finding that motility was blocked by multiple factors suggests that the blockage most likely involves the disruption of a downstream event in the signaling pathway that directs cell motility (264). The mechanism of this process is unknown, but a potential interaction between nm23 and microtubules has been reported (265). Mutations resulting in nm23 deletion and amplification have been observed in colorectal cancer (266, 267), but the overall nm23 protein levels in these cancers has no correlation with metastatic potential (264).

Carcinoembryonic antigen has been shown to play a role in the enhancement of experimental hepatic metastases (268).

GENE THERAPY

TYPES

The aim of gene therapy is to induce or suppress the expression of functional genes in target cells (269). In the first authorized human gene therapy attempt, the adenosine deaminase (ADA) gene was successfully replaced in an 8-year-old boy in 1990. Two independent clinical trials have established that ADA gene therapy has contributed to therapeutic improvement of severe combined immune deficiency (SCID) (270, 271). More than 100 clinical trials have been approved to date, approximately 50% of which involve cancer patients.

Direct and indirect strategies are used for gene therapy. Direct inhibition of dominant oncogenes involves the use of antisense ribozymes or expression of recessive tumor suppressor genes. Such techniques require a high efficiency of gene transfer to tumor cells, a goal that often is difficult to achieve. In fact, the greatest difficulty in the field of gene therapy has been efficient targeting of tumor cells and adequate expression of the transgene. Delivery of genes is accomplished by several means. One of the more efficient delivery systems is that of cationic liposomes containing the gene of interest, packaged in adeno-associated virus-based plasmids (272) or as phosphothiorate oligonucleotides (273). To avoid delivery problems, a third form of direct gene therapy that requires only intermediate efficiencies of gene transfer (1 to 10%) is that of cytotoxic prodrugs, such as the herpes simplex virus thymidine kinase (HSVtk). Once delivery is accomplished, tumor cells are killed by giving patients ganciclovir.

Indirect gene therapy involves the use of vaccines (see review elsewhere [274]), which can consist of DNA or RNA molecules encoding tumor antigens such as CEA or allogeneic MHC. In addition, genetically modified tumor vaccines promote immuno-modulation of cancer cells, which is achieved by introducing genes, such as IL-12 or GM-CSF, that promote immune responses to augment antitumor reactions (275). This approach has been attempted successfully with genes coding for lymphokines (276–278), cytokines (279–282), class I MHC antigens, and foreign antigens (283–285). Bone marrow-derived dendritic cells from the patient can be exposed to the antigen and reinfused (286, 287). These cells then present the antigen to naive T cells, which will react against the tumor.

POTENTIAL APPLICATIONS

The rationale for the use of therapeutic agents in patients stems first from observations in cell lines and in nude mice. In colon cancer, effort has been directed toward inherited forms of the disease, such as FAP. Inactivation of the APC gene is responsible for the FAP syndrome and is one of the earliest events in colorectal tumorigenesis. Other tumor suppressor genes that are possible candidates for use in gene therapy in colon carcinomas include DCC and p53. The introduction of functional copies of these genes into human colon cancer cell lines has reversed the tumorigenic phenotype (288, 289).

Genes encoding the antihuman colon carcinoma monoclonal antibody on a retroviral vector and subsequently introduced into human colon cancer cells induced antibody-dependent cell-mediated cytotoxicity against both themselves and unmodified parental cells (290). In addition, human colon cancer cells transfected with genes encoding two TNF-α receptors were killed by recombinant TNF (291).

Tracing the fate of cells subjected to gene therapy has allowed investigators to ascertain that relapse after autologous bone marrow transplant is the result of reinfusion of surviving tumor cells in the marrow (292). In a mouse model, radiolabeled antisense oligonucleotides against the c-myc oncogene were used in vivo to detect mammary tumor uptake by noninvasive imaging (293).

CONCLUSION

Molecular pathology has provided invaluable insight into the pathogenesis of several gastrointestinal disorders. Application of molecular techniques, in both experimental and surgical settings, is bound to become the cornerstone of modern pathology practice in the years to come.

ACKNOWLEDGMENTS

Special thanks to Laura Aisenman for invaluable assistance in the preparation of the manuscript; Giulia Cangi, Rajesh Mishra, and Jane Hayword for assistance with references and figures; and Drs. Arthur Mercurio, Cristina Magi Galluzzi, Giorgio Inghirami, and Harvey Goldman for helpful discussions.

REFERENCES

1. Lynch HT, Watson P, Smyrk TC, et al. Colon cancer genetics. Cancer (Supplement) 1992;70:1300–1312.
2. Jessup JM, Steele GJ, Thomas P, et al. Molecular biology of neoplastic transformation of the large bowel: Identification of two pathways. Surg Oncol Clin North Am 1994;449–477.
3. Hamelin R, Flejou J-F, Muzeau F, et al. TP53 gene mutations and p53 protein immunoreactivity in malignant and premalignant Barrett's esophagus. Gastroenterology 1994;107: 1012–1018.
4. Loda M. Polymerase chain reaction-based methods for the detection of mutations in oncogenes and tumor suppressor genes. Hum Pathol 1994;25:564–571.
5. Stork PJS, Loda M, Bosari S, et al. Detection of K-ras mutations in pancreatic and hepatic neoplasms by non-isotopic mismatched polymerase chain reaction. Oncogene 1991;6:857–862.
6. Manam S, Nichols WW. Multiplex polymerase chain reaction amplification and direct sequencing of homologous sequences: Point mutation analysis of the ras genes. Anal Biochem 1991;199: 106–111.
7. Bos JL, Fearon ER, Hamilton SR, et al. Prevalence of ras gene mutations in human colorectal cancers. Nature 1987;327:293–297.
8. Mullis KB, Faloona FA. Specific synthesis of DNA in vitro via a polymerase-catalyzed chain reaction. Methods Enzymol 1987;155: 335–350.
9. Loda M, Fiorentino M, Meckler J, et al. Hepatitis C virus reinfection in orthotopic liver transplant patients with or without concomitant hepatitis B infection. Diagn Mol Pathol 1996;5:81–87.
10. Stanta G, Schneider C, Mies CM. RNA extracted from paraffin-embedded human tissues is amenable to analysis by PCR amplification. Biotechniques 1991;11:304–308.
11. Svoboda-Newman SM, Greenson JK, Singleton TP, et al. Detection of hepatitis C by RT-PCR in formalin fixed paraffin embedded tissue from living transplant patients. Diagn Mol Pathol 1997;6:123–129.
12. Buchman G. A novel method using dUMP-containing primers and uracil DNA glycosylase. PCR Methods Appl 1993;3:28–31.
13. Wu DR, Wallace RB. The ligation amplification reaction (LAR)-amplification of specific DNA sequences using sequential rounds of template-dependent ligation. Genomics 1989;4:560–569.
14. Walker GT, Little MC, Nadeau JG, et al. Isothermal in vitro amplification of DNA by a restriction enzyme/DNA polymerase system. Proc Natl Acad Sci USA 1992;89:392–396.
15. Guatelli JC, Whitfield KM, Kwoh DY, et al. Isothermal, in vitro amplification of nucleic acids by a multienzyme reaction modeled after retroviral replication. Proc Natl Acad Sci USA 1990;87:1874–1878.
16. Wilcox JN. Fundamental principles of in situ hybridization. J Histchem Cytochem 1993;41:1725–1733.
17. DeLellis RA. In situ hybridization techniques for the analysis of gene expression: Applications in tumor pathology. Hum Pathol 1994;25: 580–585.
18. McManus AP, Gusterson BA, Pinkerton CR, et al. Dianosis of Ewing's sarcoma and related tumours by detection of chromosome 22q12 translocations using fluorescence in situ hybridization on tumour touch imprints. J Pathol 1995;176:137–142.
19. Beck JL, Hopman AH, Feitz WF, et al. Numerical aberrations of chromosomes 1 and 7 in renal cell carcinomas as detected by interphase cytogenetics. J Pathol 1995;176:123–135.
20. Persons DL, Hartmann LC, Herath JF, et al. Interphase molecular cytogenetic analysis of epithelial ovarian carcinomas. Am J Pathol 1993;142:733–741.
21. Misra DN, Dickman PS, Yunis EJ. Fluorescence in situ hybridization (FISH) detection of MYCN oncogene amplification in neuroblastoma using paraffin-embedded tissue. Diagn Mol Pathol 1995;4: 128–135.
22. Nuovo GJ. PCR in situ hybridization. Protocols and applications. New York: Raven Press, 1992.
23. Komminoth P, Long AA. In-situ polymerase chain reaction. An overview of methods, applications and limitations of a new molecular technique. Virchows Arch [B] 1993;64:67–73.
24. Pease AC, Solas D, Sullivan EJ, et al. Light-generated oligonucleotide arrays for rapid DNA sequence analysis. Proc Natl Acad Sci USA 1994;91:5022–5026.

25. Frank TS, Svoboda-Newman SM, Hsi ED. Comparison of methods for extracting DNA from formalin-fixed paraffin sections for nonisotopic PCR. Diagn Mol Pathol 1996;5:220–224.

26. Shibata D. Extraction of DNA from paraffin-embedded tissue for analysis by polymerase chain reaction: New tricks from an old friend. Hum Pathol 1994;25:561–563.

27. Mies CM. Molecular biological analysis of paraffin-embedded tissues. Hum Pathol 1994;25:555–560.

28. Ausubel FM, Brent R, Kingston RE, et al. Current protocols in molecular biology. New York: John Wiley & Sons, 1994.

29. Hermiston ML, Wong MH, Gordon JI. Forced expression of E-cadherin in the mouse intestinal epithelium slows cell migration and provides evidence for nonautonomous regulation of cell fate in a self-renewing system. Genes Dev 1996;10:985–996.

30. Morgan BA, Izpisua-Belmonte JC, Duboule D. Targeted misexpression of Hox-4.6 in the avian limb bud causes apparent homeotic transformation. Nature 1992;358:236–239.

31. Greenberg NM, DeMayo F, Finegold MJ, et al. Prostate cancer in a transgenic mouse. Proc Natl Acad Sci USA 1995;92:3439–3443.

32. Shuldiner AR. Transgenic animals. N Engl J Med 1995;334:653–655.

33. Majzoub JA, Muglia LJ. Knockout mice. N Engl J Med 1996;334:904–906.

34. Gu H, Marth JD, Orban PC, et al. Deletion of a DNA polymerase β gene segment in T cells using cell type-specific gene targeting. Science 1994;265:103–106.

35. Kuhn R, Lohler J, Rennick D, et al. Interleukin-10-deficient mice develop chronic enterocolitis. Cell 1993;75:263–274.

36. Sadlack B, Merz H, Schorle H, et al. Ulcerative colitis-like disease in mice with a disrupted interleukin-2 gene. Cell 1993;75:253–261.

37. Vivona AA, Shpitz B, Medline A, et al. K-ras mutations in aberrant crypt foci, adenomas and adenocarcinomas during azoxymethane-induced colon carcinogenesis. Carcinogenesis 1993;14:1777–1781.

38. Togo S, Shimada H, Kubota T, et al. Host organ specifically determines cancer progression. Cancer Res 1995;55:681–684.

39. Brem H, Folkman J. Analysis of experimental antiangiogenic therapy. J Pediatr Surg 1993;28:445–450.

40. Cao Y, Chen C, Weatherbee JA, et al. gro-beta, a -C-X-C- chemokine, is an angiogenesis inhibitor that suppresses the growth of Lewis lung carcinoma in mice. J Exp Med 1995;182:2069–2077.

41. Yokouchi Y, Sakiyama J-I, Kuroiwa A. Coordinated expression of Abd-B subfamily genes of the HoxA cluster in the developing digestive tract of chick embryo. Dev Biol 1995;169:76–89.

42. Bonner CA, Loftus SK, Wasmuth JJ. Isolation, characterization, and precise physical localization of human CDX1, a caudal-type homeobox gene. Genomics 1995;28:206–211.

43. De Vita G, Barba P, Odartchenko N, et al. Expression of homeobox-containing genes in primary and metastatic colorectal cancer. Eur J Cancer 1993;29A:887–893.

44. Frumkin A, Pillemer G, Haffner R, et al. A role for CdxA in gut closure and intestinal epithelia differentiation. Development 1994;120:253–263.

45. Reuter R. The gene serpent has homeotic properties and specifies endoderm versus ectoderm within the Drosophila gut. Development 1994;120:1123–1135.

46. Wysocka-Diller J, Aizemberg GO, Macagno ER. A novel homeobox cluster expressed in repeated structures of the midgut. Dev Biol 1995;171:439–447.

47. Staehling-Hampton K, Hoffman FM. Ectopic decapentaplegic in the Drosophila midgut alters the expression of five homeotic genes, dpp, and wingless, causing specific morphological defects. Dev Biol 1994;164:502–512.

48. Sebastio G, D'Esposito M, Montanucci M, et al. Modulated expression of human homeobox genes in differentiating intestinal cells. Biochem Biophys Res Commun 1987;146:751–756.

49. Wolgemuth DJ, Behringer RR, Mostoller MP, et al. Transgenic mice overexpressing the mouse homeobox-containing gene Hox-1.4 exhibit abnormal gut development. Nature 1989;337:464–467.

50. Pollock RA, Jay G, Bieberich CJ. Altering the boundaries of Hox 3.1 expression: Evidence for anitpodal gene regulation. Cell 1992;71:911–923.

51. Lechago J, Shah IA. The endocrine digestive system. In: Kovacs K, Asa SL, eds. Boston: Blackwell Scientific 1991;458–477.

52. Stork PJS. Signal transduction in endocrine cells (editorial). Endocr Pathol 1995;6:247–251.

53. Frucht H, Gazdar AF, Park JA, et al. Characterization of functional receptors for gastrointestinal hormones on human colon cancer cells. Cancer Res 1992;52:1114–1122.

54. Baldwin GS, Zhang QX. Measurement of gastrin and transforming growth factor a messenger RNA levels in colonic carcinoma cell lines by quantitative polymerase chain reaction. Cancer Res 1992;51:2262–2267.

55. Johnson LR, Guthrie PD. Stimulation of DNA synthesis by big and little gastrin (G-34 and G-17). Gastroenterology 1976;71:599–602.

56. Tielmans Y, Axelson J, Sundler F, et al. Serum gastrin concentration affects the self replication rate of the enterochromaffin-like cells in the rat stomach. Gut 1992;31:274–278.

57. Hirschowitz BI, Griffith J, Pellegrion D, et al. Rapid regression of enterochromaffin-like cell gastric carcinoids in pernicious anemia after antrectomy. Gastroenterology 1992;102:1409–1418.

58. Odell WD, Charters AC, Davidson WD, et al. Radioimmunoassay for human gastrin using unconjugated gastrin as an antigen. J Clin Endocrinol Metab 1968;28:1840–1842.

59. Bardram L. Progastrin in serum from Zollinger-Ellison patients: An indicator of malignancy? Gastroenterology 1990;98:1420–1426.

60. Rehfield JF, Hilsted L. Gastrin and cancer. Adv Clin Chem 1991;29:239–262.

61. Heyd J, Livni N, Gerbet D, et al. Gastrin-producing ovarian cystadenocarcinoma: Sensitivity of secretion and SMS 201-995. Gastroenterology 1989;47:464–467.

62. Van Solinge WW, Nielsen FC, Friis-Hansen L, et al. Expression but incomplete maturation of progastrin in colorectal carcinomas. Gastroenterology 1993;104:1099–1107.

63. Wank SA, Pisegna JR, de Weerth A. Cholecystokinin receptor family. Molecular cloning, structure, and functional expression in rat, guinea pig, and human. Ann NY Acad Sci 1994;713:49–66.

64. Wank SA, Harkins R, Jensen RT, et al. Purification, molecular cloning, and functional expression of the cholecystokinin receptor from rat pancreas. Proc Natl Acad Sci USA 1992;89:3125–3129.

65. Bold RJ, Ishizuka J, Townsend CM, et al. Biomolecular advances in gastrointestinal hormones. Arch Surg 1993;128:1268–1273.

66. Kleveland PM, Waldum HL. The gastrin receptor assay. Scand J Gastroenterol 1991;26:62–69.

67. Presti ME, Gardner JD. Receptor antagonists for gastrointestinal peptides. Am J Physiol 1993;264:G399–G406.

68. Narayan S, Chicone L, Singh P. Characterization of gastrin binding to colonic mucosal membranes of guinea pigs. Mol Cell Biochem 1992;112:163–171.

69. Lefkowitz RJ. G protein in medicine. N Engl J Med 1995;332:186–187.

70. Montminy MR, Gonzalez GA, Yamamoto KK. Regulation of cAMP-inducible genes by CREB. Trends Neurosci 1990;13:184–188.

71. Montminy MR, Gonzalez GA, Yamamoto KK. Characteristics of the cAMP response unit. Metabolism 1990;9:6–12.

72. Watson S, Durrant L, Elston P, et al. Inhibitory effects of the gastrin receptor antagonist (L365,260) on gastrointestinal tumor cells. Cancer 1991;68:1251–1260.

73. Ishizuka J, Martinez J, Townsend CMJ. The effect of gastrin on growth of human stomach cancer cells. Ann Surg 1992;215:528–535.

74. Townsend CMJ, Ishizuka J, Thompson JC. Gastrin trophic effects on transplanted colon cancer cells. In: Walsh JH, ed. Gastrin. New York: Raven Press, 1990;407–417.

75. Beauchamp RD, Townsend CMJ, Sing P, et al. Proglumide, a gastrin receptor antagonist, inhibits growth of colon cancer and enhances survival in mice. Ann Surg 1985;202:303–309.

76. Goyal RK, Hirano I. The enteric nervous system. N Engl J Med 1996;334:1106–1114.

77. Schuchardt A, D'Agati V, Larsson-Blomberg L, et al. Defects in the kidney and enteric nervous system of mice lacking the tyrosine kinase receptor Ret. Lancet 1994;367:380–383.

78. Romeo G, Ronchetto P, Luo Y, et al. Point mutations affecting the tyrosine kinase domain of the RET proto-oncogene in Hirschsprung's disease. Nature 1994;367:377–378.

79. Hofstra RM, Landsvater RM, Ceccherini I, et al. A mutation in the

RET proto-oncogene associated with multiple endocrine neoplasia type 2B and sporadic medullary thyroid carcinoma. Nature 1994; 367:375–376.

80. Huizinga JD, Thuneberg L, Kluppel M, et al. W/kit gene required for interstitial cells of Cajal and for intestinal pacemaker activity. Nature 1995;373:347–349.

81. Hosoda K, Hammer RE, Richardson JA, et al. Targeted and natural (piebald-lethal) mutation of endothelin-B receptor gene produce megacolon associated with spotted coat color in mice. Cell 1994;79: 1267–1276.

82. Baynash AG, Hosoda K, Glaid A, et al. Interaction of endothelin-3 with endothelin-B receptor is essential for development of epidermal melanocytes and enteric neurons. Cell, 1994;79:1277–1285.

83. Puffenberger EG, Hosoda K, Washington SS, et al. A missense mutation of the endothelin-B receptor gene in multigenic Hirschsprung's disease. Cell 1994;79:1257–1266.

84. Florio T, Rim C, Hershberger RE, et al. The somatostatin receptor SSTR1 is coupled to phosphotyrosine phosphatase activity in CHO-K1 cells. Mol Endocrinol 1994;8:1289–1297.

85. Fearon ER, Cho KR, Nigro JM, et al. Identification of a chromosome 18q gene that is altered in colorectal cancers. Science 1990;247: 49–56.

86. Horowitz JM, Yandell DW, Park SH, et al. Point mutational inactivation of the retinoblastoma antioncogene. Science 1989;243: 937–940.

87. Wiggs J, Nordenskjold M, Yandell D, et al. Prediction of the risk of hereditary retinoblastoma using DNA polymorphism within the retinoblastoma gene. N Engl J Med 1988;318:151–157.

88. Malkin D, Li FP, Strong LC, et al. Germ line p53 mutations in a familial syndrome of breast cancer, sarcomas, and other neoplasms. Science 1990;250:1233–1238.

89. Li FP, Garber JE, Friend SH, et al. Recommendations on predictive testing for germ line p53 mutations among cancer-prone individuals. J Natl Cancer Inst 1992;84:1156–1160.

90. Garber JE, Goldstein AM, Kantor AF, et al. Follow-up study of twenty-four families with Li-Fraumeni syndrome. Cancer Res 1990; 51:6094–6097.

91. Birch JM, Harvey AL, Blair V, et al. Cancer in the families of children with soft tissue sarcoma. Cancer 1990;66:2239–2248.

92. Housman D. Human DNA polymorphism. N Engl J Med 1995;332: 318–320.

93. Yandell DW, Campbell TA, Dayton SH, et al. Oncogenic point mutations in the human retinoblatoma gene: Their application to genetic counseling. N Engl J Med 1989;321:1689–1695.

94. Meltzer SJ, Mane SM, Wood PK, et al. Activation of c-Ki ras in human gastrointestinal dysplasias determined by direct sequencing of polymerase chain reaction products. Cancer Res 1990;50: 3627–3630.

95. Haggitt R. Barrett's esophagus, dysplasia, and adenocarcinoma. Hum Pathol 1994;25:983–992.

96. Jankowski J, McMenemin R, Yu C, et al. Proliferating cell nuclear antigen in oesophageal disease: Correlation with transforming growth factor alpha expression. Gut 1992;33:587–591.

97. Hong MK, Laskin WB, Herman BE, et al. Expansion of the Ki-67 proliferative compartment correlates with degree of dysplasia in Barrett's esophagus. Cancer 1995;75:423–429.

98. Nikulasson S, Andrews CWJ, Goldman H, et al. Sucrase-isomaltase expression in dysplasia associated with Barrett's esophagus and chronic gastritis. Int J Surg Pathol 1995;2:281–286.

99. Brito MJ, Filipe MI, Linehan J, et al. Association of transforming growth factor alpha (TGFα) and its precursors with malignant change in Barrett's epithelium: Biological and clinical variables. Int J Cancer 1995;60:27–32.

100. Jankowski J, McMenemin R, Hopwood D, et al. Abnormal expression of growth regulatory factors in Barrett's oesophagus. Clin Sci 1991;81:663–668.

101. Lapertosa G, Baracchini P, Fulcheri E, et al. Assessment of proliferating cell nuclear antigen expression in dysplastic intestinal type Barrett's esophagus. Pathologica 1994;86:174–179.

102. Wu GD, Beer DG, Moore JH, et al. Sucrase-isomaltase gene expression in Barrett's esophagus and adenocarcinoma. Gastroenterology 1993;105:837–844.

103. Jankowski J. Altered gene expression of growth factors during

oesophageal tumorigenesis. Gastroenterol Clin Biol 1994;18: D40–D45.

104. Schneider PM, Casson AG, Levin B, et al. Mutations of p53 in Barrett's esophagus and Barrett's cancer: A prospective study of ninety-eight cases. J Thorac Cardiovasc Surg 1996;111: 323–333.

105. Zhuang Z, Vortmeyer AO, Mark EJ, et al. Barrett's esophagus: Metaplastic cells with the loss of heterozygosity at the APC gene locus are clonal precursors to invasive adenocarcinoma. Cancer Res 1996; 56:1961–1964.

106. International Agency for Research on Cancer. Infection with Helicobacter pylori. IARC Monogr Eval Carcinog Risks Hum 1994;61: 177–240.

107. Blaser MJ, Parsonnet J. Parasitism by the "slow" bacterium Helicobacter leads to altered gastric homeostasis and neoplasia. J Clin Invest 1994;94:4–8.

108. Blaser MJ. Hypotheses on the pathogenesis and natural history of Helicobacter pylori-induced inflammation. Gastroenterology 1992; 102:720–727.

109. Hansson L-E, Nyren O, Hsing AW, et al. The risk of stomach cancer in patients with gastric or duodenal ulcer disease. N Engl J Med 1996;335:242–249.

110. Parsonnet J. Helicobacter pylori in the stomach—a paradox unmasked (editorial). N Engl J Med 1996;335:278–280.

111. Cahill RJ, Sant S, Beattie S, et al. Helicobacter pylori and increased epithelial cell proliferation: A risk factor for cancer. Eur J Gastroenterol Hepatol 1994;6:1123–1127.

112. Lynch DAF, Mapstone NP, Clarke AMT, et al. Cell proliferation in Helicobacter pylori-associated gastritis and the effect of eradication therapy. Gut 1995;36:346–350.

113. Brenes F, Ruiz B, Correa P, et al. Helicobacter pylori causes hyperproliferation of the gastric epithelium: Pre- and post-eradication indices of proliferating cell nuclear antigen. Am J Gastroenterol 1993;88:1870–1875.

114. Correa P, Fox JG. Gastric cancer and Helicobacter pylori. In: Pajares JM, Pena AS, Malfertheiner P, eds. Helicobacter pylori and gastroduodenal pathology. New York: Springer, 1993;239–243.

115. Correa P, Fox J, Fontham E, et al. Helicobacter pylori and gastric carcinoma. Cancer 1990;66:2569–2574.

116. Goldstone AR, Quirke P, Dixon MF. Helicobacter pylori infection and gastric cancer (review). J Pathol 1996;179:129–137.

117. Lee A, Fox JG, Otto G, et al. A small animal model of human Helicobacter pylori active chronic gastritis. Gastroenterology 1990; 99:1315–1323.

118. Fox JG, Li X, Cahill RJ, et al. Hypertrophic gastropathy in Helicobacter felis-infected wild-type C57BL/6 mice and p53 hemizygous transgenic mice. Gastroenterology 1996;110:155–166.

119. Sachar DB. Cancer risk in inflammatory bowel disease: Myths and metaphors. In: Riddell RH, ed. Dysplasia and cancer in colitis. New York: Elsevier Science, 1991;5–9.

120. Ekbom A, Helmick C, Zack M, et al. Ulcerative colitis and colorectal cancer. N Engl J Med 1990;323:1228–1233.

121. Brentnall TA, Haggitt RC, Rabinovitch PS, et al. Risk and natural history of colonic neoplasia in patients with primary sclerosing cholangitis and ulcerative colitis. Gastroenterology 1996;110: 331–338.

122. Levin B. Ulcerative colitis and colon cancer: Biology and surveillance. J Cell Biochem 1992;(Supplement) 16G:47–50.

123. Riddell RH, Goldman H, Ransohoff DF, et al. Dysplasia in inflammatory bowel disease: Standardized classification with provisional clinical applications. Hum Pathol 1983;14:931–968.

124. Burmer GC, Rabinovitch PS, Haggitt RC, et al. Neoplastic progression in ulcerative colitis: Histology, DNA content, and loss of a p53 allele. Gastroenterology 1992;103:1602–1610.

125. Burmer GC, Levine DS, Kulander BG, et al. c-Ki-ras mutations in chronic ulcerative colitis and sporadic colon carcinoma. Gastroenterology 1990;99:416–420.

126. Burmer GC, Loeb LA. Mutations in the c-Ki-ras oncogene during progressive stages of human colon carcinoma. Proc Natl Acad Sci USA 1989;86:2403–2407.

127. Vogelstein B, Fearon ER, Hamilton SR, et al. Genetic alterations during colorectal tumor development. N Engl J Med 1988; 319:525–532.

128. Brentnall TA, Crispin DA, Ravinovitch PS, et al. Mutations in the p53 gene: An early marker of neoplastic progression in ulcerative colitis. Gastroenterology 1994;107:369–378.

129. Kastrinakis WV, Ramchurren N, Rieger KM, et al. Increased incidence of p53 mutations is associated with hepatic metastases in colorectal neoplastic progression. Oncogene 1995;11:647–652.

130. Andrews CW, O'Hara CJ, Goldman H, et al. Sucrase-isomaltase expression in chronic ulcerative colitis and dysplasia. Hum Pathol 1992;23:774–779.

131. Cartwright CA, Coad CA, Egbert BM. Elevated c-src tyrosine kinase activity in premalignant epithelia of ulcerative colitis. J Clin Invest 1994;93:509–515.

132. D'Emilia JC, Mathey-Prevot B, Jaros K, et al. Preneoplastic lesions induced by myc and src oncogenes in a heterotopic rat colon. Oncogene 1991;6:303–309.

133. Mombaerts P, Mizoguchi E, Grusby MJ, et al. Spontaneous development of inflammatory bowel disease in T cell receptor mutant mice. Cell 1993;75:275–282.

134. Quinlan RM, Recht A. Cancer of the esophagus. In: Cancer manual. Osteen RT, ed. Boston: American Cancer Society, 1996;356–364.

135. Stemmermann G, Heffelfinger SC, Noffsinger A, et al. The molecular biology of esophageal and gastric cancer and their precursors: Oncogenes, tumor suppressor genes, and growth factors. Hum Pathol 1994;25:968–981.

136. Huang Y, Meltzer SJ, Yin J, et al. Altered messenger RNA and unique mutational profiles of p53 and Rb in human esophageal carcinomas. Cancer Res 1993;53:1889–1894.

137. Liu Q, Yan YX, McClure M, et al. MTS-1 (CDKN2) tumor suppressor gene deletions are a frequent event in esophagus squamous cell cancer and pancreatic adenocarcinoma cell lines. Oncogene 1995;10:619–622.

138. Nakagawa H, Zukerberg L, Togawa K, et al. Human cyclin D1 oncogene and esophageal squamous cell carcinoma. Cancer 1995;76:541–549.

139. Chang F, Syrjänen S, Shen Q, et al. Screening for human papillomavirus infections in esophageal squamous cell carcinomas by in situ hybridization. Cancer 1993;72:2525–2530.

140. Mayer RJ, Beazley RM, DeLaney TF. Cancer of the stomach. In: Cancer manual. Osteen RT, ed. Boston: American Cancer Society, 1996;365–375.

141. Correa P. Helicobacter pylori and gastric carcinogenesis. Am J Surg Pathol 1995;19:S37–S43.

142. Shino Y, Watanabe A, Yamada Y, et al. Clinicopathologic evaluation of immunohistochemical E-cadherin expression in human gastric carcinomas. Cancer 1995;76:2193–2201.

143. Mulder JW, Kruyt PM, Sewnath M, et al. Colorectal cancer prognosis and expression of exon-v6-containing CD44 proteins. Lancet 1994;344:1470–1472.

144. Washington K, Gottfried MR, Telen MJ. Expression of the cell adhesion molecule CD44 in gastric adenocarcinomas. Hum Pathol 1994;25:1043–1049.

145. Deans G, Parks T, Rowlands B, et al. Prognostic factors in colorectal cancer. Br J Surg 1992;79:608–613.

146. Anonymous. Adjuvant therapy for patients with colon and rectal cancers. Consensus statement. JAMA 1990;8:1–25.

147. Bishop JM. The molecular genetics of cancer. Science 1987;235:305–311.

148. Bos JL. The Ras gene family and human carcinogenesis. Mutat Res 1988;195:255–271.

149. Ruderman J. MAP kinase and the activation of quiescent cells. Curr Opin Cell Biol 1993;5:207–213.

150. Alessi DR, Smith R, Keyse SM. The human CL100 gene encodes a Tyr/Thr-protein phosphatase which potently and specifically inactivates MAP kinase and suppresses its activation by oncogenic ras in Xenopus oocyte extracts. Oncogene 1993;8:2015–2020.

151. Galaktionov K, Lee AK, Eckstein J, et al. Cdc25 phophatases as potential human oncogenes. Science 1995;269:1575–1577.

152. Kumagai A, Dunphy WG. Regulation of the cdc25 protein during the cell cycle in Xenopus extracts. Cell 1992;70:139–151.

153. Guan KL, Hakes DJ, Wang Y, et al. A yeast protein phosphatase related to the vaccina virus VH1 phosphatase is induced by nitrogen starvation. Proc Natl Acad Sci USA 1992;89:12175–12179.

154. Kwak SP, Hakes DJ, Martell KJ, et al. Isolation and characterization of a human dual specificity protein tyrosine phosphatase gene. J Biol Chem 1994;5:3596–3604.

155. Keyse SM, Emslie EA. Oxidative stress and heat shock induce a human gene encoding a protein-tyrosine phosphatase. Nature 1992;359:644–647.

156. Sun H, Cherles CH, Lau LF, et al. MKP-1 (3CH134), an immediate early gene product, is a dual specificity phosphatase that dephosphorylates MAP kinase in vivo. Cell 1993;75:487–493.

157. Loda M, Capodieci P, Mishra R, et al. Expression of mitogen-activated protein kinase phosphatase-1 in the early phases of human epithelial carcinogenesis. Am J Pathol 1996;149:1553–1564.

158. Nigro JM, Baker SJ, Preisinger AC, et al. Mutations in the p53 gene occur in diverse human tumour types. Nature 1989;342:705–708.

159. Greenblatt M, Bennett W, Hollstein M, et al. Mutations in the p53 tumor suppressor gene: Clues to cancer etiology and molecular pathogenesis. Cancer Res 1994;54:4855–4878.

160. Waldman T, Lengauer C, Kinzler KW, et al. Uncoupling of S phase and mitosis induced by anticancer agents in cells lacking p21. Nature 1996;381:713–716.

161. Bosari S, Viale G. The clinical significance of p53 aberrations in human tumors. Virchows Arch 1996;427:229–241.

162. Rodrigues NR, Rowan A, Smith MEF, et al. p53 mutations in colorectal cancer. Proc Natl Acad Sci USA 1990;87:7555–7559.

163. Bosari S, Viale G, Roncalli M, et al. p53 gene mutations, p53 protein accumulation and compartmentalization in colorectal adenocarcinoma. Am J Pathol 1995;147:790–798.

164. Scott N, Quirke P. Molecular biology of colorectal neoplasia. Gut 1993;34:289–292.

165. Bertorelle R, Esposito G, Del Mistro A, et al. Association of p53 gene and protein alterations with metastases in colorectal cancer. Am J Surg Pathol 1995;19:463–471.

166. Donehower LA, Garvey M, Slagle BL. Mice deficient for p53 are developmentally normal but susceptible to spontaneous tumours. Nature 1992;356:215–221.

167. Harvey M, McArthur MJ, Montgomery CA, et al. Spontaneous and carcinogen-induced tumorigenesis in p53-deficient mice. Nat Genet 1993;5:225–229.

168. Sands A, Donehower LA, Bradley A. Gene-targeting and the p53 tumor-suppressor gene. Mutat Res 1994;307:557–572.

169. Clarke AR, Gledhill S, Hooper ML, et al. p53 dependence of early apoptotic and proliferative responses within the mouse intestinal epithelium following gamma-irradiation. Oncogene 1994;9:1767–1773.

170. Jen J, Kim H, Piantadosi S, et al. Allelic loss of chromosome 18q and prognosis in colorectal cancer. N Engl J Med 1994;331:213–221.

171. Keino-Masu K, Masu M, Hinck L, et al. Deleted in colorectal cancer (DCC) encodes a netrin receptor. Cell 1996;87:175–185.

172. Hahn SA, Schutte M, Hoque AT, et al. DPC4, a candidate tumor suppressor gene at human chromosome 18q21.1. Science 1996;271:350–353.

173. Shibata D, Reale MA, Lavin P, et al. Loss of DCC expression and prognosis in colorectal cancer. N Engl J Med 1996;335:1727–1732.

174. Lees E. Cyclin-dependent kinase regulation. Curr Opin Cell Biol 1995;7:773–780.

175. Coleman T, Dunphy W. Cdc2 regulatory factors. Curr Opin Cell Biol 1994;6:877–882.

176. Sherr C, Roberts J. Inhibitors of mammalian G1 cyclin-dependent kinases. Genes Dev 1995;9:1149–1163.

177. Gu Y, Turck C, Morgan D. Inhibition of Cdk2 activity in vivo by an associated 20K regulatory subunit. Nature 1993;366:707–710.

178. Harper JW, Adami GR, Wei N, et al. The p21 Cdk-interacting protein Cip1 is a potent inhibitor of G1 cyclin-dependent kinases. Cell 1993;75:805–816.

179. El-Deiry WS, Tokino T, Velculescu VE, et al. WAF1, a potential mediator of p53 tumor suppression. Cell 1993;75:817–825.

180. Xiong Y, Hannon G, Zhang H, et al. p21 is a universal inhibitor of the cyclin kinases. Nature 1993;366:701–704.

181. Noda A, Ning Y, Venable S, et al. Cloning of senescent cell-derived inhibitors of DNA synthesis using an expression screen. Exp Cell Res 1994;211:90–98.
182. Polyak K, Lee M, Erdjement-Bromage H, et al. Cloning of p27kip1, a cyclin-dependent kinase inhibitor and a potential mediator of extracellular antimitogenic signals. Cell 1994;79:59–66.
183. Toyoshima H, Hunter T. p27, a novel inhibitor of G1-cyclin-cdk protein kinase activity, is related to p21. Cell 1994;78:67–74.
184. Matsuoka S, Edwards M, Bai C, et al. p57KIP2, a struturally distinct member of the p21CIP1 Cdk inhibitor family is a candidate tumor suppressor gene. Genes Dev 1995;9:650–662.
185. Lee M, Reynisdottir I, Massague J. Cloning of p57KIP2, cyclin-dependent kinase inhibitor with unique domain structure and tissue distribution. Genes Dev 1995;9:639–649.
186. Serrano M, Gòmez-Lahoz E, DePinho R, et al. Inhibition of Ras-induced proliferation and cellular transformation by p16 Ink4. Science 1995;267:249–252.
187. Quelle D, Ashmun R, Hannon G, et al. Cloning and characterization of murine p16INK4a and p15INK4b genes. Oncogene 1995;11:635–643.
188. Hannon GJ, Beach D. p15INK4B is a potential effector of TGF-ß-induced cell cycle arrest. Nature 1994;371:257–261.
189. Jen J, Harper W, Bigner S, et al. Deletion of p16 and p15 genes in brain tumors. Cancer Res 1994;54:6353–6358.
190. Guan K, Jenkins C, Nichols M, et al. Growth suppression by p18, a p16Ink4/Mts1- and Mts2-related Cdk6 inhibitor, correlates with wild-type pRb function. Genes Dev 1994;8:2939–2952.
191. Chan F, Zhang J, Cheng L, et al. Identification of human and mouse p19, a novel CDK4 and CDK6 inhibitor with homology to p16ink4. Mol Cell Biol 1995;15:2682–2688.
192. Hirai H, Roussel M, Kato J, et al. Novel INK4 proteins, p19 and p18, are specific inhibitors of the cyclin D-dependent kinases CDK4 and CDK6. Mol Cell Biol 1995;15:2672–2681.
193. Guan K, Jenkins C, Li Y, et al. Molecular cloning of the CDK6 inhibitor p20 and demonstration of the opposite effects of cyclin on the two CDK inhibitor families' binding to CDKs. Mol Biol Cell 1996;7:57–70.
194. Sheaff RJ, Roberts JM. Lesson in p16 from phylum Falconium. Curr Biol 1995;5:28–31.
195. Dulic V, Kaufmann W, Wilson S, et al. p53-dependent inhibition of cyclin-dependent kinase activities in human fibroblasts during radiation-induced G1 arrest. Cell 1994;76:1013–1023.
196. El-Deiry W, Tokino T, Waldman T, et al. Topological control of p21WAF1/CIP1 expression in normal and neoplastic tissues. Cancer Res 1995;55:2910–2919.
197. Kawamat AN, Morosetti R, Miller C, et al. Molecular analysis of the cyclin-dependent kinase inhibitor gene p27/kip1 in human malignancies. Cancer Res 1995;55:2266–2269.
198. Ponce-Castañeda V, Lee M, Latres E, et al. p27Kip1: Chromosomal mapping to 12p12-12p13.1 and absence of mutations in human tumors. Cancer Res 1995;55:1211–1214.
199. Pietenpol J, Bohlander S, Sato Y, et al. Assignment of the human p27Kip1 gene to 12p13 and its analysis in leukemias. Cancer Res 1995;55:1206–1210.
200. Pagano M, Tam SW, Theodoras AM, et al. Role of the ubiquitin-proteasome pathway in regulating abundance of the cyclin-dependent kinase inhibitor p27. Science 1995;269:682–685.
201. Loda M, Cukor B, Tam SW, et al. Increased proteasome-dependent degradation of the cyclin-dependent kinase inhibitor p27 in aggressive colorectal carcinomas. Nat Med 1997;3:231–234.
202. Gold LI, Korc M. Expression of transforming growth factor β1,2, and 3 mRNA and protein in human cancers. Digestive Surgery 1994;11:150–156.
203. Massague J. TGFb signaling: Receptors, transducers and MAD proteins. Cell 1996;85:947–950.
204. Glick AB, Weinberg WC, Wu IH, et al. Transforming growth factor β1 suppresses genomic instability independent of a G1 arrest, p53, and Rb. Cancer Res 1996;56:3645–3650.
205. Barnard JA, Warwick GJ, Gold LI. Localization of transforming growth factor-β isoforms in the normal murine small intestine and colon. Gastroenterology 1993;105:67–73.
206. Eppert K, Scherer SW, Ozcelik H, et al. MADR2 maps to 18q21 and encodes a TGFβ-regulated MAD-related protein that is functionally mutated in colorectal carcinomas. Cell 1996;86:543–552.
207. Garrigue-Antar L, Souza RF, Vellucci VF, et al. Loss of transforming growth factor β type II receptor gene expression in primary human esophageal cancer. Lab Invest 1996;75:263–272.
208. Jessup JM, Lavin PT, Andrews CWJ, et al. Sucrase-isomaltase is an independent prognostic marker for colorectal carcinoma. Dis Colon Rectum 1995;38:1257–1264.
209. Andrews CW, Jessup JM, Goldman H, et al. Localization of tumor-associated glycoprotein DF3 in normal, inflammatory, and neoplastic lesions of the colon. Cancer 1993;72:3185–3190.
210. Cox EC. Bacterial mutator genes and the control of spontaneous mutations. Annu Rev Genet 1976;10:135.
211. Leach FS, Nicolaides NC, Papadopoulos N, et al. Mutations of mut S homolog in hereditary nonpolyposis colorectal cancer. Cell 1993;75:1215–1225.
212. Fishel R, Lescoe MK, Rao MR, et al. The human mutator homolog MSH2 and its association with hereditary nonpolyposis colon cancer. Cell 1993;75:1027–1038.
213. Liu B, Parsons RE, Hamilton SR, et al. hMSH2 mutations in hereditary nonpolyposis colorectal cancer kindreds. Cancer Res 1994;54:4590–4594.
214. Aaltonen LA, Peltomaki P, Leach FS, et al. Clues to the pathogenesis of familial colorectal cancer. Science 1993;260:812–816.
215. de Wind N, Dekker M, Berns A, et al. Inactivation of the mouse MSH 2 gene results in mismatch repair deficiency, methylation tolerance, hyperrecombination, and predisposition to cancer. Cell 1995;82:321–330.
216. Peltomaki P, Aaltonen LA, Sistonen P, et al. Genetic mapping of a locus predisposing to human colorectal cancer. Science 1993;260:810–819.
217. Kolodner RD. Mismatch repair: Mechanisms and relationship to cancer susceptibility. Trends Biochem 20:397–402.
218. Wijnen J, Vasen H, Kahn PN, et al. Seven new mutations in hMSH2, an HNPCC gene, identified by denaturing gradient gel electrophoresis. Am J Hum Genet 56:1060–1066.
219. Lothe RA, Peltomaki P, Meling GI, et al. Genomic instability in colorectal cancer: Relationship to clinicopathological variables and family history. Cancer Res 1993;53:5849–5852.
220. Ionov, Y, Peinado AMS, Shibata D, et al. Ubiquitous somatic mutations in simple repeated sequences reveal a new mechanism for colonic carcinogenesis. Nature 1993;363:558–561.
221. Kane MF, Loda M, Gaida GM, et al. Methylation of the hMLH1 promoter correlates with lack of expression of hMLH1 in sporadic colon tumors and mismatch repair defective human tumor cell lines. Cancer Res 1997;57:808–811.
222. Reitmar AH, Redston M, Cai JC, et al. Spontaneous intestinal carcinomas and skin neoplasms in MSH2-deficient mice. Cancer Res 1996;56:3842–3849.
223. Kinzler KW, Vogelstein B. Lessons from hereditary colorectal cancer. Cell 1996;87:159–170.
224. Baba S, Ando H, Nakamura Y. Identification of germ line mutation of APC gene in possible carriers of familial adenomatous polyposis (FAP). Anticancer Res 1994;14:2189–2192.
225. Morin PJ, Vogelstein B. Apoptosis and APC in colorectal tumorigenesis. Proc Natl Acad Sci USA 1996;93:7950–7954.
226. Eckert WA, Jung C, Wolff G. Presymptomatic diagnosis in families with adenomatous polyposis using highly polymorphic dinucleotide CA repeat markers flanking the APC gene. J Med Genet 1994;31:442–447.
227. Ando H, Miyoshi Y, Nagase H, et al. Detection of 12 germ-line mutations in the adenomatous polyposis coli gene by polymerase chain reaction. Gastroenterology 1993;104:989–993.
228. Tops CMJ, Wijnen JT, Griffioen G, et al. Presymptomatic diagnosis of familial adenomatous polyposis by bridging DNA markers. Lancet 1989;2:1361–1363.
229. Park JG, Han HJ, Kang MS, et al. Presymptomatic diagnosis of familial adenomatous polyposis coli. Dis Colon Rectum 1994;37:700–707.
230. Dunlop MG, Wyllie AH, Steel CM, et al. Linked DNA markers for presymptomatic diagnosis of familial adenomatous polyposis. Lancet 1991;337:313–316.

231. Grobbelaar JJ, Oosthuizen CJJ, Madden MV, et al. The use of DNA markers in the pre-clinical diagnosis of familial adenomatous polyposis in families in South Africa. S Afr Med J 1995;85: 269–271.

232. Moser AR, Pitot HC, Dove WF. A dominant mutation that predisposes to multiple intestinal neoplasia in the mouse. Science 1990; 247:322–324.

233. Su L-K, Kinzler KW, Vogelstein B, et al. Intestinal neoplasia caused by a mutation in the murine homolog of the APC gene. Science 1992;256:668–670.

234. Dietrich WF, Lander ES, Smith JS, et al. Genetic identification of mom-1, a major modifier locus affecting min-induced intestinal neoplasia in the mouse. Cell 1993;75:631–639.

235. Kennedy AR, Beazer-Barclay Y, Kinzler KW, et al. Suppression of carcinogenesis in the intestines of min mice by the soybean-derived Bowman-Birk inhibitor. Cancer Res 1996;56:679–682.

236. Korsmeyer ST, Waldmann TA. Immunoglobulin genes: Rearrangement and translocation in human lymphoid malignancy. J Clin Immunol 1984;4:1–11.

237. O'Connor NT, Wainscoat JS, Weatherall DJ, et al. Rearrangement of the T cell receptor beta-chain gene in the diagnosis of lymphoproliferative disorders. Lancet 1985;1:1295–1297.

238. Southern EM. Detection of specific sequences among DNA fragments separated by gel electrophoresis. J Mol Biol 1975;98:503.

239. Isaacson PG. Recent advances in the biology of lymphomas. Eur J Cancer 1991;27:795–802.

240. Cunningham D, Rosin RD, Baron JH, et al. Polymerase chain reaction for detection of dissemination in gastric lymphoma. Lancet 1989;1:695–697.

241. Diss TC, Peng H, Wotherspoon AC, et al. Brief report: A single neoplastic clone in sequential biopsy specimens from a patient with primary gastric-mucosa-associated lymphoid-tissue lymphoma and Sjogren's syndrome. N Engl J Med 1993;329:172–175.

242. Freeman C, Berg JW, Cutler SJ. Occurrence and prognosis of extranodal lymphomas. Cancer 1972;29:252–260.

243. Isaacson PG, Wright DH. Extranodal malignant lymphoma arising from mucosa-associated lymphoid tissue. Cancer 1984;53:2515–2524.

244. Isaacson PG, Spencer J. Malignant lymphoma of mucosa-associated lymphoid tissue. Histopathology 1987;11:445–462.

245. Addis BJ, Hyjek E, Isaacson PG. Primary pulmonary lymphoma. A re-appraisal of its histogenesis and its relationship to pseudolymphoma and interstitial pneumonia. Histopathology 1988; 13:1–17.

246. Spencer J, Diss TC, Isaacson PG. Primary B cell gastric lymphoma. A genotypic analysis. Am J Pathol 1989;135:557–564.

247. Isaacson PG. Lymphomas of mucosa-associated lymphoid tissue (MALT). Histopathology 1990;16:617–619.

248. Wotherspoon AC, Pan L, Diss TC, et al. A genotypic study of low grade B-cell lymphomas, including lymphomas of mucosa associated lymphoid tissue (MALT). J Pathol 1990;162:135–140.

249. Van Krieken JH, Raffeld M, Raghoebier S, et al. Molecular genetics of gastrointestinal non-Hodgkin's lymphomas: Unusual prevalence and pattern of c-myc rearrangements in aggressive lymphomas. Blood 1990;76:797–800.

250. Du M, Peng H, Singh N, et al. The accumulation of p53 abnormalities is associated with progression of mucosa-associated lymphoid tissue lymphoma. Blood 1995;86:4587–4593.

251. Peng H, Chen G, Du M, et al. Replication error phenotype and p53 gene mutation in lymphomas of mucosa-associated lymphoid tissue. Am J Pathol 1996;148:643–648.

252. Sander CA, Yano T, Clark HM, et al. p53 mutation is associated with progression in follicular lymphomas. Blood 1993;82:1994–2004.

253. Gaidano G, Ballerini P, Gong JZ, et al. p53 mutation in human lymphoid malignancies associated with Burkitt lymphoma and chronic lymphocytic leukaemia. Proc Natl Acad Sci USA 1991;88: 5413–5418.

254. Baldini L, Fracchiolla NS, Cro LM, et al. Frequent p53 gene involvement in splenic B-cell leukaemia/lymphomas of possible marginal zone origin. Blood 1994;84:270–278.

255. Isaacson PG, Matutes E, Burke M, et al. The histopathology of splenic lymphoma with villous lymphocytes. Blood 1994;84:3828–3834.

256. Zetter BR. The cellular basis of site-specific tumor metastasis. N Engl J Med 1990;322:605–612.

257. Tarin D, Matsumura Y. Recent advances in the study of tumour invasion and metastasis. J Clin Pathol 1994;47:385–390.

258. Juliano RL, Varner JA. Adhesions molecules in cancer: The role of integrins. Curr Opin Cell Biol 1993;5:812–818.

259. Hynes RO. Integrins: Versatility, modulation, and signaling in cell adhesion. Cell 1992;69:11–25.

260. Tsukita S, Itoh A, Nagafuchi A, et al. Submembranous junctional pacque proteins include potential tumor suppressor molecules. J Cell Biol 1993;123:1049–1053.

261. Birchmeir W, Weidner KM, Hulsken J, et al. Molecular mechanisms leading to cell junction (cadherin) deficiencies in invasive carcinomas. Semin Cancer Biol 1993;4:231–239.

262. Chao C, Lotz MM, Clarke AC, et al. A function for the integrin $\alpha 6$ $\beta 4$ in the invasive properties of colorectal carcinoma cells. Cancer Res 1996;56:4811–4819.

263. Pignatelli M. E-cadherin: A biological marker of tumor differentiation (editorial). J Pathol 1993;171:81–82.

264. Kantor JD, McCormick B, Steeg PS, et al. Inhibition of cell motility after nm23 transfection of human and murine cells. Cancer Res 1993;53:1971–1973.

265. Biggs J, Hersperger E, Steeg PS, et al. A Drosophila gene that is homologous to a mammalian gene associated with tumor metastasis codes for a nucleoside diphosphate kinase. Cell 1990;63: 933–940.

266. Leone A, Seeger RC, Hong CM, et al. Evidence for nm23 RNA overexpression, DNA amplification, and mutation in aggressive childhood neuroblastomas. Oncogene 1993;8:855–865.

267. Wang Patel U, Hgosh L, Bannerjee S. Mutation in the nm23 gene associated with metastasis in colorectal cancer. Cancer Res 1993;53: 717–720.

268. Gangopadhyay A, Bajenova O, Kelly TM, et al. Carcinoembryonic antigen induces cytokine expression in Kupffer cells: Implications for hepatic metastases from colorectal cancer. Cancer Res 1996;56: 4805–4810.

269. Crystal RG. Transfer of genes to humans: Early lessons and obstacles to success. Science 1995;270:404–410.

270. Blaese RM, Culver KW, Miller AD, et al. T lymphocyte-directed gene therapy for ADA-SCID: Initial trial results after four years. Science 1995;270:475–480.

271. Bordignon C, Notarangelo LD, Nobili N, et al. Gene therapy in peripheral blood lymphocytes and bone marrow for ADA-immunodeficient patients. Science 1995;270:470–475.

272. Vieweg J, Boczkowski D, Robertson KM, et al. Efficient gene transfer with adeno-associated virus-based plasmids complexed to cationic liposomes for gene therapy of human prostate cancer. Cancer Res 1995;55:2366–2372.

273. Askari FK, McDonnell WM. Antisense-oligonucleotide therapy. N Engl J Med 1996;334:316–318.

274. McDonnell WM, Askari FK. DNA vaccines (review). N Engl J Med 1996;334:42–45.

275. Gilboa E. Immunotherapy of cancer with genetically modified tumor vaccines (review). Semin Oncol 1996;23:101–107.

276. Sun WH, Kreisle BA, Phillips AW, et al. In vivo and in vitro characteristics of interleukin 6-transfected B16 melanoma cells. Cancer Res 1992;52:5412–5415.

277. Tepper RI, Pattengale PK, Leder P. Murine interleukin-4 displays potent anti-tumor activity in vivo. Cell 1989;57:503–512.

278. Fearon ER, Pardoll DM, Itaya T, et al. Interleukin-2 production by tumor cells bypasses T-helper function in the generation of an antitumor response. Cell 1990;60:397–403.

279. Vieweg J, Gilboa E. Gene therapy approaches in urologic oncology (review). Surg Clin North Am 1995;4:203–218.

280. Colombo MP, Ferrari G, Stoppacciaro A, et al. Granulocyte colony-stimulating factor gene transfer suppresses tumorigenicity of a murine adenocarcinoma in vivo. J Exp Med 1991;173:889–897.

281. Asher AL, Mule JJ, Kasid A, et al. Murine tumor cells transduced with the gene for tumor necrosis factor-alpha. Evidence for paracrine immune effects of tumor necrosis factor against tumors. J Immunol 1991;146:3227–3234.

282. Gansbacher B, Bannerji R, Daniels B, et al. Retroviral vector-

mediated gamma-interferon transfer into tumor cells generates potent and long lasting antitumor immunity. Cancer Res 1990;50: 7820–7825.

283. Fearon ER, Itaya T, Hunt B, et al. Induction in a murine tumor of immunogenic tumor variants by transfection with a foreign gene. Cancer Res 1988;48:2975–2980.

284. Wallich R, Bulbuc N, Hammerling GJ, et al. Abrogation of metastatic properties of tumour cells by de novo expression of H-2K antigens following H-2 gene transfection. Nature 1985;315: 301–305.

285. Hui K, Grosveld F, Festenstein H. Rejection of transplantable AKR leukaemia cells following MHC DNA-mediated cell transformation. Nature 1984;311:750–752.

286. Porgador A, Snyder D, Gilboa E. Induction of antitumor immunity using bone-marrow generated dendritic cells. J Immunol 1996;156: 2918–2926.

287. Porgador A, Gilboa E. Bone-marrow generated dendritic cells pulsed with a class I-restricted peptide are potent inducers of cytotoxic T lymphocytes. J Exp Med 1995;182:255–260.

288. Baker SJ, Markowitz S, Fearon ER, et al. Suppression of human colorectal carcinoma cell growth by wild-type p53. Science 1990; 249:912–915.

289. Tanaka K, Oshimura M, Kikuchi R, et al. Suppression of tumorigenicity in human colon carcinoma cells by introduction of normal chromosome 5 or 18. Nature 1991;349:340–342.

290. Primus FJ, Finch MD, Masci AM, et al. Self-reactive antibody expression by human carcinoma cells engineered with monoclonal antibody genes. Cancer Res 1993;53:3355–3361.

291. Isobe K, Fan ZH, Emi N, et al. Gene transfer of TNF receptor for treatment of cancer by TNF. Biochem Biophys Res Commun 1994;202:1538–1542.

292. Brenner MK, Rill DR, Moen RC, et al. Gene-marking to trace origin of relapse after autologous bone marrow transplantation. Lancet 1993;341:85–86.

293. Dewanjee MK, Ghafouripour AK, Kapadvanjwala M, et al. Noninvasive imaging of c-myc oncogene messenger RNA with Indium-111-antisense probes in a mammary tumor-bearing mouse model. J Nucl Med 1994;35:1054–1063.

9

CELL PROLIFERATION AND KINETICS OF THE GASTROINTESTINAL EPITHELIUM

Guido Biasco, Gian Maria Paganelli, Mario Miglioli, and Luigi Barbara

METHODS TO STUDY CELL PROLIFERATION KINETICS
EPITHELIAL PROLIFERATION IN THE NORMAL GASTROINTESTINAL TRACT
FACTORS INFLUENCING CELL PROLIFERATION IN THE GASTROINTESTINAL TRACT
CELL PROLIFERATION IN PATHOLOGIC CONDITIONS
INFLAMMATION AND ACUTE MUCOSAL DAMAGE
PRECANCER AND CANCER

CLINICAL APPLICATIONS OF GASTROINTESTINAL CELL KINETICS
CELL PROLIFERATION OF THE GASTRIC MUCOSA AS A MARKER OF CYTOPROTECTION
BIOLOGY OF PRECANCEROUS LESIONS
IDENTIFICATION OF INDIVIDUALS AT HIGH RISK OF CANCER DEVELOPMENT
INTERMEDIATE ENDPOINT IN PILOT CHEMOPREVENTION STUDIES
INDICATION OF ADJUVANT TREATMENTS
CHRONOMODULATED CHEMOTHERAPY

The epithelium of the gastrointestinal mucosa undergoes a continuous renewal. In normal conditions, a huge number of cells is exfoliated daily throughout the lumen of the alimentary tract, from the mouth to the anus. These cells are immediately replaced by new cells from the stem cell compartment. The equilibrium between cell production and cell loss is essential for mucosal integrity. A defect in cell production leads to the development of mucosal erosions or ulcers, whereas mucosal hyperplasia and polyp formation is the result of an excess in newborn cells. The disequilibrium between cell production and loss is the pathologic event at the basis of morphologic and functional abnormalities of the gastrointestinal mucosa. In a biologic system with a high turnover rate, a defect in cell differentiation or the loss of the control of cell proliferation is associated with either weakening of mucosal defense mechanisms or enhancement of pre-existing genetic abnormalities that can precede cancer development. The latter issue is of outstanding importance, because proliferative abnormalities were identified in several diseases and conditions with an enhanced risk of gastrointestinal cancer. For instance, epithelial hyperproliferation can be the first phenotypical expression of the carcinogenic process in the gastrointestinal mucosa.

METHODS TO STUDY CELL PROLIFERATION KINETICS

In the study of cell kinetics in the gastrointestinal tract, it is not always easy to compare data obtained by different investigators, because study protocols and methods are not the same and are designed to explore different aspects of cell proliferation. The cell proliferation cycle is divided into four phases: premitotic rest (G1), DNA synthesis (S), postmitotic rest (G2), and mitosis (M). Moreover, cells in one pool theoretically are able to proliferate but are temporarily out of the proliferative cycle (G0). Whenever the request of newborn cells increases, two mechanisms are activated: the shortening of G1 and the recruitment of cells from G0 (1). The cell proliferation pattern can be studied by using several techniques, each of which explores different aspects of cell and tissue kinetics (Table 9.1).

The information obtained by one technique or another must be considered complementary. Several studies are carried out by means of in vitro uptake of DNA precursors on mucosal specimens, which also allows the histologic identification of proliferating (labeled) cells. The most widely used are the techniques of uptake of tritiated thymidine (^{3}H-dThd) or bromodeoxyuridine (BrdU), followed by autoradiography or immunochemistry, respectively. In these methods, the main kinetic parameter is the percentage of proliferating cells on the total number of epithelial cells, defined as the labeling index (LI). The LI represents the rate of cells that are in the S phase during contact with the DNA precursor. Studies involving humans are usually carried out in vitro by incubating biopsy specimens in culture media containing the DNA precursor, because of the possibly hazardous in vivo use of these compounds. The need for incubation procedures limits the expansion of these assays to many laboratories.

This limit is overcome by the immunohistochemical assays of proliferation-associated antigens, which do not require tissue incubation. The historically first antigen of this series is that recognized by the antibody Ki-67 on frozen tissue specimens. This antigen, however, is expressed by cells in every phase of the proliferative cycle (6); therefore, it offers only vague information on cell re-

TABLE

9 . 1   Widely Used Methods to Study Cell Kinetics in the Gastrointestinal Tract

Method	Technique	Target	Reference
Mitoses count	Histology	M phase	2
Metaphase arrest	Histology	Cell production rate	3
Tritiated thymidine ([³H]dThd) labeling	Autoradiography	S phase	4
Bromodeoxyuridine (BrdU) labeling	Immunohistochemistry	S phase	5
Ki-67 labeling	Immunohistochemistry	G_1 to M phases	6
Proliferating cell nuclear antigen (PCNA) expression	Immunohistochemistry	Mainly S phase (late G_1 to early G_2 phases)	7
Flow ctyometry	Automatic cell sorting and computer analysis	DNA content; cell cycle phases by extrapolation	8
Ornithine decarboxylase (ODC) activity	Biochemistry	Polyamine activity	9
Nuclear organizer region stain (Ag-NOR)	Histochemistry	rRNA synthesis	10

newal pattern. More recently, monoclonal antibodies were raised against the proliferating cell nuclear antigen (PCNA), an auxiliary protein of DNA polymerase δ that is maximally expressed throughout S phase, from late G1 to early G2. These antibodies can be used in fixed and paraffin-embedded specimens (11–13).

All of the abovementioned techniques are based on proliferating cell count on histologic specimens, which is a tedious and time-consuming procedure. Automation in cell kinetics measurements is preferred by many investigators. Multiparametric flow cytometry allows analysis of the DNA content and ploidy of up to thousands of cells per second. An estimate of the percentage of cells in S phase is also possible by means of computer algorithms (14). Finally, another widely used technique is the assay of ornithine decarboxylase (ODC) activity in the mucosa. ODC is the rate-limiting enzyme in the polyamine synthesis and is expressed in large amounts by proliferating cells. This technique gives results comparable to those obtained by BrdU immunostaining (15).

EPITHELIAL PROLIFERATION IN THE NORMAL GASTROINTESTINAL TRACT

The epithelial stem cell compartment is located differently in the different sites of the gastrointestinal tract. The mucosa of the mouth, pharynx, and esophagus consists of squamous, nonkeratinized epithelium. Proliferating cells are located in a single or few layers of cells on the basal membrane, covered by two to four layers of spinous cells (Fig. 9.1). Cells differentiate and migrate upward through an intermediate layer (large spinous cells) and a superficial layer (flattened cells), where they are extruded from the surface (16).

The mucosa of the stomach is formed by cylindric elements and more specialized cells. The epithelia of the gastric body and fundus and antrum are identical; nevertheless, deeper glandular structures are quite different. The glands of the gastric body and fundus consist mainly of parietal (HCl-secreting) and zymogen (pepsinogen-secreting) cells; enterochromaffin-like (ECL-like) cells are present in the deepest zone of the mucosa. Cells that form

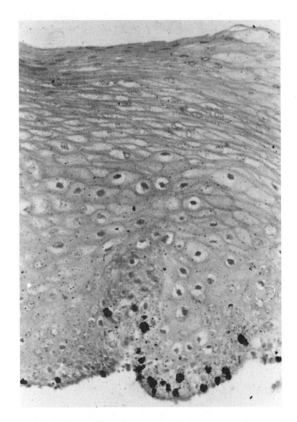

Figure 9.1 Cell proliferation in the human esophagus. In normal conditions, proliferating cells (highlighted by the nuclei with black granules) are located in the basal layers of the epithelium (autoradiography of biopsies incubated for 1 hour with tritiated thymidine, ×400).

the antral glands are either mucous or endocrine, gastrin-producing "G" cells and somatostatin-producing "D" cells. In the stomach, the proliferative compartment is located in the neck of glands both in the body and fundus (Fig. 9.2A) and in the antrum (Fig. 9.2B). From this zone, most cells move toward the surface; a few migrate toward deepest mucosal layers (17, 18). As a matter of fact, cell loss and programmed cell death (apoptosis) take place in both the surface epithelium and the glands. The integrity of the glandular component is therefore maintained by continuous input of newborn cells that migrate downward, and at the same time differentiate into mucous (in the antrum) or parietal cells (in the body and fundus). The other cell populations (G, S, or zymogen) seem to have a different proliferation turnover (19).

The mucosa of the small intestine, from the duodenum to the ileum, is formed by four types of specialized cells (columnar, mucous, Paneth, and enteroendocrine). All types derive from a stem cell compartment located in the deepest part of the glandular crypts (20) (Fig. 9.3). As in the other parts of the gastrointestinal tract, upward cell migration and differentiation occur.

The same behavior can be found in the mucosa of the large intestine (Fig. 9.4). The three types of differentiated cells—columnar (absorbent), goblet (mucous), and argentaffin (enteroendocrine)—derive from the same precursor (21). The proliferative zone is located in the lower one third of the colonic glands, and usually proliferating cells can be seen up to the lower two thirds of the crypt (21). The migration of cells from the base to the surface and exfoliation takes 3 to 8 days, whereas enteroendocrine cells undergo a slow renewal, from 35 to 100 days (22–24). Cell renewal in the sigmoid colon and in the rectum is probably slower than that of the other segments of the large intestine (25).

The goal of several studies in animals and in humans was to evaluate the proliferation rate, the duration of the cell cycle and of its various phases, and the turnover time of the various tissues of the gastrointestinal tract. Table 9.2 summarizes the results of some of these studies. Data available are remarkably different from one study to another, as a consequence of differences in methods and experimental conditions.

FACTORS INFLUENCING CELL PROLIFERATION IN THE GASTROINTESTINAL TRACT

Several studies involving animals have documented circadian variations of DNA synthesis and cell proliferation in the stomach and intestine (26, 27). In humans, two studies demonstrated that the highest proliferative activity of rectal mucosa occurs in the morning hours (3 AM to 12 PM) (28, 29).

Feeding can also influence gastric cell renewal. In dogs, food ingestion leads to an increase in the labeling index of mucosal cells (30). This kinetic modification usually follows a reduction of the height of glandular foveolae. It has been hypothesized that feeding leads to an exfoliation of surface epithelial cells, thus leading to a proliferative response with compensatory significance. Factors inducing such a response could be either chalone or gastrin release induced by food ingestion and gastric distention (31).

Long-term fasting reduces cell proliferation and induces epithelial hypoplasia of the small intestinal mucosa, whereas refeeding

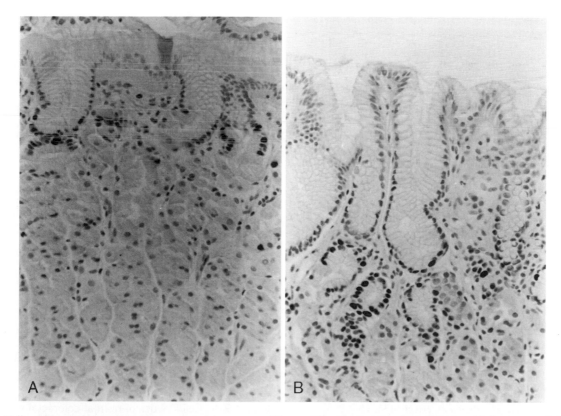

Figure 9.2 Cell proliferation in normal human gastric mucosa. The proliferative compartment (cells with brown nuclei) is located in the neck of glands both in the body-fundus (**A**) and in the antrum (**B**) (immunohistochemistry on sections of biopsies incubated for 1 hour with bromodeoxyuridine, ×300).

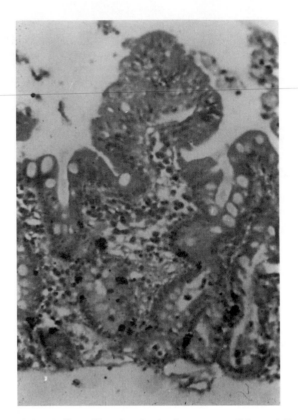

Figure 9.3 Cell proliferation in the human small bowel. Proliferating cells are located in the bottom of the glands (brown nuclei: immunolabeling with PC10 monoclonal antibody antiproliferating cell nuclear antigen [PCNA]; ×300).

leads to increased turnover and restoration of mucosal integrity, in both animals and humans (32–35).

Dietary components probably play an important role in modulating cell proliferation of the mucosa of the large bowel. It has been demonstrated that vegetarian Seventh-Day Adventists have a slow cell renewal of their rectal mucosa (36). On the contrary, expansion of the proliferative compartment was found in patients with high fecal levels of deoxycholic and lithocholic acid, which are overproduced in association with high-fat diets (37, 38).

Several hormones can influence the turnover of normal epithelium of the gastrointestinal tract. Gastrin stimulates cell proliferation in the gastric body and fundus but not in the antrum (39, 40). This hormone also affects cell proliferation in the colon and rectum. As a matter of fact, cell proliferation abnormalities similar to those observed in patients at increased risk of colorectal cancer were found in patients with endogenous hypergastrinemia (41). This finding supports other clinical evidence of a relationship between hypergastrinemia and neoplasms of the colon and rectum (42).

Other gastrointestinal hormones, such as cholecystokinin and secretin, showed no effect on gastric and duodenal cell proliferation (43, 44). Serotonin administration affects cell turnover of normal jejunum in the rat; at a low dose, it stimulates cell proliferation, whereas high doses have an inhibitory effect (45).

The effect of prostaglandin (PG) administration on gastric epithelial cell proliferation has been studied in animal models. PG can increase the cell proliferation rate and raise the surface mucous cell population (46). It has been suggested that endogenous PG production is one of the cytoprotective mechanisms of gastric mucosal repair.

Similarly, epidermal growth factor (EGF) increases DNA synthesis and prevents the occurrence of acute gastric damage induced by aminosalicylic acid (ASA) (47). EGF stimulates the activity of the enzyme ornithine decarboxylase (ODC) in the stomach and duodenum of newborn mice (47). Because ODC is required for RNA synthesis and cell growth, the induction of ODC activity by EGF may be important for the trophic effect of EGF. In particular, it has been demonstrated that EGF stimulates DNA synthesis through an effect similar to pentagastrin (47). EGF given parenterally increases DNA synthesis in a dose-dependent manner, while preventing the occurrence of acute gastric damage induced by aspirin (47). Moreover, cold-restraint stress in rats results in inhibition of gastric cell renewal, but ulcers appear several hours before any evident decrease of cell proliferation (48). An increase in EGF is observed under these stress conditions. These data lead to the hypothesis that EGF could be responsible for the delay of the decrease of cell proliferation as compared to the development of ulcers. Resection of salivary glands removes the major endogenous source of EGF, therefore reduces DNA synthesis and leads to a remarkable increase of stress-induced lesions and greater inhibition of DNA synthesis (47).

After extensive small bowel resection, enhanced replication and migration of the epithelial cells can be observed in the remaining

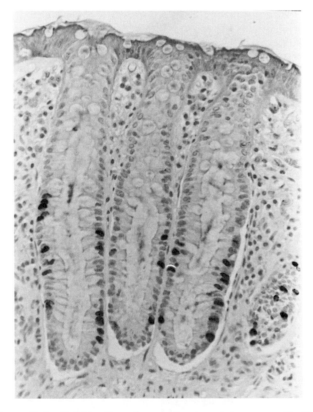

Figure 9.4 Cell kinetics of normal colorectal mucosa. Proliferating cells (brown nuclei) are located in the lower two thirds of the glands (immunohistochemistry on sections of biopsies incubated for 1 hour with bromodeoxyuridine, ×300).

TABLE 9.2	Summary of Proliferative Parameters in Normal and Diseased Gastrointestinal Mucosa of Man

	I_S (%)	I_M (%)	T_{G1} (h)	T_S (h)	T_{G2} (h)	T_C (h)	T_{OT} (h)	T_{PD} (h)
Esophageal mucosa								
Control (basal layer)	10.0			10.6			4.5	
Esophagitis	10.9							
Barrett's epithelium	23.3			10.0			<2.0	
Cancer	7.6			22.0			>10.0	
Gastric mucosa								
Normal cardia	13.1	1.3						
Normal fundus	4.2–14.0	0.8–1.0	62.0	6.1–10.0	1.0–4.0	48.0–72.0		
Normal antrum	12.8–16.0	0.36–1.4		7.6		65.4		79–122
Atrophic gastritis (fundus)	14.0–19.0			16.0	1.0–6.0	>30.0		
Atrophic gastritis (antrum)	19.9	2.9						
Intestinal metaplasia	19.0	1.0		14.0–18.0	1.6	34.0		30–46
Cardia in gastric cancer	20.1	2.1						
Fundus in gastric cancer	13.4							
Antrum in gastric cancer	16.2							
Cancer								29–204
Zollinger-Ellison syndrome	15.7	0.8	36.0	6.0	1.0	45.0		
Small intestine								
Normal duodenum		2.36				45.0–48.0		
Normal jejunum	13.0–38.0				1.5	42.0–48.0		
Ileal conduit			22.0	11.0	1.0–2.0	24.0–36.0		
Duodenum-jejunum with ileal conduit		5.1				21.0–22.0		
Sprue		5.2						
Large intestine								
Normal colon (in vivo)	12.0–18.0		14.0	11.0–20.0	1.0 6.0	40.0	72.0–96.0	
Normal rectum (in vivo)	18.0–25.0			9.0–14.0	2.0	~24.0–48.0	96.0–192.0	
Normal rectum (in vitro)	1.0–17.0			7.0–11.0		77.0–90.0	58.0–87.0	
Active ulcerative colitis	12.9–24.0			9.2		34.0		
Quiescent ulcerative colitis	8.1–18.9							
Rectal adenoma (in vitro)	23.0			7.4–12.0			32.0	
Rectal adenoma (in vivo)	2.0			15.0			>40.0	
Cancer (in vivo)	13.0–33.0	1.1–2.9		14.0			26.0–144.0	
Cancer (in vitro)	4.0–32.0	0.3–2.8		19.0			30.0–177.0	

I_S, percentage of cells in S phase; I_M, percentage of cells in M phase; T_{G1}, duration of G_1 phase; T_S, duration of S phase; T_{G2}, duration of G_2 phase; T_C, cell cycle time; T_{OT}, turnover time; T_{PD}, cell doubling time.

gut, causing a compensatory mucosal hyperplasia (49, 50). The factors mediating the adaptation of resected small bowel seem to be gastrin and enteroglucagon (51, 52).

Age seems to affect the cell proliferation pattern of the large intestine. In subjects older than 65 years, expansion of the proliferative compartment is similar to that observed in patients with colorectal adenomas or cancer. This finding gives credence to epidemiologic evidence of increasing cancer risk with increasing age (53–55).

Finally, enemas, which are used routinely for colon cleansing before endoscopic or surgical procedures, can affect colorectal cell proliferation (56, 57). It is important to consider this evidence when planning and evaluating proliferation studies in the large intestine in man.

CELL PROLIFERATION IN PATHOLOGIC CONDITIONS

INFLAMMATION AND ACUTE MUCOSAL DAMAGE

As a rule, both acute and chronic inflammation lead to an increase in epithelial cell turnover. This is due only in part to a direct stimulus to the proliferative compartment. The main event is an increase in cell proliferation rate in response to increased cell loss. Esophagitis, gastritis, celiac disease, ulcerative colitis, and Crohn's disease are all characterized by an increased cell turnover rate and an increased pool of proliferating cells in the inflamed mucosa.

A sequence of events is thought to occur in active inflammation as a function of the size of cell loss and the need of repair (1). The first event is a shortening of G1 phase of the cell cycle, the second is a recruitment of cells from G0 phase, and the third is an increase in the number of divisions of each cell leaving the proliferative compartment. Each of these mechanisms leads ultimately to the production of several new cells.

The increase in the number of divisions per cell unit has an additional consequence: the expansion of the proliferative compartment. This pattern is further enhanced if the migration rate of newborn cells toward the surface is too high to allow cells to differentiate. This finding implies that cells that are still proliferating are found at the epithelial surface. With cessation of the inflammatory stimulus, cell turnover rate and the size of the proliferative compartment usually decrease and can revert to normal.

Studies in patients with severe esophagitis demonstrated enhanced cell turnover in the basal layer of the epithelium (58). This proliferative pattern is associated with thickening of the layer and increased papillary length. These features are the hallmark of increased cell loss.

The presence of *Helicobacter pylori* induces inflammation of the gastric mucosa. In Helicobacter-induced gastritis, cell turnover is increased in the neck of the gastric glands (59). In some cases, dividing cells are present even in the mucosal surface (Fig. 9.5). With eradication of bacteria, the histology and proliferative pattern revert to normal (60).

Celiac disease is associated with an increased cell loss induced by gluten, an increase of cell proliferation, a shortening of the cell cycle time, an increase of migration rate, and an expansion of the proliferative compartment throughout the entire crypt (61). When intestinal mucosa is no longer in contact with gluten, its morphologic pattern reverts to normal (62).

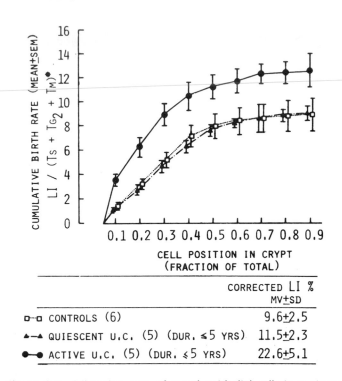

	CORRECTED LI % MV±SD
□--□ CONTROLS (6)	9.6±2.5
▲--▲ QUIESCENT U.C. (5) (DUR. ≤5 YRS)	11.5±2.3
●--● ACTIVE U.C. (5) (DUR. ≤5 YRS)	22.6±5.1

Figure 9.6 Migration rate of rectal epithelial cells in patients with active or quiescent ulcerative colitis and hospital controls. In active inflammation, migration rate from the bottom of the glands to the mucosal surface is increased as compared to the quiescent phase of colitis, where migration is similar to that observed in controls. Data computed on autoradiographs of biopsy sections incubated for 1 hour with tritiated thymidine, given a "standard" 9-hour duration of S phase (Biasco G et al., unpublished observations).

In some cases, chronicity is part of the natural history of the disease. In chronic gastritis, an expansion of the proliferative compartment has been observed (63, 64). The migration rate of epithelial cells in ulcerative colitis is increased in the active inflammation phase (Fig. 9.6). An enlargement of the proliferative compartment of the colorectal mucosa can persist also in quiescent phases of ulcerative colitis, in the absence of active inflammation (65–67). These proliferative abnormalities could be the consequence of the development of a genetic defect amplified by an increased cell turnover rate (68). On the other hand, DNA-synthesizing cells on the mucosal surface are prone to the action of genotoxic agents possibly present in the luminal microenvironment of the gut (69). This information can explain the increased risk of cancer development that usually is found in patients with chronic inflammation of the gastrointestinal mucosa.

The sequence of events involved in acute mucosal damage and repair has been studied extensively in animal models using the administration of nonsteroidal anti-inflammatory drugs (NSAID). Aspirin can reduce cell turnover rate by means of the inhibition of the enzyme cyclooxygenase and the impairment of prostaglandin production (70). The result is decreased cell proliferation in the stem cell compartment (71). When erosions or ulcers have formed and the action of the drug ceases, repair occurs by means of an increase of cell proliferation (72).

Results in humans seem to confirm this sequence. The short-term administration of low doses of aspirin causes a decrease in the

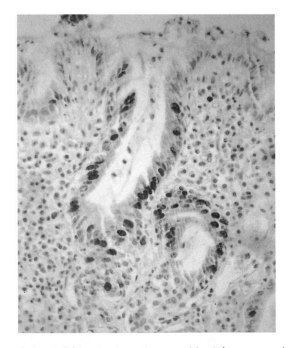

Figure 9.5 Cell kinetics in active gastritis. A larger number of proliferating cells (brown nuclei) with respect to normal are visible up to the mucosal surface (immunohistochemistry on sections of biopsies incubated for 1 hour with bromodeoxyuridine, ×400). (See color plate.)

gastric foveolar height, in both the antrum and the body-fundus (73). The event is associated with a decrease in the BrdU-labeling index, more evident in the body-fundus than in the antrum, which could represent an inhibition of the hyperproliferative compensatory mechanism of the mucosa. On the contrary, chronic NSAID administration results in an increase in the cell turnover rate, perhaps through endogenous PG production, which is one of the cytoprotective mechanisms of gastric mucosal repair (74, 75). These findings have been demonstrated only in animal models.

PRECANCER AND CANCER

According to the current hypothesis, the progression from normal gastrointestinal mucosa to cancer is a stepwise process. The occurrence of abnormalities and the rate of progression are under the influence of genetic and environmental factors. The beginning of the process leading to neoplasia does not necessarily mean the development of cancer, however. In fact, the probability of developing cancer progressively decreases as neoplastic transformation goes on. An example is colorectal adenomas—the principle preneoplastic lesions of the large bowel that rarely become malignant (76).

Cell proliferation errors can represent the earliest changes in this process. These errors can be present, even in the absence of morphologic alterations of the gastrointestinal mucosa, and are then maintained. As an example, an error in the control of cell growth occurs early in apparently normal mucosa and generally persists up to the development of neoplasia (77). The distribution of early mucosal changes is probably more widespread than that of advanced lesions (78). Moreover, some evidence indicates that early lesions could revert to normal (79).

An abnormal cell proliferation has been extensively demonstrated in experimental carcinogenesis (68, 80–83). During treatment with N-methyl-N'-nitro-N-nitrosoguanidine (MNNG) in animal models of gastric carcinogenesis, the number of proliferating cells per pyloric crypt column and the width of the proliferative zone increases. Therefore, the number of epithelial cells in each column and the thickness of the pyloric mucosa increase significantly (84). In ACI rats, which are susceptible to gastric chemical carcinogenesis, the administration of MNNG induces an increase in cell proliferation rate and an upward shift of the proliferative compartment before development of cancer (69). In resistant Buffalo rats, pyloric cells do not increase after treatment with MNNG. This experiment suggests not only the existence of genetic susceptibility to cancer development, but also that an increase in proliferating cells is one of the earliest changes.

Similar conclusions can be drawn from studies on colorectal carcinogenesis. Thurnherr and colleagues (85) gave CF1 mice weekly injections of dimethylhydrazine (DMH). This treatment induced colonic carcinomas in 90% of the animals after 86 days. The autoradiographic analysis of normal-appearing crypts after injection with tritiated thymidine showed that, after 45 days of treatment, the proliferating cell compartment expanded toward the superficial mucosal layers. The overall number of proliferating cells at that time was not changed. After 87 days of treatment, the total number of proliferating cells was also increased.

In man, expansion of the proliferative compartment and an increased number of proliferating cells have been observed in epidemiologic and clinical conditions that place the affected individual at increased risk of development of gastrointestinal cancer.

Precancerous lesions of the esophagus were well studied in Linxian, China, where there is a high incidence of esophageal cancer.

Progressive expansion of the proliferative compartment is associated with thickening of the basal epithelial layer and then with hyperplasia and dysplasia. By contrast, in a low-risk Chinese region, Jaoxian, no enlargement of the proliferative compartment was found (86, 87).

A high frequency of labeled cells in the upper portions of gastric glands has been observed in patients with chronic atrophic gastritis (63, 64). Another finding in subjects with expansion of the proliferative compartment is the presence of fetal antigens in their mucosa (64). These antigenic abnormalities are not present in patients affected by gastritis without any expansion of the proliferative compartment (64).

Cell proliferation abnormalities can also be observed in histologic precancerous lesions, such as gastric dysplasia (88–90). Increasing hyperproliferation is associated with the progression of dysplasia (89). With the highest grades of dysplasia comes a shift of the area, with the maximal proliferation up to the surface epithelium (90, 91).

An excess of proliferating cells in the upper two fifths of colorectal crypts is considered an early biologic marker of risk of cancer of the large bowel (Fig. 9.7). This marker was designated as the øh value by Lipkin et al. (92). Rectal biopsies of patients with ulcerative colitis often show an increase in the øh value (93). The distribution of patients according to the øh suggested the existence of two groups of patients, both with øh higher than controls (68). This abnormality does not seem to be related to the duration of the disease. Tissue specimens with higher values show also an abnormal antigenic expression, suggesting a loss of cell differentiation (93, 94). This result suggests that high øh values could be the hallmark of a particularly high derangement of cell proliferation and differentiation with precancerous significance.

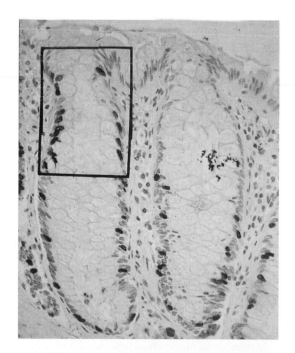

Figure 9.7 Colonic mucosa, autoradiography after incubation for 1 hour with tritiated thymidine (×300). Proliferating cells are abnormally present in the most superficial part of the gland on the left. The frame evidences the upper two fifths of the crypt. The percentage of proliferating cells in this zone is defined as the øh value. (See color plate.)

The apparently normal rectal mucosa of patients with adenoma or carcinoma of the large bowel shows an increase in the labeling index and expansion of the proliferative compartment (78–80). The degree of kinetic alteration is related to the size of adenomas, their degree of dysplasia, and the risk of recurrence after polypectomy (82, 83, 95). Similarly, patients who undergo surgery for colon cancer and show high øh values in their colorectal mucosa seem to be more susceptible to new adenomas or cancer recurrence, whereas patients with values similar to the controls do not seem to have this excess risk (96). Patients with hyperplastic polyps, which are not associated with increased risk of cancer, do not show any expansion of the proliferative zone in the colorectal mucosa (81).

In cancer tissue, the proliferative indices are usually increased and/or altered relative to normal mucosa. Several authors have suggested the use of these indices as prognostic factors in order to define a population at high risk of recurrence after radical surgery. Cytofluorometric measurements of DNA content demonstrated that aneuploidy is associated with risk of recurrence in esophageal carcinoma (97), as well as in colorectal carcinoma (98–100). Some authors suggest an inverse correlation of DNA abnormalities of colorectal tumors with survival (101). Others did not find any correlation between the Ki-67 labeling index and Dukes' stage and other pathologic variables (102). Gastric carcinoma may have a lower turnover rate than normal surrounding mucosa (103), and the proliferative activity seems to be higher only in poorly differentiated and advanced stage lesions (103, 104). The proliferative index at the site of invasion is higher than that in the central region (104).

CLINICAL APPLICATIONS OF GASTROINTESTINAL CELL KINETICS

Several methods are available for the study of gastrointestinal cell kinetics, and it is possible to take biopsy specimens from most areas of the gastrointestinal tract. Therefore, the clinical application of mucosal cell proliferation is the focus of ongoing studies.

CELL PROLIFERATION OF THE GASTRIC MUCOSA AS A MARKER OF CYTOPROTECTION

Most evidence in the literature suggests that an increased cell proliferation rate is tightly linked to the development of gastric mucosal protection (105). The protective action can be obtained through preservation or direct stimulus of the proliferative region, or through the activation of the mechanisms of response to a damaging agent (47, 106). Therefore, cell renewal in the gastric mucosa can be regarded as a marker of cytoprotection; in studies designed to evaluate the cytoprotective effect of a given substance, investigators could use cell kinetics as a marker of efficacy.

BIOLOGY OF PRECANCEROUS LESIONS

Findings of cell kinetics studies play a role in determining the biologic significance of morphologic lesions of the gastrointestinal mucosa. This issue was investigated in patients with ulcerative colitis in whom histologic findings were uncertain for dysplasia (107). Flow cytometry has been used in a surveillance program for colorectal cancer in patients affected by the disease. Aneuploidy

seems to be related to the development of dysplasia and can be considered a marker of neoplastic change of the mucosa (108).

IDENTIFICATION OF INDIVIDUALS AT HIGH RISK OF CANCER DEVELOPMENT

As mentioned previously, among subjects with previous adenoma or cancer, those showing an abnormal cell kinetics pattern in their apparently normal mucosa have a high risk of recurrence of neoplasia (95, 96). The proliferative assay of colorectal mucosa has been proposed to screen first-degree relatives of patients affected by familial polyposis coli (109). The identification of the individual level of cancer risk by means of cell kinetics can be useful in planning different strategies of surveillance and follow-up of high-risk population groups. Any kinetic method has its own biases and measurement variability (110); as with the other intermediate endpoints used in cancer research, cell proliferation biomarkers still need complete validation (111).

INTERMEDIATE ENDPOINT IN PILOT CHEMOPREVENTION STUDIES

Because proliferative abnormalities are an early event in the process of carcinogenesis, some authors suggest they can be used as intermediate biomarkers of cancer risk in pilot studies designed to test the efficacy of potential chemopreventive compounds (112, 113). Studies in human subjects demonstrated that some dietary or pharmacologic supplementation are able to reduce cell proliferation abnormalities with precancerous significance in the colon and rectum. These supplements include calcium (1500 to 2000 mg daily) (79, 114, 115); vitamins A, C, and E (116); ω-3 fatty acids (117), and sodium butyrate (118).

INDICATION OF ADJUVANT TREATMENTS

In the last decade, work has been carried out to search for new variables to implement the information provided by pathologic tumor stage, from a clinical as well as a biologic point of view. The importance of tumor cell kinetics as a prognostic index has been pointed out by several authors, and on the basis of this evidence, it has been suggested that cell proliferation can give information on therapeutic strategies, such as adjuvant (postsurgical) chemotherapy or radiotherapy.

CHRONOMODULATED CHEMOTHERAPY

The evidence of circadian variations of mucosal proliferation is the basis of nonconventional drug administration schedules, intensifying drug dose when proliferation rate in the normal tissue is lower. Moreover, despite tumors showing some degree of residual circadian cytokinetic modulation, the possibility of exploiting a cytokinetic asynchrony between tumor host tissue is feasible (119). Preclinical and clinical studies of colorectal cancer indicate that treatment schedules with chronomodulated infusion of fluoropyrimidines can obtain higher response rates with minor toxicity compared to other schedules as well as to conventional continuous infusion (120, 121).

REFERENCES

1. Wright NA, Alison MR. The biology of epithelial cell populations (volume 2). Oxford: Clarendon Press 1984:599–633.
2. Scully RE, Kempson RL, Norris HL. Mitosis counting. Hum Pathol 1976;7:481–484.
3. Sharp JG, Wright NA. Comparison of tritiated thymidine and metaphase arrest techniques of measuring cell production in rat intestine. Dig Dis Sci 1984;29:1153–1158.
4. Caro LG, Van Tubergen RP, Kolb J. High-resolution autoradiography. I. Methods. J Cell Biol 1962;15:173–188.
5. Gratzner HG. Monoclonal antibody to 5-bromo- and 5-iododeoxy-uridine: A new reagent for detection of DNA replication. Science 1982;218:474–475.
6. Gerdes J, Lemke H, Baisch H, et al. Cell cycle analysis of a cell proliferation-associated human nuclear antigen defined by the monoclonal antibody Ki-67. J Immunol 1984;133:1710–1715.
7. Waseem NH, Lane DP. Monoclonal antibody analysis of the proliferating cell nuclear antigen (PCNA). Structural conservation and the detection of a nucleolar form. J Cell Sci 1990;96:121–129.
8. Dressler LG, Bartow SA. DNA flow cytometry in solid tumors. Semin Diagn Pathol 1989;6:55–82.
9. Pegg AE. Polyamine metabolism and its importance in neoplastic growth and as a target for chemotherapy. Cancer Res 1988;48:759–774.
10. Ploton D, Menager M, Jeanneson P, et al. Improvement in the staining and in the visualization of the argyrophylic proteins of the nucleolar organiser region at the optical level. Histochem J 1986;18:5–14.
11. Paganelli GM, Biasco G, Santucci R, et al. Labeling patterns of bromodeoxyuridine and PCNA in human rectal biopsies. Cancer Res 1992;33:37.
12. Richter F, Richter A, Yang K, et al. Cell proliferation in rat colon measured with bromodeoxyuridine, proliferating cell nuclear antigen and ^{3}H-thymidine. Cancer Epidemiol Biomarkers Prev 1992;1:561–566.
13. Risio M, Candelaresi GL, Rossini FP. Bromodeoxyuridine intake and proliferating cell nuclear antigen expression throughout the colorectal tumor sequence. Cancer Epidemiol Biomarkers Prev 1993;2:363–368.
14. Paganelli GM, Lalli E, Facchini A, et al. Flow cytometry and in vitro tritiated thymidine labelling in normal rectal mucosa of patients at high risk of colorectal cancer. Am J Gastroenterol 1994;89:220–224.
15. Paganelli GM, Saccoccio G, Brandi G, et al. Correlation between bromodeoxyuridine labelling and ornithine decarboxylase levels in normal rectal mucosa of patients with colorectal adenoma. Cancer Lett 1991;59:221–224.
16. Lipkin M. Proliferation and differentiation of normal and diseased gastrointestinal cells. In: Johnson LR, ed. Physiology of the gastrointestinal tract. New York: Raven Press, 1987:255–284.
17. Lipkin M, Sherlock P, Bell B. Cell proliferation kinetics in the gastrointestinal tract of man. II. Cell renewal in stomach, ileum, colon and rectum. Gastroenterology 1963;45:721–729.
18. Hattori T, Fujita S. Tritiated thymidine autoradiographic study on cellular migration in the gastric gland of the golden hamster. Cell Tissue Res 1976;172:171–184.
19. Willems G, Lehy T. Radioautographic and quantitative studies on parietal and peptic cell kinetics in the mouse. Gastroenterology 1975;69:416–426.
20. Chang WWL, Leblond CP. Origin, differentiation and renewal of the four main epithelial cell types in the mouse small intestine. V. Unitarian theory of the origin of the four epithelial cell types. Am J Anat 1974;141:537–562.
21. Chang WWL, Leblond CP. Renewal of the epithelium in the descending colon of the mouse. I. Presence of three populations: vacuolated-columnar, mucous and argentaffin. Am J Anat 1971;131:73–100.
22. Cole JW, McKalen A. Observations of cell renewal in human rectal mucosa in vivo with thymidine-H^3. Gastroenterology 1961;41:122–125.
23. Lipkin M, Bell B, Sherlock P. Cell proliferation kinetics in the gastrointestinal tract of man. I. Cell renewal in colon and rectum. J Clin Invest 1963;42:767–776.
24. Deschner EE, Lipkin M. An autoradiographic study of the renewal of argentaffin cells in human rectal mucosa. Exp Cell Res 1966;43:661–665.
25. Lipkin M, Quastler H. Cell retention and incidence of carcinoma in several portions of the gastrointestinal tract. Nature 1962;194:1198–1199.
26. Scheving LE, Burns ER, Pauly JE, et al. Circadian variation and cell division of the mouse alimentary tract, bone marrow and corneal epithelium. Anat Rec 1978;191:479–486.
27. Scheving LE, Tsai TH, Scheving LA. Chronobiology of the intestinal tract of the mouse. Am J Anat 1983;168:433–465.
28. Buchi KN, Moore JG, Hrushesky WJM, et al. Circadian rhythm of cellular proliferation in the human rectal mucosa. Gastroenterology 1991;101:410–415.
29. Marra G, Anti M, Percesepe A, et al. Circadian variations of epithelial cell proliferation in human rectal crypts. Gastroenterology 1994;106:982–987.
30. Willems G, Vansteenkiste Y, Smets P. Effect of food ingestion on the proliferation kinetics in the canine fundic mucosa. Gastroenterology 1971;61:323–327.
31. Bertrand P, Willems G. Induction of antral gastrin cell proliferation by refeeding of rats after fasting. Gastroenterology 1980;78:918–924.
32. Williamson RCN, Malt RA. Relative importance of luminal and systemic factors in the control of intestinal adaptation. In: Appleton DR, Sunter JP, Watson AJ, eds. Cell proliferation in the gastrointestinal tract. Tunbridge Wells: Pitman Medical, 1980;230–243.
33. Biasco G, Callegari C, Lami F, et al. Intestinal morphological changes during oral refeeding in a patient previously treated with total parenteral nutrition for small bowel resection. Am J Gastroenterol 1984;79:585–588.
34. Guedon G, Schmitz J, Lerebours E, et al. Decreased brush border hydrolase activities without gross morphologic changes in human intestinal mucosa after prolonged total parenteral nutrition of adults. Gastroenterology 1986;90:373–378.
35. Pironi L, Paganelli GM, Miglioli M, et al. Morphologic and cytoproliferative patterns of duodenal mucosa in two patients after long-term total parenteral nutrition: Changes with oral refeeding and relation to intestinal resection. JPEN J Parenter Enteral Nutr 1994,18:351–354.
36. Lipkin M, Uehara K, Winawer S, et al. Seventh-day Adventist vegetarians have a quiescent proliferative activity in colonic mucosa. Cancer Lett 1985;26:139–144.
37. Stadler J, Yeung KS, Furrer R, et al. Proliferative activity of rectal mucosa and soluble fecal bile acids in patients with normal colons and in patients with colonic polyps or cancer. Cancer Lett 1988;38:315–320.
38. Biasco G, Paganelli GM, Owen RW, et al. Faecal bile acids and colorectal cell proliferation. Eur J Cancer Prev 1991;1 (Suppl. 1):63–68.
39. Hansen OH, Pedersen T, Larsen JK, et al. Effect of gastrin on gastrin mucosal cell proliferation in man. Gut 1976;17:536–541.
40. Casteleyn PP, Dubrasquet M, Willems G. Opposite effects of gastrin on cell proliferation in the antrum and other parts of the upper gastrointestinal tract in the rat. Dig Dis 1977;22:798–804.
41. Biasco G, Brandi G, Renga M, et al. Is there a relationship between hypergastrinemia and colorectal cancer risk? Rectal cell proliferation in Zollinger-Ellison syndrome. Am J Gastroenterol 1995;90:1355–1356.
42. Palmer Smith J, Wood JG, Solomon TE. Elevated gastrin levels in patients with colon cancer or adenomatous polyps. Dig Dis Sci 1989;34:171–174.
43. Johnson LR, Guthrie P. Effect of cholecystokinin and 16,16-dimethyl-prostaglandin E$_2$ on RNA and DNA of gastric and duodenal mucosa. Gastroenterology 1976;70:59–65.
44. Kawai K, Murakami M, Sasaki S, et al. Cell kinetics of superficial epithelial cells of mouse gastric mucosa (abstract). Gastroenterology 1983;84:1204.
45. Tutton PJM. The influence of serotonin on crypt cell proliferation in the jejunum of rats. Virchows Arch [B] 1974;16:79–87.
46. Goodlad RA, Madgwick AJ, Moffatt MR, et al. Prostaglandin and the gastric epithelium: Effects of misoprostol on gastric epithelial cell proliferation in the dog. Gut 1989;30:316–321.

47. Konturek S. Role of growth factors in gastroduodenal protection and healing of peptic ulcers. Gastroenterol Clin North Am 1990; 19:41–65.
48. Greant P, Delvaux G, Willems G. Influence of stress on epithelial cell proliferation in the gut mucosa of rats. Digestion 1988;40:212–218.
49. Hanson WR, Osborne JW, Sharpe JG. Compensation by the residual intestine after intestinal resection in the rat: Influence of amount of tissue removed. Gastroenterology 1977;72:692–700.
50. Williamson RCN, Bucklotz TW, Malt RA. Humoral stimulation of cell proliferation in small bowel after transection and resection in rats. Gastroenterology 1978;75:249–254.
51. Junghanns K, Kaess H, Dorner M, et al. The influence of resection of the small intestine on gastrin levels. Surg Gynecol Obstet 1975;140: 27–29.
52. Sagor GR, Al-Mukhtar MYT, Ghatei MA, et al. The effect of altered luminal nutrition on cellular proliferation and plasma concentrations of enteroglucagon and gastrin after small bowel resection in the rat. Br J Surg 1982;69:14–18.
53. Deschner EE, Godbold J, Lynch HT. Rectal epithelial cell proliferation in a group of young adults. Influence of age and genetic risk for colon cancer. Cancer 1988;61:2286–2290.
54. Roncucci L, Ponz de Leon M, Scalmati A, et al. The influence of age on colonic epithelial cell proliferation. Cancer 1988;62: 2373–2377.
55. Paganelli GM, Santucci R, Biasco G, et al. Effect of sex and age on rectal cell renewal in humans. Cancer Lett 1990;53:117–121.
56. Lehy T, Abitbol JL, Mignon M. Influence de la préparation rectale par lavement sur la prolifération cellulaire dans la muqueuse rectale normale de l'homme. Gastroenterol Clin Biol 1984;8:216–221.
57. Lipkin M, Enker WE, Winawer SJ. Tritiated thymidine labeling of rectal epithelial cells in 'non-prep' biopsies of individuals at increased risk for colonic neoplasia. Cancer Lett 1987;37:153–161.
58. Livstone EM, Sheahan DG, Behan J. Studies of esophageal epithelial cell proliferation in patients with reflux esophagitis. Gastroenterology 1977;73:1315–1319.
59. Cahill RJ, Sant S, Beattie S, et al. Helicobacter pylori and increased epithelial cell proliferation: A risk factor for cancer. Eur J Gastroenterol Hepatol 1994;6:1123–1128.
60. Cahill RJ, Beattie S, Hamilton H, et al. Eradication of Helicobacter pylori decreases the risk for cancer (abstract). Gastroenterology 1994;106:A1020.
61. Wright NA, Watson A, Morley A, et al. Cell kinetics in flat (avillous) mucosa of the human small intestine. Gut 1973;14:701–710.
62. Trier JS, Browning TH. Epithelial cell renewal in cultured duodenal biopsies in celiac sprue. N Engl J Med 1970;283:1245–1250.
63. Biasco G, Paganelli GM, Brillanti S, et al. Cell renewal and cancer risk of the stomach: Analysis of cell proliferation kinetics in atrophic gastritis. Acta Gastroenterol Belg 1989;52:361–366.
64. Lipkin M, Correa P, Mikol YB, et al. Proliferative and antigenic modifications in epithelial cells in chronic atrophic gastritis. J Natl Cancer Inst 1985;75:613–619.
65. Biasco G, Santini D, Marchesini F, et al. Kinetics of the mucous cells of the rectum in patients with chronic ulcerative colitis. In: Rozen P, Eidelman S, Gilat T, eds. Gastrointestinal cancer: Advances in diagnostic techniques and therapy. Frontiers of gastrointestinal research, volume IV. Basel: Karger, 1979:65–72.
66. Biasco G, Miglioli M, Minarini A, et al. Rectal cell renewal as a biological marker of cancer risk in ulcerative colitis. In: Sherlock P, Morson BC, Barbara L, et al., eds. Precancerous lesions of the gastrointestinal tract. New York: Raven Press, 1983;261–271.
67. Bleiberg H, Mainguet P, Galand P, et al. Cell renewal in the human rectum: In vitro autoradiographic study on active ulcerative colitis. Gastroenterology 1970;58:851–855.
68. Biasco G, Paganelli GM, Miglioli M, et al. Rectal cell proliferation and colon cancer risk in ulcerative colitis. Cancer Res 1990;50: 1156–1159.
69. Ohgaki H, Tomihari M, Sato S, et al. Differential proliferative response of gastric mucosa during carcinogenesis induced by N-methyl-N'-nitro-N-nitrosoguanidine in susceptible ACI rats, resistant Buffalo rats, and their hybrid F1 cross. Cancer Res 1988;48: 5275–5279.
70. Vane JR. Inhibition of prostaglandin synthesis as a mechanism of action of aspirin-like drugs. Nature 1971;231:232–235.
71. Levi S, Goodlad RA, Lee CY, et al. Inhibitory effect of non-steroidal anti-inflammatory drugs on mucosal cell proliferation associated with gastric ulcer healing. Lancet 1990;336:840–843.
72. Helpap B, Hattori T, Gedigk P. Repair of gastric ulcer: A cell kinetic study. Virchows Arch [A] 1981;392:159–170.
73. Biasco G, Paganelli GM, Di Febo G, et al. Cell-kinetic alterations induced by aspirin in human gastric mucosa and their prevention by a cytoprotective agent. Digestion 1992;51:146–151.
74. Yeomans ND, St John DJB, deBoer WGRM. Regeneration of gastric mucosa after aspirin-induced injury in the rat. Dig Dis Sci 1973;18: 773–780.
75. Eastwood GL, Quimby GF. Effect of chronic aspirin ingestion on epithelial proliferation in rat fundus, antrum, and duodenum. Gastroenterology 1982;82:852–856.
76. Muto T, Bussey HJR, Morson BC. The evolution of cancer of the colon and rectum. Cancer 1975;36:2251–2270.
77. Lipkin M. Phase 1 and phase 2 proliferative lesions in diseases leading to colon cancer. Cancer 1974;34:878–888.
78. Terpstra OT, van Blankenstein M, Dees J, et al. Abnormal pattern of cell proliferation in the entire colonic mucosa of patients with colon adenoma or cancer. Gastroenterology 1987;92:704–708.
79. Lipkin M, Newmark H. Effect of added dietary calcium on colonic epithelial cell proliferation in subjects at high risk for familial colon cancer. N Engl J Med 1985;313:1381–1384.
80. Ponz de Leon M, Roncucci L, Di Donato P, et al. Pattern of epithelial cell proliferation in colorectal mucosa of normal subjects and of patients with adenomatous polyps or cancer of the large bowel. Cancer Res 1988;48:4121–4126.
81. Risio M, Coverlizza S, Ferrari A, et al. Immunohistochemical study of epithelial cell proliferation in hyperplastic polyps, adenomas, and adenocarcinomas of the large bowel. Gastroenterology 1988;94: 899–906.
82. Risio M, Lipkin M, Candelaresi GL, et al. Correlations between rectal mucosa cell proliferation and the clinical and pathological features of nonfamilial neoplasia of the large intestine. Cancer Res 1991;51: 1917–1921.
83. Paganelli GM, Biasco G, Santucci R, et al. Rectal cell proliferation and colorectal cancer risk level in patients with non-familial adenomatous polyps of the large bowel. Cancer 1991;68:2451–2454.
84. Deschner EE, Tamura K, Bralow SP. Early proliferative changes in rat pyloric mucosa induced by N-methyl-N'-nitro-N-nitrosoguanidine. Front Gastrointest Res 1984;4:25–31.
85. Thurnherr N, Deschner EE, Stonehill EH, et al. Induction of adenocarcinomas of the colon in mice by weekly injections of 1,2-dimethylhydrazine. Cancer Res 1973;33:940–945.
86. Muñoz N, Lipkin M, Crespi M, et al. Proliferative abnormalities of the oesophageal epithelium of Chinese populations at high and low risk for oesophageal cancer. Int J Cancer 1985;36:187–189.
87. Yang GC, Lipkin M, Yang K, et al. Proliferation of esophageal epithelial cells in individual in Linxian, China. J Natl Cancer Inst 1987;79:1241–1246.
88. Ming SC, Bajtai A, Correa P, et al. Gastric dysplasia: Significance and pathological criteria. Cancer 1984;54:1794–1801.
89. Rubio CA, Hirota T, Itabashi T. Atypical mitoses in elevated dysplasias of the stomach. Pathol Res Pract 1985;180:372–376.
90. Hattori T. Histological and autoradiographic study on development of grade III lesion (dysplasia grade III) in the stomach. Pathol Res Pract 1985;180:36–44.
91. Ohelert W. Biological significance of dysplastic epithelium and gastritis. In: Herfarth C, Schlag P, eds. Gastric cancer. Berlin: Springer, 1979:99–105.
92. Lipkin M, Blattner WE, Fraumeni Jr JF, et al. Tritiated thymidine (øp, øh) labeling distribution as a marker for hereditary predisposition to colon cancer. Cancer Res 1983;43:1899–1904.
93. Biasco G, Lipkin M, Minarini A, et al. Proliferative and antigenic properties of rectal cells in patients with chronic ulcerative colitis. Cancer Res 1984;44:5450–5454.
94. Paganelli GM, Higgins PJ, Biasco G, et al. Abnormal rectal cell proliferation and p52/p35 protein expression in patients with ulcerative colitis. Cancer Lett 1993;73:23–28.
95. Anti M, Marra G, Armelao F, et al. Rectal epithelial cell proliferation patterns as predictors of adenomatous colorectal polyp recurrence. Gut 1993;34:525–530.

96. Scalmati A, Roncucci L, Ghidini G, et al. Epithelial cell kinetics in the remaining colorectal mucosa after surgery for cancer of the large bowel. Cancer Res 1990;50:7937–7941.

97. Sugimachi K, Ida H, Okamura T, et al. Cytophotometric DNA analysis of mucosal and submucosal carcinoma of the esophagus. Cancer 1984;53:2683–2687.

98. Banner BF, Chacho MS, Roseman DL, et al. Multiparameter flow cytometric analysis of colon polyps. Am J Clin Pathol 1987;87:313–318.

99. Goh HS, Jass JR. DNA content and the adenoma-carcinoma sequence in the colorectum. J Clin Pathol 1986;39:387–392.

100. Schutte B, Reynerds MJ, Wiggers T, et al. Retrospective analysis of the prognostic significance of DNA content and proliferative activity in large bowel carcinoma. Cancer Res 1987;47:5494–5496.

101. Armitage NC, Robias RA, Evans DF, et al. The influence of tumor cell DNA abnormalities on survival in colorectal cancer. Br J Surg 1985;72:828–830.

102. Shepherd NA, Richman PI, England J. Ki-67 derived proliferative activity in colorectal adenocarcinoma with prognostic correlations. J Pathol 1988;155:213–219.

103. Wright NA, Britton DR, Bone G, et al. Cell proliferation in gastric carcinoma: A stathmokinetic study. Cell Tissue Kinet 1977;10:429–438.

104. Kikuyama S, Kubota T, Watanabe M, et al. Cell kinetic study of human carcinomas using bromodeoxyuridine. Cell Tissue Kinet 1988;20:1–6.

105. Takeuchi K, Johnson LR. Effect of cell proliferation on healing of gastric and duodenal ulcers in rats. Digestion 1986;32:92–100.

106. Uribe A, Johansson C. Endogenous prostaglandins as regulators of cell proliferation (letter). Lancet 1990;336:1073.

107. Melville D, Northover JMA. Flow cytometry in ulcerative colitis. In: Rossini FP, Lynch HT, Winawer SJ, eds. Recent progress in colorectal cancer: Biology and management of high risk groups. Amsterdam: Elsevier Science, 1991:299–302.

108. Lofberg R, Brostrom O, Karlen P, et al. Colonoscopic surveillance in total ulcerative colitis: A 15-year follow-up study. Gastroenterology 1990;99:1021–1031.

109. Lipkin M, Blattner WA, Gardner EJ, et al. Classification and risk assessment of individual with familial polyposis, Gardner syndrome and familial non polyposis colon cancer from [³H]dThd-labeling patterns in colonic epithelial cells. Cancer Res 1984;44:4201–4207.

110. Einspahr J, Alberts DS, McGee D, et al. Evaluation of the reproducibility of [³H]thymidine labeling index determinations in crypt organ culture in normal subjects and patients with resected colorectal adenomas and cancer (abstract). Cancer Res 1990;31:233.

111. Schatzkin A, Freedman LS, Schiffman MH, et al. Validation of intermediate end points in cancer research. J Natl Cancer Inst 1990;82:1746–1752.

112. Lipkin M. Biomarkers of increased susceptibility to gastrointestinal cancer: New application to studies of cancer prevention in human subjects. Cancer Res 1988;48:235–245.

113. Lippmann SM, Lee JS, Lotan R, et al. Biomarkers as intermediate end points in chemoprevention trials. J Natl Cancer Inst 1990;82:555–560.

114. Rozen P, Fireman Z, Fine N, et al. Oral calcium suppresses increased rectal epithelial proliferation of persons at risk of colorectal cancer. Gut 1989;30:650–655.

115. Wargovich MJ, Isbell G, Shabot M, et al. Calcium supplementation decreases rectal epithelial cell proliferation in subjects with sporadic adenomas. Gastroenterology 1992;103:92–97.

116. Paganelli GM, Biasco G, Brandi G, et al. Effect of vitamin A, C and E supplementation on rectal cell proliferation in patients with colorectal adenomas. J Natl Cancer Inst 1992;84:47–51.

117. Anti M, Marra G, Armelao F, et al. Effect of ω-3 fatty acids on rectal mucosal cell proliferation in subjects at risk for colon cancer. Gastroenterology 1992;103:883–891.

118. Scheppach W, Sommer H, Kirchner T, et al. Effect of butyrate enemas on the colonic mucosa in distal ulcerative colitis. Gastroenterology 1992;103:51–56.

119. Hrushesky WJM, Bjarnason GA. Circadian cancer therapy. J Clin Oncol 1993;11:1403–1417.

120. Wesen C, Hrushesky WJM, Roemeling R, et al. Circadian modification of intra-arterial 5-fluoro-2′-deoxyuridine infusion rate reduces its toxicity and permits higher dose intensity. J Infus Chemother 1992;2:69–75.

121. Lévi F, Misset JL, Brienza S, et al. A chronopharmacologic phase-II clinical trial with 5-fluorouracil, folinic acid, and oxaliplatin using an ambulatory multichannel programmable pump. Cancer 1992;69:893–900.

PART II

Disorders Common to the Gastrointestinal Tract

10 EMBRYOLOGY AND DEVELOPMENTAL DISORDERS

Jihad Hayek, Harvey Goldman, and Harry B. W. Kozakewich

ESOPHAGUS

EMBRYOLOGY

During organogenesis, in the third to eighth week, the primitive gut is formed secondary to cephalocaudal and lateral folding of the embryo and incorporation into it of the dorsal portion of the yolk sac cavity lined by endoderm. The midgut, i.e., the middle portion of the primitive gut, connects to the extraembryonic yolk sac via the vitelline duct; the hindgut connects to the allantois. From the primitive foregut, the esophagus and respiratory tract start out as a single endoderm-derived tube (Fig. 10.1). During the fourth week, a laryngotracheal groove appears in the floor of the foregut caudal

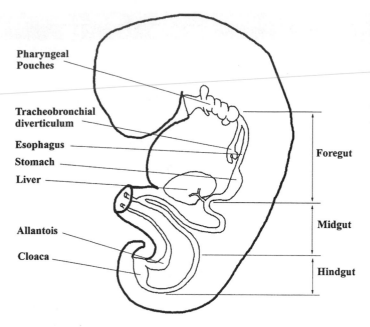

Figure 10.1 Schematic drawing of the embryon during the fifth week showing endodermal derivatives, including the primitive gut.

to the pharyngeal pouches. This groove is later converted into the "laryngotracheal tube" by the growth of a septum from converging tracheoesophageal folds of each side of the foregut wall during the fifth week (1, 2). Interposed between the laryngeal opening and the stomach is a short esophagus that lengthens dorsally secondary to the increase of the thoracic cavity, development of lung buds, and migration of the heart ventrally and caudally. Recent evidence challenges this development sequence, however, and suggests that the respiratory system develops as a ventral outgrowth from the region of the pharyngeal floor with elongation proceeding caudally (3, 4).

Upper esophageal striated muscle derives from pharyngeal arch mesoderm and is supplied by recurrent laryngeal branches of the vagus nerves. Lower esophageal smooth muscle derives from splanchnic mesoderm and is innervated by autonomic neurons originating from the neural crest. By the eight week of embryonic life, the esophageal ciliated epithelium is gradually replaced by squamous epithelium through birth.

ANOMALIES RELATED TO SIZE, POSITION, AND SHAPE

CONGENITAL ABSENCE

Acardiac fetuses often show anomalies related to foregut development, including congenital absence of the esophagus, replaced by a fibrous cord or trachea with stratified squamous epithelial lining of its posterior wall (2).

SHORT ESOPHAGUS

Congenital short esophagus occurs rarely and results in a congenital hiatal hernia. The stomach is pulled upward and is constricted into an hour-glass shape by the diaphragm. The intrathoracic gastric

portion, to be distinguished from metaplastic Barrett's esophagus, receives its arterial blood supply from branches of the descending thoracic aorta, rather than from the celiac artery (5).

ESOPHAGEAL ATRESIA AND RELATED LESIONS

TRACHEOESOPHAGEAL FISTULA WITH AND WITHOUT ESOPHAGEAL ATRESIA

This complex of anomalies traditionally has been attributed to failure of complete separation of the posteriorly located esophagus from the anteriorly placed trachea or as a result of faulty development of the already separate tracheobronchial tube and esophagus (2–4, 6). The incidence of tracheoesophageal fistula is 1 in 3000 to

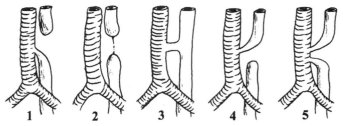

Figure 10.2 Types of esophageal atresia and tracheoesophageal fistulas (10).

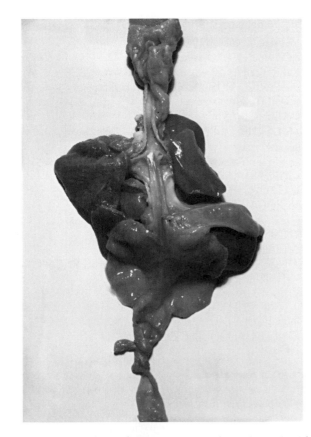

Figure 10.3 Esophageal atresia (proximal esophagus) with fistula between lower esophagus and tracheal carina (Swenson type 1, Kluth type IIIb).

TABLE 10.1	Most Frequent Variants of Esophageal Atresia and Tracheoesophageal Fistula			
		Frequency (12)	Swenson Classification (10)	Gross Classification (11)
Esophageal atresia with distal tracheoesophageal fistula		86.5%	Type I	Type C
Esophageal atresia without tracheoesophageal fistula		7.7%	Type 2	Type A
Tracheoesophageal fistula without esophageal atresia, commonly referred to as "H" type		4.2%	Type 3	Type E
Esophageal atresia with proximal tracheoesophageal fistula		0.8%	Type 4	Type B
Esophageal atresia with proximal and distal tracheoesophageal fistula		0.7%	Type 5	Type D

4500 live births, of which 20% are premature. Esophageal atresia is more frequent in cases of polyhydramnios, secondary to inability of the fetus to swallow the amniotic fluid. Cases of esophageal membranous atresia probably result from failure of esophageal recanalization after excessive epithelial proliferation and defective growth of endodermal cells. Possible associated anomalies (over 50%) include cardiovascular malformations, such as Fallot's tetralogy; anorectal agenesia; atresia or stenosis of small intestine; renal or musculoskeletal anomalies; and Down's syndrome. Tracheoesophageal fistulas are the most common component of the VACTERL association (*v*ertebral or *v*ascular defects, *a*nal atresia, *c*ardiac anomalies, *t*racheo-*e*sophageal fistula with esophageal atresia, *r*enal anomalies, and *l*imb, especially radial, defects) (7). Most of the cases are sporadic, with a subsequent risk among siblings of 0.56%, and possible familial occurrence (8).

There are several classifications of tracheoesophageal fistulas, and Kluth described 10 types and 88 subtypes (9–11). Five major groups are identified (Table 10.1; Figs. 10.2 and 10.3) and are used to describe the common cases on an anatomic basis (10, 12). The most frequent form of tracheoesophageal fistula is between the trachea or a bronchus, frequently the right, and the distal esophageal segment (Swenson type 1). The proximal separate esophageal segment, located posterior to the trachea, is blind-ended and dilated. The mucosal lining of the fistula is pseudostratified columnar or squamous, and submucosal mixed glands similar to tracheobronchial glands are present.

LARYNGOTRACHEOESOPHAGEAL CLEFT

This rare condition is related to tracheoesophageal fistula and esophageal atresia. Depending on the level and extent of the cleft, different types (Table 10.2; Fig. 10.4) have been described (13, 14).

ESOPHAGEAL BRONCHUS

In this unusual condition seen with other associated anomalies (mostly cardiac), a main bronchus arises from the esophagus and the corresponding lung arterial supply originates from the pulmonary artery, in contrast to the aberrant systemic arterial blood supply in cases of pulmonary sequestration (15).

ESOPHAGEAL STENOSIS

Stenoses secondary to webs (membranous) or cartilaginous rings encircling the esophagus are generally considered to be congenital

TABLE 10.2	Types and Extent of Laryngotracheoesophageal Cleft	
	Cleft Involving	Surgical Correction
Type I	Larynx, posterior cricoid midline	Unnecessary
Type II	Upper trachea	Required
Type III	Whole trachea up to carina	Required
Type IV	Trachea and one or both main bronchi	Required

and easily separated from acquired strictures resulting from peptic esophagitis that may develop rapidly (16). The webs, usually treatable by dilation, are mainly composed of mucosa and submucosa, affect the upper esophagus, and are seen predominantly in women (17). In contrast, the cartilaginous rings usually occur in the distal esophagus, more frequently in infants and children, causing segmental stenosis (about 2.5 cm in length), and may be considered as choristomas, heterotopias, esophageal sequestrations, or as part of the bronchopulmonary foregut malformation complex (18).

CYSTS AND DUPLICATIONS

The congenital cystic lesions are classified by anatomic site, embryology, and epithelial lining, and can be separated into three basic groups: bronchogenic cysts, intramural esophageal cysts, and dorsal enteric cysts (19–21). They have been referred to as enteric duplications, mediastinal cysts of foregut origin, gastrocytoma of the spinal cord, duplication cysts, tubular duplication, bronchogenic cysts, tracheobronchial cysts, esophageal cysts, mediastinal gastric cysts, neurenteric cysts, and enterogenic cysts.

BRONCHOGENIC CYSTS

Aberrant bronchial budding from the foregut can result in formation of cystic structures typically lined by ciliated mucus-secreting columnar epithelium and containing cartilage, smooth muscle, and seromucinous glands in their walls. They usually occur as isolated lesions in the mediastinum, along the tracheobronchial

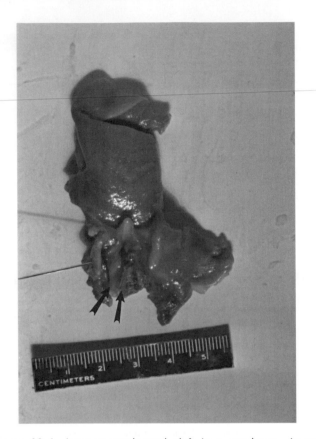

Figure 10.4 Laryngoesophageal cleft in a newborn. *Arrows,* edges of cleft.

tree with occasional communication to it, within the lung, and rarely in the abdomen or in subcutaneous tissues of the neck or chest (22, 23).

INTRAMURAL ESOPHAGEAL CYSTS

These cysts probably result from inadequate recanalization of the rapidly proliferating esophageal epithelium during embryogenesis or fusion of longitudinal folds, and develop within the esophageal wall with secondary intraluminal or extrinsic bulging and no association with cartilage or vertebral defects. Their shape is often elongate (Fig. 10.5). Their wall is thick with multiple muscle layers and ganglia, hence considered by some authors as intramural duplication. Their mucosa is usually of mixed nature, with respiratory and gastric fundic type mucosa but thick and thin squamous, cuboidal, or transitional epithelia can be seen. Mucosal ulceration is frequent and fistulization may occur.

NEURENTERIC CYSTS AND DUPLICATIONS

The theory behind their occurrence is that of a dorsal intestinal fistula formation, secondary to either a split and incomplete closure in the primitive neurenteric canal (notochord) allowing the adjacent yolk sac to herniate and become adherent to the dorsal ectoderm or abnormal ectoendodermal adhesions secondary to a defective or absent intervening mesodermal tissue during embryogenesis (19, 20). These lesions affect primarily infants, occurring in

the posterior mediastinum, and sometimes in continuity with intraabdominal mesenteric spherical cystic lesions or elongate cylindric duplications (24). These duplications may or may not communicate with the lumen of the bowel, pancreatic and bile ducts, or the lungs. Their epithelial lining is commonly of respiratory and gastric types (Fig. 10.6). Among these ectoendodermal remnants are dorsal enterocutaneous fistula with anterior and posterior spina bifida, diastematomyelia, diplomyelia, or a simple mediastinal cyst. Associated vertebral anomalies, such as butterfly and hemivertebrae, fusion of vertebrae, or the presence of a bony spur in association with diastematomyelia, are common and usually are cranial to the related cysts secondary to differential spinal cord-body growth. Thorough evaluation of infants with neurenteric cysts is required to exclude such associations. Neural elements may also be found about the cyst wall or at its vertebral attachment via a tubular tract or fibrous cord. These cysts may be found incidentally or are noted along with secondary compression symptoms, such as respiratory distress or digestive symptoms, vascular compression, pain, and hemorrhage, especially if the cyst contains acid-secreting gastric mucosa. Occasionally, mediastinal and abdominal cysts communicate across the diaphragm. All layers—muscularis propria with myenteric plexuses, submucosa, muscularis mucosa, and mucosa—are usually identifiable. The epithelial lining is frequently of gastric type, but it may be composed of small intestinal, colonic, squamous, or respiratory types, with occasional pancreatic tissue islands. Hence, the possibility of ulceration within the cyst wall or perforation into adjacent organs can have disastrous consequences.

DOUBLE ESOPHAGUS

In newborns as well as adults, a tubular structure connects the pharynx to the gastric cardia or the normal esophagus via a fistula (25).

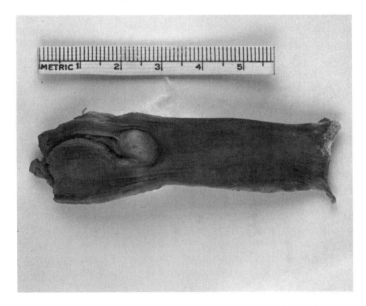

Figure 10.5 Esophageal intramural cyst in a 17-day-old infant that died of meningitis.

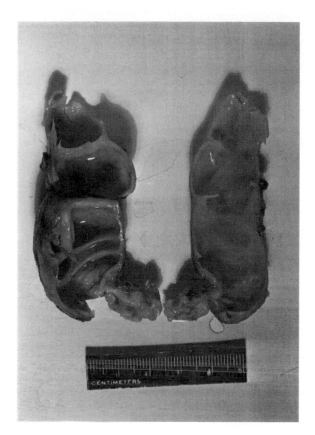

Figure 10.6 Esophageal duplication in a 5-week-old male infant. Mucosa was a mixture of squamous and gastric types.

OTHER BRONCHOPULMONARY FOREGUT MALFORMATIONS

Pulmonary sequestrations are occasionally associated with bronchogenic cysts located between the sequestration and the esophagus, probably resulting from residual nests of tissue along the migratory path. This finding suggests a common embryologic origin (18, 26).

MISCELLANEOUS DISORDERS

DIVERTICULA

Three rare types of congenital esophageal diverticula are described: (*a*) hypopharyngeal-esophageal, arising posteriorly from the same region as pulsion diverticula in adults, but with a complete muscular wall; (*b*) diverticula of the midesophagus usually associated with the tracheoesophageal fistula/esophageal atresia complex; (*c*) epiphrenic diverticula of the lower esophagus as part of the dorsal intestinal duplication complex.

IDIOPATHIC MUSCULAR HYPERTROPHY

Hypertrophy of the muscularis propria involving usually the lower one third, but occasionally the whole length, of the esophagus has been reported in children in association with typical hypertrophic pyloric stenosis or segmental muscular hypertrophy elsewhere in the alimentary tract. It has also been described in men over the age of 40 years (27).

HETEROTOPIA

Heterotopic gastric mucosa in the upper esophagus is usually recognized as an "inlet" patch in the otherwise white mucosa (see Chapter 30); heterotopic gastric mucosa in the lower esophagus is associated with chalasia (Fig. 10.7). In addition, ciliated columnar cells, sebaceous glands, thyroid tissue, and ectopic cartilage have also been described in the esophageal wall, especially in premature neonates.

HAMARTOMAS

Vascular malformations are rare in the esophagus, but they may be seen in association with hereditary hemorrhagic telangiectasia (Osler-Rendu-Weber disease). Cystic hygroma (cavernous lymphangioma) of the neck may involve the esophagus and other adjacent organs.

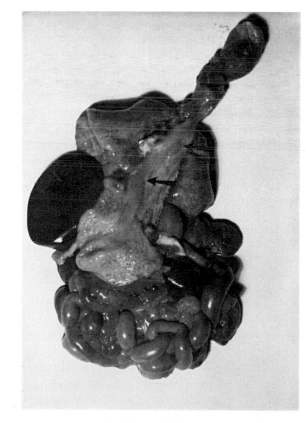

Figure 10.7 Ectopic gastric mucosa associated with chalasia in a 3-week-old infant. Note dilated esophagus and ectopic gastric mucosa in esophagus (*arrow*).

STOMACH

EMBRYOLOGY

During the fourth week of embryogenesis, the tubular stomach, located at the distal part of the foregut, shows a slight fusiform dilation. This enlargement is oriented in the median plane and continues for the following 2 weeks. The stomach enlarges ventrally less than dorsally, resulting in formation of a dorsal "greater curvature." With a slow 90° rotation in a clockwise direction around its longitudinal axis, the long axis of the stomach becomes transverse to the long axis of the body. Accompanying its rotation, the left vagus nerve supplies the anterior wall of the adult stomach and the right vagus nerve supplies the posterior wall. Similarly, the dorsal mesogastrium is carried to the left and forms the omental bursa or lesser sac of peritoneum (1, 28).

ANOMALIES RELATED TO SIZE, POSITION, AND SHAPE

CONGENITAL ABSENCE AND MALPOSITION

Absence of the stomach is reported in abnormal acardiac stillbirths. In addition, it may be located intrathoracically, as seen in cases of anencephaly or in association with a congenital left diaphragmatic hernia, or inverted with the cardia lower than the pylorus with or without diaphragmatic eventration.

DEXTROPOSITION

Dextroposition occurs in complete visceral situs inversus with 1:6000 to 1:8000 incidence or in association with other syndromes. An isolated form is rare, and two types have been described: type I with the stomach behind the liver, and type II with the stomach above the liver and associated with diaphragmatic eventration (29).

MICROGASTRIA

Congenital microgastria or hypoplasia is extremely rare and is thought to occur secondary to lack of its differential growth from the primitive foregut. The stomach keeps its "tubular" or fetal structure and persists in the midline without development of curvatures or rotation. Commonly associated with microgastria are an incompetent cardiac sphincter and a dilated esophagus (30). It may be an isolated phenomenon or part of the Asplenia with Cardiovascular Anomalies Syndrome of Ivemark (31). Feeding in the upright position is the possible treatment rather than surgery in these infants, who usually have a short life expectancy (32).

PYLORIC ATRESIA AND RELATED CONDITIONS

PYLORIC ATRESIA

Pyloric atresia is rare; approximate incidence is 1 in 1 million births (33). It may be complete or partial. In the complete form, the stomach is either totally occluded by an imperforate mucosal and submucosal diaphragm or blindly ended with pyloric aplasia and its fibrous replacement. The complete atresia is an autosomal recessive disorder (34), whether isolated or reported in association with epidermolysis bullosa (35, 36) and trisomy 21. It probably

results secondary to local vascular injury. Symptoms noted soon after birth include nonbilious vomiting, stomach distention, and scaphoid lower abdomen. Treatment involves ablation of the diaphragm or resection of the aplastic pylorus and gastroduodenal anastomosis.

ANTRAL WEB

Congenital pyloric and antral webs or membranes represent, in most cases, the partial form of pyloric atresia. The mucosal diaphragm has a central or an eccentric orifice and is lined by squamous or glandular epithelium. The cause is unknown, but it probably occurs owing to fusion of the developing mucosal folds or failure of recanalization of the gastric lumen during embryogenesis. The condition manifests clinically in childhood if the orifice is small. The majority of cases, however, are detected in adults, and some cases are probably acquired lesions secondary to peptic ulceration (37–39). Treatment usually involves surgical intervention, with or without pyloroplasty, but endoscopic ablation of membranes or diet modification have been described.

CONGENITAL/INFANTILE HYPERTROPHIC PYLORIC STENOSIS

Pyloric stenosis is the most common disorder requiring abdominal surgery in the first 6 months of life. The incidence varies, about 1 in 250 live births, with highest frequency reported in whites; it is rare in persons of Chinese descent (40). Typically, a 3- to 4-week old infant develops projectile, nonbilious vomiting followed by a voracious appetite, visible peristalsis during a test feed, gradual dehydration and constipation, occasionally jaundice, and hypochloremic alkalosis (41). Clinically, the hypertrophic pylorus is palpable, after vomiting or gastric aspiration, as an "olive-like" hypogastric mass. The diagnosis is confirmed by ultrasonic or radiologic evaluation (Fig. 10.8). The treatment of choice is surgical after fluid and electrolytes balance correction. The surgical procedure, Ramstedt pyloromyotomy, consists of dividing the ring of the hypertrophied pyloric circular muscle by a longitudinal

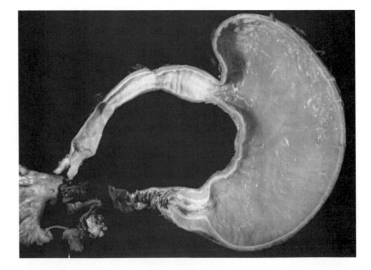

Figure 10.8 Pyloric stenosis with thickened pyloric muscle and narrow lumen in a 2-month-old infant.

incision through the anterior serosa down to the submucosa to release the obstruction. It has an excellent prognosis with rare long-term sequelae (42). Conservative medical therapy with anticholinergic drugs (atropine, scopolamine methyl nitrate) is performed, especially in Scandinavian countries, although it is not popular because it requires extended hospitalization with higher morbidity and mortality.

Pathologically, the pylorus is increased in length and diameter with thickened hypertrophic and hyperplastic circular muscle in addition to mucosal edema and inflammation (42). The stomach is dilated and the antrum is hypertrophic. Peptic ulcers may occur in long-standing cases, associated with "coffee grounds" vomiting or massive hemorrhage. Theories about the etiology of pyloric stenosis are extensive (41). It is believed to be familial with polygenic pattern of nonmendelian sex-modified inheritance, fourfold male predominance, and higher incidence in children of an affected female. It has been reported in association with esophageal atresia, hiatus hernia, partial thoracic stomach, malrotation, phenylketonuria, maternal myasthenia gravis, Hirschsprung's disease, polycystic kidneys, Smith-Lemli-Opitz syndrome, Cornelia deLange Amsterdam dwarf syndrome, trisomy 18, long arm deletion 21, Turner's syndrome (XO), XYY gonadal dysgenesis, chromosomal mosaicism, and rubella embryopathy. Other factors reported to affect its expression are being a first-born male, high birth weight, breast feeding, blood group (B, O, or AB), and season variations, with peaks in spring and autumn. Recent studies (43–46) have shown a deficiency of vasoactive intestinal peptide, enkephalin, neuropeptide Y, substance P, and nitric oxide in the circular muscle, but not in the myenteric plexus, considered as a possible underlying cause of the pyloric hypertrophy. Previous pathogenetic hypotheses, including pylorospasm, decrease and immaturity of myenteric plexus ganglion cells (47), changes in cardiac/skeletal muscle enzyme ratios, and effects of maternal gastrin, are currently less accepted.

Adult hypertrophic pyloric stenosis is occasionally seen in young to middle-aged adults. With symptomatology similar to that of the infantile form, this condition is considered by some to be a late manifestation of the congenital form of pyloric stenosis (41, 48, 49). Its exact incidence and etiology, however, are still unknown.

CYSTS AND DUPLICATIONS
GASTRIC DUPLICATION

Gastric duplications are cystic or tubular lesions surrounded by smooth muscle that is continuous with the muscle of the stomach (50, 51), excluding esophageal dorsal enteric or neurenteric cysts and diverticula. Adherence and fusion of proliferating gastric longitudinal folds during fetal life has been suggested as an underlying mechanism to their formation (52). The lining of duplications, unless destroyed by inflammation, usually represents a mixture of epithelia, gastric most frequently, with possible pancreatic heterotopia. These lesions occur most often along the greater curvature in children, typically infants, and can be detected incidentally or manifest as bleeding, vomiting with extrinsic compression and obstruction, perforation, or fistulization into adjacent organs. Most of the cystic lesions range in size from 3 to 6 cm and less than 12 cm, and the tubular forms communicate with the stomach (Fig. 10.9). Associated malformations include vertebral

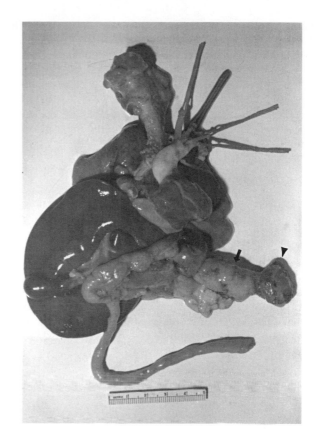

Figure 10.9 Gastric duplication attached to stomach *(tailed arrow)*. Rounded portion of its duplication *(right arrow)* was above diaphragm and contained respiratory tissue.

anomalies, other foregut complete duplication or malformations, but most frequently esophageal duplication.

DIVERTICULA

Gastric diverticula, mostly acquired in adults, communicate with the gastric lumen and have a thin wall containing few strands of smooth muscle and covered by serosa. True congenital gastric diverticula with full muscular walls that manifest in childhood may be considered gastric duplications.

CONGENITAL DOUBLE PYLORUS

Two pyloric channels connecting the stomach and the duodenum and separated by a septum are the usual findings. Most reported cases are acquired and considered gastroduodenal fistulas secondary to ulceration. Rare congenital septa with mucosa, submucosa, and occasional ectopic pancreatic tissue may be considered a special form of communicating tubular gastric duplication (53).

MISCELLANEOUS DISORDERS
SPONTANEOUS RUPTURE OF THE STOMACH

Several mechanisms may cause spontaneous gastric perforation in infancy, but the most common factors are trauma or infection. A localized congenital gastric muscular defect has been reported, however, and may be the underlying lesion. This theory has been challenged because retraction of ruptured muscle fibers surrounding the perforation may occur (54, 55).

HETEROTOPIA (SEE CHAPTER 25)

Pancreatic heterotopia is common in adults, but it can affect children, manifesting as peptic ulcer or intermittent pyloric obstruction.

HAMARTOMAS (SEE CHAPTERS 14 AND 26)

Adenomyomas are mucosal and submucosal hamartomatous malformations of glands and smooth muscle that may occur anywhere in the stomach and duodenum but are found mostly in the lower part of the stomach and the pyloric antrum. Gastric Peutz-Jeghers polyps have branching, polypoid structure, with a central core of smooth muscle fibers and connective tissue, that is similar to that seen in the small and large intestine but with secretory cells and tubules of pyloric gland type. Angiomas represent occasional causes of occult gastrointestinal blood loss and chronic anemia. Gastric lymphangiomas are rare.

INTESTINES

EMBRYOLOGY

The small and large intestines derive from the distal or caudal portion of the foregut, midgut, and hindgut, parts of the endodermal tube formed secondary to craniocaudal and lateral embryonal folding and incorporation of the dorsal part of the yolk sac into the embryo about the fourth week. The duodenum, proximal to the hepatic bud or bile duct origin, is formed by the foregut portion distal to the stomach, and its vascular supply comes from the celiac truncus. Its portion distal to the bile duct, as well as the jejunum, ileum, cecum, ascending colon, and proximal one half or two thirds of the transverse colon, derive from the midgut, supplied by the superior mesenteric artery. During the fifth week of embryonic life, the midgut is a U-shaped loop and is suspended by dorsal mesentery around the superior mesenteric artery. The loop apex communicates with the vitelline duct or yolk stalk, which is rapidly decreasing in size. During the sixth week, the midgut growth causes its "physiologic herniation" into the umbilical cord, resulting from the lack of space within the small abdominal cavity partially filled by the large liver and the two "meso- and metanephroi" sets of kidneys (1, 28). The cranial limb of the midgut loop lengthens, faster than the caudal limb, and coils, giving rise to the jejunum and most of the ileum. The caudal limb shows the cecal enlargement or diverticulum, which is conical to this point, with the tapered end forming the appendix. In addition to this growth, the midgut loop rotates 90° counterclockwise around the superior mesenteric artery (from a ventral view). Subsequently, the cecum is located to the left of the mesenteric artery and the duodenum to its right. Meanwhile, the peritoneal coelum or abdominal cavity capacity increases, an additional progressive counterclockwise 180° rotation of the midgut starts, while the midgut starts sliding back into the abdomen between the 10th and 12th weeks of embryonic life. The small intestine returns first, and its loops fill the central region.

The colon follows and occupies the periphery, with the cecum being last to return into the right iliac fossa, anterior to the duodenum and the superior mesenteric artery, and below the liver. At this stage, the colon has an almost straight oblique position between the spleen and the right iliac fossa. Later, the colon angulates where it crosses the duodenum, to which it becomes fixed and forms the hepatic flexure as the liver decreases in size. The distal transverse colon, descending colon, and sigmoid colon, derivatives of the hindgut supplied by the inferior mesenteric artery, further occupy the left abdominal periphery, thus completing the colonic "picture frame" around the small bowel. The rectum and proximal anal canal also derive from the hindgut; their formation is discussed in the following section. The gut muscular wall and serosa derive from the splanchnic mesoderm.

The lumen of the intestines, namely the duodenum around the hepatic bud, is transiently obliterated by epithelial proliferation and subsequently recanalized by vacuolation, toward the end of the embryonic period. Most of the duodenum, pressed against the right posterior abdominal wall by the colon, becomes retroperitoneal. Similarly, the ascending and descending colon mesentery fuses with the parietal peritoneum. The transverse colon mesentery fuses with part of the greater omentum and forms the transverse mesocolon. The sigmoid colon retains its mesentery free, the sigmoid mesocolon. The fan-shaped mesentery of the small bowel has a broad base of attachment to the posterior wall extending obliquely from the duodenojejunal junction to the ileocecal area.

ANOMALIES RELATED TO SIZE, POSITION, AND SHAPE

SHORT BOWEL

A congenital short small intestine may be seen incidentally or, more often, in association with gastroschisis or omphalocele, intestinal malrotation, duplication, and atresia (56–58).

ANOMALIES OF INTESTINAL ROTATION

Different types of abnormal, incomplete, or failed rotation of the midgut are described with secondary anomalies of fixation (1, 59–64).

Nonrotation

Nonrotation occurs when the midgut loop fails to rotate an additional 180° as it returns to the abdomen. The small bowel occupies the right side of the abdomen, including the duodenum that lacks its "C" configuration and lies vertically to the right of the superior mesenteric vessels. The colon is left sided and the ileum enters the cecum from the right side. Secondary nonfixation of the mesentery results in persistence of its narrow root, predisposing to volvulus and infarction. This malformation may be subclinical or may manifest in either neonatal or adult life as the only abnormality or associated with diaphragmatic hernia and exomphalos.

Mixed or Incomplete Rotation

This situation occurs when only the caudal limb of the midgut loop rotates an additional 90° beyond the first counterclockwise 90° rotation of both limbs of the midgut (see discussion of embryol-

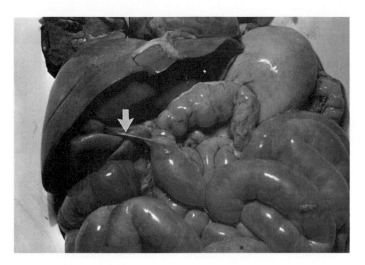

Figure 10.10 Hepatoduodenocolic band *(arrow)* causing partial obstruction of the colon in a 5-month-old infant.

ogy). As a result, the cecum is subpyloric, with partial fixation to the posterior abdominal wall by fibrous bands (Ladd's) that pass over the duodenum, occasionally causing its extrinsic obstruction (Fig. 10.10). The small bowel is right-sided with a narrow mesenteric root.

Mixed or incomplete rotation is the most common type of malrotation. Symptoms that occur in early life include bile-stained vomiting and abdominal distention, when associated with duodenal obstruction or volvulus. Intrinsic stenosis or atresia of bowel, diaphragmatic hernia, esophageal atresia, and omphalocele may accompany this anomaly, and it is seen also in association with trisomies 21, 18, 13 and other syndromes.

Reversed Rotation

This malformation occurs when the midgut loop rotates its additional 180° in an opposite clockwise fashion (see discussion of embryology). The duodenum and superior mesenteric vessels are anterior to the transverse colon, hence placed in a retroarterial mesenteric tunnel where extrinsic compression can occur. This malrotation type is rare, may be associated with situs inversus, and usually manifests in adult life. Ileocecal volvulus may also occur secondary to impaired mesenteric fixation.

SUBHEPATIC CECUM AND APPENDIX

After the physiologic herniation of the midgut loop and its rotation, the cecum returns last into the abdominal cavity, to a subhepatic location in the right iliac fossa. In 6% of fetuses, more commonly males, the cecum adheres to the liver and is subsequently retracted with it to the right upper abdominal quadrant. The importance of this anomalous position is the differential diagnosis of appendicitis.

VOLVULUS

Several congenital anomalies predispose to torsion of loops of intestine, secondary vascular ischemia, and infarction. Malrotation, as described previously, is associated with abnormal mesenteric fixation and a narrow root around which loops of intestine can easily

twist. Other factors that may contribute to volvulus with normal rotation include abnormal mesenteric fixation, herniation, gastroschisis, exomphalos, meconium ileus, peritoneal adhesions, intraabdominal vestigial fibrous bands (Fig. 10.11), or persistent omphlomesenteric duct remnants. A common example of abnormal mesenteric fixation is the "mobile cecum" seen in 10% of the population, the result of incomplete fusion of the ascending colon and/or ileal mesentery with the posterior abdominal wall. A cecal or ileocecal volvulus can result in this group of patients. Similarly, sigmoid volvulus can result from an incompletely adherent mesocolon, more frequently from an enlarged or distended loop of sigmoid colon.

INTESTINAL ATRESIA AND STENOSIS

The frequency and types of atresia and stenosis vary in different parts of the intestine. Atresia is more common in the duodenum than in the jejunum, ileum, or colon (65–67). Atresia may occur secondary to a deficient segment of bowel or an occlusive diaphragm, resulting in total interruption of bowel lumen. Similarly, different pathogenetic mechanisms have been implicated in their causation. Duodenal atresia likely results from failure of vacuolization and recanalization of the normally rapid obliterative epithelial proliferation "solid stage" that occurs during the eighth week of embryogenesis (68). Another etiologic mechanism could be the result of discordant, segmentally impaired epithelial proliferation during the rapid intestinal lengthening, producing an

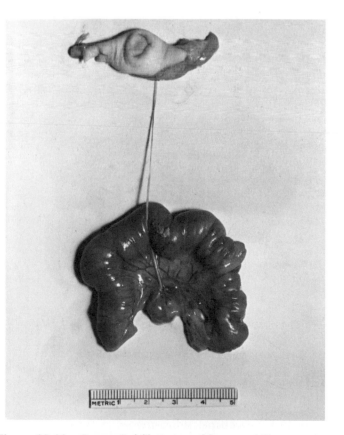

Figure 10.11 Congenital fibrous cord from umbilicus to mesentery, possibly representing obliterated vitelline vessels.

atretic or stenotic segment. Vascular injury is rarely implicated in duodenal atresia and stenosis, in contrast to the remaining intestine. In the jejunum, ileum, and colon, most atresias or stenoses result from a vascular insult occurring later during fetal life. This injury may be reflected by the presence of scarring; deposits of calcium; hemosiderin; meconium granulomas at their level, with possible meconium; squamous epithelial cells; lanugo hair; and keratin distal to it.

DUODENAL ATRESIA

Duodenal atresia occurs in 1 in 5000 live births and is the third most common cause of gastrointestinal congenital intrinsic obstruction after imperforate anus and esophageal atresia (Fig. 10.12). Atresia occurs less frequently than stenosis in its proximal portion, and it is rarely associated with jejunoileal atresia. From 25 to 30% of patients with Down's syndrome have this condition, and it is frequently associated with malrotation and annular pancreas, as well as extraabdominal abnormalities, such as esophageal atresia, tracheoesophageal fistula, anorectal anomalies, renal and cardiac malformations, and thalidomide-induced embryopathy (69).

Clinically, associated elevated levels of maternal serum α-fetoprotein and polyhydramnios (50% of cases) may be detected during pregnancy (70). Real-time ultrasonography during fetal life and neonatal abdominal radiography can identify the "double-

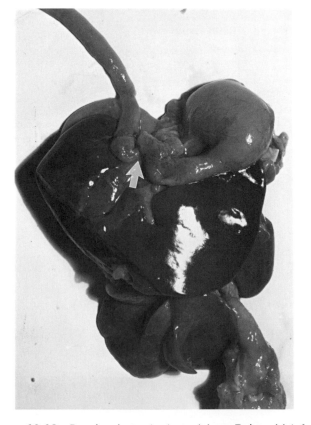

Figure 10.12 Duodenal atresia *(arrow)* in a 7-day-old infant with multiple congenital anomalies.

bubble" appearance corresponding to the distended stomach and duodenum, separated by pylorus. Neonatal postfeeding vomiting is usually bilious. With duodenal stenosis, the symptoms may be intermittent or delayed for weeks to years. Meconium may be passed. Approximately 54% of patients are premature by birth weight, and one third may become jaundiced.

Morphologically, two types of atresia may be seen: discontinuous bowel with an intermediate fibrous cord, and a gap usually replaced by pancreas (49 to 65%), or mucosa-lined membranous atresia (19 to 41%).

JEJUNAL AND ILEAL ATRESIA

Jejunoileal atresias occur less frequently than does duodenal atresia (1:6000 live births). The majority likely develop after embryogenesis secondary to ischemic injury (71), rather than because of failure of vacuolization of the fifth to eighth week intraluminal epithelial growth as seen in the duodenum (68). This hypothesis is supported by the possible identification of intestinal intraluminal bile/meconium, squamous cells, and hair distal to the atresia, intestinal infarction, and peritonitis, in the absence of intestinal perforation (72, 73).

Atresias are also described after in-utero intussusception (74), congenital syphilis with mesenteric arteritis (75), maternal shock and hypotension (76), and maternal ingestion of Cafergot (Sandoz Pharmaceutical, East Hanover, NJ) (77). The findings resemble secondary obstructions complicating postnatal necrotizing enterocolitis, and have been similarly reproduced in experimental animal studies. Atresias are rarely associated with extraabdominal malformations (78); local abnormalities predisposing to volvulus and ischemia, such as malrotation, meconium ileus, omphalomesenteric remnants, gastroschisis, or exomphalos, are frequently present (79). Nevertheless, failure of recanalization of the "solid stage" may explain the rare familial occurrence of multiple atresias with mucosal diaphragms affecting the intestine from the pylorus to the sigmoid colon (80).

Atresia frequently affects the distal ileum (36%) and proximal jejunum (31%). If the atresia is distal, the abdominal distention is more generalized and the vomiting is delayed and fecal (Fig. 10.13).

Four morphologic types are distinguished: type I—atresia with mucosa-lined diaphragm and intact muscularis propria and mesentery; type II—fibrous cord conjoining two blind-end adjacent bowel segments with loss of lumen and muscular wall continuity; type III—the most frequent, in which a V-shaped defect of mesentery is present between the two blind-ended bowel segments; and type IV—multiple atresias. In all types, the proximal intestinal segment wall is thickened and its lumen is distended by fecal material, usually without flattening of villi as may be seen with meconium ileus.

A special variety of type III atresia of distal duodenal or proximal jejunal is called "Apple peel" atresia, "maypole deformity," or "Christmas tree." It has a familial, probable autosomal recessive inheritance, and possibly is attributable to a narrow mesentery attachment, volvulus, and occlusion of the superior mesenteric artery distal to its proximal branches (81, 82). As a result, a large defect of mesentery accompanies the atresia, with the remaining short intestine coiled around the ileocecal artery, which is a branch of the patent proximal mesenteric artery.

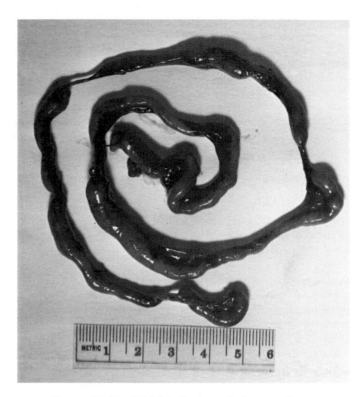

Figure 10.13 Multiple ileal atresia in a newborn.

HERNIAS, DUPLICATIONS, AND CONGENITAL DIVERTICULA

MESOCOLIC HERNIAS

Also called mesentericoparietal or paraduodenal hernias, mesocolic hernias result from an abnormal return of the midgut, after its physiologic herniation, into a defect of mesenteric attachment with formation of a retroperitoneal sac (59, 83, 84). If the descending mesocolon fails to adhere to the posterior parietal peritoneum, the small bowel can herniate into the formed sac between these layers, resulting in what is classified as a left paraduodenal hernia. Similarly, a right paraduodenal hernia can occur in a sac formed by a nonadherent ascending mesocolon and the posterior parietal peritoneum. The superior mesenteric vessels course near the orifice of the right hernia sac, whereas the inferior mesenteric vessels run near the more frequently occurring left paraduodenal hernia orifice. If a defect occurs in the transverse mesocolon, a transmesocolic or omentomesenteric parietal hernia may occur, with the middle colic artery coursing the right side of the sac orifice (Fig. 10.14). Other internal hernias may occur around the ileocecal valve, the bladder, and at the foramen of Winslow (85), independent from congenital anomalies.

These hernias are usually asymptomatic until prolapse or strangulation occur at their foramina, usually in adulthood.

DIAPHRAGMATIC HERNIAS

Agenesis of one or both leaflets of the diaphragm, defective formation with herniation, and aplasia of muscle with eventration

are congenital anomalies frequently associated with gastrointestinal and respiratory involvement. The septum transversum gives rise first to the ventral portion of the diaphragm, followed by the growth of the dorsolateral pleuroperitoneal folds, and posteromedially by a portion derived from the primitive mesentery. Hence, the thoracic and abdominal cavities are separated by the eighth to ninth weeks of gestation. When any part of these embryonic elements fail to grow, a gap is formed and, depending on the size and location, abdominal organs herniate through it, into the thoracic cavity, with secondary pulmonary hypoplasia.

Posterolateral hernias through the foramina of Bochdalek, more frequently left-sided (65 to 80%) and unilateral, are the most common, noted in 1 in 2,000 to 5,000 births (86, 87). Cyanosis and dyspnea are usually the earliest neonatal manifestation; gasping, vomiting, and eventually death occur in most untreated patients with severe pulmonary hypoplasia, worsened by intrathoracic bowel air-distention and/or incarceration. Respiratory movements and breath sounds are decreased or absent, with audible peristaltic sounds in the affected hemithorax. Right posterolateral hernias have less pulmonary implications because of interposition of the liver. Malrotation of the bowel with a narrow mesenteric root and abnormal fixation are frequently associated findings.

The outcome of surgical repair depends primarily on the degree of pulmonary hypoplasia, with improved survival by use of postoperative extracorporeal membrane oxygenation and currently limited intrauterine surgery success. Eventration of the diaphragm, secondary to muscular aplasia, occurs less frequently than posterolateral defects; usually affects males (62%); and is unilateral (85%), predominantly affecting the right side (67%). The fusion of pleura and peritoneum produces a sac that usually limits the intrathoracic protrusion of abdominal organs; hence, eventrations are most commonly subclinical, unless extensive, and may be accompanied by ipsilateral absent or paradoxic diaphragmatic movements.

HIATAL HERNIAS

These hernias occur through the esophageal hiatus, and are of the paraesophageal and sliding types. In the paraesophageal hernia, the

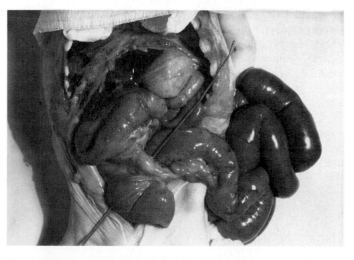

Figure 10.14 Mesenteric defect (probe) with mesenteric hernia and volvulus in an infant.

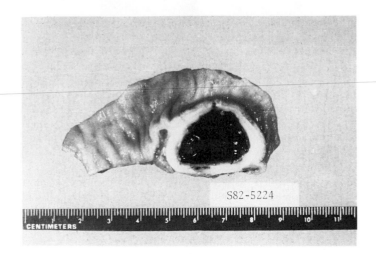

Figure 10.15 Duplication cyst of the ileum in a 10-day-old infant contains bloody mucus.

gastric fundus is intrathoracic, usually within a peritoneal sac, while the gastroesophageal junction is still below the diaphragm. In the sliding hernia, more frequent in women, the gastroesophageal junction, cardia, and part of the fundus may be intrathoracic.

RETROSTERNAL HERNIA

Parts of the transverse colon, liver, and stomach, and rarely the small bowel, pass through the foramen of Morgagni, usually on the right side (88). A peritoneal sac is identified in about 50% of cases. These patients are mostly asymptomatic until adulthood.

PERITONEOPERICARDIAL HERNIA

Less frequently, defective formation of the septum transversum results in a midline communication between the peritoneal and pericardial sacs (89). They can be associated with a supraumbilical midline defect of the abdominal wall, such as an omphalocele, a cleft of the distal sternum, and an intracardiac defect. This combination of anomalies, called pentalogy of Cantrell or thoracoabdominal ectopia cordis, may be associated with trisomy 18 (90). The associated cardiac anomalies may include a ventricular or atrial septal defect, tetralogy of Fallot, atrioventricularis communis, or a diverticulum of the left ventricle (91).

UMBILICAL HERNIAS

Congenital umbilical hernias, secondary to imperfect closure or weakness of the umbilical ring, are frequent in low-birth weight or black infants (92). Spontaneous regression is the rule by 6 to 12 months and up to 6 years. Unless the hernia is larger than 4 cm, is enlarging, and contains omentum or a part of the small intestine, surgical closure is not required.

EPIGASTRIC HERNIAS

Epigastric hernias are rare small defects of the linea alba or adjacent wall, usually with preperitoneal fat herniation, that occur between the umbilicus and the xiphoid process.

INGUINAL HERNIAS

Indirect inguinal hernias may be congenital and frequently occur in premature males, especially with cryptorchidism and hydrocele. The small intestine, or sometimes the appendix, may herniate into the sac, with risk of incarceration. This incarceration is associated with groin pain, irreducible swelling, vomiting, fever, and eventually an acute abdomen. Occasionally, the result is infarction of the ipsilateral testis or, in affected females, herniation of a fallopian tube or ovary.

DUPLICATIONS

Intestinal duplications (dorsal neurenteric cysts) may be closed cystic, ovoid, or spherical structures that vary from a few millimeters to 10 to 15 cm in diameter; they may also appear as communicating tubular, elongated structures (93). Duplications are lined by functioning intestinal mucosa with a wall composed of smooth muscle; they are always dorsal to the intestine, usually within the mesentery between the spinal cord and the intestine, and sometimes intramural. Pathogenetically, they are thought to originate secondary to abnormal recanalization of the intestinal "solid stage" lumen obliterated by epithelial proliferation, and/or persistence of outpouchings of the intestine that have been observed during embryogenesis and intrauterine intestinal ischemia (94–96). Their frequent association with vertebral clefts and rib anomalies suggests another possible explanation, such as failure of complete separation of the foregut and notochord. They communicate occasionally with the lumen of the bowel, but their surgical removal frequently requires the removal of normal bowel as well, because the vascular supply to the normal bowel usually runs along the wall of the duplication (Fig. 10.15).

Tubular duplications usually lie closely parallel to the intestine, often communicate with the lumen of the intestine in their distal portion, and share the muscular layer (Fig. 10.16). Cases of extension along entire small bowel and/or colon are reported

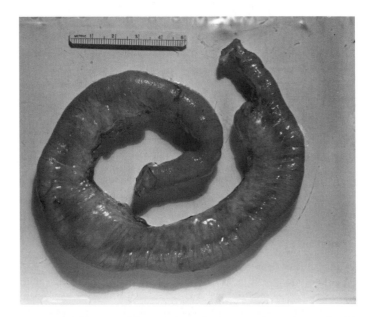

Figure 10.16 Small bowel ileal duplication in a 4-month-old infant.

(97–99). When distended by mucus accumulation, cystic or tubular duplications may cause extrinsic compression and intestinal obstruction, or provoke intussusception (mostly seen with small intramural cysts) or volvulus. Most cases affect the terminal ileum (50%) and are usually single; however, they may be associated with multiple abdominal and thoracic duplications.

Duplications of the duodenum are rare. They usually are noncommunicating, may be submucosal, are separated by only a scanty muscularis, and bulge into the lumen of the adjoining bowel. Small intestine duplications may be palpable and, because they may be partially calcified, are radiographically detectable as a curvilinear density on abdominal radiographs, and associated with intermittent pain, melena, or intussusception. Duplications of the large bowel may be associated with abnormalities of the bladder, Mullerian structures, external genitalia and urethra, or anorectal region. In one case of triplication of the entire large intestine, the patient had ovaries, but no uterus, and exstrophy of the bladder. Most duplications manifest in the newborn period or early childhood, less frequently in adult life, with 22:10 female predominance.

Duplicated ani with or without genitourinary fistula and imperforate anus may be associated with duplicated or septate bladder with double urethral openings, two uteri and duplication of the vagina, two penes or two clitora or combinations of the above, and extrapelvic anomalies. The associated abnormalities range from Meckel's diverticulum, double-headed monsters, double hemiliver with duplication of the lumbar spine but absent sacrum and anterior myelomeningocele, to an infant with four lower limbs. Renal anomalies such as horseshoe kidneys, duplex kidney, unilateral agenesis, and renal dysplasia are less frequent. Although isolated duplication can be removed surgically, even when extensive, complex malformations are harder to manage and may be fatal.

Intestinal obstruction secondary to compression of normal adjacent bowel or intussusception, pain, gastrointestinal hemorrhage, or a palpable abdominal mass are the usual clinical manifestations. Bleeding may be caused by peptic ulceration, intestinal ischemia secondary to altered blood supply by mass effect, or by intussusception. Peptic ulcers may occur within the duplication, usually at the gastrointestinal mucosal junction within the duplication or at its communication with the normal bowel. The wall of a duplication is thick and muscular, containing one, two, or even three layers of smooth muscle with identifiable Auerbach's plexuses. The mucosal lining of the duplication may be gastric, intestinal, or pseudostratified ciliated columnar mucosa with occasional heterotopic pancreatic tissue.

CONGENITAL DIVERTICULA

Identification of all layers of the bowel wall, including the muscularis propria, around the diverticula is required to differentiate true from false diverticula. The pathology of Meckel's diverticulum is discussed in the section concerning cord-related abnormalities. True "non-Meckelian" antimesenteric congenital diverticula of the small bowel are rare. Multiple upper jejunal diverticula are reported in association with multiple congenital anomalies, and represent probably unsuppressed pancreatic diverticula (100).

True diverticula of the colon affect mostly the cecum and ascending colon, and are rarely reported in infants (101). Clinical manifestations include rectal bleeding and diverticulitis, misdiagnosed as appendicitis when the diverticulum arise in the cecum. About 3% of appendiceal diverticula are congenital, with an esti-

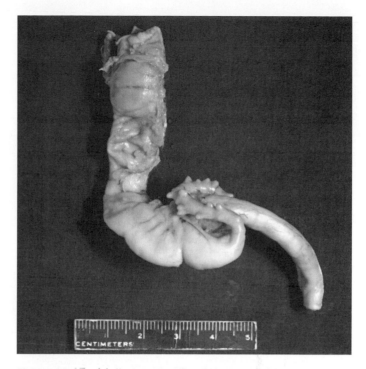

Figure 10.17 Multiple appendiceal diverticula in a patient with D trisomy.

mated incidence of 0.65% (102–104). They may be simple or multiple, as seen in the D1 trisomy syndrome (Fig. 10.17). Some of these diverticula derive from the yolk stalk or a distally placed Meckel's diverticulum.

CORD-RELATED ABNORMALITIES

OMPHALOCELE AND GASTROSCHISIS

An omphalocele or exomphalos is the persistent herniation of abdominal viscera through a defect in the umbilical and supraumbilical portions of the abdominal wall into a sac lined by peritoneum internally and amniotic membrane externally, where patches of mucoid material (Wharton's jelly) may be visible (105–108). The abdominal skin may cover the sac base, and the umbilical cord is usually attached to its apex or slightly eccentric. The umbilical arteries and vein can be seen through its mostly avascular wall. One third of patients with large omphalocele have a single umbilical artery.

Omphalocele occurs in about 1 in 6,000 live births, and traditionally, this lesion has been considered secondary to failure of normal intestinal return (10th to 12th week) into the abdominal cavity after the "physiologic hernia" into the yolk stalk. Another hypothesis cites an earlier (third week) embryogenetic defect of formation of the normal lateral folds of the ventral embryonic wall, causing secondary widening of the umbilical ring. The latter theory is supported by the frequent association of multiple organ anomalies in contrast with gastroschisis. Such malformations include vesicointestinal fistula; intestinal atresia and malrotation; imperforate anus; colonic agenesis; bladder exstrophy; defects in the sternum, diaphragm, or pericardium; central nervous system defects; and congenital heart disease (25% of cases, namely, Tetralogy of Fallot). Omphalocele may represent one manifestation of the Beckwith-

Wiedemann syndrome (109; gigantism; macroglossia; hemihypertrophy; visceromegaly, especially of the liver and kidneys; hypoglycemia; and omphalocele or umbilical hernia), or may be associated with chromosomal anomalies, e.g., trisomy 13 and 18 (110).

Omphaloceles vary in size, from a few centimeters to near absence of the anterior abdominal wall. Loops of small bowel are usually identified in the sac, and sometimes with parts of proximal colon, liver, stomach, spleen, and pancreas. A small omphalocele, less than 4 cm, is a hernia into the umbilical cord, and may be recognized only in cases complicated with intestinal obstruction and fecal fistula formation after ligation of the cord (Fig. 10.18). The wall of the sac is initially moist and transparent, and becomes dry, opaque, and somewhat friable, prone to rupture and secondary evisceration. In cases of early rupture of the exomphalos sac, before or during delivery, it is important to distinguish it from gastroschisis, based on its umbilical involvement. When vomiting occurs in an infant with an omphalocele, intestinal obstruction secondary to volvulus or adhesions should be excluded.

Gastroschisis, less common than an omphalocele, results from an extraumbilical defect of the ventral abdominal wall, lateral to the linea alba, and usually to the right of the umbilicus (106–108). A possible etiology is an abnormality of the umbilical cord, forcing the midgut to herniate through the abdominal wall. No amnioperito-

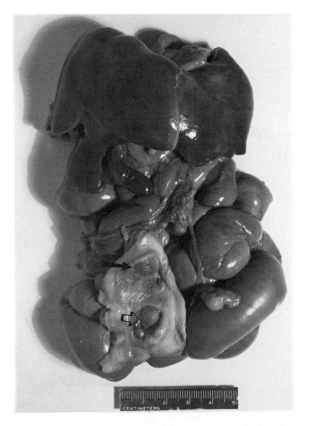

Figure 10.18 Small, gradually decreasing omphalocele *(solid arrow)* in a 45-day-old infant associated with multiple congenital anomalies including cloacal exstrophy *(hollow arrow)* where a small prolapsed bowel opening and subjacent bifid penis are seen.

neal sac is identified and the herniated organs, previously exposed to amniotic fluid, have a dull surface, thickened wall, serositis, and adhesions.

Primary surgical repair of these abdominal wall defects and closure is preferred whenever possible. Otherwise, staged closure using prosthetic materials is performed with adequate nutritional and metabolic support. Late intestinal obstruction is possible in cases associated with malrotation. Motility disturbances may follow repair of gastroschisis. Mental retardation and growth failure correlates with length of hospital stay and level of prematurity.

MECKEL'S DIVERTICULUM

Omphalomesenteric duct remnants result from an abnormal persistent patency or fibrous replacement of the vitello-intestinal or omphalomesenteric duct that connects the midgut to the yolk sac during embryogenesis. Normally, this duct becomes detached from the bowel before the physiologic herniation and subsequently regresses before the return of the bowel into the abdominal cavity. Depending on the site and extent of its patency or fibrous cord formation, different anomalies result (111, 112; Fig. 10.19).

Meckel's diverticulum results from patency of the proximal enteric end of the vitello-intestinal duct. It is the most common congenital intestinal anomaly, seen in about 2% of the general population and identified in 3.2% of patients undergoing appendectomies (113, 114). Its incidence is equal in both sexes, and higher in patients with trisomy syndromes and central nervous and cardiovascular anomalies.

The diverticulum is located on the antimesenteric border of the terminal ileum, usually 40 to 50 cm from the ileocecal valve (Fig. 10.20), although it can be situated anywhere between the cecum and rarely up to the jejunum. Its vascular supply is the proximal portion of the right omphalomesenteric artery in continuity with the superior mesenteric artery. The diverticulum can be fixed to the ileum by its mesentery, the tip usually being free, although it can be attached to the umbilicus, abdominal wall, or mesentery in 25% of cases by a fibrous cord that may contain remnants of the omphalomesenteric artery. The diverticulum length is usually between 1 and 5 cm (75%), but it can reach 26 cm. Longer diverticula that curled around the ileum and became adherent to the mesentery have been reported, as well as Pollard's case of a 90-cm long Meckel's diverticulum that extended into the umbilical cord and probably represented the entire yolk stalk. The diverticulum diameter is about 2 cm, equal to or smaller than that of the attached ileum, usually with a broad base. Its wall contains all layers of bowel. Its mucosa is predominantly ileal with gastric (43 to 81%) and pancreatic (3.2 to 5.4%) heterotopia, in addition to occasional duodenal and colonic mucosa. Eighty-five percent of represented gastric mucosa is of the fundic type (115). This heterotopia may contribute to the appearance of a nodular or bifid tip.

Most Meckel's diverticula are asymptomatic and are identified incidentally; however, 22 to 34% of diverticula cause disease, more frequently in males and during the neonatal period or childhood. The most frequent clinical manifestations are hemorrhage, intermittent or massive, and pain, unrelieved by food or antacids when gastric heterotopia is associated with ulcer formation, frequently affecting the adjacent ileal mucosa. Other presentations include intestinal obstruction secondary to intussusception (Fig. 10.21)

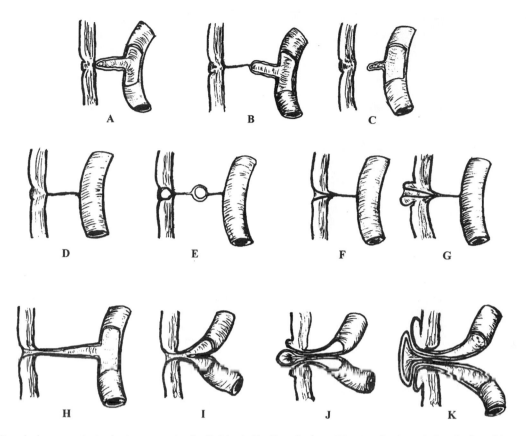

Figure 10.19 Omphalomesenteric duct remnants. **A–C.** Meckel's diverticulum (tip attached to abdominal wall in **A** and **B**). **D.** Solid fibrous cord attaching the ileum to body wall. **E.** Vitelline cysts. **F.** Umbilical sinus. **G.** Umbilical polyp. **H–K.** Umbilical fistula (**I–K.** Different degrees of ileal prolapse through patent omphalomesenteric duct).

with the diverticulum as the leading point (36.5%), or secondary to volvulus or internal hernia due to a vestigial umbilicodiverticular fibrous band. Obstruction can also result from incarceration of a herniated Meckel's diverticulum (Littre's hernia) in an inguinal (50%), umbilical, or femoral hernia. Diverticulitis is usually confused preoperatively with acute appendicitis. When diverticular rupture or infarction occur, meconium or generalized peritonitis results (116). In addition, Meckel's diverticula can harbor neoplasia, such as carcinoid tumors, adenocarcinomas, and benign and malignant stromal tumors, again more frequently in males (117). Hence, most authors favor resection of Meckel's diverticula.

OTHER OMPHALOMESENTERIC DUCT REMNANTS

Umbilical Sinus and Polyp

These lesions result from patency of the distal umbilical end of the vitello-intestinal duct, and may be associated with Meckel's diverticulum connected by a fibrous cord. The umbilical sinus is a tract that extends at a variable depth into the abdominal wall or cavity. The umbilical polyp or umbilical adenoma projects above the abdominal surface frequently with a central dimple or sinus that may extend into the abdominal wall (see Fig. 10.19). Both are lined by gastric or ileal mucosa, and occasionally contain pancreatic rests,

with mucus discharge, in contrast to umbilical granuloma formed by granulation tissue with seropurulent discharge. These lesions should be excised to avoid recurrent infections.

Umbilical Cyst

This rare lesion, also called enterocystoma, results from patency of the midportion of the vitello-intestinal duct, while the proximal ileal or distal umbilical ends involute (see Fig. 10.19). The cyst may be connected to the ileum or umbilicus with fibrous bands, and usually is located at any level in between them. Therefore, it may resemble a duplication cyst, but it can be excised without compromise of the blood supply to the intestine. Its wall contains all bowel layers and its mucosa is usually gastric.

Umbilical Fistula

This entity is also called omphaloileal fistula or patent Meckel's diverticulum, in which the entire length of the yolk stalk fails to involute and remains patent, connecting the ileum to the umbilicus. In about 20% of cases (predominantly males), prolapse of the duct or the ileum occurs, appearing as an umbilical polyp with a central opening or as a central protrusion and peripheral circumferential opening (118). If bisected, prolapsed ileal walls and lumen resemble a double-barrel, Y, or T (Figs. 10.19 and 10.22). The mucosa is ileal

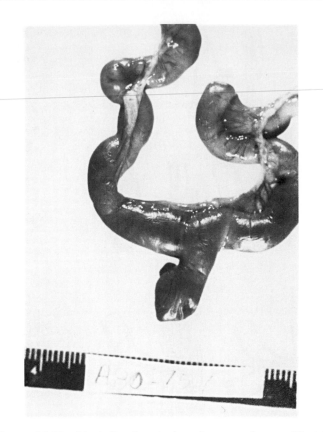

Figure 10.20 Meckel's diverticulum in a newborn with trisomy 18.

or gastric. Fecal drainage from the umbilical orifice and symptomatic intestinal obstruction with prolapse are the usual manifestations in early life and require emergency surgical repair.

AGANGLIONIC MEGACOLON

PATHOGENESIS

Also known as Hirschsprung's disease, this condition is defined by the absence of ganglion cells in a segment of bowel, usually the rectosigmoid colon, in intermuscular Auerbach's, deep submucosal Henle's, and submucosal Meissner's plexuses (119). The lack of ganglion cells results in absence of intrinsic purinergic nonadrenergic (adenosine triphosphate, serotonin, VIP, and substance P) inhibitory innervation, of which nitric oxide and nitric oxide synthase appear to be important components. The extrinsic parasympathetic cholinergic and sympathetic adrenergic innervation persists. This imbalance results in failure of relaxation of the aganglionic colon or sphincters. Another plexus of extrinsic origin in the circular muscular layer and rich in interstitial cells of Cajal has a probable pacemaker role on smooth muscle activity (120).

EMBRYOLOGY

Neurenteric ganglion cells migrate craniocaudally from the neural crest. Neuroblasts are identified within vagal nerve trunks running on the outer surface of the digestive tract by the fifth week of embryogenesis (121–123). By the 12th week, neuroblasts have reached the rectum, also innervated by the sacral crest. The

myenteric plexus is initially at the outer surface, and later is covered by formation of the outer longitudinal muscular layer. Subsequently, ganglion cells migrate through the bowel wall from the myenteric plexus to populate Henle's and Meissner's plexuses, which might explain their immature appearance and smaller size at birth. Hirschsprung's disease is considered to result from interruption of the craniocaudal migration, whether genetic in origin or secondary to intrauterine events, such as ischemia (124). Results of some animal studies suggest lack of local ganglion cell formation from the nerve trunks as an etiologic factor of Hirschsprung's disease.

CATEGORIES

Based on the extent of aganglionosis, four diagnostic groups have been identified: "short segment," the most common, affecting the rectosigmoid area; "long segment," involving a variable length of the colon but not beyond the cecum; "total colonic aganglionosis" (about 10% of cases), occasionally with involvement of ileum, jejunum, and even stomach in some cases; and "ultrashort segment," with aganglionosis of the distal one third of the rectum or considered as achalasia of the anal sphincter. The latter diagnosis is usually based on manometric rather than histologic evidence.

INCIDENCE AND GENETICS

Hirschsprung's disease is the most common motility disorder in the newborn, with an estimated incidence of 1 in 5000 live births, with

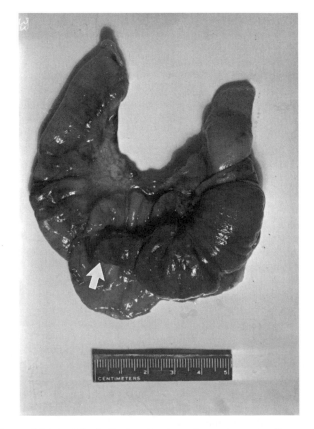

Figure 10.21 Meckel's diverticulum *(arrow)* as a leading point in an ileo-ileal intussusception in a 6-month-old infant.

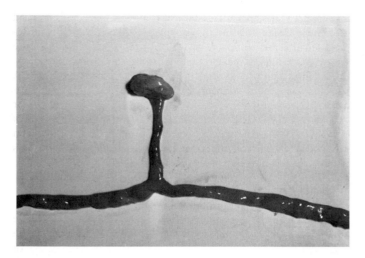

Figure 10.22 Omphalomesenteric duct extending from ileum to skin.

approximately 4% familial occurrence. A fourfold male predominance in short-segment aganglionosis has been reported (119); however, both sexes are almost equally affected in total aganglionosis (125). The disease is congenital and primarily affects the neonate, but disease onset may occur in childhood or adult life. Mothers with Hirschsprung's disease have a higher incidence of affected progeny than fathers with the disease; therefore, the disease is thought to have an autosomal recessive and sex-linked trait.

Recent studies have revealed a series of mutations, deletions and point mutations, on chromosome 10, involving the receptor tyrosine kinase gene RET, which gives rise to Hirschsprung's disease, multiple endocrine neoplasia 2A and 2B, and familial medullary carcinoma of the thyroid (126, 127). Mutations in the endothelin-receptor B and its ligand endothelin-3 (EDN-3) genes are documented in cases of Hirschsprung's disease associated with Waardenburg's syndrome (128). Another locus for Hirschsprung's disease was mapped to chromosome 13q22, and a possible genetic modifier on chromosome 21q22 in a study of Mennonite kindred with a high incidence of Hirschsprung's disease (129). Hirschsprung's disease may be associated with such malformations as Down's syndrome, congenital muscular dystrophy, congenital hypoventilation or Ondine's curse in Haddad's syndrome (130), cartilage-hair hypoplasia (131), tetrasomy 9p and 9qh with Dandy-Walker cyst (132), midline field defects similar to those in Toriello-Carey syndrome, infantile osteopetrosis, and Smith-Lemli-Opitz and Goldberg-Shprintzen syndromes (133). A rare case of Hirschsprung's disease associated with neonatal hypothalamic hamartoblastomata, holoprosencephaly, and tetramelic postaxial polydactyly was also described (134). In addition, the finding of cytomegalovirus (CMV) genomes by polymerase chain reaction in 8.8% of 72 studied cases of Hirschsprung's disease, in contrast to a total absence in control cases, raises the possibility of antenatal CMV infection as an etiologic factor (135).

CLINICAL FEATURES

The disease usually manifests as constipation or intestinal obstruction since birth, and up to 80% of cases are diagnosed within the first year of life. The remaining 20% of cases may be diagnosed in late childhood or adult life. Vomiting and progressive abdominal distention secondary to dilatation and hypertrophy of the colon proximal to the narrowed segment, or alternating constipation and diarrhea may be associated with failure to thrive and anemia.

The affected colon segment usually is narrowed; less frequently, it is of normal diameter. The transition zone is funnel-shaped distal to the proximal distended colon or small intestine (Fig. 10.23). The internal sphincter is usually involved. Zonal "skip" aganglionosis occurs rarely (136, 137).

DIAGNOSIS

The classic diagnostic approach involved taking one or more mucosal rectal biopsy specimens from 2 to 3 cm above the pectinate line that contained adequate submucosa to evaluate the presence or absence of ganglion cells in the submucosal Meissner's plexus. If no ganglion cells were observed, a full-thickness rectal biopsy was performed to confirm or negate aganglionosis, evaluating the larger Auerbach's plexus ganglion cells. The results of this approach were easier to interpret but general anesthesia was required. Now, many institutions rely primarily on mucosal suction rectal biopsies in conjunction with acetylcholinesterase staining on cryostat sections of fresh-frozen tissue, which demonstrates an increase in number and size of nerve fibers in the muscularis mucosae and often in the lamina propria. Large submucosal trunks are also seen in aganglionosis, even on hematoxylin and eosin (H & E) stains, except in total colonic aganglionosis. Thus, adequate rectal mucosal biopsies showing an absence of ganglion cells and acetylcholinesterase stain diagnostic of aganglionosis would generally exclude the necessity for a full-thickness rectal biopsy.

Ganglion cells are normally present at intervals of about 1 mm,

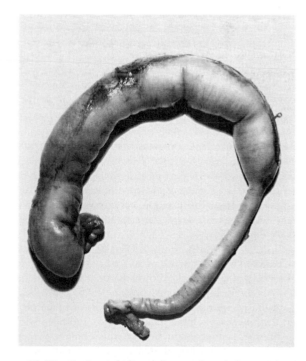

Figure 10.23 Entire colon specimen of an infant with Hirschsprung's disease and anorectal anomaly shows narrowed aganglionic distal one third with proximal dilation.

in clusters of one to five cells, and approximate density of 17 cells/mm^2 (138). These polygonal cells have abundant amphophilic cytoplasm and a round eccentric nucleus with prominent nucleolus that is less obvious on frozen section. In the rectum, a normal hypoganglionic zone extends from the pectinate line proximally for a 4- to 10-mm distance. Therefore, it is recommended to obtain biopsies 2 to 3 cm above the pectinate line. Additional higher biopsies may be helpful in assessing the length of aganglionic segment. Depending on the age of the neonate, especially in premature infants, the ganglion cells of Meissner's plexus may be difficult to identify. They appear immature, small, and with little cytoplasm and no obvious nucleolus, but their garland or horseshoe-like arrangement in small clusters around a small nerve is a clue (139). It is also advised to examine about 50 serial 4- to 5 μm-thick sections of biopsy tissue, including submucosa, and stained with H & E, in search for ganglion cells. To support the diagnosis of aganglionosis, additional techniques such as formaldehyde-induced fluorescence visualizing adrenergic fibers, antibodies to nitric oxide synthase of peptidergic nerves, S-100 protein, PGP 9.5, microtubule associated protein, and many others have been applied, but most of these techniques are reserved for research purposes (140–143). The most practical Karnovsky and Roots method or its variants demonstrate the increase of acetylcholinesterase-positive nerve fibers in the lamina propria and muscularis mucosae, where they are normally absent, or present as scarce fine twigs between the crypts (144–148). Of importance, their increase is not consistently present in cases of total colonic aganglionosis, and its evidence progresses with age.

Intraoperative seromuscular biopsy specimens should be taken during the definitive pull-through operation, allowing proper assessment of the proximal end of resection ganglion cells and the length of the aganglionic segment. Biopsies should be orientated adequately to visualize the myenteric plexus. If thick nerve trunks and ganglion cells are concomitantly present, the biopsy sample likely derives from the transitional zone. Frozen tissue should be retained, if postoperative acetylcholinesterase staining is needed.

MISCELLANEOUS DISORDERS

MECONIUM ILEUS AND RELATED CONDITIONS

About 15% of neonatal intestinal obstruction cases are attributable to meconium ileus, mostly associated with mucoviscidosis. Cystic fibrosis first manifests with meconium ileus in 15% of cases, but this disorder can also cause intermittent or complete intestinal obstruction in older patients, with impaction of fecal material in the terminal ileum and cecum, intussusception, perforation, and rectal prolapse (149–154, Fig. 10.24).

Both sexes are equally affected. Usually, the newborn fails to pass meconium within 48 hours and has a distended doughy abdomen. Radiologically, the bowel loops are distended, with ground-glass appearing contents, possible fluid levels, and focal luminal, mural, or intraperitoneal calcifications. At laparotomy or autopsy, a segment of ileum is usually dilated and filled with dark green to black viscid meconium. Distal to this segment, the terminal ileum contains gray, dried, putty-like meconium, and the colon is empty, narrow, and occasionally considered hypoplastic. Histologically, the lumen of the affected segment is filled with thick eosinophilic PAS-positive material that flattens the villi and distends

the crypts. The muscularis and serosa may be inflamed with prominent eosinophils and occasional granulomas around extravasated calcified meconium.

Meconium ileus may be associated with third trimester maternal polyhydramnios and fetal hydrops (153), or complicated by volvulus, meconium peritonitis, intestinal atresia, and occasional diverticulosis (152).

Meconium peritonitis is associated with meconium ileus in 50% of cases, but it can occur secondary to intestinal atresia, malrotation with volvulus, or hernias. It is initially a sterile, chemical peritonitis associated with fibrosis, adhesions, calcifications, and meconium granulomas. Occasionally, the meconium leak is walled-off by inflammation, forming a intraperitoneal pseudocyst, which may be seen as a mass or calcification on abdominal radiographs.

Unrelated to cystic fibrosis or Hirschsprung's disease, meconium plugs secondary to fluid restriction may cause intestinal obstruction, usually more distal, and frequently in the anorectal region. The obstruction occurs after passing normal meconium, and usually is relieved with elimination of the plug after rectal examination or contrast enema. Meconium plugs are rarely associated with mucosal ulceration, perforation, and meconium peritonitis (155).

SPONTANEOUS PERFORATION OF THE INTESTINE

Perforation of the small or large bowel is usually a complication of obstructive processes such as meconium ileus, malrotation with volvulus, intussusception, intestinal atresia, ruptured Meckel's diverticulum, and acute appendicitis, or secondary to ischemia and necrotizing enterocolitis. Spontaneous perforation of the intestine, however, is rarely determined to be the cause of neonatal peritonitis of unknown etiology.

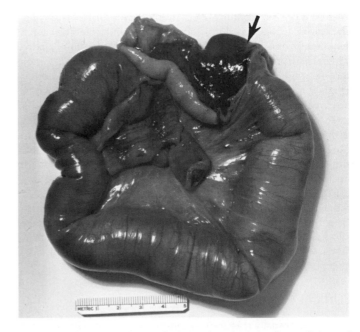

Figure 10.24 Meconium ileus and volvulus of small bowel distended by meconium *(arrow)* in a newborn with cystic fibrosis.

MICROVILLOUS INCLUSION DISEASE (SEE CHAPTER 31)

Also known as familial enteropathy or congenital microvillous atrophy, this rare familial malabsorption disease manifests at birth, worsens with oral feeding, and is associated with intractable diarrhea.

HETEROTOPIA (SEE CHAPTER 30)

Ectopic gastric and pancreatic tissue usually involves the duodenum, but it can be seen in the subserosa of the small intestine in cases of trisomy, in intestinal duplications, and in Meckel's diverticulum.

HAMARTOMAS (SEE CHAPTER 33)

Peutz-Jeghers syndrome is an autosomal dominant hamartomatous polyposis. A case of neurovascular hamartoma has been reported in Meckel's diverticulum.

Angiomas (venous malformations) of the small intestine are usually multiple, cavernous, and submucosal, and have been described as a cause of intestinal intussusception and obstruction.

CONGENITAL FIBROMATOSIS

Neonatal intestinal fibromatosis may present as a resectable solitary mass causing intestinal obstruction. The histology is that of a highly cellular benign fibroblastic proliferation. When this condition occurs as part of the syndrome of congenital generalized fibromatosis, the prognosis is less favorable. Desmoid tumors associated with Gardner's syndrome usually affect the mesentery or abdominal wall of older patients (see Chapter 18).

RECTUM AND ANUS

EMBRYOLOGY

The hindgut (caudal part of the primitive gut) ends blindly at the cloaca level, where its endoderm and the ectoderm are in contact and form the cloacal membrane (Fig. 10.25). Its most caudal part, the tailgut, is small and regresses by the sixth week. The allantois arises as a ventral diverticulum from the hindgut. By the end of the fifth week of fetal life, the mesonephric ducts enter the cranial portion of the cloaca. A mesodermal wedge, the urorectal septum, develops between the allantois and hindgut, and progresses caudally toward the cloacal membrane. This septum is completed by fusion with lateral cloacal ridges and with the cloacal membrane at the perineal body level during the seventh week. The cloaca is then divided into anterior urogenital sinus and posterior anorectal canal. The cloacal membrane is also separated into urogenital and anal membranes, with surrounding cloacal folds divided into urethral or genital folds and anal folds. The anal membrane is slightly depressed, forming the anal dimple or proctodeum, and usually ruptures by the eighth week. The pectinate line corresponds to its level, i.e., endoderm- and ectoderm-derived tissue junction. In females, the Mullerian ducts fuse to form the uterus and vagina that connects to the urogenital sinus by week 16; the urogenital membrane opens to form the vestibule. In males, the genital folds fuse and the urogenital sinus forms the urethra. The external anal sphincter is formed by fusion of developing anal tubercles with the perineal body (1).

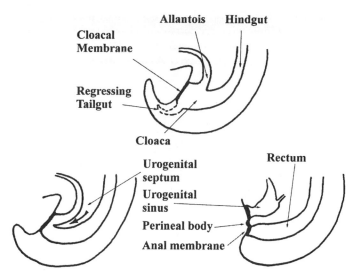

Figure 10.25 Hindgut and cloacal division that occurs between the fourth and seventh weeks of gestation.

IMPERFORATE ANUS AND RELATED ANORECTAL ANOMALIES

Anorectal anomalies is a better general term than imperforate anus to describe a broad range of malformations, likely related to abnormal development of the urorectal septum. Usually, both the rectum and the anal canal are affected. Anorectal anomalies represent common congenital, occasionally familial, malformations with an approximate incidence of 1 in 5000 births, with a slight male predominance. A true imperforate anus or membranous anal atresia, with persistence of the anal membrane, occurs rarely (156–159).

An international classification has been accepted and is useful for a clinical and surgical approach (157). Based on the termination of the rectum in relation to the levator ani muscles, with the pubococcygeal or ischial lines, respectively, on lateral or frontal radiographs as equivalent bony landmarks, these malformations can be classified as high (supralevator), intermediate, or low (translevator). Subclassification depends on the presence and site of associated fistulas between the rectum and the urogenital tract or perineum (Table 10.3; Figs. 10.26 and 10.27). Radiologic studies with contrast enhancement help to define the level of anomaly and fistulous association. The most common types are low and high anomalies.

Low anomalies are relatively more common in females, with fewer associated anomalies. Seventy-five percent of cases are associated with a fistula from the rectal pouch to the perineal skin just anterior to a covered anal dimple (Fig. 10.28). The sphincter function is normal, resulting in less morbidity and better surgical results (158).

Intermediate types, with the rectal pouch at the level of the levator ani muscle, include anal agenesis with and without fistula, and anorectal stenosis. The fistula can be rectobulbar in males, rectovestibular or rectovaginal (lower one third) in females. The internal sphincter is absent and the external sphincter is poorly formed in both sexes.

High malformations or anorectal agenesis represent the most common anomaly in males, and are associated with a rectourethral fistula in most males (Fig. 10.29) and a rectovaginal (upper two

TABLE	
10.3	**International Classification of Anorectal Anomalies**

Low (translevator)
1. Normal anal site
   a) Anal stenosis
   b) Covered anus complete
2. Perineal site
   a) Anocutaneous fistula (covered anus incomplete)
   b) Anterior perineal anus
3. At vulvar site (in females)
   a) Anovulvar fistula
   b) Anovestibular fistula
   c) Vestibular anus

Intermediate
1. Anal agenesis
   a) Without fistula
   b) With rectovestibular or rectovaginal fistula (in females)
   c) With rectobulbar fistula (in males)
2. Anorectal stenosis

High (supralevator)
1. Anorectal agenesis
   a) Without fistula
   b) With rectovaginal or rectocloacal fistula (in females)
   c) With rectourethral or rectovesical fistula (in males)
2. Rectal atresia

Miscellaneous
Imperforate anal membrane
Cloacal exstrophy
Others

Modified after Santulli TV, Kiesewetter WB, Bill AH Jr. Anorectal anomalies: A suggested international classification. J Pediatr Surg 1970;5:281.

thirds) fistula in females. The sphincteric function is abnormal, and the frequency of other associated malformations is the highest of all anorectal anomalies.

Anorectal stenosis (intermediate) and rectal atresia (high) are thought to occur as a result of vascular injury that occurs during fetal life; an intact sphincter is usually present (160).

Rectocloacal fistula or persistent cloaca is a rare condition found in female infants in which the rectum, urethra, and vagina join in a common channel leading to a single perineal orifice.

About 70% of infants with anorectal malformations have other associated congenital anomalies, such as skeletal (especially lumbo-sacral spine) and genitourinary (hydronephrosis or a double collecting system) malformations (161). Congenital heart disease and esophageal atresia with tracheoesophageal fistula occur in about one third of cases. A diagnosis of VACTERL association, occasionally part of a chromosomal (trisomy 18 and 13q deletion syndrome) anomaly, should be considered in every infant with an anorectal anomaly. Intestinal atresias, malrotations and duplications, annular pancreas, bicornuate uterus, vaginal atresia, septate vagina, absence of the rectus abdominis muscle, omphalocele, and exstrophy of the bladder and ileocecal area of the intestine are less commonly observed associated anomalies, sometimes as part of multiple complex malformation syndromes.

ENTERIC AND TAILGUT CYSTS

Single or small multiple cysts, sometimes multilocular, may occur between the coccyx or sacrum and the rectum. These cysts are called tailgut and enteric cysts or retrorectal cyst-hamartomas (162–167). These lesions derive from remnants of the normally regressed caudal postcloacal hindgut portion within the embryonic tail, from cloacal rests, sequestrated rectal duplication, or neurenteric fistulas associated with sacral anomalies or intraspinal cysts. These cysts, more common in females, manifest as an obstructive extrinsic rectal mass in infants, or later in adulthood as a retrorectal abscess or incidental

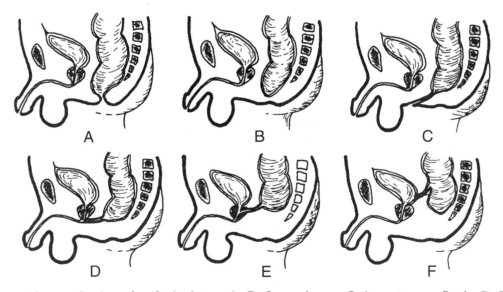

Figure 10.26   Anorectal anomalies in males. **A.** Anal stenosis. **B.** Covered anus. **C.** Anocutaneous fistula. **D.** Rectobulbar fistula. **E.** Rectourethral fistula. **F.** Rectovesical fistula.

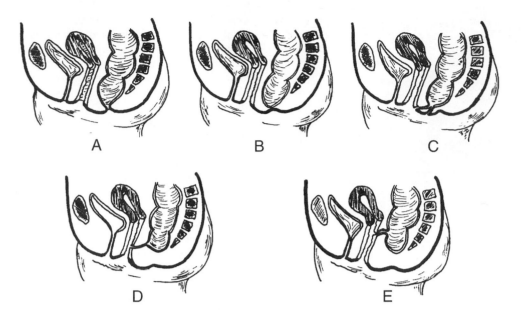

Figure 10.27 Anorectal anomalies in females. **A.** Anal stenosis. **B.** Covered anus. **C.** Anocutaneous and anovestibular fistulae. **D.** Rectovaginal fistula (intermediate). **E.** Rectovaginal fistula (high).

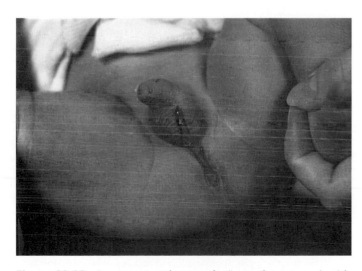

Figure 10.28 Low anorectal anomaly (imperforate anus) with anocutaneous (scrotal) fistula in a male neonate.

palpable mass. The cyst wall may contain a smooth muscle layer, resembling an intestinal duplication, especially if derived from the rectum. The mucosal lining is alimentary type, or may contain ciliated and squamous epithelia. These cysts rarely give rise to adenocarcinoma (168, 169). The differential diagnosis should include chordoma and teratoma.

MISCELLANEOUS DISORDERS

CLOACAL EXSTROPHY

Exstrophy of the cloaca is a rare complex anomaly, including an omphalocele, imperforate anus, and exstrophy of two hemibladders between which lies an everted cecum. A small colon ends blindly in

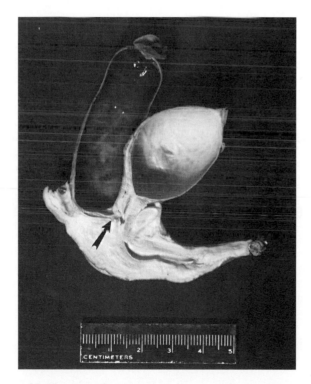

Figure 10.29 Imperforate anus in a male neonate with VACTERL association. Note blind-ended rectum on left, and suspected small rectourethral fistula *(arrow)* in this sagittal section of the pelvic organs.

the pelvis, and the terminal ileum often prolapses out of the exposed cecum (170–173). Embryologically, its origin is not totally understood. Impaired mesodermal growth of the genital or urethral folds, the genital tubercle, and the infraumbilical ventral abdominal wall is

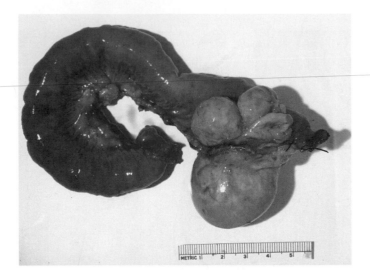

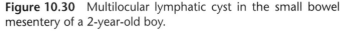

Figure 10.30 Multilocular lymphatic cyst in the small bowel mesentery of a 2-year-old boy.

thought to be the important underlying mechanism. Cloacal exstrophy results from persistence and subsequent rupture of the infraumbilical cloacal membrane during the fifth week of embryonic life, associated with incomplete urorectal septum, and exposing abnormally developed organs that derive from the cloaca, Mullerian ducts, and hindgut. The appendix may be absent, small, or duplicated. Nonfusion of the genital folds in one cephalic genital tubercle result in bifid penis or clitoris. Other anomalies, such as renal agenesis and polyhydramnios, intestinal malrotation, myelocystocele, lipomeningocele, and sacral and limb malformations are usually associated findings. Cloacal exstrophy has been reported as part of the genitourinary malformations seen in a triple 47,XXX child (174), with rare occurrence with another midline defect, a frontonasal malformation.

HETEROTOPIA

Ectopic gastric epithelium has been reported in the rectum, occasionally with salivary gland tissue, presenting as a polyp or ulcer with bleeding (see Chapter 30). In a patient with caudal regression syndrome, immature renal tissue was found in the colonic wall.

MESENTERY AND OMENTUM

MESENTERIC CYSTS (CYSTIC HYGROMA)

Mesenteric cysts are rare abdominal tumors with an estimated incidence of 1 per 100,000 to 250,000; about 820 cases of mesenteric cysts have been reported since 1507. Their pathogenesis is unclear. Growth of congenitally malformed or displaced lymphatic tissue, trauma, degeneration of lymph nodes, and improper fusion of mesenteric leaves have been suggested as possible underlying etiologic mechanisms (175–181).

Mesenteric cysts show a slight female predominance and occur at any age; peak incidence is in the fourth decade of life according to some reports, although cysts were noted in patients less than 15

years of age in some small series. The lesions may be incidental, with a palpable, slowly growing abdominal mass; occasionally, they are painful and associated with an acute abdomen, usually secondary to hemorrhage, rupture, or torsion of the cyst, and intestinal obstruction. They are known to be more mobile transversely than craniocaudally, in contrast to omental cysts, which are mobile in all directions.

These cysts can be single or multiple, uni- or multiloculated, with serous, chylous, or brown hemosiderotic contents, and varying sizes, occasionally filling the abdomen (Fig. 10.30). The ileal mesentery is most commonly involved. Three of five cases have been reported with rapid growth during pregnancy, requiring laparotomy. Histologically, the cysts are variants of cystic lymphatic malformations with endothelial lining, small bundles of smooth muscle, focal aggregates of lymphocytes, and cholesterol granulomas, and infrequently occur as nodular cellular endothelial proliferation. Cysts with mesothelial lining, and considered erroneously mesenteric cysts by location, represent benign cystic mesotheliomas. Associated sarcomas and adenocarcinoma have been reported in less than 3% of mesenteric cysts (180, 181).

Resection of the cyst, and adjacent bowel if involved, is the recommended treatment. Marsupialization and drainage with follow-up may be indicated for patients with multiple cysts.

OMENTAL CYSTS

Omental and mesenteric cysts have similar clinical manifestations and morphology, but omental cysts occur less frequently (179).

REFERENCES

1. Moore KL, Persaud TVN. The developing human: Clinically oriented embryology. 5th ed. Philadelphia: WB Saunders, 1993: 237–264.
2. Rosenthal AH. Congenital atresia of the esophagus with tracheo-esophageal fistula. Arch Pathol 1931;12:756–772.
3. Zaw-Tun HA. The tracheo-esophageal septum—fact or fantasy? Origin and development of the respiratory primordium and esophagus. Acta Anat (Basel) 1982;114:1–21.
4. O'Rahilly R, Muller F. Respiratory and alimentary relations in staged human embryos. New embryological data and congenital anomalies. Ann Otol Rhinol Laryngol 1984;93:421–429.
5. Olsen AM, Harrington SW. Esophageal hiatal hernias of the short esophagus type: Etiologic and therapeutic considerations. J Thorac Surg 1948;17:189–207.
6. Kluth D, Steding G, Seidl W. The embryology of foregut malformations. J Pediatr Surg 1987;22:389–393.
7. Evans JA, Reggin J, Greenberg C. Tracheal agenesis and associated malformations: A comparison with tracheoesophageal fistula and the VACTERL association. Am J Med Genet 1985;21: 21–34.
8. Chen H, Goei GS, Hertzler J. Family studies on congenital esophageal atresia with or without tracheo-esophageal fistula. Birth Defects 1979;15:117–144.
9. Kluth D. Atlas of esophageal atresia. J Pediatr Surg 1976;11: 901–919.
10. Swenson O, Lipman R, Fisher JH, et al. Repair and complications of esophageal atresia and tracheoesophageal fistula. N Engl J Med 1962;267:960–963.
11. Gross RE. The surgery of infancy and childhood: Its principles and techniques. Philadelphia: WB Saunders, 1953;75–102.
12. Holder TM, Cloud DT, Lewis JE, et al. IV. Esophageal atresia and tracheoesophageal fistula—a survey of its members by the Surgical

Section of the American Academy of Pediatrics. Pediatrics 1964;34: 542–549.

13. Roth B, Rose K-G, Benz-Bohm G, et al. Laryngo-tracheo-esophageal cleft. Eur J Pediatr 1983;140:41–46.

14. Ryan DP, Muehrcke DD, Doody DP, et al. Laryngotracheoesophageal cleft (type IV): Management and repair of lesions beyond the carina. J Pediatr Surg 1991;26: 962–970.

15. Lacina S, Townley R, Radecki L, et al. Esophageal lung with cardiac abnormalities. Chest 1981;79:468–470.

16. Fonkalsrud EW: Esophageal stenosis due to tracheobronchial remnants. Am J Surg 1972;124:101–103.

17. Adler RH. Congenital esophageal webs. J Thorac Cardiovasc Surg 1963;45:175–185.

18. Fowler CL, Pokorny WJ, Wagner ML, et al. Review of bronchopulmonary foregut malformations. J Pediatr Surg 1988;23:793–797.

19. Bremer JL. Dorsal intestinal fistula; accessory neurenteric canal; diastematomyelia. Arch Pathol Lab Med 1952;54:132-138.

20. Bentley JFR, Smith JR. Developmental posterior enteric remnants and spinal malformations. The split notochord syndrome. Arch Dis Child 1960;35:76–86.

21. Kirwan WO, Walbaum PR, McCormack RJM. Cystic intrathoracic derivatives of the foregut and their complications. Thorax 1973;28: 424–428.

22. Salyer DC, Salyer WR, Eggleston JC. Benign developmental cysts of the mediastinum. Arch Pathol Lab Med 1977;101:136–139.

23. Bagwell CE, Schiffman RJ. Subcutaneous bronchogenic cysts. J Pediatr Surg 1988;23:993–995.

24. Sen S, Bourne AJ, Morris LL, et al. Dorsal enteric cysts—a study of eight cases. Aust NZ J Surg 1988;58:51–55.

25. Moir JD. Combined duplication of the esophagus and the stomach. J Can Assoc Radiol 1970;21:257–262.

26. Hruban RH, Shumway SJ, Orel SB, et al. Congenital bronchopulmonary foregut malformations: Intralobar and extralobar pulmonary sequestrations communicating with the foregut. Am J Clin Pathol 1989;91:403–409.

27. Blank E, Michael TD. Muscular hypertrophy of the esophagus: Report of a case with involvement of the entire esophagus. Pediatrics 1963;32:595–598.

28. Grand RJ, Watkins JB, Torti FM. Development of the human gastrointestinal tract. Gastroenterology 1976;70:790–810.

29. Teplick JG, Wallner RJ, Levine AH, et al. Isolated dextrogastria: Report of two cases. Am J Radiol 1979;132:124–126.

30. Gorman B, Shaw DG. Congenital microgastria. Br J Radiol 1984; 57:260–262.

31. Rose V, Izukawa T, Moes CAF. Syndromes of asplenia and polysplenia. A review of cardiac and non-cardiac malformations in 60 cases with special reference to diagnosis and prognosis. Br Heart J 1975;37:840–852.

32. Velasco AL, Wolcomb GW III, Templeton Jr JM, et al. Management of congenital microgastria. J Pediatr Surg 1990;25:192–197.

33. Parrish RA, Kanavage CB, Wells JA, et al. Congenital antral membrane. Surg Gynecol Obstet 1968;127:999–1004.

34. Bar-Maor JA, Nissan S, Nevo S. Pyloric atresia: A hereditary congenital anomaly with autosomal recessive transmission. J Med Genet 1972;9:70–72.

35. Bull MJ, Norins AL, Weaver DD, et al. Epidermolysis bullosa pyloric atresia. Am J Dis Child 1992;137:449–451.

36. Chang CH, Penin EV, Bove KE. Pyloric atresia associated with epidermolysis bullosa: Special reference to pathogenesis. Pediatr Pathol Lab Med 1983;1:449–457.

37. Rhind JA. Mucosal stenosis of the pylorus. Br J Surg 1959;46: 534–540.

38. Tunell WP, Smith EI. Antral web in infancy. J Pediatr Surg 1980;15: 152–155.

39. Haddad V, Macon IV WL, Islami MH. Mucosal diaphragms of the gastric antrum in adults. Surg Gynecol Obstet 1981;152:227–233.

40. Shim WKT, Campbell A, Wright SW. Pyloric stenosis in the racial groups of Hawaii. J Pediatr 1970;70:89–93.

41. Spicer RD. Infantile hypertrophic pyloric stenosis: A review. Br J Surg 1982;69:128–135.

42. Wollstein M: Healing of hypertrophic pyloric stenosis after the Fredet-Rammstedt operation. Am J Dis Child 1922;23:511–517.

43. Tam PKH. An immunochemical study with neuron-specific-enolase

and substance P of human enteric innervation—the normal developmental pattern and abnormal deviations in Hirschsprung's disease and pyloric stenosis. J Pediatr Surg 1986;21:227–232.

44. Wattchow DA, Cass DT, Furness JB, et al. Abnormalities of peptide-containing nerve fibres in infantile hypertrophic pyloric stenosis. Gastroenterology 1987;92:443–448.

45. Malmfors G, Sundler F. Peptidergic innervation in infantile hypertrophic pyloric stenosis. J Pediatr Surg 1986;21:303–306.

46. Vanderwinder JM. Nitric oxide synthase activity in infantile hypertrophic pyloric stenosis. N Engl J Med 1992;327:511–515.

47. Friesen SR, Boley JO, Miller DR. The myenteric plexus of the pylorus: Its early normal development and its changes in hypertrophic pyloric stenosis. Surgery 1956;39:21–29.

48. Christiansen KH, Mawr B, Grantham A. Idiopathic hypertrophic pyloric stenosis in the adult: A review of the literature and the report of two cases. Arch Surg 1962;85:207–214.

49. Dye TE, Vidals VG, Lockhart CE, et al. Adult hypertrophic pyloric stenosis. Am Surg 1979;45:478–484.

50. Wieczorek RL, Seidman I, Ranson JHC, et al. Congenital duplication of the stomach: Case report and review of the English literature. Am J Gastroenterol 1984;79:597–602.

51. Abrami G, Dennison WM. Duplication of the stomach. Surgery 1961;49:794–801.

52. Bremer JL. Diverticula and duplications of the intestinal tract. Arch Pathol Lab Med 1944;38:132–140.

53. Sufian S, Ominsky S, Matsumoto T. Congenital double pylorus. A case report and review of the literature. Gastroenterology 1977; 73:154–157.

54. Meyer II JL. Congenital defect in the musculature of the stomach resulting in spontaneous gastric perforation in the neonatal period: A report of two cases. J Pediatr 1957;51:416–421.

55. McCormick WF. Rupture of the stomach in children: Review of the literature and a report of seven cases. Arch Pathol Lab Med 1959; 67:416–426.

56. Yutani C, Sakurai M, Miyaji T, et al. Congenital short intestine, a case report and review of the literature. Arch Pathol Lab Med 1973;96. 81–82.

57. Reiquam CW, Allen RP, Akers DR. Normal and abnormal small bowel lengths. An analysis of 389 autopsy cases in infants and children. Am J Dis Child 1965;109:447–451.

58. Shaw JRN, Rancroft L, Cook RCM, et al. Functional intestinal obstruction associated with malrotation and short small bowel. J Pediatr Surg 1984;19:172–173.

59. Snyder WH, Chaffin L. Embryology and pathology of the intestinal tract: Presentation of 40 cases of malrotation. Ann Surg 1954;140: 368–379.

60. Weinberger E, Winters WD, Liddell RM, et al. Sonographic diagnosis of intestinal malrotation in infants: Importance of relative positions of the superior mesenteric vein and artery. AJR Am J Roentgenol 1992;159:825–828.

61. Spigland N, Brandt ML, Yazbeck S. Malrotation presenting beyond the neonatal period. J Pediatr Surg 1990;25:1139–1142.

62. Powell DM, Othersen HB, Smith CD. Malrotation of the intestines in children: The effect of age on presentation and therapy. J Pediatr Surg 1989;24:777–780.

63. Ford EG, Senac MO, Srikanth MS, et al. Malrotation of the intestine in children. Ann Surg 1992;215:172–178.

64. Kiesewetter WB, Smith JW. Malrotation of the midgut in infancy and childhood. Arch Surg 1958;77:483–491.

65. Dykstra G, Sieber WK, Kiesewetter WB. Intestinal atresia. Arch Surg 1968;97:175–182.

66. Fonkalsrud EW, DeLorimier AA, Hays DM. Congenital atresia and stenosis of the duodenum. A review compiled from the members of the Surgical Section of the American Academy of Pediatrics. Pediatrics 1968;43:70–83.

67. Young DG, Wilkinson AW. Abnormalities associated with neonatal duodenal obstruction. Surgery 1968;63:832–836.

68. Moutsouris C. The 'solid' stage and congenital intestinal atresia. J Pediatr Surg 1966;1:446–450.

69. McBride WG. Thalidomide and congenital abnormalities. Lancet 1961;2:1358.

70. Weinberg AG, Milunsky A, Harrod MJ. Elevated amniotic fluid alpha-fetoprotein and duodenal atresia. Lancet 1975;2:496.

71. Louw JH. Jejunoileal atresia and stenosis. J Pediatr Surg 1966; 1:8–23.

72. DeLorimier AA, Fonkalsrud EW, Hays DM. Congenital atresia and stenosis of the jejunum and ileum. Surgery 1969;65:819–827.

73. Nixon HH, Tawes R. Etiology and treatment of small intestine atresia: Analysis of a series of 127 jejunoileal atresias and comparison with 62 duodenal atresias. Surgery 1971;69:41–51.

74. Adejuyigbe O, Odesanmi WO. Intrauterine intussusception causing intestinal atresia. J Pediatr Surg 1990;25:562–563.

75. Siplovich L, Davies MRQ, Kaschula ROC, et al. Intestinal obstruction in the newborn with congenital syphilis. J Pediatr Surg 1988; 23:810–813.

76. Olson LM, Flom LS, Kierney CMP, et al. Identical twins with malrotation and type IV jejunal atresia. J Pediatr Surg 1987;22:1015–1016.

77. Graham JN, Marin-Padilla N, Hoefnagel D. Jejunal atresia associated with Cafergot ingestion during pregnancy. Clin Pediatr 1983;22:226–228.

78. Collins DL, Kimura K, Morgan A, et al. Multiple intestinal atresia and amyoplasia congenita in four unrelated infants: A new association. J Pediatr Surg 1986;21:331–333.

79. Paterson-Brown S, Stalewski H, Brereton RJ. Neonatal small bowel atresia, stenosis and segmental dilatation. Br J Surg 1991;78:83–86.

80. Puri P, Guiney EJ, Carroll R. Multiple gastro-intestinal atresias in three consecutive siblings: Observations on pathogenesis. J Pediatr Surg 1985;20:22–24.

81. Blyth H, Dickson JAS. Apple peel syndrome (congenital intestinal atresia). A family study of seven index patients. J Med Genet 1969;6:275–277.

82. Seashore JH, Collins FS, Markowitz RI, et al. Familial 'apple peel' jejunal atresia: Surgical, genetic and radiographic aspects. Pediatrics 1987;80:540–544.

83. Brigham RA, Fallon WF, Saunders JR, et al. Paraduodenal hernia: Diagnosis and surgical management. Surgery 1984;96:498–502.

84. Janin Y, Stone AM, Wise L. Mesenteric hernia. Surg Gynecol Obstet 1980;150:747–754.

85. Erskine JM. Hernia through the foramen of Winslow. Surg Gynecol Obstet 1967;125:1093–1108.

86. Cope R. Congenital diaphragmatic hernia: Presentation and problems in the adult. Gastrointestinal Radiol 1981;6:157–160.

87. Benjamin DR, Juul S, Siebert JR. Congenital posterolateral diaphragmatic hernia: Associated malformations. J Pediatr Surg 1988;23:899–903.

88. Kimmelstiel RM, Holgersen LO, Hilfer C. Retrosternal (Morgagni) hernia with small bowel obstruction secondary to a Richter's incarceration. J Pediatr Surg 1987;22:996–1000.

89. Cantrell JR, Haller JA, Ravitch MM. A syndrome of congenital defects involving the abdominal wall, sternum, diaphragm, pericardium and heart. Surg Gynecol Obstet 1958;107:602–614.

90. Soper SP, Roe LR, Hoyme HE, et al. Trisomy 18 with ectopia cordis, omphalocele, and ventricular septal defect: Case report. Pediatr Pathol Lab Med 1986;5:481–483.

91. Spitz L, Bloom KR, Milner S, et al. Combined anterior abdominal wall, sternal, diaphragmatic, pericardial, and intracardiac defects: A report of five cases and their management. J Pediatr Surg 1975; 10:491–496.

92. Blumberg NA. Infantile umbilical hernia. Surg Gynecol Obstet 1980;150:187–192.

93. Grosfeld JL, O'Neill JA, Clatworthy HW. Enteric duplications in infancy and childhood: An 18-year review. Ann Surg 1970;172:83–90.

94. Favara BE, Franciosi RA, Akers DR. Enteric duplications. Thirty-seven cases: A vascular theory of pathogenesis. Am J Dis Child 1971;122:501–506.

95. Bentley JFR, Smith JR. Developmental posterior enteric remnants and spinal malformations. Arch Dis Child 1960;35:76–86.

96. Vaage S, Knutrud O. Congenital duplications of the alimentary tract with special regard to their embryogenesis. Prog Pediatr Surg 1974;7:103.

97. Gdanietz K, Wit J, Heller K. Complete duplication of the small intestine in childhood. Z Kinderchir 1983;38:414–416.

98. Weber HM, Dixon CF. Duplication of the entire large intestine (colon duplex): Report of a case. AJR Am J Roentgenol 1946;55:319–324.

99. Ravitch MM, Scott WW. Duplication of the entire colon, bladder and urethra. Surgery 1953;34:843–858.

100. Carter RA. Multiple congenital diverticula of the jejunum. Br J Surg 1959;46:586–588.

101. Andricopoulos PC, Christopoulos D. Congenital diverticula of the sigmoid colon. J R Coll Surg Edinb 1986;31:249–250.

102. Wetzig NR. Diverticulosis of the vermiform appendix. Med J Aust 1986;145:464–465.

103. Favara BE. Multiple congenital diverticula of the vermiform appendix. Am J Clin Pathol 1968;49:60–64.

104. George DH. Diverticulosis of the vermiform appendix in patients with cystic fibrosis. Hum Pathol 1987;18:75–79.

105. Yazbeck S, Ndoye, Khan AH. Omphalocele: A 25-year experience. J Pediatr Surg 1986;21:761–763.

106. deVries PA. The pathogenesis of gastroschisis and omphalocele. J Pediatr Surg 1980;15:245–251.

107. Martin LW, Torres AM. Omphalocele and gastroschisis. Surg Clin North Am 1985;65:1235–1244.

108. Duhamel B. Embryology of exomphalos and allied malformations. Arch Dis Child 1963;38:142–147.

109. Filippi G, McKusick VA. The Beckwith-Wiedemann syndrome (the exomphalos-macroglossia-gigantism syndrome). Report of two cases and review of the literature. Medicine 1970;49:279–298.

110. Soper SP, Roe LR, Hoyme HE, et al. Trisomy 18 with ectopia cordis, omphalocele, and ventricular septal defect. Pediatr Pathol Lab Med 1986;5:481–483.

111. Vane DW, West KW, Grosfeld JL. Vitelline duct anomalies. Arch Surg 1987;122:542–547.

112. Moore TC. Omphalomesenteric duct anomalies. Surg Gynecol Obstet 1956;103:569–580.

113. Soderlund S. Meckel's diverticulum in children. A report of 115 cases. Acta Chir Scand 1956;110:261–274.

114. Weinstein EC, Cain JC, ReMine WH. Meckel's diverticulum. JAMA 1962;182:251–253.

115. Capron J-P, Dupas J-L, Marti R, et al. Gastrin cells in Meckel's diverticulum. N Engl J Med 1977;297:1126.

116. Gilbert EF, Rainey Jr JR: Meconium peritonitis caused by a rupture of a Meckel's diverticulum in a newborn infant. J Pediatr 1958;53:597–601.

117. Weinstein EC, Dockerty MB, Waugh JM. Neoplasms of Meckel's diverticulum. Int Abstr Surg 1963;116:103–111.

118. Moore TC, Schumacker HE. Intussusception of ileum through persistent omphalomesenteric duct. Surgery 1952;81:278–284.

119. Bodian M, Carter CO. A family study of Hirschsprung's disease. Ann Hum Genet 1963;26:261–277.

120. Rumessen JJ, Peters S, Thuneberg L. Light and electron microscopical studies of interstitial cells of Cajal and muscle cells at the submucosal border of human colon. Lab Invest 1993;68:481–495.

121. Okamoto E, Ueda T. Embryogenesis of intramural ganglia of the gut and its relation to Hirschsprung's disease. J Pediatr Surg 1967;2:437–443.

122. Andrew A. The origin of intramural ganglia. IV. The origin of enteric ganglia: A critical review and discussion of the present state of the problem. J Anat 1971;108:169–184.

123. Kapur RP. Contemporary approaches toward understanding the pathogenesis of Hirschsprung's disease. Pediatr Pathol 1993;13:83–100.

124. Earlam R. A vascular cause for Hirschsprung's disease? Gastroenterology 1985;88:1274–1276.

125. Fekete CN, Ricour C, Martelli H, et al. Total colonic aganglionosis (with or without ileal involvement). A review of 27 cases. J Pediatr Surg 1986;21:251–254.

126. Romeo G, Ronchetto P, Luo Y, et al. Point mutations affecting the tyrosine kinase domain of the RET photo-oncogene in Hirschsprung's disease. Nature 1994;367:377–378.

127. Khairi MRA, Dexter RN, Burzynski NJ, et al. Mucosal neuroma, pheochromocytoma and medullary thyroid carcinoma: Multiple endocrine neoplasia type 3. Medicine 1975;54:89–112.

128. Omenn GS, McKusick VA. The association of Waardenburg Syn-

drome and Hirschsprung megacolon. Am J Med Genet 1979;3: 217–223.

129. Puffenberger EG, Kauffman ER, Bolk S, et al. Identity-by descent and association mapping of a recessive gene for Hirschsprung disease on human chromosome 13q22. Hum Mol Genet 1994;3: 1217–1225.

130. Verloes A, Elmer C, LaCombe D, et al. Ondine-Hirschsprung syndrome (Haddad syndrome). Further delineation in two cases and review of the literature. Eur J Pediatr 1993;152:75–77.

131. Sulisalo T, Sistonen P, Hastbacka J, et al. Cartilage-hair hypoplasia gene assigned to chromosome 9 by linkage analysis. Nat Genet 1993;3:338–341.

132. Melaragno MI, Brunoni D, Patricio F, et al. A patient with tetrasomy 9p, Dandy-Walker cyst and Hirschsprung's disease. Ann Genet 1992;35:79–84.

133. Tanaka H, Ito J, Cho K, et al. Hirschsprung's disease, unusual face, mental retardation, epilepsy and congenital heart disease: Goldberg-Shprintzen syndrome. Pediatr Neurol 1993;9:479–481.

134. Verloes A, Gillerot Y, Langhendries JP, et al. Variability versus heterogeneity in syndromal hypothalamic hamartoblastoma and related disorders: Review and delineation of the cerebro-acro-visceral early lethality (CAVE) multiplex syndrome. Am J Med Genet 1992;1:669–677.

135. Tam PK, Quint WG, van Velzen D. Hirschsprung's disease: A viral etiology? Pediatr Pathol Lab Med 1992;12:807–810.

136. Yunis E, Sieber WK, Akers DR. Does zonal aganglionosis really exist? Report of a rare variety of Hirschsprung's disease and a review of the literature. Pediatr Pathol 1983;1:33–49.

137. Kapur RP, deSa DJ, Luquette M, et al. Hypothesis: Pathogenesis of skip areas in long-segment Hirschsprung's disease. Pediatr Pathol Lab Med 1995;15:23–37.

138. Aldridge RT, Campbell PE. Ganglion cell distribution in the normal rectum and anal canal. A basis for the diagnosis of Hirschsprung's disease by anorectal biopsy. J Pediatr Surg 1986;3:475–490.

139. Yunis EJ, Dibbins AW, Sherman FE. Rectal suction biopsy in the diagnosis of Hirschsprung's disease in infants. Arch Pathol Lab Med 1976;100:329–333.

140. Nirasawa Y, Yokoyama J, Ikawa H, et al. Hirschsprung's disease: Catecholamine content, Alpha-adrenoceptors, and the effect of electrical stimulation in aganglionic colon. J Pediatr Surg 1986;21: 136–142.

141. Bishop AE, Polak JM, Lake BD, et al. Abnormalities of the colonic regulatory peptides in Hirschsprung's disease. Histopathology 1981; 5:679–688.

142. Tam PKH, Owen G. An immunohistochemical study of neuronal microtubule-associated proteins in Hirschsprung's disease. Hum Pathol 1993;24:424–431.

143. Mackenzie JM, Dixon MF. An immunohistochemical study of the enteric neural plexus in Hirschsprung's disease. Histopathology 1987;11:1055–1066.

144. Karnovsky MJ, Roots L. A 'direct coloring' thiocholine method for cholinesterases. J Histochem Cytochem 1964;12:219–221.

145. Lake BD, Puri P, Nixon HH, et al. Hirschsprung's disease. An appraisal of histochemically demonstrated acetylcholinesrerase activity in suction rectal biopsy specimens as an aid to diagnosis. Arch Pathol Lab Med 1978;102:244–247.

146. Schofield DE, Devine W, Yunis EJ. Acetylcholinesterase-stained suction rectal biopsies in the diagnosis of Hirschsprung's disease. J Pediatr Gastroenterol Nutr 1990;11:221–228.

147. Dobbins WO, Bill AH. Diagnosis of Hirschsprung's disease excluded by rectal suction biopsy. N Engl J Med 1965;272:990–993.

148. Meier-Ruge W, Lutterbeck PM, Herzog B, et al. Acetylcholinesterase activity in suction biopsies of the rectum in the diagnosis of Hirschsprung's disease. J Pediatr Surg 1972;7:11–17.

149. Donnison AB, Schwachman H, Gross RE. A review of 164 children with meconium ileus seen at the Children's Hospital Medical Center, Boston. Pediatrics 1966;37:833–850.

150. Kopel FB. Gastrointestinal manifestations of cystic fibrosis. Gastroenterology 1972;62:483–491.

151. Esterly JR, Oppenheimer EH. Pathology of cystic fibrosis: Review of the literature and comparison with 146 autopsied cases. Perspect Pediatr Pathol 1975;2:241.

152. Mullins F, Talamo R, di Sant'Agnese PA. Late intestinal complications of cystic fibrosis. JAMA 1965;192:741–746.

153. Hutchinson AA, Drew JH, Yu VYH, et al. Nonimmunologic hydrops fetalis: A review of 61 cases. Obstet Gynecol 1982;59: 347–352.

154. Oppenheimer EH, Esterley JR. Observations in cystic fibrosis of the pancreas. II. Neonatal intestinal obstruction. Bull Johns Hopkins Hosp 1962;111:1–13.

155. King A, Mueller RF, Heeley AR, et al. Diagnosis of cystic fibrosis in premature infants. Pediatr Res 1986;20:536–541.

156. Ladd WE, Gross RE. Congenital malformations of the anus and rectum: Report of 162 cases. Am J Surg 1934;23:167.

157. Santulli TV, Kiesewetter WB, Bill Jr AH. Anorectal anomalies: A suggested international classification. J Pediatr Surg 1970;5: 281–287.

158. Magnus RV, Stephens FD. Imperforate anal membrane: The anatomy and function of the sphincters of the anal canal. Aust Pediatr J 1966;2:165.

159. Partridge JP, Gough MH. Congenital abnormalities of the anus and rectum. Br J Surg 1961;49:37–50.

160. Magnus RV. Rectal atresia as distinguished from rectal agenesis. J Pediatr Surg 1968;3:593–598.

161. Smith ED. Urinary anomalies and complications in imperforate anus and rectum. J Pediatr Surg 1968;3:337–349.

162. Caropreso PR, Wengert Jr PA, Milford EH. Tailgut cyst—a rare retrorectal tumor. Dis Colon Rectum 1975;18:597–600.

163. Gius JA, Stout AP. Perianal cysts of vestigeal origin. Arch Surg 1968;57:758–768.

164. Ferry CL, Merritt Jr JW. Presacral enterogenous cyst. Ann Surg 1949;129:881–889.

165. Uhlig BE, Johnson RL. Presacral tumors and cysts in adults. Dis Colon Rectum 1975;18:581–596.

166. Campbell WL, Wolff M. Retrorectal cysts of developmental origin. AJR Am J Roentgenol 1973;117:307–313.

167. Edwards M. Multilocular retrorectal cystic disease-cyst hamartoma: Report of twelve cases. Dis Colon Rectum 1961;4:103–110.

168. Marco V, Autonell J, Farre J, et al. Retrorectal cyst-hamartomas: Report of two cases with adenocarcinoma developing in one. Am J Surg Pathol 1982;6:707.

169. Colin JF, Branfoot AC, Robinson KP. Malignant change in rectal duplication. J R Soc Med 1979;72:935–937.

170. Ben-Chaim J, Docimo SG, Jeffs RD, et al. Bladder exstrophy from childhood into adult life. J R Soc Med 1996;89:39–46.

171. Johnson TB. Extroversion of the bladder, complicated by the presence of intestinal openings on the surface of the extroverted area. J Anat Physiol 1913;48:89–106.

172. Johnston JH, Penn IA. Exstrophy of the cloaca. Br J Urol 1966;38: 302–307.

173. Zarabi CM, Rupani M. Cloacal exstrophy: A hypothesis on the allantoic origin of the distal midgut. Pediatr Pathol Lab Med 1985;4:117–124.

174. Lin HJ, Ndiforchu F, Patell S. Exstrophy of the cloaca in 47,XXX child: Review of genitourinary malformations in triple-X patients. Am J Med Genetics 1993;45:761–763.

175. Wood K. Lymphatic cysts of the mesentery: A review of the literature and a report of two cases. Br J Surg 1955;43:304–308.

176. Handelsman JC, Ravitch MM. Chylous cysts of the mesentery in children. Ann Surg 1954;140:185–193.

177. Bentley JFR, O'Donnell MB. Mesenteric cysts with malrotated intestine. Br Med J 1959;2:223–225.

178. Moore TC. Congenital cysts of the mesentery: Report of four cases. Ann Surg 1957;145:428–436.

179. Hastings N, Norris WJ. Unusual abdominal cysts in infants and children. California Med 1954;81:84–86.

180. Bliss DP, Coffin CM, Bower RJ, et al. Mesenteric cysts in children. Surgery 1994;115:571–577.

181. Liew SCC, Glenn DC, Storey DW. Mesenteric cyst. Aust NZ J Surg 1994;64:741–744.

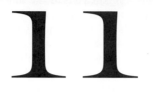

11

CHEMICAL AND PHYSICAL DISORDERS

Charles W. Andrews, Jr. and Harvey Goldman

This chapter provides detailed information on the pathogenesis of and morphologic alterations associated with gastrointestinal disorders that result from exposure to various chemical and physical agents. Related material in other parts of the book include disorders of the esophagus (see Chapter 20), disorders of the stomach (see Chapters 23 and 24), disorders of the intestines (see Chapters 30 and 31), and systemic conditions (see Chapter 19).

The mechanisms and factors involved in injury caused by chemicals, drugs, and radiation have been investigated extensively. Noteworthy are the concept of gastric cytoprotection (1–4), the elucidation of the potent actions of free radicals (5–7), the role of the effects on the microcirculation and extracellular matrix components, and the interactions of the exogenous agents

with the gut secretions and microbial flora in the production of disease (8).

MECHANISMS OF CELLULAR INJURY

Most of the deleterious effects of chemicals, drugs, and ionizing radiation are initiated by damage to the mucosal epithelial cells, either directly or mediated by vascular insufficiency. The common factors and mechanisms involved in this injury are summarized in this section. It should be stressed that the development of these lesions does not involve new biochemical reactions, but rather is due to derangements of existing processes. The pathologic features of injury are generally nonspecific and therefore do not define a particular etiology (6, 7, 9).

OXYGEN

Oxygen is of central importance in the mechanisms of cell injury. The lack of oxygen causes cell injury (e.g., ischemia), primarily by reducing oxidative phosphorylation and thus adenosine triphosphate (ATP) levels. Excess or unused cellular oxygen can be rendered toxic by the generation of free radicals, which are the highly reactive species of oxygen.

FREE RADICALS

Free radicals are chemicals with unpaired electrons and are usually the result of incomplete reduction of oxygen to water. This reaction is normally performed by the mitochondrial electron transport system and catalyzed by cytochrome oxidase. The free radicals can be induced by many chemicals and drugs and by ionizing radiation. The altered reduction of oxygen results in the generation of superoxide and hydrogen peroxide. Interaction of hydrogen peroxide with superoxide or ferrous ions produces hydroxyl radicals, which are probably the most toxic species among free radicals. Hydroxyl radicals alone, but especially in the presence of ferric ions, promote lipid peroxidation or disulfide formation of membrane proteins, leading to membrane injury and increased permeability. These changes represent the first steps in cellular damage.

Some oxygen radicals contribute to tissue damage indirectly, by causing vascular smooth muscle contraction or through interaction with endogenous nitric oxide, thereby influencing mucosal blood flow and the microvasculature (10–12). The resulting ischemia may then be one of the major causes of the ensuing tissue injury and necrosis. Free radicals can also stimulate the synthesis of other potent toxic agents, such as hypochlorous acid (9). Free radicals likely have a dominant role in the pathogenesis of cell and tissue injury, irrespective of whether it is caused by ischemia, chemicals, or physical agents.

CALCIUM

Calcium also exerts a major regulatory role in cell damage. When isolated hepatic or gastric mucosal cells are incubated in the presence or absence of calcium and of toxic concentrations of phalloidin, ethanol, or indomethacin, the viability of cells is higher in the medium with little or no calcium (13). Following membrane injury by different mechanisms, the influx of calcium from the extracellular medium is a major rate-limiting step. Calcium, however, not only comes from outside the cell, but also often is mobilized within the cell, e.g., the endoplasmic reticulum. Calcium may activate enzymes, such as phospholipases and calcium-dependent cysteine (thiol) proteases. The activated enzymes then attack the protein component of plasma membranes and other structural or enzyme proteins, thereby initiating or accelerating membrane damage. Influx also may induce immediate early genes, such as c-fos and c-jun, which through complex interactions may confer either a protective advantage to cell survival or a deleterious state leading to cell death (14).

ADENOSINE TRIPHOSPHATE

Adenosine triphosphate (ATP) production is related to the functional status of the mitochondria. Selective depletion of ATP or prevention of its synthesis are usually not sufficient to cause severe cell injury. The decrease in ATP production associated with other mitochondrial dysfunction in electron transport and membrane damage, however, leads to a loss of ion gradients, release of calcium from intracellular stores and influx from extracellular sources, and acceleration of loss of membrane integrity. This situation is aggravated by glycolysis and intracellular acidification, which are also the consequences of diminished ATP synthesis followed by alterations in the adenosine pool (15).

PROTEASES

Proteases, derived from lysosomes and activated in the cytosol, also play a major role in both cell and tissue injury (16). These enzymes, released by parenchymal cells or neutrophils that are attracted after initial cell damage, may attack the intracellular and extracellular structural proteins, cell adhesion molecules, and also activate procollagenase. The proteases are normally controlled by endogenous inhibitors, but the latter can be inactivated by free radicals, leading to the potentiation of the proteases.

CHEMICAL AND DRUG DISORDERS

Only the toxic effects of chemicals and drugs leading to inflammatory lesions are addressed in this chapter. Other chapters include discussion of the roles of chemicals in the initiation and promotion of tumors of the esophagus (see Chapters 21 and 22), of the stomach (see Chapter 27), and of the intestines (see Chapter 34).

DEFINITIONS AND CLASSIFICATION

About 50,000 chemicals are used in industry, agriculture, and households, as well as for medical purposes, including dental and veterinary use. The Merck Index lists more than 10,000 organic and inorganic chemicals that have been tested in toxicologic and/or pharmacologic evaluations, including 3000 to 4000 drugs (17). Drugs represent a subgroup of chemicals that are used in medicine for treatment, prevention, and diagnostic tests, and their effects are emphasized in this chapter. About 2 to 8% of patients receiving drugs experience some form of adverse reaction. In one study, upper gastrointestinal bleeding related to nonsteroidal anti-inflammatory drug (NSAID) use was the most frequent event requiring hospitalization, accounting for 64.6% of adverse drug-related admissions (18). Of all drug injuries noted, 18 to 33% affect one or more portions of the gastrointestinal tract (19, 20).

The actions of chemicals that are not established drugs are observed in persons with a particular addiction (e.g., ethyl alcohol) or after exposure of an accidental, occupational, or suicidal nature. The lesions tend to occur regularly and to have a standard appearance. In contrast, the effects of drugs are more variable with respect to frequency, mechanism of injury, and types of lesions.

PATHOGENESIS

The principle ways in which a chemical or drug induces injury of the gut are summarized in Table 11.1. In many situations, the specific pathogenetic event is not clearly established. This lack of specificity is particularly a problem with drugs that may act either as toxic agents or as a mediator of an immunologic reaction. Furthermore, the overall lesions observed may be attributable to a combination of the drugs with an underlying condition or with other modes of therapy, such as radiation. The intracellular factors and events involved were detailed in the preceding section on mechanisms of cellular injury. Following irreversible cell injury come the features of necrosis and reactive acute inflammation. Most lesions attributable to chemical and drug exposure undergo complete resolution, after elimination of the offending agent. From repeated exposure, however, lesions can persist in the form of erosions, ulcers, or chronic inflammatory conditions. Complications are generally uncommon and include fibrous stricture formation, deep mural necrosis leading to perforation, pseudo-obstruction from altered motility, and malabsorption.

PHYSICAL EVENTS

Some drugs cause injury by the simple entrapment of a pill or capsule in the mucosa before it has been dissolved, resulting in a localized ulceration. This type of injury is noted most often in the esophagus, less frequently in the stomach and small intestine. Such localized irritation has been observed with emepronium bromide, potassium chloride, barbiturates, tetracycline, and many other antibiotics and drugs (see subsequent section concerning the esophagus for details). Obstruction from a mass of undissolved pills, representing a type of bezoar, occurs rarely. Its development is facilitated by the attempt to take an excess number of pills and by the presence of narrowed regions of the gut.

TOXIC INJURY

This type of injury is the common mechanism for most chemicals and drugs, with effects ranging from inhibition of cell growth to necrosis. The pathogenesis of toxic injury in the gastrointestinal tract is complex and involves either direct cytotoxicity by chemicals (e.g., ethanol, HCl, ammonia, bile acids, aspirin) or indirect actions through the metabolism and release of endogenous tissue and vascular mediators of damage (e.g., free radicals and proteins). Water-soluble agents typically act directly on the cells, whereas lipid-soluble substances generally operate by the induction of free radicals. The majority of the chemicals and drugs are lipid soluble and become toxic through metabolic activation. Acetaminophen does not directly damage the liver, but during the metabolic process, toxic intermediates are formed that interact with glutathione, the endogenous protective peptide. As the concentration of hepatic glutathione decreases, the toxicity of the drug increases, leading to massive necrosis (21). The decrease of gastric mucosal glutathione by fasting also seems to contribute to the gastrotoxicity of ethanol, acrylonitrile, NSAID, and stress (22).

The indirect toxicity of a chemical to the stomach is further illustrated by the example of aspirin. Depending on the acid concentration in the stomach (the pK of aspirin is 3.5), the drug may cause mucosal injury either directly or indirectly. If the gastric pH is 3.5 or higher, most of the aspirin is not dissociated and

TABLE	
11.1	**Pathogenetic Mechanisms of Chemical and Drug Disorders**

Physical events
   Pill entrapment in mucosa
   Bezoar
Chemical injury
   Cellular toxicity
   Allergic reaction
Vascular lesions
   Hemorrhage and thrombi
   Vasoconstriction and low perfusion
   Vasculitis
Promotion of infections
Altered motility
Foreign body reactions

damages the superficial epithelium directly as a physical agent in crystallized form (8, 23). Injury is caused indirectly if the gastric acidity is below pH 3.5; most of the aspirin is lipid soluble and so is absorbed by the stomach, resulting in the formation of salicylate, which is a potent mitochondrial poison. In this case, the depletion of mucosal prostaglandins, owing to the inhibition of cyclooxygenase, is thought to be an underlying mechanism for the development of mucosal damage. Evidence of such a relationship has been established by measurements of prostaglandin E_2 (PGE_2) in residual gastric juice after administration of naproxen sodium (24).

Efforts have been made to distinguish between a direct toxic effect on the tissues and a damage that is mediated by an immunologic event. Toxic injuries are characterized by the ability to achieve reproducible lesions in animals, by a dose-related effect, by a fairly temporally specific relationship of the events, and by the development of a standard lesion. In contrast, immunologic injury is typically not regular and reproducible; it cannot be induced routinely in animals, is not dose or temporally related, and produces a lesion that may differ even within the same host. Evidence is mounting, however, that the majority of chemical and drug lesions are attributable to direct cytotoxicity or are mediated by the release of free radicals or by changes in the local microvasculature. All parts of the gut may be involved, and examples of offending agents include corrosive substances, ethanol, aspirin and other anti-inflammatory agents, and chemotherapeutic drugs.

VASCULAR LESIONS

These lesions include hemorrhages related to treatment with anticoagulants or thrombolytic agents and to drug-induced thrombocytopenia (see Chapter 19); vasculitis that can be caused by many drugs and usually is generalized, with sporadic involvement of the gastrointestinal tract (25); embolic events in the course of injection treatment of tumors or bleeding disorders (26, 27); vascular thromboses from estrogens and progesterones leading to ischemic lesions (28); and reduced splanchnic blood flow resulting from the action of vasoconstrictor, hypotensive, and hypovolemic drugs (29). (See Chapter 14 for details.)

PROMOTION OF INFECTIONS

Many antibiotics and chemotherapeutic agents are responsible for the development of pseudomembranous colitis, associated with the preferential growth of *Clostridium difficile* and elaboration of its toxins. Drugs can also lead exceptionally to agranulocytosis, favoring the appearance of neutropenic colitis, an infection resulting usually from *Clostridium septicum*. Drugs that result in more general immunosuppression allow the promotion of numerous opportunistic infections, such as herpes, cytomegalovirus, *Mycobacterium avium*, fungi, *Giardia*, and *Cryptosporidium* (see Chapter 28).

ALTERED MOTILITY

A variety of drugs acting on the nerves, ganglia, and muscles of the gut can interfere with motility, resulting in a pseudo-obstruction that is usually dominant in the colon (30). Examples include anticholinergic, antidepressant, and chemotherapeutic drugs; ganglionic blockers; and narcotics (see Chapter 13).

FOREIGN BODY DEPOSITS

These deposits are usually associated with barium and oils and are concentrated in the lower colon and rectum (31, 32) (see Figs. 30.25 and 30.26).

SYNERGISTIC EFFECTS

Many patients with advanced tumors receive multiple chemotherapeutic agents and radiation. Lesions encountered in these patients are probably a consequence of the use of multiple agents enhanced by the debilitated nature of the patients. Certain drugs, such as Adriamycin (Adria Laboratories, Dublin, OH) and actinomycin D, are radiomimetic, serving to exaggerate the radiation effects (33–35). Local, potentially toxic secretions may also act in conjunction with the chemicals and drugs to evoke the lesions; the presence of gastric acid appears to be essential for the full development of lesions attributable to ethanol and to aspirin.

GENERAL PATHOLOGIC FEATURES

All features noted in chemical and drug disorders are nonspecific, and the diagnosis depends on the history and on the exclusion of other conditions. The large variety of lesions involving the several segments of the gut have been compiled and reviewed (20, 29, 36, 37). The types of lesions are briefly described in Table 11.2. Further details are provided in subsequent sections.

HEMORRHAGES AND THROMBOSES

Solitary hemorrhages are typically fresh and concentrated in the mucosa and submucosa. They vary in size from simple streaks to relatively large hematomas, and the bigger lesions can be discerned on radiographic examination as projecting lumps. Hemorrhages are more often seen in conjunction with the inflammatory conditions, particularly gastritis and duodenitis. Venous thromboses are noted

uncommonly in patients receiving estrogens or progesterone; they usually cause local hemorrhages but exceptionally can lead to more extensive vascular insufficiency and infarction.

ULCERATIONS

This common manifestation of chemical and drug injury may represent a solitary lesion or be part of a more diffuse inflammatory condition. It can be caused by any of the pathogenetic mechanisms, including physical pressure, cytotoxic damage, vasculitis, or infection. The ulcers are usually superficial, and necrosis and a variable amount of acute inflammation are noted. Deeper ulcers and greater inflammation can be seen, especially in cases involving corrosive substances or chemotherapeutic agents. Drugs can also promote recurrences of chronic peptic ulcers of the stomach and duodenum.

APOPTOSIS

Cell death by apoptosis, although physiologic, is also produced by a variety of injurious stimuli, including drugs and radiation. Cryptal apoptotic bodies consist of single or clumps of cells surrounded by an apparent membrane that encloses dense aggregates of basophilic nuclear chromatin fragments. Increased numbers of apoptotic bodies, usually accompanied by an increase in intraepithelial lymphocytes, have been reported predominantly with antineoplastic agents and NSAID (38, 39).

INFLAMMATORY CONDITIONS

Inflammation is the typical effect seen with most chemicals and drugs in the gastroduodenal region and in the colon. The mucosa is usually diffusely involved, with variable acute inflammation and hemorrhage; erosions and ulcerations are noted in more severe cases (Fig. 11.1). A chronic inflammatory condition is rarely observed with most agents, presumably because exposure to the drugs is discontinued. It is possible that some cases of chronic antral gastritis and chronic duodenitis are attributable to repeated episodes of

TABLE 11.2	**General Pathologic Features of Chemical and Drug Disorders**

Hemorrhages and thromboses
Ulcerations
Inflammatory conditions
Apoptosis
Complications
    Perforation
    Stricture
Other features (uncommon)
    Infarction
    Pseudo-obstruction
    Foreign body deposits
    Pneumatosis

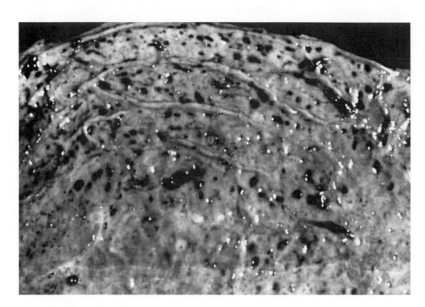

Figure 11.1 Mucosal surface of the stomach has numerous small and hemorrhagic erosions. This appearance is typical of gastric injury associated with ethyl alcohol, aspirin, other NSAID, and acute stress ulcers. (Courtesy of Dr. Karoly Balogh.)

injury from ethanol, aspirin, and other anti-inflammatory drugs, but this correlation is usually not established. Inflammatory conditions affecting the upper tract are typically limited to the mucosa, whereas those in the distal small intestine and colon can be associated with more extensive involvement and simulate cases of ischemic disease and idiopathic inflammatory bowel disease. Rare cases of enteritis and colitis with granulomas have been noted in association with diclofenac (an anti-inflammatory agent) and clofazimine (a drug used in the treatment of leprosy) (40, 41).

COMPLICATIONS

More extensive necrosis, inflammation, and fibrosis of any part of the gut can be seen in patients who have received combined chemotherapy, alone or in conjunction with radiation, for malignant tumors. Fibrous strictures from drug reactions are relatively rare but can develop in cases with deeper ulceration; they are seen most often in the esophagus from lye injury and in the distal small intestine related to potassium chloride and exceptionally to anti-inflammatory drugs.

Perforation is also uncommon and is limited to those cases involving extensive caustic damage, severe forms of colitis, and tumors. In patients with tumors, it is usually difficult or impossible to determine which effects are related to various factors, including drugs, radiation, secondary infections, or the underlying condition. Other uncommon features include vascular insufficiency and infarction of the intestines owing to vasculitis or venous thrombi, pseudo-obstruction from drug damage to the nerves or muscles of the gut, localized deposits of barium and oils, and pneumatosis coli.

CLINICAL FEATURES AND DIAGNOSIS

The particular clinical features depend on the location of the injury within the gut, the nature and extent of the lesion, and the appearance of any complications (20, 29). Symptoms in the early stages typically relate to the degree of hemorrhage, ulceration, and inflammation and are identical to those seen in cases of other etiologies. Less commonly noted are signs of obstruction related to

a fibrous stricture or a motility disorder; of malabsorption of fats, B12, or folate; and of a more severe form of enteritis or colitis that can mimic ischemic disease, Crohn disease, and ulcerative colitis. No specific features are noted on radiographic, gross endoscopic, or histologic examinations, and the diagnosis of a chemical or drug injury is reliant on the history. Endoscopic biopsies may be performed to exclude other conditions, such as recurrent tumor, infections, radiation, and the more common inflammatory conditions affecting the gut. Further details are provided in subsequent discussions of specific organ involvement.

ETIOLOGIC AGENTS

Considering the huge number of existing chemicals and drugs, it is not feasible to cite all of the reported injuries affecting the gut. Major examples are stressed, and the reader is referred to the extensive reviews on this subject for further details (20, 29, 37). In this section, the emphasis is on the causative agents and the general effects in the gastrointestinal tract. In the following section, the concentration is on the diseases involving particular segments of the gut.

Most chemicals and drugs do not uniformly affect the entire gastrointestinal tract. Caustic agents and alcohol, for example, primarily damage the esophagus and stomach. Among the steroid hormones, glucocorticoids in large doses can induce gastric and duodenal ulcers, whereas estrogens and progesterones in oral contraceptives may damage the intestinal tract. All of the NSAID cause injury to the stomach and duodenum, but some of the agents can also cause ulcers and strictures of the more distal small intestine or, rarely, the colon. The antibiotics, antineoplastic agents, and vasoactive drugs can injure any part of the tract, although the mechanism of action and nature of the lesions varies in the different regions.

Many drugs of all types can cause a vasculitis (25). Typically the result of an immunologic injury, the vasculitis tends to be generalized or have major effects in the skin, lungs, or kidneys. Involvement of the gastrointestinal tract by drug-induced vasculitis is relatively uncommon. It can lead to areas of ischemic necrosis, usually in the form of focal ulcers and rarely resulting in larger areas of infarction, and the lesions tend to be concentrated in the intestinal tract (see Chapter 14). The categories of the various chemicals and drugs, along with examples of the major alterations in the gut, are summarized in Table 11.3.

CAUSTIC AGENTS

These agents include strong alkali (lye), acids, and bleaches that are present in common household cleaning products (Table 11.4) (29, 42). The types and severity of injury have varied as the contents of preparations have changed over the years (43). Injury results from the accidental ingestion of the substances by children or from suicidal efforts, and the lesions are generally confined to the oropharynx, esophagus, or stomach (44–46). Rare cases of cleansing solutions contaminating endoscopes have caused caustic injury to the lower tract (47, 48). The location and degree of damage depend on the amount, concentration, and nature (whether crystalline or liquid) of the substance as well as the time of exposure. In general, the crystalline products tend to affect the more proximal regions and are promptly expelled, whereas the liquids reach and act throughout the esophagus and stomach.

The lesions are in the form of burns that may be limited to the mucosa and resolve rapidly or, more often, extend into the wall,

---

TABLE 11.3   Effects of Chemicals and Drugs

Category	Examples of Lesions
Caustic agents	Ulcers and strictures of esophagus and stomach
	Proctitis from enema (hydrogen peroxide)
Ethyl alcohol	Gastritis and duodenitis
	Mild effects on small intestine
	Proctitis from accidental enemas
Steroid hormones	
Glucocorticoids	Gastric and duodenal ulcers
	Promotion of infections
Estrogen and progesterone	Hemorrhage, thrombosis, and ischemia of intestines
Nonsteroidal anti-inflammatory drugs	Focal esophageal ulcers from pills
	Gastritis and duodenitis
	Focal ulcers and strictures of small intestine
	Rare colitis and proctitis (suppository)
Chemotherapeutic and immunomodulatory drugs	Ulcers and inflammation of all parts
	Synergism with radiation (Adriamycin, actinomycin D)
	Malabsorption (methotrexate, colchicine)
	Pseudo-obstruction (vincristine)
Antibiotic and antimicrobial drugs	Focal esophageal ulcers from pills
	Pseudomembranous colitis
	Malabsorption (neomycin, para-aminosalicylate)
	Other enteritis and colitis (flucytosine, clofazimine)
Anticholinergic and antidepressant drugs	Pseudo-obstruction
Anticoagulant drugs	Hemorrhages and hematomas
Cardiovascular drugs	Focal esophageal ulcers from pills (quinidine, vasopressin)
	Gastric and duodenal ulcers (reserpine, ethacrynic acid)
	Ischemic lesions of intestines (vasoconstrictor, hypovolemic, and hypotensive drugs)
	Malabsorption (methyldopa)
	Pseudo-obstruction (ganglion blockers)
Heavy metals	Focal esophageal ulcers from pills (iron salts)
	Gastric ulcers (iron and zinc salts)
	Enteritis and colitis (gold salts)
Enemas and laxatives	Proctitis from enemas (Fleet's bisacodyl, soaps)
	Cathartic colon
Miscellaneous drugs	Focal esophageal ulcers from pills
	Malabsorption and pseudo-obstruction
	Rare cases of allergic colitis
	Gastric and ileal ulcers and strictures (KCl)
	Possible ulcers of stomach and duodenum (bromocriptine, spironolactone) and pneumatosis intestinalis (lactulose and practolol)

TABLE	
11.4	**Examples of Caustic Agents**

Alkali	Acids
Sodium hydroxide	Hydrochloric acid
Potassium hydroxide	Sulfuric acid
Ammonium hydroxide	Nitric acid
Sodium metasilicate	Phosphoric acid
Sodium perborate	Acetic acid
Potassium monopersulphate	Oxalic acid
Bleaches	Fixatives
Hydrogen peroxide	Formalin
Sodium hypochlorite	Zenker's solution
	Glutaraldehyde

leading to persistent ulceration (43, 49). They manifest necrosis, reactive inflammation, and formation of granulation tissue and fibrosis in cases with deeper involvement. Early perforation from transmural involvement is uncommon, but fibrous strictures frequently develop later in the course. Also noted in the esophagus are the rare occurrence of Barrett esophagus localized to the strictured area and an increased incidence of squamous cell carcinoma (50).

Most cases of injury to the esophagus involve the liquid alkaline solutions, with effects seen throughout the middle and distal portions. Contraction of the lower sphincter protects the stomach in some instances. The esophageal squamous epithelium appears to be relatively resistant to acids, but it can be damaged by high concentrations. In contrast, both acids and alkali commonly damage the stomach, with greatest effects in the antral region. The diagnosis of caustic injury is typically afforded by the history, and treatment may include administration of glucocorticoid hormones in an attempt to limit the edema and stricture formation, and of antibiotics for secondary infections. Additional tests, including endoscopy, are performed to determine the extent of the disease, and the strictures are controlled by luminal dilation or by surgery. Other chapters provide further details on esophagitis (see Chapter 20) and gastritis (see Chapter 23).

ETHYL ALCOHOL

Extensive evidence from humans and animal experiments demonstrates that alcohol routinely damages the gastric mucosa, resulting in an acute erosive or nonerosive gastritis (51–53) (see Chapter 23). As a lipid-soluble agent, the alcohol dissolves in and damages the surface epithelial cell membranes, rendering the tissue more permeable to the back diffusion of hydrogen ions (54, 55). The ions in turn can cause vasoconstriction of the mucosal microcirculation, promoting larger areas of injury (56). The lesions are dominant in the antrum but can also involve the corpus of the stomach. Noted are a superficial necrosis, prominent edema and hemorrhages in the lamina propria, and erosions in severe cases (see Fig. 11.1). Elimination of the exposure typically leads to a prompt renewal of the mucosa and complete recovery within a few days. It is possible that repeated episodes of alcoholic injury can result in a chronic antral gastritis, although the evidence is conflicting with estimates of

incidence ranging from 3 to 10% of cases. Alcoholic patients also have an increased prevalence of chronic peptic ulcers of the antrum and duodenum (about 15 to 20%), with most cases related to the presence of hepatic cirrhosis and enhanced by shunt procedures (57); this enhancement is believed to be due to reduced inactivation of gastric acid stimulants such as histamine and gastrin by the damaged or shunted liver.

Alcohol can also affect the small intestinal mucosa (58, 59), although the changes are usually mild as a result of lesser exposure in this region, and clinical problems are uncommon. An increase in the duodenum of goblet mucous cells and gastric mucous cell metaplasia, indicative of chronic injury, has been noted. Greater enteritis, in the form of reduced villi, is usually associated with nutritional problems, such as folate deficiency. Ultrastructurally, pronounced alterations occur that resolve only partially with abstinence (59). The lower part of the intestinal tract is ordinarily not involved. Superficial proctitis has been observed after the accidental inclusion of alcohol in enema preparations (60). The diagnosis of alcoholic injury is typically established by the history, and endoscopic study may be performed to exclude other causes of hemorrhage from the upper gastrointestinal tract.

STEROID HORMONES

Considerable controversy surrounds the potential toxicity of glucocorticoid hormones in the gastrointestinal tract (61–63). They probably enhance the recurrence rate of chronic peptic ulcers and the extent of the lesions by retarding the healing process. The hormones can reduce the mucous secretion in the stomach, either directly or by inhibition of the regenerative cells, and evidence suggests a slight increase of acute gastric and small intestinal ulcer formation, particularly in the treatment of patients with rheumatoid arthritis (20, 64). It is often difficult, however, to discriminate between the actions of the steroids and those of the other medications taken by these patients; the possibility of additive effects from the drugs exists.

The ulcers are usually superficial and promptly reversible, but deeper lesions leading to perforation have been noted in the small intestine, particularly in low birth weight neonates receiving high dose levels (65, 66). Prolonged use of corticosteroids can also promote the development of secondary opportunistic infections in all parts of the gut. Infections noted most often are due to herpes, cytomegalovirus, and fungi. The appearance of these infections can worsen an underlying disorder, such as peptic ulcers and ulcerative colitis, leading to increased chance of perforation.

Estrogens and progesterone compounds, including oral contraceptive drugs, can cause ischemic lesions of the small intestine and colon (28, 67–70), although the incidence is probably low. Although more common in older patients, a reversible ischemic colitis in females 50 years of age or younger has been associated with oral contraceptive use (71). Other risk factors include cigarette smoking and systemic arterial hypertension.

The lesions usually develop in persons who have taken at least 0.5 g of the drug per day for more than 1 year. The drugs cause injury by promoting the formation of thrombi in the mesenteric arteries or veins leading to segmental areas of hemorrhage or hemorrhagic infarction of the intestines that simulate other causes of ischemic enteritis and colitis or Crohn disease (28, 72, 73). Rarely, colonic disease is more extensive and resembles ulcerative colitis (74). Use of oral contraceptive agents for greater than 6 years

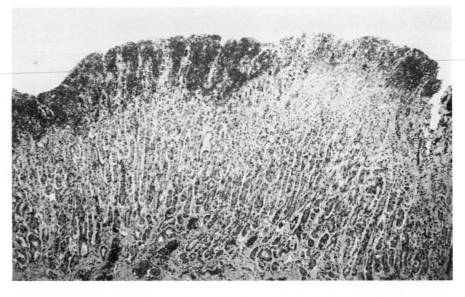

Figure 11.2 Gastric corpus mucosa in the early stage of aspirin injury, with a fragment of muscularis mucosae *(bottom).* Fresh hemorrhage is limited to the superficial foveolar region, and the corpus glands are normal. H & E, ×80. (Courtesy of Dr. Karoly Balogh.)

does appear to increase the risk of Crohn's disease but not that of ulcerative colitis (75). There is otherwise no definite evidence that these drugs promote recurrences of existing cases of idiopathic inflammatory bowel disease.

Lesions are usually reversible after elimination of the drugs, but complications including fibrous strictures and rarely bowel perforations can occur. The pathologic features are essentially identical to those seen in patients with infarction owing to vascular thromboses, and the diagnosis made on the basis of the history.

NONSTEROIDAL ANTI-INFLAMMATORY DRUGS (NSAID)

These drugs include aspirin (acetylsalicylic acid) and other salicylates, indomethacin, phenylbutazone and derivatives, and an ever expanding group of other anti-inflammatory agents that are used primarily in the treatment of rheumatoid arthritis and degenerative joint disease (Table 11.5) (76–79). Because of the large number of patients consuming these drugs, adverse effects represent a major clinical problem. In 1991 alone, more than 70 million prescriptions were written for NSAID (80). Overall, the estimated relative risk for hospitalization or death from NSAID ranges from 2.74 to 3.0 (81, 82).

The major effects of NSAID are in the gastric antrum and proximal duodenum in the form of diffuse hemorrhages, erosions, and ulcers (Figs. 11.2 and 11.3). Furthermore, these drugs can activate the recurrence of a chronic peptic ulcer in this area. Aspirin has been available for the longest time and has been investigated most extensively (20, 29, 83–86). Over 50% of patients with hemorrhage from the upper gastrointestinal tract offer a history of aspirin ingestion, and with long-term use of the drug comes increasing blood loss, possibly exceeding 10 times the normal amount in the stool. Endoscopic evidence of gastric ulcers has been noted in 20% of cases, erosions in 40%, and mucosal erythema in 75% (86). Of interest, most patients with documented blood loss or abnormal endoscopic findings do not have symptoms. Some patients exhibit a gastric adaptation, characterized by the healing of lesions despite the continued use of aspirin (87). It is possible that this healing occurs as a result of regeneration of prostaglandins in the tissues.

TABLE	
11.5	**Examples of Nonsteroidal Anti-Inflammatory Drugs (NSAID)**

Alclofenac	Meclofenamate
Aspirin	Mefenamic acid
Diclofenac	Nabumetone
Diflunisal	Naproxen
Etodolac	Niflumic acid
Fenclofenac	Oxaprozin
Fenoprofen	Oxyphenylbutazone
Floctafenine	Phenylbutazone
Flurbiprofen	Piroxicam
Glafenine	Salsalate
Ibuprofen	Sulindac
Indomethacin	Tolfenamic acid
Ketoprofen	Tolmetin

The anti-inflammatory effect of aspirin, and probably of most of the NSAID, is attributable to the inhibition of cyclooxygenase (COX) leading to reduced prostaglandin synthesis from arachidonic acid. Two isoforms of COX are COX-1, which is a constitutive enzyme, and COX-2, which is rapidly inducible and results in the production of pro-inflammatory prostaglandins (88). High concentrations of prostaglandins, especially PGE_2 and PGI_2, are present in the normal gastric and duodenal mucosa where they inhibit gastric acid secretion and increase mucous production.

The toxic action of aspirin probably involves multiple factors, including the depletion of mucosal prostaglandins; damage to the membranes of the surface epithelial cells leading to enhanced back diffusion of hydrogen ions and overall increased membrane permeability; redistribution of mucosal blood flow; decreased epithelial cell renewal; and inhibition of platelet aggregation favoring an increase in bleeding. The back diffusion is probably a vital component, because the presence of gastric acid is needed to produce the more florid lesions. The presence of other toxic agents, such as ethanol and bile salts, increases the injury caused by aspirin, whereas the administration of prostaglandins can prevent or ameliorate the lesions.

Because of the regularly observed toxicity of aspirin, a large number of alternative analgesic and anti-inflammatory drugs have been introduced and promoted. Buffered forms of aspirin and other salicylate compounds appear to cause less gastric lesions but equivalent damage to the duodenum (89), whereas the effects of acetaminophen (paramecatol) are minimal. The phenylbutazone compounds have been largely discarded because of their hematologic as well as gastrointestinal toxicity. Indomethacin and the other NSAID have all been shown to cause equivalent lesions in the stomach and duodenum, although the amount of bleeding might be less. Selective COX inhibitors, specifically COX-2 inhibitors, are being devised that represent a new pharmacologic class of NSAID that may provide anti-inflammatory and analgesic activity without gastrointestinal toxicity (90). Low-dose aspirin regimens, particularly in patients with atherosclerotic heart disease, have also been used, however; by endoscopy and biopsy, the toxic effects do not appear to be lessened (91).

The lesions that arise in association with the use of aspirin and the other NSAID are similar, revealing superficial necrosis and hemorrhage of the gastric and duodenal mucosa with focal erosions or ulcers and relatively slight inflammation. Indeed, the finding of minimal or no inflammation in the mucosa next to an ulcer helps to identify that the lesion is primarily caused by a drug rather than an established, chronic peptic ulcer in which a certain degree of inflammation is invariably present (92, 93). Elimination of the drug leads typically leads to prompt recovery with renewal of the mucosa; no definite evidence supports the idea that these drugs can cause a chronic gastritis. Other chapters provide further details on the pathology and course of gastritis (see Chapter 23) and of peptic ulcers (see Chapter 24).

Evidence that these drugs can cause necrosis and ulceration of the mucosa of the jejunum and ileum is mounting, although the exact frequency is not known (94, 95). The pathologic features are generally nonspecific, and most cases are promptly reversible. Perforation from areas of transmural necrosis and strictures from the development of significant submucosal fibrosis are infrequent

events. Several reports of strictures with a characteristic appearance of thin, concentric septate-like projections narrowing the intestinal lumen have been reported and termed "diaphragm disease." Although usually in the midportion of the small intestine or ileum, similar findings in the cecum and ascending colon have been described (94, 96, 97). Cases of the following have been recorded less frequently: enteritis with granulomas associated with diclofenac (40); colitis associated with meclofenamate, mefenamic acid, and sulfasalazine (98, 99); and proctitis secondary to the use of suppositories containing NSAID (100). There is also growing evidence that lesions of the colon, including bleeding, perforations, obstructions, and strictures, may occur with NSAID therapy (101, 102). An increased use of NSAID has also been noted over controls in patients with collagenous colitis, suggesting an etiologic role (103). Focal ulcers of the esophagus resulting from localized entrapment of pills in the mucosa have been noted after using aspirin, indomethacin, phenylbutazone, tolmetin, and various compounds containing a mixture of NSAID (104).

Overall, the diagnosis of a gut injury related to NSAID therapy is primarily determined by the history, and treatment ordinarily consists of stopping or decreasing the amount of the drug. Prostaglandins, H2-blocking agents, and other gastric protective drugs, such as sucralfate, are occasionally provided to facilitate the healing or to lessen the effects of the NSAID. Endoscopy with biopsy is often the means by which to localize the lesion, to determine the extent of the injury, and to monitor the clinical course after cessation of the drug or a reduction in its dosage.

CHEMOTHERAPEUTIC AND IMMUNOMODULATORY DRUGS

The gastrointestinal tract is regularly affected by the many drugs that are used in the treatment of malignant tumors of the gut and of the other organs and tissues of the body (Table 11.6) (20, 29, 37). Some of these drugs are also being used with increasing frequency for immunosuppressive therapy after transplantation and in patients with advanced inflammatory conditions. Because all of these agents operate primarily by the inhibition of mitotically active cells, the dominant effects are noted in the mucosal epithelial cells through-

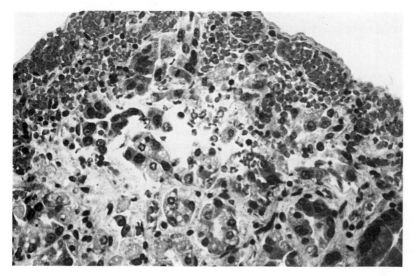

Figure 11.3 Same case as in Figure 11.2, with the luminal surface at top, shows the hemorrhage together with necrosis of the surface and foveolar (pit) epithelial cells. Inflammation is minimal at this early stage. H & E, ×200. (Courtesy of Dr. Karoly Balogh.)

TABLE 11.6	Examples of Chemotherapeutic and Immunomodulatory Drugs	
Actinomycin D	5-Fluoro-2-deoxyuridine
Adriamycin	Hydroxyurea
Bleomycin	Interleukins
Cisplatin	Methomazine
Colchicine	Methotrexate
Cyclophosphamide	Mitomycin C
Cyclosporine	Paclitaxel
Cytosine arabinoside	Procarbazine
Daunorubicin	Vinblastine
5-Fluorouracil	Vincristine

out every portion of the tract. The toxicity in the individual patients is highly variable and depends on the number of drugs used and their dosage, the time of exposure, the added effects of radiation therapy and surgery, and the extent of tumor involvement. The major lesions are ulceration and inflammation, with the greatest effects from 5-fluorouracil and its analogues as well as from combinations of drugs. Lesser amounts of injury are observed with some of the agents such as cyclophosphamide, cisplatin, and daunorubicin.

The small intestinal mucosa is probably the most sensitive region, and a reduction in mitoses and the early ultrastructural signs of cellular injury are seen about 3 hours after exposure to the drugs (105, 106). Noted are clumping of the nuclear chromatin, fragmentation of mitochondria, and dilation of the endoplasmic reticulum and Golgi region in the villous epithelial cells. The injury becomes maximal after 1 day and persists for the duration of drug usage. Damage of the villi is usually only patchy in patients receiving a single drug, whereas more extensive injury with ulceration results from the use of combination therapy. Concomitant regeneration of the epithelial cells may appear atypical, but persists until the drugs are discontinued. The mucosal epithelial cells are replenished within a few days to 2 weeks, but inflammation and vascular dilation can continue, with the potential for further bleeding, for 3 to 4 weeks (107, 108).

Some cases, particularly those involving patients in the later stages of their diseases, are compounded by the coincident development of ischemia and shock, the additive effects of radiation therapy, the promotion of complicating infections, and the progression of tumor growth (109). In such instances, it becomes difficult or impossible to sort out the particular effects of the drugs. An autopsy study revealed ulcerations of the esophagus in 55%, of the stomach in 20%, of the small intestine in 33%, and of the colon in 70% (107). Multiple lesions were noted in one third of cases, and common findings included complicating infections, pneumatosis intestinalis, and ischemic lesions. The infections are often of the opportunistic type and include *Candida* and other fungi, cytomegalovirus, and herpes virus, *Mycobacterium avium, Cryptosporidium,* and *Strongyloides.* Bleeding is frequently observed and is usually related to tumor, drug or radiation ulcers, and thrombocytopenia. Bowel perforation can occur and is typically seen in patients with extensive tumor necrosis and in individuals receiving glucocorticoid hormones; the latter may be associated with ruptured diverticula,

which is probably related to the thin walls of diverticula. Fibrous strictures are relatively uncommon and are most often located in the esophagus.

The degree of esophageal injury is relatively high, related to the aggressive treatment of tumors in the thorax, the limited size of the lumen, and the frequent combination with radiation therapy. Adriamycin and actinomycin D inhibit DNA repair and, therefore, greatly enhance the effects of radiation (33–35, 110). These agents exhibit a recall phenomenon, in which the drugs evoke further radiation-type damage after the prior administration of relatively low doses of radiation. Other drugs used that seem to increase the effects of radiotherapy in the esophagus include 5-fluorouracil, bleomycin, hydroxyurea, procarbazine, and vinblastine. After hepatic arterial infusion of such potent drugs as 5-fluor-2' deoxyuridine or 5-fluorouracil combined with mitomycin C for the treatment of malignant tumors in the liver, from 10 to 50% of the cases develop prominent necrosis of the stomach and duodenum (111–114). Significant atypia of the mucosal epithelial cells is often present, characterized by the presence of enlarged and irregularly hyperchromatic nuclei and distinguished from malignancy by noting the prominent inflammation and the lack of signs of invasion.

A variety of complicating conditions are noted in the colon, including the development of ischemic lesions secondary to shock and thromboses, pseudomembranous colitis that is typically the result of antibiotic use, and neutropenic colitis (20, 109). Neutropenic colitis occurs in patients that have agranulocytosis and is the result of a secondary infection with virulent bacteria such as C. septicum. The lesions are concentrated in the cecum (typhlitis) and right colon and reveal extensive, often transmural necrosis leading to the possibility of perforation (115–117). Examples of other effects observed in the intestines are a protein-losing enteropathy from cytosine arabinoside and from combination therapy (107), a malabsorption syndrome from methotrexate and from colchicine (118, 119), a pseudo-obstruction from vincristine (120), a toxic megacolon from methotrexate (121), and colonic perforation from paclitaxel (122, 123). Also identified is an increased prevalence of second tumor development, particularly of malignant lymphomas (124).

Various immunomodulatory drugs, such as the interferons used to treat advanced malignancies, also may cause significant and serious gastrointestinal toxicity. Acute gastric injury (125) as well as colonic perforation, ischemic necrosis, and diffuse ulceration have been reported (126).

ANTIBIOTIC AND OTHER ANTIMICROBIAL DRUGS

Some patients exhibit prompt intolerance to a variety of antibiotics, particularly erythromycin, in the form of abdominal pain, nausea and vomiting, and occasional diarrhea. This response is probably mediated by the nervous or hormonal systems, and signs of mucosal damage are rare. The major injurious effects of antibiotics are pill-induced esophagitis and pseudomembranous colitis, which are described in subsequent sections. Several drugs can induce a vasculitis, including penicillin, ampicillin, tetracycline, isoniazid, and chloramphenicol (25). Examples of other uncommon events are a malabsorption syndrome from neomycin, para-aminosalicylate, and some antimalarial agents (20); a direct toxicity leading to an ulcerative enteritis or colitis from flucytosine (127), an antifungal drug, and from clofazimine, which is used in the treatment of leprosy (41); and the lesions of the Stevens-Johnson syndrome in the esophagus from co-trimoxazole (128).

ANTIDEPRESSANT AND ANTICHOLINERGIC DRUGS

The long-term use of these drugs can retard intestinal motility and prompt the development of a pseudo-obstructive disorder (see subsequent section concerning colonic involvement).

ANTICOAGULANT DRUGS

Drug-associated gastrointestinal hemorrhage can occur in patients with reduced numbers of platelets, for example, individuals receiving chemotherapeutic agents or thrombolytic therapy. The majority of these patients, however, are receiving anticoagulant therapy. Although hemorrhages and intramural hematomas have been noted in 30 to 40% of patients receiving anticoagulants, the lesions are usually small and asymptomatic. More significant bleeding has been detected in 1.2% of patients taking heparin and 0.2% of those receiving Coumadin (DuPont, Wilmington, DE) (129). Hemorrhage is three to four times more commonly noted in males, and hematomas can occur in any part of the gut (130). One series of intestinal lesions revealed 9% in the duodenum, 59% in the jejunum, 25% in the ileum, and 7% in the colon (131).

Clinical findings may include pain, a mass, or signs of obstruction, including blockage of the pancreatic or bile ducts; massive bleeding is rare. Treatment consists mainly of cessation of the drug or a change in its dosage; surgical intervention is rarely required for a persistent obstruction. Esophageal submucosal hemorrhage and an associated dissection has been reported in a patient treated with thrombolytic therapy for myocardial infarction (132).

CARDIOVASCULAR DRUGS

Many drugs used in the treatment of cardiac diseases and that act primarily on vessels can cause damage in the gastrointestinal tract (Table 11.7) (20, 29, 37, 133). The principle mechanisms involved are a sustained vascular spasm, volume depletion, or hypotension leading to reduced splanchnic blood flow. These effects can result in the development of ischemic lesions that mainly involve the small intestine and colon, and it is probable that the drug effects are facilitated by the underlying cardiac and vascular disorders. In these instances, it is often difficult to sort out the damage caused by the

TABLE	
11.7	**Examples of Cardiovascular Drugs**

Alpha-adrenergic blockers	Ethacrynic acid
Antihypertensive drugs	Ganglion blockers
Catecholamines	Methyldopa
Calcium channel blockers	Methylsergide
Digoxin	Quinidine
Diuretics	Reserpine
Ergot compounds	Vasopressin

drugs (e.g., digoxin, diuretics, and antihypertensive medications) from the direct effects of heart failure (134, 135). The lesions are usually observed in elderly patients, reflecting the populations taking these drugs, and are relatively infrequent. Most often noted are patchy areas of hemorrhage or hemorrhagic infarction that are confined to the mucosa or submucosa; deeper involvement leading to strictures or perforation is rare. Nevertheless, any damage with hemorrhage can seriously affect patients who already have significant cardiac disease.

A variety of other effects from the cardiovascular drugs have been noted. The vasoconstrictive action of vasopressin is greatest in patients who receive the drug in a selective artery for the control of some other cause of bleeding, but vasoconstriction can also develop after systemic administration (20, 136). The ergot compounds, including ergotamine tartrate and ergonovine, are largely used in the treatment of migraine. Although they are generally safe, examples of ischemic enteritis and colitis with rare perforations and strictures have been recorded (137–139). The use of ergot drugs as suppositories can cause localized ulcers of the rectum and anal region that resemble those seen in the solitary rectal ulcer syndrome, but the lesions heal promptly (140). Gastric bleeding has been observed in about 5% of patients receiving ethacrynic acid alone and in 10% of cases with added glucocorticosteroids (129). Reserpine is linked with an increased recurrence of chronic peptic ulcers, probably related to enhanced gastric acid production (29, 141). Methyldopa can cause a reversible colitis that is associated with a rash and peripheral eosinophilia and is thought to result from an immunologic reaction (142). Examples of other lesions include pill-induced esophagitis from quinidine and vasopressin (104), rare cases of vasculitis from several of the drugs (25), malabsorption from methyldopa (143), and pseudo-obstruction from calcium channel blockers (144, 145).

HEAVY METALS

The native form of the metals is inert, but damage to the gastrointestinal tract occurs infrequently from some of the salts, principally those of iron and gold. Iron compounds, such as ferrous sulfate, appear to cause injury by a physical attachment of the pills to the mucosa, leading to localized ulceration. These effects are seen most often in the esophagus (104) and exceptionally involve the stomach (146, 147) and the small intestine (148). Most of the lesions are superficial and promptly reversible, but deeper ulcers resulting in fibrous strictures have been recorded, mainly in the small intestine.

Gold salts are used in the treatment of rheumatoid arthritis, and injuries to the gastrointestinal tract have been noted following both the parenteral and oral administration of several medications, including the thiomalate, thiosulfate, thioglucose, thiopropanolsulfate, and triethylphosphine compounds (149–153). The lesions are rare, with only about 30 cases reported by 1986, are usually seen in women, and are localized to the small intestine and colon. They typically begin within 3 months after the start of drug therapy, and the total dosage received by the patients is less than 500 mg. Because of the short exposure, the occasional association with a rash and peripheral eosinophilia, and the response to cromolyn sodium in some cases, the gold injuries are thought to have an allergic basis, but the exact mechanism of the injury is not known (154). The patients typically present with abdominal pain, fever, and diarrhea, which can range from watery to hemorrhagic, probably reflecting the severity of the lesions. The pathologic features vary from scattered mucosal petechiae to widespread inflammatory involvement of the small intestine and/or colon, the latter simulating ulcerative colitis. Mortality rate, once reported to be 25%, has declined sharply in recent years with the prompt recognition and treatment of the disorder.

Reactions to other metals are rare. Noted have been a gastritis with focal ulcers owing to zinc sulfate pills, a foreign body reaction to mercury derived from a broken thermometer in the intestine, and an inflammatory mass of the cecum following intraperitoneal installation of radioactive zirconium phosphate (29). Bismuth does not cause damage to the gut, but the inclusion of salicylates in some of the proprietary compound products can be injurious (155).

ENEMAS AND LAXATIVES

The effects of the various enema solutions and laxatives and the cathartic bowel condition are detailed in Chapter 30. Briefly summarized, laxatives are associated with the increased deposition of macrophages containing a lipofuscin-type of pigment in the lamina propria of the colonic mucosa (see Figs. 30.14 and 30.15); when pronounced, this deposition results in a uniformly dark brown surface and is termed melanosis or pseudomelanosis coli (156–158). Patients have no symptoms or other deleterious effects. More extensive use of laxatives, however, can cause damage to the muscle and intrinsic nervous tissue of the colon leading to mucosal atrophy and shortening of the segment, called the cathartic colon (159, 160).

Most preparatory enemas in current use lead to increased edema in the lamina propria but do not otherwise damage the mucosa (161). A mild and reversible proctitis has been noted in association with enemas containing Fleet's solution and especially bisacodyl salts (162, 163) (see Fig. 30.16). More remarkable lesions with the potential for fistulae and perforations have been attributed to cleansing enemas (164, 165) and to the accidental inclusion of hydrogen peroxide (166) or ethyl alcohol (60). Rarely, rectal prolapse may occur after using oral cathartics (167).

MISCELLANEOUS DRUGS

Many other drugs of all types can injure the gastrointestinal tract. These drugs are cited briefly here and are addressed in greater detail in subsequent sections on specific organ involvement.

Enteric-coated potassium chloride can cause ulcerations of the esophagus, stomach, and small intestine, and the action is probably related to the localized entrapment of the pills in the mucosa and to the sustained release of the toxic substances from the special capsules (168–170). Compared to other pills, potassium chloride is more often associated with deeper ulcers leading to fibrous strictures of both the esophagus and small intestine (171). As a result of this complication, this particular form of medication is no longer administered regularly. Emepronium bromide, an anticholinergic drug commonly used in England, is one of the more frequent causes of pill-induced esophagitis (104, 171, 172). Focal ulcers are seen, but the lesions are generally reversible and rarely lead to complications. Many other drugs can produce similar ulcers of the esophagus associated with localized attachment of the pill and injury to the mucosa: barbiturates, chloral hydrate, pantogar, estramustine phosphate, alprenolol chloride, ascorbic acid, and ™Clinitest tablets (29). (See subsequent section on specific organ involvement in the esophagus.)

Other examples of drug damage to the gut, described subsequently, include gastric ulcers from bromocriptine and spironolactone; rare reports of colitis from isotretinoin, cocaine, and penicillamine; malabsorption from diphenylhydantoin, chloribrate, and cholestyramine; and a pseudo-obstructive disorder from morphine, clonidine, omeprazole, cimetidine, amanita toxin, and loperamide. Rare cases of pneumatosis intestinalis related to practolol and in a patient with ulcerative colitis receiving lactulose have been recorded, but a definite association has not been established (29, 173).

SPECIFIC ORGAN INVOLVEMENT

Most chemicals and drugs can affect multiple portions of the gastrointestinal tract, although the dominant actions may be more restrictive. For each of the gut segments described in this section, the major injuries caused by every subgroup of agents are briefly reviewed, more complete information is provided on the lesions that are concentrated or peculiar to the region, and the clinical and diagnostic applications are considered. Elsewhere in this text, additional details are available concerning the esophagus (see Chapter 20), the stomach (see Chapters 23 and 24), and the intestines (see Chapters 30 and 31).

ESOPHAGUS

The most common type of drug damage in the esophagus is that resulting from the focal entrapment of a pill in the mucosa, leading to a localized burn and ulceration (Table 11.8) (104, 171, 172, 174–177). This injury can be caused by a wide variety of drugs, and the only common feature is the relatively large size of many of the pills. Most such drug-related damage described in the United States is attributable to antibiotics, whereas emepronium bromide is more often noted as a causative factor in the United Kingdom. Development of the lesions is facilitated by the ingestion of multiple tablets,

TABLE 11.8	**Causes of Pill-Induced Esophagitis**
Antibiotics	Miscellaneous drugs
Clindamycin	Alprenol chlorine
Doxycycline	Ascorbic acid
Erythromycin	Barbiturates
Lincomycin	Chloral hydrate
Minocycline	Clinitest tablets
Oxytetracycline	Cromolyn
Penicillin	Emepronium bromide
Tetracycline	Estramustine phosphate
Tinidazole	Ferrous salts
Anti-inflammatory drugs	Pantogar
Aspirin	Potassium chloride
Indomethacin	Quinidine
Phenylbutazone	Vasopressin
Tolmetin	
Combinations	

Modified from Lewis JH. Gastrointestinal injury due to medicinal agents. Am J Gastroenterol 1986; 81:819–834.

inadequate consumption of liquids, taking the medication while supine, and the presence of cardiomegaly or any intrinsic narrowing of the esophagus. The lesions can involve any part but tend to be concentrated in the lower half, and they usually appear as a single, well-circumscribed ulcer with adjacent edema of the mucosa, without evidence of a more diffuse esophagitis.

Patients typically present with burning pain, and dysphagia related to the prominent edema is observed in about 20% of cases. The ulcers can be readily identified by endoscopic study, and the diagnosis is ordinarily established by finding residual fragments of the pill, which is uncommon, or simply by the history. The histologic features of the ulcers are entirely nonspecific, revealing necrosis and acute inflammation in the active phase and granulation tissue and regenerative epithelium in the healing stage. The differential diagnosis includes the common form of peptic esophagitis, which reveals a diffuse inflammation and always involves the distal portion, and other causes of localized ulceration, such as infections. Mucosal biopsies of the ulcer edge and intact mucosa can help to identify the extent of the inflammation and the presence of herpes viral inclusions (178). Most pill induced ulcers are superficial and heal promptly. Deeper lesions leading to perforation or to stricture formation are uncommon in the esophagus, and usually attributable to potassium chloride.

The local injection of sclerosing agents has been used recently to treat esophageal varices, particularly in patients with advanced cirrhosis (20, 179–181). Examples of sclerosants used include ethanolamine oleate, polidocanol, and sodium tetradecyl sulfate. These substances regularly produce vascular thrombi and necrosis leading to ulceration and fibrosis. The degree of damage varies widely, probably reflecting the strengths of the agents and the experience with the procedure. Persistent ulcers are seen in only 2 to 6% of patients in some series and in 15 to 20% in others. Most lesions heal spontaneously, but transmural necrosis and perforation occur in 1 to 5% of patients and fibrous strictures in 1 to 7%. Other alterations include the presence of mucosal bridges and hematomas as well as the appearance of minor motor abnormalities.

The other causes of chemical and drug injury in the esophagus are less common and were detailed in the discussion of etiologic agents. Included are caustic damage that is mainly from strong alkaline (lye) solutions (29, 42, 43); ulceration from chemotherapeutic drugs, such as actinomycin D, Adriamycin, and 5-fluorouracil, often in conjunction with radiation effect and secondary opportunistic infections (33–35, 110); and rare allergic reactions as part of the Stevens-Johnson syndrome, which represents erythema multiforme involving the mucous membranes (e.g., from the antibiotic co-trimoxazole) (128). Injury from most antibiotics, NSAID, vasoactive drugs, and inorganic salts are attributed to the direct effects of the pills on the mucosa.

STOMACH AND DUODENUM

The major causes of chemical and drug injury in these areas are ethyl alcohol (51–53), aspirin (83–86), indomethacin, and the other NSAID (76–79). These drugs regularly damage the mucosa leading to hemorrhage with minimal inflammation, erosions, and ulcers (Figs. 11.1 to 11.3; see Fig. 23.2). They also enhance recurrences of chronic peptic ulcers in these regions. The lesions of acute gastritis and duodenitis are confined to the mucosa and heal promptly after cessation of the offending agent. It is possible, however, that some cases of chronic antral gastritis are related to repeated episodes of alcohol or drug-induced injury.

Patients typically present with burning epigastric pain and bleeding, and the diagnosis is ordinarily provided by the history. The differential diagnosis includes other causes of acute or chronic gastritis and duodenitis, principally peptic disease, stress lesions, and *Helicobacter pylori* infection. Endoscopic examination can help to determine the extent of the disease, to identify infectious agents, and to monitor the clinical course (178). Treatment consists mainly of eliminating the toxic agent, and can be facilitated by the use of H2-blocking drugs, prostaglandins, and other gastric protective medications. Other chapters provide complete details on gastritis (see Chapter 23), stress lesions and peptic ulcers (see Chapter 24), and duodenitis (see Chapter 30).

Both corticosteroid hormones and reserpine are associated with an increased frequency and recurrence rate of chronic peptic ulcers (62, 141). Ulcer formation has also been noted in patients with acromegaly who received high doses of bromocriptine and in individuals with hepatic cirrhosis treated with spironolactone (182, 183); however, because the ulcers may be related to the underlying clinical conditions, the causative effect of these drugs has not been clearly established (29). The H2-blocking agents, such as cimetidine and ranitidine, lead to a sustained reduction in gastric acid, and concerns have been expressed about the potential promotion of infections and tumors. The promotion of infections and tumors, however, has not as yet proven to be a problem. Non-ulcer dyspepsia associated with histologic and ultrastructural abnormalities of the antrum and duodenal mucosa has been described in patients receiving chronic fluoride supplementation for osteoporosis and Paget's disease of bone (184, 185). During the infusion of chemotherapeutic agents (5-fluorouracil and derivatives) into the hepatic artery for the treatment of malignant tumors in the liver, some of the substances can enter the branches supplying the stomach and duodenum. Lesions occur in 10 to 50% of the cases and consist usually of ulcerations with significant atypia of the epithelial cells and uncommon perforations (111–114).

Other examples of effects in this region were described in the previous discussion of etiologic agents and include caustic injury in the stomach from either strong alkaline solutions or acids (29, 42) (see Chapter 23); hematomas from reduced platelets or anticoagulant drugs (129–131); bleeding from ethacrynic acid, abetted by corticosteroids (20, 129); and gastric ulcers from ferrous salts, zinc sulfate, and potassium chloride (29, 146, 147, 168–171). Rarely observed in the stomach are the extension of the sclerosing agents used in the treatment of esophageal varices and the formation of bezoars from sticky substances, such as sucralfate and cholestyramine (20, 186).

JEJUNUM AND ILEUM

Most of the chemical and drug injuries affecting the small intestine were described in the discussion of etiologic agents and so are briefly reviewed here. The caustic agents do not ordinarily reach this region, and the effects of ethyl alcohol and of most antibiotics are minimal. The prolonged use of corticosteroid hormones favors the development of secondary infections and other ulcers; results of one study showed that 10% of small bowel perforations were related to these drugs (65). Aspirin and all of the other NSAID can damage the mucosa, leading to focal ulcers and to occasional strictures or the formation of fibroconnective septae, "diaphragm disease" (94–97).

TABLE 11.9	Examples of Drugs That Cause Malabsorption

Antimalarial drugs	Methotrexate
Cholestyramine	Methyldopa
Clofibrate	Neomycin
Colchicine	Para-aminosalicylate
Diphenylhydantoin	Phenformin
Metformin	

Modified from Lewis JH. Gastrointestinal injury due to medicinal agents. Am J Gastroenterol 1986; 81:819–834.

TABLE 11.10	Examples of Drugs That Cause Pseudomembranous Colitis

Ampicillin	Minocycline
Amoxicillin	Nafcillin
Carbenicillin	Neomycin
Cephalosporins	Oxacillin
Chloramphenicol	Oxytetracycline
Chlorpropamide[a]	Penicillin
Clindamycin	Rifampin
Deoxycycline	Sulfamethoxazole-trimethoprim
Dicloxacillin	Sulfasalazine[a]
Erythromycin	Streptomycin
Gentamicin	Tetracycline
Lincomycin	Ticarcillin
Metronidazole	Tinidazole
Miconazole	

Modified from Lewis JH. Gastrointestinal injury due to medicinal agents. Am J Gastroenterol 1986; 81:819–834.

[a]Nonantibiotic drug.

The small intestinal mucosa is readily damaged by chemotherapeutic agents, with focal lesions noted from single agents and more extensive damage resulting from combined therapy (105–108). Furthermore, these cases are often complicated by secondary infections, shock, and tumor growth, and it may be difficult to discern the particular effect of the drug.

Ischemic lesions can result from vascular thrombi attributable to estrogens and progesterone compounds (28, 67–71), from vasculitis related to use of many drugs (25), and from a variety of agents used in the treatment of vascular and cardiac disorders (20, 29, 36, 133). The latter consist of vasoconstrictors such as vasopressin and ergots, of digoxin and antiarrhythmic drugs, and of the potential hypovolemic and hypotensive agents, including diuretics and blocking drugs (134–140). The lesions range from reversible hemorrhages of the mucosa to more extensive infarction of the bowel wall, and it is often difficult to distinguish the drug actions from the effects of the underlying cardiac condition. Most of the ischemic lesions subside without sequelae, and perforations and strictures are relatively infrequent.

A malabsorptive disorder involving fats and B12 or folates has been observed with a variety of drugs (Table 11.9) (20, 187). The possible mechanisms involved are a direct injury to the mucosal epithelial cells and a motility derangement favoring the promotion of excess bacteria and bile salt deconjugation, but the actual events are usually not known. The disorder is typically mild and promptly reversible, and chronic effects are not seen. Cyclosporine can cause a transient ileus that is eliminated by reduction of the dosage (188). Rare cases of granulomatous inflammation associated with diclofenac and clofazimine have been recorded (40, 41). Other examples of small intestinal injury include hematomas from anticoagulant drugs (129–131), ulcers and strictures from enteric-coated potassium chloride pills (168–171), and rare cases of enteritis and colitis associated with flucytosine (127) and gold salts (149–153).

COLON AND RECTUM

The most common type of drug damage in the large intestine is pseudomembranous colitis resulting from the use of antibiotics and other antimicrobial drugs (Table 11.10) (20, 29, 189, 190). Practically all of the antibiotics can be associated with this condition. In the early 1950s, severe cases of colitis owing to *Staphylococcus aureus* were noted from the use of penicillin, tetracycline, chloramphenicol, and neomycin, particularly in postoperative patients, but this organism has been controlled and is no longer a major problem (191). Current cases involve selective overgrowth of C. difficile in the colonic lumen and the effects of its toxins. The precise mechanism is not known and probably involves both the cytotoxic and vasoconstrictive effects of the different toxins. The timing is

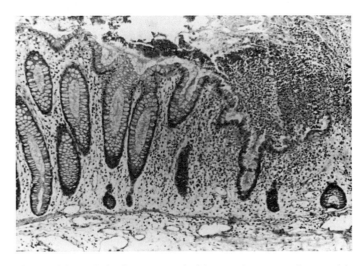

Figure 11.4 Colonic mucosal biopsy in a patient with antibiotic–associated pseudomembranous colitis reveals the characteristic early lesion. Biopsy specimen taken from the edge of a gross membrane shows the junction of the normal mucosa *(left)* with the exuberant acute inflammation reaction. The latter is concentrated in the superficial part of the mucosa and consists of a massive infiltrate of neutrophils and fibrin in the dilated crypts and on the surface *(upper right)*. The remaining mucosa and submucosa *(bottom)* are edematous. H & E, ×80. (Reprinted with permission from Goldman H, Antonioli DA. Mucosal biopsy of the rectum, colon, an distal ileum. Hum Pathol 1982;13:981–1012.)

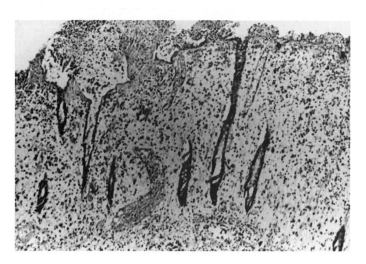

Figure 11.5 Colonic mucosa from a later stage of antibiotic–associated pseudomembranous colitis, with luminal surface at top. Extensive necrosis and inflammation involve the entire mucosa (compare to Figure 11.4). The surface is diffusely eroded and inflamed. H & E, ×80. (Reprinted with permission from Goldman H, Antonioli DA. Mucosal biopsy of the rectum, colon, an distal ileum. Hum Pathol 1982;13:981–1012.)

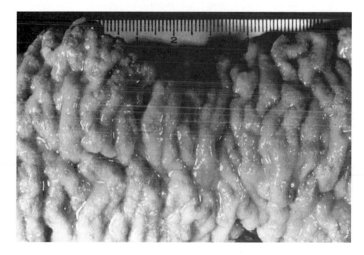

Figure 11.6 Mucosal surface of colon in a patient with severe pseudomembranous colitis. Pronounced edema results in the appearance of prominent folds rather than the normal haustra. Tiny patches of inflammatory membranes are scattered throughout the tissue surface.

highly variable, with some cases appearing after only a single dose of the drug and about one third occurring after the medicine is stopped. Diarrhea is present in all cases and is associated with colitis and hemorrhage in 20%; about 30% of lesions are limited to the right side of the colon. A nonpseudomembranous colitis with bloody diarrhea also occurs in patients receiving penicillin derivatives, usually for an upper respiratory infection. C. difficile toxin has not been found and a hypersensitivity mechanism is postulated as the mode of action (192).

The characteristic lesions in membranous cases can be identified at endoscopy, revealing small, slightly raised yellow membranes

(193). Biopsy specimens taken from the edges of the early lesions are distinctive, revealing a sharply defined area of extreme acute inflammation (Fig. 11.4), whereas examination of older lesions shows a more diffuse inflammation that is similar to other forms of colitis, particularly of ischemic colitis (Fig. 11.5) (193–197). The diagnosis is established by a positive assay for the toxin, and treatment consists of removal of the offending drug and, in severe cases, administration of vancomycin or metronidazole (198).

Most lesions rapidly subside, although recurrences are noted in 20% of patients. More severe examples leading to toxic megacolon have been observed, particularly in cases before the etiology and therapy were known, but also in current cases that are unrecognized or compounded by other conditions (Figs. 11.6 and 11.7). These lesions show greater necrosis and extreme edema of the colonic wall and usually necessitate a colectomy (199). (See also a discussion of antibiotic-associated colitis in Chapter 28 and of the role of secondary C. difficile infection in ulcerative colitis and Crohn disease in Chapter 29 [200].)

A pseudo-obstructive disorder with major effects in the colon has been noted in association with a variety of anticholinergic, antidepressant, and other drugs (Table 11.11) (29, 30, 120, 144, 201–207). These changes typically occur after prolonged use of the drugs and are thought to be caused by damage to the myenteric plexus or muscles in the colonic wall (208) (see Chapter 13). Other types of drug-related colonic damage were described in those sections concerning etiologic agents and the jejunum and ileum and are briefly reviewed in this part.

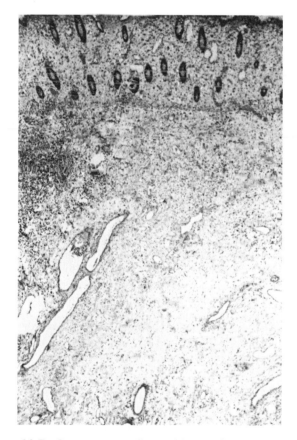

Figure 11.7 Same case as Figure 11.6, with mucosa at top. Edema greatly expands the submucosa. H & E, ×31.

TABLE 11.11	Examples of Drugs That Cause Pseudo-Obstruction

Anticholinergic drugs	Miscellaneous drugs
Benztropine	Calcium channel blockers
Trihexyphenidryl	Cimetidine
Antidepressant drugs	Clonidine
Amitriptyline	Hexamethonium
Chlorpromazine	Loperamide
Imipramine	Methadone
Nortriptyline	Morphine
Thioridazine	Omeprazole
Trifluoperazine	Oxprenolol
	Pentolinium
	Vincristine

Long-term use of corticosteroids can promote secondary infections, such as herpesvirus and cytomegalovirus in cases of ulcerative colitis, whereas estrogens and progesterone drugs infrequently cause vascular thrombi and ischemic lesions of the small and large intestines that can simulate cases of Crohn disease and ulcerative colitis (28, 67–74). The NSAID do not ordinarily affect the colon, but rare cases of colitis, stricture, and diaphragms have been noted (96–98, 101, 102), and a proctitis can be seen after the use of suppositories containing salicylates (100). In many other isolated reports, colitis occurred in association with rashes and eosinophilia and was considered to be of an allergic etiology; included are cases related to isoretinonin (209), penicillamine (37), methyldopa (142), clofazimine (41), and sulfasalazine (99). These allergic manifestations are generally reversible and do not cause strictures, although severe cases with toxic megacolon have been observed.

Patients receiving chemotherapeutic and immunosuppressive drugs often exhibit colonic lesions that can be attributed to the primary agents but more frequently are related to other factors, including the development of the following: secondary opportunistic infections, pseudomembranous colitis from the concomitant administration of antibiotics, ischemic lesions from thrombi or low perfusion, neutropenic colitis in cases with agranulocytosis, and tumor necrosis (20, 107, 109). Indeed, multiple factors are probably involved in the formation of many of the lesions.

Proctitis resulting from the use of enema solutions containing cleansing agents and the accidental presence of ethyl alcohol and hydrogen peroxide and cleansing solutions remaining on endoscopes have been described (47, 48, 60, 164–166). The other effects of enemas and laxatives were summarized previously and are detailed in Chapter 30 (161–163). Localized reactions to barium and to oils can result in nodule formation that is usually in the rectum (31, 32); these reactions are also described in Chapter 30. Other examples of drug damage in the large intestine include hematomas from anticoagulants (129–131); focal ulcers of the rectum and anal region from suppositories containing ergot compounds (140); ischemic lesions of the small and large intestines from other vasoconstrictor, hypovolemic, and hypotensive agents (37, 133–138); allergic reactions to gold salts (149–153); colonic

strictures in children with cystic fibrosis taking high-dose pancreatic enzyme supplements (210, 211); and possibly pneumatosis intestinalis from lactulose and practolol (29, 173). In other reports, colitis was attributed to cocaine and to other narcotics that were hidden in the tract but accidently released as well as to their general use. These responses may be mediated by localized vasoconstriction (212, 213).

RADIATION EFFECTS AND INJURY

Biologic substances tend to decay, resulting in the production of less stable atomic nuclei and in the release of radiation energy, either in the form of electromagnetic waves or of particulate matter (Table 11.12). Sources of radiation include cosmic rays, the earth's crust, building materials, and substances within our bodies such as phosphorus in the bones; accidental exposure as a result of occupational hazards and nuclear explosions; and the cumulative effects of radiographic diagnostic tests and radiotherapy (214, 215). The amount of radiation due to background sources has been estimated to be about 0.1 rad per year. By far, the most significant source is that from radiation therapy. Such therapy may be instituted in the treatment of various disorders of the gastrointestinal tract, principally tumors, and also of neoplasms of adjacent structures including especially the lungs, lymph nodes, genital structures, and urinary bladder.

GENERAL ASPECTS

TYPES OF RADIATION

The two forms of radiation are electromagnetic waves and particles (see Table 11.12). The electromagnetic waves have no mass or electrical charge, and each type has its own wavelength and frequency; examples include electrical, radio, and light waves; cosmic rays; and gamma rays, including x-rays. They tend to penetrate tissue deeply but generally have low to moderate energy. Radiation particles have mass and variable charges, and include beta particles (electrons), protons, alpha particles (helium nuclei), and neutrons. The particles generally exhibit higher energy and less penetration of tissues. The most commonly involved type of radiation involves x-rays, which are low- or moderate-energy photons (i.e., a type of gamma rays) and are characterized by relatively high penetration of tissue, measured as several centimeters to a meter or more. Less frequently involved types of radiation include alpha particles, which are high energy, slow moving helium nuclei with low penetration in tissue, typically less than a few millimeters but of high local intensity; and beta particles, which are rapidly moving, moderate- or low-energy electrons with an intermediate penetration, usually several millimeters to a few centimeters in tissue.

MECHANISMS OF RADIATION INJURY

Unlike chemical and biologic agents, there are no structural barriers at the tissue and cellular levels to the penetration of most forms of radiation (214). An initial atomic collision ("direct hit") between the radiation wave or particle and the macromolecules, concentrated in the cellular nuclei, results in either the excitation or the ionization (from the release of an electron) of the molecules, and ultimately the energy is dissipated as heat. The released electrons can collide with other molecules ("indirect hit") causing further damage, and some radiation forms, such as neutrons, act solely by this mechanism. Because most of the body substance is composed of water, extensive ionization and dissociation of its molecules also occur, causing the further production of free radicals, including uncharged hydrogen atoms and hydroxyl groups as well as charged molecules of water and hydrogen peroxidase. The mechanisms of action of the unstable free radicals were described previously (see Mechanisms of Cellular Injury).

Although all macromolecules within the cells and in the tissues are theoretically targeted by the radiation, the effects on the nuclear DNA are more lasting and productive of the greatest damage (214, 216). With the exception of germ cells and lymphocytes, very high doses of radiation (over 10,000 rad) are needed to kill cells that are in interphase. In contrast, the largest effect of radiation occurs during the G2 (postsynthesis gap) and M (mitotic) phases of the cell cycle and, therefore, is noted in cells that are continually dividing, such as most hematopoietic and epithelial cells.

The induced changes occur primarily as a result of large-scale structural alterations, such as chromosomal deletions, rearrangements, and recombinations. In addition to immediate cytotoxic effects and inhibition of cell replication, radiation injury also induces a so-called humoral tissue response, which results in alterations of the homeostasis maintained by endogenous mediators. Changes in levels of prostaglandins, prostacyclin, and other eicosanoids probably mediate most of the effects, such as vasodilatation, increased vascular permeability, and chemotaxis. This humoral component of the radiation response forms the rationale for anti-inflammatory drug therapy during radiotherapy (217). The mechanism responsible for chronic changes, such as fibrosis, are complex and incompletely understood. Multiple interrelated cellular and molecular events involving such systems as the fibroblastic/fibrocyte compartment and cytokines lead to a fibrotic response (218).

MEASUREMENTS OF RADIATION

The quantity of radiation to which a patient is exposed can be measured in terms of roentgens (R), with one R producing 2.08 x

10^9 electrons and an equal number of positive charges when passing through and ionizing 1 cc of air. The standard, and more useful, measure of the effect of radiation is in the form of the doses or units of absorption, known as rad; 1 rad equals 100 ergs of energy absorbed per 1 g of tissue. Another frequently used standard is the Gray (Gy), representing the absorbed radiation dose equal to 100 rad. The term rem is used to compare the biologic effects of the various radiation types, with the number of rem equal to the number of rad times the relative biologic effectiveness (RBE). At a practical level, the RBE for x-rays is 1, resulting in an equivalence of rad and rem, whereas the RBE and number of rem is greater for the particulate types of radiation.

RADIATION SENSITIVITY OF THE GASTROINTESTINAL TRACT

During the radiotherapy of tumors, the deleterious effects of radiation on the normal tissues can be restricted by using divided or fractionated doses of no more than 800 to 1000 rad per week. To estimate the potential severity of the radiation, tolerance doses for the various human tissues have been empirically obtained (219). These doses are usually expressed as the incidence of toxic damage occurring after 5 years; the dose that would be expected to affect 1 to 5% of persons is termed the "minimal tolerance dose," and the dose that would affect 25 to 50% of patients by that time is the "maximum tolerance dose." The minimal and maximum tolerance doses that have been calculated for the human gut are 6000 to 7500 in the esophagus, 4500 to 5000 in the stomach, 4500 to 6500 in the small intestines and colon, and 5500 to 8000 in the rectum. These tolerance doses relate mainly to the effects on the more sensitive elements of each of these organs, namely the epithelia and the vascular endothelial cells. Less appears to be known about the doses for some of the later effects, principally the proliferative vascular changes and tumor induction (220, 221).

The potential for significant tissue injury depends not only on the innate sensitivity, but also on the particular dose applied. Consequently, although the esophagus and rectum may seem more resistant, these areas often receive high tumoricidal doses and therefore represent sites of major radiation damage. Furthermore, it has been suggested that the radiation damage may be promoted by

| TABLE | | | | | | | |
| 11.12 | **Types of Radiation** | | | | | | |

Type	Major Source	Substance	Atomic Mass	Charge	Relative Feature	
					Energy	Tissue Penetration
Electromagnetic waves						
Cosmic rays	Background	Photon	0	0	Low	Deep
Gamma rays	Isotope	Photon	0	0	to	Deep
X-rays	Machine	Photon	0	0	Moderate	Deep
Particulate matter						
Beta	Isotope	Electron	0.00055	−1	Moderate	Intermediate
Proton	Isotope	Proton	1	+1	Moderate	Intermediate
Alpha	Isotope	Helium nucleus	4	+2	High	Superficial
Neutron	Isotope	Neutron	1	0	High	Superficial

TABLE	
11.13	Histologic Features of Radiation Injury

Acute (early) features
    Epithelial cell degeneration
    Mucosal and submucosal edema
    Small and reversible ulcerations
Chronic (late) features
   Common
     Telangiectasia
     Atypical fibroblasts
     Submucosal fibrosis
     Large and persistent ulcerations
   Uncommon
     Vascular inflammation and intimal thickening
     Deep mural necrosis
     Development of secondary tumors

a variety of conditions, including prior surgery to the area, poor nutrition, concomitant use of chemotherapeutic agents, and the presence of preexisting chronic inflammatory or vascular disorders (222). Patients infected with HIV have been noted to manifest a heightened sensitivity to radiotherapy, resulting in excessive acute and chronic tissue reactions (223). Overall, the incidence of significant radiation damage to the gut is not known; with recognition of the tolerance doses for each area and the use of fractionation, it can be kept to minimal levels (224). Clearly, the theoretic potential for damage is lessened by the reduced survival of many of the patients with tumors.

GENERAL PATHOLOGIC FEATURES

The principle effects of radiation are largely related to interactions with the nuclear DNA, especially in dividing cells, resulting either in the stoppage of mitosis and death of the cell or in the production of a mutation (214, 215). These changes can be potentiated by the concomitant administration of radiomimetic drugs such as Adriamycin, actinomycin D, and bleomycin (33–35). The cellular alterations noted are a simplification of the surface membrane structures, vacuolization of the mitochondria and other cytoplasmic organelles, and aberrations in the chromosomal number and components (225). Of interest, a delay or latency period may occur between radiation exposure and death of the cell, typically seen after doses under 1000 rad. Also, cells with enlarged nuclei can persist for several weeks, presumably because of continued nuclear synthesis but lack of mitoses.

Less clear is the understanding of mutational events, which include the initiation of tumors. It is probable that most of the radiation effects are ameliorated or totally reversed by the actions of reparative enzymes such as nucleases within the cells and by the regeneration of the surviving, unaffected cells, but these built-in protective mechanisms can be overcome by repeated radiation exposure. Some interaction between the radiation and the tissues always occurs, and it is useful to separate and classify those changes at a cellular level that are not accompanied by any important tissue

or functional derangement as "radiation effect." When destruction of tissue is more significant, with permanent structural and clinical sequela, it is termed "radiation injury."

TOTAL BODY IRRADIATION

For whole body irradiation in excess of 500 rad, a particular sequence of events, involving the gastrointestinal tract, has been established (226, 227). An initial and transient phase is characterized by significant nausea and vomiting, which is attributed to an effect on the central nervous system. Then, after a few days, significant destruction of the gastrointestinal mucosa as well as the bone marrow elements occurs, leading in most cases to fatality. The gastrointestinal tract shows extensive destruction and ulceration of the mucosa, which is a consequence of damage to the regenerative epithelial cells in all components. With lower doses of total body radiation, the effects are milder and reversible after a few weeks. This situation is usually seen in patients being prepared for bone marrow transplantation, and the changes are maximal in the small intestinal mucosa, which is the region of the gut that is most sensitive to radiation.

LOCALIZED RADIATION

The changes noted after localized radiation are separated into early or acute and late or chronic stages (Table 11.13) (228–232). There is a prompt elimination of the lymphocytes, which are concentrated in the lamina propria of both the small and large intestines, whereas the other inflammatory cells persist. The other early effects involve the mucosal epithelial cells, principally the mitotic cells, and the vascular endothelial cells (225, 233, 234). These cells initially show irregular enlargement of their nuclei with increased chromatin. This change leads to reduced maturation and a simplification of the surface epithelial structures, such as blunting of the small intestinal villi.

Coincident with the cellular alterations of the endothelial cells is an increase in permeability resulting in the transfer of edema fluid, mainly into the submucosa. This edematous fluid is often accompanied by large quantities of fibrin formation. It is interesting that in the stomach, the chief and parietal cells appear to be more sensitive than the mitotic cells in the neck region. Indeed, external irradiation has been used to reduce their content in patients with peptic ulcer disease; unfortunately, this effect was transient, as the cell population is replenished from the surviving neck mitotic cells. The only gross alterations noted at this early stage are a swelling of the mucosa and submucosa, attributed to the increased vascular permeability, and small areas of ulceration. With relatively low doses of irradiation, all of these early effects are reversible and not associated with any significant sequelae (225).

With increasing doses of radiation, there is persistence and extension of the ulcerations. Additional features include the irregular dilation of the small vessels (telangiectasia) (Fig. 11.8); a progressive increase in granulation tissue and collagen formation that is in excess of the amount expected from the inflammatory response (Fig. 11.9); and the appearance of fibroblasts with enlarged, irregular, and hyperchromatic nuclei, termed "atypical fibroblasts" (see Fig. 23.24). In some cases, there is also endothelial inflammation and an increase in muscle and fibroblastic proliferation in the small arteries and veins, leading to narrowing of their lumina (Fig. 11.10) (235, 236). The other mesenchymal elements

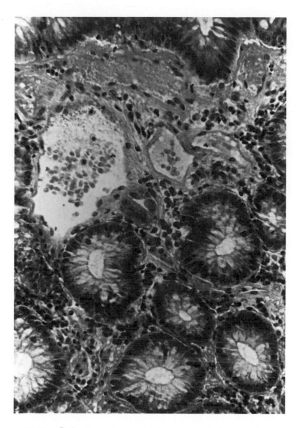

Figure 11.8   Colonic mucosal biopsy, with luminal surface at top, reveals the effects of radiation. Prominent dilation of venules (telangiectasia) and increased fibrous tissue are evident in the superficial part of the lamina propria. No increase in inflammatory cells is evident. H & E, ×200.

and nervous tissue in the gut wall are relatively radioresistant but can be secondarily damaged (220). The later effects of irradiation are a consequence of these progressive changes in the epithelia resulting in atrophy, in the fibrosis leading to stricture formation, and in the vascular narrowing occasionally associated with thrombosis causing secondary ischemic damage. Grossly, the tissues involved may show narrowing from the strictures, foci of mucosal destruction and ulceration, and secondary areas of ischemic necrosis in the form of localized fistulae or more extensive infarction. This change in morphology can lead to the problems of intestinal obstruction and exceptionally to focal areas of perforation.

SECONDARY FEATURES

Many patients with radiation injury are debilitated or immunosuppressed as a result of their underlying tumors and/or the effects of the drug and radiation therapy. This state can result in the appearance of a variety of opportunistic infections in the gastrointestinal tract, associated mainly with herpes and cytomegalovirus, and with numerous types of fungi and protozoa. Indeed, the overall damage to the gut and the patient may consist of a complex mixture of the effects from the chemical, radiation, and infectious agents; of nutritional deficiencies and metabolic disturbances; and of residual or recurrent tumor.

DEVELOPMENT OF TUMORS

A potential late effect of radiation is the development of a secondary tumor of the epithelial or stromal elements in the gastrointestinal tract (237–239). This effect is limited by the relatively poor survival of many of the patients as a result of their primary tumors, especially of the lungs, and also by the fact that radiation is a relatively weak mutagen as a result of its high cytotoxic effect. Nevertheless, it has been estimated that about 3% of carcinomas appearing in the gut may be a consequence of prior radiation, with 2.5% related to natural and accidental radiation exposure and 0.5% related to cumulative diagnostic and therapeutic radiation (240, 241). Indeed, caution has been expressed about the use of repeated radiographic tests in patients with chronic inflammatory disorders of the intestines. The suggestion that radiation could induce dysplastic lesions of the epithelium, similar to that seen in ulcerative colitis, has not been substantiated (242, 243). Rather, the epithelial changes noted, consisting of irregular glands with mildly hyperchromatic nuclei (Fig. 11.11), typically appear early in the course following radiation exposure and are reversible. Overall, the increased risk of neoplasms developing in the gut following radiation appears to be slight and mainly involving the large intestine, but additional long-term surveillance programs are needed.

The exact mechanism by which radiation causes neoplasms is not established. On the basis of studies in humans and animals, there is considerable support for the suggestion that the mechanism

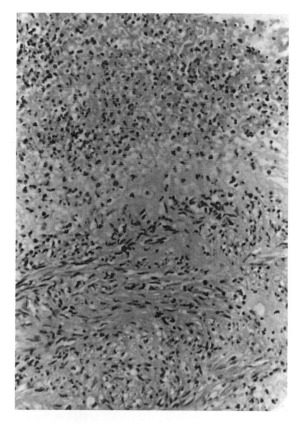

Figure 11.9   Section of an ulcer in a case of radiation damage. Necrosis and acute inflammation are evident in the top portion and fibrous tissue is prominent at the base of the lesion. H & E, ×80.

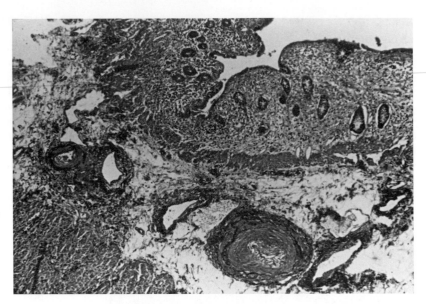

Figure 11.10 Section of colonic wall in a patient with radiation colitis. *Top,* Atrophic mucosa. *Lower right,* Narrowed artery owing to fibromuscular proliferation of its intima in the submucosa (lower right). *Lower left,* A portion of the muscularis propria. Van Gieson elastic stain, ×31. (Courtesy of Dr. Karoly Balogh.)

involves direct DNA mutations that are oncogenic (214). Alteratively, the mutations may favor the activation of viral proto-oncogenes or the radiation can lead to immunosuppression, fostering the promotion of tumors.

CLINICAL FEATURES

The presenting symptoms and signs of radiation injury are determined by the particular segment of gut involved and the pathologic stage (224, 244, 245). They relate mainly to the presence of luminal obstruction and focal ulcerations and exceptionally to the development of fistulae and perforation. Aside from pain, most often noted are dysphagia with lesions of the esophagus and gastric cardia, abdominal distention and diarrhea with involvement of the intestines, and masses or peritoneal signs with cases of deep mural necrosis. The clinical diagnosis is typically determined by the history, and radiographic tests and endoscopy with biopsy may be used to exclude complications of any associated surgery and to detect other disorders, particularly infections and recurrent tumor (246). In addition, in patients with a remote history of radiation, the late complications including secondary cancers must be distinguished from the other common inflammatory and neoplastic disorders of the gastrointestinal tract that can occur in any patient.

The treatment is largely supportive and abetted by the use of various anti-inflammatory and radioprotective drugs (247–251). Endoscopic manipulations and surgical intervention are reserved for patients with permanent fibrotic strictures, fistulae, and deep ulcerations that do not otherwise resolve (252–254).

DIAGNOSIS AND DIFFERENTIAL DIAGNOSIS

All of the features noted in cases of radiation injury are nonspecific; the prominent granulation tissue and fibrosis, atypical fibroblasts, and vascular changes have been observed in more ordinary wounds (232). This lack of specificity is compounded, in many instances, by the patients having underlying disorders or receiving adjuvant therapy that may lead to some of these alterations, such as mucosal atrophy and ulceration and increasing fibrosis. The diagnosis is secured by noting the combination of the history with compatible

morphologic features. In many instances, because the irradiation was given for a prior tumor, tissue examination is performed to distinguish between the presence of tumor elements and the nonspecific features of radiation damage. In such cases, it is extremely important to appreciate the cellular and particularly the nuclear alterations that may be seen in the epithelial cells, fibroblasts, and endothelial cells as a consequence of the radiation (216). Making this distinction can be especially difficult in small endoscopic biopsies, and great caution must be applied in their assessment. The differential diagnosis of radiation injury includes the presence of residual or recurrent tumor; other causes of mucosal destruction such as concomitant drugs, nutritional problems, or infection; and the coincidental development of ischemic damage, particularly in older patients.

SPECIFIC ORGAN INVOLVEMENT

ESOPHAGUS

Radiation damage to the esophagus typically occurs in patients who have received radiotherapy for tumors of the esophagus and contiguous structures such as the lungs, mediastinal lymph nodes, and thymus (255–258). Injury and functional effects are common because of the frequent use of radiation therapy for these tumors and the relatively narrow lumen of the esophagus. The early changes consist mainly of submucosal edema and focal, superficial ulcerations that are largely reversible after several weeks. Radiographic evidence of a chronic narrowing, owing to a fibrous stricture and often associated with persistent ulceration, has been noted in up to 30% of patients (224, 259). Any part of the esophagus can be involved, related to the site of maximal radiation exposure, but the lesions tend to be more common in the proximal and middle thirds because of the greater dependence on radiotherapy for lesions in these areas. Rare complications include the presence of more extensive mural necrosis, the development of fistulae that can extend into the bronchi or aorta and of diverticula, and perforation leading to a mediastinitis. The appearance of mucosal bridges, similar to the inflammatory pseudopolyps in patients with chronic colitis, has also been noted; these bridges consist of a core of inflamed lamina propria covered by hyperplastic squamous epithelium (260). Motility disorders have also been documented by manometry and dynamic studies years after radiation treatment (261).

The diagnosis of radiation-induced esophagitis depends primarily on the history and on the exclusion of other disorders. The latter include reflux esophagitis, if the lesion is concentrated in the distal portion; esophagitis related to infections or retained pills that tend to be more circumscribed; and residual or recurrent tumor. The development of secondary tumors related to the radiation is rare; these lesions are mainly squamous cell carcinomas and appear more than 10 years after the original therapy (258, 262–264). Considering the scant number of cases and the lack of any distinguishing features, however, it is difficult to be certain that they are related to the radiation. Alternatively, they may represent de novo tumors that occur in a tissue that is prone to carcinoma formation. Support for the role of radiation in the etiology of tumor development is provided by noting that the original tumor was not in the esophagus and that the patient has no other risk factors, such as a history of excess smoking and ethanol consumption (258). (See Chapters 20 to 22 for further details.)

STOMACH

Low-dose irradiation to reduce the parietal and chief cells was used in patients with peptic ulcer disease who were considered poor candidates for surgery (265, 266). Because the effect is transient and usually reversed by regeneration after a few weeks to months, however, this technique is no longer in vogue (see Chapter 23 for details). More extensive radiation damage to the stomach is uncommon, compared to other parts of the gut (224, 267), principally because high-dose radiation therapy is used infrequently for treating most tumors of the stomach and its contiguous structures. Also, the functional consequences may be less dramatic because of the relative spaciousness of the gastric lumen. The types of lesions are standard and include focal ulcerations, which are usually superficial, and fibrous strictures, particularly in naturally narrow regions such as the cardia and pylorus (268, 269). Rarely observed are cases with more extensive mural necrosis, fistulae, and perforation. The diagnosis is

based primarily on the history and on the exclusion of other common gastric conditions, such as ordinary gastritis, peptic ulcer disease, infections, and recurrent tumor.

Of interest, published information on the subject of secondary, radiation-associated tumors is scant. Primary gastric carcinomas and lymphomas are relatively common lesions, and their occurrence could easily mask the appearance of a radiation-induced lesion. Overall, most of the cases with significant radiation injury to the stomach were recorded many years ago, when the therapeutic instruments and techniques were in the developmental stage. With modern procedures, including greater attention to dose and tissue shielding, the occurrence of radiation effects on the stomach has been greatly reduced (224). (See also Chapter 23.)

SMALL INTESTINE

This region of the gastrointestinal tract is the most sensitive to radiation and the most extensively investigated (220, 271–276). Because primary malignant neoplasms of the small intestine are rare, with the exception of lymphomas, most cases of radiation enteritis occur in patients who have had radiotherapy for tumors involving the mesentery and retroperitoneum, including lymphomas, germ cell tumors, Wilms' tumor, neuroblastoma, and other mesenchymal lesions. In addition, parts of the mobile small bowel, and especially the fixed terminal ileum, may be exposed to radiation administered in the treatment of pelvic tumors of the genital organs and urinary bladder. A decreasing order of sensitivity from the proximal duodenum to the distal ileum has been claimed, but all regions are subject to damage (277, 278). Predisposing and potentiating factors include the fixation of a segment of intestine, typically a consequence of previous surgery; the concomitant administration of chemotherapy; and the presence of cardiovascular disease limiting the vascular supply to the gut (222).

Acute injury to the small intestine after radiation is probably a regular event, but the lesions are usually mild, reversible, and not productive of major clinical problems (224). The occurrence is dose dependent, with 90% development in patients receiving more than 3000 rad, 40% with 1000 to 3000 rad, and 20% with less than 1000

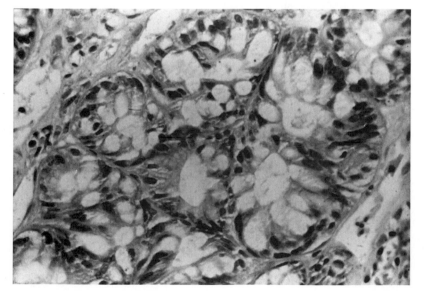

Figure 11.11 Colonic mucosal biopsy sample in a patient with radiation colitis. Note the focus of closely packed glands that vary in size and mucin production. The nuclei of the epithelial cells are generally small and lack prominent pleomorphism or hyperchromatism. H & E, ×200.

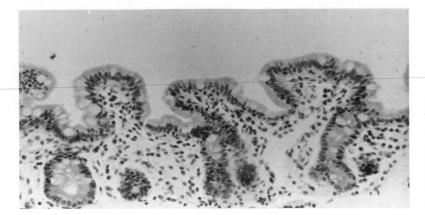

Figure 11.12 Jejunal mucosal biopsy sample shows features of chronic radiation injury, with luminal surface at top. Villi are shortened, and most epithelial cells are goblet mucous rather than absorptive cells. Crypts are probably of normal height but reduced in number. Absence of hyperplasia is striking, compared to most cases of enteritis attributable to other causes (e.g., celiac disease). H & E, ×80.

rad (232). The very early changes in the small intestinal mucosa were described by Trier and Browning (225). Observed within 12 hours of a dose of 2500 to 3000 rad were inhibition of the epithelial cell mitoses, clumping and enlargement of their nuclei, and shortening of the columnar absorptive cells. This change led to villous shortening by 7 days, but restitution began by day 14. There was also depletion of the mucosal lymphocytes, whereas the other inflammatory cells persisted. Ultrastructural studies showed shortening of the microvilli, vacuolization of the mitochondria, and nuclear aggregation in the affected epithelial cells. These changes offer an explanation for the transient gastrointestinal symptoms noted in most patients after radiation. No further problems usually arise beyond this period; in a minority of the cases, patients have small ulcers associated with prominent edema, which can be appreciated on radiographic examination (279). More severe involvement during the acute stage is rarely observed.

The development of chronic radiation enteritis is highly variable. It was noted in 5 of 14 (36%) children who had received high doses of radiation, and all 5 had evidence of acute disease (280). Most other series, mainly in adults, have failed to demonstrate any direct relation to prior acute damage, although the incidence of chronic disease has varied from 0.5 to 17%, with a general projected average of 5.2% (222, 224). In addition, delay between the radiation exposure and the appearance of chronic enteritis can be considerable and variable, ranging from 1 to 6 years (245, 270, 271), and it is thought that these changes are principally attributed to the vascular thickening leading to a localized area of vascular insufficiency.

Once the chronic lesion is established, it progresses and may lead to further complications (about 40% of patients) (281). Most often seen is a localized area of intestinal obstruction, owing to a fibrous stricture with overlying ulceration or to peritoneal adhesions, the latter related to prior surgery and/or to radiation damage of the mesentery. Less frequently, occurring in about 15 to 20% of the chronic cases, are fistulae, which usually communicate with another segment of small intestine but can also connect with the colon and other hollow viscera such as the urinary bladder. Cases with more extensive infarction and perforation are observed rarely (282).

An uncommon finding is the persistence of the villous loss in the small intestinal mucosa leading to a prolonged malabsorption disorder (283–285). Possible causes include persistent damage to the dividing epithelial cells in the crypts, abetted by vascular insufficiency, and a stagnant bowel favoring the appearance of a bacterial proliferation syndrome. In such cases, the mucosa typically shows significant shortening but not a complete loss of the villi (286), and the crypts are normal or slightly reduced in height (Fig. 11.12). This appearance is in marked contrast to the mucosa in most other causes of enteritis and malabsorption, such as celiac disease, which involves prominent, reactive hyperplasia of the crypts. The difference reflects the primary sites of the injury, which is the crypt in radiation disease and the villous epithelial cells in celiac disease. The pattern of primary crypt damage is relatively uncommon and has been observed also in vascular insufficiency, some drug injuries, possibly severe nutritional deficiency in infants, and a rare hereditary form (246, 287).

The diagnosis of radiation enteritis is typically established by the history (222, 245, 270). Radiographic, endoscopic, and biopsy examinations may be required to identify or exclude other disorders that can occur in these patients, particularly the effects of drugs, infections, and tumor. As in other parts of the gut, treatment is supportive, with surgical intervention reserved for cases involving persistent areas of obstruction and fistulae (244, 245, 251–254). There does not appear to be any significant increase in small intestinal carcinomas following radiation exposure, although several examples of angiosarcomas have been reported after pelvic irradiation (288). (See Chapter 31 for further discussion of radiation enteritis.)

COLON AND RECTUM

Although this region of the gut is relatively radioresistant, the incidence of radiation damage is high because of the high doses of radiation used to treat tumors in this area and to the fixed position of the sigmoid colon and rectum (224, 276, 289–292). Radiation at moderate doses is used as adjuvant therapy for many rectal carcinomas, but most damage occurs in patients receiving therapy for tumors of adjacent structures, including the uterus and cervix, prostate, testes, and urinary bladder. After treatment of testicular tumors, damage to the transverse colon was noted in 16% of patients receiving 4500 rad and 37% of those exposed to 6000 rad (293). Radiotherapy of cervical carcinoma is associated with about a 10% incidence of chronic damage to the large intestine, with rectal lesions seen in 50% and other colonic involvement in 75% of cases (294).

As in other parts of the gastrointestinal tract, the acute changes at a clinical level, occurring after treatment with 4000 rad or more, tend to be mild and disappear after therapy is discontinued (224, 295). Nevertheless, persistent histologic features were demonstrated in a sequential study of rectal mucosal biopsies taken from patients who received 5000 to 8800 rad for pelvic malignancies (234). The biopsy specimens obtained during treatment revealed loss of epithelial cell mitoses, enlarged nuclei, and a focal fibroblastic proliferation in the lamina propria; the vessels appeared to be normal at this stage. In contrast, biopsies taken after 4 months showed intact epithelial cells, subintimal fibrosis of the arterioles, telangiectasia of the capillaries and venules, endothelial cell degeneration, and greater fibrosis of the lamina propria with distortion of the crypts. Further studies are needed to determine whether persistent alterations at a mucosal level presage the future development of chronic radiation damage. In some cases, the collagen deposition is concentrated in the region beneath the surface epithelium, simulating the lesion noted in collagenous colitis (see Fig. 11.8). The crypts may also reveal a proliferation that mimicks dysplasia, but there is a lack of prominent pleomorphism or hyperchromasia of the epithelial cell nuclei (see Fig. 11.11) and the glandular alteration eventually disappears.

Evidence of chronic damage to the colon and rectum is seen in up to 10% of patients exposed to high doses of radiation and typically appears after 6 to 12 months. Usually noted are a chronic active colitis limited to the lower colon and rectum or a localized ulcer on the anterior wall of the rectum (244, 295–297). The latter is seen most often after treatment of cervical carcinoma and may be associated with a rectovaginal fistula. Obstruction owing to an inflammatory or fibrous stricture occurs in only 1 to 4% of cases (Fig. 11.13) (290). Rarely observed are examples of more extensive colitis and colitis cystica profunda (224, 298). The diagnosis is typically provided on the basis of the history, and the early edematous features can be well visualized by radiographic examination (279). Because of the ease of access, endoscopy and biopsies are often obtained and permit exclusion of other disorders, especially infections and recurrent tumor. It may be difficult to distinguish the chronic active colitis seen in cases involving radiation therapy from that noted in chronic ulcerative colitis. In such instances, the findings of patchy involvement, the vascular features, and the increased collagen help to support the diagnosis of radiation colitis or proctitis (234, 216).

There appears to be an increased risk of carcinoma (238, 241, 299–306), and possibly of lymphoma (307), of the colon and rectum after radiation exposure. This subject has been studied in patients treated for gynecologic malignancies, in whom the risk factor for carcinoma was estimated to be 2.0 to 3.6 (238). In most cases, tumors arise more than 10 years after the radiation, usually in the rectosigmoid region (238–300). Mucinous or colloid carcinomas are noted more frequently; in one study, they represented 58% in contrast to 10% of tumors unrelated to radiation (302). Further support for a link between radiation and colon cancer is provided by noting an increase in tumor incidence in persons exposed to atomic explosions and to radium at work (221, 227, 241, 308, 309). Overall, the number of cases from medical uses of radiation is probably less than 1%, but this percentage becomes significant when one considers that almost 150,000 new cases of large bowel carcinoma occur each year in the United States. For comparison, the cases of carcinoma complicating ulcerative colitis also constitute about 1% of the total. Accordingly, high-risk groups such as patients who were treated for gynecologic tumors, and possibly for other neoplasms, might be considered candidates for a surveillance program, especially after 10 years. Unlike patients with ulcerative colitis, however, the prior development of a dysplastic lesion that can

help to identify patients with early or preinvasive tumors has not been definitely identified in patients with radiation-induced malignancies.

OTHER PHYSICAL INJURY

THERMAL EFFECTS

Systemic alterations in temperature, in the form of hyperthermia or hypothermia, can be associated with effects on gastrointestinal function, principally on acid secretion and motility. These effects appear to be mediated by the autonomic nervous system. When hyper- or hypothermia is prolonged, lesions may arise that usually are associated with a stressful situation, including acute stress ulcers of the stomach and duodenum (see Chapter 24) and mucosal areas of hemorrhagic necrosis of the intestines (see Chapter 14); these changes are probably related to sustained reductions in splanchnic circulation. Most effects of systemic temperature alterations are transient, and any complications are neither long term nor permanent.

Local areas of thermal damage to the tissue are noted as a result of freezing or application of lasers. The introduction of freezing solutions into the gastric lumen was attempted in an effort to reduce acid secretion (310–312) (see Chapter 23), and more recently, lasers have been used in an attempt to obliterate sites of mucosal bleeding.

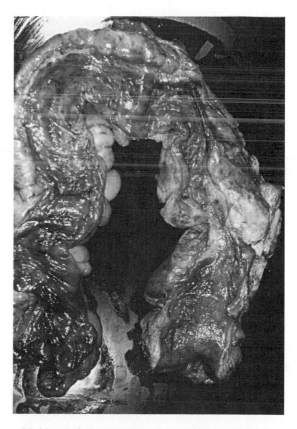

Figure 11.13 Colon segment, with a small portion of attached terminal ileum *(lower left)*, in a patient with radiation colitis. A localized fibrotic stricture in the descending colon portion is noted *(right)*. (Courtesy of Dr. Karoly Balogh.)

In either case, the result is local areas of coagulative necrosis, typically confined to the mucosa. When carefully conducted, this procedure is not associated with any deeper areas of necrosis or complications. Because of the highly localized nature of the lesion, there is no potential for any chronic effects.

TRAUMA

The segments of the gastrointestinal tract can be injured by blunt trauma or penetrating wounds. Depending on the location and severity of the wounds, possible effects include hematomas with the potential for obstruction and perforations leading to inflammation of adjacent serous cavities or other structures.

Iatrogenic lesions can occur in association with balloons to compress varices, rigid dilators to expand strictured areas, and endoscopic and radiographic procedures. Complications of flexible endoscopy are uncommon, probably related to the superficial nature of the biopsies. Hemorrhage most often occurs with removal of polyps with long stalks, and the rare perforations tend to be seen in cases with deep ulcerations (see Chapter 3).

REFERENCES

1. Robert A. Cytoprotection by prostaglandins. Gastroenterology 1979;77:761–767.
2. Terano A, Ota S, Hiraishi H, et al. Gastric cytoprotection: Morphological perspectives. Acta Pathol Jpn 1993;43:2–10.
3. Wallace JL. Non-steroidal anti-inflammatory drug gastropathy and cytoprotection: Pathogenesis and mechanisms re-examined. Scand J Gastroenterol 1992;27(Suppl 192):3–8.
4. Szabo S. Mechanisms of gastric mucosal injury and protection. J Clin Gastroenterol 1991;13(Suppl 2):S21–34.
5. Szabo S. Biology of disease-pathogenesis of duodenal ulcer disease. Lab Invest 1984;51:121–147.
6. Pihan G, Regillo C, Szabo S. Free radicals and lipid peroxidation in ethanol- or aspirin-induced gastric mucosal injury. Dig Dis Sci 1987;32:1395–1401.
7. Cotran RS, Kumar V, Robbins SL. Robbins pathologic basis of disease. 5th ed. Philadelphia: WB Saunders, 1994:1–34.
8. Szabo S, Spill WF, Rainaford KD. Non-steroidal anti-inflammatory drug-induced gastropathy: Mechanisms and management. Med Toxicol Adverse Drug Exp 1989;4:77–94.
9. Werns S, Lucchesi BR. Free radicals and ischemic tissue injury. Trans Pharmacol Sci 1990;11:161–166.
10. Kusterer K, Pihan G, Szabo S. Role of lipid peroxidation in gastric mucosal lesions induced by HCl, NaOH or ischemia. Am J Physiol 1987;252:G811–G816.
11. Whittle BJR, Lopez-Bolmonte J. Actions and interactions of endothelins, prostacyclin and nitric oxide in the gastric mucosa. J Physiol Pharmacol 1993;44:91–107.
12. Stark ME, Szurszewski JH. Role of nitric oxide in gastrointestinal and hepatic function and disease. Gastroenterology 1992;103:1928–1949.
13. Xu YL, Spill W, Szabo S. Time and temperature-dependent toxicity of indomethacin to isolated gastric mucosal cells. Proceeding of the International Conference on Gastroenterology and Biology, Los Angeles, 1988.
14. Morley P, Hogan MJ, Hakim AM. Calcium-mediated mechanisms of ischemic injury and protection. Brain Pathol 1994;4:37–47.
15. Mozsik G, Javor T. A biochemical and pharmacological approach to the genesis of ulcer disease. A model study of ethanol-induced injury to gastric mucosa in rats. Dig Dis Sci 1988;33:92–105.
16. Weiss SJ. Tissue destruction by neutrophils. N Engl J Med 1989;320:365–376.
17. The Merck Index. 12th ed. Rahway: Merck and Co, 1996.
18. Huic M, Mucolic V, Vrhovac B, et al. Adverse drug reactions resulting in hospital admission. Int J Clin Pharmacol Ther 1994;32:675–682.
19. Benson Jr JA. Gastroenterology reactions to drugs. Am J Dig Dis 1971;16:357–362.
20. Lewis JH. Gastrointestinal injury due to medicinal agents. Am J Gastroenterol 1986;81:819–834.
21. Smilkstein MJ, Knapp GL, Kulig KW, et al. Efficacy of oral N-acetylcysteine in the treatment of acetaminophen overdose. Analysis of the national multicenter study (1976 to 1985). N Engl J Med 1988;319:1557–1562.
22. Dupur D, Roza A, Szabo S. The role of endogenous nonprotein and protein sulfhydryls in gastric mucosal injury and protection. In: Szabo S, Pfieffer C, eds. Ulcer disease: New aspects of pathogenesis and pharmacology. Boca Raton FL: CRC Press Inc, 1989:421–432.
23. Domschke S, Domschke W. Gastroduodenal damage due to drugs, alcohol and smoking. Clin Gastroenterol 1984;13:405–437.
24. Sarosiek J, Marcinkiewicz M, Parolisi S, et al. Prostaglandin E2 content in residual gastric juice reflects endoscopic damage to the gastric mucosa after naproxen sodium administration. Am J Gastroenterol 1996;91:873–878.
25. McAllister Jr HA, Mullick FG. The cardiovascular system. In: Riddell RH, ed. Pathology of Drug-Induced and Toxic Diseases. London: Churchill Livingstone, 1982:207–210.
26. Bradley III EL, Goldman ML. Gastric infarction after therapeutic embolization. Surgery 1976;79:421–424.
27. Shapiro N, Brandt L, Sprayregan S, et al. Duodenal infarction after therapeutic gelfoam embolization of a bleeding duodenal ulcer. Gastroenterology 1981;80:176–180.
28. Tedesco FJ, Volpicelli NA, Moore FS. Estrogen- and progesterone-associated colitis: A disorder with clinical and endoscopic features mimicking Crohn's colitis. Gastrointest Endosc 1982;28:247–249.
29. Riddell RH. The gastrointestinal tract. In: Riddell RH, ed. Pathology of drug-induced and toxic diseases. London: Churchill Livingstone, 1982:515–606.
30. Anuras S, Shirazi SS. Colonic pseudoobstruction. Am J Gastroenterol 1984;79:525–532.
31. Lewis JW, Kerstein MD, Koss N. Barium granuloma of the rectum: An uncommon complication of barium enema. Ann Surg 1975;181:418–423.
32. Mazier WP, Sun MK, Robertson, WG. Oil-induced granuloma (oleoma) of the rectum: Report of four cases. Dis Colon Rectum 1978;21:292–294.
33. Hagemann RF, Concannon JP. Mechanism of intestinal radiosensitization by actinomycin D. Br J Radiol 1973;46:302–308.
34. Phillips TL, Fu KK. Quantification of combined radiation therapy and chemotherapy effects on critical normal tissues. Cancer 1976;37:1186–1200.
35. Rubin P. Late effects of chemotherapy and radiation therapy. Radiation Oncol Biol Phys 1984;10:5–34.
36. Lee FD. Drug-related pathological lesions of the intestinal tract. Histopathology 1994;25:303–308.
37. Cappell MS, Simon T. Colonic toxicity of administered medications and chemicals. Am J Gastroenterol 1993;88:1684–1699.
38. Anilkumar TV, Sarraf CE, Hunt T, et al. The nature of cytotoxic drug-induced death in murine intestinal crypts. Br J Cancer 1992;65:552–558.
39. Lee FD. Importance of apoptosis in the histopathology of drug related lesions in the large intestine. J Clin Pathol 1993;46:18–122.
40. Baert F, Hart J, Blackstone MO. A case of diclofenac-induced colitis with focal granulomatous change. Am J Gastroenterol 1995;90:1871–1873.
41. Karat ABA. Long-term follow-up of clofazimine (Lamprene) in the management of reactive phases of leprosy. Lepr Rev 1975;46(Suppl):105–109.
42. Loeb PM, Eisenstein AM. Caustic injury to the upper gastrointestinal tract. In: Sleisenger MH, Fordtran JS, eds. Gastrointestinal Disease: Pathophysiology, Diagnosis, Management. 5th ed. Philadelphia: WB Saunders, 1993:293–298.
43. Kikendall JW. Caustic ingestion injuries. Gastroenterol Clin North Am 1991;20:847–857.
44. Tewfik TL, Schloss MD. Ingestion of lye and other corrosive agents—a study of 86 infants and child cases. J Otolaryngol 1980;9:72–77.
45. Allen R, Thoshinsky M, Stallone R, et al. Corrosive injuries of the stomach. Arch Surg 1970;100:409.

46. Davis LL, Raffensperger J, Novak GM. Necrosis of the stomach secondary to ingestion of corrosive agents: Report of three cases requiring total gastrectomy. Chest 1972;62:48–51.

47. West AB, Kuan SF, Bennick M, et al. Glutaraldehyde colitis following endoscopy: Clinical and pathological features and investigation of an outbreak. Gastroenterology 1995;108:1250–1255.

48. Durante L, Zulty JC, Israel E, et al. Investigation of an outbreak of bloody diarrhea: Association with endoscopic cleaning solution and demonstration of lesions in an animal model. Am J Med 1992;92:476–480.

49. Cello JP, Fogel RP, Boland CR. Liquid caustic ingestion: Spectrum of injury. Arch Intern Med 1980;140:501–504.

50. Appelqvist P, Salmo M. Lye corrosion carcinoma of the esophagus: A review of 63 cases. Cancer 1980;45:2655–2658.

51. Wynn-Williams A. Effects of alcohol on gastric mucosa. Br Med J 1956;1:256.

52. Valencia-Parparcen J. Alcoholic gastritis. Clin Gastroenterol 1981;10:389.

53. Laine L, Weinstein WM. Histology of alcoholic hemorrhagic "gastritis": A prospective evaluation. Gastroenterology 1988;94:1254–1262.

54. Davenport HW. Back diffusion of acid through the gastric mucosa and its physiological consequences. In: Glass GBJ, ed. Progress in gastroenterology, vol 2. New York: Grune and Stratton, 1970.

55. Smith BM. Permeability of the human gastric mucosa: Alteration by acetylsalicylic acid and ethanol. N Engl J Med 1971;285:216.

56. Szabo S, Pihan G, Trier JS. Alterations in blood vessels during gastric injury and protection. Scand J Gastroenterol 1986;22(Suppl 125):92–96.

57. Bode JCH. Alcohol and the gastrointestinal tract. Adv Intern Med Pediatr 1980;45:1–75.

58. Persson J. Alcohol and the small intestine. Scand J Gastroenterol 1991;26:3–15.

59. Millan MS, Morris GP, Beck IT, et al. Villous damage induced by suction biopsy and by acute ethanol intake in normal human small intestine. Dig Dis Sci 1980;75:513.

60. Herreiros JM, Munioin MA, Sanchez S, et al. Alcohol-induced colitis. Endoscopy 1983;15:121–122.

61. Conn HO, Blitzer BL. Nonassociation of adrenocorticosteroid therapy and peptic ulcer. N Engl J Med 1976;294:473–479.

62. Messer J, Reitman D, Sacks HS, et al. Association of adrenocorticosteroid therapy and peptic ulcer disease. N Engl J Med 1983;309:21–24.

63. Conn HO, Poynard T. Corticosteroids and peptic ulcer: Meta-analysis of adverse events during steroid therapy. J Intern Med 1994;236:619–632.

64. Prillaman WW, Hurst DC, Ball GV, et al. Intestinal complications in rheumatoid arteritis and their relationship to corticosteroid therapy. J Chron Dis 1974;27:475.

65. Remine SG, McIlrath DC. Bowel perforation in steroid-treated patients. Ann Surg 1990;192:581–586.

66. O'Neil EA, Chwals WJ, O'Shea MD, et al. Dexamethasone treatment during ventilator dependency: Possible life-threatening gastrointestinal complications. Arch Dis Child 1992;67(1 spec no):10–11.

67. Kilpatrick ZM, Silverman JF, Betancourt E, et al. Vascular occlusion of the colon and oral contraceptives. N Engl J Med 1968;278:438–440.

68. Brennan MF, Clarke AM, MacBeth WAAG. Infarction of the midgut associated with oral contraceptives: Report of two cases. N Engl J Med 1969;279:1213–1214.

69. Cotton PB, Thomas ML. Ischemic colitis and the contraceptive pill. Br Med J 1971;3:27–28.

70. Hoyle M, Kennedy A, Prior AL, et al. Small bowel ischaemia and infarction in young women taking oral contraceptives and progestational agents. Br J Surg 1977;64:533–537.

71. Deana DG, Dean PJ. Reversible ischemic colitis in young women. Association with oral contraceptive use. Am J Surg Pathol 1995;19:454–462.

72. Gelfand MD. Ischemic colitis associated with a depot synthetic progesterone. Dig Dis Sci 1972;17:275–277.

73. Rhodes JM, Cockel R, Allan RN, et al. Colonic Crohn's disease and use of oral contraception. Br Med J 1984;288:595–596.

74. Bontils S, Hervoir V, Girodet J, et al. Acute spontaneously recovering ulcerating colitis (ARUC): Report of 6 cases. Dig Dis Sci 1977;22:429–436.

75. Boyko EJ, Theis MK, Vaughan TL, et al. Increased risk of inflammatory bowel disease associated with oral contraceptive use. Am J Epidemiol 1994;140:268–278.

76. Lanza FL. Gastrointestinal toxicity of newer NSAIDs. Am J Gastroenterol 1993;88:1318–1323.

77. Caselli M, LaCorte R, DeCarlo L, et al. Histological findings in gastric mucosa in patients treated with non-steroidal anti-inflammatory drugs. J Clin Pathol 1995;48:553–555.

78. Quinn CM, Bjarnason I, Price AB. Gastritis in patients on non-steroidal anti-inflammatory drugs. Histopathology 1993;23:341–348.

79. Henry D, Dobson A, Turner C. Variability in the risk of major gastrointestinal complications from nonaspirin nonsteroidal anti-inflammatory drugs. Gastroenterology 1993;105:1078–1088.

80. Eberhart CE, Dubois RN. Eicosanoids and the gastrointestinal tract (review). Gastroenterology 1995;109:285–301.

81. Bollini P, Garcia Rodriguez LA, Gutthann SP, et al. The impact of research quality and study design on epidemiologic estimates of the effect of nonsteroidal anti-inflammatory drugs on upper gastrointestinal tract disease. Arch Intern Med 1992;152:1289–1295.

82. Gabriel SE, Jaakimainen RL, Bombardier C. Risk for serious gastrointestinal complications related to use of nonsteroidal anti-inflammatory drugs: A meta-analysis. Ann Intern Med 1991;115:787–796.

83. Kuiper DH, Overholt BF, Fall DJ, et al. Gastroscopic findings and fecal blood loss following aspirin administration. Am J Dig Dis 1969;14:761.

84. Roderick PJ, Wilkes HC, Meade TW. The gastrointestinal toxicity of aspirin: An overview of randomised controlled trials. Br J Clin Pharmacol 1993;35:219–226.

85. Metzger WH, McAdam L, Bluestone R, et al. Acute gastric mucosal injury during continuous or interrupted aspirin ingestion in humans. Am J Dig Dis 1976;21:963–968.

86. Silvoso GR, Ivey KJ, Butt JH, et al. Incidence of gastric lesions in patients with rheumatic disease on chronic aspirin therapy. Ann Intern Med 1979;91:517.

87. Olivero JJ, Graham DY. Gastric adaptation to nonsteroidal anti-inflammatory drugs in man (review). Scand J Gastroenterol 1992(Suppl):193:53–58.

88. Raz A, Wych A, Needleman P. Temporal and pharmacological division of fibroblast cyclooxygenase expression into transcriptional and translational phases. Proc Natl Acad Sci USA 1989;86:1657–1661.

89. Lima MAS. Duodenal ulcers associated with salsalate therapy. Gastrointest Endosc 1986;32:356–357.

90. Masferrer JL, Isakson PC, Seibert K. Cyclooxygenase-2 inhibitors. A new class of anti-inflammatory agents that spare the gastrointestinal tract. Gastroenterol Clin North Am 1996;25:363–372.

91. Leivonen M, Sipponen P, Kivilaakso E. Gastric changes in coronary-operated patients with low-dose aspirin. Scand J Gastroenterol 1992;27:912–916.

92. McDonald WC. Correlation of mucosal histology and aspirin intake in chronic gastric ulcer. Gastroenterology 1973;65:381.

93. Hamilton SR, Yardley JH. Endoscopic biopsy diagnosis of aspirin-associated chronic gastric ulcers. Gastroenterology 1980;78:1178.

94. Bjarnason I, Price AB. The small and large intestinal pathologies of non-steroidal anti-inflammatory drug ingestion. Ann Pathol 1994;14:326–332.

95. Allison MC, Howatson AG, Torrance CJ, et al. Gastrointestinal damage associated with the use of nonsteroidal anti-inflammatory drugs. N Engl J Med 1992;327:749–754.

96. Halter F, Weber B, Huber T, et al. Diaphragm disease of the ascending colon. Association with sustained-release diclofenac. J Clin Gastroenterol 1993;16:74–80.

97. Haque S, Haswell JE, Dreznick JT, et al. A cecal diaphragm associated with the use of nonsteroidal anti-inflammatory drugs. J Clin Gastroenterol 1992;15:332–335.

98. Doman DB, Goldberg HJ. A case of meclofenamate sodium-induced colitis. Am J Gastroenterol 1986;81:1220–1221.

99. Schwartz AG, Targan SR, Saxon A, et al. Sulfasalazine-induced exacerbation of ulcerative colitis. N Engl J Med 1982;306:409–412.

100. Lanthier P, Detry R, Debongnic JL, et al. Solitary rectal lesions due to suppositories containing acetylsalicylic acid and paracetamol. Gastroenterol Clin Biol 1987;11:250–253.
101. Davies NM. Toxicity of nonsteroidal anti-inflammatory drugs in the large intestine. Dis Colon Rectum 1995;38:1311–1321.
102. Robinson MH, Wheatley T, Leach IH. Nonsteroidal anti-inflammatory drug-induced colonic stricture. An unusual cause of large bowel obstruction and perforation. Dig Dis Sci 1995;40:315–319.
103. Riddell RH, Tanaka M, Mazzoleni G. Non-steroidal anti-inflammatory drugs as a possible cause of collagenous colitis: A case-control study. Gut 1992;33:683–686.
104. Mason SJ, O'Meara TF. Drug-induced esophagitis. J Clin Gastroenterol 1981;3:115.
105. Trier JS. Morphologic alterations induced by methotrexate in the mucosa of the human proximal intestine. I. Serial observations by light microscopy. Gastroenterology 1962;42:295–305.
106. Trier JS. Morphologic alterations induced by methotrexate in the mucosa of human proximal intestine. II. Electron microscopic observation. Gastroenterology 1962;43:407–424.
107. Slavin RE, Dias MA, Sarai R. Cytosine arabinoside induced gastrointestinal toxic alterations in sequential chemotherapeutic protocols. A clinico-pathologic study of 33 patients. Cancer 1978;42:1747–1759.
108. Mitchell EP, Schein PS. Gastrointestinal toxicity of chemotherapeutic agents. Semin Oncol 1982;9:52–64.
109. Velanovich V, LaPorta AJ, Garrett WL, et al. Pseudomembranous colitis leading to toxic megacolon associated with antineoplastic chemotherapy. Report of a case and review of the literature. Dis Colon Rectum 1992;35:369–372.
110. Boal DK, Newburger PE, Teele RL. Esophagitis induced by combined radiation and adriamycin. AJR Am J Roentgenol 1979;132:567–570.
111. Petras RE, Hart WR, Bukowski RM. Gastric epithelial atypia associated with hepatic arterial infusion chemotherapy. Its distinction from early gastric carcinoma. Cancer 1985;56:745–750.
112. Jewell LD, Fields AL, Murray CJW, et al. Erosive gastroduodenitis with marked epithelial atypia after hepatic infusion chemotherapy. Am J Gastroenterol 1985;80:421–424.
113. Doria MI, Doria LK, Faintuch J, et al. Gastric mucosal injury after hepatic arterial infusion chemotherapy with floxuridine. A clinical and pathologic study. Cancer 1994;73:2042–2047.
114. Kwee WS, Wils JA, Schlangen J, et al. Gastric epithelial atypia complicating hepatic arterial infusion chemotherapy. Histopathology 1994;24:151–154.
115. Wagner ML, Rosenberg HS, Fernbach DJ, et al. Typhlitis: A complication of leukemia in childhood. AJR Am J Roentgenol 1970;109:341–350.
116. Koep LJ, Peters TG, Starzi TE. Major colonic complications of hepatic transplantation. Dis Colon Rectum 1979;22:218–220.
117. Ryan ME, Morrissey JF. Typhlitis complicating methimazole-induced agranulocytosis. Gastrointest Endosc 1983;29:299–302.
118. Craft AW, Kay HEM, Lawson DM, et al. Methotrexate-induced malabsorption in children with acute lymphoblastic leukemia. Br Med J 1977;4:1511–1512.
119. Race TF, Paes IC, Faloon WW. Intestinal malabsorption induced by oral colchicine. Comparison with neomycin and cathartic agents. Am J Med Sci 1970;259:32–41.
120. Sandler SG, Tobin W, Henderson ES. Vincristine-induced neuropathy. A clinical study of fifty leukemic patients. Neurology 1968;19:367–374.
121. Atherton LD, Leib ES, Kaye MD. Toxic megacolon associated with methotrexate therapy. Gastroenterology 1984;86:1583–1588.
122. Hruban RH, Yardley JH, Donehower RC, et al. Taxol toxicity. Epithelial necrosis in the gastrointestinal tract associated with polymerized microtubule accumulation and mitotic arrest. Cancer 1989;63:1944–1950.
123. Rose PG, Piver MS. Intestinal perforation secondary to paclitaxel. Gynecol Oncol 1995;57:270–272.
124. Hoover R, Fraumeni JF. Drug-induced cancer. Cancer 1981;47:1071–1080.
125. Rubin JT, Lotze MT. Acute gastric mucosal injury associated with the systemic administration of interleukin-4. Surgery 1992;111:274–280.
126. Rahman R, Bernstein Z, Vaickus L, et al. Unusual gastrointestinal complications of interleukin-2 therapy. J Immunother Emphasis Tumor Immunol 1991;10:221–225.
127. White CA, Traube J. Ulcerating enteritis associated with flucytosine therapy. Gastroenterology 1982;83:1127–1129.
128. Heer M, Altorfer J, Burger H-R, et al. Bullous esophageal lesions due to cotrimoxazole: An immune-mediated process? Gastroenterology 1985;88:1954–1957.
129. Jick H, Porter J. Drug-induced gastrointestinal bleeding. Report from The Boston Collaborative Drug Surveillance Program, Boston University Medical Center. Lancet 1978;2:87–89.
130. Avent ML, Canaday BR, Sawyer WT. Warfarin-induced intramural hematoma of the small intestine. Clin Pharmacol Ther 1992;1:632–635.
131. Herbert DC. Anticoagulant therapy and the acute abdomen. Br J Surg 1968;55:353–357.
132. Jishi F, Sissons CE, Silverstone EJ, et al. Oesophageal dissection after thrombolytic treatment for myocardial infarction. Thorax 1992;47:835–836.
133. Granger DN, Richardson PDI, Kvietys PR, et al. Intestinal blood flow. Gastroenterology 1980;78:837–863.
134. Ferrer MI, Bradley SE, Wheeler HO, et al. The effect of digoxin in the splanchnic circulation in ventricular failure. Circulation 1965;32:524.
135. Lely AH, van Enter CHJ. Non-cardiac symptoms of digitalis intoxication. Am Heart J 1972;83:149–152.
136. Renert WA, Button KF, Fuld SL, et al. Mesenteric venous thrombosis and small bowel infarction following infusion of vasopressin into the superior mesenteric artery. Radiology 1972;102:299–302.
137. Greene FL, Ariyan S, Stansel HC. Mesenteric and peripheral vascular ischemia secondary to ergotism. Surgery 1977;81:176–179.
138. Stillman AE, Weinberg M, Mast WC, et al. Ischemic bowel disease attributable to ergot. Gastroenterology 1977;72:1336–1337.
139. Wormann B, Hochter W, Seib HJ, et al. Ergotamine-induced colitis. Endoscopy 1985;17:165–166.
140. Eckardt VF, Kanzler G, Remmele W. Anorectal ergotism: Another cause of solitary rectal ulcers. Gastroenterology 1986;91:1123–1127.
141. Hollister LE. Hematemesis and melena complicating treatment with raulwolfia alkaloids. Arch Intern Med 1957;99:218–221.
142. Graham CF, Gallagher K, Jones JK. Acute colitis with methyldopa. N Engl J Med 1981;304:1044–1046.
143. Shneerson JM, Gazzard BG. Reversible malabsorption caused by methyldopa. Br Med J 1977;2:1456–1457.
144. Mantzoros CS, Prabhu AS, Sowers JR. Paralytic ileus as a result of diltiazem treatment. J Intern Med 1994;235:613–614.
145. Krevshy B, Maurer AH, Niewiarowski T, et al. Effect of verapamil on human intestinal transit. Dig Dis Sci 1992;37:919–924.
146. Filpi RG, Majd M, LoPresto JM. Reversible gastric stricture following iron ingestion. South Med J 1973;66:845–846.
147. Carne–Ross IP. Pyloric stenosis and sustained-release iron tablets. Br Med J 1976;2:642–643.
148. Knott LH, Miller RC. Acute iron intoxication with intestinal infarction. J Pediatr Surg 1978;13:720–721.
149. Stein HB, Urowitz MB. Gold-induced enterocolitis: Case report and literature review. J Rheumatol 1976;3:21.
150. Teodorescu V, Bauer J, Lichtiger, S, et al. Gold-induced colitis: A case report and review of the literature. Mt Sinai J Med 1993;60:238–241.
151. Nisar M, Winfiedl J. Gold-induced colitis and hepatic toxicity in a patient with rheumatoid arthritis. J Rheumatol 1994;21:938–939.
152. Jackson CW, Haboubi NY, Whorwell RJ, et al. Gold-induced enterocolitis. Gut 1986;27:452–456.
153. Geltner D, Sternfeld M, Becker SA, et al. Gold-induced ileitis. J Clin Gastroenterol 1986;8:184–186.
154. Martin DM, Goldman JA, Gilliam J, et al. Gold-induced eosinophilic enterocolitis: Response to oral cromolyn sodium. Gastroenterology 1981;80:1567–1570.
155. Gorbach SL. Bismuth therapy in gastrointestinal diseases. Gastroenterology 1990;99:863–875.
156. Wittoesch JH, Jackman RJ, MacDonald JR. Melanosis coli: General review and study of 887 cases. Dis Colon Rectum 1958;1:172.
157. Muller–Lissner SA. Adverse effects of laxatives: Fact and fiction. Pharmacology 1993;47(Suppl 1):138–145.

158. Geboes K, Spiessens C, Nijs G, et al. Anthranoids and the mucosal immune system of the colon. Pharmacology 1993;47(Suppl 1): 49–57.
159. Smith B. Pathology of cathartic colon. Proc R Soc Med 1972;65:288.
160. Urso FP, Urso MJ, Lee CH. The cathertic colon: Pathological findings and radiological/pathological correlation. Radiology 1975; 116:557.
161. Pockros PJ, Foroozan P. Golytely lavage versus standard colonoscopy preparation. Effect on normal colonic mucosal histology. Gastroenterology 1985;88:845–848.
162. Meisel JL, Bergman D, Graney D, et al. Human rectal mucosa: Proctoscopic and morphological changes caused by laxatives. Gastroenterology 1977;62:1274.
163. Leriche M, Devroede G, Sanchez G, et al. Changes in the rectal mucosa induced by hypertonic enemas. Dis Colon Rectum 1978;21: 227–236.
164. Hardin RD, Tedesco FJ. Colitis after Hibiclens enema. J Clin Gastroenterol 1986;8:572–575.
165. Jonas G, Mahoney A, Murray J, et al. Chemical colitis due to endoscopic cleansing solutions: A mimic of pseudomembranous colitis. Gastroenterology 1988;95:1403–1408.
166. Meyer CT, Brand M, DeLuca VA, et al. Hydrogen peroxide colitis: A report of three patients. J Clin Gastroenterol 1981;3:31–35.
167. Korkis AM, Miskovitz PF, Yurt RW, et al. Rectal prolapse after oral cathartics. J Clin Gastroenterol 1992;14:339–341.
168. Weiss SM, Rutenberg HL, Paskin DL, et al. Gut lesions due to slow-release KCl tablets. N Engl J Med 1977;262:111.
169. Lambert JR, Newman A. Ulceration and stricture of the esophagus due to oral potassium chloride (slow release tablet) therapy. Am J Gastroenterol 1980;4:508
170. Barloon T, Moore SA, Mitros FA. A case of stenotic obstruction of the jejunum secondary to slow-release potassium. Am J Gastroenterol 1986;81:192 194.
171. Collins FJ, Matthews HR, Baker SE, et al. Drug-induced esophageal injury. Br Med J 1979;1:1673.
172. Barrison JIG, Trewby PN, Kane SP. Esophageal ulceration due to emepronium bromide. Endoscopy 1980;12:197.
173. Thein SL, Asquith P. Pneumatosis coli: Complication of practolol. Br Med J 1977;1:268.
174. Doman JB, Ginsberg AL. The hazard of drug-induced esophagitis. Hosp Pract 1981;16:17.
175. Winckler K. Tetracycline ulcers of the oesophagus. Endoscopy, histology and roentgenology in two cases, and review of the literature. Endoscopy 1981;13:225–228.
176. Kikendall JW. Pill-induced esophageal injury. Gastroenterol Clin North Am 1991;20:835–845.
177. Bott S, Prakach C, McCallum RW. Medication-induced esophageal injury: Survey of the literature. Am J Gastroenterol 1987;82: 758–763.
178. Goldman H, Antonioli DA. Mucosal biopsy of the esophagus, stomach, and proximal duodenum. Hum Pathol 1982;13:423–448.
179. Evans DMD, Jones DB, Cleary BK, et al. Oesophageal varices treated by sclerotherapy: A histopathological study. Gut 1982;23: 615–620.
180. Sidhu SS, Bal C, Karak P, et al. Effect of endoscopic variceal sclerotherapy on esophageal motor functions and gastroesophageal reflux. J Nucl Med 1995;36:1363–1367.
181. Sugawa C. Perforation after endoscopic injection sclerotherapy for bleeding gastric varices. Surg Endosc 1994;8:1257.
182. Wass JAH, Thorner MO, Besser GM, et al. Gastrointestinal bleeding in patients on bromocriptine. Lancet 1976;2:851.
183. Goodman MJ. Gastric ulceration induced by spironolactone. Lancet 1977;1:752.
184. Gupta IP, Das TK, Susheela AK, et al. Fluoride as a possible aetiological factor in non-ulcer dyspepsia. J Gastroenterol Hepatol 1992;7:355–359.
185. Das TK, Susheela AK, Gupta IP, et al. Toxic effects of chronic fluoride ingestion on the upper gastrointestinal tract. J Clin Gastroenterol 1994;18:194–199.
186. Goldstein SS, Lewis JH, Rothstein R. Intestinal obstruction due to bezoars. Am J Gastroenterol 1984;79:313–318.
187. Faloon WW. Drug production of intestinal malabsorption. NY State J Med 1970;70:2189–2192.
188. Cohen DJ, Loertscher R, Rubin MF, et al. Cyclosporin: A new immunosuppressive agent for organ transplantation. Ann Intern Med 1984;101:667–682.
189. Tedesco FJ, Barton RW, Alpers HD. Clindamycin-associated colitis. Ann Intern Med 1974;81:429–433.
190. Bartlett JG, Chang TW, Gurwith M, et al. Antibiotic-associated pseudomembraneous colitis due to toxin-producing clostridia. N Engl J Med 1978;198:531–534.
191. Goulston SJM, McGovern VJ. Pseudomembranous colitis. Gut 1965;6:207–212.
192. Moulis H, Vender RJ. Antiobiotic-associated hemorrhagic colitis. J Clin Gastroenterol 1994;18:227–231.
193. Gebhard RL, Gerding DN, Olson MM, et al. Clinical and endoscopic findings in patients early in the course of Clostridium difficile-associated pseudomembranous colitis. Am J Med 1985;78: 45–48.
194. Medline A, Shin DH, Medline NM. Pseudomembranous colitis associated with antibiotics. Hum Pathol 1976;7:693–703.
195. Jaimes EC. Lincocinamides and the incidence of antibiotic-associated colitis. Clin Ther 1991;13:270–280.
196. Totten MA, Gregg JA, Fremont-Smith P, et al. Clinical and pathological spectrum of antibiotic-associated colitis. Am J Gastroenterol 1978;69:311–319.
197. Goldman H, Antonioli DA. Mucosal biopsy of the rectum, colon, and distal ileum. Hum Pathol 1982;13:981–1012.
198. Bartlett JG. Treatment of Clostridium difficile colitis. Gastroenterology 1985;89:1192–1195.
199. Schnitt SJ, Antonioli DA, Goldman H. Massive mural edema in severe pseudomembranous colitis. Arch Pathol Lab Med 1983;107: 211–213.
200. Trynka YM, LaMont JT. Association of Clostridium difficile toxin with symptomatic relapse of chronic inflammatory bowel disease. Gastroenterology 1980;80:693–696.
201. Faulk DL, Anuras S, Christensen J. Chronic intestinal pseudo-obstruction. Gastroenterology 1978;74:922–931.
202. Warnes H, Lehmann HE, Ban TA. Adynamic ileus during psychiatric medication. Can Med Assoc J 1967;96:1112–1113.
203. Milner G. Gastro-intestinal side-effects of psychotropic drugs. Med J Aust 1969;2:153–155.
204. Evans DL, Rogers JF, Peiper SC. Intestinal dilatation associated with phenothiazine therapy: A case report and literature review. Am J Psychiatry 1979;136:970–972.
205. Bauer GE, Hellestrand KJ. Pseudoobstruction due to clonidine. Br Med J 1976;1:769.
206. Butterfield WC. Surgical complications of narcotic addiction. Surg Gynecol Obstet 1972;134:237.
207. Spira IA, Rubenstein R, Wolff D, et al. Fecal impaction following methadone ingestion simulating acute intestinal obstruction. Ann Surg 1975;181:15–19.
208. Smith B. The neuropathology of the alimentary tract. London: Edward Arnold, 1972.
209. Martin P, Manley PN, Depew WT, et al. Isotretinonin-associated proctosigmoiditis. Gastroenterology 1987;93:606–609.
210. Pawel BR, de Chadarevian JP, Franco ME. The pathology of fibrosing colonopathy of cystic fibrosis: A study of 12 cases and review of the literature. Hum Pathol 1997;28:395–399.
211. MacSweeney EJ, Oades PJ, Buchdahl R, et al. Relation of thickening of colon wall to pancreatic-enzyme treatment in cystic fibrosis. Lancet 1995;345:752–756.
212. Brown DN, Rosenholtz MJ, Marshall JB. Ischemic colitis due to cocaine abuse. Am J Gastroenterol 1994;89:1558–1561.
213. Gourgoutis G, Das G. Gastrointestinal manifestations of cocaine addiction. Int J Clin Pharmacol Ther 1994;32:136–141.
214. Little JB. Cellular, molecular, and carcinogenic effects of radiation. Hematol Clin North Am 1990;7:337–352.
215. Rubin P, Casarett GW, eds. Clinical radiation pathology. Philadelphia: WB Saunders, 1968.
216. Fajardo LF, Berthrong M. Radiation injury in surgical pathology. Part I. Am J Surg Pathol 1978;2:159–199.
217. Michalowski AS. On radiation damage to normal tissues and its treatment. II. Anti-inflammatory drugs. Acta Oncol 1994;33: 139–157.
218. Rodemann HP, Bamberg M. Cellular basis of radiation-induced fibrosis. Radiother Oncol 1995;35:83–90.
219. Rubin P, Cassarette GW. A direction for clinical radiation pathology.

In: Vaeth JN, ed. Frontiers of radiation therapy and oncology, vol. 6. Baltimore: University Park Press, 1972:1–16.

220. Bloomer WD, Hellman S. Normal tissue responses to radiation therapy. N Engl J Med 1975;293:80–83.

221. Committee on the Biological Effects of Ionizing Radiation. The effects on populations of exposures to low levels of ionizing radiation. Washington D.C.: National Academy Press, 1980:367–372.

222. Sher ME, Bauer J. Radiation-induced enteropathy. Am J Gastroenterol 1990;85:121–128.

223. Costleigh BJ, Miyamoto CT, Micaily B, et al. Heightened sensitivity of the esophagus to radiation in a patient with AIDS. Am J Gastroenterol 1995;90:812–814.

224. Novak JM, Collins JT, Donowitz M, et al. Effects of radiation on the human gastrointestinal tract. J Clin Gastroenterol 1979;1:9–39.

225. Trier JS, Browning TH. Morphologic response of the mucosa of human small intestine to x-ray exposure. J Clin Invest 1966;45:194.

226. Key CR. Studies of the acute effects of the atomic bombs. Hum Pathol 1971;2:475–484.

227. Prasad KN. Radiation syndrome in human radiation biology. Hagerstown: Harper & Row, 1972:176–183.

228. Warren S, Friedman NB. Pathology and pathologic diagnosis of radiation lesions in the gastrointestinal tract. Am J Pathol 1942;18:499–507.

229. Friedman NB. Effects of radiation on the gastrointestinal tract, including the salivary glands, the liver and the pancreas. Arch Pathol Lab Med 1942;34:749–787.

230. Mulligan RM. The lesions produced in the gastrointestinal tract by irradiation. Am J Pathol 1942;18:515–525.

231. Ackerman LV. The pathology of radiation effect of normal and neoplastic tissue. AJR Am J Roentgenol 1972;14:447–459.

232. Berthrong M, Fajardo LF. Radiation injury in surgical pathology. II. Alimentary tract. Am J Surg Pathol 1981;5:153–178.

233. Tarpila S. Morphological and functional response of human small intestine to ionizing radiation. Scand J Gastroenterol 1971;6(Suppl 12):1–52.

234. Haboubi NY, Schofield PF, Rowland PL. The light and electron microscopic features of early and late phase radiation-induced proctitis. Am J Gastroenterol 1988;83:1140–1144.

235. Kirkpatrick JB. Pathogenesis of foam cell lesions in irradiated arteries. Am J Pathol 1967;50:291–309.

236. Hasleton PS, Carr N, Schofield PF. Vascular changes in radiation bowel disease. Histopathology 1985;9:517–534.

237. Sadove M, Block M, Rossof HH, et al. Radiation carcinogenesis in man: Primary neoplasms in fields of prior radiation. Cancer 1981;48:1139–1143.

238. Sandler RS, Sandler DP. Radiation-induced cancers of the colon and rectum: Assessing the risk. Gastroenterology 1983;84:51–57.

239. Lieber MR, Winans CS, Griem ML, et al. Sarcomas arising after radiotherapy for peptic ulcer disease. Dig Dis Sci 1985;30:593–599.

240. Jablon S, Bailas III JC. The contribution of ionizing radiation to cancer mortality in the United States. Prev Med 1980;9:219–226.

241. Schottenfeld D. Radiation as a risk factor in the natural history of colorectal cancer (editorial). Gastroenterology 1983;84:186–190.

242. Shamsuddin AKM, Elias EG. Rectal mucosa. Malignant and premalignant changes after radiation therapy. Arch Pathol Lab Med 1981;105:150–151.

243. Haggitt RC, Appelman HD, Correa P, et al. Dysplasia in Crohn's disease (letter). Arch Pathol Lab Med 1982;106:308–309.

244. Coia LR, Myers RJ, Tepper JE. Late effects of radiation therapy on the gastrointestinal tract. Int J Radiat Oncol Biol Phys 1995;31:1213–1236.

245. Roswit B. Complications of radiation therapy: The alimentary tract. Semin Roentgenol 1974;9:51–63.

246. Goldman H. Gastrointestinal mucosal biopsy. New York: Churchill Livingstone, 1996.

247. Wiseman JS, Senagore AJ, Chaudry IH. Methods to prevent colonic injury in pelvic radiation. Dis Colon Rectum 1994;37:1090–1094.

248. Carroll MP, Zera RT, Roberts JC, et al. Efficacy of radioprotective agents in preventing small and large bowel radiation injury. Dis Colon Rectum 1995;38:716–722.

249. Nicolopoulos N, Mantidis A, Stathopoulos E, et al. Prophylactic administration of indomethacin for irradiation esophagitis. Radiother Oncol 1985;3:23–28.

250. Montana GS, Anscher MS, Mansbach CM, et al. Topical application of WR-2721 to prevent radiation-induced proctosigmoiditis. A phase I/II trial. Cancer 1992;69:2826–2830.

251. Kao MS. Intestinal complications of radiotherapy in gynecologic malignancy: Clinical presentation and management. Int J Gynaecol Obstet 1995;49(Suppl);S69–S75.

252. Pricolo VE, Shellito PC. Surgery for radiation injury to the large intestine. Variables influencing outcome. Dis Colon Rectum 1994;37:675–684.

253. Otchy DP, Nelson H. Radiation injuries of the colon and rectum. Surg Clin North Am 1993;73:1017–1035.

254. Sher ME, Bauer J. Radiation-induced enteropathy. Am J Gastroenterol 1990;85:121–128.

255. Seamen WB, Ackerman LV. The effect of radiation on the esophagus. Radiology 1957;68:534–540.

256. Jennings FL, Arden A. Acute radiation effects on the esophagus. Arch Pathol Lab Med 1960;69:407.

257. Chowhan NM. Injurious effects of radiation on the esophagus. Am J Gastroenterol 1990;85:115–120.

258. Vanagunas A, Jacob P, Olinger E. Radiation-induced esophageal injury: A spectrum from esophagitis to cancer. Am J Gastroenterol 1990;85:808–812.

259. Goldstein HM, Rogers LF, Fletcher GH, et al. Radiological manifestations of radiation-induced injury to the normal upper gastrointestinal tract. Radiology 1975;117:135–140.

260. Papazian A, Capron J-P, Ducroix J-P, et al. Mucosal bridges of the upper esophagus after radiotherapy for Hodgkin's disease. Gastroenterology 1983;84:1028–1031.

261. Seeman H, Gates JA, Traube M. Esophageal motor dysfunction years after radiation therapy. Dig Dis Sci 1992;37:303–306.

262. Goffman TE, McKeen EA, Curtis RE, et al. Esophageal carcinoma following irradiation for breast cancer. Cancer 1983;52:1808–1809.

263. Sherril DJ, Grishkill BA, Galae FS, et al. Radiation-associated malignancies of the esophagus. Cancer 1984;54:726–728.

264. Fekete F, Mosnier H, Belghiti J, et al. Esophageal cancer after mediastinal irradiation. Dysphagia 1994;9:289–291.

265. Levin E, Clayman CB, Palmer WL, et al. Observations on the value of gastric radiation in the treatment of duodenal ulcer. Gastroenterology 1957;32:42.

266. Clayman CB, Palmer WL, Kirsner JB. Gastric irradiation in the treatment of peptic ulcer. Gastroenterology 1968;55:403.

267. Kellum JM, Jaffe BM, Calhoun T, et al. Gastric complications after radiotherapy for Hodgkin's disease and other lymphomas. Am J Surg 1977;134:314–317.

268. Hamilton FE. Gastric ulcer following radiation. Arch Surg 1947;55:394–399.

269. Goldgraber MB, Rubin CE, Palmer WL, et al. The early gastric response to irradiation: A serial biopsy study. Gastroenterology 1954;27:1–20.

270. Schier J, Symmonds RE, Dahlin DC. Clinicopathologic aspects of actinic enteritis. Surg Gynecol Obstet 1964;119:1019–1025.

271. Wellwood JM, Jackson BT. The intestinal complications of radiotherapy. Br J Surg 1973;60:814–818.

272. Churnratanakul S, Wirzba B, Lam T, et al. Radiation and the small intestine. Future perspectives for preventive therapy. Dig Dis Sci 1990;8:45–60.

273. Husebye E, Hauer-Jensen M, Kjorstad K, et al. Severe late radiation enteropathy is characterized by impaired motility of proximal small intestine. Dig Dis Sci 1994;39:2341–2349.

274. O'Brien PH, Jenette JM, Garvin AJ. Radiation enteritis. Am Surg 1987;53:501–504.

275. Yeoh EK, Horowitz M. Radiation enteritis. Surg Gynecol Obstet 1987;165:373–376.

276. Schofield PF. Radiation damage of the bowel. In: Taylor I, ed. Progress in surgery. Edinburgh: Churchill Livingstone, 1987:142–156.

277. Abrahamson R. Radiation ileitis. Arch Surg 1960;81:55–59.

278. Burn JI. Radiation duodenitis. Proc R Soc Med 1971;64:395–396.

279. Mason GR, Dietrich P, Friedland GW, et al. The radiological findings in radiation-induced enteritis and colitis. Clin Radiol 1970;21:232–247.

280. Donaldson SS, Jundt S, Ricour C, et al. Radiation enteritis in

children. A retrospective review, clinicopathologic correlation, and dietary management. Cancer 1975;35:1167–1178.

281. Galland RB, Spencer J. The natural history of clinically established radiation enteritis. Lancet 1985;1:1257–1258.

282. Dencker H, Holmdahl KH, Lunderquist A, et al. Mesenteric angiography in patients with radiation injury of the bowel after pelvis irradiation. AJR Am J Roentgenol 1972;114:476–481.

283. Greenberger NJ, Isselbacher KJ. Malabsorption following radiation injury to the gastrointestinal tract. Am J Med 1964;6:450–456.

284. Tankel HI, Clark DH, Lee FD. Radiation enteritis with malabsorption. Gut 1965;6:560–569.

285. Duncan W, Leonard JC. The malabsorption syndrome following radiotherapy. Q J Med 1965;34:319–329.

286. Wiernik G. Changes in the villous pattern of the human jejunum associated with heavy irradiation damage. Gut 1966;7:149–153.

287. Whitehead R. Mucosal biopsy of the gastrointestinal tract. 5th ed. Philadelphia: WB Saunders, 1996.

288. Wolov RB, Sato N, Azumi N, et al. Intra-abdominal "angiosarcomatosis" report of two cases after pelvic irradiation. Cancer 1991;67: 2275–2279.

289. May J, Lowenthal J. Irradiation injury to the colon. Gut 1965;6: 444–447.

290. Villasanta U. Complications of radiotherapy for carcinoma of the uterine cervix. Am J Obstet Gynecol 1974;119:727–732.

291. Sedgwick DM, Howard GCW, Ferguson A. Pathogenesis of acute radiation injury to the rectum. Int J Colorect Dis 1994;9:23–30.

292. Schmitz RM, Chao JH, Bartolome JS. Intestinal injuries to irradiation of carcinoma of the cervix of the uterus. Surg Gynecol Obstet 1984;138:29–32.

293. Friedman M. Calculated risks of radiation injury of normal tissue in the treatment of cancer of the testis. In: Proceedings of the Second National Cancer Conference, New York. The American Cancer Society. National Cancer Institute. USPHS Federal Science Agency, 1952:390–400.

294. Stockbrine MF, Hancock JE, Fletcher GH. Complications in 831 patients with squamous cell carcinoma of the intact uterine cervix treatment with 3000 rads or more whole pelvis irradiation. AJR Am J Roentgenol 1970;108:293–304.

295. Gelfand MD, Tepper M, Katz LA, et al. Acute radiation proctitis in man. Gastroenterology 1968;54:401–411.

296. Babb RR. Radiation proctitis: A review. Am J Gastroenterol 1996; 91:1309–1311.

297. Gilensky NH, Burns DG, Barbezat GO, et al. The natural history of radiation-induced proctosigmoiditis: An analysis of 88 patients. Q J Med 1983;202:40–53.

298. Ng WK, Chan KW. Postirradiation colitis cystica profunda. Case report and literature review. Arch Pathol Lab Med 1995;119:1170–1173.

299. Smith JC. Carcinoma of the rectum following irradiation of cancer of the cervix. Proc R Soc Med 1962;55:701–702.

300. Black WC, Ackerman LV. Carcinoma of the large intestine as a late complication of pelvic radiotherapy. Clin Radiol 1965;16: 278–281.

301. MacMahon CE, Rowe JW. Rectal reaction following radiation therapy of cervical carcinoma: Particular reference to the subsequent occurrence of rectal carcinoma. Ann Surg 1971;173:264–269.

302. Castro EB, Rowen PP, Quan SHQ. Carcinoma of large intestine in patients irradiated for carcinoma of cervix and uterus. Cancer 1973;31:45–52.

303. Shirouzu K, Isomoto H, Morodomi T, et al. Clinicopathologic characteristics of large bowel cancer developing after radiotherapy for uterine cervical cancer. Dis Colon Rectum 1994;7:1245–1249.

304. Cunningham MD, Wilhoite R. Radiation-induced carcinoma of the transverse colon: Report of a case. Dis Colon Rectum 1973;16: 145–148.

305. Qizilbash AH. Radiation-induced carcinoma of the rectum: A late complication of pelvic irradiation. Arch Pathol Lab Med 1974;98: 118–121.

306. O'Connor TW, Rombeau JL, Levine HS, et al. Late development of colorectal cancer subsequent to pelvic irradiation. Dis Colon Rectum 1979;22:123–128.

307. Sibly TG, Keane RM, Lever JV, et al. Rectal lymphoma in radiation injured bowel. Br J Surg 1985;72:879–000.

308. Gilbert ES, Marks S. An analysis of the mortality of workers in a nuclear facility. Radiat Res 1979;79:122–148.

309. Kato H, Schull WJ. Studies of the mortality of A-bomb survivors. VII. Mortality, 1950–1978: Part I. Cancer mortality. Radiat Res 1982; 90:395–432.

310. McIlrath DC, Hallenbeck GA. Review of gastric freezing. JAMA 1964;190:715.

311. Barnes HB, Collins CH, Jones TI, et al. Morphology of human stomach after therapeutic freezing. Arch Surg 1964;90:358.

312. Perry GT, Dunphy JV, Brain RC, et al. Gastric freezing for duodenal ulcer. A double blind study. Gastroenterology 1964;47:6.

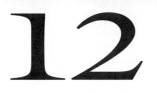

12 | ALLERGIC DISORDERS

Harvey Goldman

This chapter presents the major manifestations of the allergic disorders due to food sensitivity that affect the various parts of the gastrointestinal tract. A discussion of eosinophilic gastroenteritis, including both the allergic and nonallergic forms, is also included. Details of the normal structure and function of the immunologic system are contained in Chapter 6, and some of the allergic conditions are presented in part in the specific chapters dealing with inflammatory diseases of the esophagus (see Chapter 20), the stomach (see Chapter 23), and the intestines (see Chapters 30 and 31). Reactions to non-food substances, including chemicals and drugs, are discussed in Chapter 11.

GENERAL ASPECTS

CLINICAL FEATURES AND TERMINOLOGY

Persons react to ingested foods for a variety of reasons (Table 12.1), including the presence of heavy metals and other toxic chemicals; food poisoning owing to pathogenic bacteria and their exotoxins; selective enzyme deficiencies, such as primary lactose intolerance; celiac disease (gluten enteropathy); and other more generalized malabsorptive disorders. An abnormal response may also occur in patients with anorexia nervosa and psychologic disorders, and may result simply from a dislike of a particular food. All of these conditions and circumstances must be excluded before considering the possibility that the patient has a specific allergic reaction or sensitivity to an ingested food substance.

Allergic disorders attributable to food sensitivity are seen most often in infants and children (1, 2), but they may occur in persons of all ages, especially in young adults (3, 4). Indeed, a delay in

making the diagnosis of an allergic condition, sometimes up to several months or years, is not unusual in an adult patient, principally because of the failure to consider the diagnostic possibility.

The specific diagnosis of a food allergy or sensitivity affecting the gastrointestinal tract depends on a combination of compatible clinical and pathologic features, the exclusion of other potential causes such as infections and various malabsorptive diseases, and the beneficial response to an elimination diet or to treatment with corticosteroid hormones. The patient often exhibits an elevation of the peripheral blood eosinophil count and a rise in the serum level of IgE, but other more specific tests to support an allergic basis are ordinarily not available. Ideally, the diagnosis should be substantiated by an oral rechallenge with the suspected food allergen, noting the return of symptoms and/or the reappearance of alterations in a mucosal biopsy specimen. Such documentation has been achieved in selected cases, especially in those involving sensitivity to cow's milk protein (5), but it has proven difficult in more generalized cases of allergic gastroenteritis to establish the particular allergens involved. Furthermore, in most cases of allergic proctitis, the association with a single allergen, such as milk or soy protein, seems so secure that it is not always standard clinical practice to perform a rechallenge study (6).

A variety of terms are used to connote different aspects of allergic diseases of the gut related to foods based on the particular antigens and pathogenetic mechanisms involved, the distribution of the lesions in the different segments of the alimentary tract, and the overall severity and behavior of the lesions. Thus, if the disorder appears to be related to a single food allergen, such as cow's milk, soy, or wheat protein, the disease is often referred to by the particular etiologic agent as well as the distribution of the lesions if known

225

TABLE	
12.1	**Causes of Food Reactions in the Gut**

Allergic diseases
Contamination by toxic chemicals
Infectious food poisoning
Malabsorptive disorders
Anorexia nervosa
Psychologic reactions

(7–11). For example, terms used include cow's milk protein-allergy, -sensitivity, -hypersensitivity, -intolerance, -enteritis, or -colitis. When the disorder involves multiple antigens and is associated with more widespread effects in the gut segments, it usually is referred to as eosinophilic gastroenteritis or allergic gastroenteropathy (12–15). It is important to sort out the mucosal form of eosinophilic gastroenteritis, which has a definite or presumed allergic etiology, from the mural type, which lacks an allergic basis. Because of considerable overlap in the antigens and pathogenetic mechanisms and ambiguity in the use of the term of eosinophilic gastroenteritis, it is useful to divide the allergic cases affecting the gut into two major groups based primarily on the dominant localization of the lesions: (*a*) Allergic gastroenteritis, in which the lesions may affect any part of the gut but tend to be concentrated in the esophagus, stomach, and proximal small intestine; and (*b*) Allergic proctitis or colitis, in which the lesions are predominantly or solely present in the large bowel (2). This separation helps to explain the functional effects and overall clinical behavior of the allergic disorders.

PATHOGENETIC MECHANISMS

The potential immunologic mechanisms involved in gastrointestinal allergy (16) are summarized in Table 12.2, and further details are provided in Chapter 6. The levels of serum antibodies of the IgG class to food proteins are often elevated and associated with IgE antibodies, in both the serum and the gut lumen, in patients with food allergy. No constant correlation exists, however, between the presence of food antibodies and the activity of the allergic condition. Most cases of food allergy involve the type I or immediate hypersensitivity form of immunologic reaction. This mechanism is supported by an elevation of the serum IgE level and a positive radioallergosorbent (RAST) test to numerous food substances, including cow's milk protein, eggs, fish, soy, nuts, and wheat. Patients also frequently exhibit other signs of type I reaction, such as asthma, rhinitis, and urticaria. Furthermore, an increase in IgE-producing plasma cells has been identified in the gut mucosa by immunohistochemical staining in selected cases, including those involving milk protein allergy affecting the small intestines (17, 18) and a subset of cases of ulcerative proctitis and colitis that responded to antiallergic medication (19–21). Injury probably results from the triggering of the IgE-coated mast cells in the gastrointestinal mucosa, leading to their release of histamine, prostaglandins, and other inflammatory mediators.

The type III or humoral form of immunologic mechanism is involved in a minority of the food-related allergic cases and is characterized by the presence of circulating and mucosal immune complexes that consist of foreign protein, complement, and immunoglobulins of the IgG and IgM classes. A delayed type of hypersensitivity with activated lymphocytes has also been demonstrated in a few cases, but it is not thought to be a dominant factor, at least as a primary cause, of gastrointestinal allergy. The exact immunologic mechanism is usually not documented in an individual clinical case, but it may be inferred by the speed of onset of symptoms after exposure to the food protein: short duration is supportive of a type I reaction and a more prolonged start is indicative of a humoral or other delayed reaction. Also, the immediate reactions are often associated with similar signs of hypersensitivity in the respiratory tract and skin.

One of the major histologic features of allergic reactions is the presence of abundant eosinophils, and both mast cell mediators (22, 23) and lymphokines released from activated lymphocytes (24, 25) are known to attract and to affect the migration of eosinophils in tissues. The eosinophils may act as a scavenger of immune complexes, but they also release products, such as eosinophil granule protein, that are directly toxic to the tissues (26–29).

ALLERGIC EFFECTS IN OTHER ORGANS

Numerous attempts have been made to relate food allergy to the development of diseases of various organ systems, alone or in conjunction with gastrointestinal disease (16). It appears, however, that a strong association exists only for the occurrence of pulmonary symptoms and cutaneous disorders that are seen in about 50% of patients with allergic gastroenteritis. In most cases, the symptoms are those that would be expected in a type I or immediate hypersensitivity reaction, including wheezing, rhinorrhea, and urticaria. Although still debated, it is thought that some cases of eczema or atopic dermatitis have an allergic basis, and a beneficial response to milk-free and egg-free diets has been noted.

EOSINOPHILIC GASTROENTERITIS

Eosinophilic gastroenteritis or gastroenteropathy is a generic term used in the past to indicate a disorder characterized by tissue damage and a prominent reaction with eosinophils. Abundant eosinophils can be seen in many conditions, and it is imperative that one exclude from consideration more specific disorders such as reflux esophagitis, parasitic infections, toxic reactions to drugs, idiopathic inflammatory bowel disease, and the various collagen vascular disorders. The remaining cases of eosinophilic gastroenteritis are categorized according to three distinct forms (mucosal, mural, and serosal) based on their dominant location in the gut wall (Table 12.3) (12, 30).

MUCOSAL TYPE

In this form of eosinophilic gastroenteritis, the injury is concentrated in the mucosal layer, although the inflammation may extend into the upper submucosa. The lesions are often multiple and can be seen in any part of the gut, including the esophagus, stomach (particularly the antrum), and both the small and large intestines. Patients typically present with some combination of malabsorption, iron deficiency anemia, and a protein-losing gastroenteropathy, and allergy is likely an etiologic factor in these cases (12, 13, 15, 31, 32).

This mucosal form of eosinophilic gastroenteritis is described in detail subsequently (see Allergic Gastroenteritis).

MURAL TYPE

This form of eosinophilic gastroenteritis is characterized by the localization of tissue injury and inflammatory reaction with abundant eosinophils in the submucosa and muscularis propria (33). The mural type is more common in children, but it can occur in any age group (34). The lesions may affect any part of the gut, but more often they are noted in the gastric antrum, usually in the prepyloric region, and in the distal small intestine. Lesions are most often single and produce an obstructive mass (35, 36); exceptionally, there may be extensive ulceration and necrosis leading to perforation, especially in the intestines (37–39). This mural type is unrelated to the mucosal form of eosinophilic gastroenteritis, no evidence exists of an allergic component in its etiology, and the pathogenesis of the mural lesions is not known.

Considering the inflammatory nature of the lesion, an infectious cause has often been considered but not proven, and there is no regular evidence of a vasculitis. Despite the uniform histologic findings, the lesions are likely a heterogenous lot and may prove to have a varied etiology. In the past, the term "eosinophilic granuloma" has been applied to some of these lesions, particularly those involving the stomach. Use of this term is not optimal, however, because there are no granulomas and no relation between this mural form of eosinophilic gastroenteritis and the entity of Langerhans cell histiocytosis, which can include isolated lesions, called eosinophilic granuloma.

PATHOLOGIC FEATURES AND DIAGNOSIS

Surgery is usually required because of the obstructive symptoms and the uncertainty of the nature of the mass lesion (30, 40). The diagnosis is made on the basis of the histologic finding of a nonspecific inflammatory reaction with many eosinophils as well as on the exclusion of other specific disorders. The lesions are usually single and consist of an ill-defined mass, from a few to several centimeters in diameter, that is located in the wall of the affected portion of the gut (33–35); the overlying mucosa may show focal ulceration. Histologic examination reveals extensive inflammation with a dominance of mature eosinophils (Fig. 12.1) and either patchy or confluent areas of liquefactive or coagulative necrosis. The eosinophilic reaction may encircle areas of necrosis, but there are no increase in macrophages or presence of well-formed granulomas. Uncommonly, the necrosis may be more severe and extend through the gut wall, resulting in a perforation, especially in lesions of the intestines (38, 39).

DIFFERENTIAL DIAGNOSIS

At a clinical level, the major considerations are a tumor of the gut wall, such as a leiomyoma or leiomyosarcoma, and a chronic inflammatory condition with stricture formation. Before rendering a diagnosis of the mural form of eosinophilic gastroenteritis, it is imperative that other disorders associated with mural necrosis and a prominent eosinophilic inflammatory reaction are considered, including toxic reactions to some chemicals and drugs and, especially, chronic parasitic infections, such as anisakiasis and that attributable to strongyloides. Accordingly, stool examination and

---

TABLE 12.2   Immunologic Mechanisms in Gastrointestinal Food Allergy

Type of Reaction	Occurrence in GI Allergy	Mechanism of Injury
I. Immediate hypersensitivity Anaphylactic reaction	Yes	Degranulation of Ig+E-coated mast cell
II. Cytotoxic reaction	No	—
III. Humoral immunity Immune complex disease	Probable	Deposition of immune complexes, causing activation of complement
IV. Cell-mediated immunity Delayed hypersensitivity	Probable	Release of lymphokines from activated lymphocytes

---

TABLE 12.3   Types of Eosinophilic Gastroenteritis

Type	Location of Disease	Etiology	Functional Effect
Mucosal	Mucosa	Allergic	Bleeding, protein loss, and malabsorption
Mural	Submucosa and muscularis propria	Unknown	Mass lesion resulting in obstruction and rare perforation
Serosal	Serosa	Unknown	Ascites

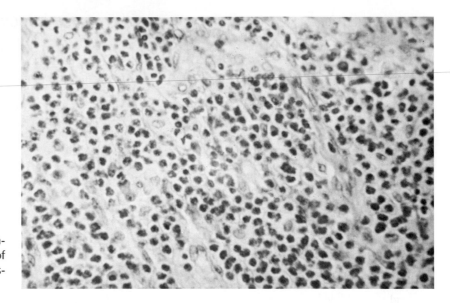

Figure 12.1   Mural type of eosinophilic gastroenteritis. Section of the lesion shows a large sheet of mature eosinophils admixed with small blood vessels. H & E, ×400.

multiple tissue sections must be surveyed for worm fragments and eggs. Crohn disease may manifest with obstruction owing to an inflammatory stricture in any part of the gut and can be associated with a significant eosinophilic infiltrate. Features supportive of Crohn disease include the presence of inflammatory sinus tracts and fistulae, the appearance of multiple lesions in the distal ileum and colon, signs of chronic enteritis in the form of prominent pyloric metaplasia and neuronal hyperplasia, and the identification of well-formed granulomas. Other less common conditions associated with a prominent tissue eosinophilia include occasional tumors, amyloidosis, and chronic granulomatous disease, all of which show other characteristic features on histologic examination.

Finally, just about any condition affecting the gut can be complicated by the unexplained appearance of numerous eosinophils in the inflammatory reaction. For example, some cases of ordinary peptic ulcer disease of the gastric antrum or duodenum reveal a sensational eosinophilic response (Fig. 12.2), and no correlation exists between this finding and the overall behavior of the lesion (41). The mural form of eosinophilic gastroenteritis is probably not a single entity; it simply describes a particular type of inflammatory mass without an apparent cause. In making the diagnosis, it is exceedingly important to stress the mural nature of the lesion to avoid confusion with the allergy-associated mucosal form of eosinophilic gastroenteritis.

SEROSAL TYPE

This rarest of the types of eosinophilic gastroenteritis is characterized by diffuse eosinophilic infiltrates of the gut serosa and a prominent ascites (12, 30, 42). Its etiology is unknown and it is unlikely that this form represents a single entity. Indeed, considering its rarity and uncertain nature, one could question whether the condition is deserving of a special name. It should be separated from the mucosal and mural forms of eosinophilic gastroenteritis, because none of these types are related.

ALLERGIC GASTROENTERITIS

DEFINITIONS

The term "allergic gastroenteritis" is used to encompass those cases of food allergy in which the lesions are often multiple and can affect any part of the gut from the esophagus to the colon. The severity of the disease is highly variable and appears to depend on the magnitude of the food allergens involved. Thus, in cases attributable to a single food substance, such as cow's milk or soy protein, patients typically present with less severe disease, possibly reflecting an early diagnosis, and the disorder is readily reversed by an elimination diet. Conversely, in cases involving multiple food allergens, the clinical course is more protracted and the patients often require corticosteroid therapy. Indeed, the particular constellation of offending food substances may not be completely identified in 50% of these more severe cases (2). Because of the differences in behavior, many investigators have preferred to designate the milder and more restrictive cases according to the particular offending food, such as cow's milk protein or soy protein allergy (or sensitivity), and to use the term eosinophilic gastroenteritis (or gastroenteropathy) for the more complex cases. As noted previously, the latter would correspond to the mucosal form of eosinophilic gastroenteritis in contrast to the mural and serosal forms (12).

The author prefers to use the collective term of allergic gastroenteritis for both the milder and the severe cases for the following reasons: (a) the pathologic pattern of injury in the mucosa is identical, consisting of epithelial and glandular degeneration with a prominence of eosinophils; (b) the distribution of lesions in the gut is the same; (c) the pathogenetic mechanisms involved appear to be similar or, at least, overlap; (d) no differences in frequency of other allergic symptoms in the patients and their families are noted; (e) the other differences in clinical features and laboratory results simply reflect the degree of injury to the mucosa and the duration of the disorder; and (f) it is possible to avoid the use of the generic term of eosinophilic gastroenteritis and the potential confusion between the mucosal and mural forms. Admittedly, in some cases, an allergic etiology is not firmly established; these are included because of the lack of any other known cause, the similarity in their clinical and pathologic features to the definite allergic cases, and their beneficial response to corticosteroid therapy.

CLINICAL AND LABORATORY FEATURES

The disorder can affect persons of either gender and of all ages, but it is more commonly seen in children and young adults. The patients typically present with some combination of bleeding or iron deficiency anemia, a protein-losing state, and malabsorptive symptoms (12, 15, 31). In a study of 38 cases in children (2), the major presenting symptoms were growth failure with diarrhea and vomiting in 26, anemia in 6, asthma in 3, the hyper-IgE syndrome in 2, and overt rectal bleeding in only 1 case. Overall, diarrhea was noted in 67%, vomiting in 51%, weight loss in 40%, abdominal pain in 33%, and rectal bleeding in 25% of the patients; symptoms were noted more commonly in the older children, probably reflecting the longer duration of the illness. A history of other allergic manifestations in the patients and their families is present in about 50% of cases and mainly includes asthma, rhinitis, and eczema. Occasionally, the patients have dominant symptoms referable to involvement of a particular part of the upper tract and clinical features that simulate ordinary peptic esophagitis (43, 44) or hypertrophic pyloric stenosis (45).

In the majority of cases, the peripheral blood eosinophil count is elevated at some time; counts may range from 5 to 15%. An increase in the serum IgE levels is noted in about three quarters of cases and is often associated with an abnormal RAST test. Anemia of the iron deficiency type is present in one quarter to one half of patients and is usually mild. As with the clinical features, the abnormal laboratory test results are more commonly noted in the older children and adults. Other signs of malabsorption and mucosal injury present in about one third of cases include excess protein excretion, reduced serum albumin and IgG, abnormal lactose and xylose tolerance tests, and prominence of gastric and intestinal folds by radiographic and endoscopic examinations.

Patients with disease related to one or two food allergens, such as cow's milk and soy protein, typically respond promptly to an elimination diet and experience no recurrences (46, 47). Most patients, especially children, appear to lose the capacity to react to the food substances after several years. This loss of sensitivity is possibly attributable to maturity in the development of the mucosal immune system, resulting in more effective production of IgG and IgA that may neutralize ingested antigens and a reduction in the synthesis of IgE. In contrast, in cases involving multiple antigens and those in which the offending foods cannot be completely identified, patients require corticosteroid or other immunosuppressive therapy and are prone to multiple relapses (48). Exceptionally, affected adults become refractory to medical therapy and develop sustained malabsorption, leading to a rare death from allergic disease.

GENERAL PATHOLOGIC FEATURES AND DIAGNOSIS

The lesions of allergic gastroenteritis are usually multiple and can affect any part of the gut; they are least common in the colon and rectum (49). Although most investigators and clinical studies have concentrated on disease of the small bowel (13, 17), lesions are often present and frequently more prominent in the esophagus and the stomach, especially the antral portion (50). The reason for the localization of the lesion in an individual case is not known, and the finding of disease in a particular tissue site does not indicate any special pathogenesis but rather determines the clinical features observed and the area that should be subjected to selective biopsy.

Lesions in allergic gastroenteritis have generally the same pathologic features, regardless of their location in the gut, and differ only in severity. Focal disease is observed in individuals with a single food allergen such as cow's milk protein and more extensive involvement is noted in patients with disease attributable to multiple antigens (so-called mucosal form of eosinophilic gastroenteritis). The lesions always affect the mucosa and are characterized by variable degrees of epithelial damage and an inflammatory infiltrate that is typically rich in mature eosinophils. The eosinophils are not only present in the lamina propria, but also extend into the epithelial layers on the surface and in the glands. The lesions may be patchy, especially in the small intestine, and multiple sections may be needed

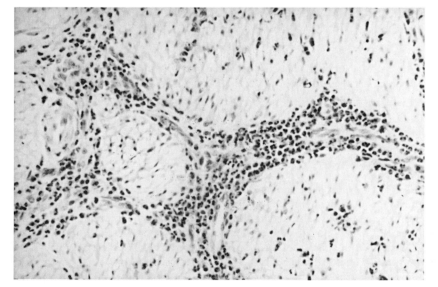

Figure 12.2 Chronic peptic ulcer of the stomach. Section of muscularis propria beneath the ulcer reveals clumps of eosinophils insinuated between the muscle bundles. H & E, ×100.

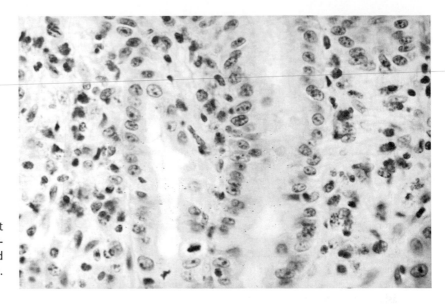

Figure 12.3 Gastric antral mucosa in a patient with healing allergic gastroenteritis. Note regenerating gastric pits with several mitoses *(center)* and persistence of eosinophils in the lamina propria. H & E, ×400.

for identification (13). Occasionally, the lesions are more extensive and confluent, resulting in prominent edema of the mucosal folds, which can be visualized by endoscopic and radiographic examinations of the stomach and intestines (51). Ulceration of the surface of the mucosa is rarely present (52); when seen, however, it is important to consider and exclude disorders that more frequently have ulceration, such as infections, idiopathic inflammatory bowel disease, and tumors. The inflammation may extend into the submucosa, but the deeper parts of the gut wall are not involved. Neutrophils are rarely prominent and usually are restricted to the cases with ulceration. An increase in plasma cells, especially those producing IgE, and in mast cells have been noted in the lamina propria of the intestines in some cases (17, 18). No regular increase occurs in the numbers of other mononuclear inflammatory cells in the lamina propria.

Although the presence of abundant eosinophils is a characteristic finding, the number of eosinophils is not always striking. This variability is a particular problem in the analysis of the intestinal mucosa, which normally contains some eosinophils in the lamina propria (53, 54) and in which only a significant increase, with aggregates, should be considered abnormal. Ideally, quantitative methods should be applied, but such analysis is not readily available in ordinary clinical practice. It is probably best to rely on evidence of epithelial damage and extension of the eosinophils into the epithelial layer for the more precise diagnosis of an allergic lesion. With healing of the lesions, following an elimination diet or the use of corticosteroid therapy, comes prompt regeneration of the epithelium, which may exhibit numerous mitoses, although the eosinophilic infiltrate in the lamina propria may linger for several days (Fig. 12.3).

The diagnosis of allergic gastroenteritis depends on several factors: the exclusion of other disorders that have a prominent eosinophilic reaction, as described in the section on differential diagnosis (Table 12.4); the finding of compatible clinical, laboratory, and pathologic features; and the beneficial response to an elimination diet or to corticosteroid therapy. Food rechallenges are often recommended but are rarely a part of standard clinical practice, probably because of the ready availability of alternative formulas and diets (6, 46, 47). The cases attributable to a single or

TABLE	
12.4	**Causes of Increased Numbers of Eosinophils in the Gut Mucosa**

Allergic disease
Reflux esophagitis
Toxic reactions to chemicals and drugs
Parasitic infections
Idiopathic inflammatory bowel diseases
   Ulcerative colitis
   Crohn disease
Collagenous colitis and lymphocytic colitis
Vasculitis
Amyloidosis
Chronic granulomatous disease
Tumors

to two food allergens are effectively eliminated by a dietary change. Relapses are more likely in cases involving to multiple antigens. The recurring lesions are identical in appearance to the original disease and usually involve the same portions of the gut. Despite repeated recurrences, the development of fibrosis, glandular atrophy, or other signs of chronic disease has not been described in cases of allergic gastroenteritis.

SPECIFIC ORGAN FEATURES AND DIFFERENTIAL DIAGNOSIS

It is important to re-emphasize that a prominent eosinophilic infiltrate in the gut mucosa is not a specific feature and, by itself, is not indicative of an allergic disorder (55). Mucosal injury with an exaggerated eosinophilic response can be seen in many other conditions of the gastrointestinal tract (see Table 12.4), including reflux esophagitis (56–58), toxic reactions to some chemicals and drugs such as gold salts (59), parasitic infections (60), the idiopathic inflammatory bowel diseases of ulcerative colitis and Crohn disease (61–63), chronic granulomatous disease (64), connective tissue disorders (65), amyloidosis, and some tumors (4).

ESOPHAGUS

The notion that the esophagus is rarely involved in food allergy (66–68) was apparently due to a lack of examination of the esophagus. At least in children, frequent and sometimes extensive lesions have been noted in the esophageal mucosa (2, 43, 58). These lesions usually coexist with disease affecting other parts of the gut, such as the stomach and small intestine, but occasionally are the dominant feature in a case of allergic gastroenteritis. Esophageal involvement has been established in the severe form of allergic gastroenteritis, but its frequency in the milder cases involving a single antigen is not known.

The lesions are concentrated in the distal esophagus, which may reflect the tendency for this area to be selectively sampled during endoscopic biopsy. Characteristic findings include basal zone hyperplasia of the squamous epithelial layer and a pronounced infiltrate of mature eosinophils within the epithelium (Fig. 12.4). Usually large numbers of eosinophils are also found in the lamina propria, but it is more difficult to evaluate this criterion because such cells may be present in this compartment in the normal esophagus (54).

The major differential diagnosis is reflux esophagitis, a more common disorder that reveals the identical histologic features of basal zone hyperplasia (69) and infiltration of eosinophils within the squamous epithelium (56–58). The diagnosis of esophageal involvement in allergic gastroenteritis is supported by an elevated blood eosinophil count and the finding of mucosal lesions in other parts of the gut, such as the gastric antrum and small intestine. In contrast, patients with reflux esophagitis have a normal blood eosinophil count, lack lesions in other parts of the tract, and show abnormalities in a pH probe and manometric examination of the esophagus. Other causes of esophagitis, including various infections and injury from entrapped pills, typically reveal more focal lesions and are not usually associated with a prominent eosinophilic reaction.

STOMACH

The stomach, particularly the antral portion, is a common site for the appearance of allergic lesions, which are often pronounced in this region (2, 50, 70). This prominence was first noted in children but appears to occur also in adults. The cause of this preferential localization is not known, but it is clear that gastric antral lesions can contribute to the blood loss and excess protein excretion observed in patients with allergic disease. Because the gastric lesions seem to be more consistently found than disease in other parts of the gut, mucosal biopsy of the gastric antrum has proven to be an effective tool in the identification of patients with food allergy. Gastric involvement is noted in both mild (single food allergen) and severe forms of allergic gastroenteritis.

The mucosal lesions generally are more pronounced in the antrum than in the corpus or fundus of the stomach. Milder lesions are typically seen in patients with disease attributable to a single allergy such as cow's milk protein, and consist of the presence of numerous eosinophils in the lamina propria and focal extension of the eosinophils into the surface and glandular epithelium (Fig. 12.5). Occasionally, the lesions are patchy, perhaps reflecting a mild insult or partial treatment, and examination of multiple samples of the antrum may be required. More often, and especially in the severe cases of allergic gastroenteritis, the gastric lesions are florid and reveal a diffuse and significant infiltrate of eosinophils, which may form aggregates and extend into the regions of the muscularis mucosae and upper submucosa (Figs. 12.6 and 12.7). An associated finding is greater destruction of the surface and glandular epithelium with the presence of clusters of eosinophils within the lumina of the gastric foveolae (pits). Exceptionally, there is significant mucosal edema and surface erosions (Fig. 12.8), which can be visualized by using endoscopic and radiographic examinations (51). Small foci of intestinal metaplasia have been observed in chronic cases, but atrophic gastritis ordinarily does not develop.

Lesions of the corpus and fundic mucosa tend to be more focal and milder in appearance, consisting of only a small number of eosinophils in the lamina propria and rare extension of the eosinophils into the epithelial layer; the corpus mucosa is typically normal in milder cases involving a single food allergen. Only a rare

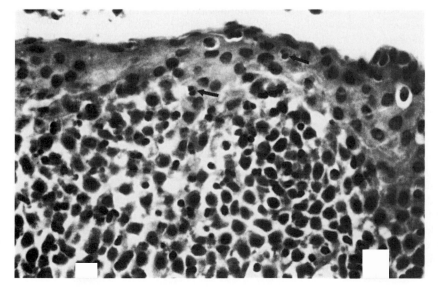

Figure 12.4 Esophageal mucosa in allergic gastroenteritis. Note significant basal zone hyperplasia of the squamous epithelium, as well as many eosinophils within the epithelial layer (*arrows*). H & E, ×400.

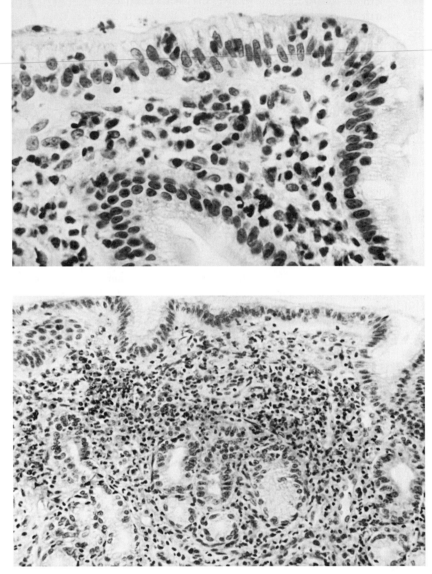

Figure 12.5 Gastric antral mucosa in allergic gastroenteritis. Numerous eosinophils are present in the lamina propria, and there is focal extension into the surface epithelial layer *(top right)*. H & E, ×400.

Figure 12.6 Gastric antral mucosa in allergic gastroenteritis. An extensive infiltrate of eosinophils is associated with damage of the gastric glands. H & E, ×100.

eosinophil is noted in the lamina propria of the normal gastric mucosa, and the cells do not penetrate the epithelial layer.

An additional advantage of looking for evidence of allergic disease in the gastric antrum is that few disorders due to other causes have a similar histologic appearance. Thus, although a prominent eosinophilic infiltrate can be seen in the gastric mucosa in some cases of parasitic infections, vasculitis, Crohn disease, amyloidosis, and occasional tumors, these disorders can be distinguished readily by finding other, more specific features. Patients in whom gastritis is related to more common etiologic elements, specifically alcohol, medications, and bile reflux, lack an inflammatory reaction, and histologic analysis in cases attributable to H. pylori reveal many neutrophils and mononuclear cell types without a prominence of eosinophils. Occasional cases of any gastritis and the mucosa adjacent to a chronic peptic ulcer may reveal scattered clusters of eosinophils in the lamina propria, causing particular concern in a mucosal biopsy sample; in such cases, however, the eosinophils rarely extend into the epithelium and glandular lumina.

Enlarged gastric folds can be observed in both adults and

children with Menetrier disease (71), but these folds are invariably confined to the proximal stomach in contrast to the antral localization in allergic disease. As described previously (see the section concerning eosinophilic gastroenteritis), the mural form commonly affects the gastric antrum. This disorder, however, is characterized by an inflammatory mass that is concentrated in the wall of the stomach, with at most a focal ulceration of the overlying mucosa. In contrast to allergic disease, there is no diffuse injury of the gastric mucosa or signs of damage to other parts of the gut mucosa; these patients demonstrate no elevation of the serum IgE level or other signs of allergy.

SMALL INTESTINE

Lesions are commonly noted in the small intestinal mucosa in patients with either mild (single food allergen) or severe allergic gastroenteritis (12–15, 31, 32). The lesions are noted most often in the duodenum and jejunum and least often in the ileum, but this distribution may reflect in part the access by endoscopy and selective biopsy of the more proximal portion of the small bowel. The allergic lesions in the small intestine are most often focal, even in severe cases involving multiple antigens, and numerous biopsy samples are usually required for their detection (13).

Characteristic findings include partial blunting of the villi, a focal infiltrate of eosinophils in the lamina propria of the villous cores, and extension of a few eosinophils into the surface epithelial layer (Fig. 12.9). In addition, the number of lymphocytes in the surface layer may be increased, and the epithelium often shows evidence of damage in the form of a less well-formed brush border, corresponding to a shortening and diminution of the microvilli, and the presence of numerous small lipid vacuoles in the cytoplasm (53). The lipid nature of these vacuoles is ordinarily inferred by the lack of reaction with various mucin stains, but electron microscopic studies have substantiated this finding.

These milder lesions usually exhibit only slight crypt hyperplasia and no great increase of other inflammatory cells in the lamina propria. More advanced lesions are observed in about 10% of the cases and reveal greater shortening or complete loss of the villi together with more pronounced damage of the surface epithelium, crypt hyperplasia, and mononuclear inflammatory cells in the lamina propria and surface epithelial layer (Figs. 12.10 and 12.11). The amount of eosinophils in these advanced lesions is variable, ranging from just a few small clusters to a diffuse infiltrate.

Trying to establish allergic disease in the small intestine is problematic. A small number of eosinophils is normally present in the lamina propria, both between the crypts and in the villous cores (53, 54). In the absence of quantitative measurements, which ordinarily are not performed (55, 72), only the presence of a considerable increase of eosinophils with the formation of large clusters or aggregates and their extension into the epithelial layer together with signs of epithelial damage can be considered evidence of an active enteritis that may be associated with allergic disease. Furthermore, the number of eosinophils in an allergic lesion is highly variable, and some patients, including those with marked villous shortening, do not demonstrate a conspicuous eosinophilic

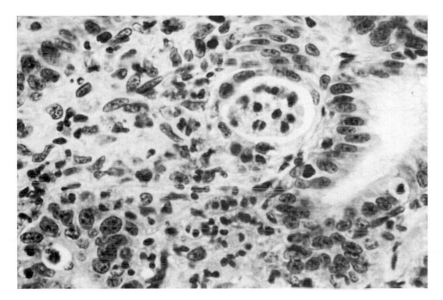

Figure 12.7 Gastric antral mucosa in allergic gastroenteritis. Note the damaged gastric pit with numerous eosinophils within its lumen. H & E, ×400. (Reprinted with permission from Goldman H, Antonioli DA. Mucosal biopsy of the esophagus, stomach, and proximal duodenum. Hum Pathol 1982;13:423–448.)

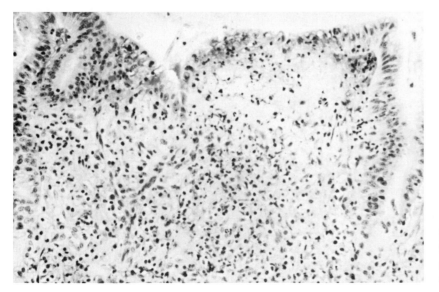

Figure 12.8 Gastric antral mucosa in allergic gastroenteritis. Extensive destruction of the glands, edema, and superficial erosion can result in grossly enlarged folds. H & E, ×60.

infiltrate. This variability in the number of eosinophils is a special problem in the evaluation of the relatively small mucosal biopsy specimens. Finally, even in the presence of significant tissue eosinophilia, the histologic findings are not specific because an equivalent increase in eosinophils can be seen in many other conditions affecting the small bowel mucosa. Accordingly, the diagnosis of allergic disease affecting the small intestine must always be made in accord with compatible clinical and laboratory features. As described previously, it may prove useful to add examination of the gastric antrum and, perhaps, the esophageal mucosa in such cases, because the differential diagnosis is more limited in these areas.

In patients with allergic disease of the small intestine resulting in malabsorption or a protein-losing enteropathy, the principal differential diagnoses are celiac disease (gluten enteropathy), prolonged infections, and a variety of immunologic disorders (see Chapter 31). The stool and biopsy samples should be examined for evidence of a protozoan or helminthic infection, and toxic reactions to ingested chemicals and drugs should be excluded. In celiac disease and in tropical sprue, the lesions are always diffuse, and observation of a focal lesion in a mucosal biopsy specimen can exclude these disease processes. Conversely, occasional cases of allergic disease are associated with diffuse lesions with variable quantities of eosinophils, and the distinction from celiac disease may require a trial of a gluten-free diet. Crohn disease may also show an increase of mucosal eosinophils, but usually as an accompaniment to signs of more extensive damage with ulcerations, sinuses, and strictures, as well as occasional granulomas. In addition, pathologic changes in Crohn disease are most often concentrated in the distal ileum and colon. Patients with vascular-connective tissue disorders, such as lupus erythematosus and polyarteritis nodosum, may disclose an increase in eosinophils that is typically located as an inflammatory band just above the muscularis mucosae (65). Exceptionally, cases of allergic disease of the small bowel develop superficial ulcerations (52) simulating refractory sprue or an occult lymphoma, and an operative biopsy may be required for the distinction.

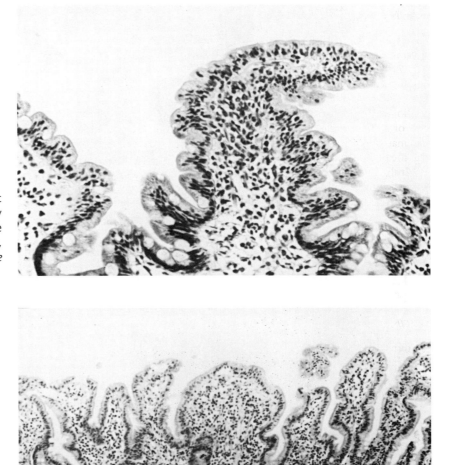

Figure 12.9 Small intestinal mucosa in allergic gastroenteritis. A mild lesion is characterized by focal and partial shortening of the villi. A large cluster of eosinophils is noted in the lamina propria, with focal extension into the epithelial layer *(left side of villus)*. H & E, ×400.

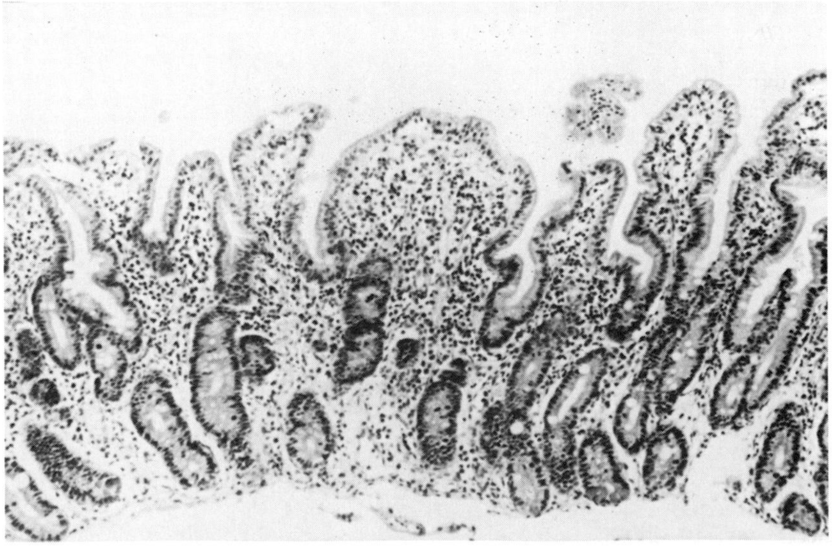

Figure 12.10 Small intestinal mucosa in allergic gastroenteritis. Note more diffuse and significant shortening of the villi and crypt hyperplasia. H & E, ×100.

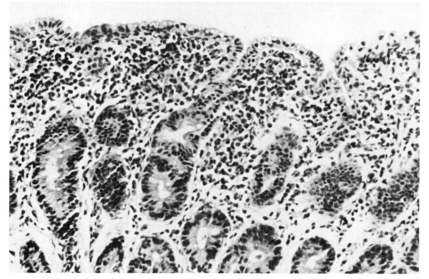

Figure 12.11 Small intestinal mucosa in allergic gastroenteritis. Complete loss of villi and flattening and degeneration of the surface epithelium simulates the appearance of active celiac disease (gluten enteropathy). H & E, ×250.

COLON AND RECTUM

The large bowel shows the least amount of involvement in generalized allergic gastroenteritis, whether due to a single or to multiple antigens. The lesions are typically minor, consisting of patchy infiltrates of eosinophils in the lamina propria and only rare damage of the surface and crypt epithelium. Patients usually experience no functional disturbances that can be directly related to the involvement of the colonic mucosa, and both endoscopic and radiographic examinations of the large intestine are typically normal in patients with the diffuse form of allergic gastroenteritis (2).

It should be stressed, however, that both the rectum and colon can be involved with food sensitivity, but such cases are usually limited to this region and are not associated with disease affecting the upper part of the gastrointestinal tract. These cases are described in the following section.

ALLERGIC PROCTITIS AND COLITIS

DEFINITIONS

The terms "allergic proctitis" and "allergic colitis" are applied for those cases in which the lesions are predominantly confined or limited to the large intestine. The majority of patients are infants and young children; only isolated reports describe disease involving the colon, alone or in conjunction with ileitis, in adults.

CHILDHOOD CASES

CLINICAL AND LABORATORY FEATURES

Isolated food allergy affecting the rectum and colon is probably the leading cause of colitis in infants (1). Most cases are attributable to cow's milk protein (7, 8, 10, 73, 74), alone or together with soy protein (9, 10, 75), and patients respond promptly to an elimination of these foods from the diet. Although rechallenge studies have been recommended (5), they ordinarily are not performed because of the clear association with the offending foods and the ready availability

of alternative formulas (6, 46, 47). Most patients lose the particular food sensitivity after several years and appear to be able to ingest the substance without problems as adults.

The disorder, which appears to be more common in males than in females, manifests in all patients before the age of 2 years and in most in the first 6 months of life (1). In a personal series of 15 childhood cases (2), the average age at onset was 5 months and the median age was 2 months. Most patients have overt rectal bleeding, alone or together with diarrhea. Other symptoms including vomiting, abdominal pain, and weight loss are uncommon, and only a rare patient or family member reveals allergic symptoms referable to other organ systems. The blood eosinophil count is usually elevated to levels of 10 to 20%, but the serum IgE level shows only a mild increase and RAST tests are typically negative. Anemia is also uncommon, and it is probable that the low frequency of general symptoms and of abnormal laboratory tests is related to the very young age of the patients. Compared to persons with allergic gastroenteritis, patients with allergic proctitis and colitis are generally younger, present with more rectal bleeding and diarrhea, and have a lesser incidence of other symptoms and altered laboratory results. Also, cases of allergic colitis more often are associated with a single antigen and, therefore, affected patients fare better.

PATHOLOGIC FEATURES

Most of the information about allergic proctocolitis has been obtained by examination of rectal mucosal biopsies, but findings of limited studies suggest equivalent involvement in the colonic mucosa (1, 2, 10, 75). The exact distribution of the disease, whether patchy or diffuse and whether concentrated in the left portion or more universally, however, is not known. The abnormal findings are generally similar in the rectal and colonic mucosa and consist mainly of a diffuse increase of eosinophils in the lamina propria and very focal damage of the surface epithelium and crypts (Fig. 12.12) (76). The area of epithelial injury is usually very small and may be limited to one or two crypts in a biopsy sample, emphasizing the need to examine multiple levels of such specimens. The injured epithelium is associated with an almost pure eosinophilic reaction, with eosinophils noted in the epithelial layer and rarely in the crypt

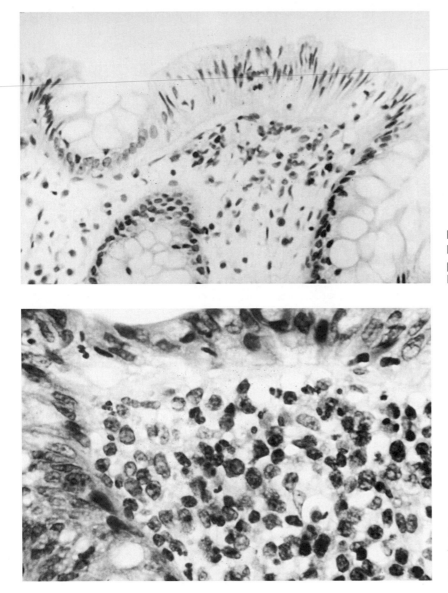

Figure 12.12   Rectal mucosa in allergic proctitis. Note the cluster of eosinophils in the upper lamina propria with extension into the surface epithelium. H & E, ×400.

Figure 12.13   Rectal mucosa in allergic proctitis. An infiltrate of eosinophils is evident in the lamina propria, with extension into the crypt *(left)* and surface *(top)* epithelium. H & E, ×400.

lumina (Fig. 12.13). More advanced cases are less often detected and show an even greater increase of eosinophils, which may extend into the region of the muscularis mucosae and upper submucosa, and more necrosis with a neutrophilic reaction. The overall mucosal architecture remains normal, and signs of a chronic colitis (77) are not seen. The underlying bowel wall is not involved. Because the mucosal lesions in the colon and rectum are generally mild, there are usually no gross abnormalities and radiographic studies typically are normal. Endoscopic examination also usually yields normal findings or may reveal scattered petechiae or a rare erosion.

Exceptionally, mucosal biopsies of the small intestine show a minor abnormality, which is not clinically significant. Usually no alterations in the mucosa of the proximal gut are present in cases of allergic proctitis or colitis.

DIAGNOSIS AND DIFFERENTIAL DIAGNOSIS

Similar to the small intestine (see previous section concerning allergic gastroenteritis), it may be difficult to evaluate the finding of

eosinophils in the colonic mucosa because a variable number are present in the normal lamina propria (55, 78, 79). One study revealed a 40-fold difference in the number of eosinophils noted within the lamina propria of normal persons, comparing biopsy results from several regions of the United States (80), with a greater number seen in southern cities. Also, it is possible to encounter an occasional eosinophil in the surface epithelium of the colonic mucosa in an otherwise normal person. In a comparative evaluation of the results of rectal biopsy in children with allergic proctitis, children with infections, and normal subjects, the finding of greater than 60 eosinophils per 10 high power fields and infiltration of the muscularis mucosae by eosinophils were the two features that best correlated with patients with allergic proctitis and colitis (81). The penetration of eosinophils into the surface and crypt epithelium can be seen in infections and in other colitides, but this feature is usually more prominent, and other inflammatory cells such as neutrophils are lacking in most cases of allergic proctitis or colitis. As with allergic disease in other parts of the gut, the diagnosis of allergic proctitis requires finding compatible clinical and biopsy features and the exclusion of other causes of colitis, notably infections. It is not sufficient to relate the onset of disease to the introduction of a new food to the patient, because this timing may be merely coincidental. The diagnosis ordinarily is confirmed by noting the clinical resolution after withdrawal of the offending food.

The principal differential diagnoses in these young patients with allergic proctitis are infections and the obstructive type of colitis that can occur in association with aganglionic megacolon. Colonic infections are often associated with more diffuse lesions and a greater neutrophilic reaction, which may be evident in the dysenteric stool; eosinophils are rarely a dominant feature. Nevertheless, it is prudent to exclude an infectious cause of proctitis or colitis by appropriate stool examination before making a diagnosis of allergic disease. The colitis that may complicate aganglionosis usually reveals relatively bland hemorrhagic necrosis without prominent tissue eosinophilia, and the primary diagnosis is secured by noting the absence of submucosal ganglia in the constricted portion.

An increase in mucosal eosinophils is commonly noted in patients with chronic ulcerative colitis and Crohn disease of the colon (61), but also present are other features of chronic colitis, such as irregular crypt architecture, with budding and atrophy, and Paneth cell metaplasia (77, 78). Furthermore, the idiopathic inflammatory bowel diseases are rare in patients younger than age 5 years. Other conditions that can affect the colonic mucosa and be associated with tissue eosinophils include some of the vasculitides and chronic granulomatous disease (64), which are distinguished by the finding of more specific features. Patients with necrotizing enterocolitis typically are much sicker and often reveal signs of obstruction or peritonitis.

ADULT CASES

Allergic disease related to food sensitivity that is limited to the colon or to the colon and ileum is rare in adults.

ULCERATIVE PROCTITIS AND COLITIS

In a subset of patients originally thought to have idiopathic ulcerative colitis, studies revealed an increased number of IgE-producing plasma cells and mast cells in the mucosa (19). The lesions were concentrated in the rectum, and the patients responded selectively to antiallergic medications with a reduction in symptoms and the number of mucosal inflammatory cells. Similar prolifera-

tions of IgE-bearing cells have been noted in other cases of proctitis and colitis (20, 21), but the provocative antigens are not known, and no long-term follow-up studies have been performed. It is not evident whether or not the allergic lesions are primary and whether the antigens are foods or other substances.

ISOLATED CASES

Isolated reports describe presumed allergic disease in adolescents and adults that seems to be confined to the colon (82, 83) or to the ileum and colon (84–86). Some cases appear to involve the mural form of eosinophilic gastroenteritis (see previous section), which can affect and be limited to the intestines, and such cases must be sorted out because they do not have an allergic etiology. Those patients in whom allergy is an etiologic factor present with abdominal pain and diarrhea, which may be bloody, and the peripheral eosinophil count is elevated. Enlarged folds and an inflamed mucosal surface are demonstrated by radiographic and endoscopic examination, and mucosal biopsy specimens typically show mucosal damage with an intense eosinophilic reaction; more than 60 eosinophils per single high-power field have been noted (83, 86). The gross lesions usually are segmental, but no extensive biopsy studies have been conducted to determine whether the cases can have more diffuse disease. Although the particular food allergen is usually not known, the patients typically respond to antiallergic therapy with complete recovery.

As described previously, many other causes of enteritis and colitis can have a prominent eosinophilic infiltrate in the mucosa, and these factors must be excluded before a diagnosis of allergic disease can be entertained. Considering the age of the patient and the apparent segmental distribution of the lesions, the principal differential diagnoses are Crohn disease, parasitic infections, and an occult lymphoma in the underlying wall of the intestine. Other common disorders that may manifest with segmental lesions of the colon include ischemic colitis and diverticular disease, but these diseases are not associated with a prominent eosinophilic reaction.

MUCOSAL BIOPSY

The general techniques and uses of endoscopy and endoscopic biopsy are described in Chapter 3. These procedures are invariably performed in cases of gastrointestinal food allergy to assist in the process of diagnosis and to monitor the course following therapy

TABLE 12.5 | Biopsy of Allergic Gastroenteritis in Children

Tissue	Cases Biopsied (%)	Positive Biopsies (%)	Marked Aleration (%)
Esophagus	39	60	53
Gastric corpus	55	52	10
Gastric antrum	58	100	73
Small intestine	89	79	12
Rectum	21	13	0

Modified from Goldman H, Proujansky R. Allergic proctitis and allergic gastroenteritis in children: Clinical and mucosal biopsy features in 53 cases. Am J Surg Pathol 1986; 10:75–86.

(53, 54, 78). The allergic lesions are essentially confined to the mucosa, but they often are focal, creating the need for multiple samples and the examination of several levels of a biopsy specimen.

The biopsy results in a series of 38 cases of allergic gastroenteritis in children are summarized in Table 12.5 (2). Although biopsy of the small intestine, including the duodenum and proximal jejunum, is performed most commonly, the lesions usually are focal and of a mild degree. In contrast, disease of the gastric antrum can be documented in a higher percentage of cases, even with only a single biopsy, and the lesions tend to be more florid. Considering also that the differential diagnosis of an eosinophilic infiltrate appears to be more limited in the stomach, it would seem that an antral biopsy should be the procedure of choice when trying to establish whether a patient has an allergic disorder. It is important that the antral mucosa be selectively sampled, because lesions in the gastric corpus or fundus are usually sparse.

Allergic disease of the esophagus is more common than formerly thought. The features observed in esophageal mucosal biopsy samples are similar to those seen in association with the more prevalent disorder of reflux esophagitis, resulting in the need to use other tests such as pH probe or manometric studies to distinguish the two conditions in uncertain cases. Of help, the blood eosinophil count is normal in patients with reflux esophagitis and is elevated in most patients with allergic gastroenteritis.

In allergic gastroenteritis, rectal and colonic involvement is uncommon in the absence of lesions in the proximal part of the gut, and it is unlikely that biopsy samples of the large bowel need be obtained in affected patients. Conversely, the colon and rectum are preferentially involved in allergic proctitis, and biopsy of this area yields abnormal findings in patients that present with rectal bleeding or prominent diarrhea, especially in infants.

REFERENCES

1. Jenkins HR, Pincott JR, Soothill JF, et al. Food allergy: The major cause of infantile colitis. Arch Dis Child 1984;59:326–329.
2. Goldman H, Proujansky R. Allergic proctitis and allergic gastroenteritis in children: Clinical and mucosal biopsy features in 53 cases. Am J Surg Pathol 1986;10:75–86.
3. Cello JP. Eosinophilic gastroenteritis—A complex disease entity. Am J Med 1979;87:1097–1104.
4. Lee C-M, Changchien C-S, Chen P-C, et al. Eosinophilic gastroenteritis: 10 years experience. Am J Gastroenterol 1993;88:70–74.
5. Goldman AS, Anderson Jr DW, Sellers WA, et al. Milk allergy. I. Oral challenge with milk and isolated milk proteins in allergic children. Pediatrics 1963;32:425–443.
6. Sumithran E, Iyngkaran N. Is jejunal biopsy really necessary in cow's milk protein intolerance? Lancet 1972;2:1122–1123.
7. Grybowski JD. Gastrointestinal milk allergy in infants. Pediatrics 1967;40:354–360.
8. Shiner M, Ballard J, Brook CGD, et al. Intestinal biopsy in the diagnosis of cow's milk protein intolerance without acute symptoms. Lancet 1975;2:1060–1063.
9. Ament M, Rubin CE. Soy protein—Another cause of the flat intestinal lesion. Gastroenterology 1972;62:227–234.
10. Halpin RC, Byrne WJ, Ament ME. Colitis, persistent diarrhea and soy protein intolerance. J Pediatr 1977;91:404–410.
11. Eastham EJ, Walker WA. Adverse effects of milk formula ingestion on the gastrointestinal tract. An update. Gastroenterology 1979;70:364–374.
12. Klein NC, Hargrove RL, Sleisenger MH, et al. Eosinophilic gastroenteritis. Medicine 1970;49:299–319.
13. Leinbach GE, Rubin CE. Eosinophilic gastroenteritis: A simple reaction to food allergens? Gastroenterology 1970;59:874–889.
14. Jacobson LB. Diffuse eosinophilic gastroenteritis: An adult form of allergic gastroenteropathy. Report of a case with probable protein-losing enteropathy. Am J Gastrenterol 1970;54:580–588.
15. Waldmann TA, Wochner RD, Laster L, et al. Allergic gastroenteropathy. N Engl J Med 1967;276:761–769.
16. Stern M, Walker WA. Food allergy and intolerance. Pediatr Clin North Am 1985;32:471–492.
17. Shiner M, Ballard J, Smith ME. The small intestinal mucosa in cow's milk allergy. Lancet 1975;1:136–140.
18. Rosekrans PC, Meijer CG, van der Wal AM, et al. Use of morphometry and immunohistochemistry of small intestinal biopsy specimens in the diagnosis of food allergy. J Clin Pathol 1980;33:125–130.
19. Rosekrans PC, Meijer CG, van der Wal AM, et al. Allergic proctitis: A clinical and immunopathological entity. Gut 1980;21:1017–1023.
20. Heatley RV, Calcroft BJ, Fifield R, et al. Immunoglobin E in rectal mucosa of patients with proctitis. Lancet 1975;2:1010–1012.
21. Murdock DL, Piris J. Immunoglobulin E in non-specific proctitis and ulcerative colitis. Studies with a monoclonal antibody. Digestion 1983;25:201–204.
22. Ogawa H, Kunkel SL, Fantone JC, et al. Comparative study of eosinophil and neutrophil chemotaxis and enzyme release. Am J Pathol 1981;105:149–155.
23. Uden AM, Palmblad J, Lindgren JA, et al. Effects of novel lipoxygenase products on migration of eosinophils and neutrophils in vitro. Int Arch Allergy Immunol 1983;72:91–93.
24. Weller PF, Dvorak JA, Whitehouse WC. Human eosinophil stimulation promoter lymphokine: Production by antigen stimulated lymphocytes and assay with a new electro-optical technique. Cell Immunol 1978;40:91–102.
25. Hirashima M, Tashiro K, Skata K, et al. Isolation of an eosinophil chemotactic lymphokine as a natural mediator for eosinophil chemotaxis from concanavalin A-induced skin reaction sites in guinea-pigs. Clin Exp Immunol 1984;57:211–219.
26. Gleich GH, Frigas E, Leogering DA, et al. Cytologic properties of the eosinophil major basic protein. J Immunol 1979;123:2925–2927.
27. Dvorak AM. Ultrastructural evidence for release of major basic protein-containing crystalline cores of eosinophil granules in vivo: Cytotoxic potential in Crohn's disease. J Immunol 1980;125:460–462.
28. Weller PF, Lee, CW, Foster DW, et al. Generation and metabolism of 5-lipoxygenase pathway leukotrienes by human eosinophils: Predominant production of leukotriene C4. Proc Natl Acad Sci USA 1983;80:7626–7630.
29. Keshavarzian A, Saverymuttu SH, Tai P-C, et al. Activated eosinophils in familial eosinophilic gastroenteritis. Gastroenterology 1985;88:1041–1049.
30. Talley NJ, Shorter RG, Zinsmeister AR. Eosinophilic gastroenteritis: A clinicopathological study of patients with disease of the mucosa, muscle layer, and subserosal tissues. Gut 1990;31:54–58.
31. Greenberger NJ, Tennenbaum L, Ruppert RD. Protein-losing enteropathy associated with gastrointestinal allergy. Am J Med 1967;43:777–784.
32. Kuitunen P, Visakorpi JK, Savilahti E, et al. Malabsorption syndrome with cow's milk intolerance. Arch Dis Child 1975;50:351–356.
33. Ureles AL, Alschibaja T, Lodico D, et al. Idiopathic eosinophilic infiltration of the gastrointestinal tract, diffuse and circumscribed. A proposed classification and review of the literature, with two additional cases. Am J Med 1961;30:899–908.
34. Jona JZ, Belin RP, Burke JA. Eosinophilic infiltration of the gastrointestinal tract in children. Am J Dis Child 1976;130:1136–1139.
35. Johnstone JM, Morson BC. Eosinophilic gastroenteritis. Histopathology 1978;2:335–348.
36. Caldwell JH, Mekhjian HS, Hurtubise PE, et al. Eosinophilic gastroenteritis with obstruction. Immunological studies of seven patients. Gastroenterology 1978;74:825–829.
37. Russell JY, Evangelow G. Eosinophilic infiltration of the stomach and duodenum complicated by perforation. Postgrad Med J 1965;41:30–33.
38. Felt-Bersma RJ, Neuwissen SG, van Velzen D. Perforation of the small intestine due to eosinophilic gastroenteritis. Am J Gastroenterol 1984;79:442–445.
39. Lysey J, Eid A. Eosinophilic gastroenteritis with small bowel perforation. J Clin Gastroenterol 1986;8:694–695.

40. Higgins GA, Lamm ER, Yutzy LV. Eosinophilic gastroenteritis. Arch Surg 1966;92:476–483.

41. Scolapio JS, DeVault K, Wolfe JT. Eosinophilic gastroenteritis presenting as a giant gastric ulcer. Am J Gastroenterol 1996;91:804–805.

42. Levinson JD, Romanathan VR, Nozick JH. Eosinophilic gastroenteritis with ascites and colon involvement. Am J Gastroenterol 1977;68:603–607.

43. Katz AJ, Goldman H, Flores AF, et al. Esophageal involvement in allergic (eosinophilic) gastroenteritis (abstract). Gastroenterology 1985;88:1438.

44. Kelly KJ, Lazenby AJ, Rowe PC, et al. Eosinophilic esophagitis attributed to gastroesophageal reflux: Improvement with an amino acid-based formula. Gastroenterology 1995;109:1503–1512.

45. Snyder JD, Rosenblum N, Wershil B, et al. Pyloric stenosis and eosinophilic gastroenteritis in infants. J Pediatr Gastroenterol Nutr 1987;6:543–547.

46. Zeiger RS, Heller S, Mellon M, et al. Effectiveness of dietary manipulation in the prevention of food allergy in infants. J Allergy Clin Immunol 1986;78:224–238.

47. Sogn D. Medications and their use in the treatment of adverse reactions to foods. J Allergy Clin Immunol 1986;78:238–243.

48. Katz AJ, Twaroq FJ, Zeiger RS, et al. Milk-sensitive and eosinophilic gastroenteropathy: Similar clinical features with contrasting mechanisms and clinical course. J Allergy Clin Immunol 1984;74:72–78.

49. Matsushita M, Hajiro K, Morita Y, et al. Eosinophilic gastroenteritis involving the entire digestive tract. Am J Gastroenterol 1995;90:1868–1870.

50. Katz AJ, Goldman H, Grand RJ. Gastric mucosal biopsy in eosinophilic (allergic) gastroenteritis. Gastroenterology 1977;73:705–709.

51. Teele RL, Katz AJ, Goldman H, et al. The radiographic features of eosinophilic gastroenteritis (allergic gastroenteropathy) of childhood. Am J Radiol 1979;132:575–580.

52. Lucak BK, Sansaricq C, Snyderman SE, et al. Disseminated ulcerations in allergic eosinophilic gastroenterocolitis. Am J Gastroenterol 1978;77:248–252.

53. Perera DR, Weinstein WM, Rubin CE. Small intestinal biopsy. Hum Pathol 1975;6:157–217.

54. Goldman H, Antonioli DA. Mucosal biopsy of the esophagus, stomach, and proximal duodenum. Hum Pathol 1982;13:423–448.

55. Lowichik A, Weinberg AG. A quantitative evaluation of mucosal eosinophils in the pediatric gastrointestinal tract. Mod Pathol 1996;9:110–114.

56. Winter HS, Madara JL, Stafford, RJ, et al. Intraepithelial eosinophils: A new diagnostic criterion for reflux esophagitis. Gastroenterology 1982;83:818–823.

57. Brown LF, Goldman H, Antonioli DA. Intraepithelial eosinophils in endoscopic biopsies of adults with reflux esophagitis. Am J Surg Pathol 1984;8:899–905.

58. Lee RG. Marked eosinophila in esophageal mucosal biopsies. Am J Surg Pathol 1986;9:475–479.

59. Martin DM, Goldman JA, Gilliam J, et al. Gold-induced eosinophilic enterocolitis: Response to oral cromolyn sodium. Gastroenterology 1981;80:1567–1570.

60. Walker NI, Croese J, Clouston AD, et al. Eosinophilic enteritis in northeastern Australia. Pathology, association with Ancylostoma caninum, and implications. Am J Surg Pathol 1995;19:328–337.

61. Heatley RV, James PD. Eosinophils in rectal mucosa. Gut 1978;20:787–791.

62. Saul SH. The watery diarrhea-colitis syndrome. A review of collagenous and microscopic/lymphocytic colitis. Int J Surg Pathol 1993;1:65–82.

63. Jawhari A, Talbot IC. Microscopic, lymphocytic and collagenous colitis. Histopathology 1996;29:101–110.

64. Ament ME, Ochs HD. Gastrointestinal manifestations of chronic granulomatous disease. N Engl J Med 1973;288:382–387.

65. DeSchryver-Kecskemeti K, Clouse RE. A previously unrecognized subgroup of "eosinophic gastroenteritis." Association with connective tissue diseases. Am J Surg Pathol 1984;8:171–180.

66. Dobbins JW, Sheahan DG, Behar J. Eosinophilic gastroenteritis with esophageal involvement. Gastroenterology 1977;72:1312–1316.

67. Picus D, Frank PH. Eosinophilic esophagitis. AJR Am J Roentgenol 1981;136:1001–1003.

68. Matzenger MA, Daneman A. Esophageal involvement in eosinophilic gastroenteritis. Pediatr Radiol 1983;13:35–38.

69. Weinstein WM, Bogoch ER, Bowes KL. The normal esophageal mucosa. A histologic reappraisal. Gastroenterology 1975;68:40–44.

70. Reimann H-J, Lewin J. Gastric mucosal reactions in patients with food allergy. Am J Gastroenterol 1988;83:1212–1219.

71. Baker A, Volberg F, Summer T, et al. Childhood Menetrier's disease: Four new cases and discussion of the literature. Gastrointest Radiol 1986;11:131–134.

72. Peckkio M, Savilahti E, Kuitunen P. Morphometric and immunohistochemical study of jejunal biopsies from children with intestinal soy allergy. Fin Eur J Pediatr 1981;137:63–69.

73. Wilson JF, Lahey ME, Heiner DC. Studies on iron metabolism. V. Further observations on cow's milk-induced gastrointestinal bleeding in infants with iron-deficiency anemia. J Pediatr 1974;84:335–344.

74. Walker-Smith JA, Harrison M, Kilby A, et al. Cow's milk-sensitive enteropathy. Arch Dis Child 1978;53:375–380.

75. Powell GK. Milk and soy-induced enterocolitis of infancy. J Pediatr 1978;93:553–561.

76. Odze RD, Bines J, Leichtner AM, et al. Allergic protocolitis in infants: A prospective clinicopathologic biopsy study. Hum Pathol 1993;24:668–674.

77. Surawicz CM, Belic L. Rectal biopsy helps to distinguish acute self-limited colitis from idiopathic inflammatory bowel disease. Gastroenterology 1984;86:104–113.

78. Goldman H, Antonioli DA. Mucosal biopsy of the rectum, colon and distal ileum. Hum Pathol 1982;13:981–1012.

79. Levine DS, Haggitt RC. Normal histology of the colon. Am J Surg Pathol 1989;13:966–984.

80. Pascal RR, Gramlich TL. Geographic variations of eosinophil concentration in normal colonic mucosa. Mod Pathol, In press.

81. Winter HS, Antonioli DA, Fukagawa N, et al. Allergy-related proctocolitis in infants: Diagnostic usefulness of rectal biopsy. Mod Pathol 1990;3:5–10.

82. Naylor AR, Pollett JE. Eosinophilic colitis. Dis Colon Rectum 1985;28:615–618.

83. Moore D, Lichtman S, Lentz J, et al. Eosinophilic gastroenteritis presenting in an adolescent with isolated colonic involvement. Gut 1986;27:1219–1222.

84. Haberkern CM, Christie DL, Haas EE. Eosinophilic gastroenteritis presenting as ileocolitis. Gastroenterology 1978;74:896–899.

85. Schulze K, Mitros FA. Eosinophilic gastroenteritis involving the ileocecal area. Dis Colon Rectum 1979;72:47–50.

86. Tedesco FJ, Huckaby CB, Hamby-Allen M, Ewing GC. Eosinophilic ileocolitis. Dig Dis Sci 1981;26:943–948.

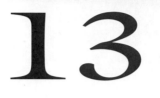

13 MOTOR AND MECHANICAL DISORDERS

Frank A. Mitros

The evaluation of patients with gastrointestinal motility disorders is one of the most frustrating areas of medicine. This frustration is shared by pathologists, gastroenterologists, and surgeons. It must be stated at the outset that, with the exception of Hirschsprung disease, it is unusual for a pathologist using morphologic methods to be able to contribute significantly to the understanding of a motility problem. In a small percentage of cases, the disorder can be successfully categorized as a myopathy or neuropathy. In a somewhat larger number of cases, the pathologic process can be recognized as occurring secondary to some systemic illness. In a distressingly large number of cases, the disorder escapes specific categorization.

Although the study of the gastrointestinal tract has been an area of intense interest to pathologists for many years, that interest, until recently, has been superficial, that is, limited largely to the mucosa. Although the smooth muscle and controlling neural apparatus constitute the bulk of the alimentary tube, these areas are relatively poorly studied, at least with regard to changes in human disease processes. Many of the diseases studied so carefully through the use of mucosal biopsy are caused by underlying neuromuscular dysfunction. Gastroesophageal reflux and its consequences and the small-intestinal mucosal alterations in the stasis syndromes are two examples. As always, the morphologically oriented pathologist

must struggle to gain an appreciation of the normal anatomy to better understand some of the changes seen in the disease process. For this reason, the following section provides a brief overview of normal gastrointestinal tract anatomy, concentrating on peculiarities of various segments.

NORMAL ANATOMY

With the exception of the proximal esophagus, the muscle of the gastrointestinal tract is smooth muscle. The myocytes of the gastrointestinal tract average about 500 to 700 μ in length and 6 μ in thickness; they are capable of as much as a fourfold change in length. The general organization comprises an inner circular layer and an outer longitudinal layer. Although some regional variations occur, the circular layer tends to be the thicker of the two. This fact is not surprising, because the circular layer controls the luminal diameter, and its rhythmic contractions provide the main propulsive force to move luminal contents.

More is understood about the physiology of gastrointestinal motility than about its morphology; these aspects are beyond the province of this chapter. Suffice it to say that myogenic, neural, and hormonal influences must be integrated; the muscle provides the

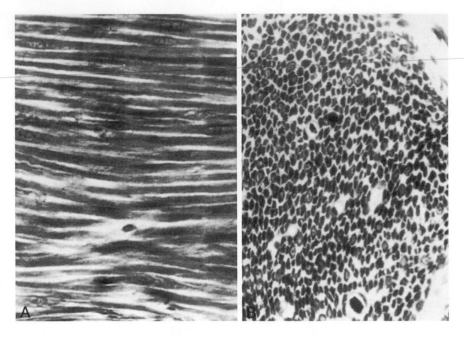

Figure 13.1 Well-oriented longitudinal **(A)** and cross **(B)** sections of the circular muscular layer of jejunum reveal a striking uniformity of the myocytes. Pericellular connective tissue is scant (trichrome, ×132).

major impetus for coordinated movement, and the neural and hormonal influences provide the fine tuning. A striking degree of uniformity in cell size is evident in the normal muscularis propria, and only scant collagen is present around the individual smooth muscle cells. These features are best appreciated in a carefully oriented cross section through the muscle fibers (Fig. 13.1).

The neural control of the gastrointestinal tract is exercised at three levels: the central nervous system, the prevertebral ganglia, and the intrinsic intramural neural structures. The intrinsic intramural neural structures are the most amenable to study by morphologic methods; nevertheless, our knowledge is scanty. The intramural plexuses have two well-known components, the submucosal plexus (Meissner) and the myenteric plexus (Auerbach). The standard histologic section provides only a slitlike window for viewing the wonders of these plexuses (Fig. 13.2).

The techniques pioneered by Barbara Smith (2) and applied to human motility disorders by Schuffler and Jonak (3) provide new insight into these structures. Briefly, frozen sections of formalin-fixed bowel are cut on a sledge microtome in a plane tangential to the serosal surface at 50 μ until the plane of the myenteric plexus is reached. This plane is recognized by the trained eye by the crisscrossing of the muscle fibers of the two layers of the muscularis propria. These sections are then stained with a silver stain by a careful and experienced technologist. Unfortunately, this staining method is difficult to perform. When used successfully, the results are extraordinary (Figs. 13.3 and 13.4). The appearance of the ganglia is radically different from that in standard sections, and the interconnections between the ganglia can begin to be appreciated. Neurons are crudely categorized into argyrophil and argyrophobe, although a good deal more heterogeneity is immediately obvious. The argyrophilic neurons stain darkly because of their large number of neurofilaments; the argyrophilic cells stain a light brown and tend to be indistinct (4). Glial cells are not well visualized. The functional correlates of this variable argyrophilia are not understood. Because of its more diffuse nature, the submucosal plexus is not amenable to such study.

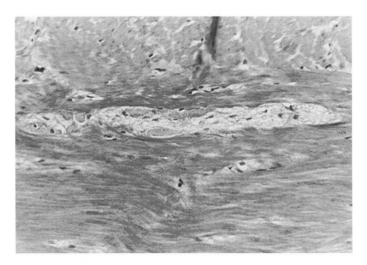

Figure 13.2 The standard view in a longitudinal section of colon provides only a glimpse at the myenteric plexus. Several mature ganglion cells and nerve fibers are visible (H & E, ×66).

The segments of the gastrointestinal tract vary greatly with regard to the structure and presumably the function of the plexuses. Specialized structures, such as thickened bundles of nerve fibers ("shunt fascicles"), are being recognized in human tissues (5). Much experience clearly is needed to understand and interpret these various neural structures in the human disease process. Because the silver techniques are difficult to perform and interpret and are not readily available in most centers, it is uncertain that they will ever play a major role in diagnostic pathology.

Standard immunoperoxidase techniques, particularly those involving use of antibodies against S-100 protein and neuron-specific enolase (NSE), are widely available and are now being used to examine a number of practical problems (6). The neurons can be identified with certainty even in difficult situations, and the nerve bundles are readily apparent (Fig. 13.5). Surprises remain in store for anyone beginning to apply these stains to the neuromuscular structures of the gut. Numerous cells of apparent neural origin occupy a substantial position in the muscular layers (Fig. 13.6). These mysterious structures, which have largely eluded the notice of even the most observant surgical pathologist, are the interstitial cells of Cajal (6–10). The function of these cells is unknown, but they likely play a major role in a number of human diseases.

It is important to examine some of the features of the muscular and neural apparatus that are peculiar to the individual segments of the gastrointestinal tract, because the differences can interfere with interpretation of surgical specimens.

Esophagus

The esophagus contains abundant skeletal muscle, which forms the typical circular and longitudinal layers proximally. The circular layer extends intact somewhat beyond the longitudinal layer into the middle third, where an admixture with smooth muscle occurs. It is not certain that these fibers are strictly under voluntary control; the myenteric plexus is present even in areas composed largely of skeletal muscle. The physiologically distinctive and important lower esophageal sphincter is not readily recognizable morphologically, showing only subtle ultrastructural differences from the surrounding smooth muscle. The muscularis mucosae of the esophagus is extraordinarily thick (200 to 400 µm), which often leads to a startling appearance and some concern in peroral biopsies. As is true of its counterpart in the rest of the gastrointestinal tract, nothing is known of its function. Ganglia tend to be small and are often located outside the plane of the large nerve bundles (parafascicular ganglia). The final peculiarity of the esophagus is the virtual absence of a submucosal neural plexus.

Stomach

The muscularis propria of the stomach is distinctive, in that it contains a third layer, the inner oblique layer, which appears to be in continuity with the lower esophageal sphincter; it diminishes the distal portion of the stomach. The circular layer exists only up to the pylorus, whereas the longitudinal layer is continuous with that of the duodenum. The muscle of the antrum is quite thick. The pyloric sphincter prevents duodenal reflux and acts as a barrier to the distal passage of the large food particles.

Small Intestine

Despite its great physiologic complexity with regard to motility, the structure of the neuromuscular portion of the small intestine is simple and uniform throughout. No obvious specializations of the muscularis propria or neural plexuses are observed on standard hematoxylin and eosin (H & E) sections. The muscularis mucosae does send numerous smooth muscle cells up into the lamina propria of the villi, which alter the villous configuration and surface area. The muscle of the ileocecal valve has a distinctive configuration, and routinely shows some excess collagen encircling individual muscle cells at its free edge (Fig. 13.7).

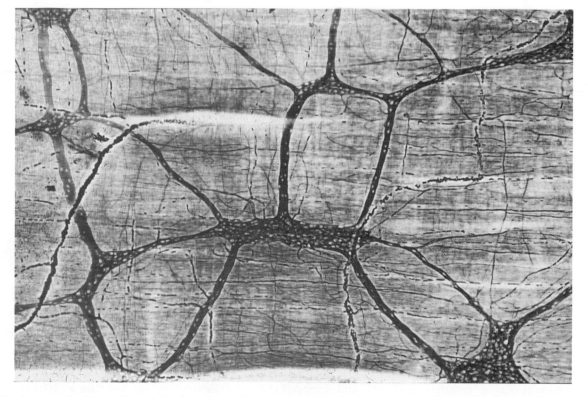

Figure 13.3 Myenteric plexus of normal colon viewed in a 50-µm section in the tangential plane. Note the variability of the ganglia and their complex connections (silver stain, ×16). (See color plate.)

COLON AND APPENDIX

The most obvious specialization in the colon is the formation of three taeniae coli by the longitudinal layer; these taeniae are present from cecum to proximal rectum. They can lead to a deceptive idea about the thickness of the external layer on longitudinal sections. A definite increase in collagen is normally present around myocytes in the taeniae, which can lead to a mistaken impression of fibrosis (Fig. 13.8). Muscle fibers of the longitudinal layer, particularly the taeniae, may pass into the circular layer and fuse with it. The study of the neuromuscular structures of the appendix provides little or no useful information about the nerve or muscle in other sections of the gastrointestinal tract.

ANALYTIC METHODS

Because the smooth muscle cells can change length and thickness greatly and rapidly under physiologic and nonphysiologic conditions (surgical excision, death, formalin fixation), absolute values of length and thickness of the muscularis propria are of little use. To

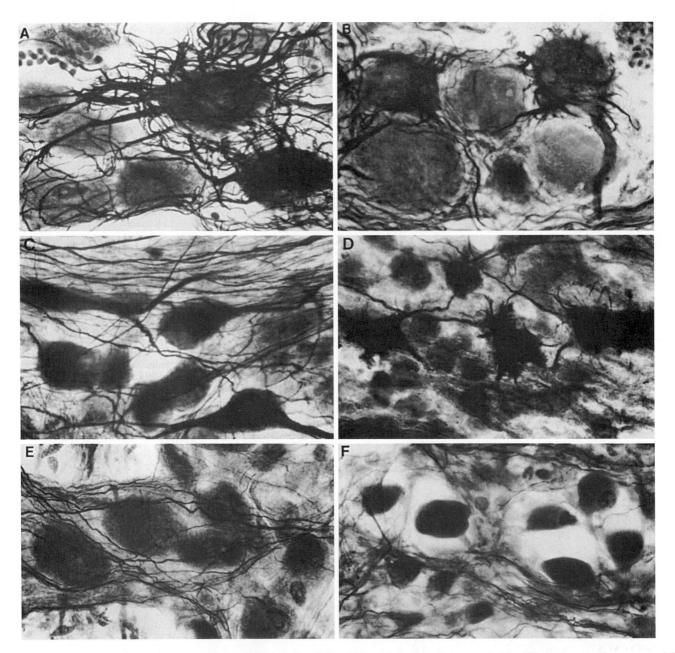

Figure 13.4   The normal esophagus, with complex argyrophilic **(A)** and rounded argyrophobic **(B)** neurons. The argyrophilic neurons of normal jejunum are smaller and less complex **(C)**; the argyrophilic neurons of normal colon are small and irregular in shape **(D)**. The normal argyrophobic neurons of jejunum **(E)** and of colon **(F)** have few visible processes (silver stain, ×1360). (Reprinted with permission from Krishnamurthy S, Schuffler MD. Pathology of neuromuscular disorders of the small intestine and colon. Gastroenterology 1987;93:610.)

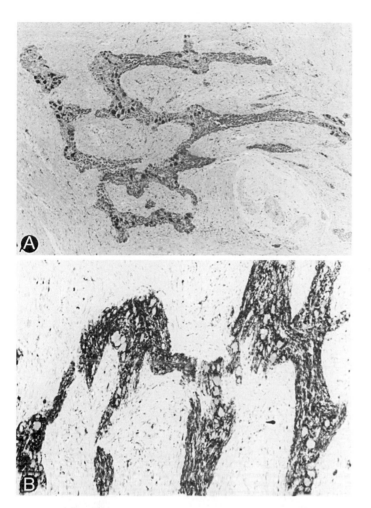

Figure 13.5 **A,** Neurons and nerve fibers are well appreciated in this 6-μm tangential section of normal colon (immunoperoxidase, NSE, ×16). **B,** Nerve fibers interconnecting ganglia in tangential section of normal colon. Immunologic methods are more widely available and less technically demanding than silver stain methods, but experience in their interpretation needs to be gained (immunoperoxidase, S-100, ×25).

examine the neuromuscular apparatus, the segment of gut is opened fresh and pinned out flat on paraffin or corkboard. Both longitudinal and cross sections are taken. In addition, tangential sections (mucosa, submucosa, and mesentery trimmed away) may provide an opportunity for an interesting perspective on the myenteric plexus. Formalin-fixed tissue is saved for potential examination in referral centers with experience in performing and interpreting silver-stained sections of plexus. Standard trichrome techniques are useful in evaluating the integrity of the smooth muscle.

MECHANICAL OBSTRUCTION

The major mechanical problem affecting the gastrointestinal tract is obstruction. Mechanical obstruction implies that a readily definable structural alteration is compromising luminal diameter and hindering passage of intestinal contents. The small intestine and the colon

are the two major segments involved. For the pathologist confronted with a specimen from a patient with intestinal obstruction, the chief tasks are identifying and defining this structural alteration and determining the degree of secondary damage to the involved segment.

CAUSES AND EFFECTS

The causes of obstruction are legion, but historically, the two most common have been hernia and adhesions (see Fig. 13.4). Because hernias are now promptly recognized and repaired, they have

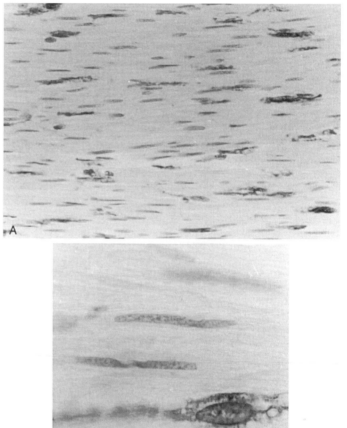

Figure 13.6 **A,** The interstitial cells of Cajal, which stain with both NSE and S-100, occupy a substantial portion of the muscularis propria throughout the gastrointestinal tract (immunoperoxidase, S-100, ×100). **B,** The nuclei of these cells are shorter and more rounded than those of the myocytes. The cytoplasm may be branched, and appears pale and slightly vacuolated on H & E sections (immunoperoxidase, S-100, ×330).

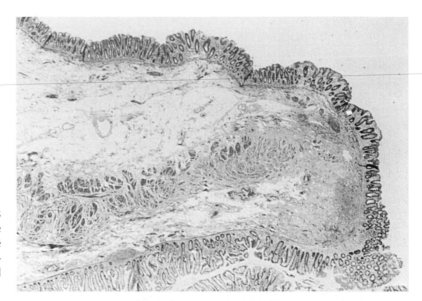

Figure 13.7 Section of normal ileocecal valve reveals ileal mucosa *(bottom)* and colonic mucosa *(top)*. The attenuated muscle fibers at the tip of the ileocecal valve are richly invested by collagen fibers, giving an appearance that can be confused with damage seen in visceral myopathies (trichrome, ×4).

become a less common cause of obstruction. The concomitant increase in abdominal surgery, however, has led to an increased frequency of adhesions as a cause of obstruction (11, 12). Volvulus, intussusception, inflammatory conditions (including diverticulitis), foreign bodies, and congenital malformations are other reasonably common causes of obstruction (12, 13).

Once obstruction occurs, the accumulation of secretions, swallowed food and air, and interference with absorption lead to distention. As noted previously, the structure of the intestine allows for remarkable distensibility. When the pressure within the obstructed loops reaches that in the arterial circulation, strangulation occurs, causing ischemic damage to the bowel and possible bacterial penetration and infection because of loss of structural integrity (13, 14). This pathophysiologic sequence accounts for the clinical manifestations of obstruction, the key symptoms of which are pain, vomiting, and obstipation. The pain tends to be episodic and colicky; when constant, it suggests strangulation and its consequences. The temporal relationship of the onset of vomiting to that of the pain can provide a clue as to the level of obstruction, as can the character of the vomitus. Feculent vomiting implies a lesion in the middle or lower small intestine; the term "feculent" is a misnomer, however, because the character of the dark, foul-smelling material reflects stasis with rapid bacterial overgrowth and decomposition of intestinal contents. Obstipation can be partial or complete, reflecting the character of the obstruction. Distention is the main physical sign. Hyperactive high-pitched peristaltic rushes and metallic tinkling sounds are commonly heard. Absence of peristaltic sounds implies peritoneal irritation.

SPECIAL FORMS OF OBSTRUCTION

Several specific forms of mechanical obstruction deserve further note. Intussusception is a particularly common cause of intestinal obstruction in children. One portion of the gastrointestinal tract (the intussusceptum) invaginates into a more distal segment (the intussuscipiens), and the ischemic compromise that results may necessitate operative intervention (Fig. 13.9). About 80% of childhood intussusceptions are ileoileal (15). The lymphoid tissue in

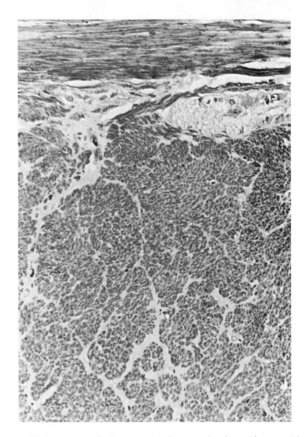

Figure 13.8 Muscularis propria of normal colon. Along with the ileocecal valve, the taeniae coli *(bottom)* physiologically contain abundant collagen, around both individual myocytes and groups of myocytes (trichrome, ×66).

Peyer patches is often prominent (Fig. 13.10). A response to a viral infection has been postulated, but the lymphoid prominence may be merely physiologic.

Intussusception in adults is more ominous. An obvious cause usually is identified, and typically is a tumor mass, which may be malignant (Fig. 13.11). This cause is particularly true with colocolic intussusception, a rare occurrence.

Volvulus results from a twisting of the bowel on itself, which produces a simultaneous closed-loop obstruction and proximal

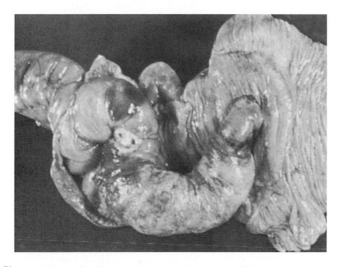

Figure 13.9 Ileoileal intussusception in a child. The intussuscepted bowel *(center)*, seen just proximal to the ileocecal valve, shows evidence of ischemic damage.

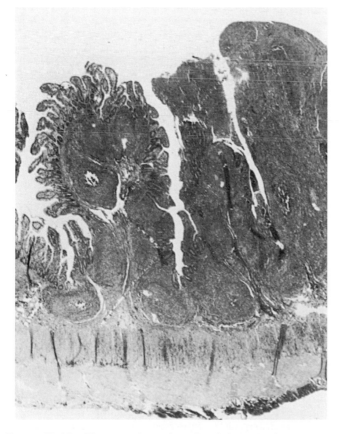

Figure 13.10 The prominent lymphoid tissue in this intussuscepted ileum shows ischemic damage, characterized by mucosal erosion *(right)* and hemorrhage in the wall and serosa (H & E, ×5).

open-loop obstruction (14). Characteristically, the degree of distention is enormous. Because this phenomenon requires a long mesenteric attachment, its sites of occurrence are predictable. Areas of predilection, roughly in order of descending frequency, include sigmoid, cecum, small bowel (all or a portion thereof), stomach, and (rarely) transverse colon. Sudden onset of pain and rapid distention are characteristic signs (14).

Intraluminal mechanical obstruction may result from gallstone impaction. So-called gallstone ileus is thought to result from bouts of cholecystitis with formation of a cholecystoenteric fistula (usually cholecystoduodenal). The stone must be of a size (about 3 cm) that will cause obstruction; such stones typically occur in the ileum. Enteroliths formed spontaneously in the gastrointestinal tract may act in a similar manner; they are recognized by their occurrence in the absence of gallbladder disease (14). Other intraluminal causes of obstruction include bezoars (usually mixtures of hair and vegetable material), parasites (*Ascaris, Taenia, Trichuris*), and ingested foreign bodies (12).

Apart from the offending lesion (adhesive band, tumor) and the ischemic damages, the neuromuscular apparatus of the gastrointestinal tract is usually unremarkable. In long-standing cases of incomplete mechanical obstruction, dilatation and muscular hypertrophy do occur (Fig. 13.12). Results of experimental studies support the hypertrophic response of intestinal smooth muscle in the presence of obstruction (16, 17).

The term "intestinal pseudo-obstruction" denotes a syndrome in which patients have typical signs and symptoms of intestinal obstruction (as just described) but no typical mechanical lesion can be demonstrated.

PSEUDO-OBSTRUCTION

CHRONIC DISORDERS

The focus of recent interest has been on chronic cases, most of which are secondary to disease processes that are systemic and can affect the neuromuscular apparatus of the gastrointestinal tract. The prime example of such disease processes is scleroderma, but many diseases

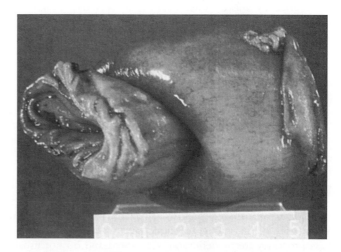

Figure 13.11 This intussusception of small bowel in an adult was the result of a submucosal mass (not shown) formed by a metastasis from a large–cell undifferentiated carcinoma of the lung. The proximal entering segment is at left.

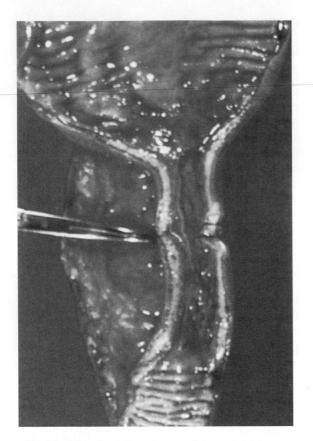

Figure 13.12   This slowly forming small-bowel stricture secondary to Crohn disease resulted in both dilatation and hypertrophy of the muscularis propria in the proximal segment of small intestine *(top)*.

behave in a similar way (see below). An ever-increasing number of cases appear to involve primary disorders of the neuromuscular apparatus. Previously undescribed lesions affecting the smooth muscle of the myenteric plexus have been recognized and are discussed in several excellent reviews (4, 16–26). Of the primary diseases affecting muscle or nerve, both familial and sporadic forms have been described (Table 13.1) (19, 23). Whether the majority of such cases affect muscle or nerve is not clear. Because lesions within the enteric nervous system are more difficult to identify morphologically than those affecting smooth muscle, it is likely that many neuropathies go unrecognized. Likewise, many early reports clearly document cases in which chronic intestinal pseudo-obstruction was recognized clinically but no pathologic lesions were identified (27–30). This inability to detect a lesion may merely reflect the lack of availability for the refined morphologic techniques such detection requires.

ACUTE DISORDERS

Acute forms of intestinal pseudo-obstruction also exist and are known more commonly as adynamic ileus or Ogilvie syndrome. These processes are by definition self-limited and do not usually come to the attention of the morphologic pathologist. Briefly, adynamic ileus is a common form of functional obstruction. To one degree or another, it follows virtually every abdominal operation. In addition, trauma, peritonitis, ischemia, spinal cord injury, and systemic infection can produce the distention and absence of peristaltic sounds characteristic of ileus. The nature and severity of the underlying disease determine the outcome. A particular form of acute pseudo-obstruction limited to the colon has been referred to as Ogilvie syndrome (31, 32). Affected patients, predominantly men, are often in the sixth decade of life. Again, various underlying disease processes are involved, including trauma (operative and

TABLE	
13.1	**Primary Intestinal Pseudo-obstruction**

Myopathies
  Familial forms
    Autosomal dominant (type I)
    Autosomal recessive (types II and III)
  Sporadic cases
Neuropathies
  Familial forms
    Autosomal recessive
    Autosomal dominant
  Sporadic cases
    Degenerative, noninflammatory
    Degenerative, inflammatory
    Isolated axonopathy
    Idiopathic constipation

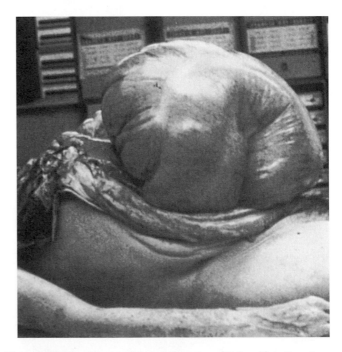

Figure 13.13   Unusually prominent colonic dilatation in an autopsy of a patient with pseudo-obstruction, a testimony to remarkable distensibility of the gastrointestinal tract and to the potentially lethal nature of these disease processes. (Courtesy of Dr. C.E. Foucar, Presbyterian Hospital, Albuquerque, NM).

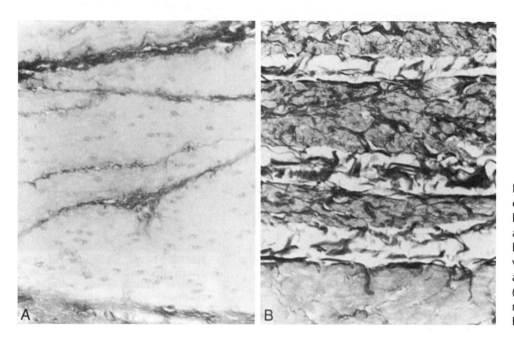

Figure 13.14 A, Normal intrafascicular collagen in a control urinary bladder. **B,** Increased intrafascicular and pericellular collagen in the urinary bladder from a patient with familial visceral myopathy; elastic fibers may also be increased (trichrome, ×325). (Courtesy of Dr. S.M. Bonsib, Department of Pathology, University of Iowa Hospitals and Clinics, Iowa City, IA.)

nonoperative), infection, myocardial infarction, and respiratory or renal failure. Other than dilatation and its consequences, there are no morphologic lesions in adynamic ileus or in Ogilvie syndrome.

CLINICAL FEATURES

In the chronic forms of pseudo-obstruction, the symptoms are, by definition, those associated with mechanical obstruction. In most cases, these symptoms begin in childhood and recur over a prolonged period; a few patients do not begin to have symptoms until middle age, and some patients are asymptomatic. Abdominal distention, pain, and vomiting predominate. The degree of distention varies but is usually quite significant and can be enormous when substantial portions of the small intestine and colon are involved (Fig. 13.13). Loud borborygmi and succussion splashes are common. Vomiting is of high volume. The pain is usually epigastric or periumbilical and correlates with the degree of distention. Alternating diarrhea and constipation, rather than obstipation, is the rule. This diarrhea may reflect small-bowel bacterial overgrowth, an important factor in many patients (see discussion of prognosis and therapy) (24). These patients often lose from 15 to 30 kg of body weight prior to diagnosis.

PRIMARY INTESTINAL PSEUDO-OBSTRUCTION

MYOPATHY

Visceral myopathy is characterized by degeneration, thinning, and fibrous replacement of the smooth muscle of the gastrointestinal tract; involvement of the muscle of the urinary tract has also been documented in some cases (Fig. 13.14) (33).

Familial Cases

The majority of cases of visceral myopathy tend to be familial (23–25, 30–42). The histologic appearance of the affected gastrointestinal segments tends to be similar in all affected families. The pattern of distribution of the involved segments, the presence or absence of gastrointestinal manifestations, and the mode of inheritance, however, have led to the recognition of several subtypes (14).

Type I, apparently the most common (27–29, 36, 41, 43–45), is characterized by autosomal dominant inheritance (43–45). Esophageal dilatation, megaduodenum, redundant colon, and megalocystis are common findings, megaduodenum in particular. The onset of symptoms usually occurs after the first decade of life, but more than 50% of affected family members are asymptomatic. Uterine inertia has been observed on occasion. In one family, members of three generations have had dysplastic nevus syndrome and multiple basal cell carcinomas in addition to the myopathy (46).

Type II familial visceral myopathy is characterized by autosomal recessive inheritance (35, 37–39). Findings include distinct gastric dilatation, as well as slight dilatation of the entire small intestine, which often has diverticula. More than 75% of the patients are symptomatic, and symptoms tend to manifest during the teenage years. Abdominal pain tends to be severe, and ptosis and external ophthalmoplegia are common.

Type III familial visceral myopathy is also autosomal recessive (34). The entire gastrointestinal tract, from esophagus to rectum, is significantly dilated. The symptoms of intestinal pseudo-obstruction, however, tend not to appear until middle age. No areas of involvement of muscle outside the gastrointestinal tract have been noted.

Sporadic Cases

Clear-cut cases of visceral myopathy that are apparently nonfamilial have been reported (23, 47, 48). Because some affected family members may be asymptomatic, and because an accurate family history can be difficult to obtain, care must be exercised before considering a case to be sporadic. In general, these cases tend to resemble the autosomal recessive familial type III visceral myopathy (14), in that they tend to have severe involvement of the entire gastrointestinal tract. Megalocystis may be present.

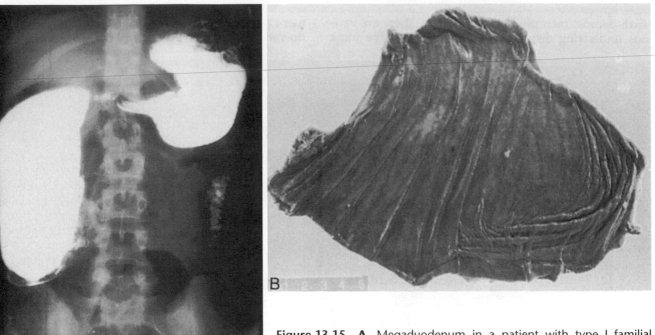

Figure 13.15 A, Megaduodenum in a patient with type I familial visceral myopathy; the massive dilatation of duodenum terminated just proximal to the ligament of Treitz. **B,** Massively dilated duodenum from a patient with visceral myopathy.

Pathologic Features

The morphologic appearance of the visceral myopathies is distinctive. The gross appearance, other than the dilatation, is unremarkable (Fig. 13.15); this dilatation tends to be segmental, particularly in the more common type I. The histologic appearance is characteristic (4, 42). The process of smooth muscle degeneration and fibrosis involves the muscularis propria but tends to spare the muscularis mucosae, although some cases with muscularis mucosae involvement have been reported (49). The longitudinal layer is usually involved more severely, and the damage may be limited to this layer (Fig. 13.16). The circular layer alone may be involved in sporadic cases (Fig. 13.17). Striking variability in the diameter of the muscle fibers is best appreciated on carefully oriented cross sections (Fig. 13.18). As the degeneration of muscle fibers continues and dense collagen is laid down around the damaged fibers, a honeycomb appearance results. This characteristic feature, referred to as vacuolar change (Fig. 13.19), distinguishes the myopathies from other forms of muscle fibrosis. The scarring of the muscularis propria in conditions such as scleroderma (see below), ischemia (Fig. 13.20), and Crohn disease (Fig. 13.21), tends to obliterate completely the muscle fibers in the affected areas and shows no preferential involvement of the longitudinal layer. Recognition of mild lesions requires careful attention to proper orientation and use of trichrome stains.

Electron microscopy confirms the smooth muscle degeneration and collagen deposition but provides no further insight into the nature of the damage. The myenteric plexus structures are normal as seen with light microscopy, electron microscopy, silver stains, and acetylcholinesterase stains in the visceral myopathies (4, 42).

Prognosis and Therapy

The treatment of these disorders is symptomatic. Of paramount importance is the consideration of small-intestinal bacterial overgrowth. This process can result in striking alteration in small-intestinal mucosal architecture (Fig. 13.22), leading to significant malabsorption with steatorrhea (50). In fact, one member of a type II family died of inanition after years of being considered to have "refractory sprue"; at autopsy, the characteristic fibrosis of visceral myopathy was evident. Patients with type I myopathy have a relatively good prognosis, perhaps related to the relatively limited area of involvement; their disease process is amenable to surgery, such as side-to-side duodenojejunostomy or partial resection of the duodenum. It is imperative that these patients receive antibiotic therapy, given the large volume of bacteria in these static bowels and the consequent high incidence of postoperative peritonitis (51). Patients with type II and III and sporadic visceral myopathy have a poorer prognosis. Often their demise is an indirect result of their severe nutritional difficulties, but in some, the cause of death is more mysterious (47).

NEUROPATHY

Visceral neuropathy is characterized by damage directed against the neural apparatus, with sparing of the smooth muscle structures. Some neuropathies may be recognized by noting decreased numbers of neurons on standard H & E sections, which necessitates fastidious neuron-counting techniques (52). In some cases, neurons may contain intranuclear inclusions visible on standard sections (52). In most cases, damage to the neurons or interconnecting

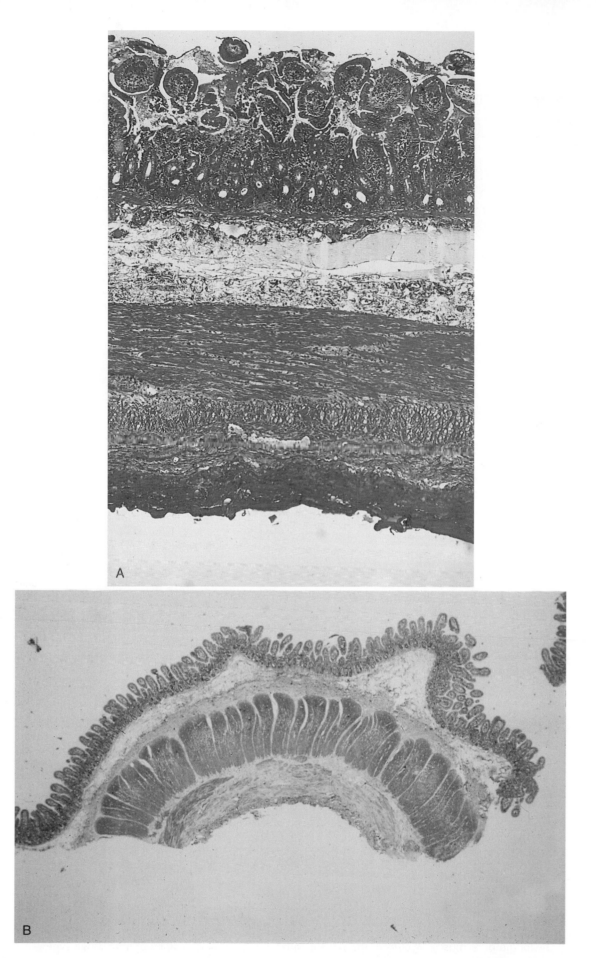

Figure 13.16 **A,** Cross section of duodenum from type I familial visceral myopathy (trichrome, ×16). **B,** Longitudinal section of jejunum from a patient with type II familial visceral myopathy (trichrome, ×8). Both show involvement limited to the longitudinal layer of the muscularis propria *(bottom)*, which is the typical early pattern. (See color plate.)

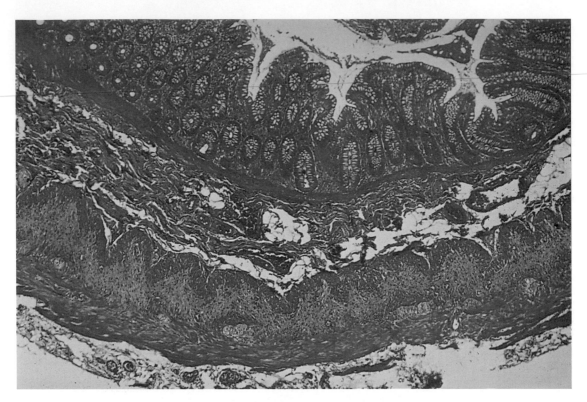

Figure 13.17   Colon from a child with sporadic visceral myopathy, who mistakenly carried a diagnosis of Hirschsprung disease for many years. Ganglion cells were intact, but the circular layer of the muscularis propria *(bottom)* was clearly damaged. This pattern of distribution is not typical of familial visceral myopathy (trichrome, ×25). (See color plate.)

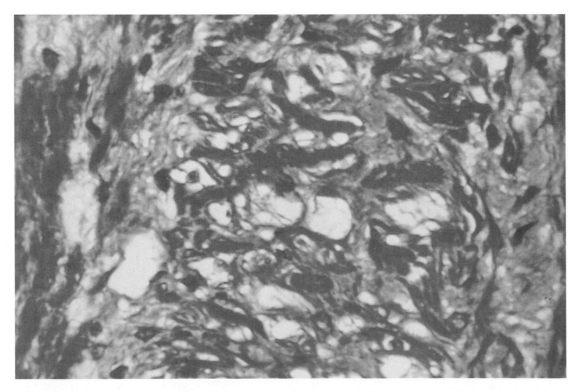

Figure 13.18   The longitudinal muscle layer from this patient with type I familial visceral myopathy shows typical vacuolar change (trichrome, ×100). (See color plate.)

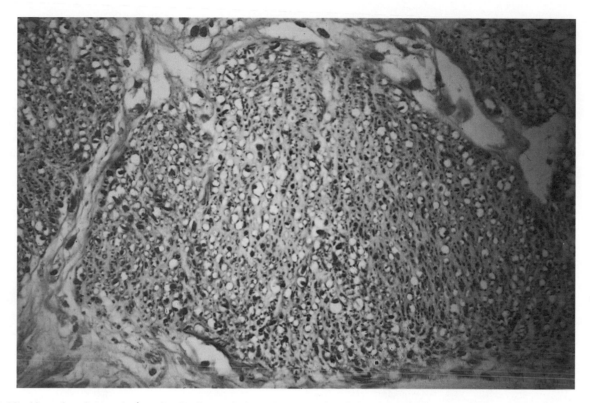

Figure 13.19 Vacuolar change in longitudinal muscle layer in type II familial visceral myopathy. In this advanced lesion, myocyte enlargement and vacuolization are prominent; individual cells are surrounded by collagen (trichrome, ×400). (See color plate.)

nerve bundles cannot be appreciated without the use of the technically difficult silver stain techniques described previously (3). The portions of the neural apparatus outside the gut that are important for controlling the movement of the gut are not amenable to ready morphologic analyses. These factors have probably led to a significant underrecognition of neural causes of motility disorders. Involvement of the central, autonomic, or peripheral nervous system elsewhere may offer some clue to the neural nature of the problem, but this is not always the case. One suggestion has been that there might be different motility patterns appreciable manometrically in the neuropathic versus myopathic processes (52–54), a hypoactive pattern being suggestive of myopathy and a hyperactive pattern being suggestive of neuropathy.

Familial Cases

Schuffler and colleagues (52) described a family with neuropathy that significantly affected the movement of the gastrointestinal tract. They noted two siblings with intestinal pseudo-obstruction who had neurologic abnormalities, including mild autonomic deficiency and denervation hypersensitivity of pupillary and esophageal smooth muscle. Inheritance is apparently recessive (13). The number of neurons in the Auerbach plexus was strikingly decreased compared with that of control subjects, and about one third of these remaining neurons contained characteristic eosinophilic intranuclear inclusions (Fig. 13.23). These inclusions do not resemble viral inclusions and were shown to be a proteinaceous and filamentous material by histochemical and electron microscopic analyses. Eosinophilic intranuclear inclusions were also found in Meissner plexus neurons, as well as in neurons of the brain, spinal cord, dorsal

root, and celiac plexus ganglion. Subsequently, similar inclusions have been noted by several observers in the neurons of patients with a variety of neurologic diseases but without significant gastrointestinal dysfunction (4, 55–57). This phenomenon has been referred to as neuronal intranuclear inclusion disease. In the family described by Schuffler and coworkers, the plexus was free of inflammatory cells; silver stains revealed a decrease in both argyrophilic and argyrophobic neurons and significantly decreased numbers of fibers in the nerve tracts.

Another family with an apparently autosomal recessive mode of inheritance for what appears to be a visceral neuropathy has been reported (58). Four siblings with pseudo-obstruction and malabsorption were also noted to have mental retardation and basal calcification. Silver staining showed a diminution in the number of argyrophilic neurons in the colon and some apparent damage to the argyrophobe neurons.

Two families with an autosomal dominant mode of transmission have also been reported (59, 60). The area of involvement seems to center on the myenteric plexus of the small intestine. Neurons appeared degenerated and decreased in number; no inclusions were noted. Some nerve fibers showed swelling and scattered beading, appreciable only on the silver stains. No evidence of extraintestinal involvement was reported.

Sporadic Cases

Given the difficulties in identifying lesions within the enteric and extraenteric nervous system previously described, it is likely that a large number of patients with gastrointestinal motility disorders will

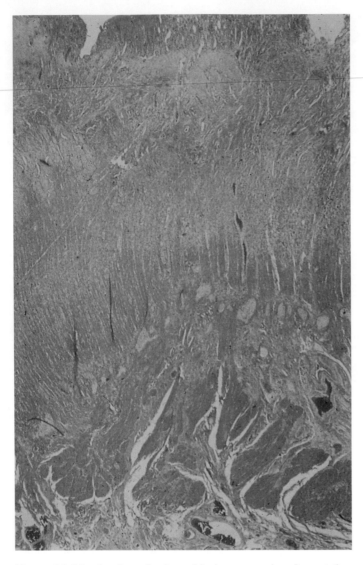

Figure 13.20   Section of colon with the mucosal surface at the top. Ischemic colonic stricture, with focally transmural fibrosis; individual degenerating fibers and vacuolar change are not present (trichrome, ×25). (See color plate.)

Degenerative inflammatory neuropathies appear to represent a more varied array of conditions. The morphologic hallmark of the condition is a lymphocytic and plasma cell infiltrate within the myenteric plexus (Fig. 13.25). Some cases appear to be idiopathic (61–63), although care is needed to exclude the paraneoplastic syndrome (64) or infection, e.g., Chagas disease (65, 66), or cytomegalovirus (67, 68) in which the myenteric plexus may have a similar appearance. This problem demonstrates the difficulties in distinguishing idiopathic pseudo-obstruction from pseudo-obstruction secondary to systemic diseases. Indeed, this separation is artificial to a good degree, but it must remain so until the pathophysiologic mechanisms of the "idiopathic" cases are understood more completely. In addition to these types of cases, findings in a curious case of rapidly progressive and lethal pseudo-

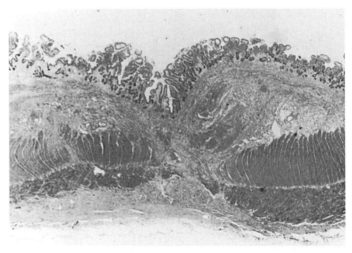

Figure 13.21   Section of small intestine with the mucosal surface at the top. Abrupt focus of transmural fibrosis (center) in a stricture of small intestine secondary to Crohn disease (trichrome, ×3.3).

eventually prove to have neural lesions. Krishnamurthy and Schuffler have done much in recent years to begin to clarify this situation; their provisional classification is used subsequently to consider this group of diseases (4).

Degenerative noninflammatory neuropathies show two basic patterns of damage. In the first type, the disease process centers on the colon, where even H & E-stained sections reveal a decreased number of neurons in the Auerbach plexus (3). This abnormality is also apparent with silver staining; additional findings include fragmentation and loss of axons as well as glial proliferation. Many neurons are swollen and have a decreased number of processes. Many of the remaining processes are thickened and have areas of swelling along their length (Fig. 13.24). In the second type, characteristic findings include a central pallor to argyrophil and argyrophobe neurons on silver staining, some disorganization, but no dendritic swellings or glial proliferation (4).

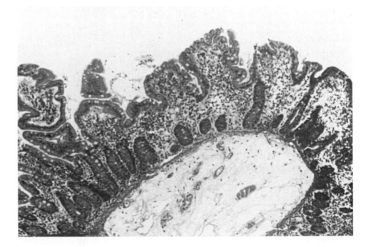

Figure 13.22   Partial and patchy villous atrophy, from the jejunum of a patient with scleroderma. Small-bowel bacterial overgrowth can be a major problem, regardless of the cause of the motility disturbance (H & E, ×25).

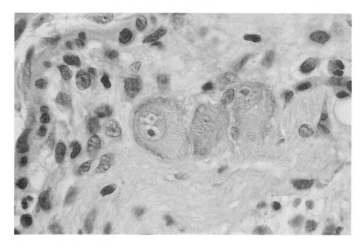

Figure 13.23 The round eosinophilic intranuclear inclusion within the ganglion cell, which is seen in some forms of familial visceral neuropathy (H & E, ×250). (See color plate.)

obstruction included normal neurons on silver sections but peculiar beading and fragmentation of axons (69). This variant has been referred to as an isolated axonopathy (4).

The problem of severe idiopathic constipation (70), also know as Arbuthnot Lane disease (71), can be considered a distinct subset of sporadic visceral neuropathy. This condition, one of the more common motility disorders encountered in the average pathology laboratory, almost exclusively affects young women who have a prolonged history of severe constipation but do not seem to have significant alimentary tract involvement beyond the colon. The severity of the constipation often results in colectomy. Colectomy specimens show little change in standard sections except for the occasional occurrence of melanosis coli. Silver stains reveal a distinctive abnormality consisting of reduced numbers of argyrophilic neurons in colonic myenteric plexuses that are otherwise populated by large numbers of cells with prominent nuclei of variable size and faint cytoplasm (Fig. 13.26); these cells are thought to represent either glial cells or abnormal (? immature) neurons. Because these patients with severe constipation have had at least some laxative usage, questions arise concerning whether or not the myenteric plexus changes represent the effect of the laxatives, i.e., "cathartic colon" (72, 73). One response is that the very existence of "cathartic colon" must be questioned (70), because heavy users of laxatives probably all have some pre-existing disorder of the neuromuscular apparatus awaiting definition. Another response is that the changes described in this characteristic clinical situation are not those seen in patients with the other motility disorders described in this chapter who may have equally impressive histories of laxative use.

SECONDARY INTESTINAL PSEUDO-OBSTRUCTION (TABLE 13.2)

Patients with secondary intestinal pseudo-obstruction are identified as those individuals with certain reasonably well-defined conditions

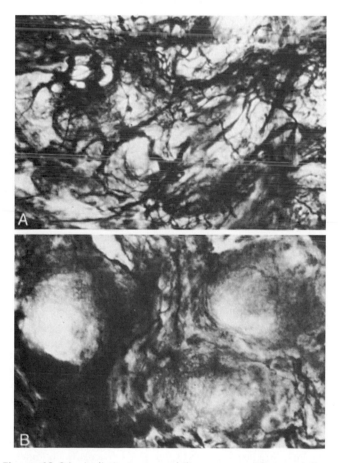

Figure 13.24 Indistinct argyrophilic neurons with axonal disorganization **(A)** and swollen degenerating argyrophilic neurons **(B)** from the ileum of a patient with degenerative noninflammatory neuropathy (silver stain, ×1360). (Reprinted with permission from Krishnamurthy S, Schuffler MD. Pathology of neuromuscular disorders of the small intestine and colon. Gastroenterology 1987;93:610.)

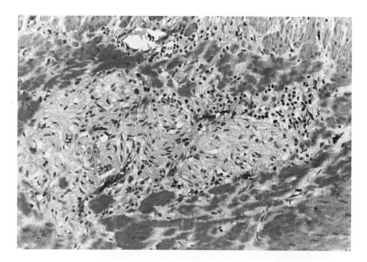

Figure 13.25 Myenteric plexus from a patient with degenerative inflammatory neuropathy. Note the lymphocytic and plasma cell infiltrate, along with decreased numbers of neurons (H & E, ×50).

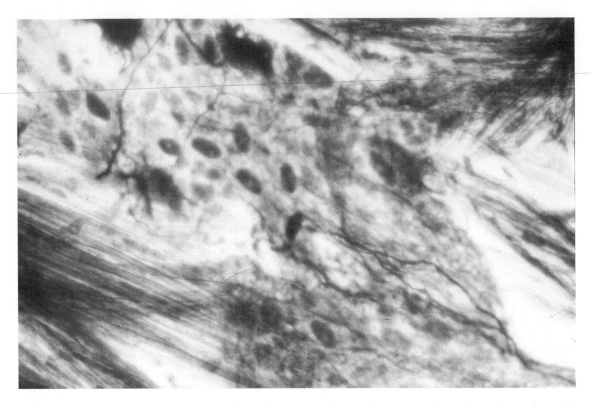

Figure 13.26   Colonic myenteric plexus in severe idiopathic constipation with increased numbers of poorly staining cells and decreased numbers of normal argyrophilic neurons (silver stain, ×100). (Section preparation courtesy of Dr. M.D. Schuffler.) (See color plate.)

or systemic diseases that cause the motility problem observed in the gastrointestinal tract (18, 19). Admittedly, the categorization as to primary and secondary is somewhat arbitrary. Some diseases considered primary or idiopathic will certainly be determined as occurring secondary to some other process as our understanding expands. Likewise, the motility problems present in such well-known clinical entities as Hirschsprung disease or Parkinson disease have traditionally been considered among the secondary causes of pseudo-obstruction (18, 19) although a cogent argument can be made for considering them under the classification of primary visceral neuropathies. Of the many conditions associated with damage to the neuromuscular apparatus of the gastrointestinal tract, those the morphologic pathologist is most likely to encounter are scleroderma, diabetes mellitus, and Hirschsprung disease.

MUSCLE DISEASES

Scleroderma

Scleroderma, or progressive systemic sclerosis, is the most common of the diseases affecting the musculature of the gastrointestinal tract to such a degree as to cause a clinically significant motility disorder (23, 74). The frequent occurrence of gastrointestinal involvement in scleroderma is well known (75–77); about 50% of patients have some significant gastrointestinal problem. All portions of the gastrointestinal tract can be involved, but esophageal problems predominate.

The clinical features usually allow ready distinction from the primary visceral myopathies, but significant morphologic differences are apparent as well (42, 74). Although both scleroderma and

the primary myopathies can involve the entire muscularis propria, the longitudinal layer often is preferentially involved in the latter. In scleroderma, the circular muscle is the layer most often affected (Fig. 13.27). In scleroderma, the collagenous replacement of the muscle tends to be nearly complete, often with an abrupt line of demarcation with adjacent normal muscle. In fact, this phenomenon accounts for the peculiar square-mouthed diverticula that are characteristic of sclerodermatous involvement of the colon (Fig. 13.28) (78). These diverticula differ from the more common banal diverticula that are herniations of mucosa through muscularis propria. The vacuolar change described previously is not present. Indeed, the presence of the broad swaths of scarring and the frequent observation of vascular abnormalities have led some authors to postulate on an ischemic component of the sclerodermatous gut (79, 80).

Much of the clinically obtained biopsy material in patients with scleroderma reveals only those disease processes secondary to the impaired musculature, namely, the consequences of gastroesophageal reflux (esophagitis and Barrett esophagus) or the small-intestinal villous architectural abnormalities secondary to bacterial overgrowth. Pseudo-obstruction with muscle damage has also been seen in association with dermatomyositis/polymyositis and systemic lupus erythematosus (SLE); in SLE particularly, an underlying vasculitis is the pathogenetic mechanism (18).

Myotonic Dystrophy and Progressive Muscular Dystrophy

In both myotonic dystrophy and in progressive muscular dystrophy, signs and symptoms suggestive of pseudo-obstruction may be present (4, 18, 81–83). Some swelling, atrophy, and degeneration of smooth muscle fibers have been reported, but a clear picture of the morphologic alterations of the muscularis propria has not yet emerged.

Ceroidosis

Ceroidosis of the gastrointestinal tract, or the "brown bowel syndrome," results from the deposition of a granular light-brown, lipofuscin-like pigment within the myocytes of the musculature of the gastrointestinal tract (Fig. 13.29). Both muscularis mucosae and muscularis propria of any segment may be involved. Ultrastructural examination reveals osmiophilic granular aggregates of electron-dense material containing myelin figures associated with abnormal distorted mitochondria (84). Deposition of ceroid pigment, which is associated with lack of vitamin E, is seen in many processes associated with malabsorption, including celiac disease, Whipple disease, and chronic pancreatitis (85, 86). Whether or not the deposition of this pigment is ever a marker for a disease process primarily damaging smooth muscle is not clear (87).

Small-Intestinal Diverticulosis

Small-intestinal diverticulosis, the most prominent area of involvement being the jejunum, may be the marker for a variety of disease processes affecting the neuromuscular apparatus (Fig. 13.30). In

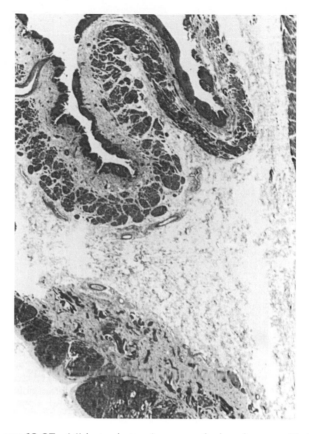

Figure 13.27   Mid-esophagus in a case of scleroderma, with the mucosal surface at the top. Fibrous replacement of the smooth muscle is almost complete in the circular layer of the muscularis propria (trichrome, ×7).

TABLE	
13.2	**Secondary Intestinal Pseudo-obstruction**

Diseases affecting smooth muscle
   Collagen vascular disease (chiefly scleroderma)
   Muscular dystrophies
   Ceroidosis
   Jejunal diverticulosis
   Amyloidosis
Diseases affecting neural structures
   Developmental abnormalities
      Hirschsprung disease
      Neuronal dysplasia
   Chagas' disease
   Parkinson disease
   Familial autonomic dysfunction
   Jejunal diverticulosis
   Amyloidosis
Endocrine disorders
   Diabetes mellitus
   Hypothyroidism
   Hypoparathyroidism
   Pheochromocytoma
Pharmacologic agents
Miscellaneous
   Jejunoileal bypass
   Radiation
   Eosinophilic gastroenteritis
   Diffuse lymphoid infiltration

those cases involving damaged muscle, the abnormal areas may resemble those seen in either the familial visceral myopathies or scleroderma (88). The diverticula tend to result from the out-pouching of a segment of jejunal wall with transmural fibrosis (4). In those patients with scleroderma-like changes in the muscle, scleroderma usually is not clinically overt, but the frequency of Raynaud phenomenon is high. Jejunal diverticulosis can also occur in association with lesions affecting the myenteric plexus. In such instances, herniations of mucosa and submucosa similar to the false diverticula commonly seen in the colon are produced. Some cases of diverticulosis apparently occur secondary to known neurologic disease processes, such as Fabry disease (89); in other cases, changes affecting the myenteric plexus, shown using silver staining, are similar to some of those seen in association with the familial visceral neuropathies (4). Interestingly, small-intestinal diverticula can occur in patients with type II visceral myopathy (35). The commonly encountered duodenal diverticula, which are usually single or few in number, are not usually associated with motility problems.

Amyloidosis

In a manner analogous to that of jejunal diverticulosis, amyloidosis can involve both the muscular and neural structures of the gut, leading to severe motility problems (4, 18, 90–92). The effect on

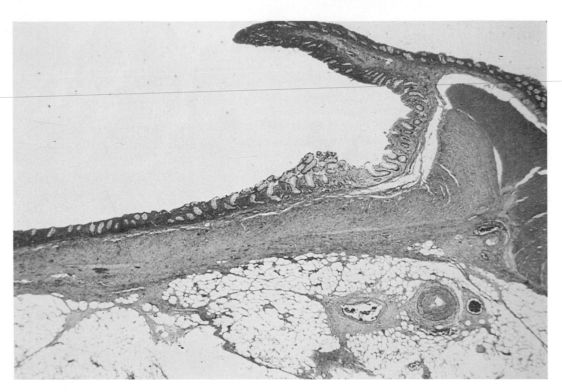

Figure 13.28   Mucosal surface at the top. Transmural obliteration and fibrosis of muscle in the colon in scleroderma. One mesenteric artery has abnormal intimal proliferation (trichrome, ×700). (See color plate.)

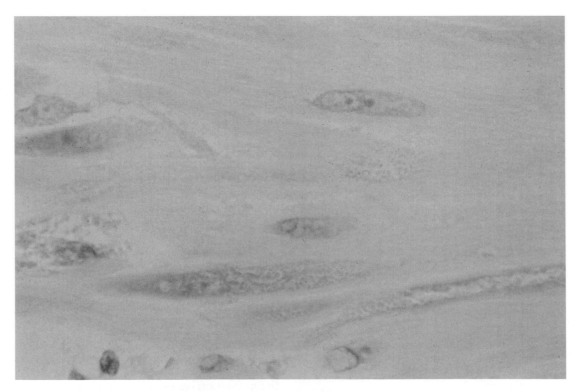

Figure 13.29   Ceroidosis of the bowel. Most myocytes in the muscularis propria contain fine granular brown pigment (H & E, ×200). (See color plate.)

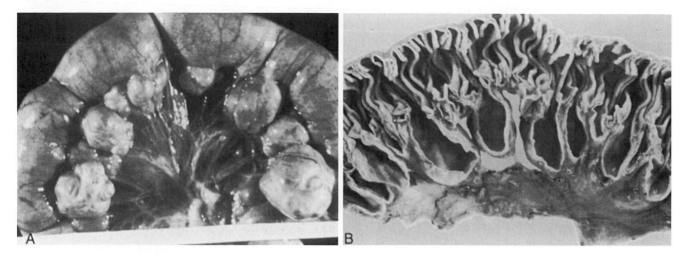

Figure 13.30 A, Jejunal diverticulosis. In this case, the diverticula occur on the mesenteric side. **B,** Opening the bowel revealed large diverticula with relatively large mouths.

muscle usually predominates. The clinical picture is dominated by features typical of amyloidosis. Within the wall of the gastrointestinal tract, large deposits of amyloid can be found in the muscularis propria and can even lead to gross mural thickening (Fig. 13.31). Although the gastrointestinal tract is frequently involved in amyloidosis, clinically significant pseudo-obstruction occurs in the minority of cases.

NEURAL DISEASES

Hirschsprung Disease

The clinical and morphologic features of Hirschsprung disease are well established (93). The process is one of aganglionosis, which affects only the distal portions of the colon (94). The striking majority of patients have the so-called short segment form, in which the disease extends proximally from the rectum no further than the sigmoid. The so-called ultra-short segment form is limited to the region of the anal sphincter, and is defined manometrically rather than morphologically. One theory is that some cases of ultra-short segment Hirschsprung are really neuronal intestinal dysplasia. The long-segment form may extend through much of the colon, but does not involve the ileum or proximal small intestine. In total colonic aganglionosis, the entire colon and some small intestine may be involved.

Although Hirschsprung disease typically manifests in the neonate or young child, as many as 10% of cases first come to diagnosis in patients who are adults. The disease shows a striking male predominance (about 80%), with the exception of total colonic aganglionosis, in which the sex incidence is roughly equal.

Severe constipation is the most typical symptom, but patients may also experience abdominal distention (owing to feces or gas) and a tight anal sphincter. The proximal, normally innervated colon is dilated, whereas the distal aganglionic segment is narrow. Symptoms and the endoscopic and histologic signs of colitis may appear, presaging the appearance of a form of enterocolitis that constitutes an emergency in these patients (95).

Several points need to be emphasized. The involved aganglionic segment is distal, within 2 cm of the pectinate line. In an area

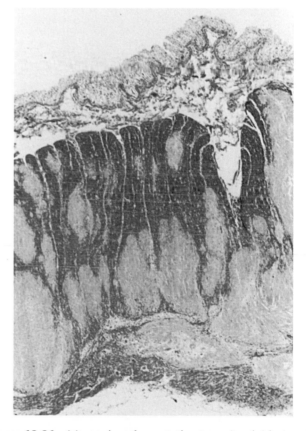

Figure 13.31 Mucosal surface at the top. Amyloidosis with multiple large, pale-staining deposits of amyloid in the muscularis propria and myenteric plexus in a patient with pseudo-obstruction syndrome (trichrome, ×8).

in the distal colon, ganglion cells are quite sparse physiologically, both in the submucosal and myenteric plexus (96). Because of this zone of hypoganglionosis, the usual recommendation is to take a biopsy sample 2 cm above the pectinate line. Ideally, additional biopsy sampling even further from the pectinate line (5 cm) should

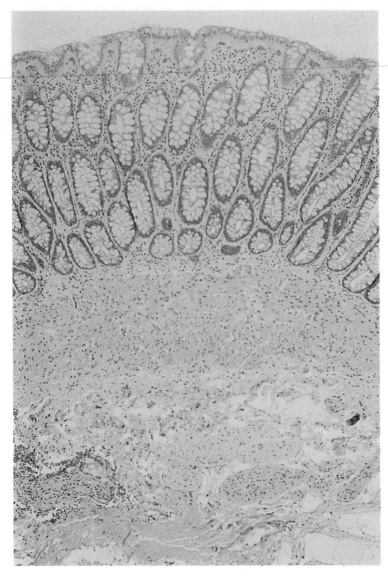

Figure 13.32   Rectal biopsy in Hirschsprung disease. Note the absence of submucosal ganglion cells and the thick nerve bundles in the submucosa (H & E, ×20). (See color plate.)

be included, and blocked separately. This additional sampling may not be practical in a small sick neonate.

The first biopsy in a patient suspected of having Hirschsprung disease is usually a rectal suction biopsy, which should be as deep as is consistent with the safety of the patient. Ideally, the sample is serially sectioned, although step sections may be more practical. The ganglion cells are about 1 mm apart and occur in clusters of from one to five cells (96). The greatest value of H & E sections is in identifying the unequivocal presence of neurons in the submucosal plexus, which effectively excludes Hirschsprung disease in that segment. Prominent hypertrophied neural bundles may also be present (Fig. 13.32). It must be emphasized that failure to identify ganglion cells in such a biopsy specimen does not establish the diagnosis of Hirschsprung disease.

The use of the acetylcholinesterase stains greatly enhances the utility of the rectal suction biopsy (97–99). In patients with Hirschsprung disease, histologic analysis demonstrates hyperplasia of the parasympathetic fibers in the lamina propria and in the muscularis mucosae, and numerous thick, tangled neural fibers are seen between the crypts (Fig. 13.33); normal subjects have only a few positively staining wisps. The hyperplasia of these fibers may not

be evident in neonates, but the test is quite reliable in the older infant and child. Unfortunately, the acetylcholinesterase stain needs to be performed on frozen tissue and can be technically difficult to perform.

The seromuscular biopsy provides a larger sample, and includes the myenteric plexus, where the density of ganglion cells is considerably greater than that in the submucosal plexus. H & E sections (frozen or paraffin embedded) usually suffice. Currently, these seromuscular biopsies, both frozen and paraffin embedded, are used most frequently at the time of the definitive operation to confirm the diagnosis made by prior rectal biopsy, manometry, and other clinical information. They also establish the area of transition to normally ganglionated colon.

Hirschsprung disease is also associated with some vascular abnormalities, typically a form of fibromuscular dysplasia (100).

Neuronal Intestinal Dysplasia

Neuronal intestinal dysplasia is similar in many aspects to Hirschsprung disease, and is the second most common cause of severe colonic motility disorders in infants and children (94). In some series, its incidence is nearly equal to that of Hirschsprung disease (101), although comparable rates of occurrence have not been the experience in most centers in the United States.

Neonatal intestinal dysplasia (NID) shares with Hirschsprung disease the presence of abnormal parasympathetic fibers, manifested by abnormal acetylcholinesterase staining in rectal biopsies (94). This abnormal staining pattern shows the thick tangled fibers in the lamina propria. Unlike Hirschsprung disease, however, ganglion cells are present in NID and, in fact, are remarkably prominent (Fig. 13.34). The ganglia are about three times the normal size, and the giant ganglia contain increased numbers of neurons (seven or more).

Two major subtypes of NID have been described: type A and type B. Type B is by far more common than type A (102). Children with type B NID have severe constipation. Type A NID is typically seen in children less than 6 months of age. The clinical picture of type A is dominated by diarrhea and bloody stools. Type A is caused by immaturity or hypoplasia of the sympathetic innervation of the gut (94).

Finally, some evidence suggests that NID and Hirschsprung disease may coexist (103). The dysplasia is usually found in the segment proximal to the area with classic aganglionosis. This coexistence may explain the occasionally poor outcome after definitive surgery (104).

Chagas Disease

The syndrome of intestinal pseudo-obstruction has long been known to be associated with Chagas disease. Chagas disease, caused by infection with the parasitic agent *Trypanosoma cruzi*, is limited to South America. The associated damage to the myenteric plexus has been shown to be related to an immunologic reaction to this agent (66). Esophageal involvement is common, resulting in achalasia; megacolon is also common. The organisms are not visualized in the plexus. Rather, findings include plasma cell and lymphocytic infiltrates of the myenteric plexus with the loss of neurons, as well as secondary hypertrophy of the muscular layers (4).

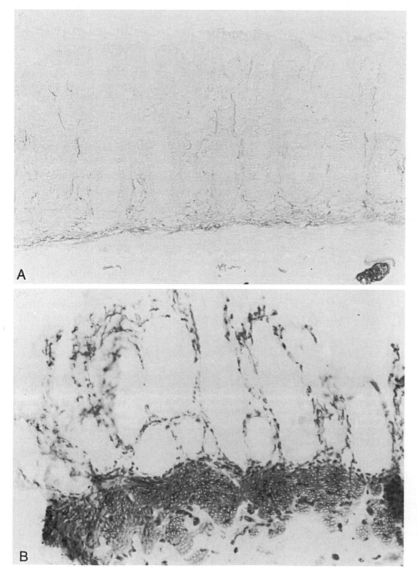

Figure 13.33 A, Normal colonic mucosa (surface at the top) contains only delicate twigs of parasympathetic fibers in the lamina propria between the crypts; staining of the muscularis mucosae is light (acetylcholinesterase, ×40). **B,** In the aganglionic colonic segment in Hirschsprung disease, the parasympathetic fibers form thick, ramifying branches in the lamina propria, and staining in the muscularis mucosae is intense (acetylcholinesterase, ×40).

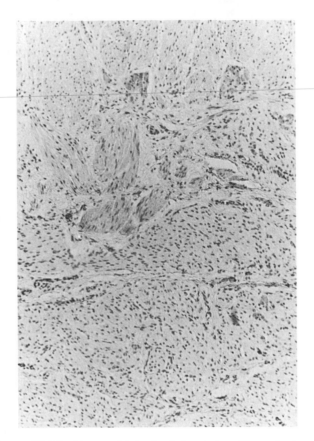

Figure 13.34 Neuronal intestinal dysplasia with a giant ganglion, occupying a substantial portion of the colonic muscularis propria in this case *(bottom)*. Fragments of muscle are seen *(top)* (H & E, ×25).

Parkinson Disease

Pseudo-obstruction has been reported to occur in patients with Parkinson disease (105–108), although the effect of therapeutic anticholinergic agents in these patients has not been excluded (18). A distinct morphologic lesion has not been described.

Other Neural Diseases

Familial autonomic dysfunction (109) and Shy-Drager syndrome (110) have widespread neurologic consequences that have been implicated in motility disorders (4, 18). Some damage to enteric neurons may occur in association with these disease processes (111), but diagnosis rests primarily on the associated clinical findings.

As described previously, jejunal diverticulosis and amyloidosis in some instances may interfere with gastrointestinal motility because of damage to the myenteric plexus.

ENDOCRINE DISORDERS

Many gastrointestinal hormones have profound effects on the secretions and motility of the gastrointestinal tract, including gastrin, cholecystokinin, secretin, glucagon, vasoactive intestinal polypeptide, gastric inhibitory peptide, motilin, enterogastrone, somatostatin, and substance P (112). Although it seems certain that many of these substances play pivotal roles in the motility disorders

of the gastrointestinal system, progress similar to that made recently (see above) in understanding clinicopathologic correlates of the enteric neural and muscular system has not been made with regard to the enteric endocrine system. The following discussion includes only the effects on the gastrointestinal tract of known systemic disorders.

Diabetes Mellitus

Diabetes mellitus, because of its frequency, is one of the most common disorders thought to be related to gastrointestinal motility disorders. There are a number of mechanisms by which the gastrointestinal tract is affected. Foremost among these mechanisms is visceral autonomic neuropathy, although some role may be played by microangiopathy, an altered electrolyte state, increased susceptibility to secondary infections, and abnormal production of insulin and glucagon (113). Subclinical involvement of the esophagus is common; when esophageal disease is clinically apparent, it usually presents as typical reflux esophagitis. Esophageal candidiasis is common. Gastroparesis can be a more disabling problem. Huge atonic stomachs may necessitate surgical intervention; no characteristic lesion is seen in the neuromuscular apparatus. Some investigators have described changes in the autonomic nerves and in the prevertebral ganglia (114). The impaired motility resulting from such damage can lead to small-bowel overgrowth and diarrhea. Care must be taken to exclude celiac disease, which appears with an increased frequency in diabetic patients (115). Constipation can also be a problem in individuals with diabetes mellitus, but no specific lesion has been found in the colon.

Hypothyroidism

Intestinal pseudo-obstruction can be significant in patients with hypothyroidism and may precede other symptoms of the disorder (116). Colonic distention may be striking, and the muscularis propria may show an infiltration by mucopolysaccharide (117).

Other Endocrine Disorders

Hypothyroidism (118) and pheochromocytoma (119) have been associated with pseudo-obstruction, although uncommonly. The effect of pheochromocytoma on motility is probably the result of catecholamine production by the tumor.

PHARMACOLOGIC AGENTS

A variety of pharmacologic agents can have a profound effect on gastrointestinal motility, and may produce the clinical picture of pseudo-obstruction. Foremost among these agents are the phenothiazines, tricyclic antidepressants, ganglionic blockers, clonidine, and antiparkinsonian medications (18). Naturally occurring toxins, such as that of *Amanita phalloides*, can also dramatically alter motility (18).

MISCELLANEOUS LESIONS

Megacolon may develop after jejunoileal bypass (120); it appears in some way to be related to an effect of the altered bacterial flora in the blind loop draining into the colon (121).

A variety of disease processes with obvious alterations in the muscle wall may present as pseudo-obstruction. Eosinophilic gastroenteritis (122) is a well-known process in which the motility problem may predominate. Likewise, the fibrosis and alteration of the intestinal musculature seen in radiation injury may have a similar effect (123). A peculiar lymphoid infiltrate of the muscularis propria resulting in pseudo-obstruction has recently been described (124).

CONCLUSION

Much needs to be learned about the structure and function of the enteric neuromuscular apparatus. Although standard techniques are sufficient for examination of the smooth muscle, those necessary for examination of the enteric nervous system are difficult at best. The silver stain techniques used in examining the myenteric plexus are capricious and require experience and expertise for proper interpretation. As recognition and knowledge of these diseases grow, the widespread application of readily available immunoperoxidase techniques should add several pieces to the puzzle. Although many of the devastating primary forms of pseudo-obstruction are rare, more subtle alterations of the neuromuscular apparatus are common. A greater understanding of such processes could conceivably have a substantial effect on our perceptions of such common diseases as reflux esophagitis and diabetes. The long-neglected study of neural and muscular morphology of the gastrointestinal tract certainly deserve greater attention.

REFERENCES

1. Christensen J, Wingate DL. A guide to gastrointestinal motility. Bristol, UK: Wright and Sons, 1983;1–214.
2. Smith BF. The neuropathology of the alimentary tract. London: Edward Arnold, 1972;3–16.
3. Schuffler MD, Jonak Z. Chronic intestinal pseudo-obstruction caused by a degenerative disorder of the myenteric plexus: The use of Smith's method to define the neuropathy. Gastroenterology 1982; 82:476–486.
4. Krishhnamurthy S, Schuffler MD. Pathology of neuromuscular disorders of the small intestine and colon. Gastroenterology 1987; 93:610–639.
5. Kumar D, Phillips SF. Human myenteric plexus: Confirmation of unfamiliar structures in adults and neonates. Gastroenterology 1989; 96:1021–1028.
6. Mackenzie JM, Dixon MF. An immunohistochemical study of the enteric neural plexi in Hirschsprung's disease. Histopathology 1987; 11:1055–1066.
7. Fausson-Pellegrini M. Comparative study of interstitial cells of Cajal. Acta Anat 1987;130:109–126.
8. Rumessen JJ, Thuneberg L. Pacemaker cells in the gastrointestinal tract: Interstitial cells of Cajal. Scand J Gastroenterol Suppl 1996; 216:82–94.
9. Sanders KKM. A case for interstitial cells of Cajal as pacemakers and mediators of neurotransmission in the gastrointestinal tract. Gastroenterology 1996;111:492–515.
10. Kobayahi S, Suzuki M, Endo T, et al. Framework of the enteric nerve plexuses: An immunocytochemical study in the guinea pig jejunum using antiserum to S-100 protein. Arch Histol Cytol 1986;49: 159–188.
11. Ellis H. The causes and prevention of intestinal adhesions. Br J Surg 1982;69:241–243.
12. Mucha P. Small intestinal obstruction. Surg Clin North Am 1987; 67:597–620.
13. Fielding LP, Welch JP. Intestinal obstruction. New York: Churchill Livingstone, 1987;32–41, 153–162.
14. Berk JE. Bockus gastroenterology. Philadelphia: WB Saunders, 1985;2056–2092.
15. Orloff MV. Intussusception in children and adults. Surg Gynecol Obstet 1956;102:313–329.
16. Gabella G. Hypertrophy of intestinal smooth muscle. Cell Tissue Res 1975;163:199–214.
17. Brent L. The response of smooth muscle cells in the rabbit colon to anal stenosis. Pathology 1973;5:209–218.
18. Faulk DL, Anuras S, Christensen J. Chronic or intestinal pseudo-obstruction. Gastroenterology 1978;74:922–931.
19. Anuras S, Christensen J. Recurrent or chronic intestinal pseudo-obstruction. Clin Gastroenterol 1981;10:177–190.
20. Golladay ES, Byrne WJ. Intestinal pseudo-obstruction. Surg Gynecol Obstet 1981;153:257–273.
21. Hirsh EH, Brandenburg D, Hersh T, et al. Chronic intestinal pseudo-obstruction. J Clin Gastroenterol 1981;3:247–254.
22. Hans JB, Meyers WC, Andersen DK. Chronic primary intestinal pseudo-obstruction. Surgery 1981;89:175–182.
23. Schuffler MD, Rohrmann CA, Chaffee RG. Chronic intestinal pseudo-obstruction. Medicine 1981;60:173–196.
24. Schuffler MD. Chronic intestinal pseudo-obstruction syndromes. Med Clin North Am 1981;65:1331–1358.
25. DeLorenzo C, Hyman PE. Gastrointestinal motility in neonatal and pediatric practice. Gastroenterol Clin North Am 1996;25: 203–224.
26. Abell TL, Werkman RF. Gastrointestinal motility disorders. Am Fam Physician 1996;53:895–902.
27. Weis W. Zu Atiologie des Megaduodenums. Dtsch Z Chir 1938;251; 317–330.
28. Law DH, Ten Eyck EA. Familial megaduodenum and megacystis. Am J Med 1962;33:911–922.
29. Newton WT. Radical enterectomy for hereditary megaduodenum. Arch Surg 1968;96:549–553.
30. Byrne WJ, Cipel L, Euler AR. Chronic idiopathic intestinal pseudo-obstruction syndrome in children. J Pediatr 1970;90:585–589.
31. Vanek VW, Al-Salti M. Acute pseudo obstruction of the colon (Ogilvie's syndrome). Dis Colon Rectum 1986;29:203–210.
32. Anuras S, Shirazi SS. Colonic pseudo-obstruction. Am J Gastroenterol 1984;79:525–532.
33. Bonsib SM, Fallon B, Mitros FA, et al. Urological manifestations of patients with visceral myopathy. J Urol 1984;132:1112–1116.
34. Anuras S, Mitros FA, Milano A, et al. A familial visceral myopathy with dilatation of the entire gastrointestinal tract. Gastroenterology 1986; 90:385–390.
35. Anuras S, Mitros FA, Nowak TV. A familial visceral myopathy with external ophthalmoplegia and autosomal recessive transmission. Gastroenterology 1983;84:346–353.
36. Faulk DL, Anuras S, Garner GD, et al. A familial visceral myopathy. Ann Intern Med 1978;89:600–606.
37. Ionasescu V. Oculogastrointestinal muscular dystrophy. Am J Med Genet 1983;15:103–112.
38. Ionasescu V, Thompson SH, Ionasescu R. Inherited opthalmoplegia with intestinal pseudo-obstruction. J Neurol Sci 1983;59: 215–228.
39. Ionasescu V, Thompson SH, Aschenbrenner C, et al. Late onset oculogastrointestinal muscular dystrophy. Am J Med Genet 1984; 18:781–788.
40. Jacobs E, Andichvili D, Perissino A, et al. A case of familial visceral myopathy with atrophy and fibrosis of the longitudinal muscle layer of the entire small bowel. Gastroenterology 1979;77:745–750.
41. Lewis TD, Daniel EE, Sarna SK, et al. Idiopathic intestinal pseudo-obstruction: Report of a case with intraluminal studies of mechanical and electrical activity, and response to drugs. Gastroenterology 1978;74:107–111.
42. Mitros FA, Schuffler MD, Teja K, et al. Pathology of familial visceral myopathy. Hum Pathol 1983;13:825–833.
43. Schuffler MD, Lowe MC, Bill AH. Studies of idiopathic intestinal pseudo-obstruction. Clinical and pathological studies. Gastroenterology 1977;73:327–338.
44. Schuffler MD, Pope CE. Studies of idiopathic intestinal pseudo-obstruction. II. A hereditary hollow visceral myopathy: Family studies. Gastroenterology 1977;73:339–344.
45. Shaw A, Shaffer H, Teja K, et al. A perspective for pediatric surgeons: Chronic idiopathic intestinal pseudo-obstruction. Pediatr Surg 1979; 14:719–727.

46. Foucar CE, Lindholm J, Anuras S, et al. A kindred with dysplastic nevus syndrome associated with visceral myopathy and multiple basal cell carcinomas. Lab Invest 1985;52:23A.

47. Anuras S, Mitros FA, Shirazi SS, et al. Cardiac arrest in two children with nonfamilial chronic intestinal pseudo-obstruction on total parenteral nutrition. J Pediatr Gastroenterol 1982;1:137–144.

48. Puri P, Lake BD, Gorman F, et al. Megacystic microcolon intestinal hypoperistalsis syndrome: A visceral myopathy. J Pediatr Surg 1983;18:64–68.

49. Alstead EM, Murphy MN, Flanagan AM, et al. Familial autonomic visceral myopathy with degeneration of muscularis mucosae. J Clin Pathol 1988;41:424–429.

50. Schuffler MD, Kaplan LR, Johnson L. Small intestinal mucosa in pseudo-obstruction syndromes. Am J Dig Dis 1978;23:821–830.

51. Anuras S, Shirazi S, Faulk DL, et al. Surgical treatment in familial visceral myopathy. Ann Surg 1979;189:306–310.

52. Schuffler MD, Bird TD, Sumi SM, et al. A familial neuronal disease presenting as intestinal pseudoobstruction. Gastroenterology 1978;75:889–898.

53. Schuffler MD, Rohrmann CA, Templeton FE. The radiological manifestations of idiopathic intestinal pseudoobstruction. AJR Am J Roentgenol 1976;127:729–736.

54. Summers RW, Anuras S, Green J. Jejunal manometry patterns in health, partial intestinal obstruction, and pseudoobstruction. Gastroenterology 1983;85:1290–1300.

55. Palo J, Haltia M, Carpenter S, et al. Neurofilament subunit-related proteins in neuronal intranuclear inclusions. Ann Neurol 1984;15:322–328.

56. Patel H, Norma MG, Perry TL, et al. Multiple system atrophy with neuronal intranuclear hyaline inclusions. J Neurol Sci 1985;67:57–65.

57. Monoz-Garcia D, Ludwin SK. Adult onset neuronal intranuclear hyaline inclusion disease. Neurology 1986;36;785–790.

58. Cockel R, Hill EE, Rushton DI, et al. Familial steatorrhea with calcification of the basal ganglia and mental retardation. Q J Med 1973;168:771–783.

59. Roy AD, Bharucha H, Nevin NC, et al. Idiopathic intestinal pseudo-obstruction: A familial visceral neuropathy. Clin Genet 1980;18:291–297.

60. Mayer EA, Schuffler MD, Rotter JI, et al. Familial visceral neuropathy with autosomal dominant transmission. Gastroenterology 1986;91:1528–1535.

61. Erskine JM. Acquired megacolon, megaesophagus and megaduodenum with aperistalsis: A case report. Am J Gastroenterol 1963;40:588–600.

62. Horoupian DS, Kim Y. Encephalomyeloneuropathy with ganglionitis of the myenteric plexuses in the absence of cancer. Ann Neurol 1982;11:628–631.

63. Arista-Nasr J, Gonzalez-Romo M, Keirns C, et al. Diffuse lymphoplasmacytic infiltration of the small intestine with damage to nerve plexus. A cause of intestinal pseudo-obstruction. Arch Pathol Lab Med 1993;117:812–819.

64. Schuffler MD, Baird HW, Fleming CR, et al. Intestinal pseudoobstruction as the presenting manifestation of small cell carcinoma of the lung: A paraneoplastic neuropathy of the gastrointestinal tract. Ann Intern Med 1983;98:129–134.

65. Earlam RJ. Gastrointestinal aspects of Chagas' disease. Dig Dis Sci 1972;17:559–571.

66. Wood JN, Hudson L, Jessell TM, et al. A monoclonal antibody defining antigenic determinants on subpopulations of mammalian neurones and Trypanosoma cruzi parasites. Nature 1982;296:34–38.

67. Press MF, Riddell RH, Ringus J. Cytomegalovirus inclusion disease: Its occurrence in the myenteric plexus of a renal transplant patient. Arch Pathol Lab Med 1980;104:580–583.

68. Sonsino E, Mouy R, Foucaud P, et al. Intestinal pseudo-obstruction related to cytomegalovirus infection of the myenteric plexus. N Engl J Med 1984;311:196–197.

69. Krishnamurthy S, Schuffler MD, Belic L, et al. An inflammatory axonopathy of the myenteric plexus causing rapidly progressive intestinal pseudo-obstruction. Gastroenterology 1986;90:754–758.

70. Krishnamurthy S, Schuffler MD, Rohrmann CA, et al. Severe idio-

pathic constipation is associated with a distinctive abnormality of the colonic myenteric plexus. Gastroenterology 1985;88:26–34.

71. Preston DM, Hawley RR, Lennard-Jones JE, et al. Results of colectomy for severe idiopathic constipation in women (Arbuthnot Lane's disease). Br J Surg 1984;71:547–552.

72. Smith B. Effect of irritant purgatives on the myenteric plexus in man and mouse. Gut 1968;9:139–143.

73. Smith B. Pathologic changes in the colon produced by anthraquinone purgatives. Dis Colon Rectum 1973;16:455–458.

74. Schuffler MD, Beegle RG. Progressive systemic sclerosis of the gastrointestinal tract and hollow visceral myopathy: Two distinguishable disorders of intestinal smooth muscle. Gastroenterology 1979;77:664–671.

75. Poirier TJ, Rankin GB. Gastrointestinal manifestations of progressive systemic sclerosis based on a review of 364 cases. Am J Gastroenterol 1972;58:30–44.

76. Goldgraber MB, Kirsner JB. Scleroderma of the gastrointestinal tract. Arch Pathol Lab Med 1957;64:255–265.

77. D'Angelo WA, Fries JF, Masi AT, et al. Pathologic observations in systemic sclerosis (scleroderma). Am J Med 1969;46:428–440.

78. Heinz ER, Steinberg AJ, Sackner MA. Roentgenographic and pathologic aspects of intestinal scleroderma. Ann Intern Med 1983;59:822–826.

79. Norton WL, Nardon JM. Vascular disease in progressive systemic sclerosis (scleroderma). Ann Intern Med 1970;73;317–324.

80. Morson BC. Gastrointestinal pathology. London: Blackwell Scientific, 1979;694–695.

81. Nowak TV, Ionasescu V, Anuras S: Gastrointestinal manifestations of the muscular dystropies. Gastroenterology 1982;82:800–810.

82. Leon SH, Schuffler MD, Kettler M, et al. Intestinal pseudo-obstruction as a complication of Duchenne's muscular dystrophy. Gastroenterology 1986;90:455–459.

83. Brunner HG, Hamel BC, Rieu P, et al. Intestinal pseudo-obstruction in myotonic dystrophy. J Med Genet 1992;29:791–793.

84. Horn T, Svendsen LB, Johansen A, et al. Brown bowel syndrome. Ultrastruct Pathol 1985;8:357–361.

85. Braustein H. Tocopherol deficiency in adults with chronic pancreatitis. Gastroenterology 1961;40:224–231.

86. Fox B. Lipofuscinosis of the gastrointestinal tract in man. J Clin Pathol 1967;20:806–813.

87. Foster CS. The brown bowel syndrome: A possible smooth muscle mitochondrial myopathy? Histopathology 1979;3:1–17.

88. Krishnamurthy S, Kelly MM, Rohrmann CA, et al. Jejunal diverticulosis: A heterogenous disorder caused by a variety of abnormalities of smooth muscle or myenteric plexus. Gastroenterology 1983;85:538–547.

89. Friedman LS, Kirkham SE, Thistlehwaite JR, et al. Jejunal diverticulosis with perforation as a complication of Fabry's disease. Gastroenterology 1984;86:558–563.

90. Legge DA, Wollaeger EE, Carlson HC. Intestinal pseudoobstruction in systemic amyloidosis. Gut 1970;11:764–767.

91. Wald A, Kichler J, Mendelow H. Amyloidosis and chronic intestinal pseudoobstruction. Dig Dis Sci 1981;26:462–465.

92. Tada S, Iida M, Yao T, et al. Intestinal pseudo-obstruction in patients with amyloidosis: Clinicopathologic differences between chemical types of amyloid protein. Gut 1993;34:1412–1417.

93. Holschneider AM. Hirschsprung's disease. New York: Thieme-Stratton, 1982;62–71.

94. Holschneider AM, Meier-Ruge W, Ure BM. Hirschsprung's disease and allied disorders — A review. Eur J Pediatr Surg 1994;4:260–266.

95. Elhalaby EA, Teitelbaum DH, Coran AG, et al. Enterocolitis associated with Hirschsprung's disease: A clinical histopathological correlative study. J Pediatr Surg 1995;30:1023–1027.

96. Aldridge RT, Campbell PE. Ganglion cell distribution in the normal rectum and anal canal. A basis for the diagnosis of Hirschsprung's disease by anorectal biopsy. J Pediatr Surg 1968;3:475–490.

97. Lake BD, Puri P, Nixon HH, et al. Hirschsprung's disease: An appraisal of histochemically demonstrated acetylcholinesterase activity in suction rectal biopsy specimens as an aid to diagnosis. Arch Pathol Lab Med 1978;102:244–247.

98. Morikawa Y, Donahoe PK, Hendren WH. Manometry and histochemistry in the diagnosis of Hirschsprung's disease. Pediatrics 1979;63:865–871.

99. Kobayashi H, Wang Y, Hirakawa H, et al. Intraoperative evaluation of extent of aganglionosis by a rapid acetylcholinesterase histochemical technique. J Pediatr Surg 1995;30:248–252.

100. Taguchi T, Tanaka K, Ikeda K. Fibromuscular dysplasia of arteries in Hirschsprung's disease. Gastroenterology 1985;88:1099–1103.

101. Meier-Ruge W. Epidemiology of congenital innervation defects of the distal colon. Virchows Arch 1992;420:171–177.

102. Ryan DP. Neuronal intestinal dysplasia. Semin Pediatr Surg 1995; 4:22–25.

103. Moore SW, Laing D, Kaschula ROC, et al. A histological grading system for the evaluation of co-existing NID with Hirschsprung's disease. Eur J Pediatr Surg 1994;4:293–297.

104. Banani SA, Forootan HR, Kumar PV. Intestinal neuronal dysplasia as a cause of surgical failure in Hirschsprung's disease: A new modality for surgical management. J Pediatr Surg 1996;31:572–574.

105. Feinstat T, Testnk H, Schuffler MD, et al. Megacolon and neurofibromatosis: A neuronal intestinal dysplasia. Gastroenterology 1984; 86:1573–1579.

106. Demos TC, Blonder J, Schey WL, et al. Multiple endocrine neoplasia (MEN) syndrome type IIB: Gastrointestinal manifestations. AJR Am J Roentgenol 1983;140:73–78.

107. Lewitan A, Nathanson L, Slade WR. Megacolon and dilatation of the small bowel in Parkinsonism. Gastroenterology 1951;17: 367–374.

108. Caplan LH, Jacobson JG, Rubenstein BM, et al. Megacolon and volvulus in Parkinson's disease. Radiology 1965;85:73–78.

109. Grossman HJ, Limosani MA, Short M. Megacolon as a manifestation of familial autonomic dysfunction. J Pediatr 1956;49:289–296.

110. Shy GM, Drager GA. A neurological syndrome associated with orthostatic hypotension. Arch Neurol 1960;2:511–516.

111. Smith B. The neuropathology of pseudo-obstruction of the intestine. Scand J Gastroenterol 1982;17(Suppl 71):103–109.

112. Ouyang A, Cohen S. Effects of hormones on gastrointestinal motility. Med Clin North Am 1981;65:111–127.

113. Yang R, Arem R, Chan L. Gastrointestinal tract complications of diabetes mellitus. Arch Intern Med 1984;144:1251–1256.

114. Hensley GT, Soergel KH. Neuropathologic findings in diabetic diarrhea. Arch Pathol Lab Med 1968;85:587–597.

115. Green PA, Wollaegen EE, Sprague RG. Diabetes mellitus associated with non-tropical sprue: Report of 4 cases. Diabetes 1962;11: 388–392.

116. Chadha JS, Ashby SW, Cowan WK. Fatal intestinal atony in myxoedema. Br Med J 1969;3:398–401.

117. Abbassi AA, Douglas RC, Bissell GW, et al. Myxedema ileus: A form of intestinal pseudo-obstruction. JAMA 1975;234:181–183.

118. Taybi H, Keele D. Hypoparathyroidism: A review of the literature and report of two cases in sisters, one with steatorrhea and intestinal pseudo-obstruction. AJR Am J Roentgenol 1962;88:432–442.

119. Mullen JP, Cartwright RC, Tisherman SE, et al. Case report: Pathogenesis and pharmacologic management of pseudo-obstruction of the bowel in pheochromocytoma. Am J Med Sci 1985;290:155–158.

120. Barry RE, Benfield JR, Nicell P, et al. Colonic pseudo-obstruction: A new complication of jejunoileal bypass. Gut 1975;16:903–908.

121. Barry RE, Chow AW, Billesdon J. Role of intestinal microflora in colonic pseudo-obstruction complicating jejunoileal bypass. Gut 1977;18:356–359.

122. Johnstone JM, Morson BC. Eosinophilic gastroenteritis. Histopathology 1978;2:335–348.

123. Berthrong M, Fajardo LF. Radiation injury in surgical pathology. Part II. Alimentary tract. Am J Surg Pathol 1981;5:153–178.

124. McDonald GB, Schuffler MD, Kadin ME, et al. Intestinal pseudoobstruction caused by diffuse lymphoid infiltration of the small intestine. Gastroenterology 1985;89:882–889.

14

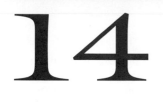

Vascular Disorders

D. Bruce Baird and H. Thomas Norris

HEMORRHAGIC NECROSIS
STRESS ULCERATION
ATHEROEMBOLIC INJURY
RADIATION INJURY

OTHER DISORDERS
EFFECT OF CHRONIC NARROWING OF SPLANCHNIC
VESSELS

In this chapter, we attempt to cover the vast number of diseases in vessels found throughout the gastrointestinal tract. Pathologic factors as diverse as emboli into the orifices of major arteries to vasculitis occurring in the smallest vessels all have a profound effect on the functioning of an organ. The gastrointestinal tract is not exempt from these changes. Resource material for this discussion is drawn predominantly from those references that have provided new knowledge during the last 10 to 15 years.

Symptoms referable to abnormalities of the gastrointestinal vasculature provide three main types of clinical findings: pain, obstruction to flow of gastrointestinal contents, and hemorrhage. One major advance has been in the greater definition of the site of bleeding.

DIAGNOSIS OF GASTROINTESTINAL BLEEDING

Dramatic changes have occurred in the last decade in the diagnosis and management of gastrointestinal tract bleeding. In the past, the cause and source of gastrointestinal bleeding often remained obscure even after extensive study. With the widespread application of fiberoptic endoscopy and advances in radiologic techniques, fewer cases now occur in which the cause of the gastrointestinal bleeding remains obscure or occult (1).

A three-step approach is often used to investigate suspected gastrointestinal bleeding. The first step in determining the source of bleeding is taking an adequate history and performing a thorough physical examination. Included in the examination is confirmation that the patient has actually experienced a gastrointestinal hemorrhage. A guaiac test for occult blood is used for this purpose.

Once gastrointestinal hemorrhage has been established, the next step is to determine whether the source of bleeding is from the upper or lower gastrointestinal tract. For purposes of this discussion, the dividing point of these two areas will be the ligament of Treitz. An upper gastrointestinal source of bleeding, that is, proximal to the ligament of Treitz, is suggested clinically by hematemesis. If the clinical situation is unclear, gastric aspiration may help to confirm the source of bleeding. A gastric aspirate positive for blood suggests an upper tract source; whereas a negative study suggests a lower tract source.

The third step is to identify, as closely as possible, the specific site of bleeding. The approach usually includes endoscopy, followed by contrast radiography, radionuclide scans, and/or arteriography, or a combination of these methods. With contemporary endoscopic techniques, the source of the current upper gastrointestinal bleeding can be identified by endoscopy in 70 to 90% of patients (2).

As noted previously, the presence of occult blood in the stools or a negative gastric aspirate suggests lower gastrointestinal bleeding. In patients with lower gastrointestinal bleeding (colonic hemorrhage), flexible fiberoptic sigmoidoscopy should be the first procedure undertaken, although appropriate patient preparation is essential to ensure a successful outcome. The development of newer

and smaller endoscopes has made examination of infants and children a practical diagnostic procedure.

Radiologic evaluation usually begins with plain film radiographs to exclude bowel obstruction and/or free intraabdominal gas. This examination is followed by upper gastrointestinal tract studies, small bowel series, or barium enemas, depending on the suspected source of hemorrhage. Radiologic evaluation may be of limited usefulness in the diagnosis of certain vascular disorders; however, a double-contrast barium study may still detect bleeding lesions that are predominantly submucosal and thus difficult to see at the time of colonoscopy.

Radionuclide studies have the advantage of documenting the presence of active bleeding in the gastrointestinal tract, although they may provide only general information about the location of its source. These studies are especially of benefit when the bleeding is intermittent or subacute. Radionuclide studies certainly help in determining the appropriate timing of angiographic studies.

With the increased use of the flexible endoscope to ascertain the source of bleeding, angiography is chosen less often as a diagnostic tool. In certain situations, however, such as when massive bleeding makes endoscopy impossible, angiography continues to be a useful diagnostic procedure. Angiography can detect active bleeding with flow rates as low as 0.5 ml/min, although the accuracy increases with the rate of bleeding. Angiography has a special role in demonstrating lesions that may not be bleeding currently but are caused by abnormal vessels, e.g. vascular malformations, telangiectasias, and hemangiomas. In addition, angiography plays an important role in the treatment of certain vascular disorders; the infusion of either vasoconstrictive agents such as vasopressin or substances used in embolization therapy has either significantly decreased or stopped bleeding in certain cases.

During upper gastrointestinal tract endoscopy, the cause of bleeding usually can be placed in one of two categories. The first category includes mucosal lesions, such as erosions, ulcerations, esophagitis, gastritis, and tears (Mallory-Weiss tears). The second major category comprises bleeding from upper gastrointestinal tract varices.

The major vascular causes of lower gastrointestinal bleeding include hemorrhoids, fissures, acute diverticulitis, and ischemic colitis. In patients 60 years of age and older, angiodysplasia is the most frequent cause.

Therapy can also be accomplished during the endoscopic examination. Therapeutic interventions include the neodymium: yttrium-aluminum-garnet (Nd:YAG) laser, the heater probe, and electrocoagulation.

All of these advances have resulted in a general benefit to the patient. The site of bleeding can be ascertained with greater accuracy. Whereras it had been assumed that gastrointestinal bleeding usually came from one specific single site, use of the flexible endoscope has shown that multiple potential sites or sources of bleeding can be found in upwards of one third of cases. With advances in technique and instruments, therapeutic endoscopy is being used with greater frequency during active bleeding. If these therapeutic attempts fail, definitive surgery may result in a cure.

METHODS OF EXAMINATION OF SPECIMENS

The type of vascular lesions affecting the gastrointestinal tract may be obvious. When the type of vascular lesion is not readily apparent, however, specific types of studies are often helpful. The input of the clinician, surgeon, and radiologist with regard to the suspected type of lesion is essential before the studies are undertaken.

INJECTION STUDIES OF BLOOD VESSELS

The documentation and demonstration of the various vascular abnormalities of the gastrointestinal tract may require a variety of approaches. It is not difficult to make the diagnosis on a histopathologic basis once the lesion has been found. Finding the lesion is often the most challenging aspect of the examination for the pathologist. Special techniques may not be necessary. The most important part of the examination is close visual inspection of the mucosal surface. Most vascular abnormalities are less than 1 cm in diameter.

A variety of injection techniques are useful in the study of vascular lesions. The best special studies leave the specimen in a state that allows subsequent radiologic and histologic analysis. These techniques demand that the vasculature be flushed with a solution to remove as much of the blood and small clots as possible. The artery to the specimen is cannulated, and this vessel is flushed until no clots are seen coming from the adjacent vein. Approximately 200 to 300 ml of warm saline or heparinized saline are usually effective; occasionally, over 500 ml of solution is necessary.

GELATIN-BARIUM MIXTURE

Infusion of a mixture of gelatin and barium yields a specimen that is amenable to both radiologic and pathologic techniques (3, 4). This mixture usually allows filling of the capillaries. The mixture is prepared by adding 3 ml of liquefied phenol and 2 ml of liquefied 2-octanol to 600 ml of hot tap water. This solution is placed in a blender and 100 g of Knox type 2136 gelatin is added slowly and blended for 1 minute. Then, 400 g of micropaque powder is added and blended for 2 minutes. This mixture is allowed to gel overnight and then is stored in the refrigerator. The solution is rewarmed and infused into the appropriate artery at the patient's systolic pressure. (This solution will not reliquefy if it has come in contact with formalin.) If the vein does not fill, the vein is then subsequently infused with the same solution at similar pressures. Monastral red or monastral blue can be added to the injection mixture in order to study the distribution of individual vessels. The specimen is then fixed in 10% formalin for 24 hours before appropriate radiologic and histopathologic studies are undertaken.

Whether or not the specimen has been injected, close examination of the mucosa is essential. Inspection may demonstrate small erosions or ulcerations. Pinpoint hemorrhages and small petechial lesions may be the only changes present on the surface. Occasionally, the lesions are linear. The presence of tiny clots on the surface of the mucosa is an extraordinarily helpful marker for the location of bleeding lesions. The judicious application of India ink to suspected lesions on the mucosa allows the examiner to return to the areas of interest and concern without causing significant morphologic alteration, such as can occur with the use of pins and other sharp objects. India ink also helps to localize the suspected area of abnormality in histologic section.

SILICONE RUBBER

Injection of silicone rubber or silicone rubber with a radiopaque material added to it is another useful technique (5). The injected specimen is refrigerated at 4.5°C for 24 hours, dehydrated in ethyl alcohol, and cleared in methyl salicylate. The result is a transparent specimen with an accentuated vascular bed. Although these specimens are very good for radiographic imaging, they yield less than optimal results when studied histologically.

OTHER TECHNIQUES

Another method is the injection of the specimen using 5 ml of "biologic" colloidal carbon suspension filtered through Whatman paper No. 1 (Peliken, Hanover, Germany) (6).

A variety of other techniques have been used, especially during surgery, when location of the malformation is a concern. One such technique is the intraoperative injection of indigo carmine solution into the appropriate artery, which has been cannulated (6). Methylene blue has also been used intraoperatively (7).

LYMPHATICS

Demonstration of the lymphatics of the gastrointestinal tract is a more challenging project. One of the authors (Norris) has had success only on an experimental basis when substances rich in lipid, such as melted butter, were placed in the lumen of the small bowel during in vivo studies. The appearance of the lipid substance in the serosal lacteals was observed. Results of one study suggest the use of cedar oil mixed with a dye (color in oil) such as Prussian blue can be helpful when attempting to delineate lymphatic vessels (8).

ANATOMY OF GASTROINTESTINAL VASCULATURE

Although the anatomy of the vasculature—arterial, venous and lymphatic—was studied extensively in the past, new diagnostic techniques and new therapeutic procedures have stimulated renewed interest in this subject. The vascular anatomy of the gastrointestinal tract is well described in in Chapter 2, and several articles offer a detailed review of the subject (9–12). These reviews emphasize the presence of a substantial anastomotic network involving both the arteries and the veins of the gastrointestinal tract. The extensive arterial anastomotic network and collateral circulation provide significant protection against ischemic episodes. The marginal artery of Drummond in the colon is one such anastomotic connection. This artery is derived from the middle colic branch of the superior mesenteric artery and the ascending division of the left colic branch of the inferior mesenteric artery.

The extensive anastomotic and collateral circulation present in the gastrointestinal venous network usually is not evident without alteration in the pathophysiologic conditions within the portal venous system. With increased portal venous pressure, changes in venous blood flow patterns occur. Significant variation in the position of veins has an impact on the segment of bowel that develops acquired venous abnormalities. Whereas the larger veins usually are located in the submucosa, occasionally they are located in the lamina propria. This situation is especially true at the junction

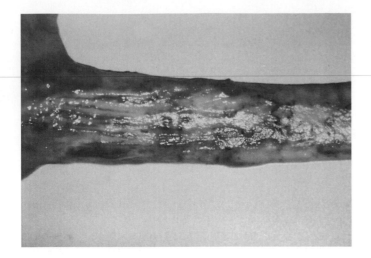

Figure 14.1 Esophageal varices. The dilated and tortuous veins are best demonstrated by turning the specimen inside out. (See color plate.)

of the esophagus and stomach. It is these areas that are thought to first manifest varices after an increase in portal venous pressure occurs.

ACQUIRED AND CONGENITAL VASCULAR MALFORMATIONS

Varices

ASSOCIATED WITH PORTAL HYPERTENSION OF HEPATIC ORIGIN

Pathophysiology

Varices are dilated veins, the result of increased pressure in vessels that are collateral connections between the portal and systemic venous circulation. Hayes et al. (13) point out that portal hypertension develops when the pressure in the portal venous system exceeds the normal range of 10 to 15 mm Hg, and becomes clinically important when portal venous pressure is above 15 mm Hg. The liver has a dual blood supply, receiving about 1 L/min through the hepatic portal vein and the hepatic artery. The hepatic portal vein supplies 75% of the hepatic blood flow. Functional interactions as well as anatomic connections occur between these two vascular systems. An increase in blood flow through one circuit produces an increase in vascular resistance in the other. The consequence of portal hypertension is the development of an abnormal collateral venous circulation between the portal and systemic venous systems.

Location

Esophagus   The anastomosis that is most important clinically is at the lower end of the esophagus (Fig. 14.1). Although several risk factors for bleeding from esophageal varices have been suggested, the reasons for variceal rupture and hemorrhage are not completely understood (14–16). Suggested risk factors include variceal size, portal pressure, variceal wall tension, and the severity of associated liver dysfunction (14).

The level of portal pressure does not correlate directly with the risk of initial bleeding but does correlate with the tendency to re-bleed. Measurement of the pressure within esophageal varices has been performed and has not been shown to be of benefit in evaluating the risk of bleeding. The role of variceal wall tension is also disputed and uncertain (14). Bleeding occurs in approximately one third of patients with varices (16).

Spence speculates that the lower esophagus is the site of varix formation because of a unique anatomic variation in the 2 to 5 cm above the esophagogastric junction (17). Here, the veins lie mainly in the lamina propria. In the stomach and proximal esophagus, the veins lie mainly within the submucosa. The close proximity of the veins in the esophagogastric junction to the lumen of the gastrointestinal tract with loss of structural support results in varix formation with increase in portal venous pressure (Fig. 14.2).

Esophageal varices are caused most frequently by portal hypertension associated with alcoholic cirrhosis. Varices ultimately develop in 90% of cirrhotic patients (16). Other causes of varices are discussed subsequently. Bleeding esophageal varices associated with alcoholic liver disease is a grave sign; greater than one third of these patients die soon after hospital admission for massive upper gastrointestinal hemorrhage (18).

Other Sites   Varices may develop at other sites in patients with portal hypertension. Using CT scanning, Cho and colleagues (19) identified patients with varices and cirrhosis and found the following frequencies of involvement: coronary veins of lesser omentum, 80%; esophageal, 45%; paraumbilical, 43%; abdominal wall, 30%; perisplenic, 30%; retrogastric, 27%; paraesophageal, 22%; omental, 20%; retroperitoneal-paravertebral, 18%; mesenteric, 10%; splenorenal, 10%; and gastrorenal, 7%. Varices other than those located in the esophagus are rarely associated with significant hemorrhage.

Portal hypertension may be so great that varices occur in the colon (Fig. 14.3), frequently on the right side of the colon. Rarely, the colonoscopist may be confronted with vascular malformations that appear to be varices but actually are capillary hemangiomas (20). A unique anastomosis between portal veins on the right side of the colon and the right ovarian veins has been documented (21). Although the majority of colonic varices occur in relation to portal hypertension, colonic varices occurring in families with no evidence of portal hypertension have been described in isolated reports (22). These occurrences may represent inherited venous dysplastic disorders.

An infrequent complication that occurs in patients with gastrointestinal stomas is the development of stomal varices. These patients have associated alcoholic or other forms of cirrhosis (23). Conservative treatment of the stomal varices appears to be most appropriate in these cases. Because the bleeding from the stomal varices frequently is mild, it may require only observation or adjustment of the stomal appliance.

ASSOCIATED WITH PORTAL HYPERTENSION OF EXTRAHEPATIC ORIGIN

Diseases other than cirrhosis cause varix formation. Included in this group are certain extrahepatic disorders associated with portal hypertension, specifically, thrombosis or cavernous transformation of the portal vein and schistosomiasis (24). These conditions may lead to the development of varices via increased portal blood pressure. The pattern and consequences of bleeding associated with varices secondary to extrahepatic portal hypertension are distinctly different from those in patients in whom the varices are the result of hepatic disease. Recurrent bleeding episodes are common. Although the incidence of recurrent bleeding is high, the incidence of exsanguination as a consequence of initial or recurrent bleeding varices is low. There is a reasonable success rate with treatment by classic shunting procedures, in children 5 years of age and older and in adults, and a negligible increase in true encephalopathy. In addition to portal vein thrombosis, splenic vein thrombosis can also lead to generalized portal hypertension (25). Hepatic vein thrombosis and pyleophlebitis are additional causes of varices.

In diseases other than alcoholic cirrhosis, the development of portal hypertension may occur in a segmental fashion, with only isolated portions of the portal venous system being involved. This pattern is particularly well documented in patients that have ileal varices after surgery for ulcerative colitis (26). Additional examples of segmental varices are those that occur in other unusual locations, such small intestinal varices occurring in sites of postoperative intestinal adhesions (27) in patients with portal hypertension. The bleeding points were traced to mucosal erosions over large submucosal varices within the bowel. Rarely, tumor invasion of specific areas of the colonic vasculature has also resulted in varix formation (28).

HEMORRHOIDS

The development of hemorrhoids may signal the presence of portal hypertension from both cirrhotic and noncirrhotic causes. A complete case evaluation is therefore necessary before hemorrhoid surgery is undertaken.

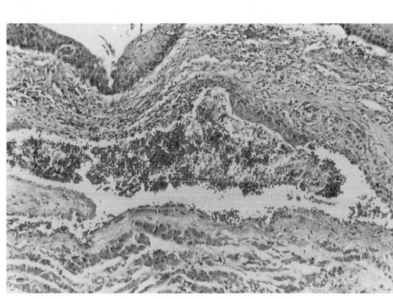

Figure 14.2 Esophageal varix, low-power photomicrograph. An unusually large dilated and congested vein is located immediately beneath the epithelium (×40).

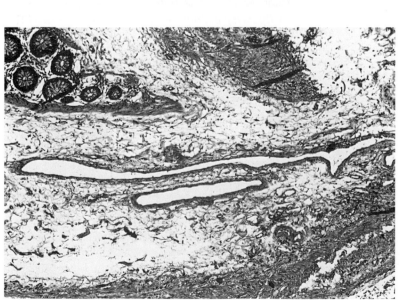

Figure 14.3 Colon varix. The vein in the submucosa collapsed during dissection (×20).

VASCULAR ABNORMALITIES OF THE GASTROINTESTINAL TRACT

CLASSIFICATION

Vascular anomalies affecting the gastrointestinal tract are extraordinarily rare (29), with estimated rates of incidence of 1 in 14,000 individuals. A great deal of confusion has been generated over this subject because of the lack of a consistent and uniform classification for these lesions. Developments in radiology over the last two decades have further confused the picture by the introduction of radiologic terms to lesions that may represent one or more pathologic entities. Camilleri et al. have proposed a new classification of vascular anomalies of the intestine (29).

For the sake of clinical utility, an even simpler classification could be used clinically. Such a classification is proposed (Table 14.1). The latter classification is similar to that proposed by Moore et al. in 1976 (30).

The majority of vascular malformations of the gastrointestinal tract fall into two main groups: angiodysplasias or telangiectasias. Hemangiomas are discussed subsequently, as well as in Chapter 18.

ARTERIOVENOUS MALFORMATIONS

Angiodysplasia

Vascular ectasias occur most frequently on the right side of the colon. They are also referred to, regrettably, as angiomas (31). They are all arteriovenous malformations (Fig. 14.4). These lesions are usually irregularly shaped clusters of ectatic small arteries, small

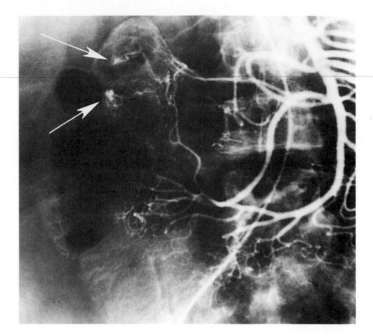

Figure 14.4   Angiogram of angiodysplasia of the colon. Note two tuft-like collections of contrast media *(arrows)* as well as prominent early draining veins in the hepatic flexure. (Reprinted with permission from Johnsrude IS, Jackson DC. A practical approach to angiography, 2nd ed. Boston: Little, Brown, 1987.)

TABLE 14.1	Proposed Classification of Vascular Abnormalities of the Gastrointestinal Tract

Malformations
  Arteriovenous malformations
  Telangiectasia
    Acquired
      Calcinosis-Raynaud-sclerodactyly-telangiectasia (CRST) syndrome
    Hereditary
      Hereditary hemorrhagic telangiectasia (Osler-Weber-Rendu)
      Turner syndrome
Disorders of connective tissue affecting blood vessels
  Pseudoxanthoma elasticum
  Ehlers-Danlos syndrome
Hemangioma
  Capillary hemangioma
  Cavernous hemangioma—single or diffuse
  Mixed capillary—cavernous hemangioma
  Diffuse intestinal hemangiomatosis
  Universal (miliary) hemangiomatosis
  Blue rubber bleb nevus syndrome
  Peutz-Jegher syndrome
  Klippel-Trenaunay-Weber syndrome
Angiosarcoma and Kaposi's sarcoma

veins, and their capillary connections. They are multiple, rather than single, and usually are less than 5 mm in diameter (Fig. 14.5). Microscopically, angiodysplastic lesions are dilated, distorted, thin-walled vessels (small arteries, capillaries, and veins) (Fig. 14.6). The amount of smooth muscle in the vessel wall is quite variable. The vessel wall can become so thinned that it appears to be composed only of endothelium. Elastic tissue stains may demonstrate the loss of elastic tissue in small arteries as they become incorporated into the ectatic mass (Fig. 14.7). Markedly dilated submucosal vasculature is the most consistent abnormality and presumably the earliest change identified. More advanced lesions involve the mucosa (32).

Because the major portion of the lesion is often submucosal, endoscopic mucosal biopsies are often not diagnostic. Characteristic histopathologic findings of angiodysplasia are only identified in 31 to 60% of endoscopically obtained biopsies. As a result of the low diagnostic yield and the risk of inducing hemorrhage, mucosal biopsy is not generally recommended for the purpose of diagnosis (33).

Angiodysplastic lesions are found most frequently on the right side of the colon, i.e., the cecum and ascending colon, in elderly patients. Lesions occur with less frequency in the jejunum and stomach and may be the cause of bleeding at these sites in younger patients, including adolescents (34). They are not associated with angiomatous lesions of the skin or other viscera. In the past, hemorrhage in association with diverticulosis was thought to be the major cause of gastrointestinal hemorrhage in older patients (5). With the advent of selective gastrointestinal angiography, colonic angiodysplasia has gained a predominant role as the cause of lower gastrointestinal bleeding in the elderly (28). Angiodysplasias are probably the most frequent cause of recurrent lower gastrointestinal tract bleeding after age 60. Angiodysplastic lesions may present as acute colonic hemorrhage or, more often, as chronic blood loss, leading to iron deficiency anemia. Gastric lesions tend not to cause persistent hemorrhage after an initial bleed. Colonic angiodysplasia may be associated with aortic valve stenosis, but no other somatic features have been recognized.

Renal insufficiency appears more prevalent in patients with gastric angiodysplasia (34).

The etiology of angiodysplasia is unknown, but the lesions are considered degenerative lesions (35). One common speculation is

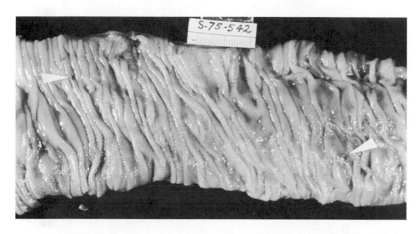

Figure 14.5   Segment of colon with two angiodysplastic lesions. Surface representation may be merely localized areas of discoloration *(arrows)*.

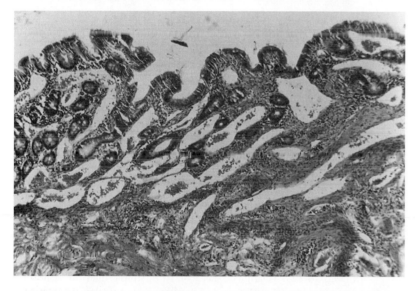

Figure 14.6   Histologic section of angiodysplasia of the colon. The abnormal vessels involve both the mucosa and the submucosa (×100).

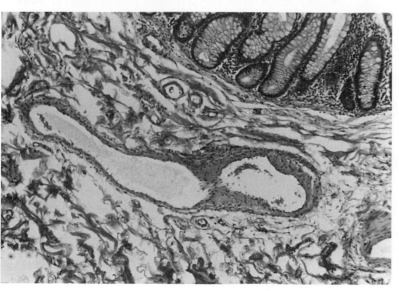

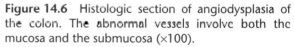

Figure 14.7   Arteriovenous malformation in the submucosa of colon of a patient with angiodysplasia. Elastic tissue stains can confirm the transition from artery to vein in many of these cases (×150).

that chronic intermittent increases in intraluminal pressure cause obstruction to the submucosal veins as they pierce the muscular layer of the bowel resulting in increased pressure within the vessels and consequent dilation (31). Angiography is the mainstay of diagnosis, although colonoscopic diagnosis (36, 37) with coagulation of the lesion is feasible. Angiodysplastic lesions cannot be detected by using air-contrast barium enemas. Controversy continues over the frequency of angiodysplastic lesions in the colon. Results of some studies indicate these lesions are common. Some reports document that as many as 25% of patients 60 years of age and older have these lesions and are without any evidence of bleeding (31, 35). Other studies deny finding these lesions in control patients (3). An excellent review of the clinical and pathologic features of angiodysplasia by Foutch was published in 1993 (33).

Submucosal Arteriovenous Malformation

Arteriovenous malformations may become rather large and remain localized to the submucosa (Figs. 14.8 to 14.11). These lesions, which rarely involve the muscular layer, may be a cause of significant gastrointestinal bleeding (6).

TELANGIECTASIA

Telangiectasia is a localized dilation of arterioles, capillaries, and venules. Multiple lesions may occur in the gastrointestinal tract in Osler-Weber-Rendu syndrome and Turner syndrome. Acquired lesions occur in the calcinosis-Raynaud-sclerodactyly-telangiectasia (CRST) syndrome.

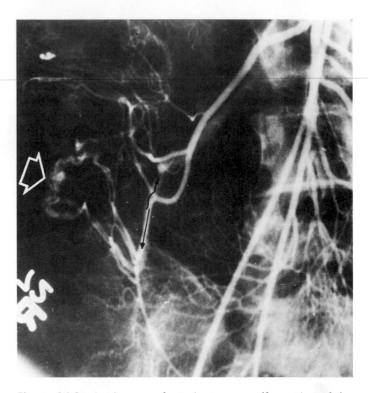

Figure 14.9   Angiogram of arteriovenous malformation of the cecum *(open arrow)*. The arterial branch is quite prominent *(straight arrow)* and premature venous return is present *(curved arrow)*. (Reprinted with permission from Johnsrude IS, Jackson DC. A practical approach to angiography, 2nd ed. Boston: Little, Brown, 1987.)

Congenital Lesions: Osler-Weber-Rendu Disease and Turner Syndrome

Hereditary hemorrhagic telangiectasia (Osler-Weber-Rendu disease) is inherited as an autosomal dominant disorder. These telangiectasias occur in many places including the skin, mucous membranes, and internal organs, resulting in recurrent hemorrhage (Fig. 14.12). Telangiectasias arise from simple dilation of normal vascular structures because of congenital thinning of the muscular coat and/or elastic fibers in the arteriolar walls. The vascular lesions may be stellate or nodular. They are punctate, red to purple, noncompressible, and vary in diameter from 1 to 4 mm. The mucocutaneous lesions usually become clinically apparent in the second and third decades of life. An early symptom is epistaxis, which can occur in childhood. Gastrointestinal bleeding occurs in about 15% of patients. It is usually chronic and manifests later in life, usually in the fourth decade. It should be noted that vascular anomalies also occur in other organs: the meninges, spinal cord, eye, liver, and genitourinary tract. Arteriovenous malformations also occur in this disease. Fibrosis and atypical cirrhosis of the liver have been reported in these patients (38). Hemorrhagic defects are also associated with Osler-Weber-Rendu syndrome (39).

Turner syndrome (ovarian dysgenesis) is associated with gastrointestinal hemorrhage from telangiectasia that may be found throughout the small and large bowel and mesentery but occurs most frequently in the small intestine. These vascular lesions tend to regress spontaneously; therefore, a conservative approach is generally warranted (29).

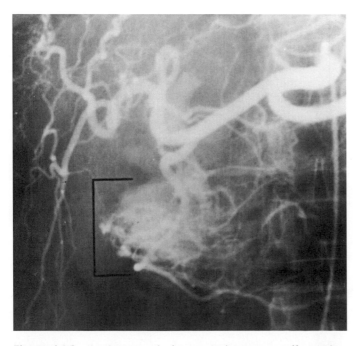

Figure 14.8   Angiogram of a large arteriovenous malformation of the duodenum. (Reprinted with permission from Johnsrude IS, Jackson DC. A practical approach to angiography, 2nd ed. Boston: Little, Brown, 1987.)

Acquired Lesions: CRST Syndrome

Telangiectasias are also present in systemic sclerosis, especially the calcinosis-Raynaud-sclerodactyly-telangiectasia (CRST) variant. Lesions arise most frequently found on the hands, lips, face, and tongue. Gastrointestinal hemorrhage may result from telangiectasias located in the stomach, rectum, and colon (29). Frequently,

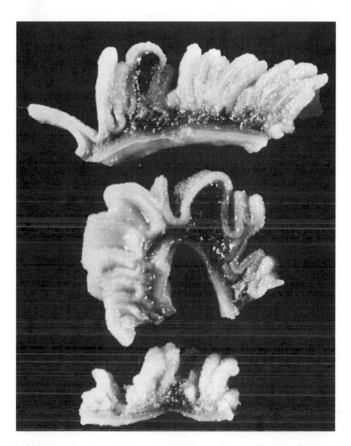

Figure 14.10 Arteriovenous malformation of the small bowel. This vascular lesion was predominantly in the submucosa.

endoscopy with electrocoagulation, heater probe, or Nd:YAG laser can adequately treat these lesions.

DISORDERS OF CONNECTIVE TISSUE AFFECTING BLOOD VESSELS

Pseudoxanthoma Elasticum

Pseudoxanthoma elasticum is associated with marked clinical variability, attributable to genetic heterogeneity. This disorder is thought to occur because of deranged elastin metabolism, affecting many tissues, including the heart, kidneys, skin, mucosa, eyes, and blood vessels in the gastrointestinal tract. Hemorrhage, the most frequent finding in individuals with gut involvement, may occur in childhood. Bleeding from the stomach is frequent and is the result of spontaneous vascular rupture. Failure of calcified vessels to contract after injury may prolong the hemorrhagic episode. The gastric and rectal mucosa has a characteristic endoscopic appearance. Angiography demonstrates abnormal tortuous, narrowed mesenteric vessels and vascular malformations within the gastrointestinal tract (29).

Ehlers-Danlos Syndrome

The Ehlers-Danlos syndrome is another group of disorders characterized by marked variation in severity because of genetic heterogeneity. These patients have defective collagen synthesis. The gastrointestinal involvement includes spontaneous rupture of arteries in the gastrointestinal tract and dilation of the bowel wall at all levels of the gastrointestinal tract. Hemorrhage from the gastrointestinal tract can also result from hiatal hernia or peptic ulceration (29).

UNCOMMON VASCULAR LESIONS

Congenital Arteriovenous Malformations

Congenital arteriovenous malformations occur anywhere in the body and have been reported to occur in the colon (31). Gastric malformations (Dieulafoy disease) is another rare condition in which massive gastric hemorrhage can occur (40). Dieulafoy disease

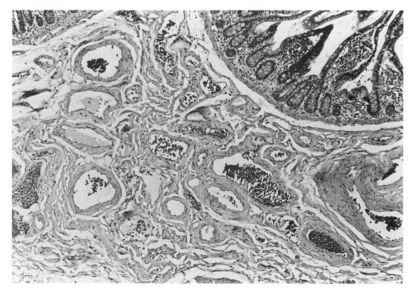

Figure 14.11 Photomicrograph of the arteriovenous malformation of the small bowel shown in Figure 14.10. Distinctly abnormal vascular complex composed of moderate-sized arteries and veins is present in the submucosa. Many of the vessels are ectatic and filled with blood. Elastic tissue stains demonstrate the transition from arteries to veins (×40).

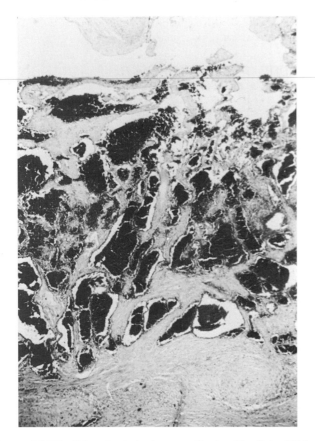

Figure 14.12 Telangiectasia in a patient with Osler-Weber-Rendu disease. The vessels are lined by endothelium and are quite dilated. Hyalinized material is present between the vascular spaces (×40).

is characterized by an unusually large tortuous artery that courses through the submucosa (41). This condition typically occurs in middle-aged and elderly men, although younger men and women can be affected. Reilly and Al-Kawas recently reviewed and discussed the diagnosis and management of 177 cases of upper gastrointestinal hemorrhage due to Dieulafoy lesion (42) (see Chapter 23 for further details).

Aneurysms

Aneurysms can occur in the human gastrointestinal tract. They are rare and usually involve the small bowel (Fig. 14.13).

Gastric Antral Vascular Ectasia

Gastric antral vascular ectasia presents a unique picture to the endoscopist or pathologist at gross examination because of nearly parallel red stripes traversing the top of the mucosal folds of the gastric antrum. Because of this unique pattern, the lesion was referred to as "watermelon stomach" by Jabbari and colleagues (43). In a study of 45 patients with watermelon stomach, Gostout et al. demonstrated the following: 71% were women; the average age was 73 years; 89% of patients presented with occult gastrointestinal bleeding and 62% were transfusion dependent; 62%

of patients had associated autoimmune connective tissue disorders; and 18% had associated liver disease (44). Histologically, gastric antral vascular ectasia is characterized by dilated mucosal capillaries, mucosal capillary thrombosis, and mucosal fibromuscular hyperplasia, often with hyalinization (45). Gastric antral vascular ectasia is clinically and pathologically similar to portal hypertensive gastropathy, but distinction of these two entities has important therapeutic implications (46). Both entities are associated with mucosal hemorrhage, occult blood loss, and liver disease. Distinguishing features include the striped distribution of mucosal hemorrhage in gastric antral vascular ectasia in contract to portal hypertensive gastropathy. The proximal stomach is usually affected in a portal hypertensive gastropathy, whereas the antrum is usually affected in gastric antral vascular ectasia. The submucosal vasculature is most commonly dilated in portal hypertensive gastropathy, whereas the mucosal vasculature is abnormal in gastric antral vascular ectasia (46).

TUMORS AND TUMOR-LIKE PROLIFERATIONS OF VESSELS

HEMANGIOMAS

CLASSIFICATION, PATHOLOGY, AND LOCATION

Whether hemangiomas found in the gastrointestinal tract are true neoplasms or represent hamartomas continues to be a subject for debate. (This issue is not addressed in this discussion.) Hemangiomas are usually classified into three types: cavernous, capillary, or mixed. Most hemangiomas are small, varying in size from a few millimeters to 1 to 2 cm, although larger lesions do occur. Bleeding from these lesions is usually slow, producing anemia or melena from occult blood loss. Rarely, large hemangiomas cause massive hemorrhage. Grossly, the large hemangiomas are usually polypoid or moundlike, reddish purple lesions seen through the mucosa. Histologically, numerous dilated, irregular blood-filled spaces within the mucosa and submucosa are encountered (Figs. 14.14 and 14.15). Occasionally, these lesions extend through the muscular layer into the serosal surface. As would be expected, the channels are lined by flat endothelial cells.

Intestinal hemangiomas are rare and not hereditary. They account for about 10% of all benign small-intestinal tumors. The majority of hemangiomas are solitary localized lesions; approximately 40% of cases involve multiple lesions. Most hemangiomas of the small bowel occur in the jejunum and ileum (29). Capillary hemangiomas are usually single lesions. Cavernous hemangiomas can often give the appearance of varices, especially in the colon (20); cavernous hemangiomas occasionally occur in the anus (47). Histologic confirmation of hemangiomas using tissue obtained by mucosal biopsy is often difficult because of the amount of hemorrhage that may occur with this procedure. Therefore, the appearance during endoscopy takes on even greater importance (48). Hemangiomas of the stomach (49) and of the esophagus (50–52) have also been reported, but they arise infrequently.

A unique form of colonic hemangioma is the cavernous hemangioma of the rectum. This lesion usually is not associated with other gastrointestinal hemangiomas, but it may be extensive, involving the entire rectum or portion of the rectosigmoid (31).

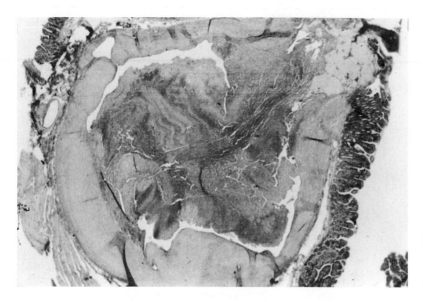

Figure 14.13 Aneurysm of the small bowel. Aneurysm formation of the gastrointestinal tract is extraordinarily rare but appears to have a predilection for the small bowel (×10).

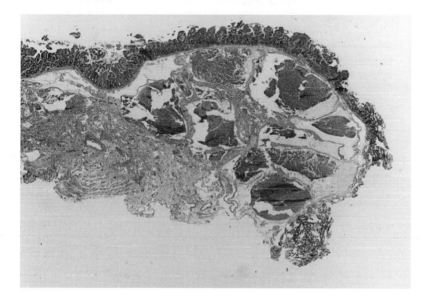

Figure 14.14 Submucosal cavernous hemangioma of the small bowel. Many thin-walled, dilated, blood filled vessels are present within the submucosa (×10).

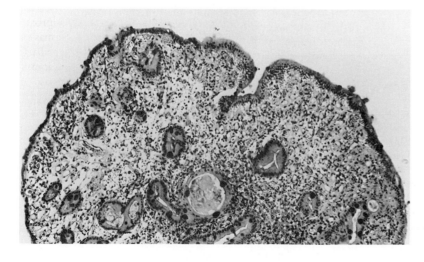

Figure 14.15 Capillary hemangioma of the large bowel. This lesion was identified as a "polyp" endoscopically. Microscopically, the mucosa is expanded by numerous small, blood-filled vessels (×100).

SYNDROMES INVOLVING GASTROINTESTINAL HEMANGIOMAS

Diffuse Intestinal Hemangiomatosis

Diffuse intestinal hemangiomatosis is an entity in which as many as 100 lesions involving the stomach, small bowel, and colon are encountered. Bleeding or anemia in childhood usually leads to the diagnosis of these conditions. Patients often present with hemangiomas of the skin and soft tissue of the head and neck, and the gastrointestinal hemangiomas may be large enough to cause intussusception (31). In diffuse neonatal hemangiomatosis, angiography is probably the most reliable means of detecting the lesion (53).

Universal (Miliary) Hemangiomatosis

This extraordinarily rare syndrome, which usually is fatal in infancy, is associated with hundreds of hemangiomas involving all organs (31).

Blue Rubber Bleb Nevus Syndrome

The blue rubber bleb nevus syndrome (cutaneous and intestinal cavernous hemangioma) was recognized in the last century because of the association of cutaneous vascular nevi, intestinal lesions, and gastrointestinal bleeding. The lesions in this syndrome are unique. The hemangiomas vary in diameter from 0.1 to 5.0 cm, are blue and raised, and have a wrinkled surface. Direct pressure on the lesion causes emptying of the blood, leaving a wrinkled sac. These lesions occur most frequently in the small bowel but may be present in any part of the gastrointestinal tract. In the colon, they typically arise on the left side and in the rectum. Microscopically, they are cavernous hemangiomas (29, 31).

Peutz-Jegher Syndrome

In this syndrome, intestinal hemangiomas without the presence of intestinal polyps has been reported. These cases are thought to represent incomplete penetrance of the gene responsible for the syndrome (29).

Klippel-Trenaunay-Weber Syndrome

This sporadic disorder of children and young adults is characterized by soft tissue and bony hypertrophy, varicose veins, and port wine hemangiomas, which may be unilateral; it is not an inherited disorder. Klippel-Trenaunay-Weber syndrome is accompanied by atresia, hypoplasia, or obstruction of the deep venous system. Involvement of the gastrointestinal tract is manifest by vascular malformations of the mixed or cavernous hemangioma type (29, 54).

MALIGNANT VASCULAR TUMORS

Kaposi sarcoma and angiosarcoma are the two malignant lesions usually associated with the vasculature. The occurrence of angiosarcoma within the gastrointestinal tract is rare. Although involvement of the gastrointestinal tract by Kaposi sarcoma is also rare, it is a common finding in patients with acquired immunodeficiency syndrome (AIDS).

KAPOSI SARCOMA

Kaposi sarcoma develops in 20 to 30% of all AIDS patients (55) and is seen almost exclusively in homosexual men with AIDS (56). The incidence of Kaposi sarcoma in HIV/AIDS patients is estimated to be at least 20,000 times that of the general population (57). In studies of 33 and 50 patients with AIDS and Kaposi sarcoma, 51% and 40%, respectively, had lesions consistent with gastrointestinal involvement identified during endoscopy of the upper gastrointestinal tract and/or flexible sigmoidoscopy (58, 59). In these studies, endoscopically visualized lesions were histopathologically positive for Kaposi sarcoma in only 41% and 23% of cases, respectively. The low yield of mucosal biopsy is likely attributable to a submucosal location of the tumor. In an endoscopic study of Mediterranean Kaposi sarcoma, a type of non-AIDS associated Kaposi sarcoma, 82% of affected patients had gastric involvement (60). In an autopsy study of HIV-infected patients, 86% of patients with Kaposi sarcoma had gastrointestinal involvement (61). Although gastrointestinal involvement by Kaposi sarcoma in AIDS patients is relatively common, morbidity is low, with 80% of lesions remaining clinically silent (58). Although patients with gastrointestinal Kaposi sarcoma have a significantly worse prognosis than those patients without gastrointestinal involvement, the less favorable prognosis is secondary to an overall greater decrease in immunity rather than a direct effect of the Kaposi sarcoma (56, 58).

At endoscopy, the lesions of Kaposi sarcoma have been described as macular, angiodysplastic with a uniform appearance, polypoid, volcano-like, and maculopapular (62). Histologically, Kaposi sarcoma is composed of neoplastic spindle cells in which erythrocytes are incorporated within "vascular" clefts between the cells. Hemorrhage and hemosiderin may be present. Intracytoplasmic eosinophilic hyaline globules can often be identified (Fig. 14.16). The small bowel is affected more frequently than the colon, rectum, or stomach (63, 64).

PRIMARY ANGIOSARCOMA

Primary angiosarcomas of the gastrointestinal tract are rare. Angiosarcoma has been reported to occur following irradiation, most frequently involving the terminal ileum (65, 66).

LYMPHANGIOMAS

Lymphangiomas of the gastrointestinal tract are also extremely rare. They usually present as submucosal polypoid lesions with cystically dilated lymph vessels seen on microscopic examination (67). By colonoscopy, they appear as smooth, soft polypoid lesions on a broad base (68). Lymphangiomas have also been reported in the esophagus (69), stomach, and jejunum (70). They seem to appear more frequently in the small intestine than in the large intestine, although they occasionally are encountered in the colon as a result of barium enema examination.

VASCULITIS

GENERAL CONSIDERATIONS

No subject is more confusing and challenging than vasculitis. Review of the extensive amount of literature on this subject may add credence to the hypothesis that the amount written about an entity

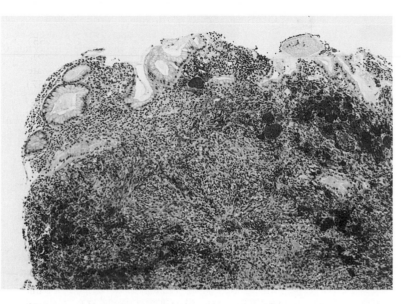

Figure 14.16 Kaposi sarcoma of the stomach. A spindle cell proliferation with blood-filled spaces and hemorrhage fills the submucosa and focally extends into the mucosa (×100).

is inversely correlated with the amount that is actually known about that entity. Much confusion surrounding the topic of vasculitis is attributable to the lack of a uniformly accepted classification system for this group of diseases. Without such a system, different names have been given to the same disease and the same name has been given to different diseases by various investigators. Some classifications are based on the size of the predominant vessel involved; other classifications are based on the most serious clinical expression, that is, the predominant site or location when a variety of vessels are involved. Some of the difficulty in classification of the vasculitides stems from significant overlap in clinical manifestations of each of these diseases. In addition, the pathogenesis of the vasculitides is also incompletely understood. Significant advances in knowledge about this group of diseases, however, such as the discovery of antineutrophil cytoplasmic autoantibodies (ANCA), contribute to the understanding and possibly classification of this group of diseases. As a result, multiple classification systems have been proposed (71–75), each with its strengths and weaknesses and its proponents and opponents. In an attempt to standardize classification nomenclature, an international consensus conference was held in Chapel Hill, North Carolina (76). At this conference, the major categories of vasculitis were named and defined. This classification system, although well accepted, also has its weaknesses, which have been pointed out by multiple investigators (71, 77, 78).

Any discussion of vasculitis would not be complete without at least a brief consideration of antineutrophil cytoplasmic autoantibodies (ANCA). ANCA is a heterogeneous group of autoantibodies targeting antigens in neutrophils, monocytes, and endothelial cells (79). ANCA are typically identified by indirect immunofluorescence. Two major patterns of positivity are observed: cytoplasmic or cANCA and perinuclear or pANCA. cANCA are directed against proteinase 3 in about 90% of cases, whereas pANCA is directed against myeloperoxidase in about 40% of cases (80). Proteinase 3 and myeloperoxidase are present in neutrophil and monocyte lysosomes. Both cANCA and pANCA are significantly associated with vasculitis. The specificity of cANCA for biopsy-proven Wegener granulomatosis is approximately 90%. The sensitivity depends on the extent and activity of the disease; the sensitivity is

approximately 50% for patients in the initial phase of Wegener granulomatosis and close to 100% for patients with active generalized disease (80). Myeloperoxidase ANCA is associated with microscopic polyarteritis and Churg-Strauss syndrome. Sixty percent of patients with microscopic polyarteritis have myeloperoxidase ANCA (80) and 75% of patients with Churg-Strauss syndrome have this autoantibody (81). ANCA may play a major role in the pathogenesis of some cases of vasculitis and many theories relative to the specific pathogenic mechanisms of ANCA in vasculitis have been suggested (79–83).

Systemic vasculitis predominantly involves skin, muscle, peripheral nervous tissue, and kidneys. Approximately 25% of patients with systemic vasculitis have gastrointestinal involvement, characterized clinically by abdominal pain, diarrhea, hemorrhage, and occasionally intestinal perforation (84).

The fundamental pathologic consequence of vasculitis is ischemia to the area supplied by the involved vasculature. If the vessels of the mucosa and submucosa are affected, then there is mucosal ischemia with erosions, ulceration, transmural infarction, and ultimately perforation.

Pneumatosis intestinalis has been associated with almost all diseases caused by vasculitis that affect the gastrointestinal tract. With the loss of mucosal integrity, enteric organisms gain access to the bowel wall (85). The etiology of the vasculitic process is based on clinical as well as histologic data. The histologic response, however, can be a guide in establishing the diagnosis.

HISTOLOGIC FEATURES AND DIFFERENTIAL DIAGNOSIS

Diseases that affect the gastrointestinal tract and are associated with involvement of the vessels by a vasculitic process are listed in Table 14.2.

Polyarteritis nodosa is characterized by acute inflammation and fibrinoid necrosis of the medium-sized and small arteries. In this disorder, lesions are found in all stages of development.

In the Churg-Strauss syndrome, characteristic features include necrotizing vasculitis of small arteries and veins with extravascular

TABLE	
14.2	Diseases with Vasculitic Processes That Affect the Gastrointestinal Tract

Polyarteritis nodosa
Churg-Strauss syndrome
Henoch-Schönlein purpura
Systemic lupus erythematosus
Rheumatoid disease
Wegener granulomatosis
Hemolytic-uremic syndrome
Enterocolic lymphocytic phlebitis

granulomas and infiltration of the vessels and perivascular tissue with eosinophils.

The distinction, microscopically, between classic polyarteritis nodosa and Churg-Strauss syndrome depends on the size of the vessel involved. In polyarteritis nodosa, the vessels involved are usually medium-sized and small arteries, whereas in Churg-Strauss, the involved vessels are small arteries and veins. In polyarteritis nodosa, the cellular infiltrate is predominantly neutrophilic leukocytes; eosinophils predominate in Churg-Strauss syndrome.

Henoch-Schönlein purpura is an example of hypersensitivity vasculitis involving predominantly the small arterioles and capillaries in children. Deposition of immunoglobulins, predominantly IgA, complement components, and fibrin have been noted in involved vessels in the gastrointestinal tract.

Severe necrotizing vasculitis affecting the small and medium-sized arteries of the submucosa is frequently encountered in individuals with systemic lupus erythematosus. Fibrinoid necrosis occurs; and the inflammatory infiltrate, although perivascular, is composed of both neutrophils and eosinophils.

Vasculitis is a common manifestation in rheumatoid disease. Small arteries and arterioles are involved in Wegener granulomatosis. Histologically, the coagulative or liquefactive necrotizing epithelioid granulomas in Wegener granulomatosis differ morphologically from the more fibrinoid necrotizing (allergic) epithelioid and eosinophilic granulomas seen in Churg-Strauss syndrome. The diagnosis is made by finding characteristic histologic lesions in the small arteries and veins. The involved vessel, often located adjacent to the granuloma, undergoes fibrinoid necrosis with mononuclear cell infiltration.

DIAGNOSTIC UTILITY OF MUCOSAL BIOPSY AND OTHER STUDIES

It is often difficult to make the diagnosis of vasculitis on the basis of mucosal biopsy (86) (Fig. 14.17). It is possible, however, to document necrotizing arteritis when the biopsy sampling is deep enough to include portions of the submucosa (Fig. 14.18). Necrotizing vasculitis affects the bowel in polyarteritis, lupus erythematosus, rheumatoid arthritis and Henoch-Schönlein purpura. Typical findings include involvement of the small arteries or veins in the wall with patchy necrosis and inflammation of the overlying mucosa. Smaller biopsy samples may be too superficial to demonstrate the

vasculitis. Patients with hemolytic uremic syndrome may have focal areas of significant mucosal edema and hemorrhage that are even evident on gross endoscopic examination. In hypersensitivity angiitis, bowel biopsy, of both large and small intestines, demonstrates extravascular tubercular granulomas without necrosis.

The use of ^{111}In-granulocyte scanning may provide significant additional information when studying the involvement of the gastrointestinal tract by collagen vascular disease (87). This procedure, although not used commonly, helps to establish the diagnosis of gastrointestinal vasculitis.

VASCULITIC LESIONS IN THE GASTROINTESTINAL TRACT

POLYARTERITIS NODOSA

Polyarteritis nodosa causes a variety of changes in the gastrointestinal tract. Involvement of the mesenteric artery can lead to aneurysm formation and occasionally rupture with exsanguination (88). In polyarteritis nodosa, approximately two thirds of the patients have symptomatology referable to the gastrointestinal tract (89). The manifestations of gastrointestinal involvement all relate to the ischemia caused by occlusion of the affected vessels.

Frequently reported findings include mesenteric infarction with gut ischemia and perforation (90), necrotizing vasculitis of the gallbladder and appendix (91), gastrointestinal ulceration, intraluminal hemorrhage, perforation, and pyloric obstruction, with localized or diffuse gangrene (89). Polyarteritis nodosa can cause ulceration in any part of the gut, but the jejunum is affected most frequently (92). Ischemic colitis has been reported in association with polyarteritis nodosa (93, 94), the degree of involvement ranging from diffuse to quite isolated and specific (95).

SYSTEMIC LUPUS ERYTHEMATOSUS

Systemic lupus eryhtematosus is associated with a variety of gastrointestinal manifestations; however, mesenteric arteritis and serositis occur frequently (96). Serositis occurs in 60 to 70% of patients with systemic lupus erythematosus. Serositis takes a variety of forms, including peritoneal inflammation, adhesions between bowel loops, perihepatitis, and perisplenitis. Small-vessel arteritis leads to involvement of the small bowel by lupus enteritis. Because of the difficulty in making this diagnosis, some cases have mistakenly been diagnosed as Crohn disease (97). In addition to lupus enteritis, lupus gastritis, ischemic colitis, and esophagitis have been reported (98). To further complicate the picture, arteritis of the mesenteric arteries has also been reported in association with lupus. Intestinal venulitis is thought to be a possible explanation for the protein-losing enteropathy seen in some of these patients (99). Considerable overlap occurs in the complications of systemic lupus erythematosus and polyarteritis as they affect the gastrointestinal tract (100).

RHEUMATOID ARTHRITIS

The vasculitis associated with rheumatoid arthritis can lead to involvement of the colon (101) with gastrointestinal bleeding, intraperitoneal bleeding, ischemic mucosal ulceration, small and large bowel infarction, and bowel perforation (102, 103). Occasionally, patients with rheumatoid arthritis develop a proliferative endarteritis, characterized by intimal proliferation without vessel wall necrosis or inflammation (103). The gastrointestinal manifestations of collagen vascular diseases were reviewed by Bassel and Harford (92).

HYPERSENSITIVITY ANGIITIS

Churg-Strauss Syndrome

The classic features of this syndrome are systemic vasculitis in the setting of bronchial asthma and eosinophilia. Although the lungs, peripheral nerves, and skin are most frequently involved, involvement of the gastrointestinal tract does occur (104–107). Gastrointestinal complications range from gastric ulceration to pseudopolyp formation in the colon.

Although some authors consider Churg-Strauss syndrome a distinct entity, others consider it a subdivision of polyarteritis nodosa. Necrotizing extravascular granulomas arc usually not seen in association with polyarteritis nodosa. A history of asthma is the rule in patients with Churg-Strauss syndrome, but asthma is encountered only infrequently in polyarteritis nodosa. Differentiating Churg-Strauss syndrome from Wegener granulomatosis also may be difficult. In this case, clinical history also plays a large role, because a history of asthma and allergic rhinitis is typical in Churg-Strauss syndrome and is noted infrequently in persons with Wegener granulomatosis.

Allergic Granulomatous Angiitis

Involvement of the bowel by allergic granulomatous angiitis has been reported (107). Part of this spectrum is the finding of eosinophilic infiltration in the gastrointestinal tract (108). This process can be diffuse or localized and perhaps, therefore, is a part of the disease spectrum of the Churg-Strauss syndrome. In the infiltrative form, the affected segment of bowel shows an ill-defined transmural thickening simulating intestinal lymphoma or Crohn

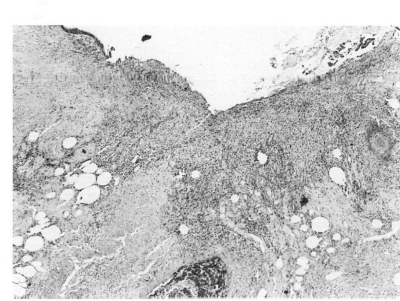

Figure 14.17   Base of colonic ulcer in a patient with periarteritis nodosa. The vessels with definitive vasculitis are present in the deeper portions of the ulcer (×20).

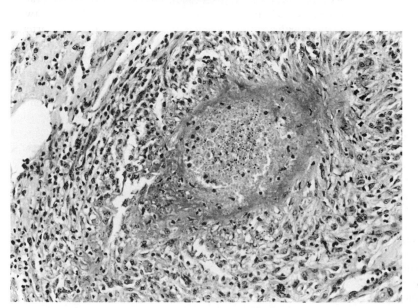

Figure 14.18   High-power view of the colon shown in Figure 14.17 demonstrates severe vasculitis and the development of fibrinoid necrosis in the wall as well as infiltration by a variety of inflammatory cells (×100).

disease. The lesions may be multiple. This process has been referred to as diffuse eosinophilic infiltration, eosinophilic gastroenteritis, and eosinophilic granuloma. In the circumscribed form, a well-delineated and polypoid mass can be encountered, commonly confined to the submucosa. This form is not associated with blood eosinophilia or an allergic history and is currently referred to as inflammatory fibroid polyp or eosinophilic granuloma. Controversy exists over whether these two presentations reflect two separate and unrelated conditions or are part of the same spectrum. The infiltrative form can be found in either the small or the large bowel. Microscopically, the hallmark of both presentations is an eosinophilic infiltrate admixed with a variety of chronic inflammatory cells, including plasma cells, lymphocytes, and histiocytes within a loose network of vascularized fibroblastic connective tissue. Granulomatous nodules occasionally are encountered. Omental nodules show the same histologic picture. See also Chapter 12 for further details.

HENOCH-SCHÖNLEIN PURPURA

Henoch-Schönlein purpura is characterized by a nontraumatic, nonthrombocytopenic hemorrhagic diathesis resulting in bleeding at the joints, skin, and viscera singly or in combination. Purpuric lesions can arise in the gastrointestinal tract; occasionally, intussusception of the ileum or ileocecal region has been associated with Henoch-Schönlein purpura (109). Superficial ulceration can occur with the development of a pseudomembrane. Although Henoch-Schönlein purpura may involve any portion of the gastrointestinal tract, the jejunum and ileum are affected most frequently. Complications include massive bleeding (110), intussusception, infarction with perforation (111), and chronic small-bowel obstruction. The primary lesion is found in the small arteries, arterioles, and capillaries. The colon is also involved in this disease (112).

On endoscopy, if the stomach is involved, coalescing erythematous lesions are encountered with large areas of purpura (113). Further studies in patients with Henoch-Schönlein purpura have documented the presence of IgA and C3 by immunofluorescence examination in the small-bowel (duodenum and proximal jejunum) blood vessels (114).

WEGENER GRANULOMATOSIS

Wegener granulomatosis is a disease of unknown etiology characterized by necrotizing granulomatous lesions of the upper or lower respiratory tract, vasculitis, and glomerulonephritis. Wegener granulomatosis rarely affects the gastrointestinal tract, although involvement in virtually all areas of the gastrointestinal tract has been reported (84, 115, 116). Clinically, patients with gastrointestinal involvement complain of a blood-stained mucous diarrhea. Gastrointestinal symptoms are responsive to appropriate therapy (116). Wegener reported an ulcerating necrotizing process in the ileum, colon, and rectum with marked edema and leukocyte infiltration in the submucosa. Hashikata and Nishioka (117) also reported multiple gastric ulcers occurring in association with Wegener granulomatosis. The process can progress to small bowel perforation (118) when intense necrotizing vasculitis is present (119). Occasionally, the process can be confused with ulcerative colitis (120, 121).

HEMOLYTIC-UREMIC SYNDROME

The hemolytic-uremic syndrome consists of microangiopathic hemolytic anemia, acute renal failure, and thrombocytopenia following a prodromal illness of gastroenteritis or upper respiratory infection. Signs and symptoms referable to the gastrointestinal tract, including abdominal pain, abdominal tenderness, or peritoneal signs, frequently herald the beginning of this syndrome. Symptoms can be so severe that patients undergo laparotomy. When the colon is resected, hemorrhagic infarction is usually encountered, with full-thickness hemorrhage and necrosis of the colon wall. Extensive fibrin thrombi and fibrinoid necrosis can be seen in the capillaries of the peritoneum and submucosa of the colon (122). In some cases, only the mucosa and submucosa are involved. Clinical presentations include bloody diarrhea or a pseudomembranous colitis-like picture (123). Currently, it is believed that the degree of gastrointestinal involvement in this syndrome is underestimated. Basically, two histologic forms occur in the colon: ischemic or pseudomembranous colitis. Some researchers think that ischemic colitis may precede the full development of hemolytic uremic syndrome (124). Late manifestations of the hemolytic-uremic syndrome include persistent colitis as well as bowel stenosis (125).

Hemolytic-uremic syndrome needs to be differentiated from appendicitis, ulcerative colitis, cecal polyp, pseudomembranous colitis, and intussusception (126–128). This disease entity may be due to a localized, Schwartzman-type of reaction with deposition of fibrin strands on the capillary endothelium (126).

ENTEROCOLIC LYMPHOCYTIC PHLEBITIS

Saraga and Costa (129) described this entity in three patients with intestinal ischemic necrosis and extensive lymphocytic phlebitis associated with thrombosis. Their patients presented with various clinical manifestations, including abdominal pain, nausea, vomiting, rectal bleeding, ileus, fever, and leukocytosis. Areas of ischemic necrosis were found in the small and large bowel. The lymphocytic phlebitis was characterized by marked and extensive venous lymphocytic infiltration with thrombosis and focal fibrinoid necrosis. Veins of all calibers were diseased, but submucosal venules were involved most conspicuously; the arteries were not diseased. None of these patients had evidence of systemic vasculitis. Follow-up ranged from 4 months to 5 years, with no recurrence necessitating re-operation. The etiology and pathogenesis of this entity are unknown.

ULCERATION OF THE STOMACH

Virtually all diseases thought to be caused by vasculitis have caused changes in the stomach that include erosions, stress ulcers, and peptic ulcer disease.

DIFFERENTIATION FROM OTHER DISEASES ASSOCIATED WITH VASCULITIS

A significant overlap exists when considering patients with rheumatoid disease and gastrointestinal symptoms and patients with such gastrointestinal diseases as ulcerative colitis and Crohn disease that also have arthritic symptoms (130). Rheumatoid disease is often associated with lesions in the gut, which are caused by arteritis. The arteritis can affect the alimentary tract at any point, resulting in erosion, ulceration, bleeding, perforation, infarction, and gangrene. Peptic ulcers are an extremely common finding; next in frequency are ischemic ulcers of the intestine, which can either bleed or perforate. If the lesions are of the larger arteries, segmental or extensive bowel gangrene can occur. Malabsorption also occurs in patients with rheumatoid arthritis.

Involvement of the gut in systemic lupus erythematosus occurs frequently, but less so than in polyarteritis nodosa. The lesions are again similar because of the arteritis that occurs. Ileus may occur along with an acute abdomen from bowel ischemia, infarction, or perforation. In lupus, an appendicitis-like picture or terminal ileitis that can mimic Crohn disease has been reported. Also, patients with systemic lupus erythematosus may manifest an ulcerative colitis-like condition.

The differential diagnostic picture is further complicated in that patients with systemic lupus erythematosus may be partially immunosuppressed. In this clinical setting, cytomegalovirus can cause mechanical occlusion of small vessels with ulceration of the overlying mucosa.

ISCHEMIC DISEASES

GENERAL CONSIDERATIONS

The focus of the following sections is on one of the more frequent causes of bowel disease, ischemia, and its most severe consequence, infarction. The principal causes of bowel ischemia are (a) occlusion of the arteries supplying an area, (b) occlusion of the veins supplying an area, and (c) low flow states in which a specific mechanical factor cannot be implicated or can be implicated only minimally.

PATHOPHYSIOLOGIC EFFECTS OF ISCHEMIA

Significant decrease in blood flow can elicit three types of responses in the human gastrointestinal tract. If the episode is transient, focal mucosal necrosis occurs, followed by restitution of tissue architecture. No significant loss of tissue is associated with this response. If the episode is of greater magnitude, the patient develops ulceration of the gastrointestinal tract but recovers from the acute episode with healing by fibrosis and resultant stricture formation, which usually develops 6 to 8 weeks after the initial episode. If the episode is severe, transmural infarction with perforation and peritonitis often results.

The pathophysiologic effects of ischemia depend on the severity of the episode, the length of time an effect lasts, and the amount of tissue involved. The episodes generally fall into two main categories: acute and chronic presentations. In the acute form, there is a dramatic loss of function of the segment of the gastrointestinal tract affected. Clinical signs and symptoms also mirror the acute nature of the insult. In the acute presentations, a single specific etiologic agent can usually be identified. In the chronic form, the changes in pathophysiology are more diffuse. In the more chronic forms, a variety of factors are all at work at the same time. In the older adult, atherosclerosis of vessels is frequently one of several factors that are at work concomitantly.

NOMENCLATURE AND CLASSIFICATION

Because transmural infarcts of the duodenum, stomach, and esophagus are rare, classifications usually relate only to infarcts of the small bowel and of the large intestine. Transmural infarcts of the small and large intestines are usually classified as follows: (a) those due to superior mesenteric artery occlusion; (b) those due to inferior mesenteric artery occlusion, mesenteric vein thrombosis, or arteritis; and (c) those due to nonocclusive causes (131).

A new classification has been proposed: (a) acute intestinal ischemia with either arterial occlusion or nonocclusion, (b) chronic arterial obstruction, and (c) focal ischemia of the small bowel or colon (132).

As with all ischemic processes, the metabolic needs of the organ are not being met by the blood supply with concomitant loss of function. With either classification, the literature relating to this subject is often listed under the topic of acute mesenteric ischemia (131).

GENERAL PATHOLOGY

Histologic consequences of ischemia are quite uniform, whatever the cause. The mucosa is the most sensitive to the ischemia because of its high oxygen demands. The mucosa responds with the usual response to any deprivation of oxygen supply, namely, increases in vascular permeability, edema formation, and concomitant coagulative necrosis with sloughing of the devitalized tissue. The earliest morphologic changes are seen just beneath the surface epithelium, where coagulation necrosis of the lamina propria occurs (Fig. 14.19). The vessels of the lamina propria become congested. In the small bowel, the earliest changes are seen in the lamina propria beneath the tip of the villus (133). The ischemic process is initially limited to the mucosa, where there is edema formation in the lamina propria and loss of integrity of the microvasculature of the lamina propria with extravasation of erythrocytes. Necrosis of the epithelium is readily apparent. These changes in the mucosa can be followed by similar changes in the submucosa, the muscular layer, and the serosa as the process extends into the wall of the bowel. If the process is sufficiently severe, transmural infarction occurs.

In the least severe forms of bowel ischemia, bloody diarrhea may be the only presenting symptom. In the more severe forms, abdominal pain and the presence of occult blood may herald the presence of the condition. In the most severe form, full-fledged signs and symptoms of tissue necrosis with perforation are usually present. Recent developments in angiography have significantly altered the natural history of the disease, because earlier diagnosis is the most important factor in lowering mortality. Angiography is also playing a therapeutic role, because it is the method by which vasodilating drugs are infused in an attempt to modify the degree of occlusion.

ETIOLOGY OF BOWEL INFARCTS

Acute occlusion of the superior mesenteric artery causes 50% of transmural gastrointestinal infarcts (98). Thrombosis and embolism are equally responsible for such occlusion (Fig. 14.20). The degree of revascularization after embolectomy, endarterectomy, or bypass graft is hard to estimate, even when using sophisticated studies such as fluorescein injection and Doppler monitoring. Second-look operations are often planned for 12 to 24 hours after definitive surgery.

Twenty-five percent of all bowel infarcts are attributable to occlusion of the inferior mesenteric artery, mesenteric vein throm-

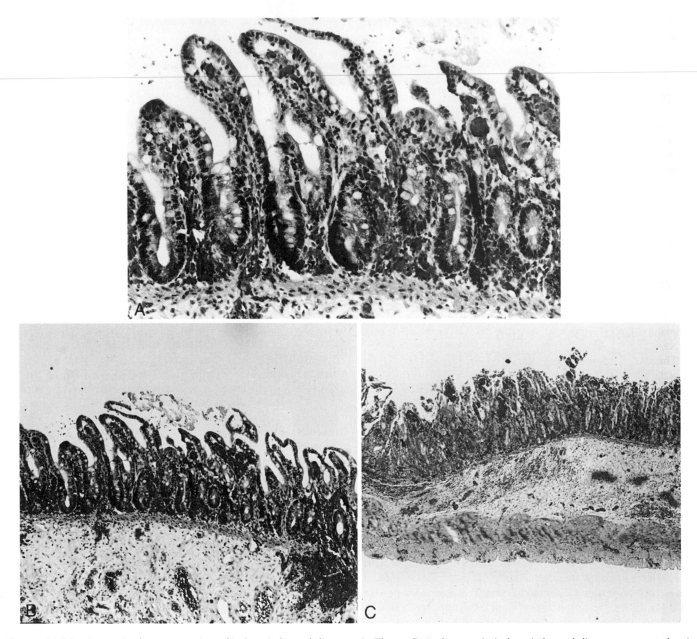

Figure 14.19   Stages in the progression of ischemic bowel disease. **A,** The earliest changes in ischemic bowel disease occur at the tip of the villus, just beneath the epithelium. The vessels become congested, the adjacent lamina propria develops edema, and erythrocytes extravasate into the lamina propria (×100). **B,** With early necrosis of the mucosal layer, the submucosa becomes edematous and the vasculature becomes congested (×40). **C,** Later stage in ischemic bowel disease. The mucosa and superficial submucosa are necrotic and beginning to slough. The remainder of the wall of the gastrointestinal tract is edematous, congested, and undergoing the earliest stages of necrosis (×20).

bosis, or arteritis. Occlusion of the inferior mesenteric artery rarely leads to colonic infarction when it is on an atherosclerotic basis. Most cases of infarction have followed ligation for aortic aneurysm surgery.

A variety of factors may cause thrombosis or compression of the superior mesenteric vein. One of the most frequent is a portion of the bowel becoming incorporated into an irreducible hernia (Fig. 14.21). Extension of a thrombus from the portal vein,

especially with rapidly enlarging hepatic tumors, can also cause venous infarcts. In many cases, however, no specific predisposing cause is found.

Nonocclusive infarction accounts for 25% of the infarcts of the small and large bowel. The pathogenesis of infarction without occlusion is more complicated than that associated with occlusion. Although this process affects small and large bowel, it can also cause similar changes in the upper gastrointestinal tract. These pathologic lesions are often grouped under the heading of ischemic bowel disease.

ISCHEMIC BOWEL DISEASE

SPECTRUM AND CLINICAL FEATURES

In recent studies, investigators have continued to define the concept and clarified the spectrum of ischemic bowel disease. Ischemic bowel disease results from a sequence of changes after anoxia. The etiology is multifactorial, involving the state of the vessels, the duration of the anoxic or hypoxic episode, and the virulence of bacteria located in the lumen of the affected gastrointestinal tract (133).

Profound changes occur in the hemodynamics of the bowel wall. Complete occlusion is usually absent and thromboembolic phenomena are seen only rarely. Ischemic bowel disease affects any age group and can be found in any area of the gastrointestinal tract. The pathogenesis of this lesion depends on supplying enough blood to prevent complete death of the involved segment but insufficient blood flow to meet the metabolic needs of the injured bowel. After necrosis, there is bacterial invasion as the mucosal barrier becomes ineffective.

The basic pathologic response is coagulative necrosis. The mucosal layer, the layer of the gastrointestinal tract most susceptible to anoxia, is affected first. The spectrum of ischemic bowel disease includes the entities listed in Table 14.3.

The clinical picture in chronic arterial obstruction is extraordinarily complex. The disease itself is rare (134, 135). Postprandial pain, weight loss, and disturbances of bowel habits do not occur in all cases. What is well accepted, however, is that when significant atherosclerosis is present in the vessels supplying the gastrointestinal tract, severe atherosclerosis also affects many other organs.

The small bowel has better collateral circulation than the large bowel. Hence, focal ischemia in the large intestine is encountered more frequently. Initial studies of patients with intestinal arterial occlusion have shown that no relationship exists between intestinal

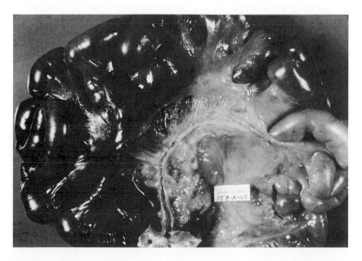

Figure 14.20 Infarct of the small bowel. Severe atherosclerosis is present around the orifice of the superior mesenteric artery *(bottom center).*

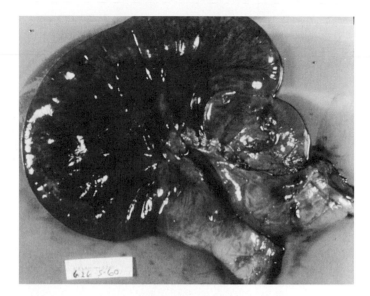

Figure 14.21 Venous infarct of the small bowel caused by an adhesive band. The venous portion of the vasculature is affected first. Significant congestion occurs before the arterial blood supply is compromised.

TABLE	
14.3	**Entities of Ischemic Bowel Disease**

Ischemic colitis
Necrotizing enterocolitis of the premature infant
Hemorrhagic necrosis of the gastrointestinal tract
Pseudomembranous enterocolitis
Staphylococcal enterocolitis
Radiation enterocolitis, delayed form
Uremic colitis
Potassium-induced stenotic ulcer
Stress ulceration
Atheroembolic injury

performance when studied by measuring insorptive and exsorptive functions and the degree of potential chronic ischemia suggested by angiographic findings (136). Results of later studies showed that a decrease in the intramural pH below the usual pH of 6.86 is a good indicator of early colonic ischemia (137). The symptomatology, diagnosis, and therapy of ischemic intestinal syndromes have been extensively reviewed (134, 135).

EXPERIMENTAL STUDIES

Most of our knowledge of intestinal blood flow has been obtained from invasive techniques used in a variety of experimental models and rarely in man. With invasive techniques, total blood flow to the small intestine is estimated to be 500 to 600 ml/min. The need for a noninvasive clinical method of measuring intestinal blood flow

(138) was met by the development of transcutaneous Doppler ultrasound, which allows the identification of intestinal arteries and the measurement of blood flow within them with minimal distress to the patient (138). Similar rates of flow were obtained using this noninvasive method.

Physiologic challenge indicates that blood flow can increase by more than 100% following a meal. Studies using noninvasive techniques in pathologic states are ongoing. Studies of ischemia show that the spectrum of clinical situations encountered on the basis of this entity are more complex than previously thought (132).

Many alterations in blood flow in the gastrointestinal tract occur during shock. The amount of tissue perfused and the volume and distribution of blood flow through the gastrointestinal tract change dramatically, specifically: (a) less than 50% of the bowel perfused during normal conditions is perfused during shock, and (b) of greater importance, the decrease in perfusion is not equitably distributed to all layers (139). The mucosa and submucosa, the layers of the bowel with the highest metabolic demands, suffer a disproportional decrease in both area perfused and volume of blood flowing through the area. Only 20% of the mucosa and submucosa perfused during normal conditions is perfused during shock, and the volume of blood flow through the mucosa and submucosa in shock is decreased to 16% of normotensive levels. These changes in hemodynamics are similar to those encountered in aquatic animals that are able to dive to great depths (the diving reflex).

PROPOSED MECHANISMS OF PATHOGENESIS

Three different perspectives have been brought to the question of pathogenesis. The first implicates the superoxide radical as the initiator (140). The second perspective focuses on changes in intracellular calcium homeostasis (141). The third brings the perspective of the action of platelet-activating factor and endotoxin when it is administered intraarterially (142).

Superoxide Radicals

The superoxide radical concept is championed by Granger and Parks. This concept offers further insight into the biochemical basis of ischemia and is the concept that has received the most recent study (140).

Parks and Granger and their coworkers have implicated the superoxide radical generated during reperfusion of the ischemic bowel as the culprit (143). Before they conducted their studies, hypoxia per se was considered the cause. The superoxide radical, an unstable and cytotoxic form of molecular oxygen, is thought to alter vascular permeability of the endothelial cell and cause necrosis of the epithelial cells by peroxidation of the cell membranes. The source and action of the superoxide radical is thought to be quite different from its well-known role in the neutrophil-mediated acute inflammatory response (144). The basic change that these investigators identified following ischemia was an increase in vascular permeability.

The major source of the superoxide radical in the ischemic bowel appears to be the enzyme xanthine oxidase (145). The liver and small intestine are the two richest sources of this enzyme in the human. Interestingly, in the small bowel, most of the enzyme is concentrated in the villus tip. In this model, the necessary substrate is hypoxanthine. The amount of xanthine oxidase present in the large intestine is smaller than that in the small bowel (146).

Intracellular Calcium Homeostasis

This concept implicating changes in intracellular calcium homeostasis is derived from studies looking at the pathogenesis of experimental stress ulceration in the stomach and its amelioration with drugs (147, 148). The effects of these changes relative to ischemic injury have received significant attention, because it has been shown that the significant increase in intracellular calcium that occurs with ischemia perhaps plays a primary role in mediating irreversible ischemic injury (141).

Intraarterial Platelet-Activating Factor and Bacterial Endotoxin

The third concept resulted from an attempt to develop another experimental model that mimicked necrotizing enterocolitis of the premature infant. This model, developed by Gonzalez-Crussi and Hsueh (142), is the first model in which vascular hypoperfusion, exsanguination, or other mechanisms of decreased blood flow are not used (142). This experimental model is produced by the intraaortic injection of synthetic platelet-activating factor or a combination of platelet-activating factor and bacterial endotoxin in the rat (149).

THERAPEUTIC CONSIDERATIONS

A variety of pharmacologic agents have been tested to determine whether they enhance or reduce the pathologic changes that occur in ischemic bowel disease. It appears that indomethacin may potentiate bowel ischemia, whereas prostaglandin E_1 (PGE_1) and ibuprofen may have a significant effect on decreasing the degree of bowel necrosis (150). The manner in which prostaglandins are protective of mucosa appears to involve several different and complex mechanisms, including production of a shielding, gelatinous layer formed by mucus and exfoliated surface epithelial cells; flow of mucosal fluid in the lumen, which dilutes noxious agents; and a rapidly healing superficial mucosal layer that quickly reconstitutes the physical barrier between the lumen and the lamina propria (151).

Slow calcium channel blockers, such as verapamil, prevent or significantly attenuate the experimentally produced stress ulcers in the stomach (147, 148).

Investigations using experimental models of necrotizing enterocolitis have shown that both polycythemia and increased blood viscosity may add to the risk of developing necrotizing enterocolitis (152).

ENTITIES OF ISCHEMIC BOWEL DISEASE
ISCHEMIC COLITIS

In the 1960s, Marston et al. (153) described three syndromes that resulted from ischemic processes in the colon. The clinical course depended on the degree of pathologic change in the visceral arteries supplying the colon, the duration of hypotension, and the virulence of bacteria present in the bowel lumen. In the most severe form, transmural infarction developed. In the intermediate form, healing by fibrosis resulted in colonic stricture; in the least severe form, bloody diarrhea developed, with subsequent healing and restitution of normal structure.

The gross pathology of the ischemic portion demonstrates mucosal ulceration and severe congestion beneath the surface. In addition, the distance between the mucosa and the muscular layers is expanded because of edema formation. Microscopically, the picture is that of coagulative necrosis with severe congestion beneath the necrotic epithelium. The process frequently extends into the submucosa with extensive edema formation. Pseudopolyp formation is the hallmark of the disease. Pseudopolyps are the result of focal severe edema of the mucosa and submucosa. During barium enema studies, they can be seen as indentations of the barium column (Fig. 14.22). The most frequent area of involvement in ischemic colitis is the splenic flexure—the watershed or anastomotic area between the superior and inferior mesenteric arteries. In addition to transient, strictured, and gangrenous forms, ischemic colitis can also present as megacolon in the elderly (154).

Ischemic colitis in the elderly can mimic ulcerative colitis and granulomatous colitis clinically (155). Studies indicate that as many as 75% of patients 50 years of age and older who initially are thought to have ulcerative colitis, Crohn colitis, or nonspecific colitis have ischemic bowel disease (156). (See Chapter 29 for further information.)

NECROTIZING ENTEROCOLITIS OF THE PREMATURE INFANT

In the past, this entity was thought to result from perinatal gastrointestinal ischemia, which facilitated the invasion of enteric bacteria in an underdeveloped gastrointestinal tract, which had, as yet, little immune protective mechanism. Results of later studies challenged these traditional thoughts about the pathogenesis and introduced data supporting the predominant role of an infectious agent (157). Controlled studies, unfortunately, have demonstrated no consistent risk factor among infants with necrotizing enterocolitis when compared with unaffected infants. Current thought indicates that neonatal necrotizing enterocolitis appears to be a single pathologic response whereby the immature intestine reacts to injury. The immature bowel may only have a limited manner in which it can respond to injury, and the unique mucosal pathologic response may be initiated by multiple factors or microbiologic agents acting either alone or in concert (157).

The incidence of necrotizing enterocolitis is dramatically increased in premature infants. The disease usually first manifests between the third and the tenth day of life. The diagnosis can be confirmed clinically only by radiographic demonstration of abnormal intestinal bacterial gas formation or pneumatosis intestinalis. Currently, considerable debate centers on the importance of composition and the rate of administration of milk in the subsequent development of necrotizing enterocolitis. Likewise, ischemia as a risk factor is still undergoing intensive reinvestigation. Many organisms have been associated with necrotizing enterocolitis including *Escherichia coli, Klebsiella, Enterobacter, Pseudomonas, Salmonella, Clostridium perfringens, Clostridium difficile,* and a variety of viruses (and their toxins).

Necrotizing enterocolitis develops only if a threshold of injury sufficient to initiate intestinal necrosis is exceeded (158). The three leading events still continue to be intestinal ischemia, colonization by pathogenic bacteria, and excess protein substrate in the intestinal lumen. Whether a single event or multiple events are necessary is not clear. Certainly, the premature infant appears at higher risk than the full-term infant of normal birth weight. The role of umbilical catheters in the pathogenesis of this disease through formation of thrombi that embolize, while considered in the past, is currently

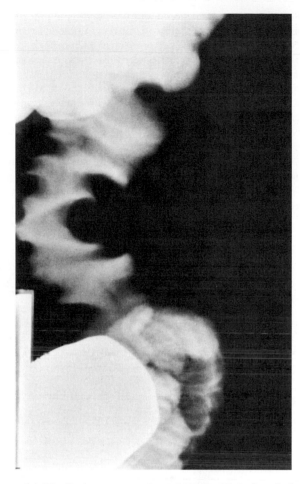

Figure 14.22 Barium enema in a patient with ischemic bowel disease. The barium column is irregular because of numerous indentations caused by focal edema of the mucosa and submucosa—the thumbprint sign.

receiving relatively little attention. Infants of less than 28 weeks gestation and those with low birth weights (less than 1500 g) are reported to have increased mortality rates due to this disease (159).

Necrotizing enterocolitis has occurred immediately after cardiac surgery, placing more emphasis on the theory that local perfusion inadequacy plays a predominant role in the pathogenesis of this disease (160). Necrotizing enterocolitis has also been observed in older infants, children, and adolescents. Unfortunately, this diagnosis is usually made only at autopsy. The majority of these patients had either an altered immune state or evidence of low flow situations or hypoxemia (161).

Recent studies reveal no increased incidence of necrotizing enterocolitis in infants receiving early enteral feeding (162). When the mesenteric veins are examined, bubbles of gas are a frequent finding. Attempts are being made to find methods of measuring the amount of hydrogen in exhaled breath in hopes that an earlier diagnosis of necrotizing enterocolitis will be possible (157).

Microscopically, coagulative necrosis is the hallmark of the disease process. The initial stages are characterized by congestion in the lamina propria, followed by extravasation of erythrocytes into the lamina propria and submucosal congestion. The ischemic process then continues with necrosis of the submucosa. By this time, the mucosa is severely infarcted and ulcerated. The process then continues with coagulative necrosis of the subjacent layers. The degree of involvement of the bowel by pneumatosis can be extensive. These findings may be lost if the tissue is not handled properly and promptly after surgical removal.

Stricture formation also occurs in association with this disease. Stricture usually forms within 5 to 8 weeks after the acute episode. Externally, the stricture is easy to demonstrate; after opening the bowel, significant dilation of the proximal intestine is plainly visible (Fig. 14.23).

Necrotizing enterocolitis most frequently affects the ileum and ascending colon. The ascending colon is the location of most frequent stricture formation. Histologically, the degree of fibrosis is often difficult to appreciate with hematoxylin and eosin stains;

however, with trichrome stains, the degree of fibrosis is readily apparent. The end stage of necrotizing enterocolitis may be the development of colonic atresia (163).

PSEUDOMEMBRANOUS COLITIS

That pseudomembranous colitis can follow the administration of a variety of antibiotics and is associated with the toxin of C. difficile has been appreciated since the mid-1970s (164). Evidence indicates that pseudomembranous colitis continues to be attributable to the administration of antibiotics (165); however, other organisms seem also to be able to cause pseudomembranous colitis (Yersinia) (166). There continues, however, to be a spectrum of patients who develop pseudomembranous colitis unassociated with antibiotic therapy (167). Whether these cases result from an initial episode of low perfusion or from bacterial toxins remains speculative. The pseudomembrane is a reflow phenomenon in which injured vessels respond with acute inflammation when circulation is re-established. (See Chapter 28 for additional information.)

HEMORRHAGIC NECROSIS

Not all ischemic processes occurring in the gastrointestinal tract result in a primary symptom complex. Some years ago, Ming summarized cases of hemorrhagic necrosis of the gastrointestinal tract studied at autopsy occurring as secondary phenomenon in patients with severely compromised cardiovascular status, shock, or severe infection (168). The histologic picture is identical to that previously described. At autopsy, small areas of hemorrhagic necrosis frequently are encountered (Fig. 14.24). Microscopically, once again, severe coagulative necrosis of the mucosa is present (Fig. 14.25).

STRESS ULCERATION

The pathogenesis of stress ulceration in the stomach is still controversial. The leading etiologic factor in the development of this phenomenon appears to be mucosal ischemia associated with cellular hypoxia, but the cause may be multifactorial (169) (Fig. 14.26). (See Chapter 24 for additional details.)

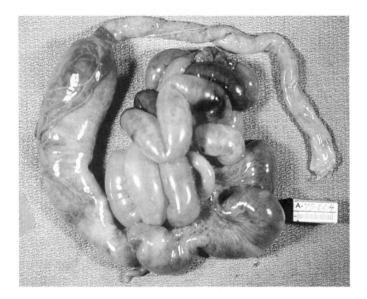

Figure 14.23 Necrotizing enterocolitis of the premature infant. Gross specimen shows an area of stenosis with dilated bowel proximal to this area. The patient experienced an episode of necrotizing enterocolitis 5 weeks before death. (See color plate.)

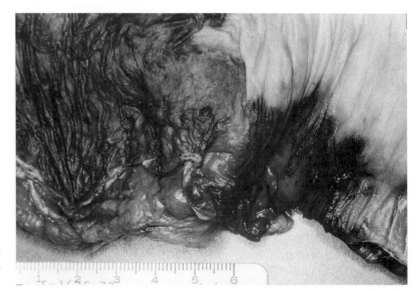

Figure 14.24 Hemorrhagic necrosis of the bowel. The degree of involvement and necrosis varies from area to area within the bowel.

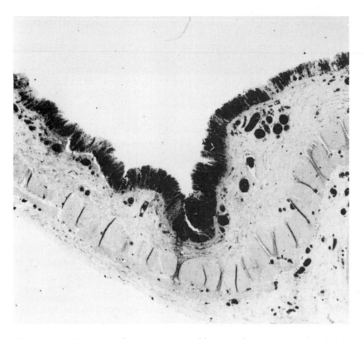

Figure 14.25 Histologic section of hemorrhagic necrosis of the bowel. The mucosa is severely congested and necrotic. The submucosa is congested and edematous. The deeper layers, however, are viable (×20).

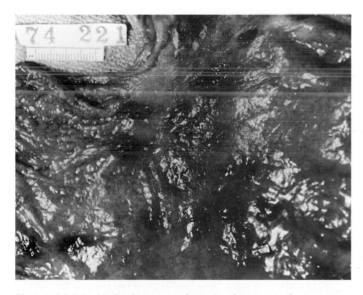

Figure 14.26 Multiple stress ulcers in the stomach represent another form of ischemic bowel disease.

ATHEROEMBOLIC INJURY

Atheroemboli result from release of atheromatous debris from an atheromatous plaque. Anticoagulant drugs, vascular surgery, and invasive radiologic procedures are the most common precipitating events resulting in the dissemination of atheroemboli (170). Dissemination may also occur spontaneously (171). The gastrointestinal tract is reported to be involved in 20% of cases of systemic atheroemboli (172).

The clinical presentation of gastrointestinal atheroemboli is varied. Patients may be asymptomatic or present with abdominal pain, hemorrhage, diarrhea, ulceration, stricture with obstruction, infarction, and/or perforation (171, 173–175). Histologically, atheroemboli are characterized by the presence of cleft-like spaces in submucosal arterioles. Other findings include associated thrombosis or giant cell reaction, an infiltrate of eosinophils in the immediately adjacent tissue, and overlying ulceration and necrosis or fibrosis with stricture formation.

Cheville and colleagues (176) described a patient who had multiple inflammatory colonic polyps associated with atheroemboli. Four patients have been reported with atheroemboli identified within adenomatous polyps (171, 170). O'Briain et al. theorized that atheroemboli localization to adenomatous polyps could be the result of anatomic variations in the arterial supply of the polyp that might favor lodgement of emboli within their stalks, or perhaps that submucosa is included in polypectomy specimens but frequently is absent in biopsy samples of flat colonic mucosa (171). The association of adenomatous polyps with atheroemboli might also be secondary to the fact that adenomatous polyps are frequently subjected to biopsy and the "chance" association of these two entities would be more frequently identified in this tissue (Fig. 14.27).

RADIATION INJURY

Radiation has a wide variety of effects on the gastrointestinal tract from the esophagus through the large intestine (177). Although mucosal injury is a frequent consequence, the ability of the mucosa to regenerate often leaves this area of the gastrointestinal tract without sequelae. Clinically, however, ischemic necrosis with concomitant massive fibrosis are sequelae of radiation injury, the picture mimicking ischemic injury to the gastrointestinal tract (177). Microvascular effects are profound (178). (See Chapter 11 for more information.)

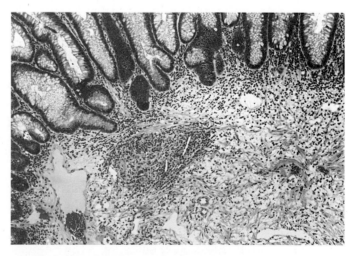

Figure 14.27 Colonic adenomatous polyp with clinically unsuspected submucosal intravascular atheroemboli. Atheroemboli appear as cleft-like spaces in submucosal arterioles (arrow) of this adenomatous polyp (×40).

OTHER DISORDERS

Other causes of gastrointestinal ischemia have been associated with the release of potassium chloride into the small bowel in the form of nonenteric-coated tablets (179, 180). McMahon and coworkers reiterated the injurious effect of these supplements (181) (see Chapter 11). Chronic uremia has also been associated with ischemic colitis (182). This disease frequently occurs after bilateral nephrectomy or renal transplantation (182, 183) (see Chapter 19). Finally, as reported previously (184, 185), various species and toxins of staphylococci have also been associated with enterocolitis. Ischemia is thought to play a significant role in the mechanism of pathogenesis.

EFFECT OF CHRONIC NARROWING OF THE SPLANCHNIC VESSELS

Partial obstruction of the celiac artery and superior mesenteric artery has been associated with the clinical syndrome of chronic intestinal ischemia. The histopathologic consequences of this obstruction have been documented and include erosions of the stomach and duodenum (186, 187).

REFERENCES

1. Hyams JS, Leichtner AM, Schwartz AN. Recent advances in diagnosis and treatment of gastrointestinal hemorrhage in infants and children. J Pediatr 1985;106:1–9.
2. Raskin JB. Upper gastrointestinal hemorrhage. Early diagnostic approaches. Comp Ther 1983;9:31–34.
3. Baer JW, Ryan S. Analysis of cecal vasculature in the search for vascular malformations. AJR Am J Roentgenol 1976;126:394–404.
4. Pounder DJ, Rowland R, Pieterse AS, et al. Angiodysplasias of the colon. J Clin Pathol 1982;35:824–829.
5. Talman EA, Dixon DS, Gutierrez FE. Role of arteriography in rectal hemorrhage due to arteriovenous malformations and diverticulosis. Ann Surg 1979;190:203–213.
6. Crawford ES, Roehm JOF, McGavran MH. Jejunoileal arteriovenous malformation: Localization for resection by segmental bowel staining techniques. Ann Surg 1980;191:404–409.
7. Fogler R, Golembe E. Methylene blue injection: An intraoperative guide in small bowel resection for arteriovenous malformation. Arch Surg 1978;113:194–195.
8. Papamiltiades MN. Injection of lymphatics: With colored cedar oil; with plastic. Stain Technol 1961;36:241–246.
9. Hamilton SR. Structure of the colon. Scand J Gastroenterol Suppl 1984;93:13–23.
10. Williams DB, Payne WS. Observations on esophageal blood supply. Mayo Clin Proc 1982;57:448–453.
11. Bulkley GB, Womack WA, Downey JM, et al. Characterization of segmental collateral blood flow in the small intestine. Am J Physiol 1985;249 (Gastrointest Liver Physiol 12):G228–G235.
12. Granger DN, Barrowman JA. Microcirculation of the alimentary tract. I. Physiology of transcapillary fluid and solute exchange. Gastroenterology 1983;84:846–868.
13. Hayes PC, Shepherd AN, Bouchier IAD. Medical treatment of portal hypertension and esophageal varices. Br Med J [Clin Res] 1983;287:733–736.
14. Korula J. Variceal bleeding. Can it be prevented? Postgrad Med 1995;98(6):131–138.
15. MacMathuna PM. Mechanisms and consequences of portal hypertension. Drugs 1992;44 (Suppl 2):1–13.
16. McCormick PA. Pathophysiology and prognosis of oesophageal varices. Scand J Gastroenterol 1994;29 (Suppl 207):1–5.
17. Spence RAJ. The venous anatomy of the lower oesophagus in normal subjects and in patients with varices: An image analysis study. Br J Surg 1984;71:739–744.
18. Navab F, Schiller TD, Slaton D. Management of variceal hemorrhage. South Med J 1984;77:1302–1307.
19. Cho KC, Patel YD, Wachsberg RH, et al. Varices in portal hypertension: Evaluation with CT. Radiographics 1995;15:609–622.
20. Lieberman DA, Krippaehne WW, Melnyk CS. Colonic varices due to intestinal cavernous hemangiomas. Dig Dis Sci 1983;28:852–858.
21. Cello JP, Crass RA, Federle MP. Colonic varices: An unusual source of lower gastrointestinal hemorrhage. West J Med 1982;136:252–255.
22. Hawkey CJ, Amar SS, Daintith HAM, et al. Familial varices of the colon occurring without evidence of portal hypertension. Br J Radiol 1985;58:677–679.
23. Grundfest-Broniatowski S, Fazio V. Conservative treatment of bleeding stomal varices. Arch Surg 1983;118:981–985.
24. Grauer SE, Schwartz SI. Extrahepatic portal hypertension: A retrospective analysis. Ann Surg 1979;189:566–571.
25. Roder OC. Splenic vein thrombosis with bleeding gastroesophageal varices: Reports of two splenectomized cases and review of the literature. Acta Chir Scand 1984;150:265–268.
26. Ricci RL, Lee KR, Greenberger NJ. Chronic gastrointestinal bleeding from ileal varices after total proctocolectomy for ulcerative colitis: Correction by mesocaval shunt. Gastroenterology 1980;78:1053–1058.
27. Moncure AC, Waltman AC, Vandersalm TJ, et al. Gastrointestinal hemorrhage from adhesion-related mesenteric varices. Ann Surg 1976;183:24–29.
28. Granqvist S. Colonic varices caused by carcinoid tumor. Gastrointestinal Radiol 1984;9:269–271.
29. Camilleri M, Chadwick VS, Hodgson HJF. Vascular anomalies of the gastrointestinal tract. Hepatogastroenterology 1984;31:149–153.
30. Moore JD, Thompson NW, Appelman HD, et al. Arteriovenous malformations of the gastrointestinal tract. Arch Surg 1976;111:381–389.
31. Boley SJ, Brandt LJ, Mitsudo SM. Vascular lesions of the colon. Adv Intern Med 1984;29:301–326.
32. Sharma R, Gorbien MJ. Angiodysplasia and lower gastrointestinal tract bleeding in elderly patients. Arch Intern Med 1995;155:807–812.
33. Foutch PG. Angiodysplasia of the gastrointestinal tract. Am J Gastroenterol 1993;88:807–818.
34. Clouse RE, Costigan DJ, Mills BA, et al. Angiodysplasia as a cause of upper gastrointestinal bleeding. Arch Intern Med 1985;145:458–461.
35. Boley SJ, Sammartano R, Adams A, et al. On the nature and etiology of vascular ectasias of the colon: Degenerative lesions of aging. Gastroenterology 1977;72:650–660.
36. Stamm B, Heer M, Buhler H, et al. Mucosal biopsy of vascular ectasia (angiodysplasia) of the large bowel detected during routine colonoscopic examination. Histopathology 1985;9:639–646.
37. Max MH, Richardson JD, Flint LM, et al. Colonoscopic diagnosis of angiodysplasias of the gastrointestinal tract. Surg Gynecol Obstet 1981;152:195–199.
38. Martini GA. The liver in hereditary haemorrhagic telangiectasia: An inborn error of vascular structure with multiple manifestations: A reappraisal. Gut 1978;19:531–537.
39. Ahr DJ, Rickles FR, Hoyer LW, et al. Von Willebrand's disease and hemorrhagic telangiectasia: Association of two complex disorders of hemostasis resulting in life-threatening hemorrhage. Am J Med 1977;62:452–457.
40. Mower GA, Whitehead R. Gastric hemorrhage due to ruptured arteriovenous malformation (Dieulafoy's disease). Pathology 1986;18:54–57.
41. Katz PO, Salas L. Less frequent causes of upper gastrointestinal bleeding. Gastrointest Clin North Am 1993;22:875–889.
42. Reilly HF, Al-Kawas FH. Dieulafoy's lesion. Diagnosis and management. Dig Dis Sci 1991;36(12):1702–1707.
43. Jabbari M, Cherry R, Lough JO, et al. Gastric antral vascular ectasia: The watermelon stomach. Gastroenterology 1984;87:1165–1170.
44. Gostout CJ, Viggiano TR, Ahlquist DA, et al. The clinical and endoscopic spectrum of the watermelon stomach. J Clin Gastroenterol 1992;15(3):256–263.
45. Suit PF, Petras RE, Bauer TW, et al. Gastric antral vascular ectasia. Am J Surg Pathol 1987;11(10):750–757.

46. Lingenfelser T. Editorial: The stomach in cirrhosis. The legend of proteus retold. J Clin Gastroenterol 1993;17(2):92–96.

47. Sweeney K, Petrelli N, Herrera L, et al. Cavernous hemangioma of the anus. J Surg Oncol 1984;27:286–288.

48. Pontecorvo C, Lombardi S, Mottola L, et al. Hemangiomas of the large bowel. Report of a case. Dis Colon Rectum 1983;26:818–820.

49. Oswalt CE, Kasal NG. Gastric hemangioma in a 15-year-old girl. Texas Med 1983;79:37–39.

50. Govoni AF. Hemangiomas of the esophagus. Gastrointest Radiol 1982;7:113–117.

51. White IL, Dunkelman D. Obstructive cervical esophageal hemangioma. Ear Nose Throat J 1981;60:324–327.

52. Hanel K, Talley NA, Hunt DR. Hemangioma of the esophagus: An unusual cause of upper gastrointestinal bleeding. Dig Dis Sci 1981;26:257–263.

53. Stillman AE, Hansen RC, Hallinan V, et al. Diffuse neonatal hemangiomatosis with severe gastrointestinal involvement: Favorable response to steroid therapy. Clin Pediatr 1983;22:589–591.

54. Ghahremani GG, Kangarloo H, Volberg F, et al. Diffuse cavernous hemangioma of the colon in the Klippel-Trenaunay syndrome. Radiology 1976;118:673–678.

55. Gill PS: Phase I/II trials of α-interferon alone or in combination with zidovudine as maintenance therapy following induction chemotherapy in the treatment of acquired immunodeficiency syndrome-related Kaposi's sarcoma. Semin Oncol 1991;18(5)Suppl 7:53–57.

56. Friedman SL. Gastrointestinal and hepatobiliary neoplasms in AIDS. Gastroenterol Clin North Am 1988;17(3):465–487.

57. Beral V, Peterman TA, Berkelman RL, et al. Kaposi's sarcoma among persons with AIDS: A sexually transmitted infection? Lancet 1990; 335:123–128.

58. Parente F, Cernuschi M, Orlando G, et al. Kaposi's sarcoma and AIDS: Frequency of gastrointestinal involvement and its effect on survival. A prospective study in a heterogeneous population. Scand J Gastroenterol 1991;26:1007–1012.

59. Friedman SL, Wright TL, Altman DF. Gastrointestinal Kaposi's sarcoma in patients with acquired immunodeficiency syndrome. Endoscopic and autopsy findings. Gastroenterology 1985;89: 102–108.

60. Kolios G, Kaloterakis A, Filiotou A, et al. Gastroscopic findings in Mediterranean Kaposi's sarcoma (non-AIDS). Gastrointestinal Endosc 1995;42(4):336–339.

61. Lee WA, Hutchins GM. Cluster analysis of the metastatic patterns of human immunodeficiency virus-associated Kaposi's sarcoma. Hum Pathol 1992;23:306–311.

62. Weber JN, Carmichael DJ, Boylston A, et al. Case report. Kaposi's sarcoma of the bowel, presenting as apparent ulcerative colitis. Gut 1985;26:295–300.

63. Bianco J, Pratt-Bianco L. Kaposi's sarcoma of the rectum: A case report. Mt Sinai J Med 1983;50:278–280.

64. Weprin L, Zollinger R, Clausen K, et al. Kaposi's sarcoma: Endoscopic observations of gastric and colon involvement. J Clin Gastroenterol 1982;4:357–360.

65. Chen KTK, Hoffman KD, Hendricks EJ. Angiosarcoma following therapeutic irradiation. Cancer 1979;44:2044–2048.

66. Nanus DM, Kelsen D, Clark DGC. Radiation-induced angiosarcoma. Cancer 1987;60:777–779.

67. Nakagawara G, Kojima Y, Mai M, et al. Lymphangioma of the transverse colon treated by transendoscopic polypectomy: Report of a case and review of literature. Dis Colon Rectum 1981;24:291–295.

68. Camilleri M, Satti MB, Wood CB. Cystic lymphangioma of the colon: Endoscopic and histologic features. Dis Colon Rectum 1982;25: 813–816.

69. Liebert Jr CW. Symptomatic lymphangioma of the esophagus with endoscopic resection. Gastrointest Endosc 1983;29:225–226.

70. Colizza S, Tiso B, Bracci F, et al. Cystic lymphangioma of stomach and jejunum: Report of one case. J Surg Oncol 1981;17:169–176.

71. Leu HJ. Classification of vasculitides. Vasa 1995;24(4):319–324.

72. Alpern RJ. Southwestern internal medicine conference: Vasculitis—it's time to reclassify. Am J Med Sci 1995;309(4):235–248.

73. Lie JT. Vasculitis 1815–1991: Classification and diagnostic specificity (Dunlop-Dottridge lecture). J Rheumatol 1991;19:83–89.

74. Cohen Tervaert JW, Kallenberg C. Neurologic manifestations of systemic vasculitides. Rheum Dis Clin North Am 1993;19:913–940.

75. Jorrizo JL. Classification of vasculitis. J Invest Dermatol 1993; 100(1):106S–110S.

76. Jennette J, Falk RJ, Andrassy K, et al. Nomenclature of systemic vasculitides. Proposal of an international consensus conference. Arthritis Rheum 1994;37(2):187–192.

77. Guillevin L, Lhote F. Distinguishing polyarteritis nodosa from microscopic polyangiitis and implications for treatment. Curr Opin Rheumatol 1995;7:20–24.

78. Lie J. Nomenclature and classification of vasculitis: Plus ça change, plus c'est la même chose [editorial]. Arthritis Rheum 1994;37: 181–186.

79. Gross WL, Csernok E, Helmchen U. Antineutrophil cytoplasmic autoantibodies, autoantigens, and systemic vasculitis. APMIS 1995: 103:81–97.

80. Gross WL, Schmitt WH, Csernok E. ANCA and associated diseases: Immunodiagnostic and pathogenetic aspects. Clin Exp Immunol 1993;91:1–12.

81. Cohen Tervaert JW, Stegeman CA, Brouwer E, et al. Anti-neutrophil cytoplasmic antibodies: A new class of autoantibodies in glomerulonephritis, vasculitis and other inflammatory disorders. Neth J Med 1994;45:262–272.

82. Gross WL, Csernok E. Immunodiagnostic and pathophysiologic aspects of antineutrophil cytoplasmic antibodies in vasculitis. Curr Opin Rheumatol 1995;7:11–19.

83. Jennette JC, Ewert BH, Falk RJ. Do antineutrophil cytoplasmic autoantibodies cause Wegener's granulomatosis and other forms of necrotizing vasculitis? Rheum Dis Clin North Am 1993;19(1):1–14.

84. Camilleri M, Pusey CD, Chadwick VS et al. Gastrointestinal manifestations of systemic vasculitis. Q J Med 1983;52(206):141–149.

85. Kleinman P, Meyers MA, Abbott G, et al. Necrotizing enterocolitis with pneumatosis intestinalis in systemic lupus erythematosus and polyarteritis. Radiology 1976;121:595–598.

86. Goldman H, Antonioli DA. Mucosal biopsy of the rectum, colon, and distal ileum. Hum Pathol 1982;13:981–1012.

87. Keshavarzian A, Saverymuttu SH, Chadwick VS, et al. Noninvasive investigation of the gastrointestinal tract in collagen-vascular disease. Am J Gastroenterol 1984;79:873–877.

88. Han SY, Jander HP, Laws HL. Polyarteritis nodosa causing severe intestinal bleeding. Gastrointest Radiol 1976;1:285–287.

89. Harvey MH, Neoptolemos JP, Fossard DP. Abdominal polyarteritis nodosa—a possible surgical pitfall? Br J Clin Pract 1984;38:282–283.

90. Gorton M, John Jr JF. Polyarteritis overlap syndrome with extensive bowel infarction. Am J Gastroenterol 1980;74:153–156.

91. Fayemi AO, Ali M, Braun EV. Necrotizing vasculitis of the gallbladder and the appendix. Similarity in the morphology of rheumatoid arteritis and polyarteritis nodosa. Am J Gastroenterol 1977;67: 608–612.

92. Bassel K, Harford W. Gastrointestinal manifestations of collagen-vascular diseases. Semin Gastrointest Dis 1995;6(4):228–240.

93. Lee EL, Smith HJ, Miller GL, et al. Ischemic pseudomembranous colitis with perforation due to polyarteritis nodosa. Am J Gastroenterol 1984;79:35–38.

94. Wood MK, Read DR, Kraft AR, et al. A rare cause of ischemic colitis: Polyarteritis nodosa. Dis Colon Rectum 1979;22:428–433.

95. Meyer GW, Lichtenstein J. Isolated polyarteritis nodosa affecting the cecum. Dig Dis Sci 1982;27:467–469.

96. Hoffman BI, Yatz WA. The gastrointestinal manifestations of systemic lupus erythematosus: A review of the literature. Semin Arthritis Rheum 1980;9:237–247.

97. Gladman DD, Ross T, Richardson B, et al. Bowel involvement in systemic lupus erythematosus: Crohn's disease or lupus vasculitis? Arthritis Rheum 1985;28:466–470.

98. Zizic TM, Shulman LE, Stevens MB. Colonic perforations in systemic lupus erythematosus. Medicine 1975;54:411–425.

99. Weiser MM, Andres GA, Brentjens JR, et al. Systemic lupus erythematosus and intestinal venulitis. Gastroenterology 1981;81: 570–579.

100. Zizic TM, Classen JN, Stevens MB. Acute abdominal complications of systemic lupus erythematosus and polyarteritis nodosa. Am J Med 1982;73:525–531.

101. Burt RW, Berenson MM, Samuelson CO, et al. Rheumatoid vasculitis of the colon presenting as pancolitis. Dig Dis Sci 1983;28: 183–188.

102. Tsai JT. Perforation of the small bowel with rheumatoid arthritis. South Med J 1980;73:939–940.

103. McCurley TL, Collins RD. Intestinal infarction in rheumatoid arthritis. Arch Pathol Lab Med 1984;108:125–128.

104. Chumbley LC, Harrison EG, DeRemee RA. Allergic granulomatosis and angiitis (Churg-Strauss Syndrome)—Report and analysis of 30 cases. Mayo Clin Proc 1977;52:477–484.

105. Guillevin L, Le Thi HD, Godeau P, et al. Clinical findings and prognosis of polyarteritis nodosa and Churg-Strauss angiitis: A study in 165 patients. Br J Rheumatol 1988;27:258–264.

106. Fraioli P, Barberis M, Rizutto G. Gastrointestinal presentation of Churg-Strauss syndrome. Sarcoidosis 1994;11:42–45.

107. Modigliani R, Muschart JM, Galian A, et al. Allergic granulomatous vasculitis (Churg-Strauss Syndrome): Report of a case with widespread digestive involvement. Dig Dis Sci 1981;26(3):264–270.

108. Suen KC, Burton JD. The spectrum of eosinophilic infiltration of the gastrointestinal tract and its relationship to other disorders of angiitis and granulomatosis. Hum Pathol 1979;10:31–43.

109. Case records of the Massachusetts General Hospital: Weekly clinicopathological exercises. Case 14-1980. N Engl J Med 1980;302:853–858.

110. Weber TR, Grosfeld JL, Bergstein J, et al. Massive gastric hemorrhage: An unusual complication of Henoch Schönlein purpura. J Pediat Surg 1983;18:576–578.

111. Smith HJ, Krupski WC. Spontaneous intestinal perforation in Schönlein-Henoch purpura. South Med J 1980;73:603–606.

112. Novy SB, Weaver RM, Jensen KM, et al. Henoch-Schönlein purpura of the colon: An unusual gastrointestinal manifestation. South Med J 1977;70:884–886.

113. Goldman LP, Lindenberg RL. Henoch-Schönlein purpura. Gastrointestinal manifestations with endoscopic correlation. Am J Gastroenterol 1981;75:357–360.

114. Morichau-Beauchant M, Touchard G, Maire P, et al. Jejunal IgA and C3 deposition in adult Henoch-Schönlein purpura with severe intestinal manifestations. Gastroenterology 1982;82:1438–1442.

115. Geraghty J, MacKay IR, Smith DC. Intestinal perforation in Wegener's granulomatosis. Gut 1986;27:450–451.

116. Haworth SJ, Pusey CD. Severe intestinal involvement in Wegener's granulomatosis. Gut 1984;25:1296–1300.

117. Hashikata Y, Nishioka K. Multiple gastric ulcers in Wegener's granulomatosis. A follow-up report (letter). Dermatologica 1983;166:325–327.

118. McNabb WR, Lennox MS, Wedzicha JA. Small intestinal perforation in Wegener's granulomatosis. Postgrad Med J 1982;58:123–125.

119. Oddis CV, Schoolwerth AC, Abt AB. Wegener's granulomatosis with delayed pulmonary and colonic involvement. South Med J 1984;77:1589–1591.

120. Kedziora JA, Wolff M, Chang J. Limited form of Wegener's granulomatosis in ulcerative colitis. AJR Am J Roentgenol 1975;125:127–133.

121. Sokol RJ, Farrell MK, McAdams AJ. An unusual presentation of Wegener's granulomatosis mimicking inflammatory bowel disease. Gastroenterology 1984;87:426–432.

122. Smith CD, Schuster SR, Gruppe WE, et al. Hemolytic-uremic syndrome: A diagnostic and therapeutic dilemma for the surgeon. J Pediatr Surg 1978;13:597–604.

123. Case records of the Massachusetts General Hospital: Weekly clinicopathological exercises. Case 12-1981. N Engl J Med 1981;304:715–721.

124. Kawanami T, Bowen A, Girdany BR. Enterocolitis: Prodrome of the hemolytic-uremic syndrome. Radiology 1984;151:91–92.

125. Sawaf H, Sharp MJ, Youn KJ, et al. Ischemic colitis and stricture after hemolytic-uremic syndrome. Pediatrics 1978;61:315–316.

126. Whitington PF, Friedman AL, Chesney RW. Gastrointestinal disease in the hemolytic-uremic syndrome. Gastroenterology 1979;76:728–733.

127. Dillard RP. Hemolytic-Uremic syndrome mimicking ulcerative colitis: Lack of early diagnostic laboratory finding. Clin Pediatr 1983;22:66–67.

128. Tochen ML, Campbell JR. Colitis in children with the hemolytic-uremic syndrome. J Pediatr Surg 1977;12:213–219.

129. Saraga EP, Costa J. Idiopathic entero-colic lymphocytic phlebitis. A cause of ischemic intestinal necrosis. Am J Surg Pathol 1989;13(4):303–308.

130. Hawkins C. Rheumatic diseases and the alimentary tract. Practitioner 1978;220:59–65.

131. Ottinger LW. Mesenteric ischemia. N Engl J Med 1982;307:535–537.

132. Marston A. Ischaemia. Clin Gastroenterol 1985;14:847–862.

133. Norris HT. Reexamination of the spectrum of ischemic bowel disease. In: Norris HT, ed. Pathology of the colon, small intestine, and anus. New York: Churchill-Livingstone, 1983;109–120.

134. Brandt LJ, Boley SJ. Ischemic intestinal syndromes. Adv Surg 1981;15:1–45.

135. Boley SJ, Brandt LJ, Veith FJ. Ischemic disorders of the intestines. Curr Probl Surg 1978;15:1–85.

136. Marston A, Clarke JMF, Garcia-Garcia J, et al. Alimentary and pancreas: Intestinal function and intestinal blood supply: A 20-year surgical study. Gut 1985;26:656–666.

137. Fiddian-Green RG, Amelin PM, Herrmann JB, et al. Prediction of the development of sigmoid ischemia on the day of aortic operations: Indirect measurements of intramural pH in the colon. Arch Surg 1986;121:654–660.

138. Qamar MI, Read AE. Intestinal blood flow (editorial). Q J Med 1985;56:417–419.

139. Norris HT, Sumner DS. Distribution of blood flow to the layers of the small bowel in experimental cholera. Gastroenterology 1974;66:973–981.

140. Granger DN, Parks DA. Role of oxygen radicals in the pathogenesis of intestinal ischemia. Physiologist 1983;26:159–164.

141. Cheung JY, Bonventre JV, Malis CD, et al. Calcium and ischemic injury. N Engl J Med 1986;314:1670–1676.

142. Gonzalez-Crussi F, Hsueh W. Experimental model of ischemic bowel necrosis: The role of platelet-activating factor and endotoxin. Am J Pathol 1983;112:127–135.

143. Parks DA, Granger DN, Bulkley GB, et al. Soybean trypsin inhibitor attenuates ischemic injury to the feline small intestine. Gastroenterology 1985;89:6–12.

144. McCord JM, Roy RS. The pathophysiology of superoxide: Roles in inflammation and ischemia. Can J Physiol Pharmacol 1982;60:1346–1352.

145. Bulkley GB, Kvietys PR, Parks DA, et al. Relationship of blood flow and oxygen consumption to ischemic injury in the canine small intestine. Gastroenterology 1985;89:852–857.

146. Parks DA, Bulkley GB, Granger DN. Role of oxygen-derived free radicals in digestive tract diseases. Surgery 1983;94:415–422.

147. Wait RB, Leahy AL, Nee JM, et al. Verapamil attenuates stress-induced gastric ulceration. J Surg Res 1985;38:424–428.

148. Ogle CW, Cho CH, Tong MC, et al. The influence of verapamil on the gastric effects of stress in rats. Eur J Pharmacol 1985;112:399–404.

149. Hsueh W, Gonzalez-Crussi F, Arroyave JL. Platelet-activating factor-induced ischemic bowel necrosis: An investigation of secondary mediators in its pathogenesis. Am J Pathol 1986;122:231–239.

150. Grosfeld JL, Kamman K, Gross K, et al. Comparative effects of indomethacin, prostaglandin E_1, and ibuprofen on bowel ischemia. J Pediatr Surg 1983;18:738–742.

151. Lacy ER. Prostaglandins and histological changes in the gastric mucosa. Dig Dis Sci 1985;30:83S–94S.

152. Dunn SP, Gross KR, Scherer LR, et al. The effect of polycythemia and hyperviscosity on bowel ischemia. J Pediatr Surg 1985;20:324–327.

153. Marston A, Pheils MT, Thomas M, et al. Ischaemic colitis. Gut 1966;7:1–15.

154. Margolis IB, Faro RS, Howells EM, et al. Megacolon in the elderly: Ischemic or inflammatory? Ann Surg 1979;190:40–44.

155. Eisenberg RL, Montgomery CK, Margulis AR. Colitis in the elderly: Ischemic colitis mimicking ulcerative and granulomatous colitis. AJR Am J Roentgenol 1979;133:1113–1118.

156. Brandt L, Boley S, Goldberg L, et al. Colitis in the elderly: A reappraisal. Am J Gastroenterol 1981;76:239–245.

157. Kliegman RM, Fanaroff AA. Necrotizing enterocolitis. N Engl J Med 1984;310:1093–1103.

158. Kosloske AM. Pathogenesis and prevention of necrotizing entero-

colitis: A hypothesis based on personal observation and a review of the literature. Pediatrics 1984;74:1086–1092.

159. Cikrit D, Mastandrea J, West KW, et al. Necrotizing enterocolitis: Factors affecting mortality in 101 surgical cases. Surgery 1984;96: 648–655.

160. Silane MF, Symchych PS. Necrotizing enterocolitis after cardiac surgery. A local ischemic lesion? Am J Surg 1977;133:373–376.

161. Moss TJ, Adler R. Necrotizing enterocolitis in older infants, children, and adolescents. J Pediatr 1982;100:764–766.

162. Otertag SG, LaGamma EF, Reisen CE, et al. Early enteral feeding does not affect the incidence of necrotizing enterocolitis. Pediatrics 1986;77:275–280.

163. Beardmore HE, Rodgers BM, Outerbridge E. Necrotizing enterocolitis (ischemic enteropathy) with the sequel of colonic atresia. Gastroenterology 1978;74:914–917.

164. Tedesco FJ, Barton RW, Alper DH. Clindamycin-associated colitis: A perspective study. Ann Intern Med 1974;81:429–433.

165. Parry MF, Rha CK. Pseudomembranous colitis caused by topical clindamycin phosphate. Arch Dermatol 1986;122:583–584.

166. Brown R, Tedesco FJ, Assad RT, et al. *Yersinia* colitis masquerading as pseudomembranous colitis. Dig Dis Sci 1986;31:548–551.

167. Moskovitz M, Bartlett JG. Recurrent pseudomembranous colitis unassociated with prior antibiotic therapy. Arch Intern Med 1981; 141:663–665.

168. Ming SC. Hemorrhagic necrosis of the gastrointestinal tract and its relation to cardiovascular status. Circulation 1965;32:332–341.

169. Pruitt Jr BA, Goodwin Jr CW. Stress ulcer disease in the burned patient. World J Surg 1981;5:209–222.

170. Freund NS. Cholesterol emboli in a colonic polyp. J Clin Gastroenterol 1994;19(3):231–233.

171. O'Briain DS, Jeffers M, Kay EW, et al. Bleeding due to colorectal atheroembolism. Diagnosis by biopsy of adenomatous polyps or of ischemic ulcer. Am J Surg Pathol 1991;15(11):1078–1082.

172. Taylor NS, Gueft B, Lebowich RJ. Atheromatous embolization: A cause of gastric ulcers and small bowel necrosis. Gastroenterology 1964;47(1):97–103.

173. Mulliken JB, Bartlett MK. Small bowel obstruction secondary to atheromatous embolism: A case report and review of the literature. Ann Surg 1971;174(1):145–150.

174. Turnbull RG, Hayashi AH, McLean DR. Multiple spontaneous intestinal perforations from atheroemboli after thrombolytic therapy: a case report. Can J Surg 1994;37(3):325–328.

175. Blundell JW. Small bowel stricture secondary to multiple cholesterol emboli. Histopathology 1988;13:459–472.

176. Cheville J, Mitros FA, Vanderzalm G, et al. Atheroemboli-associated polyps of the sigmoid colon. Am J Surg Pathol 1993;17(10):1054–1057.

177. Berthrong M, Fajardo LF. Radiation injury in surgical pathology. Part II. Alimentary tract. Am J Surg Pathol 1981;5:153–178.

178. Carr ND, Pullen BR, Hasleton PS, et al. Microvascular studies in human radiation bowel disease. Gut 1984;25:448–454.

179. Allen AC, Boley SJ, Schultz L, et al. Potassium-induced lesions of the small bowel. II. Pathology and pathogenesis. JAMA 1965;193: 1001–1006.

180. Leijonmarck CE, Raf L. Ulceration of the small intestine due to slow-release potassium chloride tablets. Acta Chir Scand 1985;151: 273–278.

181. McMahon FG, Akdamar K, Ryan JR, et al. Upper gastrointestinal lesions after potassium chloride supplements: A controlled clinical trial. Lancet 1982;2:1059–1061.

182. Aubia J, Lloveras J, Munne A, et al. Ischemic colitis in chronic uremia. Nephron 1981;29:146–150.

183. Margolis DM, Etheredge EE, Garza-Garza R, et al. Ischemic bowel disease following bilateral nephrectomy or renal transplant. Surgery 1977;82:667–673.

184. Bass JW. The spectrum of staphylococcal disease: From Job's boils to toxic shock. Postgrad Med 1982;72:58–64, 69–73, 75.

185. Gruskay JA, Abbasi S, Anday E, et al. Staphylococcus epidermidis-associated enterocolitis. J Pediatr 1986;109:520–524.

186. Force T, MacDonald D, Eade OE, et al. Ischemic gastritis and duodenitis. Dig Dis Sci 1980;25:307–310.

187. Allende HD, Ona FV. Celiac artery and superior mesenteric artery insufficiency. Unusual cause of erosive gastroduodenitis. Gastroenterology 1982;82:763–766.

15 | DISORDERS OF THE ENDOCRINE SYSTEM

Enrico Solcia, Carlo Capella, Roberto Fiocca, Fausto Sessa, Stefano La Rosa, and Guido Rindi

A manifold population of endocrine cells is scattered in the epithelium lining the gastric and the intestinal crypts and villi. Together with endocrine cells scattered in other endodermal derivatives such as the pancreas, biliary tree, lung, thyroid, and urethra, gut endocrine cells form the so-called diffuse endocrine system (DES).

Studies of endocrine cells largely depend on selective detection of these cells by refined morphologic techniques staining endocrine granules, histochemical techniques for secretory peptides or amines, and electron microscopy. In order to study the entire endocrine cell population of a tissue sample, Grimelius' silver, synaptophysin, neuron-specific enolase (NSE), or chromogranins immunohistochemistry are the techniques of choice (1–5). These techniques, however, are of little help when attempting to identify the exact type of endocrine cell. This goal is better achieved by means of hormone immunohistochemistry and, less frequently, by electron microscopy.

As a rule, secretory granules of endocrine cells are concentrated in the basal part of the cytoplasm, whereas the Golgi complex is supranuclear. In the pyloric and intestinal mucosa, most cells reach the lumen in a narrow, specialized area showing tufts of microvilli, coated vesicles, and a centriole; it is likely that this area acts as a receptor surface facing luminal contents. Such a pattern suggests some functional polarity of the cell. In the fundic mucosa, endocrine cells lack luminal contacts and show less evident polarity (6).

Secretory granules are released at the basal surface of the cell or along the lower part of its lateral surface, where intervening cells may form interstitial spaces and canaliculi. In the upper (juxtaluminal) part of the epithelium, these spaces are closed by junctional complexes with neighboring cells. Granule release at the luminal surface has never been observed.

Both endodermal and neuroectodermal origins of gut endocrine cells have been considered. Their origin from nerve cells, first proposed by Danisch, has been supported by Pearse and coworkers, who suggested the involvement of neural crests or neurally programmed cells of epiblastic origin (7). Results of graft experiments accurately performed in embryos, however, show that gut endocrine cells are not derived from neural crests or the epiblast (8). At present, an endodermal origin seems likely.

TABLE 15.1   Human Gastroenteropancreatic Endocrine Cells

| | | | Stomach | | Intestine | | | | | |
| | | | | | Small | | | | Large | |
Cell	Main Product	Pancreas	Oxyntic	Antral	Duodenum	Jejunum	Ileum	Appendix	Colon	Rectum
P	Unknown	f	+	+	+	f	f		f	f
EC	5-HT + peptides [a]	f	+	+	+	+	+	+	+	+
D	Somatostatin	+	+	+	+	f	f	+	f	+
L	GLI+PYY				f	+	+	+	+	+
A	Glucagon	+	a							
PP (F/D$_1$)	Pancreatic peptide	+			a					
B	Insulin	+								
X	Unknown		+							
G	Gastrin			+	+					
ECL	Histamine		+							
CCK	Cholecystokinin				+	+	f			
S	Secretin				+	+				
GIP	GIP				+	+	f			
M	Motilin				+	+	f			
N	Neurotensin				f	+	+			

Key: f, few; a, fetus and newborn; CCK, cholecystokinin; G, gastrin; GIP, gastric inhibitory polypeptide; GLI, glucagon-like immunoreactants: glicentin, glucagon-37, glucagon-29; PP, pancreatic peptide; PYY, PP-like peptide with N-terminal tyrosine amide; EC, enterochromaffin; ECL, enterochromaffin-like; 5-HT, 5-hydroxytryptamine.

[a]Substance P, neurokinins, opioids, guanylin, and other peptides.

Because of sequence homologies among gut hormonal peptides, reliable immunohistochemical localization of secretory products in gut endocrine cells can be obtained only by using antisera or monoclonal antibodies of well-characterized sequence specificity. The identification of different cell types among gut endocrine cells depends, on (a) the detection of hormone or prohormone and related fragments in the cell; (b) the ultrastructural characterization of the cell itself, with special reference to its secretory granules, and (c) the co-localization of different hormonal (such as glicentin and PYY in intestinal L cells) and nonhormonal products (chromogranins, membrane glycoproteins, and various enzymes) stored in the same granules. As many as 15 gastroenteropancreatic (GEP) endocrine cells were considered in the Lausanne 1977 classification, and its subsequent revisions (9, 10). This classification, improved according to additional immunocytochemical investigations (11–19), is presented in Table 15.1. The main structural and histochemical features of the various cell types are summarized in Table 15.2.

GENERAL ASPECTS OF ENDOCRINE CELL HYPERPLASIA AND TUMORS

DIAGNOSIS

Endocrine cells of the gut may increase in number and become hyperplastic while remaining intraglandular, as scattered elements or forming rows, tubules, microacini, and micronodules (20).

Sometimes, budding of small clusters of hyperplastic endocrine cells from the base of glandular epithelium is found. Minute extraglandular micronodules made up of small clusters of endocrine cells, usually surrounded by a thin basement membrane and barely exceeding the size of the glands, may be found in the lamina propria of the mucosa, especially in areas of chronic inflammation (21). Reactive proliferation of endocrine cells surviving gland damage and entrapped in the connective tissue might be involved in the genesis of such micronodules. Only occasionally have all intermediate patterns between hyperplastic micronodules and frank endocrine tumors, including enlargement and fusion of the micronodules with loss of basement membrane, been observed, especially in a pathologic condition of the stomach called microcarcinoidosis, characterized by numerous intramucosal foci of hyperplasia, dysplasia, and tumor growth (20).

In most cases, the histologic features of endocrine tumors in the gut are distinctive enough to permit their identification. Pseudoglandular (tubuloacinar) structures with true lumina, however, may be prominent in some tumors, such as somatostatin cell tumors, which on purely histologic grounds may be difficult to distinguish from usual adenomas and adenocarcinomas (22, 23). Distinguishing some endocrine tumors with solid sheets or broad trabeculae and atypical changes from solid carcinomas with moderate atypia may also be difficult. Selective staining techniques for endocrine granules, such as Grimelius' silver and lead-hematoxylin, are helpful in proving the endocrine nature of such tumors. The immunohistochemical detection of neuron-specific enolase (NSE), protein gene product 9.5 (PGP 9.5) chromogranins, and specific glycoproteins of secretory granule membrane may also provide useful and more specific markers of endocrine tumors (24–28). In particular, chromogranins A, B, and C, a family of anionic intragranular proteins, possibly involved in hormone posttranslational biosynthesis, storage, and release, seem closely related to the argyrophil and basophilic component of secretory granules, detected by selective stains such as Grimelius' silver, lead-hematoxylin, or masked metachromasia (5).

Endocrine peptides and monoamines are the most specific markers of gut endocrine tumors and represent useful tools for their characterization and classification. The immunohistochemical detection of hormones and related prohormones allows precise correlation of tumor cell differentiation and function with tumor-associated hyperfucntional syndromes (14, 20, 27, 29–31). Because

of the frequent occurrence in the same tumors of multiple cell types producing different hormones, problems may arise in classifying endocrine tumors purely on functional grounds. Thus, it seems opportune to restrict the use of functional labelings as, gastrinoma, vipoma, or somatostatinoma to those tumors that, in addition to showing the appropriate peptide in tumor cells, also develop a related hyperfunctional syndrome (Table 15.3). Tumors lacking any hyperfunctional syndrome may be classified on the basis of the prevalent tumor cell type (as, for instance, gastrin [G] cell tumor, somatostatin [D] cell tumor, G/D-cell tumor, or enterochromaffin-like [ECL] cell tumor) or even on the basis of more conventional morphologic criteria, such as histologic pattern,

TABLE 15.2   Main Histochemical and Ultrastructural Features of Human Gastroenteropancreatic Endocrine Cells

Cell	Hormone Histochemistry	Other Stains	Secretory Granule Ultrastructure		
			Size	Shape	Inner Structure
P		Grimelius, chg A	100-150	Round	Thin-haloed
EC	Serotonin	Grimelius, chg A, PbH	150-500	Pleomorphic	Heavily osmiophilic
D	Somatostatin	Davenport's silver, PbH	200-400	Round	Poorly osmiophilic, homogeneous
L	Glicentin/glucagon-37, PYY	PbH, Grimelius, chg C > A	150-300	Round	Solid, fairly dense
A	Glucagon (C-t IR)	Grimelius, chg A > C	200-350	Round	Target-like
PP	Pancreatic-polypeptide	Grimelius, chg C, A	D_1: 40-200	Round	Homogeneous, fairly dense
			F: 200-400	Variable	Variable
B	Insulin	Aldehyde fuchsin	200-400	Round	Vesicular with crystalloids
X		PbH, Grimelius	160-280	Round	Solid, fairly dense
ECL	Histamine, serotonin	Grimelius, chg A	160-300	Round	Vesicular, coarsely granular core
G	Gastrin (Non C-t IR)	Grimelius, chg A	150-350	Round	Vesicular, flocculent core
CCK	Cholecystokinin (Non-C-t IR)		150-250	Round	Thin-haloed, fairly dense
S	Secretin	Grimelius, chg A	200-350	Round to angular	Solid to target-like
GIP	Gastrin Inhibitory polypeptide		200-300	Round	Solid, fairly dense
M	Motilin		150-220	Round	Solid, fairly dense
N	Neurotensin	Grimelius, chg A	250-350	Round	Solid, fairly dense

Key: PbH, lead-hematoxylin; chg, chromogranin; C-t IR, C-terminal immunoreactivity; >, heavier staining than.

TABLE 15.3   Main Gut-Related Endocrine Syndromes

Syndrome	Increased Blood Hormone(s)	Symptoms	Cause
Carcinoid	5-HT, substance P, kallikrein-bradykinin	Red-blue flushing, diarrhea	EC-cell argentaffin carcinoid
Atypical	Histamine, 5-HT/5-HTP; ↑ by gastrin	Red flushing	ECL-cell argyrophil carcinoid
Zollinger-Ellison or gastrinoma	Gastrin; ↑ by secretin	Peptic ulcer, hyperchlorhydria	G-cell tumor
G-cell hyperfunction	Gastrin; ↓ by secretin, ↑ by meal	Peptic ulcer, hyperchlorhydria	G-cell hyperplasia
Somatostatinoma	Somatostatin	Diabetes, steatorrhea, cholelithiasis	D-cell tumor
Glucagonoma	Glucagon	Skin rash, diabetes	A-cell tumor
Verner-Morrison or Vipoma	VIP, PHM, PP	Watery diarrhea, hypokalemia, and/or hypochlorhydria (WDHA)	Epithelial endocrine or neurogenic vipoma

Key: VIP, vasoactive intestinal peptide; PHM, peptide with N-terminal histidine and C-terminal methionine; ↑, enhanced; ↓, decreased; 5-HT, 5-hydroxytryptamine; 5-HTP, 5-hydroxytryptophan.

TABLE 15.4 Cytologic and Clinicopathologic Characterization of Gut Endocrine Tumors in 239 Cases

	Cases No	Cases %	Site	Prevalent Cell Type	Main Hormonal Products	Associated Syndrome or Pathologic Condition
Well differentiated						
Gastric ECL-cell tumor (or carcinoid)	50	20.9	Body/fundus	ECL	Histamine 5-HT/5-HTP	Atypical carcinoid syndrome, A-CAG, G-cell hyperplasia, ZES/MEN-1
Gastrin-cell tumor	35	14.6	Duodenum, antrum, jejunum	G	Gastrin	ZES, ECL-cell growths
Somatostatin-cell tumor	12	5	Duodenum, antrum	D	Somatostatin	Neurofibromatosis
PP-cell tumor	1	0.4	Duodenum	PP	Pancreatic polypeptide	
Gangliocytic paraganglioma	5	2	Duodenum	D, PP	Somatostatin, PP	
EC-cell tumor (argentaffin carcinoid)	75	31.3	Appendix, small and large intestine, stomach	EC	5-HT, tachykinins	Carcinoid syndrome
L-cell tumor (hindgut trabecular carcinoid)	35	14.6	Rectum, appendix	L	Glicentin, glucagon 37, GLP-1, GLP-2, PP, PYY	
Inappropriate tumors	2	0.8	Stomach, jejunum		ACTH-MSH, VIP	Cushing or VIPoma syndrome
Mixed endocrine-exocrine tumors	3	1.2	Stomach, rectum			
Undefined tumors	4	1.6	Duodenum, jejunum, stomach			
Poorly differentiated						
Small-intermediate cell carcinoma	17	7.1	Stomach, duodenum, colon-rectum	Protoendocrine	Variable	Variable

Key: MSH, melanocyte-stimulating hormone; CAG, chronic atrophic gastritis; ZES, Zollinger-Ellison syndrome; MEN-1, multiple endocrine syndrome, type 1. Other abbreviations, see Tables 15.1 and 15.3.

reactivity to silver techniques, site of origin, and so forth (e.g., gastric argyrophil carcinoid, rectal trabecular carcinoid, or intestinal argentaffin carcinoid).

CLASSIFICATION

A classification of gut endocrine tumors into foregut (stomach, pancreas, duodenum, and upper jejunum), midgut (lower jejunum, ileum, appendix, cecum), and hindgut (colon, rectum), with considerable clinicopathologic differences among the three groups, was introduced decades ago by Williams and Sandler (32) and supported recently by hormone histochemical studies (30). In the case of foregut tumors, the utility of such a classification in practical diagnostic work remains limited by its failure to characterize individual tumor entities with well-defined histologic, cytologic, hormonal, and/or clinicopathologic profiles. Although, because gut endocrine tumors express cell types and hormones that are largely coherent with those expressed by their tissues of origin, knowledge of the exact site of origin is often of help in suggesting the nature of the tumor, to be ascertained by subsequent histochemical and ultrastructural investigations. Thus, midgut tumors are mostly 5-hydroxytryptamine (5-HT) and substance

P-producing argentaffin EC-cell carcinoids, whereas hindgut tumors show mainly glicentin/glucagon-37-, PP-, and or PYY-producing L cells. Pyloric and duodenal tumors are mainly gastrin and somatostatin cell tumors. Finally, argyrophil ECL cells largely predominate in gastric argyrophil carcinoids arising in the body-fundus mucosa (14, 33).

A general classification of carcinoids based on structural patterns developed by Soga and Tazawa (34) comprises four pure patterns (A, solid nest or insular; B, trabecular; C, glandular; and D, undifferentiated) and several mixed patterns (A+C, A+B, B+C, B+D, A+B+C). The various structural patterns have been found to correlate to the primary site of the tumor. For instance, A or A+C patterns largely prevail in the ileum and appendix, and B and B+C patterns prevail in the rectum. At least in part, structural patterns are linked with the endocrine cell type(s) composing the tumor growth, for instance, A-type carcinoids are, as a rule, EC-cell carcinoids (34, 35), whereas rectal trabecular carcinoids are mainly L-cell tumors (36). In patients with metastatic disease, these structural patterns are associated with significantly different survival rates (37).

Thus, combining information regarding the site and structural patterns of a gut endocrine tumor may provide useful information, although it can hardly fulfill all the requirements for fruitful clinicopathologic correlation. For practical purposes, the classification of gut endocrine tumors in Table 15.4, covering most available histopathologic, histochemical, ultrastructural, and clinicopathologic data, is recommended.

PROGNOSIS

With respect to gut endocrine tumors, factors known to be of prognostic relevance include site, size, multicentricity, angioinvasions, level of local tissue invasion, regional lymph node or distant metastases, histologic pattern, histochemical profile, clinical symptoms (with special reference to functional syndromes), and association with other neoplasms.

The better outcome of appendiceal tumors and, to some extent, rectal tumors in comparison with colonic, midgut, or foregut tumors is well known (38–40). This more favorable outlook results in part from their smaller size, and lower invasive level and spread at the time of discovery. The good prognosis of tumors less than 1 cm in size is well documented; most tumors 2 or 2.5 cm in diameter or larger have shown malignant behavior (40–42).

At all levels in the gut, patients with tumors that invade only the mucosa-submucosa or muscularis propria ("superficially invasive" or "intramural" tumors) show better survival than those with tumors invading the gastrointestinal wall deeply (serosa or beyond). In the extensive study of Hajdu and coworkers (40), less than 1% of "superficially invasive" tumors metastatized and caused death, whereas of the deeply invasive tumors, 85% metastatized and 65% were fatal. None of 32 carcinoids (mostly intestinal) confined to the mucosa-submucosa showed associated metastatic disease, whereas 7% of 29 tumors invading the muscularis propria and 69% of 13 lesions showing serosal involvement demonstrated metastatic spread (43). None of 45 patients who had intramural carcinoids died in the 5-year period after excision of the tumor, whereas of the 39 patients with tumor that extended into the serosa or beyond, only 2 (5%) lived longer than 5 years (44).

At the end of their study, Hajdu and colleagues reported that the survivors included 50% of patients presenting with metastases restricted to regional lymph nodes, but only 8% of patients with distant metastases. In patients with metastatic disease, both the anatomic site of the primary tumor and the histologic pattern of the tumor were significantly and independently correlated with survival. In particular, mixed A+C, pure A, pure B, mixed A+B, other mixed types, pure C, and pure D patterns ranked in a progressively decreasing order of median survival time (37).

In general, patients with endocrine tumors diagnosed because of clinical symptoms have a poorer prognosis than those in whom the tumor (most often an intramural lesion) is discovered by chance during clinical examination (44). In particular, the prognosis is less favorable for individuals with tumors associated with hyperfunctional syndromes than for those lacking the syndrome. Coexistence of other malignant neoplasms has been found in as many as 29% of patients with carcinoids of the small intestine, a fact that may greatly influence survival rates (38, 41, 43).

In the large Tumor Registry series analyzed by Godwin (39), 5% of carcinoids in the appendix were nonlocalized (1.4% in the series of Moertel et al. [38]), 14% in the rectum and rectosigmoid, 55% in the stomach (17 to 39% in the review by Brodman and Pai [45]), 64% in the ileum and jejunum, and 71% in the colon; 5-year relative survival rates were 99%, 83%, 52%, 54%, and 52%, respectively.

In general, the following criteria should be considered for a diagnosis of gut endocrine tumors with malignant potential: (a) tumor size above 1 cm (larger tumors are more aggressive); (b) wall invasion (invasion beyond the submucosa is associated with higher malignant potential); (c) structural atypia with prevalence of broad solid areas, sometimes with central necrosis, usually associated with cytologic atypia; (d) cellular atypia with reduced nuclear cytoplasmic ratio, irregular distribution of chromatin and evident nucleoli; (e) more than two mytoses per 10 HPF (high power field = ×400); (f) increased Ki-67-positive nuclei counts (> 50 per 10 HPF or more than 2% of tumor cells); (g) evidence of angioinvasion and invasion of perineural spaces; (h) cellular dedifferentiation, as assessed by loss of granular markers immunoreactivity or argyrophilia despite retention of immunoreactivity for cytoplasmic general markers; (i) nuclear P53 protein accumulation detected by immunohistochemistry.

GASTRIC ARGYROPHIL (ECL CELL) GROWTHS ARISING IN NONANTRAL MUCOSA

The association between multiple ECL-cell argyrophil carcinoids, diffuse chronic atrophic gastritis restricted to the body fundus (A-CAG), and hypergastrinemia (with or without pernicious anemia) is well recognized (46–48). The same type of tumor growth has been identified in hypergastrinemic patients with multiple endocrine neoplasia type 1 and Zollinger-Ellison syndrome (MEN-1-ZES) (49). In addition, multiple gastric ECL-cell carcinoids have been found in aged rats with severe hypergastrinemia induced by life-long treatment with inhibitors of acid secretion or by subtotal gastric resection sparing the antrum (50–52). In keeping with the known gastrin-dependence of ECL cells, these experimental observations support the hypothesis that hypergastrinemia plays a major role in the pathogenesis of ECL-cell tumors (6, 53). ECL-cell tumors, however, arise exclusively in aged (about 2 years old), inbred rats. Studies by Lee et al. (54) showed that such aged, inbred rats bear a trait for multiple endocrine tumor development. In addition, a few precarcinoid lesions and even one occasional carcinoid (55) were observed in untreated normogastrinemic, age-matched animals. These observations suggest that factors other then hypergastrinemia may be required to transform ECL cells (49). This conclusion is further supported by the frequent, spontaneous insurgence of malignant ECL-cell carcinoids in normogastrinemic *Mastomys natalensis,* a South African rodent bearing an as yet undefined genetic trait for the development of these and other extragastric tumors (56, 57).

Hypergastrinemia-promoted carcinoids arising in hypergastrinemic patients, either with chronic atrophic gastritis of type A (A-CAG) or with MEN-ZES (see following paragraphs), are frequently if not constantly accompanied by a variety of nonneoplastic ECL-cell growths (20, 58). The different patterns of endocrine growths have been classified in a system covering hyperplastic, potentially preneoplastic, and early neoplastic lesions (59, 60). A sequential appearance of hyperplastic, dysplastic, and neoplastic lesions was demonstrated in Mastomys rendered hypergastrinemic by sustained antisecretory drug treatment, but not in normogastrinemic controls (61). This result suggests that the sequence can be fully reproduced only when the trophic effects of

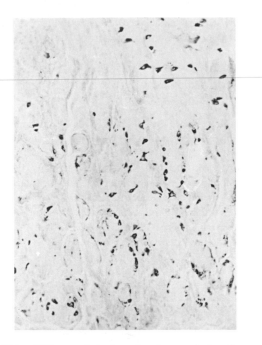

Figure 15.1 Diffuse, chain-forming hyperplasia of argyrophil cells in the oxyntic glands of a patient with antropyloric G cell hyperplasia and hyperfunction (see Fig. 15.5) (Grimelius silver, ×110).

gastrin act in conjunction with transforming factor(s) (genetic or other). ECL-cell carcinoids arising sporadically in the stomach of normogastrinemic patients are not associated with hyperplastic or dysplastic changes (see discussion of ECL cell tumors for details).

HYPERPLASTIC CHANGES

Hyperplastic changes of gastric endocrine cells occur relatively frequently, although no significant tumorigenic potential has been linked to these changes (49, 59, 62).

SIMPLE OR DIFFUSE HYPERPLASIA

This entity is defined as an increase in endocrine cells of more than twice the standard deviation with respect to age- and sex-matched controls. The cells remain scatterd as single elements or as less than five cell aggregates, and they are often hypertrophic (Fig. 15.1). Diffuse hyperplasia is found regularly in patients with ZES or gastrin cell hyperplasia and hyperfunction. It may also be observed, however, at lower rates, in ordinary duodenal ulcer patients or other clinical conditions not associated with marked hypergastrinemia.

LINEAR HYPERPLASIA

This type of hyperplasia is characterized by linear sequences of five or more cells lying inside the basement membrane of the gastric glands (Figs. 15.1 and 15.2); as a mean, at least two lines per linear millimeter of mucosa are found. This change is usually observed in severely hypergastrinemic subjects, such as patients with ZES or pernicious anemia. Linear hyperplasia may be regarded as a focal or widespread exaggeration of simple hyperplasia, leading to accumu-

lation of endocrine cells at the bottom of oxyntic glands or hyperplastic mucous-neck glands.

MICRONODULAR HYPERPLASIA

This entity is diagnosed when clusters of five or more endocrine cells not exceeding 150 μm (usually 50 to 100 μm) in diameter are observed, with at least one cluster per linear millimeter of mucosa, as a mean. Micronodular hyperplasia, usually combined with linear hyperplasia, is a regular finding in diffuse (autoimmune) type chronic atrophic gastritis of the corpus-fundus (type A CAG), which is usually associated with severe hypergastrinemia, with or without pernicious anemia (see Fig. 15.2). Endocrine cell clustering may also result from focal gland atrophy without absolute increase of endocrine cell density (simple clustering or micronodular pseudohyperplasia), such as occurs in normogastrinemic or mildly hypergastrinemic *H. pylori* gastritis with or without gastric ulcer, dyspepsia, or cancer. Focal micronodular pseudohyperplasia is not associated with linear or diffuse hyperplasia unless it coexists with hypergastrinemia. Hypergastrinemia is usually moderate and may occur secondary to the hypochlorhydria caused by confluent multifocal atrophy of acidopeptic glands (63–66). Pseudohyperplastic micronodules differ from true hyperplastic micronodules in that they are smaller (mean size about 50 μm) and are composed mainly of small cells showing rather pycnotic nucleous, scarce cytoplasm with few, small nondiagnostic secretory granules, hypotrophic Golgi and endoplasmic reticulum, but abundant microfilaments and residual bodies (66).

ADENOMATOID HYPERPLASIA

This entity is characterized by a collection of five or more micronodules that are adherent but have interposing basement membranes and thin strands of lamina propria. This lesion is found more often in a background of extensive micronodular hyperplasia related to either atrophic gastritis or MEN-ZES (52, 67, 68). Adenomatoid hyperplasia is considered a focal exaggeration of micronodular hyperplasia and does not differ substantially from the latter in its morphology and tumorigenic potential.

DYSPLASTIC GROWTHS

Dysplastic or precarcinoid growths are lesions of more than 150 μm and less than 500 μm in diameter, formed by moderately atypical endocrine cells that usually have enlarged nuclei and show reduced reactivity for tests detecting secretory granules or their contents. Because of their small size, dysplastic growths are deeply scattered in the mucosa, escape endoscopic observation, and invariably are first diagnosed histologically. Although considered precursors of carcinoids, dysplastic growths are always intramucosal and do not infiltrate beyond muscularis mucosa. Their detection, however, should encourage careful endoscopic reinvestigation, with extensive bioptic sampling in search of possible neoplasia. In fact, although in exceptional cases dysplastic lesions have been found in the absence of carcinoids, coexistence of both dysplastic and hyperplastic lesions is the rule when multiple carcinoids arise in MEN-ZES or A-CAG patients with severe hypergastrinemia (62, 69). These findings, together with the frequent occurrence of argyrophil cell hyperplasia in the absence of dysplasia in the gastric mucosa of carcinoid-free hypergastrinemic patients, point to the dysplastic growths as "spy lesions" or "markers" of occult carcinoids.

The following histologic patterns are recognized:

Enlarged micronodules: expansile growths of more than 150 μm in size

Adenomatous micronodules: one or more collections of at least five micronodules (often enlarged) closely adherent to each other with interposition of basement membranes only, mimicking the back-to-back pattern of colonic or gastric exocrine adenomas

Fused micronodules: characterized by the disappearance of the intervening basal membrane between adjacent micronodules

Microinfiltrative lesions: microinfiltration of the lamina propria by endocrine cells filling the space between glands

Nodules with newly formed stroma: gives some hint of trabecular or microlobular structure

WELL-DIFFERENTIATED ENDOCRINE TUMORS (ARGYROPHIL ECL-CELL CARCINOIDS)

Histopathologically, gastric endocrine tumors are currently classified, on the basis of their differentiation status, as well differentiated or poorly differentiated (70). Mixed endocrine-exocrine forms have been reported only exceptionally. Well-differentiated tumors are addressed in this discussion; details of poorly differentiated tumors are provided later in this chapter.

In the past literature, endocrine tumors of the stomach accounted for about 0.3% of all gastric tumors and 3% of all gastrointestinal endocrine tumors (39, 71). According to more recent series, however, the incidence ranges from 11 to 41% of all gastrointestinal endocrine tumors (39, 62, 68, 71–74). This evidence outlines the fact that the incidence of gastric endocrine tumors, with special reference to small, well-differentiated, gastrin-dependent ECL-cell tumors, may have been underestimated (39, 71), and suggests that their occurrence is not such a rare event in clinical gastroenterologic practice. The remarkable increase in the incidence of gastric endocrine tumors is likely related to the widespread use of endoscopy and to the increased awareness of such lesions.

Gastric argyrophil tumors are diagnosed as ECL-cell tumors when most tumor cells show the following: strong argyrophilia by both Grimelius' and Sevier-Munger's technique (Figs. 15.3 and 15.4) and positive immunoreactivity for chromogranin A, in the absence of reactivity for the argentaffin or diazonium tests for serotonin, and no or only occasional immunoreactivity for hormonal products (62, 75). Indeed, minor tumor subpopulations expressing serotonin, gastrin, somatostatin pancreatic polypeptide (PP), or α-hCG have been detected in a minority of tumor cells. Histamine immunohistochemical analysis, although promising, so far has not been suitable for routinely processed specimens (76). The ECL nature of argyrophil tumors is ultimately assessed by electron micros-

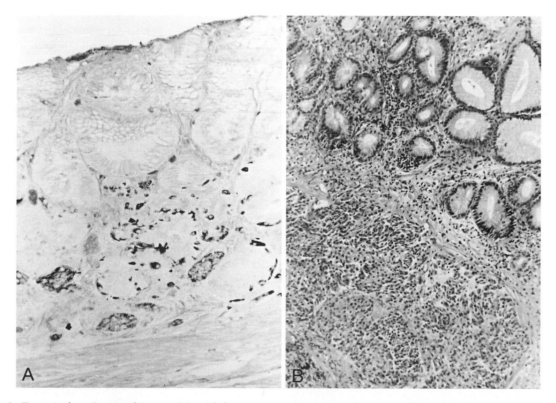

Figure 15.2   A, Type A chronic atrophic gastritis with hypergastrinemia. Irregular hyperplasia of endocrine forming intraglandular chains and extraglandular micronodules in the deep sclero-atrophic mucosa. Note lack of endocrine cells in the hyperplastic foveolae forming the upper half of the mucosa (Grimelius silver, ×150). **B,** Microcarcinoid in the deep, atrophic mucosa covered by polypoid foveolar hyperplasia (hematoxylin & eosin, ×110).

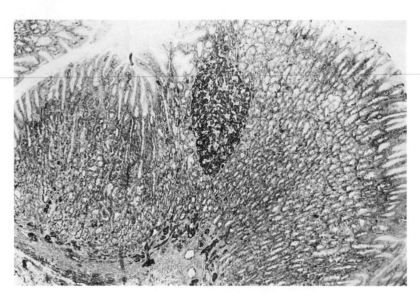

Figure 15.3 Hypertrophic gastropathy in multiple endocrine neoplasia (MEN) type I with parathyroid adenoma, pancreatic and duodenal gastrinomas (with ZES), and gastric carcinoidosis. A microcarcinoid and numerous hyperplastic micronodules are selectively stained with Sevier-Munger's silver in the superficial-middle part and basal part, respectively, of the mucosa (×65).

copy, revealing features variably fitting those described for ECL-cell granules, such as irregular to round cores and adherent to detached, smooth to wavy membranes (see Fig. 15.4C) (47, 53, 77). Large secretory granules with round cores of regular, punctate-cerebroid structure also are frequently observed and interpreted as a pathologic variant of ECL-cell granules (74, 78–80). In addition, granules resembling those of other gastric endocrine cell types (P, X, G, and EC) may be identified at ultrastructural analysis.

Histologically, the most diffuse structural pattern is variably composed of microlobules and trabeculae (62) only in part fitting Soga and Tazawa A, B, or mixed AB types (34). Microacinar-microtubular structure with small lumina, somehow mimicking tubular glands of normal gastric mucosa filled by tumor cells and corresponding to Soga's type C structure, is observed in a minority of cases (62). Similarly, the thin elongated strands of trabecular Soga type B structure may be observed; it accounted for 18% of 46 cases we reported (62). Moderately enlarged trabeculae and lobules are reported in 50% of investigated cases of sporadic ECL cell arising independently from MEN-ZES or A-CAG (62). In general, tumors associated with the latter conditions show no significant cellular atypia and only occasional mitoses (< 2 per 10 HPF), whereas "sporadic" tumors show moderate cellular atypia and increased number of mitoses (2 to 9 per 10 HPF). Useful markers of the malignant potential of well-differentiated ECL tumors are a tumor size larger then 1 cm and invasion of the muscularis propria. In addition, a careful clinicopathologic assessement of the background disease may also help in predicting tumor behavior.

Three clinicopathologic subtypes of gastric endocrine tumors have been characterized: type 1, associated with diffuse chronic atrophic gastritis of autoimmune or A type (A-CAG); type 2, associated with hypertrophic gastropathy (HG), usually in conjunction with multiple endocrine neoplasia of type 1 and Zollinger-Ellison syndrome (MEN-1-ZES); type 3 sporadic, not associated with specific gastric pathology.

AUTOIMMUNE-CHRONIC ATROPHIC GASTRITIS (A-CAG)-ASSOCIATED TUMORS

According to the most recent series available (83), ECL-cell tumors account for most, if not all, well-differentiated endocrine tumors arising in a background of diffuse atrophic gastritis (see Fig. 15.2B) with prevalence of female patients (71%) in the seventh decade of life (mean age of 63 years). A-CAG, usually coupled with achlorhydria with or without pernicious anemia, is diagnosed from samples of non-tumor gastric mucosa. Hypergastrinemia or evidence of antral gastrin cell hyperplasia is observed in all cases of A-CAG. ECL-cell hyperplastic changes are invariably detected and, frequently, dysplastic growths are also found (see previous discussion) when carcinoid tumors coexist. In our study (83), gastric mucosa of 55 cases was available for extensive evaluation of nonneoplastic ECL-cell growths. ECL-cell hyperplasia was present in all 55 cases and dysplasia was identified in 66%.

A-CAG-associated carcinoids are frequently multiple and multicentric. Of 152 cases studied, endoscopy revealed that 87 (57%) had more than two growths endoscopically identified and removed (57%), 6 had two, and 59 (39%) were apparently single (83).

Tumor histology is generally bland with mild or even absent cellular atypia and mitoses (see Fig. 15.4). Tumor size is generally small; in our series, 77% of lesions were less than 1 cm in diameter and 19% were between 1 and 1.5 cm (83). Wall invasion is normally limited to mucosa or submucosa. Of 67 cases evaluated, 18 (27%) lesions invaded the mucosa only, 43 (64%) the mucosa and submucosa, and only 6 the muscularis propria (81). The deeply invasive tumors had a mean diameter of 1.4 cm. Metastases were exceptional (Table 15.5) and survival was excellent. Review of the pertinent literature (62) revealed results in which just 17 of 197 CAG-associated tumors showed metastases, only 4 of which were distant. In our series (83), only 2 of 41 cases had metastases (one to regional lymph nodes and one to the liver). At follow up of 144 patients, survival with tumor was reported for as long as 16 years and no tumor-related death was observed (83).

MEN AND ZE SYNDROME (MEN-ZES)-ASSOCIATED TUMORS

This type of well-differentiated ECL-cell tumor is rare and represents a mere 6% (12 of 191 cases) in our study series (83). These tumors generally develop in patients in the fifth decade of life and shows no sex prevalence. Hypertrophic hypersecretory gastropathy with high levels of circulating gastrin are critical diagnostic findings. In all cases, ECL-cell hyperplasia and dysplasia were noted in the surrounding nontumor mucosa (see Fig. 15.3). Of 12 cases studied, 11 involved multiple and multicentric tumors and in only one case was a single tumor identified (83). Findings of tumor histology and cytology are always bland in the absence of significant mitoses. Tumors were between 1 and 1.5 cm in diameter in eight patients and were limited to the mucosa/submucosa in 10 (83). Metastases to local lymph nodes were observed in three patients, one of whom also had distant metstases. Patients' survival has been excellent, with tumor persistence reported for as long as 25 years and only one tumor-related death (83). Incidentally, patients with MEN-1-ZES more frequently succumb to the more aggressive coexisting gastrin-producing tumor.

SPORADIC TUMORS

Sporadic ECL tumors are generally solitary growths arising in a context of gastric mucosa devoid of significant pathologic change except for gastritis (other than A-CAG). Rare multiple tumors have been observed (83). Although less frequent than CAG-associated tumors, sporadic tumors are more common than MEN-ZES-associated tumors and account for 14% of cases (27 of 191) in our series (83). Of these 27 tumors, 20 occurred in male patients in the sixth decade of life. As a rule, neither hypergastrinemia nor gastrin-dependent ECL-cell hyperplasia are observed. In one exceptional case, such findings were ascribed to a gastrin cell subpopulaton found in the tumor itself (83).

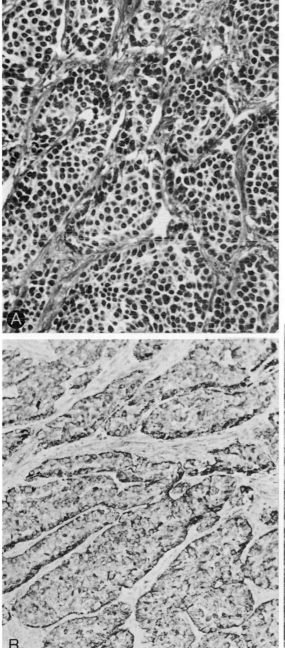

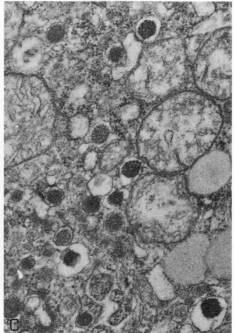

Figure 15.4 **A,** Invasive, submucosal part of a gastric argyrophil carcinoid metastatic to the liver, coupled with atypical carcinoid syndrome. Monomorphic tumor cells form trabeculae and microlobules that are strongly argyrophilic **(B)** (**A,** hematoxylin & eosin, ×220; **B,** Grimelius silver, ×140). **C,** Electron microscopy shows vesicular granules containing a fairly dense core, often with coarsely granular substructure (×28,000).

TABLE

15.5   Invasive Behavior and Metastatic Potential of Gastric Endocrine Tumors

Type	Number	Deepest Level of Wall Invasion				Metastatic			
		m	sm	mp	s	Local	Distant	Total	%
ECL cell tumor									
CAG-associated	152	18	43	6	0	1	1	2	5
MEN-ZES	12	2	8	1	0	3	1	3	30
Sporadic	27	0	4	4	9	10	9	12	75
G cell tumor	2	1	0	1	0	0	0		0
Small-intermediate cell tumor	12	0	0	4	8	6	6	12	100
Total	205	21	55	16	17	20	17	29	36

Key: m, mucosa; sm, submucosa; mp, muscularis propria; s, serosa; CAG, chronic atrophic gastritis; MEN-ZES, multiple endocrine neoplasia-Zollinger-Ellison syndrome.

Data from Rindi G, Bordi C, Rappel S, et al. Gastric carcinoids and neuroendocrine carcinomas: Pathogenesis, pathology, and behavior. World J Surg 1996;20:168–172.

Tumor histology may be relatively bland (see Fig. 15.4), although in a significant proportion of cases (5 of 10 cases described previously [62]), moderate cellular atypia with nuclear pleomorphism, evident nucleoli, hyperchromasia, and significant mitoses (2 to 9 per 10 HPF) were found. These lesions also showed a peculiar structure with broader solid aggregates and trabeculae. Of 27 tumors studied, the mean diameter was 3.2 cm; only 8 lesions (30%) were smaller than 1 cm in diameter. Deep wall invasion is frequently observed in sporadic tumors. In our series, 53% of tumors reached the serosa and, overall, 76% invaded at least the muscularis propria (83). Sporadic tumors have a definite metastatic potential. Metastases to local lymph nodes were observed in 10 of 14 patients and distant metastases were detected in 9 of 13. Tumor-related death was reported in 7 of 26 patients followed (83). In consideration of their aggressive behavior, sporadic ECL tumors that do not actually show metastases or deep wall invasion should nevertheless be regarded as at high risk for low grade malignancy, especially when 2 cm or more in diameter.

An "atypical carcinoid syndrome" with red cutaneous flushing and without diarrhea has been reported in association with sporadic gastric carcinoids, usually coupled with liver metastases and production of histamine and/or 5-hydroxytryptophan (84–86), a secretory pattern clearly reminiscent of ECL cells (6, 87). A dermatosis with the pattern of acanthosis nigricans has been found in association with a malignant sporadic ECL-cell tumor (88). Whether ECL-cell products had any role in the genesis of the dermatosis, which subsided after tumor excision, remains uncertain.

GASTRIN CELL GROWTHS

GASTRIN CELL HYPERPLASIA

Gastrin (G)-cell hyperplasia is known to occur in the pyloric mucosa of patients with peptic ulcer disease (often recurrent and resistant to medical therapy), hyperchlorhydria, and severe food-stimulated hypergastrinemia (6, 22, 89–92). In several cases (Fig. 15.5), the average number of G-cells per millimeter of pyloric mucosa (counted in 5-μm thick histologic sections) from muscularis muco-

sae to luminal surface ranged from 140 to 250, in comparison with 40 to 90 in control subjects who lacked G-cell hyperfunction and peptic ulcer disease. Borderline cases between severely hyperfunctioning, massive G-cell hyperplasia and common duodenal ulcer disease lacking G-cell hyperplasia and hypergastrinemia were also observed. Antral gastrin cell hyperplasia/hyperfunction has been well documented also in infants and children with severe peptic disease (93–97). In some of these cases, an increased ratio of antral G and somatostatin-producing (D) cells was demonstrated suggesting a lack of inhibitory control by D cells as potential pathogenetic factor (95, 97). The increased G/D ratio could be attributed to either increased G cell numbers or reduced numbers of D cells.

Bombesin, which is present in intrinsic nerves running in the lamina propria adjacent to the pyloric G cell (98), might have a role in the genesis of this primary G-cell hyperplasia. In fact, bombesin treatment has been found to stimulate gastrin cell proliferation (99). Secondary G-cell hypertrophy, hyperplasia, and hyperfunction have been reported in the pyloric mucosa of achlorhydric patients with type A CAG, with or without pernicious anemia (100–103).

Other factors to consider in connection with gastrin cell hyperplasia are H. pylori infection and the chronic inflammatory cell infiltrate that the infection creates in the antral mucosa and immediate vicinity of the G cells. Ammonia produced by the bacterium is thought to impair acid-mediated suppression of gastrin release, thus causing relative G-cell hyperstimulation and hypergastrinemia in duodenal ulcer and some ulcer-like dyspepsia patients (104). Studies involving the use of isolated perfused canine antrum have shown that the T-lymphocyte products interleukin-2 and γ-interferon stimulate gastrin release (105). A similar action should also be exerted by tumor necrosis factor (TNFα) and interleukin-8 (IL-8), which are released by gastric epithelial cells as well by mucosal inflammatory cells attracted and activated by H. pylori (106–108).

GASTRIN CELL TUMORS

Gastrin cell tumors, i.e., tumors showing a prevalent population of gastrin cells or tumors with any proportion of gastrin cells associated with ZES, represent the largest group in reported series of endocrine tumors arising in the upper small intestine (109–111) (see Fig. 15.5). In our series of 33 cases of tumors in the duodenum and jejunum, they prevailed in males (23 of 33 cases, 70%) and in 28 of 33 (85%) cases, the tumor was located in the proximal duodenum. A similar prevalence for the first portion of the duodenum has been reported elsewhere (112) and can be traced in some previous studies, although this is not outlined by the authors (109, 113).

Zollinger-Ellison syndrome (ZES) with hypergastrinemia, gastric acid hypersecretion, and fulminant ulcer diathesis is the sole syndrome of endocrine hyperfunction consistently observed in association with duodenal and upper-jejunal endocrine tumors (109, 111, 114, 115). ZES was detected in 14 cases (14 of 56 [25%]) of our patients with duodenojejunal tumors, or 42% of those with gastrin cell tumors, three of whom had type 1 multiple endocrine neoplasia (MEN-1) syndrome. In the past, in an extensive review of all cases recorded in the ZES registry, 103 of 800 patients (13%) were found to have duodenal wall tumors, whereas the majority of patients had a pancreatic tumor (116). More recent studies have shown a higher incidence of duodenal tumors, possibly related to improved diagnostic tools (111, 115, 117). In fact, duodenojejunal gastrinomas frequently are small; in only 3 of our 13 cases, the tumors were larger than 1 cm and none exceeded 1.5 cm. As a consequence, they are often missed unless carefully sought during endoscopy or surgery and may be responsible for paraduodenal metastases of apparently undiscovered primaries (114, 118). These metastases may well have been occult microgastrinomas located in a ring of the duodenal bulb removed during previous gastric surgery, as suggested by the frequent occurrence of such tumors in juxtapyloric duodenal mucosa. In this context, it seems of interest that all appropriately investigated cases of duodenal tumors associated with MEN-1-ZES involved gastrin-producing tumor cells, whereas many pancreatic tumors associated with this syndrome lacked immunohistochemical evidence of gastrin production (49, 113, 119, 120).

Thirty of our 35 cases (86%) of gastrointestinal (2 pyloric, 30 duodenal and 3 jejunal) gastrin cell tumors were apparently "nonfunctioning." All were located in the duodenal bulb. No systematic preoperative measurements of serum gastrin and gastric acid secretion had been performed in most patients, five of whom had

ordinary peptic ulcer disease and one with diarrhea cured by tumor surgery. Preoperative diagnosis and functional characterization of these tumors at a clinical level is particulary difficult because the small, very well-differentiated gastrin cell tumors arising in the duodenal bulb may cause milder peptic ulcer disease than the usual ZES caused by pancreatic gastrinomas.

Tumors associated with overt ZES differ from their apparently nonfunctioning counterpart in arising earlier in life (mean age at diagnosis is 38.8 years, as opposed to 66.1 years) and having a higher incidence of metastatic (3 of 14 cases as against none), deeply infiltrative (7 of 14, as against 3 of 19), and nonbulbar cases (5 of 14, as opposed to none). All these findings suggest a different natural history of the gastrin cell tumors in the two conditions. Nonfunctioning tumors represent a particularly benign disease, whereas ZES tumors have low-grade malignant potential, especially when arising at sites where gastrin cells are not normally present, such as in the jejunum or pancreas (15, 111). Metastases in regional lymph nodes have been reported in 4 of 8 cases of duodenal gastrinomas with ZES-MEN-1 syndrome (113), in 25% of 103 cases of duodenal tumors with ZES, 24% of which also had MEN-1 syndrome (116), and in 2 of 3 cases of jejunal gastrinomas (111). Interestingly, local lymph node metastases seem to have little influence on survival of patients with ZES (117, 118, 121). In a study focusing on metastatic rate and survival in patients with ZES (116), no difference was found in the frequency of metastases to lymph node(s) when comparing primary pancreatic (48%) and duodenal (49%) tumors. On the contrary, in the same study, the frequency of metastases to the liver found in patients with pancreatic gastrinomas was significantly higher than that noted in patients with duodenal gastrinomas (52% vs. 5%).

An overall malignancy rate of 38 to 54% has been reported in ZES cases involving duodenal tumors (116, 117) as compared to 70 to 71% in pancreatic gastrinomas (117, 122). The 10-year survival rate of patients with duodenal gastrinomas is significantly different (94% vs. 59%) from that of patients with pancreatic gastrinoma (117). The less favorable prognosis associated with pancreatic gastrinomas is probably related to the larger size and more frequent association with hepatic metastases. In this context, it is interesting to recall a highly significant correlation of primary tumor size with the occurrence of liver metastases, and that no significant indepen-

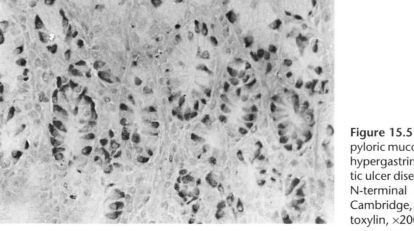

Figure 15.5 Gastrin cell hyperplasia in the pyloric mucosa of a patient with food-enhanced hypergastrinemia, hyperchlorhydria, and peptic ulcer disease. Same patient as in Figure 15.1; N-terminal gastrin-34 antiserum A30 (CRB, Cambridge, U.K.) (immunoperoxidase-hematoxylin, ×200).

dent effect of the anatomic site on development of liver metastases exists when data are analyzed after adjusting for tumor size (117).

Macroscopically, both functioning and nonfunctioning G-cell tumors appear more frequently as a slightly polypoid lesion that may be misinterpreted as an ectopic pancreas, an ectopic gastric mucosa, an inflammatory process, or some other type of polyp (123). Histopathologically, the cells are uniform with scanty cytoplasm, arranged in broad gyriform trabeculae and vascular pseudorosettes (type B2 pattern) (111), with predominant immunoreactivity for gastrin. Other peptides detected in tumor cell subpopulations are cholecystokinin, pancreatic polypeptide (PP), neurotensin, somatostatin, insulin, and the α-chain of human chorionic gonadotropin (110). Interestingly, somatostatin, which is known to inhibit gastrin release from gastrinomas, has been detected in only 3 of 14 ZES tumors of our series, whereas it was present in 10 of 19 nonfunctioning tumors.

Multifocal, intraepithelial growths forming chains or micronodules of endocrine cells, sometimes with mild atypia and in direct continuity with tumor growth, have been found in the deep crypts of intestinal mucosa adjacent to gastrin cell tumors. These findings, which are especially prominent in MEN/ZES cases, strongly support the concept that such tumors originate from differentiated intraepithelial endocrine cells (124, 125).

Gastrin cell tumors arise infrequently in the antropyloric mucosa and, in rare cases, are associated with hypergastrinemia and peptic ulcer disease (126–129). In two such cases in our series, one patient had a solitary 2-cm large tumor associated with peptic ulcer and the other patient had a clinically silent G-cell tumor.

SOMATOSTATIN CELL GROWTHS

Increased density of somatostatin D cells, coupled with a decreased G/D-cell ratio, probably due to longstanding hyperchlorhydria, has been observed in the pyloric mucosa of patients with gastrinoma (103). An increased number of somatostatin cells has also been reported in the crypts of the small intestine affected by celiac disease (130). Holle and colleagues described a case of extreme, possibly congenital, somatostatin cell hyperplasia of the gastroduodenal mucosa, coupled with dwarfism, obesity, and goiter, apparently occurring as a result of severe longstanding somatostatin cell hyperfunction (131).

Duodenal tumors composed of well-differentiated somatostatin D cells have also been reported (111, 132). In none of these cases did the patient develop the full-blown "somatostatinoma" syndrome (diabetes mellitus, diarrhea, steatorrhea, hypo- or achlorhydria, anemia, and gallstones) that has been described in association with some pancreatic D cell tumors (133), although some patients reportedly did have diabetes and/or gallstones (132, 134). In our 53 cases of duodenal tumors, 11 of the lesions showed numerous somatostatin cells, with few or no other endocrine cell types. Eight of the 11 tumors arose at, or very close to the ampulla of Vater, which had already been reported as a preferential location for such tumors (109–111, 132, 135). This positioning explains their frequent association with obstructive biliary disease.

A significant number of duodenal somatostatin cell tumors were discovered in patients with cutaneous neurofibromatosis (109, 132, 135), including 2 of our 11 cases. Some of these patients also

have a pheocromocytoma involving one or both adrenal glands, a clinical situation that can have considerable implications for complicated patient management (135, 136). Data from our series and from three series described in the literature (132, 135, 137) demonstrated that somatostatin cell tumors affect females only slightly more frequently than males (21 versus 17 cases) and manifest at a mean age of 45.2 years (range 29 to 83 years).

Histologically, these tumors usually exhibit a mixed architectural pattern with a predominant tubuloglandular (type C) component admixed with a variable proportion of insular and trabecular areas (Fig. 15.6A). Psammoma bodies have been seen mostly within glandular spaces. The glandular pattern and psammoma bodies in some cases have been so prominent that these tumors were originally misdiagnosed as adenocarcinomas. Unlike carcinomas, however, the somatostatin cell tumors are composed of uniform cells with rather bland nuclei, and few mitotic figures can be seen. It may be difficult to make the correct diagnosis because Grimelius' silver stain and chromogranin A immunostain are negative in about 50% of cases. The presence of somatostatin in tumor cells can be proven by immunohistochemical studies (Fig. 15.7B). Although most tumors show an intense immunoreactivity for somatostatin in clearly prevalent populations of the tumor cells, some tumors show minor cell populations with positive staining for calcitonin, pancreatic polypeptide, insulin, glucagon, and ACTH (111, 138). In addition, the apical cytoplasms of tubuloacinar structures bind WGA and PNA lectins (139) and express epithelial membrane antigen (EMA).

Ultrastructural examination demonstrates large, moderately electron-dense secretory granules that range from 250 to 550 nm in greatest diameter and are similar to those found in normal D cells of the intestinal mucosa (see Fig. 15.7C). The psammoma bodies appear as well-demarcated circular or coral-like structures made up of small crystalline needle-shaped structures arranged in radial fashion. They are located in the lumen of glandlike structures that are lined by D cells showing apical intestinal type microvilli.

Despite their rather bland histologic appearance, somatostatin cell tumors are often malignant (5 of 11 of our cases, 11 of 16 cases of 131, and 2 of 8 cases of 136). Malignant somatostatin cell tumors are ≥ 2 cm in diameter (131); invade such areas as the duodenal wall, the sphincter of Oddi, and/or the head of the pancreas; and can metastasize to both paraduodenal lymph nodes and the liver.

GANGLIONEUROMATOUS PARAGANGLIOMA

This rare tumor (Fig. 15.8) results from an admixture of the following: (a) polygonal, round, or columnar epithelial endocrine cells arranged in solid nests and ribbons, resembling more nonargentaffin carcinoids than nonchromaffin paragangliomas, (b) mature ganglion cells, and (c) Schwann-like spindle cells forming small fascicles or enveloping nerve cells and axons (111, 140, 141). These tumors are slightly more common in males than in females, and affected patients range in age from 23 to 80 years, with an average of 54 years (140). Association with neurofibromatosis (142) and with somatostatin cell tumor (143) have been reported.

Most tumors develop in the submucosa (with or without a mucosal component and infiltration of the muscularis propria) of the duodenum, especially in the periampullary region. Less often,

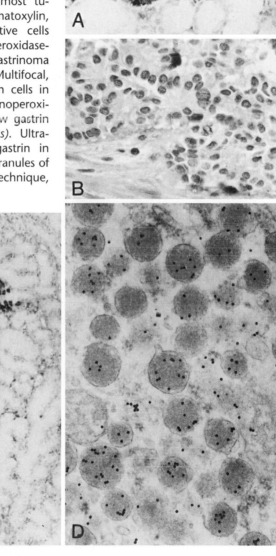

Figure 15.6 Multiple duodenal gastrinomas and gastrin cell hyperplasia in a ZES patient. Gastrin-immunoreactivity of most tumor cells (**A,** immunoperoxidase-hematoxylin, ×150) and rare CCK-immunoreactive cells (**B,** serum AB01 from CRB, immunoperoxidase-hematoxylin, ×280) in a small gastrinoma growing in the Brunner gland area. Multifocal, chain-forming hyperplasia of gastrin cells in nontumor Brunner glands (**C,** immunoperoxidase-hematoxylin, ×110); note a few gastrin cells in the deep crypts *(top links).* Ultrastructural immunolocalization of gastrin in small (about 180 nm) round, solid granules of a tumor cell (**D,** immunogold technique, ×45,000).

tumors arise in the upper jejunum (144) and stomach (145). Grossly, the majority of the lesions represent small, sessile or pedunculated, polypoid growths.

Somatostatin cells were present in the epithelial endocrine component of this tumor detected in five patients in our series as well as in 10 tumors investigated by Hamid et al. (146). In addition, PP cells and rare glucagon or insulin cells have been detected in ganglioneuromatous paragangliomas, suggesting that they may be a hamartia of the pancreatic anlage (140, 146). However, somatostatin and PP cells are normally present in the human adult ampullary glands and in fetal duodenal mucosa. Moreover, scattered insulin and PP cells have been detected in 5 to 25% of the duodenal endocrine tumors investigated (109, 111), none of which showed a neuromatous component or intrapancreatic heterotopia. These findings suggest that a potential for pancreatic hormone expression is, to some extent, inherent to duodenal endocrine tumors, independent of type and origin.

The "endodermal-neuroectodermal" complexes in fetal duodenum described by van Campenhout and reputed to be homologous with the "neuroinsular" complexes reported in the pancreas (147) may offer an alternative explanation for the histogenesis of paragangliomas. In fact, abundant endocrine cells, probably originating from endodermal epithelium, have been found to colonize the stroma between human intestinal epithelium and muscularis propria during early fetal life (148). Such neuroendocrine complexes, like those described in the appendix (149), may

well represent the starting point for an endocrine tumor with associated neuromatous growth.

Benign behavior distinguishes ganglioneuromatous paragangliomas from purely endocrine tumors, such as gastrin and somatostatin cell lesions that arise in the same area and are known to have some malignant potential. In occasional cases, however, local lymph node metastases, attributable to the endocrine component of the lesion, have been reported (150, 151).

EC-CELL TUMORS (ARGENTAFFIN CARCINOIDS)

EC-cell tumors, namely tumors almost exclusively composed by serotonin-producing enterochromaffin (EC) cells, account for

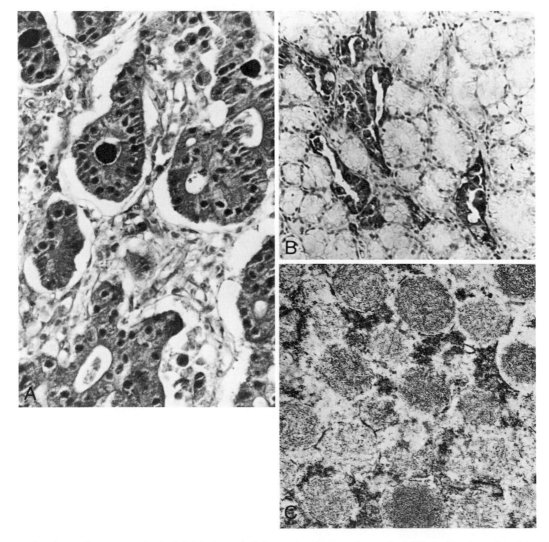

Figure 15.7 Duodenal D cell tumor with cholelithiasis and diabetes (somatostatinoma). **A,** Type C, microglandular arrangement of tumor cells with cytoplasmic granules and intraluminal psammoma bodies stained with lead-hematoxylin (×230). **B,** Somatostatin-immunoreactivity of tumor cells apparently arising from Brunner glands (immunoperoxidase-hematoxylin, ×150). **C,** Large, poorly dense, D-type granules filling the cytoplasm of a tumor cell. Electron microscopy specimen fixed in routine, non-buffered formol (×28,000).

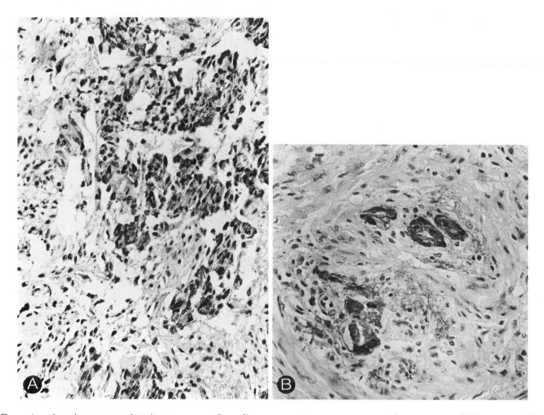

Figure 15.8 Two duodenal neuroendocrine tumors. Ganglioneuromatous component in one case **(A)** surrounds solid nests and cords of PP-immunoreactive epithelial cells (ganglioneuromatous paraganglioma), whereas in the second case **(B)**, it envelops microglands formed of somatostatin-immunoreactive epithelial cells (neurosomatostatinoma) (immunoperoxidase-hematoxylin; **A,** ×150, **B,** ×175).

nearly all endocrine tumors arising in the ileum, appendix, and Meckel's diverticulum; for the majority of those arising in the jejunum and cecum; and for a restricted few of those occurring in the duodenum, stomach, distal colon, rectum, pancreas, biliary tree, and lung.

SMALL INTESTINE

EC-cell tumors of the small intestine (Fig. 15.9) were found during 0.65% of all autopsies performed at the Mayo Clinic. Most of these lesions (133 of 137 cases) were incidental findings, and only 9% showed metastases. On the other hand, 52 of the 72 surgical cases from the same clinic were clinically symptomatic and nearly all were metastatic. Fifty-seven percent of the symptomatic patients had intermittent intestinal obstruction (41). The well-known "carcinoid syndrome," with cutaneous flushing, diarrhea, fibrous thickening of the endocardium and valves of the right heart, etc, was found in only 14 patients (7% of the whole series of 209), all of whom had metastases, mostly in the liver (41). In most series, the tumors are distributed about equally between males and females. Patients range in age from the third to tenth decade, with a peak in the sixth and seventh decades.

The small intestinal tumor, multiple in about 30% of the cases (41, 152), usually appears as a deep mucosal-submucosal nodule with apparently intact or slightly eroded overlying mucosa. Deep infiltration of the muscular wall and peritoneum is a frequent finding. Extensive involvement of the mesentery stimulates consid-

erable fibroblastic or desmoplastic reaction with consequent angulation, kinking of the bowel, and obstruction of the lumen. Thus, obstruction, the most frequent and significant among presenting symptoms, is only shown by an invasive and relatively advanced disease. Infarction of the involved loop of the bowel may occur as a result of adhesions, volvulus, or occlusion of the mesenteric blood vessels. Moreover, mesenteric arteries and veins located away from the tumor may be thickened and their lumen narrowed or even occluded by a peculiar elastic sclerosis, which may lead to ischemic lesions of the intestine (153, 154).

A close relationship was found between the size of the primary tumor and the incidence of metastases; when lesions measured less than 1 cm in diameter, 1 to 2 cm, and 2 cm or more, metastases were found in 2%, 50%, and 80%, respectively (41). The depth of invasion into intestinal wall is also significant in this respect, as no metastases were found in 17 "superficially invasive" tumors, whereas evidence of metastatic disease was noted in 23 of 26 cases in which the tumor was described as "deeply invasive" (40).

Solid, somewhat rounded nests of closely packed tumor cells, often with peripheral palisading, constitute the typical, highly diagnostic (type A) histologic pattern in most argentaffin EC-cell tumors of the midgut (34). In the same cases, rosette type, glandlike structures are detected within the solid nests. This variant of the fundamental structure, designated as mixed insular+glandular (A+C) structure, seems prognostically more favorable than the pure type A structure (37). In areas of deep invasion with abundant desmoplastic reaction, the cell nests may be oriented into cords and files. Most tumor cells are intensely argyrophilic, lead-hematoxylin-positive and reactive with chromogranin A and B antibodies. In four of four cases in our experience, various numbers of tumor cells were also reactive for prostatic acid phosphatase. Tumor cells staining for calbindin-D28k have also been reported in well-differentiated, classic insular carcinoids of the ileum and appendix (155).

The identification of tumor cells as EC cells can be accomplished using different histochemical methods for serotonin, including argentaffin, diazonium, formaldehyde-induced fluorescence, and immunohistochemical tests. Because serotonin occurs in some non-EC cells and related tumors (15, 148), electron microscopic examination of serotonin-immunoreactive tumors (particularly those failing to react with the argentaffin test) can confirm their EC cell nature by detecting characteristic pleomorphic, intensely osmiophilic granules (see Fig. 15.9B) (6, 20).

Substance P and other tachykinins such as eledoisin, physalemin, kassinin neurokinins, and substance K, are reliable markers of a fraction of intestinal EC cells as well as of midgut EC cell tumors (156, 157); foregut EC cells and related tumors remain mostly unreactive. Small populations of enkephalin, somatostatin, gastrin, ACTH, calcitonin, motilin, neurotensin, glucagon/glicentin, and PP/PYY immunoreactive cells, unassociated with pertinent hyperfunctional signs, have been reported in some ileal and jejunal tumors mostly composed of EC cells (156, 158). Dopamine and norepinephrine have also been detected, in addition to serotonin, in a type A (insular) argentaffin carcinoid of the ileum (159). In many cases

of ileal argentaffin EC-cell tumors, however, no other hormone apart from serotonin and substance P or related tachykinins can be detected (156).

Several growth factors and related receptors that have been localized in tumor cells of midgut carcinoids include transforming growth factor-α (TGFα) and epidermal growth factor (EGF)-receptor, insulin-like growth factor-I (IGF-I) and IGF-I receptors, platelet-derived growth factor (PDGF), transforming growth factor-β (TGFβ), basic fibroblast growth factor (bFGF), and acidic fibroblast growth factor (aFGF) (160–162). Some of these growth factors, such as TGFα, exert a proliferative effect, reflected by an increased mitotic index and significantly increased DNA levels in primary cell cultures of midgut carcinoids. This finding favors an autocrine regulatory function of this factor (162). A similar growth-promoting role in midgut carcinoid tumor cells is assigned to IGF-I (161). PDGF, TGFβ, bFGF, and aFGF seem to be mainly involved in tumor stromal reaction, inducing stromal desmoplasia (161, 162), by acting on receptors expressed on fibroblasts or stimulating the promotion of new vasculature and tumor progression (161).

Neural adhesion molecule (NCAM), a member of the immunoglobulin superfamily of cell adhesion molecules, is highly expressed in human midgut carcinoid tumors, with special reference to those tumors that in vitro grow in large clusters with loose attachment to the matrix (161). Because NCAM has not been demonstrated in normal gut endocrine cells, the novel expression of

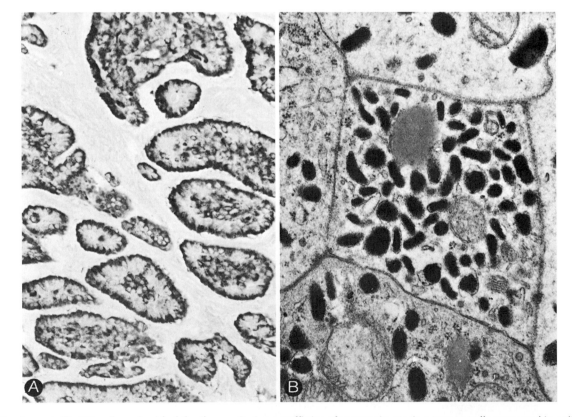

Figure 15.9   Argentaffin EC-cell carcinoid of the ileum. **A,** Argentaffinity of serotonin-storing tumor cells arranged in solid nests with peripheral palisading (Masson-Fontana method, ×150). **B,** Ultrastructure of tumor cells to show medium-sized, rod to pyriform, heavily osmiophilic granules characteristic of EC1 cells. Substance P immunoreactivity of tumor cells was obtained in paraffin sections (×28,000).

this adhesion molecule in carcinoid tumors may be of importance for growth and metastases of these tumors.

We have not found p53 accumulation in eight of eight ileal EC-cell tumors, and other studies confirm that this protein is not implicated in the pathogenesis of these tumors (163). Few data have been reported in the literature on the assessment of proliferative activity of EC cell tumors. A low frequency of mitoses and moderate cellular atypia independent of their malignant behavior are common findings. In one study (164), in which the proliferative activity was determined by means of flow cytometry and Ki-67 immunostaining on a variety of gastroenteropancreatic endocrine tumors, including three midgut carcinoids, high proliferative activity was associated with unfavorable clinical outcome. In another study, Kujari et al. (165) demonstrated that the mean proliferative DNA index of 16 endocrine tumors of the gut, including 4 small intestinal tumors, was not predictive of prognosis and survival. The mean percentage of Ki-67-positive cells that we detected in 12 of our cases of small intestinal EC-cell tumors (all malignant cases) was 1.9 (ranging from 0.4 to 5.5) with no obvious relationship with behavior.

In flow cytometric studies, Tsushima and colleagues (166) demonstrated that DNA nuclear content of small-intestinal carcinoids (53 of 56 of which were primary lesions of the ileum) is typically DNA diploid or tetraploid. Nuclear DNA content did not correlate significantly with clinicopathologic characteristics of carcinoids and with patient survival or tumor progression. The predominance of DNA diploidy of small-intestinal carcinoids, however, was consistent with the overall hypothesis that DNA diploid malignancies are in general less aggressive clinically.

In one study, the overall 5-year survival rate of patients with small bowel carcinoids was 60%, and the 10-year survival rate was 43% (152). In patients with no liver metastases, the 5- and 10-year survival rates were 72% and 60%, respectively, as opposed to 35% and 15% for patients with liver metastases. These findings demonstrate the relatively slow rate of growth of some EC-cell tumors. Metastases are generally confined to the regional lymph nodes and liver. Extraabdominal metastases were found in only 0.5% of the cases reported by Moertel et al. (41). The involved sites included pleura and bone marrow.

APPENDIX

Most endocrine tumors of the appendix have been shown to be EC-cell argentaffin tumors (carcinoids) of type A or A+C structure (34) that likely derive not from the intraepithelial endocrine cells, but from subepithelial neuroendocrine complexes (167, 168). This view is supported by the finding that S-100 protein-positive Schwann-like (sustentacular) cells are an integral component of appendicular EC-cell tumors (169), whereas they are lacking in ileal and colonic EC-cell tumors, which develop from EC cells of the mucosal crypts (168). The intimate relationship of subepithelial endocrine cells of the appendix and related argentaffin tumors with nerves of Meissner's plexus, which has been confirmed by ultrastructural investigations, could result from in vivo release of neurotrophic factors from hyperplastic or neoplastic EC cells. Interestingly, as mentioned previously, IGF-I and TGFα have been detected in some argentaffin carcinoids (161, 170) and IGF-I has been found to be released by tumor EC cells in vitro (170). Because rat fetal cholinergic neurons demonstrate the presence of both

IGF-I and EGF-receptors, IGF-I and TGFα may be considered substances with potential neurotrophic effect.

Most appendiceal EC-cell carcinoids are small (usually less than 1 cm) tumors, discovered incidentally at pelvic or gallbladder surgery (38) or found in patients undergoing surgery because of symptoms of acute appendicitis (171). The carcinoid syndrome is rarely observed in association with EC-cell tumors of the appendix. When it manifests, it usually is associated with widespread metastases of the tumor, predominantly to the liver or retroperitoneum (172, 173). In many series, carcinoid tumors of the appendix are reported to occur more frequently in females than in males. This incidence may be influenced by the greater number of incidental appendicectomies performed in women during gynecologic and gallbladder operations. Appendiceal EC-cell tumors have been reported in all age groups. They account for about 50% of all benign and malignant tumors of the appendix and show predilection (71%) for the tip of the organ.

Most tumors display muscular and lymphatic invasion or perineural involvement; two thirds of the cases in Moertel's series also showed invasion of the peritoneum, possibly through endolymphatic growth (38). Despite these signs of apparent aggressiveness, and in contrast with ileal carcinoids, appendiceal endocrine tumors rarely show lymph node or distant metastases. The reported frequency of metastases from these tumors lies between 1.4 and 8.8% (38, 39, 172-176). According to one study, in all cases of metastasis, the size of the primary tumor was greater than 2 cm (38). In an analysis of 414 cases from the literature, MacGillivray et al. (177) found that both tumor size greater than 2 cm (p < 0.0001) and invasion of the mesoappendix (p < 0.0001) were significantly related to the presence of metastasis in the entire group. In those patients with tumors smaller than 2 cm, mesoappendiceal invasion was significantly associated with metastasis (p < 0.0001). Location of tumors at the base of the appendix with involvement of the surgical margin or of the cecum is an unfavorable prognostic feature, requiring at least a partial cecectomy to avoid residual tumor or subsequent recurrence (178).

With the exception of the presence of S-100-positive sustentacular cells in appendiceal tumors, no relevant histologic, cytologic, or cytochemical differences have been detected between most ileal and appendiceal EC-cell tumors, despite their very different clinical behavior. At both sites, argentaffin EC-cells producing both serotonin and substance P usually are arranged in solid nests with some peripheral palisading (type A structure), occasionally with microlumina (type A+C).

The second, much less common, group of appendiceal endocrine tumors is composed of nonargentaffin L-cell tumors producing glicentin-related peptides (enteroglucagons) and PP/PYY, and showing a characteristic trabecular pattern (179–181). These tumors, which generally are only 2 to 3 mm in diameter, are the appendiceal counterpart of L-cell tumors found, most frequently, in the rectum. They arise from L cells, which together with EC and somatostatin cells, are a regular component of the crypt epithelium of normal appendix.

COLON

Argentaffin carcinoid tumors of the colon are associated with clinical symptoms similar to those present in patients with colonic carcinoma, including abdominal pain, diarrhea, rectal bleeding, and palpable abdominal mass. In one series (182), the average age of patients was 58 years. The carcinoid syndrome has been identified in only 3 to 5% of reported cases (182, 183). The majority of tumors are detected in the right colon (182, 183) and are larger than carcinoids of the small intestine, appendix, and rectum. The average size was 4.9 cm in cases reviewed by Berardi (182). A difference in size was found between metastatic and nonmetastatic tumors measuring 6.1 cm and 4.7 cm on average, respectively. The size of the tumor did also correlate with the presence of clinical symptoms. In our series of five cases of right colon endocrine tumors, all five had lesions with histologic, cytologic, and cytochemical features that were identical to those of ileal EC-cell tumors, including the absence of protein S-100-positive sustentacular cells.

Colonic argentaffin tumors are frequently malignant: local spread of the tumors was found in 44% of patients and distant metastases in 38% (183). The reported 5-year survival rate was 25% and the 10-year survival rate was 10%.

L-CELL TUMORS (HINDGUT TRABECULAR CARCINOIDS)

These tumors typically arise in the rectum (Fig. 15.10); a few have been reported in the appendix (see above), the colon, the pelvic soft tissue posterior to the rectum (from rectal duplication, occasionally), or the ileum. Endocrine tumors similar to rectal L-cell tumors have also been found in the middle ear (184). Endocrine tumors of the rectum account for 12 to 27% (14.7% of our 238 cases) of all gastrointestinal endocrine tumors (39, 44). Among our 33 cases, the age of the patients ranged from 28 to 76 years with an average age of 52 years, which is identical to that reported by Caldarola and coworkers (185) in their series of 147 cases. Constipation is one of the main complaints of patients bearing this type of tumor; other symptoms include rectal bleeding, change in bowel habits, and pain. No definite hyperfunctional syndrome has been identified in association with L-cell tumors producing "enteroglucagon" (glucagon 37, glicentin, GLP 1, GLP 2) and PP/PYY-related hormonal peptides. The classical carcinoid syndrome has been reported only exceptionally in association with rectal endocrine tumors, which proved to be of serotonin-producing argentaffin type (186). Some rectal endocrine tumors have been reported in the large bowel of patients with ulcerative colitis (187) or Crohn disease (188). In association with these conditions, the tumors tend to be multiple (189).

The majority of hindgut endocrine tumors are diagnosed during investigation for other gastrointestinal disease, when asymptomatic and measuring 1 cm or less in diameter. The rectal endocrine tumors appear as submucosal nodules, often with apparently intact overlying epithelium and sometimes with polypoid appearance (185). Small lesions are movable, whereas larger lesions tend to be somewhat fixed to the rectal wall. In the series reported by Caldarola et al. (185), the tumor was found 4 to 13 cm above the dentate line in 99% of cases and on the anterior or lateral rectal walls in 85% of cases. The majority of rectal endocrine tumors are small lesions. In a 1962 review of the literature, Bates found cases involving 234 tumors that measured less than 1 cm, 77 between 1 and 2 cm, and 45 more than 2 cm in diameter, with recorded malignancy rates of 1.7%, 10%, and 82%, respectively (190). An overall malignancy rate of 11 to 15% has been calculated in some

studies (39, 191). Recognized malignancy criteria include a size greater than 2 cm (189), invasion of the muscularis propria (192), presence of more than 2 mitoses per 10 high power (×400) microscopic fields, and DNA aneuploidy (193).

Histologically, L-cell tumors are characterized by a predominance of a type B ribbon pattern, often admixed with type C (tubuloacini or broad, irregular trabeculae with rosettes) and only occasionally with areas of type A solid nest structures. These patterns are different from those of EC-cell tumors in which the type A architectural pattern is prevalent. Among rectal carcinoids derived from surgical pathology files and investigated immunohistochemically, 48 (77%) displayed more or less abundant glucagon/glicentin and/or PP/PYY immunoreactivities typical of intestinal L-cells (see Fig. 15.10A and B), whereas only 21 (32%) showed serotonin immunoreactivity and 12 (18%) showed somatostatin immunoreactivity, usually in only few cells (36, 158, 194–197). Glucagon-29, glucagon-37, glicentin, proglucagon cryptic fragments, PYY, PP, and pro-PP icosapeptide all proved to be useful immunohistochemical markers of rectal L-cell tumors (36). Although there is a prevalence of L cells in these tumors, minority populations of substance P, insulin, enkephalin, beta-endorphin, neurotensin, α-hCG, and motilin immunoreactive cells have also been identified (36, 158, 191, 195, 198). Eighty-two of 85 colorectal carcinoids tested showed immunoreactivity for prostatic acidic phophatase, a finding that is unusual in other gut endocrine tumors and possibly is related to the common origin of rectum and prostate from cloacal hindgut (191). Thus, L cells seem to represent the dominant tumor cell component in rectal endocrine tumors and to be positively related to type B or B+C structure. A relationship between type A solid nest areas of both rectal and colonic tumors and serotonin-producing EC cells has also been noted (36).

Whereas in eight submucosal L-cell tumors with a diameter ≤ 2 cm we determined that percentage of Ki-67 (MIB1 antibody)-labeled nuclei never exceeded 2%, a tumor measuring 3 cm in diameter and invading the muscularis propria showed 7.5% labeled nuclei. In addition, in a study to determine the DNA content of 22 rectal carcinoids by cytomorphometry of paraffin-embedded tissues, Tsioulias et al. (193) reported that three of the tumors with synchronous or metachronous metastases showed aneuploid DNA pattern. These findings suggest that both proliferation markers and DNA ploidy pattern may be factors of significant value.

The patients with rectal endocrine tumors generally have a good prognosis, showing a 5-year survival rate of 89%, which is better than the overall survival rate of 62% for patients with ileal carcinoids (178). All tumors less than 1 cm can be treated by either fulguration or wide full-thickness excision. For lesions 1 to 2 cm in diameter, a wide local excision should be performed. Radical treatment for rectal endocrine tumors is indicated only for lesions greater than 2 cm that invade the muscularis externa (199).

ECTOPIC HORMONE-PRODUCING ENDOCRINE TUMORS

Differentiated endocrine tumors producing ectopic hormones, such as calcitonin (200, 201), adrenocorticotropic hormone/melanocyte-stimulating hormone (ACTH/MSH) (202–206), growth hormone (GH), GH-releasing factor (GRF) (207, 208),

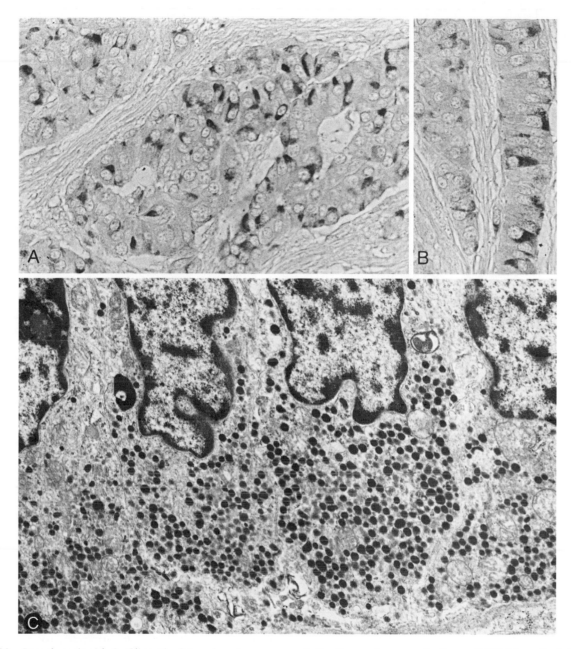

Figure 15.10   Rectal carcinoid. **A,** Glicentin C-terminus immunoreactivity of many tumor cells. Serum R4804 from Prof. N. Yanaihara (Schizuoka, Japan) (immunoperoxidase, ×360). **B,** Pancreatic polypeptide immunoreactive cells in a tumor trabecula (immuno-peroxidase, ×360). **C,** Round to slightly angular secretory granules filling the basal cytoplasm of tumor cells aligned perpendicularly in a trabecula (electron microscopy, ×13,700).

vasoactive intestinal peptide (VIP) (209), and related hyperfunctional syndromes, are rarely observed in the gut. Minority populations of inappropriate cells, including insulin, ACTH, calcitonin, GRF, human chorionic gonadotropin (hCG), and related α-chain, in the absence of pertinent functional or pathologic signs, have been found more frequently (31, 111, 159, 194, 210, 211). Given that β-endorphin-, β-lipotropin-, pro-αMSH- (12), and corticotropin releasing hormone (CRF)- (212) immunoreactive endocrine cells have been observed in normal human intestine, finding β-endorphin or CRF-producing tumors in the rectum (194) or in the colon (213) is not necessarily "inappropriate." Moreover,

although in man, VIP is confined to nerves, VIP-producing epithelial endocrine cells have been reported in the gut of other species (214).

OTHER GUT ENDOCRINE TUMORS

Tumors lacking functional or cytologic characterization are frequently diagnosed by pathologists as "carcinoids," especially "non-

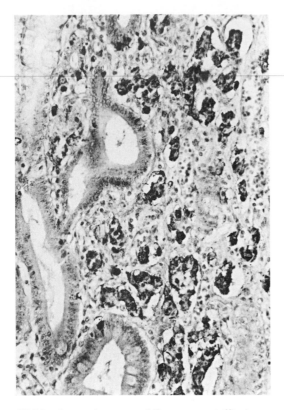

Figure 15.11 Strongly argyrophil nonargentaffin tumor cords and small nests arising from duodenal crypts in a patient with ZE syndrome due to pancreatic gastrinoma. PP and neurotensin immunoreactivity was obtained in some cells. Diagnosis: argyrophil nonargentaffin carcinoid with PP and neurotensin cells (Grimelius silver, ×150).

argentaffin carcinoids." Most such tumors, when appropriately investigated with the help of antigen unmasking techniques, fit in one of the tumor entities listed in Table 15.4. A few escape final identification, however, because of inappropriate fixation or processing of tumor tissue. These tumors should receive the generic diagnosis of "endocrine tumor" (carcinoid). Clinically nonfunctioning argyrophil and or chromogranin-immunoreactive tumors showing ultrastructurally small, thin-haloed granules and no known hormone reactivity are seldom observed in the stomach and duodenum.

A small mucosal-submucosal tumor composed of small, heavily argyrophilic (with both Grimelius' and Sevier-Munger's techniques) cells and arising from the crypts of the duodenal bulb has been observed in a patient with longstanding, severe hyperchlorhydria and peptic ulcer disease attributable to pancreatic gastrinoma (Fig. 15.11). PP and neurotensin immunoreactivity has been detected in some tumor cells (case 3b, 110). Scattered CCK-positive cells have been identified in three patients with duodenal gastrinomas associated with ZES (111). A glucagon-immunoreactive tumor associated with the "glucagonoma" syndrome has been reported in the duodenum (215). An endocrinologically inactive rectal trabecular endocrine tumor in which motilin cells represented the prevailing cell population has also been reported (216). Neurotensin cells have not been identified as a major neoplastic population in any of the intestinal endocrine tumors investigated (158).

POORLY DIFFERENTIATED ENDOCRINE CARCINOMAS

The occurence of small to intermediate cell carcinomas, resembling oat cell carcinomas of the lung, in the esophagus is well known (217). That at least part of these tumors (poorly differentiated neuroendocrine carcinomas) show histologic, histochemical, and ultrastructural signs of endocrine differentiaton has been recognized more recently (218–222). Similar tumors have been reported in the stomach (62, 75, 83, 223, 224), ampulla of Vater (225–227), and colon-rectum (228–233).

The mean age at presentation of these tumors is in the seventh decade (63 years for the stomach, ranging from 51 to 76 [83], 69.8 years for the esophagus, ranging from 51 to 88 [219]; and 63 years for the colon-rectum neoplasm, from 44 to 75 [231]). The majority (78%) of the esophageal tumors were located in the lower one third of the esophagus in one series (220); gastric tumors were found most frequently in the body/fundus (10 cases versus 2 cases located in the antrum) (83). The distribution of tumors in the colon-rectum resembles that of conventional adenocarcinomas (234). Poorly differentiated endocrine carcinomas generally are large (mean size: 5.4 cm for esophageal [221], 4.2 cm for gastric [83], 4.2 cm for colon rectum [six of our seven cases]) fungating or annular, partially obstructing lesions.

Using conventional light microscopy (Fig. 15.12), poorly differentiated endocrine carcinomas are characterized by small to intermediate-sized, round to spindle-shaped cells with indistinct nucleoli and scanty cytoplasm arranged in poorly defined solid nests and sheets, often with necrotic centers (Soga's type D structure). The neoplastic cells are supported by a delicate fibrovascular stroma with little or no inflammatory reaction. The mitotic rate is brisk, ranging from 8 to 86 mitotic figures per 10 HPF. Vascular and perineural invasion are detected in most tumors. Scattered argyrophilic cells or cell processes were observed in many cases in which Grimelius' silver was used for staining. The cells of poorly differentiated endocrine carcinomas are strongly positive for cytosolic endocrine markers (NSE and PGP 9.5), and are poorly positive or negative for endocrine granules markers (chromogranins and hormones) (83, 233). Serotonin and appropriate or inappropriate hormonal peptides (calcitonin, ACTH, etc) have been detected in a few tumors. p53 protein nuclear accumulation was detected in two of our six cases of colorectal tumors and four of five cases of gastric tumors. High (10% or more positive cells) Ki-67-labeling index is a constant finding in these tumors. Ultrastructurally, a few, small (100 to 200 nm in diameter) secretory granules resembling those of immature "protoendocrine" cells of early fetal development (235) have been observed, often concentrated in thin cell processes not seen with conventional light-microscopic study (75, 236).

The majority of tumors reported to date have not been associated with an overt endocrine syndrome, even when hormone-like immunoreactivities were detected in tumor tissue, possibly because of the scarce amount of hormone produced or because inactive prohormones, rather than active molecular species, were produced. Among the rare cases of functioning tumors, a case of mixed squamous/small cell carcinoma of the esophagus producing vasoactive intestinal peptide (VIP) and a WDHA (watery diarrhea, hypokalemia, achlorhydria) syndrome (237), and a case of combined small cell carcinoma, choriocarcinoma, hepatoid carcinoma, and tubular adenocarcinoma of the ascending colon associated with Cushing's syndrome (238) deserve mention. All tumors studied in the various sites had histologic signs suggestive of high malignancy (high mitotic rate, deep mural infiltration, angioinvasion, neuroinvasion). Metastasis occurred in most cases (11 of 11 esophageal [239], 12 of 12 gastric [83], 22 of 22 colorectal [233]), and most patients (10 of 10 with esophageal [239], 9 of 13 with gastric [83], 12 of 17 with colorectal tumors [233]) died within 1 to 21 months of diagnosis.

In fact, these poorly differentiated carcinomas with focal signs of abortive endocrine differentiation appear to display the same aggressive behavior as poorly differentiated carcinomas lacking endocrine differentiation. More or less extensive areas of squamous or glandular differentiation may also be found in such tumors (83, 221, 233), suggesting that we are dealing essentially with undifferentiated tumor cells undergoing focal, and often abortive, multidirectional differentiation. Endocrine differentiation seems to occur more frequently, however, in keeping with the early development of endocrine cells from the immature gut epithelium (235). Interestingly, 4 of 5 (229) and 13 of 22 (233) poorly differentiated colorectal endocrine carcinomas developed in tubular or villous adenomas. This fact, according to the concept just expressed, may be interpreted as a propensity for rare colonic adenomas to undergo

anaplastic transformation with multidirectional, but predominantly endocrine, differentiation.

ENDOCRINE-EXOCRINE TUMORS

Sporadic differentiation of one or more lines of endocrine cells inside nonendocrine neoplasms of the gut has been observed frequently, e.g., in 13% of gastric carcinomas (240), 9% of the intestinal adenomas (241), and in about 5 to 10% of all colorectal carcinomas (242). Endocrine cells either do not occur or are rare in squamous cell carcinoma of the esophagus; they can, however, be detected in adenocarcinomas, including those associated with Barrett's metaplasia. The cells are usually argyrophil and contain the same peptides found in gastric adenocarcinomas, including serotonin, somatostatin, gastrin, and glucagon (243). Endocrine cells occur more frequently in association with mucopeptic, rather than foveolar, growths of the stomach (244) and more often with diffuse than with glandular carcinomas (245, 246). As a rule, the lines of endocrine cell differentiation are coherent with the exocrine cell lines, both occurring in the normal tissue mimicked by the tumor growth.

No apparent change of tumor prognosis or clinical behavior has been reported for most of these tumors, compared with histologically similar tumors of the same site lacking endocrine cells (247).

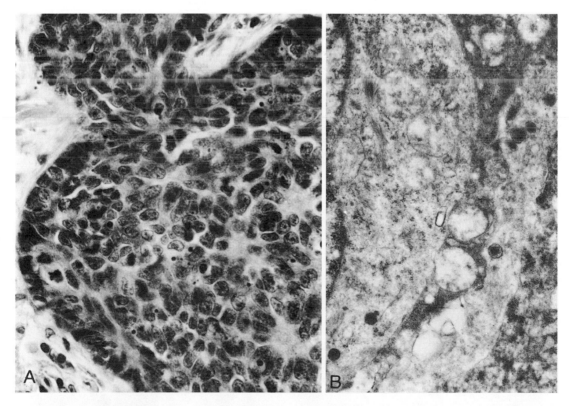

Figure 15.12 A, Small to intermediate cell endocrine carcinoma of the stomach. Note arrangement of tumor cells to form some rosette-like structures and attempts at peripheral palisading. No hormone reactivity was obtained apart from scattered hCG immunoreactivity (hematoxylin & eosin, ×400). **B,** Ultrastructure of the same tumor to show a few, small protoendocrine granules (×14,000).

Their endocrine component, however, may well account for some sign of clinical hyperfunction occasionally reported in association with ordinary carcinoma, such as the skin melanosis associated with a MSH-producing gastric papillary adenocarcinoma (248) or the ZES resulting from a gastrin-producing mucinous cystoadenocarcinoma of the ovary (249).

Amphicrine cells showing both exocrine and endocrine granules in their cytoplasm, often at opposite poles of the cell, as a result of simultaneous differentiation toward endocrine and exocrine lines have been reported in adenocarcinomas of the stomach, intestine, appendix, and esophagus (250–252).

Another known lesion is the mixed endocrine-exocrine tumor in which the endocrine component forms a major cell population, either intimately and diffusely admixed with the nonendocrine component (combined tumors) or occurring in separate areas of the same tumor (composite tumors).

COMBINED TUMORS

In gastric combined tumors (Fig. 15.13), the endocrine cells (including gastrin, somatostatin, enterochromaffin, and ECL cells) frequently are associated with "poorly differentiated" (diffuse type) scirrhous and mucin-producing growths (253, 254). A mucin-producing tubular carcinoma resembling pyloric glands has also been reported (255). In cases of scirrhous argyrophil carcinoma, the authors have also investigated the nonendocrine component and found either group II (mostly in absence of group I) pepsinogen, a known marker of pyloric type mucopeptic differentiation, or intestinal crypt markers (244). The lysozyme, M2-glycoprotein antigen, and gastrin immunoreactivities observed in these combined tumors (253, 254) also suggest pyloric gland or intestinal crypt differen-

tiation. Interestingly, in "early" gastric cancers, argyrophil cells have been found more often in deeply situated mucopeptic or intestinal crypt growths than in juxtaluminal foveolar growths of either glandular or diffuse (signet-ring) type (244, 256).

Abundant endocrine cells occur more rarely in well-differentiated intestinal adenocarcinomas (257). Investigators have observed diffusely infiltrating goblet cell carcinomas, with or without signet-ring change, containing numerous endocrine cells (245, 258). These lesions, which have been found in association with ulcerative colitis (259), may represent the more malignant counterpart of the so-called goblet cell carcinoid (251, 260–263), goblet cell carcinoma (261), goblet cell adenocarcinoid (264), adenocarcinoid/mucinous carcinoid (265), or crypt cell carcinoma (266) frequently observed in the appendix, but sometimes found also in the ileum (251), duodenum (267), and periampullary region (268). The appendiceal goblet cell carcinoid is a low-grade microglandular and cord-forming tumor showing goblet, columnar, lysozyme-producing, and secretory component-producing cells, as well as endocrine cells of EC, L, or D type, and often represent up to 30% of tumor cells. Electron microscopic studies (261) revealed the presence of cells displaying synchronous exocrine and endocrine differentiation (amphicrine cells) (252).

Goblet cell carcinoids of the appendix are rare tumors that are less common than conventional carcinoids. The mean age at presentation is 58 years, with slight preference for males (269). In many cases, the goblet cell carcinoid is not recognized macroscopically and instead represents an incidental histologic finding. In other cases, the tumor forms localized nodules or areas of induration of the appendix, and in 22% of cases, tumor spread extends beyond the appendix, with evidence of both lymphatic and transcelomatic spread producing metastatic tumor in the peritoneum, ileocolic

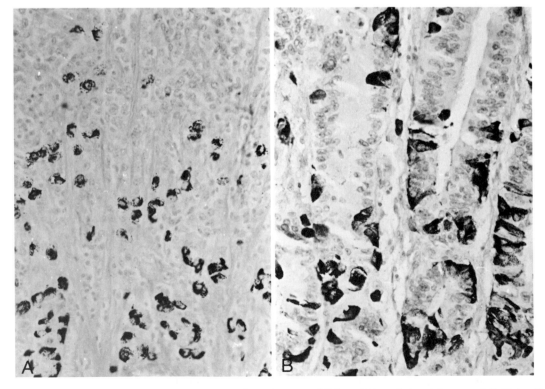

Figure 15.13   Argyrophil endocrine cells in gastric combined carcinomas of diffuse **(A)** and glandular type **(B)** (Grimelius silver, ×220).

lymph nodes, and ovary (269, 270). Goblet cell carcinoids have more aggressive behavior compared with true appendiceal carcinoids (260, 263, 269). The 5-year actuarial survival rate for the series reported by Warkel et al. (264) was 80%, and Edmonds et al. (265) found that 11 of 86 patients reported to have goblet cell carcinoids had died and three others had recurrent disease. Results of most studies demonstrate that appendectomy is adequate treatment for a small, well-differentiated goblet cell carcinoid discovered incidentally in appendectomy specimens and is still confined to the appendiceal wall. Individuals with less-differentiated tumors and those with tumors that have spread beyond the appendiceal wall should undergo right hemicolectomy.

Composite Tumors

Composite adenocarcinoma-carcinoid or glandular-carcinoid tumors have been observed in the large intestine (188, 271–274), small intestine (275), ampulla of Vater (276), stomach (277–281), and esophagus (282). By means of appropriate histochemical and ultrastructural investigations, it is important to distinguish the endocrine component of composite tumors from trabecular and solid carcinomas showing areas of peripheral palisading or basaloid patterns that mimic histologically an endocrine growth but lack histochemical and ultrastructural signs of true endocrine differentiation. Interestingly, keratin immunostaining may show a dotlike distribution in the endocrine component of composite tumors that contrasts with the ringlike pattern shown by the exocrine component of the same tumor (280). Prognosis of composite tumors depends on the stage and grade of the carcinomatous component of the lesion.

Acknowledgments

Supported by Grants from the Italian Ministry of University and Research (E.S. and C.C.) and Ministry of Health (IRCCS Policlinico San Matteo).

References

1. Grimelius L. A silver nitrate stain for α2 cells in human pancreatic islets. Acta Soc Med Upsal 1968;73:243–270.
2. Solcia E, Capella C, Vassallo G. Lead-haematoxylin as a stain for endocrine cells. Significance of staining and comparison with other selective methods. Histochemistry 1969;20:116–126.
3. Bishop AE, Polak JM, Facer P, et al. Neuron-specific enolase: A common marker for the endocrine cells and innervation of the gut and pancreas. Gastroenterology 1982;83:902–915.
4. Lloyd RV, Wilson BS. Specific endocrine tissue marker defined by a monoclonal antibody. Science 1983;222:628–630.
5. Rindi G, Buffa R, Sessa F, et al. Chromogranin A, B and C immunoreactivities of mammalian endocrine cells. Distribution, distinction with the argyrophil component of secretory granule. Histochemistry 1986;85:19–28.
6. Solcia E, Capella C, Vassallo G, et al. Endocrine cells of the gastric mucosa. Int Rev Cytol 1975;42:223–286.
7. Pearse AGE, Polak JM. The diffuse neuroendocrine system and the APUD concept. In: Bloom SR, ed. Gut hormones. Edinburgh: Churchill Livingstone, 1978;33–39.
8. Le Douarin NM. The embryological origin of the endocrine cells associated with the digestive tract: Experimental analysis based on the use of a stable cell marking technique. In: Bloom SR, ed. Gut hormones. Edinburgh: Churchill Livingstone, 1978;49–56.
9. Solcia E, Polak JM, Pearse AGE, et al. Lausanne 1977 classification of gastroenteropancreatic endocrine cells. In: Bloom SR, ed. Gut hormones. Edinburgh: Churchill Livingstone, 1978;40–48.
10. Solcia E, Creutzfeldt W, Falkmer S, et al. Human gastroenteropancreatic endocrine-paracrine cells: Santa Monica 1980 classification. In: Lechago J, Grossman MI, Walsh JH, eds. Cellular basis of chemical messangers in the digestive system. New York: Academic Press, 1981;159–165.
11. Fiocca R, Sessa F, Tenti P, et al. Pancreatic polypeptide (PP) cells in the PP-rich lobe of the human pancreas are identified ultrastructurally and immunocytochemically as F cells. Histochemistry 1983;77:511–523.
12. Sjolund K, Sanden G, Hakanson R, et al. Endocrine cells in human intestine: An immunocytochemical study. Gastroenterology 1983;85:1120–1130.
13. Bottcher G, Sjolund K, Ekblad E, et al. Coexistence of peptide YY and glicentin immunoreactivity in endocrine cells of the gut. Regul Pept 1984;8:261–266.
14. Solcia E, Capella C, Buffa R, et al. Cytology of tumours in the gastroenteropancreatic and diffuse (neuro)endocrine system. In: Falkmer S, Hakanson R, Sundler F, eds. Evolution and tumour pathology of the neuroendocrine system. Amsterdam: Elsevier, 1984;453–480.
15. Solcia E, Capella C, Buffa R, et al. Endocrine cells of the digestive system. In: Johnson LR, ed. Physiology of the gastrointestinal tract, 2nd ed. (Johnson LR, ed), Raven Press, New York, 1986:111–130.
16. Usellini L, Buchan AMJ, Polak JM, et al. Ultrastructural localization of motilin in endocrine cells of human and dog intestine by the immunogold technique. Histochemistry 1984;81:363–368.
17. Usellini L, Capella C, Frigerio B, et al. Ultrastructural localization of secretin in endocrine cells of the dog duodenum by the immunogold technique. Comparison with ultrastructurally characterized S cells of various mammals. Histochemistry 1984;80:435–441.
18. Usellini L, Capella C, Solcia E, et al. Ultrastructural localization of gastric inhibitory polypeptide (GIP) in a well characterized endocrine cell of canine duodenal mucosa. Histochemistry 1984;80:85–89.
19. Usellini L, Capella C, Malesci A, et al. Ultrastructural localization of cholecystokinin in endocrine cells of the dog duodenum by the immunogold technique. Histochemistry 1985;83:331–336.
20. Solcia E, Capella C, Buffa R, et al. Endocrine cells of the gastrointestinal tract and related tumors. Pathobiol Ann 1979;9:163–203.
21. Feyrter F. Uber die peripheren endokrinen (parakrinen) Drusen des Menschen. Wien-Dusseldorf: W. Maudrich, 1953.
22. Solcia E, Capella C, Buffa R, et al. Pathology of the Zollinger-Ellison syndrome. In: Fenoglio CM, ed. Progress in surgical pathology, vol. 1. New York: Masson, 1980;119–133.
23. Dayal Y, Nunnemacher G, Doos WG, et al. Psammomatous somatostatinomas of the duodenum. Am J Surg Pathol 1983;7:656–665.
24. Carlei F, Polak JM. Antibodies to neuron-specific enolase for the delineation of the entire diffuse neuroendocrine system in health and disease. Semin Diagn Pathol 1984;1:59–70.
25. O'Connor DT, Burton D, Deftos LH. Immunoreactive human chromogranin A in diverse polypeptide producing human tumors and normal endocrine tissues. J Clin Endocrinol Metab 1983;57:1084–1086.
26. Lloyd RV, Warner TFC, Mervak T, et al. Immunohistochemical detection of chromogranin and neuron-specific enolase in pancreatic endocrineneoplasms. Am J Surg Pathol 1984;8:607–614.
27. Solcia E, Capella C, Buffa R, et al. Antigenic markers of neuroendocrine tumors: Their diagnostic and prognostic value. In: Fenoglio CM, Weinstein RS, Kaufman N, eds. New concepts in neoplasia as applied to diagnostic pathology. Baltimore: Williams & Wilkins, 1986;242–261.
28. Wiedenmann B, Franke WW, Kuhn C, et al. Synaptophysin: A novel marker protein for neuro-endocrine cells and neoplasms. Proc Natl Acad Sci USA 1986;83:3500–3504.
29. Wilander E, Grimelius L, Lundquist G, et al. Polypeptide hormones in argentaffin and argyrophil gastroduodenal endocrine tumors. Am J Pathol 1979;96:519–530.
30. Alumets J, Sundler F, Falkmer S, et al. Neurohormonal peptides in endocrine tumors of the pancreas, stomach and upper small intestine. I. An immunohistochemical study of 27 cases. Ultrastruct Pathol 1983;5:55–72.

31. Dayal Y, Wolfe H. Regulatory substances in clinically nonfunctioning gastrointestinal carcinoids. In: Falkmer S, Hakanson R, Sundler F, eds. Evolution and tumour pathology of the neuro-endocrine system. Amsterdam: Elsevier, 1984;497–517.

32. Williams ED, Sandler M. The classification of carcinoid tumours. Lancet 1963;1:238–239.

33. Solcia E, Capella C, Buffa R, et al. The contribution of immunohistochemistry to the diagnosis of neuroendocrine tumors. Semin Diagn Pathol 1984;1:285–296.

34. Soga J, Tazawa K. Pathologic analysis of carcinoids. Histologic reevaluation of 62 cases. Cancer 1971;28:990–998.

35. Dawson IMP. The endocrine cells of the gastro-intestinal tract and the neoplasms which arise from them. In: Morson BC, ed. Pathology of the gastrointestinal tract. Curr Top Pathol 1976;63:222–258.

36. Fiocca R, Rindi G, Capella C, et al. Glucagon, glicentin, proglucagon, PYY, PP and proPP-icosapeptide immunoreactivities of rectal carcinoid tumors and related non-tumor cells. Regul Pept 1981;17:9–29.

37. Johnson LA, Lavin P, Moertel CG, et al. Carcinoids: The association of histologic growth pattern and survival. Cancer 1983;51:882–889.

38. Moertel CG, Dockerty MB, Judd ES. Carcinoid tumors of the vermiform appendix. Cancer 1968;21:270–278.

39. Godwin JD. Carcinoid tumors. An analysis of 2837 cases. Cancer 1975;36:560–569.

40. Hajdu S, Winawer SJ, Myers WPL. Carcinoid tumors. A study of 204 cases. Am J Clin Pathol 1974;61:521–528.

41. Moertel CG, Sauer H, Dockerty MB, et al. Life history of the carcinoid tumor of the small intestine. Cancer 1961;14:901–912.

42. Greenwood SM, Huvos AG, Erlandson RA, et al. Rectal carcinoid and rectal adenocarcinoma: A case report and review of the literature. Dis Colon Rectum 1974;17:644–655.

43. Zeitels J, Naunheim K, Kaplan EL, et al. Carcinoid tumors. A 37 year experience. Arch Surg 1982;117:732–737.

44. Zakariai YM, Quan SH, Hajdu SI. Carcinoid tumors of the gastrointestinal tract. Cancer 1975;35:588–591.

45. Brodman HR, Pai BN. Malignant carcinoid of the stomach and distal esophagus. Review of literature and case report. Dig Dis Sci 1968;13:677–681.

46. Capella C, Polak JM, Timson CM, et al. Gastric carcinoids of argyrophil ECL cells. Ultrastruct Pathol 1980;1:411–418.

47. Borch K, Renvall H, Liedberg G. Gastric endocrine cell hyperplasia and carcinoid tumors in pernicious anemia. Gastroenterology 1985;88:638–648.

48. Carney JA, Go VLW, Fairbanks VF, et al. The syndrome of gastric argyrophil carcinoid tumors and nonantral gastric atrophy. Ann Intern Med 1988;99:761–766.

49. Solcia E, Capella C, Fiocca R, et al. Gastric argyrophil carcinoidosis in patients with Zollinger-Ellison syndrome due to type I multiple endocrine neoplasia. A newly recognized association. Am J Surg Pathol 1990;14:503–515.

50. Poynter D, Pick CR, Harcourt RA, et al. Association of long lasting unsurmountable histamine H2 blockade and gastric carcinoid tumors in the rat. Gut 1985;26:1284–1295.

51. Havu N. Enterochromaffin-like cell carcinoids of gastric mucosa in rats after life-long inhibition of gastric secretion. Digestion 1985;5(suppl 1):42–55.

52. Matsson H, Havu N, Brautigam J, et al. Partial gastric corpectomy results in hypergastrinemia and development of gastric enterochromaffin-cell carcinoids in the rat. Gastroenterology 1991;100:311–319.

53. Håkanson E, Ekelund M, Sundler F. Activation and proliferation of gastric endocrine cells. In: Falkmer S, Hakanson R, Sundler F, eds. Evolution and tumor pathology of the neuroendocrine system. Amsterdam: Elsevier, 1984;371–398.

54. Lee AK, DeLellis RA, Blount M, et al. Pituitary proliferative lesions in aging male Long-Evans rats. A model of mixed multiple endocrine neoplasia syndrome. Lab Invest 1982;47:595–602.

55. Maika JA, Scher S. Spontaneous gastric carcinoid tumour in an aged Sprague-Dawley rat. Vet Pathol 1989;26:88–90.

56. Snell K, Stewart H. Malignant argyrophil gastric carcinoids of Praomys (Mastomys) natalensis. Science 1968;163:470.

57. Capella C, Solcia E, Snell KC. Ultrastructure of endocrine cells and argyrophil carcinoids of the stomach of Praomys (Mastomys) natalensis. J Natl Cancer Inst 1973;50:1471–1485.

58. Bordi C, Gabrielli M, Missale G. Pathological changes of endocrine cells in atrophic gastritis. Arch Pathol Lab Med 1978;102:129–135.

59. Solcia E, Bordi C, Creutzfeld W, et al. Histopathological classification of nonantral gastric endocrine growths in man. Digestion 1988;41:185–200.

60. Solcia E, Fiocca R, Villani L, et al. Hyperplastic, dysplastic and neoplastic enterochromaffin-like-cell proliferations of the gastric mucosa: Classification and hystogenesis. Am J Surg Pathol 1995;19(S1):S1–S7.

61. Nilsson O, Wangberg B, Johansson L, et al. Rapid induction of enterochromaffin-like tumors by histamine 2-receptor blockade. Am J Pathol 1993;142:1173–1185.

62. Rindi G, Luinetti O, Cornaggia M, et al. Three subtypes of gastric argyrophil carcinoid and the gastric neuroendocrine carcinoma: A clinicopathologic study. Gastroenterology 1993;104:994–1006.

63. Havu N, Maaroos HI, Sipponen P. Argyrophil cell hyperplasia associated with chronic corpus gastritis in gastric ulcer disease. Scand J Gastroenterol 1991;26(Suppl 186):90–94.

64. Solcia E, Fiocca R, Villani L, et al. Morphology and pathogenesis of endocrine hyperplasias, precarcinoid lesions and carcinoids arising in chronic atrophic gastritis. Scand J Gastroenterol 1991;26(Suppl 180):146–159.

65. Solcia E, Fiocca R, Havu N, et al. Gastric endocrine cells and gastritis in patients receiving long-term omeprazole treatment. Digestion 1992;51:82–92.

66. Lamberts R, Creutzfeldt W, Struber HG, et al. Long-term omeprazole therapy in peptic ulcer disease: Gastrin, endocrine cell growth, and gastritis. Gastroenterology 1993;104:1356–1370.

67. Bordi C, Bertele A, Davighi MC, et al. Clinical and pathological associations of argyrophil cell hyperplasias of the gastric mucosa. Appl Pathol 1984;2:282–291.

68. Sjoblom SM, Sipponen P, Miettinen M, et al. Gastroscopic screening for gastric carcinoids and carcinoma in pernicious anemia. Endoscopy 1988;20:52–56.

69. Solcia E, Rindi G, Fiocca R, et al. Distinct patterns of chronic gastritis associated with carcinoids and cancer and their role in tumorigenesis. Yale J Biol Med 1992;65:793–804.

70. Bishop AE, Power RF, Polak JM. Markers of neuroendocrine differentiation. Pathol Res Pract 1988;183:119–128.

71. McDonald RA. A study of 356 carcinoids of the gastrointestinal tract. Am J Med 1956;21:867–878.

72. Mizuma K, Shibuya H, Totsuka M, et al. Carcinoid of the stomach: A case report and review of 100 cases reported in Japan. Ann Chir Gynaecol 1983;72:23–27.

73. Solcia E, Fiocca R, Sessa F, et al. Morphology and natural history of gastric endocrine tumors. In: Håkanson R, Sundler F, eds. The stomach as an endocrine organ. Amsterdam: Elsevier, 1991;473–498.

74. Rindi G. Clinicopathologic aspects of gastric neuroendocrine tumors. Am J Pathol 1995;19(S1):S20–S29.

75. Solcia E, Capella C, Sessa F, et al. Gastric carcinoids and related endocrine growths. Digestion 1986;35(Suppl 1):3–22.

76. Sundler F, Eriksson B, Grimelius LI, et al. Histamine in gastric carcinoid tumors: Immunocytochemical evidence. Endocr Pathol 1992;3:23–27.

77. Capella C, Finzi G, Cornaggia M, et al. Ultrastructural typing of gastric endocrine cells. In: Håkanson R, Sundler F, eds. The stomach as an endocrine organ. Amsterdam: Elsevier, 1991;27–51.

78. Iwafuchi M, Hidenobu W, Noboru Y, et al. Immunohistochemical and ultrastructural characteristics of gastric carcinoids. Biomed Res 1983;4(Suppl):307–314.

79. Creutzfeld W. The achlorhydria-carcinoid sequence: Role of gastrin. Digestion 1988;39:61–79.

80. Bordi C, D'Adda T, Azzoni C, et al. Hyperplasia of gastric endocrine cells in the human oxyntic mucosa. In: Håkanson R, Sundler F, eds. The stomach as an endocrine organ. Amsterdam: Elsevier, 1991;403–424.

81. Bordi C, Yu JY, Baggi MT, et al. Gastric carcinoids and their precursor lesions. A histologic and immunohistochemical study of 23 cases. Cancer 1991;67:663.

82. Rappel S, Altendorf-Hofmann A, Stolte M. Prognosis of gastric carcinoid tumours. Digestion 1995;56:455–462.

83. Rindi G, Bordi C, Rappel S, et al. Gastric carcinoids and neuroendocrine carcinomas: Pathogenesis, pathology and behavior. World J Surg 1996;20:168–172.

84. Roberts LJ, Bloomgarden ZT, Marney SR, et al. Histamine from a gastric carcinoid provocation by pentagastrin and inhibition by somatostatin. Gastroenterology 1983;84:272–275.

85. Sandler M, Snow PJD. An atypical carcinoid tumor secreting 5-hydroxytryptophan. Lancet 1958;1:137–139.

86. Oates JA, Sjoerdsma A. A unique syndrome associated with secretion of 5-hydroxytryptophan by metatsatic gastric carcinoids. Am J Med 1962;32:333–342.

87. Håkanson R, Owman CH, Sjöberg NO, et al. Amine mechanisms in enterochromaffin-like cells of gastric mucosa in various mammals. Histochemie 1970;21:189–220.

88. Hage E, Hage J. A gastric carcinoma identified as a gastric ECL-OMA associated with acanthosis nigricans. In: Fujita T, ed. Endocrine gut and pancreas. Amsterdam: Elsevier, 1976:359–363.

89. Solcia E, Capella C, Vassallo G. Endocrine cells of the stomach and pancreas in states of gastric hypersecretion. Rendic Gastroenterol 1970;2:147–158.

90. Polak JM, Stagg B, Pearse AGE. Two types of Zollinger-Ellison syndrome: Immunofluorescent, cytochemical and ultrastructural studies of the antral and pancreatic gastrin cells in different clinical states. Gut 1972;13:501–512.

91. Keuppens F, Willems G, Degraef J, et al. Antral gastrin cell hyperplasia in patients with peptic ulcer. Ann Surg 1980;191:276–281.

92. Friesen SR, Tomita T. Pseudo-Zollinger-Ellison syndrome: Hypergastrinemia, hyperchlorhydria without tumor. Ann Surg 1981;194:481–491.

93. Zaatar R, Younoszai MK, Mitros F. Pseudo Zollinger Ellison syndrome in a child presenting with anemia. Gastroenterology 1987;92:508–512.

94. De Giacomo C, Fiocca R, Villani L, et al. Omeprazole treatment of severe peptic disease associated with antral G cell hyperfunction and hyperpepsinogenemia I in an infant. J Pediatr 1990;117:989–993.

95. Annibale B, Bonamico M, Rindi G, et al. Antral gastrin cell hyperfunction in children. Gastroenterology 1991;101:1547–1551.

96. Oderda G, Fiocca R, Villani L, et al. Gastrin cell hyperplasia in childood Helicobacter pylori gastritis. Eur J Gastroenterol Hepatol 1993;5:13–16.

97. Rindi G, Annibale B, Bonamico M, et al. Helicobacter pylori infection in children with antral gastrin cell hyperfunction. J Pediatr Gastroenterol Nutr 1994;19:152–158.

98. Buffa R, Solovieva I, Fiocca R, et al. Localization of bombesin and GRP (gastrin-releasing peptide) sequences in gut nerves or endocrine cells. Histochemistry 1982;76:457–467.

99. Lehy T, Accardy JP, Labeille D, et al. Chronic administration of bombesin stimulates antral gastrin cell proliferation in the rat. Gastroenterology 1983;84:914–919.

100. Creutzfeldt W, Arnold R, Creutzfeldt C, et al. Gastrin and G-cells in the antral mucosa of patients with pernicious anaemia, acromegaly and hyperparathyroidism and in a Zollinger-Ellison tumour of the pancreas. Eur J Clin Invest 1971;1:461–479.

101. Stockbrugger R, Larsson LI, Lundqvist G, et al. Antral gastrin cells and serum gastrin in achlorhydria. Scand J Gastroenterol 1977;12:209–213.

102. Solcia E, Frigerio B, Capella C. Gastrin and related endocrine cells modulating gastric secretion. In: Rehfeld JF, Amdrup E, eds. Gastrin and the vagus. London: Academic Press, 1979;31–39.

103. Arnold R, Hülst MV, Neuhof CH, et al. Antral gastrin producing G-cells and somatostatin-producing D-cells in different states of gastric acid secretion. Gut 1982;23:285–291.

104. El-Omar E, Penman I, Ardill JES, et al. A substantial number of non-ulcer dyspepsia patients have the same abnormality of acid secretion as duodenal ulcer patients. Gut 1995;36:534–538.

105. Teichmann RK, Pratschke E, Grab J, et al. Gastrin release by interleukin-2 and γ-interferon in vitro. Can J Physiol Pharmacol 1986;64 (Suppl 62).

106. Naoch LA, Bosma NB, Jansen J, et al. Mucosal tumor necrosis factor-α, interleukin-1b, and interleukin-8 production in patients with Helicobacter pylori infection. Scand J Gastroenterol 1994;29:425–429.

107. Golodmer EH, Soll AH, Walsh JH, et al. Release of gastrin from cultured canine G-cells by interferon-γ and tumor necrosis factor-α (abstract). Gastroenterology 1993;104:A89.

108. Teichmann RK, Andress HJ, Gycha S, et al. Immunologic mediated gastrin release (abstract). Gastroenterology 1983;84:1333.

109. Stamm B, Hedinger E, Saremaslani P. Duodenal and ampullary carcinoid tumors. A report of 12 cases with pathological characteristic, polypeptide content and relation to the MEN1 syndrome and von Recklinghausen's disease (neurofibromatosis). Virchows Arch 1986;498:475–489.

110. Burke AP, Federspiel BH, Sobin LH, et al. Carcinoids of the duodenum. A histologic and immunohistochemical study of 65 tumors. Am J Surg Pathol 1989;13:828–837.

111. Capella C, Riva C, Rindi G, et al. Histopathology, hormone products and clinico-pathologic profile of endocrine tumors of the upper small intestine. A study of 44 cases. Endocr Pathol 1991;2:92–110.

112. Thom AK, Norton JA, Axiotis CA, et al. Localization, incidence and malignant potential of duodenal gastrinomas. Surgery 1991;110:1086–1093.

113. Pipeleers-Marichal M, Somers G, Willems G, et al. Gastrinomas in the duodenum of patients with multiple endocrine neoplasia type 1 and with Zollinger-Ellison syndrome. N Engl J Med 1990;322:723–727.

114. Thompson NW, Vinik AI, Eckauser FE. Microgastrinomas of the duodenum: A cause of failed operations of the Zollinger-Ellison syndrome. Ann Surg 1989;209:396–404.

115. Jensen RT, Gardner JD. Gastrinoma. In: Go VLW, DiMagno EP, Gardner JD, et al., eds. The pancreas, biology, pathobiology and disease. 2th ed. New York. Raven Press, 1993;931–978.

116. Hofmann JW, Fox PS, Milwaukee SDW. Duodenal wall tumors and the Zollinger-Ellison syndrome. Arch Surg 1973;107:334–338.

117. Weber HC, Venson DY, Lin JT, et al. Determinants of metastatic rate and survival in patients with Zollinger-Ellison syndrome: A prospective long term study. Gastroenterology 1995;108:1637–1649.

118. Delcore Jr R, Cheung LY, Friesen SR. Outcome of lymph node involvement in patients with the Zollinger-Ellison syndrome. Ann Surg 1988;208:291–298.

119. Klöppel G, Willemer S, Stamm B, et al. Pancreatic lesions and hormonal profile of pancreatic tumors in multiple endocrine neoplasia type 1. An immunocytochemical study of nine patients. Cancer 1986;57:1824–1832.

120. Bordi C, De Vita O, Pilato FP, et al. Multiple islet cell tumors with predominance of glucagon-producing cells and ulcer disease. Am J Clin Pathol 1987;88:153–161.

121. Stabile BE, Passaro E. Benign and malignant gastrinoma. Am J Surg 1985;149:1144–1150.

122. Ellison EH, Wilson SD. The Zollinger-Ellison syndrome; reappraisal and evolution of 260 registered cases. Ann Surg 1964;160:512–528.

123. De Schryver-Kecskemeti K, Clouse RE, Kraus FT. Surgical pathology of gastric and duodenal neuroendocrine tumors masquerading clinically as common polyps. Semin Diagn Pathol 1984;1:5–12.

124. Lundqvist M, Eriksson B, Öberg K, et al. Histogenesis of a duodenal carcinoid. Pathol Res Pract 1989;184:217–222.

125. Rindi G, Grant SGN, Yangou Y, et al. Development of neuroendocrine tumours in the gastrointestinal tract of transgenic mice. Am J Pathol 1990;136:1349–1363.

126. Larsson LI, Ljungberg O, Sundler F, et al. Antropyloric gastrinoma associated with pancreatic nesidioblastosis and proliferation of islets. Virchows Arch 1973;360:305–310.

127. Soulé JC, Potet F, Mignon FC, et al. Syndrome de Zollinger-Ellison dû à un gastrinome gastrique. Arch Fr Mal Appar Dig 1976;65:215–225.

128. Bhagavan BS, Hofkin GA, Woel GM, et al. Zollinger-Ellison syndrome. Ultrastructural and histochemical observations in a child with endocrine tumorlets of gastric antrum. Arch Pathol Lab Med 1974;98:217–222.

129. Farley DR, van Heerden JA, Grant CS, et al. Extrapancreatic gastrinomas. Arch Surg 1994;129:506–512.

130. Sjölund K, Alumets J, Berg NO, et al. Duodenal endocrine cells in adult coeliac disease. Gut 1979;20:547–552.

131. Holle GE, Spann W, Eisenmenger W, et al. Diffuse somatostatin-immunoreactive D-cell hyperplasia in the stomach and duodenum. Gastroenterology 1986;91:733–739.

132. Dayal Y, Tallberg KA, Nunnemacher G, et al. Duodenal carcinoids in patients with and without neurofibromatosis. Am J Surg Pathol 1986;10:348–357.

133. Krejs GJ, Orci L, Conlon JM, et al. Somatostatinoma syndrome. Biochemical, morphologic and clinical features. N Engl J Med 1979;301:285–292.

134. Taccagni GL, Carlucci M, Sironi M, et al. Duodenal somatostatinoma with psammoma bodies: An immunohistochemical and ultrastructural study. Am J Gastroenterol 1986;81:33–37.

135. Griffiths DFR, Jasani B, Newman GR, et al. Glandular duodenal carcinoid. A somatostatin rich tumor with neuroendocrine associations. J Clin Pathol 1984;37:163–169.

136. Cantor AM, Rigby CC, Beck PR, et al. Neurofibromatosis, pheochromocytoma and somatostatinoma. Br Med J 1982;285:1618–1619.

137. Burke AP, Sobin LH, Shekitka KM, et al. Somatostatin-producing duodenal carcinoids in patients with Von Recklinghausen's neurofibromatosis: A predilection for black patients. Cancer 1990;65:1591–1595.

138. Dayal Y, Ganda OP. Somatostatin-producing tumors. In: Dayal Y, ed. Endocrine pathology of the gut and pancreas. Boca Raton: CRC Press, 1991;241–277.

139. Ranaldi R, Bearzi I, Cinti S. Ampullary somatostatinoma. An immunohistochemical and ultrastructural study. Pathol Res Pract 1988;183:8–16.

140. Perrone T, Sibley RK, Rosai J. Duodenal gangliocytic paraganglioma. An immunohistochemical and ultrastructural study and a hypothesis concerning its origin. Am J Surg Pathol 1985;9:31–41.

141. Burke AP, Helwig EB. Gangliocytic paraganglioma. J Clin Pathol 1989;92:1–9.

142. Kheir SM, Halpern NB. Paraganglioma of the duodenum in association with congenital neurofibromatosis. Cancer 1984;53:2491–2496.

143. Stephens M, Williams GT, Jasani B, et al. Synchronous duodenal neuroendocrine tumors in Von Recklingausen's disease. A case report of coexisting gangliocytic paraganglioma and somatostatin rich glandular carcinoid. Histopathology 1987;11:1331–1340.

144. Savio OS, Gonzales BN, Cortes FG, et al. Paraganglioma non cromafinico del yeyuno. Rev Cubana Chir 1974;13:497–505.

145. Delmarre J, Potet F, Capron JP. Chémodectoma gastrique. Etude d'un cas et revue di la littérature. Arch Fr Mal Appar Dig 1975;64:339–346.

146. Hamid QA, Bishop AE, Rode J, et al. Duodenal gangliocytic paragangliomas: A study of 10 cases with immunohistochemical neuroendocrine markers. Hum Pathol 1986;17:1151–1157.

147. van Campenhout E. Contribution au probleme des connexions neuro-entoblastiques. Acad R Med Belg 1940;5:189–201.

148. Solcia E, Capella C, Fiocca R, et al. The gastroenteropancreatic endocrine system and related tumors. Gastroenterol Clin North Am 1989;18:671–693.

149. Rode J, Dhillon AP, Papadaki L, et al. Neurosecretory cells of the lamina propria of the appendix and their possible relationship to carcinoids. Histopathology 1982;6:69–79.

150. Büchler M, Malfertheiner P, Baczako K, et al. A metastatic endocrine-neurogenic tumor of the ampulla of Vater with multiple endocrine immunoreaction. Malignant paraganglioma? Digestion 1985;31:54–59.

151. Inai K, Kobuke T, Yonehara S, et al. Duodenal gangliocytic paraganglioma with lymph node metastasis in a 17-year-old boy. Cancer 1989;63:2540–2545.

152. Strodel WE, Talpos G, Eckhauser F, et al. Surgical therapy for small bowel carcinoid tumors. Arch Surg 1983;191:391–397.

153. Anthony PP, Druy RAB. Elastic vascular sclerosis of mesenteric blood vessels in argentaffin carcinoma. J Clin Pathol 1970;23:110–118.

154. Qizilbash AH. Carcinoid tumors, vascular elastosis and ischemic disease of the small intestine. Dis Colon Rectum 1977;20:554–560.

155. Katsetos CD, Jami MH, Krishna L, et al. Novel immunohistochemical localization of 28000 molecular-weight (Mr) calcium binding protein (Calbindin-D28K) in enterochromaffin cells of the human appendix and neuroendocrine tumors (carcinoids and small cell carcinomas) of the midgut and foregut. Arch Pathol Lab Med 1994;118:633–639.

156. Mårtensson H, Nobin A, Sundler F, et al. Endocrine tumors of the ileum. Cytochemical and clinical aspects. Pathol Res Pract 1985;180:353–363.

157. Bishop AE, Hamid QA, Adams C, et al. Expression of tachykinins by ileal and lung carcinoid tumors assessed by combined in situ hybridization, immunocytochemistry and radioimmunoassay. Cancer 1989;63:1129–1137.

158. Yang K, Ulrich T, Chen GL, et al. The neuroendocrine products of intestinal carcinoids. Cancer 1983;51:1918–1926.

159. Goedert M, Otten U, Suda K, et al. Dopamine, norepinephrine and serotonin production by an intestinal carcinoid tumor. Cancer 1980;45:104–107.

160. Chaudry A, Papanicolau V, Öberg K, et al. Expression of platelet-derived growth factor and its receptors in neuroendocrine tumors of the digestive system. Cancer Res 1992;52:1006–1012.

161. Ahlman H, Wangberg B, Nilsson O. Growth regulation in carcinoid tumors. Endocr Metab Clin North Am 1993;2:889–915.

162. La Rosa S, Chiaravalli AM, Capella C, et al. Immunohistochemical localization of acidic fibroblast growth factor in normal human enterochromaffin cells and related gastrointestinal tumors. Virchows Arch 1996;430:117–124.

163. Wang DG, Johnstone C, Anderson N, et al. Overexpression of the tumour suppressor gene p53 is not implicated in neuroendocrine tumour carcinogenesis. J Pathol 1995;175:397–401.

164. von Herbay A, Sieg B, Schürmann G, et al. Proliferative activity of neuroendocrine tumours of the gastroenteropancreatic endocrine system: DNA flow cytometric and immunohistological investigations. Gut 1991;32:949–953.

165. Kujari H, Joensuu H, Klemi P, et al. A flow cytometric analysis of 23 carcinoid tumors. Cancer 1981;61:2517–2520.

166. Tsushima K, Nagorney DM, Weiland LH, et al. The relationship of flow cytometric DNA analysis and clinicopathology in small-intestinal carcinoids. Surgery 1989;105:366–373.

167. Masson P. Carcinoids (argentaffin-cell tumors) and nerve hyperplasia of the appendicular mucosa. Am J Pathol 1928;4:181–211.

168. Lundqvist M, Wilander E. A study of the histopathogenesis of carcinoid tumours of the small intestine and appendix. Cancer 1987;60:201–206.

169. Moyana TN, Satkunam N. A comparative immunohistochemical study of jejunoileal and appendiceal carcinoids. Implications for histogenesis and pathogenesis. Cancer 1992;70:1081–1082.

170. Nilsson O, Wangberg B, Theodorsson E, et al. Presence of IGF-I in human midgut carcinoid tumours. An autocrine regulator of carcinoid tumour growth? Int J Cancer 1992;51:1–9.

171. Ryden SE, Drake RM, Ralph A, et al. Carcinoid tumors of the appendix in children. Cancer 1975;36:1538–1542.

172. Glasser CM, Bhagavan BS. Carcinoid tumours of the appendix. Arch Pathol Lab Med 1980;104:272–275.

173. Thirlby RC, Kasper CS, Jones RC. Metastatic carcinoid tumor of the appendix: Report of a case and review the literature. Dis Colon Rectum 1984;24:42–46.

174. Anderson JR, Wilson BG. Carcinoid tumours of the appendix. Br J Surg 1985;72:545–546.

175. Bowman GA, Rosenthal D. Carcinoid tumours of the appendix. Am J Surg 1983;146:700–703.

176. Syracuse DC, Perzin KH, Price JB, et al. Carcinoid tumours of the appendix. Mesoappendiceal extension and nodal metastases. Ann Surg 1979;190:58–63.

177. MacGillivray D, Heaton KB, Rushin JM, et al. Distant metastases from carcinoid tumour of the appendix less than one centimeter in size. Surgery 1992;111:466–471.

178. Thompson GB, van Heerden H, Martin JK, et al. Carcinoid tumours of the gastrointestinal tract: Presentation, management and prognosis. Surgery 1985;98:1054–1063.

179. Iwafuchi M, Watanabe H, Ajioka Y, et al. Immunohistochemical and ultrastructural studies of twelve argentaffin and six argyrophil carcinoids of the appendix vermiformis. Hum Pathol 1990;21:773–780.

180. Shaw PAV, Pringle JH. The demonstration of a subset of carcinoid tumours of the appendix by in situ hybridization using synthetic probes to proglucagon mRNA. J Pathol 1992;167:375–380.

181. Solcia E, Fiocca R, Rindi G, et al. The pathology of the gastrointes-

tinal endocrine system. Endocrinol Metab Clin North Am 1993;22:795–821.

182. Berardi RS. Carcinoid tumors of the colon (exclusive of the rectum). Dis Colon Rectum 1972;15:383–391.

183. Rosenberg JM, Welch JP. Carcinoid tumors of the colon. Am J Surg 1985;149:775–779.

184. Azzoni C, Bonato M, D'Adda T, et al. Well-differentiated endocrine tumours of the middle ear and of the hindgut have immunohistochemical and ultrastructural features in common. Virchows Arch 1995;426:411–418.

185. Caldarola VT, Jackman RJ, Moertel GC, et al. Carcinoid tumors of the rectum. Am J Surg 1964;107:844–849.

186. Gross M. Tumeurs carcinoides du rectum. Helv Chir Acta 1968;35:239–248.

187. Gledhill A, Hall PA, Cruse JP, et al. Enteroendocrine cell hyperplasia, carcinoid tumours and adenocarcinoma in long-standing ulcerative colitis. Histopathology 1986;10:501–508.

188. Hock YL, Scott LW, Grace RH. Mixed adenocarcinoma/carcinoid tumour of large bowel in a patient with Crohn's disease. J Clin Pathol 1993;46:183–185.

189. McNeely B, Owen DA, Pezim M. Multiple microcarcionoids arising in chronic ulcerative colitis. Am J Clin Pathol 1992;98:112–116.

190. Bates Jr HR. Carcinoid tumors of the rectum. Dis Colon Rectum 1962;5:270–278.

191. Federspiel BH, Burke AP, Sobin LH, et al. Rectal and colonic carcinoids. A clinicopathologic study of 84 cases. Cancer 1990;65:135–140.

192. Orloff M. Carcinoid tumor of the rectum. Cancer 1971;28:175–180.

193. Tsioulias G, Muto T, Kubota Y, et al. DNA ploidy pattern in rectal carcinoid tumors. Dis Colon Rectum 1991;34:31–36.

194. Alumets J, Alm P, Falkmer S, et al. Immunohistochemical evidence of peptide hormones in endocrine tumors of the rectum. Cancer 1981;48:2409–2415.

195. Fiocca R, Capella C, Buffa R, et al. Glucagon-, glicentin- and pancreatic polypeptide-like immunoreactivities in rectal carcinoids and related colorectal cells. Am J Pathol 1980;100:81–92.

196. O'Brian DS, Dayal Y, De Lellis RA, et al. Rectal carcinoids as tumors of the hindgut endocrine cells. A morphological and immunohistochemical analysis. Am J Surg Pathol 1982;6:131–142.

197. Wilander E, Portela-Gomes G, Grimelius L, et al. Enteroglucagon and substance P-like immunoreactivity in argentaffin and argyrophil rectal carcinoids. Virchows Arch 1977;25:117–124.

198. Moyana TN, Satkunam N. Crypt cell proliferative micronests in rectal carcinoids. An immunohistochemical study. Am J Surg Pathol 1993;17:350–356.

199. Jetmore AB, Ray JE, Garhright Jr JB, McMullen KM, et al. Rectal carcinoids. The most frequent carcinoid tumor. Dis Colon Rectum 1992;35:717–725.

200. Cattan D, Pappo E, Dervichian M, et al. Tumeur carcinoide de l'intestin grêle avec métastases hépatique riches en thyrocalcitonine associée a un adénome benin à cellule C de la glande thyroide. Arch Fr Mal Appar Dig 1973;62:141–150.

201. Weder W, Saremaslani P, Maurer R. Calcitoninbildendes duodenalkarzinoid bei neurofibromatose von Recklingausen. Schweiz Med Wschr 1983;113:885–892.

202. Johnson W, Waisman J. Carcinoid tumor of the vermiform appendix with Cushing's syndrome. Cancer 1971;27:681–686.

203. Miller T, Bernstein J, Var Herle A. Cushing's syndrome cured by resection of appendiceal carcinoid. Arch Surg 1971;103:770–773.

204. Hirata Y, Sakamoto N, Yamamoto H, et al. Gastric carcinoid with ectopic production of ACTH and b-MSH. Cancer 1976;37:377–385.

205. Marcus FS, Friedman MA, Callen PW, et al. Successful therapy of an ACTH-producing gastric carcinoid APUD tumor. Cancer 1980;46:1263–1270.

206. Heitz PU, Klöppel G, Polak JM, et al. Ectopic hormone production by endocrine tumors: Localization of hormones at the cellular level by immunohistochemistry. Cancer 1981;48:2029–2037.

207. Leveston SA, McKeel W, Buckley PJ, et al. Acromegaly and Cushing's syndrome associated with a foregut carcinoid tumor. J Clin Endocrinol Metab 1981;53:682–689.

208. Spero M, White EA. Resolution of acromegaly, amenorrhea-galactorrhea syndrome, and hypergastrinemia after resection of jejunal carcinoid. J Clin Endocrinol Metab 1985;60:392–395.

209. Capella C, Polak JM, Buffa R, et al. Morphological patterns and diagnostic criteria of VIP-producing endocrine tumours: A histological, histochemical, ultrastructural and biochemical study of 32 cases. Cancer 1983;52:1860–1874.

210. Dayal Y, Lin HD, Tallberg K, et al. Immunocytochemical demonstration of growth hormone-releasing factor in gastrointestinal and pancreatic endocrine tumors. Am J Clin Pathol 1986;85:13–20.

211. Bostwick DG, Quan R, Hoffman AR, et al. Growth-hormone releasing factor immunoreactivity in human endocrine tumors. Am J Pathol 1984;117:167–170.

212. Kawahito Y, Sano H, Kawata M, et al. Local secretion of corticotropin-releasing hormone by enterochromaffin cells in human colon. Gastroenterology 1994;106:859–865.

213. Upton GV, Amatruda TI. Evidence for the presence of tumor peptides with corticotropin-releasing factor-like activity in the ACTH ectopic syndrome. N Engl J Med 1971;285:419–424.

214. Larsson LI, Polak JM, Buffa R, et al. On the immunocytochemical localization of the vasoactive intestinal polypeptide. J Histochem Cytochem 1979;27:936–938.

215. Roggli VL, Judge DM, McGavran MH. Duodenal glucagonoma: A case report. Hum Pathol 1979;10:350 353.

216. Gronstad K, Grimelius L, Ekman R, et al. Disseminated rectal carcinoid tumours with production of immunoreactive motilin. Endocr Pathol 1992;3:194–200.

217. McKeown F. Oat cell carcinoma of the esophagus. J Pathol Bacteriol 1952;64:889–891.

218. Tateishi R, Taniguchi K, Horai T, et al. Argyrophil cell carcinoma (apudoma) of the esophagus: A histopathologic entity. Virchows Arch 1976;371:283–294.

219. Reyes CV, Chejfec G, Jao W, et al. Neuroendocrine carcinomas of the esophagus. Ultrastruct Pathol 1980;1:367–376.

220. Briggs JC, Ibrahim NBN. Oat cell carcinoma of the esophagus: A clinico-pathological study of 23 cases. Histopathology 1983;7:261–277.

221. Mori M, Matsukuma A, Adachi Y, et al. Small cell carcinoma of the esophagus. Cancer 1989;63:564–573.

222. Law SY, Fok M, Lam KY, et al. Small cell carcinoma of the esophagus. Cancer 1994;79:2894–2899.

223. Chejfec G, Gould V. Malignant gastric neuroendocrinomas. Hum Pathol 1977;8:433–440.

224. Sweeney EC, McDonnel L. Atypical gastric carcinoids. Histopathology 1980;4:215–224.

225. Zamboni G, Franzin G, Bonetti F, et al. Small cell neuroendocrine carcinoma of the ampullary region. A clinicopathologic, immunohistochemical, and ultrastructural study of three cases. Am J Surg Pathol 1990;14:703–713.

226. Lee CS, Macher D, Rode J. Small cell carcinoma of the ampulla of Vater. Cancer 1992;70:1502–1504.

227. Sarker AB, Hoshida Y, Akagi S, et al. An immunohistochemical and ultrastructural study of a case of small-cell neuroendocrine carcinoma in the ampullary region of the duodenum. Acta Pathol Jpn 1992;42:529–535.

228. Gould VE, Chejfec G. Neuroendocrine carcinomas: Ultrastructural and biochemical evidence of their secretory function. Am J Surg Pathol 1978;2:31–38.

229. Mills SE, Allen Jr MS, Cohen AR. Small-cell undifferentiated carcinoma of the colon. A clinicopathological study of five cases and their association with colonic adenomas. Am J Surg Pathol 1983;7:643–651.

230. Schwartz AM, Orenstein JM. Small cell undifferentiated carcinoma of the rectosigmoid colon. Arch Pathol Lab Med 1985;109:629–632.

231. Wick MB, Weatherby RB, Weiland LH. Small cell neuroendocrine carcinoma of the colon and rectum. Clinical, histologic, and ultrastructural study and immunohistochemical comparison with cloacogenic carcinoma. Hum Pathol 1987;18:9–21.

232. Sarsfield P, Anthony PP. Small cell undifferentiated ("neuroendocrine") carcinoma of the colon. Histopathology 1990;16:357–363.

233. Gaffey MJ, Mills SE, Lack E. Neuroendocrine carcinoma of the colon

and rectum. A clinicopathologic, ultratsructural and immunohistochemical study of 24 cases. Am J Surg Pathol 1990;14:1010–1023.

234. Capella C, Heitz PU, Höfler H, et al. Revised classification of neuroendocrine tumours of the lung, pancreas and gut. Virchows Arch 1995;425:547–560.

235. Capella C, Hage E, Solcia E, et al. Ultrastructural similarity of endocrine-like cells of the human lung and some related cells of the gut. Cell Tissue Res 1978;186:25–37.

236. Gould VE, Jao W, Chejfec G, et al. Neuroendocrine carcinomas of the gastrointestinal tract. Semin Diagn Pathol 1984;1:13–18.

237. Watson KJR, Shulkes A, Surallwood RA, et al. Watery diarrhea-hypokalemia-achlorhydria syndrome and carcinoma of the esophagus. Gastroenterology 1988;88:798–803.

238. Onishi R, Sano T, Nakamura Y, et al. Ectopic adrenocorticotropin syndrome associated with undifferentiated carcinoma of the colon showing multidirectional neuroendocrine, exocrine and squamous differentiation. Virchows Arch 1996;427:537–542.

239. Nichols GL, Kelsen DP. Small cell carcinoma of the esophagus. The Memorial Hospital experience 1970 to 1987. Cancer 1989;64: 1531–1533.

240. Azzopardi JG, Pollock DJ. Argentaffin and argyrophil cells in gastric carcinoma. J Pathol 1963;86:443–451.

241. Bosman FT. Neuroendocrine cells in non-neuroendocrine tumours. In: Falkmer S, Håkanson R, Sundler F, eds. Evolution and tumor pathology of the neuroendocrine system. Amsterdam: Elsevier, 1984;519–543.

242. Arends JW, Wiggers T, Verstijnen C, et al. The occurrence and clinicopathological significance of serotonin immunoreactive cells in large bowel carcinoma. J Pathol 1986;149:97.

243. Bosman FT, de Bruine A. Endocrine cells in nonendocrine tumors of the gut and pancreas. In: Dayal Y, ed. Boca Raton: CRC Press, 1991;319–338.

244. Fiocca R, Villani L, Tenti P, et al. Characterization of four main cell types in gastric cancer. Foveolar, mucopeptic, intestinal columnar and goblet cells: An histopathologic, histochemical and ultrastructural study of "early" and "advanced" tumours. Pathol Res Pract 1987; 182:308–325.

245. Kubo I, Watanabe H. Neoplastic argentaffin cells in gastric and intestinal carcinomas. Cancer 1971;27:447–454.

246. Proks C, Feit V. Gastric carcinoma with argyrophil and argentaffin cells. Virchows Arch 1982;395:201–206.

247. Smith DM, Haggit RC. The prevalence and prognostic significance of argyrophil cells in carcinomas of the colon and rectum. Am J Surg Pathol 1984;8:123–128.

248. Waldum HL, Burhol PG, Johnson JA, et al. MSH-producing gastric tumour. Acta Hepatol Gastroenterol 1977;24:386–388.

249. Cocco AE, Conway SJ. Zollinger-Ellison syndrome associated with ovarian mucinous cystoadenocarcinoma. N Engl J Med 1978;298: 144–146.

250. Ratzenhofer M, Aubock L. The amphicrine (endoexocrine) cells in the human gut with a short reference to amphicrine neoplasia. Acta Morphol Acad Sci Hung 1980;28:37–58.

251. Höfler H, Klöppel G, Heitz PU. Combined production of mucus, amines and peptides by goblet-cell carcinoids of the appendix and ileum. Pathol Res Pract 1984;178:555–561.

252. Chejfec G, Capella C, Solcia E, et al. Amphicrine cells dysplasias and neoplasias. Cancer 1985;56:2683–2689.

253. Pradé M, Bara J, Gadenne C, et al. Gastric carcinoma with argyrophilic cells: Light microscopic, electron microscopic, and immunohistochemical study. Hum Pathol 1982;13:588–592.

254. Tahara E, Hisao I, Nakagami K, et al. Scirrhous argyrophil cell carcinoma of the stomach with multiple production of polypeptide hormones, amine, CEA, lysozyme, and HCG. Cancer 1982;49: 1904–1915.

255. Soga J, Tazawa K, Aizawa O, et al. Argentaffin cell adenocarcinoma of the stomach: A atypical carcinoid? Cancer 1971;28:1904–1915.

256. Tahara E, Ito H, Shimamoto F, et al. Argyrophil cells in early gastric carcinoma: An immunohistochemical and ultrastructural study. J Cancer Res Clin Oncol 1982;103:187–202.

257. Ulich TR, Cheng L, Glover H, et al. A colonic adenocarcinoma with argentaffin cells. An immunoperoxidase study demonstrating the presence of numerous neuroendocrine products. Cancer 1982;51: 1483–1489.

258. Shousha S. Signet ring cell adenocarcinoma of rectum: A histological, histochemical and electron microscopic study. Histopathology 1982; 6:341–350.

259. Lyss AP, Thompson JJ, Glick JN. Adenocarcinoid tumor of the colon arising in preexisting ulcerative colitis. Cancer 1981;48:833–839.

260. Subbuswamy SG, Gibbs NM, Ross CF, et al. Goblet cell carcinoid of the appendix. Cancer 1974;34:338–344.

261. Abt AB, Carter SL. Goblet cell carcinoma of the appendix. Arch Pathol Lab Med 1976;100:301–306.

262. Park K, Blessing K, Kerr K, et al. Goblet cell carcinoid of the appendix. Gut 1990;31:322–324.

263. Anderson NH, Somerville JE, Jonhnston CF, et al. Appendiceal goblet cell carcinoids: A clinicopathological and immunohistochemical study. Histopathology 1991;18:61–65.

264. Warkel RL, Cooper PH, Helwig EB. Adenocarcinoid: a mucin producing tumor of the appendix. A study of 39 cases. Cancer 1978;42:2781–2793.

265. Edmonds P, Merino MJ, Li Volsi VA, et al. Adenocarcinoid (mucinous carcinoid) of the appendix. Gastroenterology 1984;86: 302–309.

266. Isaacson P. Crypt cell carcinoma of the appendix (so-called adenocarcinoid tumour). Am J Surg Pathol 1981;5:213–224.

267. Burke AP, Lee YK. Adenocarcinoid (goblet cell carcinoid) of the duodenum presenting as a gastric outlet obstruction. Hum Pathol 1990;21:238–239.

268. Jones MA, Griffith LM, West AB. Adenocarcinoid tumor of the periampullary region: A novel duodenal neoplasm presenting as biliary tract obstruction. Hum Pathol 1989;20:198–200.

269. Berardi RS, Lee SS, Chen HP. Goblet cell carcinoids of the appendix. Surg Gynecol Obstet 1988;13:81–86.

270. Klein EA, Rosen MH. Bilateral Krukenberg tumors due to appendiceal mucinous carcinoid. Int J Gynecol Pathol 1996;15:85–88.

271. Bates Jr HR, Belter LF. Composite carcinoid tumour (argentaffin adenocarcinoma) of the colon: Report of two cases. Dis Colon Rectum 1967;10:467–470.

272. Hernandez FL, Reid JD. Mixed carcinoid and mucous-secreting intestinal tumors. Arch Pathol Lab Med 1969;88:489–496.

273. Klappenbach RS, Kurman RJ, Sinclair CF, et al. Composite carcinoma-carcinoid tumors of the gastrointastinal tract. A morphologic, histochemical and immuohistochemical study. Am J Clin Pathol 1988;84:137–143.

274. Moyana TN, Qizilbash AH, Murphy F. Composite glandular-carcinoid tumors of the colon and rectum. Report of two cases. Am J Surg Pathol 1988;12:607–611.

275. Goldberg SL, Toker C. Composite tumor of small intestine. Mt Sinai J Med NY 1976;43:153–156.

276. Shah IA, Schlageter MO, Boehm N. Composite carcinoid-adenocarcinoma of ampulla of Vater. Hum Pathol 1990;21:1188–1190.

277. Parks TG. Malignant carcinoid and adenocarcinoma of the stomach. Br J Surg 1970;57:377–379.

278. Rogers LW, Murphy RC. Gastric carcinoid and gastric carcinoma. Morphologic correlates of survival. Am J Surg Pathol 1979; 3:195–202.

279. Yamashina M, Flinner RA. Concurrent occurrence of adenocarcinoma and carcinoid tumor of the stomach: A composite tumor or collision tumors? Am J Clin Pathol 1985;83:233–236.

280. Ulich TR, Kollin M, Lewin KJ. Composite gastric carcinoma. Report of a tumor of the carcinoma-carcinoid spectrum. Arch Pathol Lab Med 1988;112:91–93.

281. Caruso ML, Pilato FP, D'Adda T, et al. Composite carcinoid-adenocarcinoma of the stomach associated with multiple gastric carcinoids and nonantral gastric atrophy. Cancer 1989;64:1534–1539.

282. Chong FK, Graham JH, Madoff IM. Mucin-producing carcinoid (composite tumor) of upper third of esophagus: A variant of carcinoid tumor. Cancer 1979;44:1853–1859.

16 IMMUNODEFICIENCY DISORDERS AND THEIR EFFECTS ON THE GASTROINTESTINAL TRACT

David F. Keren and Jeffrey S. Warren

The gastrointestinal tract is lined by a delicate mucosal surface that is exposed to a barrage of infectious agents and potentially toxic chemicals daily. An elaborate mucosal immune system (see Chapter 6) has evolved to prevent these agents from gaining a foothold throughout this surface. Although the mucosal immune system exhibits a number of tissue-specific and compartment-specific features, the gastrointestinal tract is affected by many systemic immunodeficiency diseases. Immunodeficiency diseases may be congenital or acquired; may affect the humoral immune system, the cellular immune system, or both; and may affect the nonspecific phagocytic host defense. We review these immune deficiencies with an emphasis on their relationship to the gastrointestinal tract.

CONGENITAL IMMUNODEFICIENCY SYNDROMES

X-LINKED (BRUTON) AGAMMAGLOBULINEMIA (XLA)

X-linked (recessive) agammaglobulinemia is the most common type of congenital immunodeficiency disease that results in a complete, or nearly complete absence of plasma cells. This disorder occurs in approximately 1 of 100,000 live male births (1). Although these boys are unable to produce immunoglobulins, they are usually well for the first 6 months of life, after which they begin to suffer from recurrent pyogenic infections, recurrent gastrointestinal infections (e.g., *Giardia lamblia*), and atypical responses to infections with various enteroviruses (e.g., paralytic poliomyelitis from live virus vaccines and chronic meningoencephalitis secondary to persistent enteroviral infections) as transplacentally acquired maternally-derived IgG concentrations decline. Plasma cells that contain IgM can be found within the lamina propria of normal infants very early in life. Within 3 to 6 months following birth, these IgM-containing plasma cells are superseded by IgA-containing cells (2). Patients with XLA possess virtually no detectable plasma cells within the lamina propria.

The fundamental defect in XLA results in B cell precursors that are unable to complete their maturation to mature B cells and plasma cells (3). The underlying "defect" has recently been identified as a series of mutations in a gene located in Xq22 that encodes a tyrosine kinase (4). The btk gene (Bruton [or B cell] tyrosine kinase) contains a 20-kb segment of DNA that encodes mRNA normally expressed in all B lymphocytes (including pre-B cells in the bone marrow) and myeloid cells (5, 6). Several mutations have been described, but the relationship between a particular alteration in the btk gene and immunoglobulin production is complex, thus clouding the precise relationship between a given defect and specific immunologic consequences (7). The btk gene is not expressed in T lymphocytes (8). Not surprisingly, patients with XLA have low

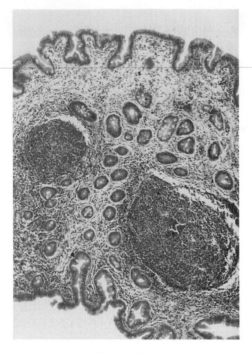

Figure 16.1 Prominent lymphoid nodules in small intestinal biopsy from patient with common variable immunodeficiency syndrome. Villi appear shortened, due in part to the orientation of the biopsy (H & E, ×100). (See color plate.)

levels or undetectable levels of both the mRNA and the specific tyrosine kinase in their B lymphocytes (9). Although the gene is believed to be involved in signal transduction, the mechanism by which the decrease in functional enzyme interferes with B cell maturation is not yet known (10).

Patients with XLA possess serum IgG concentrations of less than 2 g/L, whereas IgA and IgM are usually undetectable. The fact that granulocytes are also deficient in cytoplasmic Bruton's tyrosine kinase may account for the observation that some patients with XLA are neutropenic (11). Neutropenia in XLA patients may be especially pronounced during episodes of acute infection (8).

Most patients with XLA possess markedly decreased concentrations of circulating B lymphocytes. In the bone marrow, however, pre-B lymphocytes are present (12–14). The few mature B lymphocytes that can be detected in the circulation are typically devoid of CD21, a cell surface-associated marker of B lymphocyte maturity. Available data suggest that btk encodes a tyrosine kinase that is critical to B cell maturation. Study of the btk gene has led to the observation that there is considerable variability in the number of B lymphocytes that circulate in the peripheral blood (15). The peripheral blood T lymphocytes are present in normal concentrations and the ratio of helper (CD4)/suppressor (CD8) T cells is normal (16, 17).

In patients with XLA, the lymphoid tissue is atrophic and lacks germinal centers. The gastrointestinal tract is virtually devoid of plasma cells, whereas T lymphocyte zones in lymph nodes and Peyer patches are normal.

In contrast to the thought that XLA was not associated with increased incidence of neoplasia, Van der Meer and colleagues reported a 30-fold increase in the occurrence of colorectal carci-

noma and recommended screening even young individuals for this complication (18).

TRANSIENT HYPOGAMMAGLOBULINEMIA OF INFANCY (THI)

The incidence of THI is poorly defined because most cases are likely to go unrecognized. As many as 20% of infants may have modest delays in the development of "normal" immunoglobulin concentrations (19). Serum immunoglobulin concentrations remain low in THI patients until 3 to 5 years of age, when they spontaneously rise to normal concentrations. Some of these children suffer from recurrent pyogenic infections. In a study by Cano et al., 13 such children possessed a mean serum IgG of 0.27 G/L (controls had 0.75 G/L) (20). Patients with THI possess normal concentrations of peripheral blood B lymphocytes, but experience a transient depression in CD4 T lymphocyte levels. Depressed CD4-positive T lymphocyte concentrations rise in parallel with their serum immunoglobulin concentrations (21).

OTHER AGAMMAGLOBULINEMIA SYNDROMES

Very rare cases of pre-B cell deficiency and autosomal recessive agammaglobulinemia have also been described. These syndromes occur in males and females (22). As in XLA patients, these individuals often suffer from recurrent pyogenic infections after about 3 to 18 months of age, lack circulating B lymphocytes, and possess normal numbers of circulating T lymphocytes (23).

COMMON VARIABLE IMMUNODEFICIENCY DISEASE (CVID)

Patients with CVID are usually young to middle-aged adults who develop recurrent pyogenic sinopulmonary infections, sequelae of such recurrent infections (e.g., chronic obstructive lung disease

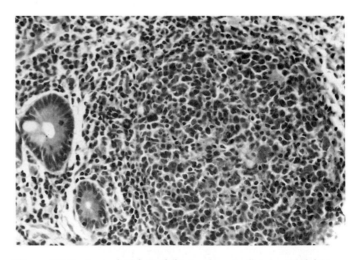

Figure 16.2 Lymphoid nodule in the small intestinal biopsy from a patient with common variable immunodeficiency syndrome. Note the lack of a mantle zone of lymphocytes and how the nodule blends irregularly with the surrounding lamina propria (H & E, ×250). (See color plate.)

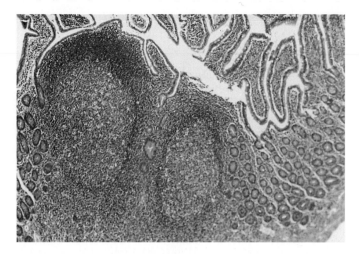

Figure 16.3   Prominent lymphoid nodules in tissue sample from small intestinal biopsy from a patient with blind loop syndrome and bacterial overgrowth. Note the prominent zone of small lymphocytes that surrounds the nodules (H & E, ×60). (See color plate.)

and/or bronchiectasia), recurrent herpes infections, diarrhea (often associated with *G. lamblia*), and in some patients, atypical enteroviral infections similar to those seen in patients with XLA. CVID is a heterogeneous group of disorders. In addition to mostly sporadic cases, autosomal dominant, autosomal recessive, and X-linked patterns of inheritance have been described (6, 24). The disease has a prevalence of about 1:100,000 and has been associated with HLA A1 B8 DR3 haplotypes in some, but not all, families (25). Although giardiasis is not the only cause of malabsorption in CVID patients (see subsequent discussion), it can lead to severe protein depletion if untreated (26). Quantification of serum immunoglobulins is the most useful laboratory screening method in these patients. Despite the presence of low concentrations of immunoglobulins, patients tend to develop autoimmune and inflammatory disorders that include inflammatory bowel disease, hemolytic anemia, thrombocytopenia, and pernicious anemia. The incidence of gastric carcinoma (about fifty-fold) and lymphoma (seen more often in female patients than in male patients) is dramatically increased (27).

Whereas most immunologic diseases are accompanied by few or minor morphologic features discernible on routine histologic analysis, patients with CVID have striking gastrointestinal nodular lymphoid hyperplasia, as well as splenomegaly and diffuse lymphadenopathy (Fig. 16.1) (28). In some cases, the gastrointestinal lymphoid hyperplasia is sufficiently prominent that it can be visualized on upper gastrointestinal radiographs. These nodules usually lack the prominent mantle layer of smaller lymphocytes and instead exhibit germinal centers that are ragged and blend irregularly into the surrounding connective tissue (Fig. 16.2). Nodular lymphoid hyperplasia is not specific to CVID. Grossly apparent nodular lymphoid hyperplasia may be seen in conditions that are associated with intestinal bacterial overgrowth (e.g., blind loop syndrome). In contrast to nodular lymphoid hyperplasia associated with CVID, however, a prominent mantle zone of smaller lymphocytes surrounds the germinal center and abundant plasma cells are present in the lamina propria (Fig. 16.3) (29). The lamina propria contains few plasma cells, a feature that is best appreciated by immunohistochemical staining of the routine paraffin-embedded

tissue for IgG, IgA, and IgM (Fig. 16.4). Noncaseating granulomas, as occur in Crohn disease, may be found along the gastrointestinal tract and in other locations. In addition to lymphoid nodules and occasional granulomas, some CVID patients possess atrophic villi. The pathogenesis of this finding is not known. The villus epithelial cells can produce secretory component, implying that the regulation of this component of the mucosal immune system is immunoglobulin-independent. Approximately 25% of patients classified as having CVID have atrophic gastritis (30).

The heterogeneity of CVID is emphasized by studies of the immunoglobulin content of lamina propria plasma cells in the small intestinal lamina propria. Some patients possess no detectable IgA-containing plasma cells and no serum IgA. These patients are the most likely to develop *G. lamblia*, *Campylobacter jejuni*, and *Candida albicans* infections (30) (Fig. 16.5). Patients deficient

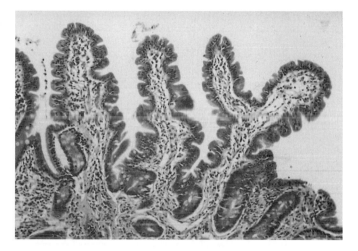

Figure 16.4   Jejunal biopsy specimen from a patient with common variable immunodeficiency syndrome shows shortened villi with relatively few plasma cells in the lamina propria. A cluster of indistinct microorganisms over the middle villus suggests the possibility of giardiasis (see Fig. 16.5) (H & E, ×100). (See color plate.)

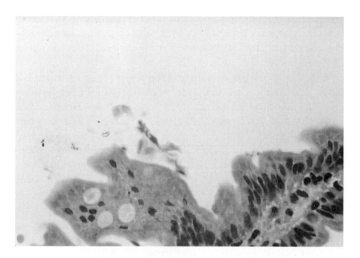

Figure 16.5   Prominent cluster of Giardia lamblia atop villus from a patient with common variable immunodeficiency syndrome (H & E, ×400). (See color plate.)

only in serum IgG are unlikely to experience diarrhea or malabsorption.

The concentration of peripheral blood B lymphocytes is usually normal or in the low normal range. B lymphocytes from CVID patients are morphologically immature but can produce immunoglobulin following stimulation. Because immature B lymphocytes appear to be functionally intact and because stimulation of T lymphocytes (via T-cell receptors) in many cases results in subnormal transcription and secretion of interferon-γ, interleukins (IL)-2, -4, and -5, as well as subnormal expression of CD40 ligand, the "fundamental defect" in at least some cases of CVID appears to reside in CD4-positive T lymphocytes (31). A defect in the heavy chain switch mechanism has been described in a patient with isolated deficiency of IgG and IgA (32), and some patients possess a defect in the expression of μ-chain by B lymphocytes (33). The latter finding is likely attributable to a lack of appropriate signaling from T lymphocytes.

Some CVID patients exhibit a decrease in the numbers of CD4 cells; others possess normal CD4 cell numbers, but increased numbers of CD8 cells (34–36). Patients in the subgroup who possess decreased concentrations of CD4 lymphocytes often possess significantly elevated serum concentrations of tumor necrosis factor, which may be important in the immunopathogenesis of their disease (37). A small number of CVID patients has had recovery of normal immunoglobulin levels following treatment with cimetidine. These patients tend to be individuals with excessive numbers of CD8 lymphocytes in their peripheral blood (38, 39). Other reports have noted the lack of appropriate lymphokine stimulation in patients with CVID. Indeed, stimulation of lymphocytes from patients with CVID by antigen, mitogens, IL-2, or IL-6 can facilitate the maturation of B lymphocytes from these patients (40–43). A defect in the early phase of the T-cell receptor-mediated activation has been hypothesized for patients with decreased T cell proliferative responses or production of IL-2 or interferon-γ (44). Still other reports cite a subset of cases with a depressed expression of CD 40 ligand (glycoprotein 39 [gp39]), a ligand expressed by CD4 T lymphocytes that is thought to be important in T-B cell interactions (45, 46).

When CVID occurs in early childhood, distinction from XLA can be difficult in the subset of patients that have decreased circulating B lymphocytes. In these patients, analysis of X chromosome inactivation of female relatives can reveal whether the deficiency is part of an X-linked process or is a sporadic occurrence of CVID (47).

Although the genetics of CVID are yet to be elucidated in detail, interesting links with other immunodeficiencies imply a genetic connection. For instance, CVID is sometimes found in families that have selective IgA deficiency in siblings or in subsequent generations (48). Acquired CVID has also been reported both after phenytoin therapy and in renal transplant patients following immunosuppressive therapy (49–51).

Intravenous gammaglobulin (IVGG) replacement has been the mainstay of therapy for these patients. Although responses to this therapy are variable, differences likely relate to the heterogeneity of the condition itself (52). Recently, administration of polyethylene glycol-conjugated IL-2 was shown to have a positive effect on helper T cells and immunoglobulin production in patients with CVID, offering hope that IVGG may be replaced in some patients (53).

HYPER-IgM IMMUNODEFICIENCY

This X-linked (or occasionally autosomal recessive) immunodeficiency results from a defect in the ability for heavy chain genes to switch from production of μ to the other isotypes (54). Similar to XLA, these individuals are highly susceptible to bacterial infections. Unlike most XLA patients, however, they also develop problems with opportunistic infections. Recurrent bacterial infections may be severe. This disease is most commonly an X-linked inherited disorder, but sometimes it is acquired (55). The infections result from the significantly decreased or absent IgG, IgA, and IgE. Both IgM and IgD levels are elevated (56).

Recent studies link hyper-IgM syndrome to the CD40 ligand gene that is present on the long arm of the X chromosome (57). The ligand, gp39, is present on activated T cells, interacts with the B lymphocyte CD40 surface receptor, and triggers both B lymphocyte proliferation and differentiation (58). Conflicting study results suggest the involvement of an intrinsic defect in B lymphocytes from patients with the hyper-IgM immunodeficiency syndrome (59). Further, stimulation of the CD40 receptor alone was not able to produce IgA or IgG switching, although IgE was produced. These observations suggest the possibility of two or more defects in this group of patients; the CD40 ligand deficiency and an intrinsic B cell defect (60).

Histologically, the lamina propria contains plasma cells that exclusively contain IgM (61). The elevated levels of serum IgM may relate to antigenic stimulation of the mucosal lymphoid tissues. The lymphoid nodules in the submucosa of the colon are morphologically primary follicles (61). Because of the impaired humoral immune response, these patients are particularly predisposed to cryptosporidium infections that result in diarrhea and cholangitis (62). Indeed, cryptosporidium-related cholangitis occurs with surprising frequency in these individuals, occasionally leading to cirrhosis. Giardiasis is another important cause of diarrhea in hyper-IgM immunodeficiency patients (63). Esophageal fungal infections, including histoplasmosis, have been reported (64).

Many of these patients have been treated with gammaglobulin replacement therapy. In one case, a 5-month-old infant with hyper-IgM immunodeficency syndrome received a bone marrow transplant from his sister that resulted in restoration of CD40 ligand (65). The patient's family included two maternal uncles who died at 6 months and 2 years of age, respectively, with protracted diarrhea, and a first cousin with the same disease now requires a liver transplantation.

SELECTIVE IgA DEFICIENCY

This most common of all congenital immunodeficiency diseases has an incidence of about 1 in 700, yet it is not often detected because individuals with selective IgA deficiency are usually asymptomatic. The condition is defined by a serum IgA concentration of less than 50 mg/L, normal IgG and IgM levels, and an intact cellular immune system (66). Although most individuals with this condition are clinically well, some have gastrointestinal infections, gluten-sensitive enteropathy, sinopulmonary problems, or autoimmune disease (67–69). The number of circulating B lymphocytes with surface IgA is often decreased (70), although surface marker analysis is not needed to make the diagnosis of selective IgA deficiency.

Some patients with selective IgA deficiency develop anti-IgA antibodies. Because of the potential for anaphylaxis in these cases, great care must be taken when providing these patients with blood products. Removal of IgA from platelets and other preparations may be necessary for sensitized individuals (71). Anti-IgA antibodies develop in as many as 20% of patients with serum IgA <0.05 mg/L and tend to remain constant with time (72).

IgA-containing plasma cells are lacking in the lamina propria (Fig. 16.6). Because of a compensatory increase in IgM and normal gut intraepithelial T cell function, these patients usually do not experience significant gastrointestinal infections (73). The IgM produced in the lamina propria is able to bind to secretory component and is secreted by the surface epithelium into the gut lumen (74).

Selectively IgA-deficient patients usually do not exhibit a clear-cut mode of inheritance for the defect. Some kindreds display autosomal dominant or recessive inheritance, but this pattern of

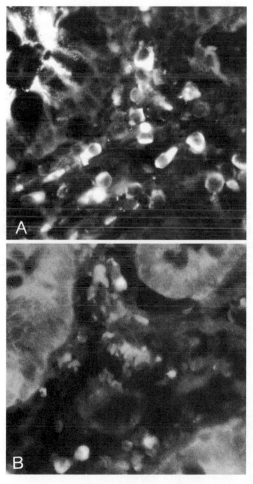

Figure 16.6.   A, Dark-field photomicrograph of normal human lamina propria stained with fluorescein-conjugated anti-human IgA. Numerous plasma cells stain, and staining is prominent in the surface of the crypt epithelium. **B,** Dark-field photomicrograph of IgA-deficient human lamina propria stained with fluorescein-conjugated anti-human IgA. No plasma cells stain, and no staining is noted in the surface of the crypt epithelium. (See color plate.)

inheritance is not the rule. Results of a study of Swedish kindreds with CVID and selective IgA deficiency casts doubt on previous claims of a linkage with specific major histocompatibility complex (MHC) regions (53, 75, 76).

Selective IgA deficiency may be acquired, especially in patients receiving penicillamine or phenytoin. This deficiency, thought to be attributable to enhanced suppressor T cells, is reversed by discontinuing the medication (77).

In the mid-1970s, Strober et al. (78) described a patient who was not able to produce secretory component (necessary for transport of IgA or IgM across the epithelium into the gut lumen). This patient suffered from chronic intestinal candidiasis. Biopsy of the small bowel revealed normal numbers of IgA plasma cells, and serum concentrations of IgA were normal. The patient was successfully treated with bovine colostrum.

Although most cases of IgA deficiency require therapy only for specific infections, some individuals with recurrent infections and IgG2 or IgG3 deficiency in addition to the IgA deficiency have benefited from immunoglobulin replacement therapy (79).

HYPERIMMUNOGLOBULIN E SYNDROME (JOB SYNDROME)

This rare condition involves both prominent physical features and defects in lymphoid and myeloid cells. Clinical presentation usually reflects recurrent, prominent "cold" abscesses in the skin, on mucosal surfaces, and within viscera. The so-called cold abscesses are caused by staphylococci, although fungal infections, including cryptococcosis, have also been reported. Cold abscesses appear to result from a defect in monocyte and neutrophil chemotaxis that has been associated with decreased γ-interferon production (80). The defects in neutrophil and monocyte chemotaxis may be related to inhibitory factors. Gammaglobulin therapy has been successful in ameliorating symptoms in isolated cases (81).

Physical features of note include a protruding jaw, hypertelorism, and cranial synostosis (82). Osteoporosis is a prominent feature in some patients and can lead to pathologic fractures. The bone loss and fractures are the result of mononuclear cell activation with bone resorption mediated by locally secreted cytokines (83). Serum IgE concentration is elevated and that of IgG is normal or depressed. A poor response to polysaccharide antigens is present in some, but not all of these patients (84).

A few interesting cases of Job syndrome and gastrointestinal manifestations have been reported. The main gastrointestinal manifestation is mucocutaneous candidiasis. Although these patients often have decreased IgA levels, it is not clear that this finding relates to the mucocutaneous candidiasis (85). The disease mimicks Crohn disease, with perirectal abscesses and granulomatous colitis (86). One patient had well-documented cryptococcosis confined to the colon and perirectal tissues, and another patient had histoplasma budding yeasts in the cecum and ileum (87). In yet another case, focal transmural purulent necrosis in the ascending colon was present adjacent to a perforation. Cultures of this area revealed *Enterobacter cloacae* and *Bacteroides fragilis* (88). These observations imply that the mucosal surfaces of the colon may be as susceptible as the skin with regard to the poor response to bacterial infections. This diagnosis should be suspected when viewing perirectal or colonic abscesses in the clinical setting of an individual

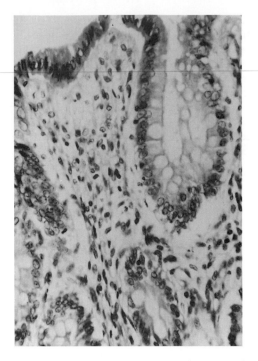

Figure 16.7 Appendix from a patient with SCID. The lamina propria is devoid of plasma cells (H & E, ×400). (See color plate.)

with skin abscesses. Seeking a history of "cold" abscesses and measuring serum IgE concentration are recommended.

A possibly related disorder, with dramatically elevated levels of IgE, has been reported in four related male infants. All of the infants developed intractable diarrhea, recurrent infections, an exfoliative skin rash, and insulin-dependent diabetes. All four cases were fatal. This condition is apparently inherited as an X-linked recessive trait (89).

HYPERIMMUNOGLOBULIN D SYNDROME

Infants with this relatively recently recognized condition present with recurrent attacks of high spiking fevers, often accompanied by abdominal pain, diarrhea, vomiting, headache, arthralgia, lymphadenopathy, and splenomegaly (90). The attacks persist for up to 1 week and occur once every month or two. Most patients have been from Europe (91). As the name implies, the children exhibit a polyclonal increase in IgD, usually greater than 100 U/mL (92). Males and females are affected equally, and family studies demonstrate an autosomal recessive pattern of inheritance. The etiology of the periodic febrile attacks is unknown, but the episodes correlate with elevations of C-reactive protein, IL-6, interferon-γ, and soluble type-II phospholipase A2 (PLA2) (93, 94). Although no therapy for this condition is currently available, the frequency and severity of attacks decline as the patients age (91).

SEVERE COMBINED IMMUNODEFICIENCY (SCID)

As with CVID, SCID is a heterogeneous condition characterized by varied pathogeneses and modes of inheritance. The fact that SCID

is about three times more common in males than females reflects the fact that the most frequent mode of inheritance is the X-linked form of the disease (6). The severity of the deficiency varies depending on the mutation (95). The various forms of SCID have in common a dramatic clinical presentation in which infants die of bacterial, viral, or fungal infections, unless they undergo bone marrow transplantation soon after birth. Because these infants are deficient in both cellular and humoral immunity, gammaglobulin replacement therapy alone is insufficient to protect them from the opportunistic infections that often lead to their demise. Autosomal recessive, X-linked, and sporadic forms of SCID have been reported (96, 97).

Children with SCID typically present within the first 3 months of life with failure to thrive. The small number of viable lymphocytes present in a blood transfusion are sufficient to initiate graft-versus-host disease (GVHD) in these profoundly defenseless infants (98, 99). All blood products received by these infants must be irradiated. Even in the absence of transfusion, some infants develop fatal graft-versus-host disease that has been mediated by viable maternal lymphocytes that have traversed the placenta and entered the fetal circulation (99). The entire mucosa in these individuals is deficient in both B and T cell functions, and the lamina propria is devoid of plasma cells (Fig. 16.7). Interepithelial lymphocytes are rarely seen in histologic sections (Fig. 16.8), and the appendix lacks lymphoid follicles (Fig. 16.9).

Graft-versus-host disease (GVHD) occurs in children with SCID and individuals who receive bone marrow transplantation. In acute GVHD, gastrointestinal manifestations include diarrhea and abdominal pain. Histologically, rectal crypts show focal apoptotic cell loss as well as abscesses (100). In the lamina propria, lymphocytic infiltration occurs. After 3 months, chronic GVHD is found in a minority (10%) of patients who had acute GVHD and in some individuals who never suffered from the acute disease (101). These patients experience difficulty swallowing, reflux esophagitis, diarrhea, malabsorption, and abdominal pain (100). Histologically, the esophagus exhibits a variety of findings from minor vacuolization of basal epithelial cells to frank ulceration with prominent lymphocytes and plasma cell infiltrates. In the small bowel, changes in the lamina propria usually are minimal, although a moderate increase in the

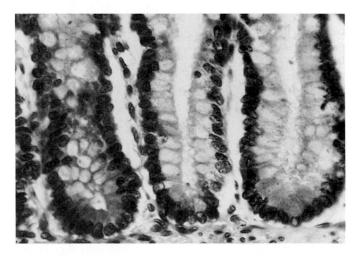

Figure 16.8 Small intestine from a patient with SCID. Only rare intraepithelial lymphocytes are seen (H & E, ×400). (See color plate.)

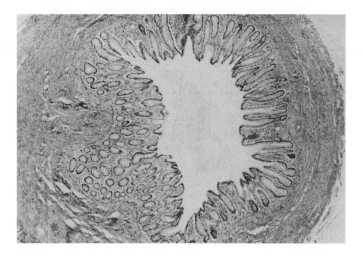

Figure 16.9   Low-power view of appendix from a patient with SCID. Note total lack of lymphoid follicles (H & E, ×60). (See color plate.)

numbers of plasma cells may be noted. Injury to the submucosal endothelium and smooth muscle cells has also been observed (100).

In most patients with SCID, the primary defect is in the T cell lineage. Serum IgG, IgA, and IgM levels are absent and lymphopenia is remarkable. The numbers of B cells in the peripheral blood vary depending on the subtype of SCID. For instance, patients with X-linked SCID have a maturation arrest that affects their B lymphocytes. These cells express markers usually present on precursor cells: CD1c, CD38, and CD23 (102–104). In the X-linked form of SCID, the deficiency is linked to a mutation of the γ-chain of interleukin receptors for IL-2, IL-4, IL-11, and IL-15, resulting in a profound maturation arrest of T cells and B cells (105, 106).

The less common autosomal recessive forms of SCID have several causes. The most frequent deficiency is of adenosine deaminase (ADA) found in 20% of patients with SCID (about 50% of the autosomal recessive cases) (107). Rarely, this ADA deficiency has resulted in immunodeficiency presenting in adult life, suggesting that partial ADA deficiency can deteriorate with time (108). Less common forms of autosomal recessive SCID include deficiency of purine-nucleoside phosphorylase that results in increased accumulation of deoxyguanosine (109), and ZAP-70 deficiency, which is associated with defects in the T cell antigen receptor signal (110).

Bone marrow transplantation is the mainstay of therapy for these children. Bone marrow restoration has led not only to improved peripheral immunologic capacity in these children, but also to restoration of IgA plasma cells in the lamina propria (110–113). Because of the importance of bone marrow transplants for these children, some HLA mismatches have been attempted, and in some cases, have been successful (114).

DiGeorge Syndrome (Congenital Thymic Aplasia)

In DiGeorge syndrome, humoral immunity is basically intact, but cell-mediated immunity is impaired. Babies with DiGeorge syndrome have physical features that allow the condition to be suspected at birth: low-set ears, hypertelorism, micrognathia, and an "antimongoloid" slant of the eyes. Many DiGeorge patients exhibit conotruncal cardiac abnormalities. When these findings are present, it is important to monitor serum calcium levels, because affected babies can develop hypocalcemic tetany within a few days of birth. Because of failure of the thymus gland to develop properly (see subsequent discussion), chest radiographic findings include a diminished or absent thymic shadow.

During the twelfth week of fetal development, there is interference with the development of the third and fourth pharyngeal pouches that give rise to the thymus gland. DiGeorge syndrome is associated with translocation of a portion of the proximal long arm of chromosome 22 (115, 116). Despite the lack of a grossly identifiable thymus gland, patients with DiGeorge syndrome have some CD3 T lymphocytes in their peripheral blood. Although some patients do recover sufficient T cell function with time, other patients have been treated with thymic transplantation or even implants from fetal thymus glands (17, 117).

Gastrointestinal complications occur in a minority of these patients (118). Children with DiGeorge syndrome may develop chronic rotavirus infection in which the virus persists in the liver or the kidneys (119). Chronic infection with enterovirus has been reported to cause chronic, persistent diarrhea in some of these patients (120).

Ataxia Telangiectasia (AT)

Ataxia telangiectasia is an autosomal recessive disease that manifests in children with gait disturbance and telangiectasias (121). The majority of patients with AT have low concentrations of serum IgA, IgG2, and IgE, and experience recurrent respiratory tract infections that may be associated with their ineffective cellular immunity.

DNA from patients with AT is particularly susceptible to damage from ionizing radiation. The proportion of peripheral blood lymphocytes bearing γ/δ antigen receptors is increased (122). Instability of DNA renders patients with AT susceptible to increased risk for developing neoplasms.

Wiskott-Aldrich Syndrome (WAS)

This X-linked recessive immunodeficiency has a classic presentation that includes eczema, thrombocytopenia, and recurrent bacterial and viral infections (123, 124). Although carriers of the disease are clinically well, DNA probes can be used to identify the defective gene in the proximal portion of the short arm of the X chromosome (Xp11.23) (125, 126). Several mutations have been identified in the WAS gene (127). Screening protocols have been developed to allow identification of missense, nonsense, and frameshift mutations (128).

Serum IgA and IgE levels are increased, the IgG level is normal, and IgM levels and isohemagglutinins usually are absent (129). Antibodies that are produced are catabolized more rapidly than normal (130). As children mature, lymphocyte (T cell) numbers and function gradually decline.

Although bone marrow transplantation using HLA siblings has been the treatment of choice for these boys, cord blood transplantation has also achieved favorable results (131, 132).

ACQUIRED IMMUNODEFICIENCY SYNDROME (AIDS)

CLINICAL AND PATHOLOGIC FEATURES OF HIV INFECTION

Human immunodeficiency virus (HIV) is the virus associated with the acquired immunodeficiency syndrome (AIDS). HIV is spread by sexual contact, exposure to blood or blood products, exposure to body fluids, and vertical transmission from mother to child (133, 134). Although men having sex with men and intravenous drug users still account for the majority of clinical AIDS cases in the United States, the rate of heterosexually acquired AIDS has shown an extraordinary increase (135, 136). In addition, approximately 20% of babies born to HIV-infected women are HIV-positive.

As of November 24, 1995, over 500,000 cases of clinical AIDS had been reported in the United States to the Centers for Disease Control (CDC) (137). In 1993, the CDC reported that the number of new cases of AIDS among Hispanic and African Americans exceeded those among white Americans (135–137), and the shift of the epidemic to the minority communities continues. Clearly, efforts to educate the public and populations at risk are failing to slow the spread of this disease.

HIV is a member of the lentivirus subfamily of retroviruses, which are RNA viruses that use the enzyme reverse transcriptase to transcribe viral RNA into proviral DNA in the host. The gp120 viral envelope glycoprotein attaches to the CD4 molecule on CD4-positive T lymphocytes (138). Other cell surface proteins (e.g., CKR-5, fusin) are also important to HIV-1 infection. By its use of reverse transcriptase, the viral RNA is integrated into the host DNA as proviral DNA and resides there during a latent period that can last for years. During this time, viral particles are produced and infect other lymphocytes. The number of active replicating viruses is directly related to the number of CD4-positive lymphocytes (139). Eventually, CD4 lymphocytes are depleted (< 200 per microliter) to the extent that the patient exhibits an extraordinary inability to resist the onslaught of opportunistic microorganisms. In addition, the host defenses of the individual are unable to prevent the development of lymphoproliferative and neoplastic (e.g., Kaposi sarcoma) disorders (possibly initiated by Epstein-Barr and other viruses). Despite the presence of their profound immune susceptibility, these patients exhibit a striking polyclonal increases in immunoglobulins (140). The massive polyclonal increase in IgG finds its way into the intestinal fluids. Normally, 75 to 80% of intestinal immunoglobulins are secretory IgA. In HIV-infected patients, however, the proportion of IgA and IgG are roughly equivalent (Table 16.1). The IgA in these patients is predominantly monomeric, as opposed to the dimeric secretory IgA present normally. These features suggest considerable leakage of serum immunoglobulins into the intestinal lumen (141).

Usually, about 80 to 90% of lamina propria plasma cells produce IgA. In HIV-infected patients, however, IgM-producing plasma cells account for slightly more than 35% of the lamina propria plasma cells (141). IgG plasma cells are as uncommon in HIV-infected patients as in controls (< 5%), indicating that the IgG in intestinal fluids derives from exudation from the serum rather than from local secretion. These immunologic features are consistent with widespread damage to the mucosal surface of the bowel. In the epithelium of the intestinal mucosa, CD4 lymphocytes are depleted continually until they are virtually absent in patients with AIDS

(142). Lamina propria lymphocytes, which usually are CD4 positive, are predominantly CD8 positive (see Chapter 6).

GASTROINTESTINAL PATHOLOGY IN HIV AND AIDS

The gastrointestinal tract is a major site of entry of the virus (rectal transmission) into the body. It is also a major location for the development of opportunistic infections that result in the malabsorption and diarrhea noted in at least 50% of HIV-positive patients (143, 144). Initial uptake of the virus may occur via tears in rectal mucosa, uptake by M cells overlying lymphoid follicles, or direct infection of the rectal epithelium (145–147). Infection of the surface epithelium by HIV may in itself be responsible for the villous atrophy, blunting, and hyperplastic crypts seen in some AIDS patients who have no demonstrable opportunistic infection (148). Other manifestations that have been lumped into HIV enteropathy include proctocolitis, focal ulcers, and lymphoid hyperplasia (149, 150). The damage may be caused by the virus itself, activation of lymphokines by T lymphocytes, or by the T lymphocytes themselves (151). Although proctocolitis, focal ulcers, and lymphoid hyperplasia have been termed HIV enteropathy, it remains a diagnosis of exclusion and may represent yet unidentified pathogens in patients whose intestinal mucosa happens to contain identifiable HIV.

The most common gastrointestinal manifestation in AIDS patients is diarrhea; the second most common manifestation is esophagitis. The altered immune system in HIV-infected patients renders them susceptible to a plethora of gastrointestinal manifestations from candida esophagitis to Kaposi sarcoma (152). Infants with AIDS are particularly prone to develop diarrhea and malnutrition (153). Esophageal symptoms include odynophagia, dysphagia, and retrosternal chest pain (154). Candida esophagitis is, by far, the most common cause of esophageal symptoms followed by cytomegalovirus (CMV) esophagitis, herpes simplex virus (HSV) esophagitis, idiopathic esophagitis and ulcers, and Kaposi sarcoma (Table 16.2) (154). The percentage of cases involving CMV and HSV may be underestimated when histopathologic analysis is the only basis of identification. Viral esophagitis should be suspected when erosions or ulcers are present. Additional tissue sections may be helpful because the pathognomonic CMV-infected cells are often

TABLE 16.1	Immunoglobulins in Intestinal Fluid of HIV-Infected Patients		
Immunoglobulin	HIV-Infected	Controls
IgA	288 ± 68	158 ± 69
IgG	321 ± 70	33 ± 19
IgM	53 ± 22	7 ± 6

Modified from Janoff EN, Jackson S, Wahl SM, et al. Intestinal mucosal immunoglobulins during human immunodeficiency virus type I infection. J Infect Dis 1994;170:299–307.

Data from 39 HIV-infected patients and 10 controls expressed as microgram/ml ± standard error.

TABLE 16.2	Etiology of Esophageal Symptoms in Patients with AIDS

Etiology	Percent of Esophagitis Cases
Candida species	64%
Cytomegalovirus	11%
Herpes simplex virus	10%
Idiopathic esophagitis/ulcers	5%
Kaposi's sarcoma	8%

Data modified from Laine L, Bonacini M. Esophageal disease in human immunodeficiency virus infection. Arch Intern Med 1994;154:1577–1582.

Percentages derived as a summary of data from Bonacini M, Young T, Laine L. The causes of esophageal symptoms in human immunodeficiency virus infection: A prospective study of 110 patients. Arch Intern Med 1991;151:1567–1572; Connolly GM, Hawkins D, Harcourt-Webster JN, et al. Oesophageal symptoms, their causes, treatment, and prognosis in patients with the acquired immunodeficiency syndrome. Gut 1989;30:1033–1039; Smith PD, Eisner MS, Manischewitz JF, et al. Esophageal disease in AIDS is associated with pathologic processes rather than mucosal human immunodeficiency virus type 1. J Infect Dis 1993;167:547–552.

difficult to find (158). Special studies, such as polymerase chain reaction, are more sensitive than routine histology in identifying CMV, but false positives from contaminant saliva or blood limit the usefulness of this expensive test (159).

In part because of its ubiquity, Candida albicans is one of the most common infections of the gastrointestinal tract in these patients; less often, *C. tropicalis* and *C. glabrata* have been identified as etiologic agents of esophagitis in these patients (160). Although most often involving the upper gastrointestinal tract (mouth, pharynx, and esophagus), Candida can involve the small bowel and colon, resulting in necrotizing enterocolitis and death (161). Because of the prevalence of Candida esophagitis (occurring in as many as 40% of AIDS patients), some clinicians recommend initial empiric antifungal therapy and perform endoscopy only in those individuals who continue to have symptoms for 1 to 2 weeks (154). Although Candida species, CMV, and HSV are the infectious processes most often responsible for the esophagitis in patients with AIDS, other agents, including Cryptosporidium, *Histoplasma capsulatum*, *Pneumocystis carinii*, *Cryptococcus neoformans*, Mycobacteria species, and Epstein-Barr virus, should be considered (154, 162–164).

The most common cause of systemic bacterial infections in HIV/AIDS patients is *Myocbacterium avium-intracellulare* (165). This bacterium usually enters the body through the gastrointestinal tract; therefore, it is not surprising that it frequently involves the small intestine and hepatobiliary tract (166). Infection usually develops relatively late in the course of HIV disease, when the CD4 lymphocyte count is less than 60 per microliter (167). Patients often develop diarrhea and malabsorption, and may complain of abdominal pain. The duodenum is the most common site of involvement; usually, the stomach and duodenal bulb are uninvolved (168). Grossly and histologically, the disease closely resembles Whipple disease. The lamina propria is filled with foamy, PAS-positive macrophages (168, 169), resulting in a clubbed appearance of the villi on gross examination. M. avium intracellulare is easily distin-

guished from Whipple disease because the foamy macrophages are strongly acid fast-positive in the former and are acid fast-negative in the latter (Fig. 16.10). In addition, the typical antigenic pattern seen in patients with Whipple disease is absent from the mycobacterium-infected duodenum (170, 171). Lastly, polymerase chain reaction for *Tropherema whippelii* can help to make the distinction, but performing this study would be costly overkill.

Proctocolitis and anal ulceration have been largely associated with HSV and CMV (172, 173). Although both of these pathogens can be found throughout the gastrointestinal tract their presence does not necessarily imply their involvement in local disease (174). When it is associated with pathology, CMV will often cause colitis with focal ulcerations (175).

Enteritis owing to bacterial and fungal pathogens is significantly more common in patients with AIDS than in immunologically competent individuals. This difference may relate to the decreased gastric acid secretion and decreased motility of the bowel in many patients with AIDS (176, 177); these two major, albeit nonspecific, host defense mechanisms help to prevent colonization of intestinal mucosa by enteropathogens (100). Shigella, Salmonella, Campylobacter, and Clostridium all occur with increased frequency in patients with AIDS compared to control individuals, and when they occur, the consequences are more likely to be grave than in immunocompetent hosts (100, 178). Enterocolitis can also be found in patients with disseminated histoplasmosis, Cryptococcus, or pneumocystis (100, 179, 180). In those individuals, focal ulcerations with demonstrable microorganisms are often found (181).

A less common cause of enteritis is microsporidiosis caused by *Enterocytozoon bieneusi* (100, 182, 183). Histologic findings may show the microorganisms within vacuoles in the surface epithelium. The surface epithelium may be separated from the basement membrane (100).

Cryptosporidium is the most common enteric infection in AIDS patients (Fig. 16.11). It occurs throughout the gastrointestinal tract (including the biliary tract) and accounts for about 20% of infections in patients with gastrointestinal symptoms (184, 185). Cryptosporidia are small, 2 to 5-µm, spherical microorganisms on

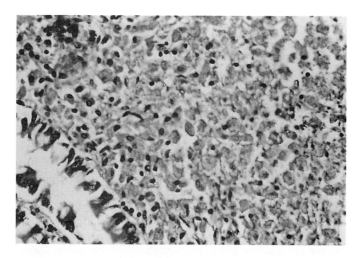

Figure 16.10 Small intestine from a patient with AIDS. Foamy macrophages fill the lamina propria in this patient with M. avium-intracellulare infection (H & E, ×250). (See color plate.)

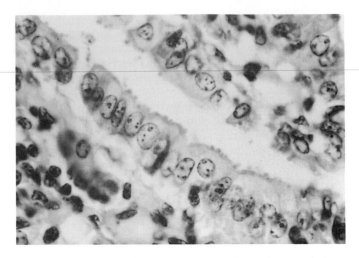

Figure 16.11 Extensive involvement of the surface epithelium by cryptosporidia in this case of simian AIDS (H & E, ×600). (See color plate.)

the luminal surface of epithelial cells. Their basophilia allows their detection on routine hematoxylin and eosin (H & E) sections. The small intestine and colon are the most common sites of involvement. Usually the cryptosporidia are seen over the villus epithelium with involvement of the crypt surfaces associated with large burdens of the microorganism (186). Usually, affected patients have increased number of eosinophils, neutrophils, and plasma cells in the lamina propria. The presence of cryptosporidia is associated with villous atrophy and crypt hyperplasia; less commonly, crypt abscesses form (186). Colonic cryptosporidia are less likely to be associated with inflammatory features than those found in the small bowel, but here too, patchy inflammation with crypt abscesses may be seen (186). The organisms may be detected on biopsy, in duodenal aspirates, and in stool samples. The cysts can be detected in stool when using an acid-fast method. Note that the cryptosporidia in tissue do not stain with acid-fast, but can be shown to advantage with a Giemsa stain (100).

DISORDERS OF THE PHAGOCYTIC SYSTEM

Along the normal gastrointestinal tract, the lamina propria contain large numbers of phagocytic cells. Beekin et al. reported that human colon contains about 2,000,000 eosinophils, 1,500,000 macrophages, and 200,000 neutrophils per gram of mucosa (187). They further demonstrated that these cells were able to actively phagocytize bacteria (187). Although eosinophils are usually thought of in terms of their role in allergic conditions, they are both actively phagocytic and able to migrate across intestinal epithelium in response to specific chemotactic gradients (188). Decreased numbers of phagocytic cells can occur as primary deficiencies or, more commonly, represent complications of therapy for neoplasia. As with immunologic deficiencies, impairment in phagocytic cell response results in increased susceptibility to common microorganisms that are usually disposed of, or processed by, these cells. Cancer patients receiving chemotherapy often develop transient, profound granulocytopenia and become exquisitely susceptible to infections with microorganisms of low intrinsic pathogenicity, such as As-

pergillus species. Aside from these obvious iatrogenic causes of phagocyte deficiency, a variety of defects have been characterized that result in increased susceptibility to infections with microorganisms of low pathogenicity.

LEUKOCYTE ADHESION DEFECTS

Initiation of the phagocyte response requires binding of the phagocytic cell to endothelium. β2 integrins are a family of leukocyte adhesion molecules expressed on cell surfaces that allow phagocytes to bind endothelial surfaces during inflammation. Neutrophils and monocytes have at least three types of cell surface β2 integrins on their surfaces: Mo1 (also called Mac-1, CD11b, or CR3), lymphocyte-associated antigen (LFA-1 or CD11a), and p150,95 (or CD11c). These β2 integrins adhesion molecules have unique α-chains (CD11a, CD11b, CD11c) and a common β-chain (CD18). β2 integrins bind to intercellular adhesion molecule-1 (ICAM-1) for LFA-1 (CD11a) and to surface-associated iC3b for Mac-1 (CD11b) and p150,95 (CD11c) (189).

Rare cases of complete or partial absence of Mo-1, LFA-1, and p150,95 have been reported. The fundamental defect in leukocyte adhesion deficiency (LAD) is a mutation in the gene that encodes CD18. CD18 gene expression is required for CD11/CD18 to translocate to cell surfaces. Patients with LAD typically experience a delay in umbilical cord separation after birth, severe gingivitis, periodontitis, and delayed wound healing. A variety of infections can be found in these patients, and they experience a persistent leukocytosis with white blood cell counts as high as 150,000/ml (190). The key laboratory features for the diagnosis of LAD are the inability of phagocytes to adhere to testing surfaces and the lack of CD11/CD18 on phagocyte membranes. Clinical manifestations of Hirschsprung disease have been reported in a child with LAD with a defect in the expression of CD18 (191).

MYELOPEROXIDASE DEFICIENCY

Myeloperoxidase (MPO) deficiency occurs in 1 in 2100 individuals and results from a defect in packaging MPO into azurophilic granules. Molecular studies have defined point mutations in some patients (192, 193). Because individuals with MPO deficiency exhibit a variable reduction in MPO activity, people with mild cases manifest no clinical symptoms. In the 50% of MPO-deficient patients who exhibit no detectable MPO activity, an impairment in ability to clear Candida species and a variety of bacterial skin infections have been reported (194). Gastrointestinal manifestations are not common complications of this condition. Neutrophils from these patients exhibit increased phagocytic capacity as well as an enhanced respiratory burst with exaggerated production of hydrogen peroxide.

CHRONIC GRANULOMATOUS DISEASE

Chronic granulomatous disease (CGD) occurs in 1 in 1,000,000 people. Several modes of inheritance have been described including an X-linked, autosomal dominant and an autosomal recessive mode. Normally, in phagocytes, electrons generated from the hexose-monophosphate shunt catalyze the reduction of molecular oxygen (O_2) to superoxide anion (O_2^-). Reduction of O_2 to superoxide anion O_2^- is catalyzed by an enzyme complex named NADPH oxidase. The NADPH oxidase-associated electron transport chain includes cytochrome b_{558}, flavin adenine dinucleotide (FAD) and a membrane quinone, and several regulatory proteins. A variety of mutations in various subunits of the NADH complex have been described.

Clinically, CGD is more severe than MPO deficiency. Before the age of 1 year, individuals with CGD often present with lung abscesses, pneumonia, hepatic abscesses, osteomyelitis, and recurrent granulomatous soft tissue infections. The granulomas appear to form in response to the inability of phagocytes to inactivate inflammatory mediators. This ineffective phagocytosis results in a prolonged recruitment of inflammatory cells. Typically, infections are caused by *Staphylococcus aureus* and Gram-negative bacilli. It is uncommon for CGD patients to have gastrointestinal abnormalities (195–198).

Flow cytometry, which has replaced the nitroblue tetrazolium test in many centers, takes advantage of fluorescent dyes, such as dihydrorhodamine 123 and $2',7'$-dichlorofluorescein, that are reduced when exposed to hydrogen peroxide (H_2O_2). The lack of H_2O_2 (dismutation product of superoxide anion) prevents the change in the fluorescent dyes by the CGD cells (199, 200).

CHEDIAK-HIGASHI SYNDROME

The Chediak-Higashi syndrome is a rare disorder of leukocyte migration, inadequate natural killer cell function, loss of cytotoxic T cell function, and impaired macrophage activation that results in an increased susceptibility to bacterial infections (201). It is an autosomal recessive disease in which affected cells contain giant granules. These granules are fused primary and secondary granules because of abnormal microtubule assembly. In addition to the neutrophil dysfunction, these patients demonstrate a variety of neurologic defects and may exhibit partial oculocutaneous albinism.

Chediak-Higashi patients are usually neutropenic and may present with gingivitis and periodontitis. Gastrointestinal disease is uncommon. Some of these individuals respond favorably to ascorbate. Chemotherapy has been used with some early success to ameliorate the macrophage responses, but eventually, patients become refractory to this therapy. Successful treatment has been reported using HLA-identical bone marrow transplantation (202).

CYCLIC NEUTROPENIA

Cyclic neutropenia is a cyclic disorder of hematopoiesis that manifests with episodes of fever and infections involving pyogenic microorganisms because of increased susceptibility resulting from the relatively short half-life of neutrophils. Other blood cells circulate for a longer time and do not influence the host defense in these patients. The problem may be the result of ineffective growth factor-receptor binding interactions (203). Typically, neutropenia occurs every several weeks. During these periods, patients experience fever, mucosal infections, and lymphadenopathy. Children have more pronounced manifestations than adults. Whereas splenectomy and/or steroid therapy were occasionally effective, granulocyte-colony stimulating factor (G-CSF) has proven useful in the treatment of this disease (204). The circulating neutrophils in patients treated with G-CSF produce normal amounts of important cytokines, including IL-1β, IL-8, and tumor necrosis factor-α (204). Even without therapy, however, monocytes that are present when the neutrophil count decreases seem to protect the patients from most serious infections.

Rarely, Crohn disease has been associated with cyclic neutropenia. In one case, exacerbations of the inflammatory bowel disease preceded a further decline in the number of circulating neutrophils. It is unlikely that the neutropenia itself has any relationship to the pathogenesis of Crohn disease in this case (205).

DISORDERS OF THE COMPLEMENT SYSTEM

Patients with deficiencies of complement components have an increased frequency of autoimmune disease. The explanation for this relationship is unclear, but it may involve genetic linkages between complement genes and genes that predispose to autoimmune disease. Alternatively, the impaired antigen elimination that can occur as a result of complement deficiency may result in unusually prolonged antigen exposure, which in turn may result in development of an immunologically mediated inflammatory response (206).

The most common complement deficiency is of C2. The carrier rate in the general population is 1.2%. In some studies, 50% of patients with homozygous C2 deficiency exhibit signs of autoimmune disease, and most C2 deficient patients have an increased susceptibility to pyogenic bacterial infection. Those rare individuals who have C1 subunit deficiencies (C1q, C1r, C1s) also may present with autoimmune disease (especially systemic lupus erythematosus) and pyogenic infections (especially meningitis). Some individuals with low C1q levels also suffer from hypogammaglobulinemia.

C4 deficiency is extremely rare because there are two distinct genetic loci where C4 molecules are encoded. Thus, it is highly unusual for an individual to have mutations at both loci. Heterozygotes have normal levels of C4. Even heterozygotes, however, have an increased incidence of autoimmune disease, including chronic active hepatitis. Because of its key role in both the classical and alternative pathways of complement activation, deficiency of C3 results in profound infectious complications in most of the patients. Some individuals also exhibit autoimmune disease, including SLE and vasculitis. Deficiency of properdin is sex-linked and has been associated with meningococcal infections.

Deficiencies of terminal complement components C5 to C9 may lead to recurrent and/or chronic meningococcal or gonococcal infections. A smaller number of these individuals display autoimmune disease susceptibility than those individuals with the complement deficiencies noted previously (207, 208).

The most serious gastrointestinal complication in patients with a complement abnormality is the bowel edema associated with deficiency of the complement regulatory protein of C1 esterase (C1 esterase deficiency—C1INH). These individuals have hereditary or acquired angioedema. Because about one half of the normal concentration of C1INH is required to prevent spontaneous activation of C1, even heterozygotes suffer occasional attacks. An attack of angioedema caused by C1INH deficiency typically results in swelling of an extremity (e.g., hand) and can manifest with swelling of the face or larynx. Laryngeal edema can lead to suffocation. The bowel edema that can also occur can lead to severe abdominal pain, sometimes followed by diarrhea. Because C1INH also controls important components of the coagulation system, including the Hageman factor, clotting factor XIa, kallikrein, and plasmin, these aspects of its deficiency may complicate the comple-

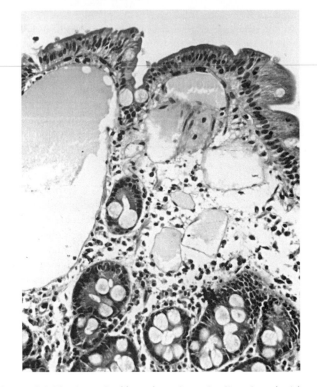

Figure 16.12   Intestinal lymphangiectasia. (Reprinted with permission from Keren DF. Immunology and immunopathology of the gastrointestinal tract. Chicago: ASCP Press, 1980.)

ment activation. During attacks of angioedema, patients often have decreased levels of C2 and C4 in the peripheral blood; C3 levels usually are normal.

INTESTINAL LYMPHANGIECTASIA AND IMMUNODEFICIENCY

Intestinal lymphangiectasia is often accompanied by loss of both protein and lymphocytes into the gut lumen (Fig. 16.12). Because of the malabsorption that most of these patients experience, they may be considered to have another more common condition, such as celiac disease (209). Malabsorption is a more frequent complication than that of recurrent infections in these patients.

Lymphocyte analyses have revealed decreased numbers of CD4 (helper) T lymphocytes, CD8 (suppressor/cytotoxic) T lymphocytes, and a decrease in circulating B lymphocytes in some patients with intestinal lymphangectasia. The decrease in CD8 cells has been reported to be more substantial than that of the CD4 cells, leading to an increase in the CD4/CD8 ratio (210). Not surprisingly, the number of intraepithelial lymphocytes is decreased (211). The T lymphocytes present, however, have normal cellular functions (212). Because the lesions may be focal, endoscopically directed biopsies are needed to obtain appropriate specimens for histologic evaluation (213).

REFERENCES

1. Springer TA, Dustin ML, Kishimoto TK, et al. The lymphocyte function-associated LFA-1, CD2 and LFA-3 molecules: Cell adhesion receptors of the immune system. Annu Rev Immunol 1987;5: 223–252.
2. Perkkio M, Savilahti E. Time of appearance of immunoglobulin-containing cells in the mucosa of the neonatal intestine. Pediatr Res 1980;14:953–995.
3. Conley ME, Brown P, Pickard AR. Expression of the gene defect in X-linked agammaglobulinemia. N Engl J Med 1986;315:564–567.
4. Vetrie D, Vorechovsky I, Sideras P, et al. The gene involved in X-linked agammaglobulinaemia is a member of the src family of protein-tyrosine kinases. Nature 1993;361:226–233.
5. Puck JM. Molecular and genetic basis of X-linked immunodeficiency disorders. J Clin Immunol 1994;14:81–89.
6. Rosen FS, Cooper MD, Wedgwood RJP. The primary immunodeficiencies. N Engl J Med 1995;333:431–440.
7. Kornfeld SJ, Good RA, Litman GW. Atypical X-linked agammaglobulinemia (letter). N Engl J Med 1994:331:349–350.
8. Buckley RH. Breakthroughs in the understanding and therapy of primary immunodeficiency. Pediatr Clin North Am 1994;41: 665–690.
9. Tsukada S, Saffran DC, Rawlings DJ, et al. Deficient expression of a B cell cytoplasmic tyrosine kinase in human X-linked agammaglobulinemia. Cell 1993;72:279–290.
10. Tsukada S, Rawlings DJ, Witte ON. Role of Bruton's tyrosine kinase in immunodeficiency. Curr Opin Immunol 1994;6:623–630.
11. Kozlowski C, Evans DI. Neutropenia associated with X-linked agammaglobulinemia. J Clin Pathol 1991;44:388–390.
12. Pearl ER, Vogler LB, Okos AJ, et al. B lymphocyte precursors in human bone marrow: An analysis of normal individuals and patients with antibody-deficiency states. J Immunol 1978;120: 1169–1175.
13. Conley ME. B cells in patients with X-linked agammaglobulinemia. J Immunol 1985;134:3070–3074.
14. Schwaber J. Pre-B cells in X-linked agammaglobulinemia. Birth Defects 1983;19:177–182.
15. Saffran DC, Parolini O, Fitch-Hilgenberg ME, et al. Brief report: A point mutation in the SH2 domain of Bruton's tyrosine kinase in atypical X-linked agammaglobulinemia. N Engl J Med 1994;330: 1488–1491.
16. Aiuti F, Pandolfi F, Fiorilli M, et al. Monoclonal antibody analysis of T cell subsets in 40 patients with immunodeficiencies. J Clin Immunol 1982;2:81S–89S.
17. Reinherz EL, Cooper MD, Schlossman SF. Abnormalities of T cell maturation and regulation in human beings with immunodeficiency disorders. J Clin Invest 1981;68:699–705.
18. van der Meer JW, Weening RS, Schellekens PT, et al. Colorectal cancer in patients with X-linked agammaglobulinaemia. Lancet 1993;341:1439–1440.
19. McGeady SJ. Transient hypogammaglobulinemia of infancy: Need to reconsider name and definition. J Pediatr 1987;110:47–50.
20. Cano F, Mayo DR, Ballow M. Absent specific viral antibodies in patients with transient hypogammaglobulinemia of infancy. J Allergy Clin Immunol 1990;85:510–513.
21. Siegel RL, Issekutz T, Schwaber J. Deficiency of T helper cells in transient hypogammaglobulinemia of infancy. N Engl J Med 1981; 305:1307–1313.
22. Landreth KS, Engelhard D, Anasetti C. Pre-B cells in agammaglobulinemia: Evidence for disease heterogeneity among affected boys. J Clin Immunol 1985;5:84–89.
23. Hoffman T, Winchester R, Schulkind M. Hypogammaglobulinemia with normal T cell function in female siblings. Clin Immunol Immunopathol 1977;7:364–371.
24. Smith CIE, Hammarstrom L, Lindahl M, et al. Kinetics of the spontaneously occurring common variable hypogammaglobulinemia: An analysis of two individuals with previously normal immunoglobulin levels. Clin Immunol Immunopathol 1985;37: 22–29.
25. de Asis MLB, Iqbal S, Sicklick M. Analysis of a family containing three members with common variable immunodeficiency. Ann Allergy Asthma Immunol 1996;76:527–529.

26. Dawson J, Hadgson HJF, Pepys MB, et al. Immunodeficiency, malabsorption and secretory diarrhea, a new syndrome. Am J Med 1979;67:540–546.

27. Cunningham-Rundles C, Siegal FP, Cunningham-Rundles S, et al. Incidence of cancer in 98 patients with common varied immunodeficiency. J Clin Immunol 1987;7:294–299.

28. Hermans, P. Nodular lymphoid hyperplasia of the small intestine and hypogammaglobulinemia: Theoretical and practical considerations. Fed Proc 1967;29:1606–1611.

29. Banwell JG, Kistler LA, Giannella RA, et al. Small intestinal bacterial overgrowth syndrome. Gastroenterology 1981;80:834–845.

30. Herbst EW, Armbruster M, Rump JA, et al. Intestinal B cell defects in common variable immunodeficiency. Clin Exp Immunol 1994;95:215–221.

31. Tedder TF, Crain MJ, Kubagawa H. Evaluation of lymphocyte differentiation in primary and secondary immunodeficiency diseases. J Immunol 1985;135:1786–1791.

32. Kondo N, Inoue R, Kasahara K, et al. Failure of IgG production due to a defect in the opening of the chromatin structure of I gamma1 region in a patient with IgG and IgA deficiency. Clin Exp Immunol 1995;99:21–28.

33. Mushiake K, Motoyoshi F, Kondo N, et al. mu-chain gene expression in common variable immunodeficiency. Exp Clin Immunogenet 1993;10:189–194.

34. Pandolfi F, Trentin L, San Martin JE, et al. T cell heterogeneity in patients with common variable immunodeficiency as assessed by abnormal T cell subpopulations and T cell receptor gene analysis. Clin Exp Immunol 1992;89:198–203.

35. Cunningham-Rundles C. Clinical and immunologic analyses of 103 patients with common variable immunodeficiency. J Clin Immunol 1989;9:22–33.

36. Ichikawa Y, Gonzalez EB, Daniels JC. Suppressor cells of mitogen-induced lymphocyte proliferation in the peripheral blood of patients with common variable hypogammaglobulinemia. Clin Immunol Immunopathol 1982;25:252–263.

37. Aukrust BP, Lien E, Kristoffersen AK, et al. Persistent activation of the tumor necrosis factor system in a subgroup of patients with common variable immunodeficiency—possible immunologic and clinical consequences. Blood 1996;87:674–681.

38. White WB, Ballow M. Modulation of suppressor cell activity by cimetidine in patients with common variable hypogammaglobulinemia. N Engl J Med 1985;312:198–202.

39. Segal R, Dayan M, Epstein N, et al. Common variable immunodeficiency: A family study and therapeutic trial with cimetidine. J Allergy Clin Immunol 1989;84:753–761.

40. Sneller MC, Strober W. Abnormalities of lymphokine gene expression in patients with common variable immunodeficiency. J Immunol 1990;144:3762–3769.

41. Rump JA, Jahreis A, Schlesier M, et al. Possible role of IL-2 deficiency for hypogammaglobulinaemia in patients with common variable immunodeficiency. Clin Exp Immunol 1992;89:204–210.

42. North ME, Spickett GP, Allsop J, et al. Defective DNA synthesis by T cells in acquired common variable hypogammaglobulinemia on stimulation with mitogens. Clin Exp Immunol 1989;76:19–23.

43. Adelman DC, Matsuda T, Hirano T, et al. Elevated serum interleukin-6 associated with a failure in B cell differentiation in common variable immunodeficiency. J Allergy Clin Immunol 1990;86:512–521.

44. Fischer MB, Hauber I, Eggenbauer H, et al. A defect in the early phase of T-cell receptor-mediated T-cell activation in patients with common variable immunodeficiency. Blood 1994;84:4234–4241.

45. Farrington M, Grosmaire LS, Nonoyama S, et al. CD40 ligand expression is defective in a subset of patients with common variable immunodeficiency. Proc Natl Acad Sci USA 1994;91:1099–1103.

46. Laman JD, Classen E, Noelle RJ. Immunodeficiency due to a faulty interaction between T and B cells. Curr Opin Immunol 1994;6:636–641.

47. Tsuge I, Matsuoka H, Abe T, et al. X chromosome inactivation analysis to distinguish sporadic cases of X-linked agammaglobulinemia from common variable immunodeficiency. Eur J Pediatr 1993:152:900–904.

48. Buckley RH. Assessing inheritance of agammaglobulinemia. N Engl J Med 1994;330:1526–1528.

49. Britigan BE. Diphenylhydantoin-induced hypogammaglobulinemia in a patient infected with human immunodeficiency virus. Am J Med 1991;90:524–527.

50. Travin M, Macris NT, Block JM, et al. Reversible common variable immunodeficiency syndrome induced by phenytoin. Arch Intern Med 1989;149:1421–1422.

51. Miller BW, Brennan DC, Korenblat PE, et al. Common variable immunodeficiency in a renal transplant patient with severe recurrent bacterial infection: A case report and review of the literature. Am J Kidney Dis 1995;25:947–951.

52. Mushiake K, Motoyoshi F, Kondo N, et al. Long-term follow up of patients with common variable immunodeficiency treated with intravenous immunoglobulin: Reevaluation of intravenous immunoglobulin replacement therapy. Biotherapy 1994;7:101–107.

53. Cunningham-Rundles C, Kazbay K, Hassett J, et al. Brief report: Enhanced humoral immunity in common variable immunodeficiency after long-term treatment with polytheylene glycol-conjugated interleukin-2. N Engl J Med 1994;331:918–921.

54. DiSanto JP, Markiewicz S, Gauchat J-F, et al. Brief report: Prenatal diagnosis of X-linked hyper-IgM syndrome. N Engl J Med 1994;330:969–973.

55. Brahmi Z, Lazarus KH, Hodes ME. Immunologic studies of three family members with the immunodeficiency with hyper-IgM syndrome. J Clin Immunol 1983;3:127–134.

56. Schwaber JF, Lazarus H, Rosen FS. IgM-restricted production of immunoglobulin by lymphoid cell lines from patients with immunodeficiency with hyper IgM (dysgammaglobulinemia). Clin Immunol Immunopathol 1981;19:91–97.

57. Graf D, Korthauer U, Mages HW, et al. Cloning of TRAP, a ligand for CD40 on human T cells. Eur J Immunol 1992;22:3191–3194.

58. Chu Y, Marin E, Fuleihan R, et al. Somatic mutation of human immunoglobulin V genes in the X-linked hyperIgM syndrome. J Clin Invest 1995;95:1389–1393.

59. Porat YB, Levy D, Levy J, et al. Intrinsic defect in B cells of patients with hyper-IgM syndrome. Clin Diagnostic Immunol 1995;2:412–416.

60. Saiki O, Tanaka T, Wada Y, et al. Signalling through CD40 rescues IgE but not IgG or IgA secretion in X-linked immunodeficiency with hyper-IgM. J Clin Invest 1995;95:510–514.

61. Facchetti F, Appiani C, Salvi L, et al. Immunohistologic analysis of ineffective CD40-CD40 ligand interaction in lymphoid tissues from patients with X-linked immunodeficiency with hyper-IgM. J Immunol 1995;154:6624–6633.

62. Chag HH, Shaw D, Klesius P, et al. Inability of oral bovine transfer to eradicate cryptosporidial infection in a patient with congenital dysgammaglobulinemia. Clin Immunol Immunopathol 1989;50:402–406.

63. Benkerrou M, Gougeon ML, Griscelli C, et al. Hypogammaglobulinemie G et A avec hypergammaglobulinemie M, A propos de 12 observations. Arch Pediatr 1990;47:345–349.

64. Tu RK, Peters ME, Gourley GR, et al. Esophageal histoplasmosis in a child with immunodeficiency with hyper-IgM. AJR Am J Roentgenol 1991;157:381–382.

65. Thomas C, de Saint Basile G, Le Deist F, et al. Brief report: Correction of X-linked hyper-IgM syndrome by allogeneic bone marrow transplantation. N Engl J Med 1995;333:426–429.

66. Koskinen S, Tolo H, Hirvonen M, et al. Long-term persistence of selective IgA deficiency in healthy adults. J Clin Immunol 1994;14:116–119.

67. Sadler DA, Keren DF. Surface markers and immunodeficiency disease. In: Keren DF, Hanson CA, Hurtubise P, eds. Chicago, ASCP Press, 1994.

68. Degraeff PA, The TH, Van Munster PJJ, et al. The primary immune response in patients with selective IgA deficiency. Clin Exp Immunol 1983;54:778–784.

69. Barka N, Shen GQ, Shoenfeld Y, et al. Multireactive pattern of serum autoantibodies in asymptomatic individuals with immunoglobulin A deficiency. Clin Diag Lab Immunol 1995;2:469–472.

70. Kondo N, Takao A, Li GP, et al. Immunoglobulin-secreting cells in lymphocytes of patients with IgA deficiency or hyper-IgA. Biotherapy 1994;6:279–282.

71. Sloand EM, Fox SM, Banks SM, et al. Preparation of IgA-deficient platelets. Transfusion 1990;30:322–326.

72. Koskinen S, Tolo H, Hirvonen M, et al. Long-term follow-up of anti-IgA antibodies in healthy IgA-deficient adults. J Clin Immunol 1995;15:194–198.

73. Mellander L, Bjorkander J, Carlsson B, et al. Secretory antibodies in IgA-deficient and immunosuppressed individuals. J Clin Immunol 1986;6:284–291.

74. Dura WT, Bernatowska E. Secretory component, alpha 1-antitrypsin and lysozyme in IgA-deficient children. An immunohistochemical evaluation of intestinal mucosa. Histopathology 1984;8:747–757.

75. Vorechovsky I, Zetterquist H, Paganelli R, et al. Family and linkage study of selective IgA deficiency and common variable immunodeficiency. Clin Immunol Immunopathol 1995;77:185–192.

76. Cobain TJ, French MAH, Christiansen FT, et al. Association of IgA deficiency with HLA A28 and B 14. Tissue Antigens 1983;22:151–154; Cunningham-Rundles C. Genetic aspects of immunoglobulin A deficiency. Adv Hum Genet 1990;19:235–266.

77. Dosch HM, Jason J, Gelfand EW. Transient antibody deficiency and abnormal T suppressor cells induced by phenytoin. N Engl J Med 1982;306:406–409.

78. Strober W, Krakauer R, Klaeveman HL, et al. Secretory component deficiency a disorder of the IgA immune system. N Engl J Med 1976;294:351–356.

79. Lane P, MacLennan I. Impaired lung function in patients with IgA deficiency and low levels of IgG2 or IgG3. N Engl J Med 1985;314:924–925.

80. Yokota S, Mitsuda T, Shimizu H, et al. Hyper IgE syndrome—a disease of imbalanced activation of helper T cell subsets? Arerugi 1990;39:442–451.

81. Kimata H. High-dose intravenous gamma-globulin treatment for hyperimmunoglobulinemia E syndrome. J Allergy Clin Immunol 1995;95:771–774.

82. Fanconi S, Seger RA, Willi U, et al. Oral chloramphenicol therapy for multiple liver abscesses in hyperimmunoglobulinemia E syndrome. Eur J Pediatr 1984;142:292–295.

83. Cohen-Solal M, Prieur AM, Prin L, et al. Cytokine-mediated bone resorption in patients with the hyperimmunoglobulin E syndrome. Clin Immunol Immunopathol 1995;76;76–81.

84. Sheerin KA, Buckley RH. Antibody responses to protein, polysaccharide, and phi X174 antigens in the hyperimmunoglobulin E syndrome. J Allergy Clin Immunol 1991;87:803–811.

85. Hatori M, Yoshiya M, Kurachi Y, et al. Prolonged infection of the floor of the mouth in hyperimmunoglobulinemia E (Buckley's syndrome). Report of a case. Oral Surg Oral Med Oral Pathol 1993;76:289–293.

86. Hutto JO, Bryan CS, Greene FL, et al. Cryptococcus of the colon resembling Crohn's disease in a patient with the hyperimmunoglobulinemia E-recurrent infection (Job's) syndrome. Gastroenterology 1988;94:808–812.

87. Alberti-Flor JJ, Granada A. Ileocecal histoplasmosis mimicking Crohn's disease in a patient with Job's syndrome. Digestion 1986;33:176–180.

88. Chen CM, Lai HS, Lin CL, et al. Colon perforation in a patient with hyperimmunoglobulin E (Job's) syndrome. J Pediatr Surg 1995;30:1479–1480.

89. Peake JE, McCrossin RB, Byrne G, et al. X-linked immune dysregulation, neonatal insulin-dependent diabetes, and intractable diarrhoea. Arch Dis Child 1996;74:F195–F199.

90. van der Meer JWM, Radl J, Meyer CJLM, et al. Hyperimmunoglobulinemia D and periodic fever: A new syndrome. Lancet 1984;i:1087–1090.

91. Drenth JPH, Denecker NEJ, Prieur AM, et al. Le syndrome hyperiimmunoglobuline D. Presse Med 1995;24:1211–1213.

92. Havenaar EC, Drenth JPH, Van Ommen ECR, et al. Elevated serum level and altered glycosylation of alpha1-acid glycoprotein in hyperimmunoglobulinemia D and periodic fever syndrome: Evidence for persistent inflammation. Clin Immunol Immunopathol 1995;76:279–284.

93. Drenth JPH, van Deuren M, van der Ven-Jongekrijg J, et al. Cytokine activation during attacks of the hyperimmunoglobulinemia D and periodic fever syndrome. Blood 1995;85:3583–3586.

94. Drenth JPH, Powell RJ, Brown NS, et al. Interferon-gamma and urine neopterin in attacks of the hyperimmunoglobulinaemia D and periodic fever syndrome. Eur J Clin Invest 1995;25:683–686.

95. Schmalstieg FC, Leonard WJ, Noguchi M, et al. Missense mutation in exon 7 of the common gamma chain gene causes a moderate form of X-linked combined immunodeficiency. J Clin Invest 1995;95:1169–1173.

96. Spirer Z, Zakuth V, Tzechoval E, et al. Lack of proliferation to alloantigen in a sibling of two infants with severe combined immunodeficiency (SCID). Clin Immunol Immunopathol 1982;24:286–291.

97. Gelfand EW, Dosch HM. Diagnosis and classification of severe combined immunodeficiency disease. Birth Defects 1983;19:65–72.

98. Blomquist MD, Boggards M, Hanson IC, et al. Monoclonal anti-T cell (T12) antibody treatment of graft-versus-host disease in severe combined immunodeficiency: Targeting of antibody and activation of complement on CD8+ cytotoxic T cell surfaces. J Allergy Clin Immunol 1991;87:1029–1033.

99. Appleton AL, Curtis A, Wilkes J, et al. Differentiation of maternofetal GVHD from Omenn's syndrome in pre-BMT patients with severe combined immunodeficiency. Bone Marrow Transplant 1994;14:157–159.

100. Rotterdam H, Tsang P. Gastrointestinal disease in the immunocompromised patient. Hum Pathol 1994;25:1123–1140.

101. Shulman HM, Sullivan KM, Weiden PL. Chronic graft-versus-host syndrome in man. A long-term clinicopathologic study of 20 Seattle patients. Am J Med 1980;69:204–216.

102. Small TN, Keever C, Collins N, et al. Characterization of B cells in severe combined immunodeficiency disease. Hum Immunol 1989;25:181–193.

103. Buckley RH. Breakthroughs in the understanding and therapy of primary immunodeficiency. Pediatr Clin North Am 1994;41:665–690.

104. Conley ME. Molecular approaches to analysis of X-linked immunodeficiencies. Ann Rev Immunol 1992;10:215–238.

105. Kondo M, Takeshita T, Higuchi M. Functional participation of the IL-2 receptor gamma chain in IL-7 receptor complexes. Science 1994;263:1453–1454.

106. Russell SM, Keegan AD, Harada N. Interleukin-2 receptor gamma chain: A functional component of the interleukin-4 receptor. Science 1993;262:1880–1883.

107. Ballow M, Hirschhorn R. Varicella pneumonia in a bone marrow-transplanted, immune-reconstituted adenosine deaminase-deficient patient with severe combined immunodeficiency disease. J Clin Immunol 1985;5:180–186.

108. Shovlin CL, Simmonds HA, Fairbanks LD, et al. Adult onset immunodeficiency caused by inherited adenosine deaminase deficiency. J Immunol 1994;153:2331–2339.

109. Markert ML. Purine nucleoside phosphorylase deficiency. Immunodef Rev 1991;3:45–81.

110. Chan AC, Kadlecek TA, Elder ME, et al. ZAP-70 deficiency in an autosomal recessive form of severe combined immunodeficiency. Science 1994;264:1599–1601.

111. O'Reilly RJ, Kapoor N, Kirkpatrick D, et al. Transplantation of hematopoietic cells for lethal congenital immunodeficiencies. Birth Defects 1983;19:129–137.

112. Shearer WT, Ritz J, Finegold MJ, et al. Epstein-Barr virus-associated B cell proliferations of diverse clonal origins after bone marrow transplantation in a 12 year old patient with severe combined immunodeficiency. N Engl J Med 1985;312:1151–1159.

113. Markert ML, Hershfield MS, Wiginton DA. Identification of a deletion in the adenosine deaminase gene in a child with severe combined immunodeficiency. J Immunol 1987;138:3203–3206.

114. Loechelt BJ, Shapiro RS, Jyonouchi H, et al. Mismatched bone marrow transplantation for Omenn syndrome: A variant of severe combined immunodeficiency. Bone Marrow Transplant 1995;16:381–385.

115. Fibison WJ, Budarf M, McDermid H, et al. Molecular studies of DiGeorge syndrome. Am J Hum Genet 1990;46:888–895.

116. Lupski JR, Langston C, Friedman R, et al. DiGeorge anomaly associated with a de novo Y;22 translocation resulting in monosomy del(22)(q11.2). Am J Med Genet 1991;40:196–198.

117. Mayumi M, Kimata H, Suehiro Y, et al. DiGeorge syndrome with hypogammaglobulinaemia: A patient with excess suppressor T cell activity treated with fetal thymus transplantation. Eur J Pediatr 1989;148:518–522.

118. Mulholland MW, Delaney JP, Foker JE, et al. Gastrointestinal complications of congenital immunodeficiency states. The surgeon's role. Ann Surg 1983;198:673–680.

119. Gilger MA, Matson DO, Conner ME, et al. Extraintestinal rotavirus infections in children with immunodeficiency. J Pediatr 1992;120: 912–917.

120. Wood DJ, David TJ, Chrystie IL, et al. Chronic enteric virus infection in two T-cell immunodeficient children. J Med Virol 1988;24: 435–444.

121. Rosen FS, Cooper MD, Wedgwood RJP. The primary immunodeficiencies. N Engl J Med 1984;311:235–242.

122. Carbonari M, Cherchi M, Paganelli R, et al. Relative increase of T cells expressing the gamma/delta rather than the alpha/beta receptor in ataxia-telangiectasia. N Engl J Med 1990;322:73–76.

123. Burgio GR. The Wiskott-Aldrich syndrome. Eur J Pediatr 1995;154: 261–262.

124. Sullivan KE, Mullen CA, Blaese RM, et al. A multi-institutional survey of the Wiskott-Aldrich syndrome. J Pediatr 1994;125: 876–891.

125. Goodship J, Carter J, Espanol T, et al. Carrier detection in Wiskott-Aldrich syndrome: Combined use of M27 beta for X-inactivation studies and as a linked probe. Blood 1991;77:2677–2710.

126. Kwan S, Hagemann TL, Radtke BE, et al. Identification of mutations in the Wiskott-Aldrich syndrome gene and characterization of a polymorphic dinucleotide repeat at DXS6940, adjacent to the disease gene. Proc Natl Acad Sci USA 1995;92:4706–4710.

127. Zhu Q, Zhang M, Blaese RM, et al. The Wiskott-Aldrich syndrome and X-linked congenital thrombocytopenia are caused by mutations of the same gene. Blood 1995;86:3797–3804.

128. Derry JMJ, Kerns JA, Weinberg IK, et al. WASP gene mutations in Wiskott-Aldrich syndrome and X-linked thrombocytopenia. Hum Mol Genet 1995;4:1127–1135.

129. Nahm MH, Blaese RM, Crain MJ, et al. Patients with Wiskott-Aldrich syndrome have normal IgG2 levels. J Immunol 1986;137: 3484–3487.

130. Lum LG, Tubergen DG, Corash L, et al. Splenectomy in the management of the thrombocytopenia of the Wiskott-Aldrich syndrome. N Engl J Med 1980;302:892–896.

131. Brunel V, Mozziconacci MJ, Sainty D, et al. Direct evidence for dissociated megakaryocytic chimaerism in a Wiskott-Aldrich patient successfully allografted. Br J Haematol 1995;90:336–340.

132. Kernan NA, Schroeder ML, Ciavarella D, et al. Umbilical cord blood infusion in a patient for correction of Wiskott-Aldrich syndrome. Blood Cells 1994;20:245–248.

133. Greene WC. The molecular biology of human immunodeficiency virus type 1 infection. N Engl J Med 1991;324:308–317.

134. Blattner WA. HIV epidemiology: Past, present, and future. FASEB J 1991;5:2340–2348.

135. CDC. Update: Trends in AIDS incidence, deaths, and prevalence — United States, 1996. JAMA 1997;277:874–875.

136. CDC. Update: Trends in AIDS among men who have sex with men (MSM)—United States, 1989–1994. MMWR 1995;44:401–404.

137. CDC. Update: Acquired immunodeficiency syndrome—United States, 1994. MMWR 1995;44:84–85.

138. Fauci AS. The human immunodeficiency virus: Infectivity and mechanisms of pathogenesis. Science 1988;239:617–622.

139. Danner SA, Carr A, Leonard JM, et al. A short-term study of the safety, pharmacokinetics, and efficacy of ritonavir, an inhibitor of HIV-1 protease. N Engl J Med 1995;333:1528–1533.

140. Keren DF. High-resolution electrophoresis and immunofixation. Boston: Butterworth-Heinemann, 1994.

141. Janoff EN, Jackson S, Wahl SM, et al. Intestinal mucosal immunoglobulins during human immunodeficiency virus type 1 infection. J Infect Dis 1994;170:299–307.

142. Ellakany S, Whiteside TL, Schade RR. Analysis of intestinal lymphocyte subpopulations in patients with AIDS and AIDS-related complex. Am J Clin Pathol 1987;87:356–364.

143. Johanson JS, Sonnenberg A. Efficient management of diarrhea in the acquired immunodeficiency syndrome (AIDS). Ann Intern Med 1990;112:942–948.

144. Fantini J, Yahi N, Baghdiguian S, et al. Human immunodeficiency virus infection of human intestinal epithelial cells. Mucosal Immunol Update 1994:21–13.

145. Smith PD. Role of the mucosa in human immunodeficiency virus disease. Mucosal Immunol Update 1994;2:3–6.

146. Amerongen HM, Weltzin R, Farner CM, et al. Transepithelial transport of HIV-1 by intestinal M cells: A mechanism for transmission of AIDS. J AIDS 1991;4:760–765.

147. Yahi N, Baghdiguian S, Bolmont C, et al. Recombinant gamma interferon inhibits HIV-1 and HIV-2 infection in human colon epithelial cells. Eur J Immunol 1992;22:2495–2499.

148. Ullrich R, Heise W, Bergs C, et al. Gastrointestinal symptoms in patients infected with human immunodeficiency virus: Relevance of infective agents isolated from gastrointestinal tract. Gut 1992;33: 1080–1084.

149. Kotler DP, Weaver S, Terzakis JA. Ultrastructural features of epithelial cell degeneration in rectal crypts of patients with AIDS. Am J Surg Pathol 1986;10:531–538.

150. Kotler DP, Reka S, Clayton F. Intestinal mucosal inflammation associated with HIV infection. Dig Dis Sci 1993;38:1119–1127.

151. Cummins AG, LaBrooy JT, Stanley DP. Quantitative histological study of enteropathy associated with HIV infection. Gut 1990;31: 317–321.

152. Cu-Uvin S, Flanigan TP, Rich JD, et al. Human immunodeficiency virus infection and acquired immunodeficiency syndrome among North American women. Am J Med 1996;101:316–322.

153. Kotloff KL, Johnson JP, Nair P, et al. Diarrheal morbidity during the first 2 years of life among HIV-infected infants. JAMA 1994;271: 448–452.

154. Laine L, Bonacini M. Esophageal disease in human immunodeficiency virus infection. Arch Intern Med 1994;154:1577–1582.

155. Bonacini M, Young T, Laine L. The causes of esophageal symptoms in human immunodeficiency virus infection: A prospective study of 110 patients. Arch Intern Med 1991;151:1567–1572.

156. Connolly GM, Hawkins D, Harcourt-Webster JN, et al. Oesophageal symptoms, their causes, treatment, and prognosis in patients with the acquired immunodeficiency syndrome. Gut 1989;30: 1033–1039.

157. Smith PD, Eisner MS, Manischewitz JF, et al. Esophageal disease in AIDS is associated with pathologic processes rather than mucosal human immunodeficiency virus type 1. J Infect Dis 1993;167: 547–552.

158. Goodgame RW, Genta RM, Estrada R, et al. Frequency of positive tests for cytomegalovirus in AIDS patients: Endoscopic lesions compared with normal mucosa. Am J Gastroenterol 1993;88: 338–343.

159. Persons DL, Moore JA, Fishback JL. Comparison of polymerase chain reaction, DNA hybridization, and histology with viral culture to detect cytomegalovirus in immunosuppressed patients. Mod Pathol 1991;4:149–153.

160. Laine L, Dretler RH, Conteas CN. Fluconazole compared with ketoconazole for the treatment of Candida esophagitis in AIDS: a randomized trial. Ann Intern Med 1992;117:655–660.

161. Balthazar EJ, Stern J. Necrotizing Candida enterocolitis in AIDS: CT features. J Comput Assist Tomogr 1994;18:298–300.

162. Goodman P, Pinero SS, Rance RM, et al. Mycobacterial esophagitis in AIDS. Gastrointest Radiol 1989;14:103–105.

163. Kazlow PG, Shah K, Benkow KJ, et al. Esophageal cryptosporidiosis in a child with acquired immunodeficiency syndrome. Gastroenterology 1986;91:1301–1303.

164. Kitchen VS, Helbert M, Francis ND. Epstein-Barr virus-associated oesophageal ulcers in AIDS. Gut 1990;112:65–66.

165. Smith PD, Quinn TC, Strober W, et al. Gastrointestinal infections in AIDS. Ann Intern Med 1991;116:63–77.

166. Cappell MS. Hepatobiliary manifestations of the acquired immune deficiency syndrome. Am J Gastroenterol 1991;86:1–15.

167. Horsburgh Jr CR. Mycobacterium avium complex infection in the acquired immunodeficiency syndrome. N Engl J Med 1991;324: 1332–1338.

168. Poorman JC, Katon RM. Small bowel involvement by Mycobacterium avium complex in a patient with AIDS: Endoscopic, histologic and radiographic similarities to Whipple's disease. Gastrointest Endosc 1994;40:753–759.

169. Roth RI, Owen RL, Keren DF. AIDS with Mycobacterium avium-intracellulare lesions resembling those of Whipple's disease N Engl J Med 1983;309:1324–1325.

170. Keren DF. Whipple's disease. The causative agent defined—its pathogenesis remains obscure. (Commentary) Medicine 1993;72:355–358.

171. Roth RI, Owen RL, Keren DF, et al. Intestinal infection with Mycobacterium avium in acquired immune deficiency syndrome (AIDS). Histologic and clinical comparison with Whipple's disease. Dig Dis Sci 1985;30:497–504.

172. Siegal FP, Lopez C, Hammer GS. Severe acquired immunodeficiency in male homosexuals, manifested by chronic perianal ulcerative herpes simplex lesions. N Engl J Med 1981;305:1439–1444.

173. Dieterich DT, Kotler DP, Busch DF. Ganciclovir treatment of cytomegalovirus colitis in AIDS: A randomized double-blind, placebo-controlled multicenter study. J Infect Dis 1993;167:278–282.

174. Laine L, Bonacini M, Sattler F. Cytomegalovirus and candida esophagitis in patients with AIDS. J Acquir Immune Defic Syndr Hum Retrovirol 1992;5:605–609.

175. Dieterich DT, Kotler DP, Busch DF. Ganciclovir treatment of cytomegalovirus colitis in AIDS: A randomized double-blind placebo-controlled multicenter study. J Infect Dis 1993;167:278–282.

176. Lake-Bakaar G, Quadros E, Beidas S. Gastric secretory failure in patients with AIDS. Ann Intern Med 1988;109:502–504.

177. Batman PA, Miller AR, Sedgwick PM. Autonomic denervation in jejunal mucosa of homosexual men infected with HIV. AIDS 1991;5:1247–1252.

178. Baskin DH, Lax JD, Barenberg D. Shigella bacteremia in patients with AIDS. Am J Gastroenterol 1987;82:338–341.

179. Washington K, Gottfried MR, Wilson ML. Gastrointestinal cryptococcosis. Mod Pathol 1991;4:707–711.

180. Dieterich DT, Lew EA, Bacon DJ. Gastrointestinal pneumocystosis in HIV-infected patients on aerosolized pentamidine: Report of five cases and literature review. Am J Gastroenterol 1992;87:1763–1770.

181. Clarkston WK, Bonacini M, Peterson I. Colitis due to Histoplasma capsulatum in the acquired immune deficiency syndrome. Am J Gastroenterol 1991;86:913–915.

182. Weber R, Bryan RT, Owen RL. Improved light microscopical detection of microsporidia spores in stool and duodenal aspirates. N Engl J Med 1992;326:161–166.

183. Orenstein JM, Chiang J, Steinberg W. Intestinal microsporidiosis as a cause of diarrhea in human immunodeficiency virus-infected patients: A report of 20 cases. Hum Pathol 1990;21:475–481.

184. Guarda LA, Stein SA, Cleary K, et al. Human cryptosporidiosis in the acquired immune deficiency syndrome. Arch Pathol Lab Med 1983;107:562–566.

185. Rene E, Marche C, Regnier B. Intestinal infections in patients with acquired immunodeficiency syndrome: A prospective study in 132 patients. Dig Dis Sci 1989;34:773–780.

186. Clayton F, Heller T, Kotler DP. Variation in the enteric distribution of cryptosporidia in acquired immunodeficiency syndrome. Am J Clin Pathol 1994;102:420–425.

187. Beeken W, Northwood I, Beliveau C, et al. Phagocytes in cell suspensions of human colon mucosa. Gut 1987;28:976–980.

188. Resnick MB, Colgan SP, Parkos CA, et al. Human eosinophils migrate across an intestinal epithelium in response to platelet-activating factor. Gastroenterology 1995;108:409–416.

189. Hogg N. The leukocyte integrins. Immunol Today 1989;10:111–114.

190. Repo H. Defects in phagocytic functions. Ann Clin Res 1987;19:263–279.

191. Rivera-Matos IR, Rakita RM, Mariscalco MM, et al. Leukocyte adhesion deficiency mimicking Hirschsprung disease. J Pediatr 1995;127:755–757.

192. Kizaki M, Miller CW, Selsted ME, et al. Myeloperoxidase (MPO) gene mutation in hereditary MPO deficiency. Blood 1994;83:1935–1940.

193. Nauseef WM, Brigham S, Cogley M. Hereditary myeloperoxidase deficiency due to a missense mutation of arginine 569 to tryptophan. J Biol Chem 1994;269:1212–1216.

194. Kusenbach G, Rister M. Myeloperoxidase deficiency as a cause of recurrent infections. Klin Padiatr 1985;197:443–445.

195. Okamura N, Malawista SE, Roberts RL, et al. Phosphorylation of the oxidase-related 48K Phosphorprotein family in the unusual autosomal cytochrome-negative and X-linked cytochrome-positive types of chronic granulomatous disease. Blood 1988;72:811–816.

196. Curnutte JT. Classification of chronic granulomatous disease. Hematol Oncol Clin North Am 1988;2:241–252.

197. Ezerowitz RAB, Phil D, Dinauer MC, et al. Partial correction of the phagocyte defect in patients with X-linked chronic granulomatous disease by subcutaneous interferon gamma. N Engl J Med 1988;319:146–151.

198. Gallin JI, Buescher ES, Seligmann BE, et al. Recent advances in chronic granulomatous disease. Ann Intern Med 1983;99:657–674.

199. Stelzer GT, Robinson JP. Flow cytometric evaluation of leukocyte function. Diagn Clin Immunol 1988;5:223–231.

200. Roberts RL, Ohno Y, Gallin JI. Staining of eosinophils with nitroblue tetrazolium in patients with chronic granulomatous disease. Pediatr Res 1986;20:378–380.

201. Baetz K, Isaaz S, Griffiths GM. Loss of cytotoxic T lymphocyte function in Chediak-Higashi syndrome arises from a secretory defect that prevents lytic granule exocytosis. J Immunol 1995;154:6122–6131.

202. Haddad E, Le Deist F, Blanche S, et al. Treatment of Chediak-Higashi syndrome by allogenic bone marrow transplantation: Report of 10 cases. Blood 1995;85:3328–3333.

203. Hammond WP, Chatta GS, Andrews RG, et al. Abnormal responsiveness of granulocyte-committed progenitor cells in cyclic neutropenia. Blood 1992;79:2536–2539.

204. Marcolongo R, Zambello R, Trentin L, et al. Childhood onset cyclic neutropenia: G-CSF therapy restores neutrophil count but does not influence superoxide anion and cytokine release by neutrophils. Br J Haematol 1995;89:277–281.

205. Lamport RD, Katz S, Eskreis D. Crohn's disease associated with cyclic neutropenia. Am J Gastroenterol 1992;87:1638–1642.

206. West CD. The complement profile in clinical medicine. Inherited and acquired conditions lowering the serum concentrations of complement component and control proteins. Complement Inflammation 1989;6:49–64.

207. Natata M, Hara T, Aoki T, et al. Inherited deficiency of the ninth component of complement: An increased risk of meningococcal meningitis. J Pediatr 1989;114:260–264.

208. Vossen JM. Bone marrow transplantation in the treatment of primary immunodeficiencies. Ann Clin Res 1987;19:285–292.

209. Nazer HM, Abutalib H, Hugosson C, et al. Intestinal lymphangiectasia masquerading as coeliac disease. Ann Trop Paediatr 1991;11:349–355.

210. Arato A, Savilahti E, Balogh L. The distribution of lymphocyte subpopulations in an infant with primary intestinal lymphangiectasia. Acta Paediatr Hung 1992;32:309–317.

211. Bretagne JF, Gosselin M. Immunological study in primary intestinal lymphangiectasia. Digestion 1994;55:59–64.

212. Yamamoto H, Tsutsui T, Mayumi M, et al. Immunodeficiency associated with selective loss of helper/inducer T cells and hypogammaglobulinaemia in a child with intestinal lymphangiectasia. Clin Exp Immunol 1989;75:196–200.

213. Bereket A, Lowenheim M, Blethen SL, et al. Intestinal lymphangiectasia in a patient with autoimmune polyglandular disease type I and steatorrhea. J Clin Endocrinol Metab 1995;80:933–935.

17

LYMPHOPROLIFERATIVE DISORDERS OF THE GASTROINTESTINAL TRACT

Peter G. Isaacson

T-CELL LYMPHOMA UNASSOCIATED WITH ENTEROPATHY HISTIOCYTIC AND MYELOPROLIFERATIVE LESIONS OF THE GASTROINTESTINAL TRACT

HISTIOCYTIC SARCOMA (TRUE HISTIOCYTIC LYMPHOMA)
GRANULOCYTIC SARCOMA

The intestinal tract is a major lymphoid organ in its own right, containing more lymphoid tissue than the entire complement of peripheral lymph nodes. In contrast to peripheral lymph nodes, which deal with antigens transported from remote sites via afferent lymphatics, gut or mucosa-associated lymphoid tissue (MALT) has evolved specifically to protect permeable mucosa that is in direct contact with antigens of the external environment. (The structure and function of MALT is described in Chapter 6.) In light of the structural and functional differences between MALT and peripheral nodal tissue, it is not surprising that the lymphoproliferative disorders that occur in these lymphoid compartments also differ. These differences have been further accentuated by the formulation of the MALT lymphoma concept (see subsequent section).

When discussing lymphoproliferative disorders, it is customary to describe nonneoplastic conditions as a group distinctly separate from the lymphomas. For the pathologist, however, the principal importance of nonneoplastic lymphoid hyperplasias and related conditions lies in their distinction from lymphoma, which they can closely simulate. Therefore, in this chapter, the nonneoplastic lymphoproliferative disorders are discussed in the context of their differential diagnosis of the various lymphomas.

PRIMARY GASTROINTESTINAL LYMPHOMA

DEFINITION

Because lymphomas arising in peripheral lymph nodes frequently disseminate to the gastrointestinal tract, strict criteria for the diagnosis of primary gastrointestinal lymphoma are necessary. On the other hand, if these criteria are too strict, the result is underdiagnosis of these tumors. The definition proposed by Dawson et al. (1), which requires that a primary gastrointestinal lymphoma is limited to the stomach or intestine and its contiguous lymph nodes, is probably too strict. An operational definition, which states that a gastrointestinal lymphoma is considered "primary" when the tumor presents with the bulk of the disease in the gastrointestinal tract, is less restrictive and more practical.

INCIDENCE

The gastrointestinal tract is the most common site of primary extranodal lymphoma (30 to 50% of cases) (2). The overall incidence of gastrointestinal lymphoma varies considerably with respect to geography; in western countries, lymphoma accounts for 4 to 18% of all non-Hodgkin lymphomas (3), whereas in the Middle East, 25% of lymphomas, the most common malignancy excluding skin cancer, arise in the gastrointestinal tract (4). Variation also exists between individual western countries, for example, the incidence of gastric lymphoma in northeastern Italy is 12-fold higher than that in England and Wales (5).

SITES

In the West, the most common site of primary gastrointestinal lymphoma is the stomach, followed by the small intestine (2). In the Middle East, the reverse is true, with most lymphomas arising in the small intestine. In both geographic regions, esophageal and colonic lymphomas are rare.

STAGING

Although determining the best system for staging primary gastrointestinal lymphomas is controversial, the Musshoff modification (6) of the Ann Arbor system is generally preferred. In this system, stage I_E indicates that the lymphoma is confined to the wall of the stomach or intestine; stage II_{1E} indicates that contiguous lymph nodes are involved,; stage II_{2E} indicates noncontiguous regional nodes are involved; and stages III, III_S, and IIII_{E+S} refer, respectively, to involvement of lymph nodes on both sides of the diaphragm or the spleen. A conference convened specifically to address the problem of staging gastrointestinal lymphoma yielded some suggested modifications to the Musshoff system (7).

THE MALT LYMPHOMA CONCEPT

GENERAL PRINCIPLES

In 1983, Isaacson and Wright (8) noted that just as nodal lymphomas recapitulated the histologic features of normal nodal tissue, certain low grade B-cell gastrointestinal lymphomas recapitulated the features of Peyer patches or MALT. These observations were later extended to include a wide variety of extranodal lymphomas, many of which arose in other mucosal sites (9). The lymphomas were characterized by reactive B-cell follicles around which, in the distribution of the marginal zone, were the neoplastic B-cells that extended into the mucosa invading individual glands. The resulting lymphoepithelial lesions were thought to be the neoplastic equivalent of the normal MALT lymphoepithelium that forms the dome over Peyer patches (10). The MALT lymphomas, as they came to be called, not only were histologically quite different from nodal low grade B-cell lymphomas, but also differed in their clinical characteristics.

ACQUIRED MALT

An inherent paradox in the MALT lymphoma concept is that almost all sites at which MALT lymphomas occur are normally devoid of lymphoid tissue. The stomach, the most common site of MALT lymphoma, is a graphic example. Moreover, MALT lymphomas are rare in the terminal ileum, which contains the greatest concentration of normally occurring MALT. This paradox has been explained by the observation that gastric MALT lymphoma, like similar lymphomas of other extranodal sites, is invariably preceded by chronic inflammation, which results in the acquisition of organized MALT. The chronic inflammatory conditions concerned almost invariably have an autoimmune component. Thus, in the stomach, most if not all MALT lymphomas are preceded by chronic gastritis associated with *Helicobacter pylori*. Although an infectious condition, this type of chronic gastritis is associated with autoimmune phenomena (11) and, typically, is characterized by the accumulation of MALT in the gastric mucosa (12–14). These observations may help to explain the differences in the types of lymphoma that arise in the gastrointestinal tract from those that arise in peripheral lymph nodes.

CLASSIFICATION OF PRIMARY GASTROINTESTINAL NON-HODGKIN LYMPHOMA

Among the differences between nodal and extranodal lymphomas in general, perhaps the most striking is the vanishingly rare incidence of primary extranodal Hodgkin disease. The gastrointestinal tract is no exception in this respect. Hence, any classification of primary gastrointestinal lymphoma can be confined to the non-Hodgkin lymphomas. Until the advent of the revised European American lymphoma (REAL) classification (15), classifications of non-Hodgkin lymphomas did not distinguish some extranodal lymphomas, including those that account for most of the gastrointestinal lymphomas. The classification in Table 17.1 is essentially a regrouping of lymphomas listed in the REAL classification to reflect their occurrence in the gastrointestinal tract.

B-cell lymphomas account for the majority of gastrointestinal lymphomas, and most of these lesions are of MALT type. Gastric MALT lymphomas have been studied most intensively and are the paradigm for this group. Low-grade MALT lymphomas may undergo high-grade transformation, and in a significant proportion of apparently primary high-grade lymphomas, a residual low-grade MALT component can be identified. It is problematic whether those high-grade lymphomas in which no low-grade MALT component is present are biologically different from high-grade MALT lymphomas. Current evidence suggests that they are not. Immunoproliferative small intestinal disease is a specific subtype of MALT lymphoma distinguished by its epidemiology and association with the synthesis of abnormal immunoglobulin (Ig) α-heavy chain. Of the other B-cell lymphomas that arise in the gut, mantle cell lymphoma, which gives rise to the condition known as lymphomatous polyposis, and Burkitt lymphoma, which tends to involve the ileocecal region, are the most important. Other types of low-grade B-cell lymphomas that commonly arise in lymph nodes may arise in the gastrointestinal tract but do so infrequently. The gut is also a favored site for the origin of lymphomas associated with immunodeficiency-related lymphoproliferative disorders.

Primary gastrointestinal T-cell lymphomas are less common than B-cell tumors. Enteropathy-associated T-cell lymphoma (EATL), which appears to arise from a distinctive intestinal cytotoxic intraepithelial T cell, is the most important member of this group.

LOW-GRADE B-CELL GASTRIC MALT LYMPHOMA

The evolution of the MALT lymphoma concept has been based in large part on observations of low-grade gastric B-cell lymphomas, because not only is the stomach by far the most common site of these tumors, but also, at least until recently, gastrectomy was the preferred treatment. This has resulted in the availability of sufficient tissue to permit detailed studies of the pathology and cell biology of gastric MALT lymphoma, which has yielded information that may then be applied to the group of MALT lymphomas as a whole.

Helicobacter pylori AND GASTRIC MALT LYMPHOMA

The paradox of lymphoma arising in the stomach, where there is normally no lymphoid tissue, could be explained by the fact that MALT-type lymphoid tissue is acquired as the result of H. pylori infection (12–14). Indeed, some investigators have gone so far as to suggest that lymphoid tissue accumulates in the gastric mucosa only as a result of this infection. Although it is undoubtedly true that H pylori infection is responsible for the presence of gastric mucosal lymphoid tissue in most cases, other causes, notably Sjögren syndrome, have subsequently been identified (16). A considerable body of evidence, however, links H. pylori and gastric lymphoma. H. pylori can be detected in more than 90% of cases of low-grade gastric MALT lymphoma (17), and an early epidemiologic study (5) showed that in at least one area, namely northeastern Italy, the incidence of gastric lymphoma is extraordinarily high as is the prevalence of H. pylori infection in the community. Subsequently, a more formal epidemiologic study (18) confirmed the link between H. pylori and gastric lymphoma by showing that patients with gastric lymphoma were significantly more likely to be infected with H. pylori than a matched group of patients with other forms of lymphoma. Even more concrete evidence for the etiologic role of H. pylori derived from cell biology experiments showing that the growth of neoplastic B cells from low-grade gastric MALT lymphoma can be stimulated by tumor-specific strains of H. pylori (19).

TABLE	
17.1	**Primary Gastrointestinal Non-Hodgkin Lymphoma**

B cell
  Mucosa-associated lymphoid tissue (MALT)-type (including
    immunoproliferative small intestinal disease (IPSID))
    Low grade
    High grade with or without a low-grade component
  Mantle cell (lymphomatous polyposis)
  Burkitt
  Other types corresponding to lymph node equivalents
  Immunodeficiency related
    Post-transplant
    Acquired (AIDS)
    Congenital
T cell
  Enteropathy associated
  Other types not associated with enteropathy

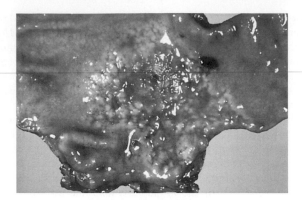

Figure 17.1 Macroscopic appearance of low-grade gastric MALT lymphoma. A superficial infiltrate of lesion contains numerous ulcers. (See color plate.)

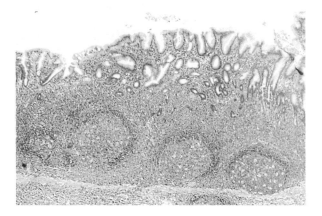

Figure 17.2 Low-grade gastric MALT lymphoma. Multiple reactive B-cell follicles are surrounded by lymphomatous infiltrate. (See color plate.)

Interestingly, it is not the neoplastic B cells that react to H. pylori, but rather the intratumoral T cells, which then indirectly stimulate the growth of the tumor by a contact-mediated mechanism (20). In light of these studies, numerous patients with low-grade gastric MALT lymphoma have been treated successfully by eradication of H. pylori with appropriate antibiotics (21–28).

INCIDENCE

For many years, because of their clinical indolence, many if not most low-grade gastric MALT lymphomas were called "pseudolymphomas," and for this reason, the true incidence of this tumor is difficult to estimate. This difficulty is compounded by the geographic variation in the incidence of gastric lymphoma mentioned previously. Some evidence exists that the incidence of gastric lymphoma is rising (29).

CLINICAL PRESENTATION

Low-grade gastric lymphoma occurs predominantly in patients 50 years of age and older, but cases have been reported in individuals as young as 7 years of age. The male-to-female ratio is approximately 1.5 : 1. Patients usually complain of nonspecific dyspepsia and other peptic ulcer-like symptoms; only rarely are cancer-related symptoms

and signs of severe abdominal pain with an abdominal mass present. Similarly, the endoscopic findings are usually those of nonspecific gastritis and/or a peptic ulcer, the presence of a mass again being unusual. The depth of invasion by the tumor is difficult to estimate from endoscopic examination alone, however, and other investigations, such as endoscopic sonography, may show a surprising degree of invasion.

Staging procedures show that most cases of low-grade gastric MALT lymphoma are at stage I_E or II_E. Extraabdominal dissemination is unusual, although in one study, bone marrow involvement was reported in 10% of patients (26).

MACROSCOPIC APPEARANCE

Gastric lymphoma most often involves the antrum, but it may occur in any part of the stomach. It is usually a flat infiltrative lesion (Fig. 17.1), sometimes associated with one or more ulcers. Large masses are less common.

HISTOPATHOLOGY (30)

Nonneoplastic, reactive B-cell follicles are an integral component of the tumor; the lymphomatous infiltrate tends to concentrate around these follicles, in the marginal zone, from which it spreads diffusely

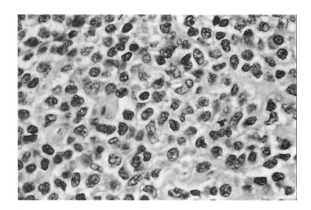

Figure 17.3 Centrocyte-like cells of low-grade gastric MALT lymphoma. (See color plate.)

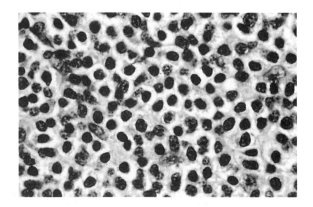

Figure 17.4 Low-grade gastric MALT lymphoma characterized by a "monocytoid" cytologic appearance. (See color plate.)

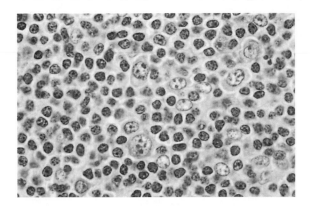

Figure 17.5 Cells of this low-grade gastric MALT lymphoma closely resemble small lymphocytes. Note scattered larger transformed cells. (See color plate.)

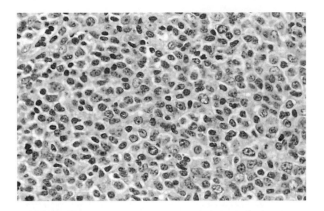

Figure 17.6 Low-grade gastric MALT lymphoma. Numerous nucleated blasts are scattered among the centrocyte-like cells. (See color plate.)

into the mucosa (Fig. 17.2). The neoplastic B cells are small and show considerable cytologic variation both within an individual case and between cases. These cells usually are characterized by a narrow rim of cytoplasm around small nuclei with a distinctly irregular outline (Fig. 17.3). They resemble the centrocytes (small cleaved cells) of the follicle center and have been called centrocyte-like (CCL). The lymphoma cells may accumulate more abundant pale-staining cytoplasm leading to a monocytoid appearance (Fig. 17.4) or they more closely resemble unremarkable small lymphocytes (Fig. 17.5). Typically, larger transformed nucleolated blasts are scattered through the infiltrate; at times, these blasts can be numerous, leading to problems with grading the lymphoma (Figs. 17.5 and 17.6).

A highly characteristic feature of low-grade gastric MALT lymphoma is the presence of lymphoepithelial lesions formed by the invasion of individual glands or surface epithelium by CCL or monocytoid lymphoma cells that displace or destroy the glandular epithelium, which then often shows an eosinophilic or "oncocytic" degenerative change (Figs. 17.7 and 17.8). The number of these lesions is variable, but they usually are easy to find; their presence in a lymphoproliferative lesion of the stomach is highly suggestive, although not on its own diagnostic of, MALT lymphoma. Lymphoepithelial lesions probably represent the neoplastic equivalent

of the lymphoepithelium that characterizes MALT. There appears to be a specific "tropism" of the MALT lymphoma cells for glandular epithelium; in less dense mucosal infiltrates, lymphoma cells often concentrate around glands, even though actual lymphoepithelial lesions are not formed. Plasma cell differentiation is present in approximately one third of cases and tends to concentrate beneath the surface epithelium (Fig. 17.9). In some cases, plasma cell differentiation can be so significant as to suggest a diagnosis of plasmacytoma, and careful examination is required to reveal the lymphoid component of the tumor. The plasma cells may be large with abundant cytoplasm packed with eosinophilic immunoglobulin, sometimes in crystal form. Escape of this immunoglobulin may lead to massive extracellular accummulation of eosinophilic material (Fig. 17.10). Immunoglobulin inclusions may displace the nucleus, lending a signet ring appearance to the lymphoma cells that can lead to a mistaken diagnosis of carcinoma. This diagnosis is also suggested sometimes by a goblet cell change of the gastric epithelium that can be induced by the lymphomatous infiltrate (31) (Fig. 17.11).

Reactive B-cell follicles are an essential component of gastric MALT lymphoma, and the smallest lymphomatous focus is typically found in the marginal zone of a reactive follicle. MALT lymphoma cells tend specifically to colonize these follicles in a complex way

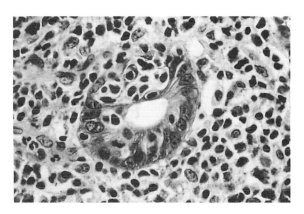

Figure 17.7 A lymphoepithelial lesion in a low-grade gastric MALT lymphoma. (See color plate.)

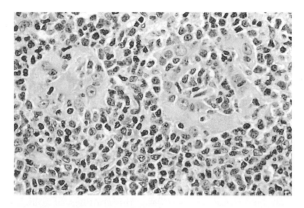

Figure 17.8 Lymphoepithelial lesions in low-grade gastric MALT lymphoma, accompanied by eosinophilic degeneration of the epithelium. (See color plate.)

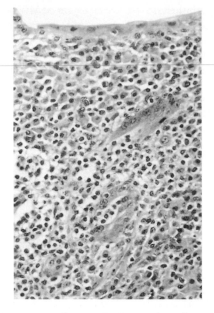

Figure 17.9 Low-grade gastric MALT lymphoma. Note the plasmacytic differentiation of the cells beneath the surface epithelium. (See color plate.)

(32). They may simply replace the entire follicle, which results in a vaguely nodular appearance to the tumor as a whole (Fig. 17.12), or specifically colonize the follicle centers with preservation of the mantle zone (Fig. 17.13). This colonization may be accompanied by blastic transformation or plasma cell differentiation (Fig. 17.14) of the intrafollicular lymphoma cells and can lead to a remarkable resemblance to follicular lymphoma.

MULTIFOCALITY OF GASTRIC MALT LYMPHOMA

In gastrectomy specimens, small foci of lymphoma can often be identified some distance from the main tumor. The smallest of these foci consists of a single reactive follicle with a lymphomatous marginal zone. Using the "Swiss role" technique to create a map of the tumor, it has been shown that most, if not all, gastric MALT lymphomas are multifocal (33).

BIOPSY APPEARANCES

The typical features of gastric MALT lymphoma described previously are not as easily observed in small endoscopic biopsy samples. Reactive follicles may be difficult to define, especially if there is any crush artifact, and the characteristic cytologic appearances of the lymphoma cells can be distorted. The presence of a dense lymphoid infiltrate extending beyond the immediate borders of identifiable follicles should raise the suspicion of lymphoma, and under these circumstances, careful evaluation of the cytology of the cells and a search for lymphoepithelial lesions is indicated. Immunohistochemical analysis (see subsequent discussion) can be helpful in identifying the confines of follicles, the presence of lymphoepithelial lesions, and the presence of immunoglobulin light chain restriction. Despite these difficulties, it should be stressed that histologic criteria remain the most im-

portant in the biopsy-based diagnosis of gastric lymphoma. Although molecular evidence for monoclonality may be obtained using the polymerase chain reaction (PCR) (34), a diagnosis of gastric lymphoma should never be made unless the histologic findings are compatible (28).

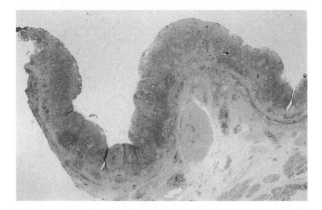

Figure 17.10 Low-grade gastric MALT lymphoma with extensive extracellular pools of eosinophilic immunoglobulin. (See color plate.)

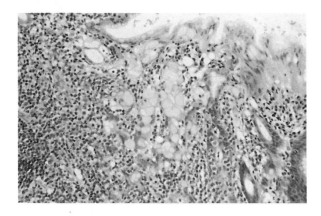

Figure 17.11 Goblet cell change of the epithelium in a low-grade gastric MALT lymphoma, not to be confused with signet ring cell carcinoma. (See color plate.)

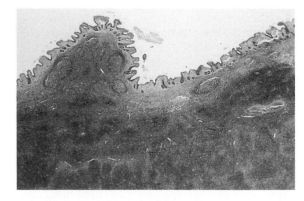

Figure 17.12 Follicular colonization, type I. Reactive follicles are surrounded, partially replaced, and finally completely replaced by lymphoma cells, leading to an overall nodular pattern. (See color plate.)

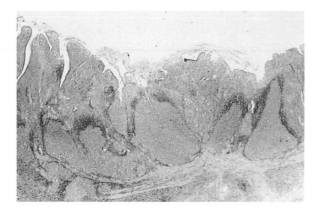

Figure 17.13 Follicular colonization, type II. Colonized follicle centers are greatly expanded, with retention of mantle zones. (See color plate.)

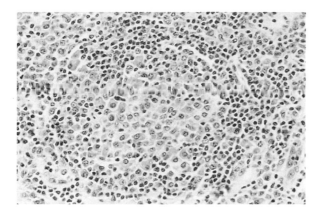

Figure 17.14 Follicular colonization, type III. The cells that have colonized the reactive follicle center have undergone plasma cell differentiation. (See color plate.)

LYMPH NODE INVOLVEMENT

In its early stages, lymph node involvement by gastric MALT lymphoma may manifest only with subtle widening of marginal zones. Later manifestations include more obvious infiltration of the interfollicular area and, finally, effacement of the entire node (Fig. 17.15). The cells in the lymph nodes show the same cytologic variation as in the stomach, and both plasma cell differentiation and follicular colonization may be seen.

DISTANT SPREAD

Although distant spread is uncommon, dissemination to the bone marrow, small intestine, liver, and spleen have been recorded. Lymphoma in the spleen has been observed preferentially to localize in the marginal zone (35) (Fig. 17.16).

IMMUNOHISTOCHEMISTRY

The immunophenotype of low-grade gastric MALT lymphoma is outlined in Table 17.2. This immunophenotype is shared by marginal zone B cells and supports the histologic inferences that these cells are the normal cell counterparts of MALT lym-

phoma. Especially useful in establishing the diagnosis are the demonstration of pan B-cell antigens, which, together with the use of anticytokeratins, is helpful in identifying lymphoepithelial lesions (Fig. 17.17), and the demonstration of immunoglobulin light chain restriction as an indicator of monoclonality (Fig. 17.18).

MOLECULAR GENETICS

Monoclonal rearrangement of the immunoglobulin heavy chain gene has been confirmed in low-grade gastric MALT lymphoma by both Southern blotting and PCR (34). Further investigations of the immunoglobulin genes have shown mutations that indicate that the lymphoma originates from post-follicular B cells and that antigen selection occurs in some cases (36, 37). A significant number of replication errors have been noted in low-grade gastric MALT lymphomas (38) and, interestingly, some of these errors are shared by adjacent nonlymphomatous, but chronically inflamed, mucosa. Additionally, c-myc mutations (39), but not translocations, and p53 mutations (40), without loss of heterozygosity, have been identified in 50% and 15% of cases, respectively. Trisomy 3 has been demonstrated in 60% of patients with low-grade gastric MALT lymphoma (41).

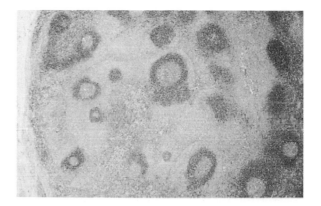

Figure 17.15 Gastric lymph node involved by low-grade MALT lymphoma shows infiltration of marginal zones and interfollicular areas. (See color plate.)

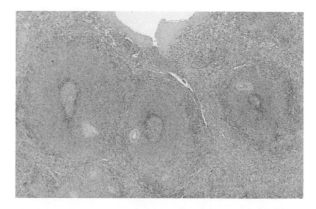

Figure 17.16 Splenic involvement in a case of low-grade gastric MALT lymphoma. Tumor cells localize in splenic marginal zones. (See color plate.)

CLINICAL BEHAVIOR

The behavior of low-grade MALT lymphoma is quite different from that of comparable nodal lymphomas. The nodal lymphomas usually are already widely disseminated, with bone marrow involvement, at diagnosis. They run a slowly progressive course, often terminating after 7 to 10 years with high-grade transformation. In contrast, low-grade MALT lymphomas are usually localized at the time of diagnosis and seldom involve the bone marrow. Their course is marked by local recurrences and limited dissemination, often to other mucosal sites. Although relapse-free survival is similar to that associated with nodal low-grade lymphoma, relatively few patients die of their disease. In a large series reported by Cogliatti et al. (42), the survival rates after a variety of treatment protocols were 91% at 5 years and 75% at 10 years. Pathologic stage is the most important prognostic variable.

DIFFERENTIAL DIAGNOSIS

"PSEUDOLYMPHOMA"

This well-entrenched term is included in this discussion only to dismiss it. Difficulty in distinguishing between extreme lymphoid hyperplasia and low-grade lymphoma in gastric lesions, compounded by the favorable clinical behavior of low-grade gastric lymphoma, led to its emergence. Neither the meaning, the precise histopathology, nor the clinical significance of "pseudolymphoma" are clear. Careful histologic analysis coupled with modern immunohistochemical and molecular genetic methods almost always permit the distinction between lymphoid hyperplasia. When making this distinction proves impossible, the pathologist should delay making a definitive diagnosis rather than conveying a false sense of security with the use of a meaningless term.

CHRONIC FOLLICULAR GASTRITIS

The histologic appearances of this condition, which is caused by H. pylori, can closely simulate those of lymphoma (Fig. 17.19). Within a dense mucosal lymphoid infiltrate are numerous hyperplastic B-cell follicles. These follicles are often associated with poorly formed marginal zones and the marginal B cells may infiltrate the

TABLE 17.2	Immunophenotype of Low-Grade Gastric MALT Lymphoma Compared to Marginal Zone B Cells	
	MALT Lymphoma	Marginal Zone
Ig	M+ D–	M+ D–
CD20	+	+
CD10	–	–
CD5	–	–
CD23	–	–
CD21	+	+
CD35	+	+
CD43	+/–	–

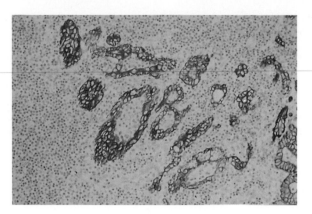

Figure 17.17 Low-grade gastric MALT lymphoma stained with anticytokeratin, which highlights lymphoepithelial lesions. (See color plate.)

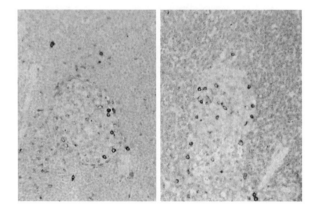

Figure 17.18 Low-grade gastric MALT lymphoma stained with anti-κ *(left)* and anti-λ *(right)* light chains. There is λ-light chain restriction of the tumor cells that surround a polytypic reactive follicle center. (See color plate.)

epithelium of individual gastric glands, forming structures bearing a close resemblance to lymphoepithelial lesions of MALT lymphoma. Eosinophilic degeneration or destruction of glandular epithelium are not present, however. Moreover, the lymphocytic infiltrate is confined to the follicles and their immediately proximate marginal zone; between the follicles, the mucosa is infiltrated by plasma cells and histiocytes rather than sheets of CCL or monocytoid lymphocytes characteristic of MALT lymphoma. The differential diagnosis between follicular gastritis and low-grade MALT lymphoma presents a particular problem in endoscopic gastric biopsies. For this reason, a system of grading the lymphocytic infiltrate has been proposed (21) (Table 17.3).

The demonstration of immunoglobulin light chain restriction using immunohistochemistry is extremely useful in confirming a diagnosis of lymphoma. Unfortunately, with the exception of those cases in which there is plasma cell differentiation, this technique is difficult to perform in small, often partly crushed biopsy specimens. PCR for the demonstration of monoclonal rearrangement of the immunoglobulin gene heavy chain can be applied to DNA extracted from paraffin-embedded biopsy material. This technique is useful only to support histologic findings, because both false-negative and false-positive results are common (28, 34, 43).

LYMPHOID HYPERPLASIA ASSOCIATED WITH A CHRONIC PEPTIC ULCER

Numerous B-cell follicles are sometimes present in the base of a chronic peptic ulcer and the adjacent mucosa. The follicles are not associated with marginal zones and are well demarcated from the surrounding relatively sparse infiltrate of plasma cells, other inflammatory cells, and fibroblasts. In resection specimens, scarring associated with a peptic ulcer typically extends through the muscularis propria, whereas when the ulcer is caused by lymphoma, the muscularis is usually intact.

OTHER LOW-GRADE LYMPHOMAS

With the exception of mantle cell lymphoma (see subsequent discussion), low-grade B-cell lymphomas other than MALT lymphoma do not arise as primary lesions in the stomach. Nevertheless, these lymphomas often involve the stomach secondarily and may be encountered in endoscopic biopsies (44). Usually there is evidence of chronic lymphocytic leukemia (CLL) or lymphoma, most often follicular lymphoma, involving peripheral lymph nodes. In CLL, the gastric mucosa is diffusely infiltrated by small lymphocytes without a background of reactive follicles, and lymphoepithelial lesions are not a feature. The differential diagnosis of follicular lymphoma from low-grade MALT lymphoma in which follicular colonization has occurred is more problematic (32). The former is not usually associated with a significant diffuse component of the mucosal infiltrate, and lymphoepithelial lesions are not present. The cytologic appearances are clearly those of follicle center cells, as is the immunophenotype. The t(14;18) translocation so characteristic of follicular lymphoma is not a feature of MALT lymphoma.

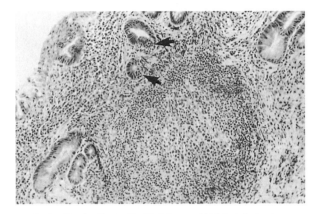

Figure 17.19 Chronic follicular gastritis due to Helicobacter-pylori infection. Note the well-defined B-cell follicle in the gastric mucosa with lymphocytic infiltration of adjacent gastric glands *(arrows)*. (See color plate.)

HIGH-GRADE B-CELL GASTRIC MALT LYMPHOMA

In most reported series, the incidence of high-grade gastric lymphoma is higher than that of the low-grade lesion. This difference may, however, be more apparent than real, because, until recently, many low-grade gastric lymphomas were labeled as "pseudolymphoma" or florid lymphoid hyperplasia and, therefore, were not included. Foci of high-grade lymphoma are sometimes present in low-grade MALT lymphoma consistent with transformation, as is well recognized in nodal low-grade B-cell lymphomas (45). The extent of this secondary high-grade component varies. In some cases, it is confined to colonized follicle centers, whereas in others, sheets of transformed blasts may lie within the predominantly low-grade infiltrate. Another variant includes those lesions characterized by a predominance of high-grade lymphoma within which are small residual low-grade foci. Thus, a problem exists with the definition of high-grade MALT lymphoma, which in

TABLE 17.3	Histologic Scoring for Diagnosis of MALT Lymphoma	
Grade	Description	Histologic Features
0	Normal	Scattered plasma cells in lamina propria; no lymphoid follicles
1	Chronic active gastritis	Small clusters of lymphocytes in lamina propria; no lymphoid follicles; no LELs
2	Chronic active gastritis with florid lymphoid follicle formation	Prominent lymphoid follicles with surrounding mantle zone and plasma cells; no LELs
3	Suspicious lymphoid infiltrate in lamina propria, probably reactive	Lymphoid follicles surrounded by small lymphocytes that infiltrate diffusely in lamina propria and occasionally into epithelium
4	Suspicious lymphoid infiltrate in lamina propria, probably lymphoma	Lymphoid follicles surrounded by CCL cells that infiltrate diffusely in lamina propria and into epithelium in small groups
5	Low-grade B-cell lymphoma of MALT	Presence of dense diffuse infiltrate of CCL cells in lamina propria with prominent LELs

CCL, centrocyte-like; LEL, lymphoepithelial lesion.

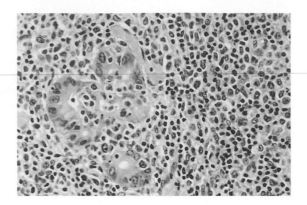

Figure 17.20   Low-grade gastric MALT lymphoma showing a lymphoepithelial lesion *(left)* and high-grade transformation *(right)*. (See color plate.)

the first instance relates to the number of high-grade (transformed) cells present. Most authors now agree that the presence of cohesive sheets of high-grade (transformed) cells, excluding those in colonized follicles, is indicative of high-grade transformation (Fig. 17.20).

A second problem is posed by those cases in which no low-grade component can be detected. These lesions, therefore, must be presumed to be high-grade gastric lymphomas de novo. Some of these lesions may still be transformed low-grade MALT lymphomas in which the low-grade component has been not been detected or has been overgrown, but there almost certainly remains a group of truly primary high-grade gastric lymphomas. It is arguable whether or not this group should be categorized as MALT lymphoma. Both high- and low-grade gastric lymphoma are related to previous H. pylori infection (18) and, given that the histologic and cytologic features of both secondary and primary high-grade gastric B-cell lymphoma are identical and no significant difference is noted in their clinical behavior (42), it seems nothing is gained by separating high-grade gastric lymphoma into MALT and non-MALT groups.

CLINICAL PRESENTATION

The mean age of patients presenting with high-grade gastric lymphoma is higher than that of patients with low-grade MALT lymphoma (64 versus 55 years), but the sex distribution is the same. The symptoms are essentially similar to those of gastric carcinoma, consisting of pain, weight loss, bleeding, etc. Endoscopic examination usually shows an obvious tumor mass. The stage of cases at presentation is equally divided between I_E and II_E. Evidence of distant spread, including bone marrow involvement, is uncommon.

MACROSCOPIC APPEARANCE

Most high-grade lymphomas are bulky tumors, but some are more diffusely infiltrative.

HISTOPATHOLOGY

The tumor usually infiltrates in cohesive sheets between glands, unlike poorly differentiated carcinoma, which destroys glands as it advances through the mucosa. A few residual follicles may be present, but this feature is not a consistent finding. Lymphoepithelial lesions are present in some cases (Fig. 17.21). The tumor cells are large with moderately abundant eosinophilic cytoplasm and vesicular nuclei containing one or more randomly distributed nucleoli. Classic centroblasts (large noncleaved cells) are not characteristic. Bizarre multinucleated cells are present in some cases.

IMMUNOHISTOCHEMISTRY

The cells often contain abundant monotypic immunoglobulin, usually IgM. The immunophenotype is not in any way distinctive, although some evidence suggests that expression of bcl-2 protein is less common than in nodal high-grade lymphomas (46). Staining with anticytokeratins may be helpful in highlighting lymphoepithelial lesions.

MOLECULAR GENETICS

Analyses of the immunoglobulin genes in high-grade gastric lymphoma with a low-grade MALT component have confirmed the clonal identity of the two lesions (47). Ongoing mutations, however, are not present in the high-grade lymphomas. High-grade gastric B-cell lymphomas show a range of c-myc mutations that is similar to that in low-grade MALT lymphoma (39), but p53 mutations, with loss of heterozygosity and expression of the protein, are more common (29% of cases) (40).

CLINICAL BEHAVIOR

Some investigators have suggested that grade is not an independent variable in the prognosis of gastric lymphoma (48). Others have argued the contrary (49). In the series of Cogliatti et al. (42), the 5-year survival rate of high-grade gastric lymphoma was 75% vs 91% for low-grade MALT lymphoma. No difference in survival was noted between those cases in which a low-grade component could be identified and those in which it could not.

GASTRIC MALT LYMPHOMA AND CARCINOMA

Synchronous gastric lymphoma and carcinoma has been described in numerous case reports, which were summarized by Wotherspoon

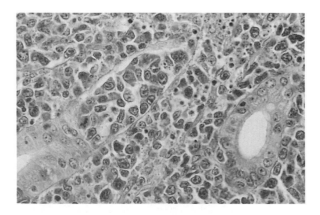

Figure 17.21   High-grade gastric (MALT) lymphoma showing a lymphoepithelial lesion. (See color plate.)

and Isaacson (50), who added seven cases of their own. A series of 190 gastric MALT lymphomas in which there were nine synchronous carcinomas (5%) has subsequently been reported by Nakamura et al. (51). These observations can be interpreted as further evidence for the role of H. pylori in both gastric carcinoma and lymphoma.

INTESTINAL MALT LYMPHOMA

With the same provisos regarding gastric B-cell lymphomas, most primary B-cell lymphomas of the intestine are of MALT type. The small intestine is by far the most common site, with colorectal lymphomas occurring only rarely (52). No pathologic or clinical difference exists between small intestinal and colorectal lymphomas. Distinction must be made between "usual" (sometimes called "western") intestinal lymphoma and immunoproliferative small intestinal disease (IPSID), which is a special type of intestinal MALT lymphoma with a restricted geographic distribution.

USUAL (WESTERN) INTESTINAL MALT LYMPHOMA

This tumor occurs with equal frequency in western countries of Europe and the USA, where it is uncommon. Intestinal lymphoma is a common disease in the Middle East, however, where it accounts for a substantial proportion of non-Hodgkin lymphoma, a particularly common malignancy in this region.

CLINICAL PRESENTATION

Most lesions occur in elderly patients and manifest with intestinal obstruction or bleeding. Inflammatory bowel disease appears to be a risk factor for colorectal lymphomas (53), but not for those lymphomatous lesions arising in the small intestine. Any level of the intestine may be involved, and the lymphomas usually occur as single ulcerating or polypoid lesions (54), although presentation at multiple sites has been described. The mesenteric lymph nodes are usually involved (stage II_E), but extraabdominal spread is not characteristic.

HISTOPATHOLOGY

The histologic features of intestinal MALT lymphoma are identical to those of the gastric MALT lymphoma (30) (Fig. 17.22). In low-grade tumors, reactive B-cell follicles are prominent and are surrounded by the lymphoma cells that show the same cytologic variation as they do in gastric lymphoma. Plasma cell differentiation is common. Lymphoepithelial lesions are usually present but they are not as numerous as in gastric lymphoma, and follicular colonization may be seen. High-grade B-cell lymphomas occur more commonly than the low-grade tumors and, as in the stomach, a low-grade MALT component may be present. Histologically, the high-grade intestinal lymphomas resemble their gastric counterparts, and they manifest the same immunohistochemical properties. No formal molecular genetic studies on intestinal MALT lymphomas have been performed.

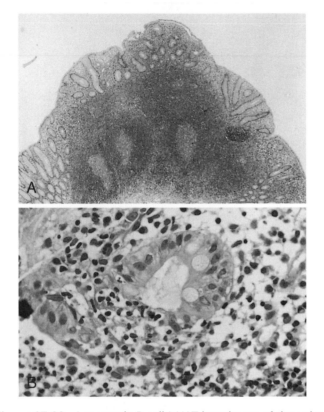

Figure 17.22   Low-grade B-cell MALT lymphoma of the colon. **A.** Mucosal infiltration around reactive follicles. **B.** Detail of lymphoepithelial lesion. (See color plate.)

CLINICAL BEHAVIOR

The clinical behavior of intestinal MALT lymphoma is not as favorable as that of gastric lymphoma. Histologic grade, stage, and resectability have all been shown to be relevant to the prognosis (52, 55). Five-year survival rates of 44 to 75% have been reported for low-grade MALT lymphoma and 25 to 37% for high-grade disease. As in the stomach, the presence or absence of a low-grade MALT component has no effect on these figures, suggesting that high-grade B-cell lymphoma of the intestine is a single biologic entity.

DIFFERENTIAL DIAGNOSIS

OTHER B-CELL LYMPHOMAS

Other types of low-grade B-cell lymphoma are more common in the intestine than in the stomach. Their differential diagnosis from MALT lymphoma is discussed later in the section on IPSID.

FOCAL LYMPHOID HYPERPLASIA

This condition (56) typically occurs in the terminal ileum and takes two forms; the more common occurs in children and young adults, and a rarer form is seen in older individuals. The first type is known by a number of names, including enteritis follicularis, cobblestone ileum, nonsclerosing ileitis, pseudopolyposis lymphatica, and terminal lymphoid ileitis. It occurs more frequently in males and may manifest as ileocecal intussusception, with appendicitis-like symp-

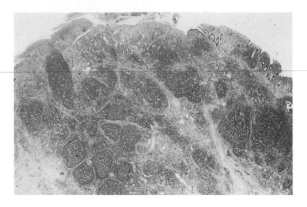

Figure 17.23 Focal lymphoid hyperplasia of terminal ileum, adult type. Note the surface ulceration with infiltration of the ileum by floridly reactive B-cell follicles. (See color plate.)

toms or with bleeding. The few histologic descriptions of this disorder cite marked hyperplasia of Peyer patches with sharply circumscribed follicles and submucosal edema. No disorganization of lymphoid tissue or invasion is evident below the submucosa and, hence, this condition bears little resemblance to lymphoma.

In the adult form (57), which is sometimes known as florid lymphoid hyperplasia of the terminal ileum, the clinical findings include chronic abdominal pain frequently associated with a right iliac fossa mass. The histologic features consist of follicular hyperplasia with associated superficial ulceration and a diffuse interfollicular lymphoplasmacytic infiltrate (Fig. 17.23). Eosinophils may be present in large numbers. This infiltrative process extends deeply into the wall of the ileum, frequently involving the serosa. The normal marginal zone component of Peyer patches participates in the hyperplasia; the result can be misidentified as part of a lymphoepithelial lesion, leading to a mistaken interpretation of the lesion as a MALT lymphoma.

DIFFUSE NODULAR LYMPHOID HYPERPLASIA OF THE INTESTINE

This rare lesion, which involves long segments of small or large intestine, occurs in two forms. The more common form (58) is associated with congenital or acquired hypogammaglobulinemia and is rarely complicated by the development of lymphoma. Histologic features include mucosal follicular hyperplasia with an inconspicuous marginal zone and no associated interfollicular infiltrate (Fig. 17.24). In the second form (59), immunoglobulin deficiency is not present and an association with lymphoma is well documented. The lymphoma is of low-grade MALT type and appears to arise in the background of the acquired lymphoid hyperplasia in common with other MALT lymphomas.

IMMUNOPROLIFERATIVE SMALL INTESTINAL DISEASE (IPSID)

This curious condition, first described by Ramot et al. in 1965 (60), is a variant of MALT lymphoma characterized by a diffuse lymphoplasmacytic (predominantly plasmacytic) infiltrate of the jejunum. The highest incidence of IPSID is in the Middle East, but

significant numbers of cases have been reported from the Cape region of South Africa (61) and there have been sporadic reports from other areas, including Greece and the Indian subcontinent. The important distinguishing feature of IPSID is the synthesis of α-immunoglobulin heavy chain, without light chain, by the plasma cells. The α-chain can be detected in the plasma or duodenal juice in approximately two thirds of cases, which has led to the term "α-chain disease." In the remaining one third of cases, the α-chain protein is synthesized but is not secreted (62).

CLINICAL PRESENTATION

This disease manifests in young patients with severe unremitting malabsorption. Typically, the lymphoma is confined to the intestine and mesenteric lymph nodes; extraabdominal spread is not present. In numerous reports, remission, or even cure, of IPSID in its early stages occurred after the administration of broad-spectrum antibiotics (63, 64). This course draws clear parallels with the response of gastric MALT lymphoma to eradication of H. pylori.

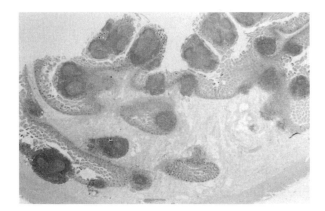

Figure 17.24 Diffuse nodular lymphoid hyperplasia of the small intestine. Multiple mucosal lymphoid nodules comprise hyperplastic B-cell follicles. (See color plate.)

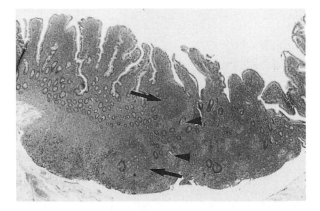

Figure 17.25 Immunoproliferative small intestinal disease (stage B). Small intestinal villi are expanded by a lymphoplasmacytic infiltrate that extends into the submucosa. Lymphoid follicles *(arrows)* and lymphoepithelial lesions *(arrowheads)* are evident. (See color plate.)

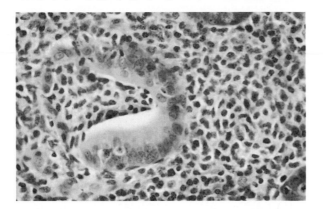

Figure 17.26 Centrocyte-like cells forming a lymphoepithelial lesion in IPSID. (See color plate.)

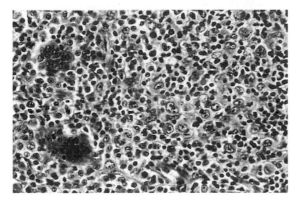

Figure 17.27 High-grade transformation in IPSID. (See color plate.)

MACROSCOPIC APPEARANCE

In most cases, diffuse even thickening of the jejunum is accompanied by enlarged mesenteric lymph nodes. Circumscribed, sometimes multiple or polypoid tumor masses may be present.

HISTOPATHOLOGY (30)

The histopathologic features of IPSID are those of low-grade MALT lymphoma with significant plasma cell differentiation. Three stages of intestinal infiltration are recognized, all of which are accompanied by involvement of the mesenteric lymph nodes. In stage A, the infiltrate is confined to the mucosa; in stage B, nodular mucosal infiltration extends into the submucosa; and in stage C, large lymphomatous masses are often complicated by high-grade transformation. The lymphoplasmacytic infiltrate of the mucosa causes broadening of the villi, but no true villous atrophy or crypt hyperplasia is seen (Fig. 17.25). The plasma cells themselves are not invasive and show no evidence of proliferation, but already present in stage A and increasing in numbers through stages B and C are lymphoepithelial lesions (Fig. 17.26) formed by the lymphoid component that comprises CCL or monocytoid cells. Reactive B-cell follicles, characteristically situated just above the muscularis mucosae, are usually prominent and it is follicular colonization that is responsible for the nodularity of the infiltrate in stage B IPSID. Transformation of high-grade lymphoma, often with bizarre high-

grade tumor cells, is a late development that occurs focally at first before forming large tumor masses (Fig. 17.27).

The mesenteric lymph nodes are involved early in the course of IPSID. Initially, mature plasma cells fill the sinuses, but later, CCL or monocytoid lymphoma cells invade the marginal zone. Follicular colonization with plasma cell differentiation is especially prominent.

IMMUNOHISTOCHEMISTRY

The mixed B-lymphocyte and plasma cell infiltrate is well demonstrated by staining with CD20, which also highlights lymphoepithelial lesions (Fig. 17.28). Studies have confirmed the synthesis of α-heavy chain without light chain by both plasma cells and lymphocytes (65, 66) (Fig. 17.29). The α-chain is almost always of the α1 subclass, but synthesis of α2 has been described in occasional cases. Immunoglobulin light chain synthesis with light chain restriction has been demonstrated in a handful of cases (67). The immunophenotype is otherwise similar to that of gastric MALT lymphoma.

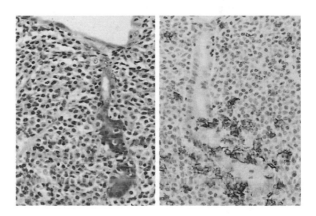

Figure 17.28 Immunproliferative small intestinal disease. Within plasma cell infiltration of mucosa is a lymphoepithelial lesion. Immunostaining with CD20 *(right)* shows CD20-positive B-cells forming the lymphoepithelial lesion in contrast to the plasma cells, which are CD20 negative. (See color plate.)

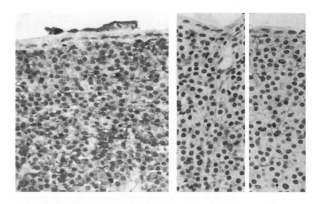

Figure 17.29 Plasmacytic infiltrate in IPSID. Staining for α-heavy chain *(left)* is positive. Staining for κ- and λ-light chains *(right)* is negative. (See color plate.)

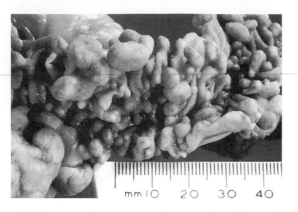

Figure 17.30 Lymphomatous polyposis (mantle cell lymphoma) of the small intestine. (See color plate.)

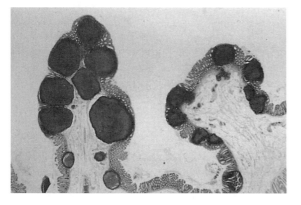

Figure 17.31 Colonic mucosa from a patient with lymphomatous polyposis. Multiple lymphomatous nodules are seen. (See color plate.)

MOLECULAR GENETICS

Southern blotting has shown that the lymphoproliferation in IPSID is monoclonal (68). Cytogenetic analyses have been performed in a few cases and have shown a variety of abnormalities, including t(9;14) and t(2;14) (69).

CLINICAL BEHAVIOR

IPSID runs a prolonged course, often over many years. It is the malabsorption rather than the neoplasm itself that is mostly responsible for the morbidity of the disease. Spread outside the abdomen with bone marrow involvement occurs only in the terminal stages usually following high-grade transformation.

PATHOPHYSIOLOGY

Just as the indolent clinical behavior coupled with its unusual histology led to the thinking that low-grade gastric MALT lymphoma was a nonneoplastic lymphoproliferative disorder (pseudolymphoma), so has the thinking been that the early stages of IPSID, during which response to antibiotics may be seen, are nonneoplastic. Both disorders, however, are monoclonal neoplasms de novo. The response of IPSID to antibiotics is in keeping with a degree of immunoresponsiveness of the tumor to a small intestinal

lumenal antigen, which is probably bacterial in nature. Unlike the stomach, in which the range of infective agents is limited, identification of a putative IPSID-associated organism within the intestinal bacterial flora is a more difficult task.

MANTLE CELL LYMPHOMA (LYMPHOMATOUS POLYPOSIS)

This condition, although relatively uncommon, is well characterized (70, 71). Most lesions occur in patients 50 years of age or older and there is no gender preponderance. Symptoms are nonspecific and include abdominal pain and melena. Barium studies or endoscopy characteristically show numerous polyps, the presence of which is confirmed in resection specimens (Fig. 17.30). Any part, or all, of the gastrointestinal tract may be involved, but the largest polyps tend to concentrate in the terminal ileum. With the increased use of endoscopy and "blind" biopsy, some mantle cell lesions are being diagnosed in a prepolypoid phase (unpublished observations). The bone marrow usually is involved at the time of clinical presentation.

HISTOPATHOLOGY (30)

The lesions initially involve preexisting lymphoid nodules, including Peyer patches, which are drawn out to form the polyps (Fig. 17.31). The lymphoma replaces the mantle zone and surrounds a "naked" follicle center (Fig. 17.32). These small lesions then fuse into larger polypoid masses exhibiting the characteristic features of mantle cell lymphoma. Naked follicle centers often persist and are selectively replaced with a consequent follicular growth pattern in all or part of the tumor. Typically, the cells are small, with a nucleus that has an irregular outline similar to that of the follicle center centrocyte (Fig. 17.33). Transformed nucleolated blasts in the so-called blastoid variant of the disease are larger cells with euchromatic smooth nuclear chromatin. Plasma cell differentiation does not occur, but invasion of individual glands with the formation of lymphoepithelial lesions may be seen.

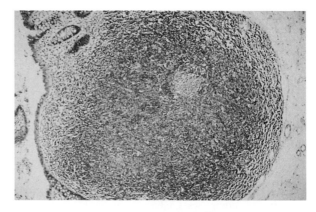

Figure 17.32 Lymphomatous polyposis (mantle cell lymphoma) of the colonic mucosa. Note neoplastic expansion of the mantle zone around a small residual reactive follicle center. (See color plate.)

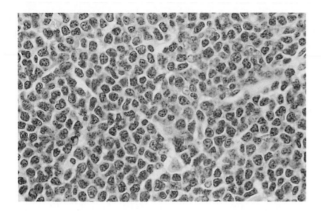

Figure 17.33 Typical cytologic appearance of mantle cell lymphoma cells. (See color plate.)

IMMUNOHISTOCHEMISTRY

The tumor cells express mature B-cell antigens and exhibit strong membrane staining for both IgM and IgD. They are usually CD5 and CD43-positive and, in almost all cases, the nuclei express cyclin D1 (72) (Fig. 17.34).

MOLECULAR GENETICS

Most mantle cell lymphomas, including those arising in the gastrointestinal tract, show t(11;14) in which there is translocation of the cyclin-D1 gene on chromosome 11 to chromosome 14 where it approximates the IgH gene. This translocation leads to upgrading of the expression of both cyclin-D1 RNA and protein.

CLINICAL BEHAVIOR

Like its nodal counterpart, gastrointestinal mantle cell lymphoma disseminates widely early in its course. Although histologically "low grade," it is an aggressive disease with a median survival of only 3 years (73).

DIFFERENTIAL DIAGNOSIS

The cells of mantle cell lymphoma can closely resemble the CCL cells of MALT lymphoma. In both tumors, reactive B-cell follicles may be seen, follicular "colonization" with a follicular growth pattern may occur, and lymphoepithelial lesions can be present (72). Thus, especially in small endoscopic biopsy specimens, the differential diagnosis between these two clinically different lymphomas can be extremely difficult. The virtual absence of transformed blasts in mantle cell lymphoma is helpful, but immunohistochemistry is the final arbiter. Nuclear expression of cyclin-D1 is never seen in MALT lymphoma and expression of CD5 is extremely rare.

BURKITT LYMPHOMA

In the Middle East, primary intestinal Burkitt lymphoma is a common disease of children (74). In Algeria, Burkitt lymphoma accounts for 46.5% of childhood non-Hodgkin lymphoma, and 60% of these lesions arise in the intestine (75). Except for its site, the features of this tumor, including its association with Epstein-Barr virus (EBV) and its molecular genetic characteristics, are identical to those of classic endemic African Burkitt lymphoma.

This form of primary gastrointestinal Burkitt lymphoma is more common in boys than in girls, and shows a peak incidence between 4 and 5 years of age. Any part of the intestine may be involved, but the disease shows a predilection for the terminal ileum; intussusception is, hence, a common mode of presentation.

The lesions vary from localized obstructing tumors to huge masses involving long lengths of intestine. Common features include retroperitoneal extension and mesenteric lymph node involvement.

The histologic appearances are those of classic African Burkitt lymphoma; lymphoepithelial lesions are not present.

In western countries, gastrointestinal lymphoma is rare in children, but the most common form, which also occurs in young adults, is equivalent to so-called nonendemic or sporadic Burkitt lymphoma. Fewer than 20% of cases are associated with EBV and the molecular genetic characteristics are similar (76, 77). The ileocecal region is again the most common site of presentation, but the histologic features may show subtle differences from endemic Burkitt lymphoma in the form of slightly greater cytologic variability with more cytoplasm in the tumor cells.

FOLLICULAR LYMPHOMA

Although the gastrointestinal tract is a frequent site of secondary involvement, primary follicular lymphoma is distinctly uncommon and only rarely arises as a primary tumor of the stomach. Occasionally, lesions arise in the small intestine, especially in the ileocecal region (78). Cases characterized by the formation of numerous polyps have been described (79).

In follicular lymphoma, the intestine is infiltrated by characteristic neoplastic follicles, accompanied by a variable interfollicular diffuse component (Fig. 17.35). Neither plasma cell differentiation nor lymphoepithelial lesions are present.

In small endoscopic biopsy samples, the differential diagnosis from MALT lymphoma with follicular colonization can be extremely difficult, even with the aid of immunohistochemistry (32). If frozen material is available, CD10 expression by neoplastic (light chain restricted) follicles is a distinctive property of fol-

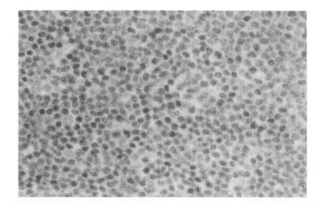

Figure 17.34 Mantle cell lymphoma (lymphomatous polyposis) stained for cyclin-D1. Most of the nuclei are positive. (See color plate.)

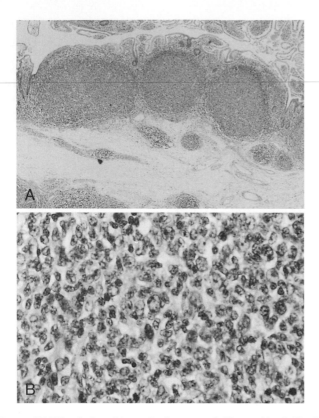

Figure 17.35   A. Small intestinal mucosa infiltrated by follicular lymphoma. **B.** Cytologic detail of this infiltrate shows a mixture of centroblasts and centrocytes. (See color plate.)

licular lymphoma. Molecular studies can be helpful in detecting bcl-2 rearrangement [t(14;18)], which is diagnostic of follicular lymphoma.

LYMPHOCYTIC LYMPHOMA (CHRONIC LYMPHOCYTIC LEUKEMIA)

Lymphocytic lymphoma rarely arises primarily in the gastrointestinal tract, but it is included in this discussion because secondary gastrointestinal involvement by chronic lymphocytic leukemia (CLL) should always be considered in the differential diagnosis of low-grade B-cell gastrointestinal lymphomas. The gastrointestinal tract is frequently involved in CLL, and endoscopic biopsy may be the first diagnostic procedure if gastrointestinal symptoms precede detection in the peripheral blood or peripheral lymph nodes. CLL is associated with a diffuse infiltrate of small lymphocytes in the mucosa with variable involvement of the deeper layers of the gastric or intestinal wall. Larger nucleolated paraimmunoblasts are characteristically present, either singly or in clusters forming proliferation centers. Reactive follicles within the infiltrate are not a consistent feature and lymphoepithelial lesions are not present.

Immunohistochemistry is, once more, important in differentiating CLL from MALT lymphoma and the other low-grade lymphomas. Expression of IgM, IgD, CD5, and CD23 are all characteristic of CLL. The immunohistochemical features that are

most helpful in distinguishing between the low-grade B-cell lymphomas that occur in the gastrointestinal tract are outlined in Table 17.4.

IMMUNODEFICIENCY-ASSOCIATED LYMPHOPROLIFERATIVE DISORDERS

Because a full discussion of this complex subject is beyond the scope of this chapter, only a brief overview follows.

Extranodal sites and, in particular, the gastrointestinal tract are the favored sites for involvement by this group of disorders. The immunodeficiency is rarely congenital (including conditions such as hereditary ataxia telangiectasia, severe combined immunodeficiency, etc.) and, more commonly, is acquired owing to human immunodeficiency virus (HIV) infection (AIDS) or therapeutic immunosuppression for purposes of organ transplantation.

The pathogenesis and pathology of these disorders are essentially similar, regardless of the specific underlying cause. Suppression of T cell-mediated immunity leads to reactivation of a latent EBV infection or, less commonly, increased susceptibility to an initial infection with the virus. Epstein-Barr virus causes blastic transformation and proliferation of B cells, which in immunocompetent individuals, is controlled by EBV-specific T cells. In the immunosuppressed individual, this B-cell proliferation is uncontrolled and leads to growth of B-cell tumor masses, which may be polyclonal in the initial stages. Subsequent changes include outgrowth of a monoclonal population and the development of clonal molecular genetic abnormalities, i.e., true lymphoma. A subgroup of Burkitt-like lymphomas seen in AIDS patients is not associated with EBV.

ACQUIRED IMMUNODEFICIENCY SYNDROME (AIDS)

Most gastrointestinal lymphoproliferative lesions in AIDS are EBV-associated large (high-grade) B-cell lymphomas (80). Their development may include a polyclonal phase, but this feature is

TABLE 17.4	Immunohistochemistry of Low Grade B-Cell Lymphomas Occurring in the Gastrointestinal Tract			
	MALT Lymphoma	Mantle Cell Lymphoma	Follicular Lymphoma	Lymphocytic Lymphoma (CLL)
Ig	M	M, D	M (G)	M, D
CD20	+	+	+	+
CD5	–	+	–	+
CD10	–	–	+	–
CD23	–	–	–	+
Cyclin D1	–	+	–	–

immaterial because, at least at present, the immunodeficiency is irreversible. The tumors occur throughout the gastrointestinal tract and are often multifocal. In most cases, the lymphoma shows rearrangement of the c-myc gene. Occasional T-cell lymphomas have been described (81). The Burkitt-like non-EBV-associated lymphomas (82) that are also seen in association with HIV disease and AIDS do not occur in the gastrointestinal tract. A few cases of low-grade MALT gastric lymphomas in AIDS patients have been reported (83).

POST-TRANSPLANT LYMPHOPROLIFERATIVE DISORDER (PTLD)

Gastrointestinal lymphoproliferative lesions are a well-recognized hazard of therapeutic immunosuppression for the purposes of organ transplantation (84, 85). The incidence of this complication and the posttransplant interval varies with the particular organ being transplanted and the choice of immunosuppressive agent(s). Because the immunosuppression can, at least to a certain degree, be controlled, it is important to recognize the phase of the disorder when it manifests.

In the early, polyclonal phase, the lesion is typically polymorphic comprising a mixture of transformed B cells, plasma cells, and small lymphocytes. With progression, the lesion of PTLD becomes more monomorphic with emergence of a monoclonal B-cell population, and is less likely to respond to modulation of the immunosuppression. The final phase is frank immunoblastic lymphoma, which is often characterized by c-myc gene rearrangement.

ENTEROPATHY-ASSOCIATED T-CELL LYMPHOMA

The long-recognized association between intestinal lymphoma and malabsorption has been the subject of ongoing controversy with respect to the cause and effect relationship, the nature of the enteropathy causing the malabsorption, and the nature of the lymphoma. It is now clear that enteropathy precedes the lymphoma rather than the reverse, although the onset of lymphoma may aggravate the malabsorption (86). The histology and distribution of the enteropathy are those of celiac disease and, in keeping with this association, objective gluten sensitivity has been formally demonstrated in 70% of a series of patients with the disorder (87). A gluten-free diet has been shown to protect against the development of lymphoma (88). These patients also share the HLA phenotype characteristic of celiac disease (89, 90) and often manifest other celiac disease-associated conditions, including dermatitis herpetiformis and splenic atrophy (91). The T-cell nature of the lymphoma has been well established in both immunophenotypic and genotypic studies (92).

CLINICAL PRESENTATION

Enteropathy-associated T-cell lymphoma (EATL) may complicate long-established celiac disease, but more often follows a short history of so-called adult onset celiac disease. This is in keeping with the protective effect of a gluten-free diet, because patients with the adult onset form of the disease are presumed, nevertheless, to have suffered from gluten sensitivity since birth. Some patients have no

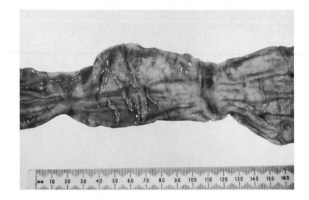

Figure 17.36 Jejunum from a patient with enteropathy-associated T-cell lymphoma. Two strictures are caused by ulcerating lymphomatous infiltration. (See color plate.)

history of gluten sensitivity, but jejunal villous atrophy and crypt hyperplasia are found after resection of the lymphoma. In a few cases, the jejunum shows only an excess of intraepithelial lymphocytes or is even normal. This finding is consistent with the small group of patients with so-called latent celiac disease in whom the enteropathy is demonstrated only after a formal gluten challenge (93).

The incidence of EATL is equal between genders and the disease usually occurs in patients 50 years of age or older. The typical presentation is that of abdominal pain and deteriorating malabsorption in a patient with established adult celiac disease. Other presentations include the apparent sudden onset of severe, usually gluten-insensitive, malabsorption or an acute abdominal emergency involving perforation or hemorrhage. Another group of patients experiences a prolonged chronic illness characterized by malabsorption and intestinal ulceration, a condition known as ulcerative jejunitis (see subsequent discussion). Enteropathy-associated T-cell lymphoma has usually already disseminated by the time of diagnosis. Common sites of involvement include mesenteric lymph nodes, liver, spleen, bone marrow, lung, and skin.

MACROSCOPIC APPEARANCE

Most lesions arise in the jejunum, but any part of the gastrointestinal tract can be involved. The lymphoma is commonly multifocal and causes multiple ulcers, strictures, or tumor nodules (Fig. 17.36); a single large lymphomatous mass is found in some patients. EATL often extends into the mesentery and mesenteric lymph nodes are commonly enlarged. In a few cases, minimal macroscopic evidence of the disease is evident in the intestine in the face of more obvious mesenteric lymph node involvement or even extraabdominal spread.

HISTOPATHOLOGY

Most cases of EATL are characterized by highly pleomorphic large, often bizarre cells (Fig. 17.37), but in others, the cells are more monomorphic immunoblasts or even small to medium-sized lymphocytes (30). Intraepithelial tumor cells may be prominent. Histologic interpretation is frequently complicated by a heavy inflammatory component, with particular prominence of eosino-

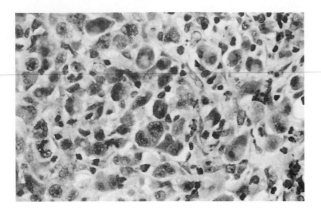

Figure 17.37 Typical histologic appearance of enteropathy-associated T-cell lymphoma. (See color plate.)

phils, and large areas of necrosis within which lymphoma cells are difficult to identify. Noncaseating epithelioid granulomas are present in some cases.

The uninvolved small intestine usually shows crypt hyperplasia with villous atrophy together with plasmacytosis of the lamina propria. An increase in intraepithelial lymphocytes is present and may be exceptionally florid (Fig. 17.38). These cells may extend into the lamina propria and merge with the lymphoma. Occasionally, the intestinal mucosa shows no abnormality or only an increase in intraepithelial lymphocytes. In these cases, it is likely that the celiac disease is effectively latent (93).

Multiple benign-appearing inflammatory mucosal ulcers of the small intestine are frequently seen in patients with EATL. Partial or complete healing of these ulcers is accompanied by scarring, which may lead to stricture formation. Healing also results in distortion of the mucosal architecture and the emergence of glands lined by cells of the ulceration-associated lineage (94) (pyloric metaplasia).

In a few patients, for reasons discussed previously, the mucosa may appear normal or show only minimal changes.

In involved mesenteric lymph nodes, the paracortex is expanded by the lymphoma cells, which may also be found within sinuses. Large areas of necrosis are present in some cases.

IMMUNOHISTOCHEMISTRY

The tumor cells in EATL are characteristically CD3+, CD4-, CD8/+, CD103+ and contain cytotoxic granules that stain with the TIA-1 antibody (95) (Fig. 17.39). The large tumor cells are frequently CD30+. This immunophenotype is closely similar to that of intraepithelial T cells and suggests that EATL may be derived from this cell population. The strikingly florid increase in intraepithelial T cells seen in some cases and the presence of intraepithelial tumor cells add weight to this suggestion.

MOLECULAR GENETICS

EATL is associated with clonal rearrangement of the TCR-β (92) and δ-chain genes, but no other reproducible gene rearrangements have been identified. TCR-δ gene rearrangement can be studied in DNA extracted from paraffin-embedded tissue; using this technique, investigators have shown that both the intraepithelial T cells

and the "inflammatory" ulcers in EATL often show monoclonal TCR-δ chain gene rearrangement in common with the lymphoma itself (96, 97).

CLINICAL COURSE

With the exception of a few cases in which resection of localized lymphoma results in a prolonged remission, the prognosis in EATL is abysmal. Gastrointestinal recurrences with perforation or hemorrhage usually follow surgery or chemotherapy.

CHRONIC ULCERATIVE JEJUNITIS AND EATL

Chronic ulcerative jejunitis (jejunoileitis) is another recognized complication of celiac disease that is closely related to EATL (98, 99). Indeed, the frequent presence of multiple "benign" ulcers in EATL, and the documentation of cases in which EATL has emerged after rendering a diagnosis of ulcerative jejunitis, have led to the suggestion that ulcerative jejunitis is a manifestation of EATL (98). The opposite view, that ulcerative jejunitis is a benign inflammatory disorder in its own right, is supported by those cases in which no morphologic evidence of lymphoma can be found despite thorough investigation (100). The TCR-δ chain rearrangement studies just mentioned (96) showed that a monoclonal neoplastic T-cell population can be present in an apparently inflammatory intestinal ulcer. Extension of these studies to cases of ulcerative jejunitis has shown that multiple ulcers in a given patient share the same monoclonal T-cell population. Results of these molecular studies strongly support the view that ulcerative jejunitis is a manifestation of EATL.

T-CELL LYMPHOMA UNASSOCIATED WITH ENTEROPATHY

In a number of case reports, authors describe apparently primary T-cell gastrointestinal lymphomas in which they found no evidence of enteropathy. In view of the variable morphology of the intestinal mucosa in EATL, the evidence for these cases must be examined critically.

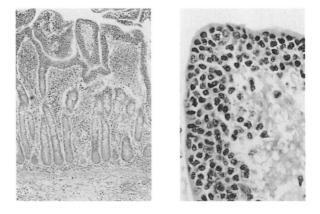

Figure 17.38 "Uninvolved" mucosa from a case of enteropathy-associated T-cell lymphoma showing florid intraepithelial lymphocytosis. (See color plate.)

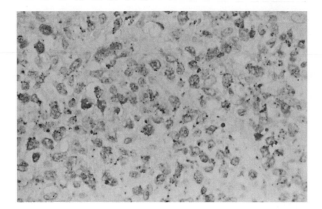

Figure 17.39 Enteropathy-associated T-cell lymphoma stained with antibody TIA-1 to show cytotoxic granules in lymphoma cells. (See color plate.)

HISTIOCYTIC AND MYELOPROLIFERATIVE LESIONS OF THE GASTROINTESTINAL TRACT

Rare cases of gastrointestinal Langerhans cell histiocytosis have been described, as have isolated cases of mast cell disease.

HISTIOCYTIC SARCOMA (TRUE HISTIOCYTIC LYMPHOMA)

Small collections and single cases of histiocytic malignancy arising in the small intestine have been described (101). These tumors manifest as large, usually single, ulcerating masses with obvious lymph node involvement. Histologically, they are polymorphic, comprising large cells with foamy cytoplasm and highly contorted nuclei, smaller more typical histiocytes, and fibroblastic sarcomatoid cells. Collectively, the cells are CD68+ with clearly neoplastic subpopulations in which the cytoplasm contains lysozyme or S-100 protein. The tumor cells thus embrace the features of both phagocytic histiocytes and interdigitating reticulum cells. The clinical behavior of these tumors has not been documented.

GRANULOCYTIC SARCOMA

Classic acute myeloid leukemia may be complicated by diffuse infiltration of the gastrointestinal tract. Less commonly, this disease results in isolated solid tumors or granulocytic sarcoma (102). Although such tumor formation is rare, when it occurs, it can easily be confused with lymphoma. The tumor cells are characterized by moderately abundant eosinophilic cytoplasm and an eccentric or central nucleus with homogeneous pale-gray chromatin. In some cases, these cells are easily confused with plasma cells. The traditional histochemical stain for ASD chloracetate esterase may be positive, but frequently is negative. Immunohistochemical staining for lysozyme, however, is usually positive in these cases. Obvious acute myeloid leukemia usually manifests soon after the diagnosis of granulocytic sarcoma, but intervals as long as 15 years have been reported.

REFERENCES

1. Dawson IMP, Cornes JS, Morson BC. Primary malignant lymphoid tumours of the intestinal tract. Report of 37 cases with a study of factors influencing prognosis. Br J Surg 1961;49:80–89.
2. Freeman C, Berg JW, Cutler SJ. Occurrence and prognosis of extranodal lymphomas. Cancer 1972;29:252–260.
3. Otter R, Bieger R, Kluin PM, et al. Primary gastrointestinal non-Hodgkin's lymphoma in a population-based registry. Br J Cancer 1989;60:745–750.
4. Azab MB, Henry-Amar M, Rougier P et al. Prognostic factors in primary gastrointestinal non-Hodgkin's lymphoma: A multivariate analysis, report of 106 cases, and review of the literature. Cancer 1989;64:1208–1217.
5. Doglioni C, Wotherspoon AC, Moschini A, et al. High incidence of primary gastric lymphoma in northeastern Italy. Lancet 1992;339:834–835.
6. Musshoff K. Klinische Stadieneinteilung der Nicht-Hodgkin-Lymphome. Strahlentherapie 1977;153:218–221.
7. Rohatiner A, d'Amore F, Coiffer B, et al. Report on a workshop convened to discuss the pathological and staging classifications of gastrointestinal tract lymphoma. Ann Oncol 1994;5:397–400.
8. Isaacson P, Wright DH. Malignant lymphoma of mucosa-associated lymphoid tissue. A distinctive type of B-cell lymphoma. Cancer 1983;52:1410–1416.
9. Isaacson P, Wright DH. Extranodal malignant lymphoma arising from mucosa-associated lymphoid tissue. Cancer 1984;53:2515–2524.
10. Spencer J, Finn T, Pulford KAF, et al. The human gut resembles a novel population of B lymphocytes which resemble marginal zone cells. Clin Exp Immunol 1985; 62:607–610.
11. Negrini R, Lisato L, Zanella I, et al. Helicobacter pylori infection induces antibodies cross-reacting with human gastric mucosa. Gastroenterology 1991;101:437–445.
12. Wyatt JI, Rathbone BJ. Immune response of the gastric mucosa to Campylobacter pylori. Scand J Gastroenterol 1988;suppl 142:44–49.
13. Stolte M, Eidt S. Lymphoid follicles in antral mucosa: immune response to Campylobacter pylori? J Clin Pathol 1989;42:1269–1271.
14. Genta RM, Hamner HW, Graham DY. Gastric lymphoid follicles in Helicobacter pylori infection: frequency, distribution, and response to triple therapy. Hum Pathol 1993;24:577–583.
15. Harris NL, Jaffe ES, Stein H, et al. A revised European-American Classification of lymphoid neoplasms: A proposal from the International Lymphoma Study Group. Blood 1994;84:1361–1392.
16. Ferraccioli GF, Sorrentino D, De Vita S, et al. B cell clonality in gastric lymphoid tissues of patients with Sjogren's syndrome. Ann Rheu Dis 1996;55:311–316.
17. Wotherspoon AC, Ortiz-Hidalgo C, Falzon MR, Isaacson PG. Helicobacter pylori-associated gastritis and primary B-cell gastric lymphoma. Lancet 1991;338:1175–1176.
18. Parsonnet J, Friedman GD, Vandersteen DP, et al. Helicobacter pylori infection and the risk of gastric carcinoma. N Engl J Med 1991;325:1127–1131.
19. Hussell T, Isaacson PG, Crabtree JE, Spencer J. The response of cells from low-grade B-cell gastric lymphomas of mucosa-associated lymphoid tissue to Helicobacter pylori. Lancet 1993;342:571–574.
20. Hussell T, Isaacson PG, Crabtree JE, Spencer J. Helicobacter pylori-specific tumour-infiltrating T cells provide contact dependent help for the growth of malignant B cells in low-grade gastric lymphoma of mucosa-associated lymphoid tissue. J Pathol 1996;178:122–127.
21. Wotherspoon AC, Doglioni C, Diss TC, Pan LX, Moschini A, de Boni M, Isaacson PG. Regression of primary low-grade B-cell gastric lymphoma of mucosa-associated lymphoid tissue after eradication of Helicobacter pylori. Lancet 1993;342:575–577.
22. Wotherspoon AC, Doglioni C, de Boni M, Spencer J, Isaacson PG. Antibiotic treatment for low-grade gastric MALT lymphoma. Lancet 1994;343:1503.
23. Weber DM, Dimopoulos MA, Anandu DP, Pugh WC, Steinbach G. Regression of gastric lymphoma of mucosa-associated lymphoid tissue with antibiotic therapy for Helicobacter pylori. Gastroenterology 1994;107:1835–1838.

24. Roggero E, Zucca E, Pinotti G, et al. Eradication of Helicobacter pylori infection in primary low-grade gastric lymphoma of mucosa-associated lymphoid tissue. Ann Intern Med 1995;122:767–769.

25. Bayerdorffer E, Neubauer A, Rudolph B, et al. Regression of primary gastric lymphoma of mucosa-associated lymphoid tissue type after cure of Helicobacter pylori infection. Lancet 1995;345:1591–1594.

26. Montalban C, Castrillo JM, Abraira V, et al. Gastric B-cell mucosa-associated lymphoid tissue (MALT) lymphoma. Clinicopathological study and evaluation of the prognostic factors in 143 patients. Ann Oncol 1995;6:355–362.

27. Blecker U, McKeithan TW, Hart J, Kirschner BS. Resolution of Helicobacter pylori-associated gastric lympho-proliferative disease in a child. Gastroenterology 1995;109:973–977.

28. Savio A, Franzin G, Wotherspoon AC, et al. Diagnosis and posttreatment follow-up of Helicobacter pylori-positive gastric lymphoma of mucosa-associated lymphoid tissue: Histology, polymerase chain reaction, or both? Blood 1996;87:1255–1260.

29. Hayes J, Dunn E. Has the incidence of primary gastric lymphoma increased? Cancer 1989;63:2073–2076.

30. Isaacson PG, Norton AJ. Extranodal lymphomas. Edinburgh, Churchill Livingstone, 1994.

31. Zamboni G, Franzin G, Scarpa A, et al. Carcinoma-like signet-ring cells in gastric mucosa-associated lymphoid tissue (MALT) lymphoma. Am J Surg Pathol 1996;20:588–598.

32. Isaacson PG, Wotherspoon AC, Diss T, Pan L. Follicular colonization in B-cell lymphoma of mucosa-associated lymphoid tissue. Am J Surg Pathol 1991;15:819–828.

33. Wotherspoon AC, Doglioni C, Isaacson PG. Low-grade gastric B-cell lymphoma of mucosa-associated lymphoid tissue (MALT) a multi-focal disease. Histopathology 1992;20:29–34.

34. Algara P, Martinez P, Sanchez L, et al. The detection of B-cell monoclonal populations by polymerase chain reaction: accuracy of approach and application in gastric endoscopic biopsy specimens. Hum Pathol 1993;24:1184–1188.

35. Du MQ, Peng HZ, Diss TC, et al. Splenic dissemination of gastric MALT lymphoma. J Pathol 1996;11A.

36. Qin Y, Greiner A, Trunk MJF, Schmausser B, Ott MM, Muller-Hermelink H-K. Somatic hypermutation in low-grade mucosa-associated lymphoid tissue-type B-cell lymphoma. Blood 1995;86:3528–3534.

37. Du M, Diss TC, Xu C, Peng H, Isaacson PG, Pan L. Ongoing mutation in MALT lymphoma immunoglobulin gene suggests that antigen stimulation plays a role in the clonal expansion. Leukemia 1996;10:1190–1197.

38. Peng H, Chen G, Du M, Singh N, Isaacson PG, Pan L. Replication error phenotype and p53 gene mutation in lymphomas of mucosa-associated lymphoid tissue. Am J Pathol 1996;148:643–648.

39. Peng HZ, Diss TC, Isaacson PG, Pan LX. C-myc gene abnormalities in mucosa-associated lymphoid tissue (MALT) lymphomas. J Pathol (in press).

40. Du M, Peng H, Singh N, Isaacson PG, Pan L. The accumulation of p53 abnormalities is associated with progression of mucosa-associated lymphoid tissue lymphoma. Blood 1995;86:4587–4593.

41. Wotherspoon AC, Finn TM, Isaacson PG. Trisomy 3 in low-grade B-cell lymphomas of mucosa-associated lymphoid tissue. Blood 1995;85:2000–2004.

42. Cogliatti SB, Schmid U, Schumacher U, et al. Primary B-cell gastric lymphoma: A clinicopathological study of 145 patients. Gastroenterology 1991;101:1159–1170.

43. Hsi ED, Greenson JK, Singleton TP, Siddiqui J, Schnitzer B, Ross CW. Detection of immunoglobulin heavy chain gene rearrangement by polymerase chain reaction in chronic active gastritis associated with Helicobacter pylori. Hum Pathol 1996;27:290–296.

44. Fischbach W, Kestel W, Kirchner T, et al. Malignant lymphomas of the upper gastrointestinal tract. Results of a prospective study in 103 patients. Cancer 1992;70:1075–1080.

45. Chan JKC, Ng CS, Isaacson PG. Relationship between high-grade lymphoma and low-grade B-cell mucosa-associated lymphoid tissue lymphoma (MALToma) of the stomach. Am J Pathol 1990;136:1153–1164.

46. Villuendas R, Piris MA, Orradre JL, et al. Different bcl-2 protein expression in high-grade B-cell lymphomas derived from lymph node or mucosa-associated lymphoid tissue. Am J Pathol 1991;139:989–993.

47. Montalban C, Manzanal A, Castrillo JM, Escribano L, Bellas C. Low-grade gastric B-cell MALT lymphoma progressing into high-grade lymphoma. Clonal identity of the two stages of the tumour, unusual bone involvement and leukaemic dissemination. Histopathology 1995;27:89–91.

48. Weingrad DN, Decosse JJ, Sherlock P, et al. Primary gastrointestinal lymphoma: a 30-year review. Cancer 1982;49:1258–1265.

49. Joensuu H, Söderström KO, Klemi PJ, Eevola E. Nuclear DNA content and its prognostic value in lymphoma of the stomach. Cancer 1987;60:3042–3048.

50. Wotherspoon AC, Isaacson PG. Synchronous adenocarcinoma and low-grade B-cell lymphoma of mucosa associated lymphoid tissue (MALT) of the stomach. Histopathology 1995;27:325–331.

51. Nakamura S, Akazawa K, Yao T, Tsuneyoshi M. Primary gastric lymphoma. A clinicopathologic study of 233 cases with special reference to evaluation with the MIB-1 index. Cancer 1995;76:1313–1324.

52. Domizio P, Owen RA, Shepherd NA, et al. Primary lymphoma of the small intestine: a clinicopathological study of 119 cases. Am J Surg Pathol 1993;17:429–432.

53. Greenstein AJ, Mullin GE, Strauchen JA, et al. Lymphoma in inflammatory bowel disease. Cancer 1992;69:1119–1123.

54. Schmid C, Vazquez JJ, Diss TC, Isaacson PG. Primary B-cell mucosa-associated lymphoid tissue lymphoma presenting as a solitary colorectal polyp. Histopathology 1994;24:357–362.

55. Radaszkiewicz T, Dragosics B, Bauer P. Gastrointestinal malignant lymphomas of the mucosa-associated lymphoid tissue: Factors relevant to prognosis. Gastroenterology 1992;102:1628–1638.

56. Fieber SS, Schaefer HJ. Lymphoid hyperplasia of the terminal ileum —a clinical entity? Gastroenterology 1966;50:83–98.

57. Rubin A, Isaacson PG. Florid reactive lymphoid hyperplasia of the terminal ileum in adults: a condition bearing a close resemblance to low-grade malignant lymphoma. Histopathology 1990;17:19–26.

58. Hermans PE, Huizenga KA, Hoffman HN, et al. Dysgamma-globulinemia associated with nodular lymphoid hyperplasia of the small intestine. Am J Med 1966;40:78–89.

59. Matuchansky C, Touchard G, Lemaire M et al. Malignant lymphoma of the small bowel associated with diffuse nodular lymphoid hyperplasia. N Engl J Med 1985;313:166–171.

60. Ramot B, Shahin N, Bubis JJ. Malabsorption syndrome in lymphoma of small intestine. A study of 13 cases. Isr J Med Sci 1965;1:221–226.

61. Price SK. Immunoproliferative small intestinal disease: a study of 13 cases with alpha heavy-chain disease. Histopathology 1990;17:7–17.

62. Rambaud JC, Modigliani R, Phuoc BK, et al. Non-secretory alpha-chain disease in intestinal lymphoma. N Engl J Med 1980;303:53.

63. Ben-Ayed F, Halphen M, Najjar T et al. Treatment of alpha chain disease. Results of a prospective study in 21 Tunisian patients by the Tunisian-French Intestinal Lymphoma Study Group. Cancer 1989;63:1251–1256.

64. Gilinsky NH, Novis BH, Wright JP, Dent DM, King H, Marks IN. Immunoproliferative small-intestinal disease: clinical features and outcome in 30 cases. Medicine 1987;66:438–446.

65. Isaacson PG, Dogan A, Price SK, Spencer J. Immunoproliferative small-intestinal disease: An immunohistochemical study. Am J Surg Pathol 1989;13:1023–1033.

66. Isaacson PG. Middle eastern intestinal lymphoma. Sem Diag Pathol 1985;2:210–223.

67. Isaacson PG, Price SK. Light chains in Mediterranean lymphoma. J Clin Pathol 1985;38:601–607.

68. Smith W, Price SK, Isaacson PG. Immunoglobulin gene rearrangement in immunoproliferative small intestinal disease (IPSID). J Clin Pathol 1987;40:1291–1297.

69. Berger R, Bernheim A, Tsapis A, Brouet J-C, Seligmann M. Cytogenetic studies in four cases of alpha chain disease. Cancer Genet Cytogenet 1986;22:219–223.

70. Isaacson PG, MacLennan KA, Subbuswamy SG. Multiple lymphomatous polyposis of the gastrointestinal tract. Histopathology 1984;8:641–656.

71. Lavergne A, Brouland J-P, Launay E, Nemeth J, Ruskone-Fourmestraux A, Galian A. Multiple lymphomatous polyposis of the gastrointestinal tract. An extensive histopathologic and immunohistochemical study of 12 cases. Cancer 1994;74:3042–3050.

72. Kumar S, Krenacs L, Otsuki T, et al. Bcl-1 rearrangement and cyclin D-1 protein expression in multiple lymphomatous polyposis. Am J Clin Pathol 1996;105:737–743.

73. Ruskone-Fourmestraux A, Aegerter P, Delmer A, Brousse N, Galian A, Rambaud JC. Primary digestive tract lymphoma: a prospective multicentric study of 91 patients. Group de Etude des Lymphomes Digestifs. Gastroenterology 1993;105:1662–1671.

74. Anaissie E, Geha S, Allam C, et al. Burkitt's lymphoma in the Middle East: A study of 34 cases. Cancer 1985;56:2539–2543.

75. Ladjadj Y, Philip T, Lenoir GM et al. Abdominal Burkitt-type lymphomas in Algeria. Br J Cancer 1984;49:503–512.

76. Pelicci PG, Knowles DM, Magrath I, Dalla-Favera R. Chromosomal breakpoints and structural alteration of the c-myc locus differ in endemic and sporadic forms of Burkitt lymphoma. Proc Natl Acad Sci USA 1986;83:2984–2988.

77. Neri A, Barriga F, Knowles DM, et al. Different regions of the immunoglobulin heavy-chain locus are involved in chromosomal translocations in distinct pathogenetic forms of Burkitt lymphoma. Proc Natl Acac Sci USA 1988;85:2748–2752.

78. LeBrun DP, Kamel OW, Cleary ML, et al. Follicular lymphomas of the gastrointestinal tract. Pathologic features in 31 cases and bcl-2 oncogenic protein expression. Am J Pathol 1992;140:1327–1335.

79. Moynihan MJ, Bast MA, Chan WC, et al. Lymphomatous polyposis. A neoplasm of either follicular mantle or germinal center cell origin. Am J Surg Pathol 1996;20:442–452.

80. Levine AM. Acquired immunodeficiency syndrome-related lymphoma. Blood 1992;80:8–20.

81. Waller EK, Ziemianska M, Bangs CD, Cleary M, Weissman I, Kamel OW. Characterization of posttreatment lymphomas that express T-cell associated markers: immunophenotypes, molecular genetics, cytogenetics and heterotransplantation in severe combined immunodeficient mice. Blood 1993;82:247–261.

82. Carbone A, Gloghini A, Gaidano G, et al. AIDS-related Burkitt's lymphoma. Morphologic and immunophenotypic study of biopsy specimens. Am J Clin Pathol 1995;103:561–567.

83. Wotherspoon AC, Diss TL, Pan L, Singh N, Whelan J, Isaacson PG. Low-grade gastric B-cell lymphoma of mucosa associated lymphoid tissue in immunocompromised patients. Histopathology 1996;28:129–134.

84. Craig FE, Gulley ML, Banks PM. Posttransplant lymphoproliferative disorders. Am J Clin Pathol 1993;99:265–276.

85. Nalesnik MA, Jaffe R, Starzl TE, et al. The pathology of posttransplant lymphoproliferative disorders occurring in the setting of cyclosporine A-Prednisone immunosuppression. Am J Pathol 1988;133:173–192.

86. Isaacson PG. Intestinal lymphoma and enteropathy. Editorial. J Pathol 1995;177:111–113.

87. Swinson CM, Slavin G, Coles EC, Booth CC. Coeliac disease and malignancy. Lancet 1983;i:111–115.

88. Holmes GKT, Prior P, Lane MR, et al. Malignancy in coeliac disease —effect of a gluten free diet. Gut 1989;30:333–338.

89. O'Driscoll BRC, Stevens FM, O'Gorman TA et al. HLA-type of patients with coeliac disease and malignancy in the west of Ireland. Gut 1982;23:662–665.

90. Howell WM, Shu Tong Leung, Jones DB, Nakshabendi I, Wright DH. HLA-DRB, DQA and DQB polymorphism in celiac disease and enteropathy associated T-cell lymphoma: common features and additional risk factors for malignancy. Hum Immunol 1995; 43:29–37.

91. Freeman HJ, Weinstein WM, Shnitka TK, Piercey JRA, Wensel RH. Primary abdominal lymphoma. Presenting manifestation of celiac sprue or complicating dermatitis herpetiformis. Am J Med 1977; 63:585–594.

92. Isaacson PG, Spencer J, Connolly CE. Malignant histiocytosis of the intestine: a T-cell lymphoma. Lancet 1985;28:688–691.

93. O'Mahony S, Vestey JP, Ferguson A. Similarities in intestinal humoral immunity in dermatitis herpetiformis without enteropathy and in coeliac disease. Lancet 1990;335:1487–1490.

94. Wright NA, Pike C, Elia G. Induction of a novel epidermal growth factor-secreting cell lineage by mucosal ulceration in human gastrointestinal stem cells. Nature 1990;343:82–85.

95. Russell GJ, Nagler-Anderson C, Anderson P, Bhan AK. Cytotoxic potential of intraepithelial lymphocytes (IELs). Presence of TIA-1, the cytolytic granule-associated protein, in human IELs in normal and diseased intestine. Am J Pathol 1993;143:350–354.

96. Alfsen GC, Beiske K, Bell H, Marton PF. Low-grade intestinal lymphoma of intraepithelial T lymphocytes with concomitant enteropathy-associated T cell lymphoma: case report suggesting a possible histogenetic relationship. Hum Pathol 1989;20:909–913.

97. Murray A, Cuevas EC, Jones DB, Wright DH. Study of the immunohistochemistry and T cell clonality of enteropathy-associated T cell lymphoma. Am J Pathol 1995;146:509–519.

98. Isaacson P, Wright DH. Malignant histiocytosis of the intestine: its relationship to malabsorption and ulcerative colitis. Hum Pathol 1978;9:661–677.

99. Jewell DP. Ulcerative enteritis. Br Med J 1983;287:1740–1741.

100. Mills PR, Brown IL, Watkinson G. Idiopathic ulcerative enteritis. Report of five cases and review of the literature. Q J Med 1980; 49:133–149.

101. Milchgrub S, Kamel OW, Wiley E, et al. Malignant histiocytic neoplasms of the small intestine. Am J Surg Pathol 1992;16:11–20.

102. Brugo EA, Marshall RB, Riberi AM, Pautasso OE. Preleukemic granulocytic sarcomas of the gastrointestinal tract. Report of two cases. Am J Clin Pathol 1977;68:616–621.

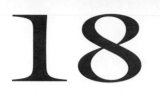

18 MESENCHYMAL TUMORS OF THE GASTROINTESTINAL TRACT

Henry D. Appelman

GENERAL FEATURES

The gastrointestinal tract is a long tube endowed with a variety of motile activities that are the responsibility of a the muscularis propria, a huge mass of smooth muscle, mainly situated in a deep bilayer. The tract also contains other smooth muscle, such as the thin bilayer that separates the mucosa from the submucosa, the muscularis mucosae. Furthermore, all layers contain blood vessels, the larger of which have considerable smooth muscle in their walls.

In addition to this impressive smooth muscle mass are other types of mesenchymal tissue. Nerves with their Schwann cell support traverse all layers and are concentrated mostly in plexuses in the muscularis propria and in the submucosa; the exception is the esophagus, in which the submucosal plexus is insignificant. Scattered adipose cells are found in the submucosa, especially in the right colon. Fibroblasts and myofibroblasts are ubiquitous. Clearly, if

there are blood vessels and lymphatic vessels, then there are endothelial cells to line them. Finally, the serosal surfaces throughout the gut are covered by mesothelium. Presumably all or some of these tissues give rise to the mesenchymal tumors of the gut, and/or the gut mesenchymal tumors presumably differentiate along the lines of these tissues. It appears however, that this assumption is only partly true, as discussed subsequently.

CELL ORIGIN AND DIFFERENTIATION: LEIOMYOMAS, SCHWANNOMAS, NERVE PLEXUS TUMORS, OR NONE OF THE ABOVE?

Two broad groups of mesenchymal tumors originate within the gastrointestinal tract. The first and smaller group contains tumors identical to those that arise in the somatic soft tissues. In this group, the benign neoplasms are composed of differentiated mesenchymal cells. Some of these lesions are typical leiomyomas, identical in every morphologic aspect to those arising elsewhere, including the uterus; most are tiny and are found in the esophagus and less frequently in the rectum. It is surprising that typical, totally differentiated leiomyomas are so rare in the stomach, small bowel, and colon, considering the mass of smooth muscle in those parts of the gut. Submucosal lipomas composed of mature adipocytes arise all throughout the gastrointestinal tract, but they are found mainly in the colon. Patients with von Recklinghausen disease may form plexiform neurofibromas anywhere in the gut, although these lesions are most common in the colon. Hemangiomas and lymphangiomas occur throughout the gut, but they are uncommon. The typical malignant counterparts, the leiomyosarcomas, the liposarcomas, the malignant schwannomas, and the angiosarcomas also arise in the gut, but they are so rare as to be curiosities. It is likely that published case reports exist for at least one of every imaginable mesenchymal tumor, both benign and malignant, that has arisen in the gastrointestinal tract, including synovial sarcoma, rhabdomyosarcoma, osteosarcoma, and malignant fibrous histiocytoma (1).

The second and far larger and more important group of mesenchymal tumors avoids the esophagus and arises in the stomach and intestines. This group comprises spindle cell and epithelioid cell tumors, which are different from typical somatic soft tissue tumors; that is, they are uniquely gastrointestinal, although a few can be found in the omentum, mesenteries, and retroperitoneum. Certainly, with all the smooth muscle in the gastrointestinal tract, it would be foolish to avoid designating all of these tumors, especially those composed of spindle cells, as smooth muscle tumors, unless there were compelling reasons to do so. The early students of gut mesenchymal tumors were no fools, because they usually referred to these tumors as leiomyomas or leiomyosarcomas (2, 3). These designations were based on the light microscopic suggestions of fibrillar cytoplasm in the cells of many of these tumors, the pericellular reticulin fibers that seemed to indicate smooth muscle differentiation, the blunt-ended nuclei that were considered at one time to be a hallmark of the smooth muscle cell, and the fact that many tumors occurred partially or completely within the muscularis propria.

The fact that some tumors contained rounded or polygonal epithelioid cells instead of, or as well as, spindled cells added confusion to the smooth muscle differentiation issue. Clearly, these rounded cells did not look like any normal mesenchymal cells of the gut and certainly did not resemble smooth muscle. Some tumors, especially those in the stomach, were composed entirely of epithelioid cells, but even these unusual tumors were also assigned smooth muscle names.

Adding to the confusion is a gastric neoplasm that contains spindle cells arranged in spectacular palisades. Who could blame any sane pathologist for deciding such a tumor was a schwannoma or a neurilemmoma? Thus, in some reports, such a subset of spindle cell palisaded gastric tumors is referenced as nerve sheath lesions of one type or another.

Interpretation of the literature concerning gastrointestinal mesenchymal tumors has long been confused by the peculiarly common misconception that the origin of a tumor is synonymous with its differentiation (4). In general, origin means cell of origin, and such cells are not known for any mesenchymal tumor anywhere in the body. In contrast, differentiation refers to the expression of adult phenotypic characteristics that exist in recognizable tissues, such as smooth or skeletal muscle, Schwann cells, endothelial cells, and adipocytes. Thus, differentiation has nothing to do with origin. In this chapter, so as not to perpetuate this confusion, the term "origin" does not refer to the cell of origin, but rather to the tissue in which a tumor develops. Most of the discussion therefore concentrates on differentiation.

Because light microscopic examination alone was not providing unimpeachable evidence of differentiation, investigators once hoped that the final decisions concerning differentiation would follow the development of electron microscopy and the immunohistochemical identification of cytoplasmic filaments or cellular proteins. Theoretically, these highly sophisticated techniques should be ready made to determine exactly what kind or kinds of differentiated cells were contained within these peculiar tumors. Regrettably, neither technique performed satisfactorily.

On electron microscopic evaluation, it appeared that most of the cells of most stromal tumors, regardless of site of origin, lacked cytoplasmic sophistication (5–12). Findings include mitochondria, occasional profiles of endoplasmic reticulum of smooth and granular type, scattered ribosomes, and an occasional filament or two, but nothing was definitive. A rare cell had some features that suggested smooth muscle differentiation, such as a few pinocytotic vesicles, or an increase in the number of cytoplasmic microfilaments, with occasional aggregation into dense bodies. A rare cell contained a subplasmalemmal linear density. None of these cells, however, came close to normal smooth muscle cells in terms of cytoplasmic differentiation.

In the cells of some tumors, suggestions of Schwann cell differentiation included elongated processes, which seemed tightly applied to each other, and bits of basement membrane (6–12). In occasional tumors, the cells contained structures that suggested nerve differentiation, including synaptic vesicles; such tumors were even designated "gastrointestinal autonomic nerve tumors" (13–18). Determining if a tumor belongs in this class, however, requires electron microscopic examination, because by light microscopy, the autonomic nerve tumors are identical to other common stromal tumors in the specific sites in which they arise. Because electron microscopic examination is expensive and time-consuming, it is infrequently used for gut stromal tumors. Therefore, in this discussion, no distinctions are made between the autonomic nerve tumors and other typical tumors.

In spite of these occasional flirtations with differentiation by electron microscopic examination, the overwhelming cellular constituents of almost all tumors were not differentiated Schwann cells, differentiated smooth muscle, or even differentiated fibroblasts. Lack of differentiation was the case for all the common stromal tumors arising in all sites.

Immunohistochemical studies have yielded conflicting results, probably because of differences in fixatives, antibodies, technologists, interpretations, and the mixes of tumors from different sites in different institutions (19–31). Most studies have demonstrated that vimentin is the common intermediate filament protein in most cells of most tumors. Stromal tumors from all sites usually have intense and diffuse immunoreactivity for vimentin. Vimentin does not help to determine cell type, however; it seems to be a nonspecific marker of stromal cells in general and is found commonly in fibroblasts and endothelial cells.

Some investigators reported prominent staining with antibodies to various actins, and much less commonly to desmin, in some tumors, suggesting muscle differentiation (23, 24, 28, 30). Others described differing reaction patterns with antibody to the S-100 protein, depending on the site of origin of the tumor (21, 22). Thus, gastric tumors were likely to have scattered S-100-positive cells, perhaps trapped Schwann cells from the myenteric plexus. The stromal tumors of the small intestine were more likely to be S-100 positive. Of note, the cells that were staining positively and the cells that were staining negatively looked exactly alike by light microscopy and apparently by electron microscopy as well. Furthermore, some tumors contained cells that stained positively with both muscle and neural markers, suggesting both smooth muscle and neural differentiation, evidence of stromal cell schizophrenia (25, 29). Some tumors had no markers at all. Further complicating matters was a report of two large, solitary small-intestinal stromal tumors in patients with von Recklinghausen disease. Ultrastructurally and immunohistochemically, these lesions were exactly the same as the common variety of small-intestinal stromal tumors from patients without the syndrome. (32) Rare tumor cells had imperfect ultrastructural smooth muscle features, although these two patients would be expected to have Schwann cell tumors (32).

These highly sophisticated approaches to the demonstration of differentiation of gastrointestinal stromal tumors indicate that these tumors, no matter where they arise, are composed predominantly of undifferentiated cells and that the benign and malignant tumors have exactly the same cellular constituents. Although the concept of a benign undifferentiated tumor is a chilling thought for traditionally oriented pathologists, it nevertheless must be accepted. This concept has a parallel in the colonic adenomas, which are named as if they are benign columnar cell tumors, when in reality, they are epithelial dysplasias composed of poorly differentiated cells, and are the usual precursors of colonic adenocarcinomas. Perhaps the common gastrointestinal stromal tumors are really stromal cell dysplasias, the benign lesions representing dysplasia that is lower in grade relative to that of the malignant lesions. Benign stromal tumors may even be the precursors for the malignant stromal tumors, particularly in the stomach and small intestine. Malignant

tumors often contain small areas that are histologically benign, and histologically benign tumors sometimes contain small areas that look malignant (33).

Because these tumors are composed of such primitive cells, it is difficult to know what to call them. By tradition, rather than by proof, they usually are designated as smooth muscle tumors and occasionally as neural tumors. The "leiomyo-" prefix is widely accepted by surgeons, radiologists, gastroenterologists, and many pathologists, and the current World Health Organization classification retains the smooth muscle designation (34). These names, however, are only nicknames or pseudonyms as far as the gut is concerned. This nomenclature does not recognize the nondifferentiated or minimally differentiated stromal cells that are the basic component of most of these tumors. Therefore, in recognition of this new reality, in this chapter, gastrointestinal neoplasms arising within the mesenchymal tissues are referred to as "mesenchymal tumors," and the specific group of tumors of undifferentiated or minimally differentiated cells is designated as "stromal tumors," be they benign or malignant. The relatively new generic name of "stromal tumor" has gradually gained greater and greater acceptance, and is now almost the standard term in the pathology literature (24–31). In fact, the entire group is now often named by its initials, GISTs, for Gastro-Intestinal Stromal Tumors. Malignant stromal tumors may also be referred to simply as "sarcomas." Specific smooth muscle or neural designations are reserved for tumors that are composed entirely of unquestionably differentiated smooth muscle cells or Schwann cells.

SITE SPECIFICITY

Specific mesenchymal neoplasms, both benign and malignant, including those composed mainly of undifferentiated cells, generally arise in specific sites (5, 35–37) (Table 18.1). Thus, the indigenous tumors are not the same in all areas of the gastrointestinal tract. Furthermore, a particular type of tumor in one site may

TABLE 18.1	Site Specificity of Gastrointestinal Mesenchymal Tumors	
Site	Generic Gastrointestinal Stromal Tumors (GISTs)	Other Mesenchymal Tumors and Tumor-Like Lesions
Esophagus	None	Leiomyomas, including seedling Granular cell tumors Fibrovascular polyps
Stomach	Benign tumors Cellular spindled cell Epithelioid cell Sarcomas Epithelioid cell Spindle cell	Inflammatory fibroid polyps
Small intestine, from duodenum through ileum	Benign spindle cell tumors with organoid pattern and skeinoid fibers Spindle cell sarcomas	Inflammatory fibroid polyps of terminal ileum
Abdominal colon	Odds and ends of sarcomas	Lipomas
Rectum	Deep intramural spindle cell tumors, both benign and malignant	Leiomyomatous polyps

be predictably benign, whereas a histologically similar, although not necessarily identical, tumor arising in a second site may be predictably malignant. This type of local variability is well known and totally accepted for stromal tumors arising in extragastrointestinal sites. For instance, certain bone tumors arise commonly in certain bones and rarely or never in other bones. Rhabdomyosarcomas of the head and neck are likely to be of the embryonal subtype, whereas those of the peripheral soft tissues more commonly have the alveolar pattern. Similarly, the esophageal mesenchyme seems capable of producing a cast of tumors different from that produced by the mesenchyme in its immediately distal neighbor, the stomach.

The following is a summary of this site specificity for gut mesenchymal tumors:

1. In the esophagus, small, typical, differentiated leiomyomas frequently arise in the two muscle layers, especially the muscularis propria. Generic stromal tumors and sarcomas are so rare that not enough data about them are available to draw any conclusions concerning behavior. Granular cell tumors occur in the esophagus more often than anywhere else in the gastrointestinal tract.

2. The stomach is the primary site for close to two thirds of all gut stromal tumors. It houses the glomus tumor almost exclusively. Epithelioid cell stromal tumors, both benign and malignant, are the most common tumors in the stomach. The next most common, the cellular spindled tumor with perinuclear vacuoles and palisades, rarely arises anywhere else in the gut. Furthermore, although gastric stromal tumors are found mostly in the body of the stomach, some arise in the cardia and fundus; others are rarely found in these areas. Thus, site specificity is evident even within this single viscus.

3. The small intestine, including the duodenum, contains about 25% of the tumors. It is the site of origin for a group of spindle cell stromal tumors with organoid vascular patterns and big lumps of modified collagen called "skeinoid fibers" (38, 39). Such tumors are not found anywhere else in the gut, except, on rare occasions, in the proximal colon.

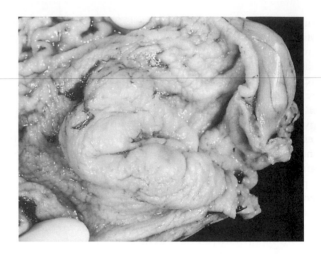

Figure 18.2 This lobulated gastric sarcoma has elevated the mucosa and produced several huge knobby folds. (See color plate.)

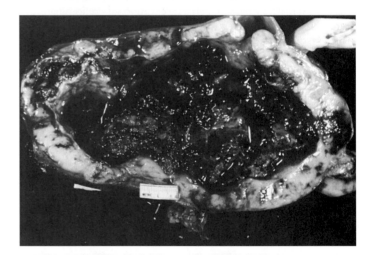

Figure 18.3 A huge small intestinal sarcoma forms a circumscribed mass mainly outside the wall of the bowel. A small ulcer *(top right center)* communicates with a giant central hemorrhagic and necrotic cavity.

Small bowel sarcomas tend to be highly cellular and composed of uniform small spindle cells (40).

4. The colon, excluding the rectosigmoid, is an unusual site for stromal tumors, so unusual in fact, that minimal data about them have been published. The colon may be the only gut site in which truly pleomorphic sarcomas arise.

5. The rectum, and, to a lesser extent, the sigmoid colon, contain two characteristic neoplasms. One is a small nodular expansion of the muscularis mucosae, the leiomyomatous polyp. The second is a deep intramural highly cellular spindle cell tumor that superficially resembles the benign spindle cell lesion in the stomach but is likely to be malignant (41).

In spite of this site specificity, current literature contains studies of stromal tumor differentiation and behavior that combine tumors from all sites. This tendency toward combination studies reflects the

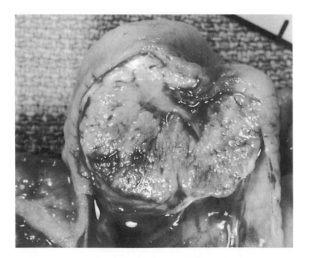

Figure 18.1 This benign, intramural gastric stromal tumor has pushed the mucosa inward and ulcerated it. (Photograph courtesy Dr. Aina Silenieks, Lincoln, NE.) (See color plate.)

rarity of these neoplasms; i.e., in order for a study from a single institution to accumulate enough tumors to achieve statistical significance, it is necessary to combine all tumors of the stomach and small and large intestines. This strategy is comparable to mixing carcinomas of esophagus, stomach, colorectum, and pancreatobiliary tract with the assumption that they are all alike, and then analyzing this mix for level of differentiation, pattern of growth and survival parameters. It is well known that carcinomas from all these sites are not the same. They differ in epidemiologic associations, genetic alterations, behavior, method of spread, and histologic features. Were a pathologist to undertake such a study and attempt to publish the results, he or she would probably quickly lose credibility. If investigators studying gut stromal tumors are to accumulate enough cases to produce significant data, they should initiate cooperative ventures involving many institutions, and then analyze these tumors by specific sites.

CLINICAL FEATURES

Much like gastrointestinal epithelial and lymphoid neoplasms, mesenchymal tumors are discovered in male and female patients mainly during the fourth through the seventh decades, with slight variation in peak incidence from one primary site to another. Signs and symptoms depend on size, site of origin, location within the wall, and whether the tumor is benign or malignant. In general, tumors in the small bowel, with its smaller diameter, are likely to cause symptoms when they are smaller than are those in the stomach, which has a much larger diameter. Thus, a relatively small intramural tumor, perhaps 1.5 to 2 cm across, arising in a part of the gut with a narrow lumen, such as the pylorus or the small bowel, may cause obstruction with pain and vomiting, whereas a similar tumor in the gastric body is usually asymptomatic. A large tumor attached to the greater curvature of the body of the stomach not involving the mucosa may cause no symptoms or may be detected as an abdominal mass during a physical examination or during self examination by the patient. A tumor that ulcerates is likely to cause bleeding, pain, or both. An intramural mass in the small intestine may form the

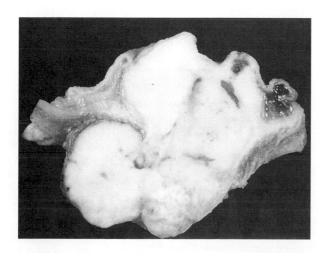

Figure 18.4   This 3-cm diameter benign stromal tumor of the duodenum has submucosal and subserosal components, separated by a constriction at the muscularis propria. At the top is the mucosa, which covers the tumor and is ulcerated in the center. (See color plate.)

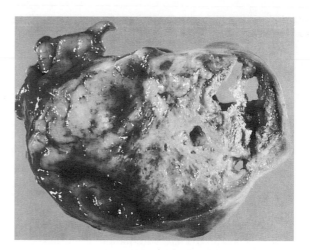

Figure 18.5   A benign gastric stromal tumor forms a circumscribed intramural nodule, which has several dark areas of hemorrhage and cysts, the result of liquefactive necrosis. (Photograph courtesy of Dr. James K. Billman, Jr., Moline, IL.) (See color plate.)

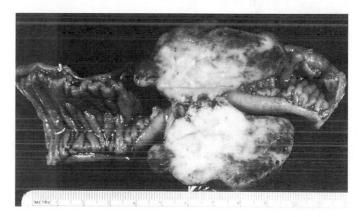

Figure 18.6   A 6.5-cm diameter malignant small bowel stromal tumor is slightly lobulated and well circumscribed and forms a mass that protrudes outward into the peritoneal cavity. The tumor has been cut across and both halves are shown. (See color plate.)

leading end of an intussusception. Weight loss is frequently associated with sarcomas, as it is with malignancies in general. Small sarcomas and those with most of their bulk projecting outside the gut may present as metastases, such as with hepatomegaly.

GROSS CHARACTERISTICS

Gut stromal tumors, regardless of site, usually are single intramural masses; most expand the wall, and some push toward the lumen, elevating the mucosa that may secondarily ulcerate (Figs. 18.1 and 18.2). Some tumors expand outwardly into the subserosa (Fig. 18.3). On occasion, especially with large gastric tumors, the mass may be almost totally outside the wall, with only a tiny attachment to the muscularis propria. Some tumors have both intramural and extramural components separated by a constriction at the muscularis propria, the "dumbbell"-shaped appearance (Fig. 18.4).

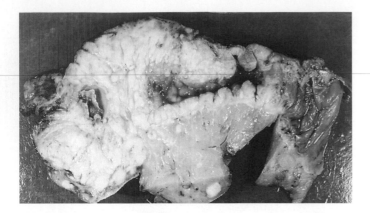

Figure 18.7 The unusual infiltrative pattern of a gut sarcoma forms a large mass on the left, and nodules that thicken the wall toward the center. The nodules in the mesentery at the bottom are metastases. (Photograph courtesy of Dr. Aina Silenieks, Lincoln, NE.) (See color plate.)

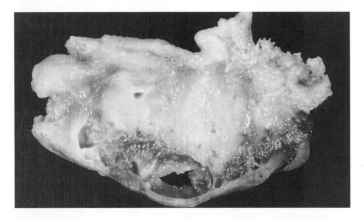

Figure 18.8 A slightly lobulated, discrete, 3-cm intramural benign jejunal stromal tumor fills the submucosa. Note the liquefactive cysts at the bottom center. (See color plate.)

Most tumors are circumscribed; even the malignant tumors are likely to have easily identified perimeters (Figs. 18.5 and 18.6). Their growth pattern is expansile. Only rarely does a tumor, usually a sarcoma, invade the gut wall or invade adjacent structures (Fig. 18.7). Most tumors are solitary, round or oval, occasionally lobulated, masses (Figs. 18.8 and 18.9).

The one predictable exception to the solitary mass appearance is the multinodular or multifocal epithelioid cell tumor of the stomach (Fig. 18.10). This tumor is associated with pulmonary chondromas and extraadrenal pheochromocytomas usually occurring in young women, a triad described by Carney (42, 43).

On cross section, esophageal leiomyomas are identical to uterine leiomyomas, because both are mature smooth muscle tumors. The generic stromal tumors in other gastrointestinal sites, however, are quite different. For instance, they do not bulge when cut across, and they do not appear whorled. Instead, the cut surface is flat and appears granular and pockmarked by vessels and patches of collagenization, lysis, and hemorrhage (Figs. 18.1, 18.4, and 18.11). At times, these degenerative changes dominate the cross-sectional appearance with the formation of cysts and broad zones of

hemorrhagic necrosis (Fig. 18.12), which may communicate with overlying ulcers (see Fig. 18.3). The sarcomas tend to be more hemorrhagic and necrotic than their benign counterparts; however, these characteristic changes may be more a manifestation of size than of malignancy, because the larger benign tumors are also extensively degenerated. The gross appearances of the benign tumors and the sarcomas may overlap to the degree that they cannot be distinguished. Large size may be a strong hint that a tumor of the small bowel is malignant, but this feature is not nearly as helpful in the stomach.

GENERAL MICROSCOPIC FEATURES

Whereas the gross characteristics of the solitary stromal tumors of stomach and intestines tend to be much the same no matter the type and the site, the microscopic features differ and are site specific. Therefore, the specific microscopic patterns are described separately within the context of the individual locations in which they occur. Before beginning these descriptions, however, some common histologic characteristics warrant discussion.

Tumors in all sites are situated within either the submucosa, the muscularis propria, or most likely, both layers (Fig. 18.13). The muscle of the muscularis tends to be hypertrophic and often hyalinized at the edges of a tumor, and muscle bundles sometimes penetrate the tumor, forming muscular septa that subdivide the mass into smaller units or lobules (Figs. 18.14 and 18.15). This lobulation is more accentuated in gastric than in intestinal tumors (Fig. 18.16). On the other hand, in an occasional small bowel stromal tumor, the muscularis propria passes through the tumor like a sling, with the fibers separated by fascicles of neoplastic spindle cells (Fig. 18.17). Sometimes, the hypertrophied muscularis completely or partially surrounds the tumor like a capsule, even blending with fibers of the muscularis mucosae. There is never a transition between normal smooth muscle and tumor cells, although often there is an interdigitation of tumor cells and muscle cells at the edges of a tumor, creating the appearance of tumor either infiltrating muscularis or arising from it. In tumors that involve the deep muscularis and extend into the adjacent soft tissues, sheets of tumor cells often push into the surrounding adipose tissue, but rarely do the cells infiltrate among the adipocytes.

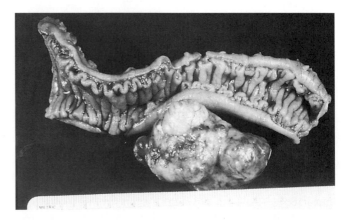

Figure 18.9 A lobulated, outwardly protruding small intestinal stromal tumor. (See color plate.)

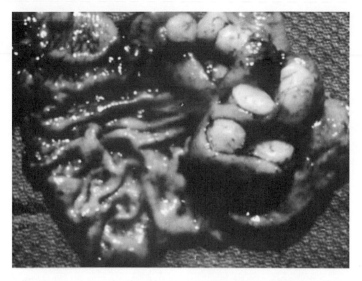

Figure 18.10 A multinodular epithelioid cell gastric tumor characteristic of Carney's triad. (Photograph courtesy of Dr. Donald Antonioli, Boston, MA.)

DIAGNOSTIC CONSIDERATIONS

BENIGN VERSUS MALIGNANT TUMORS

In general, benign and malignant tumors can be distinguished by certain histologic features, but the features differ somewhat from one primary site to another. As mentioned previously, malignant tumors often contain histologically benign areas, and benign tumors sometimes contain small foci that are histologically malignant. These findings lead to the suggestion that benign tumors are the precursors of the malignant tumors, but they also raise some problems in interpretation. For instance, it is unclear how much of a malignant component in an otherwise benign tumor imparts malignant behavior to that tumor. In a tumor that measures $5 \times 4 \times 4$ cm or 80 cm³ in which 76 cm³ are benign and 4 cm³ are malignant, is the tumor benign or malignant? At present, no data are available to answer that question.

The literature regarding criteria for malignancy is filled with studies combining tumors from all sites, so establishing criteria for each site is problematic. On the basis of analysis of tumors with proven metastases, however, the following generalizations may be made:

1. Malignant gut stromal tumors tend to be larger, more densely cellular, and more mitotically active than their benign counterparts in all locations (5, 44–46).
2. What is larger, more cellular, and more mitotically active, differs from one site to another.
3. The risk of metastasis increases with increasing size and increasing mitotic rate at all locations (47).
4. Using anaplasia as a criterion of malignancy is pointless, because these tumors, whether benign or malignant, are composed predominantly of undifferentiated cells. Highly pleomorphic sarcomas are uncommon (44, 45).
5. Gross invasion of adjacent organs is clear evidence of malignancy, but adherence to an adjacent structure is not.
6. Somewhat similar tumors occurring in different sites are

likely to behave differently. For example, a highly cellular tumor of the gastric wall composed of uniform tightly packed spindle cells arranged in fascicles and whorls is predictably benign. A cellular spindle cell tumor deep in the rectal wall is likely to recur multiple times and eventually metastasize. An epithelioid cell tumor of the stomach composed of fairly large cells with plentiful cytoplasm is predictably benign, whereas a comparable tumor of the small bowel with nearly identical cells will have a higher mitotic rate and probably metastasize. A tumor in the stomach that is 6 cm in diamter rarely metastasizes, no matter what it looks like microscopically. This statement reflects the fact that almost all 6-cm gastric stromal tumors are histologically benign. A 6-cm tumor in the small intestine will metastasize probably 50% of the time based on size alone, a reflection of the fact that one half or more small bowel stromal tumors of that size are microscopic sarcomas.

7. Microscopic invasion of the mucosa with separation of epithelial elements by stromal cells is indicative of

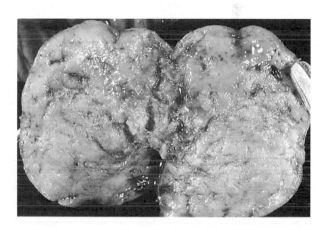

Figure 18.11 The cut surface of a typical gastric or intestinal stromal tumor is pale and pockmarked by vessels and degenerative changes. There is no whorling or gristlelike appearance, features that are typical of uterine leiomyomas. (See color plate.)

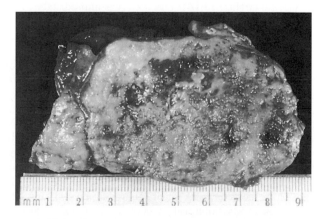

Figure 18.12 The cut surface of this benign tumor of the stomach is dominated by irregular zones of hemorrhage and necrosis. (See color plate.)

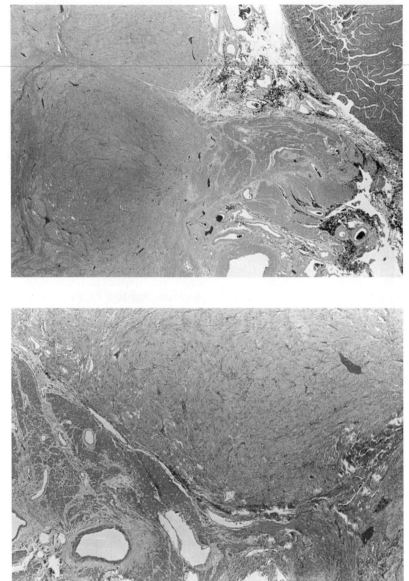

Figure 18.13   At the edge of this benign small intestinal stromal tumor, which fills the left side of the field, the muscularis propria becomes thick with the dark muscle bundles separated by pale collagen *(right center)* (×13).

Figure 18.14   At the edge of this benign small bowel tumor, which fills the upper part of this field, the muscularis propria, in the lower half of the field, is thick and partly encapsulates the tumor (×33).

malignancy (Fig. 18.18). This feature is unpredictable, however, because mucosal invasion is likely to cause ulceration, and the resultant ulcers obliterate the foci of mucosal invasion.

8. Tumor necrosis, especially acute ischemic necrosis, may be a marker of malignancy, but many benign tumors also have necrotic foci.

Therefore, no specific criteria for malignancy are applicable to all tumors arising in all sites (5, 44). In general, a few rules may be useful based on analysis of multiple morphologic features, including site, size, cellularity, mitotic rate, and invasive characteristics. In the stomach, an epithelioid cell tumor that measures over 6 cm in diameter, with small solidly packed cells and easily found mitoses, is a potentially metastasizing tumor. The same tumor, but with a diameter less than 6 cm, has a minimal metastatic risk. Also in the stomach, a densely packed spindle cell tumor with uniform cells, especially with perinuclear vacuoles, will probably not metastasize, no matter what the size. A spindle cell tumor without the vacuoles and with a high mitotic rate measuring over 6 cm across has a definite metastatic risk, which increases with increasing size. In the small intestine, or colon, any cellular spindle cell tumor with a diameter greater than 2 cm that has mitoses carries a metastatic risk. Any relatively pure epithelioid cell tumor in the small intestine is probably malignant. A deeply situated, highly cellular, spindle cell tumor of the rectum is likely to be malignant and should be treated aggressively when it is first discovered.

Mitotic rates in many metastasizing gastrointestinal sarcomas are much lower than what would be demanded for the diagnosis of a sarcoma in another primary site, such as the uterus. Leiomyosarcomas of the uterus generally have at least 5 to 10 mitoses per 10 high power fields, depending on the study. Such numbers would be extremely high for the gut, where any tumor with more than 1 mitosis per 10 high power fields is likely to be malignant. Thus, it is important to remember that the criteria for malignancy in gut

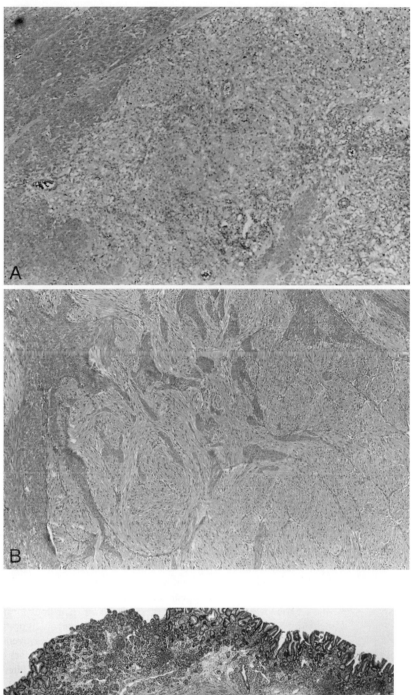

Figure 18.15   Relationships between stromal tumors and the adjacent muscularis propria. **A.** At the edge of this gastric benign tumor, the muscularis propria *(left side of the field)* forms a partial muscular capsule from which a muscular trabeculum penetrates the tumor as a septum *(lower right center)* (×53). **B.** Muscular trabeculae extend from the muscular capsule into the center of this small bowel benign tumor. The normal smooth muscle *(dark)* and the tumor cells *(light)* stain completely differently with hematoxylin and eosin (×53).

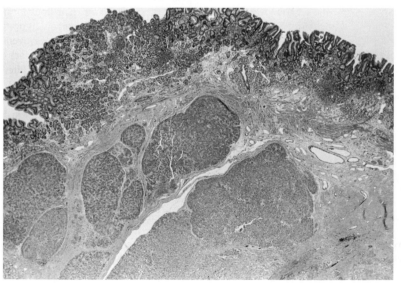

Figure 18.16   Discrete tumor lobules in the submucosal aspect of this benign gastric tumor are separated by bands of collagen (×53).

stromal tumors are not necessarily the same for stromal tumors in other sites (44).

Histologic grading systems for gastrointestinal sarcomas have been developed at different institutions based on tumor cellularity, mitoses, nuclear cytoplasmic ratio, and pleomorphism (45, 47–49). These systems seem to have some validity in their correlation with frequency or rapidity of metastases and death from tumor, at least in the institutions in which they are used. Unfortunately, systems differ from one institution to another, so it is difficult to compare them to determine which factors used in grading are truly useful predictors of behavior.

Quite often, tumors with histologically malignant areas also have areas that are equally obviously benign. These benign foci usually are situated in the submucosa, whereas the malignant foci are deeper. The factor that determines metastasizability in such cases, be it the size of the tumor as a whole or simply the size of the sarcomatous component, is not known.

Proliferation markers, such as proliferating cell nuclear antigen (PCNA) and Ki-67, correlate with behavior in some studies, but it is not clear if they are independent markers, or if they occur in tumors with other morphologic criteria of malignancy (39, 50–54). Similarly, in some studies, aneuploidy in GISTs, as determined by flow cytometry, correlated with shortened patient survival, although aneuploidy was not always an independent prognosticator; it also correlated with morphologic features, such as cell type, tumor grade, and tumor size (55–61).

Certain immunohistochemical and ultrastructural features may be helpful in distinguishing malignant from benign tumors. Results of some studies indicate that the tumors with neural (not Schwann cell) differentiation, that is, the gastrointestinal autonomic nerve tumors, or GANTs, are more likely than other tumors to be malignant (46). It appears, however, that those GANTs reported to be malignant usually have other criteria of malignancy, such as frequent mitoses or dense cellularity or large size (14, 16, 18). As a result, it is not an established fact that GANTs should be regarded as malignant, and it is also not an established fact that examining

GISTs with the electron microscope is needed, which should be welcome news for the cost-conscious managed care systems.

Finally, the need to use multiple factors or parameters to determine malignancy has led to the recognition of a group of tumors that have conflicting or overlapping features, and are thus not easily defined as either benign or malignant. Such tumors may be referred to as possessing "borderline" features or features of "undetermined malignant potential." Examples of this type of tumor include a tumor that is so unusual that no one has experience with it, a benign tumor with a small malignant component, a tumor with benign cellularity but a high mitotic rate, and a tumor with a degree of cellularity that is not easily determined to be benign or malignant. Presumably, tumors belonging to this borderline or undetermined group will eventually be categorized as pathologists gain experience with them.

The pattern of metastases for almost all sarcomas throughout the gastrointestinal tract is predictable. The two primary sites of metastasis are the liver and the peritoneal surfaces. Sometimes, the metastases are larger than the primary tumor, as occurs especially with small-intestinal sarcomas, some of which are quite small. Peritoneal studding is common, and in advanced cases, the entire peritoneal surface can be covered by large tumor nodules. Lymph node metastases do occur, but they can be demonstrated only in about 10% of the sarcomas that metastasize. Another intraabdominal site of metastasis is the retroperitoneal soft tissues, usually not clearly within lymph nodes. Rarely do gastrointestinal sarcomas metastasize outside the abdomen. When they do, they are likely to involve the lung (about 10% of cases), the subcutaneous tissues (another 10%), and anywhere else throughout the body (much lower frequency).

ROLE OF FROZEN SECTION OR GROSS INTRAOPERATIVE CONSULTATION

A surgeon who encounters a mass in the gastrointestinal tract is likely to want to know what it is, because subsequent surgical treatment may be dictated by the diagnosis. Current data suggest that the proper treatment for a gastrointestinal tract stromal tumor is gross total removal, whether the tumor is benign or malignant (37, 45, 48, 62). It is not known how wide a margin of resection is necessary, but it does not appear that a major resection, such as a total gastrectomy, offers a greater chance of cure than does local resection. The fact that the treatment of benign and malignant tumors is similar limits the role of frozen section diagnosis of gastrointestinal stromal tumors, although frozen sections and operating room consultation have certain uses.

When a tumor is submitted from the operating room for analysis, the pathologist should first measure it, because size alone can be a reasonably good predictor of behavior of a gastrointestinal stromal tumor. A frozen section can then be performed for two informational reasons, neither of which probably is critical for immediate management. The first reason is to verify that the tumor is of stromal type and not something else; however, the gross characteristics of gut stromal tumors, namely their tendency to form circumscribed intramural masses, are so different from those of any other neoplasm, that a frozen section may be unnecessary. The one exception is the tiny nodule of the muscularis propria-myenteric plexus, which can look like a metastasis from a carcinoma. The second reason for frozen section is to see if the tumor is obviously malignant; that is, if it is highly cellular and mitoses are easily

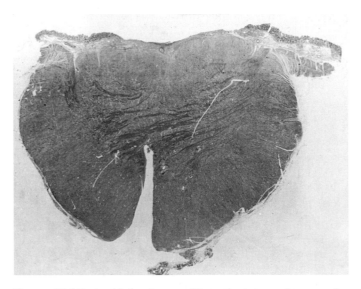

Figure 18.17 In this benign small intestinal stromal tumor, the fibers of the muscularis propria *(dark staining)* traverse the tumor like a sling (×8).

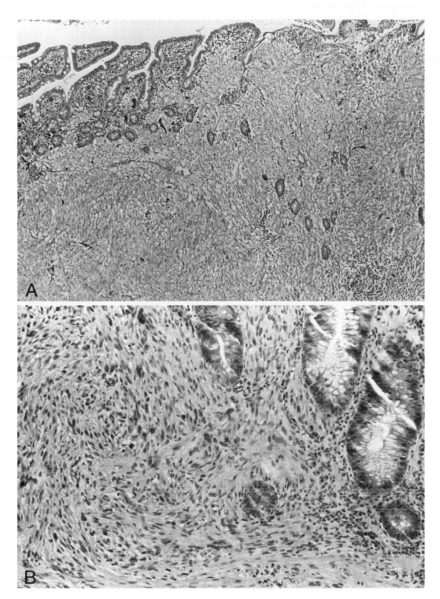

Figure 18.18 Mucosal invasion with separation of the epithelial elements by tumor cells is an excellent criterion of malignancy. **A.** Small bowel sarcoma (×53). **B.** Rectal sarcoma (×132).

identified on the frozen section. This determination may help the surgeon when he or she discusses the situation with the patient and the family after the operation, but it is not likely to dictate the definitive treatment. The information to give to the surgeon includes the fact that the tumor is stromal, whether it is obviously malignant or if the pathologist cannot tell if it is malignant, and finally, the size of the tumor as a potential prognosticator. It is important to remember that it is impossible to determine if many gastrointestinal stromal tumors are benign or malignant on the basis of frozen section alone. Too many sarcomas have very low mitotic rates, and many benign tumors characteristically are highly cellular, depending on the site of origin.

Finally, a word of caution is in order. Occasionally, the cells of an epithelioid cell tumor of the stomach form clusters or cords. On frozen section, these clusters may closely resemble a diffuse spreading carcinoma. The gross features should clarify the issues, because the carcinoma produces a diffuse mural thickening, whereas the stromal tumor forms a discrete expansile mass. If, however, the tissue sample submitted for frozen section is not the entire tumor,

error becomes more likely, because the pathologist is unable to assess the gross features. In such cases, particularly if the stromal nature of a tumor is in doubt, it is best to ask the surgeon to describe the gross characteristics.

It is clear from the foregoing discussion that the diagnosis of a gut stromal tumor and a statement as to whether or not it is malignant are really permanent section issues.

DISSECTION AND TISSUE SAMPLING

The proper gross handling of these neoplasms, regardless of type, is predicated on the fact that gross examination and sampling are critical in the determination of benignancy or malignancy. First, size is important, because of its association with metastases. Big tumors are more likely to be malignant, and the bigger the sarcoma, the greater the likelihood of metastasis. Second, adequate sampling is important, although no data are available to indicate what amount and type of sample is adequate. Such sampling probably should include mucosa over the tumor or at the edge of any ulcer in order to detect mucosal infiltration, an excellent marker of malignancy. In large tumors, most samples should be taken from the deeper aspects, where sarcomatous components are most likely found. No rules pertain to the number of sections to be examined per centimeter of tumor diameter. Personal experience has shown that examining three or four sections from any tumor, no matter the size, is sufficient to identify a tumor and to determine if it is benign or malignant. Some pathologists, however, may prefer to take more than four samples.

USE OF IMMUNOHISTOCHEMISTRY AND ELECTRON MICROSCOPY

As noted previously, the literature concerning the differentiation and behavior of the generic stromal tumors of the gut is inconsistent. These inconsistencies are based on different results of immunostaining for microfilaments and other cellular proteins, including muscle markers and neural markers, be they for Schwann cells or neurites. Furthermore, the findings of muscle or neural differentiation by electron microscopy are also inconsistent. Personal experience has led to several conclusions and recommendations. After receiving many cases of GISTs in consultation, including trays of negative immunostains that frustrate the contributors because of the inability of the tumor cells to stain like muscle or Schwann cells, it is clear that the cells of most GISTs stain with nothing other than antibody to vimentin, which does not help to define differentiation. For some cases, there are even electron photomicrographs of primitive spindle cells with no differentiation. For such cases, the conclusion to draw is that immunostaining and/or electron microscopy is not necessary or helpful. Extensive experience shows also that the cells of both benign and malignant stromal tumors have much the same immunohistochemical and ultrastructural characteristics; they are mainly undifferentiated cells. No highly sophisticated examination is better than careful light microscopic examination in telling if a tumor is benign or malignant. Furthermore, these techniques are expensive and time-consuming, and despite the potential value of whatever information these ancillary techniques may offer, it is best to evaluate all GISTs by H & E light microscopy alone, obviating immunostaining and ultrastructural examination.

MESENCHYMAL TUMORS PECULIAR TO SPECIFIC SITES IN THE GASTROINTESTINAL TRACT

ESOPHAGUS

LEIOMYOMA

The esophagus is the only site within the gut, in which, with few exceptions, the common mesenchymal tumors are typical, classic, ordinary leiomyomas (35, 36). Most of these lesions arise within the muscularis propria, although occasional leiomyomas develop within the muscularis mucosae. An exhaustive survey of the world's literature on smooth muscle tumors of the esophagus through 1971 was compiled by Seremetis et al., and these data are still valid (63). They reported that more than 50% of leiomyomas arose in the lower one third with about 30% in the middle third and the rest in the upper one third of the esophagus. This distribution, however, probably reflects the location of the large, often symptomatic tumors, and it corresponds to the relative amounts of smooth muscle within the muscularis propria: the lower one third consists totally of smooth muscle, the middle one third is mostly smooth muscle, and the proximal portion is mainly skeletal muscle.

Most esophageal leiomyomas are tiny, subclinical lesions that lie within one of the muscle layers, and the majority arise in the region of the esophagogastric junction, mainly on the esophageal side. Such tiny tumors have been designated as "seedling leiomyomas" (64). They occur in the esophagus of close to 10% of adults, and they may be multiple (Fig. 18.19). The large leiomyomas are likely to produce symptoms of dysphagia or pain, depending on their size and whether they obstruct the lumen.

In most reported clinical cases, the leiomyomas have been 5 cm in diameter or less, but occasional giant tumors occur, some weighing over 1000 g. Some leiomyomas become calcified. Grossly, on cut section, esophageal leiomyomas are pale or white, firm, rubbery, whorled, and well circumscribed. Histologically, the esophageal leiomyoma contains normal appearing or hypertrophic smooth muscle cells arranged in fascicles or whorls. The tiny seedling lesions look like localized expansions of the muscularis. In

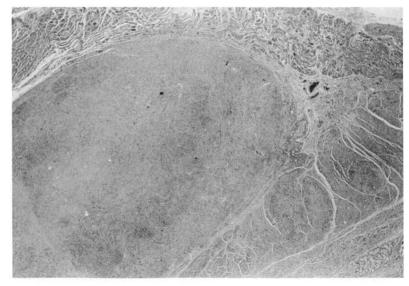

Figure 18.19 Three seedling leiomyomas of the esophageal muscularis propria, a large one on the left and two smaller ones on the right.

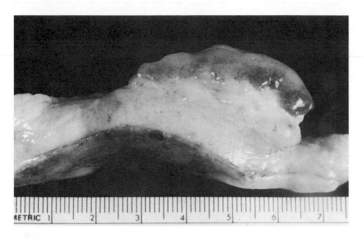

Figure 18.20 A giant fibrovascular polyp of the esophagus on cross-section. This 9-cm long structure was attached to the high cervical esophagus by the pedicle on the right.

fact, it is impossible at times to tell a tiny seedling leiomyoma from a bundle of hypertrophic smooth muscle, especially in the upper-middle part of the esophagus where skeletal and smooth muscle fibers are mixed in the muscularis propria.

Circumferential leiomyomas have been reported. These lesions probably are examples of an entity known as diffuse leiomyomatosis of the esophagus, a rare disorder, mainly of young women, who have long-standing dysphagia (36, 65–68). In this condition, the lower esophagus and usually the proximal stomach have an eccentric nodular thickened muscularis propria that looks like a confluence of leiomyomas. Occasionally, such cases have been associated with vulvar leiomyomas as well.

SARCOMA

In their literature review, Seremetis et al. unconvered only 40 published reports of esophageal sarcomas compared to 838 cases of leiomyoma (63). Not many sarcomas have been reported since that time, and there are definitely no large series (69–71). In fact, the largest published series contain only 10 and 13 cases (72, 73). As is true for the generic gut stromal tumors, clear-cut ultrastructural and immunohistochemical demonstration of smooth muscle differentiation or any other differentiation in these reported sarcomas is lacking. Many or even most of these cases resemble the pseudosarcomatous variants of squamous cell carcinoma in terms of clinical presentation, patient sex and age, location in the esophagus predominantly in the middle third, gross polypoid characteristics, and prognosis. For instance, cases of esophageal leiomyosarcoma with adjacent or overlying squamous cell carcinoma have been reported, suggesting that these are really examples of polypoid pseudosarcomatous squamous cell carcinoma (70). Therefore, although there is no reason to expect that sarcomas of the esophagus do not occur, they are probably even more uncommon than the number of published cases implies. A true sarcoma of the esophagus should be a malignant spindle cell neoplasm with mitoses and variable pleomorphism that has definite ultrastructural and/or immunohistochemical characteristics that are purely mesenchymal; it should invade and/or metastasize purely as a mesenchymal tumor, and have no squamous cell carcinoma at the margin or overlying it.

On the basis of a literature review, it is obvious that few tumors meet these requirements.

A few cases of rhabdomyosarcoma of the esophagus have been reported, perhaps as many as five (74). Such few cases contribute no important data, and therefore, warrant no further discussion.

GIANT FIBROVASCULAR (FIBROLIPOMATOUS) POLYP OF THE ESOPHAGUS

One of the most unusual mesenchymal proliferations of the gut is a long, slender polyp arising from the upper esophagus behind the cricoid cartilage and filling the lumen for various numbers of centimeters, sometimes all the way to the gastric cardia (36, 75) (Fig. 18.20). These lesions occur in patients presenting with gradually evolving dysphagia. The core of such polyps is expanded lamina propria composed of a loose stellate and spindle cell proliferation in a myxoid rather than vascular stroma (Fig. 18.21). Lobules of adipose tissue cells are scattered in this peculiar stroma; in fact, in some polyps, adipose tissue is so prominent that they have been termed "fibrolipoma." Furthermore, descriptions of these tumors and tumors designated simply as lipomas of the esophagus overlap so much so that they may even be variants of the same lesion (36, 76). These lumps are usually called "giant fibrovascular or fibrolipomatous polyps." Although what they are remains unclear, giant fibrovascular polyps are exclusively an esophageal phenomenon. They may be stromal neoplasms, like lipomas, or mesenchymal redundancies or even vascular aberrations. Whatever their essence, they are benign, although they have become huge before they produce symptoms, hence the "giant" designation. Another remarkable feature is the relatively short duration of symptoms that many of the patients experience, considering the size of these polyps, probably the result of slow growth that allows the esophageal wall to compensate for the expanding intralumenal mass and the pliability of these soft tumors (36, 77). In a few reported cases, regurgitation of the polyp led to impaction on the larynx and asphyxiation.

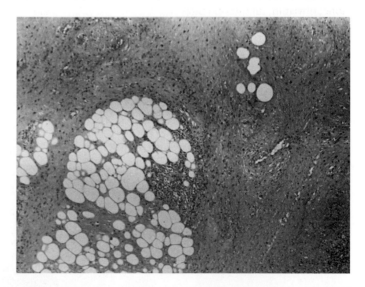

Figure 18.21 The stroma of giant fibrovascular esophageal polyps contains a mixture of adipose, myxoid, and heavily collagenized tissues with inflammatory cells (×80).

These lesions are so rare that they usually appear in single case reports, sprinkled equally within the radiologic, surgical, and gastroenterologic literature. In their detailed book on the pathology of the esophagus, Enterline and Thompson state that they have never seen a case (76). At the University of Michigan, we have seen only three cases, one from within our own patient population and two as consultations. The radiologic archives of the Armed Forces Institute of Pathology produced only 16 cases that were reported in 1996 (77).

STOMACH

BENIGN CELLULAR SPINDLED CELL STROMAL TUMOR

This tumor is composed of spindle cells arranged in whorls or cartwheels or fascicles, often with spectacular nuclear palisades (78) (Figs. 18.22 and 18.23). Usually, the cells are uniform and monotonous, but some tumors contain enlarged forms. Broad areas of liquefaction and hyalinization are likely present, so that very cellular areas alternate with sparsely cellular foci, the latter making the palisades even more prominent. In most tumors, many of the cells have a single vacuole that compresses or indents the nucleus at one pole (Fig. 18.24). These vacuoles may be artifactual, because they do not exist when the tumors are viewed ultrastructurally or in frozen sections. Peculiarly, these perinuclear vacuoles do not occur in sarcomas, so they seem to be quite specific benign markers. In those tumors with some cellular pleomorphism, the larger cells contain larger vacuoles. Mitotic figures are scattered throughout, but usually are no more frequent than 1 per 10 high power fields. The only tumor of this histologic appearance that has been reported to metastasize measured 17 cm across and had 5 mitoses per 50 high power fields. It was composed of uniform spindled cells that looked bland, but it lacked the palisades and the perinuclear vacuoles. A few of these lesions have recurred in operative beds 15 years or more

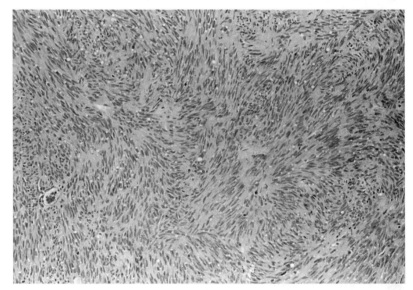

Figure 18.22   Benign cellular spindle cell tumor of the stomach. The uniform spindle cells are arranged in fascicles and in palisade (×132).

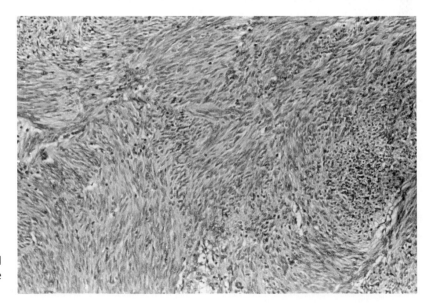

Figure 18.23   Benign cellular spindle cell stromal tumor of the stomach. These spindle cell fascicles have a storiform pattern (×132).

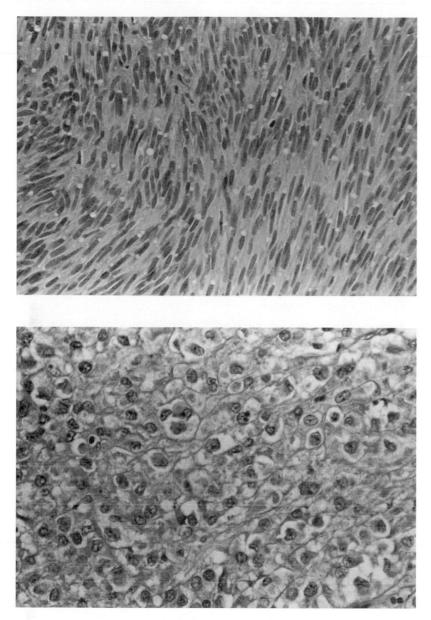

Figure 18.24 Benign cellular spindle cell tumor of the stomach. Many of these uniform spindle cells have round clear vacuoles indenting the nucleus at one pole (×330).

Figure 18.25 Benign epithelioid cell stromal tumor of the stomach. Many of the rounded cells have clear peripheral cytoplasm and condensed darker cytoplasm adherent to the nuclei (×330).

after the original resection, and the recurrences looked exactly like the primary lesions.

BENIGN AND MALIGNANT EPITHELIOID CELL STROMAL TUMORS

In the early 1960s, Martin et al. from France, and Stout from the United States, identified a group of gastric stromal tumors that contained rounded or polygonal cells, many of which had clear cytoplasm (79, 80). Stout coined the name "leiomyoblastoma," a noncommittal term that had neither benign or malignant connotations, because Stout was not certain how these tumors behaved (80). It now appears that in the stomach, epithelioid cell stromal tumors are as common as the cellular spindle cell tumors. The clear cytoplasm is actually an artifact of fixation (7). After formalin fixation, the cells contain a small amount of eosinophilic cytoplasma condensed about the nuclei, but on frozen section, the cells have eosinophilic cytoplasm and are not clear (Fig. 18.25). Also, no electron microscopic features correlate with the cytoplasmic clearing.

Few tumors are composed totally of epithelioid cells (62); most have a mixture of epithelioid and plump spindle cells (Fig. 18.26). Multinucleated cells and cells with giant nuclei are common and are found in the benign rather than the malignant tumors (Fig. 18.27). These tumors are often multinodular, and commonly contain different types of cells and different patterns of growth in different nodules (Fig. 18.28).

The epithelioid cells are usually arranged in sheets, but occasionally there is a prominent perivascular orientation, suggesting a recapitulation of vascular smooth muscle (62) (Fig. 18.29). As a result, areas within these tumors may resemble glomus tumors or hemangiopericytomas. Liquefaction and hyalinization are common features (Fig. 18.30).

The malignant variants, or epithelioid sarcomas, contain smaller cells with less cytoplasm than do the benign lesions

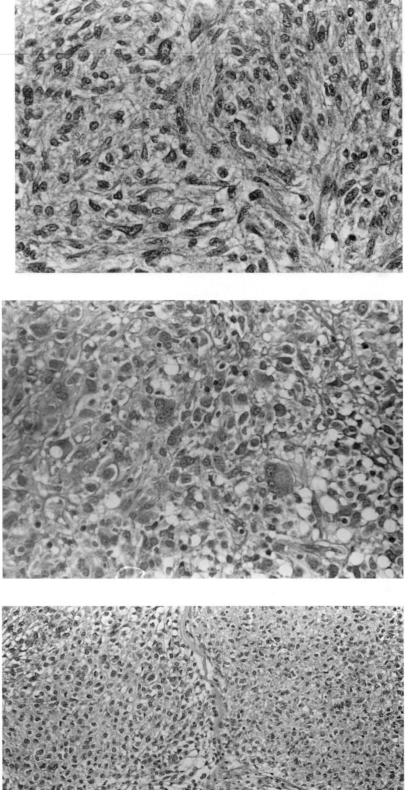

Figure 18.26   Benign epithelioid cell gastric stromal tumor. This field reveals a mixture of epithelioid cells and plump spindle cells (×330).

Figure 18.27   Cellular pleomorphism with variable nuclear sizes and multinucleated giant cells are common in the benign, but not the malignant, epithelioid cell gastric tumors (×330).

Figure 18.28   An example of variation in growth pattern and cellular composition in adjacent lobules of a benign epithelioid cell gastric stromal tumor. The lobule at the left has only epithelioid cells, whereas the lobule on the right has a mixture of epithelioid and plump spindle cells (×132).

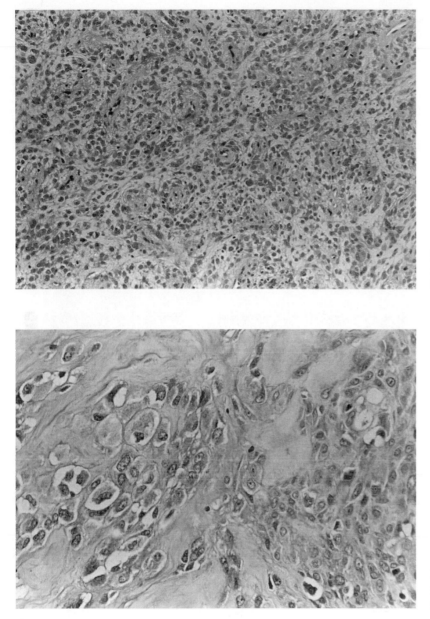

Figure 18.29   The perivascular or perithelial pattern of growth in a benign gastric epithelioid cell stromal tumor (×132).

Figure 18.30   Broad zones of hyalinization separate cell strands, clusters, and sheets in a benign gastric epithelioid cell tumor (×330).

(Fig. 18.31). The sarcoma cells are also more uniform, and multinucleated and pleomorphic cells are unusual. Furthermore, the epithelioid cells in the sarcomas frequently form small clusters or groupings resembling alveoli, often embedded in an acid mucopolysaccharide-rich stroma. In some sarcomas, foci of small, tightly packed palisaded spindle cells in a comparable stroma also are found. Frequently, both benign and malignant appearing areas are present in the same tumor.

Both epithelioid leiomyomas and leiomyosarcomas typically arise in the body of the stomach, but peculiarly, almost half of the sarcomas arise in the cardia and fundus and rarely in the antrum, whereas almost half of the benign tumors arise in the antrum but rarely occur in the proximal stomach. A subset of the epithelioid sarcomas constitutes one of the components of a multiorgan abnormality occurring mainly in young women described originally by Carney (43, 44). In this syndrome, the gastric epithelioid sarcoma tends to occur as multiple, usually small, discrete tumor lumps that have a microscopic organoid appearance and a low metastatic rate. Some investigators have reported that some of the Carney tumors have the electron microscopic features of autonomic nerve tumors (81, 82). The other components of the syndrome are pulmonary chondromas and extraadrenal functioning paragangliomas.

The epithelioid cell composition of a benign gastric tumor really does not impart to that tumor any unusual qualities that make it different from other benign gastric stromal tumors. They look the same grossly, although as mentioned subsequently, the epithelioid sarcomas differ somewhat from other gastric sarcomas from a prognostic standpoint.

SPINDLE CELL SARCOMAS

In addition to the epithelioid cell sarcomas is a group of sarcomas of large size and various microscopic patterns, usually composed of

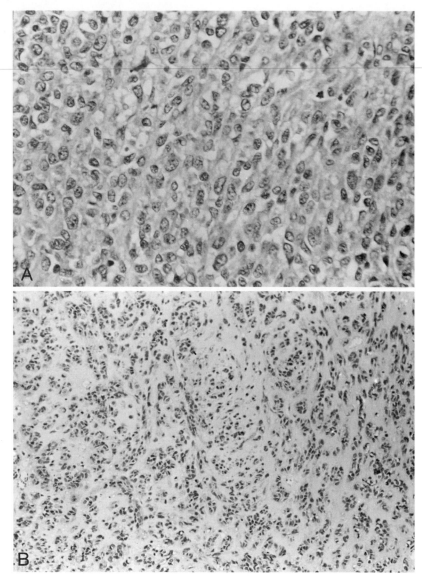

Figure 18.31 Gastric epithelioid cell sarcomas. **A.** This tumor contain cells that are smaller, have less cytoplasm, and are thus more tightly packed than does the comparable benign epithelioid cell tumor. Compare with Figure 18.22 (×330). **B.** In this field, the cells are clustered in a pale stroma full of acid mucopolysaccharide (×132).

spindle cells, sometimes with considerable pleomorphism and invariably with a high mitotic rate (37, 49, 83) (Fig. 18.32). These tumors are so diverse that it has not been possible to subdivide them on the basis of specific histologic patterns or to accumulate sufficient numbers of patients with tumors of any one pattern to generate statistically significant data. As a result, they are grouped together in a generic sarcoma category.

These spindle cell sarcomas are highly aggressive tumors that metastasize rapidly and widely throughout the abdomen. Patients with these tumors have a median survival of only about 9 to 10 months after diagnosis, whereas patients with sarcomas of epithelioid cell type have a median survival of slightly over 5 years (79, 83). In contrast to the epithelioid cell sarcomas, these spindle cell sarcomas do not contain areas that are histologically benign.

Efforts have been made to grade sarcomas of the stomach based on cellularity, mitoses, and pleomorphism. These grading systems vary from one study to another, so attempting to compare them is a nearly impossible task. In some of these studies, it appears that some benign cellular spindle cell tumors and some benign epithe-lioid cell tumors have been included among the sarcomas, especially the low grade sarcomas, further confounding the data.

SMALL INTESTINE

DISTRIBUTION AND COMPOSITION OF STROMAL TUMORS

Stromal tumors occur throughout the small bowel, perhaps somewhat more frequently in the ileum than in the jejunum. A disproportionately large number occur in the duodenum, considering its short length. Stromal tumors arising in Meckel diverticula have been reported, although some of these lesions may be sarcomas of the ileum with central cavitation and others may actually be tumors of the diverticulum itself.

Stromal tumors in the small bowel, including the duodenum, are quite different from those that occur in the stomach. Almost all are composed of spindle cells; predominantly epithelioid cell tumors are rare (Fig. 18.33).

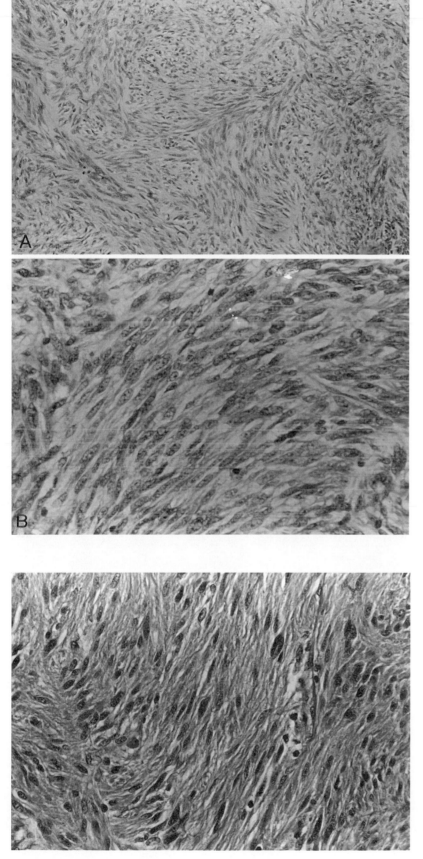

Figure 18.32   Spindle cell gastric sarcoma with storiform arrangement. **A.** Low power (×132); **B.** High power of the large spindle cells. Two mitoses are evident in this field *(top and bottom center)* (×330).

Figure 18.33   The typical benign stromal tumor of small intestine has spindle cells with plentiful fibrillar cytoplasm (×330).

BENIGN VERSUS MALIGNANT TUMORS

In the benign tumors, the spindle cells tend to be organized into short fascicles, and often the fascicles are separated into small nodules by fine fibrovascular septa, creating a distinctly organoid appearance (5, 35) (Fig. 18.34). This organization is more likely present in the submucosal aspect of a tumor than deeper within the lesion, but some, especially small tumors, may be completely organoid. Benign small bowel tumors frequently contain dense hyaline balls or blobs that lie among the cells in no particular orientation, but they tend to be more obvious and more numerous deeper in the tumor (Fig. 18.35). Ultrastructurally, these blobs are clumps of abnormal collagen fibers that have been given the name of "skeinoid fibers" by Min because of their ultrastructural resemblance to skeins of yarn (32, 38). Whether they are produced by the tumor cells is not known, but the tumor cells lack well-developed synthetic ultrastructural features, suggesting that these fibers are made by other cells. Sarcomas do not have either the organoid growth pattern or the skeinoid fibers, unless they contain histologically benign areas.

The spindle cells of the benign tumors are long and have plentiful cytoplasm, which may appear longitudinally fibrillar (see Fig. 18.33). Sarcomas have smaller, shorter, plumper, spindle cells with less cytoplasm, which resemble the cells of the mesenchymal condensations about the central epithelial core in the embryonic gut (Fig. 18.36). As a result of this difference in cell size, sarcomas are more cellular than are their benign counterparts, and cellularity seems to be the most important distinguishing feature. In the benign tumors, a search of 100 high power fields may not yield a single mitosis. In the sarcomas, mitoses also may be rare, so that a tumor with no more than 1 mitosis per 20 high power fields is capable of metastasis if the cellularity and cell type are characteristic of sarcoma (39, 40, 44, 45). Pleomorphism in small intestinal sarcomas is not common (39, 40, 44). Small intestinal dumbbell-shaped tumors may have benign areas in the submucosa, while the component outside the intestinal wall may have a completely sarcomatous appearance. Purely epithelioid tumors in the small intestine are likely to be malignant, no matter their cellularity or mitotic counts.

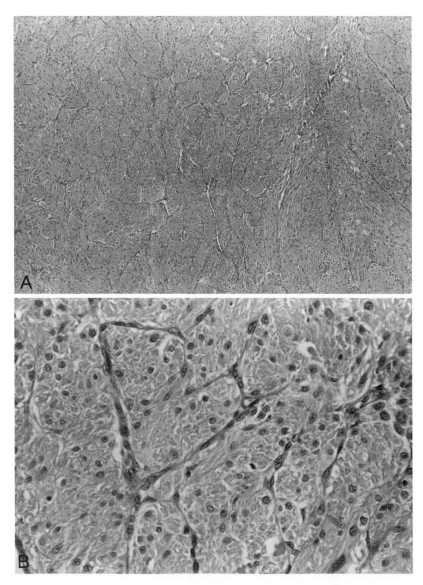

Figure 18.34 Many benign small intestinal stromal tumors have this organoid pattern with short cell fascicles surrounded by thin vascular septa. **A.** Low power (×53); **B.** High power (×330).

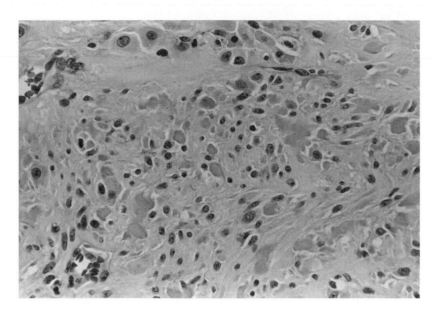

Figure 18.35 Collagen blobs (skeinoid fibers) are frequently interspersed randomly among the cells in benign small bowel stromal tumors and in benign areas of sarcomas (×330).

Limited data address the question of whether duodenal stromal tumors are identical to those in the jejunum and ileum. For that matter, no published data reveal if jejunal and ileal tumors are the same. In a study of 20 purely duodenal stromal tumors, all sarcomas had the cellularity just described (39). Tumors larger than 5 cm across that had mitotic counts of more that 2 per 50 high power fields metastasized, although some smaller tumors and some with fewer mitoses also metastasized. In contrast, results of a study combining jejunal and ileal tumors demonstrated that all tumors 7 cm or more across with mitotic counts of 4 or more per 50 high power fields metastasized (40). Thus, duodenal sarcomas may be somewhat smaller and less mitotically active than their more distal counterparts, which is another example of site specificity.

COLON AND RECTUM

BENIGN AND MALIGNANT STROMAL TUMORS OF THE ABDOMINAL COLON

The colon, exclusive of the rectum, is an unusual site for stromal tumors. In the largest series of sarcomas of the intestines reported to date, covering the period from 1911 to 1974, Akwari et al. reported 106 small bowel tumors and 26 rectal tumors, but only 15 tumors that arose in the abdominal colon (45). These tumors are so unusual that they typically are grouped together with small intestinal tumors or with rectal tumors, yet the tumors in each of these sites differ from those in the other sites. So few data on colonic stromal tumors are available that little is known of their behavior and appearance (84–86). Most seem to arise in the ascending and transverse colon, fewer in the sigmoid colon. Most reported tumors are considered by the authors to be malignant, rather than benign, which is consistent with the greater number of colonic sarcomas than benign stromal tumors in our practice.

In general, the colonic sarcomas appear to be highly aggressive tumors that either metastasize soon after diagnosis or are discovered well after metastasis has occurred.

Grossly, some colonic sarcomas grow as multiple confluent nodules in a longitudinal fashion, a pattern virtually never encountered elsewhere in the gut (Fig. 18.37). Most, however, seem to produce the solid or lobulated localized mass appearance characteristic of gastrointestinal sarcomas in other sites. Benign stromal tumors are generally smaller than sarcomas and are circumscribed single nodules, comparable in gross appearance to those in the stomach and small intestine.

Compared to rectal sarcomas, which tend to be fairly uniform in cell composition, colonic sarcomas are likely to be pleomorphic with variably sized and shaped cells and nuclei, bizarre mitotic figures, and a more haphazard, rather than fascicular, growth pattern (Fig. 18.38). A few look like small intestinal sarcomas and a few look like rectal sarcomas. The benign tumors are less cellular and contain uniform, long spindle cells with plenty of cytoplasm. In a study of 19 colonic stromal tumors, metastasis and death from tumor correlated with microscopic (not gross) infiltration of the colonic wall, mucosal invasion, and mitotic counts of over 5 per 50 high power fields. Adjuvant treatment with either radiation or chemotherapy or both reduced the risk of metastasis and death, although this study was not controlled for treatment regimen (86).

Appendiceal stromal tumors are too uncommon to warrant discussion.

DEEP INTRAMURAL STROMAL TUMORS OF THE RECTUM AND ANUS

A small group of spindle cell tumors arise in the rectum, generally in the muscularis propria, often extending into the submucosa, and in the deep anal soft tissues (41, 87–92). Because they are often large tumors and involve rectum and anus in continuity, they are grouped together as arising in the anorectum. About 50% of these tumors recur after initial and subsequent excisions, and only after several recurrences over a number of years do metastases occur (41, 87, 88). Thus, behavioral studies of rectal tumors are incomplete unless follow-up continues for many years, probably 5 years at a minimum. It is not clear if this clinical story is a manifestation of the tumor's intrinsic growth capabilities and/or simply a result of inadequate local excision. The natural history of many anorectal tumors thus differs from those arising in the proximal colon, which tend to metastasize earlier after they are discovered. In one study, the

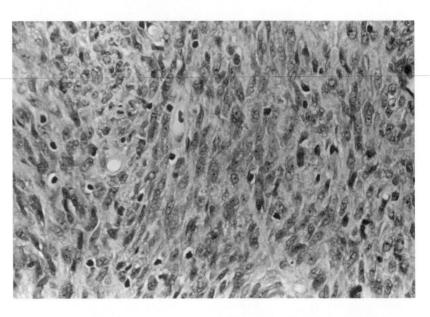

Figure 18.36 The small intestinal sarcomas are composed of smaller, uniform, more crowded cells than are the benign tumors. Compare with Figure 18.30 (×330).

median survival for 14 colonic sarcomas was only about 2 years, whereas that for rectal sarcomas was more than 10 years (85). When first observed, these neoplasms are composed of long, slender uniform spindle cells with dark nuclei (Fig. 18.39A). The cells are arranged in small fascicles. Mitotic figures are usually present but in low frequency. The cells are densely packed together so that the tumors resemble the cellular leiomyomas of the stomach, but they lack the palisades and perinuclear vacuoles of the gastric tumors. With each recurrence, the cells tend to become shorter and even more tightly packed, the nuclei become more vesicular rather than dark, mitotic figures become more frequent, and the fascicles become broader and sheetlike. Also, with subsequent recurrences, epithelioid cells are likely to appear, either scattered or in clusters. Occasionally, at initial presentation, the tumor has the full-blown malignant features or a biopsy specimen contains areas of mucosal infiltration, an indication of malignancy. These characteristics suggest that highly cellular spindle cell tumors deep in the rectal wall should be treated aggressively, rather than by wide local excision, at initial presentation (89). This treatment plan may decrease local recurrence, but it may not affect survival (90, 92).

Less cellular tumors, presumably the benign counterparts of these progressively worsening sarcomas, also appear in the deep rectal wall and are characterized by their smaller size, circumscription, larger cells, less dense cellularity, and virtually absent mitotic figures (41, 88) (Fig. 18.39B). It has been suggested that large rectal tumors considered to be benign initially may recur if they are inadequately excised, but whether these lesions are really benign or are just less cellular sarcomas is not known.

LEIOMYOMA OF THE MUSCULARIS MUCOSAE OF THE RECTUM AND SIGMOID COLON (LEIOMYOMATOUS POLYP)

The muscularis mucosae of the gastrointestinal tract is a continuous layer of smooth muscle with inner circular and outer longitudinal components, comparable to those in the much thicker muscularis

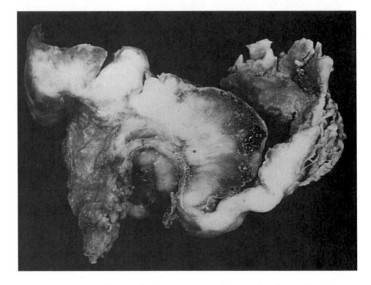

Figure 18.37 This colonic sarcoma forms both a dominant mass and extensive diffuse mural thickening, a picture rarely seen outside the colon.

propria. This muscle has considerable bulk, yet it is surprising that only one tumor arises predictably from this layer with any frequency; it is confined to the rectum and sigmoid colon where it produces a rounded elevation or bump, seen by the endoscopist as a small sessile polyp (92). These leiomyomatous polyps, with a median size of only about 5 to 6 mm, are too small to produce symptoms. Rare polyps have grown to as large as 1.5 cm in diameter. The age and sex distribution is much the same as that for patients who have routine lower endoscopic examinations, because these asymptomatic lumps are detected as incidental findings.

Other than the esophageal leiomyomas, this rectal nodule is the only other tumor of the gastrointestinal tract composed of typical, often hypertrophic mature smooth muscle. The muscularis mucosae seems to undergo a nodular expansion in which the smooth muscle cells lose their normal bilayer orientation and form small bundles that seemingly go off in all directions (Figs. 18.40 and 18.41). These nodules are covered by normal or slightly attenuated colonic mucosa.

TINY STROMAL TUMORS OF THE MUSCULARIS PROPRIA/MYENTERIC PLEXUS INTERFACE

One of the more common GISTs is a tiny spindle cell nodule situated in the muscularis propria in the region of the myenteric plexus (Fig. 18.42) (35, 37). These proliferations rarely exceed 1 cm in diameter, and they are not malignant. It is common for both the myenteric nerves and the smooth muscle fibers of the muscularis propria to be enveloped by the tumor cells that may even appear to wrap around nerve twigs. The tumor cells are uniform and spindled, arranged in short fascicles, and interdigitate with the

smooth muscle cells (Fig. 18.43). Calcification and hyalinization are common.

Compared to other stromal tumors that differ by site, these tiny tumors look exactly the same no matter where they occur. Immunohistochemically, they are no different than other spindle cell gastrointestinal tract stromal tumors. Occasional cells contain S-100 protein, but most do not. Such positively staining cells may be trapped myenteric Schwann cells.

The surgical pathologist with a heavy caseload usually sees these tiny spindle cell nodules in a frozen section. Surgeons find them protruding from the mesenteric surface anywhere in the gut, but usually the small bowel or stomach. When discovered during a laparotomy performed to determine the resectability of a neoplasm, usually a carcinoma, and before definitive resection, metastases need to be excluded. To the surgeon, this small lump is suspect as a peritoneal metastasis. As a result, the major significance of these tumors is that they constitute a frozen section diagnostic problem.

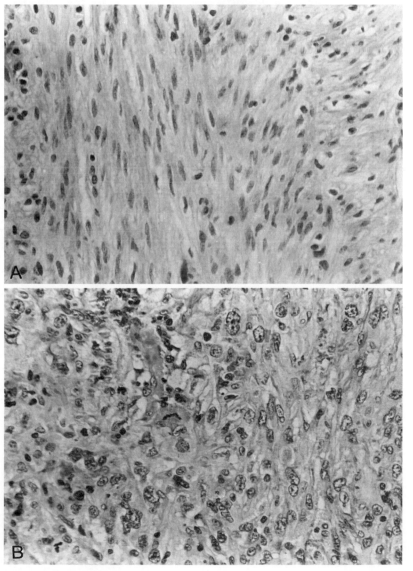

Figure 18.38   A. A benign colonic stromal tumor with uniform spindle cells. **B.** A sarcoma with pleomorphism, a mitosis, and a mixture of spindled and epithelioid cells. (**A** and **B,** ×330.)

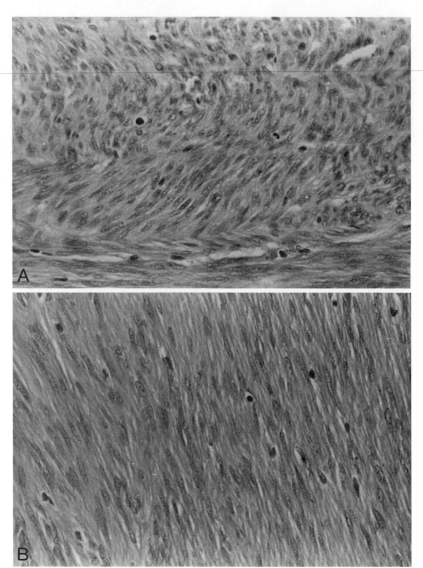

Figure 18.39   A. A rectal sarcoma with the tightly packed spindle cells. Note the mitoses at the left and right center. **B.** A benign rectal stromal tumor with less cellularity. (**A** and **B,** ×330).

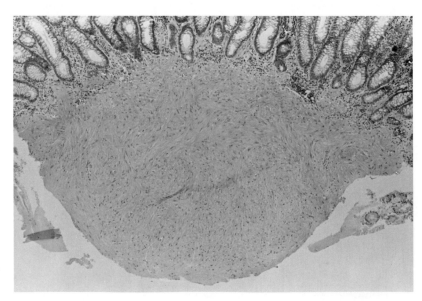

Figure 18.40   The leiomyomatous polyp of the rectosigmoid muscularis mucosae typically forms a ball of typical smooth muscle beneath the mucosa (×53).

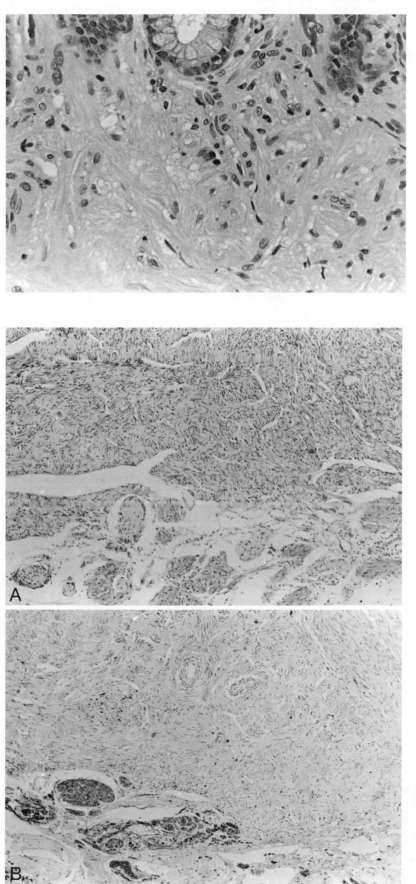

Figure 18.41 High-power view of a rectosigmoid leiomyomatous polyp. The spindle cells of the tumor are located immediately beneath the base of the crypts (×330).

Figure 18.42 The tiny stromal tumor of the myenteric plexus-muscularis propria. **A.** A myenteric nerve at the periphery *(lower left corner)* is partially surrounded by the tumor situated mainly in the upper half of the field. The darker bundles at the lower edge of the field are muscularis propria (×83). **B.** This section is stained for S-100 protein, which strongly stains the nerve at the lower left corner, but is only positive in scattered cells within the tumor, possibly trapped Schwann cells. The tumor cells otherwise do not contain stainable S-100 (×83).

TUMORS AND TUMOR-LIKE PROLIFERATION COMMON TO THE ENTIRE GASTROINTESTINAL TRACT

LESIONS OF ADIPOSE TISSUE

LIPOMAS AND LIPOSARCOMAS

Lipomas have been found in all levels of the gastrointestinal tract, but the colon, especially the right side, seems to be the most common site (93–98). These circumscribed intramural yellow masses attenuate the overlying mucosa (Fig. 18.44). The mucosa overlying the larger lesions may be ulcerated and have secondary fibrotic and hemorrhagic changes at the ulcer base. Occasional lipomas are pedunculated, and, as a result, may cause intussusception with intestinal obstruction. Not surprisingly, big tumors are more likely than smaller lesions to produce bleeding, pain, or obstruction. Rare cases of multiple lipomas occur, and sometimes, especially in the small intestine, these lumps are so numerous that the condition has been termed "lipomatosis" (99). Many lipomas are discovered as incidental findings during endoscopic procedures and are amputated completely at that time. Biopsy specimens of large tumors, if taken deeply enough, usually yield the characteristic solid sheet of submucosal adipocytes.

Microscopically, these submucosal masses of rather uniform adipose cells compress the muscularis mucosae and often cause thinning of the overlying mucosa. In the occasional case involving an ulcer, sclerotic septa may penetrate the tumor from the base of the ulcer. Some lesions may be associated with atypical-appearing granulation tissue with proliferating, somewhat pleomorphic spindled and stellate cells that superficially resemble liposarcoma (100) (Fig. 18.45). Right-sided colonic lipomas tend to be covered by a mucosa that is identical to that found in hyperplastic polyps.

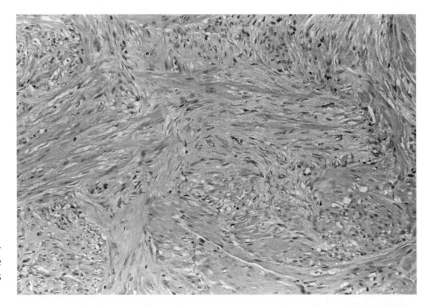

Figure 18.43 High-power view of the tumor in Figure 18.42. The pale tumor cells interdigitate with the darker staining smooth muscle fibers of the muscularis propria (×330).

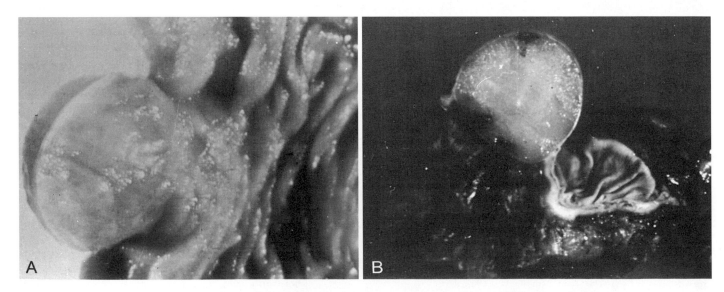

Figure 18.44 Two submucosal lipomas that form circumscribed yellow nodules. **A.** An ileal tumor. **B.** A colonic tumor. (Photograph courtesy of Dr. Donald Antonioli, Boston, MA.)

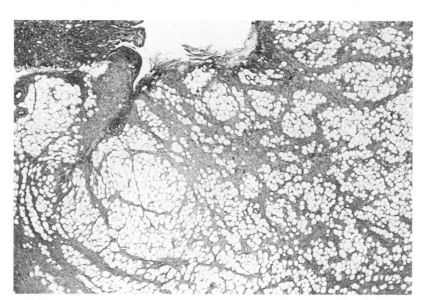

Figure 18.45 This ulcerated lipoma of the duodenum is criss-crossed by granulation tissue and fibrous septa, radiating from the base of the ulcer at the top center (×13).

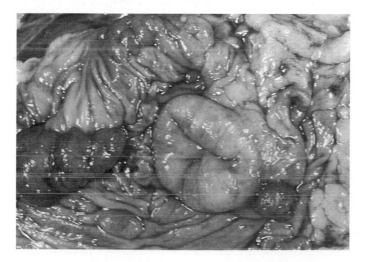

Figure 18.46 Lipomatous hypertrophy of the ileocecal valve; the huge puckered valve is in the center. The large polyps to the left and right of this big pale valve are adenomas of the colonic mucosa. Smaller adenomas are present above and below the valve.

Descriptions of gastrointestinal lipomas are especially prevalent in the radiologic literature because of a set of fairly characteristic features, including pliability, allowing for changing shape of the tumor, and the low density as noted in computed tomographic studies.

A few gastrointestinal liposarcomas have been reported (101). Whether these lesions are really liposarcomas or epithelioid cell stromal tumors with clear cytoplasm is not always clear.

LIPOMATOUS HYPERTROPHY (LIPOMATOSIS, LIPOHYPERPLASIA) OF THE ILEOCECAL VALVE

The ileocecal valve is a slender projection of smooth muscle from the inner muscularis propria covered on one side by ileal mucosa, on the other side by colonic mucosa, and on the tip by a variable-sized area of peculiar transitional mucosa with features of both small intestine

and colon. Usually, the submucosa on both sides of this muscular projection contains adipose tissue. On occasion, this adipose tissue becomes excessive, producing a large, protruding ileocecal valve that grossly resembles the uterine cervix or a set of huge pouting yellow lips (102, 103) (Fig. 18.46).

As the big valve protrudes into the cecal lumen, it can produce a dramatic radiographic filling defect resembling a neoplasm, even a cecal carcinoma, which seems to be the reason for the notoriety of this aberration. Now that colonoscopy has essentially replaced colonic barium studies, this condition no longer has such importance. The endoscopists seem to recognize it readily. At times, an endoscopist will retrieve tissue from one of these lips for biopsy, which demonstrates adipose tissue covered by normal mucosa, a picture identical to that in a biopsy of a lipoma.

Patients may have nonspecific clinical problems, such as constipation or abdominal pain, presumably the reasons for performing the radiographic or endoscopic studies, but it does not seem that the big valves cause such symptoms. In most cases, the hypertrophic valves are found incidentally during endoscopy, barium studies, or resections for other problems. Intestinal obstruction and bleeding from an ulcerated valve have been reported, but these cases are truly unusual.

No one knows why excess adipose tissue occurs in these valves. Obesity is not an explanation; more people with lipomatous hypertrophy are slender than obese. That patients with this condition are more commonly middle-aged women may suggest a hormonal process is at work. Perhaps these valves are simply exaggerations of the norm that fall outside of the two standard deviation level of confidence.

VASCULAR AND PERIVASCULAR LESIONS
GLOMUS TUMORS

This benign neoplasm is composed of uniform round cells that ultrastructurally are mature smooth muscle cells. In the gut, almost all glomus tumors occur within the stomach, especially the antral region, where they appear grossly as intramural, rather circumscribed masses (36, 37, 104–106). A few have been found in the esophagus and even fewer in the small intestine. Most tumors are

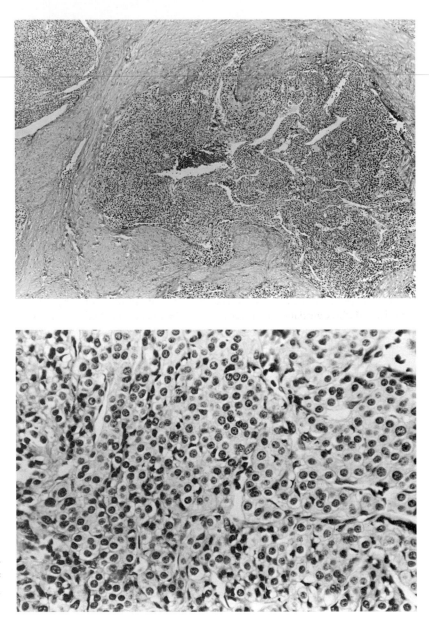

Figure 18.47   A gastric glomus tumor. Several nodules of neoplasm are separated by hypertrophic smooth muscle septa from the muscularis propria. Note the elongated and angulated vascular channels in the nodules (×53).

Figure 18.48   High-power view of a gastric glomus tumor. Cells are uniform and round and have pale or clear cytoplasm. Compare these cells with the cells of the epithelioid leiomyoma in Figure 18.22 at the same magnification (×330).

about 2 to 2.5 centimeters across, but they may grow to 4 cm in diameter. The bigger glomus tumors are likely to be ulcerated.

Microscopically, glomus tumors lie mostly within the muscularis propria, where they form nodules separated by bands of hypertrophic, often collagenized smooth muscle (Fig. 18.47). The mucosa is never infiltrated. The tumor cells are monotonous, round cells with central uniform nuclei and pale to clear cytoplasm (Fig. 18.48). The cells are arranged in sheets, cords, or clusters, usually intimately applied to the walls of capillaries, some of which may be peculiarly angulated or dilated. Structurally, these tumors look exactly like their counterparts in the skin. The major differential diagnosis for such a small intramural round cell tumor is an epithelioid cell stromal tumor. Grossly, glomus tumors are so small that they probably never reach the size of metastasizing epithelioid stromal tumors. Histologically, the major differences involve the uniformity of the cells in the glomus tumor, where each cell is almost

exactly the same as the one next to it. In contrast, the cells of the epithelioid cell stromal tumor are larger and more variable. Furthermore, the characteristic perivascular orientation of the glomus cells is only rarely encountered in epithelioid cell stromal tumors, and, then, only in a few small foci.

OTHER VASCULAR TUMORS

Angiomas, both of blood vascular and lymphatic types, occur in the gut and look exactly like angiomas elsewhere in the body; some have cavernous channels, some have small capillary channels arranged in lobules, some have thicker walled vessels, and some have various mixtures of these characteristics (37, 107–110). Some angiomas are small, whereas others involve long segments of bowel, especially in the colon. Gastrointestinal angiosarcomas are so rare that meaningful discussion is impossible.

Early reports of gastrointestinal hemangiopericytomas, arising especially in the stomach, apparently described mostly epithelioid cell tumors, including sarcomas, which had prominent perivascular orientation as described previously. Rarely, however, a real hemangiopericytoma does occur within the gut (111). Finally, Kaposi's sarcoma involving the bowel has gained recent headlines because of its occurrence in AIDS (see discussion in Chapters 14 and 16).

INFLAMMATORY FIBROID POLYPS

Inflammatory fibroid polyp (IFP) is the name given collectively to a group of expansile, mainly submucosal lumps that arise in all levels of the gut and contain a mixture of spindled cells, small vessels, and inflammatory cells (37, 112–127). Careful analysis of these lesions suggests they may not be as homogenous as the common name implies.

Inflammatory fibroid polyps occur mainly in the distal stomach or pylorus and the distal ileum; they have been found in the esophagus, colon, more proximal small intestine, and more proximal stomach, but too rarely to have accumulated any meaningful clinical and pathologic data. In one report, ileal IFPs were described as being an important cause of small intestinal obstruction in Malawi in Africa, suggesting specific geographic influences (125). Another report described a family with what is an apparent inherited tendency to form ileal and gastric IFPs, some of which are multiple and recurrent (124). Table 18.2 compares the IFPs in the two most common locations.

The gastric lesions usually arise immediately proximal to or even overlying the pyloric sphincter musculature, where they produce sessile lumps, although a few pedunculated tumors have been reported. Because the lesions are small (median size of about 1.5 cm), most have been discovered incidentally in asymptomatic individuals, in individuals with symptoms not clearly the result of the tumor, or during laparotomies or endoscopy. Occasional tumors as large as 4 to 5 cm across have been described, and some of them occasionally produce gastric outlet obstruction. Some gastric IFPs have overlying ulcers, but symptoms apparently do not correlate with the presence or absence of an ulcer. IFPs may be more common in patients with atrophic gastritis, including those with pernicious anemia.

The gastric tumors tend to fill the superficial submucosa and have a sharp lower border deeper in that layer; they rarely involve the muscularis propria. Superficially, they spread apart or splay the bundles of the muscularis mucosae and infiltrate the base of the mucosa where they separate the glands (Fig. 18.49). In one study, several tumors were described as totally mucosal, suggesting origin in mucosa. This finding has been substantiated in other studies and in this author's experience.

These tumors are composed of plump spindled cells and inflammatory cells, usually including many eosinophils. The spindled cells and eosinophils tend to form concentric layers about small, thin-walled vessels that are usually seen in cross-sectional profiles (Fig. 18.50).

The terminal ileal IFPs differ from the gastric lesions. Most importantly, they are larger. Because of their size, they tend to produce symptoms, most frequently the result of intussusception with intestinal obstruction as the pedunculated tumor forms the leading edge of the internal hernia (Figs. 18.51 and 18.52). Furthermore, as a result of these gross characteristics, the ileal polyps usually are extensively ulcerated. The ileal IFPs tend to be transmural, filling the submucosa, replacing the muscularis propria, and often having a large subserosal component as well (Fig. 18.53). These tumors look like excessive granulation tissue, and compared to the gastric lesions, they are likely to have more edematous stroma, more elongated than rounded vascular profiles, a cell population likely to be more stellate than spindled, no prominent perivascular laminations, and a mixed inflammatory cell population more mixed, including plasma cells and lymphocytes, as well as eosinophils (Fig. 18.54). Occasionally, ileal IFPs have highly proliferative central foci with many mitoses and nuclear hyperchromatism. Such areas may resemble sarcoma superficially.

Peculiarly, the esophageal IFPs usually resemble those in the terminal ileum, whereas those in the colon tend to look more like the IFPs in the stomach.

The histogenesis of these lesions has not been clarified to date. They have been called collectively "inflammatory fibroid polyps," in an attempt to indicate that they are inflammatory and not neoplastic. Of course, this nomenclature implies that some type of inflammation is the stimulus, but none has been identified to date. In ultrastructural and immunohistochemical studies of the gastric and

TABLE 18.2	Comparison of Inflammatory Fibroid Polyps in Stomach and Ileum	
Characteristic Features	Stomach	Ileum
Age at presentation	Mid sixth decade	Mid sixth decade
Sex distribution	Males slightly greater than females	Males slightly greater than females
Site	Prepyloric	Terminal
Size	75% 3 cm or less	Greater than 2 cm (median 4+ cm)
Symptoms	None. Occasional outlet obstruction if over 2.5 cm	Intestinal obstruction (intussusception)
Upper border	Mucosa, infiltrating	Muscularis mucosae, extensions into mucosa
Lower border	Submucosa, sharp	Muscularis propria or subserosa, infiltrating
Microscopic appearance	Perivascular	Loose like granulation tissue
Associations	? Atrophic gastritis ? Pernicious anemia	None

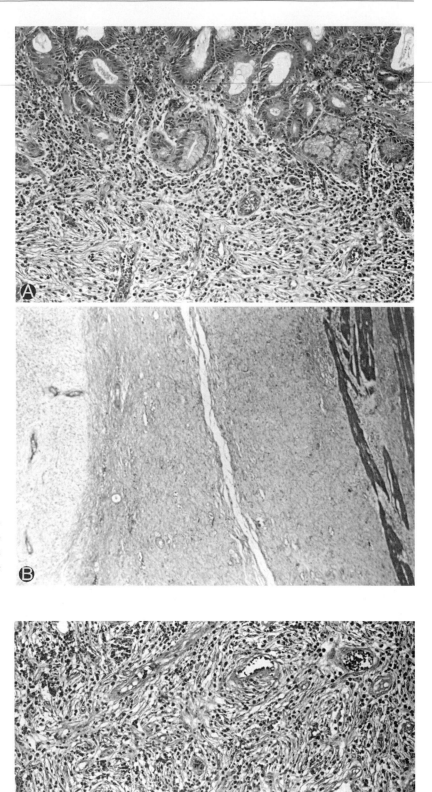

Figure 18.49   The gastric inflammatory fibroid polyp (IFP). **A.** Invasion of the base of the mucosa by the tumor cells (×132). **B.** The pale tumor on the left has a sharp lower border in the submucosa *(center)*. The muscularis propria is at right (×33).

Figure 18.50   Gastric IFP. Perivascular orientation of spindled and inflammatory cells (×132).

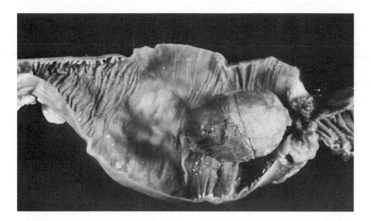

Figure 18.51 Ileal IFP. A typical gross polypoid lesion within a dilated segment of bowel.

small intestinal tumors, the stellate and spindle cells have features of fibroblasts and myofibroblasts, and there is also a population of macrophages, findings that correlate quite well with the granulation tissue appearance (119, 121–123, 125–127).

TUMORS OF NERVE TISSUE

As mentioned previously, many gut stromal tumors, particularly the gastric spindle cell tumor with the spectacular palisades, are periodically reported as some type of nerve sheath tumor, using names such as neurofibroma, neurilemmoma, schwannoma, neuroma, or their malignant counterparts. Apparently most of these reports describe tumors that are really identical to the indigenous stromal tumors, so it is meaningless to redescribe them here in a separate part of this chapter. Classic schwannomas with capsules, both palisading and microcystic spindle cell proliferation patterns, typical sclerotic blood vessels, and degenerative changes are too rare in the gastrointestinal tract to be of concern. In a report from Japan, the authors described 23 gastric and 1 colonic spindle cell tumors, designated as schwannomas, that seemed to involve the myenteric plexus and stained positively with antibodies to S-100 protein. These tumors, however, had a storiform rather than a palisaded growth pattern, were not encapsulated, and also stained positively with antibody to glial fibrillary acidic protein, all findings that are not typical of schwannomas (128). Another series of almost identical tumors was reported from Finland and the United States (129). Because tumors of this type have not been substantiated in other studies, and these tumors lack some of the typical features of peripheral nerve schwannomas, their identity is not clear. Nevertheless, occasional nerve sheath and nervous tissue tumors do involve the gastrointestinal tract, three of which are detailed in the following sections.

INTRAMURAL NEUROFIBROMA

Patients with von Recklinghausen multiple neurofibromatosis commonly have gastrointestinal involvement, sometimes taking the form of neurofibromas of the plexiform pattern characterized by expansion of nerves by spindle cells and collagen bundles all loosely arranged in a mucopolysaccharide-rich stroma (Fig. 18.55). Less commonly, diffuse neurofibromas extend from the submucosa

across the muscularis mucosae into the mucosa where they expand the mucosa and distort the crypts, producing a picture resembling the mucosa in incipient juvenile polyps (Fig. 18.56). The occurrence of a typical neurofibroma of the gastrointestinal tract in the absence of von Recklinghausen disease is too rare to discuss. It is important to remember that gut stromal tumors of typical or usual type also may occur in patients with von Recklinghausen multiple neurofibromatosis (32, 130). Malignancies or nerve sheath sarcomas have been reported as arising in the gut in association with von Recklinghausen disease, but documentation of their nerve sheath differentiation is uniformly poor (131).

GANGLIONEUROMA AND GANGLIONEUROMATOSIS

Within the alimentary tract, mainly in the colon, occasional proliferations of nerves, their associated Schwann cells, and ganglion cells occur in any or all plexuses and in other sites, including the mucosa. Such lesions have been designated as ganglioneuromas, although they vary considerably from the solid tumors of the same name that occur in the retroperitoneum and mediastinum (Fig. 18.57). Although ganglion cells normally do not reside within the gastrointestinal tract mucosa, such proliferations occasionally involve the mucosa, often secondary to submucosal plexus lesions. When these proliferations are confined to mucosa, the result is the formation of polyps or plaques (132–138). In such mucosal lesions, the Schwann cells and neurites extend among the epithelial elements, be they glands, pits, or crypts, separating them and often distorting them, resulting in branching or dilated or bizarre-shaped tubules situated in a hypercellular expanded lamina propria (133). Such distortion also resembles that encountered in juvenile polyps. Mixed with the Schwann cells are variable numbers of ganglion cells, sometimes clustered, sometimes isolated, and, in occasional lesions, very difficult to find. In a few instances, only the nerve and Schwann cell proliferations are present without ganglion cells, which encourages the use of the designation "neuroma."

The pattern of bowel wall, including mucosal involvement, has

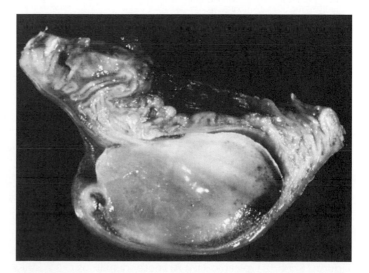

Figure 18.52 This ileal IFP forms the leading edge of an intussusception, which is captured in the distal segment of ileum. The cross section of the tumor is pale and glistening. (Photograph courtesy of Dr. Mahendra Ranchod, San Jose, CA.)

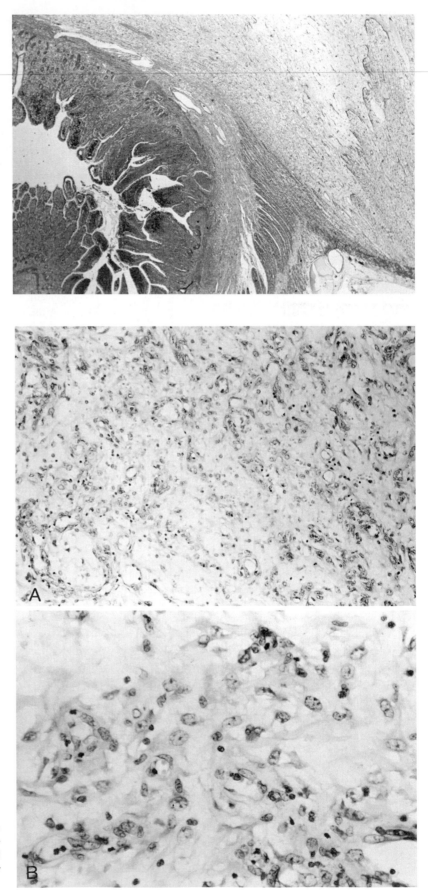

Figure 18.53   The ileal IFP fills the submucosa *(top)* and gradually replaces the muscularis propria *(right)* (×13).

Figure 18.54   A typical ileal IFP. **A.** Loose edematous, highly vascularized stroma resembles granulation tissue (×132). **B.** High-power view of the stellate and spindle cells with the superimposed inflammatory cells and the prominent capillaries (×330).

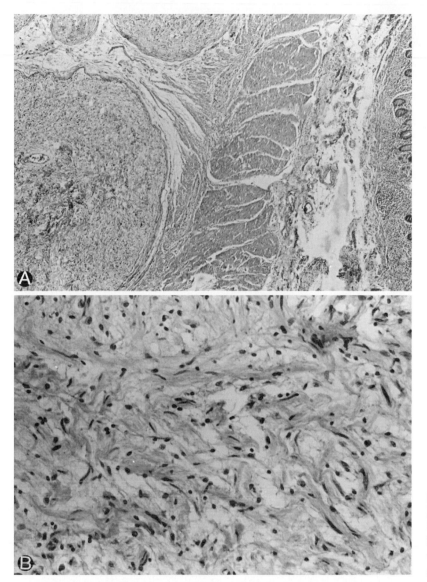

Figure 18.55 Plexiform neurofibroma of the small bowel in a patient with von Recklinghausen disease. **A.** Low-power view of the typical expansion of the nerves in the gut wall forming nodules (×33). **B.** High-power view of the loose spindle cells and collagen bundles (×330).

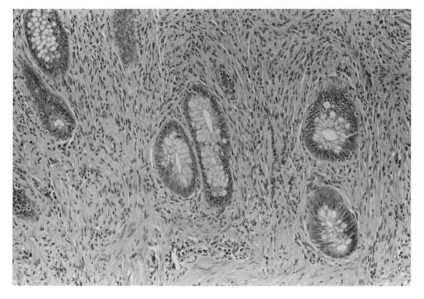

Figure 18.56 A diffuse colonic mucosal neurofibroma in a case of von Recklinghausen disease. The crypts are widely separated by the spindle cell proliferation (×132).

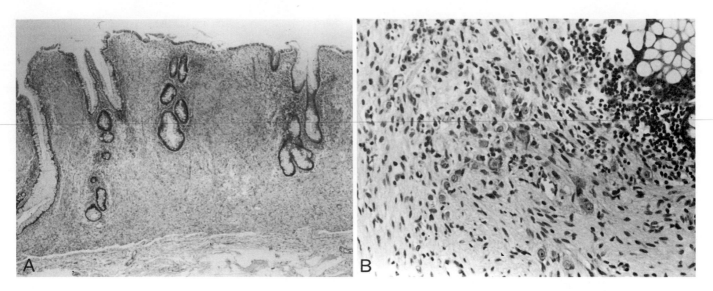

Figure 18.57 Ganglioneuroma of the colon. **A.** The colonic lamina propria is expanded by a spindle cell proliferation, and the crypts are spread widely apart and are grotesquely distorted (×53). **B.** High-power view of one of these foci. The lamina propria expansion is attributable mainly to the spindle cells, which are Schwann cells, but ganglion cells are present as well (×265).

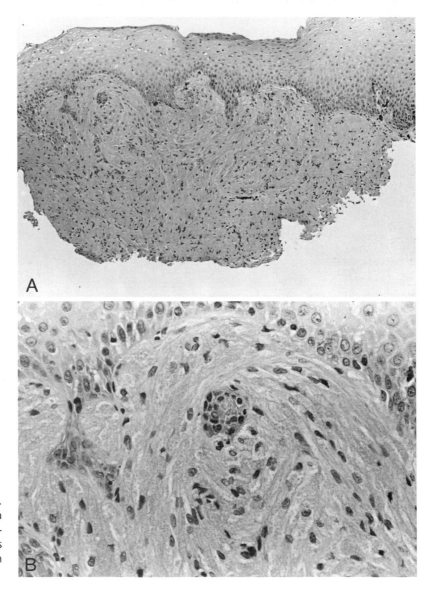

Figure 18.58 Granular cell tumor of the esophagus. **A.** Immediately beneath the saw-tooth epithelium is a nodule of spindle cells, the fascicles of which interdigitate with the deeply projecting squamous prongs (×83). **B.** High-power view of the spindle cells with granular cytoplasm (×330).

led to a plethora of descriptors, including "polypoid," "nonpolypoid," and "diffuse" ganglioneuromatosis, and "solitary" ganglioneuroma, which seems to be synonymous with "localized" ganglioneuromatosis (133). These lesions, and generally certain specific modifications, have been described as common manifestations of MEN, type IIb syndrome, and rarely of von Recklinghausen disease (132–134). For instance, the solitary polypoid lesions do not seem to be part of any syndrome. By contrast, when multiple polyps arise, they have been associated with multiple juvenile polyps, colonic adenomas, a cecal carcinoma, multiple cutaneous lipomas, and Cowden syndrome, as well as other complex multiorgan disorders (132–138). It is those lesions that involve the nerve plexuses as well as all other layers of the bowel that are likely to be part of either the MEN IIb or von Recklinghausen syndromes.

GRANULAR CELL TUMORS

Granular cell tumors of the gastrointestinal tract are exactly like their namesake in the skin or mouth (36, 37, 139–143). These intramural nodules produce sessile lumps when viewed from the mucosal aspect. Granular cell tumors are composed of uniform plump spindled or epithelioid cells stuffed with coarse eosinophilic cytoplasmic granules. The granules are PAS-positive after diastase digestion, and, on electron microscopic analysis, are giant lysosomes filled with a mixture of granular and membranous material, essentially intracellular junk. The spindle cells are arranged in packets or blunt fascicles. Also, like their counterparts elsewhere, the cells of the gastrointestinal granular cell tumors stain positively with the antibody to the S-100 protein.

Granular cell tumors have been found in all sites in the gut, but most arise in the esophagus where they are likely to be associated with an overlying squamous mucosal alteration that may be hyperplastic, even to the point of pseudoepitheliomatous hyperplasia. In some cases, the epithelium actually may be thinner than normal (Fig. 18.58). The cells of the granular cell tumor usually fill the lamina propria and hug the base of the squamous epithelium. Thus, a full-thickness mucosal biopsy is likely to pick up the diagnostic cells. In other gastrointestinal sites, the tumorous granular cells create submucosal masses, replace the muscularis mucosae, and extend into the lamina propria. This pattern of mucosal infiltration is common only to the granular cell tumors, diffuse neurofibromas, ganglioneuromas, the gastric variants of inflammatory fibroid polyps, and the sarcomas.

In the esophagus, about two thirds of the granular cell tumors occur in the lower segment, with the remaining one third split evenly between the upper and the middle esophageal segments. The size of the tumor correlates with symptoms, which consist principally of dysphagia or pain. Tiny granular cell tumors are often found serendipitously during upper endoscopy in asymptomatic patients.

REFERENCES

1. Nojima T, Gebhardt MC, Mankin HJ, et al. Extraosseous osteosarcoma presenting with intestinal hemorrhage: Case report and literature review. Hum Pathol 1986;17:85–87.
2. Stout AP. Tumors of the stomach, Section VI, Fiscule 21. Atlas of tumor pathology. Washington, D.C.: Armed Forces Institute of Pathology, 1953.
3. Golden T, Stout AP. Smooth muscle tumors of the gastrointestinal tract and retroperitoneal tissues. Surg Gynecol Obstet 1941;73:784–810.
4. Mills SE. Editorial: Sometimes we don't look like our parents. Mod Pathol 1995:8:347.
5. Appelman HD. Smooth muscle tumors of the gastrointestinal tract. What we know that Stout didn't know. Am J Surg Pathol 1986;10(Suppl.):83–99.
6. Brown EF, Banner BF, Gould VE. Differential diagnosis of gastrointestinal schwannomas and leimyomas: A detailed histologic study with electron microscopic correlation. Lab Invest 1984;50:7A.
7. Cornog Jr JL. Gastric leiomyoblastoma: A clinical and ultrastructural study. Cancer 1974;34:711–719.
8. Hajdu, SI, Erlandson RA, Paglia MA. Light and electron microscopic studies of a gastric leiomyoblastoma. Arch Pathol Lab Med 1972;93:36–41.
9. Knapp RH, Wick MR, Goellner JR. Leiomyoblastomas and their relationship to other smooth-muscle tumors of the gastrointestinal tract. Am J Surg Pathol 1984;8:449–461.
10. Salazar H, Totten RS. Leiomyoblastoma of the stomach—an ultrastructural study. Cancer 1970;25:176–185.
11. Weiss RA, Mackay B. Malignant smooth muscle tumors of the gastrointestinal tract. Ultrastruct Pathol 1981;2:231–240.
12. Welsh RA, Meyer AT. Ultrastructure of gastric leiomyoma. Arch Pathol Lab Med 1969;87:71–81.
13. Walker P, Dvorak AM. Gastrointestinal autonomic nerve (GAN) tumor. Ultrastructural evidence for a newly recognized entity. Arch Pathol Lab Med 1986;110:309–316.
14. Herrera GA, Cerezo L, Jones JE, et al. Gastrointestinal autonomic nerve tumors. "Plexosarcomas." Arch Pathol Lab Med 1989;113:846–853.
15. Antonioli DA. Gastrointestinal autonomic nerve tumors. Expanding the spectrum of gastrointestinal stromal tumors. Arch Pathol Lab Med 1989;113:831–833.
16. Lauwers GY, Erlandson RA, Casper ES, et al. Gastrointestinal autonomic nerve tumors. A clinicopathological, immunohistochemical, and ultrastructural study of 12 cases. Am J Surg Pathol 1993;17:887–897.
17. Segal A, Carello S, Caterina P, et al. Gastrointestinal autonomic nerve tumors: A clinicopathological, immunohistochemical and ultrastructural study of 10 cases. Pathology 1994;26:439–447.
18. Shanks JH, Harris M, Banerjee SS, et al. Gastrointestinal autonomic nerve tumours: A report of nine cases. Histopathology 1996;29:111–121.
19. Evans DJ, Lampert JA, Jacobs M. Intermediate filaments in smooth muscle tumors. J Clin Pathol 1986;36:57–61.
20. Donner L, deLanerolle P, Costa J. Immunoreactivity of paraffin-embedded normal tissues and mesenchymal tumors for smooth muscle myosin. Am J Clin Pathol 1983;80:677–681.
21. Mazur MT, Clark HB. Gastric stromal tumors: Reappraisal of histogenesis. Am J Surg Pathol 1983;7:507–519.
22. Pike AM, Appelman HD, Lloyd RV. Cell markers in gastrointestinal stromal tumors. Hum Pathol 1988;19:830–834.
23. Saul SH, Rast ML, Brooks JJ. The immunohistochemistry of gastrointestinal stromal tumors. Am J Surg Pathol 1987;11:464–473.
24. Franquemont DW, Frierson HF Jr. Muscle differentiation and clinicopathologic features of gastrointestinal stromal tumors. Am J Surg Pathol 1992;16:947–954.
25. Hurlimann J, Gardiol D. Gastrointestinal stromal tumours: An immunohistochemical study of 165 cases. Histopathology 1991;19:311–320.
26. Ma CK, Amin MB, Kintanar E, et al. Immunohistologic characterization of gastrointestinal stromal tumors: A study of 82 cases compared with 11 cases of leiomyomas. Mod Pathol 1993;6:139–144.
27. Miettinen M, Virolainen M, Maarit Sarlomo Rikala. Gastrointestinal stromal tumors—value of CD34 antigen in their identification and separation from true leiomyomas and Schwannomas. Am J Surg Pathol 1995;19:207–216.
28. Monihan JM, Carr NJ, Sobin LH. CD 34 immunoexpression in stromal tumours of the gastrointestinal tract and in mesenteric fibromatoses. Histopathology 1994;25:469–473.
29. Newman PL, Wadden C, Fletcher CDM. Gastrointestinal stromal tumours: Correlation of immunophenotype with clinicopathological features. J Pathol 1991;164:107–117.

30. Ueyama T, Guo K-J, Hashimoto H, et al. A clinicopathologic and immunohistochemical study of gastointestinal stromal tumors. Cancer 1992;69:947–955.

31. van de Rijn M, Hendrickson MR, Rouse RV. CD34 expression by gastrointestinal tract stromal tumors. Hum Pathol 1994;25:766–771.

32. Schaldenbrand JD, Appelman HD. Solitary solid stromal gastrointestinal tumors in von Recklinghausen's disease with minimal smooth muscle differentiation. Hum Pathol 1984;15:229–232.

33. Appelman HD. Mesenchymal tumors of the gut: Historical perspectives, new approaches, new results, and does it make any difference? In Goldman H, Appelman HD, Kaufman N, eds. Gastrointestinal pathology. International Academy of Pathology Monograph Series. Baltimore: Williams & Wilkins, 1990.

34. Jass JR, Sobin LH, Watanabe H. The World Health Organization's histologic classification of gastrointestinal tumors. A commentary on the second edition. Cancer 1990;66:2162–2167.

35. Appelman HD. Stromal tumors of the esophagus, stomach and duodenum. In: Appelman HD, ed. Pathology of the esophagus, stomach, and duodenum. Contemporary issues in surgical pathology. New York: Churchill Livingstone, 1984.

36. Lewin KJ, Appelman HD. Mesenchymal tumors and tumor-like proliferations of the esophagus, tumors of the esophagus and stomach, volume 18, chapter 6. Third series. Atlas of tumor pathology. Washington, D.C.: Armed Forces Institute of Pathology, 1996.

37. Lewin KJ, Appelman HD. Mesenchymal tumors and tumor-like proliferations of the stomach, tumors of the esophagus and stomach, volume 18, chapter 14. Third series. Atlas of tumor pathology. Washington, D.C.: Armed Forces Institute of Pathology, 1996.

38. Min K-W. Small intestinal stromal tumors with skeinoid fibers. Clinicopathological, immunohistochemical, and ultrastructural investigations. Am J Surg Pathol 1992;16:145–155.

39. Goldblum JR, Appelman HD. Stromal tumors of the duodenum. A histologic and immunohistochemical study of 20 cases. Am J Surg Pathol 1995;19:71–80.

40. Tworek JA, Appelman HD, Singleton TP, et al. Stromal tumors of the jejunum and ileum. Mod Pathol, In press.

41. Haque S, Dean PJ. Stromal neoplasms of the rectum and anal canal. Hum Pathol 1992;23:762–767.

42. Carney JA. The triad of gastric epithelioid leiomyosarcoma, functioning extra-adrenal paraganglioma and pulmonary chondroma. Cancer 1979;43:374–382.

43. Carney JA. The triad of gastric epithelioid leiomyosarcoma, pulmonary chondroma and functioning extra-adrenal paraganglioma: A five-year review. Medicine 1983;62:159–169.

44. Ranchod M, Kempson RL. Smooth muscle tumors of the gastrointestinal tract and retroperitoneum. Cancer 39:255–262, 1977.

45. Akwari OE, Dozois RR, Weiland LH, et al. Leiomyosarcoma of the small and large bowel. Cancer 1978;42:1375–1384.

46. Rosai J. Ackerman's surgical pathology. 8th ed. St. Louis: Mosby, 1996:645–647, 691–693.

47. Shiu MH, Farr GH, Papachristou DN, et al. Myosarcomas of the stomach: Natural history, prognostic factors and management. Cancer 1982;49:177–187.

48. Evans HL. Smooth muscle tumors of the gastrointestinal tract. A study of 56 cases followed for a minimum of 10 years. Cancer 1985;56:2242–2250.

49. Lindsay PC, Ordonez N, Raaf JH. Gastric leiomyosarcomas: Clinical and pathological review of fifty patients. J Surg Oncol 1981;18:399–421.

50. Amin MB, Ma CK, Linden MD, et al. Prognostic value of proliferating cell nuclear antigen index in gastric stromal tumors. Correlation with mitotic count and clinical outcome. Am J Clin Pathol 1993;100:428–432.

51. Franquemont DW, Frierson HF Jr. Proliferating cell nuclear antigen immunoreactivity and prognosis of gastrointestinal stromal tumors. Mod Pathol 1995;8:473–477.

52. Ray R, Tahan SR, Andrews C, et al. Stromal tumor of the stomach: Prognostic value of the PCNA index. Mod Pathol 1994;7:26–30.

53. Sbaschnig RJ, Cunningham RE, Sobin LH, et al. Proliferating-cell nuclear antigen immunocytochemistry in the evaluation of gastsrointestinal smooth-muscle tumors. Mod Pathol 1994;7:780–783.

54. Yu CC-W, Fletcher CDM, Newman PL, et al. A comparison of proliferating cell nuclear antigen (PCNA) immunostaining, nucleolar organizer region (AgNOR) staining, and histological grading in gastrointestinal stromal tumours. J Pathol 1992;166:147–152.

55. Cooper PN, Quirke P, Hardy GJ, et al. A flow cytometric, clinical, and histological study of stromal neoplasms of the gastrointestinal tract. Am J Surg Pathol 1992;16:163–170.

56. Cunningham RE, Federspiel BH, McCarthy WF, et al. Predicting prognosis of gastrointestinal smooth muscle tumors. Role of clinical and histologic evaluation, flow cytometry, and image analysis. Am J Surg Pathol 1993;17:588–594.

57. El-Naggar AK, Ro JY, McLemore D, et al. Gastrointestinal stromal tumors: DNA flow-cytometric study of 58 patients with at least five years of follow-up. Mod Pathol 1989;2:511–515.

58. Kiyabu MT, Bishop PC, Parker JW, et al. Smooth muscle tumors of the gastrointestinal tract. Flow cytometric quantitation of DNA and nuclear antigen content and correlation with histologic grade. Am J Surg Pathol 1988;12:954–960.

59. Lerma E, Oliva E, Tugues D, et al. Stromal tumours of the gastrointestinal tract: A clinicopathological and ploidy analysis of 33 cases. Virch Arch 1994;424:19–24.

60. Shimamoto T, Haruma K, Sumii K, et al. Flow cytometric DNA analysis of gastric smooth muscle tumors. Cancer 1992;70:2031–2034.

61. Tsushima K, Rainwater LM, Goellner JR, et al. Leiomyosarcomas and benign smooth muscle tumors of the stomach: Nuclear DNA patterns studied by flow cytometry. Mayo Clin Proc 1987;62:275–280.

62. Appelman HD, Helwig EB. Gastric epithelioid leiomyoma and leiomyosarcoma (leiomyoblastoma). Cancer 1976;38:708–728.

63. Seremetis MG, Lyons WS, DeGuzman VC, et al. Leiomyomata of the esophagus: An analysis of 838 cases. Cancer 1976;38:2166–2177.

64. Takubo K, Nakagawa H, Tsuchiya S, et al. Seedling leiomyoma of the esophagus and esophagogastric junction zone. Hum Pathol 1981;12:1006–1010.

65. Enterline H, Thompson J. Pathology of the esophagus. New York: 1984:169–171.

66. Fernandas JP, Mascarenhas MJ, da Costa JC, et al. Diffuse leiomyomatosis of the esophagus. Dig Dis Sci 1975;20:684–690.

67. Heald J, Moussalli H, Hasleton PS. Diffuse leiomyomatosis of the oesophagus. Histopathology 1986;10:755–759.

68. Kabuto T, Taniguchi K, Iwanaga T, et al. Diffuse leiomyomatosis of the esophagus. Dig Dis Sci 1980;25:388–391.

69. DeMeester TR, Skinner DB. Polypoid sarcomas of the esophagus. A rare but potentially curable neoplasm. Ann Thorac Surg 1975;20:405–417.

70. Gaede JT, Postlethwait RW, Shelburne JD, et al. Leiomyosarcoma of the esophagus. Report of two cases, one with associated squamous cell carcinoma. J Thorac Cardiovasc Surg 1978;75:740–746.

71. Rainer WG, Brus R. Leiomyosarcoma of the esophagus; review of the literature and report of 3 cases. Surgery 1965;58:343–350.

72. Caldwell CB, Bains MS, Burt M. Unusual malignant neoplasms of the esophagus. Oat cell carcinoma, melanoma, and sarcoma. J Thorac Cardiovasc Surg 1981;101:100–107.

73. Levine MS, Buck JL, Pantongrag-Brown L, et al. Leiomyosarcoma of the esophagus: Radiographic findings in 10 patients. AJR Am J Roentgenol 1996;167:27–32.

74. Vartio T, Nickels J, Hockerstedt K, et al. Rhabdomyosarcoma of the oesophagus. Virchows Arch 1980;386:357–361.

75. Patel J, Kieffer RW, Martin M, et al. Giant fibrovascular polyp of the esophagus. Gastroenterology 1984;87:953–956.

76. Enterline H, Thompson J. Pathology of the esophagus. New York: Springer, 1984:172–173.

77. Levine MS, Buck JL, Pantongrag-Brown L, et al. Fibrovascular polyps of the esophagus: Clinical, radiographic, and pathologic findings in 16 patients. AJR Am J Roentgenol 1996;166:781–787.

78. Appelman HD, Helwig EB. Cellular leiomyomas of the stomach in 49 patients. Arch Pathol Lab Med 1977;101:373–377.

79. Martin JF, Bazin P, Feroldi J, et al. Tumeurs myoides intra-murales de

l estomac: Considerations microscopiques a propos de 6 cas. Ann Pathol 1960;5:484–497.

80. Stout AP. Bizarre smooth muscle tumor of the stomach. Cancer 1962;15:400–409.

81. Tortella BJ, Antonioli DA, Dvorak AM, et al. Gastric autonomic nerve (GAN) tumor and extra-adrenal paraganglioma in Carney's triad. A common origin. Ann Surg 1987;205:221–225.

82. Perez-Atayde AR, Shamberger RC, Kozakewich HWP. Neuroectodermal differentiation of the gastrointestinal tumors in the Carney triad. An ultrastructural and immunohistochemical study. Am J Surg Pathol 1993;17:706–714.

83. Appelman HD, Helwig EB. Sarcomas of the stomach. Am J Clin Pathol 1977;67:2–10.

84. Tang CK, Melamed MR. Leiomyosarcoma of the colon exclusive of the rectum. Am J Gastroenterol 1975;64:376–381.

85. Meijer S, Peretz T, Gaynor JJ, et al. Primary colorectal sarcoma. A retrospective review and prognostic factor study of 50 consecutive patients. Arch Surg 1990;125:1163–1168.

86. Tworek JA, Goldblum JR, Weiss SW, et al. Stromal tumors of the colon. Mod Pathol 1997;10:66A.

87. Moyana TN, Friesen R, Tan LK. Colorectal smooth-muscle tumors. A pathologiologic study with immunohistochemistry and histomorphology. Arch Pathol Lab Med 1991;115:1016–1021.

88. Tworek JA, Goldblum JR, Weiss SW, et al. Stromal tumors of the rectum and anus. Mod Pathol 1997;10:66A.

89. Tjandra JJ, Antoniuk PM, Webb B, et al. Leiomyosarcoma of the rectum and anal canal. Aust NZ J Surg 1993;63:703–709.

90. Khalifa AA, Bong WL, Rao VK, et al. Leiomyosarcoma of the rectum —report of a case and review of the literature. Dis Colon Rectum 1986;29:427–432.

91. Sasaki K, Gutoh Y, Nakayama Y, et al. Leiomyoma of the rectum. Int J Surg 1985;70:149–152.

92. Walsh TH, Mann CV. Smooth muscle neoplasms of the rectum and anal canal. Br J Surg 1984;71:597–599.

93. Wychulis AR, Jackman CJ, Mayo CW. Submucous lipomas of the colon and rectum. Surg Gynecol Obstet 1964;118:337–340.

94. Peiser J, Ovnat A, Herz A, et al. Lipoma of the esophagus. Isr J Med Sci 1984;20:1068–1070.

95. Agha FP, Dent TL, Fiddian-Green RC, et al. Bleeding lipoma of the upper gastrointestinal tract. Am Surg 1985;51:279–285.

96. Michowitz M, Lazebnik N, Noy S, et al. Lipoma of the colon. A report of 22 cases. Am Surg 1985;51:449–454.

97. Whetstone MR, Zuckerman MJ, Saltzsterin EC, et al. CT diagnosis of duodenal lipoma. Am J Gastroenterol 1985;80:251–252.

98. Ryan J, Martin JE, Pollock DJ. Fatty tumours of the large intestine: A clinicopathological review of 13 cases. Br J Surg 1989;76:793–796.

99. Climie ARW, Wylin RF. Small-intestinal lipomatosis. Arch Pathol Lab Med 1981;105:40–42.

100. Snover DC. Atypical lipomas of the colon: Report of two cases with pseudomalignant features. Dis Colon Rectum 1984;27:484–488.

101. Laky D, Stoica T. Gastric liposarcoma – a case report. Pathol Res Pract 1986;181:112–115.

102. Boquist L, Bargdahl L, Anderson A. Lipomatosis of the ileocecal valve. Cancer 1972;29:136–140.

103. Skaane P, Eide TJ, Westgaard T, et al. Lipomatosis and true lipomas of the ileocecal valve. Rofo Fortschr Geb Rongenstr Neuen Bildgeb Verfahr 1981;135:663–668.

104. Kay S, Callahan Jr WP, Murray MR, et al. Glomus tumors of the stomach. Cancer 1951;4:726–736.

105. Appelman HD, Helwig EB. Glomus tumors of the stomach. Cancer 1969;23:203–213.

106. Almagro UA, Schulte WJ, Norback DH, et al. Glomus tumor of the stomach: Histologic and ultrastructural features. Am J Clin Pathol 1981;75:415–419.

107. Okumura T, Tanoue S, Chiba K, et al. Lobular capillary hemangioma of the esophagus. A case report and review of the literature. Acta Pathol Jpn 1983;33:1303–1308.

108. Ikeda K, Murayama H, Takano H, et al. Massive intestinal bleeding in hemagiomatosis of the duodenum. Endoscopy 1980;12:306–310.

109. Kuroda Y, Katoh H, Ohsato K. Cystic lymphangioma of the colon. Report of a case and review of the literature. Dis Colon Rectum 1984;27:679–682.

110. Mills CS, Lloyd TV, Van Aman ME, et al. Diffuse hemangiomatosis of the colon. J Clin Gastroenterol 1985;7:416–421.

111. Genter B, Mir K, Strauss R, et al. Hemangiopericytoma of the colon. Report of a case and review of the literature. Dis Colon Rectum 1982;25:149–156.

112. Vanek J. Gastric submucosal granuloma with eosinophilic infiltration. Am J Pathol 1949;25:397–411.

113. Helwig EB, Ranier A. Inflammatory fibroid polyps of the stomach. Surg Gynecol Obstet 1953;96:355–367.

114. Bullock WK, Moran ET. Inflammatory fibroid polyps of the stomach. Cancer 1953;6:488.

115. Salm R. Gastric fibroma with eosinophilic infiltration. Gut 1965;6: 85–91.

116. Samter TG, Alstott DF, Kurlander GJ. Inflammatory fibroid polyps of the gastrointestinal tract. A report of 3 cases, 2 occurring in children. Am J Clin Pathol 1966;45:420–436.

117. Goldman RL, Friedman NB. Neurogenic nature of so-called inflammatory fibroid polyps of the stomach. Cancer 1967;20: 134–143.

118. LiVolsi VA, Perzin KA. Inflammatory pseudotumors (inflammatory fibrous polyps) of the esophagus. Am J Dig Dis 1975;20: 475–481.

119. Benjamin SP, Hawk WA, Turnbull RB. Fibrous inflammatory polyps of the ileum and cecum. Cancer 1977;39:1300–1305.

120. Johnstone JM, Morson BC. Inflammatory fibroid polyps of the gastrointestinal tract. Histopathology 1978;2:349–361.

121. Navas-Palacios JJ, Colina-Ruizdelgado F, Sanchez-Larren MD, et al. Inflammatory fibroid polyps of the gastrointestinal tract: An immunohistochemical and electron microscopic study. Cancer 1983;51: 1682–1690.

122. Shimer GR, Helwig EB. Inflammatory fibroid polyps of the intestine. Am J Clin Pathol 1984;81:708–714.

123. Nkanza NK, King M, Hutt MS. Intussusception due to inflammatory fibroid polyps of the ileum: A report of 12 cases from Africa. Br J Surg 1980;67:271–274.

124. Allibone RO, Nanson JK, Anthony PP. Multiple and recurrent inflammatory fibroid polyps in a Devon fanily ("Devon polyposis syndrome"): An update. Gut 1992;33:1004–1005.

125. Ishikura H, Sato F, Naka A, et al. Inflammatory fibroid polyp of the stomach. Acta Pathol Jpn 1986;36:327–335.

126. Kolodziejczyk P, Yao T, Tsuneyoshi M. Inflammatory fibrous polyps of the stomach. A special reference to an immunohistochemical profile of 42 cases. Am J Surg Pathol 1993;17:1159–1168.

127. Hui Y-Z, Noffsinger AED, Guo Q-X, et al. Delineation of the proliferative component of inflammatory fibroid polyps of the intestine. Int J Surg Pathol 1995;2:207–214.

128. Daimaru Y, Kido H, Hashimoto H, et al. Benign schwannoma of the gastrointestinal tract: A clinicopathologic and immunohistochemical study. Hum Pathol 1988;19:257–264.

129. Sarlomo-Rikala M, Miettinen M. Gastric schwannoma—a clinicopathological analysis of six cases. Histopathology 1995;27:355–360.

130. Fuller CE, Williams GT. Gastrointestinal manifestations of type I neurofibromatosis (von Recklinghausen's disease). Histopathology 1991;19:1–19.

131. Croker JR, Greenstein RJ. Malignant schwannoma of the stomach in a patient with von Recklinghausen's disease. Histopathology 1979; 3:79–85.

132. Carney JA, Go VLW, Sizemore GW, et al. Alimentary-tract ganglioneuromatosis. A major component of the syndrome of multiple endocrine neoplasias, type 2b. N Engl J Med 1976;295: 1287–1291.

133. Shekitka KM, Sobin LH. Ganglioneuromas of the gastrointestinal tract. Relation to von Recklinghausen disease and other multiple tumor syndromes. Am J Surg Pathol 1994;18:250–257.

134. d Amore ES, Manivel JC, Pettinato G, et al. Intestinal ganglioneuromatosis: Mucosal and transmural types. A clinicopathologic and immunohistochemical study of six cases. Hum Pathol 1991;22: 276–286.

135. Snover DC, Weigent CE, Summer HW. Diffuse mucosal ganglioneuromatosis of the colon associated with adenocarcinoma. Am J Clin Pathol 1981;75:225–229.

136. Mendelsohn G, Diamond MP. Familial ganglioneuromatous polyp-

osis of the large bowel. Report of a family with associated juvenile polyposis. Am J Surg Pathol 1984;8:515–520.

137. Weidner N, Flanders DJ, Mitros FA. Mucosal ganglioneuromatosis associated with multiple colonic polyps. Am J Surg Pathol 1984;8: 779–786.

138. Lashner BA, Riddell RH, Winans CS. Ganglioneuromatosis of the colon and extensive glycogenic acanthosis in Cowden's disease. Dig Dis Sci 1986;31:213–216.

139. Schwartz DT, Gaetz HP. Multiple granular cell myoblastomas of the stomach. Am J Clin Pathol 1965;44:453–457.

140. Calhoun T, Odelowo EOO, Ali S, et al. Granular cell myoblastoma:

Another unusual esophageal lesion. J Thorac Cardiovasc Surg 1975; 69:472–475.

141. Johnston J, Helwig EB. Granular cell tumors of the gastrointestinal tract and perianal region—a study of 74 cases. Dig Dis Sci 1981;26: 807–816.

142. Vuyk HD, Snow GB, Tiwari RM, et al. Granular cell tumor of the proximal esophagus: A rare disease. Cancer 1985;55: 445–449.

143. Coutinho DS, Soga J, Yoshikawa T, et al. Granular cell tumors of the esophagus: A report of two cases and review of the literature. Am J Gastroenterol 1985;80:758–762.

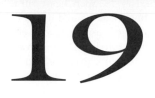

399

The focus of this chapter is on diseases of other organs and systemic disorders that may affect multiple portions of the alimentary tract (1). Some of these conditions are presented in detail in other parts of the book, and only the salient findings are reviewed in the following discussion.

DISEASES OF OTHER ORGANS AND SYSTEMS

Nonspecific or constitutional symptoms referable to the gastrointestinal tract are exceedingly common in diseases affecting other organs and tissues in the body. Anorexia, nausea, vomiting, abdominal pain that often is crampy, and either diarrhea or constipation may herald the onset of the diseases and persist for a variable time. These symptoms also are commonly seen in persons experiencing stressful situations (2). They are thought to be related to stimulation of the autonomic nervous system components and to the effects of mediators, such as prostaglandins, that are released as part of an inflammatory reaction. In addition, the gastrointestinal tract is a common site for the development of opportunistic infections (3–7) and drug reactions (8–11) that may be attributed to diseases of other organs and their therapies.

CARDIOVASCULAR SYSTEM
ISCHEMIC DISEASE

The most common effects of ischemic disease on the gastrointestinal tract are seen in cases of cardiac failure and of shock, as well as in those involving occlusive lesions of the mesenteric vessels. The resulting lesions range from mucosal necrosis to transmural infarction of the intestines (12–15). Ischemic damage may also be seen in cases of disseminated intravascular coagulation, in which the cause is probably low blood flow rather than obstruction of the small vessels, as well as in patients with vasculitis, which may be associated with many systemic conditions (16, 17). Rarely, fibromuscular dysplasia, a disease characterized by nonatherosclerotic, noninflammatory thickening of the arterial media, involves the large and/or medium-sized mesenteric vessels in a multicentric fashion and leads to ischemic damage of the gastrointestinal tract (18, 19). These subjects are discussed in Chapter 14.

LYMPHANGIECTASIA

In some patients with sustained high central venous pressure, such as may occur in constrictive pericarditis and in valvular lesions of the right side of the heart, the elevated pressure may be transmitted retrograde to the mesenteric and intestinal lymphatic system, resulting in marked dilation of the lacteals and a leakage of protein-rich fluid into the gut lumen (20, 21). The appearance of a tissue sample obtained during small intestinal mucosal biopsy is usually normal, except for diffuse dilation of the lymphatics in the lamina propria, but distinguishing this finding from the effects of a traumatized sample is sometimes difficult (22, 23). The condition must also be separated from primary lymphangiectasia, which is more common in children, and in which the mucosa reveals focal malformations of the small lymphatic vessels. This topic and the overall subject of protein-losing enteropathy is addressed in Chapter 31.

EFFECTS OF CARDIAC SURGERY

Gastrointestinal complications secondary to open heart surgery (or transplantation) are uncommon, but are associated with a high mortality rate (24). The pathologic change is usually related either to the trauma and stress of the procedure or to the effects of vascular insufficiency. Hemorrhage due to esophageal, gastric, or duodenal "stress" type erosions or ischemic necrosis in any part of the gastrointestinal tract may occur because of the low flow state (25). Exacerbation of diverticular disease has also been reported. The effect of transplant-related immunosuppressive therapy is covered in Chapter 16.

RESPIRATORY SYSTEM

Hypoxemia for whatever reason can facilitate the development of or worsen any ischemic injury of the intestines. Patients with chronic obstructive lung disease (COPD) have an increased incidence of peptic ulcers of the duodenum (26), which likely is related to the appearance of hypercapnia, which results in the stimulation of excess gastric acid secretion (27). Peptic ulcers also occur with increased incidence in COPD patients with α_1-antitrypsin deficiency (28). Some patients with bronchial carcinoid tumors and oat cell carcinomas develop a paraneoplastic syndrome characterized by watery diarrhea. The syndrome is attributable to the release of serotonin and other ectopic hormones from the tumors, which leads to hypermotility of the gut musculature and a reduced transit time.

KIDNEYS AND URINARY SYSTEM
ACUTE RENAL FAILURE

Gastrointestinal complications of acute renal failure are mainly attributable to the effects of hypotension, stress, and multiple organ failure. Hemorrhage from gastric or duodenal erosions/ulcers are typical (29). Rarely, the ulcers perforate and lead to an acute abdomen. Morphologically, the lesions are typical "stress" type ulcers as described in Chapter 24.

UREMIA

A variety of injuries that affect the gastrointestinal tract are commonly seen in patients with chronic renal disease (30), including patients who have received hemodialysis and renal allografts (31–33). From a pathogenetic point of view, however, it is difficult to know whether the effects are attributable to the uremia itself or to soluble blood-borne products related to hemodialysis or transplantation (34). Uremic patients, in general (up to 60%), may develop mucosal and submucosal hemorrhages, gastric and duodenal erosions, and hemorrhagic vascular ectasias, but it is still unclear if the incidence of peptic ulcer disease is increased in these patients (35). The hemorrhages frequently are multiple, are seen more often in the stomach and duodenum (36, 37), and are thought to be related to bleeding abnormalities, such as platelet dysfunction, that are present in patients with renal failure; a prominent telangiectasia has been noted in the gastric mucosa in some of the transplant patients (38). Multiple small ulcers are also noted in the upper tract and small intestine (39), whereas they tend to be solitary and larger in the colon, with most occurring in the cecum (40, 41). Multiple factors are probably involved in the genesis of the ulcers (37, 42, 43), including damage to the gastric mucosal barrier by urea resulting in increased back diffusion of acid, secondary hyperparathyroidism leading to increased acid secretion, and bacterial conversion of the urea in the gut lumen to ammonia, which might be irritating to the intestinal mucosa. Larger areas of hemorrhage and necrosis with variable inflammation may be seen in the intestines, and these lesions most closely resemble ischemic disease (44).

Renal transplant patients may develop similar mucosal hemorrhages, particularly in the early postoperative period, but they also have a propensity for nonocclusive vascular ischemia, increased complications of diverticular disease, bacterial peritonitis, and even pseudomembranous colitis. The ischemic effects are related in part to acute fluid loss, but defects in coagulation may also play a role. Exacerbation of diverticulitis is a serious and not uncommon potential sequelae that may be related to the effects of immunosuppressive therapy (45). The pseudomembranes in renal failure-associated colitis tend to be larger than those seen in typical antibiotic-associated colitis, and a constant pathogen has not been identified in the uremic cases. No correlation exists between the occurrence of these various lesions and the type and duration of the renal disease or the severity of the renal failure.

The clinical presentation depends on the type and distribution of the lesions and includes some combination of bleeding, abdominal pain, and diarrhea. Most of the lesions regress with the initiation of treatment of the renal failure, but some persist. Complications include significant hemorrhage (39, 43), perforation (46), and obstruction from fibrous stricture formation. The histologic features of the uremic lesions are nonspecific, and the diagnosis depends on the compatible clinical information and on the exclusion of other causes.

SECONDARY INFECTIONS

Patients receiving immunosuppressive therapy for renal disease or after transplantation can also develop opportunistic infections of the gut (47). Infections in the esophagus are mainly due to herpes and candida (48). Infections in the intestines may be due to herpes and candida as well as cytomegalovirus (49); bacteria, such as salmonella; other fungi (4); and uncommon parasites, such as Cryptosporidium (50) and Strongyloides (51) in the intestine. Accordingly, when encountering an ulcer or inflammatory condition of the intestine in a patient with chronic renal disease, the possible causes are the uremic lesion per se, ischemic disease, an opportunistic infection, or a drug effect. In such cases, mucosal biopsy can help to detect the lesions and to identify the particular infectious agents (23, 52–54).

DISEASES COMMON TO THE KIDNEYS AND GASTROINTESTINAL TRACT

Both organs are involved in a variety of systemic disorders, and this combination is particularly prominent in those diseases with a vasculitic component (17, 55) or with an infiltrative lesion, such as amyloidosis (56). Indeed, when the major lesions are in the kidney, aspiration biopsy of the rectum, which is less traumatic than a renal biopsy, is often chosen as a means to look for evidence of vasculitis (57) or amyloid deposits (58) in the submucosal vessels. The more common causes of the vasculitis affecting the smaller vessels of the two organs are lupus erythematosus (59, 60), rheumatoid arthritis (61, 62), and Henoch-Schönlein purpura (63). In the hemolytic

uremic syndrome, evidence of antecedent inflammatory disease of the intestinal tract is characterized by the presence of significant edema and hemorrhages in the mucosa and wall (64–66) (see Chapter 14). An IgA type of glomerulonephritis has been noted in some patients with a chronic enteritis, such as celiac disease (67, 68), and it is thought that this type of glomerulonephritis results from an increased circulation of the immunoglobulin and immune complexes.

COMPLICATIONS OF URETEROENTEROSTOMY

Techniques for diverting urine from diseased or malignant urinary bladders generally fall into three categories: ureterosigmoidostomy, isolated ileal bladder, and antirefluxing colonic conduits (69, 70).

Ureterosigmoidostomy (i.e., ureter implanted into the sigmoid colon) has been a popular method of urinary diversion since the early 1900s, particularly for infants with extrophy of the urinary bladder and/or other obstructive lesions of the cloacogenic area. Most of the problems with this technique are related to the admixture of urine with fecal stream and fecal bacteria. Slight inflammation and crypt hyperplasia of the adjacent colonic mucosa results as well as the occasional formation of small inflammatory polyps, although these changes typically have no clinical significance (71, 72). In addition, early complications include peritonitis, pyelonephritis, and distal ureteral obstruction. Finally, it has been demonstrated that the colonic mucosa adjacent to the ureteral openings is exceptionally prone to the later development of neoplasm, including adenomas and adenocarcinoma (72–76). The tumors usually appear in patients between the ages of 15 and 25 years, manifesting with either rectal bleeding or, more often, signs of ureteral obstruction. It appears that fecal bacteria act on urinary components (such as nitrates), which are transformed into active carcinogens (nitrosamines) that have malignant-transforming potential. The gross and histologic features of the neoplasms are identical to those seen in the colon in general, and the prognosis after surgical resection depends on the presence and the extent of invasion by the carcinoma. For those patients that still have the ureters connected to the colon, periodic endoscopic examination with mucosal biopsy is recommended to look for epithelial dysplasia (77, 78) (Fig. 19.1). In this regard, we have observed unusual positions of the ureter, such as in the transverse colon, and a radiologic study of the urinary system should be obtained soon after ureterosigmoidostomy to determine the exact location of the ureteral implants.

Following the recognition of this neoplastic complication, ureterosigmoidostomy is no longer used and has been replaced by the creation of the ileal bladder in patients requiring diversion of the urinary system (79, 80). This procedure preserves renal function and is not associated with metabolic disturbances or other problems related to the fecal stream, such as the increased risk of malignancy. The ileal mucosa, with time, typically shows villous shortening, increased chronic inflammation, dilated cystic crypts, mucin pools, and fibrosis. Other complications include obstruction, stomal problems related to surgical technique, renal calculi, and pyelonephritis (81).

The antirefluxing colonic conduit, another form of ureteral preservation, is used less often. This technique involves using a segment of colon as an isolated conduit rather than in continuity with the fecal stream (79). The thicker musculature of the colon

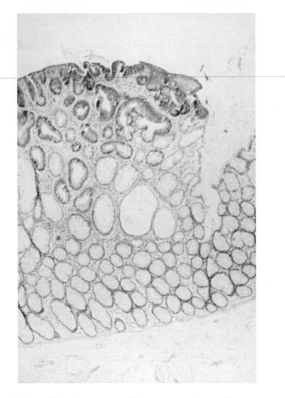

Figure 19.1   Colonic mucosal biopsy specimen from area next to ureteral orifice in a patient with ureteral implant in the sigmoid colon. A superficial focus of adenomatous epithelium *(top left and center)* represents glandular dysplasia (H & E, ×100).

is more adaptable to the prevention of reflux, as occurs in ileal conduits, and has dramatically decreased the incidence of pyelonephritis.

HEMATOLOGIC SYSTEM

HEMORRHAGIC (COAGULATION) DISORDERS

Patients with bleeding and coagulation disorders of all causes may manifest spontaneous hemorrhages in any part of the gastrointestinal tract. The lesions in the primary bleeding disorders usually regress promptly; examples of massive bleeding or obstruction from an intramural hematoma are rare.

Up to 20% of patients with hemophilia may present with bleeding (82). Occasionally, intramural bleeding may be severe enough to cause obstruction, from luminal narrowing and rigidity, or intussusception. Most patients with gastrointestinal manifestations, however, show hemorrhage limited to the submucosal space, particularly in the upper gastrointestinal tract.

Hemolytic uremic syndrome (acute renal failure, microangiopathic anemia, and thrombocytopenia) is a bleeding disorder that involves predominantly children, although adults may be affected as well, especially after therapy with certain antineoplastic agents such as bleomycin (83, 84). Up to 90% of affected patients develop gastrointestinal symptoms. Colonic involvement is commonly observed because of thrombosis of the submucosal and intramural blood vessels resulting in hemorrhage and ischemic necrosis. This disorder is thought to be related to the bacterial cytotoxin effect on

vascular endothelium, which results in intravascular thrombosis and hemorrhage. E. coli (0157:H7), Campylobacter, Shigella, and Salmonella organisms have all been implicated in the development of this disorder (84). Potential complications include transmural ischemic necrosis, toxic megacolon, and stricture formation in the long term.

Thrombotic thrombocytopenic purpura is a bleeding disorder (angiopathic anemia, thrombocytopenia, renal insufficiency, fever, central nervous system effects) that may involve the gastrointestinal tract in up to 10 to 20% of patients. The clinical findings are similar to those associated with hemolytic uremic syndrome, including hemorrhage, vascular thrombosis, and an acute "ischemic" colitis-like syndrome (85–86).

SICKLE CELL ANEMIA

Patients with sickle cell disease are prone to developing ischemic lesions of the intestines (87), which are more commonly located in the watershed area of the distal transverse colon and splenic flexure. These lesions are thought to result from or to be facilitated by the abnormal sickling and hyperviscosity of the blood. As with other instances of a sickle cell crisis, the intestinal disease is often precipitated by a state of dehydration. The lesions usually are superficial and respond to medical therapy, consisting of hydration and antibiotics; surgical resection is rarely needed.

IRON DEFICIENCY ANEMIA

The rate of iron absorption is normally controlled by the concentration of protein-bound iron in the surface epithelial cells of the proximal small intestine (88). In the common causes of iron deficiency anemia, namely chronic bleeding and poor nutrition, reduction in the amount of iron in the surface cells leads to an increased rate of absorption, but is not accompanied by any structural change at a histologic level. This control mechanism is altered in the abnormal state of primary hemochromatosis, in which iron absorption continues despite the saturated levels in the epithelial cells (see subsequent section concerning hepatic disease for further details). The Plummer-Vinson syndrome is characterized by the presence of iron deficiency anemia and by numerous squamous-lined webs in the proximal esophagus (89) that are prone to malignant transformation (see Chapters 13 and 20).

MEGALOBLASTIC ANEMIA

The anemias related to deficiencies of folic acid and vitamin B12 are characterized by megaloblastic proliferation of all actively growing cells, including not only the immature blood cells but also many of the epithelial cells in the body (90). This epithelial change can be readily appreciated in the gut, particularly in the stomach and the small intestine (91–93). Present in the gastric pits and in the intestinal crypts and low part of the villi are big rounded cells that contain enlarged and immature-appearing nuclei (Fig. 19.2). These megaloblastic cells are distinguished from ordinary regeneration by the larger size of the nuclei and the relative diminution of the amount of cytoplasm, and from neoplastic cells by the lack of hyperchromasia and pleomorphism. There is also an overall reduction in the number of mitoses. The intestinal villi are often partially blunted in cases of folate deficiency, but it is not completely clear whether this alteration can lead to a functional problem itself or is a sign of an underlying condition, such as celiac or tropical sprue, that is responsible for the nutrient problem. It is noteworthy, in this regard, that most patients with tropical sprue can be treated simply with folate, resulting in complete resolution of the histologic lesion as well as the functional effect (94). These changes in the small intestine are also observed in cases of vitamin B_{12} deficiency due to pernicious anemia and are not associated with clinical problems (91), supporting the notion that they are of a secondary nature. No gross changes or complications result from the megaloblastic proliferations, whatever the cause, and the lesions promptly regress when the folate or B_{12} deficiency is corrected. (See Chapter 23 for details of the pathology of pernicious anemia in the stomach.)

POLYCYTHEMIA

In patients with primary polycythemia, thrombosis can occur in the portal and mesenteric veins leading to hemorrhage and infarction of the intestines (16). The abnormal clotting is probably related to the hyperviscosity of the blood that may be present in patients with this condition. The lesions typically involve the deeper parts of the wall, including the muscularis propria and the serosal layer, and surgery is ordinarily required. The specific diagnosis is provided by finding venous thrombi in the mesenteric and mesocolic tissues that are not in the field of the infarction and by the pertinent clinical information. The features of hemorrhagic infarction of the intestine are otherwise nonspecific and can be seen in the advanced phase of ischemic disease due to reduced flow or occlusion of the arterial system and in other common causes of venous obstruction, such as a volvulus, hernia, and peritoneal adhesions (see Chapter 14).

LEUKEMIA AND LYMPHOMA

The gastrointestinal tract is commonly affected in cases of leukemia, either directly by the tumor or by the various complications of the disease (coagulation defects) and its therapy (drug toxicity, immunosuppression) (95, 96). These effects are more often observed in

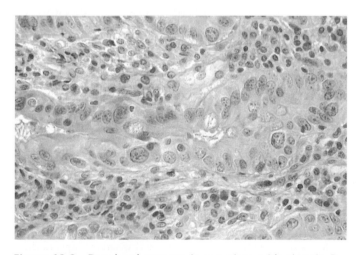

Figure 19.2 Duodenal mucosa in a patient with vitamin B_{12} deficiency and megaloblastic anemia. Many crypt cells show enlarged and occasionally multilobed nuclei typical of megaloblastic change. The biopsy also revealed subtotal villous shortening and increased lamina propria lymphocytes and plasma cells (H & E, ×400). (See color plate.)

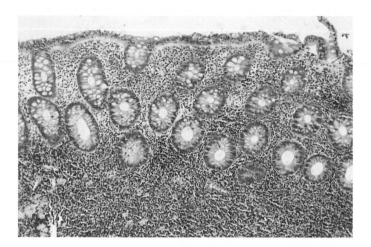

Figure 19.3 Colonic mucosa in a patient with chronic lymphocytic leukemia (CLL). The lamina propria is diffusely infiltrated with numerous small, monotonous appearing, well-differentiated lymphocytes pushing and separating the crypts from the base of the mucosa (H & E, ×100). (See color plate.)

the aggressive types of leukemia, including the myelogenous and acute lymphoblastic forms. Gut involvement has been noted in up to 50% of leukemia patients at autopsy (97). The tumor infiltrates are usually multifocal, can affect all parts of the alimentary tract, and often are concentrated in the submucosal and mucosal layers (Fig. 19.3). They vary in size from microscopic foci to several centimeters in diameter, and the larger nodules, which are soft tan to pale yellow, and are frequently associated with a central ulceration on the mucosal aspect. Infiltrates may also develop polypoid or diffuse masses, however, which may significantly narrow the lumen and cause obstruction or intussusception. The lesions are often a source of hemorrhage into the lumen, and perforation of the bowel wall can occur when extensive necrosis is present, a circumstance that may be facilitated by treatment of the tumor. Obstruction by the tumor itself is uncommon; more often, it is related to the effects of therapy leading to prominent edema or fibrosis.

As a result of the leukemic infiltration and destruction of the marrow elements and of the potent therapeutic drugs used, secondary effects appear in many tissues of the body. All parts of the gastrointestinal tract are involved, consisting of fresh hemorrhages, toxic injuries (98, 99), which are more often noted in the small intestine (see Chapter 11), and increased infections with the common appearance of opportunistic type (100, 101) and with unusual forms such as neutropenic colitis (102) (see Chapter 28). In addition, patients that have received bone marrow transplants may develop a graft-versus-host reaction (103), resulting in inflammation and ulceration of the stomach and small intestine in the acute form (104–106), and more focal lesions of the proximal esophagus (107) and intestines (103, 108), in the chronic type (see Chapters 5 and 16).

Malignant lymphoma can involve the gastrointestinal tract in several forms. Primary tumors (109, 110) may be solitary or diffuse. The latter type is more common in the small intestine, where it may cause a malabsorptive state (111), either from contiguous spread of tumors arising in the mesenteric lymph nodes, or as part of a generalized dissemination (112) (see Chapter 17).

Gastrointestinal complications may also be seen in patients with myelodysplastic syndromes. The bleeding results in part from defective thrombosis but also occurs as a secondary effect of portal hypertension, which develops from infiltration of the liver with extramedullary hematopoiesis, or by direct involvement of the bowel wall (usually submucosa) by extramedullary hematopoiesis.

Plasma cell tumors may also directly involve the gastrointestinal tract, aside from its indirect effect by systemic or localized amyloidosis (see later section and Chapter 13). Plasmacytomas may involve any portion of the gastrointestinal tract, and may cause bleeding or pain (113). Extracellular deposits of immunoglobulin (IgM) may occur in the small intestinal mucosa in patients with Waldenstrom macroglobulinemia (114). These deposits stain positively with the PAS stain and in this manner may simulate Whipple disease morphologically (see Chapter 31).

ENDOCRINE SYSTEM

Many of the effects noted in the gastrointestinal tract as a result of endocrine diseases involve changes in motility (see Chapter 13 for greater detail).

HYPERTHYROIDISM

Hyperthyroidism may be associated with hypermotility of the gut (115, 116), resulting in rapid gastric emptying (117), reduced transit time, and the appearance of watery diarrhea or steatorrhea in up to 75% of patients. Steatorrhea may result in decreased calcium absorption attributable to decreased absorption of fat-soluble vitamins A, D, E, and K (118). No constant structural changes occur in the mucosa and wall of the bowel (119, 120), and the functional effects are believed to be due to the rapid transit. Other effects of hyperthyroidism (thyrotoxicosis) on the gastrointestinal system include an association with superficial chronic gastritis and hypergastrinemia, which is due in part to an increased number and sensitivity of gastric gastrin-producing cells. Acid levels, however, usually are normal in this setting. Contrary to popular belief, thyrotoxicosis does not increase the risk of peptic ulcer disease, and whether the incidence of chronic atrophic gastritis is increased in this disorder is controversial. An interesting association has been noted between Graves disorder and ulcerative colitis (121). Up to 4% of ulcerative colitis patients develop Graves disease, usually before the onset of colitis. When present, Graves disease may aggravate the symptoms of collitis and render the disease refractory to therapy.

HYPOTHYROIDISM

In contrast to patients with hyperthyroidism, hypothyroid patients show a delay in gastric emptying and reduced intestinal and colonic motility (116, 122), which may lead to gastric bezoar formation, ileus, volvulus, constipation, or even megacolon. Myxedema patients show defective sphincter function, which often leads to reflux esophagitis (123). In severe cases of myxedema, edema and mild inflammation of the intestinal wall may be found (124). Malabsorption may also occur, and appears to be related to stasis and bacterial proliferation in the small intestine. The intestinal mucosa usually is normal; the jejunum may demonstrate patchy inflammation, which is probably related to the excess bacteria.

A chronic atrophic gastritis with reduced acid secretion is seen in some cases of hypothyroidism related to Hashimoto thyroiditis. Patients frequently have serum antibodies to thyroglobulin, intrinsic factor (125), and gastric parietal cells, and are at risk for the later development of pernicious anemia. An association with ulcerative colitis has also been shown with Hashimoto thyroiditis.

THYROID NEOPLASMS

Patients with medullary carcinoma of the thyroid, either isolated or as part of a multiple endocrine neoplasia syndrome (MEN), may have prominent watery diarrhea (126). No morphologic changes occur in the intestinal mucosa, and the diarrhea is thought to result from the release of ectopic hormones from the tumor leading to hypermotility of the gut. In this regard, calcitonin, which is the natural hormone of these tumors, does not have a stimulatory effect on the bowel muscle. MEN syndromes are autosomal dominant disorders that may involve the gastrointestinal tract either by the direct effects of tumor formation or by the effects of functionally active peptides produced by tumors elsewhere in the body (127, 128). A full discussion of MEN is beyond the scope of this book, but the major gastrointestinal manifestations of these tumor syndromes are summarized in Table 19.1.

PARATHYROID DISEASES

Patients with untreated hyperparathyroidism frequently have gastrointestinal symptoms, including nausea and vomiting, abdominal pain, and either diarrhea or constipation (129, 130). The effects are likely attributable mainly to hypercalcemia, which can lead to increased acid secretion, and may explain the incidence of peptic ulcers of the duodenum in about 15% of patients (131). Ectopic calcifications may also appear, but they typically are microscopic and cause no clinical problem. Patients with hypoparathyroidism may develop malabsorption, perhaps associated with stagnant bowel. A rare syndrome with hypoparathyroidism, Addison disease, and atrophic gastritis has been reported (132). Hypoparathyroidism has also recently been described in association with intestinal lymphangiectasia (133).

ADRENAL DISEASES

Up to 50% of patients with Addison disease present with a variety of gastrointestinal symptoms, including anorexia, weight loss, abdominal pain, and diarrhea resulting in dehydration (134). Rare cases are thought to have an immunologic basis, in which inflammatory lesions leading to atrophy are noted in the adrenal cortex and in other endocrine tissues, including the thyroid and parathyroid. These rare cases frequently are associated with atrophic gastritis and pernicious anemia (125, 132). Patients with pheochromocytomas often have nonspecific gastrointestinal symptoms. Uncommonly, these patients experience severe constipation leading to megacolon or an enterocolitis, which is thought to occur as a result of the vasoconstrictive action of the excess circulating catecholamines (135).

DIABETES MELLITUS

Up to 75% of patients with diabetes mellitus (136–139) demonstrate changes in gastrointestinal structure and function, most of which are thought to be mediated by damage to the enteric nervous

TABLE 19.1	Gastrointestinal Manifestations of MEN Syndromes	

MEN Syndrome	Clinical and Pathologic Features	Mechanism
MEN 1		
Hyperparathyroidism (adenoma)	Peptic ulcer, abdominal pain, constipation	↑ Serum Ca
Pituitary adenoma	Gastric ulcer, acromegaly → colon adenomas	↑ ACTH
		↑ Growth hormone
Islet cell tumor (Gastrinoma)	Diarrhea, steatorrhea	VIP oversecretion, hypergastrinemia → parietal cell
	Peptic ulcer disease	hyperplasia → ↓ ph, pancreatic enzyme inactivation
	Z-E syndrome	
MEN 2A		
Thyroid medullary carcinoma	Watery diarrhea, ileus	Calcitonin, +/− VIP hypersecretion, serotonin, ↓ K^+, ? altered motility
Hyperparathyroidism (hyperplasia)	Peptic ulcer, abdominal pain, constipation	↑ Serum Ca
Pheochromocytoma	Abdominal pain	? Impaired motility
Gastrinoma (rare)	Diarrhea, steatorrhea	VIP oversecretion, hypergastrinemia → parietal cell
	Peptic ulcer disease	hyperplasia → ↓ ph, pancreatic enzyme inactivation
	Z-E syndrome	
MEN 2B		
Thyroid medullary carcinoma	Watery diarrhea, ileus	Calcitonin, +/− VIP hypersecretion, serotonin, ↓ K^+, ? altered motility
Pheochromocytoma	Abdominal pain	? Impaired motility
Mucosal neuromas	Pain, constipation, megacolon	Neuromotility disturbance
	Intestinal ganglioneuroma	
	↑ Achalasia	
	↑ Adenomas/adenocarcinoma	

system. No close correlation exists, however, between the appearance of most of these effects and the duration and severity of the diabetes or the presence of a peripheral neuropathy. A decrease in the contractibility of the esophageal musculature and reduced pressure of the lower esophageal sphincter have been observed, but these changes do not usually have any clinical significance (140), except for perhaps mild reflux-related symptoms in a few patients. The stomach can become atonic leading to poor emptying and marked dilation, and this dilation is seen more often in patients with decompensated disease (gastroparesis diabeticorun) (141, 142). If this condition is not corrected, pressure damage can result in an acute form of gastritis with flattening and erosions of the mucosa, thinning of the wall, and potential perforation. The features of chronic gastritis affecting the proximal stomach have been noted in about two thirds of the patients with diabetes (143), and this presentation is associated with reduced acid secretion, a decreased incidence of duodenal peptic ulcers (144), and with frank pernicious anemia in about 5% of cases. Whether the gastric disease is due to an immunologic injury as in ordinary atrophic gastritis or is the result of repeated episodes of gastric dilation is not known. At present, the role of H. pylori in the etiology of diabetes-induced gastritis is unclear (145, 146).

Patients with diabetes also experience periodic episodes of watery diarrhea and crampy abdominal pain (136–139, 147, 148). This symptom pattern appears to be more common in young patients with the insulin-dependent form of diabetes, is often associated with other complications including peripheral neuropathy, and is thought to be due to a motility disturbance. Steatorrhea and other signs of malabsorption can also develop; possible causes include hypomotility of the small bowel leading to stasis and bacterial proliferation, associated inflammation or tumor of the exocrine pancreas, and obstruction of the bile duct by gallstones. In addition, it has been suggested that celiac disease is more common in persons with diabetes (149), but this association is not certain. Patchy, nonspecific inflammatory changes noted in the small intestinal mucosa are probably related to the bowel stasis (150, 151). Although abnormalities are not typically seen in the ganglia and nerves of the intestinal wall by ordinary histologic examination, special studies with silver stains have revealed changes in these neural structures in some cases (147, 152) (see Chapter 13).

HYPOTHALAMIC AND PITUITARY DISEASE

Disorders of the hypothalamic pituitary areas, including pituitary neoplasms, affect the gastrointestinal tract only infrequently, and usually are related to one of the MEN syndromes. Of particular note is that acromegaly, a condition resulting from excessive growth hormone production, is associated with an unusual incidence of intestinal adenomas and cancers (mainly stomach and colon) (153).

REPRODUCTIVE SYSTEM

DISEASES OF CONTIGUOUS TISSUES

Because of its close proximity, lesions of the pelvic organs and tissues can impact on the intestinal tract, and the effects are most commonly noted in the sigmoid colon and rectum. Various inflammatory conditions and neoplasms of the uterine adnexa may compress on or extend into the wall of the distal intestine, and prostatic carcinoma can directly invade the rectum. This invasion may result in a localized obstruction or bleeding, the latter caused by pressure effects on the mucosa or actual invasion of this layer by tumor. Mucosal biopsy can help in the determination and typing of the secondary cancers and in their distinction from primary intestinal lesions. It should be noted, however, that the histology of some of the pelvic tumors, such as the mucinous types in the ovary, can be very similar or identical to colonic lesions, and the separation may depend on the results of immunocytochemical and ultrastructural studies and the gross distribution of the tumor. For example, prostatic carcinomas usually can be identified by the presence of prostate-specific antigen and the prostate fraction of acid phosphatase, and ovarian tumors may lack the characteristic terminal webs that are present in colonic adenocarcinomas. In addition, lesions may develop in the bowel as a result of radiation and drug therapy of genital tract cancers; these effects are described in Chapter 11. Endometriosis commonly affects the intestinal tract and the lesions are most often present in the serosa and muscularis propria of the sigmoid colon and rectum (154), where they may invoke a prominent fibrous tissue and smooth muscle response (see Chapter 30).

EFFECTS OF PREGNANCY AND EXOGENOUS HORMONES

Nausea and vomiting are characteristic symptoms of early pregnancy and are also noted in association with use of exogenous estrogens or the contraceptive pill. No structural changes occur in the gastrointestinal tract, and the effects are probably mediated through the nervous system. In addition, heartburn is commonly observed during pregnancy and is thought to be attributable to the action of the hormones leading to a reduced lower esophageal sphincter pressure (155). The expansion of the uterus resulting in an increase of the intraabdominal pressure may be a contributing factor in the later stages of the pregnancy. No evidence exists to suggest that the pregnancy is the cause of clinically significant peptic esophagitis, although it may worsen a preexisting condition. Constipation is a frequent problem during the late stage of pregnancy and is related to pressure from the enlarged uterus and/or the ingestion of supplemental calcium medications. Following multiple pregnancies with vaginal deliveries, some women develop damage to and weakening of the wall separating the posterior vagina and the rectum. This situation may lead to protrusion of the rectal wall into the vagina at the time of straining and may result in intermittent episodes of constipation and fecal incontinence. No constant abnormalities are noted in the rectal mucosa, and the prolapse can be surgically corrected. Extensive clinical investigations have not revealed any deleterious effects of the pregnancy on the course of patients with ulcerative colitis and Crohn disease (156). Other uncommon effects of increased estrogen levels may occur during pregnancy but are more often noted with sustained use of the contraceptive pill or other exogenous hormones in older patients. These effects include the sporadic appearance of intestinal hemorrhages and inflammation (157, 158) (see Chapter 11), and the promotion of thromboses (see Chapter 14).

SKIN DISEASES

A variety of inflammatory and bullous diseases of the skin are associated with pathologic changes in the gastrointestinal tract,

either as a common manifestation of a systemic disease, such as diabetes or scleroderma, or associated with either a primary disease in the skin itself (dermatitis herpetiformis) or in the gut (inflammatory bowel disease) (159). The focus of this section is on those conditions that occur with significant frequency in the gut and are not covered elsewhere in this text. Tumors of the epidermis and skin appendages can affect the anal canal and are described in Chapter 36. Some patients with acrodermatitis enteropathica develop diarrhea in association with nonspecific inflammation of the small intestinal mucosa (160); this condition is discussed in Chapter 31.

BULLOUS DISORDERS

A variety of proliferative and bullous conditions of the skin may rarely involve the esophagus, especially the upper portion. Examples include pemphigus vulgaris (161), bullous pemphigoid (162), epidermolysis bullosa (163–168), Stevens-Johnson syndrome, dermatitis herpetiformis, and erythema multiforme (167, 169). Pemphigus, pemphigoid, and epidermolysis bullosa commonly involve the esophagus with symptoms of dysphagia and odynophagia and appear morphologically similar in the esophageal squamous mucosa as they do in the skin. In all forms, bullae may remain intact or separate leading to the formation of erosions, ulcerations, and eventually fibrosis and stricture formation if left untreated (see Chapter 20).

DERMATITIS HERPETIFORMIS

This condition shows a strong association with celiac disease (see Chapter 31), probably because of genetic concordance (169–171). In about two thirds of the patients with this skin condition, abnormalities are noted in the mucosa of the proximal small intestine (169–173), ranging from patchy villous blunting to complete loss of the villi. In severe cases of dermatitis herpetiformis, patients demonstrate signs of malabsorption and respond to a gluten-free diet (174, 175). Most patients with dermatologic eruptions have no intestinal problems and, therefore, a jejunal mucosal biopsy should be performed only in symptomatic patients. It has been reported that the skin lesions may also regress in patients consuming a gluten-free diet (176), but this effect has not been firmly established. Recent studies have revealed a variant of dermatitis herpetiformis in which the cutaneous IgA deposition is in the form of a linear band at the epidermal-dermal junction rather than the usual granular deposition at the tips of the dermal papillae. This subtype is referred to as linear-IgA bullous dermatosis, and limited studies have shown that this subtype is associated with only minimal abnormalities in jejunal structure and no functional problems (177).

ERYTHEMA MULTIFORME

This common skin disorder is characterized clinically by the presence of multiple small red papules and vesicles, and histologically by lymphocytic infiltrates around small vessels in the upper dermis, together with a variable degree of epidermal necrosis. The disease is called the Steven-Johnson syndrome when it affects mucosal surfaces such as the lips, oral cavity, and conjunctiva. Rarely, the alimentary tract is involved, most often affecting the distal half of the esophagus (167, 168). Present on the surface of the esophageal mucosa are small white patches, ranging in size from 2 to 5 mm in diameter, which resemble monilial infection. Histologic examination reveals a superficial ulceration and intraepithelial inflammation and individual cell necrosis of the adjacent intact squamous epithelium. Lesions have been noted on occasion in the mucosa of the small and large intestines and reveal foci of crypt epithelial destruction with mononuclear inflammatory cells but a paucity of neutrophils in the lamina propria (48, 178). Patients with the esophageal lesion may experience dysphagia and those with intestinal lesions often have abdominal pain and bloody diarrhea. The lesions typically regress and local complications in the gut are not observed.

KÖHLMEIER-DEGOS DISEASE

This rare disorder is characterized by the appearance of multiple vasculitic lesions of the skin, referred to as malignant atrophic papulosis, and subsequent spread to many other tissues of the body (179, 180). Lesions of the intestines have been noted in about 60% of cases and consist of fibrinoid necrosis of small arteries and veins together with a predominantly lymphocytic infiltrate around the vessels in the early stage and the development of intimal proliferation and organized thrombi in advanced cases. This degree of involvement results in areas of ischemic necrosis and ulceration of the intestine, which often proceeds to perforation of the bowel (181).

RHEUMATOLOGIC AND CONNECTIVE TISSUE DISEASES

Rheumatologic and connective tissue diseases often involve the gastrointestinal tract in the form of chronic inflammation and by the effects of vasculitis. Most of these disorders, such as scleroderma, are covered in other chapters. This section addresses those conditions that necessitate elaboration of the topic.

Congenital and acquired disorders with primary effects in the connective tissues, including the Ehlers-Danlos syndrome (182, 183), pseudoxanthoma elasticum (184, 185), Fabry disease (186–188), systemic sclerosis (189–191), mixed connective tissue disease (192), and visceral myopathies (193–195), can damage the musculature of the various parts of the alimentary tract. In particular, involvement with systemic sclerosis is common, and the effects include esophageal dysmotility and injury to the lower esophageal sphincter, which favor the development of peptic esophagitis, stasis of the small intestine leading to bacterial proliferation and steatorrhea, and the appearance of megacolon (196, 197). All of these connective tissue disorders promote hypomotility and the formation of diverticula (188, 198, 199), which is especially prominent in the small intestine. In addition, the gut may uncommonly be affected in systemic cases of myositis (200) and some degenerative diseases of the skeletal (201, 202) muscles (see Chapter 13). The gut is also a common target organ for the effects of the systemic vasculitides (17), such as lupus erythematosus (59, 60, 203, 204) and periarteritis nodosum (205) (see Chapter 14). The gastrointestinal manifestations of Behçet disease are described in Chapters 20 and 30.

RHEUMATOID ARTHRITIS

Gastrointestinal abnormalities are observed in about 25% of patients with long-standing rheumatoid arthritis and are due mostly to the occurrence of a necrotizing vasculitis affecting the medium-size and small arteries (61, 62, 206–210). The vascular lesions are mild and are asymptomatic in most cases (211), but they can lead to the development of mucosal hemorrhages, focal ulcers, and exceptionally to larger areas of infarction, mainly of the intestines (62, 208). Rarely, patients may present with a pancolitis. Because the pathologic features are otherwise nonspecific, the diagnosis depends on the clinical information and on the exclusion of other causes of vasculitis. Additional problems may appear that are related to the long-term use of medications, including ulcerations of the stomach and duodenum from aspirin (212), corticosteroids (213) and other antiinflammatory agents (9), and an enteritis or colitis from gold salts (214–216) (see Chapter 11). Patients with rheumatoid arthritis are also prone to the formation of secondary amyloidosis and the deposits frequently involve the gastrointestinal tract. Rectal biopsies are often performed in patients with suspected vasculitis or amyloidosis. These as well as biopsies from other sites should be of the larger aspiration type to ensure that an adequate sample of submucosa is obtained (57).

REACTIVE ARTHRITIS

This term is used to describe a group of inflammatory disorders that fall under the term "seronegative spondylarthropathy," such as psoriatic arthritis, Reiter syndrome, and ankylosing spondylitis as well as arthritides associated with inflammatory bowel disease (217, 218). All these conditions share features of arthritis with bowel inflammation (217). Up to 50% of patients with these disorders show subclinical histologic inflammation, and many present with diarrhea before the onset of the arthritis. Given that the arthritic features occur occasionally after a bout of infectious colitis, such as in Reiter syndrome, one suggestion is that a reaction to bacteria such as Chlamydia and Salmonella may be related to the etiology of the arthropathy. Endoscopy has revealed patchy areas of inflammation and small erosions in the mucosa of the colon and distal ileum that are not associated with drug therapy or significant intestinal symptoms (219). In one series, gross lesions were noted in 30% and microscopic alterations of acute and chronic inflammation in 61% of patients with seronegative spondylarthropathy (220). It was suggested by the authors of that study that the gut disease might be the primary event, but its cause is not known. As yet, in only a few cases have patients developed the classic form of idiopathic inflammatory bowel disease, particularly those with psoriatic arthritis.

SJÖGREN SYNDROME

Abnormalities of the alimentary tract are occasionally noted in patients with the Sjögren syndrome (221), and the effects are more common in the esophagus and stomach. It is important to separate the changes that are related to glandular inflammation from those of systemic sclerosis, which may coexist in these patients. Atrophy and chronic inflammation of the esophageal glands are commonly present and, together with similar effects in the salivary glands and oral cavity, may lead to dysphagia. Esophageal motility may be reduced, but this effect is more prominent in patients with systemic sclerosis. Esophageal webs have been noted in up to 10% of patients (222). An atrophic gastritis, with reduced gastric acid secretions and the presence of parietal cell antibodies, is observed in most patients with Sjögren syndrome. Dysfunction of the intestinal muscle and the development of steatorrhea are seen only in individuals with associated systemic sclerosis. Isolated reports describe the occurrence of celiac disease, enteritis, and colitis that are thought to have a vasculitic basis, and colonic ulcers in patients with this syndrome.

POLYMYOSITIS-DERMATOMYOSITIS

This condition, characterized by inflammatory myopathy, muscle weakness, and a violaceous rash (dermatomyositis) may affect the gastrointestinal tract through its effects on the musculature, particularly in the upper aerodigestive tract (cricopharynx), leading to disturbances in motility. Rarely, patients develop vasculitis, which results in colonic inflammation, ulceration, and perforation (223). Some investigators suggest the incidence of cancer is increased in association with this disorder (224).

PANCREAS, BILIARY TRACT, AND LIVER

CYSTIC FIBROSIS

This condition, also referred to as mucoviscidosis, is characterized by the presence of abnormally viscid mucus that results in the obstruction of small ducts, with major effects noted in the bronchi and lungs and in the pancreas (225). Patients tend to develop multiple infections and chronic inflammatory disease, and steatorrhea often appears as a consequence of chronic pancreatitis and maldigestion of lipids. This effect may be enhanced by biliary obstruction leading to a reduction of bile salts, because patients with cystic fibrosis also have an increased incidence of gallstones. Lesions are noted less commonly in other ducts and glands, including the small bile ductules in the liver and the intestinal mucosa.

Meconium ileus, a complication noted mainly in newborns and infants, consists of one or more areas of obstruction of the small intestine caused by a partially solidified admixture of thick mucus and fecal contents (226). The lesions are more common in the distal half of the small intestine, can be from one to several centimeters in length, and reveal evidence of mucosal damage that likely is due to a pressure effect from the luminal mass. Histologic features include hemorrhage and necrosis of the mucosa that may slough, followed by a stage of granulation tissue and the presence of hardened crystalline fecal material, which frequently evokes a foreign body giant cell reaction. It is probable that superficial lesions limited to the mucosa are capable of complete regression. The ulcers can extend deep into the submucosa and the muscularis propria and may be associated with marked fibrosis leading to permanent stricture formation. Indeed, cystic fibrosis is perhaps a major cause of atresia of the jejunum (227) (see Chapter 10).

Prominence of luminal mucus and enlarged goblet cells occasionally seen in older children with the disease can lead to distention and obstruction of narrow regions, such as the appendix (see Chapter 35). The size of the goblet mucous cells, as visualized in small intestinal and colonic mucosal biopsies, had been considered as a test for the diagnosis of cystic fibrosis (228), but the variability of the measurements proved excessive and there was considerable overlap with specimens obtained from control patients without the disease (229).

OTHER PANCREATIC AND BILIARY DISEASES

Lipid maldigestion and steatorrhea are common findings in patients with long-standing chronic pancreatitis and those with pancreatic

ductal obstruction caused by tumor or calculi. These signs are due simply to the reduced secretion or excretion of the pancreatic enzymes and is associated in the very severe cases with maldigestion of proteins and carbohydrates as well. The mucosa of the small intestine usually is normal, but patchy areas of inflammation may result from pooling of the undigested nutrients and secondary bacterial proliferation. Obstruction of the common bile duct for any reason can lead to a reduction in the excretion of bile salts, which also favor the development of steatorrhea. The fat maldigestion that occurs in these various disorders can further result in a deficiency of vitamin K and the appearance of fresh hemorrhages in the gastrointestinal tract. A variety of endocrine hyperplasias and tumors of the pancreas, including those that produce gastrin, glucagon, pancreatic polypeptides, and somatostatin, can affect the gastrointestinal tract predominantly via the hormone effects on gut motility (see Chapter 15).

HEPATIC DISEASES

Patients with acute liver disease such as viral hepatitis typically present with nausea, vomiting, and abdominal pain. Despite the manifestation of these constitutional symptoms, no alterations in the gastrointestinal tract are observed. Disorders associated with chronic cholestasis may be associated with the development of steatorrhea, probably related to a decrease in excretion of the bile salts by the liver. This effect may be seen in patients with any type of cirrhosis, but it is more prominent in individuals with primary biliary cirrhosis. Patients with primary biliary cirrhosis also appear to have an increased frequency of celiac disease (230). Patients with primary sclerosing cholangitis have a high incidence of ulcerative colitis (60 to 100%) and may even present with the biliary disease before the onset of colitis (231). Recent studies also suggest that after ileal pouch-anal anastomosis for ulcerative colitis, the incidence of pancreatitis is elevated in patients with primary sclerosing cholangitis (232).

Hemorrhages in all parts of the gastrointestinal tract, ranging from scattered petechiae to extensive bleeding, are often noted in patients with chronic liver disease. They are seen mainly in cases of acute or chronic disease with extensive hepatic necrosis and are related to a decrease in synthesis of clotting factors such as prothrombin. A reduction in platelets, which occurs in cases involving sustained portal hypertension and hypersplenism and in some patients with circulating antibodies to the thrombocytes, can also contribute to the formation of gut hemorrhage.

Cirrhosis of any etiology may induce pathologic changes in the gut in a significant number of patients (233–235). An increase in the incidence of duodenal peptic ulcers is observed in patients with cirrhosis, particularly in those who have had a portacaval shunt, and is thought to be due to reduced degradation of gastric secretagogues, such as histamine and gastrin. Other disorders of the gastrointestinal tract that are attributed to cirrhosis and its major etiologic factor of alcoholic disease include esophageal and gastric varices, the Mallory-Weiss tear of the esophagogastric junction, gastritis, and portal venous thrombosis leading to bowel infarction. Patients with cirrhosis may develop a form of reactive gastritis characterized by foveolar hyperplasia, epithelial regenerative changes, and a marked proliferation and ectasia of mucosal blood vessels that is difficult to distinguish from gastric antral vascular ectasia syndrome (236, 237). More often, findings include a mild proliferation and dilatation of capillaries in the superficial lamina propria, with or without fibrin thrombi, in any portion of the gut mucosa, but especially in the stomach and colon (congestive gastropathy or colopathy) believed to be secondary to chronic portal hypertension and increased vascular pressures (Fig. 19.4). These areas may appear as erythematous patches or vascular ectasia to the endoscopist and occasionally bleed extensively.

HEMOCHROMATOSIS

In the advanced stage of both the primary and secondary forms of hemochromatosis, iron deposits are noted in the parenchymal cells throughout the body. These deposits are evident in the epithelial cells of the gut and appear to be especially prominent in the parietal cells of the stomach (238), but they are not associated with any sign of injury (Fig. 19.5), and no structural change is evident to account for the increased rate of iron absorption by the small intestine in the

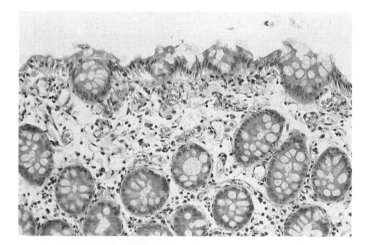

Figure 19.4 Colonic mucosa in a patient with advanced cirrhosis and portal hypertension. The lamina propria shows edema and marked proliferation of capillary sized blood vessels mainly in the superficial portion of the mucosa. Microhemorrhages are seen in other areas as well (H & E, ×200). (See color plate.)

primary type (88, 239). Hemosiderin deposits are frequently noted within the macrophages in the lamina propria of the normal intestine (240) and are present in increased numbers in patients with hemosiderosis and with the secondary form of hemochromatosis.

VITAMIN DISORDERS

Symptoms referable to multiple vitamin deficiencies are often noted in the various malabsorptive disorders (241), which are discussed in Chapter 31.

FAT-SOLUBLE VITAMINS

VITAMIN K DEFICIENCY

A deficiency in vitamin K for whatever reason leads to a decrease in the formation of prothrombin and other essential clotting factors by the liver. The possible result is the appearance of fresh hemorrhages in all parts of the body (242). The effects on the gastrointestinal tract are variable and often unpredictable, and the lesions may occur in any part of the tract and range from focal petechiae of the mucosal and serosal surfaces to larger areas of hemorrhage with extensive bleeding into the gut lumen. No special features permit their distinction from other causes of spontaneous hemorrhage in the bowel, and the diagnosis relies on the demonstration of a condition that could cause the vitamin depletion and on the exclusion of other causes of hypothrombinemia. The hemorrhages typically regress with the correction of the vitamin disorder, and complications such as ulceration, fibrous structure, and perforation of the bowel are not observed. Residual foci of hemosiderin-filled macrophages may persist in the tissues for a short period of time, but they eventually disappear; the finding of such macrophages in the lamina propria is not diagnostic because they may be seen also in normal persons.

DISORDERS OF OTHER FAT-SOLUBLE VITAMINS

It has been suggested that the brown bowel syndrome, which is characterized by the deposition of a lipofuscin-type pigment in the intestinal wall, might be caused by a deficiency in vitamin E, but this

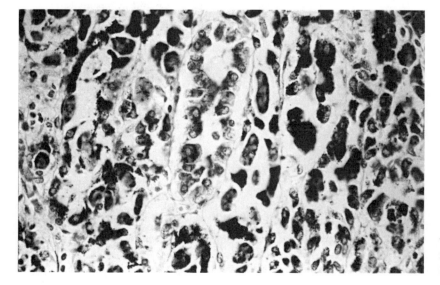

Figure 19.5 Gastric corpus mucosa in a patient with hemochromatosis demonstrates marked deposition of iron in the parietal cells (Prussian blue reaction for iron, ×250).

has not been clearly established (see subsequent section on depositions). Deficiencies in vitamins A and D have no direct effects on the gastrointestinal tract. Hypervitaminosis D may be associated with symptoms that are largely related to the upper tract and that are thought to be due to hypercalcemia and its stimulatory effect on gastric acid secretion.

WATER-SOLUBLE VITAMINS

PELLAGRA

This disorder of niacin deficiency, which usually follows a decrease in oral intake, is particularly prevalent in developing counties. It is also noted occasionally in persons with poor or unusual nutritional habits such as alcoholics, food faddists, and the elderly. The deficiency leads to an interference with the normal renewal of the epithelia in many parts of the body, and the most marked effects are noted in the skin, oral cavity, and intestinal tract (243). This involvement in the gastrointestinal tract can result in focal ulcers or more extensive and confluent lesions of the small intestine and colon, and the patients typically present with abdominal pain and bloody diarrhea. The character of the inflammation is nonspecific, and the intact mucosa of the small intestine may show milder changes in the form of villous shortening and increased inflammatory cells (244). It is often difficult, however, to distinguish these morphologic features from those of concurrent intestinal infections, which are also common in persons from poor societies. Indeed, both conditions may coexist in the same patient. Furthermore, the effects in pellagra may be compounded by the presence of deficiencies of other B vitamins and by the development of secondary infections that are often attributable to opportunistic agents. The lesions are shallow and resolve with specific vitamin therapy, unless there is associated infection or tropical sprue (245). Local complications are rare. The diagnosis of pellagra is often overlooked initially in western countries because of its relative rarity and the nonspecific nature of the lesions. Diagnosis depends on the recognition of other features of the disease, including dermatitis and mental confusion; the exclusion of infections and other known causes of intestinal lesions; and, ultimately, the response to treatment with niacin.

DISORDERS OF OTHER WATER-SOLUBLE VITAMINS

Deficiencies of thiamine, riboflavin, and pyridoxine do not cause direct injury to the gastrointestinal tract, but they may worsen the intestinal lesions of pellagra. Cases of folic acid and B_{12} deficiency are associated with a megaloblastic proliferation of the epithelial cells that is most prominent in the stomach and small intestine (91–93) (see preceding discussion of diseases of the hematologic system). The features of scurvy, resulting from vitamin C deficiency, include the appearance of hemorrhage and delay in wound healing, but prominent effects in the gastrointestinal tract are rare.

DEPOSITIONS

The term "depositions" is used to signify the presence in the tissues of an excessive amount of a normal or endogenous component of the body or the appearance of an abnormal or exogenous substance. The diseases involved are often referred to as storage disorders, particularly when they have a hereditary basis. The

deposited material is variable and includes examples of proteins, lipids, carbohydrates, minerals, and pigments. Some of the conditions are unique to the gastrointestinal tract, but most can affect multiple tissues in the body. Of the latter, the deposits in the gut may be an incidental finding, yet this area can serve as an accessible site for its diagnosis, or may lead to significant disease of the alimentary tract. (See also the discussion of malabsorptive disorders in Chapter 31.)

CONDITIONS THAT MAY SIMULATE STORAGE DISEASES

In the consideration of a storage disease, it is necessary to exclude more common conditions such as localized xanthomatous reactions (246–248) and clusters of muciphages (53, 249) in the lamina propria. Xanthomas or xanthelasmas represent the accumulation of neutral lipid and cholesterol within macrophages and are usually visualized grossly as tiny yellow nodules or streaks on the mucosal surface (Fig. 19.6). They are thought to form as a consequence of mucosal hemorrhage in patients with severe inflammatory diseases and are seen most often in the stomach (246), particularly the proximal remnant after surgery for peptic ulcer disease, and in the duodenum (248). These lesions may appear as small nodules or polyps to the endoscopist.

Foamy macrophages due to the inclusion of organisms with prominent lipid capsules are also seen in Whipple disease and in infection with Mycobacterium avium complex (249) (Fig. 19.7). Muciphages are macrophages that contain mucus in their cytoplasm

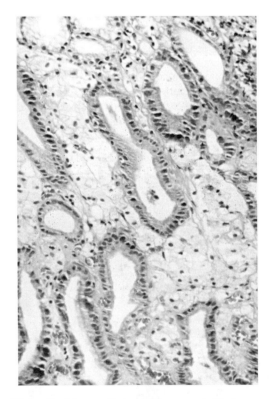

Figure 19.6 Gastric xanthoma. Numerous finely vacuolated (foamy) macrophages are evident within the lamina propria. The epithelium is intact (H & E, ×250).

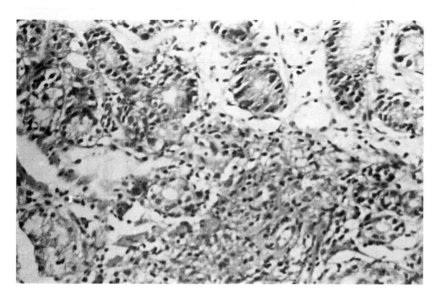

Figure 19.7   Gastric mucosa in a patient with acquired immunodeficiency syndrome. A collection of enlarged, slightly vacuolated macrophages is present in the lower right portion. Acid-fast stain revealed many bacilli of Mycobacterium avium complex (H & E, ×400).

and are observed most frequently in the large intestine (250). Although the appearance of muciphages was once considered a sequelum of laxative use or of a prior inflammatory condition, they are seen almost invariably in the lamina propria of normal persons of all ages, particularly in the rectum (Fig. 19.8). The vacuoles in muciphages tend to be large and irregularly shaped and their nature is identified readily by the periodic acid-Schiff (PAS) reaction and other stains for mucus.

Rarely, the cells of a granular cell tumor (so-called "myoblastoma") may be mistaken for enlarged macrophages. Their cytoplasm, without vacuoles, has a distinctly granular appearance and stains faintly with the PAS reaction. The characteristics of pigmented macrophages are discussed subsequently in the section on lipid pigment disorders. In this regard, an increase in macrophages containing a lipofuscin type pigment in the lamina propria is often present in patients with chronic granulomatous disease; the pigment is restricted to these cells, and there may be other signs of the disease in the form of inflammation and granulomas. The distinctive pathologic features of some of these disorders and depositions are summarized in Table 19.2.

LIPOPROTEIN DISORDERS

TANGIER DISEASE

This disease is characterized by a reduction in the serum levels of the high-density α-lipoproteins and of cholesterol and by the deposition of cholesterol esters in the phagocytic cells of several organs, including the liver, spleen, bone marrow, lymph nodes, and the gut (251). Affected patients are able to synthesize apoproteins in the intestinal epithelium and to form chylomicrons, but they appear to have a defect in catabolism (252). The patients may present with hepatosplenomegaly, signs of a peripheral neuropathy, and, occasionally, diarrhea. Usually no steatorrhea develops because α-lipoproteins are not involved in lipid absorption. Lesions are noted in the small intestine and colon and consist of tiny yellow nodules, less than a few millimeters in diameter, on the mucosal surface. Histologic study reveals finely vacuolated, lipid-laden macrophages and some free lipid in the lamina propria (253, 254) (Fig. 19.9).

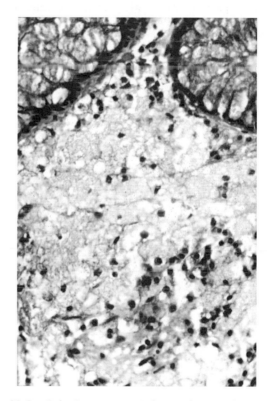

Figure 19.8   Colonic mucosa. A large cluster of mucin-filled macrophages (muciphages) is visible in the lamina propria, just beneath the surface epithelium. The cytoplasmic vacuoles are coarser than those due to lipids (PAS reaction, ×400).

Because of the identical appearance of xanthomatous lesions, the specific diagnosis of Tangier disease depends on the blood lipid findings and other clinical features. Muciphages commonly present in the lamina propria of the large intestine in normal persons are readily distinguished by their coarser vacuoles and positive reactions for mucin in the cytoplasm. Lipid-filled macrophages may also be seen in association with other storage diseases, such as the glycolipid

| TABLE 19.2 | Pathologic Features of Disorders Associated with or Simulating Lamina Propria Macrophage Infiltrates | |

Disorder/Cell Type	Cytoplasmic Content	Diagnostic Features/Stains
Xanthoma	Neural lipid/cholesterol	Yellow streak, central bland nuclei, Oil Red O+, mucin–
Muciphage	Mucin	Coarse large cytoplasmic vacuoles, mucin+, PASD+, Alb ph2.5+
Whipple disease	Bacteria	Extracellular lipid, pink foamy macrophages, small granules, PAS+ granules/rods, +/– gram+, EM intra- and extracellular rods
MAI	Bacteria	AFB+, PAS+
Melanosis	Lipofuscin-like pigment	Finely granular brown pigment, superficial lamina propria, PAS+
Hemosiderosis/chromatosis	Iron	Intra/extracellular dark refractile pigment, Prussian blue+
Pseudolipomatosis	Air	Spaces with no cell lining or lined by fibroblasts/stromal cells
Chronic granulomatous disease	Lipofuscin-like substance	Refractile pigments on H+E, enlarged macrophages (clusters), deep lamina propria, light golden-brown pigment, Oil Red O+, PAS+
Signet ring carcinoma	Mucin	Eccentric hyperchromatic atypical nuclei, macrovesicular cytoplasm, mucin+, PAS+
Malakoplakia	Lysosomes and Michaëlis Guttman bodies	PAS+ macrophages, Prussian blue+, Ca+ stain+
Histiocytosis X	Normal constituents	Macrophages with finely granular cytoplasm, rare vacuoles, no pigments, associated eosinophils
Barium granuloma	Barium	Submucosal macrophages, faint brown/pale green crystals refractile, not birefringent, PAS–
Granular cell tumor	Giant lysosomes	Coarse granular cytoplasm, PAS+, S-100+

MAI, Myobacterium avium intracellulare; AFB, acid fast bacteria; PAS, periodic acid Schiff; Ca+ calcium; Alb pH 2.5, Alcian blue pH 2.5; EM, electron microscopy.

disorders, but close examination usually reveals deposits in other mesenchymal elements and in nerves as well.

ABETALIPOPROTEINEMIA

This disease is caused by a failure to form β-lipoproteins, which are required for optimal absorption of lipids in the gut. This failure results in the absence of these lipoproteins in the blood as well as a marked reduction in the levels of triglycerides and a general diminution in other lipids (255, 256). Additional features include the presence of steatorrhea, which usually begins in early childhood, acantholytic red blood cells attributable to defects in the lipid membrane, and neurologic lesions involving the cerebellum, basal ganglia, retina, and peripheral nerves (257). The patients are capable of normal intraluminal digestion of lipids, the transport of triglycerides and monoglycerides, and their reesterification within the absorptive cells of the small intestine. The defect lies in the inability to form normal chylomicrons, and the lipids are not excreted from the epithelial cells into the lymphatics. The structural alterations in the gastrointestinal tract are limited to the small intestine, and most of the information has been based on results of jejunal mucosal biopsies (258–260). The villi are of normal dimension, but accumulation of lipid within the covering absorptive cells is striking and the mucosal lymphatics are collapsed (Fig. 19.10). The lipid is seen as rounded vacuoles of irregular size and their

nature can be confirmed by fat stains, such as Oil Red O, on nondehydrated histologic sections and by ultrastructural study. The appearance of the villous epithelial cells is similar to that seen in normal persons after a recent lipid-rich meal, but the biopsy samples are obtained in fasted patients. No damage to the epithelial cells or other abnormalities in the mucosa are evident. The diagnosis is determined by the distinctive blood lipid and other clinical features, and small intestinal biopsy is performed mostly for investigative purposes. Because lipid absorption through the portal venous route appears to be unaffected, medium-chain triglycerides can be used in treatment (see Chapter 31 for further details).

GLYCOLIPID STORAGE DISEASES

Several inherited disorders of lipid and carbohydrate metabolism are associated with deposits of substances in many tissues of the body (261, 262), and the materials are most often localized in the phagocytic cells, other mesenchymal cells, and neurons (Table 19.3). The diseases are rare, usually due to deficiencies of lysosomal enzymes, and mostly transmitted as autosomal recessive conditions. Although the gastrointestinal tract is often involved, the lesions typically are small and usually are not productive of local problems in the gut (263). In the examination of intestinal biopsy specimens from patients with these storage diseases with depositions in the macrophages and nervous tissue elements, the appearance at light microscopy may be relatively nonspecific (264, 265). The macrophages most often reveal a foamy cytoplasm related to the presence of numerous closely packed small vacuoles, and the identification of the specific contents usually requires application of other techniques, such as histochemical and ultrastructural studies (266). Indeed, because of the nonspecificity of the results obtained with intestinal biopsies, this technique has been largely supplanted by other procedures for the purpose of the primary diagnosis (267). Studies of the specific enzyme content of circulating leukocytes and of biopsies of the skin, conjunctiva, and skeletal muscles have been used (268).

GANGLIOSIDOSES (269, 270)

Prominent lipid deposits have been observed in rectal biopsy specimens from patients with GM-gangliosidosis, β-galactosidase-neuraminidase deficiency, Tay-Sachs disease, and Sandhoff disease. Lipid bodies, both free in the cytoplasm or as membrane-bound

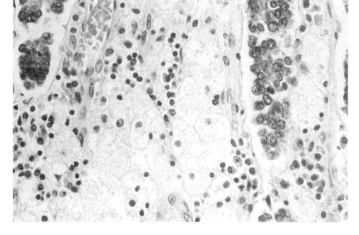

Figure 19.9   High-power view of the basal portion of a colonic mucosal biopsy from a patient with Tangier disease. The lamina propria is replaced with numerous macrophages containing clear bubbly cytoplasm similar to muciphages (H & E, ×400). (See color plate.)

cytosomes, are seen in unmyelinated axons, Schwann cells, endothelial cells, fibroblasts, and plasma cells (266). The cytosomes range in size from 0.3 to 1.0 μm in diameter. No lipid deposits are evident in the muscle cells or in the macrophages. The lipid deposition is probably present in other parts of the gastrointestinal tract but is not associated with any clinical problems.

SULFATIDOSES

In metachromatic leukoencephalopathy, free lipid bodies without cytosomes are present in the cytoplasm of Schwann cells (266). The macrophages in the lamina propria may contain inclusions that stain with toluidine blue and other metachromatic stains (261, 264, 265). Other mesenchymal cells or axons usually are not involved, and gastrointestinal symptoms are typically absent.

FABRY DISEASE

This sex-linked lysosomal storage disease affects males with major involvements of the skin, kidneys, heart, and nervous system (186). Mild gastrointestinal symptoms are noted in most patients and male family members, and appear to be related to reduced motility (186, 187). Delayed gastric emptying may develop, leading to early satiety and bacterial proliferation in the small intestine, which in turn results in more significant diarrhea and steatorrhea. The abnormal deposition can cause weakening of the muscularis propria and favors the formation of small bowel diverticula (188). Abundant lipid deposits are noted in may tissue elements of the gut, including macrophages, endothelial cells, smooth muscle, ganglia, axons, and Schwann cells (187, 271) (see also Chapter 13).

NIEMAN-PICK DISEASE

Lipid bodies are often present in macrophages, other mesenchymal cells, and the ganglia of the gut, but motility problems are observed only rarely (266, 272). The deposits range in size from 0.2 to 1.7 μm in diameter and have a variable appearance, including homogeneous and laminated bodies and those with a central lucency.

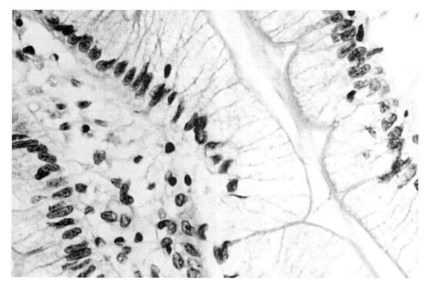

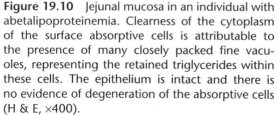

Figure 19.10   Jejunal mucosa in an individual with abetalipoproteinemia. Clearness of the cytoplasm of the surface absorptive cells is attributable to the presence of many closely packed fine vacuoles, representing the retained triglycerides within these cells. The epithelium is intact and there is no evidence of degeneration of the absorptive cells (H & E, ×400).

TABLE 19.3 Storage Diseases of Gastrointestinal Tract: Nature and Localization of Deposits

Disorder	Chemical	Location of Deposit[d]			
		Macrophage	Muscle	Nerve/Ganglia	Other[e]
Glycolipids					
Gangliosidoses[a]	Ganglioside	0	0	+	+
Metachromatic leukoencephalopathy	Sulfatide	+	0	0	Rare
Fabry disease	Ceramide trihexoside	+	+	+	+
Nieman-Pick	Sphingomyelin	+	+	+	+
I-cell disease	Mucolipid	0	0	Rare	+
Lipid pigments					
Melanosis	Lipofuscin	++	0	0	0
Neuronal forms[b]	Lipofuscin	++	+	Rare	+
Brown bowel disease	Lipofuscin	+	++	+	+
Other					
Wolman disease	Cholesterol ester	+	0	0	0
Mucopolysaccharidoses[c]	Heparin + other sulfates	0	0	0	+
Mannosidosis	Oligosaccharides	+	+	+	+
Cystinosis	Cystine	+	0	0	0

[a]Includes GM$_1$ and GM$_2$ (Tay-Sachs and Sandhoff) types.

[b]Changes most marked in infantile type (Batten) and rare in adult form (Kufs).

[c]Includes Hurler (type I), Hunter (II), and Sanfillipo (III) types.

[d]Present (++ or +), rare, or absent (0).

[e]Other mesenchymal elements, including Schwann cells, fibroblasts, and endothelial cells.

MUCOLIPIDOSES

Lipid bodies and enlarged lysosomes have been noted in Schwann cells, fibroplasts, and endothelial cells of patients with I-cell disease (266). Only rarely are axons involved, and no alteration of the ganglia or macrophages occurs. Gastrointestinal disease does not develop.

LIPID PIGMENT DISORDERS

Ceroid or lipofuscin pigment represents the undigestible residue of lipid oxidation and peroxidation reactions within the cells. The pigment is not affected by the dehydration procedures and reacts with the Sudan fat stain in paraffin-embedded sections. It also stains with acid-fast stains and with the periodic acid-Schiff (PAS) reaction and has a bright yellow autofluorescence. This substance, often referred to as "wear and tear" pigment, accumulates in the parenchymal cells of the body in direct relation to aging. Scattered macrophages containing lipofuscin pigments are seen in the lamina propria of normal persons (273, 274). Conditions associated with increased deposition of these pigments or with their appearance in abnormal locations have been termed ceroidosis or lipofuscinosis. The presence of increased macrophages containing a lipofuscin-type pigment in the lamina propria has also been noted in association with chronic granulomatous disease.

NEURONAL CEROID LIPOFUSCINOSIS

These rare lysosomal storage diseases include the infantile and juvenile forms of Batten disease and the adult type of Kufs disease. They are characterized by the deposition of pigment in many cells of the body, with major involvement of the central nervous system and retina; the changes are most dramatic in the infantile type. Because the particular enzyme deficiency is not known, the diagnosis often depends on biopsies of skeletal muscle (268) and the rectum (275). Pigment deposition within the macrophages of the lamina propria is prominent and can be readily detected by light microscopy; compared to the normal, the macrophages occur in clusters and the granules appear larger and coarser. Less amounts of pigment are seen in the Schwann cells, muscle cells, and endothelial cells. The axons are involved only rarely, and the ganglia are uninvolved. Electron microscopy reveals lipid bodies of variable density and configuration and membrane-bound cytosomes that range up to 3.5 μm in diameter. Similar distribution of the pigment but of lesser concentration is noted in the juvenile type, whereas the adult form is associated with sparse pigment only in the neurons. The cause of the lipofuscin deposition in these disorders is not known, and the structural findings are not entirely specific. Ceroid deposits are seen in macrophages in patients with chronic granulomatous disease and those with melanosis coli; more widespread pigment is noted in individuals with the brown bowel syndrome. The diagnosis of the Batten and Kufs diseases depends on the compatible clinical features aided by the ultrastructural characteristics. Symptoms referable to the gastrointestinal tract do not occur.

BROWN BOWEL SYNDROME

This rare acquired disorder is characterized by the abundant deposition of lipofuscin pigment in the bowel smooth muscle leading to the appearance of dark brown tissues (276–278). It is observed most commonly in the small intestine, but it may affect the stomach and colon and, exceptionally, the entire tract. This condition is typically seen in association with a variety of malabsorptive disorders (277, 279, 280), including cystic fibrosis, celiac disease, biliary cirrhosis, biliary atresia, and Crohn disease, and is thought to be a consequence of fat malabsorption and vitamin E deficiency (281). This vitamin, α-tocopherol, is an antioxidant, and it is postulated that its absence may promote an increase in lipid oxidation and the excess formation of the lipofuscin pigment. It is not clear, however, why the bowel condition should occur so infrequently in view of the common occurrence of malabsorption of fat-soluble vitamins in the underlying diseases. Usually no clinical problems are directly related to the brown bowel, although a decrease in contractibility has been rarely observed. The pigment deposition is most prominent in the smooth muscle cells of the muscularis mucosa and propria, and lesser amounts are seen in the macrophages, ganglia, nerves, and vessel walls. The staining characteristics are typical for lipofuscin and include positive reactions with Sudan black in dehydrated sections, with acid-fast stains, and with the periodic acid-Schiff (PAS) technique. The pigment exhibits a bright yellow autofluorescence and does not react with stains for iron or other minerals.

Ultrastructural studies have revealed that the lipid pigment is concentrated in the perinuclear Golgi region of the muscle cells (277, 282). Enlarged and deformed mitochondria are also noted, and it has been suggested that an alteration in these organelles may be important in the genesis of the pigment lesion (276, 282).

A lipofuscin deposition may be seen in macrophages of normal persons and of patients with melanosis coli and chronic granulomatous disease, and more widespread distribution in other mesenchymal cells and nerves is noted in individuals with Batten disease. None of these conditions, however, reveals the extreme deposition in the muscle that is diagnostic of the brown bowel syndrome.

MELANOSIS COLI

This condition is characterized by the presence of a lipofuscin-like pigment in the macrophages of the lamina propria throughout the rectum, colon, and appendix (283). (See also Chapter 30.)

OTHER STORAGE DISEASES

WOLMAN DISEASE

This disease, which occurs as a result of a deficiency in lysosomal acid phosphatase, is characterized by the appearance of increased serum cholesterol and enlargement of the liver and spleen (284). Deposits of cholesterol esters are located in the lymphoid tissues and phagocytic cells, including the macrophages in the lamina propria of the gastrointestinal tract (285). No lipid deposits are found in the other mesenchymal cells or neurons in the gut wall, and gastrointestinal symptoms are not present. Similar lesions of cholesterol deposits limited to the macrophages may be seen in localized xanthomatous reactions, which are more common in the stomach, and in Tangier disease. The diagnosis of Wolman disease is based on the blood lipid findings and on the determination of the specific enzyme deficiency in leukocytes.

MUCOPOLYSACCHARIDOSES

Deposits of heparin sulfate have been found in rectal biopsy samples from patients with some of these disorders, including the Hurler, Hunter, and Sanfilippo types (266, 286). Membrane-bound vacu-

oles are noted in fibroblasts, plasma cells, endothelial cells, and occasional Schwann cells, but they appear to be absent in muscle, nerves, ganglia, and macrophages. Most of the vacuoles are vacant; others show a dispersed granular or globular material. No gastrointestinal symptoms accompnay these disorders.

MANNOSIDOSIS

This disorder is characterized by the presence of mannose-containing oligosaccharides in the lysosomes of many cells in the body, including nerves, muscle, fibroblasts, and macrophages (268). The deposits are in the form of small membrane-bound bodies with fibrillar material or vacuoles with scant granules. No specific effects on gut function have been described.

CYSTINOSIS

Alterations have been noted in thin-section electron microscopic studies of jejunal mucosal biopsy material (287), including the appearance of angular spaces that conform to the size and shape of cystine crystals within the macrophage and ground substance of the lamina propria and the occasional presence of vacuoles in the absorptive epithelial cells. This condition does not result in gastrointestinal disease.

GLYCOGEN STORAGE DISEASES

Several forms, with principal involvement of the liver, heart, and skeletal muscles, have been described. In the gut, the striated muscle of the upper esophagus is uncommonly affected, leading to poor contractility and dysphagia, and glycogen deposits are rarely noted in the smooth muscles of the intestines (288).

IRON STORAGE

Hemochromatosis is discussed in the preceding section concerning hepatic diseases.

OTHER PIGMENT DEPOSITIONS

Melanin-like depositions are occasionally noted in other areas of the gastrointestinal tract, such as the esophagus, duodenum, distal ileum, and even in the gallbladder (289). Melanosis esophagi is a rare condition with black pigmentation of the mucosa, usually affecting the distal one third. This condition is due to increased numbers of basal layer melanocytes, which normally are present in up to 10% of patients (290).

Melanosis duodeni occurs secondary to the accumulation of ferrous sulfate in cytoplasmic membrane-bound lysosomal bodies in villous lamina propria macrophages (Fig. 19.11). Patients are asymptomatic and the condition is discovered incidentally at the time of endoscopy and usually appears as "speckled" duodenum. This condition is thought to be related to blood products from bleeding peptic ulcers combined with sulfur from ingested food or drugs. Prussian blue stain is typically negative, however (291).

Melanosis ilei is also a rare brown-black or gray-black pigmentation of the distal ileum that may be associated with melanosis coli or occur as an isolated finding. The pigment occurs in

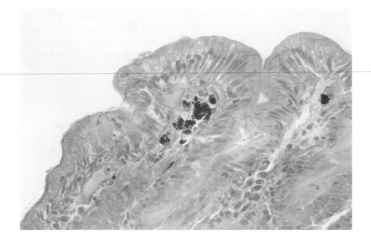

Figure 19.11 High-power view of the tips of two duodenal villi in a patient with melanosis duodeni ("speckled duodenum"). Dark pigment is present within lamina propria macrophages predominantly in the superficial aspects of the villi. This pigment does not usually stain positive with Prussian blue (H & E, ×400). (See color plate.)

macrophages, usually adjacent to Peyers patches, and is believed to consist of an accumulation of aluminum and magnesium-rich silicate particles due to inhaled dust or ingested materials (289). Pseudomelanin deposition has been noted in the duodenal mucosa (see discussion of melanosis coli in Chapter 30). Carbon and other exogenous pigments are occasionally seen in the normal gut mucosa and are especially concentrated in lymphoid nodules (292, 293).

AMYLOIDOSIS

DEFINITION AND TYPES

Amyloid in its pure form is a specific fibrous protein. It appears as an interlacing network of fibrils with a diameter of 7.5 to 10 nm that can be recognized with certainty by ultrastructural examination (56). In tissues, amyloid is coupled to glycoproteins, which constitute about 10% of the deposits, and this property allows for the more rapid and economic identification of the amyloid by special histochemical stains at the light microscopic level. The most specific of these reactions is the Congo Red stain, which, when viewed with polarized light, reveals the characteristic apple-green birefringence of amyloid.

Traditionally, amyloidosis has been separated into the systemic or generalized type, which in turn may be primary or secondary to long-standing inflammatory diseases, a localized form in which the amyloid is limited to a single organ or system, and special categories that are associated with various neoplasms and hereditary diseases (294). The preexisting inflammatory diseases include chronic infections, rheumatoid arthritis, and Crohn disease. Despite the identical morphologic features of amyloid in all of these types, distinct chemical and antigenic differences allow for a newer, more exact biochemical classification of amyloidosis based on the dominant fibrillar protein (295, 296). Thus, the amyloid is composed of immunoglobulin light chains and is referred to as the AL-type in primary systemic amyloidosis and in B-cell neoplasms, including multiple myeloma, whereas a different protein called amyloid-

associated or AA type is seen in the secondary systemic cases associated with chronic inflammatory disorders and in familial Mediterranean fever. Many of the localized and neuropathic forms contain a prealbumin as the major constituent of the amyloid, and this type of proteinaceous substance occurs both in the familial form of amyloidosis (AF) and in senile amyloidosis (AS). Of interest, the purely localized form of amyloidosis does not normally occur in the gastrointestinal tract. Rather, the amyloid occurs as part of the systemic disease; it most commonly affects the small vessels and infrequently is associated with larger infiltrates in the tissues of the gut, leading to local functional problems.

PATHOPHYSIOLOGY AND CLINICAL FEATURES

With the exception of the rarer hereditary forms (297, 298), amyloidosis tends to be more common in middle-aged and older persons, with the latter more typical of the primary systemic type (299–301). It has been estimated from autopsy studies that amyloid involvement of the gastrointestinal tract is present in more than 75% and possibly in all cases of systemic amyloidosis. In most cases, however, the amyloid deposits are patchy and generally limited to the small vessels, and either no symptoms are referable to the gut or just rare episodes of bleeding occur. Clinical problems can develop with greater and more widespread involvement of the vessels and with the appearance of infiltrates of amyloid in the nervous and muscular tissues (302–304). These problems are characterized by: (*a*) more frequent and severe hemorrhages (305–307), resulting from fragility and rupture of affected vessels; (*b*) focal ulcers, which are more commonly noted in the stomach (308–310) and colon (311, 312), probably caused by localized ischemia as a further consequence of the damaged vessels; and (*c*) reduced motility from amyloid deposits in the enteric muscles and nerves (298, 300, 313, 314). The motor disturbances have been noted in all parts of the tract and include reduced contractions of the distal esophagus with occasional formation of megaesophagus, prolonged emptying time and outlet obstruction of the stomach, and an increase in the transit time, which may result in dilatation of the intestine (see also Chapter 13). Malabsorption also may develop (315, 316) as a result of stasis and bacterial proliferation in the small intestine (317). Clinical symptoms depend on the particular problem and consist of upper or lower tract bleeding, those of peptic disease, and either diarrhea or constipation. Rarely, amyloid may manifest as a solitary mass in the gastrointestinal tract.

PATHOLOGY

The histologic appearance of amyloid is the same in all forms of amyloidosis (318). With the standard hematoxylin and eosin (H & E)-stained sections, this homogenous pink, hyaline substance may contain small slitlike spaces due to a cracking of the material during the tissue preparation. Histochemical stains based on attached carbohydrates are used to distinguish amyloid from other proteins, and these techniques include metachromatic dyes such as toluidine blue and crystal violet, the fluorochrome thioflavin, and, most specifically, the Congo Red stain with polarized light to show the apple-green birefringence. The amyloid glycoprotein also stains faintly with the periodic acid-Schiff (PAS) reaction, but it is negative with various lipid and mineral stains. The amyloid deposits are most often concentrated in the media of the small arteries and arterioles in any part of the bowel wall, and these are readily detected in biopsy samples that include the submucosa (Fig. 19.12). A patchy or diffuse infiltrate in the lamina propria and submucosa is noted occasionally in severe cases. This pattern of amyloid deposition might also be the result of trauma sustained during the biopsy procedure, which leads to an escape of amyloid from the blood vessels.

In patients with motility problems, the amyloid is also observed in the region of the muscularis mucosae and propria and ganglia, and the infiltrates range in amount from fine strands to extensive replacement of the muscle (Fig. 19.13). In severe cases, amyloid may cause gross alterations in the form of a thickened intestinal wall with a waxy appearance, and nodular masses of amyloid may project into the gut lumen (319–321). Gross changes are otherwise lacking in most cases of amyloidosis or reveal the effects of complications, such as ulcers and dilation. Infrequently, amyloidosis may develop in a patient with Crohn disease (322). Authors of one study suggest that the predominant pattern of amyloid deposition in the bowel

wall depends on the etiology of the deposits (muscularis in the AL-type and lamina propria in the AA-type), but this variability is yet to be confirmed (318).

DIFFERENTIAL DIAGNOSIS

The diagnosis of amyloidosis depends simply on its identification in a biopsy or other tissue sample by using special histochemical staining or ultrastructural examination (323). The differential is related to the particular location of the amyloid deposits. In the vascular walls, the amyloid must be distinguished from the very common changes of arteriosclerosis that also result in the appearance of a pink hyaline thickening of the media. The amyloid infiltrates in the muscle need to be separated from collagen, which is seen in systemic sclerosis and in the later stages of intestinal myopathies. Furthermore, in cases of secondary amyloidosis with mucosal damage, it may be necessary to sort out the effects that are

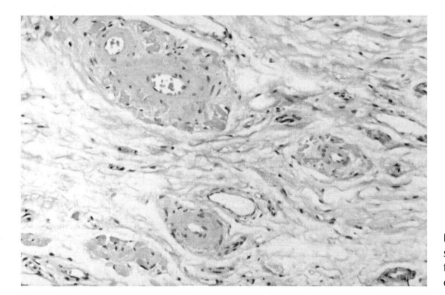

Figure 19.12 Colonic submucosa in a patient with systemic amyloidosis. Note the hyaline thickening of the small vessel media and some free strands outside of the vessels (H & E, ×250).

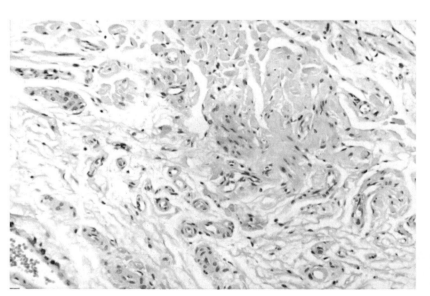

Figure 19.13 Colonic muscularis propria in an individual with systemic amyloidosis. Prominent infiltrate of hyaline amyloid material replaces the muscle fibers (H & E, ×100).

directly attributable to the amyloid disorder and those of the underlying disease and its therapy.

MUCOSAL BIOPSY

Mucosal biopsy of the rectum is the preferred choice to establish the diagnosis of systemic amyloidosis, whether of the primary or secondary types, because the rectum is readily accessible and the procedure is associated with minimal discomfort and a high rate of detection (58, 316, 324–326). This preference for biopsy applies to patients that have no clinical problems attributable to the gastrointestinal tract, which represent the majority of the cases, and include those individuals that have suspected amyloid disease in an internal organ, such as the liver or kidney. Because the aim of the procedure is to obtain a sample of arteries, the biopsy must be of the aspiration type to ensure the inclusion of a large portion of submucosa. It is essential that the special stains be applied in all cases to achieve the highest sensitivity. It has been estimated that in patients with systemic amyloidosis that is not associated with clinically significant gut involvement, amyloid is detected in the rectal biopsy in about 80 to 85% of cases. The deposits in some instances may be minimal and unassociated with any apparent thickening of the arterial walls on standard H & E sections. The question has arisen, however, as to whether the finding of amyloid restricted to the vessel walls in elderly patients can always be considered evidence of significant disease. In this regard, the senile cardiovascular type of amyloidosis is a fairly common condition in such patients and is often asymptomatic. The possibility, therefore, exists that the finding of amyloid in the submucosal vessels of older patients is simply a reflection of aging. This issue has not yet been resolved.

Mucosal biopsy is occasionally performed to determine the presence of amyloid in other parts of the gastrointestinal tract, particularly in patients with signs of mucosal inflammation or ulceration and in those with malabsorption. It is important to ensure that the sample includes the submucosal vessels. Positive results have been obtained from biopsy specimens from all parts of the tract, including the stomach (309, 327) and small intestine (328). In fact, recent data suggest that 100% of duodenal biopsy samples may be positive in affected patients. Acquisition of tissue from the duodenum is laborious and uncomfortable for the patient, however, compared to obtaining rectal tissue by sigmoidoscopy (329).

GRANULOMATOUS DISORDERS

Many conditions of varied etiology are associated with granulomatous inflammation in the gastrointestinal tract (Table 19.4) (330). The most common disorders are infections (see Chapter 28) and Crohn disease (see Chapter 29). Other chapters include discussion of foreign body reactions with granulomas in the esophagus (Chapter 20), the stomach (Chapter 23), and the intestines (Chapter 30). The following section briefly reviews some of the common disorders and provides details on those disorders that are not covered fully in other parts of the book.

Granulomas are broadly defined as a nodular collection of macrophages (or histiocytes) that are often hypertrophied and may be fused to form multinucleated giant cells. Variable features present in some granulomas include necrosis of the liquefactive, coagulative,

TABLE	
19.4	**Granulomatous Disorders of Gastrointestinal Tract**

Infections
  Chlamydial
  Bacterial: Yersinia, Mycobacteria (human, avium), Campylobacter, syphilis
  Fungal: Histoplasma, Blastomyces, Cryptococcus, Phycomyces
  Helminthic: Schistosoma, Anisakidae, other worms
Crohn disease
Foreign body reactions
  Food, feces, and mucin
  Suture, talc, and starch
  Barium and oils
Miscellaneous
  Isolated granulomas (especially of stomach)
  Sarcoidosis
  Malakoplakia
  Chronic granulomatous disease of childhood
  Langerhans cell histiocytosis
  Reaction to carcinoma
  Granulomatous vasculitis

Modified from Haggitt RC. Granulomatous diseases of the gastrointestinal tract. In: Ioachim HL, ed. Pathology of granulomas. New York: Raven Press, 1983; 257–305.

or caseous types; other inflammatory cells including neutrophils, eosinophils, and lymphocytes; signs of repair and fibrosis; and inclusions of all sorts within the macrophages. Also apparent within the granuloma may be the particular causative agent, such as a microorganism or foreign material.

Granulomas should not be confused with lymphoid nodules, which are composed of mature lymphocytes surrounding a germinal center. Occasionally noted is an enlargement of the cytoplasm of the germinal center cells so that they appear more epithelial, but these cells can be recognized by their restricted location to the center of the lymphoid nodule. Other structures that may be mistaken for granulomas, particularly in tangential sections, include ganglia and nerves, the fibrous sheath around the crypts, and foci of disrupted or hypertrophied muscle cells. Clusters of macrophages containing mucin (muciphages) or lipid substances (foam cells) and isolated giant cells should also be distinguished from well-formed granulomas (see Figs. 19.6 and 19.8). Lipogranulomas are observed in lymph nodes and consist of poorly circumscribed collections of lipid vacuoles of variable size both within and between macrophages. They probably result from the drainage of oils and other lipid substances that are absorbed from the bowel or released from fatty areas that are damaged by many diseases, including tumors. The macrophages in lipogranulomas do not typically have an enlarged or epithelial appearance.

INFECTIONS

Granulomas are a characteristic feature of tuberculosis; yersinial infections; several fungal diseases, such as histoplasmosis, blastomycosis, cryptococcosis, and phycomycosis; and the parasitic disorders of schistosomiasis and anisakiasis (330). They may also be seen in some cases of infection related to the Myobacterium avium complex in immunosuppressed patients (249), although the inflammatory reaction is often severely inhibited, resulting in just the presence of only small clusters of granular macrophages in most instances, as well as in reactions to intestinal worms (331, 332). Granulomas are noted only rarely in other infections, including lymphogranuloma venereum and related chlamydial infections (333, 334), in Campylobacter infection of the intestines (335), and in syphilis (336). Whipple disease occasionally is associated with a granulomatous reaction (337); the granulomas usually form in lymph nodes but less often are present in the bowel wall. Staining with the PAS reaction is not conclusive, but the organisms can be identified by ultrastructural study or their presence inferred by the immunohistochemical demonstration of a typical bacterial antigen profile (see Chapter 31). Malakoplakia is discussed subsequently.

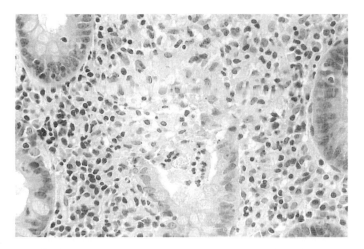

Figure 19.14 Colonic mucosal biopsy in a patient with chronic-active ulcerative colitis. A mucin granuloma adjacent to a ruptured crypt protrudes into the lumen. Mucicarmine stain was positive within the macrophages that form the granuloma (H & E, ×400). (See color plate.)

CROHN DISEASE

Granulomas are present in about 50% of cases of Crohn disease and may be located in any layer of the bowel wall (338, 339). They are also noted in the regional lymph nodes in about 15 to 20% of cases and uncommonly in distant sites such as the liver or even the skin. The granulomas are typically devoid of necrosis, except when associated with extensive fat necrosis or with foreign material, and they may be poorly formed (see Chapter 29).

FOREIGN BODY GRANULOMAS

The most common reactions are attributable to fecal material at sites of perforation, to mucin from ruptured crypts (Fig. 19.14), and to suture material. These as well as other foreign body reactions are summarized in Chapter 30.

ISOLATED GRANULOMAS

Solitary or multiple granulomas without an apparent cause can be seen occasionally in any part of the alimentary tract, usually in the mucosal layer. It is important, in these situations, to exclude granulomas that are related to ruptured crypts or to foreign materials, and multiple sections of the tissue block may be needed. It follows that the sporadic granuloma could occur in some disease that is not expected to be associated with its presence, such as ulcerative colitis; fortunately, this event is rare. The finding of a granuloma in the gut, therefore, must be considered in context with the other morphologic and clinical features of a case. Isolated granulomatous inflammation most often involves the stomach (340, 341), which is described in Chapter 23 (Fig. 19.15).

SARCOIDOSIS

This granulomatous disorder of unknown etiology most often affects the lungs, hilar lymph nodes, and spleen (342, 343). Multiple tissues in the body may be involved, but it typically spares the gastrointestinal tract; disease limited to or starting in the gut is extremely rare. Before 1960, investigators tended to ascribe most cases of granulomas in the tract to sarcoidosis if they did not have

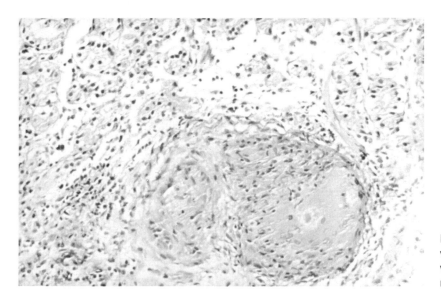

Figure 19.15 Gastric antral mucosa in a patient with isolated granulomas of the stomach. Several well-circumscribed granulomas are located in the mucosa (H & E, ×100).

overt evidence of infection or Crohn disease. This assignment proved to be incorrect, and the diagnosis of gastrointestinal sarcoidosis now depends on finding coexisting disease in a more characteristic location in the body.

PATHOLOGY

Most lesions that have been described occurred in the stomach (344–350), but instances of esophageal involvement (351) and generalized intestinal disease (352–355) have also been reported. Colonic involvement is extremely rare, and the small intestine may also be affected, but usually indirectly by involvement of adjacent lymph nodes. Changes include thickened mucosal folds, pyloric obstruction, or diffuse ulceration, which can be visualized by radiographic and endoscopic examination. Biopsies typically reveal multiple noncaseating granulomas. The granulomas are concentrated in the mucosa and submucosa, and are composed of enlarged or epithelioid macrophages, which often contain laminated calcific inclusions within the cytoplasm. An admixture of lymphocytes and eosinophils is often noted at the periphery of the granulomas, with some fibrinoid material in the center but no areas of caseous necrosis. The adjacent mucosa may reveal signs of a more diffuse chronic inflammation.

DIFFERENTIAL DIAGNOSIS

The diagnosis of gastrointestinal sarcoidosis depends on the thorough exclusion of other causes of granulomatous inflammation and on the presence of the disease in another typical organ system, such as the lung. It must be distinguished from infections such as tuberculosis by appropriate stains and cultures and from Crohn disease, which would reveal other characteristic lesions in the intestines. Within the stomach, isolated granulomatous gastritis must also be considered in the absence of evidence of systemic disease. Because sarcoidosis of the gastrointestinal tract is rare, all other causes of granulomas, including local foreign body reactions, must be eliminated before rendering this diagnosis.

CHRONIC GRANULOMATOUS DISEASE
DEFINITION, ETIOLOGY, AND CLINICAL FEATURES

This rare X-linked or autosomal recessively inherited disorder of phagocytic function is characterized by the appearance of multiple and recurrent infections in infants and children (356, 357). The phagocytic leukocytes lack the ability to generate hydrogen peroxide and are unable to eliminate catalase-positive bacteria (such as *Staphylococcus aureus*) and fungi. Patients typically manifest chronic infections with abscesses of many organs, including the lymph nodes, skin, lungs, liver, bones, ears, and sinuses, and they often have enlargement of the lymph nodes, liver, and spleen. The diagnosis is established by a negative nitroblue-tetrazolium assay and other tests showing reduced bactericidal activity in the leukocytes. Gastrointestinal problems that occur in about 25% of patients include gastritis and pyloric obstruction (358), vitamin B_{12} deficiency with an abnormal Schilling test that is usually not corrected by the addition of intrinsic factor (359), persistent perineal abscesses, and occasional cases of steatorrhea and of diffuse colitis that may mimic Crohn disease or ulcerative colitis (360).

PATHOLOGY

The pathologic reaction of chronic granulomatous disease is the result of pyogenic infections leading to necrosis and abscess formation and the frequent development of granulomas, the latter caused by the inability of the macrophages to catabolize the intracellular microorganisms (361). Necrotizing lesions with deep ulcers and inflammatory sinus tracts have been noted in the stomach, colon, and perianal region (356, 357). The granulomas in these areas are often sparse and poorly formed, and there is usually a marked infiltrate of eosinophils. Patients with colitis can develop multiple ulcers and inflammatory pseudopolyps, simulating Crohn disease, or diffuse acute and chronic inflammation of the mucosa only, simulating ulcerative colitis. Of interest, the responsible microorganisms are typically not detectable in the gut lesions by special stains or cultures. In most patients with chronic granulomatous disease, including those without overt necrotizing lesions in the gastrointestinal tract, additional abnormalities are noted in the intact mucosa. These changes can be identified by performing jejunal and rectocolonic biopsies (23, 356).

Clusters of enlarged macrophages, ranging in size from 50 to 100 μm in diameter, typically are located adjacent to the muscularis mucosae in the basal portion of the lamina propria. Their cytoplasm contains vacuoles and a golden-brown, lipofuscin-type pigment, which stains positively with fat stains and the periodic acid-Schiff (PAS) reaction. When abundant, the macrophages can extend between and separate the bases of the crypts from the muscularis mucosae, and isolated cells are occasionally noted in the submucosa. Rectal biopsy has also demonstrated the appearance of granulomas, in the absence of cryptitis, and an overall increase in inflammatory cells in the lamina propria and submucosa, including mononuclear cell types, neutrophils, and eosinophils, in about 50% of cases studied.

DIFFERENTIAL DIAGNOSIS

The diagnosis of chronic granulomatous disease depends ultimately on the demonstration of the impaired bactericidal action of the macrophages or neutrophilic leukocytes. The inflammatory and ulcerative lesions of the stomach and colon must be distinguished mainly from primary granulomatous infections by appropriate stains and cultures, and from inflammatory bowel disease by the absence of necrotizing lesions in other tissues and organs. Primary immunodeficiency disorders may be associated with secondary infections of the gut, but these conditions frequently involve the small intestine and opportunistic agents are not associated with a granulomatous reaction (362). Scattered macrophages containing a lipofuscin-type pigment are seen in the colonic mucosa of normal persons, are usually more prominent in the superficial lamina propria, and are more abundant in cases of melanosis coli, but they do not form clusters or nodules and are typically very sparse or absent in the small intestinal mucosa. Although prominent macrophages with lipid pigments are observed in association with some storage disorders, such as Batten disease and in the brown bowel syndrome, these conditions reveal more widespread depositions in the nerves and muscle cells. Many other storage diseases and other conditions associated with lipid-filled macrophages can be distinguished by their absence of PAS-positive pigments (see previous section concerning depositions.) Foamy macrophages containing PAS-positive material are also seen in Whipple disease and in infection with Mycobacterium avium complex, but they do not reveal refractile pigments in standard histologic sections.

MALAKOPLAKIA

DEFINITION, ETIOLOGY, AND CLINICAL FEATURES

This rare disorder is characterized by the development of soft plaque-like lesions and the distinctive appearance of mineralized inclusions within macrophages (363, 364). Thought to be due to an acquired defect in the lysosomal function of monocytic-phagocytic cells, the condition results in the promotion of infections that usually are caused by enteric organisms such as E. coli or klebsiella (365, 366). The exact deficiency has not been established, although it has been suggested that the error might be corrected by the use of cholinergic agonists (367). The disease is seen most frequently in the urinary tract (368), but it may affect almost any tissue in the body (364). Involvement of the gastrointestinal tract ranks second

in order of distribution (369); most reports cite the occurrence of malakoplakia in the colon (370–376), with rare instances in the esophagus, stomach (377), small intestine, and appendix. The intestinal disease is often associated with extension into the regional lymph nodes, mesentery, and retroperitoneum. In contrast to disease of the urinary tract, which is more common in older women, gut involvement affects both sexes equally and all age groups, including children. Rare associations with other colonic disorders, such as ulcerative colitis (378), adenomas, and carcinoma (375) have been noted. Presenting symptoms are mainly related to the colonic disease and include fever, bleeding, and the appearance of masses in the bowel and retroperitoneum. The disease persists and often results in such complications as bowel obstruction, perforation, and fistula formation.

PATHOLOGY

The colon is involved in the majority of cases; isolated disease of the upper tract or small intestine is rare. Grossly, several distinct forms exist. One type presents as a sessile or polypoid mass with or without ulceration and usually in the rectosigmoid. Other masslike lesions occur anywhere in the colon but they usually are associated with carcinoma. In fact, in these cases, up to 30% of patients have a coexistent carcinoma (379). Rarely, a diffuse type of colonic malakoplakia may occur.

The early lesions are soft, flat, yellow-to-tan nodules on the mucosal surface. Scattered small plaques have been noted in the stomach, whereas those in the intestines tend to coalesce into larger masses or more diffuse lesions (Fig. 19.16). The intestinal lesions also extend into the wall and this extension may promote bowel perforation and fistula formation. The histologic features are distinctive (366, 380–383), revealing masses of enlarged macrophages that contain characteristic inclusions. Present in all of these cells is an abundance of enlarged membrane-bound lysosomes, ranging in size from 1 to 3 μm in diameter, which stain positively with the periodic acid-Schiff reaction (Fig. 19.17). In addition, many of the macrophages contain the diagnostic Michaëlis-Gutmann bodies, which probably evolve from the mineralization of the lysosomes. These bodies, measuring 2.5 to 9.5 μm in

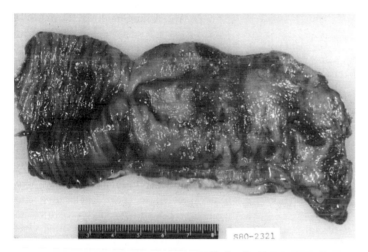

Figure 19.16 Malakoplakia of the colon. The mucosal surface is effaced by the presence of numerous soft plaques with central areas of ulceration.

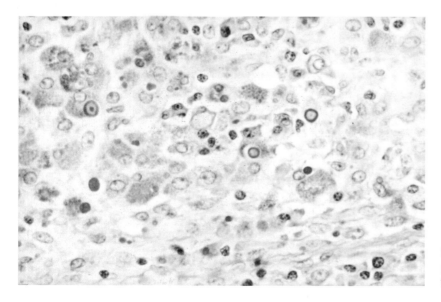

Figure 19.17 Malakoplakia of colon. Note the prominent phagolysosomes within the cytoplasm of the macrophages (PAS reaction, ×400).

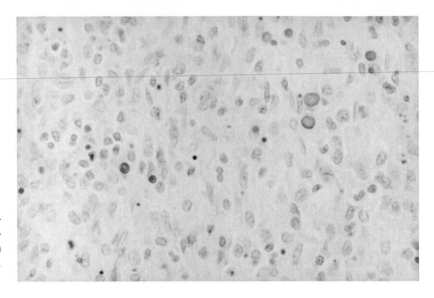

Figure 19.18   Malakoplakia of colon. The Michaëlis-Guttman inclusions in the macrophages are highlighted by the deposition of iron. Stains for calcium may also be used (Prussian blue reaction for iron, ×400).

diameter, are composed of a central matrix of glycolipid material and an outer mineral layer that reacts with stains for iron and calcium (Fig. 19.18). In some cases, typical inclusions are difficult to find and require a careful search. Other nonspecific inflammatory cell types may be present in the tissues adjacent to the masses of macrophages, particularly neutrophils.

DIFFERENTIAL DIAGNOSIS

The diagnosis of malakoplakia is based on finding masses of macrophages that contain the characteristic Michaëlis-Gutmann inclusion bodies within their cytoplasm. Although at the clinical or gross level the disorder may resemble chronic infections, Crohn disease, and tumors with multiple soft nodules, such as lymphomas, the distinction can be readily made by microscopic examination. Many other conditions are associated with a prominence of macrophages, but none have the distinctive mineralized inclusions.

LANGERHANS CELL HISTIOCYTOSIS
DEFINITION AND TERMINOLOGY

This uncommon condition noted in children is characterized by the proliferation of dendritic cells in several tissues of the body (384–388). It appears that most of these cells represent Langerhans cells, based on electron microscopic evidence of Birbeck granules and on the results of immunocytochemical techniques (389). Depending on the overall severity and distribution of the lesions, the disease has been divided into three forms: the localized eosinophilic granuloma (unifocal disease), the Hand-Schuller-Christian type with prominent depositions (multifocal disease), and the disseminated Letter-Siwe form. The term "eosinophilic granuloma" has also been used variably to describe lesions of the gastrointestinal tract that are not related to the histiocytic disorder or even to a granulomatous condition (330); it has been applied to unusual polyps such as the inflammatory fibroid polyp and to the mural form of eosinophilic gastroenteritis.

PATHOLOGY

Within the digestive tract, the histiocytic lesions most commonly affect the major bile ducts and ductules within the portal tracts of the liver, leading to their destruction and the frequent development of a biliary cirrhosis (390, 391). This type of sequelae may result in reduced bile salt excretion and the appearance of diarrhea and, rarely, steatorrhea. In a personal review of fatal cases of Langerhans cell histiocytosis, small collections of dendritic cells were observed in the lamina propria of the small intestine in 50% of the patients. This clustering of dendritic cells had been noted previously (392) but usually does not have any clinical significance. The cells, arranged in a compact cluster, are enlarged and have a finely granular cytoplasm with only rare vacuoles. The intestinal mucosa shows no other signs of inflammation or evidence of damage. These nodular lesions, also detected in mucosal biopsies of the stomach (393) and rectum (394), should be distinguishable from other conditions with accumulation of macrophages in the lamina propria by the absence of prominent vacuoles or pigments.

MISCELLANEOUS GRANULOMATOUS CONDITIONS

Granulomas are occasionally observed in the bowel wall and draining lymph nodes in the vicinity of carcinomas (330, 395). These lesions possibly occur in response to tumor antigens. They have also been noted rarely in association with some forms of vasculitis (396).

REFERENCES

1. Sack TL, Sleisenger MH. Effects of systemic and extra-intestinal disease on the gut. In: Sleisenger MH, Fordtran JS, eds. Gastrointestinal disease, 4th ed. Philadelphia: WB Saunders, 1989:488–528.
2. Lennard-Jones JE. Functional gastrointestinal disorders. N Engl J Med 1983;308:431–435.
3. Hinnant KL, Rotterdam HZ, Bell ET, et al. Cytomegalovirus infection of the alimentary tract: A clinicopathological correlation. Am J Gastroenterol 1986;81:944–950.

4. Rosen PP. Opportunistic fungal infections in patients with neoplastic diseases. Pathol Annu 1986;11:255–315.
5. Ament ME, Rubin CE. Relation of giardiasis to abnormal intestinal structure and function in gastrointestinal immunodeficiency syndromes. Gastroenterology 1972;62:216–226.
6. Casemore DP, Sands RL, Curry A. Cryptosporidium species—a "new" human pathogen. J Clin Pathol 1985;38:1321–1336.
7. Dworkin B, Wormser GP, Rosenthal WS, et al. Gastrointestinal manifestations of the acquired immunodeficiency syndrome: A review of 22 cases. Am J Gastroenterol 1985;80:774–778.
8. Riddell RH. The gastrointestinal tract. In Riddell RH, ed. Pathology of drug-induced and toxic diseases. New York: Churchill Livingstone, 1982:515–606.
9. Pemberton RE, Strand LJ. A review of upper gastrointestinal effects of the newer non-steroidal anti-inflammatory agents. Dig Dis Sci 1979;24:53–64.
10. Fortson WC, Tedesco FJ. Drug-induced colitis—a review. Am J Gastroenterol 1984;79:878–883.
11. Lewis JH. Gastrointestinal injury due to medicinal agents. Am J Gastroenterol 1986;81:819–834.
12. Williams LF Jr. Vascular insufficiency of the intestines. Gastroenterology 1971;61:757–777.
13. Whitehead R. The pathology of ischemia of the intestines. Pathol Annu 1976;11:1–52.
14. Alschibaja T, Morson BC. Ischemic bowel disease. J Clin Pathol 1977;11:68.
15. Swerdlow SH, Antonioli DA, Goldman H. Intestinal infarction: A new classification (letter). Arch Pathol Lab Med 1981;105:218.
16. Norris HT. Reexamination of the spectrum of ischemic bowel disease. In: Norris HT, ed. Pathology of the colon, small intestine, and anus. New York: Churchill Livingstone, 1983;109–120.
17. Camilleri M, Pusey CD, Chadwick VS, et al. Gastrointestinal manifestations of systemic vasculitis. Q J Med 1983;206:141–149.
18. Harrison EG, Hung JC, Bernatz PE. Morphology of fibromuscular dysplasia of the renal artery in renovascular hypertension. Am J Med 1994;43:97–112.
19. Furie DM, Tien RD. Fibromuscular dysplasia of arteries of the head and neck. Imaging findings. AJR AM J Roentgenol 1994;162:1205–1209.
20. Nelson DL, Blaese RM, Strober W, et al. Constrictive pericarditis. Intestinal lymphangiectasia, and reversible immunologic deficiency. J Pediatr 1975;86:548–554.
21. Strober W, Cohen LS, Waldmann TA, et al. Tricuspid regurgitation. A newly recognized cause of protein-losing enteropathy, lymphocytopenia, and immunologic deficiency. Am J Med 1968;44:842–850.
22. Asakura H, Miura S, Morashita T et al. Endoscopic and histopathological study on primary and secondary intestinal lymphangiectasia. Dig Dis Sci 1981;26:312–320.
23. Dobbins WO III. Small bowel biopsy in malabsorptive states. In: Norris HT, ed. Pathology of the colon, small intestine, and anus. New York: Churchill Livingstone, 1983:121–165.
24. Aranha GV, Pickleman J, Pifarre R, et al. The reasons for gastrointestinal consultation after cardiac surgery. Am Surg 1984;50:301–304.
25. Steed DL, Brown B, Reilly JJ, et al. General surgical complications in heart and heart-lung transplantation. Surgery 1985;98:739–745.
26. Glick DL, Kern F Jr. Peptic ulcer in chronic obstructive bronchopulmonary disease. A prospective clinical study of prevalence. Gastroenterology 1964;47:153–160.
27. Ellison LT, Ellison RG, Carter CH, et al. The role of hypercapnia and hypoxia in the etiology of peptic ulceration in patients with chronic obstructive pulmonary emphysema. Am Rev Resp Dis 1964;89:909–916.
28. Langman MJS, Cooke AR. Gastric and duodenal ulcer and their associated diseases. Lancet 1976;1:680.
29. Bumaschny E, Doglio G, Pusajo J, et al. Postoperative acute gastrointestinal tract hemorrhage and multiple-organ failure. Arch Surg 1988;123:722–726.
30. Mason EE. Gastrointestinal lesions occurring in uremia. Ann Intern Med 1952;37:96–105.
31. Berg B, Groth CG, Magnusson G, et al: Gastrointestinal complications in 248 kidney transplant recipients. Scand J Urol Nephrol 1975;(Suppl 29):19–20.
32. Archibald SD, Jirsch DW, Bear RA. Gastrointestinal complications of renal transplantation. 2. The colon. Can Med Assoc J 1978;119:1301–1314.
33. Franzin G, Musola R, Mencarelli R. Morphological changes of the gastroduodenal mucosa in regular dialysis in uremic patients. Histopathology 1982;6:429–437.
34. Ala-Kaila K, Kekki M, Paronen I, et al. Serum gastrin in chronic renal failure: Its relation to acid secretion, G-cell density, and upper gastrointestinal findings. Scand J Gastroenterol 1989;24:939.
35. Merrill JP, Hampers CL. Uremia. N Engl J Med 1970;282;953.
36. Musola R, Franzin G, Mora R, et al. Prevalence of gastroduodenal lesions in uremic patients undergoing dialysis and after transplantation. Gastrointest Endosc 1984;30:343–346.
37. Tani N, Harasawa S, Suzuki S, et al. Lesions of the upper gastrointestinal tract in patients with chronic renal failure. Gastroenterol Jpn 1980;15:480.
38. Cunningham JT. Gastric telangiectasias in chronic hemodialysis patients: a report of six cases. Gastroenterology 1981;81:1131–1133.
39. Shepard AMM, Stewart WK, Wormsley KG. Peptic ulceration in chronic renal failure. Lancet 1973;1:1357–1359.
40. Sutherland DER, Chan FY, Fouchar E, et al. The bleeding cecal ulcer in transplant patients. Surgery 1979;86:386–398.
41. Huded F, Posner GL, Tick R. Non-specific ulcer of the colon in a chronic hemodialysis patient. Am J Gastroenterol 1982;77:913–916.
42. Dinoso VP Jr, Murthy SNS, Saris AL, et al. Gastric and pancreatic function in patients with end-stage renal disease. J Clin Gastroenterol 1982;4:321–324.
43. Franzin G, Musola R, Mencarelli R. Changes in the mucosa of the stomach and duodenum during immunosuppressive therapy after renal transplantation. Histopathology 1982;6:439–449.
44. Diamond SM, Emmett M, Henrich WL. Bowel infarction as a cause of death in dialysis patients. J Am Med Assoc 1987;256:2545–2547.
45. Scheff RT, Zuckerman G, Harter II, et al. Diverticular disease in patients with chronic renal failure due to polycystic kidney disease. Ann Intern Med 1980;92:202.
46. Bischel MD, Reese T, Engel J. Spontaneous perforation of the colon in a hemodialysis patient. Am J Gastroenterol 1980;74:182–184.
47. Komorowski RA, Cohen EB, Kauffman HM, et al. Gastrointestinal complications in renal transplant recipients. Am J Clin Pathol 1986;86:161–167.
48. Watts SJ, Alexander LC, Fawcett K, et al. Herpes simplex esophagitis in a renal transplant patient treated with Cyclosporine A: A case report. Am J Gastroenterol 1986;81:185–188.
49. Franzin G, Muolo A, Griminelli T. Cytomegalovirus inclusions in the gastroduodenal mucosa of patients after renal transplantation. Gut 1981;22:698–701.
50. Weisburger WR, Hutcheon DF, Yardley JH, et al. Cryptosporidiosis in an immunosuppressed renal transplant recipient with IgA deficiency. Am J Clin Pathol 1979;72:473–478.
51. Ainley CC, Clarke DG, Timothy AR, et al. Strongyloides stercoralis hyperinfection associated with cimetidine in an immunosuppressed patient: Diagnosis by endoscopic biopsy. Gut 1986;27:337–338.
52. Goldman H, Antonioli DA. Mucosal biopsy of the esophagus, stomach and proximal duodenum. Hum Pathol 1982;13:423–448.
53. Goldman H, Antonioli DA. Mucosal biopsy of the rectum, colon and distal ileum. Hum Pathol 1982;13:981–1012.
54. Goldman H. Gastrointestinal mucosal biopsy. New York: Churchill Livingstone, 1996.
55. Burke AP, Sobin LH, Virmani R. Localized vasculitis of the gastrointestinal tract. Am J Surg Pathol 1995;19:338–349.
56. Cohen AS. Amyloidosis. N Engl J Med 1967;277:522–530; 574–583; 628–637.
57. Tribe CR, Scott DGI, Bacon PA. Rectal biopsy in the diagnosis of systemic vasculitis. J Clin Pathol 1981;34:843–850.
58. Gafni J, Sohar E. Rectal biopsy for the diagnosis of amyloidosis. Am J Med Sci 1960;240:332–336.
59. Gore RM, Marn CS, Ujiki GT, et al. Ischemic colitis associated with systemic lupus erythematosus. Dis Colon Rectum 1983;26:449–451.
60. Wood ML, Foulds IS, French MA. Protein-losing enteropathy due to systemic lupus erythematosus. Gut 1984;25:1013–1015.
61. Burt RW, Berenson MM, Samuelson CO, et al. Rheumatoid vasculitis of the colon presenting as pancolitis. Dig Dis Sci 1983;28:183–188.

62. McCurley TL, Collins RD. Intestinal infarction in rheumatoid arthritis. Three cases due to unusual obliterative vascular lesion. Arch Pathol Lab Med 1984;108:125–128.
63. Morichau-Beauchant M, Touchard G, Maire P, et al. Jejunal IgA and C3 deposition in adult Henoch-Schönlein purpura with severe intestinal manifestations. Gastroenterology 1982;82:1438–1442.
64. Lieberman E. Hemolytic-uremic syndrome. J Pediatr 1972;80:1–16.
65. Tochen ML, Campbell JR. Colitis in children with the hemolytic-uremic syndrome. J Pediatr Surg 1977;12:213–217.
66. Whitington PF, Friedman AL, Chesney RW. Gastrointestinal disease in the hemolytic-uremic syndrome. Gastroenterology 1979;76:728.
67. Helin H, Mastonen J, Reunala T, et al. IgA nephropathy associated with celiac disease and dermatitis herpetiformis. Arch Pathol Lab Med 1983;107:324–327.
68. Katz A, Dyck RF, Bear RA. Celiac disease associated with immune complex glomerulonephritis. Clin Nephrol 1979;11:39–44.
69. Resnick MI, Caldamone AA. The use of large and small bowel in urologic surgery. Urol Clin North Am 1986;13:(2).
70. Chiou RK, Taylor RJ, Mays SD. Has the pendulum swung too far for continent diversion? A case for the ileal conduit. Semin Urol 1993;11:99.
71. Lasser A, Acosta AE. Colonic neoplasms complicating ureterosig-moidostomy. Cancer 1975;35:1218–1222.
72. Ali MH, Satti MB, Al-Nafussi A. Multiple benign colonic polypi at the site of ureterosigmoidostomy. Cancer 1984;53:1006–1010.
73. Kille JN, Glick S. Neoplasia complicating ureterosigmoidostomy. Br Med J 1967;4:783–784.
74. Whitaker RH, Rugle RCB, Dow D. Colonic tumors following ureterosigmoidostomy. Br J Urol 1971;43:562–575.
75. Ansell ID, Vellacott KD. Colonic polyps complicating ureterosigmoidostomy. Histopathology 1980;4:429–436.
76. Cipolla R, Garcia RL. Colonic polyps and adenocarcinoma complicating ureterosigmoidostomy: Report of a case. Am J Gastroenterol 1984;79:453–457.
77. Stewart M, Macrae FA, William CB. Neoplasia and ureterosigmoidostomy: A colonoscopy survey. Br J Surg 1982;69:414–416.
78. Sterling JR, Uehling DT, Gilchrist KW. Value of colonoscopy after ureterosigmoidostomy. Surgery 1984;96:784–790.
79. Shokeir AA, Ghoneim MA. Further experience with the modified ileal ureter. J Urol 1995;154:45.
80. Kalbe T, Amelung F, Mohring K, et al. Prevention of colon tumors following urinary diversion by antagonizing of nitrosamines or separation of feces and urine? Invest Urol 1994;5:239.
81. Byard RW, Phillips GE, Ahmed S. Pathologic features of the ureteroileal anastomosis in ileal conduits in childhood. Hum Pathol 1993;24:189.
82. Dodds WJ, Spitzer RM, Friedland GW. Gastrointestinal roentgenographic manifestations of hemophilia. AJR Am J Roentgenol 1970;110:412.
83. Sun CC, Hill JL, Combs JW. Hemolytic-uremic syndrome: Initial presentation mimicking intestinal intussusption. Pediatr Pathol 1983;1:415.
84. Neill MA, Agosti J, Rosen H. Hemorrhagic colitis with Escherichia coli 0157:H7 preceding adult hemolytic uremic syndrome. Arch Intern Med 1985;145:2215.
85. Lichtin AE, Silberstein LE, Schrieber AD. Thrombotic thrombocytopenic purpura with colitis in an elderly woman. JAMA 1986;225:1435.
86. Jacobs WA. Acute thrombotic thrombocytopenic purpura and cholecystitis. J Emerg Med 1985;2:265.
87. Gage TP, Gagnier JM. Ischemic colitis complicating sickle cell crisis. Gastroenterology 1983;84:171–174.
88. Astaldi G, Meardi G, Lisino T. The iron content of jejunal mucosa obtained by Crosby biopsy in haemochromatosis and haemosiderosis. Blood 1966;28:70–82.
89. Chisholm M, Ardran GM, Callender ST, et al. Iron deficiency and autoimmunity in postcricoid webs. Q J Med 1971;40:421–423.
90. Graham RM, Rheault MH. Characteristic cellular changes in epithelial cells in pernicious anemia. J Lab Clin Med 1954;43:235–245.
91. Foroozan P, Trier JS. Mucosa of the small intestine in pernicious anemia. N Engl J Med 1967;277:553–559.
92. Hermos JA, Adams WM, Liu YK, et al. Mucosa of the small intestine in folate-deficient alcoholics. Ann Intern Med 1972;76:959–965.
93. Bianchi A, Chipman DW, Dreskin A, et al. Nutritional folic acid deficiency with megaloblastic changes in the small bowel epithelium. N Engl J Med 1970;282:859–861.
94. Lindenbaum J. Tropical enteropathy. Gastroenterology 1973;64:637–652.
95. Fromke VL, Weber LW. Extensive leukemic infiltration of the gastrointestinal tract in chronic lymphosarcoma cell leukemia. Am J Med 1974;56:879–882.
96. Dewar GJ, Lim CNH, Michalyshyn B. Gastrointestinal complications in patients with acute and chronic leukemia. Can J Surg 1981;24:67–71.
97. Winton RR, Gwynn AM, Robert JC, et al. Leukemia and the bowel. Med J Aust 1975;4:89.
98. Smith FP, Kisner DL, Widerlite L, et al. Chemotherapeutic alteration of small intestinal morphology and function: A progress report. J Clin Gastroenterol 1979;1:203.
99. Gwavava NJT, Pinkerton CR, Glasgow JFT, et al. Small bowel enterocyte abnormalities caused by methotrexate treatment in acute lymphoblastic leukaemia of childhood. J Clin Pathol 1981;34:790–795.
100. Bodey GP: Fungal infections complicating acute leukemia. J Chronic Dis 1966;19:667–687.
101. Strayer DS, Phillips GB, Barker KH, et al. Gastric cytomegalovirus infection in bone marrow transplant patients: An indication of generalized disease. Cancer 1981;48:1478–1483.
102. Kies MS, Luedke DW, Boyd JF, et al. Neutropenic enterocolitis. Cancer 1979;43:730–734.
103. McDonald GB, Shulman HM, Sullivan KM, et al. Intestinal and hepatic complications of human bone marrow transplantation. Part I. Gastroenterology 1986;90:460–477.
104. Snover DC, Weisdorf SA, Vercolotti GM, et al. A histopathologic study of gastric and small intestinal graft-versus-host disease following allogeneic bone marrow transplantation. Hum Pathol 1985;16:387–392.
105. Spencer GD, Shulman HM, Mayerson D, et al. Diffuse intestinal ulceration after marrow transplantation: A clinicopathologic study of 13 patients. Hum Pathol 1986;17:621–633.
106. Thornung D, Howard JD. Epithelial denudement in the gastrointestinal tracts of two bone marrow transplant recipients. Hum Pathol 1986;17:560–566.
107. McDonald GB, Sullivan KM, Schuffler MD, et al. Esophageal abnormalities in chronic graft-vs-host disease in humans. Gastroenterology 1981;80:914–921.
108. Sale GE, Shulman HM, McDonald JB, et al. Gastrointestinal graft-versus-host disease in man: A clinicopathologic study of the rectal biopsy. Am J Surg Pathol 1979;3:291–300.
109. Isaacson PG, Spencer J, Connolly CE, et al. Malignant histiocytosis of the intestine: A T-cell lymphoma. Lancet 1985;2:688–691.
110. Isaacson PG. Gastrointestinal lymphoma. Hum Pathol 1994;25:1020–1029.
111. Ramot B. Malabsorption due to lymphomatous disease. Ann Rev Med 1971;22:19.
112. Appelman HD, Hirsch SD, Schnitzer B, et al. Clinicopathologic overview of gastrointestinal lymphomas. Am J Surg Pathol 1985;9(Suppl):71–83.
113. Rao KG, Yaghmai J. Plasmacytoma of the large bowel. A review of the literature and a case report of multiple myeloma involving the rectosigmoid. Gastrointest Radiol 1978;3:225.
114. Bohus R, Waltzer WC, Frischer Z, et al. Retroperitoneal hemorrhage with abscess formation complicating Waldenstrom macroglobulinaemia. Int Urol Nephrol 1985;17:255.
115. Scarf M. Gastrointestinal manifestations of hyperthyroidism. J Lab Clin Med 1936;21:1253–1258.
116. Miller LJ, Gorman CA, Go VLW. Gut-thyroid interrelationships. Gastroenterology 1978;75:901–911.
117. Bock OAA, Witts LJ. Gastric acidity and gastric biopsy in thyrotoxicosis. Br Med J 1963;2:20–24.
118. Shafer RB, Prentiss RA, Bond JH. Gastrointestinal transit in thyroid disease. Gastroenterology 1984;86:852.
119. Thomas FB, Caldwell JH, Greenberger NJ. Steatorrhea in thyrotoxicosis. Relation to hypermotility and excessive dietary fat. Ann Intern Med 1973;78:669.
120. Hellesen C, Friis T, Larsen E, et al. Small intestinal histology,

radiology and absorption in hyperthyroidism. Scand J Gastroenterol 1969;4:169–175.

121. Modebe O. Autoimmune thyroid disease with ulcerative colitis. Postgrad Med J 1986;62:475.

122. Wells I, Smith B, Hinton M. Acute ileus in myxoedema. Br Med J 1977;1:211–212.

123. Eastwood GL, Braverman LE, White EM, et al. Reversal of lower esophageal sphincter hypotension and esophageal aperistalsis after treatment for hypothyroidism. J Clin Gastroenterol 1982;4:307.

124. Case records of the Massachusetts General Hospital. N Engl J Med 1965;272:1118–1127.

125. Irvine WJ. The association of atrophic gastritis with autoimmune thyroid disease. Clin Endocrinol Metab 1975;4:351.

126. Carney JA, Hayles AB. Alimentary tract manifestations of multiple endocrine neoplasia, type 2b. Mayo Clin Proc 1977;52:543.

127. Solcia E, Capella C, Fiocca R, et al. The gastroenteropancreatic endocrine systems and related tumors. Gastroenterol Clin North Am 1989;18:671.

128. Schimke RN. Multiple endocrine neoplasia: How many syndromes? Am J Med Genet 1990;37:375.

129. Eversmann JJ, Farmer RG, Brown CH, et al. Gastrointestinal manifestations of hyperparathyroidism. Arch Intern Med 1967;119:605–609.

130. Gardner EC Jr, Hersh T. Primary hyperparathyroidism and the gastrointestinal tract. South Med J 1981;74:197–199.

131. Linos DA, van Heerden JA, Abboud CF, et al. Primary hyperparathyroidism and peptic ulcer disease. Arch Surg 1978;113:384–386.

132. Morse WI, Cochrane WA, Landrigan P, et al. Familial hypoparathyroidism with pernicious anemia, steatorrhea and adrenocortical insufficiency. N Engl J Med 1961;264:1021–1026.

133. O'Donnell D, Myers AM. Intestinal lymphangiectasia with protein-losing enteropathy, toxic copper accumulation and hypoparathyroidism. Aust NZ J Med 1990;20:167.

134. Tobin MV, Aldridge SA, Morris AI, et al. Gastrointestinal manifestations of Addison disease. Am J Gastroenterol 1989;84:1302–1305.

135. Rosati LA, Augur Jr NA. Ischemic enterocolitis in pheochromocytoma. Gastroenterology 1971;60:581–585.

136. Goyal RK, Spiro HM. Gastrointestinal manifestations of diabetes mellitus. Med Clin N Am 1971;55:1031–1044.

137. Scarpello JHB, Sloden GE. Diabetes and the gut. Gut 1978;19:1153–1162.

138. Taub S, Mariani A, Barkin JS. Gastrointestinal manifestations of diabetes mellitus. Diabetes Care 1979;2:437.

139. Feldman M, Schiller LR. Disorders of gastrointestinal motility associated with diabetes mellitus. Ann Intern Med 1983;98:378–384.

140. Hollis JB, Castell DO, Braddon RL. Esophageal function in diabetes mellitus and its relation to peripheral neuropathy. Gastroenterology 1977;73:1098–1102.

141. Marshak RH, Maklansky D. Diabetic gastropathy. Am J Dig Dis 1964;9:366–370.

142. Liavag I, Tonjum S. Gastric retention in diabetes mellitus. Acta Chir Scand 1971;137:593.

143. Angervall L, Dotevall G, Lehmann KE. The gastric mucosa in diabetes mellitus: Functional and histopathological study. Acta Med Scand 1961;169:339–349.

144. Dotevall G. Incidence of peptic ulcer disease in diabetes mellitus. Acta Med Scand 1959;164:463.

145. Simon L, Tornoczky J, Toth M, et al. The significance of Campylobacter pylori infection in gastroenterologic and diabetic practice. Orv Hetil 1989;130:1325.

146. Barnett JL, Behler EM, Appelman HD, et al. Campylobacter pylori is not associated with gastroparesis. Dig Dis Sci 1989;34:1677.

147. Hensley GT, Soergel P. Neuropathologic findings in diabetic diarrhoea. Arch Pathol Lab Med 1968;85:857–897.

148. Malins JM, Mayne N. Diabetic diarrhoea: A study of 13 patients with jejunal biopsy. Diabetes 1969;18:858–866.

149. Walsh CH, Cooper BT, Wright AD, et al. Diabetes mellitus and coeliac disease: A clinical study. Q J Med 1978;185:89–100.

150. Drewes VM, Olsen S. Histological changes in the small bowel in diabetes mellitus: A study of peroral biopsy specimens. Acta Pathol Microbiol Scand 1965;63:478–480.

151. Riecken EO, Zennek A, Lay A, et al. Quantitative study of mucosal structure, enzyme activities and phenylalanine accumulation in jejunal biopsies of patients with early and late onset diabetes. Gut 1979;20:1001–1007.

152. Smith B. Neuropathology of the oesophagus in diabetes mellitus. J Neurol Neurosurg Psychiatry 1974;37:1151–1154.

153. Ezzat S, Melmed S. Are patients with acromegaly at increased risk for neoplasm? J Clin Endocrinol Metab 1991;72:245.

154. Spjut HJ, Perkins DE. Endometriosis of the sigmoid colon and rectum. AJR Am J Roentgenol 1959;82:1070.

155. Murphy EJ, Murphy P. Gastrointestinal aspects of pregnancy. J Int Med Res 1978;6(Suppl 1):1–5.

156. Vender RJ, Spiro HM. Inflammatory bowel disease and pregnancy. J Clin Gastroenterol 1982;4:231–249.

157. Bernardino ME, Lawson TL. Discrete colonic ulcers associated with oral contraceptives. Am J Dig Dis 1976;21:503–506.

158. Tedesco FJ, Volpicelli NA, Moore FS. Estrogen- and progesterone-associated colitis: A disorder with clinical and endoscopic features mimicking Crohn colitis. Gastrointest Endosc 1982;28:247–249.

159. Marks J. The relationship of gastrointestinal disease and the skin. Clin Gastroenterol 1983;12:693–712.

160. Kelly R, Davidson GP, Townley RR, et al. Reversible intestinal mucosal abnormalities in acrodermatitis enteropathica. Arch Dis Child 1976;51:219.

161. Eliakim R, Goldin E, Livskin R, et al. Esophageal involvement in pemphigus vulgaris. Am J Gastroenterol 1988;83:155–157.

162. Sharon P, Green ML, Rachmilewitz D. Esophageal involvement in bullous pemphigoid. Gastrointest Endosc 1978;24:122–123.

163. Orlando RC, Bozymski EM, Briggaman RA. Epidermolysis bullosa: Gastrointestinal manifestations. Ann Intern Med 1974;81:203–206.

164. Rabinowitz BN, Coldwell JG, Jegathnesan S. Epidermolysis bullosa and gastrointestinal anomalies. J Pediatr 1979;95:488.

165. Johnston DE, Koehler RE, Balfe DM. Clinical manifestations of epidermolysis bullosa dystrophica. Dig Dis Sci 1981;26:1144–1149.

166. Agha FP, Francis IR, Ellis CN. Esophageal involvement in epidermolysis bullosa dystrophica: Clinical and roentgenographic manifestations. Gastrointest Radiol 1983;8:111–117.

167. Zweiban B, Cohen H, Chandrasoma P. Gastrointestinal involvement complicating Stevens Johnson syndrome. Gastroenterology 1986;91:469–472.

168. Heer M, Altorfer J, Burger H-R, et al. Bullous esophageal lesions due to cotrimoxazole: An immune-mediated process? Gastroenterology 1985;88:1954–1957.

169. Brow JR, Parker F, Weinstein WM, et al. The small intestinal mucosa in dermatitis herpetiformis. I. Severity and distribution of the small intestinal lesion and associated malabsorption. Gastroenterology 1971;60:355–361.

170. Scott BB, Losowsky MS. Patchiness and duodenal-jejunal variation of the mucosal abnormality in coeliac disease and dermatitis herpetiformis. Gut 1976;17:984–992.

171. Katz SI, Hall RP III, Lawley TJ, et al. Dermatitis herpetiformis: The skin and the gut. Ann Intern Med 1980;93:857–874.

172. Fry L, Seah PP, Harper PG, et al. The small intestine in dermatitis herpetiformis. J Clin Pathol 1974;27:817–824.

173. Kosnai I, Karpati S, Savilahti E, et al. Gluten challenge in children with dermatitis herpetiformis: A clinical, morphological and immunohistological study. Gut 1986;27:1464–1470.

174. Weinstein WM, Brow JR, Parker F, et al. The small intestinal mucosa in dermatitis herpetiformis. II. Relationship of the small intestinal lesion to gluten. Gastroenterology 1971;60:362–369.

175. Gawkrodger DJ, Blackwell JN, Gilmour HM, et al. Dermatitis herpetiformis: Diagnosis, diet and demography. Gut 1984;25:151–157.

176. Leonard J, Haffendon G, Tucker W, et al. Gluten challenge in dermatitis herpetiformis. N Engl J Med 1983;308:816–819.

177. de Franchis R, Primignani M, Cipolla M, et al. Small bowel involvement in dermatitis herpetiformis and in linear-IgA bullous dermatosis. J Clin Gastroenterol 1983;5:429–436.

178. Crawford GM, Luikart RH II. Erythema multiforme with colitis. JAMA 1949;140:780–781.

179. Degos R. Malignant atrophic papulosis. Br J Dermatol 1979;100:21–35.

180. Case records of the Massachusetts General Hospital. N Engl J Med 1980;303:1104–1111.

181. Atchabahian A, Laisné MJ, Riche F, et al. Small bowel fistulae in Degos' disease: A case report and literature review. Am J Gastroenterol 1996;91:2208–2211.

182. Bain NH. Ehlers-Danlos syndrome: Case report. Am J Gastroenterol 1977;67:167–170.

183. Sigurdson E, Stern HS, Houpt J, et al. The Ehlers-Danlos syndrome and colonic perforation. Report of a case and physiologic assessment of underlying motility disorder. Dis Colon Rectum 1985;28:962–966.

184. Goodman RM, Smith EW, Paton D, et al. Pseudoxanthoma elasticum: A clinical and histopathological study. Medicine 1963;42:297–334.

185. Cocco AE, Grayer DL, Walker BA, et al. The stomach in pseudoxanthoma elasticum. JAMA 1969;210:2381–2382.

186. Flynn DM, Lake BD, Boothby DB, et al. Gut lesions in Fabry disease without a rash. Arch Dis Child 1972;47:26–33.

187. O'Brien BD, Schnitka TK, McDougall R, et al. Pathophysiologic and ultrastructural basis for intestinal symptoms in Fabry disease. Gastroenterology 1982;82:957–962.

188. Friedman LS, Kirkham SE, Thistlethwaite JR, et al. Jejunal diverticulosis with perforation as a complication of Fabry disease. Gastroenterology 1984;86:558–563.

189. Hoskins LC, Norris HT, Gottlieb LS, Zamcheck N. Functional and morphologic alterations of the gastrointestinal tract in progressive systemic sclerosis (scleroderma). Am J Med 1962;33:459–470.

190. Peachey RD, Creamer B, Pierce JW. Sclerodermatous involvement of the stomach and the small and large bowel. Gut 1969;10:285–292.

191. Poirer TJ, Rankin GB. Gastrointestinal manifestations of progressive systemic scleroderma based on a review of 364 cases. Am J Gastroenterol 1972;58:30–44.

192. Marshall JB, Kretschmar JM, Gerhardt DC, et al. Gastrointestinal manifestations of mixed connective tissue disease. Gastroenterology 1990;98:1232–1238.

193. Schuffler MD, Lowe MC, Bill AH. Studies of idiopathic intestinal pseudoobstruction. I. Hereditary hollow visceral myopathy: Clinical and pathological studies. Gastroenterology 1977;73:327–338.

194. Anuras S, Crane SA, Faulk DL, et al. Intestinal pseudoobstruction. Gastroenterology 1978;74:1318–1324.

195. Faulk DL, Anuras S, Christensen J. Chronic intestinal pseudoobstruction. Gastroenterology 1978;74:922–931.

196. Orringer MB, Dabich L, Zarafonetis CJ, et al. Gastroesophageal reflux in esophageal scleroderma: Diagnosis and implications. Ann Thorac Surg 1976;22:120–130.

197. Cohen S, Laufer I, Snape WJ, et al. The gastrointestinal manifestations of scleroderma: Pathogenesis and management. Gastroenterology 1980;79:155–166.

198. Compton R. Scleroderma with diverticulosis and colonic obstruction. Am J Surg 1969;118:602–606.

199. Krishnamurthy S, Kelly MM, Rohrmann CA, et al. Jejunal diverticulosis. A heterogeneous disorder caused by a variety of abnormalities of smooth muscle or myenteric plexus. Gastroenterology 1983;85:538–547.

200. Kleckner FS. Dermatomyositis and its manifestations in the gastrointestinal tract. Am J Gastroenterol 1970;53:141–146.

201. Nowak TV, Ionasescu V, Anuras S. Gastrointestinal manifestations of the muscular dystrophies. Gastroenterology 1982;82:800–810.

202. Leon SH, Schuffler MD, Kettler M, et al. Chronic intestinal pseudoobstruction as a complication of Duchenne muscular dystrophy. Gastroenterology 1986;90:455–459.

203. Brown CH, Shirey EK, Haserick JR. Gastrointestinal manifestations of systemic lupus erythematosus. Gastroenterology 1956;31:649–666.

204. Hoffman BI, Katz WW. The gastrointestinal manifestations of systemic lupus erythematosus: A review of the literature. Semin Arthritis Rheum 1980;9:237–247.

205. Wood MK, Read DR, Kraft AR, et al. A rare cause of ischemic colitis—polyarteritis nodosa. Dis Colon Rectum 1979;22:428.

206. Adler RH, Norcross BM, Lockie L. Arteritis and infarction of the intestine in rheumatoid arthritis. JAMA 1962;180:921–926.

207. Bywaters EGL, Scott JT. The natural history of vascular lesions in rheumatoid arthritis. J Chron Dis 1963;16:905–914.

208. Bienenstock H, Minick CR, Rogoff B. Mesenteric arteritis and intestinal infarction in rheumatoid disease. Arch Intern Med 1967;119:359–364.

209. Petterson T, Wegelius O, Skrituars B. Gastrointestinal disturbances in patients with severe rheumatoid arthritis. Acta Med Scand 1970;188:139.

210. Lindsay MK, Tavadia HB, Whyte AS, et al. Acute abdomen in rheumatoid arthritis due to necrotizing arteritis. Br Med J 1973;2:592–593.

211. Marcolongo R, Bayell PF, Montagnani M. Gastrointestinal involvement in rheumatoid arthritis: A biopsy study. J Rheumatol 1979;6:163–173.

212. Silvoso GR, Ivey KJ, Butt JH, et al. Incidence of gastric lesions in patients with rheumatic disease on chronic aspirin therapy. Ann Intern Med 1979;91:517–520.

213. Prillaman WW, Hurst DC, Ball GV, et al. Intestinal complications in rheumatoid arteritis and their relationship to corticosteroid therapy. J Chron Dis 1974;27:475–481.

214. Sckolnick BR, Katz LA, Kozower M. Life-threatening enterocolitis after gold salt therapy. J Clin Gastroenterol 1979;1:145–148.

215. Reinhart WH, Kapeller M, Halter F. Severe pseudomembranous and ulcerative colitis during gold therapy. Endoscopy 1983;15:70–72.

216. McCormick PA, O'Donoghue D, Lemass B. Gold-induced colitis: Case report and literature review. Irish Med J 1985;78:17–18.

217. Cuvelier C, Barbatis C, Mieflants H, et al. Histopathology of intestinal inflammation related to reactive arthritis. Gut 1987;28:394.

218. Mielants H, Veys EM, Cuvelier C, et al. HLA-B27 related arthritis and bowel inflammation. J Rheumatol 1985;12:294.

219. Cuvelier C, Barbatis C, Mielants H, et al. Histopathology of intestinal inflammation related to reactive arthritis. Gut 1987;28:394–401.

220. DeVos M, Cuvelier C, Mielants N, et al. Ileocolonoscopy in seronegative spondylarthropathy. Gastroenterology 1989;96:339–344.

221. Sheikh SH, Shaw-Stiffel TA. The gastrointestinal manifestations of Sjogren syndrome. Am J Gastroenterol 1995;90:9–14.

222. Tsjanos EB, Chiras CD, Drosos AA, et al. Esophageal dysfunction in patients with primary Sjögren syndrome. Ann Rheum Dis 1985;44:610.

223. DeMerieux P, Verity A, Clements PJ, et al. Esophageal abnormalities and dysphagia in polymyositis and dermatomyositis. Clinical, radiographic and pathologic features. Arthritis Rheum 1983;26:9612.

224. Lukhanpal S, Bunch TW, Ilstrup DM, et al. Plymyositis-dermatomyositis and malignant lesions: Does an association exist? Mayo Clin Proc 1986;61:645.

225. Park RW, Grand RJ. Gastrointestinal manifestations of cystic fibrosis: A review. Gastroenterology 1981;81:1143–1161.

226. Jeffrey I, Durrans D, Wells M, et al. The pathology of meconium ileus equivalent. J Clin Pathol 1983;36:1292–1297.

227. Carpenter HM. Pathogenesis of congenital jejunal atresia. Arch Pathol Lab Med 1962;73:390–396.

228. Hage E, Anderson FU. Light and electron microscopic studies of rectal biopsies in cystic fibrosis. Acta Pathol Microbiol Scand 1972;80A:345.

229. Neutra MR, Grand RJ, Trier JS. Glycoprotein synthesis, transport, and secretion by epithelial cells of human rectal mucosa. Normal and cystic fibrosis. Lab Invest 1977;36:535–546.

230. Logan RFA, Ferguson A, Finlayson NDC, et al. Primary biliary cirrhosis and celiac disease. An association? Lancet 1978;1:230–233.

231. Loftus EV, Sandborn WJ, Tremaine WJ, et al. Primary sclerosing cholangitis is associated with nonsmoking: A case-control study. Gastroenterology 1996;110:1496–1502.

232. Brentnall TA, Haggitt RC, Rabinovitch PS, et al. Risk and natural history of colonic neoplasia in patients with primary sclerosing cholangitis and ulcerative colitis. Gastroenterology 1996;110:331–338.

233. Kozarek RA, Botoman VA, Bredfeldt JE, et al. Portal colopathy: Prospective study of colonoscopy in patients with portal hypertension. Gastroenterology 1991;101:1192–1197.

234. Iredale JR, Ridings P, McGinn FP, et al. Familial and idiopathic colonic varices: An unusual cause of lower gastrointestinal hemorrhage. Gut 1992;33:1285–1288.

235. Parikh SS, Desai SB, Prabhu SR, et al. Congestive gastropathy: Factors influencing development, endoscopic features, Helicobacter

pylori infection, and microvessel changes. Am J Gastroenterol 1994;
89:1036–1042.

236. D'Amico G, Montabano L, Traina M, et al. Natural history of congestive gastrophy in cirrhosis. Gastroenterology 1990;99:1558–1564.

237. McCormack TT, Sims J, Eyre-Brook I, et al. Gastric lesions in portal hypertension: Inflammatory gastritis or congestive gastropathy? Gut 1985;26:1226–1232.

238. Conte D, Velio P, Brunelli L, et al. Stainable iron in gastric and duodenal mucosa of primary hemochromatosis patients and alcoholics. Am J Gastroenterol 1987;82:237–240.

239. Powell LW, Campbell CB, Wilson E. Intestinal mucosal uptake of iron and iron retention in idiopathic haemochromatosis as evidence for a mucosal abnormality. Gut 1970;11:727–731.

240. Steckman M, Bozymski EM. Hemosiderosis of the duodenum. Gastrointest Endosc 1983;29:326–327.

241. Robbins SL, Cotran RS, Kumar V. Nutritional disease. In: Pathologic basis of disease, 3rd ed. Philadelphia: WB Saunders, 1984;399–429.

242. Ansell JE, Kumar R, Deykin D, et al. The spectrum of vitamin K deficiency. JAMA 1979;238:40–42.

243. Spivak JL, Jackson DL. Pellagra: An analysis of 18 patients and review of the literature. Johns Hopkins Med J 1977;140:295–309.

244. Mehta SK, Kaur S, Avastni G, et al. Small intestinal deficiency in pellagra. Am J Clin Nutr 1979;25:545–549.

245. Cook GC. Etiology and pathogenesis of postinfective tropical malabsorption (tropical sprue). Lancet 1984;1:721–723.

246. Domellof L, Eriksson S, Helander HF, et al. Lipid islands in the gastric mucosa after resection for benign ulcer disease. Gastroenterology 1977;72:14–18.

247. Drude RB, Balart LA, Herrington JP, et al. Gastric xanthoma: Histological similarity to signet ring cell carcinoma. J Clin Gastroenterol 1982;4:217–221.

248. Coletta U, Stargill BC. Isolated xanthomatosis of the small bowel. Hum Pathol 1985;16:422–424.

249. Roth RI, Owen RZ, Keren DF, et al. Intestinal infection with Mycobacterium avium in acquired immune deficiency syndrome (AIDS). Histological and clinical comparison with Whipple disease. Dig Dis Sci 1985;30:497–504.

250. Azzopardi JG, Evans DJ. Muciprotein-containing histiocytes (muciphages) in the rectum. J Clin Pathol 1966;19:368–374.

251. Herbert PN, Forte T, Heinen RJ, et al. Tangier disease. N Engl J Med 1978;299:519–521.

252. Glickman RM, Green PHR, Lees RS, et al. Apolipoprotein A-I synthesis in normal intestinal mucosa and in Tangier disease. N Engl J Med 1978;299:1424–1427.

253. Bale PM, Clifton-Bligh P, Benjamin BNP, et al. Pathology of Tangier disease. J Clin Pathol 1971;24:609–616.

254. Ferrans VJ, Fredrickson DS. The pathology of Tangier disease: A light and electron microscopic study. Am J Pathol 1975;78:101.

255. Isselbacher KJ, Scheig R, Plotkin GR, et al. Congenital beta-lipoprotein deficiency: A hereditary disorder involving a defect in the absorption and transport of lipids. Medicine 1964;43:347–361.

256. Gotto A, Levy R, John K, et al. On the protein defect in a-beta-lipoproteinemia. N Engl J Med 1971;284:813–818.

257. Kayden HJ. Abetalipoproteinemia. Annu Rev Med 1972;23:285–296.

258. Dobbins III WO. An ultrastructural study of the intestinal mucosa in congenital beta-lipoprotein deficiency with particular emphasis upon the intestinal absorptive cell. Gastroenterology 1966;50:195–210.

259. Greenwood N. The jejunal mucosa in two cases of A-beta-lipoproteinemia. Am J Gastroenterol 1976;65:160–162.

260. Delpre G, Kadish U, Glantz I. Endoscopic assessment in abetalipoproteinemia (Bassen-Kornzweig syndrome). Endoscopy 1978;10:59–62.

261. Landing BH, Silverman FN, Craig JM, et al. Familial neurovisceral lipidosis. Am J Dis Child 1964;108:503–522.

262. Brady RO. The genetic mismanagement of complex lipid metabolism. Bull NY Acad Med 1971;47:173–182.

263. Adachi M, Volk BW, Schneck L, et al. Fine structure of the myenteric plexus in various lipidoses. Arch Pathol Lab Med 1969;87:228–241.

264. Bodian M, Lake BD. The rectal approach to neuropathology. Br J Surg 1963;50:702–714.

265. Den Tandt WR, Vio PM, Eggermont E. Intestinal biopsy in lysosomal storage disease (letter). Lancet 1974;2:1149.

266. Yamano T, Shimada M, Okada S, et al. Ultrastructural study of biopsy specimens of rectal mucosa. Its use in neuronal storage diseases. Arch Pathol Lab Med 1982;106:673–677.

267. Brett EM, Lake BD. Reassessment of rectal approach to neuropathology in childhood: Review of 307 biopsies over 11 years. Arch Dis Child 1975;50:753.

268. Carpenter S, Karpati G. Lysosomal storage in human skeletal muscle. Hum Pathol 1986;17:683–703.

269. O'Brien JS. Generalized gangliosidosis. Handbook Clin Neurol 1970;10:462–483.

270. Volk BW, Adachi M, Schneck L. The gangliosidoses. Hum Pathol 1975;6:555–569.

271. Rowe JW, Gilliam JI, Warthin TA. Gastrointestinal manifestations of Fabry disease. Ann Intern Med 1974;81:628–631.

272. Dinari G, Rosenbach Y, Grunebaum M, et al. Gastrointestinal manifestations of Niemann-Pick disease. Enzyme 1980;25:407–412.

273. Ansanelli Jr V, Lane N. Lipochrome ("ceroid") pigmentation of the small intestine. Ann Surg 1957;146:117–123.

274. Fox B. Lipofuscinosis of the gastrointestinal tract in man. J Clin Pathol 1967;20:806–813.

275. Rapola J, Santavuori P, Savilahti E. Suction biopsy of rectal mucosa in the diagnosis of infantile and juvenile types of neuronal ceroid lipofuscinoses. Hum Pathol 1984;15:352–360.

276. Foster CS. The brown bowel syndrome: A possible smooth muscle mitochondrial myopathy? Histopathology 1979;3:1–17.

277. Gallagher RL. Intestinal ceroid deposition—"brown bowel syndrome." A light and electron microscopic study. Virchows Arch 1980;389:145–151.

278. Hosler JP, Kimmel KK, Moeller DD. The "brown bowel syndrome": A case report. Am J Gastroenterol 1982;77:854–855.

279. Papp JP, Farmer RG, Hawk WA. Ceroid deposition of the small intestine associated with regional enteritis. Cleve Clin Q 1969;30:189–194.

280. Lambert JR, Luk SC, Pritzker KPH. Brown bowel syndrome in Crohn disease. Arch Pathol Lab Med 1980;104:201–205.

281. Bauman MB, Di Mase JD, Oshi F, et al. Brown bowel and skeletal myopathy with vitamin E depletion in pancreatic insufficiency. Gastroenterology 1968;54:93–100.

282. Horn T, Svendsen LB, Johansen A, et al. Brown bowel syndrome. Ultrastruct Pathol 1985;8:357–361.

283. Wittoesch JH, Jackman RJ, MacDonald JR. Melanosis coli: General review and study of 887 cases. Dis Colon Rectum 1958;1:172–180.

284. Lough J, Fawcett J, Wiegensberg B. Wolman disease: An electron microscopic, histochemical and biochemical study. Arch Pathol Lab Med 1970;89:103–110.

285. Partin JC, Schubert WK. Small intestinal mucosa in cholesterol ester storage disease. A light and electron microscope study. Gastroenterology 1969;57:542–558.

286. Dorfman A, Matalon R. The mucopolysaccharidoses (a review). Proc Natl Acad Sci USA 1976;73:630–637.

287. Morecki R, Paunier L, Hamilton JR. Intestinal mucosa in cystinosis. Arch Pathol Lab Med 1968;86:297–307.

288. Sidbury Jr JB, Heick HM. Glycogen storage diseases: A review with emphasis on gastrointestinal manifestations. South Med J 1968;61:915–922.

289. Ghadially FN, Walley VM. Melanoses of the gastrointestinal tract. Histopathology 1994;25:197–207.

290. Geller A, Aguilar II, Burgart L, et al. The black esophagus. Am J Gastroenterol 1995;90(12):2210–2212.

291. Pounder DJ, Ghadially FN, Mukherjee TM, et al. Ultrastructure and electron-probe X-ray analysis of the pigment in melanosis duodeni. J Submicrosc Cytol Pathol 1982;14:389–400.

292. Shephard NA, Crocker PR, Smith AP, et al. Exogenous pigment in Peyer patches. Hum Pathol 1987;18:50–54.

293. Urbanski SJ, Arsenault L, Green FHY, et al. Pigment resembling atmospheric dust in Peyer patches. Mod Pathol 1989;2:222–226.

294. Kyle RA, Bayrd ED. Amyloidosis: Review of 236 cases. Medicine 1975;54:271–299.

295. Cohen AS. An update of clinical pathologic and biochemical aspects of amyloidosis. Int J Dermatol 1981;20:515.

296. Glenner GG. Amyloid deposits and amyloidosis: The beta-fibrilloses. N Engl J Med 1980;302:1283–1292; 1333–1343.

297. Mordechai R, Sohar E. Intestinal malabsorption: First manifestation of amyloidosis in familial Mediterranean fever. Gastroenterology 1974;66:446–449.

298. Steen LE, Oberg L. Familial amyloidosis with polyneuropathy: Roentgenological and gastroscopic appearance of gastrointestinal involvement. Am J Gastroenterol 1980;78:417–420.

299. Chernenkoff RM, Costopoulos LB, Bain GO. Gastrointestinal manifestations of primary amyloidosis. Can Med Assoc J 1972;106:567–569.

300. Patel SA, Al-Haddadin D, Schoop J, et al. Gastrointestinal manifestations of amyloidosis: A case of diverticular perforation. Am J Gastroenterol 1993;88(4):578–582.

301. Lee JG, Wilson JA, Gottfried MR. Gastrointestinal manifestations of amyloidosis. South Med J 1994;87(2):243–247.

302. Gilat T, Revach M, Sohar E. Deposition of amyloid in the gastrointestinal tract. Gut 1969;10:98.

303. Monteiro JG. The digestive system in familial amyloidotic polyneuropathy. Am J Gastroenterol 1973;60:47.

304. Kumar SS, Appavu SS, Abcarion H, et al. Amyloidosis of the colon. Report of a case and review of the literature. Dis Colon Rectum 1983;26:541–544.

305. Jarnum S. Gastrointestinal haemorrhage and protein loss in primary amyloidosis. Gut 1965;6:14–18.

306. Levy DJ, Franklin GO, Rosenthal WS. Gastrointestinal bleeding and amyloidosis. Am J Gastroenterol 1982;77:422–426.

307. Figler TJ, Keshavarzian A, Nand S, et al. Retroperitoneal amyloidosis, factor IX and X deficiency, and gastrointestinal bleeding. Abdom Imaging 1996;21(3):266–268.

308. Brom B, Bonks S, Marks IN. Ischemic colitis, gastric ulceration, and malabsorption in a case of primary amyloidosis. Gastroenterology 1969;57:319–323.

309. Yamada M, Hatakeyama S, Tsukagoshi H. Gastrointestinal amyloid deposition in AL (primary or myeloma-associated) and AA (secondary) amyloidosis. Diagnostic value of a gastric biopsy. Hum Pathol 1985;16:1206–1211.

310. Walley VM. Amyloid deposition in a gastric arteriovenous malformation. Arch Pathol Lab Med 1986;110:69–71.

311. Perarnau JM, Raabe JJ, Courrier A, et al. A rare etiology of ischemic colitis—amyloid colitis. Endoscopy 1982;14:107–109.

312. Vernon SE. Amyloid colitis. Dis Colon Rectum 1982;25:728–730.

313. Battle WM, Rubin MR, Cohen S, et al. Gastrointestinal motility dysfunction in amyloidosis. N Engl J Med 1979;301:24–25.

314. Wald A, Kichler J, Mendelow H. Amyloidosis and chronic intestinal pseudoobstruction. Dig Dis Sci 1981;26:462–465.

315. Herskovic T, Bartholomew LG, Green P, et al. Amyloidosis and malabsorption syndrome. Arch Intern Med 1964;114:629–633.

316. Schmidt H, Fruehmorgan P, Riemann JF, et al. Mucosal suggillations in the colon in secondary amyloidosis. Endoscopy 1981;13:181–183.

317. Kawaguchi M, Koizumi F, Shimao M, et al. Protein-losing enteropathy due to secondary amyloidosis of the gastrointestinal tract. Acta Pathol Jpn 1993;43(6):333–339.

318. Rocken C, Saeger W, Linke RP. Gastrointestinal amyloid deposits in old age—report on 110 consecutive autopsical patients and 98 retrospective bioptic specimens. Pathol Res Pract 1994;190:641–649.

319. Hunter AM, Campbell IW, Borsey DDG, et al. Protein-losing enteropathy due to gastrointestinal amyloidosis. Postgrad Med J 1979;55:822.

320. Johnson DH, Guthrie TH, Tedesco FJ, et al. Amyloidosis masquerading as inflammatory bowel disease with a mass lesion simulating malignancy. Am J Gastroenterol 1982;77:141–145.

321. Jensen K, Raynor S, Rose SG, et al. Amyloid tumors of the gastrointestinal tract: A report of two cases and review of the literature. Am J Gastroenterol 1985;80:784–786.

322. Fitchen JH. Amyloidosis in granulomatous ileocolitis. N Engl J Med 1975;292:352–353.

323. Shousha S, Lowdell CP, Bull TB, et al. Secondary amyloidosis of the gastrointestinal tract: An electron microscopic study. Hum Pathol 1985;16:596–601.

324. Fentum PH, Turnberg LA, Wormsley KG. Biopsy of the rectum as an aid to the diagnosis of amyloidosis. Br Med J 1962;1:364.

325. Kyle A, Spencer RJ, Dahlin DC. Value of rectal biopsy in the diagnosis of primary systemic amyloidosis. Am J Med Sci 1966;251:501–506.

326. Coughlin GP, Remer RG, Grant AK. Endoscopic diagnosis of amyloidosis. Gastrointest Endosc 1980;26:154.

327. Ohno F, Numata Y, Yamano T, et al. Gastroscopic biopsy of the stomach for the diagnosis of amyloidosis. Gastroenterol Jpn 1982;17:415–421.

328. Green PA, Higgins JA, Brown AL Jr, et al. Amyloidosis: Appraisal of intubation biopsy of the small intestine in diagnosis. Gastroenterology 1961;41:452–456.

329. Tada S, Iida M, Iwashiba MD, et al. Endsoscopic and biopsy findings in the upper digestive tract in patients with amyloidosis. Gastrointest Endosc 1990;36:10.

330. Haggitt RC. Granulomatous diseases of the gastrointestinal tract. In: Ioachim HL, ed. Pathology of granulomas. New York: Raven Press, 1983;257–305.

331. Kojima Y, Sakuma H, Izumi R, et al. A case of granuloma of the ascending colon due to penetration of Trichuris trichiura. Gastroenterol Jpn 1981;16:193–196.

332. Vafai M, Mohit P. Granuloma of the anal canal due to Enterobius vermicularis. Report of a case. Dis Colon Rectum 1983;26:349–350.

333. Geller SA, Zimmerman MJ, Cohen A. Rectal biopsy in early lymphogranuloma venereum proctitis. Am J Gastroenterol 1980;74:433–435.

334. Quinn TC, Goodell SE, Mhrtichion E, et al. Chlamydia trachomatis proctitis. N Engl J Med 1981;305:195–200.

335. Surawicz CM, Belic L. Rectal biopsy helps to distinguish acute self-limited colitis from idiopathic inflammatory bowel disease. Gastroenterology 1984;86:104–113.

336. Surawicz CM, Goodell SE, Quinn TC, et al. Spectrum of rectal biopsy abnormalities in homosexual men with intestinal symptoms. Gastroenterology 1986;91:651–659.

337. Cho C, Linscheer WG, Hirschkorn MA, et al. Sarcoid-like granuloma as an early manifestation of Whipple disease. Gastroenterology 1984;87:941–947.

338. Surawicz CM, Meisel JL, Ylvisaker T, et al. Rectal biopsy in the diagnosis of Crohn disease: Value of multiple biopsies and serial sectioning. Gastroenterology 1981;80:66–71.

339. Petri M, Poulson SS, Christensen K, et al. The incidence of granulomas in serial sections of rectal biopsies from patients with Crohn disease. Acta Pathol Microbiol Immunol Scand 1982;90:145–147.

340. Shapiro JL, Goldblum JR, Petras RE. A clinicopathology study of 42 patients with granulomatous gastritis. Is there really an "idiopathic" granulomatous gastritis? Am J Surg Pathol 1996;20:462–470.

341. Weinstock JV. Idiopathic isolated granulomatous gastritis: Spontaneous resolution without surgical intervention. Dig Dis Sci 1980;25:233–235.

342. Israel HL, Stones M. Sarcoidosis: Clinical observations on 160 cases. Arch Intern Med 1958;102:766–776.

343. James DG, Neville E, Siltzbach LE, et al. A worldwide review of sarcoidosis. Ann NY Acad Sci 1976;278:321–334.

344. Ectors EL, Dixon MF, Geboes KJ, et al. Granulomatous gastritis: A morphological and diagnostic approach. Histopathology 1993;23:55–61.

345. Berens DL, Montes M. Gastric sarcoidosis. NY State J Med 1975;75:1290–1293.

346. Konda J, Ruth M, Sassaris M, et al. Sarcoidosis of the stomach and rectum. Am J Gastroenterol 1980;73:516.

347. Tobi M, Kobrin I, Ariel I. Rectal involvement in sarcoidosis. Dis Colon Rectum 1982;25:491–493.

348. Tinker MA, Viswanathan B, Laufer H, et al. Acute appendicitis and pernicious anemia as complications of gastrointestinal sarcoidosis. Am J Gastroenterol 1984;79:868–872.

349. Chinitz MA, Brandt LJ, Frank MS, et al. Symptomatic sarcoidosis of the stomach. Dig Dis Sci 1985;30:682–688.

350. Roth D, West B, Madison J, et al. Gastric carcinoma in a patient with sarcoidosis of the gastrointestinal tract. Am J Gastroenterol 1994;89(9):1589–1591.

351. Polachek AA, Matre WJ. Gastrointestinal sarcoidosis: Report of a case involving the esophagus. Am J Dig Dis 1964;9:429–433.

352. Popovic OS, Brkic S, Bojic P, et al. Sarcoidosis and protein losing enteropathy. Gastroenterology 1980;78:119–125.

353. Rauf A, Davis P, Levendoglu H. Sarcoidosis of the small intestine. Am J Gastroenterol 1988;83:187–189.

354. Sprague R, Harper P, McClain S, et al. Disseminated gastrointestinal sarcoidosis. Case report and review of the literature. Gastroenterology 1984;87:421–425.

355. Stampfl DA, Grimm IS, Barbot DJ, et al. Sarcoidosis causing duodenal obstruction. Case report and review of gastrointestinal manifestations. Dig Dis Sci 1990;35(4):526–532.

356. Ament ME, Ochs HD. Gastrointestinal manifestations of chronic granulomatous disease. N Engl J Med 1973;288:382–387.

357. Werlin SL, Chusid MJ, Caya J, et al. Colitis in chronic granulomatous disease. Gastroenterology 1981;82:328–331.

358. Griscom NT, Kirkpatrick JA, Girdany JA, et al. Gastric antral narrowing in chronic granulomatous disease of childhood. Pediatrics 1974;54:456–460.

359. Harris BH, Boles ET. Intestinal lesions in chronic granulomatous disease of childhood. J Pediatr Surg 1973;5:955–956.

360. Sloan JM, Cameron CHS, Maxwell RJ, et al. Colitis complicating chronic granulomatous disease. A clinicopathological case report. Gut 1996;38:619–622.

361. Hopkins PJ, Bemiller LS, Curnutte JT. Chronic granulomatous disease: Diagnosis and classification at the molecular level. Clin Lab Med 1992;12:277–304.

362. Ament ME, Ochs HD, Davis SD. Structure and function of the gastrointestinal tract in primary immunodeficiency syndromes: A study of 39 patients. Medicine 1973;52:227–248.

363. Damjanov I, Katz SM. Malakoplakia. Pathol Annu 1981;16:103–126.

364. McClure J. Malakoplakia. J Pathol 1983;140:275–330.

365. Yunis EJ, Estevez JM, Pinson GJ, et al. Malakoplakia: Discussion of pathogenesis and report of three cases including one of fatal gastric and colonic involvement. Arch Pathol Lab Med 1967;83:180–187.

366. Lewin KJ, Fair WR, Steibigel RT, et al. Clinical and laboratory studies into the pathogenesis of malakoplakia. J Clin Pathol 1976;29:354–363.

367. Abdou NI, NaPombejara C, Sagawa A, et al. Malakoplakia: Evidence for monocyte lysosomal abnormality correctable by cholinergic agonist in vitro and in vivo. N Engl J Med 1977;297:1413–1418.

368. Melicow MM. Malakoplakia. J Urol 1957;78:33–40.

369. Ranchod M, Kahn LB. Malakoplakia of the gastrointestinal tract. Arch Pathol Lab Med 1972;94:90–97.

370. DiSilvio TV, Bartlett EF. Malakoplakia of the colon. Arch Pathol Lab Med 1971;92:167–171.

371. De LaGarza T, Nunez-Rasilla V, Alegre-Palafox R, et al. Malakoplakia of the colon. Dis Colon Rectum 1973;16:216–233.

372. MacKay EH. Malakoplakia in ulcerative colitis. Arch Pathol Lab Med 1978;102:140–145.

373. Miranda D, Vuletin JC, Kauffman SL. Disseminated histiocytosis and intestinal malakoplakia. Arch Pathol Lab Med 1979;103:302–308.

374. McClure J. Malakoplakia of the gastrointestinal tract. Postgrad Med J 1981;57:95–103.

375. Moran CA, West B, Schwartz IS. Malacoplakia of the colon in association with colonic adenocarcinoma. Am J Gastroenterol 1989;84:1580–1582.

376. Cipolletta L, Bianco MA, Fumo F, et al. Malacoplakia of the colon. Gastrointest Endosc 1995;41(3):255–258.

377. Nakabayashi H, Ito T, Izutsu K, et al. Malakoplakia of the stomach: Report of a case and review of the literature. Arch Pathol Lab Med 1978;102:136–139.

378. Ng IO, Ng M. Colonic malacoplakia: Unusual association with ulcerative colitis. J Gastroenterol Hepatol 1993;8(1):110–115.

379. Sandmeier D, Guillou L. Malakoplakia and adenocarcinoma of the caecum: A rare association. J Clin Pathol 1993;46(10):959–960.

380. Lewin KJ, Harell GS, Lee AS, et al. Malakoplakia: An electron microscopic study. Demonstration of bacilliform organisms in malakoplakic macrophages. Gastroenterology 1974;66:28–45.

381. Chaudhry AP, Saigal KP, Intengan M, et al. Malakoplakia of the large intestine found incidentally at necropsy: Light and electron microscopic features. Dis Colon Rectum 1979;22:73–81.

382. McClure J, Cameron CHS, Garrett R. The ultrastructural features of malakoplakia. J Pathol 1981;134:13–25.

383. Stevens S, McClure J. The histochemical features of the Michaelis-Gutmann body and a consideration of the pathophysiological mechanisms of its formation. J Pathol 1982;137:119–127.

384. Newton WA Jr, Hamoudi AB. Histiocytosis: A histologic classification and clinical correlation. Perspect Pediatr Pathol 1973;1:251.

385. Lahey ME. Histiocytosis X—an analysis of prognostic factors. J Pediatr 1975;87:184–189.

386. Oberman HA. Idiopathic histiocytosis: A clinicopathologic study of 49 cases and review of the literature. Pediatrics 1981;28:307–327.

387. Jaffe R, Wollman MR, Kocoshis S, et al. Pathological cases of the month. Langerhans' cell histiocytois with gastrointestinal involvement. Am J Dis Child 1993;147(1):79–80.

388. Egeler RM, D'Angio GJ. Langerhans cell histiocytois. J Pediatr 1995;127(1):1–11.

389. Mierau GW, Favara BE, Brennan JM. Electron microscopy of histiocytes. Ultrastruct Pathol 1982;3:137–142.

390. Parker JW, Lichtenstein L. Severe hepatic involvement in chronic disseminated histiocytosis X. Am J Clin Pathol 1963;40:624–632.

391. Landing BH, Wells TR, Reed GB, et al. Diseases of the bile ducts in children. In: Gall EA, Mostofi FK, eds. The liver. Baltimore: Williams & Wilkins, 1973;503–509.

392. Keeling JW, Harris JT. Intestinal malabsorption in infants with histiocytosis X. Arch Dis Child 1973;48:350–354.

393. Iwofuchi M, Watanabe H, Shiratsuka M. Primary benign histiocytosis of the stomach. A report of a case showing spontaneous remission after 5½ years. Am J Surg Pathol 1990;14:489–496.

394. Lee RG, Braziel RM, Stenzel P. Gastrointestinal involvement in Langerhans cell histiocytosis (histiocytosis X): Diagnosis by rectal biopsy. Mod Pathol 1990;3:154–157.

395. Gregorie HB, Otherson H, Moore MP. The significance of sarcoid-like lesions in association with malignant neoplasms. Am J Surg 1962;104:577–586.

396. Churg J, Strauss L. Allergic granulomatosis, allergic angiitis and periarteritis nodosa. Am J Pathol 1951;27:277–301.

PART III

ESOPHAGUS

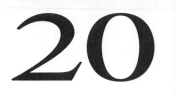
The esophagus is affected in a wide variety of inflammatory and other nonneoplastic disorders. Pathologists are often involved in the diagnosis of esophagitis when examining specimens from endoscopic biopsy, surgical resection, and autopsy. Pathologic recognition of the specific cause of esophagitis is often difficult, and the situation is confounded by the relatively common occurrence of multifactorial esophagitis. This chapter emphasizes the pathologic findings that are helpful in differential diagnosis.

PATHOLOGIC FINDINGS

Esophagitis means inflammation of the esophagus and connotes the presence of inflammatory cells, which are easily recognized by light microscopy. Esophagitis has numerous causes, only a few of which involve diagnostic histopathologic findings. Evidence of severe injury in the form of erosion and ulceration is sometimes present in patients with esophagitis, and any injury is usually followed by a

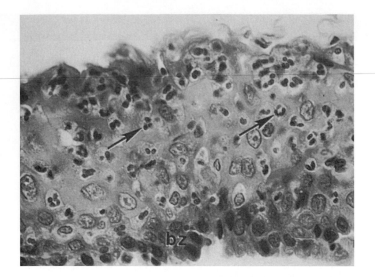

Figure 20.1 Active esophagitis. The squamous epithelium is heavily infiltrated by neutrophils *(arrows)* and thinned because of erosion of the superficial layers. The basal zone (bz) is reactive with hyperchromatic nuclei, and the epithelium is immature, as manifested by enlarged nuclei with prominent nucleoli in the prickle cell layer.

stereotyped repair process with similar histopathologic findings, regardless of the cause.

Active esophagitis is characterized by infiltration of the squamous epithelium by polymorphonuclear leukocytes, usually neutrophils (Fig. 20.1). In addition, accompanying findings include congestion with dilated blood vessels ("vascular lakes") in the lamina propria and epithelial edema characterized by enlargement and clearing of cells and of the spaces between them. The repair process consists in part of epithelial proliferation. The histopathologic findings in this reactive epithelial response to injury include thickening of the basal zone with increased mitotic figures; elongation and increased numbers of lamina propria papillae; and the presence at the luminal surface of immature ovoid squamous epithelial cells with enlarged nuclei. These features represent reactive epithelial changes (Fig. 20.2).

Chronic esophagitis cannot be defined well pathologically because of ambiguity in the use of the term *chronic*. On the one hand, lymphocytes and plasma cells, generally regarded as chronic inflammatory cells, are a common histopathologic finding in the lamina propria. Chronic inflammation can persist long after active esophagitis and its clinical symptoms have resolved and therefore may relate poorly to the patient's clinical status. In this situation, application by the pathologist of the term "chronic esophagitis" seems inappropriate to the patient's resolved symptoms. On the other hand, active esophagitis can persist clinically and become chronic in the temporal sense, but biopsies may continue to show predominantly acute inflammation, particularly in the epithelium. Again, in this situation, use by the pathologist of chronic esophagitis does not portray accurately the clinical circumstances with ongoing acute injury. Because of these ambiguities, the term should probably not be used for pathologic findings without qualification. Clinical chronic esophagitis connotes recurrent or persistent disease and is usually associated with reflux esophagitis;

it can include histologic findings of Barrett esophagus and/or peptic stricture.

Severe injury in active esophagitis can lead to epithelial destruction. *Erosion* refers to less than full-thickness destruction of the epithelium such that the superficial layers are absent but the deeper layers, including the basal zone, remain (see Fig. 20.1). The deeper layers of the epithelium commonly show active inflammation with neutrophils, and luminal fibroinflammatory exudate is frequently present. If sufficient time has elapsed between onset of injury and time of tissue sampling, reactive epithelial changes accompany erosion.

An *ulcer* results from severe injury and is characterized by complete loss of the epithelium (Fig. 20.3). After ulceration, the lamina propria or even deeper layers of the esophageal wall are exposed to the luminal contents. In an *acute ulcer* of recent occurrence, the base consists of necrotic tissue and debris with active inflammation and exudate. With time, the repair occurs, involving processes characterized by epithelial regeneration and growth of granulation tissue into the base, with fibrosis and scarring. Continuation of injury along with the repair processes results in an *active chronic ulcer* (see Fig. 20.3). Re-epithelization manifests by a layer of immature epithelial cells migrating from the periphery of the ulcer. When a layer of epithelium covers the ulcer but the mucosa has not been reconstituted, the term *healing ulcer* can be applied. Completion of mucosa reconstitution results in a *healed ulcer*, but reactive epithelial changes may persist for some time.

The importance of these definitions of active esophagitis, erosion, and ulcer relates to the complications of esophagitis. Generally, severe hemorrhage, perforation, and stricture formation occur as a result of ulceration. Hemorrhage and perforation are produced by the ulceration itself, whereas stricture formation results from the deposition of scar tissue as part of the repair process. Thus,

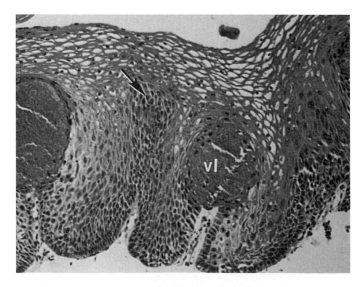

Figure 20.2 Reactive epithelial changes and vascular lakes in esophageal squamous epithelium. The vascular papillae *(arrow)* are elongated, extending approximately three fourths of the thickness of the epithelium. Vascular lakes (vl) are formed by dilated vascular papillae with congestion. The basal zone (which can be delineated by the absence of staining with periodic acid-Schiff [PAS] stain) is of normal thickness in this example.

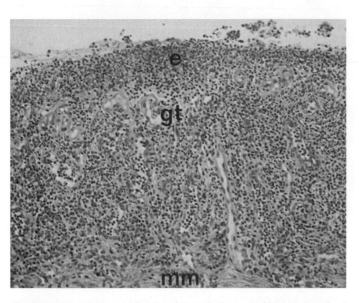

Figure 20.3 Active chronic ulcer of the esophagus. Luminal fibrinoinflammatory exudate (e) overlies inflamed granulation tissue (gt) which occupies the region of the lamina propria on the luminal side of the muscularis mucosae (mm). An ulcer in the esophagus has full-thickness loss of the squamous epithelium but does not necessarily extend into the muscularis mucosae, in contrast to other regions of the gastrointestinal tract, because of the layer of lamina propria connective tissue between the epithelium and smooth muscle.

recognition of the early stages of injury in endoscopic biopsy specimens may lead to therapy, which can prevent the development of ulceration, whatever the cause of the injury, and its complications.

NORMAL HISTOLOGIC VARIANTS

GLYCOGENIC ACANTHOSIS

Glycogenic acanthosis appears as white mucosal plaques. Specimens showing prominent glycogenic acanthosis (Fig. 20.4A) are frequently submitted for histologic study as "leukoplakia." The plaques consist of large clusters of enlarged clear cells grouped together in the upper layers of the thickened squamous epithelium. The cells contain abundant glycogen, much of which is removed during histologic processing. The result is a clear appearance, unless fixative to preserve glycogen (e.g., Carnoy fluid) or frozen section is used. The reason for the development of clusters of such cells is unknown.

"Balloon cells" are enlarged squamous epithelial cells that resemble the cells of glycogenic acanthosis but have translucent, rather than clear, cytoplasm in hematoxylin and eosin (H & E)-stained sections (Fig. 20.4B). Balloon cells can be seen to contain plasma proteins when examined by immunohistochemical methodology and appear to develop as a result of increased permeability of the cell membrane, attributable to injury. The nuclei are often pyknotic. Balloon cells can be found in the middle or superficial layers of the squamous epithelium, depending on the nature of the epithelial injury: with chronic gastroesophageal reflux, the balloon cells are typically in the middle layers, whereas with infectious esophagitis and acute chemical injury the balloon cells are usually superficial. Balloon cells can be distinguished easily from glycogenic acanthosis by absence of the periodic acid-Schiff (PAS) staining characteristics of glycogen.

ECTOPIC SEBACEOUS GLANDS

Ectopic sebaceous glands in the lamina propria have been found to produce endoscopically visible nodules. The histopathologic appearance of the glands themselves is similar to that of sebaceous glands in the skin.

MELANOCYTIC PROLIFERATION

Melanocytes are present in the basal layer of the squamous epithelium. In some patients, melanocytic proliferation occurs with melanocytes in all layers of the epithelium, as well as melanin-containing macrophages in the lamina propria. This melanocytic proliferation is seen grossly or endoscopically as a small pigmented area, most commonly in the midesophagus.

ESOPHAGITIS DUE TO INFECTIOUS AGENTS

The esophagus is affected by a variety of infectious agents (Table 20.1). These agents have various portals of entry into the esophagus, including the mucosal surface, the vascular and lymphatic systems, and direct extension from adjacent mediastinal structures. The site of esophageal infection is influenced by both characteristics of the agent and host factors. The organisms are presented individually in this discussion although in many patients with infective esophagitis, more than one agent is identifiable by microbiologic and histopathologic methods; these cases represent mixed infections. This potential for mixed infections is particularly important in immunocompromised patients, including those with human immunodeficiency virus (HIV) infection and acquired immunodeficiency syndrome (AIDS).

FUNGAL ESOPHAGITIS

Fungal infections of the esophagus can be considered in two categories: those caused by organisms with little inherent pathogenicity but occurring with underlying abnormality in the host (opportunistic fungi) and those caused by organisms with inherent pathogenicity (pathogenic fungi). The opportunistic fungal infections are by far the more commonly encountered.

OPPORTUNISTIC FUNGAL ESOPHAGITIS

Candidal Esophagitis (Figs. 20.5 to 20.9)

Candidal (monilial) esophagitis is usually due to *Candida albicans* or occasionally *Candida tropicalis* or *krusei*. *Candida (Torulopsis) glabrata,* which has distinguishing histopathologic characteristics (see Fig. 20.9), also produces esophagitis in rare cases.

Candidal esophagitis is usually an opportunistic infection that occurs in association with some abnormality in the host. The

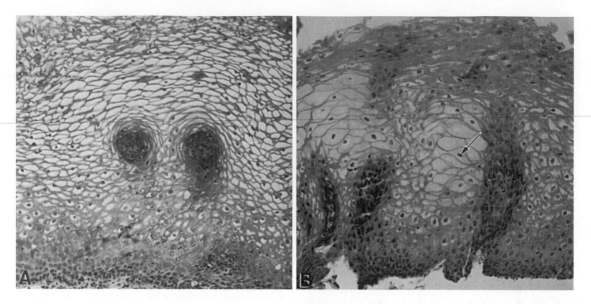

Figure 20.4 Glycogenic acanthosis and balloon cells in esophageal squamous epithelium. **A.** Glycogenic acanthosis has thickened squamous epithelium with increased numbers of enlarged cells characterized by clear cytoplasm that contains glycogen (demonstrable by PAS stain). **B.** Balloon cells are enlarged squamous epithelial cells with translucent cytoplasm due to the presence of plasma proteins, which signify increased cellular permeability related to injury. The plasma proteins can be demonstrated by immunohistochemical methods. The cytoplasm of balloon cells stains poorly with PAS stain, in contrast to glycogenic acanthosis. The nuclei are often pyknotic (*arrow*). The squamous epithelium with balloon cells is usually of normal thickness. (Same magnification in parts A and B.)

TABLE 20.1 Usual Localizations of Infectious Agents in the Esophagus

Agent	Lumen Only	Squamous Epithelium	Ulcer Bed and/or Mural Structures
Fungi			
Opportunistic fungi		X	X
Candida			
Aspergillus			
Phycomycetes			
Pathogenic fungi			X
Histoplasma			
Blastomyces			
Sporothrix			
Paracoccidioides			
Viruses			
Herpes virus, viral exanthems		X	
Human immunodeficiency virus			
Epstein-Barr virus			
Human papilloma virus			
Cytomegalovirus			X
Bacteria			
Opportunistic bacteria		X	X
Tuberculous and nontuberculous mycobacteria			X
Miscellaneous bacteria	X	X	X
Spirochetes			
Treponema pallidum			X
Parasites			
Ascaris	X		
Amoeba			X
Echinococcus			X
Cysticercus			
Trichinella			
Filaria			

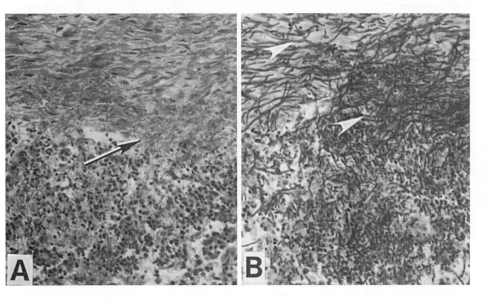

Figure 20.5 Candidal esophagitis. **A.** With hematoxylin and eosin stain, layers of accumulated squamous epithelial debris with numerous bacteria *(arrow)* and inflammatory cells are obvious, but the *Candida* organisms are difficult to visualize. **B.** With PAS stain of the same tissue fragment as shown in part A, large numbers of candidal pseudohyphae *(arrowhead)* are evident throughout the tissue. (Same magnification in parts A and B.)

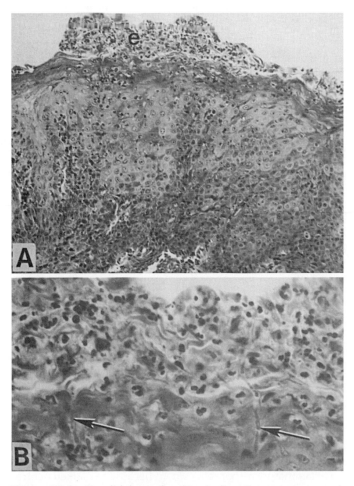

Figure 20.6 Candidal esophagitis. **A.** Reactive squamous epithelium with intraepithelial neutrophils and luminal fibrinoinflammatory exudate (e) containing *Candida* are present. **B.** Candida pseudohyphae *(arrows)* extend into the superficial layers of the squamous epithelium beneath the exudate.

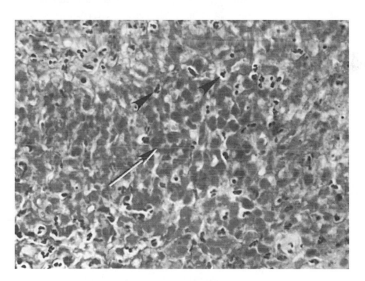

Figure 20.7 Candidal esophagitis with characteristic "mummified" necrotic tissue. The outlines of necrotic squamous epithelial cells are evident *(arrow)* and contrast with intact neutrophils *(arrowheads)*. Although no *Candida* organisms are identified in this field, they were evident in an adjoining area of the tissue. This histopathologic appearance should lead to a careful search for *Candida* with the use of a stain for fungi.

systemic conditions favoring the development of candidiasis in general and esophageal candidiasis in particular include medication with broad-spectrum antibacterial antibiotics, systemic steroids, cytotoxic chemotherapy for cancer, immune suppression after organ transplantation, AIDS, postoperative state, and low birth weight. Local esophageal injury further promotes the fungal infection.

The yeasts are commensal inhabitants of the gastrointestinal tract, including the mouth and oropharynx, in a sizable percentage of persons. The organisms appear to reach the esophagus by being swallowed, but clinically evident oral thrush is absent in many

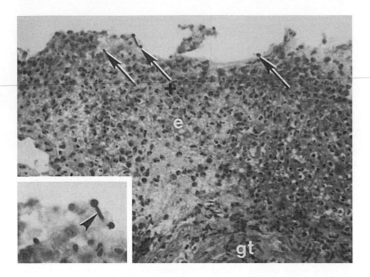

Figure 20.8 Candidal colonization of esophageal ulcer. The fibrinoinflammatory exudate (e) overlying inflamed granulation tissue (gt) contains scattered yeast forms of *Candida (arrows)* in this PAS-stained section. The inset shows the area indicated by the plus (+) sign, where pseudohyphal formation *(arrowhead)* is evident in one *Candida* yeast.

patients with candidal esophagitis. Pre-existing abnormality in the esophageal mucosal surface predisposes to the infection.

The clinical spectrum of candidal esophagitis has been categorized into acute, subacute, and chronic forms. The most common form is acute candidal esophagitis, which typically occurs in the lower esophagus of compromised patients and is of sudden onset. With progression of the infection into the esophageal wall, the acute form may lead to disseminated candidiasis. Rare examples of perforation have been reported. Esophageal stenosis may result from spasm, mucosal edema, and a thick pseudomembrane composed of *Candida,* accumulated squamous epithelial debris, and fibrinoinflammatory exudate (see Fig. 20.5). Local treatment of acute candidal esophagitis often results in resolution with no sequelae. Occasionally, however, patients develop an esophageal stricture late in the course, probably attributable to fibrosis resulting from previous extension of the infectious and inflammatory process into the esophageal wall or submucosal glands.

Subacute candidal esophagitis is uncommon. This form seems to occur as indolent, often asymptomatic, infection in patients who are not apparently compromised. The subacute form is usually first recognized when the patient presents with complaints resulting from an esophageal stricture and/or intramural pseudodiverticulosis. The strictures are most common in the upper esophagus and are said to be more pliant than strictures due to other factors. Intramural pseudodiverticulosis, as the name implies, is recognized on barium contrast studies by the presence of what appear to be multiple small diverticula within the wall of the esophagus. Autopsy cases of intramural pseudodiverticulosis show *Candida* involving the ducts of submucosal glands with hyperplasia of the squamous epithelium. Obstruction, dilatation, inflammation, and destruction of the glands result, producing outpouchings communicating with the esophageal lumen, which are filled by barium and produce the characteristic radiographic appearance. The association among the occurrence in the upper esophagus of large numbers of submucosal

glands, *Candida*-related strictures, and intramural pseudodiverticulosis has suggested a pathogenetic relationship to some authors. Disseminated candidiasis rarely results from subacute candidal esophagitis.

Chronic candidal esophagitis is rare. This form generally occurs with chronic mucocutaneous candidiasis associated with a variety of cell-mediated immunologic deficits. Granulomatous inflammation in response to *Candida* sometimes occurs. Fibrous esophageal strictures may occur, but esophageal narrowing due to inflammation and spasm are more common. Disseminated candidiasis resulting from chronic candidal esophagitis is uncommon.

The histopathologic features of candidal esophagitis have great variability (see Figs. 20.5 to 20.9). *Candida* may appear as budding yeast forms or pseudohyphae; they may be few or numerous. The esophageal tissue may show necrosis, ulceration, erosion, or intact epithelium. The severity of inflammatory response is also variable, depending on patient capabilities. The yeast and pseudohyphae may invade the esophageal tissue to variable depths, or the organisms may show no evidence of invasion.

Candida organisms are basophilic in H & E-stained sections. Even when numerous, the organisms are difficult to visualize in the midst of inflammatory exudate and debris. As a result, routine use of a stain for fungi (PAS, which may be conveniently included in

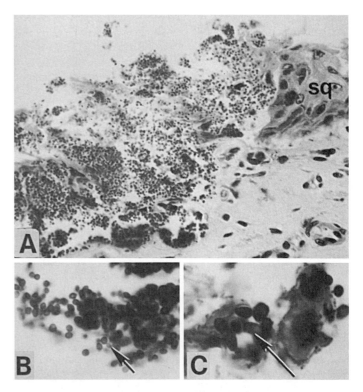

Figure 20.9 Esophagitis due to *Candida (Torulopsis) glabrata.* **A.** Small, round yeasts characteristic of *C. glabrata* extend through the squamous epithelium (sq) into the lamina propria. No inflammatory response is evident because of marked neutropenia induced by cytotoxic chemotherapy in the patient. **B.** High-power view of *C. glabrata.* Budding of one yeast is evident *(arrow).* **C.** *Candida albicans,* at the same magnification as in part B, illustrating larger size, ovoid shape, and the presence of pseudohyphae *(arrow),* which are not evident in *C. glabrata.*

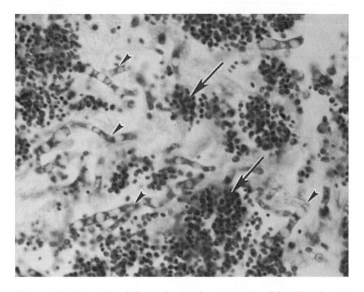

Figure 20.10 Mixed fungal esophagitis. *Candida (Torulopsis) glabrata (arrows)* and *Aspergillus (arrowheads)* in necrotic tissue from esophageal biopsy of a patient receiving intensive cytotoxic chemotherapy.

combination with alcian blue, pH 2.5, or methenamine silver) is recommended, particularly when inflammation is identified (see Fig. 20.5). The yeast forms of *C. albicans, tropicalis,* and *krusei* are oval. Buds frequently extend from the yeast cells (blastospores) and may elongate to produce nonseptate pseudohyphae under conditions that inhibit cell division but not growth. The pseudohyphae may grow to striking lengths and interdigitate to form large clumps of organisms. The pseudohyphal form of the organism usually occurs in invaded tissue, although yeast forms can also invade. With colonization and invasion, the proportion of the organisms in the pseudohyphal form increases with the age of the lesion.

C. albicans, tropicalis, and *krusei* cannot be differentiated in histopathologic sections; *C. albicans* is most common. *C. (Torulopsis) glabrata,* however, is smaller than the other species and tends to occur as large masses of round, budding yeast without pseudohyphae (see Fig. 20.9). *Candida* organisms are usually accompanied by numerous bacteria. Sometimes histopathologic evidence of other fungi (Fig. 20.10) or of viral esophagitis (Fig. 20.11) is also found (see subsequent discussions of fungal and viral esophagitis). Occasionally, the squamous epithelium is intact, with *Candida* in a mass along the luminal surface (see Fig. 20.6). Pseudohyphae often extend into the superficial layers of the epithelium, which shows active inflammation and reactive epithelial changes. The pseudohyphae appear to anchor the fungal mass, which may be quite thick because of the presence of accumulated layers of squamous epithelial debris. Erosion of the invaded epithelium is sometimes present. More commonly, complete epithelial loss with ulceration is present, manifested by fibrinoinflammatory exudate containing neutrophils, necrotic debris, and inflamed granulation tissue.

The exudate in the base of an ulcer often contains budding yeast without pseudohyphae or evidence of tissue invasion (see Fig. 20.8). Large fungal masses are sometimes attached to the ulcer base. The presence of "mummified" necrotic tissue with intact inflammatory cells (see Fig. 20.7) should heighten the suspicion of

Candida; staining of additional sections is recommended if the organisms are not demonstrated on initial examination of specimens containing necrotic tissue with this appearance.

From a clinical and therapeutic standpoint, a fact of major importance concerning candidal esophagitis is that it may serve as a portal of entry for disseminated candidiasis. Biopsy histopathology plays a role in assessing the risk of dissemination, along with the clinical characteristics of the patient, and may influence the decision to undertake systemic as opposed to local antifungal therapy. For this reason, in addition to the diagnosis of *Candida* esophagitis, a biopsy report should provide the clinician with an indication of the numbers of fungi, their morphologic form (e.g., yeast or pseudohyphae), the nature of the specimen in which the organisms are located (e.g., exudate or tissue), the severity of the inflammatory response, and the depth of invasion if present. The significance of *Candida* is often unclear, however, because colonization may occur after other forms of esophageal injury, e.g., gastroesophageal reflux. Furthermore, the problem of sampling affects assessment of invasion in biopsy specimens. Biopsies are sometimes undertaken after therapy for candidal esophagitis for assessment of efficacy.

Aspergillus and Phycomycetes Esophagitis

Aspergillus esophagitis and Phycomycetes esophagitis are two rare forms of opportunistic esophagitis caused by unrelated organisms. They are considered together in this discussion because of similarities in their clinical and pathologic features. *Aspergillus* infections may be caused by any one of several species, including *A. fumigatus, A. niger,* and *A. flavus.* Phycomycetes (mucormycosis) infection includes fungi from the genera *Absidia, Rhizopus,* and *Mucor.* Esophageal infections with these organisms are essentially limited to severely compromised hosts. Esophageal infection appears to result

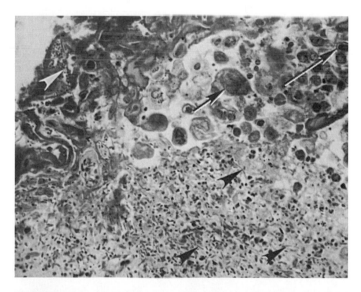

Figure 20.11 Mixed fungal and viral esophagitis. Candidal esophagitis is evident with budding yeast *(white arrowhead)* in squamous epithelium and pseudohyphae *(black arrowheads)* in lamina propria beneath squamous epithelium with herpes inclusions *(arrows).* The characteristic inclusions have a peri-inclusion halo *(long arrow)* in some cells and occur in multinucleated epithelial giant cells *(short arrow).*

from either direct mucosal involvement from the lumen after swallowing of inhaled organisms or involvement of the esophageal wall after extension from contiguous structures, or after blood-borne dissemination. Esophageal infection is usually associated with involvement of other portions of the gastrointestinal tract or widely disseminated disease.

Aspergillus in tissue is characterized by septate hyphae with dichotomous branching that produces acute angles (see Fig. 20.10; Fig. 20.12). Phycomycetes show broad irregular nonseptate hyphae with obtuse to right-angle branches. Both types of organisms may be difficult to identify in H&E-stained sections, but they stain well with methenamine silver. Fungal cultures permit specification.

Both types of organisms have a predilection for blood vessel invasion (see Fig. 20.12). Arterial involvement produces thrombosis and infarction with coagulative necrosis. The presence of infarcted tissue in the esophagus of an immunocompromised patient, therefore, should lead to a careful search for these types of organisms. The organisms may also be found in ulcerated tissue. Because infections with *Aspergillus* and Phycomycetes

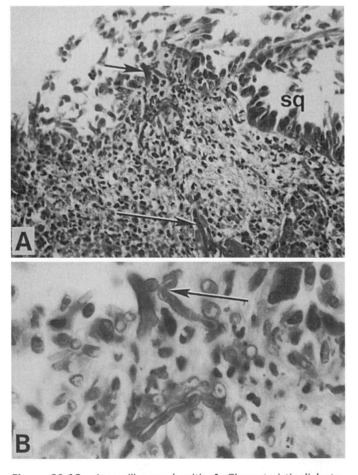

Figure 20.12 *Aspergillus* esophagitis. **A.** Characteristic dichotomously branching septate hyphae *(short arrow)* of *Aspergillus* infiltrate degenerating squamous epithelium (sq) and the lamina propria with blood vessel invasion *(long arrow)*. **B.** High-power view of the area indicated by the short arrow in part A. Dichotomous branching *(arrow)* is evident.

occur in severely compromised patients, inflammatory response is often minimal. Additional infectious agents may also be present (see Fig. 20.10).

PATHOGENIC FUNGAL ESOPHAGITIS

Pathogenic fungi reported to involve the esophagus include *Histoplasma capsulatum, Blastomyces dermatitidis* (North American blastomycosis), *Sporothrix schenckii,* and *Paracoccidioides brasiliensis* (South American blastomycosis), but esophageal infection by pathogenic fungi is rare. For example, in an autopsy series of 120 cases of disseminated histoplasmosis, esophageal involvement was found in only two patients, although in other series, prevalence figures were as high as 13%.

Esophageal infection by pathogenic fungi generally occurs in apparently normal individuals during the course of disseminated disease. Disseminated infections with pathogenic fungi can also occur in immunocompromised hosts exposed in endemic areas. The primary site from which esophageal involvement occurs is usually the lungs, and both direct extension and hematogenous spread to the esophagus are possible. Primary esophageal involvement by pathogenic fungi has not been demonstrated convincingly. Patients generally have extrinsic compression, stricture, mass, or ulceration of the esophagus. Organisms cannot be demonstrated in endoscopic biopsy specimens unless mucosal involvement is present.

Histoplasmal esophagitis usually develops by extension from involved subcarinal lymph nodes. Intracellular yeasts in histiocytes occur in granulomatous inflammation, and active inflammation with neutrophils is sometimes present. In H & E-stained sections, the yeasts appear small, with an artifactual clear area between the cell wall and retracted cytoplasm, which was misinterpreted as a capsule (hence, "*capsulatum*"). PAS and methenamine silver stain the cell wall and demonstrate the true size of the yeast. Biopsy diagnosis of histoplasmal esophagitis depends upon demonstration of the organisms in the base of ulcerated areas. Culture is important because of the problem of sampling.

Blastomycotic esophagitis has been reported to have histopathologic features similar to those seen in the skin, a squamous-lined surface that is commonly affected in disseminated disease. The squamous epithelium often shows pseudoepitheliomatous hyperplasia. The yeasts are large and usually extracellular. The cytoplasm is retracted from the capsule. Acute inflammation, necrosis, and granulomatous inflammation are common; but the organisms are often difficult to find. As a result, culture is important in diagnosis.

VIRAL ESOPHAGITIS

Viruses that infect the esophagus are included in Table 20.1.

HERPES ESOPHAGITIS (SEE FIGS. 20.11 AND 20.13 TO 20.15)

This form of viral esophagitis is generally due to herpes simplex virus type I (except in neonates). The portal of entry is uncertain, but swallowing of infected saliva has been suggested. The virus can be harbored in the salivary glands, and some patients have herpetic gingivostomatitis as a possible source.

Herpes esophagitis is usually an opportunistic infection, although it can occur in patients without apparent underlying disease.

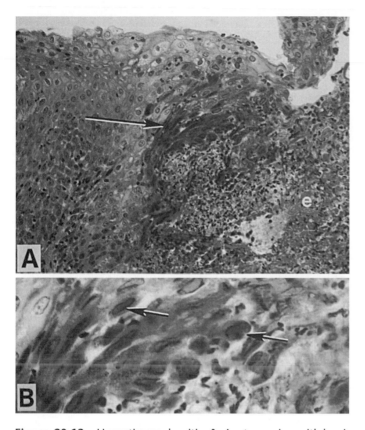

Figure 20.13 Herpetic esophagitis. **A.** Acute erosion with luminal fibrinoinflammatory exudate (e) has herpetic inclusions characteristically located in the squamous epithelial cells at the periphery *(arrow).* **B.** High-power view of area indicated by the arrow in part A. Typical herpes inclusions are evident in squamous epithelial cells *(arrows).*

Infections with other pathogens and of other organs are commonly associated with herpetic esophagitis. The major clinical importance of herpetic ulcers lies often in their being a portal of entry for bacteria and fungi (see Fig. 20.11), and individual epithelial cells have been shown to have dual infection with herpesvirus and *Candida.* Herpes esophagitis is often asymptomatic such that antemortem diagnosis was uncommon in the past; in some patients, however, odynophagia or dysphagia leads to endoscopic investigation, including biopsy and/or cytology. Strictures rarely develop.

Esophageal involvement is common in disseminated herpes simplex virus infection in neonates. Because the infection is usually acquired intrapartum, type 2 virus is most often involved. If the neonate survives, esophageal stenosis is common.

Herpes infection of the esophagus usually results in ulcer formation. Specimens properly taken from the edges and base of the ulcer show both squamous epithelium and fibroinflammatory exudate containing neutrophils (Fig. 20.13). Granulation tissue is typically absent because of the acute nature of the ulcers. The epithelium contains the histopathologic evidence of herpetic infection in the form of smudgy "ground-glass" eosinophilic to amphophilic intranuclear inclusions. The inclusions show a range of morphologic features (Fig. 20.14), some filling the nucleus to the nuclear membrane (Cowdry type B) and others having a halo-like clear area between them and the chromatin clumped against the

nuclear membrane (Cowdry type A). The epithelial cells that contain inclusions sometimes are enlarged and multinucleated. Loss of cohesion of the infected cells with hyalinization of the cytoplasm is often seen.

The inclusion-bearing epithelial cells are usually confined to the area immediately adjacent to the ulcer (see Fig. 20.13). In rare cases, herpes can be identified in the connective tissue bed of an esophageal ulcer. Occasionally, inclusions are found in biopsy samples of intact epithelium or endoscopically visible intraepithelial vesicles, which appear to represent preulcerative lesions. When epithelial virus inclusions are identified, the differential diagnosis includes the other types of viral infections that involve squamous epithelium, particularly varicella (see Table 20.1 and the following section).

Immunohistochemical studies using specific anti-herpes simplex virus type 1 and 2 antibodies can be used to confirm herpetic esophagitis (Fig. 20.15). In addition, immunohistochemical studies demonstrate that herpetic antigens are present in epithelial cells that do not have recognizable inclusions. This finding supports the observation that inclusion formation occurs relatively late in the development of the infection. As a result, herpetic esophagitis may not be recognizable histopathologically because inclusions are absent, but more commonly this situation results from the problem of sampling.

Histopathologic diagnosis depends on the detection of characteristic inclusions. Specimens, therefore, must include squamous epithelium from the periphery of the ulcer to ensure that inclusions are found (see Table 20.1). Owing to the problem of sampling, multiple specimens, brush cytology, and viral cultures can increase the likelihood of diagnosis. Because herpetic ulcers are portals of entry for other organisms, particularly candida (see Fig. 20.11), stains for fungi should be used routinely in assessment of biopsy specimens with herpetic esophagitis. Viral and fungal cultures and smears taken at the time of endoscopy are also helpful. Bacteria are

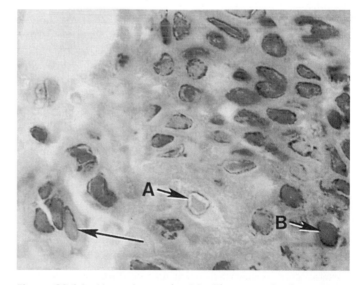

Figure 20.14 Herpetic esophagitis. The range in the appearance of herpetic inclusions in squamous epithelium is evident Cowdry type A *(arrow A)* and Cowdry type B *(arrow B)* are illustrated along with a multinucleated epithelial giant cell (long arrow) with inclusions.

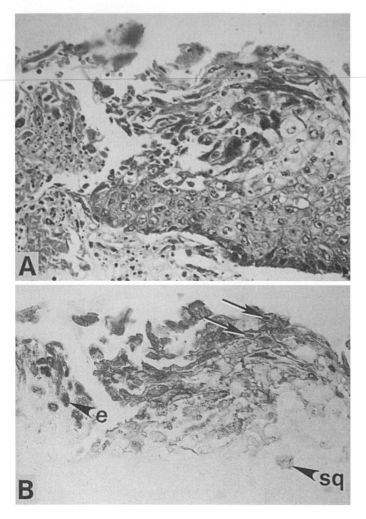

Figure 20.15 Herpetic esophagitis. **A.** H & E-stained section demonstrates degenerating squamous epithelium with ill-defined viral inclusions. **B.** Immunoperoxidase stain for herpes simplex virus antigens in serial section adjoining section shown in part A. Antigen is evident in necrotic cellular debris in the fibrinoinflammatory exudate (e) and the cytoplasm of squamous epithelial cells without inclusions (sq), as well as in intranuclear inclusions themselves *(arrows).*

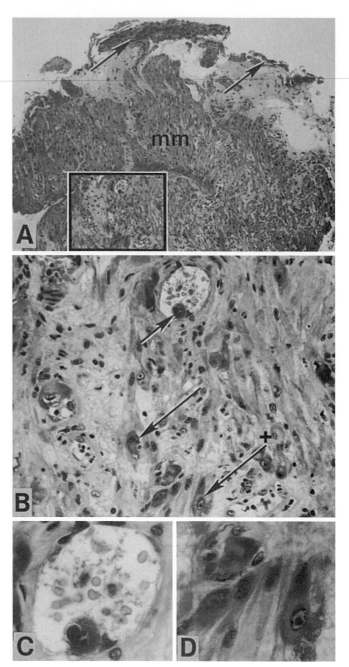

Figure 20.16 Cytomegaloviral (CMV) esophagitis. **A.** Acute ulcer with necrotic debris *(arrows)* extends into muscularis mucosae (mm). **B.** High-power view of the area enclosed by the box in part A. Characteristic inclusions of cytomegalovirus are present in the lumen of capillaries *(short arrow)* and smooth muscle cells *(long arrows).* **C.** High-power view of the area indicated by the short arrow in part B. The CMV inclusion involves an endothelial cell. **D.** High-power view of the area indicated by the long arrow with a plus (+) sign in part B. An early CMV inclusion is evident in a smooth muscle cell.

often identifiable in herpetic ulcers, which can serve as the portal of entry for bacterial infections. The significance of bacteria, however, is difficult to determine because simple colonization can occur.

CYTOMEGALOVIRUS ESOPHAGITIS (FIG. 20.16)

As with herpes esophagitis, cytomegalovirus (CMV) infection of the esophagus is generally an opportunistic infection. CMV esophagitis usually occurs along with generalized CMV infection. The portal of entry is uncertain, but it may be through viremia with localization in areas of previous esophageal injury, as well as from infected saliva in the esophageal lumen. CMV appears to be a secondary infecting agent in many cases, and its role in producing primary esophageal injury is often open to question. Systemic and esophageal infections with other organisms frequently accompany CMV esophagitis. Antemortem diagnosis usually results from

endoscopy and biopsy of an immunocompromised patient with odynophagia or dysphagia.

Ulceration is a common finding in CMV esophagitis. Specimens of the ulcer base generally show fibrinoinflammatory exudate containing neutrophils and inflamed granulation tissue with characteristic inclusions. The enlarged cells in capillary walls that show inclusions often bulge into the vessel lumen, but the infected cells may be pericytes as well as endothelial cells. Smooth muscle cells of the muscularis mucosae and fibrocytes in connective tissue also appear to be involved in some cases (see Fig. 20.16). In addition to being enlarged (cytomegaly), the affected cells have an enlarged nucleus, frequently with a purple inclusion surrounded by a clear halo, resulting in an "owl's eye" appearance. Cytoplasmic inclusions are often evident. The cells with distinctive inclusions are characteristic of CMV infection, but other enlarged cells in the specimen frequently contain only rudimentary inclusions. In some cases, fully developed inclusions are not found despite a careful search. Immunohistochemical analysis with anti-CMV antibodies is especially helpful in such cases. The epithelium in biopsy specimens taken from the periphery of the ulcer shows reactive changes and sometimes active inflammation, but not inclusions (see Table 20.1).

Histopathologic diagnosis depends on the detection of characteristic inclusions. In contrast to herpetic esophagitis, in which the inclusions are usually in the epithelium at the periphery of the ulcer, CMV inclusions are in the ulcer base. Tissue specimens, therefore, must include samples of both the base and the periphery of an ulcer. Because infected cells that have not yet formed an inclusion cannot always be distinguished confidently from reactive cells in ulcers with other causes, viral cultures and immunohistochemical studies for CMV can be helpful. Specimens with CMV should be evaluated for histopathologic evidence of other organisms, especially herpesvirus and *Candida* in patients with AIDS.

ESOPHAGITIS ASSOCIATED WITH VARICELLA, RUBELLA, AND VARIOLA

Clinical involvement of the esophagus by the viral exanthem varicella has been reported, and autopsy histopathologic analysis indicates that the esophageal lesions are similar to those in the squamous epithelium of the skin. Early abnormalities include degeneration of the basal zone of the epithelium, characterized by swelling with rarefaction and vacuolization of the cytoplasm. In larger lesions, the basal layer separates from the lamina propria. Acidophilic nuclear inclusions, cytoplasmic inclusions, and occasional giant epithelial cells are also seen.

Involvement of the esophagus in congenital rubella has also been reported. Multinucleated squamous epithelial cells with intranuclear inclusions were present, but the reported case is subject to criticism because the electron-microscopic features of the viral particles were different from those of the usual rubella.

Esophageal involvement by variola (smallpox) is now of only historical interest.

ESOPHAGITIS DUE TO HIV AND EPSTEIN-BARR VIRUS

Aphthous ulcers have been found in patients with HIV-1 infection, and viral particles have been identified by electron microscopy of the lesions. As a consequence, HIV-1 infection of the esophagus with ulceration has been suggested to occur during the early phases of HIV infection and seroconversion. A recent report of five patients with HIV-1 infection suggested that Epstein-Barr virus can also infect the squamous epithelium of the esophagus and contribute to esophageal ulceration in patients with AIDS. Esophageal symptoms, especially dysphagia, are common in patients with AIDS. Esophageal abnormalities in such patients can be attributed to a variety of causative factors, including infections by *Candida*, herpesvirus, and CMV.

HUMAN PAPILLOMAVIRUS INFECTION OF THE ESOPHAGUS

Squamous papillomas with koilocytic change occur rarely. Confirmation of human papillomavirus can be obtained by immunohistochemistry or in situ hybridization.

BACTERIAL ESOPHAGITIS

Bacteria are often present in specimens with histopathologic evidence of ulceration, but usually represent secondary infectious agents, either alone (Fig. 20.17) or with fungi or viruses. Bacterial colonization of the esophageal epithelium can also occur with obstruction due to a variety of factors (Fig. 20.18). Primary bacterial infections appear to be rare in the antibiotic era, except in severely compromised hosts, but they can be an occult source of bacteremia.

OPPORTUNISTIC BACTERIAL ESOPHAGITIS

Great attention has been focused on opportunistic fungal and viral esophagitis in severely compromised patients. Bacteria, however, are primary pathogens in opportunistic esophageal infections, accounting for about 10 to 15% of cases of infective esophagitis. Esophagitis attributable to a single species of bacteria and to mixed bacterial flora have been described. Implicated bacteria include a wide variety of gram-positive and gram-negative organisms, but bacterial esophagitis with bacteremia usually involves gram-positive bacteria. Antecedent esophageal injury probably contributes to the pathogenesis of the esophageal infection.

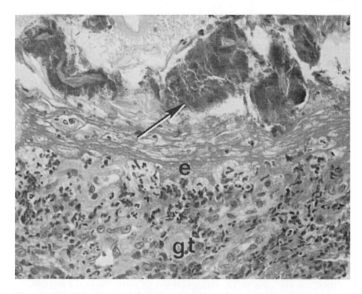

Figure 20.17 Bacterial colonization of esophageal ulcer. An active chronic ulcer with inflamed granulation tissue (gt) and luminal fibrinoinflammatory exudate (e) contains bacterial colonies *(arrow)* in the luminal debris.

Opportunistic bacterial esophagitis is characterized histopathologically by numerous bacteria extending into the lamina propria and involving blood vessels with necrosis of the squamous epithelium (Fig. 20.19). The absence of inflammation in the face of numerous organisms is a striking feature caused by granulocytopenia in some patients, but acute inflammation may be present in nonneutropenic patients.

MYCOBACTERIAL ESOPHAGITIS

Mycobacterium tuberculosis infection involving the esophagus is rare. Portals of entry include direct extension from tuberculous pharyngitis; direct extension from mediastinal lymph nodes or the vertebral column; and the vascular system in disseminated (miliary) tuberculosis. Mucosal involvement as a primary site or after swallowing infected sputum is rare (only 25 of 16,489 autopsy patients in one series). Endoscopically, esophageal tuberculosis may be characterized by ulceration or a mass lesion. Complications include obstruction and tracheobronchial fistula.

Specimens may show the range of histopathologic findings in tuberculosis, including nonspecific inflammation as well as caseating granulomas with epithelioid histiocytes and multinucleated giant cells. The differential diagnosis includes other causes of esophagitis as well as other diseases characterized by granulomas. Identification of acid-fast bacilli in histopathologic sections or culture of *M. tuberculosis* from the esophagus is diagnostic. In patients without mucosal involvement, however, biopsy specimens are unable to show histopathologic evidence of the underlying tuberculosis because of the shallow depth of the specimens.

Mycobacterium avium-intracellulare occasionally involves the esophagus in patients with AIDS.

ACTINOMYCES ISRAELI ESOPHAGITIS

Actinomyces organisms are anaerobic gram-positive bacteria that are frequently normal flora in the oronasopharynx, including the

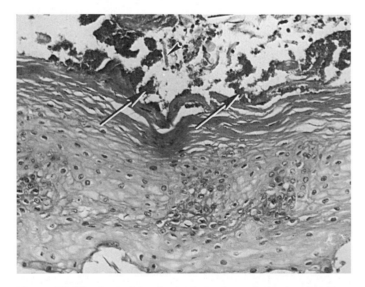

Figure 20.18 Bacterial colonization of esophageal epithelium in a patient with esophageal obstruction due to external compression. Numerous bacteria *(arrows)* are present on the luminal surface, but with no evidence of inflammatory response. The luminal debris also contains food material *(arrowhead)*.

gingiva and tonsils. Both primary and secondary infections of the esophagus by *Actinomyces* have been reported. Primary mucosal involvement may result from swallowing a foreign body, which produces injury to the epithelium and allows entry of the organism. Invasion into the esophageal wall can then occur, with formation of sinus tracts and abscesses, particularly in the upper esophagus. Secondary involvement of the esophagus occurs by extension from hilar lymph nodes and the vertebral column or by hematogenous dissemination.

Diagnosis depends on recognition of "sulfur granules," the small yellow bodies representing colonies of the organisms, or histopathologic identification of the intertwined thin, branching filaments. The filaments at the periphery of the colonies are club-shaped, with an enlargement at the end. Fibrinoinflammatory exudate with neutrophils usually surrounds the colonies, and granulation tissue representing the fistula tract may also be present. Differential diagnosis includes colonies of other bacteria in tissue (botryomycosis) and the Splendore-Hoeppli phenomenon (bacterial colonies surrounded by eosinophilic material). *Actinomyces* may appear in esophageal specimens as a contaminant, probably from the oronasopharynx; careful consideration should precede a diagnosis of esophageal involvement by the organism.

MISCELLANEOUS BACTERIAL ESOPHAGITIS

Historically, esophageal infections have been attributed to *Corynebacterium diphtheriae, Salmonella typhosa,* and *Shigella.* A case of esophageal infection by *Lactobacillus acidophilus* has been reported, although the clinical setting and features of the infection resembled candidal esophagitis. Whipple disease can involve the esophagus (Fig. 20.20).

SPIROCHETAL (SYPHILITIC) ESOPHAGITIS

Clinically evident *Treponema pallidum* infection involving the esophagus is extremely rare (two cases in 7000 patients in one series). When it occurs, it is generally in the acquired, rather than the congenital, form of syphilis. Primary lesions (chancres) of the esophagus are unusual. Secondary lesions occur in the esophagus as part of the generalized involvement but are rarely identified because the skin lesions usually dominate the clinical findings. The secondary lesions are superficial and usually heal. Tertiary lesions in the esophagus are uncommon but are more likely to undergo biopsy because they manifest clinically. Four main types of lesions have been described: ulcers due to ischemia resulting from endarteritis; active syphilitic lesions that have extended directly into the esophagus from adjacent organs or lymph nodes; submucosa gummas, which may enlarge and rupture into the esophageal lumen; and strictures due to scarring that resulted from healing of the first three types of lesions.

Specimens may show a range of findings, from necrosis in gummas, which is indistinguishable from caseous necrosis of tuberculosis, to intact squamous epithelium, with characteristic vasculitis in the lamina propria and submucosa. As in syphilis involving other body sites, the vasculitis shows a prominent perivascular accumulation of plasma cells. The lumen of an affected artery is often obliterated (hence "endarteritis"). Spirochetes may be demonstrable in primary and secondary lesions with silver impregnation techniques, such as the Dieterle stain; tertiary lesions lack spirochetes. Therefore, diagnosis of syphilis involving the esophagus usually depends on the presence of the characteristic vasculitis in

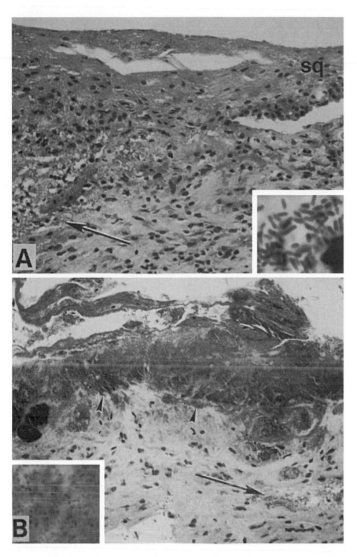

Figure 20.19 Opportunistic bacterial esophagitis. **A.** Escherichia coli esophagitis. Necrotic squamous epithelium (sq) contains numerous bacteria, which extend into the lamina propria *(arrow)*. **Inset.** Bacilli at high magnification. Tissue Gram staining showed gram-negative bacilli, and the patient's blood cultures were positive for *E. coli,* which indicated bacteremic bacterial esophagitis. No inflammatory response to the infection is evident because of the patient's profound neutropenia, resulting from cytotoxic chemotherapy. **B.** Streptococcal esophagitis. Extensive erosion of the squamous epithelium is evident with a large mass of bacteria *(arrowheads)* involving the lamina propria. Blood vessels *(arrow)* contain bacteria. **Inset.** Small cocci were gram-positive on tissue Gram stain. No inflammatory response to the infection is evident.

the setting of a compatible clinical and serologic picture, rather than demonstration of spirochetes in specimens, because the tertiary lesions are most commonly encountered.

PARASITIC ESOPHAGITIS

Esophageal involvement by parasitic infections is extremely uncommon in developed countries. The most common parasitic involve-

ment is by Chagas disease, which produces reactive changes in the squamous epithelium as a consequence of stasis after denervation. *Ascaris* passes through the lumen of the esophagus as part of its life cycle. (Maggots can also be identified in the lumen.) Mucosal involvement by amebiasis can occur. The esophageal wall can be affected by *Echinococcus, Cysticercus, Trichinella,* and *Filaria.*

ESOPHAGEAL INJURY DUE TO EXOGENOUS CHEMICALS

LYE, ACIDS, DETERGENTS, AND OTHER HOUSEHOLD PRODUCTS

Ingestion of lye, acids, or nonphosphate detergents, either accidentally or as a suicide attempt, often produces dramatic injury to the esophagus. Although endoscopy is often chosen as a means to assess the severity of injury, biopsies are rarely performed. When biopsy is undertaken, the specimens usually show only hemorrhagic, necrotic tissue and fibrinoinflammatory exudate, representing the effects of the chemical and the inflammatory response to the injury. If the patient survives, evidence of repair processes, including granulation tissue and regenerating epithelium, can be found in biopsy specimens. Autopsy specimens may show a range of findings that depend on the time course until the patient's death. Surgical specimens most commonly result from resection of strictures, which are characterized by transmural scarring, often with ongoing ulceration even

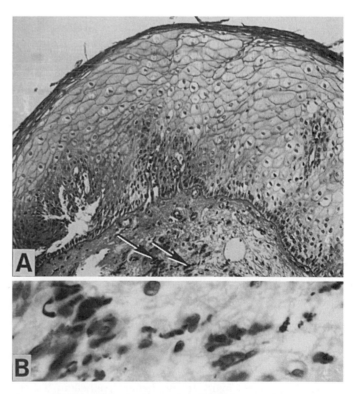

Figure 20.20 Whipple disease involving the esophagus. **A.** PAS staining shows characteristic PAS-positive granules in histiocytes in the lamina propria *(arrows)*. **B.** High-power view of the area indicated by the arrows in part A. PAS-positive granules are identical to those found in the small intestinal biopsy specimen of the patient.

years after the initial injury. The lye-injured esophagus is associated with increased risk of squamous carcinoma. Less serious esophageal injury (Fig. 20.21) can result from ingestion of a variety of household products. The nature and severity of the injury depend on the chemical constituents.

DRUG CONTACT

Esophageal ulceration and/or inflammation have been reported with a large number of drugs (Table 20.2). Direct contact with the mucosa is the usual mechanism of injury. Delay in esophageal passage of tablets is common in normal individuals at recumbency, particularly the elderly; ingestion of medications just before lying down or with small fluid volume increases the risk of slow passage. Patients with structural abnormalities of the esophagus are at particular risk. Extrinsic compression associated with left atrial enlargement from mitral valve disease and intrinsic structural abnormalities such as a neoplasm, stricture, and hiatal hernia are predisposing factors. Motility abnormalities with increased lower esophageal sphincter pressure (e.g., achalasia) and abnormal peristalsis (e.g., scleroderma and diffuse esophageal spasm) may also delay passage of medication.

The formulation of the drug is an important factor in esophageal injury: large tablets, capsules, and tablets with hygroscopic agents to accelerate disintegration are more likely to remain in the esophagus and release the contained drug. The chemical nature of the drug affects the potential for injury when the drug is released: the ulcerogenic nature of potassium chloride is well known, whereas dissolved doxycycline HCl, tetracycline HCl, and ferrous sulfate have acidic pH, and emepronium bromide is basic. Hyperosmolality and heat generated during dissolving may also play a role in injury. Stricture formation and death due to perforation or hemorrhage may occur as complications of drug-

TABLE 20.2	Drugs Associated with Esophagitis and Ulceration

Antibiotics
  Doxycycline
  Tetracycline hydrochloride
  Oxytetracycline
  Minocycline hydrochloride
  Clindamycin phosphate
  Lincomycin hydrochloride
  Trimethoprim-sulfamethoxazole
  Erythromycin
  Chloramphenicol
  Tinadazole
  Phenoxymethyl penicillin
  Apocillin
Anti-inflammatory and related drugs
  Aspirin and aspirin-containing combination products
  Indomethacin[a]
  Ibuprofen
  Piroxicam
  Phenylbutazone
  Prednisone and prednisolone
  Diphenhydramine hydrochloride
  Cromolyn inhalant
  Theophylline
Cardiovascular drugs
  Quinidine[a]
  Alprenolol[a]
  Potassium chloride tablets[a]
Chemotherapeutic agents
  Fluorouracil
  Cytosine arabinoside
  Estramustine phosphate
Nutritional supplements
  Ferrous sulfate and
    ferrous succinate
  Ascorbic acid
  Multivitamin tablets
Miscellaneous
  Emepronium bromide
  Cimetidine
  Chloral hydrate
  Cocaine
  Phenytoin
  Kayexalate
  Acetaminophen

[a]Associated with severe ulceration, perforation, or stricture.

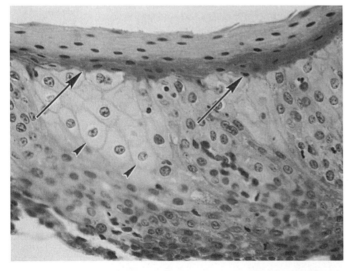

Figure 20.21 Lysol injury to esophageal epithelium. Esophageal biopsy specimen taken 4 hours after Lysol ingestion by a child shows bandlike fixation of the superficial layers of the squamous epithelium *(arrows)* with hyperchromatic nuclei and balloon cells *(arrowheads)* in the subjacent layers. Only a few neutrophils are evident.

induced injury; these complications have been reported most commonly with slow-release potassium chloride tablets. Specimens of drug-induced esophageal injury usually show evidence of nonspecific ulceration and/or esophagitis. Kayexalate (Sanofi Winthrop, New York, NY) in sorbitol, however, occasionally causes local coagulative necrosis of the mucosa. The crystals have a characteristic appearance in H & E-stained sections (Fig. 20.22) and are PAS-positive and acid-fast, which allows recognition of the cause of the injury.

With some drugs, esophagitis is attributed to other mechanisms such as immunologic or allergic injury, cytotoxic effects (see subsequent discussion of chemotherapeutic agents), and induction of gastroesophageal reflux by production of lower esophageal sphincter dysfunction (see section concerning gastroesophageal reflux).

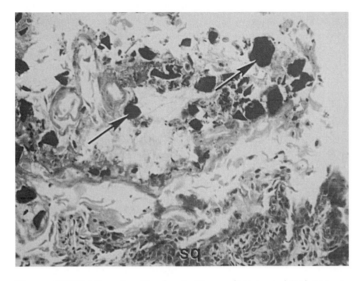

Figure 20.22 Esophagitis due to Kayexalate in sorbitol. Necrosis of the superficial layers of the squamous epithelium (sq) is present in areas containing characteristic crystals of Kayexalate *(arrows).*

SCLEROTHERAPY FOR ESOPHAGEAL VARICES

Injection of esophageal varices with a sclerosing solution under visualization through an esophagoscope was described in 1939 and is the subject of renewed interest with the use of fiberoptic instruments. The findings in the esophagus after sclerotherapy have been described in several autopsy series. Necrosis with inflammation, hemorrhage, granulation tissue, and scarring are seen, the features influenced by the time since injection and the severity of the injury (Fig. 20.23). Morrhuate can be identified histopathologically (see Fig. 20.23).

CHEMOTHERAPEUTIC AGENTS

Esophageal mucosal injury can result from the effects of various systemic chemotherapeutic agents. The basal zone of the squamous epithelium sometimes is atypical owing to cytotoxic effects on the proliferative zone (Fig. 20.24).

Further details on chemical and drug injuries of the esophagus are provided in Chapter 11.

ESOPHAGEAL TRAUMA

External trauma to the esophagus may occur with both blunt and penetrating trauma to the neck and thorax. Internal trauma can result from swallowed foreign bodies, including food and bezoars; from vomiting; and from iatrogenic injury by instruments, catheters, and tubes. Luminal hemorrhage is common, and rupture with perforation into the mediastinum may occur. Mallory-Weiss tears and hematomas at the gastroesophageal junction region may develop after emesis or aborted sneezes. Spontaneous hematomas also occur, most often proximally or at multiple sites, in patients with acquired or congenital coagulopathies.

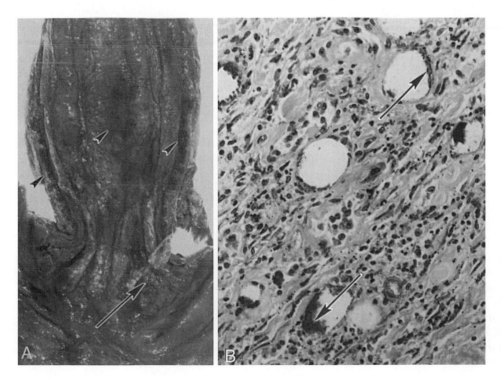

Figure 20.23 Esophageal perforation after sclerotherapy for esophageal varices. **A.** Transmural necrosis *(arrow)* is present with mural hemorrhage involving the entire distal esophagus *(arrowheads).* **B.** Morrhuate sclerosing agent in tissue. The morrhuate *(arrows)* appears golden brown and is often associated with vacuoles.

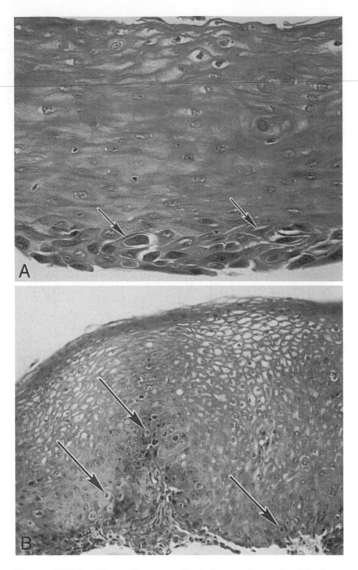

Figure 20.24 Chemotherapy effects in esophageal epithelium. **A.** In this example from a patient receiving combination chemotherapy, the basal zone *(arrows)* shows nuclear abnormalities due to the effects of cytotoxic drugs. Epithelial maturation is abnormal with ovoid immature nuclei at the luminal surface. **B.** In this example from a patient receiving Taxol (Bristol-Meyers Squibb, Princeton, NJ), many epithelial cells in the basal zone are in mitotic arrest *(arrows)*, as also occurs with colchicine. Wide dispersion of nuclear material is a characteristic finding.

These types of lesions are most commonly encountered by the pathologist at autopsy. Endoscopy is often performed in the clinical settings just mentioned, but biopsies are rarely done. In one report, the biopsy specimen of a Mallory-Weiss tear showed necrosis, hemorrhage, and inflammation. Hematomas may be mistaken for tumors on radiographic and endoscopic examination, and a biopsy specimen in one report showed blood clot with attenuated squamous epithelium. Since the advent of soft tubes, esophageal injury associated with nasogastric intubation has most commonly been attributed to gastroesophageal reflux from interference with lower esophageal sphincter (LES) function, rather than to direct mucosal

injury (see subsequent section concerning gastroesophageal reflux). Foreign body reactions, including multinucleated giant cells, can occur if foreign material is introduced into the mucosa.

ESOPHAGEAL INJURY DUE TO PHYSICAL AGENTS

RADIATION ESOPHAGITIS

The esophagus is often exposed to radiation during radiotherapy for tumors of the lung, mediastinum, or vertebral column. Radiation injury and recovery are influenced by the type of radiotherapy, the dose, the time course of administration, and a variety of patient-related factors. The spectrum of injury may range from mild degenerative changes in dividing cells and temporary hyperemia to total necrosis of the esophageal wall. Similarly, repair processes may be rapid and complete or incomplete with nonhealing ulcers and scarring. The tolerated dose of radiation is said to be about 6000 rad, given at a rate of 1000 rad per week; strictures rarely occur at this dose, but chemotherapy with Adriamycin (Adria, Columbus, OH) appears to reduce tolerance.

The components of the esophageal wall show varying degrees of radiosensitivity and resistance: the squamous epithelium and blood vessels are relatively radiosensitive, whereas smooth muscle of the muscularis mucosae and muscularis propria and fibrous connective tissue are relatively radioresistant. Within the squamous epithelium of the mucosal surface and ducts of submucosal glands, the basal zone, with its proliferating cells, is more sensitive than the superficial layers, composed of differentiated postmitotic cells. Radiation esophagitis can be classified into acute and chronic forms on the basis of the time course and pathogenetic mechanisms involved.

Acute radiation esophagitis occurs during the first few weeks after initiation of therapy as a result of the direct injurious effects of the radiation. The epithelium and blood vessels are the main sites of the abnormalities in the acute phase (Fig. 20.25). *Chronic radiation esophagitis* occurs weeks to months after irradiation; chronic fibrovascular lesions predominate, leading to ongoing ischemic necrosis, scarring, and impaired epithelial cell proliferation.

Although patients are often symptomatic during acute radiation esophagitis, biopsies are rarely performed. In the first few days after initiation of radiotherapy, the squamous epithelium shows degenerative changes, focal necrosis, and decreased mitotic figures in the basal zone. Blood vessels are dilated and congested and have swollen endothelial cells. Lamina propria and submucosal connective tissue show edema and scattered inflammatory cells. In the second week, necrosis and thinning of the epithelium is more pronounced, often with some sloughing of debris and exudate into the lumen to produce erosions with pseudomembranes. In the third and fourth weeks, the epithelial necrosis is accompanied by regeneration (see Fig. 20.25). Also, the submucosa shows chronic inflammation and increased numbers of fibroblasts.

Biopsies are sometimes undertaken in patients with chronic radiation esophagitis. As radiation esophagitis enters the chronic phase, the epithelium may show either hyperplasia with parakeratosis or atrophy. Atypical cells are sometimes seen in the basal zone. The lamina propria and submucosa show progressive fibrosis, sometimes with a homogeneous hyalinized appearance and atypical fibroblasts. The fibrosis leads to stricture formation in some patients. Inflammatory cell infiltration, usually consisting of lymphocytes and plasma cells, is typically mild. In addition, telangiectatic capillaries and thick-walled hyalinized arterioles, sometimes with intimal foam cells and luminal narrowing, may be identified. Endothelial cells are enlarged and bizarre. Chronic ulcers with nonspecific inflamed granulation tissue may develop as a result of vascular insufficiency. Hemosiderin may be seen as a result of previous hemorrhage. When submucosal glands are included in the specimen, atrophy, fibrosis, and squamous metaplasia may be seen.

The most important aspect of pathologic diagnosis of radiation esophagitis is the clinical history of previous radiotherapy. The histopathologic findings just described provide pathologic confirmation and an objective assessment of the severity of injury within the limitations of sampling. In addition, the specimen should be examined carefully for evidence of complicating factors such as superinfecting bacteria, fungi, and viruses, as well as recurrent or residual tumor.

Additional information on radiation esophagitis is in Chapter 11.

THERMAL INJURY

Heat injury to the esophageal mucosa can occur from ingestion of excessively hot food or beverages. Microwaved food has been reported to lead to such injury because of uneven heat distribution; food items may have extremely high temperatures in the center but can be swallowed because of their cooler exterior. Cold injury to the esophagus is unusual.

HIATAL HERNIA

In hiatal hernia, the upper portion of the stomach (rarely, the entire stomach, a segment of the colon, or the spleen) evaginates through the widened esophageal hiatus of the diaphragm into the thorax. It is a relatively common condition; on routine barium

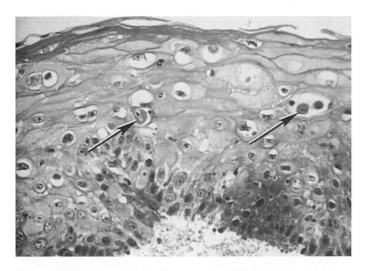

Figure 20.25 Acute radiation esophagitis. Esophageal biopsy taken during the third week of radiotherapy for mediastinal lymphoma shows degenerating epithelial cells with formation of acidophilic bodies *(arrows)* and reactive epithelial changes.

examination, hiatal hernia was found in 0.8 to 2.9% of adults. With increased intraabdominal pressure during examination, the prevalence increases to 2.1 to 11.8%; lying prone also increases the occurrence of hiatal hernia. In symptomatic patients subjected to endoscopic or manometric examination, hiatal hernia was found in 16 to 22%. Geographic variation, however, is wide. Hiatal hernia is common in Western countries and uncommon in Africa: barium examination of symptomatic Nigerians revealed hiatal hernia in only 0.39%. Western dietary habits are thought to be responsible for the difference in frequency. The prevalence of hiatal hernia increases with age. It is, however, well recognized in infants and children, with a reported prevalence of 0.62% in children undergoing barium examination.

The cause of hiatal hernia is unknown. It is likely to be environmental rather than genetic. Structurally, characteristics include separation of the diaphragmatic crura and widening of the space between the crura and the esophageal wall. Two major types of hiatal hernia are axial, or sliding, and nonaxial, or paraesophageal. Rarely, extensive scarring of the esophagus may result in retraction of the esophagus and herniation of the gastric cardia.

SLIDING HIATAL HERNIA

The sliding hiatal hernia is by far the more common type (about 95% of cases). About 60% of sliding hiatal hernias are less than 3 cm in diameter, and only 14% are more than 5 cm in diameter, according to the study by Pridie. Rare instances of herniation of the entire stomach have been reported. The herniated portion of the stomach can usually be reduced back into the abdominal cavity. The small asymptomatic hernias are merely anatomic phenomena and have no clinical significance. Most commonly, the symptoms are related to accompanying reflux esophagitis rather than to the hernia itself.

The relationship between the sliding hiatal hernia and reflux esophagitis is complex and controversial. It is evident that these two conditions often coexist but are not totally dependent on each other. Berstad et al. reported that 63% of the patients with reflux esophagitis had hiatal hernia, whereas only 8% of patients without reflux esophagitis had this condition. Conversely, 42% of patients with hiatal hernia had no esophagitis. Low pressure of the LES and a short intraabdominal segment of LES contribute to cardiac sphincter incompetence and result in gastroesophageal reflux. In the presence of hiatal hernia, the acidic fluid trapped in the hernia enters the esophagus when the LES is relaxed, accounting for delayed esophageal clearance and contributing to subsequent esophagitis. (Reflux esophagitis is discussed in detail subsequently.)

In addition to peptic esophagitis, the herniated stomach may become ulcerated, causing bleeding and perforation. Bleeding can also occur from incarcerated mucosal folds of the herniated stomach. In one report, ulceration caused aortogastric fistula. A large hernia may become incarcerated, causing obstruction: Haas et al. reported volvulus of the stomach in 21 of 138 surgically treated cases. Additional complications associated with hiatal hernia include diffuse esophageal spasm, carcinoma in the gastric cardia, cardiac arrhythmia, fibrosis of the lung, Mallory-Weiss syndrome, and intussusception of esophagus into the hernia. Rarely, rectal bleeding has been reported to occur from the colon that herniates through the diaphragmatic hiatus. Coincidental lesions with hiatal hernia include Zenker diverticulum, colonic diverticulosis, and gallstones.

PARAESOPHAGEAL HERNIA

Paraesophageal hernia constitutes about 5% of hiatal hernia cases. This condition is not age-related, the LES is not affected, and no reflux esophagitis occurs, unless a sliding hernia coexists. The herniated portion of the stomach is usually along the greater curvature. Other organs such as the small bowel, the colon, and the spleen may also enter the paraesophageal hernia. Paraesophageal hernias may be caused by previous surgery in the region of the diaphragmatic hiatus, including operations for sliding hernia: 13% of cases at the Lahey Clinic in Boston had an iatrogenic cause.

Complications of paraesophageal hernia are serious and may be fatal. They include bleeding from ulcer, obstruction, volvulus, incarceration, and strangulation of the herniated stomach. In one case, the ulcer penetrated the right ventricle of the heart, causing massive bleeding. Because of the seriousness of the complications, early surgical repair of paraesophageal hernia has been advocated.

OTHER DIAPHRAGMATIC HERNIAS

Hernias may develop at sites away from the esophageal hiatus. Congenital hernias may be symptomatic at birth and can be diagnosed in utero sonographically. They are usually located posterolaterally, involving the foramen of Bochdalek, or retrosternally, involving the foramen of Morgagni. These and other congenital diaphragmatic hernias are discussed in detail in Chapter 10. Respiratory problems are prominent in these patients because of hypoplasia of the lung in the presence of a large intrathoracic mass of abdominal organs or because of aspiration of regurgitated materials. Extracorporeal membrane oxygenation has been beneficial to these patients. Hernia may also be caused by traumatic injury to the diaphragm.

GASTROESOPHAGEAL REFLUX

Reflux esophagitis refers in general to esophageal inflammation resulting from gastroesophageal reflux, which is the regurgitation of gastric contents into the esophagus. Reflux of intestinal contents after total gastrectomy with esophagojejunostomy, however, can also produce reflux esophagitis. The specific clinical, endoscopic, radiologic, and pathologic definitions of *reflux esophagitis* are strikingly different. For example, the endoscopic definition refers to the presence of visible reddening of the mucosal surface, the result of prominent blood vessels. On the other hand, to the pathologist, "-itis" generally connotes the presence of inflammatory cells. The endoscopist is often unable to identify those patients with acute inflammatory cell infiltration of the epithelium, representing more severe injury, from those without active inflammation. As a result of the potential for confusion based on disparate definitions of *reflux esophagitis,* the phrase "changes due to gastroesophageal reflux" is used in this chapter for discussion of the histopathologic findings.

Persistent gastroesophageal reflux results from loss of effective antireflux mechanisms. These mechanisms appear to include anatomic factors at the gastroesophageal junction and diaphragmatic hiatus, but intrinsic lower esophageal sphincter tone is of cardinal importance. The specific sphincter abnormalities leading to gastroesophageal reflux are the subject of considerable investigation. In some patients, esophageal intubation, involvement of the muscularis propria by scleroderma, or a tumor at the esophagogastric junction can result in reflux. Persistent vomiting, sometimes on a psychogenic basis, can be considered as an extreme form of reflux. Reflux esophagitis is often part of a spectrum of upper gastrointestinal tract peptic disease, accompanied by gastritis and duodenitis.

Gastroesophageal reflux and reflux esophagitis are not synonymous, because "physiologic" reflux occurs in normal individuals. The development of esophagitis as a consequence of reflux depends on (a) the volume of refluxed gastric fluid, which is affected by gastric secretion, gastric emptying, and duodenogastric reflux; (b) the potency of the reflux material, which can include biliary and pancreatic secretions following duodenogastric reflux as well as hydrochloric acid and pepsin produced by the gastric epithelium; (c) the efficiency of esophageal clearing of refluxed material by gravity, peristalsis, saliva, and normal esophageal sphincter relaxation with deglutition, because the efficiency of clearing in turn determines contact time with the mucosa; and (d) the resistance of the esophageal squamous epithelium.

At the cellular level, reflux-induced squamous epithelial injury may result from damage to mucopolysaccharide intercellular cement and resultant back-diffusion of hydrogen ions, which leads to further damage. Increased cellular desquamation and increased epithelial cell turnover appear to occur in response to injury; if the severity of the injury exceeds the repair processes, inflammatory cell infiltration of the epithelium or even erosion and ulceration can result.

It is best to avoid categorization of reflux changes into "acute" and "chronic" based on the histopathologic character of the inflammatory cell infiltrate and epithelial changes because of the discordance between the histopathologic terminology and the time course of the process in the patient. For example, a biopsy diagnosis of "acute esophagitis" rendered because of the presence of neutrophils in the specimen is inappropriate in a patient with months or years of reflux esophagitis. On the other hand, the pathogenesis of peptic complications of gastroesophageal reflux can be used as a basis for classification of the histopathologic changes into high-grade and low-grade types. Peptic strictures and Barrett esophagus result from mucosal ulceration with loss of squamous epithelium and subsequent repair processes, i.e., deposition of scar tissue in the case of stricture, and re-epithelization with columnar epithelium in the case of Barrett esophagus (see subsequent section concerning Barrett esophagus). Furthermore, frank ulceration is often preceded by epithelial erosion with less than full-thickness destruction. Therefore, high-grade changes due to gastroesophageal reflux are characterized histopathologically by evidence of epithelial injury and destruction, usually accompanied by active inflammation, including neutrophils. These findings indicate severe insult to the esophageal mucosa. Less severe epithelial injury without histopathologic evidence of destruction or active inflammation but with reactive epithelial changes occurs in low-grade changes due to gastroesophageal reflux. When using this classification, however, it is important to remember that in addition to the peptic complications, gastroesophageal reflux may play a role in the pathogenesis of asthma and sudden infant death syndrome. Aspiration pneumonia may occur as a complication. As a result, the severity of the histopathologic findings may not be related to the severity or the gravity of the clinical picture.

The histopathologic changes attributable to gastroesophageal reflux are responsible for a wide spectrum of findings, ranging from subtle reactive epithelial changes to active esophagitis, peptic erosion, and ulcer. The histopathologic changes have been described in both capsule and endoscopic biopsy specimens in studies attempting to delineate clinically significant reflux or to correlate endoscopic findings in reflux esophagitis.

LOW-GRADE CHANGES

These reactive epithelial changes have received a great deal of attention since 1970, when Ishmail-Beigi et al. described "basal cell hyperplasia of the squamous epithelium" and "location of the papillae close to the epithelial surface" as "the histologic consequences of gastroesophageal reflux." Their criteria in well-oriented capsule biopsy samples taken about 2 cm above the manometrically demonstrated lower esophageal sphincter were *(a)* the basal zone comprising more than 15% of the total thickness of the epithelium and *(b)* papillae extending more than two thirds of the distance to the surface (Fig. 20.26).

Additional features of low-grade changes due to gastroesophageal reflux described by other authors include vascularization of the epithelium with dilated vessels ("lakes") at the tops of the papillae (see Fig. 20.2), increased numbers of papillae, loss of the longitudinal orientation of the surface epithelial cells due to the presence of ovoid immature cells at the surface, increased mitotic figures and incorporation of tritiated thymidine in the basal zone, and "balloon cells," i.e., enlarged translucent squamous epithelial cells that contain plasma proteins (see Fig. 20.4B). Except for balloon cells and vascular lakes, these features are morphologic consequences of increased epithelial proliferation resulting from relatively mild injury induced by reflux. By contrast, balloon cells are the result of epithelial injury with increased permeability of the cell membrane and usually occur in the midzone of the squamous epithelium in patients with chronic gastroesophageal reflux. Vascular lakes are equivalent to congestion and represent the vascular phase of the

TABLE 20.3	Epithelial Changes of Reflux Esophagitis
Histopathologic Feature	**Pathogenetic Mechanism**
Erosion/ulcer	Severe epithelial injury
Balloon cells	Epithelial injury
Vascular dilatation ("lakes") in papillae	Vascular phase of inflammatory response
Polymorphonuclear leukocytes (neutrophils/eosinophils)	Leukocytic phase of inflammatory response
Elongation of vascular papillae	Epithelial proliferation
Increased numbers of vascular papillae	Epithelial proliferation
Immature epithelial cells at luminal surface	Epithelial proliferation
Widening of basal zone of epithelium	Epithelial proliferation
Increased mitotic figures in epithelium	Epithelial proliferation

inflammatory process. The epithelial changes of reflux esophagitis are summarized in Table 20.3. The changes are similar to those induced by injury to squamous epithelium of other body sites, e.g., skin.

Very rarely, intraepithelial polymorphonuclear leukocytes may be seen as part of the spectrum of low-grade changes attributable to gastroesophageal reflux. The presence of more than a few in a biopsy specimen should lead to classification of the reflux changes as high-grade, especially if the epithelium shows injury or prominent reactive changes. Intraepithelial eosinophils (see Fig. 20.26) have been reported to be an indicator of delayed acid clearance after reflux, even in the absence of reactive epithelial changes. The lamina propria may demonstrate chronic inflammation with lymphocytes, eosinophils, plasma cells, and lymphoid aggregates and fibrosis, although the relationship of these findings to reflux-induced injury is uncertain.

The ultrastructural features of the squamous epithelium in reflux esophagitis have been described. Intracellular findings include edema, mitochondrial damage, membrane whorls, dilatation of the endoplasmic reticulum and Golgi apparatus, reduced membrane-coated granules, and occurrence of keratohyalin and parakeratotic granules. Intercellular spaces are enlarged and contain particulate debris with neutral mucosubstances. When cells are present in the intercellular spaces, they usually are lymphocytes, but neutrophils are found occasionally. The epithelial basement membranes show areas of thickening, thinning, and interruption, and anchoring fibrils are increased in number.

HIGH-GRADE CHANGES

A range of features can be seen. Active esophagitis is characterized by active inflammation and epithelial injury (see Fig. 20.1). Neutrophils usually predominate in the active inflammation when epithelial injury is severe and may be seen in both the epithelium and lamina propria. Occasionally, the heavy polymorphonuclear infil-

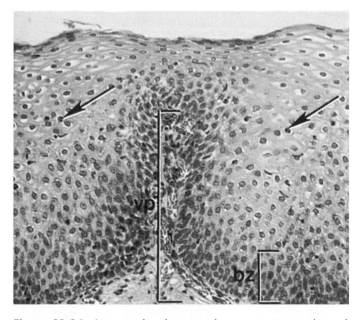

Figure 20.26 Low-grade changes due to gastroesophageal reflux. The esophageal epithelium in this biopsy taken about 3 cm above the esophagogastric junction has elongated vascular papillae (vp) and widened basal zone (bz). Scattered intraepithelial eosinophils *(arrows)* are also present.

trate consists of eosinophils producing the histopathologic finding of "eosinophilic esophagitis" (Table 20.4). The factors determining the predominant cell type in the infiltrate are unknown. Lymphocytes in intercellular spaces of the epithelium sometimes have elongated nuclei and must be distinguished from polymorphonuclear leukocytes (Fig. 20.27). Intercellular lymphocytes are sometimes numerous but even then do not appear to indicate a high-grade esophageal mucosal injury. A principal manifestation of epithelial injury is edema, which appears as widened intercellular spaces; loss of epithelial cell cohesion is sometimes evident. Epithelial cell necrosis is usually not a prominent feature, even with intense polymorphonuclear leukocytic infiltration. Reactive epithelial findings usually accompany active inflammation.

Epithelial destruction can take the form of erosion, acute ulcer, or active chronic ulcer (see Fig. 20.3). Luminal fibrinoinflammatory exudate often occurs on the surface of adjacent epithelium as well as in the eroded area and ulcer crater itself. The presence of exudate in specimens often provides evidence of erosion or an ulcer when tissue fragments showing epithelial destruction are not included. This

TABLE	
20.4	**Differential Diagnoses of Eosinophilic Infiltration of Esophageal Epithelium**

Acid-peptic reflux
Alkaline reflux
Infectious esophagitis
Eosinophilic gastroenteritis
Drug injury
Allergic esophagitis
Idiopathic eosinophilic esophagitis

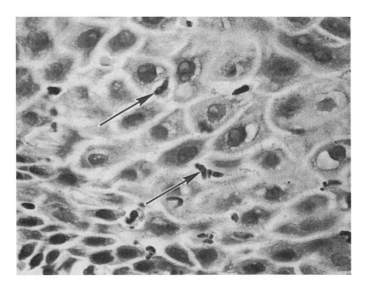

Figure 20.27 Lymphocytes in intercellular spaces of esophageal squamous epithelium. The "squiggly" nuclei and absence of cytoplasm containing granules help to distinguish lymphocytes from eosinophils and neutrophils.

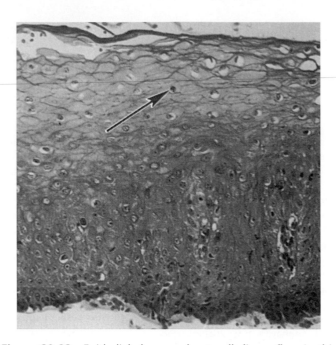

Figure 20.28 Epithelial changes due to alkaline reflux. In this patient with total gastrectomy and esophagojejunal anastomosis, the squamous epithelium contains scattered intraepithelial eosinophils *(arrow)* and has reactive epithelial changes indistinguishable from those of acid reflux.

finding can be especially helpful in biopsy specimens because of the problem of sampling. The depth of ulceration often can be determined relative to the muscularis mucosae or muscularis propria, including that in biopsy specimens from the ulcer base. Inflammatory polyps with granulation tissue and reactive epithelial changes may be seen. In extreme cases, septa may bridge the esophageal lumen, leading to a "double-barreled" appearance. Aortoesophageal fistula has also been reported as a consequence of reflux.

The utility of esophageal biopsies in the evaluation of cases of suspected gastroesophageal reflux and reflux esophagitis is controversial. Some authors report that esophageal biopsy is an excellent diagnostic tool in this clinical setting, whereas others do not support this claim. Interpretation of inflammation and reactive epithelial changes as evidence of reflux esophagitis is complicated by several factors. First, the changes are etiologically nonspecific, occurring in response to esophageal epithelial injury of *any* etiology as part of the body's stereotyped inflammatory and reparative processes. For example, the abnormalities can occur as a consequence of alkaline reflux (Fig. 20.28) as well as acid reflux, which is the usual clinical situation. From the morphologic perspective, the histopathologic features are sometimes discordant: elongated vascular tufts may occur without basal zone thickening, and balloon cells indicative of injury may be seen in the absence of reactive epithelial changes (Fig. 20.29).

Second, squamous epithelium with reactive changes is normally distributed in the distal few centimeters of esophagus, probably as a result of "physiologic" gastroesophageal reflux. Thus, interpretation of reactive epithelium as evidence of abnormality depends heavily on the site of the biopsy specimens relative to the LES. The endoscopist, therefore, plays a key role when choosing the level of the biopsy. Furthermore, at a given level, the histopathologic findings often have a nonuniform, patchy distribution around the circumference of the esophagus. Sampling, therefore, plays an important role in the biopsy findings, and the endoscopist should take multiple biopsy specimens to reduce the problem of sampling.

Third, histopathologic assessment itself is affected by the type of biopsy specimen and the histologic techniques used for embedding and sectioning. Some authors insist that only capsule biopsies are suitable for evaluation of reflux changes, whereas others find endoscopic biopsies are satisfactory. Endoscopic biopsy specimens are obtained far more often in current practice and appear to be interpretable *if* numerous step sections are cut through the specimen. With this approach, some portion of the biopsy specimen usually is sufficiently well oriented for interpretation of length of vascular papillae and width of basal zone. Furthermore, dilatation of vessels in the papillae and increased numbers of papillae can be assessed even in poorly oriented specimens; papillae appear to be increased in number when they overlap on a line perpendicular to the basal layer in en face sections.

The final point regarding histopathologic assessment is intra- and interobserver variation. This factor is addressed only superficially in most studies. In one study, problem, however, intra- and interobserver disagreement on two separate interpretations of the same specimen was 20%, even when assessment was limited to "normal" versus "abnormal."

The histopathologic features that occur as a consequence of gastroesophageal reflux-associated changes are an important aspect of the pathophysiology of reflux esophagitis. Their usefulness as a diagnostic test, however, depends on their clinical utility. Several studies conducted under carefully controlled conditions have given esophageal biopsy high marks as a diagnostic test for gastroesophageal reflux. Furthermore, in one study with 24-hour esophageal

pH monitoring of a large number of patients, the degree of exposure of the distal esophageal mucosa to gastric acid was highly correlated with length of papillae and thickness of the basal zone. On the other hand, the correlation coefficients were only .275 to .333, and wide scatter is evident in the graphs comparing the histopathologic features in each biopsy specimen with acid exposure. These results do not bode well for esophageal biopsy as a robust diagnostic test for reflux in individual patients because of poor predictive values.

In patients with gastroesophageal reflux, problems of specificity, topography of findings, specimen type, histologic processing, observer variation, and clinical correlation enter into the interpretation of esophageal biopsy specimens. Appropriate use of biopsy is determined by the goal of the endoscopist in taking the specimens. Histopathologic evidence of esophagitis and reactive epithelial changes can be attributed to many causative factors. Some biopsy tissue samples demonstrate specific features that do permit identification of the cause of the pathologic change noted (e.g., infectious esophagitis with morphologic evidence of the organisms). Biopsy cannot be used in the primary diagnosis of reflux esophagitis, but it is helpful in identifying esophagitis from other causes or due to other factors complicating reflux. In a patient with documented reflux, biopsy to evaluate the severity of the mucosal injury is inappropriate. Endoscopic examination with biopsy is best for identification of active esophagitis, erosion, or ulcer. Biopsies are also especially helpful in calling attention to patients in whom the histopathologic findings are more severe than was suggested by the endoscopic appearance. High-grade changes of gastroesophageal reflux lead to aggressive management to prevent the peptic complications of esophageal stricture and Barrett esophagus in addition to relieving symptoms. After antireflux therapy, follow-up biopsies for determining the objective response are appropriate.

BARRETT ESOPHAGUS

Barrett esophagus is the eponym applied to the columnar epithelium-lined lower esophagus, which is acquired as a complication of chronic gastroesophageal reflux. The precise prevalence of Barrett's esophagus is unknown, but in one autopsy study, 376 cases were identified per 100,000 population. Many affected persons are asymptomatic. The prevalence in patients who undergo upper gastrointestinal tract endoscopy and biopsy is about 1 to 2%, and among patients with symptoms of gastroesophageal reflux who undergo endoscopy and biopsy, the prevalence is about 10%.

The clinical importance of Barrett esophagus is enhanced by its predisposition to malignancy. Adenocarcinoma in Barrett esophagus accounts for the majority of adenocarcinomas of the esophagogastric junction and esophagus. Many patients are not known to have Barrett esophagus until they present with the complicating adenocarcinoma. Among patients with recognized Barrett esophagus, about 10% have or eventually develop adenocarcinoma; the risk is about 40 times that of the general population. In follow-up studies of patients with Barrett esophagus, however, the incidence of adenocarcinoma is low: only about 1 in 200 to 1 in 400 patient-years of follow-up.

The publication by N. R. Barrett in 1950 first called attention to the columnar epithelium-lined lower esophagus, although the condition had been identified earlier. Much of the confusion about the entity resulted from failure to appreciate the reflux-related etiology and pathogenesis, beginning with Barrett himself: he

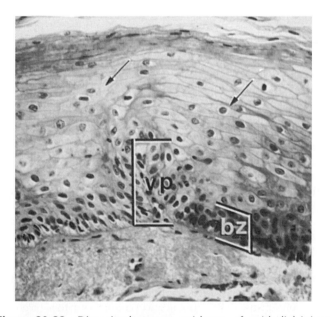

Figure 20.29 Disparity between evidence of epithelial injury and reactive changes in a patient with reflux esophagitis. Numerous balloon cells are present in the middle layers of the squamous epithelium *(arrows)*, but the vascular papillae (vp) and basal zone (bz) are of normal size.

described the columnar-lined structure as intrathoracic stomach due to congenitally short esophagus. After the columnar-lined region was demonstrated to be esophagus, Barrett proposed that the epithelium was congenital embryonic epithelium. The available evidence now indicates that Barrett esophagus is generally acquired as a consequence of chronic gastroesophageal reflux and reflux esophagitis, although a congenital origin is still proposed in a few cases.

Evidence cited as favoring gastroesophageal reflux as the cause of Barrett esophagus includes endoscopic observations with sequential biopsies showing upward migration of columnar-lined mucosa over time with continuing reflux; acquisition of Barrett mucosa with onset of gastroesophageal reflux after esophagogastrostomy following partial esophagogastrectomy; experimental studies in animal models demonstrating healing of denuded esophagus with columnar-lined mucosa in the setting of reflux; failure to identify Barrett esophagus in extensive autopsy studies of stillborns and neonates; and the absence from Barrett epithelium of gastrin-containing cells, which are present in congenital gastric heterotopia in Meckel diverticulum and gastric duplication (although gastrin and gastrin-containing cells have been identified in Barrett mucosa in other studies). Ethanol abuse and acid secretion from parietal cells in Barrett mucosa have been suggested to play a role in its etiology. Barrett esophagus has also been reported to occur after total gastrectomy, which indicates that reflux of gastric contents is not necessarily required.

The pathogenesis of Barrett esophagus has been the subject of speculation by many authors. Direct metaplasia of squamous epithelium into columnar epithelium has little good evidence to support it. On the other hand, destruction of acid-, pepsin-, and bile-sensitive squamous-lined mucosa by chronic gastroesophageal reflux followed by re-epithelization with more resistant columnar epithelium is supported by both clinical and experimental evidence. The "cell of origin" of the columnar epithelium has been debated in the literature. Migration of columnar cells from esophageal cardiac glands has been suggested on histologic grounds. Alternatively, however, migration of undifferentiated columnar progenitor cells from adjacent gastric and Barrett mucosa into an ulcerated area, followed by their differentiation to columnar epithelial cells of various types, is more consistent with the usual mechanisms of mucosal healing. Migration of squamous progenitor cells from the adjacent squamous epithelium probably occurs simultaneously, but in the abnormal milieu of ongoing reflux-induced injury, the columnar progenitor cells may have selective advantage.

Totipotentiality of the undifferentiated cells is another possible explanation, in that the cells may differentiate into either columnar or squamous cells, depending on the milieu. Proliferation of connective tissue cells occurs to form lamina propria of the Barrett mucosa. Over time, intestinalization appears to occur in the columnar epithelium, which often is initially gastric in type.

Whatever the precise mechanism, Barrett mucosa is metaplastic columnar-lined mucosa that has replaced the original squamous-lined mucosa, provides greater resistance to the effects of gastroesophageal reflux, and can undergo further metaplasia to intestinal-type differentiation. Differences among patients in severity and location of reflux-induced injury and in the characteristics of the repair process probably influence the mucosal remodeling. The dynamic nature of this pathogenetic process in turn may account for the variability of Barrett esophagus, including the topography of

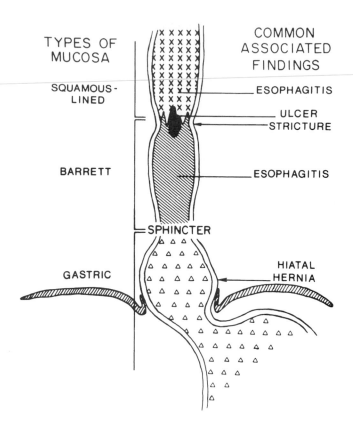

Figure 20.30 Diagrammatic representation of Barrett esophagus. The columnar-lined mucosa acquired secondary to gastroesophageal reflux extends from the lower esophageal sphincter zone into the esophagus for variable distances. Other findings associated with Barrett mucosa include ulcer, stricture, reflux esophagitis in both squamous-lined mucosa and Barrett mucosa, and hiatal hernia.

Barrett mucosa; the variable association with ulcer, stricture, and esophagitis; and the variable histopathologic features of the Barrett mucosa (see subsequent discussion).

Barrett esophagus is best considered as a morphologic (and therefore endoscopic and surgical) syndrome with a variety of possible components (Fig. 20.30). The sine qua non is columnar epithelium-lined lower esophagus. By definition, the squamocolumnar junction on the mucosal surface is located above the anatomic esophagogastric junction. Barrett mucosa can have a wide variety of topographic appearances. Classically, Barrett mucosa appears as a circumferential sheet resembling gastric mucosa without rugae that extends for variable distances into the esophagus above the lower esophageal sphincter zone; tongues, fingers, or even islands of Barrett mucosa involving only portions of the esophageal circumference occur frequently. Regardless of the topography, some portion of the Barrett mucosa generally occurs in continuity with the true gastric mucosa below it (although one exceptional case with Barrett mucosa in continuity with heterotopic gastric mucosa in the midesophagus has been reported). Islands of squamous-lined mucosa often remain within the columnar-lined region, attesting to the esophageal location.

The variable components of the Barrett syndrome are peptic ulcer, stricture, reflux esophagitis, and hiatal hernia. The Barrett ulcer is commonly seen at the squamocolumnar junction at the uppermost extent of the Barrett mucosa, but ulcers also occur within the columnar-lined region, sometimes in association with squamous-lined remnants. The Barrett stricture typically occurs at the uppermost extent of the Barrett mucosa, as a sequela of deep ulceration at that site. Occasionally, more than one stricture is seen, presumably as a result of more than one area of ulceration or repeated episodes. Spasm of the muscularis propria sometimes produces radiographic or endoscopic evidence of a stricture that is not present on a pathologic examination.

Reflux esophagitis can involve the squamous-lined mucosa above the uppermost extent of the Barrett mucosa as well as the columnar-lined mucosa itself. This finding represents the consequence of ongoing reflux of gastric contents into the esophagus (see discussion of reflux esophagitis). Hiatal hernia, characterized by extension of stomach through the diaphragmatic hiatus into the thoracic cavity, may be subtle or obvious. A key aspect of the diagnosis of Barrett esophagus is recognition that the columnar-lined esophagus may be associated with none, some, or all of the other components of the morphologic Barrett syndrome.

HISTOPATHOLOGIC FEATURES

A bewildering array of terminology for Barrett mucosa has been used in the literature because of the wide spectrum of histopathologic features that can be seen. The types of cells identified in the epithelium of Barrett mucosa include gastric-type columnar mucus-containing cells, which stain with PAS and sometimes with alcian blue, pH 2.5 (AB), and mucicarmine; intestinal-type goblet cells, which stain with PAS, AB, and mucicarmine; columnar epithelial cells with a brush border and no mucus vacuoles, similar to small-intestinal absorptive epithelial cells; Paneth cells, with their characteristic eosinophilic cytoplasmic granules; parietal and chief cells; and neuroendocrine cells, which can be argyrophil, argentaffin, and enterochromaffin, and which contain various hormones as noted by immunohistochemistry, including somatostatin, serotonin, substance P, enkephalin, and gastrin. The cell types identified by light microscopy in Barrett epithelium thus include various constituents of normal gastric and small-intestinal epithelium.

The macroscopic architecture of Barrett mucosa can include glands with deep and shallow pits, as in gastric mucosa, and villous structures resembling small-intestinal mucosa. The lamina propria of all types of Barrett mucosa can show varying severity of congestion, edema, acute and chronic inflammation, and fibrosis. These findings appear to be related to ongoing reflux-induced injury. Acute inflammation involving the epithelium is often accompanied by reactive epithelial changes that can be misinterpreted as dysplasia. Chronic inflammatory cells in the lamina propria may include plasma cells, lymphocytes, and eosinophils with scattered histiocytes and mast cells.

A variety of mucosa histopathology can be seen in any one patient, forming a mosaic or zonal arrangement of mucosal types. Barrett mucosa also shows wide variation in histopathologic appearance among patients. Although it has shortcomings owing to the arbitrary pigeonholing of specimens representing a continuum of findings, the classification shown in Table 20.5 can be used for Barrett mucosa.

Distinctive-type Barrett mucosa has a villiform configuration and cryptlike glands (Figs. 20.31A). The villous structures vary widely in appearance, and the glands vary in number. The glands are often contiguous with the muscularis mucosae, and no intervening connective tissue is present in many examples. This appearance contrasts with the findings in the usual squamous-lined esophageal mucosa and appears to be a manifestation of previous ulceration of the lamina propria with epithelial regeneration directly on the smooth muscle. The glands may show cystic dilatation, particularly with active inflammation of the epithelium resulting in gland abscesses.

The epithelium of the villous structures and glands is usually composed in large part of columnar mucous cells with PAS-staining gastric-type mucin. Goblet cells that stain with PAS, AB, and mucicarmine are both interspersed among and contiguous with the columnar mucous cells (see Fig. 20.31B). This distinctive epithelial morphologic appearance with interspersed goblet cells is identical to that of incomplete intestinal metaplasia of gastric

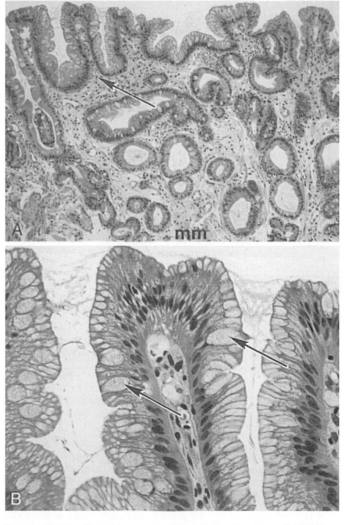

Figure 20.31 Barrett mucosa of the distinctive type. **A.** Villiform architecture *(arrow)* with subjacent glands is evident. The glands adjoin the muscularis mucosae (mm). **B.** High-power view of the area indicated by the arrow in part A. The distinctive-type epithelium is characterized by goblet cells *(arrows)* interspersed among columnar mucous cells.

mucosa, but contrasts with that of complete intestinal metaplasia, in which the columnar mucous cells are inapparent in intestinalized glands by light microscopy. The characteristic interspersed goblet cells allow histopathologic recognition of distinctive-type Barrett mucosa.

The proportion of goblet cells varies widely, and absorptive cells also accompany the goblet cells. In some examples, the intestinalized cells dominate the epithelial morphology. Paneth cells may be seen, usually in association with numerous goblet cells, small-intestinal-type columnar absorptive cells, and relatively few columnar mucous cells; these findings appear to represent advanced intestinalization. Plump columnar cells with prominent mucin vacuoles that resemble goblet cells in H & E-stained sections but do not stain with AB are seen in some cases. An array of argyrophil, argentaffin, and enterochromaffin cells is present; these endocrine cells are most numerous in the glands. A few parietal and chief cells may be scattered through the epithelium of the glands. The distinctive-type Barrett mucosa is present in the majority of adult patients with Barrett esophagus but is found less frequently in children, providing evidence for the occurrence of intestinalization over time.

Cardiac-type Barrett mucosa, as the name implies, resembles gastric cardiac mucosa (Fig. 20.32). This type of Barrett mucosa sometimes contains deep pits, which may produce a villiform configuration. Mucus-containing epithelial cells are the predominant cell type in both surface and glandular epithelium. Endocrine cells are present, and scattered parietal and chief cells can occur. Goblet cells are scarce, and if present, are widely scattered, although intestinal-type mucin staining with AB or mucicarmine can be seen in columnar mucous cells (the precise border between distinctive-type and cardiac-type Barrett mucosa is arbitrary). Features of cardiac-type Barrett mucosa that differ from those of normal gastric cardiac mucosa include glandular distortion, edema, and chronic inflammation.

Fundic-type Barrett mucosa appears to be the least common form. As the name implies, the mucosa resembles gastric fundic mucosa in having shallow pits lined by mucus-containing columnar cells and a heavy complement of parietal and chief cells in the glands. Like cardiac-type Barrett mucosa, the fundic-type mucosa often lacks a completely normal configuration, showing distorted or short glands and a villiform surface. Endocrine cells are present; intestinal differentiation is absent.

A zonal distribution of Barrett mucosa has been suggested in some patients: the distinctive-type mucosa occurs most proximally, the fundic type most distally, and the cardiac-type mucosa interposed between the other two. Studies of resection specimens, however, rather than biopsy specimens with their inherent sampling problem, revealed a mosaic distribution of the various types of mucosa.

The category of *indeterminate-type Barrett mucosa* is provided because of the wide spectrum of histopathologic features; peculiar configurations and types of epithelium are found in some patients. As a result, a particular specimen may not meet precisely the criteria of the first three categories. For example, foci of complete intestinal differentiation manifested by goblet cells and small-intestinal columnar cells without interspersed columnar mucous cells sometimes occur in Barrett mucosa that would otherwise be classified as cardiac-type or fundic-type. In other cases, small-intestinal-type mucin that stains strongly with AB occurs in columnar mucous cells in the absence of recognizable goblet cells. Because the characteristic pattern of goblet cells interspersed with columnar mucous cells is absent, categorization as distinctive-type does not seem justified,

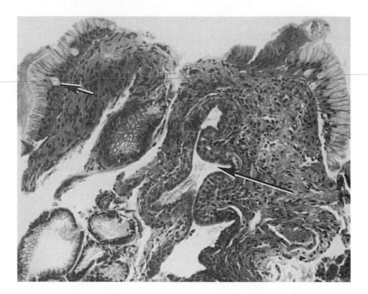

Figure 20.32 Cardiac-type Barrett mucosa. The cardiac-type epithelium is composed of columnar mucous cells, some of which have distended vacuoles *(short arrow).* The mucosal architecture is abnormal, with fibrosis and chronic inflammation in the lamina propria. The squamous-lined duct *(long arrow)* of an esophageal submucosal gland localizes the specimen to the esophagus.

although some authors accept this criterion. Biopsy sampling often plays a role in these troublesome cases, because specimens from other areas of the Barrett mucosa may show the usual distinctive-type, cardiac-type, or fundic-type mucosa. The presence of dysplasia can also lead to classification of Barrett mucosa as indeterminate type by obscuring the characteristics of the antecedent columnar epithelium.

ULTRASTRUCTURAL STUDIES

Transmission electron-microscopic studies of the epithelial and endocrine cells in Barrett mucosa have been reported. The findings confirm those of light microscopy. Scanning electron-microscopic studies produce spectacular views of the mucosal and epithelial surfaces.

HISTOPATHOLOGIC DIAGNOSIS

The diagnosis of Barrett esophagus is as much a matter of specimen site as histopathologic findings in the specimen. The pathologist examining a surgical resection specimen or autopsy specimen can identify the location of a tissue sample submitted for histology. In addition, histopathologic landmarks in the esophageal wall are available to aid in localization (e.g., esophageal submucosal glands, twisting of the muscle fibers of the muscularis propria in the lower esophageal sphincter zone). For biopsy specimens, however, the pathologist depends on the endoscopist for the site from which the specimen is taken. Mural structures are rarely accessible to mucosal biopsy. In the proper setting, mucosa with the histopathologic features of gastric cardiac or fundic mucosa represents cardiac-type or fundic-type Barrett mucosa, respectively, if the specimen was taken from a site above the anatomic esophagogastric junction. Such is not the case if the biopsy tissue was taken from the gastric cardia or a hiatal hernia pouch. Ideally, interpretation of biopsy specimens requires demonstration of the lower esophageal sphincter zone, preferably by manometry, and documentation by the endoscopist of the topography and location of the suspected columnar-lined areas, including the biopsy sites. Diagrammatic documentation by the endoscopist is particularly helpful when biopsies are taken during serial follow-up endoscopies for monitoring effects of therapy and development of dysplasia (see subsequent discussion).

Some clinical situations make diagnosis difficult. The presence of a stricture at the upper extent of the Barrett mucosa may prohibit further advancement of the endoscope so that directed biopsies can be obtained. Patients with a short segment of Barrett mucosa in the region of the esophagogastric junction pose the greatest problem in diagnosis. The definition of Barrett esophagus as columnar-lined lower esophagus acquired secondary to chronic gastroesophageal reflux does not translate easily into diagnostic criteria because the acquired pathogenesis is not often evident in the histopathologic findings.

The criteria for diagnosis of Barrett esophagus include histopathologic findings, specimen localization, and topography of the columnar-lined mucosa. The histopathologic findings are (a) the presence of distinctive-type Barrett mucosa or (b) demonstration of other columnar-lined mucosa with histopathologic features appropriate for Barrett mucosa (Table 20.5). Also needed are endoscopic localization of the biopsy site to the esophagus and endoscopic demonstration of at least a portion of the columnar-lined mucosa in continuity with gastric mucosa (see discussion of differential diagnosis).

Distinctive-type Barrett mucosa in an esophageal biopsy specimen is usually diagnostic of Barrett esophagus. In the absence of distinctive-type mucosa, appropriate histopathologic findings include the presence of any of the other types of Barrett mucosa, including cardiac-type and fundic-type. In this situation, however, endoscopic localization of the biopsy sites to the esophagus is also needed, preferably with manometric demonstration of the lower esophageal sphincter zone, which usually occurs only in research settings. Occasionally, biopsy specimens can be localized to the esophagus on the histopathologic basis of esophageal submucosal glands (not cardiac glands) with their characteristic AB-staining epithelium or their squamous-lined ducts beneath the columnar-lined mucosa in the specimen (see Fig. 20.32). The ducts alone are sometimes seen in the mucosa. Also, when circumferential biopsy samples are taken at the same level of the esophagus, the presence of

squamous-lined mucosa along with another specimen showing presumed Barrett mucosa at the same level increases confidence that the biopsy specimens were from esophagus originally lined by squamous epithelium. If gastric biopsies accompany the esophageal biopsies, the finding of intestinal differentiation in the candidate esophageal columnar-lined mucosa in the absence of gastric mucosal intestinalization provides circumstantial histopathologic evidence favoring Barrett mucosa. Finally, endoscopic demonstration of at least part of the columnar-lined mucosa in continuity with gastric mucosa favors Barrett esophagus rather than gastric heterotopia.

Additional circumstantial evidence for Barrett esophagus, which may be absent in some cases, includes demonstration of gastroesophageal reflux, demonstration of ulceration and/or a stricture at the upper extent of the columnar-lined mucosa, evidence of reflux esophagitis in the squamous-lined mucosa above the columnar-lined region, and the presence of a hiatal hernia (see Fig. 20.30).

Some authors require the presence of 2 or 3 cm of cardiac-type or fundic-type mucosa for a diagnosis of Barrett esophagus. These numeric definitions do not permit recognition of short-segment Barrett esophagus unless distinctive-type mucosa is present. Such definitions are not applicable in pediatric patients, who often lack distinctive-type mucosa and have a much shorter esophagus than do adults.

DIFFERENTIAL DIAGNOSIS

As discussed previously, the distinctive-type Barrett mucosa in an esophageal specimen is essentially diagnostic of Barrett esophagus. Other types of columnar epithelium-lined mucosa in specimens of the esophagus can represent the following:

1. *True gastric cardiac or fundic mucosa.* In this situation, the specimen was usually obtained from a hiatal hernia pouch that was mistaken for esophagus by the endoscopist or pathologist. For this reason, manometric localization of the LES zone is highly desirable in evaluating patients for Barrett esophagus but rarely is done. This type of mucosa cannot be differentiated reliably from Barrett mucosa of the cardiac or fundic type by histopathology alone.
2. *Embryonic ciliated cell rests.* These rests represent remnants of the columnar epithelium that lines the embryonic

TABLE					
20.5	**Histopathologic Classification of Barrett Mucosa**				
Category	Typical Macroscopic Configuration	Predominant Glandular Epithelial Cells	Predominant Surface Epithelial Cells	Evidence of Intestinal Differentiation
Distinctive-type	Villous structures and cryptlike glands	Columnar mucous	Goblet interspersed among columnar mucous	Goblet cells Absorptive cells Paneth cells (variable)
Cardiac-type	Glands with deep pits	Columnar mucous	Columnar mucous	Absent
Fundic-type	Glands with shallow pits	Parietal, chief	Columnar mucous	Absent
Indeterminate-type	Variable	Variable	Variable	Variable

esophagus until about the seventh fetal month, when replacement by squamous epithelium typically is completed. Such rests are incidental findings, usually in the upper esophagus of young children. Cilia can be identified on the luminal surface of the columnar epithelial cells, and the epithelium is simplistic, with only occasional well-formed glands. This type of epithelium is not seen in Barrett esophagus.

3. *Tracheobronchial remnants.* Esophageal strictures attributable to tracheobronchial remnants in the lower esophagus rarely occur (Fig. 20.33). The surface epithelium sometimes shows pseudostratified ciliated columnar epithelium of the type present in the respiratory tract, and the remnants often contain cartilage. This type of mucosa is not seen in Barrett esophagus. In many cases, squamous epithelium overlies the remnants that are located deep in the wall and are not obtainable by biopsy.

4. *Gastric heterotopia (ectopia).* Gastric epithelium or mucosa can occur in the esophagus, presumably as a result of misplacement or abnormal differentiation during embryonic development. Small foci of columnar epithelium may be interspersed in the squamous epithelium, particularly in the upper esophagus. Heterotopic mucosa can be composed of fundic-, transitional-, or antral-type glands. Peptic ulceration and adenocarcinoma can be complications of gastric heterotopia, further confusing the distinction from Barrett esophagus. The endoscopic demonstration of columnar-lined mucosa in continuity with gastric mucosa provides evidence favoring Barrett esophagus, although islands of true Barrett mucosa may be formed during the ongoing process of injury and repair in the esophagus. Interpretation of findings in the esophagogastric junction region is also complicated by the common occurrence of esophageal cardiac glands, which can be interspersed with the squamous epithelium.

The pathologist's diagnosis for biopsy specimens with columnar-lined mucosa said to be from the esophagus must take into account the endoscopist's observations. The biopsy report should indicate the type of columnar-lined mucosa and whether or not dysplasia is present or suspected if the specimen is thought to represent Barrett mucosa (see following section). Biopsy specimens showing the distinctive type of Barrett mucosa can be reported as such, e.g., "Barrett mucosa of the distinctive type. Negative for dysplasia." Specimens with cardiac- or fundic-type mucosa can be reported for interpretation in light of other clinical evidence, e.g., "Cardiac-type mucosa consistent with Barrett mucosa if the specimen was obtained from the esophagus. Negative for dysplasia." Specimens showing mucosa of other types can be reported descriptively.

DYSPLASIA AND ADENOCARCINOMA IN BARRETT MUCOSA

The association between adenocarcinoma and Barrett esophagus (Fig. 20.34) is now well recognized following publication of numerous case reports and a study series. Barrett esophagus can be termed a "premalignant condition," i.e., a clinical state that increases the risk of cancer. The factors producing the high risk are not as yet known; white men constitute the majority of patients with Barrett carcinoma, in contrast to squamous carcinoma of the

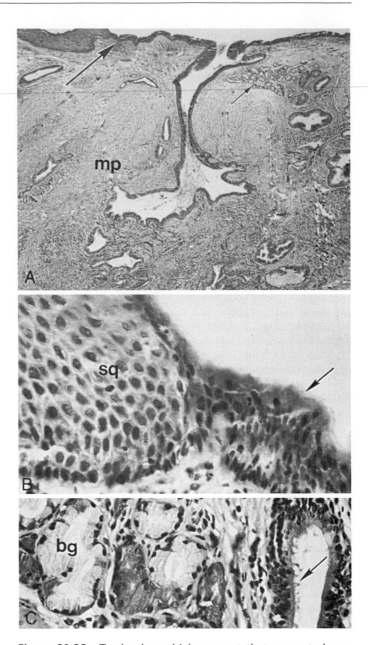

Figure 20.33   Tracheobronchial remnant that presented as a distal esophageal stricture in an adult. **A.** Ciliated respiratory epithelium is present on the esophageal luminal surface (*large arrow*) and lines cystic spaces, which extend through the muscularis propria (mp) into periesophageal soft tissue. Bronchial glands (*small arrow*) accompany the respiratory epithelium-lined structures. Islands of cartilage were present in other areas. **B.** Junction of squamous epithelium (sq) and respiratory epithelium on the esophageal luminal surface in area indicated by large arrow in upper panel. Cilia (*arrow*) are evident on the apical surface of the respiratory epithelium. **C.** Bronchial glands (bg) accompany respiratory epithelium-lined structures with ciliated epithelium (*arrow*).

esophagus, in which nonwhites predominate. The possible role of alcohol and tobacco, as in squamous carcinoma of the esophagus, has been raised. In many patients, adenocarcinoma arising in Barrett esophagus is accompanied by dysplasia (esophageal columnar intraepithelial neoplasia) in the surrounding Barrett mucosa. Sequential biopsy specimens have demonstrated development of adenocarcinoma in some patients who initially had dysplasia alone. As a result, a dysplasia-carcinoma sequence is associated with Barrett mucosa, as occurs generally in carcinogenesis involving epithelial surfaces. The natural history of dysplasia remains to be defined precisely, but based on available data, the dysplasia-adenocarcinoma sequence appears to occur over a few years. In addition to adenocarcinoma, squamous carcinoma of the esophagus has been reported in patients with Barrett esophagus.

As used here, the term "dysplasia" indicates a neoplastic abnormality. Dysplasia in Barrett mucosa is characterized histopathologically by abnormalities in mucosal architecture, epithelial characteristics, and epithelial cell cytology (Figs. 20.35 to 20.39). The presence of proliferated or bizarrely shaped glands and villiform structures is common in dysplastic Barrett mucosa, which resembles adenomas of other sites in the gastrointestinal tract. The epithelium is hypercellular, with stratified, enlarged, irregular, pleomorphic nuclei showing loss of polarity, hyperchromatism with abnormal distribution of chromatin, and prominent nucleoli. Epithelial differentiation is also abnormal, because cytoplasmic mucin is generally decreased in amount and, when present, often occurs in relatively apical vacuoles of relatively uniform size. This appearance contrasts with that of the prominent mucin in columnar cells and goblet cells of Barrett mucosa without dysplasia. The architectural and epithelial features often produce an adenomatous appearance of dysplastic Barrett mucosa. In other cases, the dysplasia has vesicular nuclei without prominent hypercellularity and stratification. The features of Barrett dysplasia are similar in many respects to dysplasia in gastric mucosa (see also Chapters 19, 20, and 25). The type of dysplastic Barrett mucosa, i.e., distinctive or cardiac, is often difficult to determine because of the replacement of the antecedent epithelium; therefore, the dysplasia is of indeterminate type.

Histopathologic assessment of dysplasia in Barrett mucosa is complicated by the occurrence of nonneoplastic reactive epithelial changes (Fig. 20.40). Reactive changes are often associated with active inflammation, owing to persistent gastroesophageal reflux with reflux esophagitis involving the Barrett mucosa. The problem of distinguishing the effects of inflammation from dysplasia is similar to that encountered with inflammatory bowel disease. Therefore, the terminology for classification of colonic biopsy specimens developed by the Inflammatory Bowel Disease-Dysplasia Morphology Study Group (see Chapter 29) is also useful for specimens of Barrett mucosa. Specimens are classified as "negative for dysplasia," "indefinite for dysplasia," or "positive for dysplasia." The negative for dysplasia category includes those specimens with reactive epithelial changes associated with active inflammation. The phrase "Indefinite for dysplasia" is applied to specimens about which there is uncertainty as to whether the epithelial abnormalities represent reactive changes or dysplasia. Uncertainty can arise from the nature of the histopathologic abnormalities or technical problems with specimen processing, such as poor orientation. The indefinite category is particularly useful in allowing pathologists to express simultaneously their concern and uncertainty about the nature of the epithelial abnormalities, thereby heightening endoscopists' awareness of the need for additional evaluation. The indefinite category can be subdivided into "probably negative," "unknown (no choice)," and "probably positive" to allow expression of the degree of concern, although intra- and interobserver variation may hinder the utility of this subdivision. Specimens with unequivocal

dysplasia are categorized as low-grade, intermediate-grade, or high-grade on the basis of the severity of the abnormalities and their reported relationship to invasive adenocarcinoma (some authors use only two grades, low and high, to attempt to improve on reproducibility of classification).

The histopathologic criteria for classifying biopsy specimens as indefinite or positive often require interpretation of epithelial

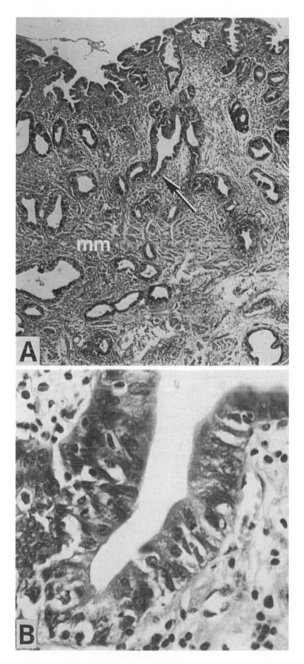

Figure 20.34 Adenocarcinoma arising in Barrett esophagus. **A.** Adenocarcinoma infiltrates the muscularis mucosae (mm) and the submucosa. The overlying Barrett mucosa has distorted glands *(arrow)* lined by dysplastic epithelium that appear to give rise to the submucosal invasion and may represent intramucosal adenocarcinoma. **B.** High-power view of the gland indicated by the arrow in part A. The epithelium is hypercellular, with stratified, cytologically atypical, irregular nuclei with loss of polarity.

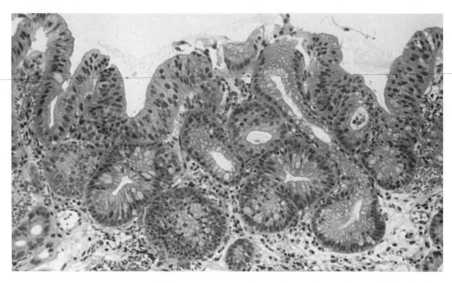

Figure 20.35 Low-grade epithelial dysplasia (esophageal columnar intraepithelial neoplasia) in Barrett mucosa of the distinctive type. The villous structures are blunt and short, and there is proliferation of glands, which are in close proximity to each other. The epithelium is mildly hypercellular, with full-thickness stratification of small and relatively uniform nuclei characterized by mild pleomorphism and loss of polarity. Mucous vacuoles are evident in the cytoplasm of the dysplastic epithelial cells.

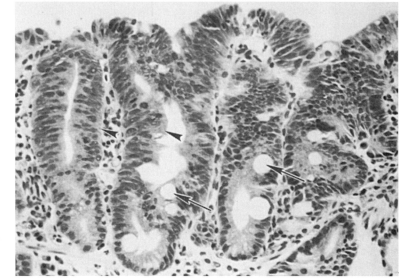

Figure 20.36 Intermediate-grade epithelial dysplasia (esophageal columnar intraepithelial neoplasia) in Barrett mucosa of the distinctive type. The mucosal architecture is characterized by relatively uniform glands with no villous structures. The dysplastic epithelium is hypercellular with full-thickness stratification *(arrowheads)* of moderately pleomorphic nuclei. Goblet cells *(arrows)* remain in the epithelium.

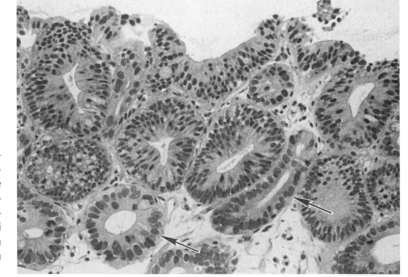

Figure 20.37 Intermediate-grade dysplasia (esophageal columnar intraepithelial neoplasia) in Barrett mucosa of the distinctive type. The mucosal architecture is characterized by glandular proliferation. The dysplastic epithelium is moderately hypercellular, with full-thickness stratification of relatively uniform small nuclei except in some glands, where nuclear enlargement with prominent nucleoli is evident *(arrows)*. Epithelial mucin content is markedly reduced.

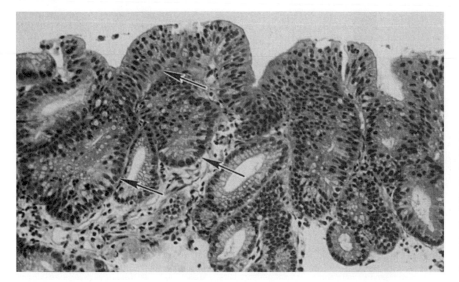

Figure 20.38 High-grade dysplasia (esophageal columnar intraepithelial neoplasia) in Barrett mucosa of the distinctive type. The mucosal architecture shows blunt villi with proliferated glands. The epithelium is markedly hypercellular with full-thickness stratification of hyperchromatic nuclei. Enlarged nuclei with prominent nucleoli are present in some areas *(arrows)*, including the surface epithelium. Epithelial mucin content is reduced.

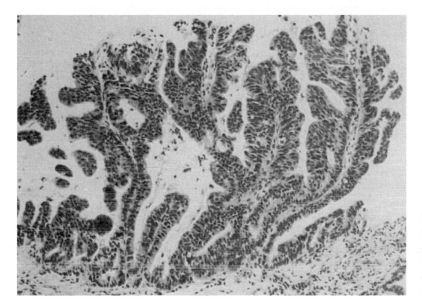

Figure 20.39 High-grade epithelial dysplasia (esophageal columnar intraepithelial neoplasia) in Barrett mucosa of indeterminate type. Bizarre villiform and papillary structures are lined by markedly hypercellular epithelium with full-thickness stratification of small, hyperchromatic and pleomorphic nuclei.

abnormalities in the context of active inflammation. If an ulcer, erosion, or more than a few neutrophils are present in the Barrett mucosa, careful consideration should precede classification of a biopsy specimen as positive. The criteria for separating high-grade, intermediate-grade, and low-grade dysplasia are also arbitrary but include severity of mucosal architectural disturbance, epithelial cellularity, and extent of stratification of nuclei, along with loss of polarity, prominent nuclear enlargement, irregularity, pleomorphism, hyperchromatism, and nucleolar enlargement. The implications of the categories for patient management are discussed in the section concerning biopsies for monitoring Barrett mucosa. The presence of mucosal invasion (intramucosal adenocarcinoma) can be difficult to distinguish from high-grade dysplasia. Such invasion (Fig. 20.41) mandates consideration of therapeutic, rather than prophylactic, esophagectomy.

Various methods have been applied to attempt to improve on the identification of dysplasia as evidence of neoplastic change in Barrett mucosa. These methods include markers of epithelial

proliferation, histochemical and immunohistochemical studies of epithelial mucin and carcinoembryonic antigen expression, assay for ornithine decarboxylase (ODC, the rate-limiting enzyme in polyamine biosynthesis), and flow cytometry and image analysis for altered total DNA content in nuclei. DNA aneuploidy and ODC activity are currently the most promising markers in the hands of some investigators.

Additional discussion of dysplasia and carcinoma in Barrett esophagus is presented in Chapter 22.

BIOPSIES FOR MONITORING BARRETT MUCOSA

Two major types of complications occur in patients with Barrett esophagus:

1. Peptic complications of ulceration, including resultant hemorrhage, penetration into mediastinal structures,

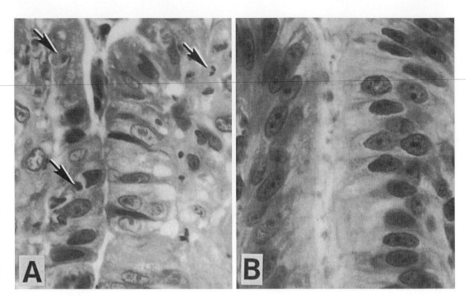

Figure 20.40 Comparison of reactive and dysplastic Barrett epithelium. **A.** Reactive epithelium. In this example, adjoining an active chronic ulcer in distinctive-type Barrett mucosa, the striking abnormalities include full-thickness stratification of vesicular nuclei with prominent nucleoli. Polymorphonuclear leukocytes *(arrows)* are present. **B.** High-grade dysplasia in Barrett mucosa of indeterminate type. The enlarged nuclei have striking cytologic abnormalities, including hyperchromatism and irregular, multiple nucleoli. (Same magnification in parts A and B.)

stricture formation, and continued upward extension of Barrett mucosa.

2. Neoplastic complication of development of dysplasia and adenocarcinoma (see previous discussion). After the diagnosis of Barrett esophagus is made, endoscopic biopsies are often obtained to monitor the effects of antireflux therapy and development of neoplasia.

With effective antireflux therapy, active inflammation, erosion, and ulceration in Barrett mucosa as well as in the squamous-lined mucosa above it decrease in severity. Biopsy evaluation of the squamous-lined region is important after therapy, as diminishing epithelial injury in the esophagus above Barrett mucosa may prevent further upward extension. Regression of Barrett mucosa and replacement by squamous-lined mucosa after antireflux surgery or after medical antireflux therapy, including use of a drug that improves LES function, has been reported but appears to be uncommon. Documentation of cases of such regression, however, is strongly dependent on localizing the biopsies to the same level of the esophagus on different occasions. Surgical manipulation of the esophagus complicates assessment of the biopsy site because of possible changes in distances from the incisors. Thus, interpretation of the obtaining of columnar-lined mucosa on one occasion and squamous-lined mucosa at a later endoscopy as evidence of regression requires caution.

Although controversial, surveillance for dysplasia and adenocarcinoma is now generally regarded as part of management of patients with Barrett esophagus. In most patients without surveillance, adenocarcinoma arising in Barrett esophagus is advanced at the time of presentation, and survival is poor. The hope of improved outcome rests on early detection and prevention of the columnar epithelial dysplasia-adenocarcinoma sequence. As a result, yearly surveillance endoscopy is often recommended on an empiric basis for patients known to have Barrett esophagus. The decision to undertake surveillance should be made only when the patient's overall physical condition would permit a "prophylactic" esophagectomy to remove Barrett esophagus with premalignancy or early malignancy. If the patient is not a candidate for treatment because

of other medical problems, surveillance is pointless. Patients should continue surveillance even if they are receiving antireflux therapy and are asymptomatic, because there is little evidence for lessening of the neoplastic predilection of Barrett mucosa by successful therapy.

The overall impact of surveillance on the incidence of and mortality from adenocarcinoma arising in Barrett esophagus remains to be assessed. In our series and those of other investigators, a sizable minority of Barrett patients with adenocarcinoma would not have been included in a surveillance program: these patients were recognized to have Barrett esophagus only after they presented with adenocarcinoma arising in it. Such patients did not have a previous history of symptomatic gastroesophageal reflux or reflux esophagitis to bring them to medical attention. Such patients cannot benefit from even an optimal surveillance program. On the other hand, the few patients in whom dysplasia and adenocarcinoma have developed during surveillance have a good outcome if esophagectomy is performed successfully. Surveillance of the large bowel is also a consideration because of several reports indicating increased prevalence of colorectal adenomas and carcinomas in patients with Barrett esophagus.

In the evaluation of dysplasia, cytologic specimens obtained by brushing as well as multiple biopsy specimens appear to be useful in sampling large surface areas of Barrett mucosa. Invasive adenocarcinoma may develop in Barrett mucosa with dysplasia, which is less severe than carcinoma in situ, and invasion may be difficult to recognize owing to the shallowness of biopsy specimens and the tendency of carcinoma to "drop off" beneath an area of dysplasia (see Fig. 20.34). As a result, confirmed high-grade dysplasia in biopsy specimens should raise the question of performing "prophylactic" esophagectomy, because about one third to one half of patients with biopsy diagnosis of high-grade dysplasia will be found to have adenocarcinoma in their esophagectomy specimen. The occurrence of synchronous adenocarcinoma and dysplasia is more frequent in patients who are found to have dysplasia when the diagnosis of Barrett esophagus is first made (prevalent cases of dysplasia) than in those in whom dysplasia develops under surveillance (incident cases of dysplasia). Expected operative morbidity and mortality in the particular patient under consideration in the hands of the clinicians managing the patient are the major determinants of outcome.

MOTOR AND RELATED DISORDERS OF THE ESOPHAGUS

ACHALASIA

This condition is characterized by two defects. First, the LES provides an impediment to flow because of spasm and/or failure of relaxation. Second, the lower two thirds of the esophagus, representing the portion with smooth muscle, shows failure of normal peristalsis with contraction but no progressive peristalsis. Investigation of the neuropathologic changes in the esophageal wall in achalasia reveals abnormalities that include decreased or absent ganglion cells in the myenteric plexus and the presence in ganglion cells of Lewy bodies of the type seen in the brain of patients with Parkinson disease. Dilatation of the middle and upper esophagus and hypertrophy of the muscularis propria (Fig. 20.42) are attributable to the functional obstruction in the distal esophagus. Findings related to previous therapy may be seen: some patients develop reflux esophagitis after dilatation (see Fig. 20.42).

Endoscopic biopsies in patients with presumed achalasia may be performed at the time of initial evaluation because of the possibility of tumor in the esophagogastric junction region as the cause of the clinical picture. In addition, patients with achalasia appear to have an increased incidence of squamous carcinoma of the esophagus, and biopsies sometimes are performed to evaluate dysplasia (see Chapter 21). Specimens show the effects of chronic stasis on the esophageal mucosa (Fig. 20.43), as also occurs with Chagas disease and above strictures of various causes. Reactive epithelial changes and balloon cells, sometimes with active inflammation, may be present. Food material, *Candida,* and bacteria are sometimes seen on the luminal surface. The pearly white mucosal surface may have a corrugated appearance, and squamous papillomas have been reported. In long-standing cases, findings may include cornification and keratinization of the surface epithelial layers.

RINGS AND WEBS

Constrictions of the esophageal lumen, found at any level of the esophagus, may be formed by mucosal rings, which do not involve the muscularis propria; muscular or contractile rings; by ringlike peptic strictures; and benign tumors. Upper esophageal webs may be found in patients without or with anemia, the latter referred to as Paterson-Kelly or Plummer-Vinson syndrome. The histopathologic findings in such webs include reactive epithelial changes with proliferation of the basal zone, elongation of vascular papillae, and parakeratosis, along with chronic inflammation, fibrosis, and

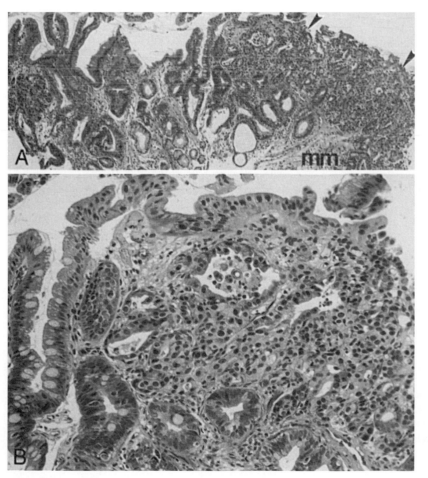

Figure 20.41 Adenocarcinoma invading lamina propria of distinctive-type Barrett mucosa. **A.** This esophageal biopsy specimen shows obliteration of Barrett glands by infiltrating adenocarcinoma *(arrowheads)* which does not breach the muscularis mucosae *(mm)* and is confined to the lamina propria. **B.** High-power view of intramucosal adenocarcinoma. The glandular architecture of the Barrett mucosa is replaced by the infiltrating glands of the adenocarcinoma involving the lamina propria.

hemosiderin deposition in the lamina propria. The nature of lower esophageal rings and webs is a matter of unresolved controversy, probably because of the variability of the pathologic findings. The "Schatzki ring" (Fig. 20.44) is reported by some authors to be located at the squamocolumnar junction; others describe the ring as lying within squamous-lined esophagus. Webs can be acquired as a result of severe esophageal injury from gastroesophageal reflux, radiation, lye-induced injury, and graft-versus-host disease.

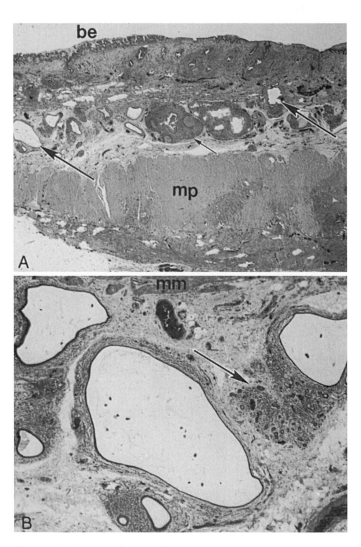

Figure 20.42 Achalasia with Barrett esophagus secondary to gastroesophageal reflux resulting from dilatation procedures and with intramural pseudodiverticulosis. **A.** Hypertrophy of the muscularis propria *(mp)* is evident. The Barrett esophagus *(be)* has cardiac-type and distinctive-type mucosa. Esophageal intramural pseudodiverticulosis is manifested by cystic dilatation of submucosal gland ducts *(large arrow)*, some of which have surrounding lymphoid tissue *(small arrow)*. **B.** Higher-power view of intramural pseudodiverticulosis. Dilatation of the squamous-lined ducts of the esophageal submucosal glands deep to the muscularis mucosae *(mm)* is accompanied by atrophy of the glands *(arrow)*.

DIVERTICULA

Traction and pulsion diverticula occur in the esophagus. Intramural pseudodiverticulosis results from cystic dilatation of the ducts of esophageal submucosal glands (see Fig. 20.42) in association with obstruction, which can result from candidiasis and other etiologies.

ESOPHAGEAL INVOLVEMENT BY SYSTEMIC DISEASES

COLLAGEN VASCULAR—CONNECTIVE TISSUE DISEASES

Esophageal motor abnormalities are a well-recognized feature of collagen vascular-connective tissue disease, particularly progressive systemic sclerosis (scleroderma), but also mixed connective tissue disease, systemic lupus erythematosus, rheumatoid arthritis, dermatomyositis, and Sjögren syndrome. Fibrous replacement of the outer layer of the muscularis propria is the characteristic finding in scleroderma. Ulcers and strictures can occur as primary manifestations of the diseases, particularly rheumatoid arthritis, ankylosing spondylitis, and Sjögren syndrome, as well as secondary to gastroesophageal reflux associated with abnormal function of the LES. The pathologic findings in the ulcers and strictures are usually etiologically nonspecific. In some cases, however, arteritis may be demonstrable. (See Chapter 19 for further details.)

CROHN DISEASE

The etiology of Crohn disease is unknown at the present time, but generalized mucosal abnormality of the gastrointestinal tract is a well-recognized characteristic of the disease. Some patients have clinically evident esophageal involvement; most have obvious evidence of Crohn disease elsewhere, but cases of only "regional esophagitis" have been reported. Crohn disease involving the esophagus generally shows the pathologic features found in other sites: discrete ulceration, fistulas, strictures, and transmural inflammation. Certain recognition depends on finding of a characteristic noncaseating epithelioid cell granuloma in the appropriate clinical setting (Table 20.6).

A wide range of pathologic abnormalities is seen in biopsy specimens, including nonspecific ulcers and active inflammation as well as characteristic granulomas, sometimes with multinucleated giant cells in the lamina propria or submucosa if it is included. Aphthoid ulcers have been reported, but biopsy specimens showed only intact squamous epithelium with acute inflammation. In one unusual case, Crohn disease of the esophagus occurred along with Barrett esophagus.

Crohn disease manifested by nonspecific ulceration or acute and chronic mucosal inflammation is difficult to identify because of the occurrence of so many other causes of esophagitis with similar or nonspecific findings that can also occur in patients who have Crohn disease (see outline at beginning of chapter). Furthermore, the shallow depth of both endoscopic and capsule biopsies precludes the specimen showing the characteristic abnormalities in the deep layers of the esophageal wall, which are important criteria for recognition of Crohn disease, especially in unusual sites.

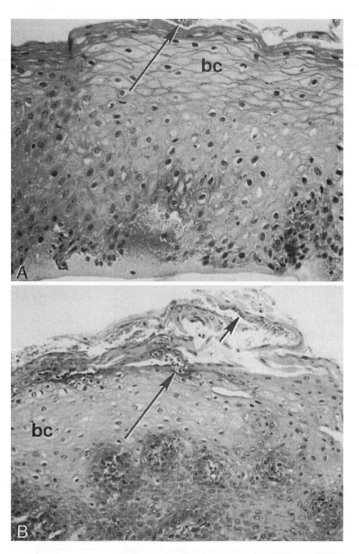

Figure 20.43 Squamous epithelial findings in achalasia. Food material (**A**, *arrow*) and bacterial colonies (**B**, *short arrow*) are present on the luminal surface. Polymorphonuclear leukocytes (**B**, *long arrow*) accompany the bacterial colonization. Balloon cells *(bc)* are present in the upper layers of the epithelium in both examples, along with reactive epithelial changes.

The chances of identifying a granuloma in specimens of Crohn disease are affected by many factors, including the occurrence of the granulomatous form of Crohn disease in the patient; the site, number, and size of the granulomas; the site, number, and size of the histopathologic specimens; the number of slides prepared; and the diligence with which the slides are examined. The differential diagnosis of granulomatous esophagitis (see Table 20.6) must be considered in patients thought to have Crohn disease involving the esophagus. (See Chapter 29 for further details.)

BEHÇET DISEASE

Recurrent ulcers of the mouth and genitalia associated with uveitis or iridocyclitis constitute Behçet disease. Differentiation from

Crohn disease is problematic. Esophageal ulcers occur in occasional patients but show only nonspecific inflammation and ulcer. Disordered esophageal motility has also been reported in association with a normal mucosal surface. (See Chapter 30 for further details.)

EOSINOPHILIC GASTROENTERITIS AND ESOPHAGITIS

Findings of esophageal involvement by eosinophilic gastroenteritis include the presence of eosinophils in any layer of the esophageal wall. Mucosal involvement is accompanied by reactive epithelial changes of basal zone proliferation and elongated vascular papillae. Of note in this regard, "eosinophilic esophagitis" is most commonly a result of gastroesophageal reflux with eosinophilic involvement of only the mucosa (see Table 20.4). Allergic esophagitis in the absence of eosinophilic gastroenteritis also occurs and involves the mucosa. Eosinophilic inflammation of the esophagus can be associated with drug injury.

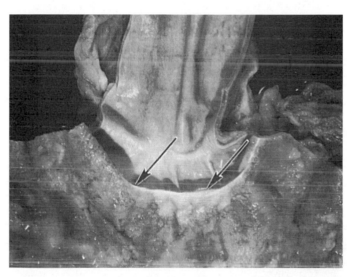

Figure 20.44 Lower esophageal ring. The shelflike circumferential ring *(arrows)* involves the esophagogastric junction and lower esophagus in this autopsy specimen, which was fixed before opening. Histopathology showed that the ring was formed of protruding mucosa and submucosa but not muscularis propria.

TABLE	
20.6	**Differential Diagnosis of Granulomatous Esophagitis**

Tuberculosis
Histoplasmosis
Blastomycosis
Foreign body reaction
Crohn disease
Sarcoidosis

TABLE	
20.7	**Dermatologic Diseases Affecting the Esophagus**

Bullous dermatoses
  Epidermolysis bullosa of the autosomal recessive dystrophic,
    acquired, and letalis types
  Pemphigus vulgaris
  Bullous pemphigoid
  Benign mucous membrane pemphigoid
  Familial benign chronic pemphigus
  Darier's disease (keratosis follicularis)
  Angina bullosa haemorrhagica
  Hailey-Hailey disease
Toxic epidermal necrolysis
Stevens-Johnson syndrome
Acanthosis nigricans
Tylosis (keratosis palmaris et plantaris)
Lichen sclerosis

DERMATOLOGIC DISEASES

Because the esophagus and skin both have squamous epithelium, it is not surprising that a variety of dermatologic diseases affect the esophagus (Table 20.7). In many patients, esophageal involvement accompanies skin disease, but occasionally, only the esophagus is affected. The findings generally resemble those in the skin (see Chapter 19). Tylosis is associated with increased incidence of esophageal carcinoma.

SARCOIDOSIS

The etiology of sarcoidosis is unknown. External compression of the esophagus by enlarged mediastinal lymph nodes as well as intrinsic involvement of the esophageal wall have been reported as causes of

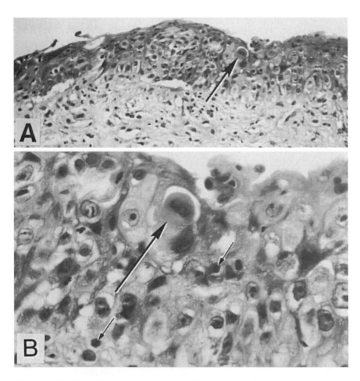

Figure 20.45 Graft-versus-host disease involving the esophagus 18 days after allogeneic bone marrow transplant. **A.** The squamous epithelium is thin, with focal detachment from the lamina propria and scattered dyskaryotic cells *(arrow)*. **B.** High-power view of the area indicated by the arrow in part A. The dyskaryotic cell *(large arrow)* has dense cytoplasm and nuclear degeneration. The epithelium is immature, with ovoid cells containing prominent nucleoli subjacent to the luminal surface. Lymphocytes *(small arrows)* representing infiltrating donor cells are present in the epithelium.

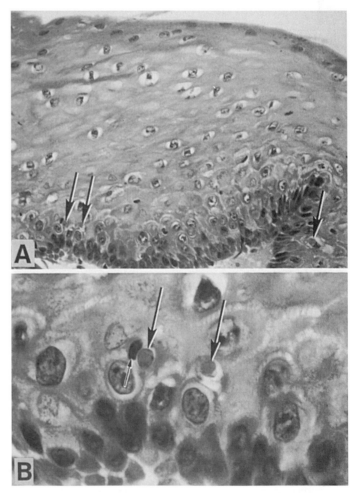

Figure 20.46 Mild graft-versus-host disease involving the esophagus 60 days after allogeneic bone marrow transplant. **A.** Epithelial maturation is abnormal, with immature cells at the luminal surface and hyperchromatic nuclei in the basal zone. Degenerating squamous epithelial cells *(arrows)* are present immediately above the basal zone. **B.** High-power view of the area indicated by arrows in part A. The degenerating epithelial cells *(large arrows)* are accompanied by a satellite donor lymphocyte *(small arrow)*.

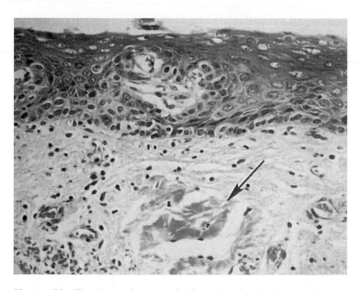

Figure 20.47   Secondary amyloidosis involving the esophagus. Amyloid *(arrow)* is present in the wall of a vein in the lamina propria.

symptoms in some patients. With intrinsic involvement, the characteristic noncaseating epithelioid cell granulomas can occur in the lamina propria and submucosa, where they are detectable by biopsy, as well as in the deeper layers of the esophageal wall. The differential diagnosis of esophageal granulomas is presented in Table 20.6. (See also Chapter 19.)

IMMUNODEFICIENCY

In addition to the variety of infectious agents that can affect the esophagus in immunocompromised patients, nonspecific ulcers have also been described.

GRAFT-VERSUS-HOST DISEASE

Esophageal squamous epithelium, like that in the skin and mucous membranes, is a target (Figs. 20.45 and 20.46). Biopsies are sometimes performed for differential diagnosis of esophageal symptoms, particularly those caused by infectious agents. (See Chapter 16 for further details.)

AMYLOIDOSIS

Esophageal involvement by amyloid is uncommon in patients with amyloidosis. Deposition in blood vessels, muscularis mucosae, and lamina propria connective tissue may occur (Fig. 20.47). Additional information is provided in Chapters 13 and 19.

CONCLUSION

The most common esophageal inflammatory disease encountered by most pathologists is reflux esophagitis. The proliferation of fiberoptic endoscopes and the widespread favorable publicity among endoscopists for the utility of esophageal biopsy in the evaluation of patients with symptoms of reflux assures the numeric superiority of reflux esophagitis for the foreseeable future.

Follow-up of patients with treated reflux esophagitis and Barrett esophagus will also continue to provide many specimens. Although the histopathologic features in reflux esophagitis are etiologically nonspecific, other forms of esophagitis do have characteristic findings. Most notable are the various forms of infective esophagitis in which morphologic evidence of the causative organism(s) may be identifiable. The emergence of AIDS in addition to immunosuppressive therapies for transplantation and neoplasia as conditions in which patients commonly have esophageal symptoms also focuses attention on infective esophagitis. Nonetheless, the pathologic characteristics of esophageal inflammation rarely establish its cause. As a result, the clinical history is likely to remain the key element for interpretation of esophagitis in specimens from biopsy, resection, and autopsy.

ADDITIONAL READINGS

General Topics

Appelman HD, ed. Pathology of the esophagus, stomach and duodenum. New York: Churchill Livingstone, 1984.

Castell DO, Johnson LF, eds. Esophageal function in health and disease. New York: Elsevier, 1983.

Enterline H, Thompson J. Pathology of the esophagus. New York: Springer, 1984.

Goldenberg SP, Wain SL, Marignoni P. Acute necrotizing esophagitis. Gastroenterology 1990;98:493.

Hill LD, ed. The esophagus: Medical and surgical management. Philadelphia: WB Saunders, 1988.

Normal Morphologic Features

Al Yassin TM, Toner PG. Fine structure of squamous epithelium and submucosal glands of human oesophagus. J Anat 1977;123:705.

Denardi FG, Riddell RH. The normal esophagus. Am J Surg Pathol 1991;15:296.

Geboes K, Desmet K. Histology of the esophagus. Front Gastrointest Res 1978;3:1–17.

Geboes K, De Wolf-Peeters C, Rutgeerts P, et al. Lymphocytes and Langerhans cells in the human oesophageal epithelium. Virchows Arch [A] 1983;401:45.

Hopwood D, Logan KR, Bouchier IAD. The electron microscopy of the normal human oesophageal epithelium. Virchows Arch [B] 1978; 26:345.

Glycogenic Acanthosis

Bender MD, Allison J, Cuartos F. Glycogenic acanthosis of the esophagus: A form of benign epithelial hyperplasia. Gastroenterology 1973;65:373.

Glick SN, Teplick SK, Goldstein J, et al. Glycogenic acanthosis of the esophagus. AJR Am J Roentgenol 1982;139:683.

Stern Z, Sharon P, Ligumsky M. Glycogenic acanthosis of the esophagus: A benign but confusing endoscopic lesion. Am J Gastroenterol 1980;74:261.

Ectopic Tissues

Bertoni G, Sassatelli R, Nigrisoli E, et al. Ectopic sebaceous glands in the esophagus: Report of three new cases and review of the literature. Am J Gastroenterol 1994;89:1884–1887.

Jabbori M, Goresky CA, Laugh J. The inlet patch: Heterotopic gastric mucosa in the upper esophagus. Gastroenterology 1985;89:352.

Marcial MA, Villafana M. Esophageal ectopic sebaceous glands: Endoscopic and histologic findings. Gastrointest Endosc 1994;40:630–632.

Wang HH, Zeroogian JM, Spechler SJ, et al. Prevalence and significance of pancreatic acinar metaplasia at the gastroesophageal junction. Am J Surg Pathol 1996;20:1507–1510.

Melanocytic Proliferation

Ghadially FN, Walley VM. Melanoses of the gastrointestinal tract. Histopathology 1994;25:197–207.

Ohashi K, Kato Y, Kanno J, et al. Melanocytes and melanosis of the oesophagus in Japanese subjects: Analysis of factors affecting their increase. Virchows Arch [A] 1990;417:137.

Sharma SS, Venkateswaran S, Chacko A, et al. Melanosis of the esophagus. An endoscopic, histochemical, and ultrastructural study. Gastroenterology 1991;100:13–16.

Tateishi R, Taniguchi H, Wada A, et al. Argyrophil cells and melanocytes in esophageal mucosa. Arch Pathol Lab Med 1974;98:87.

Fungal Esophagitis—Candida

Dutta SK, Al-Ibrahim MS. Immunological studies in acute pseudomembranous esophageal candidiasis. Gastroenterology 1978;75:292.

Knoke M, Bernhardt H. Endoscopic aspects of mycosis in the upper digestive tract. Endoscopy 1980;12:295.

Kodsi BE, Wickremesinghe PC, Kozinn PJ, et al. Candida esophagitis: A prospective study of 27 cases. Gastroenterology 1976;71:715.

Mathieson R, Dutta SK. Candida esophagitis. Dig Dis Sci 1983;28:365.

Ratton J, Hallak A, Rozen P, et al. Esophageal monilioma and mucosa bridge. Gastrointest Endosc 1982;28:114.

Runfeld W, Jenkins D, Scott BB. Unsuspected gastroesophageal candidiasis: An endoscopic study. Gut 1980;21:A895.

Scott BB, Jenkins D. Gastro-oesophageal candidiasis. Gut 1982;23:137.

Sheft DJ, Shrago G. Esophageal moniliasis: Spectrum of disease. J Am Med Assoc 1970;213:1859.

Walsh TJ, Hamilton SR, Belitsos N. Esophageal candidiasis: Managing an increasingly prevalent infection. Postgrad Med 1988;84:193–205.

Fungal Esophagitis—Torulopsis

Bentlif PS, Wiedermann B. Esophagitis caused by Torulopsis glabrata: Case report. Am J Gastroenterol 1979;71:395.

Grimley PM, Wright LD, Jennings AE. Torulopsis glabrata infection in man. Am J Clin Pathol 1965;43:216.

Fungal Esophagitis—Aspergillus and Phycomycetes

Heffernan AGA, Asper SP. Insidious fungal disease: A clinicopathologic study of secondary aspergillosis. Bull Johns Hopkins Hosp 1966;118:10.

Margolis PS, Epstein A. Mucormycosis esophagitis in a patient with the acquired immunodeficiency syndrome. Am J Gastroenterol 1994;89:1900–1902.

Whiteway DE, Virata RL. Mucormycosis. Arch Intern Med 1979;139:944.

Young RC, Bennett JE, Vogel CL, et al. Aspergillosis: The spectrum of the disease in 98 patients. Medicine 1970;49:147.

Fungal Esophagitis—Histoplasmosis

Coss KC, Wheat LJ, Conces DJ, et al. Esophageal fistula complicating mediastinal histoplasmosis: Response to amphotericin B. Am J Med 1987;83:343.

Fucci JC, Nightengale ML. Primary esophageal histoplasmosis. Am J Gastroenterol 1997;92:530–531.

Goodwin RA, Loyd JE, Des Prez RM. Histoplasmosis in normal hosts. Medicine (Baltimore) 1981;60:231.

Jenkins DW, Fisk DW, Byrd RB. Mediastinal histoplasmosis with esophageal abscess: Two case reports. Gastroenterology 1976;70:109.

Miller DP, Everett ED. Gastrointestinal histoplasmosis. J Clin Gastroenterol 1979;1:233.

Fungal Esophagitis—Other Pathogenic Fungi

Angulo A, Pollak L. Paracoccidioidomycosis. In: Baker RD, ed. The pathologic anatomy of mycoses: Human infection with fungi, actinomycetes and algae. New York: Springer, 1971;547.

Khandekar A, Moser D, Fidler WJ. Blastomycosis of the esophagus. Ann Thorac Surg 1979;30:71.

Ziliotta Jr A, Kunzle JE, Takeda FA. Paracoccidioidomycosis of the esophagus: Report of a case. Rev Inst Med Trop Sao Paulo 1980;22:261.

Viral Esophagitis—Herpes

Bastian JF, Kaufman IA. Herpes simplex esophagitis in a healthy 10-year-old boy. J Pediatr 1982;100:426.

Depew WT, Prentice RSA, Beck IT, et al. Herpes simplex ulcerative esophagitis in a healthy subject. Am J Gastroenterol 1977;68:381.

Howilder W, Goldbert HI. Gastroesophageal involvement in herpes simplex. Gastroenterology 1976;70:775.

Lightdale CJ, Wolf DJ, Marcucci RA, et al. Herpetic esophagitis in patients with cancer: Antemortem diagnosis by brush cytology. Cancer 1977;39:223.

McKay JS, Day DW. Herpes simplex oesophagitis. Histopathology 1983;7:409.

Mirra SS, Bryan JA, Butz WC, et al. Concomitant herpes-monilial esophagitis: Case report with ultrastructural study. Hum Pathol 1982;13:760.

Nash G, Ross JW. Herpetic esophagitis: A common cause of esophageal ulceration. Hum Pathol 1974;5:339.

White CL III, Hamilton SR. Immunoperoxidase localization of viral antigens in Herpes esophagitis (abstract). Lab Invest 1983;48:92A.

Viral Esophagitis—Cytomegalovirus

Allen JI, Silvis SE, Summer HW, et al. Cytomegalic inclusion disease diagnosed endoscopically. Dig Dis Sci 1981;26:133.

Chetty R, Roskell DE. Cytomegalovirus infection in the gastrointestinal tract. J Clin Pathol 1994;47:968–972.

Freeman HJ, Schnitzka TK, Pierce JRA, et al. Cytomegalovirus infection of the gastrointestinal tract in a patient with late onset immunodeficiency syndrome. Gastroenterology 1977;73:1397.

Henson D. Cytomegalovirus inclusion bodies in the gastrointestinal tract. Arch Pathol Lab Med 1972;93:477.

St. Onge G, Bezahler GH. Giant esophageal ulcer associated with cytomegalovirus. Gastroenterology 1982;83:127.

Toghill PJ, McGaughey M. Cytomegalovirus esophagitis. Br Med J 1972;2:294.

Wilcox CM, Diehl DL, Cello JP, et al. Cytomegalovirus esophagitis in patients with AIDS: A clinical, endoscopic, and pathologic correlation. Ann Intern Med 1990;113:589.

Viral Esophagitis—Viral Exanthems

Bardhan KD. Cimetidine in "chicken pox oesophagitis." Br Med J 1978;1:370.

Chatty EM, Tomeh MO, Mercer RD, et al. Congenital rubella syndrome with viral esophagitis. An electron microscopic study. Cleve Clin Q 1971;38:73.

Gill RA, Gebhard RL, Dozeman RL, et al. Shingles esophagitis: Endoscopic diagnosis in two patients. Gastrointest Endosc 1984;30:26–27.

Johnson HN. Visceral lesions associated with varicella. Arch Pathol Lab Med 1940;30:292.

Esophagitis Due to HIV and Related Viruses

Bartewlsman JFWM, Lang JMA, van Leeuwen R, et al. Acute primary HIV esophagitis. Endoscopy 1990;22:184.

Chawla SK, Ramani K, Chawla K, et al. Giant esophageal ulcers of AIDS: Ultrastructural study. Am J Gastroenterol 1994;89:411–415.

Connolly GM, Hawkins D, Harcourt-Webster JN, et al. Oesophageal symptoms, their causes, treatment, and prognosis in patients with the acquired immunodeficiency syndrome. Gut 1989;30:1033.

Kitchen VS, Helbert M, Francis ND, et al. Epstein-Barr virus associated oesophageal ulcers in AIDS. Gut 1990;31:1223.

Lafeuillade A, Mazzerbo F, Aubert L, et al. Corticosteroid-responsive giant oesophageal ulcer in AIDS. Presse Med 1990;19:1725.

Rabeneck L, Boyko WJ, McLean DM, et al. Unusual esophageal ulcers containing enveloped viruslike particles in homosexual men. Gastroenterology 1986;90:1882.

Rabeneck L, Popovic M, Gartner S. Acute HIV infection presenting with painful swallowing and esophageal ulcers. JAMA 1990;263:2318.

Schechter M, Pannain VLN, de Oliveira AV. Papovavirus-associated esophageal ulceration in a patient with AIDS. AIDS 1991;5:238.

Papillomavirus Infection of the Esophagus

Williamson AL, Jaskiesicz K, Gunning A. The detection of human papillomavirus in oesophageal lesions. Anticancer Res 1991;11:263.

Winkler B, Capo V, Reumann W, et al. Human papillomavirus infection of the esophagus. A clinicopathologic study with demonstration of papillomavirus antigen by the immunoperoxidase techniques. Cancer 1985; 55:149–155.

Opportunistic Bacterial Esophagitis

Walsh TJ, Belitsos NJ, Hamilton SR. Bacterial esophagitis in immunocompromised patients. Arch Intern Med 1986;146:1345.

Mycobacterial Esophagitis

Dow CJ. Oesophageal tuberculosis: Four cases. Gut 1981;22:234.

Eng J, Sabanathan S. Tuberculosis of the esophagus. Dig Dis Sci 1991; 36:536.

Milnes JP, Holmes GKT. Recurrent oesophageal stricture due to tuberculosis. Br Med J 1983;286:1977.

Quader Z, Co BT, Atten MJ, et al. AIDS and esophageal tuberculosis. Am J Gastroenterol 1995;90:2237–2238.

Wigley FM, Murray HW, Mann RB. Unusual manifestation of tuberculosis: TE fistula. Am J Med 1976;60:310.

Actinomycetic and Other Bacterial Esophagitis

McManus JPA, Webb JN. A yeast-like infection of the esophagus caused by Lactobacillus acidophilus. Gastroenterology 1975;68:583–586.

Poles MA, McMeeking AA, Scholes JV, et al. Actinomyces infection of a cytomegalovirus esophageal ulcer in two patients with acquired immunodeficiency syndrome. Am J Gastroenterol 1994;89:1569–1572.

Vinson PP, Sutherland CG. Esophagobronchial fistula resulting from actinomycosis. Report of a case. Radiology 1978;6:63.

Spirochetal Esophagitis

Hudson TR, Head JR. Syphilis of the esophagus. J Thorac Surg 1950; 20:216.

Stone J, Freidberg SA. Obstructive syphilitic esophagitis. JAMA 1961; 177:711.

Parasitic Esophagitis

Villanueva JL, Torre-Cisneros J, Jurado R, et al. Leishmania esophagitis in an AIDS patient: An unusual form of visceral leishmaniasis. Am J Gastroenterol 1994;89:273–275.

Zucoloto S, Derezende JM. Mucosal alterations in human chronic chagasic esophagopathy. Digestion 1990;47:138.

Esophageal Injury Due to Exogenous Chemicals

Anyanwu CH, Okonkwo PO. Oesophageal strictures induced by herbal preparation. Trans R Soc Trop Med Hyg 1981;75:864.

Burrington JD. Clinitest burns of the esophagus. Ann Thorac Surg 1975;20:400.

Dafoe CS, Ross CA. Acute corrosive esophagitis. Thorax 1969;24:291.

Lovejoy FH Jr. Corrosive injury of the esophagus in children: Failure of corticosteroid treatment reemphasizes prevention. N Engl J Med 1990;323:668.

Poelman JR, Hausman RH, Holtsma HFW. Endoscopy in lye burns of oesophagus and stomach. Endoscopy 1977;9:172.

Potter JL. Acute zinc chloride ingestion in a young child. Ann Emerg Med 1981;10:267.

Symbas PN, Vlasis SE, Hatcher CR Jr. Esophagitis secondary to ingestion of caustic material. Ann Thorac Surg 1983;36:73.

Widmer F, Aeberhard P. Acid and alkali corrosion of esophagus, stomach and duodenum. Schweiz Med Wochenschr 1982;112:742.

Drug Contact—Reviews

Bonavina L, DeMeester TR, McChesney L, et al. Drug-induced esophageal strictures. Ann Surg 1987;206:173.

Kikendall JW, Friedman AC, Oyewole MA, et al. Pill-induced esophageal injury: Case reports and review of the medical literature. Dig Dis Sci 1983;28:174.

Lee FD. Drug-related pathological lesions of the intestinal tract. Histopathology 1994;25:303–308.

Mason SJ, O'Meara TF. Drug-induced esophagitis. J Clin Gastroenterol 1981;3:115.

McCord GS, Clouse RE. Pill-induced esophageal strictures: Clinical features and risk factors for development. Am J Med 1990;88:512.

Perry PA, Dean BS, Krenzelok EP. Drug-induced esophageal injury. J Toxicol Clin Toxicol 1989;27:281.

Taha AS, Dahill S, Sturrock RD, et al. Predicting NSAID-related ulcers—assessment of clinical and pathological risk factors and importance of differences in NSAID. Gut 1994;35:891–895.

Drug Contact—Emepronium

Barrison IG, Tremby PW, Kane SP. Oesophageal ulceration due to emepronium bromide. Endoscopy 1980;12:197.

Hillman LL, Scobie BA, Pomare EW, et al. Acute esophagitis due to emepronium bromide. NZ Med J 1981;93:4.

Kenwright S, Norris ADC. Oesophageal ulceration due to emepronium bromide. Lancet 1977;1:548.

Drug Contact—Potassium

Lambert JR, Newman A. Ulceration and strictures of the esophagus due to oral potassium chloride (slow release tablet) therapy. Am J Gastroenterol 1980;73:508.

Peters JL. Benign oesophageal stricture following oral potassium chloride therapy. Br J Surg 1976;63:698.

Drug Contact—Antibiotics

Channer KS, Hollanders D. Tetracycline-induced oesophageal ulceration. Br Med J 1981;282:1359.

Delpre G, Kadish U, Stahl B. Induction of esophageal injuries by doxycycline and other pills: A frequent but preventable occurrence. Dig Dis Sci 1989;34:797.

Finet L, Saleme R, Delcenserie R, et al. Esophageal ulceration association with ingestion of dextropropoxyphene-paracetamol tablets. Gastroenterol Clin Biol 1990;14:1033.

Levine MS. Giant esophageal ulcer due to Clinoril. AJR Am J Roentgenol 1991;156:955.

Sutton DR, Gasnold JK. Oesophageal ulceration due to clindamycin. Br Med J 1977;1:1598.

Winckler K. Tetracycline ulcers of the oesophagus: Endoscopy, histology and roentgenology in 2 cases, and review of the literature. Endoscopy 1981;13:225.

Drug Contact—Miscellaneous Drugs

Abbarah TR, Fredell JE, Ellens GB. Ulceration by oral ferrous sulfate. JAMA 1976;236:2320.

Bataille C, Soumagne D, Loly J, et al. Esophageal ulceration due to indomethacin. Digestion 1982;24:66.

Bohane TD, Perrault J, Fowler RS. Oesophagitis and oesophageal obstruction from quinidine tablets in association with left atrial enlargement: A case report. Aust Paediatr J 1978;14:191.

Heller SR, Fellows IW, Ogilvie AL, et al. Non-steroidal anti-inflammatory drugs and benign oesophageal stricture. Br Med J 1982;285:167.

Kharasch S, Vinci R, Reece R. Esophagitis, epiglottitis, and cocaine alkaloid (crack)—Accidental poisoning or child abuse? Pediatrics 1990;86:117.

Santucci L, Patoia L, Fiorucci S, et al. Oesophageal lesions during treatment with piroxicam. Br Med J 1990;300:1018.

Seidner DL, Roberts IM, Smith MS. Esophageal obstruction after ingestion of a fiber-containing diet pill. Gastroenterology 1990;99:1820.

Walta DC, Giddens JD, Johnson LF, et al. Localized proximal esophagitis secondary to ascorbic acid ingestion and esophageal motor disorder. Gastroenterology 1976;70:766.

Sclerotherapy

Ayres SJ, Goff JS, Warren GH. Endoscopic sclerotherapy for bleeding esophageal varices: Effects and complications. Ann Intern Med 1983; 98:900.

Evans DMD, Jones DB, Cleary BK, et al. Oesophageal varices treated by sclerotherapy: A histopathologic study. Gut 1982;23:615.

Helpap B, Bollweg L. Morphological changes in the terminal oesophagus with varices, following sclerosis of the wall. Endoscopy 1981;13:229.

Ponce J, Froufe A, de la Morena E, et al. Morphometric study of the esophageal mucosa in patients with variceal bleeding. Hepatology 1981;1:641.

Chemotherapeutic Agents

Greco FA, Breveton HD, Kent H, et al. Adriamycin and enhanced radiation reaction in normal esophagus and skin. Ann Intern Med 1976;85:294.

Horwich A, Lokich JJ, Bloomer WP. Doxorubicin, radiotherapy, and oesophageal stricture. Lancet 1975;2:561.

Hruban RH, Yardley JH, Donehower RC, et al. Epithelial necrosis in the gastrointestinal tract associated with polymerized microtubule accumulation and mitotic arrest. Cancer 1989;63:72.

Slavin RE, Dias MP, Saral R. Cytosine arabinoside-induced gastrointestinal toxic alterations in sequential chemotherapeutic protocols. Cancer 1978;42:1747.

Esophageal Trauma

Appleton DS, Sandrasagra FA, Flower CD. Perforated esophagus: review of twenty-eight consecutive cases. Clin Radiol 1979;30:493.

Crysdale WS, Sendi KS, Yoo J. Esophageal foreign bodies in children—15 year review of 484 cases. Ann Otol Rhinol Laryngol 1991;100:320.

Farivar M. Bee sting of the esophagus. N Engl J Med 1981;305:1020.

Hunter TB, Protell RL, Horsley WW. Food laceration of the esophagus. AJR Am J Roentgenol 1983;140:503.

Meislin H, Kobernick M. Corn chip laceration of the esophagus and evaluation of suspected esophageal perforation. Ann Emerg Med 1983;12:455.

Nadi P, Ong GB. Foreign body in the esophagus: A review of 2394 cases. Br J Surg 1978;65:5.

Oldenburger D, Gundlach WJ. Intramural esophageal hematoma in a hemophiliac: An unusual cause of gastrointestinal bleeding. JAMA 1977;237:800.

Shay SS, Berendson RA, Johnson LF. Esophageal hematoma: Four new cases, a review, and proposed etiology. Dig Dis Sci 1981;26:1019.

Steadman C, Kerlin P, Crimmins F, et al. Spontaneous intramural rupture of the oesophagus. Gut 1990;31:845.

Zenone EA, Trotman BW. Boerhaave's syndrome: Spontaneous formation of an esophageal-bronchial fistula. JAMA 1977;238:2048–2049.

Radiation Esophagitis

Berthrong M, Fajardo LF. Radiation injury in surgical pathology. Part II. Alimentary tract. Am J Surg Pathol 1981;5:153.

Chowhan NM. Injurious effects of radiation on the esophagus. Am J Gastroenterol 1990;85:115–120.

Lepke RA, Libshitz HI. Radiation-induced injury of the esophagus. Radiology 1983;148:375.

Papazian A, Capron JP, Ducroix JP, et al. Mucosal bridges of the upper esophagus after radiotherapy for Hodgkin's disease. Gastroenterology 1983;84:1028.

Vanagunas A, Jacob P, Olinger E. Radiation-induced esophageal injury: a spectrum from esophagitis to cancer. Am J Gastroenterol 1990;85:808–812.

Yang ZY, Hu YH, Gu XZ. Non-cancerous ulcer in the esophagus after radiotherapy for esophageal carcinoma: A report of 27 patients. Radiother Oncol 1990;19:121.

Thermal Injury

Grana L, Ablin RJ, Goldman S, et al. Freezing of the esophagus: Histological changes and immunological response. Int Surg 1981;66:295.

Lieberman DA, Keefee EB. Esophageal burn and the microwave oven. Ann Intern Med 1982;97:137.

Stevens AE, Dove GA. Oesophageal cast: Oesophagitis. Lancet 1980;2:1279.

Hiatal Hernia

Arima T, Igarashi M, Shiraishi M, et al. Hiatal herniation of the colon in an infant. Int Surg 1988;73:196.

Berstad A, Weberg R, Froyshov LI, et al. Relationship of hiatus hernia to reflux oesophagitis: A prospective study of coincidence, using endoscopy. Scand J Gastroenterol 1986;21:55.

Cathcart RS III, Gregorie HB Jr, Holmes SL. Nonreflux complications of hiatal hernia. Am Surg 1987;53:320.

Haas O, Rat P, Christophe M, et al. Surgical results of intrathoracic gastric volvulus complicating hiatal hernia. Br J Surg 1990;77:1379.

Jonsell G. The incidence of sliding hiatal hernias in patients with gastroesophageal reflux requiring operation. Acta Chir Scand 1983;149:63.

Laforet EG. Acute hemorrhagic incarceration of prolapsed gastric mucosa. Gastroenterology 1976;70:589.

Mittal RK, Lange RC, McCallum RW. Identification and mechanism of delayed esophageal acid clearance in subjects with hiatus hernia. Gastroenterology 1987;92:130.

Pridie RB. Incidence and coincidence of hiatus hernia. Gut 1996;7:188.

Riggs W Jr. The incidence of hiatal hernia in infants and children: Results of a survey of members of the Society of Pediatric Radiology. Radiology 1976;120:451.

Sato H, Takase S, Takada A. The association of esophageal hiatus hernia with Mallory-Weiss syndrome. Gastroenterol Jpn 1989;24:233.

Gastroesophageal Reflux

Behar J, Sheahan DG. Histologic abnormalities in reflux esophagitis. Arch Pathol Lab Med 1975;99:387.

Bennett JR. Etiology, pathogenesis, and clinical manifestations of gastro-oesophageal reflux disease. Scand J Gastroenterol 1988;23(S146):67.

Bhan I, Leape LL, Ramenofsky ML. Histologic features of esophageal biopsies from children with gastroesophageal reflux. Lab Invest 1982;46:2.

Black DD, Haggitt RC, Orenstein SR, et al. Esophagitis in infants. Morphometric histological diagnosis and correlation with measures of gastroesophageal reflux. Gastroenterology 1990;98:1408.

Brand DL, Eastwood IR, Martin D, et al. Esophageal symptoms, manometry and histology before and after antireflux surgery: A long-term follow-up study. Gastroenterology 1979;76:1393.

Brown LF, Goldman H, Antonioli DA. Intraepithelial eosinophils in endoscopic biopsies of adults with reflux esophagitis. Am J Surg Pathol 1984;8:899.

Cronen P, Snow N, Nightingale D. Aortoesophageal fistula secondary to reflux esophagitis. Ann Thorac Surg 1982;33:78.

Curci M, Dibbins A. Gastroesophageal reflux in children: An underrated disease. Am J Surg 1982;143:413.

DeMeester TR, Bonavina L, Iascone C, et al. Chronic respiratory symptoms and occult gastroesophageal reflux: A prospective clinical study and results of surgical therapy. Ann Surg 1990;211:337.

Dent J, Holloway RH, Toouli J, et al. Mechanisms of lower oesophageal sphincter incompetence in patients with symptomatic gastroesophageal reflux. Gut 1988;29:1020.

Dodds WJ, Dent J, Hogan WJ, et al. Mechanisms of gastroesophageal reflux in patients with reflux esophagitis. N Engl J Med 1982;307:1547.

Eastwood GL. Histologic changes in gastroesophageal reflux. J Clin Gastroenterol 1986;(Suppl 1) 8.

Eriksen CA, Sadek SA, Cranford C, et al. Reflux oesophagitis and oesophageal transit: Evidence for a primary oesophageal motor disorder. Gut 1988;29:448.

Fink SM, Barwick KW, Winchenbach CL, et al. Reassessment of esophageal histology in normal subjects: A comparison of suction and endoscopic techniques. J Clin Gastroenterol 1983;5:177.

Funch-Jensen P, Cock K, Christensen LA, et al. Microscopic appearance of the esophageal mucosa in a consecutive series of patients submitted to upper endoscopy: Correlation with gastro-esophageal reflux symptoms and macroscopic findings. Scand J Gastroenterol 1986;21:65.

Geboes K, Desmet V, Vantrappen G, et al. Vascular changes in the esophageal mucosa: An early histologic sign of esophagitis. Gastrointest Endosc 1980;26:29.

Goodall RJR, Faris JE, Cooper DN, et al. Relationship between asthma and gastro-esophageal reflux. Thorax 1981;36:116.

Heading RC. Epidemiology of oesophageal reflux disease. Scand J Gastroenterology 1989;24 (Suppl. 168):33.

Herbst JJ, Meyers WF. Gastroesophageal reflux in children. Adv Pediatr 1981;28:159.

Himal HS. Alkaline gastritis and alkaline esophagitis: A review. Can J Surg 1977;20:403.

Hopwood D, Bateson MC, Milne G, et al. Effects of bile acids and hydrogen ion on the fine structure of oesophageal epithelium. Gut 1981;22:306.

Ishmail-Beigi F, Pope CE II. Distribution of the histological changes of gastroesophageal reflux in the distal esophagus of man. Gastroenterology 1974;66:1109.

Janisch HD, von Kleist D, Hampel KE. Intraepithelial eosinophils in esophageal reflux. Gastroenterology 1983;85:785.

Jessurun J, Yardley JH, Giardiello FM, et al. Intracytoplasmic plasma proteins in distended esophageal squamous cells (balloon cells). Mod Pathol 1988;1:175.

Kahrilas RJ. Gastroesophageal reflux disease. JAMA 1996;276:983–988.

Knuff TE, Benjamin SB, Worsham F, et al. Histologic evaluation of chronic gastroesophageal reflux. An evaluation of biopsy methods and diagnostic criteria. Dig Dis Sci 1984;29:194.

Kraus BB, Sinclair JW, Castel DO. Gastroesophageal reflux in runners—characteristics and treatment. Ann Intern Med 1990;112:429.

Mangano MM, Antonioli DA, Schnitt SJ, et al. Nature and significance of cells with irregular nuclear contours in esophageal mucosal biopsies. Mod Pathol 1992;5:191–196.

Matikamen M, Loatikainen T, Kalima T, et al. Bile acid composition and esophagitis after total gastrectomy. Am J Surg 1982;143:196.

Riddell RH. The biopsy diagnosis of gastroesophageal reflux disease, "carditis," and Barrett's esophagus, and sequelae of therapy. Am J Surg Pathol 1996;20:S31–S51.

Shoenut JP, Wieler JA, Micflikier AB, et al. Esophageal reflux before and after isolated myotomy for achalasia. Surgery 1990;108:876–879.

Shub MD, Ulshen MH, Hargrove CB, et al. Esophagitis: A frequent consequence of gastroesophageal reflux in infancy. J Pediatr 1985; 107:881.

Sonnenberg A, Lepsien G, Muller-Lissner SA, et al. When is esophagitis healed? Esophageal endoscopy, histology and function before and after cimetidine treatment. Dig Dis Sci 1982;27:297.

Tummala V, Barwick KW, Sontag SJ, et al. The significance of intraepithelial eosinophils in the histologic diagnosis of gastroesophageal reflux. Am J Clin Pathol 1987;87:43.

Tytgat GNJ, Nio CY, Schotborgh RH. Reflux esophagitis. Scand J Gastro 1990;25:1.

Wang HH, Mangano MM, Antonioli DA. Evaluation of T-lymphocytes in esophageal mucosal biopsies. Mod Pathol 1994;7:55–58.

Werdmuller BFM, Loffeld RJLF. Helicobacter pylori infection has no role in the pathogenesis of reflux esophagitis. Dig Dis Sci 1997;42:103–106.

Zaninotto G, DeMeester TR, Schweizer W, et al. The lower esophageal sphincter in health and disease. Am J Surg 1988;155:104.

Barrett Esophagus

Allan NK, Weitzner S, Scott L, et al. Adenocarcinoma arising in Barrett esophagus with synchronous squamous cell carcinoma of the esophagus. South Med J 1986;79:1036.

Banner BF, Memoli VA, Warren WH, et al. Carcinoma with multi-directional differentiation arising in Barrett esophagus. Ultrastruct Pathol 1983;4:205.

Barrett NR. The lower esophagus lined by columnar epithelium. Surgery 1957;41:881.

Berenson MM, Johnson TD, Markowitz NR, et al. Restoration of squamous mucosa after ablation of Barrett's esophageal epithelium. Gastroenterology 1993;104:1686–1691.

Blot WJ, Devesa SS, Kneller RW, et al. Rising incidence of adenocarcinoma of the esophagus and gastric cardia. JAMA 1991;265:1287.

Brand DL, Ylvisaker JT, Gelfand M, et al. Regression of columnar esophageal (Barrett) epithelium after anti-reflux surgery. N Engl J Med 1980;302:844.

Burke AP, Sobin LH, Shekitka KM, et al. Dysplasia of the stomach and Barrett esophagus: A follow-up study. Mod Pathol 1991;4:336.

Cameron AJ, Ott BJ, Payne WS. The incidence of adenocarcinoma in columnar-lined Barrett esophagus. N Engl J Med 1985;313:857.

Cameron AJ, Payne WS. Barrett esophagus occurring as a complication of scleroderma. Mayo Clin Proc 1978;53:612.

Cameron AJ, Zinsmeister AR, Ballard DJ, et al. Prevalence of columnar-lined (Barrett) esophagus. Gastroenterology 1990;99:918.

Cameron AJ, Lombay CT. Barrett's esophagus: Age, prevalence, and extent of columnar epithelium. Gastroenterology 1992;103:1241–1245.

Cameron AJ, Lombay CT, Pera M, et al. Adenocarcinoma of the esophagogastric junction and Barrett's esophagus. Gastroenterology 1995; 109:1541–1546.

Cooper JE, Spitz L, Wilkins BM. Barrett esophagus in children: A histologic and histochemical study of 11 cases. J Pediatr Surg 1987;22:191.

Dahms BB, Rothstein FC. Barrett esophagus in children: A consequence of chronic gastroesophageal reflux. Gastroenterology 1984;86:318.

DeBaecque C, Potet F, Molas G, et al. Superficial adenocarcinoma of the oesophagus arising in Barrett mucosa with dysplasia: A clinicopathological study of 12 patients. Histopathology 1990;16:213.

DeMeester TR, Atwood SEA, Smyrk TC, et al. Surgical therapy in Barrett esophagus. Ann Surg 1990;212:528.

Drewitz DJ, Sampliner RE, Garewal HS. The incidence of adenocarcinoma in Barrett's esophagus: A prospective study of 170 patients followed 4.8 years. Am J Gastroenterol 1997;92:212–215.

Fennerty MB, Sampliner RE, Way D, et al. Discordance between flow cytometric abnormalities and dysplasia in Barrett esophagus. Gastroenterology 1989;97:815.

Flejou J-F, Paraf F, Potet F, et al. p53 protein expression in Barrett's adenocarcinoma: A frequent event with no prognostic significance. Histopathology 1994;24:487–489.

Garewal HS, Sampliner R, Gerner E, et al. Ornithine decarboxylase activity in Barrett esophagus: A potential marker for dysplasia. Gastroenterology 1988;94:819.

Garewal HS, Sampliner RE, Fennerty MB. Flow cytometry in Barrett esophagus. What have we learned so far? Dig Dis Sci 1991;36:548.

Geisinger KR, Teot LA, Richter JE. A cooperative cytopathologic and histologic study of atypia, dysplasia, and adenocarcinoma in Barrett's esophagus. Cancer 1992;69:8–16.

Gottfried MR, McClave SA, Boyce HW. Incomplete intestinal metaplasia in the diagnosis of columnar lined esophagus (Barrett esophagus). Am J Clin Pathol 1989;92:741.

Griffin M, Sweeney EC. The relationship of endocrine cells, dysplasia and carcinoembryonic antigen in Barrett mucosa to adenocarcinoma of the oesophagus. Histopathology 1987;11:53.

Haggitt RC, Reid BJ, Rabinovitch PS, et al. Barrett esophagus: Correlation between mucin histochemistry, flow cytometry, and histologic diagnosis for predicting increased cancer risk. Am J Pathol 1988;131:53.

Haggitt RC. Barrett's esophagus, dysplasia, and adenocarcinoma. Hum Pathol 1994;25:982–993.

Hameeteman W, Tytgat GN, Houthoff HJ, et al. Barrett esophagus: Development of dysplasia and adenocarcinoma. Gastroenterology 1989; 96:1249.

Hamilton SR, Hutcheon DF, Ravich WJ, et al. Adenocarcinoma in Barrett esophagus after elimination of gastroesophageal reflux. Gastroenterology 1984;86:356.

Hamilton SR, Smith RRL, Cameron JL. Prevalence and characteristics of Barrett esophagus in patients with adenocarcinoma of the esophagus or esophagogastric junction. Hum Pathol 1988;19:942.

Hamilton SR, Smith RRL. The relationship between columnar epithelial dysplasia and invasive adenocarcinoma arising in Barrett esophagus. Am J Clin Pathol 1987;87:301.

Hamilton SR, Yardley JH. Regeneration of cardiac type mucosa and acquisition of Barrett mucosa after esophagogastrostomy. Gastroenterology 1977;72:669.

Hardwick RH, Shepherd NA, Moorghen M, et al. Adenocarcinoma arising in Barrett's oesophagus: Evidence for the participation of p53 dysfunction in the dysplasia/carcinoma sequence. Gut 1994;35:764–768.

Hassall E, Dimmick JE, Magee JF. Adenocarcinoma in childhood Barrett's esophagus: Case documentation and the need for surveillance in children. Am J Gastroenterol 1993;88:282–288.

Hong MK, Larkin WB, Herman BE, et al. Expansion of the Ki–67 proliferative compartment correlates with degree of dysplasia in Barrett's esophagus. Cancer 1995;75:423–429.

Iftikhar SY, James PD, Steele RJC, et al. Length of Barrett's esophagus: An important factor in the development of dysplasia and adenocarcinoma. Gut 1992;33:1155–1158.

Jaakkola A, Reinikainen P, Ovaska J, et al. Barrett's esophagus after cardiomyotomy for esophageal achalasia. Am J Gastroenterol 1994;89: 165–169.

James PD, Atkinson M: Value of DNA image cytometry in the prediction of malignant changes in Barrett oesophagus. Gut 1989;30:899.

Jauregui HO, Davessar K, Hale JH, et al. Mucin histochemistry of intestinal metaplasia in Barrett esophagus. Mod Pathol 1988;1:188.

Kalish RJ, Clancy PE, Orringer MB, et al. Clinical, epidemiologic, and morphologic comparison between adenocarcinomas arising in Barrett esophageal mucosa and in the gastric cardia. Gastroenterology 1984; 86:461.

Kortan P, Warren RE, Gardner J. Barrett esophagus in 6 patients with surgically treated achalasia. J Clin Gastroenterol 1981;3:557.

Kruse P, Boesby S, Bernstein IT, et al. Barrett's esophagus and esophageal adenocarcinoma. Endoscopic and histologic surveillance. Scand J Gastroenterol 1993;28:193–197.

Lee RG. Mucins in Barrett esophagus: A histochemical study. Am J Clin Pathol 1984;81:500.

Levine DS, Reid BJ, Haggitt RC, et al. Correlation of ultrastructural aberrations with dysplasia and flow cytometric abnormalities in Barrett epithelium. Gastroenterology 1989;96:355.

Levine DS, Rubin CE, Reid BJ, et al. Specialized metaplastic columnar epithelium in Barrett esophagus. A comparative transmission electron microscopic study. Lab Invest 1989;60:418.

Levine DS, Haggitt RC, Blount PL, et al. An endoscopic biopsy protocol can differentiate high-grade dysplasia from early adenocarcinoma in Barrett's esophagus. Gastroenterology 1993;105:40–50.

Loffeld RJLF, Ten Tije BJ, Arends JW. Prevalence and significance of Helicobacter pylori in patients with Barrett's esophagus. Am J Gastroenterol 1992;87:1598–1600.

McArdle JE, Lewin KJ, Randall G, et al. Distribution of dysplasias and early invasive carcinoma inn Barrett's esophagus. Hum Pathol 1992;23:479–482.

Menke-Pluymers MBE, Hop WCJ, Dees J, et al. Risk factors for the development of an adenocarcinoma in columnar-lined (Barrett) esophagus. Cancer 1993;72:1155–1158.

Menke-Pluymers MBE, Mulder AH, Hop WCJ, et al. Dysplasia and aneuploidy as markers of malignant degeneration in Barrett's oesophagus. Gut 1994;35:1348–1351.

Mills LR, Schuman BM, Assad RT, et al. Scanning electron microscopy of dysplastic Barrett epithelium. Mod Pathol 1989;2:112.

Montgomery EA, Hartmann D-P, Carr NJ, et al. Barrett esophagus with dysplasia. Flow cytometric DNA analysis of routine, paraffin-embedded mucosal biopsies. Am J Clin Pathol 1996;106:298–304.

Naef AP, Savary M, Ozzello L. Columnar-lined lower esophagus: An acquired lesion with malignant predisposition: Report on 140 cases of Barrett esophagus with 12 adenocarcinomas. J Thorac Cardiovasc Surg 1975;70:826.

Nikulasson S, Andrews CW Jr, Goldman H, et al. Sucrase-Isomaltase expression in dysplasia associated with Barrett's esophagus and chronic gastritis. Int J Surg Pathol 1995;4:281–286.

Paraf F, Flejou J-F, Pignon J-P, et al. Surgical pathology of adenocarcinoma arising in Barrett's esophagus. Analysis of 67 cases. Am J Surg Pathol 1995;19:183–191.

Paull A, Trier JS, Dalton MD, et al. The histologic spectrum of Barrett esophagus. N Engl J Med 1976;295:476.

Paull G, Yardley JH. Gastric and esophageal Campylobacter pylori in patients with Barrett esophagus. Gastroenterology 1988;95:216.

Pera M, Cameron AJ, Trastek VF, et al. Increasing incidence of adenocarcinoma of the esophagus and esophagogastric junction. Gastroenterology 1993;104:510–513.

Postlethwait RW, Musser AW. Changes in esophagus in one thousand autopsy specimens. J Thorac Cardiovasc Surg 1974;68:953.

Provenzale D, Kemp JA, Arora S, et al. A guide for surveillance of patients with Barrett's esophagus. Am J Gastroenterol 1994;89:670–680.

Qualman SJ, Murray RD, McClung HJ, et al. Intestinal metaplasia is age related in Barrett esophagus. Arch Pathol Lab Med 1990;114:1236.

Reid BJ, Haggitt RC, Rubin CE, et al. Observer variation in the diagnosis of dysplasia in Barrett esophagus. Hum Pathol 1988;19:166.

Reid BJ, Weinstein WM, Lewin KJ, et al. Endoscopic biopsy can detect high-grade dysplasia or early adenocarcinoma in Barrett esophagus without grossly recognizable neoplastic lesions. Gastroenterology 1988;94:81.

Reid BJ, Blount PL, Rubin CE, et al. Flow-cytometric and histological progression to malignancy in Barrett's esophagus: Prospective endoscopic surveillance of a cohort. Gastroenterology 1992;102:1212–1219.

Rice TW, Falk GW, Achkar E, et al. Surgical management of high grade dysplasia in Barrett's esophagus. Am J Gastroenterol 1993;88:1832–1836.

Robey SS, Hamilton SR, Gupta PK, et al. Diagnostic value of cytopathology in Barrett esophagus and associated carcinoma. Am J Clin Pathol 1988;89:493.

Rosengard AM, Hamilton SR. Squamous carcinoma of the esophagus in patients with Barrett esophagus. Mod Pathol 1989;2:2.

Rusch VW, Levine DS, Haggitt R, et al. The management of high grade dysplasia and early cancer in Barrett's esophagus. Cancer 1994;74:1225–1229.

Sampliner RE, Garewal HS, Fennerty MB, et al. Lack of impact of therapy on extent of Barrett esophagus in 67 patients. Dig Dis Sci 1990;35:93.

Sartori S, Nielson I, Indelli M, et al. Barrett esophagus after chemotherapy with cyclophosphamide, methotrexate, and 5-fluorouracil (CMF): An iatrogenic injury. Ann Intern Med 1991;114:210.

Schreiber DS, Apstein M, Hermos JA. Paneth cells in Barrett esophagus. Gastroenterology 1978;74:1302.

Smith RRL, Hamilton SR, Boitnott JK, et al. The spectrum of carcinoma arising in Barrett esophagus: A clinicopathologic study of 26 patients. Am J Surg Pathol 1984;8:563.

Snyder JD, Goldman H. Barrett esophagus in children and young adults: Frequent association with mental retardation. Dig Dis Sci 1990;35:1185.

Spechler SJ. Endoscopic surveillance for patients with Barrett esophagus: Does the cancer risk justify the practice? Ann Intern Med 1987;106:902.

Spechler SJ, Goyal RK, eds. Barrett esophagus: Pathophysiology, diagnosis and management. New York: Elsevier, 1985.

Spechler SJ, Schimmel EM, Dalton JW, et al. Barrett epithelium complicating lye ingestion with sparing of the distal esophagus. Gastroenterology 1981;81:580.

Spechler SJ, Goyal RK. The columnar-lined esophagus, intestinal metaplasia, and normal Barrett. Gastroenterology 1996;110:614–621.

Spechler SJ, Zeroogian JM, Antonioli DA, et al. Prevalence of metaplasia at the gastro-oesophageal junction. Lancet 1994;344:1533–1536.

Streitz JM Jr, Ellis FH Jr, Gibb SP, et al. Adenocarcinoma in Barrett esophagus: A clinicopathologic study of 65 cases. Ann Surg 1991;213:122.

Streitz JM, Andrews CW Jr, Ellis FH. Endoscopic surveillance of Barrett's esophagus. Does it help? J Thorac Cardiovasc Surg 1993;105:383–388.

Thompson JJ, Zinssen KR, Enterline HT. Barrett metaplasia and adenocarcinoma of the esophagus and gastroesophageal junction. Hum Pathol 1983;14:42.

Wang HH, Antonioli DA, Goldman H. Comparative features of esophageal and gastric adenocarcinomas: Recent changes in type and frequency. Hum Pathol 1986;17:482.

Wang HH, Sovie S, Zeroogian JM, et al. Value of cytology in detecting intestinal metaplasia and associated dysplasia at the gastroesophageal junction. Hum Pathol 1997;28:465–471.

Waring JP, Legrand J, Chinichian A, et al. Duodenogastric reflux in patients with Barrett esophagus. Dig Dis Sci 1990;35:759.

Wu GD, Beer DG, Moore JH, et al. Sucrase-isomaltase gene expression in Barrett's esophagus and adenocarcinoma. Gastroenterology 1993;105:837–844.

Younes M, Lebovitz RM, Lechago LV, et al. p53 protein accumulation in Barrett's metaplasia, dysplasia, and carcinoma: A follow-up study. Gastroenterology 1993;105:1637–1642.

Zwas F, Shields HM, Doos WG, et al. Scanning electron microscopy of Barrett epithelium and its correlation with light microscopy and mucin stains. Gastroenterology 1986;90:1932.

Achalasia

Adams CWH, Brain RHF, Trounce JR. Ganglion cells in achalasia of the cardia. Virchows Arch [B] 1976;372:75.

de Oliveira RB, Filho JR, Dantas RO, et al. The spectrum of esophageal motor disorders in Chagas' disease. Am J Gastroenterol 1995;90:1119–1124.

Gilles M, Nicks R, Skyring A. Clinical manometric, and pathologic studies in diffuse oesophageal spasm. Br Med J 1967;2:527.

Goldblum JR, Whyte RI, Orringer MB, et al. Achalasia. A morphologic study of 42 resected specimens. Am J Surg Pathol 1994;18:327–337.

Goldblum JR, Rice TW, Tichter JE. Histopathologic features in esophagomyotomy specimens from patients with achalasia. Gastroenterology 1996;111:648–654.

Marshall JB, Diaz-Arias AA, Bochna GS, et al. Achalasia due to diffuse esophageal leiomyomatosis and inherited as an autosomal dominant disorder: Report of a family study. Gastroenterology 1990;98:1358.

Qualman SJ, Haupt HM, Yang P, et al. Esophageal Lewy bodies associated with ganglion cell loss in achalasia: Similarity to Parkinson's disease. Gastroenterology 1984;87:848.

Robertson CS, Marti BAB, Atkinson M. Varicella-zoster virus DNA in the oesophageal myenteric plexus and achalasia. Gut 1993;34:299–302.

Smith B: The neurological lesion in achalasia of the cardia. Gut 1970; 11:388.

Rings and Webs

Bretagne JF, Ramee MP, Gosselin M, et al. Esophageal keratosis associated with peptic stricture. Gastroenterol Clin Biol 1982;6:869.

Eckardt VF, Adami B, Hucker H, et al. The esophagogastric junction in patients with asymptomatic lower esophageal mucosal webs. Gastroenterology 1980;79:1426.

Entwistle CC, Jacobs A. Histological findings in the Paterson-Kelly syndrome. J Clin Pathol 1965;18:408.

Goyal RK, Glancy JJ, Spiro HM. Lower esophageal ring. N Engl J Med 1970;282:1298.

Hendrix TR. Schatzki ring, epithelial junction, and hiatal hernia—an unresolved controversy. Gastroenterology 1980;79:584.

Janisch HD, Eckardt VF. Histological abnormalities in patients with multiple esophageal webs. Dig Dis Sci 1982;27:503.

Lesser PB, Moyer P, Andrews PJ, et al. Upper oesophageal ring. Ann Intern Med 1978;88:657.

Marshall JB, Kretschmar JM, Diazarias AA. Gastroesophageal reflux as a pathogenic factor in the development of symptomatic lower esophageal rings. Arch Intern Med 1990;150:1669.

Schatzki R, Gary JE. Dysphagia due to a diaphragm-like localized narrowing in the lower esophagus ("lower esophageal ring"). AJR Am J Roentgenol 1953;20:91.

Intramural Pseudodiverticulosis

Bruhlmann WF, Zollikoten CL, Maranta E, et al. Intramural pseudodiverticulosis of the esophagus: Report of seven cases and literature review. Gastrointest Radiol 1981,6:199.

Evans PR. Oesophageal intramural pseudodiverticulosis—always benign. Aust NZ J Med 1991;21:58.

Farman J, Rosen Y, Dallemand S, et al. Esophagitis cystica: Lower esophageal retention cysts. AJR Am J Roentgenol 1977;128:495.

Medeiros JF, Doos WG, Balogh K. Esophageal intramural pseudodiverticulosis: A report of two cases with analysis of similar, less extensive changes in "normal" autopsy esophagi. Hum Pathol 1988;19:928–931.

Piazza M, Palma PD. Polycystic "dystrophy" of the esophagus. Am J Clin Pathol 1977;67:307.

Voirol W, Welsh RA, Genet EF. Esophagitis cystica. Am J Gastroenterol 1973;59:446.

Collagen Vascular—Connective Tissue Disorders

Bretagne JF, Launois B, Ferrand B, et al. Rheumatoid stricture of the esophagus. Gastroenterol Clin Biol 1982;6:709.

Gutierrez F, Valenzuela JE, Ehresmann GR, et al. Esophageal dysfunction in patients with mixed connective tissue diseases and systemic lupus erythematosus. Dig Dis Sci 1982;27:592.

Kleckner FS. Dermatomyositis and its manifestations in the gastrointestinal tract. Am J Gastroenterol 1970;53:141.

Nishikai M, Asaba G, Homma M. Rheumatoid esophageal disease. Am J Gastroenterol 1977;67:29.

Orringer MB, Dabick L, Zarafonetis CJD, et al. Gastroesophageal reflux in esophageal scleroderma: Diagnosis and implications. Ann Thorac Surg 1976;22:120.

Rothstein RD. Gastrointestinal motility disoders in diabetes mellitus. Am J Gastroenterol 1990;85:782–785.

Russell ML, Friesen D, Henderson RD, et al. Ultrastructure of the esophagus in scleroderma. Arthritis Rheum 1982;25:1117.

Sheikh SH, Shaw-Stiffel TA. The gastrointestinal manifestations of Sjögren syndrome. Am J Gastroenterol 1995;90:9–14.

Zamost BJ, Hirschberg J, Ippoliti AF, et al. Esophagitis in scleroderma: Prevalence and risk factors. Gastroenterology 1987:92:421–428.

Crohn Disease

Freedman PG, Dieterich DT, Balthaza EJ. Crohn disease of the esophagus: Case report and review of the literature. Am J Gastroenterol 1984;79: 835–838.

Geboes K, Janssens J, Rutgierts P, et al. Crohn disease of the esophagus. J Clin Gastroenterol 1986;8:31–37.

LiVolsi VA, Jaretzki A. Granulomatous esophagitis: A case of Crohn's disease limited to the esophagus. Gastroenterology 1973;64:313.

Miller LJ, Thistle JL, Payne WS, et al. Crohn's disease involving the esophagus and colon: Case report. Mayo Clin Proc 1977;52:35.

Niv Y. Esophageal involvement in Crohn disease. Am J Gastroenterol 1988;83:205–206.

Taskin V, von Sohsten R, Singh B, et al. Crohn disease of the esophagus. Am J Gastroenterol 1995;90:1000–1001.

Werthamer S, Zak FG, Milailos P, et al. Granulomatous esophagitis (Crohn's disease) associated with granulomatous enterocolitis. NY State J Med 1976;76:938.

Behçet Syndrome

Chajek T, Fainaru M. Behçet's disease: Report of 41 cases. Medicine (Baltimore) 1975;54:179.

Lakhanpal S, Tani K, Lie JT, et al. Pathologic features of Behçet's syndrome: A review of Japanese autopsy registry data. Hum Pathol 1985;16: 790–795.

Lorenzetti ME, Forbes IJ, Robertsthomson IC. Oesophageal and ileal ulceration in Behçet's disease. J Gastroenterol Hepatol 1990;5:714.

Parkin JV, Wight DGD. Behçet's disease and the alimentary tract. Postgrad Med J 1975;51:260.

Eosinophilic Esophagitis

Dobbins JW, Sheahan DG, Behar J. Eosinophilic gastroenteritis with esophageal involvement. Gastroenterology 1977;72:1312.

Goldman H, Proujansky R. Allergic proctitis and gastroenteritis in children: Clinical and mucosal biopsy features in 53 cases. Am J Surg Pathol 1986;10:75–86.

Lee RG. Marked eosinophilia in esophageal mucosal biopsies. Am J Surg Pathol 1985;9:475.

Dermatologic Diseases

Barnes LM, Clark ML, Estes SA, et al. Pemphigus vulgaris involving the esophagus. A case report and review of the literature. Dig Dis Sci 1987;32:655–659.

Celinski K, Krasowska D, Pokora J, et al. Esophageal lichen planus. Endoscopy 1994;26:755–756.

Dickens CM, Hasteltine D, Walton S, et al. The oesophagus in lichen planus: An endoscopic study. Br Med J 1990;300:84.

Eliakim R, Goldin E, Livshin R, et al. Esophageal involvement in pemphigus vulgaris. Am J Gastroenterol 1988;83:155–157.

Ergun GA, Linan AN, Dannenberg AJ, et al. Gastrointestinal manifestations of epidermolysis bullosa. A study of 101 patients. Medicine 1992;71: 121–127.

Goldin E, Lijovetsky G. Esophageal involvement by pemphigus vulgaris. Am J Gastroenterol 1985;80:828–830.

Hillemeier C, Touloukian R, McCallum R, et al. Esophageal web: A previously unrealized complication of epidermolysis bullosa. Pediatrics 1981;67:678.

Itai Y, Kogure T, Okuyama Y, et al. Radiological manifestations of esophageal involvement in acanthosis nigricans. Br J Radiol 1976; 49:592.

Johnston DE, Koehler RE, Balte DM. Clinical manifestations of epidermolysis bullosa dystrophica. Dig Dis Sci 1981;26:1144.

Kahn D, Hutchinson E. Esophageal involvement in familial benign chronic pemphigus. Arch Dermatol 1974;109:718.

Renner WR, Johnson JF, Lichtenstein JE, et al. Esophageal inflammation and stricture—complication of chronic granulomatous disease of childhood. Radiology 1991;178:189.

Stewart MI, Woodley DT, Briggaman RA. Epidermolysis bullosa acquisita and associated symptomatic esophageal webs. Arch Dermatol 1991; 127:373.

Trattner A, Lurie R, Leiser A, et al. Esophageal involvement in pemphigus vulgaris: A clinical, histologic, and immunopathologic study. J Am Acad Dermatol 1991;24:233.

Weinman D, Stewart MI, Woodley DT, et al. Epidermolysis bullosa acquisita (EBA) and esophageal webs: A new association. Am J Gastroenterol 1991;86:1518–1522.

Zweiban B, Cohen H, Chandrasoma P. Gastrointestinal involvement complicating Stevens-Johnson syndrome. Gastroenterology 1986;91: 469–474.

Sarcoidosis

Cook DM, Dines DE. Sarcoidosis: Report of a case presenting as dysphagia. Chest 1970;57:84.

Davies RJ. Dysphagia, abdominal pain and sarcoid granulomata. Br Med J 1972;3:564.

Weisner RJ, Kleinman MS, Coademi JJ. Sarcoidosis of the esophagus. Am J Dig Dis 1971;16:943.

Graft-Versus-Host Disease

Ferrara JIM, Deeg HJ. Graft-versus-host disease. N Engl J Med 1991;324: 667–674.

McDonald GB, Sullivan KM, Schuffler MD, et al. Esophageal abnormality in chronic graft-versus-host disease in humans. Gastroenterology 1981; 80:914.

Slavin RE, Woodruff JM. The pathology of bone marrow transplantation. In: Sommers SC, ed. Pathology annual. New York: Appleton-Century-Crofts, 1974;312.

Amyloid

Busuttil A, More IAR, Jones DG. Amyloid deposits in the trachea and esophagus: Ultrastructural confirmation. Laryngoscope 1976; 86:850.

Heitzman EJ, Heitzman GC, Elliott CF. Primary esophageal amyloidosis: Report of a case with bleeding, perforation, and survival following resection. Arch Intern Med 1962;109:595.

Kyle RA, Bayrd ED. Amyloidosis: Review of 236 cases. Medicine 1975;54: 271.

Miller RH: Amyloid disease—an unusual cause of megalo-oesophagus. S Afr Med J 1969;43:1202.

Solanke TF, Olurin EO, Nwakonobi F, et al. Primary amyloid tumor of the oesophagus treated by colon transplant. Br J Surg 1967;54:943.

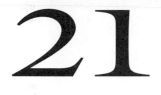

21 SQUAMOUS CELL CARCINOMA AND VARIANTS OF THE ESOPHAGUS

Chik-Kwun Tang and Si-Chun Ming

The esophagus serves as a conduit for ingested food to reach the stomach where digestive processes begin. Its function is supported by a muscular wall and a resilient multilayered squamous mucosa. Tumors are uncommon in the esophagus. The majority of tumors, about 80%, are malignant and nearly all are carcinomas. Although the caliber of esophageal lumen is small, only 2.5 cm in average diameter, the symptoms of the tumors often appear late and, at the time of diagnosis, most tumors are already advanced. Unlike other parts of the digestive tract, the esophagus has no serosa. Its central location in the chest puts it in close proximity to the vital

cardiorespiratory organs. These clinical and anatomic features have influenced the therapeutic considerations and resulted in a poor survival rate. Whereas new cases of esophageal cancer represent 0.9% of the total cancer cases in the United States in 1997, deaths from esophageal cancer account for about 2.0% of total cancer deaths (1). Among cancers of the digestive tract, esophageal cancer constitutes 5.5% of the estimated new cases and 8.9% of deaths.

Considering the fact that the esophagus is lined almost entirely with squamous epithelium, it is not surprising that squamous cell carcinoma is the dominant cancer type. The incidence of adenocarcinoma, thought to be rare in the past, has increased remarkably in recent years in the Western countries, accounting for 20 to 50% of all esophageal cancers in some reports (2, 3). Adenocarcinomas and other epithelial tumors of the esophagus are discussed in Chapter 22. The focus of this chapter is on general features of esophageal cancer and specific features of squamous cell carcinoma and its variants.

GENERAL PRINCIPLES

NORMAL ESOPHAGEAL ANATOMY

The esophagus develops from the foregut during the fourth week of embryonic life. It elongates rapidly as the stomach descends into the abdominal cavity. The esophagus in the adult is approximately 25 cm long, beginning about 15 cm from the incisor teeth and ending about 2 to 3 cm below the diaphragm. The upper esophagus is located at the midline. It shifts slightly to the left in the mediastinum so that it lays behind the left main bronchus, aortic arch, and heart. The esophagus passes through the diaphragm at the tenth thoracic vertebra, anterior and slightly to the left of the aorta. The relationship with these thoracic organs plays an important role in the clinical presentation and management of esophageal cancer.

Histologically, the esophageal wall is composed of mucosa, submucosa, and muscularis propria. Its outer layer is the adventitia, corresponding to the subserosa in other segments of the gut. The esophageal mucosa (Fig. 21.1) consists of a thick stratified squamous epithelium, a fibrovascular lamina propria and a muscularis mucosae. During embryonic life, the esophageal epithelium initially is composed of a single layer of columnar cells which are replaced by ciliated cells in the third month. At this time, superficial glands are present within the lamina propria. Because of their resemblance to the cardiac glands of the stomach and secret neutral mucus, these structures are referred to as cardiac or gastric glands. During the fourth month, squamous cells appear in the midesophagus, spreading out to cover the entire esophagus during the seventh month. Remnants of surface columnar cells and superficial glands occasionally persist after birth at both ends of the esophagus (4, 5). The deep esophageal glands, resembling minor salivary glands, are located in the submucosa. They do not appear until late fetal life and develop mainly after birth. In addition to these congenital and normally occurring columnar and glandular cells, an acquired metaplastic columnar epithelium occurs with increasing frequency in the lower esophagus. Barrett epithelium, named after the discoverer of this condition (6), is discussed fully in Chapters 20 and 22.

In the adult, the squamous epithelium is pearly white. Its upper end is continuous with pharyngeal mucosa, but its lower end is sharply demarcated from the pink velvety gastric mucosa. This squamocolumnar junction, known as Z line, defines the lower limit of esophageal epithelium. It may coincide with the cardiac orifice of the stomach (6), or 2 to 3 cm above it.

The normal squamous cells are arranged in an orderly pattern. The regenerative cells in the basal zone are cuboidal, occupying less than 20% of the thickness of the epithelium. The cells in the upper layers are larger, elliptic, and increasingly horizontal. The superficial cells appear clear because of accumulation of glycogen in the cytoplasm. Occasionally, the amount of glycogen is excessive and the cells are enlarged. The affected area may appear pale and elevated grossly. This condition is known as glycogenic acanthosis. The

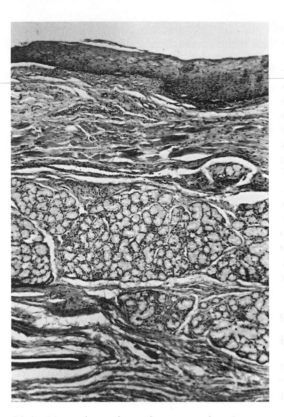

Figure 21.1 Normal esophageal mucosa showing squamous epithelium, fibrovascular lamina propria, and deep mucous glands. (Reprinted with permission from Ming SC. Pathology of esophageal cancer. In: Aisner J, Arriagada R, Green MR, Martini N, Perry MC, eds. Comprehensive textbook of thoracic oncology. Baltimore: Williams & Wilkins, 1996.)

squamous cells do not show keratosis, although they contain abundant tonofilaments. Endocrine cells and melanocytes may be present in the basal epithelium (7). Rarely, the number of melanocytes present is sufficient to cause focal brown pigmentation of the mucosa (8).

Both lamina propria and submucosa are composed of fibroadipose tissue, containing blood vessels, lymphatics, and scattered mononuclear inflammatory cells. The presence of lymphatics in these tissues facilitates early spread of cancer cells. The adventitial lymphatic vessels drain into the paraesophageal, deep cervical, posterior mediastinal, and subdiaphragmatic nodes, depending on the level of their location.

HISTOLOGIC CLASSIFICATION OF ESOPHAGEAL TUMORS

Primary esophageal tumors can be classified on the basis of cell origin into epithelial and nonepithelial tumors (9). Each category may be further subdivided into benign and malignant types. The nonepithelial tumors arise from the mesenchymal or supporting stromal tissue; most of them are benign. Sarcomas rarely arise in the esophagus; these tumors are discussed in Chapter 18. Nearly all esophageal cancers are carcinomas. Squamous cell carcinomas remain the most common type of cancer in the esophagus, although the incidence of adenocarcinomas is increasing dramatically. The types of epithelial tumors and their possible cell origins are listed in Table 21.1. The origins of most tumors are obvious. Tumors with mixed cell types may have derived from separate stem cells synchronously or metachronously. The component cell types in such composite tumors are unevenly distributed. If the tumor is derived from one stem cell with separate directions of differentiation, the component elements are intimately mixed and the tumor is called a combination tumor. The collision tumors are composed of tumors arising in adjacent but separate loci. As they grow, they merge and invade into each other at the interface.

The esophageal carcinomas have also been classified into early and advanced types. The concept of treating these cancers as separate entities was developed in China. Early carcinoma of esophagus is defined as a tumor with depth of invasion not beyond the submucosa with no lymph node involvement. In advanced carcinoma, the tumor has invaded the muscularis propria or beyond or has metastasized to the lymph nodes irrespective of the depth of invasion (10).

PATHOLOGIC STUDY

CYTOLOGY AND ENDOSCOPIC BIOPSY

The initial pathologic diagnosis of esophageal cancer is usually established by brush cytology. Details of cytologic diagnosis are presented in Chapter 4. In the high-risk region of esophageal cancer

TABLE 21.1	Type and Origin of Epithelial Tumors of Esophagus	
Tumor Type	**Origin**
Malignant Tumors	
Squamous cell carcinoma	
Ordinary squamous cell carcinoma	Squamous epithelium
Verrucous carcinoma	Squamous epithelium
Basaloid carcinoma	Squamous epithelium
Spindle cell carcinoma	Squamous epithelium
Adenocarcinoma	
Ordinary adenocarcinoma	Columnar epithelium
Adenoacanthoma	Columnar cell with metaplasia
Mucoepidermoid carcinoma	Esophageal gland duct
Adenoid cystic carcinoma	Esophageal gland duct
Choriocarcinoma	Germ cell rest
Composite tumors	
Adenosquamous carcinoma	Squamous cell with metaplasia or esophageal gland duct
Carcinosarcoma	Totipotential cell or mixed stem cells
Small cell carcinoma and carcinoid	Foregut endocrine cell
Malignant melanoma	Melanocytes
Benign tumors	
Squamous cell papilloma	Squamous epithelium
Adenoma	Columnar epithelium or duct

in northern China, a plastic catheter with an inflatable balloon attached to its distal end was used to collect cytologic specimens for mass screening (11). The catheter can be inserted easily into the esophagus. After the balloon has entered the stomach, it is inflated with air and withdrawn. The cells collected on the cotton net covering the balloon are processed for cytologic study. Tens of thousands of specimens have been collected and many early carcinomas were diagnosed and treated with excellent results.

Endoscopic biopsies are essential for clinical diagnosis and localization of the lesion. The specimens must be properly oriented in order to evaluate the depth of tumor invasion. In addition, endoscopically directed and ultrasound guided fine needle biopsy and cytology have been used for assessment of advanced tumors (12).

GROSS EXAMINATION

The surgically resected specimen is examined promptly. It should be properly oriented and measured. External inspection and palpation may reveal the extent of tumor invasion into the adventitia and neighboring organs. The location and status of lymph nodes should be recorded. The specimen is then opened longitudinally along the least involved plane to avoid cutting into the lesion. The location, size, and shape of the tumor are determined. The pathologist should pay special attention to the extent of tumor spread at its border, which may be covered by an intact mucosa, and the length of tumor-free segment toward the resection margins. The mucosa outside the main tumor should be examined carefully for any area of discoloration, plaque, erosio, or ulceration. Such lesions may turn out to be early carcinomas. Patches of red, soft, and intact mucosa in the distal esophagus may be Barrett epithelium, which is the usual seat for adenocarcinoma but may accompany squamous cell carcinoma in rare cases. Areas of ulceration, hemorrhage, and necrosis in the tumor should be recorded. Fresh tissue samples are taken for other studies and special fixations.

HISTOLOGIC STUDY

Histologic diagnosis of tumors is readily evident in most cases. Nevertheless, occasional instances of composite tumors may be encountered. For these and some poorly differentiated tumors, special stains and additional studies may be required. It is important to note the following: vascular, lymphatic, and perineural invasions; microscopic foci of metastasis in the lymph nodes; and intramural spread of the tumor away from the main lesion.

EPIDEMIOLOGY

GEOGRAPHIC DISTRIBUTION

Esophageal cancer has a world-wide distribution. Its incidence and death rates vary greatly among nations (Fig. 21.2) (13). The highest incidence areas include parts of northern China, northern Iran along the Caspian Sea, and the Transkei region of South Africa. Regional differences within these countries have also been reported. For example, in the high-risk area of Linxian in northern China, the incidence rate of esophageal cancer in men is 161.5 per 100,000, whereas in Fanxian, about 100 miles away, the incidence is only 26.5 (14). Such differences support the view that environment, not

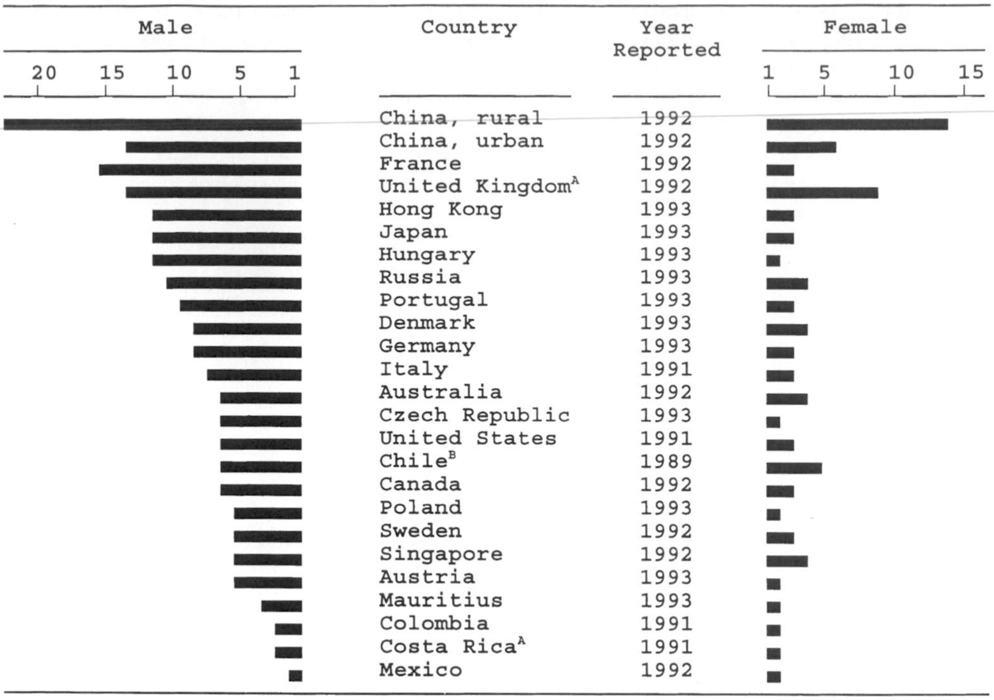

Male	Country	Year Reported	Female
20 15 10 5 1			1 5 10 15
	China, rural	1992	
	China, urban	1992	
	France	1992	
	United Kingdom[A]	1992	
	Hong Kong	1993	
	Japan	1993	
	Hungary	1993	
	Russia	1993	
	Portugal	1993	
	Denmark	1993	
	Germany	1993	
	Italy	1991	
	Australia	1992	
	Czech Republic	1993	
	United States	1991	
	Chile[B]	1989	
	Canada	1992	
	Poland	1993	
	Sweden	1992	
	Singapore	1992	
	Austria	1993	
	Mauritius	1993	
	Colombia	1991	
	Costa Rica[A]	1991	
	Mexico	1992	

Figure 21.2   Death rates for esophageal cancer per 100,000 population by sex in selected countries.

genetics or race, are significant risk factors for esophageal cancer. The mortality rate in men in urban areas of China had decreased remarkably from 31.7 in 1977 (15) to 12.6 in 1992 (12), probably because of improved food preservation and early diagnosis and treatment. Decreases have been noted also in central Asia and other high risk regions as life styles change (16).

In the United States, the incidence rate of esophageal cancer is 3.9 per 100,000 population (17). The estimated number of new cases in 1997 is 12,300 and the estimated number of deaths is 11,500, 3.1 times more in men than in women (1). From 1973 to 1992, both incidence and mortality rates have shown a slight increase, mainly in the white population, with an annual increase of 0.9 and 1.1%, respectively (17). Similar increases were noted in other Western nations, probably because of an increase in adeno-carcinoma.

AGE, SEX AND RACIAL DISTRIBUTION

The incidence of esophageal cancer increases with age, more prominent in the high risk regions (13). The age distribution in the United States is shown in Figure 21.3 (17). The incidence, mortality, and 5-year survival rates and lifetime risks of being diagnosed with and dying from esophageal cancer are shown in Table 21.2. The incidence and mortality rates are three to four times higher in males than in females in both whites and blacks, whereas the survival rates are similar between the races. The higher incidence and mortality rates in African Americans may be related to higher consumption of alcohol and tobacco (18). The survival rates are lower in blacks, although the distribution of cases at different stages of the disease is similar in both white and black patients.

ETIOLOGIC FACTORS

The etiology of esophageal cancer is unknown. Several risk factors, however, are well recognized, the significance of which varies in different areas. Multiple factors are likely involved in any particular region.

CARCINOGENS

N-nitrosamines are the only group of carcinogens recognized as effective on the esophagus (19). They have been used extensively in animal experiments (20). Low levels of nitrosamines and their precursors have been found in the food in high-risk regions in China and India (21, 22). In addition, evidence of endogenous nitrosation of amines with measurable amounts of N-nitroso compounds in the urine correlated with esophageal cancer mortality (23). The presence of n-nitroso compounds and aromatic hydrocarbons in alcoholic beverages and tobacco smoke may be responsible for the carcinogenicity of these substances (24, 25).

ALCOHOL AND TOBACCO

Excessive use of tobacco and alcohol has been considered a major risk factor for esophageal cancer in many parts of the world, including the United States, Europe, Japan, and parts of China (18, 24, 26). Carcinogens in tobacco may be directly related to esophageal cancer. The action of alcohol on esophageal carcinogenesis may be indirect, aside from possible contamination of carcinogens. Alcohol may modify the absorption or metabolism of the carcinogens, including tobacco-specific carcinogens (25). Thus, alcohol and tobacco may have synergistic effects on the development of esophageal carcinoma (27). Stopping drinking has been shown to reduce the risk of esophageal cancer 10 to 14 years later for moderate drinkers and 15 or more years later for heavy drinkers (28). Alcohol, however, is not a significant etiologic factor in Iran and northern China (29).

DIETARY FACTORS

The high-risk regions for esophageal cancer generally have poor agriculture, i.e., lacking fresh vegetables and fruit (24, 30). In northern China, ingestion of pickled vegetables and moldy food is common, and these food items may be contaminated with carcinogens (20, 31). In India, smoked meat and fish and dried vegetables are common dietary components that may contain carcinogens (22). The diet in China is often low in beta-carotene; vitamins A, B complex, C, E; and trace elements, such as selenium, molybdenum, zinc, and others (21, 32). Levels of these metals are low also in the soil in the high-risk areas, which can affect the local vegetation; e.g., soil low in molybdenum may lead to an increase in nitrates and

possibly nitrosamines in plants grown in that soil (24). Dietary supplements of vitamins and minerals have been used in China in recent years in efforts to reduce the risk of esophageal cancer. Preliminary 6-year results are inconclusive (17).

INFECTIOUS AGENTS

The pickled vegetables and moldy food eaten in the high-risk regions of China are often contaminated with fungi, such as Fusarium moniliforme and Alternaria alternata. Both of these fungi have also been found in corn, a stable food in northern China (21, 34, 35). Fumonisins from the former and alternariol monomethyl ether from the latter are mutagenic in vitro and tumorigenic in mice and rats. Human papillomavirus (HPV) induces papilloma in the esophagus (36). These papillomas are benign and rarely become malignant. N-nitrosamines induce papillomas as well as carcinomas in the rats (37). Human esophageal carcinomas are generally not associated with papillomas. Recently, using in situ hybridization techniques, HPV genomes, mostly types 16 and 18, have been

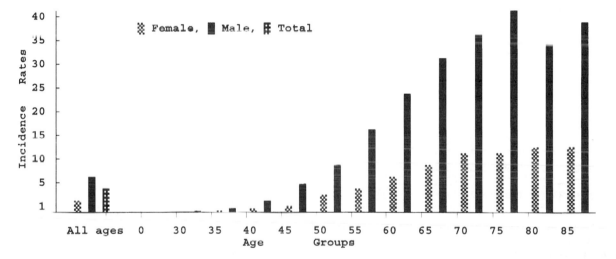

Figure 21.3 Incidence rates of esophageal cancer in the United States per 100,000 population by sex and age, 1988–1992.

| TABLE 21.2 | Incidence, Mortality, and Survival Rates and Lifetime Risks of Esophageal Cancer in U.S. Population According to Race and Sex |

	All Races			Whites			Blacks		
	T	M	F	T	M	F	T	M	F
Incidence rate (1988–1992)	3.9	6.5	1.8	3.4	5.7	1.6	9.8	16.7	4.7
Mortality rate (1988–1992)	3.5	6.0	1.5	3.0	5.3	1.2	8.3	14.8	3.7
5-year survival rate (1986–1991)	10.1	10.1	9.7	11.1	11.5	10.0	7.1	6.6	8.4
Lifetime risk (%)									
Being diagnosed with		0.71	0.26		0.66	0.25		1.26	0.49
Dying from		0.65	0.23		0.62	0.22		0.99	0.42

Data from Kosary LL, Ries LAG, Miller, et al., eds. SEER Cancer Statistical Review 1973–1992. Bethesda: NCI Publication 96–2789, 1996;181–189.

T, total; M, males; F, females.

detected in human squamous cell carcinomas from a variety of countries (38). Epstein-Barr virus has been found in an undifferentiated carcinoma with lymphoid stroma (39).

RADIATION AND THERMAL INJURY

Patients who received radiotherapy to the chest for breast carcinoma and less frequently for lymphoma may develop esophageal carcinoma many years later (40). In one report (41), 5 of 1534 (0.335%) breast carcinoma patients treated with postoperative radiotherapy and 8 of 4777 (0.17%) patients treated with surgery alone developed cancer of the thoracic esophagus.

Thermal injury resulting in chronic esophagitis after the intake of hot food, tea, or soup has been associated with esophageal cancer in China and Japan (42, 43). Hot maté drink is similarly implicated in South America (44).

GENETIC FACTORS

Patients with esophageal carcinoma may have a family history of the disease (29, 45). In general, a genetic connection appears weak. The only disease showing significant hereditary transmission is familial tylosis palmaris and plantaris, a rare autosomal dominant disease (46). It is estimated that these patients have a 90% chance of developing esophageal carcinoma by age 65 (47).

Chromosomal alterations have been detected in esophageal cancer tissue and cell lines (48, 49). The number of chromosomes ranged from 45 to 100. Y chromosome loss and numeric and structural changes of autosomes have been noted. Detailed discussions of cytogenetic changes are presented in Chapter 7.

Recent advances in molecular techniques have elicited many changes involving oncogenes and tumor suppressor genes in the esophageal carcinomas (see Chapter 13). Briefly stated, amplification and overexpression have been found for oncogenes c-myc, c-fos, c-ras, c-sis, c-raf, cyclin Dl, c-erbB, hstl, and int-2 (25, 50). Suppressor genes showing inactivation, mutation or loss of heterozygosity include p53, rb, APC, MCC, DCC and MTS-1 (25, 51). Allelic loss has also been found in loci other than those containing known suppressor genes (52). Microsatellite instability is noted in association with many carcinomas (53).

EXPERIMENTAL CARCINOGENESIS

N-nitroso compounds have been used to induce esophageal tumors in rats (20, 37). N-nitrosomethylbenzylamine produces carcinoma in 15 weeks (54). Papillomas are common (29). Precancerous lesions include epithelial hyperplasia and dysplasia (55). In the high-risk region of Linxian in northern China, the incidence rate of squamous cell carcinoma of the pharynx and upper esophagus in farm-raised chickens was 175.8 per 100,000, whereas in the nearby low-risk region of Fanxian, the corresponding incidence rate was only 18.9 (15). These rates are comparable to the incidence rate of esophageal cancer in the human population in these regions. Of note, the chickens ate scraps of food stuffs consumed by local residents and therefore were exposed to the carcinogenic effects of the contaminated agents in the food.

ASSOCIATED CONDITIONS

Esophageal cancer occurs more frequently in patients with certain other conditions affecting the esophagus. These conditions may be called precancerous, although the frequency of esophageal malignancy (usually low) varies, and the causal relationship of these conditions to carcinogenesis is not clear in most instances.

CHRONIC ESOPHAGITIS

Nonspecific chronic esophagitis is generally mild. Endoscopy and biopsy studies in China and Iran revealed that the incidence of overt chronic esophagitis was higher in the high-risk areas than in low-risk areas (56), even in young age groups. In one study in China involving persons 25 years of age or younger, chronic esophagitis was present in 43.6% of males and 35.6% of females (57). Its occurrence has been related to drinking hot beverages, smoking, and alcohol consumption (57, 58). The inflamed squamous epithelium may show foci of atrophy and dysplasia (58). Esophagitis secondary to acid or alkaline reflux may be severe and associated with columnar epithelial metaplasia and adenocarcinoma (see Chapter 22).

HIATUS HERNIA

Hiatus hernia is commonly associated with reflux esophagitis, followed by the development of Barrett epithelium and adenocarcinoma. Squamous cell carcinoma has been reported in about 1% of hernia patients (59), usually in the squamous epithelium, and occasionally in columnar epithelium (60).

BENIGN STRICTURE OF THE ESOPHAGUS

Benign stricture complicating peptic ulceration is another facet of Barrett esophagus. Adenocarcinoma has been reported in 22% of patients with stricture (61). Esophageal stricture may follow accidental ingestion of lye or other caustic liquids during childhood. Carcinomas have been reported in 0 to 4% of such patients (62), occurring many years after the ingestion of caustic chemicals (63). The carcinomas are located mostly in the midesophagus where the esophagus normally is compressed by the neighboring organs and suffers more severe injury than other parts of the esophagus.

ACHALASIA

The reported incidence of esophageal carcinoma in achalasia varies from 0 to 33 times that of the normal population (64, 65). The mean interval after the onset of symptoms of achalasia is 11.5 to 17 years (65,66). Among patients with achalasia for 30 years, 12% died of esophageal cancer (67). In one report, 1.1% of cases of esophageal carcinoma were associated with achalasia (66). The survival rates were low, probably because of late diagnosis.

PLUMMER-VINSON SYNDROME

Plummer-Vinson syndrome occurs predominantly in Scandinavian women. Its triad of symptoms are iron deficiency anemia, stomatitis, and dysphagia. Webs may be present in the esophagus.

Carcinomas develop in the pharynx and cervical esophagus, particularly at the postcricoid region in about 1.4% of the patients (68).

CELIAC DISEASE

Celiac disease affects primarily the small intestines, causing malabsorptive syndrome. Patients have a high incidence of malignancies, mainly lymphomas and gastrointestinal carcinomas, most commonly esophageal carcinoma. The prevalence is about 4 to 10% (69, 70).

ESOPHAGEAL DIVERTICULUM

Carcinoma may develop within an esophageal diverticulum, mostly of Zenker's type. The incidence is 0 to 4% (71). Cheng et al. described four cases of esophageal carcinoma that arose near the diverticulum (72). No evidence exists to suggest a causal relationship between these two entities.

PRECANCEROUS LESIONS

Precancerous lesions are pathologic lesions from which carcinoma develops through a series of cellular changes.

SQUAMOUS PAPILLOMA

Squamous papillomas are commonly found in the esophagus in rats treated experimentally with N-nitroso compounds (20). These lesions are either precancerous in that carcinomas evolve within them, or paracancerous in that they remain benign, but coexist with separate carcinomas. In humans, squamous papillomas are uncommon. When they arise, they are located mostly in the distal esophagus and may be multiple; they are caused by HPV (36). Although human esophageal squamous cell carcinomas generally are not associated with benign papillomas, HPV DNA has been demonstrated in about one half of the carcinomas, mainly of types 16 and 18 (73–75).

DYSPLASIA OF SQUAMOUS EPITHELIUM

The dysplastic epithelium is composed of abnormal pleomorphic cells in a disorderly arrangement. On the basis of the degree of the abnormalities, the dysplastic changes may be considered mild, moderate, or severe (Fig. 21.4). The precancerous nature of dysplastic epithelium is supported by two essential observations. First, dysplasia and carcinoma often coexist in continuity. Second, follow-up studies have shown the development of carcinoma in dysplastic epithelium after a variable interval. In a study in China, 66.7% of early esophageal carcinomas were accompanied by dysplastic epithelium (10). In a report from Japan, the correlation was noted in 20.1% (76). Of 73 dysplastic foci in this report, 12 were mild, 33 were moderate, and 30 were severe. In a follow-up study, 15% of severely dysplastic esophagi developed carcinoma in 1 to 12 years, whereas only 1% of hyperplastic esophagi developed carcinoma (77). The dysplastic epithelial cells can be detected by exfoliative cytology, a technique that has been used in mass survey in China. In a 15-year follow-up study of 12,693 patients with dysplastic cells, carcinoma developed in 1162 (9%) (78).

Using molecular techniques, DNA aneuploidy was detected in 50% of moderately and severely dysplastic esophageal cells, similar to that of in situ carcinoma (79). Epidermal growth factor receptor was expressed in the dysplastic tissue (80). A report on p53 immunostaining of esophageal epithelium in patients with carcinoma revealed positive staining in 1 of 3 normal epithelia, 3 of 23 hyperplastic epithelia, 4 of 11 dysplastic epithelia, and 16 of 29 early carcinoma (81). These reports indicate that dysplastic epithelium has markers of neoplastic transformation and abnormal DNA content and composition. These changes may be taken as evidence of irreversible malignancy. On the other hand, dysplasia may regress, even disappear, histologically. Further studies are needed to determine the true nature of dysplastic cells. It is likely that they are heterogeneous and should be evaluated individually.

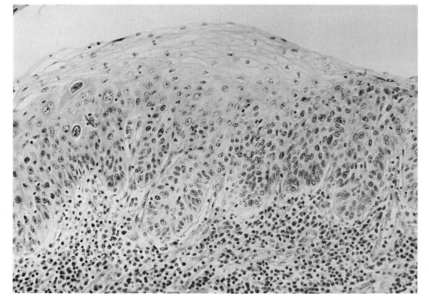

Figure 21.4 Moderate dysplasia of squamous epithelium showing pleomorphic cells with enlarged nuclei and decreased cytoplasm in lower layers of the epithelium. Cells in the left upper layers appear normal. (Reprinted with permission from Ming SC. Pathology of esophageal cancer. In: Aisner J, Arriagada R, Green MR, Martini N, Perry MC. eds. Comprehensive textbook of thoracic oncology. Baltimore: Williams & Wilkins, 1996.)

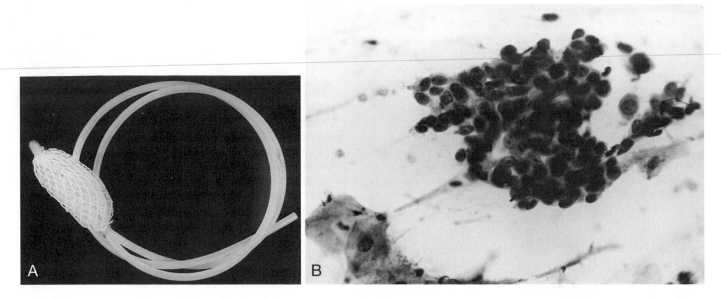

Figure 21.5 **A.** A balloon used for obtaining cytologic specimens. It is wrapped by a nylon net, which traps the superficial cells of the esophageal epithelium and tumor as the inflated balloon is gently pulled out of the esophagus. The cytologic material obtained by this technique is similar to that of a brush cytologic preparation. **B.** Cytologic appearance of a moderately differentiated squamous cell carcinoma of the esophagus. The malignant cells are characterized by reversed nuclear to cytoplasmic ratio, hyperchromatic nuclei with prominent nucleoli. A few nonneoplastic squamous cells are present for comparison. (Courtesy of K. Ni, M.D. Temple University School of Medicine, Philadelphia, PA.)

PATHOLOGY OF SQUAMOUS CELL CARCINOMA

LOCATION

The most common site of squamous cell carcinoma (SCC) of the esophagus is the middle one third, followed by the lower and upper thirds (82–87). In Linxian, China, where the high incidence of esophageal SCC is well known, a study showed that 63.3%, 24.9%, and 11.7% of SCC were found in the middle, lower, and upper thirds, respectively (84). Studies of esophageal SCC at autopsy and of surgically removed specimens have shown similar distributions. It is rare to find SCC at either end of the esophagus.

Although the pathologic features of SCC at different locations are similar, the anatomic structures surrounding the esophagus are different at different levels. Location of the tumor, therefore, is a major factor in determining the surgical management of esophageal SCC (88).

EARLY SQUAMOUS CELL CARCINOMA

Early esophageal carcinoma is defined as a tumor that has not extended beyond the submucosa and has not metastasized (84). The term "early carcinoma" has become known since the 1960s, as a result of the finding of improved survival of patients in whom esophageal SCC was detected by using balloon cytology (Fig. 21.5), many in their early stage, and treated by surgical resection (89). The improved survival rate of patients with esophageal SCC reported from China has attracted many studies (90–99). Most of the early SCC lesions were found in the middle and lower portions of the

esophagus and rarely in the upper portion and range from 0.4 to 8.5 cm in diameter (84).

The gross appearance of early carcinoma is categorized into four types. The most common early SCC is the plaque type, followed by erosive, papillary, and occult types (84). The plaque type demonstrates a platform-like structure, elevated above the adjacent esophageal mucosa. The surface is coarsely granular and white, and may show erosion. The cut surface shows a thickened zone along the surface. On histologic examination, approximately 45% are intramucosal and another 33% are submucosal; the remainder are intraepithelial (84). The erosive type is clearly demarcated and slightly depressed or, as the term indicates, eroded. The eroded surface appears granular. Microscopically, most of these lesions are intraepithelial or intramucosal; the minority are submucosal. Like the plaque type, the papillary early carcinomas are elevated above the surrounding mucosa, are clearly demarcated, and may be eroded. Unlike the plaque type, they have polypoid or papillary contours. Microscopically, more than one half of the papillary carcinomas are submucosal; the others are intramucosal or intraepithelial. The occult type is small and displays a pink or congested surface that is flat and in continuity with the normal esophageal mucosa. These subtle features are difficult to recognize grossly. All occult carcinomas are intraepithelial. Because it is virtually grossly undetectable, it may be impossible for the endoscopist to perform a precise biopsy of this lesion, missing a virtually curable stage. It may also escape the surgeon's examination when they attempt to determine the margin of resection, paving the way for recurrence.

Histologically, three types have been included in the category of early SCC, namely, intraepithelial, intramucosal, and submucosal (84). The intraepithelial carcinomas are characterized by malignant squamous cells involving the entire thickness of the squamous epithelium underlined by an intact basement membrane, hence, squamous cell carcinoma in situ (Fig. 21.6A). The irregularly arranged neoplastic cells are large, pleomorphic, or small with hyperchromatic nuclei. Mitoses are present. With the hematoxylin and eosin stain, the intact basement membrane is usually reflected by a smooth line between the neoplastic epithelium and the subjacent stroma. Usually seen in the plaque and papillary early carcinomas, the in situ SCC composed of large cells may cause the increase in thickness of the involved mucosa, either raising it above the level of the surrounding mucosa or growing downward to create buddings. The latter may cause difficulty in assessing invasion. The in situ SCC composed of small cells usually does not thicken the involved mucosa, and usually is seen in the grossly erosive type of early

carcinoma. The descriptive term "erosive", therefore, is applied to the surface appearance, i.e., grossly disrupted, and is not necessarily correlated with denuded mucosa.

Sometimes, a section obtained from the margin of infiltrating SCC carcinoma shows malignant cells above the basement membrane and in direct contact with neighboring normal squamous cells with an abrupt demarcation (see Fig. 21.6B). This change suggests spread of carcinoma cells intraepithelially rather than in situ squamous cell carcinoma (89), as the latter should show a gradual change from normal to dysplastic to frankly malignant cells (see Fig. 21.6A).

The intramucosal type of early carcinoma is characterized by infiltration of small groups of carcinoma cells in the lamina propria, but not beyond, signifying that the previously in situ SCC has already penetrated the basement membrane. The epithelium-

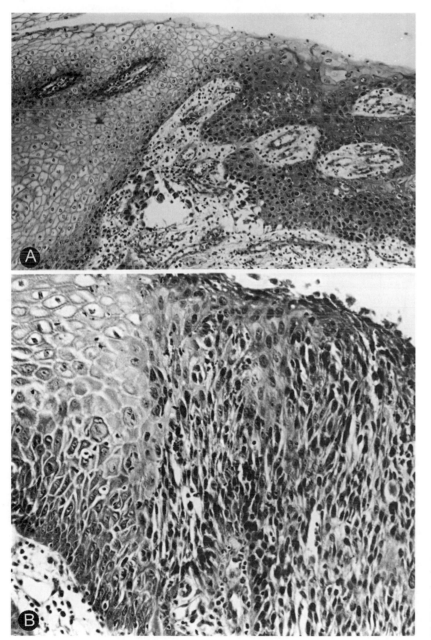

Figure 21.6 A. In situ SCC showing a gradual transition from the benign squamous epithelium on the left to the neoplastic area on the right. **B.** Intraepithelial spread of a SCC. The spreading malignant cells and the apposing nonneoplastic epithelium create a sharp demarcation.

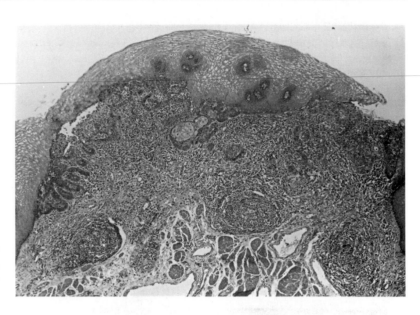

Figure 21.7 Intramucosal SCC characterized by infiltration of clusters of carcinoma in the lamina propria, associated with chronic inflammation. Note also buddings of in situ SCC.

stroma interface shows an irregular border (Fig. 21.7) as compared to the smooth outline seen in the intact basement membrane in the normal esophageal epithelium or in in situ SCC (see Fig. 21.5A).

The submucosal SCC lesions are characterized by carcinoma cells that have penetrated the muscularis mucosa into the submucosa but have not reached the muscularis proper, the invasive area showing a continuity with the intraepithelial component of the SCC. The tissue surrounding the invasive areas often shows chronic inflammation. These lesions are larger than the intraepithelial and intramucosal carcinomas.

Kitamura et al. suggested that dysplasia of the squamous epithelium is the earliest carcinoma (95). The destruction of the basement membrane underlying the in situ neoplasm, as demonstrated in an immunohistochemical study, may be a mechanism for invasion (99). Rubio et al. observed that the degree of cellular atypia and the formation of the neoplastic buds were associated with progression toward microinvasion (96).

When the intraepithelial, intramucosal, and submucosal SCC were analyzed separately and compared (90–94, 98), the results indicated that the submucosal SCC lesions were different from the intraepithelial and intramucosal SCC in that the former have shown more frequent lymph node metastases and lower survival rates compared to intraepithelial and intramucosal SCC (91–94, 98).

Sugimachi et al. recommended that a submucosal carcinoma should be excluded from the classification of early carcinoma (97). We agree and propose the use of intraepithelial, intramucosal, and submucosal categories in diagnosing esphageal SCC, because these terms are more precise than either early or superficial.

ADVANCED SQUAMOUS CELL CARCINOMA

Esophageal SCC that invades the muscularis propria and beyond belong to this category. Unfortunately, most patients have advanced SCC at the time of presentation, largely due to the lack of symptoms or signs associated with small lesions.

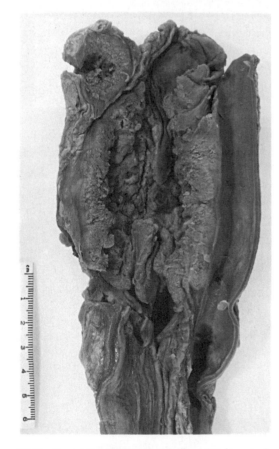

Figure 21.8 Fungating SCC. The surface is ulcerated and the cut surface shows full penetration of the esophageal wall and extension to the adventitia of the aorta. A lymph node involved by metastatic carcinoma is seen in the left upper corner. (Reprinted with permission from Ming SC. Tumors of the esophagus and stomach. Washington, DC: Armed Forces Institute of Pathology, 1973;24–26.)

Infiltrating SCC accounts for 15% of cases and is characterized by intramural infiltration of tumor; the surface of these lesions may be shallowly ulcerated. The walls infiltrated by tumor cells are rigid, although not contracted, resulting in stenosis of the lumina.

The cut surfaces of SCC show homogenous gray-white, firm to hard tissue disrupting the mucosa and infiltrating the esophageal walls. In some cases, the tumor substance is soft, presumably from the lack of fibrous tissue (the so-called medullary type). Areas of necrosis may be present, either covering the base of an ulcerated SCC or within the tumor substance. The necrotic areas are friable and chalky white or yellow. The tumor may be observed extending into the deep (adventitial) resection margin. Twenty of 50 (40%) resected esophagi for cancer showed involvement of the deep margins (101).

Microscopically, advanced esophageal SCC are divided into well-, moderately, and poorly differentiated tumors. The well-differentiated SCC lesions are composed of oval or polygonal tumor cells with oval or round nuclei and prominent nucleoli. Although disorganized, the tumor cells exhibit some degree of maturation, and invariably, keratin production in the center of tumor cell groups surrounded by the flattened keratotic cells with pyknotic nuclei, creating structures called "keratin pearls" (Fig. 21.11). Mitoses are uncommon. Cells of the moderately differentiated SCC are slightly smaller, and more pleomorphic than those of the well-differenitiated SCC. Focally, keratin may be observed. Mitoses are easily found. Although tumor cells form sheets and clusters (Fig. 21.12), trabecular patterns can be seen, characterized by ribbon-like arrangements of tumor cells. The poorly differentiated SCC are composed of extremely pleomorphic cells with variable amount of cytoplasm and bizarre nuclei with prominent nucleoli (Fig. 21.13). Virtually no keratin is present; the tumor cells vary from round, polygonal, to spindly (see Fig. 21.13B), bearing very little or no resemblance to the normal squamous cells of the esophagus. When SCC are composed predominantly of spindle cells, they are regarded as spindle cell carcinomas or sarcomatoid

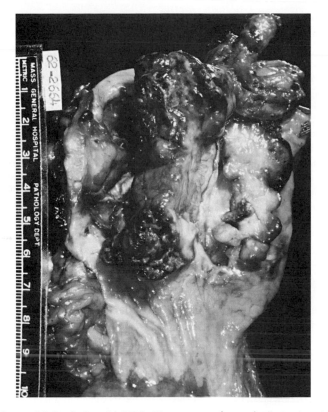

Figure 21.9 Polypoid SCC. The tumor shows large polypoid masses protruding into the lumen. The surface of the tumor is hemorrhagic, superficially ulcerated, and partly necrotic. (Reprinted with permission from Ming SC. Tumors of the esophagus and stomach. Washington, DC: Armed Forces Institute of Pathology, 1973;24–26.)

The gross appearance of advanced SCC assumes three types: fungating, ulcerative, and infiltrating (24). On the basis of their experience, researchers in China formulated a classification into medullary, fungating, ulcerative, scirrhous (stenosing), and intraluminal (polypoid) SCC (84).

The fungating SCC, the most common lesions, include those that are flat and plaquelike, or nodular and polypoid, protruding into the lumina of the esophagi, causing partial or complete obstruction (Fig. 21.8). They may be ulcerated and usually do not involve the entire circumference of the esophagi.

Polypoid SCC lesions were found in 7% of patients in the series studied by Sasajima et al. (100). These tumors are characterized by intraluminal polypoid or pedunculated lesions (Fig. 21.9). The incidence of adventitial invasion of these polypoid SCC is significantly lower than that of their nonpolypoid counterparts.

Ulcerative SCC constitutes 25% of the advanced cases. The ulcerated areas are shaggy and depressed but surrounded by flat or slightly elevated margins, which overhang over the edge of ulcer, from which the tumor may spread laterally (Fig. 21.10) to involve the adjacent tissue. The lateral spread may create a nodular appearance, over which the mucosa is intact. The vertical penetration of the esophageal wall and extension of the tumor into the surrounding organs, such as a trachea, may create a fistula.

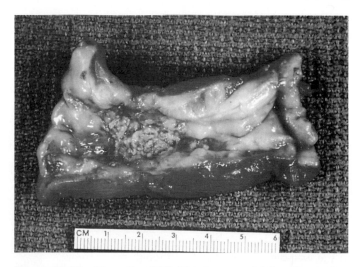

Figure 21.10 Ulcerative SCC. This tumor exhibits a large ulcer covered by necrotic material. Its edge is surrounded by slightly elevated mucosa. The cut surface of the esophageal wall is infiltrated by columns of tumor. (See color plate.)

carcinomas (see subsequent discussion). Tumor necrosis and mitoses are common.

On the basis of the features just described, the esophageal SCC are divided into grades I, II and III, representing well-, moderately, and poorly differentiated SCC, respectively (84). In a significant number of cases, however, the same tumors may show different degrees of differentiation; focal or large areas resembling papillary transitional cell carcinoma may be observed in an otherwise ordinary SCC. Apoptosis is observed in all three grades (102).

In many esophageal SCC lesions, HPV-type changes or koilocytosis are observed, leading Chang et al. to suggest that HPV is an

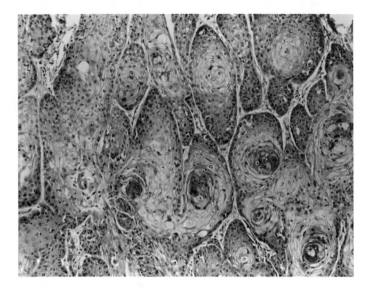

Figure 21.11   Well-differentiated (grade I) SCC characterized by sheets and islands of neoplastic squamous epithelium infiltrating the wall of the esophagus. The tumor cells show evidence of maturation and concentric layers of keratin, so-called keratin pearls.

etiologic factor (103). Further discussion of the etiology of this condition is found elsewhere in this chapter.

MULTIPLE SQUAMOUS CELL CARCINOMAS

Studies at autopsy (86) and of surgically resected esophagi for carcinoma (87, 104–107) have shown foci of squamous cell carcinoma separate from the primary SCC in 13.5 to 91.9%. Most of these separate carcinomas were intraepithelial, and less frequently, intramucosal, submucosal, or invasive (104, 105). The second lesions tended to arise proximal to the primary SCC of the lower esophagus and distal to the upper SCC (104). Pesko et al. (106) applied the following criteria for the diagnosis of multiple primary carcinoma of the esophagus: (a) The lesion shows malignant histologic features. (b) The second carcinoma shows in situ changes. (c) At least 1.5 cm of healthy esophageal tissue exists between two lesions. Using these criteria, they found that the rate of synchronous SCC was 31% (17 of 54 specimens). All 17 carcinomas were squamous, of which 10 were intraepithelial and/or submucosal and 7 invaded beyond the submucosa. In the same series, foci of dysplasia of varying degrees were found in 60% of 54 specimens, independent of the main SCC. In another series, Maeta et al. (107) found that the mean distance between the second primary and the main carcinomas was 2.6 cm.

These findings suggest that many SCC are multicentric in origin, reflecting field carcinogenesis. Yokoyama et al. (108) found a higher prevalence of multiple esophageal SCC in alcoholics with mutant aldehyde dehydrogenase 2*2 allele (ALDH2*2) than in those without this allele. The mutated ALDH2*2 results in ALDH2 enzyme inactivity. Without active ALDH2, an enzyme to eliminate the aldehyde, the blood level of the latter increases dramatically after drinking. Multiple epithelial cells of the esophagus are aldehyde-preconditioned, which may be activated with exposure to known carcinogens (e.g. smoking, etc.), to undergo an irreversible malignant change. The findings of mutated p53 suppressor gene and p53 protein accumulation in different regions of the esophagus indicate

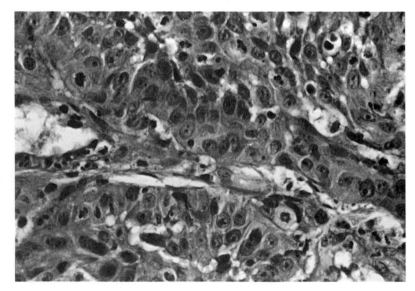

Figure 21.12   Moderately differentiated (grade II) SCC. The tumor cells are more pleomorphic than those in the well-differentiated SCC. Although many tumor cells can be recognized as squamous, keratinization is not observed. The tumor cells have relatively abundant cytoplasm and large nuclei with prominent nucleoli. Mitoses are easily found.

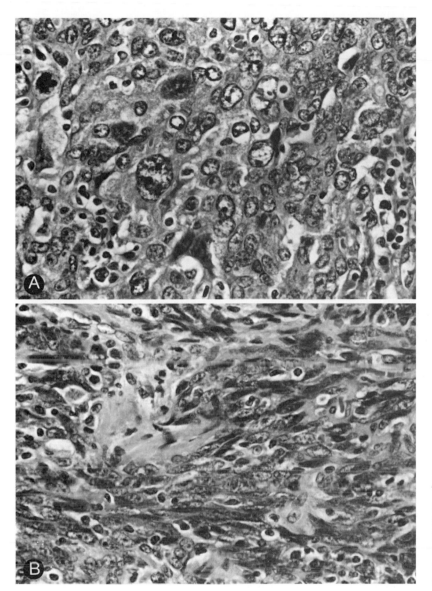

Figure 21.13   Poorly differentiated (grade III) SCC. The tumor cells vary greatly in size and shape, from polygonal, oval **(A)**, to spindly **(B).** Some tumor cells are bizarre. Mitoses are easily found. Cytologically, there is little resemblance to the normal squamous epithelial cells. If the spindle cells as seen in part B are predominant, the tumor is regarded as a spindle cell carcinoma.

that p53 alterations might be key molecular events in multifocal esophageal carcinogenesis (109).

CARCINOMAS OF THE UPPER AERODIGESTIVE TRACT ASSOCIATED WITH ESOPHAGEAL SQUAMOUS CELL CARCINOMA

Concurrent primary head and neck and gastric carcinomas can be associated with esophageal SCC (110–112). Of 339 patients with primary carcinoma of the esophagus, 11 (3.2%) had concurrent head and neck squamous cell carcinoma (110). Conversely, using endoscopy and Lugol dye, 8 of 127 (6.3%) patients with head and neck carcinomas were found to have esophageal SCC (112). Five of the 8 cases had superficial SCC. The rate of gastric carcinoma associated with esophageal SCC was 5.6% (110). Thirty nine of 1,294 patients with esophageal SCC had either synchronous or

metachronous primary carcinoma of the lung (113). The risk of a second cancer associated with esophageal carcinoma increases in patients with a family history of cancer of the upper aerodigestive tract (111).

VARIANTS OF SQUAMOUS CELL CARCINOMA

VERRUCOUS CARCINOMA

Verrucous carcinomas are rare (114, 115). They are considered a distinct entity but morphologically have the features of a very well-differentiated SCC. Grossly, verrucous carcinomas are exophytic, cauliflower-like or papillary, and white. Its color reflects the marked keratosis on the surface as observed microscopically. The superficial part of the tumor shows the characteristic papillary projections, but the deeper part is composed of islands of acanthotic squamous epithelium, compressing or infiltrating the underlying tissue (Fig. 21.14A). Most of the tumor cells are mature squamous

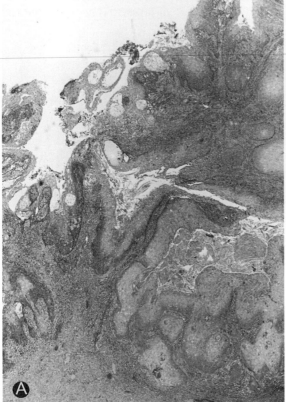

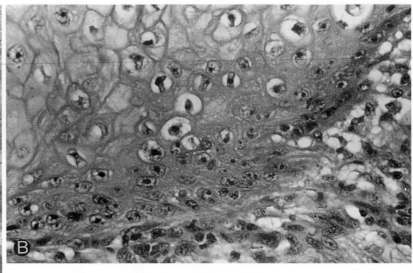

Figure 21.14   A. Low magnification of a verrucous carcinoma displaying papillary surface protruding into the lumen and a pushing component in the bottom. Keratinization is prominent. **B.** The malignant cells are characteristically found in the basal layers. Some tumor cells are vacuolated, resembling the human papilloma virus-related changes, or koilocytosis.

cells, exhibiting abundant eosinophilic cytoplasm and slightly atypical nuclei. Besides the evidence of invasion, which may not be apparent, the malignant nature is indicated by the highly atypical features of the squamous cells in the basal layer (see Fig. 21.14B). Endoscopic biopsy offers access to the superficial part of the lesion, which may not be sufficiently characteristic for a definitive diagnosis, emphasizing the importance of a close clinicopathologic correlation. Despite the well-differentiated state of verrucous carcinoma, the associated mortality rate is high (114, 115). Most patients died of complications, such as pneumonia, however.

BASALOID CARCINOMA

Basaloid carcinoma occurs in a variety of organs, including the esophagus. It is characterized microscopically by solid sheets or islands of tumor cells surrounded by basal lamina, closely resembling features of basal cell carcinomas of the skin, or by glandlike structures, resembling those of the salivary gland. The tumor cells are small, and have relatively scanty cytoplasm (Fig. 21.15), similar to cells of the basal layer of the squamous epithelium. Peripheral palisading is prominent and characteristic of basaloid carcinoma. Mitoses are frequent. Focal necrosis may be observed. The close histologic resemblance to adenoid cystic carcinoma of the salivary gland (see Fig. 21.15) has led some investigators to regard these tumors as adenoid cystic carcinoma of the esophagus (116). Because of the obvious squamous cell component observed invariably in basaloid carcinoma, including in situ changes, basaloid carcinoma is best regarded as a variant of SCC. In a recent study, Abe et al. found that 7 of 371 (1.9%) esophageal SCC fulfilled the criteria of basaloid

carcinoma (117). The ultrastructural examination confirmed the basal lamina. Immunohistochemical stains revealed staining with CK14 and CK19 in the peripheral neoplastic basal cells and basal cells of the normal squamous mucosa, and immunoreactivity of EGFR in all seven tumors. p53 was positive in five of seven cases. All tumors were aneuploid. Six of the seven patients had lymph nodes metastases; in four, the metastatic tumors showed basaloid components. The rate of lymph node metastasis suggests that basaloid carcinomas are aggressive, but their clinical behavior is difficult to determine based on a few cases (117).

SPINDLE CELL CARCINOMA AND CARCINOSARCOMA

In a small group of SCC, definite malignant squamous cells are admixed with malignant spindle tumor cells (see Fig. 21.13B) (118–121). Sometimes, the spindle cells are so prominent that they may be indistinguishable from those of a mesenchymal sarcoma. Numerous terms have been used to designate these tumors, i.e., sarcomatoid carcinoma, carcinosarcoma, metaplastic carcinoma, carcinoma with sarcomatoid changes, carcinoma with pseudosarcomatous stroma, pseudosarcoma, and spindle call carcinoma (118). The confusing terminology reflects the uncertain histogenesis, largely of the spindle cell (sarcomatoid) component. Transmission electron microscopic studies have shown desmosomes and tonofilaments in the spindle cells, indicating the epithelial nature of the spindle cells (119). Another study, however, revealed that spindle cells exhibited ultrastructural and immunologic features of pure epithelial cells, pure mesenchymal cells (i.e., fibroblasts, myofibroblasts, and fibroblastic or osteoclastic giant cells), or a mixture of both cell types (118). In another study of SCC with spindle cell component, the metastatic sites contained both carcinoma and sarcoma, or pure sarcoma (120).

Grossly, these tumors are polypoid, a feature similar to that of some polypoid SCC. The tumors may reach a diameter of 15 cm (24), with a surface that is smooth and intact or ulcerated. In some tumors, there is no sharp demarcation between the malignant spindle cell and the squamous carcinoma cell components. In others, the spindle cells may appear to be surrounding islands of ordinary SCC, without recognizable transition. Osseous, cartilaginous, and muscular tissue may be seen. Mitotic activities vary from tumor to tumor. Mixed inflammatory cells are frequently present in and around the tumor; the background may show fibrosis. Most tumors do not extend beyond the esophageal wall.

Results of light and electron microscopic and immunohistochemical studies demonstrate that these tumors are heterogeneous but can be categorized into two groups. One group consists of tumors in which both the epithelial nature of the SCC and the mesenchymal nature of the malignant spindle cell components are

proven, hence, carcinosarcomas. The other consists of tumors in which both SCC and the malignant spindle cells show epithelial markers, hence sarcomatoid carcinomas.

COMPOSITE CARCINOMAS

Some esophageal cancers show two or more cellular components (122–124). Different components either intermingle or demonstrate transition from one to another. The mixed heterogeneous cellular populations in the same tumor have been considered analogous to the different parts of a chimera (125). Perhaps it is appropriate to refer to these composite tumors as chimeric tumors. Different combinations are noted. Sugimachi et al. found glandular differentiation in 16.1% of the 310 SCC studied and suggested that the mucous gland or ducts may also be the origin of adenosquamous carcinoma (124). The carcinosarcoma, as described previously, is also a type of chimeric tumor. We observed an esophageal cancer consisting of both SCC and small cell

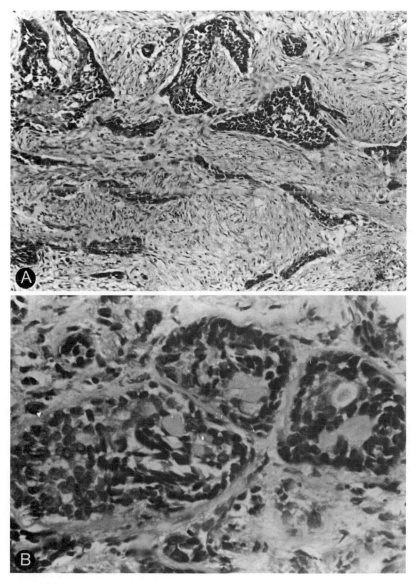

Figure 21.15 Basaloid carcinoma. **A.** This infiltrating tumor exhibits islands of tumor cells composed of scanty cytoplasm and hyperchromatic nuclei indistinguishable from those of basal cell carcinomas of the skin. Focally, squamous differentiation is observed in the central part of an island. **B.** Another example of basaloid carcinoma of the esophagus resembling adenoid cystic carcinoma of the salivary gland. The cytologic features are essentially the same as those of part A.

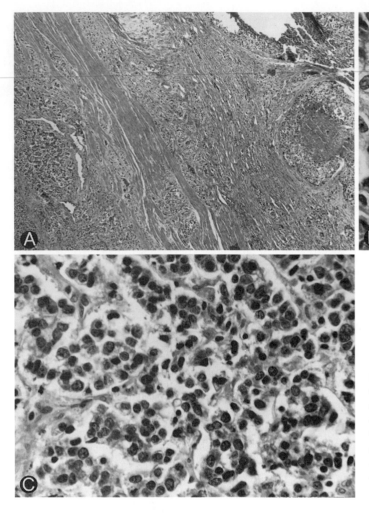

Figure 21.16 A malignant composite (or mixed) tumor composed of SCC with glandular differentiation on the right and carcinoid tumor component. On higher magnification, in the areas of SCC, the tumor cells are larger and possess more cytoplasm than those of the carcinoid components; some of these tumor cells form circular structures, strongly suggesting glandular differentiation **(B)**. The carcinoid components are characterized by ribbons or microglandular structures **(A)**; the tumor cells are relatively uniform and have scanty cytoplasm and round to oval nuclei **(C)**.

carcinoma, and a squamous cell carcinoma with focal glandular differentiation and carcinoid (Fig. 21.16).

TUMOR SPREAD AND METASTASIS

INTRAMURAL SPREAD

Extensions of SCC by direct invasion or metastasis through lymphatics within the walls of the esophagus or stomach are considered intramural spread.

The intraepithelial expansion of SCC can be recognized by a sharp demarcation between the malignant and the normal squamous cells (see Fig. 21.6B) (89). The invading malignant cells may appear singly (Fig. 21.17) or in small clusters. Another form is an intraductal spread (Fig. 21.18). Takubo et al. found that 111 of 175 (63%) SCC showed intraepithelial spread, and in 33 cases, gland duct involvement (126). The gland duct involvement may be a route to spread to deep tissue.

A clinicopathologic study showed that 24 of 201 (11.9%) patients had evidence of intramural metastasis in resected esophageal tissue (127). Beneath the mucosa, the SCC can spread along the tissue plane to a distance of 20 mm or more, as seen in the superficial spreading type of SCC or advanced cancers (Fig. 21.19) (128). Because of submucosal location and multifocality, it may be difficult for surgeons to determine adequate resection margins during surgery.

The neoplastic cells expand and invade the deep muscular tissue or form columns to vertically dissect the muscle bundles. The tumor cells continue to expand to involve the adventitia. Kawamura et al. found that the p53 expression and the labeling index of Ki-67 correlated with the depth of invasion (129).

Patients with intramural spread of tumor have a higher incidence of lymph node and distant metastases than those without such metastasis (127). Lateral spread of SCC through lymphatic channels may form satellite nodules resembling separate primary tumor. Lymphatic (Fig. 21.20), vascular, and neural invasions were found in 48.5%, 32.9%, and 26.1%, respectively, of esophageal SCC (130).

CONTIGUOUS INVOLVEMENT OF NEIGHBORING ORGANS

The vertical invasion from the superficial to the deep esophageal wall and beyond is responsible for the involvement of the adjacent tissue or organs and fistula formation.

Autopsy studies have shown an overall incidence of contiguous involvement ranging from 9.1%, 18% to over 60% (82, 85, 86). Organs involved include the trachea, bronchus, aorta, mediastinum, pericardium, pleura, and lung (86, 131), the trachea being the most frequently affected. Tracheal invasion is most often observed in tumors of the upper (proximal) one third of the esophagus. Infiltration of the tracheobronchi often leads to the development of esophagorespiratory fistulae, which are life threatening and difficult to manage (131, 132). All 41 patients with malignant tracheoesophageal fistulae died within 1 year (131). Complications from contiguous involvement depend on the organs affected. Mediastinitis, pneumonia, abscess and rupture of the aorta can be observed (85).

LYMPH NODE METASTASIS

The rates of node metastasis correlate with the depth of invasion (Table 21.3). Observations have confirmed that the intraepithelial SCC, or squamous cell carcinoma in situ, are not associated with lymph node metastasis. The high rates of lymph node metastasis in the surgically removed specimens of invasive carcinoma (87, 91) are similar to those studied at autopsy (85, 86). Regional lymph nodes typically are involved. For instance, in one report, the cervical lymph nodes were most often involved when the lesions were in the upper one third of the esophagus (82). This finding has prompted the recommendation that esophageal SCC of the

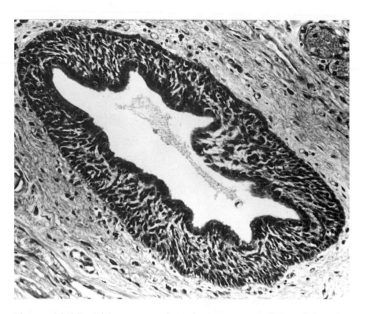

Figure 21.18 This mucous duct shows tumor cells involving the wall, but the basement membrane appears intact. The main tumor is a SCC.

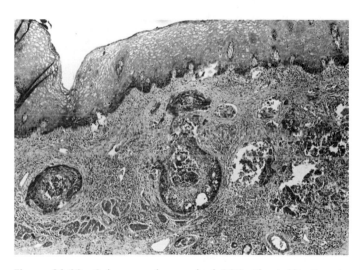

Figure 21.19 Submucosal spread of SCC. The infiltrating islands of SCC are observed in the lamina propria and submucosa. The overlying esophageal mucosa is noncancerous.

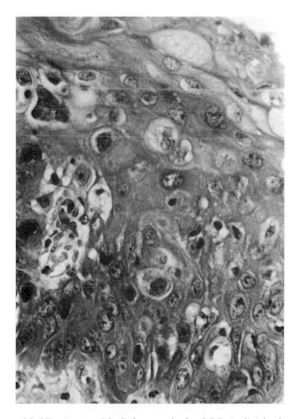

Figure 21.17 Intraepithelial spread of a SCC. Individual tumor cells are found infiltrating the nonneoplastic squamous epithelial cells. The main tumor in this case is a SCC.

upper one third be surgically treated differently than those of the middle or lower thirds (88).

HEMATOGENOUS METASTASIS

Venous invasion has not been observed in association with intraepithelial (in situ) or intramucosal esophageal SCC, but it has been noted in 27% of the submucosal SCC (93) and in 32.9 to 76.5% of advanced SCC (130, 133). Distant organ metastasis often reflects venous invasion. Autopsy studies have shown the rate of visceral metastasis to be 29.8 to 50% (85, 86). The organ most frequently involved is the lung (20 to 30%), followed by the liver (14 to 23%).

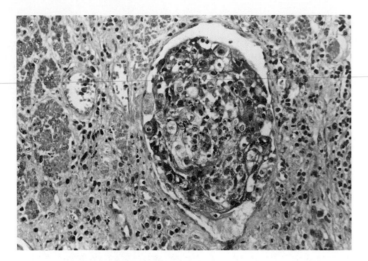

Figure 21.20 Lymphatic invasion characterized by small clusters of SCC in the lumen of lymphatics.

Bone, kidney, adrenal gland, brain, peritoneum biliary tract, skin, pancreas, etc., can also be affected.

STAGING OF ESOPHAGEAL CANCERS

The most commonly used staging system is that proposed by the American Joint Commission on Cancer (134), which is based on the status of the primary tumor (T), lymph nodes (N), and distant metastasis (M) (Table 21.4). Unlike previous versions of this staging system, the size of the primary tumor and fistula formation are not taken into account. The more aggressive submucosal lesions are grouped with the less aggressive intramucosal lesions, as T1. Although both are superficial lesions, hence, stage I disease, the presence of lymph node and/or distant metastasis upstage the submucosal SCC to advanced stages. Some investigators use N1 to denote metastasis to one to four regional lymph nodes, and N2 for five or more nodes (135). Metastasis to distant lymph nodes outside the region in which the SCC arises, e.g., abdominal lymph nodes in a SCC of the upper one third, etc., is considered distant metastasis. The staging system consists of cTMN and pTMN, for clinical and pathologic staging, respectively.

SURVIVAL RATES AND PROGNOSTIC FACTORS

SURVIVAL RATES

The overall survival rate of esophageal SCC generally is low (136–140), although the rate in China is higher (139, 140) (Table 21.5). The slightly better prognosis may be related to the high number of early carcinomas detected by mass survey in China.

PROGNOSTIC FACTORS

STAGE OF CARCINOMA

The stage of esophageal cancer at the time of diagnosis is the most important prognostic factor (84, 137, 139, 140). The 5-year survival rates of pTNM stages I, II, III and IV tumors were 83.3% to 46.3%, 26.4%, and 6.7%, respectively (84).

TUMOR SPREAD AND METASTASIS

Esophageal carcinomas with intramural spread are associated with higher rates of lymph node and distant organ metastases than those without such metastasis (127). When a comparison was made between stages II and IV diseases, the survival was significantly improved in patients with tumors that showed no intramural metastasis. The recurrence rate in tumors with positive circumferential resection margins was higher (40%) than in those with negative margins (13%) (101). The status of lymph node metastasis clearly affects the prognosis. The 5-year survival rate of patients without lymph node metastasis is about three times that of patients with nodal metastasis (84). The number of positive lymph nodes also affects the prognosis. For instance, the 18-month survival rates were 83% for N0, 53% for N1, and 43% for N2 (N0 = negative lymph node; N1 = 1 to 4 positive nodes; N2 = 5 or more lymph nodes). The 5-year survival rate in patients with blood vessel or lymphatic invasion was 0%, whereas that in patients without such spread was 15.9 and 21.9%, respectively (130).

LOCATION OF PRIMARY CARCINOMA

Contiguous involvement of the adjacent organs by esophageal SCC reduces the resectability and causes complications. The organ most frequently affected is the tracheobronchial tree, from the SCC of the upper one third of the esophagus. One possible result is the development of an esophagorespiratory fistula (85), which is not only difficult to manage but also fatal (131). SCC of the midthoracic esophagus may cause rupture of the aorta (131). Carcinomas of the lower one third frequently are associated with metastasis to the abdominal lymph nodes and visceral organs (82).

SIZE OF CARCINOMA

Size is not a parameter in the TNM staging system (134). The majority of superficial SCC are small; large tumors are most likely advanced SCC. In studies correlating the size of tumor, the 5-year survival rate in patients with tumors 1 cm or less in diameter was 82.9%; that for lesions 3 to 5 cm in diameter was 27.2%. All 22 patients with tumors larger that 15 cm died within 3 years (141). The 5-year survival rate of patients with 3 cm in diameter or smaller tumors was 48%, and that of patients with larger tumors was 28.9% (84). Tumors larger than 7 cm reduce the resectability (139).

PLOIDY OF CARCINOMA CELLS

Studies of DNA ploidy in correlation with prognosis have shown controversial conclusions. Classifying the DNA content into types I to IV, Matsuura et al. (142) found that the incidence of high ploidy group (types III and IV) in advanced esophageal carcinomas was high and was associated with a poor prognosis. No significant correlation between DNA ploidy and prognosis was found in other studies, however (143, 144). Of interest is the intratumoral heterogeneity of DNA ploidy observed when different samples were examined from the same tumor (145, 146). The DNA heterogeneity raises a question as to whether the analysis based on a single sample from each tumor accurately reflects the true behavior of SCC.

MOLECULAR MARKERS

Immunohistochemical study of blood group-related antigens in superficial carcinomas showed significant correlation between immunoreactivity of Lewis a and depth of invasion. In the superficial carcinoma, there were significant correlations between immunoreactivity of Lewis x and lymph node status and between immunoreactivity of Lewis y and prognosis (147). The survival rate of patients with cancers that expressed p53 was significantly lower than those with cancers without p53 (148). SCC with high levels of both epidermal growth factor (EGF) and epidermal growth factor receptor (EGFR) were associated with a poorer prognosis than those with low levels (149). The transforming growth factor-alpha (TGF-α) has also been associated with a poor prognosis (150).

Proliferative marker MIB-1 (Ki-67) index may have prognostic significance (151, 152).

CLINICOPATHOLOGIC CORRELATION

PATHOLOGIC BASIS OF CLINICAL PRESENTATION AND DIAGNOSIS

Patients with early esophageal SCC are often asymptomatic. Using cytology, the screening procedure has resulted in accurate diagnosis. Retrospective clinicopathologic studies of early carcinomas have

---

TABLE 21.3 Esophageal Squamous Cell Carcinoma: Relation Between Depth of Tumor, Lymph Node Metastasis, and 5-year Survival

Depth of Tumor	Rate of Node Metastasis (%)	5-year Survival (%)
Intraepithelial carcinoma	0 (91–93, 98)	100 (91, 93, 98)
Intramucosal carcinoma	0–4 (90–94, 98)	83.5–100 (90, 91, 94, 98)
Submucosal carcinoma	21–47 (90–94, 98)	37.6–59.2 (90, 91, 93, 94, 98)

Numbers in parentheses are reference numbers.

TABLE 21.4 TNM Classification of Esophageal Cancer by American Joint Committee on Cancer

Stage	Primary Tumor (T)	Lymph Nodes (N)	Distant Metastasis (M)
0	Tis (carcinoma in situ)	N0 (no metastasis)	M0 (absent)
I	T1 (invasion of lamina propria or submucosa)	N0	M0
IIA	T2 (invasion of muscularis propria)	N0	M0
	T3 (invasion of adventitia)	N0	M0
IIB	T1	N1 (regional lymph node metastasis)	M0
	T2	N1	M0
III	T3	N1	M0
	T4 (invasion of adjacent structures)	Any N	M0
IV	Any T	Any N	M1 (present)

Reprinted with permission from Ming SC. Pathology of esophageal cancer. In: Aisner J, Arriagada R, Green MR, et al. Comprehensive textbook of thoracic oncology. Baltimore: Williams & Wilkins, 554.

TABLE 21.5 Overall Survival Rate of Esophageal Squamous Cell Carcinoma

Reference	1 yr	3 yr	4 yr	5 yr	10 yr	15 yr
Mandard et al. (136)		31%	25%			
Lieberman et al. (137)	68%	39%		27%		
Galandiuk et al. (138)				15.4%		
Wu and Huang (139)				30%		
Huang et al. (140)				30.2%	22.4%	18.9%

shown that, on average, about one half of the patients were asymptomatic. The diagnosis in asymptomatic patients was made during the screening examination of the upper gastrointestinal tract or during follow-up examination of ulcer diseases. The protruded or polypoid lesions were relatively apparent endoscopically, but they usually had submucosal extensions, of which about 20% had lymph node metastasis. The flat lesions usually were intraepithelial or intramucosal and were difficult to diagnose, frequently requiring the aid of the Lugol solution staining technique (153). Briefly, the iodine content in Lugol solution stains the glycogen-rich normal squamous epithelium, leaving the unstained areas as the targets for biopsy. Using this technique, Yokonyama et al. discovered superficial cancers ranging from 6 to 70 mm in diameter in 21 of 629 (3.3%) asymptomatic alcoholics and in 12 of the 21 multiple carcinomas (153). In symptomatic patients, the most common presenting symptom is dysphagia (82, 137, 138), which is attributable to obstruction and usually represents a late manifestation, because the tumors are extensive when dysphagia occurs (82). Dysphagia caused by carcinomas of the upper one third of the esophagus may present earlier than those of the lower one third because the latter region can adapt to obstruction more easily (82).

Microscopically, the well-, and moderately differentiated SCC can be diagnosed easily. The poorly differentiated or anaplastic type may be difficult to be distinguish from anaplastic adenocarcinoma, malignant melanoma, large cell lymphoma, and sarcoma. The sarcomatous component of a carcinosarcoma may be indistinguishable from leiomyosarcoma or other types of sarcoma. Adequate sampling of the representative areas of the lesions is important. Histochemical and immunohistochemical stains and transmission electron microscopy may be helpful for the differential diagnosis, depending on the situation.

In summary, efforts can be made to diagnose the more subtle but potentially curable esophageal SCC. In patients with known risk factors, head and neck cancer and upper gastrointestinal diseases, screening of the esophagus should be a routine procedure.

COMPLICATIONS AND CAUSES OF DEATH

Contiguous intramural spread and distant metastasis are primarily responsible for complications, many of which are fatal. Vertical spread results in fistula formation, which in turn causes fatal infection, such as pneumonia, mediastinitis etc., or rupture of the aorta with fatal hemorrhage. Local recurrence is an ominous sign; 44 of 45 patients who presented with recurrence died (137). Cachexia is a serious complication (84). In their autopsy study (86), Mandard et al. found that bronchopneumonia was the most common cause of death, frequently associated with esophagorespiratory fistula; other causes of death were interstitial pneumopathy, pulmonary embolism, Mendelssohn syndrome, diffuse lymphangeal carcinomatosis, anoxia through compression, hepatic and cardiovascular disease, various toxic infectious states, and cerebral metastases.

TREATMENT-INDUCED PATHOLOGIC CHANGES

Surgery, irradiation, and chemotherapy, alone or in various combinations, are therapeutic options for esophageal SCC. Surgery alone may cause complications, such as wound leakage, but does not change the morphologic appearance of the tumor. Morphologic changes can be found shortly after the completion of external beam

TABLE 21.6	Radiation and Chemotherapy-Induced Morphologic Changes	
	Radiation Alone	Radiation and Chemotherapy
Tumors		
Gross	Ulceration	Ulceration
		Fungating tumor
		Scar without cancer
Micro	Necrosis	Necrosis
	Cytoplasmic vacuolation	Cytoplasmic vacuolation
	Nuclear pyknosis	Nuclear pyknosis
	Intense keratinization with giant cell reaction	
	Enlargement of cells and nuclei	
Nonneoplastic tissue		
Micro	Mild acanthosis	
	Mild basal cell hyperplasia	
	Lymphoplasmacytic infiltrate	
	Fibrosis	

radiation (EBR), intraluminal brachytherapy (ILBT), or chemoradiotherapy (CRT) (136, 154–156) (Table 21.6).

Radiation changes have been classified into three grades (84). In grade I, focal degeneration of the tumor occurs, but the size of the tumor remains unchanged. Inflammatory cells are prominent. In grade II, the tumor becomes smaller and the border is indistinct. Microscopically, only a small number of degenerating tumor cells remain. Foreign body giant cells and neutrophils are present in the granulation tissue. In grade III, tumor cells have disappeared and the esophageal wall is thin and fibrotic. The degree of these changes is radiation dose related. The 5-year survival rate for patient showing grade I changes is 22.3%; for grade II, 32.4%; and for grade III, 37.8% (84).

REFERENCES

1. Parker SL, Tong T, Bolden S, et al. Cancer statistics, 1997. CA Cancer J Clin 1997;47:5–27.
2. Johnston BJ, Reed PI. Changing pattern of oesophageal cancer in a general hospital in the UK. Eur J Cancer Prev 1991;1:23–25.
3. Blot WJ, Devesa SS, Kneller RW, et al. Rising incidence of adenocarcinoma of the esophagus and gastric cardia. JAMA 1991;265:1287–1289.
4. Rector LE, Connerley ML. Aberrant mucosa in the esophagus in infants and in children. Arch Pathol Lab Med 1941;31:1285–1294.
5. Jabbari M, Goresky CA, Lough J, et al. The inlet patch: Heterotopic gastric mucosa in the upper esophagus. Gastroenterology 1985;89: 352–356.
6. Barrett NR. Chronic peptic ulcer of the oesophagus and esophagitis. Br J Surg 1950;38:175–182.

7. Tatcishi R, Taniguchi H, Wada A, et al. Argyrophil cells and melanocytes in esophageal mucosa. Arch Pathol Lab Med 1974;98: 87–89.

8. De la Pava S, Nigogosyan G, Pickren JW, et al. Melanosis of the esophagus. Cancer 1963;16:48–50.

9. Watanabe H, Jass JR, Sobin LH. Histological typing oesophageal and gastric tumours. In: World Health Organization. International classification of tumours. 2nd ed. Berlin: Springer, 1990;11–18.

10. Liu FS, Li L, Qu SL. Clinical and pathological characteristics of early esophageal cancer. In: Burghardt E, Holzer E, eds. Minimal invasive cancer (microcarcinoma). Clin Oncol 1982;1:539–557.

11. Shen Q. Diagnostic cytology and early detection. In: Huang GJ, Wu YK. Carcinoma of the esophagus and gastric cardia, Berlin: Springer, 1984;157–190.

12. Layfield LJ, Reichman A, Weinstein WM. Endoscopically directed fine needle aspiration biopsy of gastric and esophageal lesions. Acta Cytol 1992;36:69–74.

13. World Health Organization. 1994 Statistics Annual. Geneva: World Health Organization, 1995:D4–D396.

14. Cancer Prevention, Treatment and Research Center of the Ministry of Health. Research investigation on the mortality from malignant tumors in China. (Chinese). Beijing: People's Health Press, Beijing, 1979;96.

15. Liu BQ, Li B. Epidemiology of carcinoma of the esophagus in China. In Huang GJ, Wu YK, eds. Carcinoma of the esophagus and gastric cardia. Berlin: Springer, 1984;1–24.

16. Day NE, Varghese C. Oesophageal cancer. Cancer Surv 1994;19–20:43–54.

17. Kosary LL, Ries LAG, Miller BA, et al, eds. SEER cancer statistics Review, 1973-1992. Bethesda: National Cancer Institute, NIH Pub 96-2789, 1996:181–189.

18. Brown LM, Hoover RN, Greenberg RS, et al. Are racial differences in squamous cell esophageal cancer explained by alcohol and tobacco use?. J Natl Cancer Inst 1994;86:1340–1345.

19. Craddock VM. Aetiology of oesophageal cancer: Some operative factors. Eur J Cancer Prev 1992;1:89–103.

20. Magee PN. The experimental basis for the role of nitroso compounds in human cancer. Cancer Surv 1989;8:207–239.

21. Li MX, Cheng SJ. Etiology of carcinoma of the esophagus. In: Huang GJ, Wu YK, eds. Carcinoma of the esophagus and gastric cardia. Berlin: Springer, 1984;25–51.

22. Siddiqi MA, Tricker AR, Kumar R, et al. Dietary sources of N nitrosamines in a high-risk area for oesophageal cancer—Kashmir, India. IARC Sci Publ 1991;105:210–213.

23. Wu Y, Chen J, Ohshima H, et al. Geographic association between urinary secretion of N-nitroso compounds and oesophageal cancer mortality in China. Int J Cancer 1993;54:713–719.

24. Ming SC. Tumors of the esophagus and stomach, second series. Washington, DC: Armed Forces Institute of Pathology, 1973:24–26.

25. Hecht SS, Stoner GD. Lung and esophageal carcinogenesis. In: Aisner J, Arriagada R, Green MR, et al., eds. Comprehensive textbook of thoracic oncology. Baltimore: Williams & Wilkins, 1996;25–50.

26. Gao YT, McLaughlin JK, Blot WJ, et al. Risk factors for esophageal cancer in Shanghai, China. I. Role of cigarette smoking and alcohol drinking. Int J Cancer 1994;58:192–196.

27. Notani PN. Role of alcohol in cancers of upper alimentary tract: Use of models in risk assessment. J Epidemiol Community Health 1988;42:187–192.

28. Cheng KK, Duffy SW, Day NE, et al. Stopping drinking and risk of oesophageal cancer. Br Med J 1995;310:1094–1097.

29. Guo W, Blot WJ, Li JY, et al. A nested case-control study of oesophageal and stomach cancers in the Linxian nutrition intervention trial. Int J Epidemiol 1994;23:444–450.

30. Ghadirian P, Ekoe JM, Thouez JP. Food habits and esophageal cancer: An overview. Cancer Detect Prev 1992;16:163–168.

31. Wang YP, Han XY, Su W, et al. Esophageal cancer in Shanxi Province, People's Republic of China: A case-control study in high and moderate risk areas. Cancer Causes Control 1992;3:107–113.

32. Hu J, Nyren O, Wolk A, et al. Risk factors for oesophageal cancer in northeast China. Int J Cancer 1994;57:38–46.

33. Li JY, Taylor PR, Li B, et al. Nutrition intervention trials in Linxian, China: Multiple vitamin/mineral supplementation, cancer incidence,

34. and disease-specific mortality among adults with esophageal dysplasia. J Natl Cancer Inst 1993;85:1492–1498.

34. Liu GT, Qian YZ, Zhang P, et al. Etiological role of Alternaria alternata in human esophageal cancer. Chin Med J 1992;105: 394–400.

35. Yoshizawa T, Yamashita A, Luo Y. Fumonisin occurrence in corn from high- and low-risk areas for human esophageal cancer in China. Appl Environ Microbiol 1994;60:1626–1629.

36. Odze R, Antonioli D, Shocket D, et al. Esophageal squamous papillomas. A clinicopathologic study of 38 lesions and analysis for human papillomavirus by the polymerase chain reaction. Am J Surg Pathol 1993;17:803–812.

37. Wargovich MJ, Imada O. Esophageal carcinogenesis in the rat: A model for aerodigestive tract cancer. J Cell Biochem Suppl 1993;17F: 91–94.

38. Togawa K, Jaskiewicz K, Takahashi H, et al. Human papillomavirus DNA sequences in esophagus squamous cell carcinoma. Gastroenterology 1994;107:128–136.

39. Mori M, Watanabe M, Tanaka S, et al. Epstein-Barr virus-associated carcinomas of the esophagus and stomach. Arch Pathol Lab Med 1994;118:998–1001.

40. Fekete F, Mosnier H, Belghiti J, et al. Esophageal cancer after mediastinal irradiation. Dysphagia 1994;9:289–291.

41. Ueda M, Matsubara T, Kasumi F, et al. Possible radiation induced cancer of the thoracic esophagus after postoperative irradiation in breast cancer. J Jpn Assoc Thorac Surg 1991;39:1852–1857.

42. Hanaoka T, Tsugane S, Ando N, et al. Alcohol consumption and risk of esophageal cancer in Japan: A case-control study in seven hospitals. Jpn J Clin Oncol 1994;24:241–246.

43. Gao YT, McLaughlin JK, Gridley G, et al. Risk factors for esophageal cancer in Shanghai, China. II. Role of diet and nutrients. Int J Cancer 1994;58:197–202.

44. Muir CS, McKinney PA. Cancer of the oesophagus: A global overview. Eur J Cancer Prev 1992;1:259–264.

45. Ghadirian P. Familial history of esophageal cancer. Cancer 1985;56: 2112–2116.

46. Ashworth MT, Nash JR, Ellis A, et al. Abnormalities of differentiation and maturation in the oesophageal squamous epithelium of patients with tylosis: Morphological features. Histopathology 1991;19: 303–310.

47. Marger RS, Marger D. Carcinoma of the esophagus and tylosis. A lethal genetic combination. Cancer 1993;72;17–19.

48. Wuu KD, Wang-Wuu S. Karyotypic analysis of seven established human esophageal carcinoma cell lines. J Formos Med Assoc 1994; 3:5–10.

49. Rosenblum-Vos LS, Meltzer SJ, Leana-Cox J, et al. Cytogenetic studies of primary cultures of esophageal squamous cell carcinoma. Cancer Genet Cytogenet 1993;70:127–131.

50. Wong FH, Hu CP, Chiu JH, et al. Expression of multiple oncogenes in human esophageal carcinomas. Cancer Invest 1994;12:121–131.

51. Huang Y, Boynton RF, Blount PL, et al. Loss of heterozygosity involves multiple tumor suppressor genes in human esophagesl cancers. Cancer Res 1992;52:6525–6530.

52. Shibagaki I, Shimada Y, Wagata T, et al. Allelotype analysis of esophageal squamous cell carcinoma. Cancer Res 1994;54:2996–3000.

53. Ogasawara S, Maesawa C, Tamura G, et al. Frequent microsatellite alterations on chromosome 3p in esophageal squamous cell carcinoma. Cancer Res 1995;55:891–894.

54. Wargovich MJ, Imada O. Esophageal carcinogenesis in the rat: A model for aerodigestive tract cancer. J Cell Biochem Suppl 1993;17F: 91–94.

55. Mandal S, Stoner GD. Inhibition of N-nitrosobenzylmethyl-amine-induced esophageal tumorigenesis in rats by ellagic acid. Carcinogenesis 1990;11:55–61.

56. Monuz N, Crespi M, Grassi A, et al. Precursor lesions of esophageal cancer in high risk populations in Iran and China. Lancet 1982;1: 876–879.

57. Chang-Claude J, Wahrendorf J, Qiu SL, et al. Epidemiological study of precursor lesions of oesophageal cancer among young persons in Huixian, China. IARC Sci Publ 1991;105:192–196.

58. Jacob JH, Riviere A, Mandard AM, et al. Prevalence survey of precancerous lesions of the oesophagus in a high-risk population for

oesophageal cancer in France. Eur J Cancer Prev 1993;2:53–79.

59. Kuylenstierna R, Munck-Wikland E. Esophagitis and cancer of the esophagus. Cancer 1985;56:837–839.

60. Paraf F, Flejou JF, Potet F, et al. Esophageal squamous carcinoma in five patients with Barrett's esophagus. Am J Gastroenterol 1992;87:746–750.

61. Moghissi K, Sharpe DA, Pender D. Adenocarcinoma and Barrett's oesophagus. A clinico-pathological study. Eur J Cardio-Thorac Surg 1993;7:126–131.

62. Hopkins RA, Postlethwait RW. Cautic burns and carcinoma of the esophagus. Ann Surg 1981;194:146–148.

63. Csikos M, Horvath O, Petri A, et al. Late malignant transforrnation of chronic corrosive oesophageal strictures. Langenbecks Arch Chir 1985;365:231–238.

64. Streitz Jr JM, Ellis Jr FH, Gibb SP. Achalasia and squamous cell carcinoma of the esophagus: Analysis of 241 patients. Ann Thorac Surg 1995;59:1604–1609.

65. Meijssen MA, Tilanus HW, van Blankenstein M, et al. Achalasia complicated by oesophageal squamous cell carcinoma: A prospective study in 195 patients. Gut 1992; 33:155–158.

66. Peracchia A, Segalin A, Bardini R, et al. Esophageal carcinoma and achalasia: Prevalence, incidence and results of treatment. Hepatogastroenterology 1991;38:514–516.

67. Aggestrup S, Holm JC, Sorenson HR. Does achalasia predispose to cancer of the esophagus? Chest 1992;102:1013–1016.

68. Chisholm M, Ardran GM, Callender ST, et al. A follow-up study of patients with postcricoid webs. Q J Med 1971;40:409.

69. Holmes GKT, Stokes PL, Sorahan TM, et al. Coeliac disease, gluten-free diet and malignancy. Gut 1976;17:612–619.

70. Swinson CM, Slavin G, Coles CE, et al. Celiac disease and malignancy. Lancet 1983;1:111–115.

71. Sauvanet A, Gayet B, Lemee J, et al. Les cancers sur diverticule de l'oesophage. Presse Med 1992;21:305–308.

72. Cheng H, Ren H, Yu H, et al. Esophageal diverticulum associated with carcinoma of the esophagus—a report of four cases. Chin Med Sci J 1991;6:244–246.

73. Chang F, Syrjanen S, Shen Q, et al. Screening for human papillomavirus infections in esophageal squamous cell carcinomas by in situ hybridization. Cancer 993;72:2525–2530.

74. Benamouzig R, Pigot F, Quiroga G, et al. Human papillomavirus infection in esophageal squamous-cell carcinoma in western countries. Int J Cancer 1992;50:549–552.

75. Cooper K, Taylor L, Govind S. Human papillomavirus DNA in oesophageal carcinomas in South Africa. J Pathol 1995;175:273–277.

76. Kuwano H, Watanabe M, Sadanaga N, et al. Squamous epithelial dysplasia associated with squamous cell carcinoma of the esophagus. Cancer Lett 1993;72:141–147.

77. Shu YJ, Yuan XQ, Jin SP. Further investigation of the relationship between dysplasia and cancer of the esophagus. Chin Med J 1981;1:39–41.

78. Dawsey SM, Yu Y, Taylor PR, et al. Esophageal cytology and subsequent risk of esophageal cancer. A prospective follow-up study from Linxian, China. Acta Cytol 1994;38:183–192.

79. Itakura Y, Sasano H, Mori S, et al. DNA ploidy in human esophageal squamous dysplasias and squamous cell carcinomas as determined by image analysis. Mod Pathol 1994;7:867–873.

80. Yano H, Shiozaki H, Kobayashi K, et al. Immunohistologic detection of the epidermal growth factor receptor in human esophageal squamous cell carcinoma. Cancer 1991;67:91–98.

81. Gao H, Wang LD, Zhou Q, et al. p53 tumor suppressor gene mutation in early esophageal precancerous lesions and carcinoma among high-risk populations in Hunan, China. Cancer Res 1994;58:4342–4346.

82. Burgess HM, Baggenstoss AH, Moersch HJ, et al. Carcinoma of the esophagus: A clinicopathologic study. Surg Clin North Am 1951;31:965–976.

83. Gunnlaugsson GH, Wychulis AR, Roland C, et al. Analysis of the records of 1,657 patients with carcinoma of the esophagus and cardia of the stomach. Surg Gynecol Obstet 1970;130:997–1005.

84. Liu F-S, Wang Q-L. Squamous cell carcinoma of the esophagus. In: Ming S-C, Goldman H, eds. Pathology of the gastrointestinal tract. 1st ed. Philadelphia: WB Saunders, 1992;439–454.

85. Sons HU, Borchard F. Esophageal cancer. Autopsy findings in 171 cases. Arch Pathol Lab Med 1984;108:983–988.

86. Mandard AM, Chasle J, Marnay J, et al. Autopsy findings in 111 cases of esophageal cancer. Cancer 1981;48:329–335.

87. Mandard AM, Marnay J, Gignoux M, et al. Cancer of the esophagus and associated lesions. Detailed pathologic study of 100 esophagectomy specimens. Hum Pathol 1984;15:660–669.

88. Peters JH, Demeester TR. Esophagus and diaphragmatic hernia. In: Schwartz SI, Shires GT, Spencer FC, eds. Principles of surgery. 6th ed. New York: McGraw-Hill, 1994;1043–1122.

89. Ming SC. Pathology of esophageal cancer. In: Aisner J, Arriagada R, Green MR, Martini N, et al., eds. Comprehensive textbook of thoracic oncology. Baltimore: Williams & Wilkins, 1996;533–562.

90. Kato H, Tachimori Y, Watanabe H, et al. Superficial esophageal carcinoma. Surgical treatment and the results. Cancer 1990;66:2319–2323.

91. Yoshinaka H, Shimazu H, Fukimoto T, et al. Superficial esophageal carcinoma: A clinicopathologic review of 59 cases. Am J Gastroenterol 1991;86:1413–1418.

92. Haruma K, Tokutomi T, Tsuda T, et al. Superficial esophageal carcinoma: A report of 27 cases in Japan. Am J Gastroenterol 1991;86:1723–1728.

93. Kitamura K, Ikebe M, Morita M, et al. The evaluation of submucosal carcinoma of the esophagus as a more advanced carcinoma. Hepatogastroenterol 1993;40:236–239.

94. Hölscher AH, Bollschweiler E, Schneider PM, et al. Prognosis of early esophageal cancer. Comparison between adeno- and squamous cell carcinoma. Cancer 1995;76:178–186.

95. Kitamura K, Kuwano H, Yasuda M, et al. What is the earliest malignant lesion in the esophagus? Cancer 1996;77:1614–1619.

96. Rubio CA, Liu F-S, Zhao H-Z. Histological classification of intraepithelial neoplasias and microinvasive squamous cell carcinomas of the esophagus. Am J Surg Pathol 1989;13:685–690.

97. Sugimachi K, Kitamura K, Matsuda H, et al. Proposed new criteria for early carcinoma of the esophagus. Surg Gynecol Obstet 1991;173:303–308.

98. Sugimachi K, Ikebe M, Kitamura K, et al. Long-term results of esophagectomy for early esophageal carcinoma. Hepatogastroenterol 1993;40:203–206.

99. Baba K, Kuwano H, Kitamura K, et al. Carcinomatous invasion and lymphocyte infiltration in early esophageal carcinoma with special regard to the basement membrane. An immunohistochemical study. Hepatogastroenterol 1993;40:226–231.

100. Sasajima K, Takai A, Taniguchi Y, et al. Polypoid squamous cell carcinoma of the esophagus. Cancer 1989;54:94–97.

101. Sagar PM, Johnston D, McMahon MJ, et al. Significance of circumferential resection margin involvement after esophagectomy for cancer. Br J Surg 1993;80:1386–1388.

102. Ohbu M, Seagusa M, Okayasu I. Apoptosis and cellular proliferation in oesophageal squamous cell carcinomas: Differences between keratinizing and nonkeratinizing types. Virchows Arch 1995;427:271–276.

103. Chang F, Syrjanen S, Wang L, et al. Infectious agents in the etiology of esophageal cancer. Gastroenterology 1992;103:1336–1348.

104. Kuwano H, Ohno S, Matsuda H, et al. Serial histologic evaluation of multiple primary squamous cell carcinomas of the esophagus. Cancer 1988;61:1635–1638.

105. Nagamatsu M, Mori M, Kuwano H, et al. Serial histologic investigation of squamous epithelial dysplasia associated with carcinoma of the esophagus. Cancer 1992;69:1094–1098.

106. Pesko P, Rakic S, Miliceric M, et al. Prevalence and clinicopathologic features of multiple squamous cell carcinoma of the esophagus. Cancer 1994;73:2687–2690.

107. Maeta M, Kondo A, Shibata S, et al. Esophageal cancer associated with multiple cancerous lesions: Clinicopathologic comparisons between multiple primary and intramural metastatic lesions. Gastroenterol Jpn 1993;28:187–192.

108. Yokoyama A, Muramatsu T, Ohmosi T, et al. Multiple primary esophageal and concurrent upper aerodigestive tract cancer and the aldehyde dehydrogenase—2 genotype of Japanese alcoholics. Cancer 1996;77:1986–1990.

109. Wang LD, Zhou Q, Hong J-Y, et al. p53 protein accumulation and gene mutations in multifocal esophageal precancerous lesions from

symptom free subjects in a high incidence area for esophageal carcinoma in Hunan, China. Cancer 1996;77:1244–1249.

110. Kuwano H, Morita M, Tsutsui S-I, et al. Comparison of characteristics of esophageal squamous cell carcinoma associated with head and neck cancer and those with gastric cancer. J Surg Oncol 1991;46:107–109.

111. Morita M, Kuwano H, Ohno S, et al. Multiple occurrence of carcinoma in the upper aerodigestive tract associated with esophageal cancer: Reference to smoking, drinking and family history. Int J Cancer 1994;58:207–210.

112. Ina H, Shibuya H, Ohashi I, et al. The frequency of a concomitant early esophageal cancer in male patients with oval and oroparyngeal cancer. Cancer 1994;73:2038–2041.

113. Fekete F, Sauvanet A, Kaisserian G, et al. Associated primary esophageal and lung carcinoma: A study of 39 patients. Ann Thorac Surg 1994;58:837–842.

114. Agha FP, Weatherbee L, Sams JS. Verrucous carcinoma of the esophagus. Am J Gastroenterol 1984;79:844–849.

115. Meyerowitz BR, Shea LT. The natural history of squamous verrucous carcinoma of the esophagus. J Thorac Cardiovasc Surg 1971;61:646–649.

116. Cevar A, Jutersek A, Vidmar S. Adenoid cystic carcinoma of the esophagus. A clinicopathologic study of three cases. Cancer 1991;67:2159 2164.

117. Abe K, Sasano H, Itakura Y, et al. Basaloid-squamous carcinoma of the esophagus. A clinicopathologic, DNA ploidy, and immunohistochemical study of seven cases. Am J Surg Pathol 1996;20:453–461.

118. Balercia G, Bhan AK, Dickerson GR. Sarcomatoid carcinoma: An ultrastructural study with light microscopic and immunological correlation of 10 cases from various anatomic sites. Ultrast Pathol 1995;19:249–263.

119. Battifora H. Spindle-cell carcinoma: Ultrastructural evidence of squamous origin and collagen production by the tumor cells. Cancer 1976;37:2275–2282.

120. Kimura N, Tezuka F, Ono I, et al. Myogenic expression in esophageal polypoid tumors. Arch Pathol Lab Med 1989;113:1159–1165.

121. Ooi A, Kawahara E, Okada Y, et al. Carcinosarcoma of the esophagus. An immunohistochemical and electron microscopic study. Acta Pathol Jpn 1986;36:151–159.

122. Kuwano H, Sadanaga N, Watanabe M, et al. Oesophageal cancer composed of mixed histological types. Eur J Surg Oncol 1996;22:225–231.

123. Newman J, Antonakopoulos N, Darnton SJ, et al. The ultrastructure of esophageal carcinoma: Multidirectional differentiation. A transmission electron microscopic study of 13 cases. J Pathol 1992;167:193–198.

124. Sugimachi K, Sumiyoski K, Nozoe T, et al. Carcinogenesis and Histogenesis of esophageal carcinoma. Cancer (Suppl) 1995; 75:1440–1445.

125. Marx J. Tumors: A mixed bag of cells. Science 1982;215:275–277.

126. Takubo K, Takai A, Takayama S, et al. Intraductal spread of esophageal squamous cell carcinoma. Cancer 1987;59:1751–1757.

127. Takubo K, Sasajima K, Yamashita K, et al. Prognostic significance of intramural metastasis in patients with esophageal carcinoma. Cancer 1990;65:1816–1819.

128. Soga J, Tanaka O, Sasaki K, et al. Superficial spreading type carcinoma of the esophagus. Cancer 1982;56:1641–1645.

129. Kawamura T, Goseki N, Koike M, et al. Acceleration of proliferative activity of esophageal squamous cell carcinoma with invasion beyond the mucosa. Immunohistochemical analyses of Ki-67 and p53 antigen in relation to histologic findings. Cancer 1996;77:843–849.

130. Sarbia M, Porschen R, Borchard F, et al. Incidence and prognostic significance of vascular and neural invasion in squamous cell carcinomas of the esophagus. Int J Cancer 1995;61:333–336.

131. Gschossmann JM, Bonner JA, Foote RL, et al. Malignant tracheoesophageal fistula in patients with esophageal cancer. Cancer 1993;72:1513–1521.

132. Burt M, Diehl W, Martini N, et al. Malignant esophagorespiratory fistula: Management options and survival. Am Thorac Surg 1991;52:1222–1228.

133. Theunissen PH, Borchard F, Poortvliet DC. Histopathological evaluation of esophageal carcinoma: The significance of venous invasions. Br J Surg 1991;78:930–932.

134. Beahrs OH, Henson DE, Hutter RVP, et al. Manual for staging of cancer, 4th ed. Philadelphia: JB Lippincott, 1992;57–61.

135. Skinner DB, Skinner KA. Neoplasms of the esophagus. In: Holland JF, Frei III E, Bast Jr RC, et al. (eds). Cancer medicine, 3rd ed. Philadelphia: Lea & Febiger, 1993;1382–1394.

136. Mandard A-M, Dalibard F, Mandard J-C, et al. Pathologic assessment of tumor regression after postoperative chemotherapy of esophageal carcinoma. Cancer 1994;73:2680–2686.

137. Lieberman M, Shriver CD, Bleckner S, et al. Carcinoma of the esophagus. Prognostic significance of histologic type. J Thorac Cardiovasc Surg 1995;109:130–139.

138. Galandiuk S, Herman R, Gassman JJ, et al. Cancer of the esophagus. The Cleveland Clinic experience. Ann Surg 1986; 203:101–108.

139. Wu YK, Huang GJ. Surgical treatment. In: Huang GJ, Wu YK, eds. Carcinoma of the esophagus and gastric cardia. Berlin: Springer, 1984;276–284.

140. Huang GJ, Wang LJ, Liu JS, et al. Surgery of esophageal carcinoma. Semin Surg Oncol 1985;1:74–83.

141. Iizuka T, Kato H, Watanabe H. One-hundred-and-two 5-year survivors of esophageal carcinoma after resective surgery. Jpn J Clin Oncol 1985;15:369–375.

142. Matsuura H, Kuwano H, Morita M, et al. Predicting recurrence time of esophageal carcinoma through assessment of histologic factors and DNA ploidy. Cancer 1991;67:1406–1411.

143. Edwards JM, Jones DJ, Wilkes SJL, et al. Ploidy as a prognostic indicator in esophageal squamous carcinoma and its relationship for various histological criteria. J Pathol 1989;159:35–41.

144. Ruol A, Segatin A, Panozzo M, et al. Flow cytometric DNA analysis of squamous cell carcinoma of the esophagus. Cancer 1990;65:1185–1188.

145. Sasaki K, Murakami T, Nakamura M. Intratumoral heterogeneity in DNA ploidy of esophageal squamous cell carcinomas. Cancer 1991;68:2403–2406.

146. Tsutsui S, Kuwano H, Mori M, et al. A flow cytometric analysis of DNA content in primary and metastatic lesions of esophageal squamous cell carcinoma. Cancer 1992;70:2586–2591.

147. Tauchi K, Kakudo K, Machimura T, et al. Immunohistochemical studies of blood group-related antigens in human superficial esophageal carcinomas. Cancer 1991;67:3042–3050.

148. Shimaya K, Shiozaki H, Inone M, et al. Significance of p53 expression as a prognostic factor in esophageal squamous cell carcinomas. Virchows Arch A Pathol Anat 1993;422:271–276.

149. Mukaida H, Toi M, Hirai T, et al. Clinical significance of the expression of epidermal growth factor and its receptor in esophageal cancer. Cancer 1991;68:142–148.

150. Iihara K, Shiozaki H, Tahara H, et al. Prognostic significance of transforming growth factor—α in human esophageal carcinoma. Implication for the autocrine proliferation. Cancer 1993;71:2902–2909.

151. Youssef EM, Matsuda T, Takada N, et al. Prognostic significance of the MIB-1 proliferation index for patients with squamous cell carcinoma of the esophagus. Cancer 1995;76:358–366.

152. Lam K-Y, Law S Y-K, So M K-P, et al. Prognostic implication of proliferative markers MIB-1 and PC10 in esophageal squamous cell carcinoma. Cancer 1996;77:7–13.

153. Yokoyama A, Ohmori T, Makuuchi H, et al. Successful screening for early esophageal cancer alcoholics using endoscopy and mucosal iodine staining. Cancer 1995;76:928–934.

154. Berry B, Miller RR, Luoma A, et al. Pathologic findings in total esophagectomy specimens after intracavitary and external beam radiation. Cancer 1989;64:1833–1837.

155. Akakura I, Nakamura Y, Kakegawa T, et al. Surgery of carcinoma of the esophagus with preoperative radiation. Chest 1970;57:47–56.

156. Sur M, Sur R, Cooper K, et al. Morphologic alterations in esophageal squamous cell carcinoma after preoperative high dose rate intraluminal brachytherapy. Cancer 1996;77:2200–2205.

22

ADENOCARCINOMA AND OTHER EPITHELIAL TUMORS OF THE ESOPHAGUS

Si-Chun Ming

Primary adenocarcinomas of the esophagus used to be uncommon. In reports published more than 30 years ago, about 10% of esophageal carcinomas were adenocarcinomas and only 1% were primary lesions (1). The majority of adenocarcinomas occurred in the distal esophagus. They were considered gastric lesions that invaded the esophagus secondarily. This concept has been drastically modified in recent years, particularly since the late 1970s.

It is clear now that many adenocarcinomas of the lower esophagus are primary tumors originating in the Barrett epithelium, which is described subsequently. Such tumors constitute 30 to 50% of esophageal carcinomas in some Western countries, including the United States (2–4). Squamous cell carcinoma remains the most common carcinoma of the esophagus. Other epithelial tumors are rare.

CELL ORIGIN OF ESOPHAGEAL ADENOCARCINOMA AND OTHER EPITHELIAL TUMORS

COLUMNAR EPITHELIUM OF THE ESOPHAGUS

CONGENITAL REMNANTS AND GASTRIC HETEROTOPIA

During early fetal life, the esophagus is lined by columnar cells and superficial mucous glands. Ciliated cells appear in the third month of embryonic life. Squamous cells begin to appear in the fourteenth week, spreading from the middle to both ends of the esophagus. Residual columnar cells and glands may persist into childhood and even into adult life, mainly at the upper end. Some investigators consider these tissues heterotopic gastric epithelium. The incidence of such occurrence was reported to be 11.8% in children (5) and 4 to 10% in adults (6, 7). These patches may consist of fundic type of gastric glands with chief and parietal cells and measure 0.2 to 0.3 cm to 3×5 cm (7).

BARRETT EPITHELIUM

While residual columnar cells may be present in the distal esophagus, attention has been focused on the columnar epithelium associated with hiatal hernia and reflux of gastric contents into the esophagus. This epithelium is known as Barrett epithelium because it was first described in detail by Barrett in 1950 (8, 9). Barrett originally thought that the esophagus, with columnar epithelium lining its lower portion, was a congenitally short esophagus if one defined the esophagus as the organ lined by squamous epithelium. Results of subsequent studies supported the idea that Barrett epithelium is acquired and is located within the esophagus (10). Clinical follow-up studies (11) and experiments in dogs (12) indicate a cephalad extension of the columnar epithelium from the cardiac end of the stomach, suggesting a gastric origin. If this is the only source of Barrett epithelium, it has to be invariably connected with the gastric mucosa. It is common, however, to see isolated patches of Barrett epithelium surrounded by squamous cells (13). Such an occurrence indicates that the columnar epithelium develops de novo from the residual epithelial cells in a denuded region through a metaplastic process (10, 14). This possibility is supported by an experiment in dogs in which columnar epithelium developed in an area disconnected from the gastric mucosa where the squamous mucosa had been stripped off (15). The metaplastic origin of the epithelium explains its unique histologic composition, which is distinctly different from that of the adjacent gastric cardia and the high incidence of malignant transformation in this abnormal tissue. In this regard, the congenital or ectopic gastric epithelium can be readily differentiated from the Barrett epithelium in most instances: the former is composed commonly of well-developed fundic glands, whereas the latter often shows intestinal metaplasia.

The prevalence of Barrett epithelium is 0.24 to 1.38% in patients requiring upper gastrointestinal endoscopy (16–18), 8.7% in patients with hiatal hernia, 8 to 20% in patients with reflux esophagitis, and 30 to 50% in esophagi with peptic stricture (20–22). The prevalence rate at autopsy is 1 to 2% (23). The incidence increases with age, reaching a plateau at age 70 years (17). Rarely, Barrett esophagus is found in children (24, 25); in one case, it was detected in a 3-week-old male infant with gastroesophageal

reflux (26). Barrett esophagus is more common in men than in women, with a male-to-female ratio of about 2 to 1 (17).

Grossly, the Barrett epithelium is pink and velvety, resembling the gastric mucosa, in contrast to the light gray normal squamous mucosa. Its size varies greatly, from a minute focus to diffuse involvement of the esophagus (27). In one report of 50 cases (28), the length of Barrett epithelium was 3 to 5 cm in 22 cases, 5 to 10 cm in 20 cases, and more than 10 cm in 8 cases. The mean length was about 8 cm and did not increase with age (17). Short segments of Barrett epithelium, defined as extending less than 2 cm above the esophagogastric junction (29), may not be recognized endoscopically (30). Its incidence at biopsy in two prospective studies was 9.4% and 18%, respectively (29, 30).

The histologic features of Barrett epithelium are described in detail in Chapter 20. Briefly, it has three main histologic patterns: cardiac (junctional), fundic, or intestinalized (specialized) epithelium (31), often in combination. The most distinctive form is the so-called specialized type, made of intestinal type cells commonly seen in the metaplastic glands of stomach (see Chapters 23 and 27 for details). The intestinalized epithelium (Fig. 22.1) is present in the majority of cases (32, 33) and serves as a marker for Barrett epithelium.

As in the stomach, intestinalization of the Barrett epithelium may be complete or incomplete (Fig. 22.2). The glands in the less common complete type is composed mainly of goblet and absorptive cells, resembling those of normal small intestine. The incomplete type has a mixture of goblet cells and intervening columnar mucous cells. These cells may contain low acidic sialated mucin, as is present in the normal small intestine, or strongly acidic sulfomucin, as in the colon. The columnar mucous cells resemble the foveolar mucous cells of the stomach histologically and ultrastructurally (34). Unlike the gastric foveolar cells, which have sparse short microvilli and dense mucin granules, some columnar cells of Barrett epithelium have well-developed microvilli, mixed density of

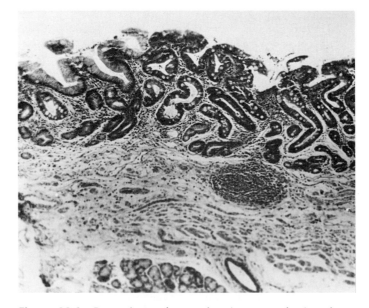

Figure 22.1 Barrett's esophagus showing metaplastic columnar epithelium and thickened muscularis mucosae. The presence of submucosal glands *(bottom)* identifies the organ as esophagus.

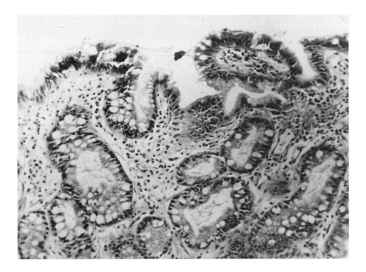

Figure 22.2   Barrett epithelium showing incomplete intestinal metaplasia with goblet cells and varying numbers of intervening columnar mucous cells. *At right,* more inflammatory cells are visible and the glands are slightly hyperplastic (×150).

mucin granules, and complex interdigitating lateral plasma membranes (Fig. 22.3). Cells showing features of both squamous and columnar cells by scanning electron microscopy were described by Shields et al. (35). In addition, Paneth cells, ciliated cells, endocrine cells, and pancreatic acinar cells may be present also (10, 14, 31, 36–38). Gastrin and pepsinogen have been found in Barrett epithelium (39).

Other features of Barrett esophagus are a thick or double-layered muscularis mucosae and the presence of muscle cells in fibrotic lamina propria (40, 41). Like the stomach, the intestinalized Barrett epithelium is the common seat of malignant transformation, and sulfomucin is a marker for precancerous potential (42, 43). Because the Barrett epithelium is a glandular epithelium, carcinomas originating in it generally are adenocarcinomas, although a few carcinomas have turned out to be squamous cell carcinomas (44, 45). Squamous cell carcinoma may also develop in the squamous epithelium outside the Barrett epithelium (46).

SUBMUCOSAL ESOPHAGEAL GLANDS

The esophagus has its own glands, which are located in the submucosa, with ducts penetrating through the squamous epithelium into the lumen of the esophagus (see Chapter 2). These esophageal glands are developed throughout late fetal life and early postpartum periods. They resemble minor salivary glands and are composed mainly of mucous cells and occasionally of serous cells. Carcinomas of esophageal gland or duct origin are rare and have distinctive features. It is possible, however, that some adenocarcinomas of the esophagus also may arise from the submucosal glands or their ducts (47).

UNCOMMON CELL TYPES OF ESOPHAGEAL EPITHELIUM

The normal esophageal squamous epithelium has scattered endocrine and melanocytes, which are not evident on routine histologic examination. Because the esophagus is a foregut organ, its endocrine cells are argyrophilic and not argentaffinic. Tateishi et al. (48) found argyrophilic cells in 14 of 50 esophagi. The melanocytes were present in 2.5 to 8% of cases when Fontana's silver stain was used and in 11.5% by dopa reaction (48, 49). These cells give rise the rare melanomas, carcinoids, and small cell carcinomas.

The proliferating basal cells of the epithelium may have the potential to differentiate into other cell types. These totipotential cells are not clearly delineated, but circumstances suggest that some epithelial tumors other than ordinary squamous cell carcinoma, such as choriocarcinoma and carcinosarcoma, may develop from them. These totipotential cells also may be responsible for columnar cell metaplasia leading to the development of Barrett epithelium and adenocarcinoma.

The types of epithelial tumors of the esophagus and their possible cell of origin are summarized in Table 21.1 (see Chapter 21).

PATHOLOGIC STUDY OF SPECIMENS

The general principles of pathologic study of esophageal tumors are discussed in Chapter 21. In regard to adenocarcinoma, the main focus of pathologic study is the establishment of the relationship

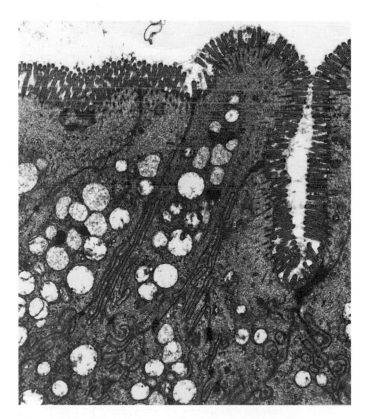

Figure 22.3   Ultrastructure of Barrett epithelium. The mucous columnar cells have well-developed microvilli and cell junctions with complex interdigitations of lateral plasma membranes. The mucin granules are mostly light with focal dense areas (×19,200). (Courtesy of Dr. Bruce Elfenbein, Temple University Hospital, Philadelphia, PA.)

between the tumor and Barrett epithelium. This task is difficult when dealing with cytologic specimens, because the identification of specific cells of Barrett epithelium is not reliable (50). When working with a biopsy specimen, knowledge of the location of the biopsy site is important. Therefore, it is essential to collaborate with the endoscopist, who has a reliable view of the biopsy site during esophagoscopy. Histologically, the presence of intestinal metaplasia, particularly the incomplete type, is strong evidence for Barrett epithelium.

The resected specimen offers additional anatomic features that may be helpful in ascertaining the nature of the epithelium. In many specimens, gastric tissue is grossly evident. Barrett mucosa is pink, soft, and movable, resembling the gastric mucosa. It usually is in direct continuity with the tumor; small patches may be present nearby. Some adenocarcinomas, particularly in the region of the esophagogastric junction or cardia, are associated with short segments of Barrett epithelium not evident at endoscopy (30, 51). Use of a dissecting microscopy has been helpful when searching for any minute focus of Barrett epithelium (14). In the histologic section of resected specimens, the structures indicative of esophageal origin are squamous epithelium, submucosal glands and their ducts (see Fig. 22.1), two-layer structure of muscularis propria, and adventitial tissue instead of serosa.

The nature of most tumors is readily appreciated microscopically. Special and immunohistologic stains on paraffin-embedded tissue may be needed to establish the diagnosis of rare or unusual tumors or to investigate molecular alterations. Because fresh tissue may be necessary for the latter, a portion of fresh specimen should be routinely quick-frozen and stored in a low-temperature freezer, if possible.

ADENOCARCINOMA

Most primary adenocarcinomas of the esophagus occur in Barrett epithelium. This origin of the tumor, if located in the distal esophagus, may be assumed, even though the benign Barrett epithelium is not present in the microscopic sections; the carcinoma may have destroyed it. When the adenocarcinoma is located in the middle (52–55) or upper (52, 56, 57) esophagus, it may be associated with gastric-type epithelium or superficial glands. These types of tissue are considered congenital remnants or ectopic tissue. Rarely, however, Barrett metaplasia may be diffuse and give rise to a carcinoma in the upper esophagus (27). In any case, the clinical and pathologic features of adenocarcinoma in the proximal regions of the esophagus do not have distinctive features.

PREVALENCE AND INCIDENCE

The prevalence of adenocarcinoma in Barrett epithelium in 17 reports reviewed from 1971 to 1985 varied from 0 to 46.5%, with an average of 13.6% among 994 patients (58). The prevalence in recent reports varied from 5 to 28% (4, 18, 59–62). In follow-up studies, the reported incidence of adenocarcinoma in Barrett esophagus varied from 1 in 52 (63) to 1 in 441 (64) patient-years (22, 28, 59, 62–68), with an estimated 30-fold to 125-fold increase in risk over that in the general population (22, 28, 65). Thus, the probability of carcinoma is higher at the time of initial diagnosis of Barrett epithelium than in later years after the presence of Barrett epithelium has been established.

The reports just mentioned came mainly from Western countries in which the incidence of adenocarcinoma has shown a steady increase because of either increased incidences of Barrett epithelium or increased awareness and better diagnostic criteria. In a report from the United Kingdom, adenocarcinoma accounts for 50% of all esophageal cancers (2). In the United States, where the incidence of adenocarcinoma has increased by 10% per year, up to one third of esophageal carcinomas are adenocarcinomas (3). In France, however, there is no increase in the incidence of esophageal adenocarcinoma (69). Barrett adenocarcinoma is uncommon in some countries. In a report from Taiwan of 450 cases of esophageal cancer, neither Barrett carcinoma nor Barrett epithelium were found (70). In another report, 10 of 1674 esophageal carcinomas were adenocarcinomas (71). Similarly, of 5481 surgically treated cases in Japan, 214 involved adenocarcinomas at the esophagogastric junction or cardia, but all esophageal carcinomas were of squamous type (72).

Barrett esophagus is more common in men than women. Male predominance is heightened in cases involving carcinoma (4, 22, 73), with a reported male-to-female ratio of 3:1 to 15:1 (4, 59, 74, 75). In some reports, nearly all of patients are men (4, 58). The mean age of patients with Barrett esophagus, be it benign or maligant, is in the early seventh decade of life (17, 73). Benign Barrett epithelium may affect children, however, and adenocarcinoma as well has been reported in this population (22, 76). Two cases reported by Cheu et al. involved 11- and 14-year-old patients (24). Unlike squamous cell carcinoma, adenocarcinoma affects whites more frequently than blacks, even in places with a predominantly black population (73, 77).

ETIOLOGY AND RISK FACTORS

The etiology of carcinoma in the Barrett epithelium is unknown. Recognized risk factors are as follows.

ACID AND ALKALINE REFLUX

Chronic gastroesophageal reflux is often more severe in patients with adenocarcinoma than in those individuals without carcinoma (3, 77). Hiatus hernia is common (75), although symptoms of reflux are present in less than one half of the patients in some reports (4). Furthermore, successful antireflux therapy does not prevent the development of carcinoma (4, 78–80). McDonald et al. reported an incidence of carcinoma of 1 in 273.8 patient-year in treated patients (78). Alkaline bile reflux from the duodenum is also present in some patients, even though the esophageal pH value may be within the normal range (81). In experiments in rats, pancreatic fluid was a more important factor than bile alone (82) (see subsequent section concerning experimental studies).

ALCOHOL AND TOBACCO

A smoking and drinking history is a common although not constant finding (75, 83, 84). Patients with esophageal adenocarcinoma smoked more for longer years and drank more than those individuals with Barrett esophagus only (85). In one report, however, 60% of patients with Barrett carcinoma had no smoking history and 47% were nondrinkers (86). Unlike squamous cell carcinoma of the esophagus, alcohol appears to be a less important factor.

DIETARY FACTORS

Raw fruits, vegetables, and dietary fibers decrease the risk of adenocarcinoma in the esophagus. Obesity increases this risk, although there is no significant association with total caloric and fat intake (87). In rat experiments, a high-fat diet increases the yield of esophageal adenocarcinoma (88).

FAMILIAL HISTORY

A familial occurrence of Barrett esophagus and adenocarcinoma has been reported. In one report (89), 6 of 24 family members had Barrett esophagus, 3 with adenocarcinoma. None of the spouses had the disease. In another report (90), Barrett esophagus was present in 7 family members, 2 with adenocarcinoma at the gastroesophageal junction. A strong family history of gastroesophageal reflux and Barrett disease was noted in four other families (91).

ASSOCIATED CONDITIONS

Associated diseases in patients with Barrett carcinoma include achalasia (92, 93), scleroderma (94–96), and Zollinger-Ellison syndrome (97, 98), all of which were accompanied by esophagitis. In those patients with scleroderma, however, long-term follow-up study did not show any significant increase in the incidence of esophageal carcinoma (95, 96). Paraf et al. described a case of Barrett carcinoma in a 51-year-old man with Muir-Torre syndrome and colonic carcinoma (99).

PRECANCEROUS LESIONS

In contrast to the lack of information on the possible etiologic factors, a number of local tissue changes have been implicated in the development of carcinoma in the Barrett epithelium. These local risk factors include epithelial dysplasia, intestinal metaplasia in the columnar epithelium, and adenoma.

INTESTINAL METAPLASIA IN BARRETT EPITHELIUM

The majority of Barrett epithelium shows intestinal metaplasia. In biopsy specimens from the distal esophagus, the presence of intestinal metaplasia is a major diagnostic marker when attempting to differentiate Barrett epithelium from gastric epithelium. Because the incidence of adenocarcinoma in such epithelium is high, the metaplastic Barrett epithelium is considered a precancerous lesion. In a study by Moghissi et al. (59), the incidence rate of esophageal adenocarcinoma in patients with Barrett epithelium was 1 in 74 person-years and 1 in 51.7 person-years in complicated Barrett epithelium, but only 1 in 1500 person-years in patients with esophagogastric reflux without Barrett epithelium.

Whereas carcinoma may be more common in extensive than in limited amounts of columnar epithelium (100, 101) (average length is around 7.4 cm [51, 60]), the size of columnar epithelium accompanying the carcinoma is variable and may be absent (51), possibly overgrown by the neoplastic tissue. On the other hand, the nature of metaplasia appears to be an important precancerous factor. Particularly important is the sulfomucin-secreting incomplete metaplasia, which commonly is present in the carcinomatous but not the benign Barrett esophagus (43).

DYSPLASIA OF BARRETT EPITHELIUM

The prevalence of dysplasia in Barrett epithelium is about 5 to 10% (68). It usually occurs in the intestinalized epithelium of the Barrett esophagus and often coexists with adenocarcinoma (4, 13, 14, 28, 42, 73, 92, 102, 103). In our experience, dysplasia was present in 12 of 16 carcinoma cases (102). Thus, dysplasia of Barrett epithelium is closely related to adenocarcinoma, and surgical resection of the involved esophagus has been advocated (28, 68, 77, 103, 105–108).

Histologic Features

Dysplasia has been divided into mild, moderate, and severe, or low and high grades. The high-grade dysplasia includes both moderate and severe dysplasia. For some authors, high-grade dysplasia also includes in situ carcinoma (73, 77). The criteria for grading of dysplasia are based on the degree of differentiation, maturation, and pleomorphism of the cells and the architectural arrangement of the cells and glands. Because the structure of Barrett epithelium resembles that of the gastric mucosa, the same criteria for dysplasia may be applied to both types of tissue (see Chapter 27).

Low-grade or mild dysplasia (Fig. 22.4) shows decreased mucus secretion, crowding of slender columnar cells with pseudostratified nuclei, and occasional mitosis. Pleomorphism is absent or mild. The glands retain the normal contour but may be enlarged. High-grade dysplasia (Figs. 22.5 and 22.6) shows moderate pleomorphism, plump cells, marked reduction of mucus secretion, and frequent mitosis. The glands may show budding, branching,

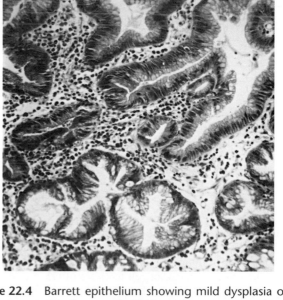

Figure 22.4 Barrett epithelium showing mild dysplasia of foveolar type epithelium, with decreased mucus secretion and pseudostratification of nuclei. Their size is relatively uniform (×150).

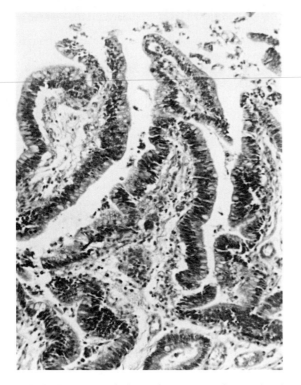

Figure 22.5 Barrett epithelium showing moderate dysplasia of intestinalized epithelium. Pseudostratification is prominent and the amount of mucus is reduced. The surface region has a villous appearance (×140).

crowding, and intraluminal infolding. Ultrastructurally, the dysplastic cells show depletion and alteration of organelles for mucus production, dilated rough endoplasmic reticulum, and accumulation of glycogen (109). In carcinoma in situ, the cells are plump and large, pleomorphism is prominent, mitosis is frequent, and the glands may be distorted. Interobserver agreement is about 90% for high-grade dysplasia and 70% for low-grade dysplasia (110). The histologic distinction between high-grade dysplasia and in situ carcinoma can be difficult, and interobserver disagreement may exist. The same difficulty is recognized with respect to gastric carcinoma, and a category of possible carcinoma is designed to include such cases. (This provision is discussed in Chapter 27.) Low-grade dysplasia should be differentiated from regenerative hyperplasia. When the changes are between reactive hyperplasia and low-grade dysplasia, the designation of "indefinite for dysplasia" has been applied. Additional information concerning dysplasia of Barrett epithelium is presented in Chapter 20.

Molecular Studies

Dysplastic Barrett epithelium shows enhanced cell proliferation and an expanded proliferating zone (111), with a shift toward the surface region of the mucosa as the histologic abnormalities increase (112). There is an increase of cell fractions in G1, S and G2/M phases of the cell cycle (113, 114). Flow cytometry of epithelium with high-grade dysplasia often reveals aneuploid and hyperploid cells (113, 115, 116). Reid (117) found aneuploidy in 63% of cases of high-grade dysplasia and 86% of carcinoma, but in only 6% of

cases of low-grade dysplasia and 4% of Barrett epithelium without dysplasia. In another report, aneuploidy was present in 2% of cases with indefinite for dysplasia, 11% with low-grade dysplasia, 44% with high-grade dysplasia, and 78% with carcinoma (114). Patients with aneuploid clones or increased G2/tetraploid cells developed esophageal adenocarcinoma in later years (113, 118). Aneuploidy is associated with chromosomal abnormalities that may precede dysplasia or carcinoma (119). Thus, these abnormalities may represent early cellular modification before actual neoplastic transformation.

The tumor suppressor gene p53 is often overexpressed in dysplastic epithelium, more often in instances of high-grade dysplasia than in those of low-grade dysplasia (120, 121). Ramel et al. (122) observed p53 expression in 5% of biopsy specimens showing Barrett epithelium negative for dysplasia, 15% showing indefinite or low-grade dysplasia, 45% with high-grade dysplasia, and 53% with evidence of carcinoma. Mutation of p53 was found in 33 to 60% of cases involving high-grade dysplasia (123, 124). Altered p53 has also been found in nondysplastic Barrett epithelium associated with carcinoma, overexpression in 50 to 60% (123, 125), and mutation in 14% (123). Allelic loss of 17p occurred in the diploid cells of dysplastic lesions either before the development of or in association with aneuploidy (126). Alteration of p53 appears to be an early event in the neoplastic progression of Barrett epithelium. See Chapters 5 and 8 for additional information on molecular alterations in dysplastic Barrett epithelium.

Dysplasia-Carcinoma Sequence and Follow-Up Studies

In Barrett epithelium, carcinoma appears to evolve through the stages of intestinal metaplasia, dysplasia, preinvasive stage of intra-

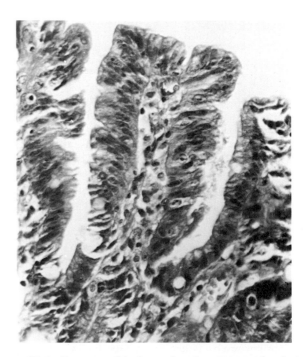

Figure 22.6 Barrett epithelium showing severe dysplasia of intestinalized epithelium. Findings include pseudostratification, reduction of mucus secretion, plump nuclei, and pleomorphism (×240).

glandular carcinoma (carcinoma in situ), and finally invasive carcinoma. In this sequence of events, dysplasia is the most immediate precancerous lesion. It was found in about 80% of cases of Barrett epithelium with carcinoma (42, 127), but in only 6% of those without carcinoma (42). The evolution from dysplasia to carcinoma is not necessarily inevitable, however, even for epithelium showing high-grade dysplasia.

The natural history of dysplasia can be evaluated by prospective follow-up studies. Few such studies have been undertaken to date. Lee reported follow-up (up to 29 month) on six patients (104). Four patients with high-grade dysplasia subsequently had esophagectomy. Three of the four esophagi had invasive carcinoma; in two, the carcinoma went through the wall. The remaining one had an adenoma. Two patients with low-grade dysplasia developed no clinical evidence of carcinoma. Similar cases were reported by other investigators (67, 77). Miros et al. (128) followed 81 patients with proven Barrett esophagus for 289.2 patient-years (mean 3.6 years). Twenty-three patients (28%) had dysplasia. Of three patients with high-grade dysplasia, two developed adenocarcinoma after 2.6 and 4.5 years; in the third, however, the high grade dysplasia regressed to low-grade dysplasia in 1.5 years. Of 10 patients with an initial diagnosis of low-grade dysplasia, 1 developed carcinoma after 4.3 years, 2 regressed after 3 and 5 years, and 7 remained unchanged. Ten patients developed low-grade dysplasia during surveillance, dysplasia regressed in 3 patients after 0.5 and 5 years, and in none of the patients did dysplasia progress. These reports indicate that dysplasia is a precancerous as well as a paracancerous process. The advanced stage of the carcinoma in short-term follow-up studies reaffirms that dysplasia is a marker for a coexisting carcinoma. Furthermore, dysplasia may regress, more often in cases involving low-grade dysplasia than in those involving high-grade dysplasia.

Clinical Significance

Because of the high incidence of associated carcinoma, the presence of aneuploid cells, and increased G2/tetraploid fractions, some investigators consider high-grade dysplasia of Barrett epithelium a neoplastic lesion encompassing in situ carcinoma (73, 77, 113). Some patients have undergone esophagectomy because of it. In the resected esophagi, invasive adenocarcinoma was present in less than one half of cases (28, 77, 104, 105, 107, 128, 129). Many of the carcinomas were in the early stage and highly curable. Reid et al. (105) reported eight cases in which esophagectomy was performed for intramucosal carcinoma in four and high-grade dysplasia in four others. In the carcinoma cases, malignancy was confirmed, but in the dysplasia cases, no carcinoma was found in the resected specimens. Two patients died postoperatively. Rice et al. described 16 patients who had esophagectomy for high-grade dysplasia (129). No invasive carcinoma was found, but 6 patients had intramucosal carcinoma. One patient died 3 months later. Early complications occurred in 7 and late complications occurred in 11 patients, with anastomotic stricture in 7 of the latter group. Complications were successfully managed for all but 2 patients.

These reports indicate that the probability of high-grade dysplasia coexisting with carcinoma is high. Serious postoperative complications may occur, however, so the question of resection for high-grade dysplasia should be evaluated carefully for each patient. A vigorous endoscopic biopsy protocol adopted by Levine et al.

presents a logical and successful approach (130). Surgical resection of Barrett esophagus is considered if the results of repeat biopsies show carcinoma or persistent high-grade dysplasia. Rusch et al. (131) carried out surgical exploration on 27 such patients whose preoperative diagnosis was carcinoma (22 cases) and high-grade dysplasia (5 cases). The postoperative diagnosis was carcinoma in all cases, including in situ carcinoma in 10. One patient had distant metastasis; the others showed neither distant nor lymph node metastasis.

The esophagus of patients with high-grade dysplasia of Barrett epithelium should be examined carefully for malignancy. Because dysplasia and carcinoma may develop anywhere in the Barrett epithelium (132), biopsies from multiple sites are required for adequate evaluation. If a carcinoma is not found by intensive search and high-grade dysplasia persists, the choice of esophagectomy versus continued surveillance with endoscopic follow-up in short regular intervals should be evaluated with regard to the possibility of grave complications of the operation, the expectation of cure, and postoperative quality of life (133). It should be noted, however, that even with multiple biopsies, it is possible to miss the carcinoma (134).

The diagnosis of low-grade dysplasia appears to have less ominous importance (104, 128), although its progression to high-grade dysplasia and carcinoma have been reported (28, 130). Furthermore, dysplasia may regress, more frequently with low-grade than with high-grade dysplasia (128).

ADENOMA

Adenomas, by definition, consist of dysplastic epithelium. The term "adenoma" is used here to denote an unequivocal benign neoplasia that does not regress. It is characterized by and differentiated from the dysplastic lesion just described by its expanding, although localized, growth resulting in a sharply demarcated interface with the surrounding tissue (Fig. 22.7). Using this criterion, we found 5 cases of adenoma in continuity with adenocarcinoma among 16

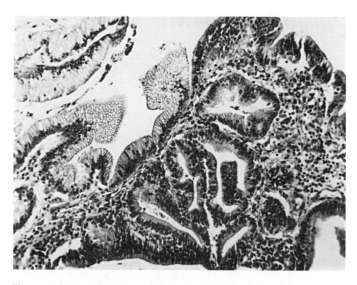

Figure 22.7 Adenoma of Barrett esophagus. *At left,* nonneoplastic Barrett epithelium is shown. Note the sharp demarcation between the two types of epithelium (×60).

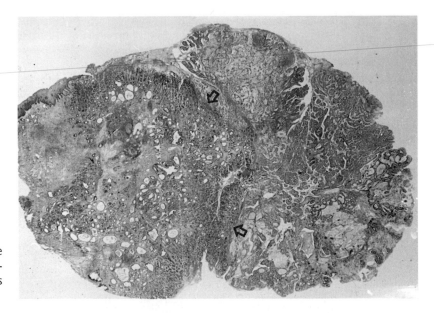

Figure 22.8   Scanning view of a nodular tumor. The right half is a moderately differentiated adenocarcinoma. The left half is an adenoma; their interface is indicated *(arrows)* (×75).

carcinomatous Barrett esophagi (102). In one case, the adenoma occupied one half of the tumor nodule, and an invasive adenocarcinoma occupied the other half (Figs. 22.8 and 22.9). A similar case was reported by Stillman and Sylman (135). Paraf et al. reported three cases of adenoma arising in Barrett epithelium (136), two associated with adenocarcinoma. In one case, multiple pedunculated and sessile lesions gave a polyposis appearance. Wong et al. also reported a case of adenomatous polyposis of the esophagus associated with adenocarcinoma (137). Thompson et al. reported eight carcinomatous cases, including two adenomas with in situ carcinomatous change (14). One adenoma resembled the villous adenoma of colon, with invasive carcinoma in it. McDonald et al. (138) described another case of multiple villous and adenomatous nodules with focal carcinoma.

EXPERIMENTAL STUDIES

Experimental induction of columnar epithelium in dog esophagus has shown that acid reflux is essential (15). The development of adenocarcinoma, however, requires reflux of intestinal contents. In rat experiments conducted by Pera et al. (139), subcutaneous injection of 2,6-dimethylnitrosomorphine induced squamous cell carcinoma in the esophagus of normal rats and adenocarcinoma in the lower esophagus of rats with glandular metaplasia after prior esophagojejunostomy. Further experiments revealed no esophageal carcinoma in rats with bile reflux alone, but the development of adenocarcinoma in 13% of rats with reflux of pancreatic fluid and in 33% of rats with both biliary and pancreatic reflux (82). Rat experiments performed by Clark et al. (88) revealed that gastroduodenal reflux alone induced inflammatory changes in the esophagus in 97% of rats, columnar metaplasia in 10%, dysplasia in 8%, and squamous cell carcinoma in 3%. When the carcinogen methyl-n-amylnitrosamine was given to the rats with gastroduodenal reflux, the incidence of esophageal carcinoma increased to 57%; 42% of the tumors were adenocarcinomas. The incidence of carcinoma further increased to 83% when the rats received a high-fat diet.

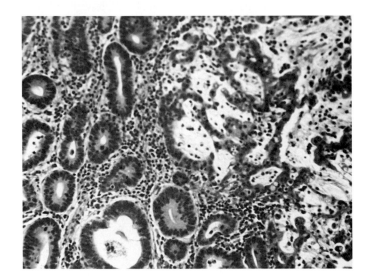

Figure 22.9   High magnification of the interface shown in Figure 22.6. The adenoma is on the left and a mucus-secreting adenocarcinoma is on the right (×150).

PATHOLOGY OF BARRETT ADENOCARCINOMA

Adenocarcinomas of the esophagus originate from the columnar epithelium of the mucosa. Tumors arising from the submucosal glands are discussed in another section.

LOCATION

Adenocarcinoma arising in Barrett epithelium occurs mostly in the distal portion of the esophagus and may invade the adjacent cardia of the stomach (21). Occasional adenocarcinomas are located in the midesophagus (140, 141). In one study, only 11 of 58 cases with adenocarcinoma in the midthoracic esophagus were associated with Barrett epithelium; the others were extensions from the stomach (142). In another report, adenocarcinoma developed in the cervical esophagus in a patient with a long history of gastric reflux and extensive Barrett epithelium (27). The adenocarcinoma in the latter regions (143, 144) may be associated with congenital remnants of superficial glands or heterotopic gastric epithelium.

GROSS MORPHOLOGY

Regardless of their tissue origin, adenocarcinomas of the esophagus have similar morphologic features. Endoscopic surveillance may not reveal gross evidence of early intramucosal or submucosal tumors (68, 105). These lesions usually are flat, but some may be polypoid and large, measuring up to 4.5 cm (145). The majority of the tumors are at an advanced stage at the time of diagnosis, showing extensive intramural and adventitial involvement (73, 102, 146). Most advanced tumors are flat and ulcerated (Fig. 22.10), and about one third are polypoid or fungating (Fig. 22.11). Diffusely infiltrative lesions in the form of linitis plastica (102, 147) as well as grossly papillary lesions (148) are rare (Figs. 22.12 and 22.13). The size of the tumors varies, up to 10 cm in length (mean 5.7 ± 1.8 cm) (149). Two separate carcinomas may be present in the same esophagus (73, 146). In many cases, benign Barrett epithelium is present in the vicinity of the tumor, usually distal to it.

MICROSCOPIC FEATURES

The majority of tumors are well or moderately differentiated tubular adenocarcinomas (Figs. 22.14 and 22.15). In their detailed description of 67 adenocarcinomas, Paraf et al. (75) reported 40% well-differentiated, 31% moderately differentiated, 15% poorly

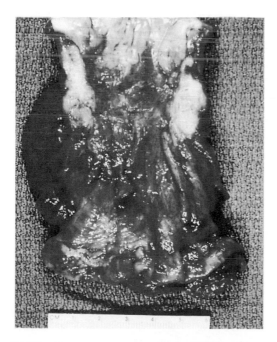

Figure 22.10 Gross appearance of an ulcerative Barrett carcinoma. Its lower end is about 2.5 to 4 cm above the cardiac orifice. The tumor was a well-differentiated adenocarcinoma and measured 2.5 cm long, 1 cm thick, and involved 5 of the 6 cm circumference of the esophagus. The congested Barrett epithelium extended from the distal esophagus to the tumor. (See color plate.)

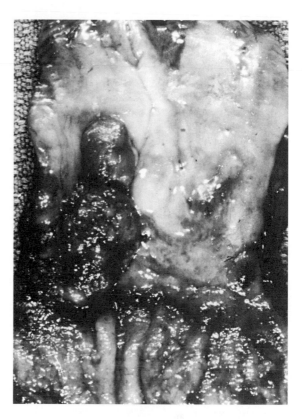

Figure 22.11 Gross appearance of a polypoid Barrett carcinoma, measuring 4.5 × 2.0 × 0.7 cm high. The surface of its lower two thirds was hemorrhagic and eroded. Barrett epithelium was present in small patches to the left of the tumor.

differentiated, 7% mucinous, and 6% signet ring cell type. The carcinoma was intramucosal in 13%, submucosal in 18%, in muscle layer in 12%, in adventitia in 33%, and involving periesophageal tissue in 24%. Papillary pattern is present in about 20% of tumors, and ciliated cells may be present as well (37).

The tumor cells secrete various types of mucin, with prominent sulfomucin in many cases. Neutral mucoprotein and pepsinogen II have also been found in about one half of the tumors at gastroesophageal junction (150). The amount of mucus in the tumor varies; some tumors have mucus pools (75). In general, the mucin is present in the lumen of the tumorous glands, but intracellular mucus goblets are few and scattered. Hormones, including gastrin, bambesin, substance P, somatostatin, serotonin, and gastrin, are present in some lesions (151). Motoyama et al. (152) reported an unusual tubular adenocarcinoma with areas showing features of choriocarcinoma, hepatoid carcinoma, and small cell carcinoma.

Vascular and perineural invasion may be present (Fig. 22.16). Lymph node metastasis occurs in one half to three quarters of cases (75), even if the tumor involves only mucosa or submucosa. The growth pattern of the tumor is nearly equally divided between expanding and infiltrative types. The diffusely infiltrative carcinoma in one of our patients was a signet-ring cell carcinoma (Fig. 22.17). Signet-ring cells have been reported previously (147). The tumor infiltration may be by single glands (Fig. 22.18). In terms of Lauren's classification used for gastric carcinoma (153) (see Chapter 27 for detailed explanation), 11 of our 16 cases were of intestinal type, 3 were diffuse type, and 2 were unclassified.

Other tumors occurring in the Barrett epithelium include squamous cell carcinoma (44, 45, 73, 154, 155), adenosquamous carcinoma, adenocarcinoid (73), carcinoid (156), and mucoepidermoid carcinoma (157). The occurrence of these tumors supports the view that Barrett epithelium may arise from totipotential cells.

The esophageal epithelium adjacent to the carcinoma shows varying degrees of reflux esophagitis. The amount of residual Barrett epithelium is variable; in fact, such tissue may be absent (14), presumably replaced by tumor cells. Dysplasia, sometimes together with in situ carcinoma, is present in most cases (14, 68, 73, 103). Occasionally, Barrett adenocarcinoma coexists with a separate squamous cell carcinoma in the squamous epithelium of the same esophagus (73, 158, 159).

STAGING

The staging system for adenocarcinoma is the same as that used for squamous cell carcinoma (see Chapter 21). Of 61 patients reported by Streitz et al. (4), 6.7% were in stage 0, 16.7% in stage I, 28.3% in stage II, 41.7% in stage III, and 6.7% in stage IV. The 5-year overall survival rate was 23.7%. Corresponding results were reported by Lerut et al. (60): stage 0 and 1, 38.3%; stage II, 20.6%; stage III, 22.2%; and stage IV, 19%. The stages of adenocarcinoma at the time of diagnosis are better in patients undergoing endoscopic surveillance. In a report by Peters et al., the tumors were in early stage in 12 of 13 surveyed patients and in only 10 of 35 nonsurveyed patients (134).

MOLECULAR STUDIES

Cytometric studies of Barrett carcinoma revealed aneuploidy in 70 to 100% of tumors (117, 160–163). Karyotypic analysis showed extensive chromosomal changes, both structurally and numerically (164–167). Loss of Y chromosome was commonly observed (162, 165–167), noted in 93% of adenocarcinomas in one study (167). (See Chapter 7 for detailed information on cytogenetic studies.)

Tumor suppressor gene p53 is overexpressed in 50 to 100% of Barrett carcinomas (120, 121, 124, 168–171). Among cases studied by Rice et al. (121), mutated p53 was present in 67% of intramural and 40% of submucosal carcinomas. Loss of heterozygosity or allelic loss of 17p, where p53 locus is located, occurred in

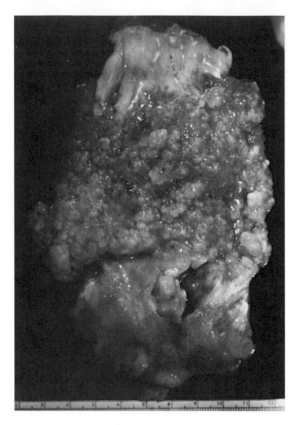

Figure 22.12   Gross appearance of a papillary adenocarcinoma of the lower esophagus. The tumor was 7 cm long, 1 cm thick, and involved the entire circumference of the esophagus. (From Ming SC. Tumors of the esophagus and stomach. Washington DC: Armed Forces Institute of Pathology, 1973.)

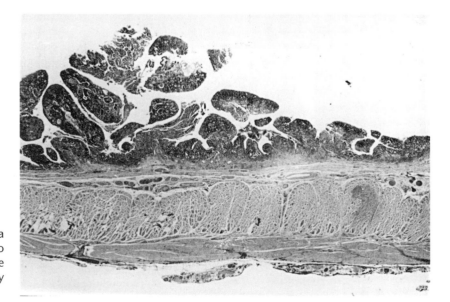

Figure 22.13   A scanning view of the carcinoma shown in Figure 22.12. The tumor is limited to the mucosa in this section. The two-layer structure of muscularis propria of the esophagus is clearly shown (×5.5).

56 to 100% of carcinomas (122, 126, 172, 173). Allelic loss of adenomatous polyposis coli (APC) gene on 5q was noted in 80% of tumors (172). Additionally, allelic loss was found on 9p (64%), 17q (56%), 13q (43%), 18q (43%), and 1p (41%) (172, 173). H-ras oncoprotein was present in 4 of 10 carcinomas and 1 of 10 Barrett epithelium (124), and c-erbB-2 was expressed in 15 to 43% of carcinomas (161, 170, 174). The presence of c-erbB-2 was related to recurrence rate and distal metastasis of the tumors (161). bcl-2 oncoprotein, an inhibitor of apoptosis, has not been detected in Barrett carcinoma or dysplastic epithelium (175).

Microsatellite instability has been detected in Barrett carcinomas; in one report (176), it was present in 7% of Barrett epithelium, 22% of adenocarcinomas, and 2% of squamous cell carcinoma. In another report, it was present in all 17 carcinomas tested (177). Only one tumor showed widespread alterations involving 45.3% of test sites, whereas the other tumors showed changes in only 0.8 to 8.1% of tested loci.

Transforming growth factor alpha (TGFα) and epidermal growth factor receptor are overexpressed in Barrett carcinoma (174, 178, 179). TGFα expression is positive more often in tubu-

lar carcinoma than in signet ring cell carcinoma (178). (See Chapter 8 for additional information on molecular changes in Barrett epithelium and adenocarcinoma.)

ADENOCARCINOMA AT THE ESOPHAGOGASTRIC JUNCTION

The majority of the tumors at the esophagogastric junction are adenocarcinomas. Squamous cell and anaplastic carcinomas constitute about 10% of tumors at this site (180). Occasional cases of adenoacanthoma, mucoepidermoid carcinoma, and double carcinomas have also been reported (181).

There is no barrier to carcinomatous invasion at the esophagogastric junction. Carcinomas can readily invade from esophagus to stomach and vice versa by contiguous intramural spread or through lymphatic channels. It had been reported that about two thirds of adenocarcinomas at the gastroesophageal junction originate in the stomach and one third in the esophagus (150, 182), but the histologic features of these carcinomas are essentially the same (183, 184). It is therefore difficult to determine the origin of the tumors, whether from esophagus or stomach, on the basis of pathologic features alone. The basis for differentiation is circumstantial, relying on such factors as the location of the center of the tumor and the presence of the specific structures of the respective organs. Clearly, these features cannot be applied to a biopsy specimen. In some cases, the specialized, incompletely intestinalized epithelium gives a reasonably reliable clue to the esophageal location of the lesion.

The misgivings of this difficulty are diminished somewhat by the observation that adenocarcinomas of the distal esophagus, esophagogastric junction, and gastric cardia so share many features pathologically and epidemiologically that they may form one entity, distinct from the squamous carcinoma of the esophagus and the adenocarcinoma of the distal stomach (14, 183–186). These features include younger age (sixth versus seventhth decade), male predominance, high incidence of smoking and drinking history, symptom complexes related to hiatal hernia and reflux esophagitis, and the low incidence of signet-ring cell carcinoma. Pathologic evidence supporting the single entity concept of the tumors is the high prevalence of Barrett epithelium in association with adenocarcinomas at the esophagogastric junction in 67% of cases with

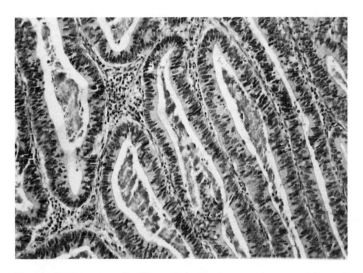

Figure 22.14 A well-differentiated adenocarcinoma of Barrett esophagus (×150).

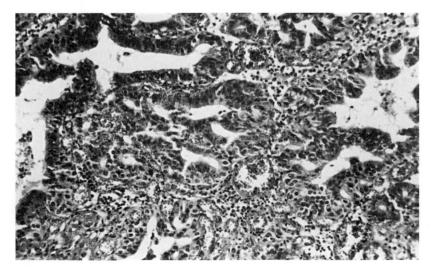

Figure 22.15 A moderately to poorly differentiated adenocarcinoma of Barrett esophagus (×150).

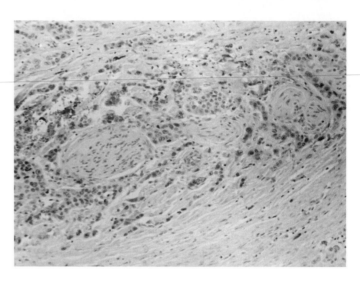

Figure 22.16 An infiltrative type of poorly differentiated adeno-carcinoma showing perineural invasion (×200).

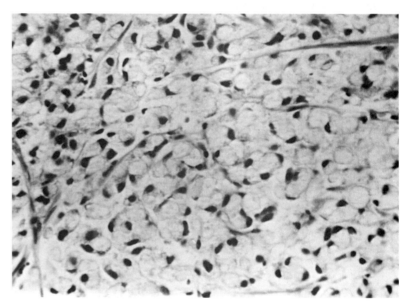

Figure 22.17 A signet-ring cell carcinoma of Barrett esophagus (×240).

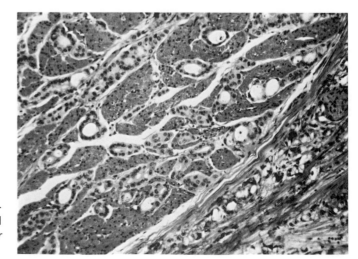

Figure 22.18 An infiltrative type of well-differentiated adenocar-cinoma showing infiltration of muscularis propria by individual glands. Signet-ring carcinoma cells are also present *(right lower corner)* (×150).

carcinomas 6 cm or less in length, but in only 17% of cases with larger tumors (187).

Commensurate with the increased incidence of adenocarcinoma of the esophagus in recent years has been an increase in the incidence of carcinoma of the cardia, reaching 50% of all gastric carcinomas in some reports (3). Barrett epithelium was present in 42% of these cases involving carcinoma in the cardia, but in only 5% of cases with carcinoma in the subcardiac region (51). The Barrett epithelium in these cases was short (average 2.7 cm, versus 7.4 cm in esophageal adenocarcinoma cases) and might not be recognized endoscopically.

SPREAD AND METASTASIS OF ADENOCARCINOMA

The routes of spread and metastasis of adenocarcinoma are similar to those of squamous cell carcinoma of the esophagus (see Chapter 21). Differences between them stem primarily from the location of the primary tumors rather than the intrinsic biology of tumor cells.

Intramural spread of adenocarcinoma may be by continuous invasion or via lymphatics. Lateral spread by lymphatics may result in the formation of disconnected nodules resembling separate primary tumors. Transmural spread of tumor occurs in 60 to 88% of Barrett carcinomas (68). Lymph node metastasis is present in 51 to 74% of adenocarcinomas (68, 75). Endoscopically surveyed patients have less metastatic nodes—26.5% in surveyed and 78% in nonsurveyed cases (60). Frequency of lymph node metastasis is related to the depth of tumor invasion. Among 43 cases reported by Clark et al. (188), nodal involvement was present in 33% of intramucosal, 67% of intramural, and 89% of transmural carcinomas. The nodes involved most commonly were at the lesser curvature of the stomach at 42%; 35% of the nodes were perihiatal, 28% periesophageal, and 21% celiac. The supraclavicular nodes are involved in 10% of cases (189). Sixty-two percent of carcinomas at the esophagogastric junction have lymph node metastasis, mostly intraabdominal (190). Thoracic nodes are involved in 7% of cases.

SURVIVAL RATES AND PROGNOSTIC FACTORS

SURVIVAL RATES

The survival rates of patients with Barrett adenocarcinoma is low, similar to those of squamous cell carcinoma (22, 68, 73, 191, 192), although longer survival time in patients with adenocarcinoma have been reported (193). The survival rates given by Sanfey et al. (194) were 34% at 2 years and 14.8% at 5 years. The overall survival rates reported by Lerut et al. (60) were 80.5% at 1 year, 62.7% at 2 years, and 58.2% at 5 years, and those described by Paraf et al. were 63%, 41%, and 32%, respectively (75). The better results in the former group might be related to the larger number of early cases, 58.9 and 43% in stages 0 to II in respective series. The mean survival time of curatively resected cases reported by Witt et al. was only 12 months (146). The medium survival time for adenocarcinoma at the gastroesophageal junction was 27 months, similar to that of squamous cell carcinoma of esophagus (192).

PROGNOSTIC FACTORS

Prognosis of esophageal adenocarcinoma is not influenced by the gross morphology or the histologic grade of the tumor. The pathologic features that influence the outcome of the disease are stage, lymph node metastasis, and the number of involved nodes by multivariant analysis (102). Overexpression and mutation of tumor suppressor genes, oncogenes, and regulators of tumor biology may also affect the outcome.

Stage of Carcinoma

The stage of esophageal cancer at the time of diagnosis is the most important prognostic factor; the higher the tumor stage, the lower the survival rate. In a report by Streitz et al. (4), the 3-year survival rates for stages 0, I, IIA, IIB, III, and IV tumors were 100%, 85.7%, 53.6%, 45%, 25.2%, and 0%, respectively. The overall 5-year survival rate was 23.7%. Favorable prognosis for early carcinoma was noted also in other reports (103, 146). Five-year survival rates reported by Lerut et al. (60) for stages 0 and I, II, III, and IV tumors were 100%, 87.5%, 22.2%, and 14%, respectively. In this regard, endoscopic surveillance results in early detection of Barrett carcinoma and increases the curability of the cancer. The depth of tumor invasion in the esophageal wall is an independent prognostic factor. Five-year survival rate of tumors limited to mucosa and submucosa was 82%, in contrast to 12% for tumors with deep invasion (75).

Lymph Node Metastasis

The survival rate is influenced by the number but not the location of involved lymph nodes. Without nodal involvement, the 5-year survival rate was 85.3%, significantly higher than 38.3% with positive nodes (60). The corresponding rates in another report were 59% and 10%, respectively (75). The survival rate is better for patients with four or less metastatic nodes than those with larger number of involved nodes (188, 192).

Molecular Status of Tumor Cells

Poor survival, tumor recurrence, depth of invasion, and the risk of lymph node metastasis in esophageal adenocarcinoma have been related to aneuploidy of the tumor cells (161, 195). Khan et al. analyzed DNA content of 30 Barrett carcinomas and found that 80% of tumors were aneuploid and 20% were diploid (163). The mean 5-year survival time was 20.4 months for diploid tumors and 10.6 months for aneuploid tumors. Overexpression of p53 is related to tumor recurrence, but not survival (170). In one report, however, survival was longer for patients with p53-positive carcinomas than for patients with p53-negative tumors—28 versus 13.5 months (196). Expression of c-erbB-2 has been related to 5-year survival rate—60% for positive tumors versus 10% for negative tumors (170).

CLINICOPATHOLOGIC CORRELATION

The prominent symptoms of esophageal adenocarcinoma are dysphagia and symptoms of gastric reflux (73, 146, 197, 198). Symptoms of reflux, however, have been found in relatively low percentage of cases of adenocarcinoma of the esophagus (194, 198, 199) and were of shorter duration than those observed in patients without malignant disease (200). Dysphagia is related to the gross pathologic features of the tumor and the level of its location. In advanced cases, additional symptoms occur, including weight loss, bleeding, fatigue, chest pain, and vomiting (146), depending on the extent of tumor invasion and the nature of complications. One patient had osteoarthropathy that disappeared after the resection of Barrett carcinoma (151).

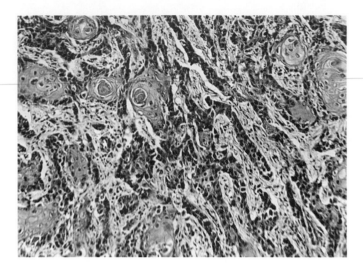

Figure 22.19   An adenoacanthoma of the esophagus showing squamous metaplasia of a poorly differentiated tubular adenocarcinoma (×200).

Adenocarcinomas, being mucosal lesions, are readily accessible for endoscopic visualization and biopsy. Most of the tumors are well or moderately differentiated, and therefore are easily diagnosed. Ultrasound-guided fine needle biopsy and cytologic examination may provide histologic confirmation of the extent of the disease, including distant metastasis (201). The question of routine systematic surveillance of Barrett esophagus by endoscopy and biopsy has been debated. Some investigators think that it is not indicated because the incidence of malignancy apparently is not as high as previously reported (65, 202).

ADENOACANTHOMA AND ADENOSQUAMOUS CARCINOMA

Adenoacanthoma and adenosquamous carcinoma are characterized by the presence of both squamous and glandular cells. These terms have been used interchangeably with mucoepidermoid carcinoma by some authors. Because they have different origin, some differentiation should be made. They should also be differentiated from the squamous cell carcinoma with pseudoglandular degeneration, which has no mucus secretion (203).

The adenoacanthoma is an adenocarcinoma with focal squamous metaplasia (Fig. 22.19). Squamous cells were seen ultrastructurally in a Barrett adenocarcinoma by Banner et al. (151). Adenoacanthomas are rare; one case each were found among 50 superficial and 133 advanced esophageal carcinomas (204). On the other hand, the adenosquamous carcinoma is basically a squamous cell carcinoma with occasional mucus-secreting glandular components. This combination occurred in 23 of 195 squamous cell carcinomas reviewed by Kuwano et al. (205). Similar observations were made by Sugimachi et al. (47), who suggested that such tumors might have arisen from the esophageal glands or ducts in addition to the squamous epithelium. In another report, adenosquamous elements, in addition to squamous cells, were found in a polypoid spindle cell carcinoma (206). The outcome of these tumors is the same as that for tumors without the minor metaplastic components.

CARCINOMAS OF THE SUBMUCOSAL ESOPHAGEAL GLAND

Two distinctive carcinomas originate from the duct system of the deep esophageal glands: mucoepidermoid carcinoma and adenoid cystic carcinoma. These tumors are rare. In one report, only one of each type was found among 1674 esophageal carcinomas (71). Some authors report an incidence range of 1 to 4% (207-210). Initially, these submucosal tumors are covered by intact mucosa (211, 212), creating a diagnostic problem for radiologic and endoscopic visualization. Dysphagia is the primary symptom. Other tumors of the major salivary glands, such as pleomorphic adenomas and acinic carcinomas, have not been documented in the esophagus.

MUCOEPIDERMOID CARCINOMA

Mucoepidermoid carcinoma is composed of both squamous and glandular cells. Mafune et al. identified 4 cases of mucoepidermoid carcinoma among 135 patients with esophageal cancer (3.1%) (210). These lesions showed sclerosing submucosal infiltration with funnel-shaped obstruction of the esophagus. Two tumors showed intraepithelial spread and two others had dysplasia of the epithelium, suggesting a possible origin of the tumors in the squamous epithelium. In one case, the mucopidermoid carcinoma was reported to have arisen in a Barrett esophagus (213). About 50% of tumors occur in the middle one third of the esophagus. As in similar tumors in the salivary gland, the squamous and mucous cells in esophageal mucoepidermoid tumors are intimately intermingled, although their relative amounts vary. The squamous cells are generally well to moderately differentiated, and show intercellular bridges, keratin, and occasional pearl formation. The mucous cells are cuboidal or columnar, forming glands or sheets. The amount of mucus varies both intracellularly and intraluminally. Large cystic areas containing extracellular secretion may be observed. Smaller intermediate cells are also present. By electron microscopy, some cells contain both keratin and secretary granules (214).

Clinically, patients typically are male and in the seventh decade. Although most tumors are resectable, the mucoepidermoid carcinomas of the esophagus are aggressive; extensive invasion and lymph node metastasis are common. The prognosis is poor, as it is with squamous cell carcinomas (210, 211, 215), unless the tumor is confined to the submucosa with no lymph node metastasis (208).

ADENOID CYSTIC CARCINOMA

Adenoid cystic carcinoma, also known as cylindroma, is believed to originate from the intercalated duct of submucosal esophageal glands (205, 216). Petursson reviewed 44 cases reported in the literature up to 1986 (217). The tumors are found mostly in the middle one third of the esophagus (209, 218), primarily in the submucosa, although they may become ulcerated or polypoid (209, 219, 220). Histologically, lesions are composed of well-defined islands of tumor cells with a cribriform pattern and many cystic spaces. Squamous cells may be present. By electron microscopy, the cysts contain replicated basement membrane and are lined by epithelial cells (216). Myoepithelial cells are also present. The tumor cells shows positive immunohistologic reaction for S-100 protein. Some tumors have a basaloid appearance and may actually be basaloid squamous carcinomas (218) (see the discussion of basaloid carcinoma in Chapter 21). Whereas some tumors appear to be relatively indolent, others tend to have widespread metastasis and a corresponding low survival rate (209, 211, 217). Clinically, the tumors occur about equally among men and women. Most patients are in the seventh decade of life.

CARCINOID AND SMALL (OAT) CELL CARCINOMA

Carcinoids and small cell carcinomas of the esophagus are tumors of neuroendocrine cells. As foregut tumors, they are usually argyrophilic. The argentaffin reaction may be positive in the carcinoid (221), but generally is negative in small cell carcinomas (222–225). Thus, the small cell carcinoma has also been called argyrophil cell carcinoma (223).

CARCINOID

Carcinoids, noted rarely in the esophagus, are composed of uniform polygonal or round cells in sheets and trabeculae (Fig. 22.20). Carcinoids are primarily submucosal tumors that arise mostly in the distal esophagus. One tumor was reported to have ACTH activity (226). In another case, mucus producing adenocarcinoma was admixed with the carcinoid tissue (221). An adenocarcinoid was reported to occur in a Barrett esophagus (73). In another case, a carcinoid in Barrett epithelium was accompanied by a separate adenocarcinoma (156).

SMALL (OAT) CELL CARCINOMA

Oat cell carcinoma of the esophagus was first recognized by McKeown (227). He reported two ulcerated tumors. One was composed of pure oat cells, but the other had a mixture of squamous and oat cells. By 1992, 150 cases of esophageal tumor had been reported (228). Second to the lung, the esophagus is the most common site for small cell carcinoma. The reported incidences among all carcinomas of the esophagus varied from 0.05 to 7.6% (223, 229–232). In 1984, Doherty et al. reviewed 66 cases and reported 6 additional cases (229). They noted that about two thirds

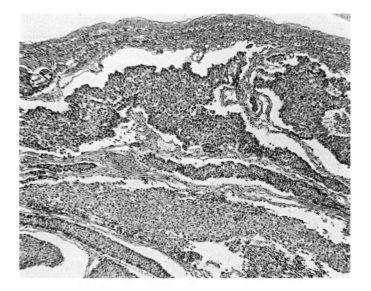

Figure 22.20   A carcinoid of the esophagus showing sheets of uniform tumor cells with hyperchromatic cells at the periphery.

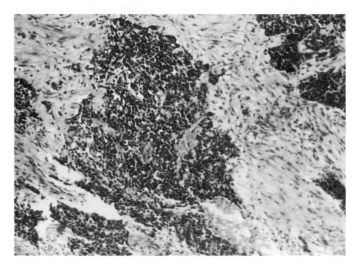

Figure 22.21   A small cell carcinoma of the esophagus. The tumor cells are markedly hyperchromatic and the cytoplasm is scanty and hardly visible at this magnification (×120).

of the tumors were pure oat cell carcinomas. The other tumors often had squamous elements, less commonly adenocarcinoma, and rarely carcinoid differentiation. The combination of different cell types prompted some investigators to raise the possibility of tumor origin from the totipotential cells in the squamous epithelium or ducts of the submucosal glands (222, 224, 233). In one case, an aberrant columnar epithelium was the presumed origin (227).

Grossly, small cell carcinomas of the esophagus are usually large fungating or ulcerated; the polypoid form is rare (224). Multiple tumors may be present in one esophagus (234). The size varies from 2.5 to 14.5 cm (223). Histologically, the tumor is composed of small cells with hyperchromatic nuclei and scanty cytoplasm (Fig. 22.21). The characteristic cell morphology allows diagnosis by cytology (225). Larger intermediate cells are present in about one half of the cases, alone or mixed with small cells (235). Neurosecretory granules are present in most lesions (227, 230–232). Some cells also have tonofilaments. Immunohistochemical reactions for neuron-specific enolase, synaptophysin, S-100 protein, and chromogranin generally are positive and serve as useful diagnostic markers (235, 236). ACTH activity is often present (221, 230–232), but Cushing syndrome has not been reported. Calcitonin was found in some tumors (231). Inappropriate antidiuretic hormone syndrome and hypercalcemia have been reported (229). Flow cytometry revealed aneuploidy and a high S-phase fraction, indicating rapid cell proliferation (231).

It has been suggested that a small cell carcinoma showing negative argyrophil reaction and no neurosecretory granules should be called non-oat cell type (237, 238). Because non-oat cell type can coexist with squamous cell carcinoma, an origin in the squamous epithelium or duct of esophageal gland was proposed for the non-oat cell type of small cell carcinoma (237). Clinically, there is no difference between the oat cell type and the non-oat cell type.

Small cell carcinomas occur mainly in the sixth to seventh decade in both sexes (231), arising most often in the middle and distal esophagus. Many tumors are in late stage with extensive dissemination at the time of diagnosis. The prognosis is poor, even when the primary growth is limited (223, 229, 230). The overall mean survival time is only 3 to 7 months (230, 231, 239, 240).

Multidrug chemotherapy may offer temporary remission (230, 231, 234, 240).

MALIGNANT MELANOMA

Primary malignant melanoma of the esophagus is rare and accounts for about 0.1% of esophageal malignant tumors (241, 242). Its existence was in doubt until the demonstration of melanocytes in the normal esophageal epithelium (48, 49). An increase in the number of melanocytes in the adjacent mucosa, in some cases, results in extensive brown pigmentation of the esophageal mucosa beyond the tumor, even involving the entire esophagus (243). The first black patient with esophageal melanoma was reported in South Africa in 1992 (244). Benign pigmented nevus has not been reported.

Primary malignant melanoma is located most frequently in the lower esophagus, rarely in the upper portion (241, 245, 246). Most tumors are large polypoid lesions (242, 246), often with a smooth surface. Dark pigmentation may be striking (241, 245). About 10% of tumors are amelanotic (245, 247). One patient had multiple nodules (248). Histologically, the tumor is characterized by marked cellularity, frequent mitosis, and the presence of intracellular as well as extracellular melanin pigments. Immunohistochemical staining for neuron-specific enolase and S-100 protein are positive. Electron microscopy reveals many melanosomes and premelanosomes, which are also present in amelanotic tumors (247). Junctional changes with melanoma cells at the base of the covering squamous epithelium are common (249, 250). In some reports, a prominent lentiginous growth pattern is described (243, 249). The presence of junctional change is considered conclusive evidence of the primary nature of the melanoma and should be sought. If the junctional change is absent, the primary nature of the tumor can be ascertained only by exclusion of other possible sources. Metastatic melanoma to the esophagus is rare, however, in contrast to the relatively high incidence of metastatic melanoma to the stomach and intestines (251).

Clinically, malignant melanoma affects males more often than females (2:1) (245). Patients range in age, from a 7-year-old boy (252), two patients in their thirties (246, 253), to the majority of patients in the sixth and seventh decades. Lymphatic metastasis is common (245). Prognosis is poor, with a 5-year survival rate of only 4.2% (241, 245). Radiotherapy and chemotherapy may be beneficial (245).

CHORIOCARCINOMA

Choriocarcinoma of the esophagus is very rare (254–258). The tumor is composed of cyto- and syncythiotrophoblasts, with some areas showing other cell types, including well-differentiated adenocarcinoma and undifferentiated cells (255–257).

Of those cases reported to date, two involved tumors that occurred in Barrett esophagus. In addition to trophoblasts, one showed yolk sac differentiation (258). Immunohistochemical stains of the tumor for human chorionic gonadotropin and human placental lactogen were positive (255). Choriocarcinomas are large and ulcerated tumors arising mainly in the lower esophagus. Extensive metastases are frequent. Other findings in patients with choriocarcinoma include increased serum and urinary gonadotropin levels (256, 257). All patients were 50 years of age or younger and both sexes were affected.

PAGET DISEASE

Rare cases of Paget disease of the esophagus have been reported. In one case involving a 60-year-old man with dysphagia (259), the resected lower esophagus showed diffuse induration. Histologically, large clear pagetoid cells were found in the squamous epithelium and glandular ducts, without stromal invasion. The pagetoid cells show focal positive reaction for epithelial membrane antigen, carcinoembryonic antigen, periodic acid Schiff reagent, and alcine blue, but negative reaction for S-100, neuron-specific enolase, and melanin. In another case involving a 59-year-old man (260), the Paget cells were in the epithelium of the upper and middle esophagus. Focal invasion by undifferentiated cells was observed. In two other cases, intraepithelial pagetoid cells were found in association with an adenosquamous carcinoma in one case (261) and a squamous cell carcinoma in the other (262).

SECONDARY AND METASTATIC TUMORS

About 3% of all carcinomas show metastasis to the esophagus at autopsy (263), mostly from primary tumors of the stomach, lung, or breast. The esophagus may be invaded directly by malignant tumors of the lung or mediastinal lymph nodes, the latter having primary lymphoma or metastatic tumors. Carcinomas of the upper stomach and hypopharynx may extend into the contiguous esophagus or metastasize to the esophageal wall by lymphatics. Antler et al. found esophageal involvement in 33 of 423 cases of lung carcinoma at autopsy, 14 by direct invasion (264). Carcinoma of the breast metastasizes to the esophagus via lymphatics and intercostal vessels, sometimes causing dysphagia and esophageal stenosis. Varanasi et al. reported four such cases (265). In most cases, dysphagia is caused by external compression by involved nodes (266). Such complications may occur many years after the diagnosis of primary carcinoma in the breast. The hematogenous route appears to be operating in the case of metastatic melanoma to the esophagus (267).

In general, metastatic tumors are submucosal, small, and asymptomatic. An intraluminal mass or large ulceration is exceedingly rare, unless the esophageal lesion is contiguous with the primary tumor. Cooney et al. reported a case of metastatic thyroid carcinoma forming an expansile intraluminal mass resembling primary esophageal carcinoma (268). In such cases, surgical resection of the metastatic tumor occasionally results in long survival (269). The exception is metastatic melanoma in the esophagus, which, like the primary melanoma, may form a large pigmented polypoid mass (270, 271). Therefore, the junctional change must be sought in order to identify the primary nature of a melanomatous lesion in the esophagus.

BENIGN TUMORS AND TUMOR-LIKE LESIONS

Benign tumors of the esophagus are mostly mesenchymal (see Chapter 18). Benign epithelial tumors, namely squamous cell papilloma and adenoma, are rare. Among 522 benign esophageal tumors reported by Schmidt et al. (272) and Plachta (273), only 14 were papillomas and 5 were adenomas, in contrast to 283 leiomyomas, 110 polyps, and 59 cysts.

SQUAMOUS PAPILLOMA

Squamous papilloma is a sessile lesion. Its papillae are composed of a central core of connective tissue covered with hyperplastic squamous cells in an orderly arrangement and without dysplastic changes. Its incidence at endoscopy is only 0.04% (274, 275). Distal esophagus is the usual site (276). Most lesions are only a few millimeters in diameter, although large papillomas (up to 6 cm in greatest dimension) have been reported (277). The majority of papillomas are single (274, 276). In one report, a 6-year-old girl had multiple papillomas in the hypopharynx and the entire length of esophagus, which regressed spontaneously in 2 years (278). Another report described a case involving a 2½-year-old boy with multiple esophageal papillomas. His mother had vulvar condyloma when the child was born (279). These cases suggest possible viral origin of the papillomas. In the past, human papillomavirus (HPV) antigen was only infrequently demonstrated in the papilloma (274, 280). More recently, however, Odze et al. found 50% positivity among 26 papillomas tested, most commonly for HPV type 16 (276). HPV has also been implicated in the development of squamous cell carcinoma (281). (See Chapter 21 for additional discussion on the relationship between squamous papilloma and squamous cell carcinoma of esophagus.)

ADENOMA

Adenomas of the esophagus arising in the Barrett esophagus have been reported (102, 136, 138, 141) and were described in the preceding discussion of precancerous lesions.

Adenomas of the submucosal esophageal gland are extremely rare. The adenoma reported by Takubo et al. (282) was a 7 mm × 8 mm submucosal tumor of midesophagus, covered by intact normal squamous epithelium, and accompanied by a separate squamous cell carcinoma. The tumor was papillary and lined with two layers of cuboid cells. No Barrett epithelium was found. In another case, the adenoma was a 1-cm cystic submucosal mass in the distal esophagus (282).

POLYPS

Polyps of the esophagus are composed of mesenchymal tissue and covered by intact squamous epithelium. The mesenchymal tissue may be fibrous, vascular, adipose, or in combination, and the polyp is named accordingly, such as fibrovascular polyp and pedunculated lipoma (284–287). Polyps can be large and may produce dramatic clinical presentation by regurgitation of the polyp. This occurrence may cause asphyxiation and even death. Inflammatory polyps have also been reported (288, 289). Benign mesenchymal lesions are discussed in Chapter 18.

CYSTS

Isolated retention cysts formed by dilated ducts of the esophageal glands are relatively common (290). They are submucosal and occur more often in the lower esophagus than elsewhere. They may form a dome-shaped bulge, but usually they are small and asymptomatic.

Duplication cysts of developmental origin are primarily extramural and connect with the esophagus only partially if at all. These cysts may be lined by esophageal, bronchial, or gastric epithelium. Rarely, the cyst lies within the esophageal wall (291). Its lining epithelium is commonly ciliated. (See Chapter 10 for details concerning congenital cysts.)

REFERENCES

1. Raphal HA, Ellis FH Jr, Dockerty MD. Primary adenocarcinoma of the esophagus: 18 year review and review of literature. Ann Surg 1966;164:785–796.
2. Johnston BJ, Reed PI. Changing pattern of oesophageal cancer in a general hospital in the UK. Eur J Cancer Prev 1991;1:23–25.
3. Blot WJ, Devesa SS, Kneller RW, et al. Rising incidence of adenocarcinoma of the esophagus and gastric cardia. JAMA 1991;265:1287–1289.
4. Streitz JM Jr, Ellis FH Jr, Gibb SP, et al. Adenocarcinoma in Barrett's esophagus. A clinicopathologic study of 65 cases. Ann Surg 1991;213:122–125.
5. Rector LE, Connerley ML. Aberrant mucosa in the esophagus in infants and in children. Arch Pathol Lab Med 1994;31:1285–1294.
6. Jabbari M, Goresky CA, Lough J, et al. The inlet patch: Heterotopic gastric mucosa in the upper esophagus. Gastroenterology 1985;89:352–356.
7. Borhan-Manesh F, Farnum JB. Incidence of heterotopic gastric mucosa in the upper esophagus. Gut 1991;32:968–972.
8. Barrett NR. Chronic peptic ulcer of the oesophagus and esophagitis. Br J Surg 1950;38:175–182.
9. Barrett NR. The lower esophagus lined by columnar epithelium. Surgery 1957;41:881–894.
10. Ozzello L, Savary M, Rooethlisberger B. Columnar mucosa of the distal esophagus in patients with gastroesophageal reflux. Pathol Annu 1977;12:41–86.
11. Borrie J, Goldwater L. Columnar cell-lined esophagus: Assessment of etiology and treatment. A 22 year experience. J Thorac Cardiovasc Surg 1976;71:825–834.
12. Bremner CG, Lynch VP, Ellis FH Jr. Barrett's esophagus: Congenital or acquired? An experimental study of esophageal mucosal regeneration in the dog. Surgery 1970;68:209–216.
13. Saubier EC, Gouillat C, Samaniego C, et al. Adenocarcinoma in columnar lined Barrett's esophagus. Analysis of 13 esophagectomies. Am J Surg 1985;150:365–369.
14. Thompson JJ, Zinsser KR, Enterline HT. Barrett's metaplasia and adenocarcinoma of the esophagus and gastroesophageal junction. Hum Pathol 1983;14:42–61.
15. Gillen P, Keeling P, Byrne PJ, et al. Experimental columnar metaplasia in the canine oesophagus. Br J Surg 1988;75:113–115.
16. Pinero R, Salomon A, Gonzalez R, et al. Esofago de Barret. Frecuencia, caracteristicas, clinicas. Endoscopicas e histologicas. G E N 1990;44:46–48.
17. Cameron AJ, Lomboy CT. Barrett's esophagus: Age, prevalence, and extent of columnar epithelium. Gastroenterology 1992;103:1241–1245.
18. Ferrando J, Reig G. esofago de Barrerr como lesion precancerosa. Rev Espan Enfermed Digest 1991;80:83–86.
19. Ribet M, Mensier E, Pruvot FR. Barrett's esophagus and adenocarcinoma. Eur J Cardio-Thorac Surg 1987;1:29–32.
20. Spechler SJ, Goyal RK. Barrett's esophagus. N Engl J Med 1986;315:362–371.
21. Naef AP, Savary M, Ozzello L. Columnar lined lower esophagus: An acquired lesion with malignant predisposition. Report on 140 cases of Barrett's esophagus with 12 adenocarcinomas. J Thorac Cardiovasc Surg 1975;70:826–834.
22. Winters C Jr, Spyrling TJ, Chobanian SJ, et al. Barrett's esophagus. A prevalent, occult complication of gastroesophageal reflux disease. Gastroenterology 1987;92:118–124.
23. Cameron AJ, Zinsmeister AR, Ballard DJ, et al. Prevalence of columnar-lined (Barrett's) esophagus. Comparison of population-based clinical and autopsy findings. Gastroenterology 1990;99:918–922.
24. Cheu HW, Grosfeld JL, Heifetz SA, et al. Persistence of Barrett's esophagus in children after antireflux surgery: Influence on follow-up care. J Pediatr Surg 1992;27:260–264.
25. Fonkalsrud EW, Ament ME. Gastroesophageal reflux in childhood. Curr Probl Surg 1996;33:1–70.
26. Robins DB, Zaino RJ, Ballantine TV. Barrett's esophagus in a newborn. Pediatr Pathol 1991;11:663–667.
27. Goodwin WJ Jr, Larson DL, Sajjad SM. Adenocarcinoma of the cervical esophagus in a patient with extensive columnar cell-lined

(Barrett's) esophagus. Otolaryngol Head Neck Surg 1983;91:446–449.

28. Hameeteman W, Tytgat GN, Houthoff HJ, et al. Barrett's esophagus: Development of dysplasia and adenocarcinoma. Gastroenterology 1989;96:1249–1256.

29. Johnston MH, Hammond AS, Laskin W, et al. The prevalence and clinical characteristics of short segments of specialized intestinal metaplasia in the distal esophagus on routine endoscopy. Am J Gastroenterol 1996;91:1507–1511.

30. Spechler SJ, Zeroogian JM, Antonioli DA, et al. Prevalence of metaplasia at the gastro-oesophageal junction. Lancet 1994;344:1533–1536.

31. Paull A, Trier JS, Dalton MD, et al. The histologic spectrum of Barrett's esophagus. N Engl J Med 1976;295:476–480.

32. Schnell T, Sontag S, Wanner J. Endoscopic screening for Barrett's esophagus (BE), esophageal adenocarcinoma (AdCA) and other mucosal changes in ambulatory subjects with symptomatic gastro-esophageal reflux (GER) (abstract). Gastroenterology 1985;88:1576.

33. Zwas F, Shields HM, Doos WG, et al. Scanning electron microscopy of Barrett's epithelium and its correlation with light microscopy and mucin stains. Gastroenterology 1986;90:1932–1941.

34. Levine DS, Rubin CE, Reid BJ, et al. Specialized metaplastic columnar epithelium in Barrett's esophagus: A comparative transmission electron microscopic study. Lab Invest 1989;60:418–432.

35. Shields HM, Sawhney RA, Zwas F, et al. Scanning electron microscopy of the human esophagus: Application to Barrett's esophagus, a precancerous lesion. Microsc Res Tech 1995;31:248–256.

36. Shreiber DS, Apstein M, Hermos JA. Paneth cells in Barrett's esophagus. Gastroenterology 1978;74:1302–1304.

37. Rubio CA, Aberg B. Stemmermann G. Ciliated cells in papillary adenocarcinomas of Barrett's esophagus. Acta Cytol 1992;36:65–68.

38. Krishnamurthy S, Dayal Y. Pancreatic metaplasia in Barrett's esophagus. An immunohistochemical study. Am J Surg Pathol 1995;19:1172–1180.

39. Mangla JC, Schenk EA, Desbaillets L, et al. Pepsin secretion, pepsinogen, and gastrin in "Barrett's esophagus": Clinical and morphological characteristics. Gastroenterology 1976;70:669–676.

40. Rubio CA, Aberg B. Further studies on the musculofibrous anomaly of the Barrett's mucosa in esophageal carcinomas. Pathol Res Pract 1991;187:1009–1013.

41. Takubo K, Sasajima K, Yamashita K, et al. Double muscularis mucosae in Barrett's esophagus. Hum Pathol 1991;22:1158–1161.

42. Schmidt HG, Riddell RH, Walther B, et al. Dysplasia in Barrett's esophagus. J Cancer Res Clin Oncol 1985;110:145–152.

43. Jass JR. Mucin histochemistry of the columnar epithelium of oesophagus: A retrospective study. J Clin Pathol 1981;34:866–870.

44. Tamura H, Schulman SA. Barrett type esophagus associated with squamous carcinoma. Chest 1971;59:330–332.

45. Resano CH, Cabrera N, Gonzalez-Cueto D, et al. Double early epidermoid carcinoma of the esophagus in columnar epithelium. Endoscopy 1985;17:73–75.

46. Rosengard AM, Hamilton SR. Squamous carcinoma of the esophagus in patients with Barrett esophagus. Mod Pathol 1989;2:2–7.

47. Sugimachi K, Sumiyoshi K, Nozoe T, et al. Carcinogenesis and histogenesis of esophageal carcinoma. Cancer 1995;75(Suppl):1440–1445.

48. Tateishi R, Taniguchi H, Wada A, et al. Argyrophil cells and melanocytes in esophageal mucosa. Arch Pathol Lab Med 1974;98:87–89.

49. De la Pava S, Nigogosyan G, Pickren JW, et al. Melanosis of the esophagus. Cancer 1963;16:48–50.

50. Fennerty MB, DiTomasso J, Morales TG, et al. Screening for Barrett's esophagus by balloon cytology. Am J Gastroenterol 1995;90:1230–1232.

51. Clark GW, Smyrk TC, Burdiles P, et al. Is Barrett's metaplasia the source of adenocarcinomas of the cardia? Arch Surg 1994;129:609–614.

52. Cederqvist C, Zielsen J, Berthelsen A, et al. Adenocarcinoma of the esophagus. Acta Chir Scand 1980;146:411–415.

53. Radigan LR, Glover JL, Shipley FE, et al. Barrett esophagus. Arch Surg 1977;112:486–490.

54. Dawson JL. Adenocarcinoma of the middle oesophagus arising in an oesophagus lined by gastric (parietal) epithelium. Br J Surg 1964;51:940–942.

55. Shimazu H, Kobori O, Shoji M, et al. Superficial carcinoma of the esophagus. Gastroenterol Jpn 1983;18:409–416.

56. Bosch A, Frias Z, Caldwell WL. Adenocarcinoma of the esophagus. Cancer 1979;43:1557–1561.

57. Davis WM, Goodwin MN Jr, Black HC Jr, et al. Polypoid adenocarcinoma of the cervical esophagus. Arch Pathol Lab Med 1060;88:367–370.

58. Ming SC. Adenocarcinoma and other epithelial tumors of the esophagus. In: Ming SC, Goldman H, eds. Pathology of the gastrointestinal tract. Philadelphia: WB Saunders, 1992:459–477.

59. Moghissi K, Sharpe DA, Pender D. Adenocarcinoma and Barrett's oesophagus. A clinico-pathological study. Eur J Cardiothorac Surg 1993;7:126–131.

60. Lerut T, Coosemans W, Van Raemdonck D, et al. Surgical treatment of Barrett's carcinoma. Correlations between morphologic findings and prognosis. J Thorac Cardiovasc Surg 1994;107:1059–1065.

61. Menke-Pluymers MB, Schoute NW, Mulder AH, et al. Outcome of surgical treatment of adenocarcinoma in Barrett's oesophagus. Gut 1992;33:1454–1458.

62. Williamson WA, Ellis FH Jr, Gibb SP, et al. Barrett's esophagus. Prevalence and incidence of adenocarcinoma. Arch Intern Med 1991;151:2212–2216.

63. Bartlesman JF, Hameeteman W, Tytgat GN. Barrett's oesophagus. Eur J Cancer Prev 1992;1:323–325.

64. Cameron AJ, Ott BJ, Payne WS. The incidence of adenocarcinoma in columnar-lined (Barrett's) esophagus. N Engl J Med 1985;313:857–859.

65. Van der Veen AH, Dees J, Blackensteijn JD, et al. Adenocarcinoma in Barrett's oesophagus: An overrated risk. Gut 1989;30:14–18.

66. Ovaska J, Miettinen M, Kivilaakso E. Adenocarcinoma arising in Barrett's esophagus. Dig Dis Sci 1989;34:1336–1339.

67. Atkinson M, Iftikhar SY, James PD, et al. The early diagnosis of oesophageal adenocarcinoma by endoscopic screening. Eur J Cancer Prev 1992;1:327–330.

68. Tytgat GN, Hameeteman W. The neoplastic potential of columnar-lined (Barrett's) esophagus. World J Surg 1992;16:308–312.

69. Launoy G, Faivre J, Pienkowski P, et al. Changing pattern of oesophageal cancer incidence in France. Int J Epidemiol 1994;23:246–251.

70. Wang JH, Hsu CP, Chen CY, et al. Primary adenocarcinoma of the esophagus. Kaohsiung J Med Sci 1991;7:363–368.

71. Lin YK, Wang LS, Fahn HJ, et al. Primary uncommon malignant tumors of the esophagus: An analysis of 30 cases. Chung Hua I Hsueh Tsa Chih (Taipei) 1995;55:463–471.

72. Iizuka T, Kato H, Watanabe H. One-hundred-and-two 5-year survivors of esophageal carcinoma after resective surgery. Jpn J Clin Oncol 1985;15:369–375.

73. Smith RRL, Hamilton SR, Boitnott JK, et al. The spectrum of carcinoma arising in Barrett's esophagus. A clinicopathologic study of 26 patients. Am J Surg Pathol 1984;8:563–573.

74. Rogers EL, Goldkind S, Iseri OA, et al. Adenocarcinoma of the lower esophagus: a disease primarily of white men with Barrett's esophagus. J Clin Gastroenterol 1986;8:613-618.

75. Paraf F, Flejou JF, Pignon JP, et al. Surgical pathology of adenocarcinoma arising in Barrett's esophagus. Analysis of 67 cases. Am J Surg Pathol 1995;19:183–191.

76. Hassall E, Dimmick JE, Magee JF. Adenocarcinoma in childhood Barrett's esophagus: Case documentation and the need for surveillance in children. Am J Gastroenterol 1993;88:282–288.

77. Skinner DB, Walther BC, Riddell RH, et al. Barrett's esophagus. Comparison of benign and malignant cases. Ann Surg 1983;198:554–566.

78. McDonald ML, Trastek VF, Allen MS, et al. Barrett's esophagus: Does an antireflux procedure reduce the need for endoscopic surveillance?. J Thorac Cardiovasc Surg 1996;111:1135–1138.

79. Sampliner RE, Fass R. Partial regression of Barrett's esophagus—an inadequate endpoint. Am J Gastroenterol 1993:88:2092–2094.

80. Hamilton SR, Hutcheon DF, Ravich WJ, et al. Adenocarcinoma in Barrett's esophagus after elimination of gastroesophageal reflux. Gastroenterology 1984;86:356–360.

81. Kauer WK, Burdiles P, Ireland AP, et al. Does duodenal reflux into the esophagus of patients with complicated GERD? Evaluation of a fiberoptic sensor for bilirubin. Am J Surg 1995;169:98–103.

82. Pera M, Trastek VF, Carpenter HA, et al. Influence of pancreatic and biliary reflux on the development of esophageal carcinoma. Ann Thorac Surg 1993:55:1386–1393.

83. Vaughan TL, Davis S, Kristal A, et al. Obesity, alcohol, and tobacco as risk factors for cancers of the esophagus and gastric cardia: Adenocarcinoma versus squamous cell carcinoma. Cancer Epidemiol Biomarkers Prev 1995;4:85–92.

84. Brown LM, Silverman DT, Pottern LM, et al. Adenocarcinoma of the esophagus and esophagogastric junction in white men in the United States: Alcohol, tobacco, and socioeconomic factors. Cancer Causes Control 1994;5:333–340.

85. Gray MR, Donnelly RJ, Kingsnorth AN. The role of smoking and alcohol in metaplasia and cancer risk in Barrett's columnar lined oesophagus. Gut 1993;34:727–731.

86. Levi F, Ollyo JB, La Vecchia C, et al. The consumption of tobacco, alcohol and the risk of adenocarcinoma in Barrett's oesophagus. Int J Cancer 1990;45:852–854.

87. Brown LM, Swanson CA, Gridley G, et al. Adenocarcinoma of the esophagus: Role of obesity and diet. J Natl Cancer Inst 1995;87:104–109.

88. Clark GW, Smyrk TC, Mirvish SS, et al. Effect of gastroduodenal juice and dietary fat on the development of Barrett's esophagus and esophageal neoplasia: An experimental rat model. Ann Surg Oncol 1994;1:252–261.

89. Jochem VJ, Fuerst PA, Fromkes JJ. Familial Barrett's esophagus associated with adenocarcinoma. Gastroenterology 1992;102:1400–1402.

90. Eng C, Spechler SJ, Ruben R, et al. Familial Barrett esophagus and adenocarcinoma of the gastroesophageal junction. Cancer Epidemiol Biomarkers Prev 1993;2:397–399.

91. Fahmy N, King JF. Barrett's esophagus: An acquired condition with genetic predisposition. Am J Gastroenterol 1993;88:1262–1265.

92. Feczko PJ, Ma CK, Halpert RD, et al. Barrett's metaplasia and dysplasia in postmyotomy achalasia patients. Am J Gastroenterol 1983;78:265–268.

93. Goodman P, Scott LD, Verani RR, et al. Esophageal adenocarcinoma in a patient with surgically treated achalasia. Dig Dis Sci 1990;35:1549–1552.

94. Recht MP, Levine MS, Katzka DA, et al. Barrett's esophagus in scleroderma: Increased prevalence and radiographic findings. Gastrointest Radiol 1988;13:1–5.

95. Segel MC, Campbell WL, Medsger TA Jr, et al. Systemic sclerosis (scleroderma) and esophageal adenocarcinoma: Is increased patient screening necessary? Gastroenterology 1985;89:485–488.

96. Katzka DA, Reynolds JC, Saul SH, et al. Barrett's metaplasia and adenocarcinoma of the esophagus in scleroderma. Am J Med 1987;82:46–52.

97. Strader DB, Benjamin SB, Orbuch M, et al. Esophageal function and occurrence of Barrett's esophagus in Zollinger-Ellison syndrome. Digestion 1995;56:347–356.

98. Symonds DA, Ramsey HE. Adenocarcinoma arising in Barrett's esophagus with Zollinger-Ellison syndrome. Am J Clin Pathol 1980;73:823–826.

99. Paraf F, Sasseville D, Watters AK, et al. Clinicopathologic relevance of the association between gastrointestinal and sebaceous neoplasms: The Muir-Torre syndrome. Hum Pathol 1995;26:422–427.

100. Ramson JM, Patel GK, Clift SA, et al. Extended and limited types of Barrett's esophagus in the adult. Ann Thorac Surg 1982;33:19–27.

101. Menke-Pluymers MB, Hop WC, Dees J, et al. Risk factors for the development of an adenocarcinoma in columnar-lined (Barrett) esophagus. The Rotterdam Esophageal Tumor Study Group. Cancer 1993;72:1155–1158.

102. Ming SC. Tumors of the esophagus and stomach. Supplement, fascicle 7, second series. Atlas of tumor pathology. Washington, DC: Armed Forces Institute of Pathology, 1985;S9–S17.

103. Rosenberg JC, Budev H, Edwards RC, et al. Analysis of adenocarcinoma in Barrett's esophagus utilizing a staging system. Cancer 1985;55:1353–1360.

104. Lee RG. Dysplasia in Barrett's esophagus. A clinicopathologic study of six patients. Am J Surg Pathol 1985;9:845–852.

105. Reid BJ, Weinstein WM, Lewin K, et al. Endoscopic biopsy can detect high-grade dysplasia or early adenocarcinoma in Barrett's esophagus without grossly recognizable lesions. Gastroenterology 1988;94:81–90.

106. Dent J. Approaches to oesophageal columnar metaplasia (Barrett's oesophagus). Scand J Gastroenterol Suppl 1989;168:60–66.

107. Edwards MJ, Gable DR, Lentsch AB, et al. The rationale for esophagectomy as the optimal therapy for Barrett's esophagus with high-grade dysplasia. Ann Surg 1996;223:585–589.

108. Heitmiller RF, Redmond M, Hamilton SR. Barrett's esophagus with high-grade dysplasia. An indication for prophylactic esophagectomy. Ann Surg 1996;224:66–71.

109. Levine DS, Reid BJ, Haggitt RC, et al. Correlation of ultrastructural aberrations with dysplasia and flow cytometric abnormalities in Barrett's epithelium. Gastroenterology 1989;96:355–367.

110. Reid BJ, Haggitt RC, Rubin CE, et al. Observer variation in the diagnosis of dysplasia in Barrett's esophagus. Hum Pathol 1988;19:166–178.

111. Jankowski J, McMenemin R, Yu C, et al. Proliferating cell nuclear antigen in oesophageal diseases; correlation with transforming growth factor alpha expression. Gut 1992;33:587–591.

112. Hong MK, Laskin WB, Herman BE, et al. Expansion of the Ki-67 proliferative compartment correlates with degree of dysplasia in Barrett's esophagus. Cancer 1995;75:423–429.

113. Reid BJ, Sanchez CA, Blount PL, et al. Barrett's esophagus: Cell cycle abnormalities in advancing stages of neoplastic progression. Gastroenterology 1993;105:119–129.

114. Robaszkiewicz M, Hardy E, Volant A, et al. Analyse du contenu cellulaire en ADN par cytometrie en flux dans les endobrachyoesophages. Etude de 66 cas. Gastroenterol Clin Biol 1991;15:703–710.

115. Reid BJ, Haggitt RC, Rubin CE. Barrett's esophagus: Correlation between flow cytometry and histology in detection of patients at risk for adenocarcinoma. Gastroenterology 1987;93:1–11.

116. James PD, Atkinson M. Value of DNA image cytometry in the prediction of malignant change in Barrett's oesophagus. Gut 1989;30:899–905.

117. Reid BJ. Barrett's esophagus and esophageal adenocarcinoma. Gastroenterol Clin North Am 1991;20:817–834.

118. Reid BJ, Blount PL, Rubin CE, et al. Flow-cytometry and histological progression to malignancy in Barrett's esophagus: Prospective endoscopic surveillance of cohort. Gastroenterology 1992;102:1212–1219.

119. Raskind WH, Norwood T, Levine DS, et al. Persistent clonal areas and clonal expansion in Barrett's esophagus. Cancer Res 1992;52:2946–2950.

120. Younes M, Lebovitz RM, Lechago LV, et al. p53 protein accumulation in Barrett's metaplasia, dysplasia, and carcinoma: A follow-up study. Gastroenterology 1993;105:1637–1642.

121. Rice TW, Goldblum JR, Falk GW, et al. p53 immunoreactivity in Barrett's metaplasia, dysplasia, and carcinoma. J Thorac Cardiovasc Surg 1994;108:1132–1137.

122. Ramel S, Reid BJ, Sanchez CA, et al. Evaluation of p53 protein expression in Barrett's esophagus by two-parameter flow cytometry. Gastroenterology 1992;102:1220–1228.

123. Gleeson CM, Sloan JM, McGuigan JA, et al. Base transitions at CpG dinucleotides in the p53 gene are common in esophageal adenocarcinoma. Cancer Res 1995;55:3406–3411.

124. Schneider PM, Casson AG, Levin B, et al. Mutations of p53 in Barrett's esophagus and Barrett's cancer: A prospective study of ninety-eight cases. J Thorac Cardiovasc Surg 1996;111:331–333.

125. Sorsdahl K, Casson AG, Troster M, et al. p53 and ras gene expression in human esophageal cancer and Barrett's epithelium: A prospective study. Cancer Detect Prev 1994;18:179–185.

126. Blount PL, Galipeau PC, Sanchez CA, et al. 17p allelic losses in diploid cells of patients with Barrett's esophagus who develop aneuploidy. Cancer Res 1994;54:2292–2295.

127. Hamilton S, Smith R, Cameron J, et al. Prevalence and characteristics of Barrett's esophagus in patients with adenocarcinoma of the esophagus or the esophagogastric junction. Hum Pathol 1988;19:942–948.

128. Miros M, Kerlin P, Walker N. Only patients with dysplasia progress to adenocarcinoma in Barrett's oesophagus. Gut 1991;32:1441–1446.

129. Rice TW, Falk GW, Achkar E, et al. Surgical management of high-grade dysplasia in Barrett's esophagus. Am J Gastroenterol 1993;88:1832–1836.

130. Levine DS, Haggitt RC, Blount PL, et al. An endoscopic biopsy protocol can differentiate high-grade dysplasia from early adenocarcinoma in Barrett's esophagus. Gastroenterology 1993;105:40–50.

131. Rusch VW, Levine DS, Haggitt R, et al. The management of high grade dysplasia and early cancer in Barrett's esophagus. A multidisciplinary problem. Cancer 1994;74:1225–1229.

132. McArdle JE, Lewin KJ, Randall G, et al. Distribution of dysplasias and early invasive carcinoma in Barrett's esophagus. Hum Pathol 1992;23:479–482.

133. Provenzale D, Kemp JA, Arora S, et al. A guide for surveillance of patients with Barrett's esophagus. Am J Gastroenterol 1994;89:670–680.

134. Peters JH, Clark GW, Ireland AP, et al. Outcome of adenocarcinoma arising in Barrett's esophagus in endoscopically surveyed and non-surveyed patients. J Thorac Cardiovasc Surg 1994;108:813–821.

135. Stillman AE, Selwyn JI. Primary adenocarcinoma of the esophagus arising in a columnar lined esophagus. Am J Digest Dis 1975;20:577–582.

136. Paraf F, Flejou JF, Potet F, et al. Adenomasarising in Barrett's esophagus with adenocarcinoma. Report of three cases. Pathol Res Pract 1992;188:1028–1032.

137. Wong RS, Temes RT, Follis FM, et al. Multiple polyposis and adenocarcinoma arising in Barrett's esophagus. Ann Thorac Surg 1996;61:216–218.

138. McDonald GB, Brand DL, Thorning DR. Multiple adenomatous neoplasms arising in columnar-lined (Barrett's) esophagus. Gastroenterology 1977;72:1317–1321.

139. Pera M, Cardesa A, Bombi JA, et al. The influence of esophagojejunostomy on the induction of adenocarcinoma of the distal esophagus in Sprague-Dawley rats by subcutaneous injection of 2,6-dimethylnitrosomorphine. Cancer Res 1989;49:6803–6808.

140. Levine MS, Caroline D, Thompson JJ, et al. Adenocarcinoma of the esophagus: Relationship to Barrett mucosa. Radiology 1984;150:305–309.

141. Jernstrom P, Brewer LA III. Primary adenocarcinoma of the mid-esophagus arising in ectopic gastric mucosa with associated hiatal hernia and reflux esophagitis (Dawson's syndrome). Cancer 1970;26:1343–1348.

142. Moghissi K, Papiri N. A clinico-pathological study of the origin of adeno-carcinoma of the mid-thoracic oesophagus and results of surgical resection. Chirurgie 1992;118:298–303.

143. Christensen WN, Sternberg SS. Adenocarcinoma of the upper esophagus arising in ectopic gastric mucosa. Two case reports and review of the literature. Am J Surg Pathol 1987;11:397–402.

144. Ishii K, Ota H, Nakayama J, et al. Adenocarcinoma of the cervical oesophagus arising from ectopic gastric mucosa. The histochemical determination of its origin. Virchows Arch [A] Pathol Anat Hispathol 1991;419:159–164.

145. Levine MS, Dillon EC, Saul SH, et al. Early esophageal cancer. AJR Am J Roentgenol 1986;146:507–512.

146. Witt TR, Bains MS, Zaman MB. Adenocarcinoma in Barrett's esophagus. J Thorac Cardiovasc Surg 1983;85:337–345.

147. Chejfec G, Jablokow VR, Gould VE. Linitis plastica carcinoma of the esophagus. Cancer 1981;51:2139–2143.

148. Ming SC, Bullough PG. Coexisting adenocarcinomas of the esophagus and of the esophagogastric junction. Am J Dig Dis 1963;8:439–443.

149. Naunheim KS, Petruska PJ, Roy TS, et al. Multimodality therapy for adenocarcinoma of the esophagus. Ann Thorac Surg 1995;59:1085–1090.

150. Sarbia M, Borchard F, Hengels KJ. Histogenetical investigations on adenocarcinomas of the esophagogastric junction. An immuno-histochemical study. Pathol Res Pract 1993;189:530–535.

151. Banner BF, Memoli VA, Warren WH, et al. Carcinoma with multi-directional differentiation arising in Barrett's esophagus. Ultrastruct Pathol 1983;4:205–217.

152. Motoyama T, Higuchi M, Taguchi J. Combined choriocarcinoma, hepatoid adenocarcinoma, small cell carcinoma and tubular adenocarcinoma in the oesophagus. Virchows Arch 1995;427:451–454.

153. Lauren P. The two histological main types of gastric carcinoma: Diffuse and so-called intestinal type carcinoma. Acta Pathol Microbiol Scand 1965;64:31–49.

154. Paraf F, Flejou JF, Potet F, et al. Esophageal squamous carcinoma in five patients with Barrett's esophagus. Am J Gastroenterol 1992;87:746–750.

155. Resano CH, Cabrera N, Gonzalez-Cueto D, et al. Double early epidermoid carcinoma of the esophagus in columnar epithelium. Endoscopy 1985;17:73–75.

156. Cary NR, Barron DJ, McGoldrick JP, et al. Combined oesophageal adenocarcinoma and carcinoid in Barrett's oesophagitis: Potential role of enterochromaffin-like cells in oesophageal malignancy. Thorax 1993;48:404–405.

157. Pascal RR, Clearfield HR. Mucoepidermoid (adenosquamous) carcinoma arising in Barrett's esophagus. Dig Dis Sci 1987; 32:428–432.

158. Allan NK, Weitzner S, Scott L, et al. Adenocarcinoma arising in Barrett's esophagus with synchronous squamous cell carcinoma of the esophagus. South Med J 1986;79:1036–1039.

159. Sheahan DG, Berman MA. Barrett's mucosa with multiple carcinomas of the esophagus and oral cavity. J Clin Gastroenterol 1986;8:103–107.

160. Rabinovitch PS, Reid BJ, Haggitt RC, et al. Progression to cancer in Barrett's esophagus is associated with genomic instability. Lab Invest 1988;60:65–71.

161. Nakamura T, Nekarda H, Hoelscher AH, et al. Prognostic value of DNA ploidy and c-erbB-2 oncoprotein overexpression in adenocarcinoma of Barrett's esophagus. Cancer 1994;73:1785–1794.

162. Krishnadath KK, Tilanus HW, van Blankenstein M, et al. Accumulation of genetic abnormalities during neoplastic progression in Barrett's esophagus. Cancer Res 1995;55:1971–1976.

163. Khan M, Bui HX, del Rosario A, et al. Role of DNA content determination by image analysis in confirmation of dysplasia in Barrett's esophagus. Mod Pathol 1994;7:169–174.

164. Rodriguez E, Rao PH, Ladanyi M, et al. 11p13-15 is a specific region of chromosomal rearrangement in gastric and esophageal adenocarcinomas. Cancer Res 1990;50:6410–6416.

165. Garewal HS, Sampliner R, Liu Y, et al. Chromosomal rearrangements in Barrett's esophagus: A premalignant lesion of esophageal adenocarcinoma. Cancer Genet Cytogenet 1989;42:281–296.

166. Rao PH, Mathew S, Lauwers G, et al. Interphase cytogenetics of gastric and esophageal adenocarcinomas. Diagn Mol Pathol 1993;2:264–268.

167. Hunter S, Gramlich T, Abbott K, et al. Y chromosome loss in esophageal carcinoma: An in situ hybridization study. Genes Chromosom Cancer 1993;8:172–177.

168. Symmans PJ, Linehan JM, Brito MJ, et al. p53 expression in Barrett's oesophagus, dysplasia, and adenocarcinoma using antibody DO-7. J Pathol 1994;173:221–226.

169. Hardwick RH, Shepherd NA, Moorghen M, et al. Adenocarcinoma arising in Barrett's oesophagus: Evidence for the participation of p53 dysfunction in the dysplasia/carcinoma sequence. Gut 1994;35:764–768.

170. Duhaylongsod FG, Gottfried MR, Iglehart JD, et al. The significance of c-erbB-2 and p53 immunoreactivity in patients with adenocarcinoma of the esophagus. Ann Surg 1995;221:677–683.

171. Casson AG, Mukhopadhyay T, Clearv KR, et al. p53 gene mutations in Barrett's epithelium and esophageal cancer. Cancer Res 1991;51:4495–4499.

172. Barrett MT, Galipeau PC, Sanchez CA, et al. Determination of the frequency of loss of heterozygosity in esophageal adenocarcinoma by cell sorting, whole genome amplification and microsatellite polymorphisms. Oncogene 1996;12:1873–1878.

173. Swift A, Risk JM, Kingsnorth AN, et al. Frequent loss of heterozygosity on chromosome 17 at 17q11.2-q12 in Barrett's adenocarcinoma. Br J Cancer 1995;71:995–998.

174. al-Kasspooles M, Moore JH, Orringer MB, et al. Amplification and over-expression of the EGFR and erbB-2 genes in human esophageal adenocarcinomas. Int J Cancer 1993;54:213–219.

175. Goldblum JR, Rice TW. bcl-2 protein expression in the Barrett's metaplasia-dysplasia-carcinoma sequence. Mod Pathol 195;8:866–869.

176. Meltzer SJ, Yin J, Manin B, et al. Microsatellite instability occurs frequently and in both diploid and aneuploid cell populations of

Barrett's-associated esophageal adenocarcinomas. Cancer Res 1994; 54:3379–3382.

177. Gleeson CM, Sloan JM, McGuigan JA, et al. Ubiquitous somatic alterations at microsatellite alleles occur infrequently in Barrett's-associated esophageal adenocarcinoma. Cancer Res 1996;56: 259–263.

178. Brito MJ, Filipe MI, Linehan J, et al. Association of transforming growth factor alpha (TGFA) and its precursors with malignant change in Barrett's epithelium: Biological and clinical variables. Int J Cancer 1995;60:27–32.

179. Jankowski J, Hopwood D, Wormsley KG. Flow-cytometric analysis of growth-regulatory peptides and their receptors in Barrett's oesophagus and oesophageal adenocarcinoma. Scand J Gastroenterol 1992; 27:147–154.

180. Webb JN, Busuttil A. Adenocarcinoma of the esophagus and of the esophagogastric junction. Br J Surg 1978;65:475–479.

181. Ming SC. Tumors of the esophagus and stomach, second series. Washington, DC: Armed Forces Institute of Pathology, 1973:44–57.

182. Potet F, Flejou JF, Gervaz H, et al. Adenocarcinoma of the lower esophagus and the esophagogastric junction. Semin Diagn Pathol 1991;8:126–136.

183. Wang HH, Antoniolli DA, Goldman H. Comparative features of esophageal and gastric adenocarcinoma: Recent changes in type and frequency. Hum Pathol 1986;17:482–487.

184. Kalish RJ, Clancy PE, Orringer MB, et al. Clinical, epidemiologic, and morphologic comparison between adenocarcinoma arising in Barrett's esophageal mucosa and in the gastric cardia. Gastroenterology 1984;86:461–467.

185. Morstyn G, Thomas RJ, Ma J, et al. Similarity between adenocarcinoma (AC) arising in Barrett's esophagus (BE) and AC arising at the cardioesophageal junction (CEJ). Proc Annu Meet Am Assoc Cancer Res 1985;26:147.

186. Duhaylongsod FG, Wolfe WG. Barrett's esophagus and adenocarcinoma of the esophagus and gastroesophageal junction. J Thorac Cardiovas Surg 1991;102:36–41.

187. Cameron AJ, Lomboy CT, Pera M, et al. Adenocarcinoma of the esophagogastric junction and Barrett's esophagus. Gastroenterology 1995;109:1541–1546.

188. Clark GW, Peters JH, Ireland AP, et al. Nodal metastasis and sites of recurrence after en bloc esophagectomy for adenocarcinoma. Ann Thorac Surg 1994;58:646–653.

189. van Overhagen H, Lameris JS, Berger MY, et al. Supraclavicular lymph node metastases in carcinoma of the esophagus and gastroesophageal junction: Assessment with CT, US, and US-guided fine-needle aspiration biopsy. Radiology 1991;179:155–158.

190. Aikou T, Shimazu H, Takao T, et al. Significance of lymph nodal metastases in treatment of esophagogastric adenocarcinoma. Lymphology 1992;25:31–36.

191. Oliver SE, Robertson CS, Logan RF. Oesophageal cancer: A population-based study of survival after treatment. Br J Surg 1992; 79:1321–1325.

192. Lieberman MD, Shriver CD, Bleckner S, et al. Carcinoma of the esophagus. Prognostic significance of histologic type. J Thorac Cardiovasc Surg 1995;109:130–138.

193. Mangla JC. Barrett's esophagus: An old entity rediscovered. J Clin Gastroenterol 1981;3:347–356.

194. Sanfey H, Hamilton SR, Smith RR, et al. Carcinoma arising in Barrett's esophagus. Surg Gynecol Obstet 1985;161:570–574.

195. Schneeberger AL, Finley RJ, Troster M, et al. The prognostic significance of tumor ploidy and pathology in adenocarcinoma of the esophagogastric junction. Cancer 1990;65:1206–1210.

196. Sauter ER, Keller SM, Erner SM. p53 correlates with improved survival in patients with esophageal adenocarcinoma. J Surg Oncol 1995;58:269–273.

197. Sjogren RW, Johnson LF, Barrett's esophagus: A review. Am J Med 1983;74:313–321.

198. Harle IA, Finley RJ, Belsheim M, et al. Management of adenocarcinoma in a columnar lined esophagus. Ann Thorac Surg 1985;40: 330–335.

199. Skinner DB. The columnar lined esophagus and adenocarcinoma. Ann Thorac Surg 1985;40:321–322.

200. Sarr MG, Hamilton SR, Marrone GC, et al. Barrett's esophagus: Its prevalence and association with adenocarcinoma in patients with symptoms of gastroesophageal reflux. Am J Surg 1985;149: 187–193.

201. van Overhagen H, Lameris JS, Berger MY, et al. Assessment of distant metastases with ultrasound-guided fine-needle aspiration biopsy and cytologic study in carcinoma of the esophagus and gastroesophageal junction. Gastrointest Radiol 1992;17:305–310.

202. Spechler SJ, Robbins AH, Rubins HB, et al. Adenocarcinoma in Barrett's esophagus. An overrated risk? Gastroenterology 1984;87: 927–933.

203. Ming SC. Tumors of the esophagus and stomach, second series. Washington, DC: Armed Forces Institute of Pathology, 1973:23–43.

204. Tauchi K, Kakudo K, Machimura T, et al. Superficial esophageal carcinoma. With special reference to basaloid features. Pathol Res Pract 1990;186:450–454.

205. Kuwano H, Ueo H, Sugimachi K, et al. Glandular or mucus secreting components in squamous cell carcinoma of the esophagus. Cancer 1985;56:514–518.

206. Orsatti G, Corvalan AH, Sakurai H, et al. Polypoid adenosquamous carcinoma of the esophagus with prominent spindle cells. Report of a case with immunohistochemical and ultrastructural studies. Arch Pathol Lab Med 1993;117:544–547.

207. Fegelman E, Law SY, Fok M, et al. Squamous cell carcinoma of the esophagus with mucin-secreting component. Mucoepidermoid carcinoma. J Thorac Cardiovasc Surg 1994;107:62–67.

208. Kuwano H, Sugimachi K, Morita M, et al. A consideration of the definition of early esophageal cancer on the basis of clinicopathologic viewpoint (Japanese). J Jpn Surg Soc 1991; 92:276–280.

209. Cerar A, Jutersek A, Vidmar S. Adenoid cystic carcinoma of the esophagus. A clinicopathologic study of three cases. Cancer 1991; 67:2159–2164.

210. Mafune K, Takubo K, Tanaka Y, et al. Sclerosing mucoepidermoid carcinoma of the esophagus with intraepithelial carcinoma or dysplastic epithelium. J Surg Oncol 1995;58:184–190.

211. Bell Thomson J, Haggitt RC, Ellis FH Jr. Mucoepidermoid and adenoid cystic carcinomas of the esophagus. J Thorac Cardiovasc Surg 1979;79:438–446.

212. Blaauwgeers JL, Allema JH, Bosma A, et al. Early adenoid cystic carcinoma of the upper esophagus. Eur J Surg Oncol 1990;16:77–81.

213. Pascal RR, Clearfield HR. Mucoepidermoid (adenosquamous) carcinoma arising in Barrett's esophagus. Dig Dis Sci 1987,32:428–432.

214. Woodard BH, Shelburne JD, Vollmer RT, et al. Mucoepidermoid carcinoma of the esophagus: A case report. Hum Pathol 1978;9: 352–354.

215. Sasajima K, Watanabe M, Takubo K, et al. Mucoepidermoid carcinoma of the esophagus: Report of two cases and review of the literature. Endoscopy 1990,22:140 143.

216. Sweeney EC, Cooney T. Adenoid cystic carcinoma of the esophagus: A light and electron microscopic study. Cancer 1980;45:1516–1525.

217. Petursson SR. Adenoid cystic carcinoma of the esophagus. Complete response to combination chemotherapy. Cancer 1986;57: 1464–1467.

218. Epstein JI, Sears DL, Tucker RS, et al. Carcinoma of the esophagus with adenoid cystic differentiation. Cancer 1984;53:1131–1136.

219. Mori M, Mimori K, Sadanaga N, et al. Polypoid carcinoma of the esophagus. Jpn J Cancer Res 1994;85:1131–1136.

220. Kim JH, Lee MS, Cho SW, et al. Primary adenoid cystic carcinoma of the esophagus: A case report. Endoscopy 1991;23:38–41.

221. Chong FK, Graham JH, Madoff IM. Mucin-producing carcinoid ("composite tumor") of upper third of esophagus: A variant of carcinoid tumor. Cancer 1979;44:1853–1859.

222. Tateishi R, Taniguchi K, Horai T, et al. Argyrophil cell carcinoma (apudoma) of the esophagus. A histopathologic entity. Virchows Arch [Pathol Anat] 1976;371:283–294.

223. Briggs JC, Ibrahim NBN. Oat cell carcinoma of the oesophagus: A clinico-pathological study of 23 cases. Histopathology 1983;7: 261–277.

224. Mori M, Matsukuma A, Adachi Y, et al. Small cell carcinoma of the esophagus. Cancer 1989;63:564–573.

225. Hoda SA, Hajdu SI. Small cell carcinoma of the esophagus. Cytology and immunohistology in four cases. Acta Cytol 1992;36:113–120.

226. Imura H, Matsukura S, Yamamoto H, et al. Studies on ectopic ACTH producing tumors. II. Clinical and biochemical features of 30 cases. Cancer 1975;35:1430–1437.

227. McKeown F. Oat cell carcinoma of the oesophagus. J Pathol 1952;64:889–891.

228. Proctor DD, Fraser JL, Mangano MM, et al. Small cell carcinoma of the esophagus in a patient with longstanding primary achalasia. Am J Gastroenterol 1992;87:664–667.

229. Doherty MA, McIntyre M, Arnott SJ. Oat cell carcinoma of esophagus: A report of six British patients with a review of the literature. Int J Radiat Oncol Biol Phy 1984;10:147–152.

230. Law SY, Fok M, Lam KY, et al. Small cell carcinoma of the esophagus. Cancer 1994;73:2894–2899.

231. Isolauri J, Mattila J, Kallioniemi OP. Primary undifferentiated small cell carcinoma of the esophagus: Clinicopathological and flow cytometric evaluation of eight cases. J Surg Oncol 1991;46:174–177.

232. Huncharek M, Muscat J. Small cell carcinoma of the esophagus. The Massachusetts General Hospital experience, 1978 to 1993. Chest 1995;107:179–181.

233. Ho KJ, Herrera GA, Jones JM, et al. Small cell carcinoma of the esophagus: Evidence for a unified histogenesis. Hum Pathol 1984;15:460–468.

234. Rosenthal SN, Lemkin JA. Multiple small cell carcinomas of the esophagus. Cancer 1983;51:1944–1946.

235. Liu YH. Clinicopathologic and immunohistochemical study on 22 cases of small cell carcinoma of the esophagus (Chinese). Chin Oncol J 1991;13:123–125.

236. Melo CR, Melo IS, Cerski CT. Small cell carcinoma of the esophagus. Clinicopathological and immunohistochemical findings in four cases. Arq Gastroenterol 1993;30:52–57.

237. Kishida H, Sodemoto Y, Ushigome S, et al. Non-oat cell small cell carcinoma of the esophagus. Report of a case with ultrastructural observation. Acta Pathol Jpn 1983;33:403–413.

238. Sato T, Mukai M, Ando N, et al. Small cell carcinoma (non-oat cell type) of the esophagus concomitant with invasive squamous cell carcinoma and carcinoma in situ. A case report. Cancer 1986;57:328–332.

239. Craig SR, Carey FA, Walker WS, et al. Primary small-cell cancer of the esophagus. J Thorac Cardiovasc Surg 1995;109:284–288.

240. Huncharek M, Muscat J. Small cell carcinoma of the esophagus. The Massachusetts General Hospital experience, 1978 to 1993. Chest 1995;107:179–181.

241. Chalkiadakis G, Wihlm JM, Morand G, et al. Primary malignant melanoma of the esophagus. Ann Thorac Surg 1985;39:472–475.

242. Stranks GJ, Mathai JT, Rowe-Jones DC. Primary malignant melanoma of the oesophagus: Case report and review of surgical pathology. Gut 1991;32:828–830.

243. Piccone VA, Klopstock R, LeVeen HH, et al. Primary malignant melanoma of the esophagus associated with melanosis of the entire esophagus. First case report. J Thorac Cardiovasc Surg 1970;59:864–870.

244. Mannell A, Hunter SJ, Hale MJ. Primary malignant melanoma of the oesophagus. Report of a case with flow cytometric DNA analysis. S Afr J Surg 1991;29:120–122.

245. Sabanathan S, Eng J, Pradhan GN. Primary malignant melanoma of the esophagus. Am J Gastroenterol 1989;84:1475–1481.

246. Prabhu SR, Puranik GV, Menezes W. Primary malignant melanoma of esophagus. Indian J Gastroenterol 1991;10:109–110.

247. Watanabe H, Yoshikawa N, Suzuki R, et al. Malignant amelanotic melanoma of the esophagus. Gastroenterol Jpn 1991;26:209–212.

248. Assor D, Santa Cruz D. Multifocal malignant melanoma of the esophagus. South Med J 1979;72:1009–1012.

249. Takubo K, Kanda Y, Ishii M, et al. Primary malignant melanoma of the esophagus. Hum Pathol 1983;14:727–730.

250. Isaacs JL, Quirke P. Two cases of primary malignant melanoma of the oesophagus. Clin Radiol 1988;39:455–457.

251. Nelson RS, Lanza C. Malignant melanoma metastatic to the upper gastrointestinal tract. Gastrointest Endosc 1978;24:156–158.

252. Basque GJ, Boline JE, Holyoke JB. Malignant melanoma of the esophagus: First reported case in a child. Am J Clin Pathol 1970;53:609–611.

253. Boulafendis D, Damiani M, Sie E, et al. Primary malignant melanoma of the esophagus in a young adult. Am J Gastroenterol 1985;80:417–420.

254. Trillo A, Accettullo LM, Yeiter TL. Choriocarcinoma of the esophagus: Histologic and cytologic findings. A case report. Acta Cytol 1979;23:69–74.

255. McKechnie JC, Fechner RE. Choriocarcinoma and adenocarcinoma of the esophagus with gonadotropin secretion. Cancer 1971;27:694–702.

256. Sasano N, Abe S, Satake O. Choriocarcinoma mimickry of an esophageal carcinoma with urinary gonadotropic activities. Tohoku J Exp Med 1970;100:153–163.

257. Kikuchi Y, Tsuneta Y, Kawai T, et al. Choriocarcinoma of the esophagus producing chorionic gonadotropin. Acta Pathol Jpn 1988;38:489–499.

258. Wasan HS, Schofield JB, Krausz T, et al. Combined choriocarcinoma and yolk sac tumor arising in Barrett's esophagus. Cancer 1994;73:514–517.

259. Nonomura A, Kimura A, Mizukami Y, et al. Paget's disease of the esophagus. J Clin Gastroenterol 1993;16:130–135.

260. Matsukuma S, Aida S, Shima S, et al. Paget's disease of the esophagus. A case report with review of the literature. Am J Surg Pathol 1995;19:948–955.

261. Norihisa Y, Kakudo K, Tsutsumi Y, et al. Paget's extension of esophageal carcinoma. Immunohistochemical and mucin histochemical evidence of Paget's cells in the esophageal mucosa. Acta Pathol Jpn 1988;38:651–658.

262. Yates DR, Koss LG. Paget's disease of the esophageal epithelium. Report of first case. Arch Pathol Lab Med 1968;86:447–452.

263. Abrams HL, Spiro R, Goldstein N. Metastases in carcinoma. Analysis of 1000 autopsied cases. Cancer 1950;3:74–85.

264. Antler AS, Ough, Y, Pitchumoni CS, et al. Gastrointestinal metastases from malignant tumors of the lungs. Cancer 1982;49:170–172.

265. Varanasi RV, Saltzman JR, Krims P, et al. Breast carcinoma metastatic to the esophagus: Clinicopathological and management features of four cases, and literature review. Am J Gastroenterol 1995;90:1495–1499.

266. Laforet EG, Kondi ES. Postmastectomy dysphagia. Am J Surg 1971;121:368–372.

267. Caputy GG, Donohue JH, Goellner JR, et al. Metastatic melanoma of the gastrointestinal tract. Results of surgical management. Arch Surg 1991;126:1353–1358.

268. Cooney BS, Levine MS, Schnall MD. Metastatic thyroid carcinoma presenting as an expansile intraluminal esophageal mass. Abdom Imaging 1995;20:20–22.

269. Oka T, Ayabe H, Kawahara K, et al. Esophagectomy for metastatic carcinoma of the esophagus from lung cancer. Cancer 1993;71:2958–2961.

270. Butler ML, Van Heertum RL, Teplick SK. Metastatic malignant melanoma of the esophagus: A case report. Gastroenterology 1975;69:1334–1337.

271. Wood CB, Wood RA. Metastatic malignant melanoma of the esophagus. Am J Dig Dis 1975;20:786–789.

272. Schmidt HW, Claggett OT, Harrison EG Jr. Benign tumors and cysts of the esophagus. J Thorac Cardiovasc Surg 1961;41:717–732.

273. Plachta A. Benign tumors of the esophagus. Review of literature and report of 99 cases. Am J Gastroenterol 1962;38:639–652.

274. Colina F, Solis JA, Munoz MT. Squamous papilloma of the esophagus. A report of three cases and review of the literature. Am J Gastroenterol 1980;74:410–414.

275. Fernandez-Rodriguez CM, Badia-Figuerola N, Ruiz del Arbol L, et al. Squamous papilloma of the esophagus: Report of six cases with long-term follow-up in four patients. Am J Gastroenterol 1986;81:1059–1062.

276. Odze R, Antonioli D, Shocket D, et al. Esophageal squamous papillomas. A clinicopathologic study of 38 lesions and analysis for human papillomavirus by the polymerase chain reaction. Am J Surg Pathol 1993;17:803–812.

277. Walker JH. Giant papilloma of the thoracic esophagus. AJR Am J Roentgenol 1978;131:519–520.

278. Frootko NJ, Rogers JH. Oesophageal papillomata in the child. J Laryngol Otol 1978;92:822–824.

279. Nuwayhid NS, Ballard ET, Cotton R. Esophageal papillomatosis: Case report. Ann Otol Rhinol Laryngol 1977;86:623–626.

280. Syrjanen K, Pyrhonen S, Aukee S, et al. Squamous cell papilloma of

the esophagus: A tumour probably caused by human papilloma virus (HPV). Diagn Histopathol 1982;5:291–296.

281. Chang F, Syrjanen S, Shen Q, et al. Screening for human papillomavirus infections in esophageal squamous cell carcinomas by in situ hybridization. Cancer 1993;72:2525–2530.

282. Takubo K, Esaki Y, Watanabe A, et al. Adenoma accompanied by superficial squamous cell carcinoma of the esophagus. Cancer 1993;71:2435–2438.

283. Rouse RV, Soetikno RM, Baker RJ, et al. Esophageal submucosal gland duct adenoma. Am J Surg Pathol 1995;19:1191–1199.

284. Ming SC. Tumors of the esophagus and stomach, second series, fascicle 7. Atlas of tumor pathology. Washington DC: Armed Forces Institute of Pathology. 1973;68.

285. Patel J, Kieffer RW, Martin M, et al. Giant fibrovascular polyp of the esophagus. Gastroenterology 1984;87:953–956.

286. Halfhide BC, Ginai AZ, Spoelstra HA, et al. Case report: A hamartoma presenting as a giant esophageal polyp. Br J Radiol 1995;68: 85–88.

287. Zonderland HM, Ginai AZ. Lipoma of the esophagus. Diagn Imag Clin Med 1984;53:265–268.

288. Eller JL, Ziter FMH, Zuck TF, et al. Inflammatory polyp: A complication in esophagus lined by columnar epithelium. Radiol 1971;98:145–146.

289. LiVolsi VA, Perzin KH. Inflammatory pseudotumors (inflammatory fibrous polyps) of the esophagus. A clinicopathologic study. Am J Dig Dis 1975;20:475–481.

290. Ming SC. Tumors of the esophagus and stomach, second series, fascicle 7. Atlas of tumor pathology. Washington DC: Armed Forces Institute of Pathology, 1973;19–22.

291. Akiyama S, Sakamoto M, Imaizumi M, et al. Esophageal cyst: A case report and review of the literature. Jpn J Surg 1980;10: 338–342.

PART IV

STOMACH

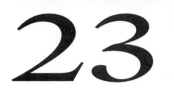

The focus of this chapter is on the inflammatory conditions that principally involve or are limited to the stomach. Gastritis that occurs in association with other disorders affecting the gut, as a primary or secondary event, is discussed in detail in other parts of the book, and so is mentioned only briefly in this chapter.

GENERAL ASPECTS

DEFINITIONS AND DISEASE LOCATION

Unless otherwise qualified, the term "gastritis" denotes an inflammatory lesion that primarily begins in the gastric mucosa. Cases of gastritis are further classified into acute and chronic forms based on

the temporal relations and clinical course (1). Acute gastritis is characterized by a sudden onset, a relatively uniform set of clinical and pathologic features, and a rapid resolution after elimination of the causative agent. In chronic gastritis, by contrast, the onset is often more insidious; the clinical course is typically protracted and occasioned by remissions and relapses; and, because cases of chronic gastritis include multiple entities, both the clinical and pathologic features are more variable (2–4). When a patient with chronic gastritis has a relapse or recurrence, there is acute inflammation in the mucosa in the form of a variable amount of necrosis and a neutrophilic reaction. It is preferable, however, to refer to this clinical picture as chronic active gastritis rather than acute gastritis.

A rough correlation exists between the cause of the gastritis and the primary or dominant location of the lesion in the stomach (5).

525

TABLE	
23.1	**Classification of Gastritis**[a]

Toxic chemicals and drugs
   Acute gastritis due to ethanol, aspirin, nonsteroidal anti-
      inflammatory drugs, and bile salts
   Postgastrectomy gastritis
   Corrosive gastritis
Infections
   Chronic antral gastritis due to Helicobacter
   Other infections
Immunologic injury
   Chronic fundic gastritis
   Allergic (eosinophilic) gastroenteritis
   Graft-versus-host disease
Radiation
Vascular diseases
   Stress gastritis and ulcer
   Gastric antral vascular ectasia
   Vasculitis
Motor and mechanical disorders
   Obstruction
   Diverticula and bezoars
   Gastric atrophy
Granulomatous conditions
   Crohn disease
   Foreign body reactions and infections
   Isolated granulomatous gastritis
   Rare—sarcoidosis, chronic granulomatous disease
Miscellaneous conditions
   Gastritis cystica profunda
   Lymphocytic gastritis
   Uremia
   Depositions

[a]Gastritis may be primary and limited to the stomach, associated with disease in other parts of the gut, or secondary to other conditions affecting the stomach.

Thus, gastritis that is due to toxic substances, such as ethanol and anti-inflammatory drugs, or to *Helicobacter pylori* infection is concentrated in the antral mucosa, whereas lesions that result from immunologic damage begin in the gastric corpus and fundus. With increased duration of disease, however, the two types of chronic gastritis may overlap in their locations. Many of the less common disorders, including infections, allergic gastritis, and the granulomatous diseases, show more major effects in the gastric antrum. Some conditions, such as antral gastritis and stress ulceration, frequently are associated with similar lesions in the proximal duodenal mucosa, probably related to the same etiologic factors and to hyperacidity affecting contiguous tissues.

CLASSIFICATION OF GASTRITIS

The preferred classification of gastritis is based mainly on its etiology and pathogenesis (Table 23.1). This listing encompasses cases in which the gastritis is the primary or sole lesion in the gut (such as the common forms of acute toxic gastritis and the various types of chronic gastritis) and those in which the gastric inflammation is often associated with lesions in other parts of the gut (e.g., allergic and infectious diseases) or occurs as a secondary event to mechanical and vascular conditions.

ACUTE TOXIC GASTRITIS

Acute gastritis is a self-limited condition that is typically confined to the antral region. It is characterized by a nonspecific acute inflammatory reaction in the mucosa with a variable degree of edema, hemorrhage, and erosions (6). Based on the presence of the latter features, such descriptive terms as "acute hemorrhagic gastritis" and "acute nonerosive versus erosive gastritis" have been applied, and these phrases relate mainly to the severity of the lesions rather than to the particular etiology (7). Because most cases of acute gastritis are attributable to the ingestion of toxic substances, such as ethanol and drugs, or to the reflux of bile salts, this condition has also been referred to as acute chemical or drug gastritis (8).

ETIOLOGY AND PATHOGENESIS

The majority of cases of acute gastritis are due to the intake of ethanol (9–11) and anti-inflammatory drugs, such as aspirin (12, 13) and nonsteroidal agents (8, 14–16). In patients lacking such a history, the injury likely results from the reflux of bile salts through an incompetent pyloric sphincter into the gastric antrum (17–20), although this circumstance is usually not documented in an individual patient. All of these substances are lipid soluble, and it is believed that they dissolve in the cytomembranes of the surface mucous cells in the antrum, damaging the mucosal barrier and facilitating the increased back-diffusion of hydrogen ions into the mucosa (21). Multiple factors are involved in the mucosal destruction, including direct damage to the surface layer of mucous cells, a reduction in the protective prostaglandins that are made in these cells (22), and a vasoconstrictive effect by the acid on the small vessels in the underlying lamina propria (see Chapter 11 for further details).

Similar mucosal lesions are seen in patients who develop stress ulceration (see Chapter 24). Although acute injury has been observed after the ingestion of *Helicobacter pylori* (23), no evidence exists as yet to incriminate this organism in the etiology of usual cases of acute gastritis. Rather, the bacterium is the major cause of chronic antral gastritis.

CLINICAL FEATURES

Patients with acute gastritis typically present with the abrupt onset of "burning" upper abdominal pain, nausea, and vomiting. The diagnosis is usually established on the basis of the clinical history (6). Overt hematemesis is noted in severe cases, and endoscopic examination is often performed to separate the erosive and nonerosive forms and to distinguish gastritis from other causes of upper tract hemorrhage, such as bleeding varices, a Mallory-Weiss tear, or a chronic peptic ulcer (24, 25). The lesion of acute gastritis is usually too superficial to be appreciated by radiographic study of the stomach.

The majority of patients respond promptly to the elimination of any toxic agents and to medications that reduce gastric acidity. Uncontrolled hemorrhage may require surgical resection or angiographic injection of vasoconstrictive substances. Most patients recover completely without sequelae, but acute gastritis can recur and it is possible that some cases of chronic antral gastritis develop after repeated exposure to toxic substances.

PATHOLOGY

Most information about acute gastritis has been obtained from endoscopic appearances and mucosal biopsy samples (4, 7, 11, 24–28), because tissue resection is rarely needed. At a macroscopic level, the milder cases show some combination of edema, erythema, scattered petechiae, and friability of the mucosal surface. The more dramatic examples reveal greater hemorrhage, ranging from multiple streaks to diffuse involvement of the mucosa, and the appearance of superficial erosions. Such cases have been termed "acute hemorrhagic gastritis" or "acute erosive gastritis." The lesions ordinarily are limited to the antrum, but they may extend into the lower part of the gastric corpus in severe cases. Patients in whom the gastritis is caused by ingestion of alcohol and drugs may have an associated duodenitis (see Chapter 30). An endoscopic study serves to identify the gastritis and/or duodenitis and to exclude a chronic peptic ulcer in these areas.

The histologic features of acute gastritis ordinarily are confined to the mucosal layer and are entirely nonspecific. The earliest lesions, established by investigative studies in animals and humans, reveal only edema, congestion, and patchy hemorrhages in the upper part of the lamina propria (27), and it is impossible to distinguish these features from the potential traumatic effects of the endoscopic procedure (Fig. 23.1). More certain features of acute toxic gastritis include regeneration and hyperplasia of the surface and foveolar (pit) mucous cells as well as the absence or only rare presence of neutrophils in the lamina propria (Fig. 23.2) (19, 28). Milder lesions are limited to the upper one third or one half of the mucosa and frequently are associated with focal dilation of the gastric pits. The underlying pyloric glands usually are not involved. In more extensive cases, greater hemorrhage and necrosis leads to the formation of patchy erosions, which represent superficial ulcers that

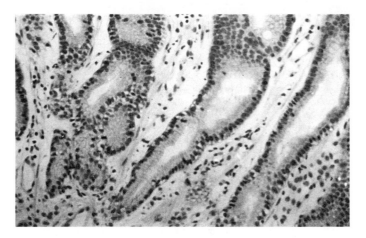

Figure 23.2 Gastric antral mucosal biopsy in a case of acute toxic gastritis. There is a prominent lengthening of the foveolae due to regeneration, with mitoses evident in the center, and no neutrophils (H & E, ×130).

are limited to the mucosal layer. Vascular congestion but no inflammation in the submucosa may be observed in severe cases. Small numbers of mononuclear inflammatory cells and occasional eosinophils are present in the lamina propria of the normal gastric antrum (29), especially in adults, and numbers of these cells are not conspicuously increased in cases of acute gastritis. Indeed, increased numbers of such cells should raise the possibilities of alternative etiologies or the presence of an underlying chronic gastritis.

The healing phase of acute gastritis is characterized by a reduction in the congestion and the transient elongation of the gastric pits, which contain scattered mitoses. Ultimately, the mucosal structure returns to normal in most cases. Following repeated attacks of acute gastritis, however, it is possible that some cases evolve into a chronic gastritis.

DIFFERENTIAL DIAGNOSIS

Because the morphologic features of acute toxic gastritis are relatively nonspecific, the diagnosis depends on the clinical history and the exclusion of a discrete ulcer or other inflammatory disorders (such as infections, allergic disease, and chronic active gastritis) that may affect the stomach. Localized ulcers, whether acute or chronic, can be discerned by endoscopic and radiographic examinations. Mucosal biopsy specimens are often obtained at the edge of the ulcers to exclude malignancy, and these samples reveal a prominent degree of mucosal inflammation in cases of chronic peptic ulcers. Conversely, only minimal or no inflammation is observed in the adjacent mucosa in most cases of acute drug-induced ulcer, such as those due to salicylates, and this information can help in suggesting the etiology of a gastric ulcer (30, 31). Patients with acute stress ulceration are usually much sicker than those with ordinary acute gastritis and frequently have multiple ulcers in the stomach and duodenum. This diagnosis is typically established by recognition of the underlying clinical condition that has precipitated the development of the stress lesions.

A greater inflammatory reaction is noted in most infectious lesions of the stomach, and their specific nature is suspected or revealed by the identification of the microorganisms or cellular

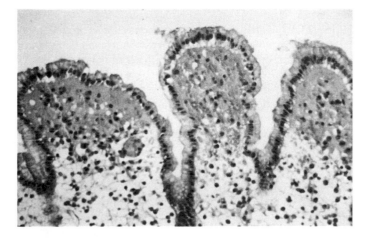

Figure 23.1 Gastric mucosal biopsy, showing fresh hemorrhages in the superficial part of the lamina propria. The surface and pit mucous cells are intact, and there is no neutrophilic reaction. Although such changes can be seen in the earliest phase of an acute toxic gastritis, they also can be the result of the endoscopic procedure alone (H & E, ×310).

inclusions of a granulomatous response. Antral involvement is common in allergic gastroenteritis, the associated lesion of which ordinarily is distinguished from acute toxic gastritis by noting the abundant eosinophilic reaction (see Chapter 12). Of further help, the peripheral blood eosinophil count is commonly elevated in cases of allergic disease, whereas it is normal in acute toxic gastritis.

CHRONIC GASTRITIS

TYPES OF CHRONIC GASTRITIS

In contrast to acute gastritis, chronic gastritis is characterized by a greater variation in etiology, the location of disease in the stomach, and the clinical features. The major types of chronic gastritis are listed in Table 23.2. The two most common forms are categorized according to their different causes and primary sites of injury into chronic fundic gastritis and chronic antral gastritis, which are identified, respectively, as type A and type B chronic gastritis (5). Other types of chronic gastritis relate to a particular pathogenesis, such as the gastritis that develops in patients that have undergone distal gastric resection and gastrojejunostomy, or to cases in which certain morphologic features are prominent, including multiple erosions (chronic erosive gastritis) or hypertrophy of the surface and foveolar area (chronic hypertrophic gastritis).

GENERAL PATHOLOGIC FEATURES

Independent of the particular type of chronic gastritis, many of the histologic alterations observed are similar. Differences relate mainly to the extent of pathologic change (Table 23.3).

TABLE 23.2	Major Types of Chronic Gastritis
	Chronic antral gastritis
	Chronic fundic gastritis
	Postgastrectomy gastritis
	Chronic erosive gastritis
	Chronic hypertrophic gastritis

TABLE 23.3	Histologic Features of Chronic Gastritis

Signs of chronic disease
  Increased mononuclear inflammatory cells and eosinophils in lamina propria, and presence of lymphoid nodules
  Loss of specialized glands
  Intestinal and pyloric gland metaplasia
  Variable hyperplasia of surface-foveolar mucous cells
  Early increase and late decrease of indigenous endocrine cells
Signs of active disease
  Epithelial cell degeneration and regeneration, with variable erosions
  Neutrophilic reaction in lamina propria and epithelial layer

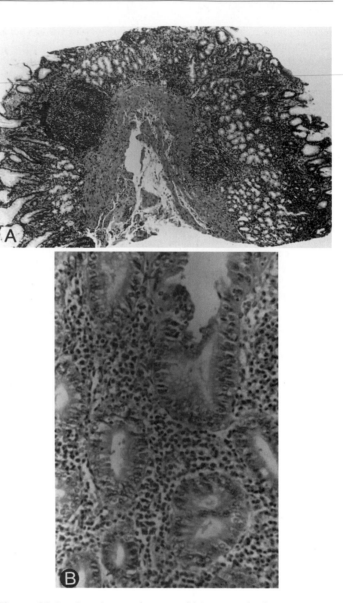

Figure 23.3   Gastric antral mucosal biopsy with chronic gastritis. **A.** There is a marked infiltrate of mononuclear inflammatory cells in the lamina propria, with lymphoid nodules adjacent to and extending into the muscularis mucosae (upper left). There is a variable loss of pyloric glands *(left and top)* (H & E, ×32). **B.** Noted are mononuclear inflammatory cells in the lamina propria, regeneration of the gastric pits, and focal infiltrates of mononuclear cells in the epithelial layer. Contrast with acute toxic gastritis in Figure 23.2 (H & E, ×100).

FEATURES OF CHRONIC DISEASE

Common features that signify the chronic nature of the lesion include increased numbers of mononuclear inflammatory cells (macrophages, lymphocytes, and plasma cells), and occasionally of eosinophils, in the lamina propria (Fig. 23.3); the appearance of lymphoid nodules, which are rare in the normal stomach; progressive destruction of the specialized glands that contain parietal and chief cells in the fundus and corpus or of the pyloric glands in the antrum, which causes thinning of the mucosal layer in the late stages of the disease; and intestinal metaplasia in all parts of the stomach and pyloric (also called pseudopyloric) metaplasia in place of the lost glands in the proximal part of the stomach (2–4, 32–36). More variable features noted in association with chronic gastritis are an increase in the indigenous endocrine cells and hyperplasia of the foveolar mucous cells. The latter feature may result in the formation of localized polyps or of diffuse hypertrophy of the mucosal surface. The lesion of chronic gastritis is confined to the mucosal layer; submucosal congestion may occur at the time of an active gastritis, but the rest of the gastric wall is unaffected.

The presence of pancreatic metaplasia in cases of chronic gastritis (37) has been described as microscopic foci of compact pancreatic acinar cells that blend with the other glands in the gastric mucosa (Fig. 23.4). Noted in all parts of the stomach as well as in the glandular area in cases of Barrett esophagus (38), the metaplasia differs from ectopic pancreas, which typically is a larger lesion, extending into the submucosa, and composed of ducts and fibrous tissue together with the acini.

FEATURES OF ACTIVE DISEASE

Active disease, often corresponding to a clinical relapse, can be superimposed on any type of chronic gastritis and is characterized by the presence of degeneration and regeneration of the epithelial cells and a neutrophilic reaction in the lamina propria and epithelial area (Fig. 23.5).

The surface is usually intact, but superficial erosions can appear in more severe cases and occasionally is the dominant feature (see subsequent discussion of chronic erosive gastritis). Active lesions always involve the surface and foveolar regions, and extend to the underlying mucosal glands in advanced cases. Depending on whether necrosis and acute inflammation are present or absent, cases can be categorized as chronic active gastritis or chronic inactive gastritis. It is best not to use the term "acute gastritis" in this setting to avoid any confusion with the separate clinical entity of acute toxic gastritis.

SPECIAL FEATURES AND TERMS

A variety of additional terms have been used to indicate the extent of the chronic gastritis in the mucosa, to portray special morphologic features, and to relate to the functional disturbances (Table 23.4). In the early stage of chronic gastritis, whether in the antrum or the corpus-fundus, the inflammation is limited to the surface and gastric pit region, and the underlying mucosal glands are either

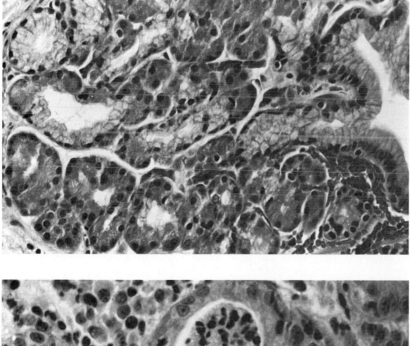

Figure 23.4 Pancreatic metaplasia in the gastric mucosa. A sheet of mature pancreatic acinar tissue with prominent zymogen granules is attached to the gastric pits (H & E, ×425). (Reproduced with permission from Goldman H. Gastrointestinal mucosal biopsy. New York: Churchill Livingstone, 1996; 95–159.)

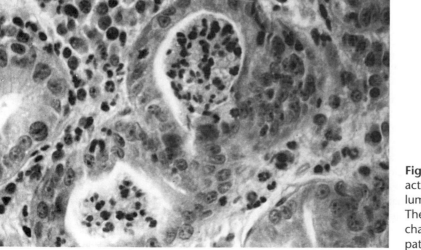

Figure 23.5 Gastric mucosal biopsy with chronic active gastritis. Many neutrophils are present in the lumen of the gastric pits and in the lamina propria. The epithelial nuclei show features of regeneration, characterized by enlargement, a stippled chromatin pattern, and prominent nucleoli (H & E, ×200).

TABLE		
23.4	**Stages of Chronic Gastritis**	

Category	Inflammation	Specialized Glands
Chronic superficial gastritis	Limited to foveolar region or upper gland area	Intact or mild decrease
Chronic atrophic gastritis	Involves full thickness of mucosa	Marked decrease to complete loss
Gastric atrophy	None or minimal	Complete loss

Pernicious anemia occurs in cases of chronic atrophic gastritis and gastric atrophy involving the corpus-fundic region.

intact or mildly affected; this lesion is referred to as chronic superficial gastritis (39). The mild lesion may persist or eventually extend, usually over a period of several years, to a stage characterized by progressive destruction of the mucosal glands, which is called chronic atrophic gastritis. Other cases show complete loss of the specialized mucosal glands with little or no inflammation and are called gastric atrophy. Although it is not usually possible to establish the sequence of histologic stages in an individual patient, the state of gastric atrophy is generally considered a final sequela of a chronic atrophic gastritis (40). The atrophic effect is typically more pronounced in those cases involving the fundus-corpus and may eventually lead to the functional disorder of primary pernicious anemia.

INTESTINAL METAPLASIA

A common and striking histologic feature of all types of chronic gastritis is the presence of intestinal cells and glands in the gastric mucosa (41). This metaplasia is seen in the majority of cases, in both the antrum and the corpus, and appears to increase in quantity in direct relation to the duration of the disease. The amount of intestinal metaplasia in chronic gastritis varies considerably from scattered foci to extensive replacement of large parts of the gastric mucosa. In early or milder cases, the lesion tends to be in the foveolar region in the upper part of the mucosa and may involve only one to a few pits. It is often focal and merges with the gastric mucous cells on the surface or in the foveolae. The advanced cases of metaplasia are more frequently associated with the atrophic forms of chronic gastritis and reveal larger and deeper areas that may extend to the mucosal base and occupy the entire mucosal thickness.

Intestinal metaplasia has been extensively investigated, allowing detailed descriptions of its ultrastructure (42, 43), enzymatic content (44, 45) and mucin histochemical characteristics (46–48). Intestinal metaplasia appears to take two major forms (complete and incomplete), based on a similarity in structure and function to the normal mucosa of the small intestine and of the colon (Table 23.5) (49–51).

In the type I (or complete) form of intestinal metaplasia, the lesion most closely resembles the small intestine and reveals numerous columnar absorptive cells; relatively fewer goblet mucous cells that contain mildly acidic mucins (such as sialomucin); a variable number of Paneth cells, which tend to be concentrated at the base of the glands; and an occasional villous surface, which usually is poorly formed (Fig. 23.6). The absorptive cells have a fully developed brush border that contains alkaline phosphatase, beta-glucuronidase, and other enzymatic markers of this region. Studies have shown that the cells are capable of lipid absorption (52, 53).

TABLE		
23.5	**Major Types of Intestinal Metaplasia**	

Feature	Type I (Complete)	Type IIB (Incomplete)
Absorptive cells	Many	Absent
Paneth cells	Present	Rare
Goblet mucous cells	Few	Many
Stains for:		
Sialomucins	Positive	Positive
Sulfomucins	Negative	Positive
Strong association with carcinoma	No	Yes

In contrast, the type IIB (or incomplete) form of intestinal metaplasia consists of a mixture of gastric foveolar and colonic type goblet mucous cells (Fig. 23.7). Both types of mucous cells contain highly acidic mucins, such as sulfomucin as well as sialomucin; the mucosal surface is generally flat; and there are no fully developed absorptive cells and only rare Paneth cells (49–51). The type IIA form of intestinal metaplasia appears to be a variant of type IIB, in which the goblet cells have sulfomucins but the foveolar cells contain mainly sialomucins. Some investigators have substituted the term type II for IIA and type III for IIB (48). Intestinal-type endocrine cells are also present in the various forms of metaplasia (54).

The areas of intestinal metaplasia are readily seen in the gastric mucosa by the ordinary H & E preparation and can be enhanced by the use of mucin stains (Fig. 23.8) (46–48). Of the many mucin stains that have been studied, those used most commonly are the periodic acid-Schiff (PAS) reaction for neutral glycoproteins, alcian blue at pH 2.5 for sialomucins and other slightly acidic mucosubstances, and alcian blue at pH 1.0 and metachromatic stains for the strongly acidic mucins. The high iron diamine stain appears to be most specific for the identification of sulfomucins (55). In the normal stomach, the surface and foveolar mucous cells are columnar, and the mucin vacuoles are relatively small and concentrated at the luminal end of the cells; the mucin stains strongly with the PAS reaction and is negative for acid substances, except for a faint staining with alcian blue at pH 2.5 in the lower part of the gastric pits in the proximal stomach. This alcian blue positivity is occasionally increased in the foveolar cells in cases of gastritis, but it is never as intense as in areas of intestinal metaplasia. The goblet mucous cells

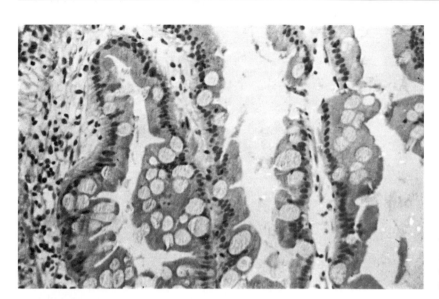

Figure 23.6 Gastric mucosa with an example of the complete (small intestinal) form of intestinal metaplasia. There are numerous goblet-type mucous cells and absorptive cells, and a villus-like structure is present at right (H & E, ×130).

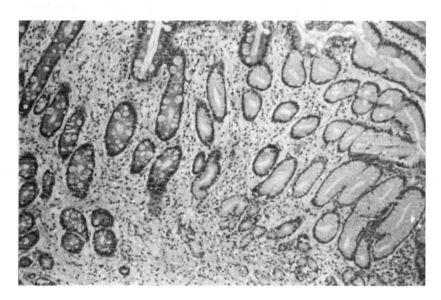

Figure 23.7 Gastric antral mucosa revealing foveolar hyperplasia on the right and the incomplete (colonic) form of intestinal metaplasia on the left. Compared to Figure 23.6, the metaplastic area shows more mucous cells and no villous configuration (H & E, ×80).

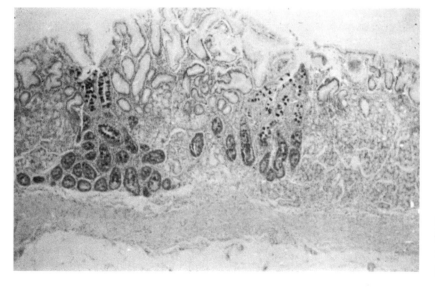

Figure 23.8 Gastric corpus mucosa with two foci of intestinal metaplasia, highlighted by a special stain for acidic mucins (alcian blue stain at pH 2.5, ×32).

of the normal intestines and of the areas of metaplasia are identical in appearance, showing a bulging of the lateral membranes due to the presence of many large mucin vacuoles that fill the cytoplasm and that extrude from the surface. The goblet mucus stains faintly with the PAS reaction, strongly with only the alcian blue at pH 2.5 in the normal small intestine and type I metaplasia, and strongly with alcian blue at both pH 2.5 and 1.0 as well as with the high iron diamine in the normal colon and type IIB metaplasia.

Despite efforts to strictly categorize the various types of intestinal metaplasia, it should be stressed that there is a spectrum, with considerable heterogeneity (46, 49). Supporting evidence includes the admixture noted in the type IIA metaplasia; the finding of contiguous, columnar foveolar cells that stain strongly for acid mucins; and the occasional identification of cells that seem to share both the neutral type and acidic type vacuoles within their cytoplasm (42).

The importance of the finding of intestinal metaplasia in the stomach is that it helps to identify a case of chronic gastritis. Furthermore, because the incidence of gastric carcinoma is increased in patients with long-standing gastritis and many of the tumors are composed of intestinal type glands (56, 57), the metaplasia was once considered a necessary precursor lesion of the tumor. It is now generally accepted, however, that the metaplasia is just one of the signs of the underlying inflammatory condition (58). Debate continues over whether the presence of metaplasia can define a subgroup of patients with chronic gastritis that are especially prone to the development of carcinoma. Metaplasia overall is too ubiquitous a lesion to be specific, but studies have shown that malignant tumors of the stomach are more often associated with the type IIB or incomplete form of intestinal metaplasia (59–64). It is probable that this form of metaplasia will also be too common to serve as a useful marker for surveillance, but prospective studies are needed to settle this issue (see Chapter 27 for further details about the structure and significance of intestinal metaplasia).

CHRONIC ANTRAL GASTRITIS

This type B or environmental form of chronic gastritis is caused by bacteria, principally H. pylori, and by other exogenous agents, and is largely confined to the antral mucosa. Prevalence increases with age and practically all persons older than age 40 years have some degree of chronic inflammatory changes in their antra. Only a minority of the population, however, has active disease or atrophy and develops a clinical disturbance.

Some cases of chronic antral gastritis were thought to result from repeated episodes of acute injury due to ethanol (9, 65) and drugs (8, 12–16) or to reflux of bile salts into the stomach (17–20, 66, 67), but these circumstances are usually not documented. Also incriminated has been the ingestion of a great deal of spicy foods (68) and smoked products, especially in countries in which such diets are a customary practice.

ROLE OF HELICOBACTER ORGANISMS

Although bacteria have for long been noted in the gastric lumen (69), one particular organism, H. pylori, is seen more often in active cases of chronic antral gastritis (35, 70–77). This agent was formerly referred to as a *Campylobacter*-like organism and also called C. pyloridis and C. pylori. It can be readily detected by histologic examination of mucosal biopsy samples, culture of gastric mucosal tissue, and a specific serologic test (71, 78–81). Furthermore, the organisms are rich in urease, which can be measured in the mucosa (80) and can also serve as the basis for a noninvasive breath test (82). Radioactively labeled urea is ingested and the quantity of tagged carbon dioxide is measured in the expired air. The Helicobacter organisms can be seen in regular H & E preparations and are enhanced by a variety of stains, including Gram, Giemsa, and especially silver stains of the Warthin-Starry or Dieterle type (Fig. 23.9) (36, 83, 84). The spiral organisms measure about 3.5 μ in length and 0.5 μ in width, and are selectively located on the surface and in the lumina of the gastric pits (85). The organisms can be destroyed by the gastric acid but survive by attaching to the surface cells beneath the mucous layer. Ultrastructural examination reveals a partial envelopment of the organisms by the surface membranes, similar to the adherence of some forms of E. coli in the intestines (86–88).

The gastric microorganisms are found in about 65 to 75% of patients with chronic antral gastritis who have active disease and in

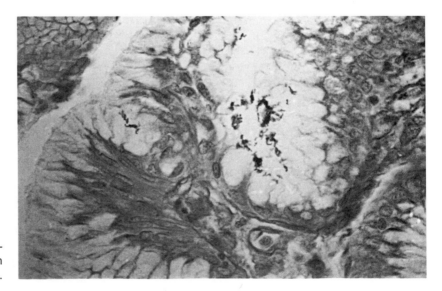

Figure 23.9 Gastric pit containing numerous *Helicobacter pylori* microorganisms, in a patient with chronic active gastritis (Dieterle silver stain, ×500).

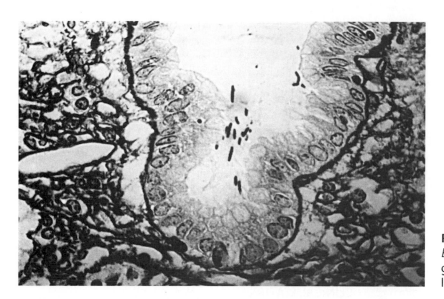

Figure 23.10 Gastric pit containing several *Helicobacter heilmanii*, in a patient with chronic active gastritis (Dieterle silver stain, ×800). The bacteria are longer than those seen in Figure 23.9.

only 5% or less of individuals with inactive disease or normal mucosa. They are also seen in asymptomatic persons who have histologic evidence of active gastritis and the prevalence increases with age (89). Of interest, the bacteria are seen in the antra of more than three quarters of patients with chronic peptic ulcers of the stomach and duodenum, and it is thought that the common factor is the presence of chronic active gastritis, which so often accompanies ulcer disease (77, 90–92). The bacteria are less often found in the gastric corpus-fundus and in the duodenal mucosa and then typically when the patient has an active antral gastritis (35, 93); in the duodenum, they are seen only in areas of gastric mucous cell metaplasia, suggesting that a specific receptor, present in such cells, may be needed for the attachment of the organism to the cell surface (94). The organisms have also been noted in the esophagus in some patients with Barrett esophagus, but only in those individuals that have associated active gastritis and bacteria in the gastric antrum (95, 96), and in areas of heterotopic gastric mucosa (97).

The appearance of H. pylori in the gastric antrum correlates best with the presence of active disease, and many studies have shown a loss of both symptoms and organisms after treatment with antimicrobial drugs, including a variety of antibiotics and bismuth-containing compounds (98–100). Furthermore, in a few recorded cases, ingestion of the organisms, either accidental (101) or by intent (23, 102), led to a gastritis with histologic confirmation of the presence of the bacteria and active inflammation in the mucosa. All of these observations support the contention that H. pylori is the dominant cause of chronic antral gastritis.

ROLE OF OTHER BACTERIA

Other bacteria have been noted in the gastric antrum, and some may represent saprophytes. One organism, measuring about 5 to 6 μ in length and more tightly spiralled than H. pylori, has been seen uncommonly in cases of chronic active antral gastritis, more so in children, and is believed to be another causative agent (103–107). The bacterium, formerly termed *Gastrospirillum hominis* and now called *Helicobacter heilmanii*, is Gram negative and is easily detected in antral smears and histologic sections (Fig. 23.10) (108, 109). These patients also respond to antibiotic therapy.

CLINICAL FEATURES

The clinical aspects of chronic antral gastritis are mainly related to the episodes of active disease and include abdominal pain and vomiting, with bleeding in severe cases. The majority of patients with chronic active gastritis affecting the antrum harbor H. pylori in the gastric mucosa, and treatment with antimicrobial agents results in a diminution or complete clearing of symptoms in most cases.

No specific functional effect can be attributed to the loss of pyloric glands in the later or atrophic stage of the disease. Atrophy, however, is occasionally associated with a reduction in the antral endocrine cells, including those that produce gastrin, and this change can result in decreased acid secretion and hypochlorhydria.

PATHOLOGY

The common features of chronic gastritis and of active disease were described in the preceding discussion of the general pathologic features (2–4, 32–36, 110). In the early stages, alterations are largely confined to the gastric pit region in the upper mucosa and consist of an increase in the amount of mononuclear inflammation in the lamina propria and a variable degree of foveolar hyperplasia (see Fig. 23.3). With advancement of the disease comes extension of inflammation into the lower part of the mucosa, a partial loss of the pyloric glands and the endocrine cells that are located in this region, the appearance of lymphoid follicles (111, 112), and a progressive replacement of the mucosa by intestinal metaplasia (see Fig. 23.6). As a result of the inflammation and the variable types of glands, the mucosal surface that ordinarily is fairly smooth in the normal antrum develops a granular appearance. Occasionally, persistence of the foveolar hyperplasia leads to the formation of localized hyperplastic polyps or to a more diffuse thickening of the mucosal surface (113).

The active phase of chronic antral gastritis is characterized by the additional presence of neutrophils in the lamina propria and glands, variable necrosis, and regeneration of the gastric pits (see Fig. 23.5); this lesion typically starts in the pit region and extends to the lower mucosa in the severe cases. The areas of intestinal metaplasia are infrequently involved with the active inflammation, suggesting that the metaplastic tissue may be resistant to the action of the injurious agents. Clusters of H. pylori are often seen on the surface and in the lumina of the superficial gastric pits at the time of active disease (see Fig. 23.9), whereas they are usually absent during the inactive phase of chronic gastritis. A close correlation exists between the presence of the bacteria and neutrophils in the mucosa. The bacteria are typically seen in association with the gastric mucous cells and uncommonly with the metaplastic intestinal cells (114).

It is not known whether the progression of the chronic gastritis to the atrophic stage is continuous or is the result of recurrent episodes of active disease. In the late stages of chronic antral gastritis, the disease often extends into the junctional area and the lower part of the gastric corpus, but the uppermost region of the stomach, including the cardia and the fundus, ordinarily shows no functional effects from this spread.

DIFFERENTIAL DIAGNOSIS

The majority of adults, and probably all persons 40 years of age or older, contain patchy areas of chronic inflammation and intestinal metaplasia in the gastric antrum; this finding alone is not usually associated with clinical problems. In contrast, most cases of chronic active gastritis reveal the presence of both H. pylori and a prominent neutrophilic infiltrate. The condition is distinguished from acute toxic gastritis by the finding of lymphoid follicles and other signs of chronic inflammation in the gastric mucosa. Chronic peptic ulcer is invariably associated with chronic inflammation in the adjacent intact mucosa, but the ulcers can be readily visualized by gross endoscopic and radiographic examinations. Other inflammatory disorders reveal more characteristic features, such as the presence of microorganisms or granulomas in other infections and a prominent eosinophilic reaction in allergic disease (see previous section concerning acute toxic gastritis for further details regarding the differential diagnosis of active gastritis).

CHRONIC FUNDIC GASTRITIS

This disorder corresponds to the type A form of chronic gastritis in which the lesion typically occurs in older persons, primarily affects the fundic and corpus mucosa, and is believed to result from an immunologic injury (5, 115). As with other forms of chronic gastritis, stages or degrees of severity range from superficial mucosal inflammation to complete atrophy of the specialized glands (39). In long-standing cases, the inflammatory lesions often spread into the antral region. Indeed, because the prevalence of chronic antral gastritis is fairly high, the two forms of chronic fundic and of chronic antral gastritis may coexist in the same patients.

ETIOLOGY AND PATHOGENESIS

Chronic fundic gastritis occurring in adults is generally considered to be a consequence of continuous immunologic damage of the mucosa (115, 116). More than 50% of patients have antibodies to components of parietal cells and intrinsic factor in the serum and gastric fluid (117, 118). There is also a common association with other diseases that are thought to have an immunologic basis, including thyroiditis and hypothyroidism, diabetes mellitus, adrenal insufficiency, Sjögren disease, and myasthenia gravis, and patients frequently have shared autoantibodies to the various tissues (119). The exact mechanism of the injury in the stomach is not known. Despite the presence of the gastric antibodies, it is not proven that

they are responsible for the initiation or even the perpetuation of the disorder; rather, the release of the antibodies could be simply secondary to the tissue damage. Furthermore, the character of the inflammatory cells in the gastric mucosa, dominated by the presence of lymphocytes and other mononuclear cells, suggests instead that a cellular type of immunologic injury may be involved. Whatever the mechanism, the gastric mucosa clearly reflects the development over the course of several years of progressive destruction of the specialized glands containing the parietal (oxyntic) and chief cells throughout the corpus and fundic region.

A rare juvenile form of primary pernicious anemia occurs in children, and its etiology is not known (120). Of interest, despite the same functional effect, atrophic mucosa is found in only some cases, whereas others show preservation of the specialized glands, suggesting that multiple factors or causes may be involved, including a biochemical blockage of the secretory process or its products.

CLINICAL FEATURES

The clinical effects are due to the loss of the cells in the specialized glands of the corpus-fundic region and become evident only in the advanced or atrophic stage of the disease (121). Damage to the chief cells leads to a reduction in the class of pepsinogens, but this change causes no functional deficit, because many other proteolytic enzymes are normally excreted by the pancreas. More major effects result from the loss of the parietal cells, leading to achlorhydria, and particularly of the intrinsic factor that is located in its cellular membranes. The latter is required for the optimal absorption of vitamin B_{12} in the ileum, following binding of the intrinsic factor to the ingested vitamin, and the loss of the factor ultimately results in the development of primary pernicious anemia. The effects of the reduced acid secretion are less striking. One result is reduced activation of the pepsinogens to pepsins, but this effect is not important, considering the alternative supply of pancreatic enzymes. Although the loss of gastric acid may permit the survival of more ingested microorganisms, theoretically favoring the appearance of more infections in the stomach and intestines, this situation has not proven to be a major problem unless the patient's immune system is otherwise compromised. Achlorhydria also causes a sustained stimulation of the gastrin-producing endocrine cells in the antrum (122), resulting in hypergastrinemia and, rarely, the appearance of multiple hyperplastic nodules of the endocrine cells and carcinoid tumors in the antrum.

The adult form typically presents in older persons, usually over age 60, in the atrophic stage of the disease with the appearance of a megaloblastic anemia. The anemia is often severe, and diagnosis depends on the findings of achlorhydria, both basal and stimulated, and of an abnormal Schilling test, which is corrected by the addition of intrinsic factor. Gastric biopsies are not ordinarily performed to establish a diagnosis because the small samples may not be representative of the entire fundic-corpus region and the functional tests are more specific. Unlike antral gastritis, the early stage of the fundic disease is not punctuated by episodes of clinically evident active gastritis. In less advanced cases, when there is still preservation of some of the specialized glands, the lesion may be inhibited or arrested by the use of corticosteroid hormones (123). The anemia responds fully to treatment by injection of B_{12}, but the patients are at some increased risk for the development of polyps and carcinoma of the stomach (124, 125), as discussed subsequently.

PATHOLOGY

The common alterations of chronic gastritis were described in the section concerning the general pathologic features (2–4, 32–36). In the early stage of the disorder, called chronic superficial gastritis,

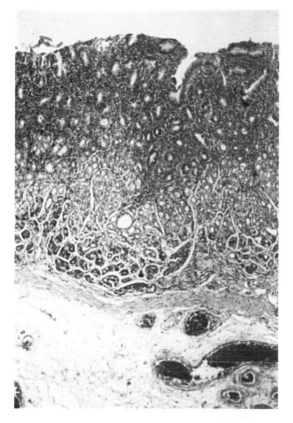

Figure 23.11 Gastric corpus mucosa with superficial chronic gastritis. The inflammation is limited to the upper half of the mucosa *(top),* and most of the specialized glands are preserved. The submucosa at the bottom is not involved (H & E, ×13).

increased numbers of mononuclear inflammatory cells are evident in the upper part of the lamina propria beneath the surface epithelium and between the gastric pits (Fig. 23.11). Damage of the superficial mucous epithelial cells and acute inflammatory reaction are usually patchy and of a slight degree. As the disease advances, typically over many years, the mononuclear and acute inflammatory reactions extend into the lower part of the mucosa with progressive destruction of the specialized glands throughout the corpus-fundic region (Fig. 23.12). Over time, the mucosa is replaced by a mixture of areas of foveolar hyperplasia and of intestinal metaplasia (see Fig. 23.7), and prominent pyloric gland metaplasia is often noted in the basal part. The disorder is referred to as chronic atrophic gastritis at this stage; cases in which findings include complete loss of the specialized glands and minimal inflammation have been termed gastric atrophy, but they probably represent the end stage of the same disorder.

The disease is limited to the mucosa; vascular congestion in the submucosa is common, but no other abnormalities of the gastric wall are noted. The mucosa is usually thinner than normal, resulting in a decrease in the size and number of the rugae and an enhanced visualization of the submucosal vessels on gross examination (Fig. 23.13) (126). In some cases, greater foveolar hyperplasia leads to the formation of multiple hyperplastic polyps (Fig. 23.14) or, rarely, to a diffuse hypertrophy of the mucosa (127, 128).

The findings in the gastric antrum in cases of chronic fundic gastritis are variable (129). Most patients have only patchy areas of chronic inflammation with intestinal metaplasia, equivalent in degree to what is seen in normal adult persons. The pyloric glands in the antrum are intact, and there is often hyperplasia of the endocrine cells (130), including those producing gastrin, that is thought to result from the sustained stimulation by the low gastric acid concentration in the lumen (Fig. 23.15). This hyperplasia occasionally leads to the formation of multiple small nodules of endocrine cells and carcinoid tumors in the antrum. In some cases of chronic fundic gastritis, in contrast, the antral mucosa reveals more widespread inflammatory changes with atrophy; it usually is not known whether this finding represents an extension of the fundic disease into the antrum or a coexistence of the two

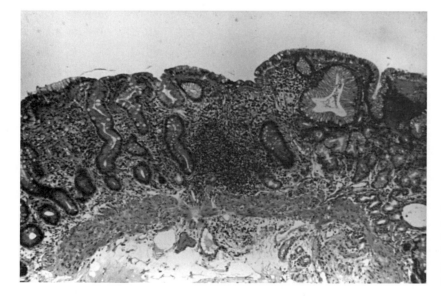

Figure 23.12 Gastric corpus mucosa in a case of chronic atrophic gastritis with primary pernicious anemia. There is a thinning of the mucosa and a complete loss of the specialized gastric glands. The mucosa is replaced by intestinal glands *(left)* and by pyloric glands *(right)* representing metaplasia. The submucosa *(bottom)* is not affected (H & E, ×32).

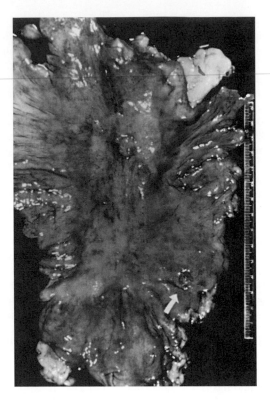

Figure 23.13 Segment of stomach with contiguous duodenum *(bottom)* in a patient with atrophic gastritis and pernicious anemia, showing absence of rugae. Two small hyperplastic polyps are visible, one at the arrow and one near top center.

forms of chronic fundic and of chronic antral gastritis in the same patient. The incidence of H. pylori in the antrum is low, even in patients with active inflammation, possibly due to the associated achlorhydria (131).

DIFFERENTIAL DIAGNOSIS

In the late atrophic stage of chronic fundic gastritis with the appearance of the megaloblastic anemia, the diagnosis is readily determined by the functional tests of gastric acid secretion and of vitamin B_{12} absorption. Considering just the histologic features, the differential is also limited because most inflammatory disorders of the stomach (such as acute toxic gastritis, chronic peptic ulcers, infections and allergic disease) primarily affect the antrum. Superficial chronic inflammation, usually very mild and associated with only rare foci of acute inflammation and of intestinal metaplasia, is occasionally seen in older persons and in patients with the late stage of chronic antral gastritis. Localized areas of atrophy of the corpus mucosa may occur overlying mural tumors and adjacent to rare helminthic infections. In cases in which mucosal polyps develop (see Fig. 23.14), it is necessary to distinguish the common hyperplastic (or regenerative) type from adenomas and carcinomas. This distinction is readily accomplished by biopsy examination. When diffuse foveolar cell hyperplasia results in enlarged rugae and an overall thickening of the mucosal surface, the differential includes tumor infiltration, both of carcinoma and of lymphoma, and Menetrier disease (132). The latter condition in its pure form shows an isolated hyperplasia of the surface-foveolar mucous cells, result-

ing in dramatic lengthening of the gastric pits, and only minimal or no inflammation; the underlying specialized glands are not affected.

POSTGASTRECTOMY GASTRITIS

ETIOLOGY AND CLINICAL FEATURES

Inflammation of the gastric corpus mucosa invariably occurs after excision or bypass of the pyloric sphincter (133, 134). Such inflammation is seen in patients who have had an antral gastrectomy and either a gastrojejunostomy (Billroth II) or a gastroduodenostomy (Billroth I) and also after just a gastrojejunostomy. The antrectomy is most often performed for the treatment of chronic peptic ulcers of either the stomach or duodenum. The gastritis is thought to result mainly from the constant reflux of the bile salts through the open stoma, causing damage to the membranes of the surface epithelial cells that allows increased back-diffusion of acid into the mucosa (135). Alternatively, because the resected antra are usually inflamed, the subsequent appearance of gastritis in the proximal stomach may simply represent an extension of the underlying inflammatory condition to this area in some cases (136).

Although all patients who have had these operative procedures develop histologic alterations, clinically apparent disease is noted in only about 10% of cases (137). The clinical features are those that would be expected in any case of active gastritis and include intermittent episodes of upper abdominal burning pain and hemorrhage, in more severe cases. Treatment is essentially medical and consists of the use of agents that reduce or neutralize gastric acid and that bind to the bile salts. The disorder of bile-induced gastritis must

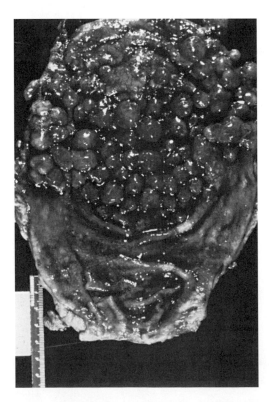

Figure 23.14 Stomach in a patient with atrophic gastritis and pernicious anemia. Note the large conglomerate of hyperplastic polyps in the corpus region *(top)*.

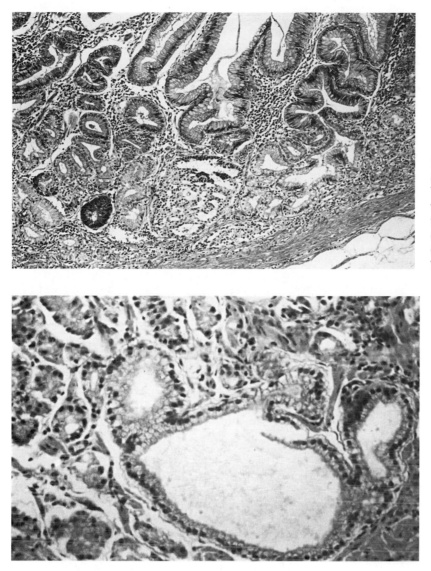

Figure 23.15 Gastric antral mucosa in a case of atrophic corpus gastritis and pernicious anemia. There is an increase in the number of endocrine cells with a large nest (microcarcinoid) in the basal portion of the mucosa. The submucosa is at the bottom (H & E, ×105). (Reproduced with permission from Goldman H. Gastrointestinal mucosal biopsy. New York: Churchill Livingstone, 1996;95–159.)

Figure 23.16 Gastric corpus mucosa in a case of postgastrectomy gastritis shows pyloric gland metaplasia with cystic glands (H & E, ×130).

be distinguished from other conditions that can occur in patients who have had an antral resection, including the dumping syndrome and a bacterial proliferation state resulting from an enlarged afferent loop of jejunum.

PATHOLOGY

The inflammatory lesion begins in the corpus mucosa just adjacent to the anastomotic stoma and may spread with time to affect much of the proximal stomach (134, 138, 139). The early features relate to the toxic effects of the bile salts and include edema, foveolar regeneration, and minimal inflammation. Later changes resemble chronic fundic gastritis and include the presence of mononuclear inflammatory cells and a loss of the specialized corpus glands, which are replaced by pyloric glands. Also noted is a focal cystic dilation of the gastric pits (Fig. 23.16). Of interest, intestinal metaplasia is observed in less than 50% of cases and is rarely a dominant feature. The atrophy of the specialized corpus glands is typically patchy in the early stage but may become confluent with increased duration; a complete loss of the glands in the corpus and fundus with the de-

velopment of pernicious anemia has only rarely been recorded. As with other types of chronic gastritis, some patients have a prominent degree of foveolar cell hyperplasia resulting in the formation of hyperplastic polyps and rarely a diffuse mucosal hypertrophy (140, 141). This proliferation may be especially prominent at the stoma and is associated with the extension of mature glands into the underlying submucosa, representing a localized form of gastritis cystica profunda. The lesion can simulate carcinoma and is described further in the discussion of gastritis cystica. Other late effects, including the predisposition to dysplasia and carcinoma, are discussed in the section concerning complications of chronic gastritis.

DIFFERENTIAL DIAGNOSIS

The diagnosis of gastritis following distal gastric resection or bypass is promptly suggested by the clinical history, but further studies are needed to exclude other causes of the recurrent pain and bleeding. Radiographic and endoscopic procedures, with biopsy if needed, are used to detect a recurrent peptic ulcer that typically is on the intestinal side of the anastomosis, to evaluate any mass lesions, and to identify other causes of inflammation and hemorrhage in the upper alimentary tract. The histologic features of the gastritis are essentially nonspecific, but the findings of prominent cystic dilation of the gastric pits, preservation of small clusters of parietal and chief cells, and relative paucity of intestinal metaplasia may help to distinguish the postgastrectomy type from other forms of chronic gastritis affecting the corpus.

CHRONIC EROSIVE GASTRITIS

In this form of chronic active gastritis, the mucosal surface is deformed by the presence of alternating areas of erosions and small polyps (142–145). The condition, also called varioliform gastritis, is characterized by diffuse involvement of the fundic-corpus region and more variable effects in the antrum. This mucosal appearance may simulate a tumor on radiographic and endoscopic examinations and may even make biopsy interpretation difficult. It is possibly a subset of other forms of chronic gastritis and is separately designated because of the special gross features and the potential confusion with carcinoma.

PATHOLOGY

Histologic study reveals multiple erosions, usually a marked acute and chronic inflammatory cell reaction that extends into and dilates the underlying glandular lumina, and pseudopolyp formation of the adjacent intact mucosa (Fig. 23.17). The polypoid areas show prominent regeneration of the gastric foveolae, which become irregular in size and shape. This appearance, together with the cystic glands, can resemble that seen in early gastric carcinoma affecting the mucosa. The nuclei of the regenerating epithelial cells are enlarged and have prominent nucleoli but, in contrast to those of tumor cells, are generally regular in size and shape and lack prominent hyperchromatism (Fig. 23.18); also, regenerative cells usually have more abundant cytoplasm. Another helpful feature is that the mucosa in chronic erosive gastritis, when it affects the corpus region, reveals partial preservation of the parietal and chief

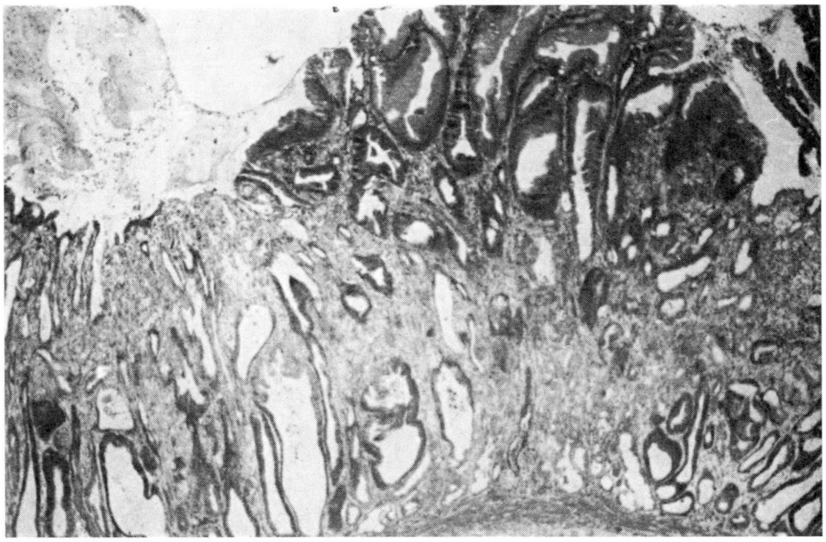

Figure 23.17   Gastric mucosa in a case of chronic erosive (varioliform) gastritis. Present are alternating areas of erosion *(left)* and foveolar hyperplasia *(right)*. Submucosa is at bottom (H & E, ×80).

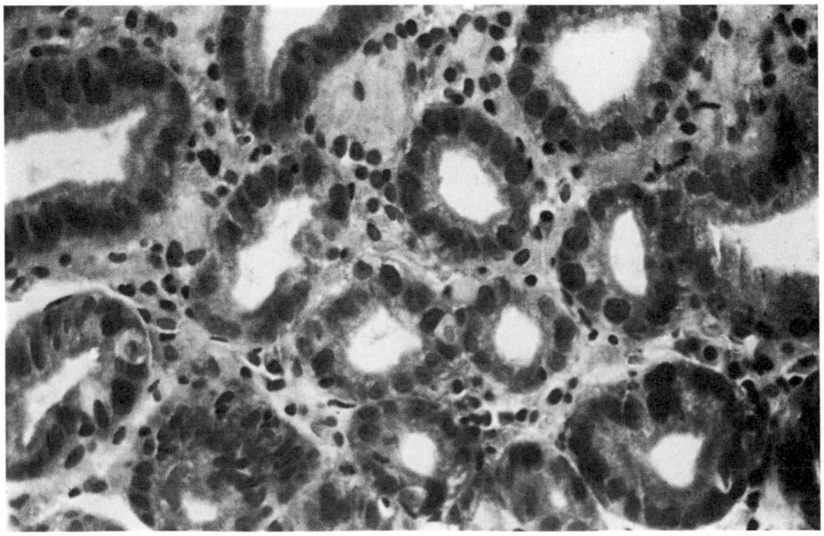

Figure 23.18   Gastric foveolae in a case of chronic erosive gastritis showing marked regeneration. The epithelial nuclei are enlarged but are mostly round and fairly regular in size and shape (H & E, ×310). Contrast with dysplastic epithelium in Figure 23.20.

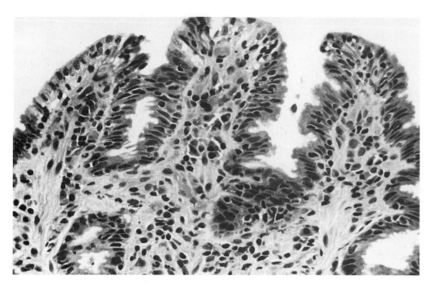

Figure 23.19 Gastric antral mucosa in a case of active celiac disease, with surface at the top. There is a marked increase of intraepithelial lymphocytes involving the surface and pit mucous layer (H & E, ×425). (Reproduced with permission from Goldman H. Gastrointestinal mucosal biopsy. New York: Churchill Livingstone, 1996;95–159.)

cells lining the inflamed and dilated glands, whereas these specialized cells are generally absent in tumor glands.

DIFFERENTIAL DIAGNOSIS

The diagnosis of chronic erosive gastritis is based on the gross appearance of the lesion and on documentation by histologic examination of its inflammatory nature. Cases of acute toxic gastritis and of stress ulceration may reveal multiple erosions and regenerative glands, but the lesions are usually limited to or dominant in the antrum in acute gastritis; in both conditions, prominent polyp formation and chronic inflammation are absent. Erosions and hyperplastic polyps can be seen in standard cases of chronic antral gastritis and chronic fundic gastritis, and the separation of chronic erosive gastritis may simply depend on the presence of both features to a significant degree.

LYMPHOCYTIC GASTRITIS

In some cases of chronic erosive (or varioliform) gastritis, findings include a significant increase in the number of lymphocytes within the epithelial layer lining the gastric surface and foveolae, particularly in those affecting the corpus region (146). Conversely, of all cases designated by biopsy as showing this lymphocytic gastritis, about 20% did not exhibit the gross thickening of the mucosa, suggesting that the lymphocytic infiltrate may represent an early or precursor lesion. Accordingly, the alternative term of lymphocytic gastritis has been offered. Cases in which hyperplasia is more prominent may be associated with a protein-losing condition (147) and there is a weak link with cases of lymphocytic colitis (148).

Similar lymphocytic lesions that are limited to the antrum are less specific because they are seen in otherwise ordinary cases of chronic antral gastritis including those associated with H. pylori infection (149, 150). Furthermore, increased numbers of lymphocytes are observed in the gastric surface-foveolar epithelium in the antrum of patients with celiac sprue, and are directly related to the presence of gluten in the diet (Fig. 23.19) (151, 152).

CHRONIC HYPERTROPHIC GASTRITIS

In this variant form of chronic gastritis, a prominent degree of hyperplasia of the surface and foveolar mucous cells results in dramatic and often diffuse hypertrophy of the involved segment of mucosa (113, 127, 128). Pronounced hyperplasia can be seen in cases of both chronic antral and chronic fundic gastritis, but the reason for its occurrence in these instances is not known. Some details are provided in the sections addressing general pathologic features and differential diagnosis of chronic fundic gastritis (see also Chapter 25 for a more complete discussion).

COMPLICATIONS OF CHRONIC GASTRITIS

Certain conditions of the stomach occur more frequently in patients with the various types of chronic gastritis. Some of the lesions are a direct consequence of the inflammatory process, such as xanthomas and hyperplastic (or regenerative) polyps, whereas others relate to an increased propensity of the chronically inflamed mucosa to develop neoplasms, including adenomas, carcinomas, carcinoid tumors, and malignant lymphoma. Chronic inflammation of the antral mucosa is also noted in patients with chronic peptic ulcers of the antrum, and the inflammatory lesion may be a necessary factor for the ulcer formation in this region (see Chapter 24).

XANTHOMA (XANTHELASMA)

These slightly raised, yellow nodules on the mucosal surface typically measure less than a few millimeters in diameter (153–157), are sessile, may be single or multiple, and are more often noted in the corpus-fundic region. The nodules are composed of a core of numerous, finely vacuolated macrophages that contain lipids within the lamina propria and are covered by normal or slightly hyperplastic epithelium (see Fig. 19.6). They are confined to the mucosa, and there is usually no other inflammation in the lesion. Although xanthomas occasionally are seen in a noninflamed stomach, they are more frequently noted in patients with chronic gastritis, particularly the postgastrectomy form (155, 156). It is thought that the lesion results from prior episodes of mucosal hemorrhage and that the lipids are derived from the destroyed blood cells. The natural course is not known, but it is probable that the nodules resolve spontaneously.

The diagnosis of xanthoma ordinarily is made on regular H & E preparations. Stains for fat, which would require frozen sections, are neither available nor needed. Lesions that might be confused with xanthomas include clusters of macrophages containing mucin (muciphages) and a granular cell tumor within the gastric mucosa. Muciphages are infrequently noted in the stomach, in contrast to their common presence in the colonic mucosa. They contain larger and more irregular cytoplasmic vacuoles that stain strongly with the periodic acid-Schiff (PAS) reaction (see Fig. 19.8). The cells of a granular cell tumor ("myoblastoma") have a distinct granular cytoplasm that stains weakly with the PAS reaction. Although signet ring cell carcinomas may manifest with sheets of cells in the lamina propria, particularly in biopsy specimens, they contain mucus and their nature is readily discerned by the highly irregular and hyperchromatic nuclei (154). Some granulomas, especially those associated with foreign bodies or *Mycobacterium avium* complex, may contain enlarged and vacuolated macrophages, but the lesions are smaller, circumscribed, and usually associated with giant cells and other inflammatory cells. Rarer causes of macrophage accumulations in the mucosa include chronic granulomatous disease of childhood, which reveals cytoplasmic pigment, and malakoplakia that has characteristic inclusions.

EPITHELIAL POLYPS

Some cases of chronic gastritis, both of the antral and of the fundic types, are associated with foveolar cell hyperplasia, which can result in the formation of localized hyperplastic (regenerative) polyps (140, 141). These polyps are more common in the proximal stomach and have been found in up to 10% of patients with chronic fundic gastritis in the atrophic stage and of the postgastrectomy cases. The polyps are usually small and sessile and have a smooth or coarsely lobulated surface (158, 159). They frequently are multiple and occasionally present with a large conglomerate of lesions that effaces the mucosal surface (see Fig. 23.14). Hyperplastic polyps are composed of a core of edematous and inflamed lamina propria and contain a variable amount of pyloric glands and of hyperplastic or actively regenerative foveolar epithelium; intestinal metaplasia may be present but usually is not prominent. The polypoid lesions are analogous to the inflammatory pseudopolyps seen in cases of chronic colitis. These and other epithelial polyps of the stomach are described more fully in Chapter 26.

Although fundic gland polyps, consisting of intact fundic mucosa with focal cystic dilation of the pits and glands, have been noted in cases of chronic gastritis, they do not occur more frequently in these conditions (160). Adenomas of the stomach, representing benign neoplasms of the gastric epithelium, generally are rare, but when they arise, they are more common in patients with chronic gastritis; they have been noted in 1% of cases in some series of postgastrectomy gastritis. Compared to hyperplastic polyps, the adenomas are typically larger, have a papillary surface contour, and contain dysplastic epithelium of the foveolar or intestinal metaplastic types. They also may contain foci of adenocarcinoma.

DYSPLASIA AND ADENOCARCINOMA

Patients with the atrophic forms of chronic gastritis are at increased risk for the development of gastric adenocarcinoma after a latent period of about 10 years (161). The prevalence in different geographic regions varies widely, however, and is probably related to the baseline frequency of such tumors in each country. In areas with a high rate of gastric carcinoma, follow-up studies of patients with gastric atrophy and pernicious anemia have revealed an 8 to 10-fold increase of tumors after 10 to 15 years of known disease (124, 125, 162). Furthermore, many cases of carcinoma of the gastric antrum are related to prior chronic gastritis due to H. pylori (163–165). Similarly, an increased frequency of carcinoma (from 1 to 5%) has been noted in the proximal stomach (referred to as stump carcinoma) 10 to 15 years after an antral resection (166–170). Again, the enhanced risk has been well documented in countries that have a high de novo rate of carcinoma, such as Scandinavia and England, whereas it has not been clearly established in the U.S.A. (171, 172). The stump tumors typically occur in the mucosa just proximal to the anastomosis, in the area in which inflammation is the greatest.

Cases of gastric adenocarcinoma of the intestinal type involving gland formation are often associated with glandular dysplasia of the adjacent nontumorous mucosa (Fig. 23.20) (173, 174). Histologic evidence of dysplasia has also been observed in the flat mucosa in advance of the formation of overt carcinoma in patients with pernicious anemia (124, 125) and in those with postgastrectomy gastritis (167, 175–177). This finding has served as the basis for the use of endoscopic and mucosal biopsy surveillance in high risk patients (178). It appears that the detection of a severe or high-grade dysplasia correlates best with tumor development (179–183), but the clinical consequence of biopsy-proven evidence of dysplasia in the absence of apparent carcinoma is not settled. Furthermore, it is not known whether the identification of dysplasia will prove more useful then the search for gross features of early and minute gastric carcinomas (161, 184, 185) (see Chapter 27).

CARCINOID TUMORS

The incidence of endocrine cell hyperplasia (129, 130, 186) and carcinoid tumors (187–192) of the antrum in patients with chronic atrophic gastritis involving the corpus and fundus has increased. This change is likely attributable to reduced or absent gastric secretion resulting in a loss of the normal negative feedback and a sustained stimulation of the antral endocrine cells, principally the gastrin producing G cells. The tumors are usually multiple and range in size from microscopic foci to a few millimeters in diameter (see Fig. 23.15); lesions larger than a centimeter are rarely observed. The hypergastrinemia may lead further to the stimulation and proliferation of the enterochromaffin-like (ECL) cells in the corpus, resulting in endocrine cell hyperplasia and tumors in this area as well (193). Functional problems from the excess hormonal secretion include effects on the peripheral vasculature and on gastrointestinal motility (see Chapter 15 for further details).

MALIGNANT LYMPHOMA

A strong association exists between the chronic gastritis due to H. pylori and the development of malignant lymphoma of the

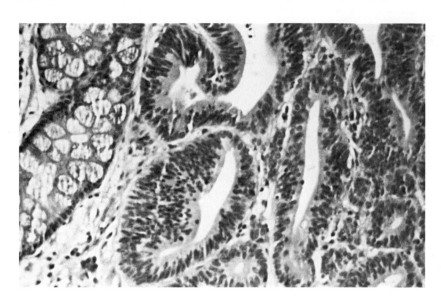

Figure 23.20 Gastric mucosa revealing glandular dysplasia *(center and right)*. Compared to regeneration (see Fig. 23.18), the dysplastic epithelium shows more variation in size and shape, prominent palisading, and hyperchromatism of the nuclei. A gland with nondysplastic intestinal metaplasia is at left (H & E, ×200).

mucosa-associated lymphocytes, termed MALToma (194, 195). It is believed that the persistent infection can lead to lymphoid hyperplasia and ultimately to tumor formation. The earlier lesions reveal only a small or no gross lesion, and may be treated successfully with antibiotic therapy (196). Biopsy can assist in the detection, revealing invasion by the atypical lymphocytes into the epithelium, but additional tests to demonstrate monoclonality and gene rearrangement are usually needed to provide a definitive diagnosis (see Chapter 17 for further details).

CORROSIVE GASTRITIS
ETIOLOGY AND CLINICAL FEATURES

This form of gastritis is due to the ingestion of highly toxic chemicals, including strong alkaline, acid, and fixative solutions (197–199). The compounds most often involved are sodium hydroxide (lye), sulfuric, nitric and hydrochloric acids, and formaldehyde. This condition follows the accidental intake of these substances, which are present in many household cleaning products, or a suicidal effort. The degree of damage depends on the amount and concentration of the toxic material; the injury may be lessened if the stomach contains food, which covers and protects part of the mucosal surface. Although alkali exert their greatest effect on the esophageal squamous mucosa, they can also damage the stomach. As a result of pylorospasm, the duodenum typically sustains no injury.

Patients present promptly with intense oropharyngeal and midepigastric pain. Other findings include hemorrhage in acute cases, peritonitis if deep mural necrosis has occurred, and signs of obstruction in patients who later develop strictures. Initial medical therapy is supportive, and surgical resection is required in patients with protracted hemorrhage, peritonitis, or obstruction (200).

PATHOLOGY

The antral region is most affected, and the lesions resemble those seen in ischemic disease of the bowel. Milder cases involve patchy or diffuse hemorrhagic necrosis of the mucosal layer which heals with just minor fibrosis in the submucosa. In more dramatic cases, greater necrosis extends into the gastric wall, which can lead to perforation, peritonitis, and potential fatality. There is reactive inflammation of a nonspecific nature, and patients with deep necrosis often develop marked fibrosis and stricture of the pyloric area. The diagnosis is provided by the clinical history; additional studies ordinarily are not required. Endoscopy is sometimes used to gauge the extent of injury or to identify the presence of a stricture (199, 201).

INFECTIONS OF THE STOMACH (TABLE 23.6)

Infections are much less common in the stomach than in the intestinal tract, perhaps because of the high concentration of hydrochloric acid. Of interest, however, patients who develop atrophic fundic gastritis and achlorhydria do not show a notable increase in the incidence of gastric infections, suggesting that additional factors are operative in this protection. As in other parts of the gut, the stomach can also be involved with opportunistic infections, which typically occur in debilitated and immunocompromised patients and in cases involving extensive necrosis related to other underlying conditions (202).

VIRAL INFECTIONS

Although the term "gastroenteritis" is often used clinically to refer to transient viral infections of the gut, such as those due to the Norwalk agent and other enteroviruses, the histologic lesions are limited to the small intestinal mucosa and the stomach is spared (203). Following an investigative study with gastroscopy, several previously normal persons developed gastritis and hypochlorhydria, which lasted for several weeks. It was postulated that gastritis and hypochlorhydria was due to viral contamination of the endoscopes. It has been shown subsequently, however, that infection with H. pylori was the likely cause (101).

TABLE

23.6   Infections of the Stomach[a]

Viral infections
  Herpes simplex[b]
  Cytomegalovirus[b]
Bacterial infections
  Helicobacter pylori and *heilmanii* in chronic antral gastritis
  Pyogenic organisms in phlegmonous and emphysematous gastritis
  Tuberculosis
  Mycobacterium avium complex[b]
  Actinomyces
  Syphilis
Fungal infections
  Candida (Monilia)[b]
  Histoplasma
  Mucor (Phycomycete)[b]
Protozoan infections
  Cryptosporidia[b]
  Toxoplasma[b]
  Giardia in fluid
Helminthic infections
  Anisakiasis
  Strongyloides[b]
  Rare—*Schistosoma*, *Ascaris*, flukes

[a] Infection may be limited to the stomach, associated with lesions in other regions of the gut, or part of a systemic spread.

[b] Usually present in immunocompromised or severely debilitated patients.

HERPESVIRUS

Infection with the herpes simplex viruses typically favors the squamous-lined mucosa of the esophagus and anal canal (204), and effects on the tissues with glandular mucosa are rare. Cases in the stomach have been noted only in immunodeficient patients, and usually are associated with more widespread herpetic infection in the body (205, 206). The lesions are similar in appearance to herpes infection elsewhere, characterized by multiple vesicles on the mucosal surface that proceed to small erosions. The diagnosis is determined by finding the typical intranuclear inclusion within the mucous epithelial cells; the multinucleated giant cells that characteristically are seen in infections of the squamous epithelium are rarely present. Little is known of the natural course of the gastric infection, and the clinical behavior depends on the underlying disorder.

CYTOMEGALOVIRUS

This virus has been demonstrated with increasing frequency in the gastric and duodenal mucosa in patients who are immunocompromised (202, 207–210). It is a frequent finding in patients with the acquired immunodeficiency syndrome and in individuals receiving immunosuppressive drugs for renal transplants and other inflammatory conditions (211, 212). Intact mucosa or a previously ulcerated area (207, 208) may be involved, and the characteristic features are the presence of the typical red intranuclear and large intracytoplasmic inclusions within the covering epithelial cells as

well as the endothelial cells and other mesenchymal cells in the lamina propria or in the granulation tissue beneath an ulcer (Fig. 23.21). As with CMV infection elsewhere in the body, it is not known whether the virus can initiate the tissue injury or is a secondary invader in an area of prior inflammation and necrosis. The virus can sustain or enhance tissue destruction, and a positive culture of the tissue, or possibly a rise in its serologic titer, is seen in such cases.

BACTERIAL INFECTIONS

Bacteria are often noted over areas of necrosis and tumors in the stomach and they are also commonly seen in patients with stress ulceration attributable to extensive body burns. It is thought that the organisms are saprophytes and that they do not contribute to the tissue injury.

HELICOBACTER PYLORI AND HEILMANII

H. pylori are found in the gastric antrum in two thirds to three quarters of patients with chronic active gastritis and chronic peptic ulcers of the stomach and duodenum. The organisms are probably the major cause of these conditions (see previous discussion of chronic antral gastritis).

ACUTE PHLEGMONOUS GASTRITIS

This rare condition is characterized by the presence of extensive and often transmural necrosis associated with intense suppuration (213–217). Most cases are due to infections with hemolytic streptococci; other organisms observed include pneumococci, staphylococci, and coliforms. This condition is seen more often in older persons, particularly in those individuals with general debility, septicemia, or shock. Patients present with pain, hematemesis, and signs of an acute abdomen; antibiotic therapy alone is insufficient and early gastric resection is required to avoid fatality. Examination of the stomach usually reveals diffuse involvement with deep red to purple tissues, prominent mural thickening, and pockets of pus that ooze from the submucosa and peritoneal surface. Histologic features include significant necrosis of all parts of the gastric wall, sloughing of the mucosa, many neutrophils and microorganisms, and thrombosis of the small blood vessels. Possibly because of the general looseness of the tissue, the inflammatory and thrombotic features are often best visualized in the submucosal layer. Unless affected areas are resected, patients develop gastric perforation and generalized peritonitis. The diagnosis is suggested by the presence of bacteria together with the acute inflammatory reaction; culture of the gastric tissue is confirmatory. Ordinary ischemic disease is rarely noted in the stomach and does not elicit as prominent an inflammatory reaction. The inflammatory lesions associated with the common disorders of acute gastritis and of chronic gastritis are limited to the mucosa, and peptic ulcers are localized conditions.

ACUTE EMPHYSEMATOUS GASTRITIS

This condition is probably a variant of phlegmonous gastritis in which the responsible microorganisms, most often *Clostridium welchii* (218), are gas-forming. Acute emphysematous gastritis is noted most often in patients with malignant tumors of the stomach and in those that have had prior corrosive damage or infarction

(219, 220). The morphologic features are similar to the phlegmonous cases except for the addition of gas-filled spaces of variable size in the gastric wall. These areas can be identified radiographically. The diagnosis is provided by the distinctive features and culture of the gastric tissue. Post-mortem tissues may reveal extensive autolysis and gas-filled spaces owing to the secondary invasion and proliferation of enteric bacteria, but there is no evidence of inflammation. Pneumatosis ordinarily is confined to the intestines and the spaces lack bacteria and neutrophils. Other conditions that may be associated with the appearance of spaces in the gastric wall include gastritis cystica profunda and mucinous carcinoma, but the mucinous nature of the contents and lining of the epithelial cells are evident.

TUBERCULOSIS

Gastrointestinal tuberculosis, uncommon in Western countries, most often affects the ileocecal region and only rarely involves the stomach (221–224). Most cases in the United States result from primary pulmonary infection, either as part of a systemic spread or by the swallowing of infective material that has been coughed up into the oral cavity. Gastric lesions have a predilection for the antral-pyloric region and are often associated with contiguous disease of the duodenum. In some cases, findings include deep ulceration with occasional fissure formation, whereas in others, marked thickening of the antral mucosa is noted. Patients typically present with signs of gastric outlet obstruction, and the radiographic and endoscopic appearances may simulate malignancy. Characteristic histologic findings include numerous granulomas in all layers of the gastric wall. Necrosis may or may not be present in the granulomas, and the diagnosis is secured by the demonstration of tubercle bacilli on acid-fast stain and by culture of the gastric tissue. The stains are more often positive in cases with caseating granulomas. The inflammation around the ulcers and fissures is otherwise nonspecific, and a fibrous stricture can develop in advanced cases. Medical therapy usually is sufficient, and surgical intervention is reserved for those patients with permanent obstruction. The overall prognosis depends on the extent of infection in the body.

The differential at a clinical and macroscopic level includes tumors, which usually are confined to the stomach but may exceptionally extend across the pyloric sphincter, and ordinary peptic ulcer disease, which typically presents with a more localized lesion and lacks fissures. The distinction from Crohn disease may be more difficult, because both disorders affect the same areas of the gut and may be associated with mural fissures and a granulomatous reaction. Of help, granulomas are present in only 50% of cases of Crohn disease and never reveal necrosis unless associated with foreign material, whereas they are always present in tuberculosis and caseation is frequently demonstrated. Ultimately, the distinction is made by finding the organism in stains or culture. Other granulomatous disorders that can affect the stomach (described in subsequent sections) include sarcoidosis; foreign body reactions; infections due to M. avium complex, syphilis, and histoplasmosis; and isolated granulomatous gastritis. Most of these conditions are associated with less tissue destruction and the granulomas are rarely of the caseating type.

MYCOBACTERIUM AVIUM COMPLEX

Infection due to M. avium intracellulare (MAI)has been described in humans and occurs exclusively in patients with the acquired immunodeficiency syndrome (AIDS) or other immunocompromised conditions (202, 225). The infection can involve multiple tissues of the body, including the liver and all portions of the gastrointestinal tract from the esophagus to the rectum. There is usually concomitant involvement of the stomach and duodenum. The lesions are concentrated in the mucosal layer and consist of small clusters of enlarged macrophages or poorly formed granulomas without necrosis in the lamina propria (see Fig. 19.7). Acid-fast stains demonstrate abundant organisms both within the macrophages and lying free in the stroma; cultures are not ordinarily required. Because the macrophages may vary considerably in amount, and can even be absent in a single tissue section, routine acid-fast stains on gut mucosal biopsy samples are recommended for all patients with AIDS. Results usually show no acute or other inflammatory reaction and a lack of tissue necrosis in the MAI

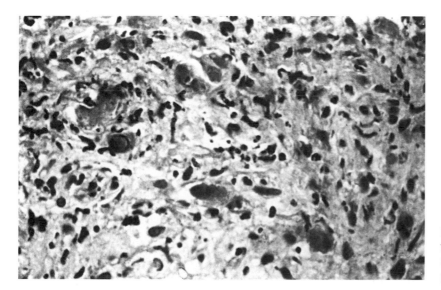

Figure 23.21 Base of a gastric ulcer showing effects of cytomegalovirus in the mesenchymal elements. There are large intranuclear and intracytoplasmic inclusions (H & E, ×500).

infections of the stomach. Additional opportunistic infections are frequently present in the gut and other body tissues, however, and the overall prognosis is poor.

ACTINOMYCOSIS

This uncommon bacterial infection of the gut is due to *Actinomyces israelii*. The lesions are noted most often in the terminal ileum, cecum, and appendix (226). The responsible organisms are filamentous, Gram-positive anaerobic bacteria that normally reside in the oral cavity, especially in the tonsillar region. They have a typical gross appearance consisting of tiny yellow "sulfur granules." Infection of the stomach is rare and usually affects the antral region (226–228). Actinomycosis is characterized by persistent ulceration with occasional fistulae and a thickened wall that resembles a tumor and requires resection. The histologic features are distinctive: a chronic abscess in the gastric wall with marked neutrophilia and numerous bacterial colonies. The diagnosis is afforded by these findings and culture of the exudate.

SYPHILIS

Some patients with early secondary syphilis have inflammatory lesions of a nonspecific nature in their gastric and colonic mucosa (229–231). The mucosa reveals acute and chronic inflammatory cells, occasional small erosions, and numerous *Treponema pallidum* spirochetes by the Warthin-Starry silver stain or the acridine orange fluorochrome stain; granulomas are not present. These patients often lack any gastrointestinal symptoms, however, and the mucosal findings are mainly observed in investigative studies; both gut and cutaneous lesions resolve after specific antibiotic therapy. More rarely, symptomatic cases of gastric syphilis occur in the late secondary and the tertiary stages of the disease (232–235). These patients present with signs of gastritis or obstruction, and the clinical suspicion, based on the gross appearance of a thickened gastric wall, is usually of a tumor. The characteristic morphologic features are expansion of the submucosal layer by inflammation and fibrosis and the presence of an obliterative endarteritis. Acute and chronic inflammation of the mucosa, which can lead to enlarged folds (236), and a hypertrophy of the muscularis propria are also observed, and

the overall gross appearance can resemble a linitis plastica stomach. Granulomatous lesions or gummas are rare, and a marked lymphoid reaction is noted on occasion (237). Because the histologic features are not absolutely specific, a high level of suspicion for the infection is needed. The diagnosis is provided by finding spirochetes in the tissue by stains or PCR analysis, either in the inflamed mucosa or in the area of the involved submucosal vessels, and by positive serology.

The differential is fairly limited and includes tumors at the gross level and conditions that are associated with prominent fibrosis, such as radiation damage and systemic sclerosis. An equivalent degree of submucosal fibrosis and vascular changes can be seen in the late stages after radiation; also evident may be atypical mesenchymal cells and pronounced ectasia of the small vessels in the mucosa. In systemic sclerosis, the fibrosis is not limited to the submucosa but extends throughout the muscularis propria. Ordinary cases of chronic gastritis lack the mural findings, and patients with peptic ulcers or Crohn disease have more localized lesions.

FUNGAL INFECTIONS

Fungi act as opportunistic agents and typically appear in debilitated or immunocompromised patients and in areas of prior necrosis (238, 239).

CANDIDIASIS (MONILIASIS)

Fungal elements of *Candida albicans* are frequently noted overlying the base of chronic peptic ulcers of the stomach (Fig. 23.22). It has been suggested that fungi enhance the degree of necrosis and that such patients have protracted disease and deeper ulcers with more perforations (240, 241). Other studies, however, have noted the fungi but failed to show any correlation with the amount of necrosis and clinical course. This issue is not completely resolved (242, 243). It has also been postulated that the number of organisms might be increased in the stomach of patients who are receiving potent medications, such as H2 blockers to reduce gastric acidity, but adequate control studies have not been performed and the deleterious effects from the presence of the fungi in these cases have not been substantiated.

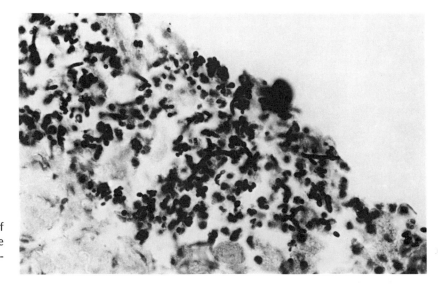

Figure 23.22   Surface of a chronic peptic ulcer of the stomach, showing necrotic material and a large number of fungal spores and pseudohyphae (periodic acid-Schiff stain, ×450).

Primary and secondary monilial infections are definitely noted in the stomach and are generally confined to patients with severe debility or an immunodeficiency condition (244–248). Such infections are more common in the esophagus but can affect any part of the gut, and multiple sites can be involved in an individual case. The lesions appear as multiple plaques or ulcers of the mucosa in any part of the stomach. Variable degrees of inflammation of a nonspecific nature are present, and the diagnosis is secured by the demonstration of the characteristic slender pseudohyphae in biopsy samples or scrapings of the mucosal lesions; cultures are ordinarily not needed. The infection can respond to specific antifungal therapy, but other types of infections may be present and the overall prognosis relates to the underlying condition.

HISTOPLASMOSIS

Rare examples of systemic spread of histoplasmosis to the gut have been described (249–252). The disease is noted most often in the intestines, but it can affect the stomach on occasion. The lesions appear as single or multiple areas of ulceration and contain numerous granulomas that are usually noncaseating. The organisms of *Histoplasma capsulatum* grow as spores in the body, are typically small and located within the macrophage or giant cell cytoplasm in the granulomas, and are best demonstrated by silver stains. The differential includes other granulomatous conditions of the stomach that may be associated with tissue destruction, principally tuberculosis and Crohn disease.

MUCORMYCOSIS (PHYCOMYCOSIS)

These infections are due to the *Mucor* agents, which are part of the Mucoraceae family in the Phycomcetes class. Gastric infection is rare, is seen only in severely debilitated or immunocompromised patients, and appears to be more prevalent in tropical regions (253–256). The lesions can affect any part of the stomach and manifest with extensive hemorrhage, necrosis, and thrombosed vessels; it may extend deep into the gastric wall, resulting in perforation. The inflammatory reaction is nonspecific and lacks granulomas, and the specific diagnosis is provided by the identification of the fungi. The organisms are relatively large hyphae that are nonseptate and have short branches; they can be seen in regular H & E preparations and are enhanced by silver stains and the periodic acid-Schiff (PAS) reaction.

PARASITIC INFECTIONS

PROTOZOAN INFECTIONS

Protozoan infections do not ordinarily occur in the stomach. In patients with achlorhydria due to atrophic gastritis who are having endoscopic examination, *Giardia lamblia* have been noted in the cytologic smears, but they do not cause gastric lesions. Patients with AIDS develop cryptosporidial infection of the small intestines, and the organism may exceptionally be found in the stomach (257, 258). Also rarely noted in AIDS patients is infection due to toxoplasmosis (259). Similarly, helminthic infestations typically occur in the intestines and only rarely affect the stomach.

ANISAKIASIS

This infection, which results from the ingestion of the larvae of the small nematode, *Anisakidae*, occurs most frequently in Asian countries where large amounts of raw fish are consumed (260–262). The disorder has been noted in the United States and typically causes a chronic lesion in the distal ileum that can resemble Crohn disease. Infection in the stomach is less common and may be associated with the acute onset of pain just a few hours after the ingestion of the larvae. Endoscopic examination at this early stage reveals mucosal swelling and inflammation as well as the organism, which has burrowed into the mucosa but is still partially present in the lumen. Most cases resolve spontaneously, but in some patients, the infection persists, with the development of necrosis and a poorly formed granulomatous reaction containing large numbers of eosinophils. The inflammation can extend into the gastric wall resulting in the appearance of a deep ulcer or a mass lesion and necessitating resection in some cases. The differential diagnosis includes other lesions that can be associated with prominent necrosis and an eosinophilic reaction, such as Crohn disease and the rare mural form of eosinophilic gastroenteritis. The specific diagnosis of anisakiasis depends on finding worm fragments in the lesion.

OTHER HELMINTHIC INFECTIONS

Rare cases of helminthic involvement of the stomach due to *Strongyloides stercoralis* (263, 264), which typically is seen in immunocompromised hosts, and to *Schistosoma mansoni* (265), have been reported. Usual findings include ulceration of the mucosa and a prominent inflammatory reaction with many eosinophils and occasional granulomas. The diagnosis requires the identification of the specific ova in the tissues or the stools. *Ascaris* (266, 267) and various flukes have also been noted rarely in the stomach.

MISCELLANEOUS CONDITIONS OF THE STOMACH

MALLORY-WEISS SYNDROME

ETIOLOGY AND CLINICAL FEATURES

The Mallory-Weiss lesion is a longitudinal tear of the mucosa at the esophagocardiac junction that is believed to be a consequence of severe retching (268–271). It is commonly observed in alcoholics, presumably because they frequently experience episodes of toxic gastritis that lead to severe vomiting. Patients typically present with heartburn or midepigastric pain and hematemesis. Upper gastrointestinal tract endoscopy is performed to sort out the various causes of hemorrhage in such patients, which include severe gastritis and ruptured esophageal or gastric varices, as well as the Mallory-Weiss tear. Medical therapy, consisting of the elimination of any toxic substances from the diet and the reduction or neutralization of gastric acid, is usually sufficient. Balloon tamponade or surgical intervention is reserved for cases involving prolonged hemorrhage and impending perforation.

PATHOLOGY

The Mallory-Weiss lesion is characteristic and reveals a longitudinal laceration of the mucosa that straddles the cardioesophageal junction (Fig. 23.23). It is usually single and measures less than 1 cm in length. The term "syndrome" is used because some patients, possibly manifesting an earlier stage of the condition, show only prominent mucosal hemorrhage in this area without the tear. The typical lesion extends into the deep part of the submucosa and is associated with marked hemorrhage from the torn vessels and later by a nonspecific acute inflammatory reaction. Healing is usually prompt and may be associated with a slight degree of submucosal fibrosis but without stricture formation. Complications are uncommon and include persistence of the lesion, which can lead to the development of a larger ulcer with greater hemorrhage, and penetration of the tear into the deeper parts of the wall, leading to perforation.

The differential is limited and consists of ulcerating lesions of the junctional area that can be seen in severe cases of reflux esophagitis and in the mucosa overlying an early carcinoma or a mural mass such as a leiomyoma of the lower esophageal and gastric cardiac regions. In all of these conditions, the ulcerated area is often larger and less consistently located right at the junction, and the typical clinical history of severe vomiting and retching is usually absent.

GASTRITIS DUE TO PHYSICAL AND CHEMICAL AGENTS

This subject has been discussed in detail previously (see sections concerning acute toxic gastritis and chronic antral gastritis, as well as Chapter 11). The major points related to the action of physical agents on the stomach follow.

RADIATION EFFECTS AND DAMAGE

Patients with severe peptic ulcer disease who are poor surgical candidates have occasionally received gastric irradiation in an attempt to reduce the number of parietal cells (272, 273). The dose is in the order of 1500 rad and the gastric injury is typically confined to the mucosa, revealing patchy or confluent areas of active gastritis and a partial reduction of the specialized glands in the fundic-corpus region. No other distinctive histologic features are noted and complications rarely develop. Patients may experience mild abdominal pain, and the gastritis can be readily seen by endoscopy and biopsy. Because the inflammatory features are entirely nonspecific, the cause of the gastritis in these cases and its distinction from the other common forms of active gastritis depend on available clinical information.

More extensive gastric damage can occur when radiation doses of 4500 rad or more are applied, alone or in conjunction with chemotherapy, for the treatment of tumors of the stomach or contiguous tissues (274, 275). The acute phase is associated with prominent edema and inflammation of the mucosa and submucosa with the development of focal erosions and sloughing of the mucosal layer. Transient obstruction from the swelling may ensue in the cardiac or pyloric regions (276). These superficial lesions usually subside without sequelae over a period of a few weeks. In some cases, gastric damage persists or recurs, with the formation of deeper ulcers that are more often in the antrum and may simulate a chronic peptic ulcer. These lesions can develop months to years after the initial radiation exposure and are thought to be mediated by damage to the vessels in the gastric wall and perigastric tissues.

The histologic findings noted in this later (subacute or chronic) phase of radiation disease include the nonspecific findings of necrosis and inflammatory cells and also the more distinctive features associated with radiation (275): a marked amount of granulation tissue and fibrosis in the submucosa that appears to be in excess of that expected from the ulcer extent; the presence of atypical fibroblasts and endothelial cells with enlarged and variably hyperchromatic nuclei (Fig. 23.24); and vascular changes consisting of any combination of an active endarteritis, thrombosis, intimal thickening, and fibrotic occlusion. Endoscopy and mucosal biopsy are often performed to distinguish among radiation or drug-induced lesions, opportunistic infections, and recurrent tumor. The diagnosis of radiation effects and disease of the stomach may be suggested by the histologic features, but also depends on the clinical history and the exclusion of other conditions.

GASTRIC FREEZING

In an attempt to reduce acid secretion, iced solutions were formerly instilled into the gastric lumen (277–279). This procedure resulted in a patchy or diffuse hemorrhagic necrosis of the mucosa and a variable but transient fall in the gastric acid concentration. It was never established whether the decreased acid was due to a reversible loss of the parietal cells or to an exaggerated back diffusion of acid through the inflamed mucosa. The mucosa healed promptly without sustained benefit to the patients. This procedure is no longer used.

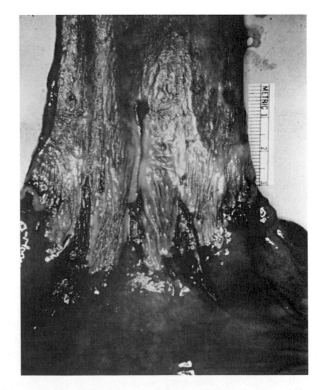

Figure 23.23   Segment of esophagus *(top)* and stomach from a patient with the Mallory-Weiss syndrome. Several longitudinal tears of the mucosa straddle the esophagocardiac junction.

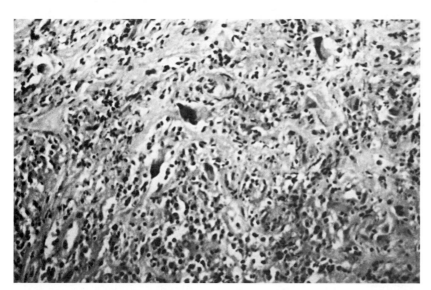

Figure 23.24 Gastric tissue in a case of radiation-induced injury. There is marked fibrosis and the presence of enlarged atypical nuclei in the mesenchymal cells (H & E, ×200).

EOSINOPHILIC GASTRITIS

The two major types of eosinophilic gastroenteritis (280) are a mucosal form, which has an allergic basis and has also been called allergic gastroenteritis (281), and a rare mural form (282). The stomach is often affected in patients with either of these conditions. Indeed, the antral mucosa is so often involved in the allergic cases that mucosal biopsy of this area is recommended to help establish the diagnosis (283) (see Chapter 12).

GASTRITIS ASSOCIATED WITH MOTOR AND MECHANICAL DISORDERS

This subject was addressed in detail in Chapter 13. The secondary inflammatory changes that complicate some of the conditions are highlighted in the following discussion.

CONGENITAL PYLORIC STENOSIS

The infants with this disorder may develop a nonspecific inflammation of the gastric mucosa as a result of obstruction and distention of the gastric lumen. Following diagnosis and surgical therapy, the mucosa reverts to normal and no complications occur. Some infant patients with allergic gastritis develop marked swelling and obstruction of the distal antrum, and this condition must be distinguished from the congenital type of pyloric obstruction (284) (see Chapters 10 and 12 for further details about congenital and allergic diseases).

DIVERTICULA OF THE STOMACH

Two major types of diverticula are noted in the stomach (285). The more common pulsion form is usually located on the posterior wall of the proximal stomach near the cardia and is thought to result from a localized congenital weakness of the wall in that area. Some mild chronic inflammation in the diverticular mucosa may be seen, but patients typically are asymptomatic. Rarely, patients develop a blockage of the diverticulum that leads to greater and active inflammation and requires surgical excision. The other type of diverticulum is found in the antrum in conjunction with a deep penetrating peptic ulcer or tumor and is invariably inflamed.

BEZOARS

Bezoars include a variety of plant products, hair, foods (such as partially digested citrus fruits), collections of drug capsules, fungal balls, and other foreign objects that might be ingested or accidentally retained after an endoscopic procedure (286, 287). The development of a large mass from the bezoar and its retention in the stomach is favored by poor digestion and is seen more often in edentulous patients and individuals who have undergone partial gastrectomy (288). Gastric inflammation usually results from the impaction of these objects on the mucosal surface leading to ulceration and rare perforation. Obstruction can occur, resulting in gastric dilation and secondary mucosal damage.

GASTRIC ATONY

A prominent dilation of the stomach can be observed in patients with various endocrine diseases and motor disorders such as systemic sclerosis. The lesion is more frequent and may be especially pronounced in patients with diabetes mellitus. This dilation results in an abdominal mass that can be appreciated by physical examination and confirmed by a radiographic flat plate. If the lesion is not decompressed, the elevated pressure can cause a hemorrhagic necrosis and inflammation of the mucosa and gastric wall, with the potential for perforation.

GASTRITIS ASSOCIATED WITH VASCULAR DISEASES

Necrosis and variable inflammation can result from diseases of the major vessels and microcirculation of the stomach (Table 23.7). Causes include ordinary ischemic disease (289, 290) and volvulus, which are uncommon in the stomach, and the effects of vasculitis and of atheromatous and foreign body emboli (291, 292) (see Chapter 14 for further details). The acute stress-induced lesions are also believed to have a vascular basis (see Chapter 24). Localized gastric ulcers with marked epithelial atypia are noted in some patients who receive instillation of chemotherapeutic agents into their hepatic arteries for the treatment of hepatic tumors (293–296).

GASTRIC ANTRAL VASCULAR ECTASIA

This rare form of gastritis is characterized by the presence of both inflammatory and vascular components in the mucosa (297–300). Most cases occur in older women. Patients typically present with chronic bleeding and iron deficiency anemia. The lesion is localized to the antral region and gross endoscopic examination reveals prominent longitudinal folds, which have striking red streaks; this appearance has been likened to the rind of a watermelon and called the "watermelon stomach." The histologic features in the mucosa are distinctive, revealing not only inflammatory cells but also an increase in the amount of fibromuscular stroma and numerous dilated blood vessels, many of which contain recent and organizing thrombi (Fig. 23.25). Other findings include congestion of the submucosal vessels, but no evidence of a vascular malformation, based on angiographic and morphologic examinations. The enlarged mucosal folds result from hypertrophy of the surface-foveolar mucous cells, and these areas also contain the prominent stroma and ectatic vessels. In some cases, thickening of the muscularis propria and/or a prolapse of the hypertrophied folds into the duodenum are observed. The lesions are treated by endoscopic cautery (301), and antral resection is not ordinarily required.

TABLE	
23.7	**Vascular Diseases of the Stomach**

Ischemic disease
Stress lesions
Small vessel diseases
   Vasculitis
   Atheromatous and foreign body emboli
   Amyloidosis
Vascular malformations
   Congestive gastropathy
   Gastric antral vascular ectasia
   Angiodysplasia
   Dieulafoy disease

The diagnosis of gastric antral vascular ectasia is based on the typical endoscopic and biopsy appearances of the mucosa, together with a compatible clinical history. In more common cases of chronic antral gastritis, the amount of fibromuscular stroma in the lamina propria is enhanced, but fewer dilated blood vessels are noted and thrombi are absent. Other conditions that can be associated with prominent mucosal thickening and the appearance of folds in the antral region are gastritis due to allergic and granulomatous diseases and infiltrative tumors, all of which have distinguishing histologic features. In Menetrier disease, the big folds are confined to the fundic-corpus region.

OTHER VASCULAR LESIONS

Large gastric varices commonly develop as a result of portal hypertension, and these cases are sometimes associated with a more widespread small vessel ectasia in the mucosa of the stomach, termed congestive gastropathy, and of other parts of the gut (302–305). A similar ectasia, consisting of dilated venules in the mucosa, is also seen in patients receiving hemodialysis or following bone marrow transplantation (306). In gastric angiodysplasia, an arteriovenous aneurysm or malformation is primarily located in the submucosa (307–309); the lesions are often multiple, found in any part of the stomach, and identified by angiographic study. Arterial aneurysms, known also as Dieulafoy disease, occur more often in younger patients, are usually present in the proximal stomach, and cause a localized ulceration (310–312). In the larger vascular lesions, the episodes of hemorrhage are often massive and demand early surgical correction.

GRANULOMATOUS DISEASES OF THE STOMACH

The major granulomatous disorders affecting the stomach are sarcoidosis, Crohn disease, infections, foreign body reactions, and isolated disease (313, 314). These conditions generally involve the antral region and are often associated with prominent mucosal and mural thickening that can simulate the gross appearance of a malignancy. The patients typically present with signs of gastritis and/or pyloric obstruction. The diagnosis of a granulomatous lesion is provided by mucosal biopsy examination.

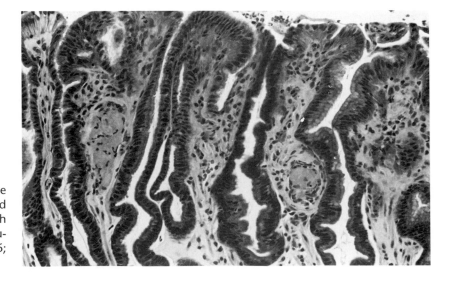

Figure 23.25 Gastric antral vascular ectasia. The lamina propria shows venules that are distended with thrombi (H & E, ×635). (Reproduced with permission from Goldman H. Gastrointestinal mucosal biopsy. New York: Churchill Livingstone, 1996; 95–159.)

Gastric infections that commonly contain distinct granulomas include tuberculosis and histoplasmosis, but we currently see many more cases that are attributable to M. avium in immunocompromised patients (see previous discussion of infections of the stomach). Foreign body granulomas may result from a variety of substances, such as suture material, talc, or starch that may be introduced during a surgical procedure; barium from a radiographic study; extravasated mucus in inflammatory and neoplastic conditions; and, surprisingly, even cereal products (313–316). The usually small foreign body lesions can be multiple and located in any part of the gastric wall from the mucosal to the serosal layers. It is now appreciated that sarcoidosis only rarely involves the stomach or other regions of the alimentary tract, and its diagnosis depends on finding concomitant disease in a more characteristic location, such as the lungs and hilar lymph nodes. In addition to a general discussion of granulomatous disorders affecting the gut, details about foreign body reactions and sarcoidosis as well as the rare effects of malakoplakia and chronic granulomatous disease of childhood in the stomach, are found in Chapters 19 and 30.

CROHN DISEASE OF THE STOMACH

In patients with established Crohn disease of the distal small intestine and the colon, microscopic alterations are noted in the gastric mucosa in about one quarter to one half of the cases (317, 318). These changes are detected in mucosal biopsy samples and consist of patchy areas of active gastritis and granulomas. Patients typically lack any symptoms referable to the gastritis, and the finding of these features does not predict that they will develop clinically significant disease in this area.

Uncommonly, Crohn disease of the intestine is associated with more major evidence of gastric involvement, characterized by the presence of single or multiple ulcers that are concentrated in the antrum and of deep mural fissures (319, 321). Granulomas without necrosis are seen in about 50% of cases (see Fig. 29.45). Also often noted is involvement of the contiguous duodenum, and these patients experience pain, bleeding, and signs of pyloric obstruction. Occasionally, the stomach is secondarily affected by a fistula that extends from a diseased area of intestine; in such cases, the gastric inflammation is minimal and is confined to the area of the fistulous opening. Isolated Crohn disease of the stomach is extremely rare, and one should be wary of making this diagnosis until intestinal disease has been demonstrated.

The diagnosis of Crohn disease of the stomach, alone or in conjunction with duodenal disease, is ordinarily suggested by the clinical history of known intestinal involvement and by the radiographic features and is supported by biopsy-proven evidence of granulomas of the inflamed areas. In the common cases of chronic peptic disease, the ulcers typically are single and no fissures or granulomas are present. The morphologic features of Crohn disease may be identical to those seen in gastric or gastroduodenal tuberculosis, and the distinction depends on the clinical history and, if needed, on culture of the lesion. The granulomas in tuberculosis may or may not show caseation, and positive stains for the tubercle bacilli are generally positive only in those cases with caseation. In isolated granulomatous gastritis, no ulceration is present and the duodenum is not affected (see Chapter 29 for additional details).

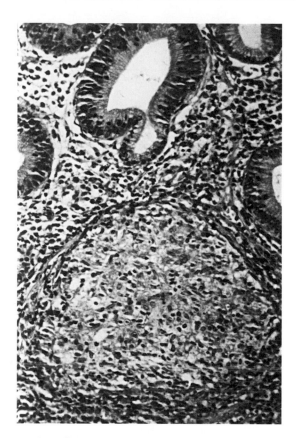

Figure 23.26 Gastric antral mucosa in a case of isolated granulomatous gastritis. A well-formed granuloma without necrosis is evident in the lamina propria *(bottom)* (H & E, ×200).

ISOLATED GRANULOMATOUS GASTRITIS

This uncommon disorder of unknown etiology is characterized by the presence of a granulomatous inflammation of the gastric antrum (322–326). It appears to be limited to the stomach and is not associated with disease in other parts of the gut or body tissues. Older persons are most often affected. Patients typically present with signs of gastritis and/or pyloric obstruction. The gastric mucosa and wall are thickened, and the radiographic and gross endoscopic appearances raise the suspicion of a tumor. Histologic study reveals numerous noncaseating granulomas that are concentrated in the mucosa (Fig. 23.26), neutrophils and increased mononuclear inflammatory cells in the intervening lamina propria, and a variable amount of hyperplasia of the surface-foveolar mucous cells (see Fig. 19.15). Typically, no ulceration is found. Additional radiographic studies of the lungs and intestines are performed to exclude more generalized granulomatous diseases. Considering the rarity of granulomatous infection in this area, culture of the gastric lesion usually is not performed. The disease is self-limited and resolves after a period of several weeks to months, without the development of a chronic gastritis or other sequelae. Although corticosteroid therapy has been used occasionally, most patients require only symptomatic relief.

The diagnosis of isolated granulomatous gastritis depends on the finding of granulomas without necrosis in a mucosal biopsy of the antrum, on the absence of more destructive lesions, such as ulcers and fissures; on negative stains for microorganisms; and on

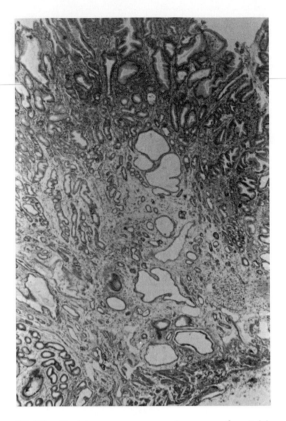

Figure 23.27   Gastric corpus mucosa in a case of gastritis cystica profunda, with luminal surface at top and small fragment of muscularis mucosae at bottom right. This condition affected the proximal gastric remnant near the stoma following a distal gastric resection. Expansion of the mucosa is mainly attributable to foveolar hyperplasia; many of the glands are cystic. There is also edema and inflammation of the lamina propria and an absence of the specialized corpus glands (H & E, ×13).

the exclusion of the other granulomatous diseases that can affect the stomach. Patients with sarcoidosis or Crohn disease usually are younger and have lesions in other more characteristic sites. Furthermore, patients with Crohn disease may have ulcers or mural fissures and involvement of the duodenum. Any of the common diseases of the antrum, such as chronic antral gastritis and chronic peptic ulcer, may be associated with a rare granuloma that is probably of the foreign body type. Perhaps the most difficult diagnosis to distinguish is a case of gastric tuberculosis that involves no apparent disease in the lungs and other parts of the gut and in which the granulomas are noncaseating and stain negatively for microorganisms. Accordingly, gastric tissue is obtained by repeat biopsy for specific culture in situations in which the patient seems unusually ill, has any other suspicious feature (such as a history of pulmonary disease, a positive tuberculin skin test, or exposure to a tuberculous patient), or fails to improve.

GASTRITIS CYSTICA PROFUNDA

Gastritis cystica profunda is a rare condition in which mature glandular epithelium extends into the tissues beneath the muscularis mucosae (327–330). It is analogous to similar conditions affecting the small and large intestines that are called respectively enteritis and colitis cystica profunda. The gastric lesion seems to be less common and usually is seen in association with an inflammatory lesion of the mucosa, such as in cases of chronic gastritis. This condition has been produced experimentally in rodents by administering high doses of salicylates, but no evidence exists to incriminate these or any other drugs in human cases. The glands typically extend into the upper part of the submucosa and rarely into the deeper parts of the gastric wall (Fig. 23.27). They usually are composed of cystic pyloric glands, which may show slight inflammation and signs of regeneration but no dysplasia of the epithelium (Fig. 23.28). The cystic change in the glands is also often noted in the mucosa. The natural course of these lesions is not known.

The most pronounced examples of this lesion have been noted in the region of the gastric stoma in patients who have had a gastroenterostomy (327). A frequent association is prominent polypoid hyperplasia of the mucosal foveolar cells, resulting in a mass lesion; this mass must be distinguished from carcinoma, which can also develop in the gastric stump of such patients (166–170). Indeed, the actual coexistence of gastritis cystica and adenocarcinoma has been noted (331, 332), and surgical resection is required in such cases.

The diagnosis of gastritis cystica is based on the identification of normal or regenerative epithelium in the misplaced glands in

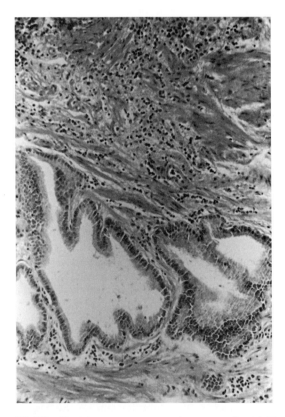

Figure 23.28   Gastric corpus mucosa in a case of gastritis cystic profunda. There is the presence of cystic glands containing mature foveolar epithelium, and associated mononuclear inflammatory cells, in the region of the disrupted muscularis mucosae (fragments at upper right and at bottom) (H & E, ×200). Contrast with dysplastic epithelium in Figure 23.20.

contrast to the expected dysplasia and prominent stroma in an invasive carcinoma. Hamartomatous polyps associated with the Peutz-Jeghers syndrome may show extension of mature glands into the gastric wall, but these polyps are multiple and involve the small intestine to a greater extent. Other conditions, such as some foreign body reactions, emphysematous gastritis, and post-mortem autolysis, can produce irregular spaces in the submucosa that may vaguely resemble dilated glandular lumina, although such spaces are readily distinguished by their lack of mucin and epithelial cell lining.

OTHER CONDITIONS

An increase in intraepithelial lymphocytes, largely representing T cells, within the surface and foveolar epithelium can be seen in association with several disorders. In the corpus and fundus, this increase is a major feature of cases of chronic erosive or varioliform gastritis (see previous discussion of lymphocytic gastritis) (146). Within the antrum, the presence of the lymphocytes is less specific and can be seen in both H. pylori infection and celiac disease (149–152). The gastric infiltrate in association with celiac disease is closely linked with the same finding in the small intestine, showing resolution following gluten withdrawal and return of the inflammation after rechallenge.

Xanthoma (or xanthelasma) of the stomach was discussed in the section concerning complications of chronic gastritis, and the topics of graft-versus-host disease (333, 334) and pseudolymphoma (335) are included in Chapters 16 and 17. The inflammatory effects of uremia (336, 337) and of amyloidosis (338, 339) as well as of other metabolic and endocrine disorders that can affect the stomach are detailed in Chapter 19.

A single case of chronic active gastritis in a child, in whom a gastric biopsy revealed pronounced fibrosis in the upper and midportions of the mucosa has been reported (340). This condition was termed "collagenous gastritis," but there was no relationship between this case and collagenous sprue or collagenous colitis. The cause of the gastritis and the significance of the collagen deposition are not known.

MUCOSAL BIOPSY

Endoscopy and mucosal biopsy of the stomach are being performed with increasing frequency to evaluate patients with gastritis and gastric ulcers (4, 32–34, 225, 341–343). The biopsies can assist in the diagnosis of gastritis and its various forms, in monitoring patients after therapy, and in the detection of complications. The technical aspects and overall discussion of the endoscopic procedure are presented in Chapter 3.

A relatively poor correlation is noted between the gross endoscopic appearances and the histologic findings in cases of acute and of active chronic gastritis, particularly in those that lack overt erosions (26, 27, 344). Accordingly, if an endoscopic study is performed in a patient with suspected gastritis but reveals only nonerosive changes, such as patchy erythema or small hemorrhages of the mucosa, biopsy should be performed to seek more certain evidence of inflammation. Cases of both acute toxic gastritis and of the active phase of a chronic gastritis reveal some mixture of necrosis, a neutrophilic reaction, and regenerative glands, and H. pylori can be readily detected. Biopsy can also assist in establishing chronic disease by noting some combination of a an increase in

mononuclear cells and the presence of lymphoid nodules in the lamina propria, of a loss of the specialized glands, and of the appearance of intestinal metaplasia. Biopsy is less helpful in establishing the stage of chronic disease, whether superficial or atrophic, because the degree of histologic damage in various biopsies can vary considerably. Even if multiple tissue samples are obtained, the results usually are still not as sensitive or reliable as the use of functional tests in the determination of the atrophic stage, especially in cases of the fundic type.

Mucosal biopsy of the stomach may suggest or provide support for the diagnosis of some of the less common causes of gastritis, such as other infections, allergic disease, and the granulomatous conditions. Involvement of the gastric antrum is noted in practically all cases of allergic gastroenteritis, revealing a prominent infiltrate of eosinophils, and mucosal biopsy of this area is recommended in the evaluation of such cases. Patients with long-standing chronic gastritis have an increased risk for the development of gastric tumors, and surveillance endoscopy with mucosal biopsy is often performed, especially in countries with a relatively high baseline incidence of carcinoma. These biopsies distinguish between hyperplastic (regenerative) polyps and adenomas and identify areas of dysplasia and early gastric carcinoma. Furthermore, biopsy may help in detecting the early development of lymphoma in patients with H. pylori infection.

REFERENCES

1. Palmer ED. Gastritis: A reevaluation. Medicine 1954;33:199.
2. Owen DA. Gastritis and duodenitis. In: Appleman HD, ed. Pathology of the esophagus, stomach, and duodenum. New York: Churchill Livingstone, 1984:37–77.
3. Appelman HD. Gastritis: Terminology, etiology, and clinicopathological correlations: another biased view. Hum Pathol 1994;25:1006–1019.
4. Goldman H. Gastrointestinal mucosal biopsy. New York: Churchill Livingstone, 1996;95–159.
5. Strickland RG, Mackay IR. A reappraisal of the nature and significance of chronic atrophic gastritis. Am J Dig Dis 1973;18:426.
6. Dagredi AE, Lee ER, Bosco DL, et al. The clinical spectrum of hemorrhagic erosive gastritis. Am J Gastroenterol 1973;60:30.
7. Weinstein WM. The diagnosis and classification of gastritis and duodenitis. J Clin Gastroenterol 1981;3(Suppl 2):7–16.
8. Cooke AR. Drug damage to the gastroduodenum. In: Sleisenger MH, Fordtran JS, eds. Gastrointestinal disease, 2nd ed. Philadelphia: WB Saunders, 1978:807–826.
9. Gottfried EB, Korsten MA, Lieber CS. Alcohol-induced gastric and duodenal lesions in man. Am J Gastroenterol 1978;70:587–592.
10. Valencia-Parparcen J. Alcoholic gastritis. Clin Gastroenterol 1981;10:389.
11. Laine L, Weinstein WM. Histology of alcoholic hemorrhagic "gastritis": A prospective evaluation. Gastroenterology 1988;94:1254–1262.
12. Langman MJS. Epidemiological evidence for the association of aspirin and acute gastrointestinal bleeding. Gut 1970;11:627.
13. Metzger WH, McAdam L, Bluestone R, Guth PH. Acute gastric mucosal injury during continuous or interrupted aspirin ingestion in humans. Am J Dig Dis 21:1976;963–968.
14. Graham DY, Smith JL. Gastroduodenal complications of chronic NSAID therapy. Am J Gastroenterol 1988;83:1081–1084.
15. Allison MC, Howatson AG, Torrance CJ, et al. Gastrointestinal damage associated with the use of nonsteroidal anti-inflammatory drugs. N Engl J Med 1992;327:749–754.
16. Henry D, Dobson A, Turner C. Variability in the risk of major gastrointestinal complications from non-aspirin non-steroidal anti-inflammatory drugs. Gastroenterology 1993;105:1078–1088.
17. Mann NS. Bile-induced acute erosive gastritis. Its prevention by

antacid, cholestyramine, and prostaglandin E2. Am J Dig Dis 1976;21:89–92.

18. Meshkinpour H, Marks JW, Schoenfield LJ, et al. Reflux gastritis syndrome: Mechanism of symptoms. Gastroenterology 1980; 79:1283.

19. Dixon MF, O'Connor HJ, Axon ATR, et al. Reflux gastritis: A distinct histopathological entity? J Clin Pathol 1986;39:524–530.

20. Niemela S, Kaittunen T, Heikkila J, et al. Characteristics of bile gastritis. Scand J Gastroenterol 1987;22:345–354.

21. Smith BM. Permeability of the human gastric mucosa: Alteration by acetylsalicylic acid and ethanol. N Engl J Med 1971;285:216.

22. Robert A. Cytoprotection by prostaglandins. Gastroenterology 1979;77:761.

23. Marshall BJ, Armstrong JA, McGechie DB, Glancy RJ. An attempt to fulfill Koch's postulates for pyloric Campylobacter. Med J Austr 1985;142:436–439.

24. Myren J, Serck-Hanssen A. The gastroscopic diagnosis of gastritis with particular reference to mucosal reddening and mucus covering. Scand J Gastroenterol 1974;9:457–462.

25. Carpenter HA, Talley NJ. Gastroscopy is incomplete without biopsy: Clinical relevance of distinguishing gastropathy from gastritis. Gastroenterology 1995;108:917–924.

26. Elta GH, Appelman HD, Behler EM, et al. A study of the correlation between endoscopic and histological diagnoses in gastroduodenitis. Am J Gastroenterol 1987;82:749–753.

27. Laine L, Weinstein WM. Subepithelial hemorrhages and erosions of human stomach. Dig Dis Sci 1988;33:490–503.

28. Quinn CM, Bjarnason I, Price AB. Gastritis in patients on non-steroidal anti-inflammatory drugs. Histopathology 1993;23: 341–348.

29. Kreunig J, Bosman FT, Kuiper G, et al. Gastric and duodenal mucosa in "healthy" individuals: An endoscopic and histological study of 50 volunteers. J Clin Pathol 1978;31:69.

30. McDonald WC. Correlation of mucosal histology and aspirin intake in chronic gastric ulcer. Gastroenterology 1973;65:381.

31. Hamilton SR, Yardley JH. Endoscopic biopsy diagnosis of aspirin-associated chronic gastric ulcers. Gastroenterology 1980;78:1178.

32. Joske RA, Finckh ES, Wood IJ. Gastric biopsy: a study of 1000 consecutive successful gastric biopsies. Quart J Med 1955;24: 269–294.

33. MacDonald WC, Rubin CE. Gastric biopsy—a critical evaluation. Gastroenterology 1967;53:143–170.

34. Whitehead SC, Truelove SC, Gear MWL. The histological diagnosis of chronic gastritis in fiberoptic gastroscope biopsy specimens. J Clin Pathol 1972;25:1.

35. Yardley JH. Pathology of chronic gastritis and duodenitis. In: Goldman H, Appelman HD, Kaufman N, eds. Gastrointestinal pathology. Baltimore: Williams & Wilkins, 1990:69–143.

36. Dixon MF, Genta RM, Yardley JH, et al. Classification and grading of gastritis. Am J Surg Pathol 1996;20:1161–1181.

37. Doglioni C, Laurino L, Dei Tos A, et al. Pancreatic (acinar) metaplasia of the gastric mucosa. Histology, ultrastructure, immunocytochemistry, and clinicopathologic correlations of 101 cases. Am J Surg Pathol 1993;17:1134–1143.

38. Wang HH, Zeroogian JM, Speckler SJ, et al. Prevalence and significance of pancreatic acinar metaplasia at the gastroesophageal junction. Am J Surg Pathol 1996;20:1507–1510.

39. Ihamaki T, Sankkonen M, Siurala M. Long term observation of subjects with normal mucosa and superficial gastritis: results of 23–27 years follow-up examinations. Scand J Gastroenterol 1978;13:771.

40. Cheli R, Giacosa A. Chronic atrophic gastritis and gastric mucosal atrophy—one and same. Gastrointest Endosc 1983;29:23–25.

41. Stemmermann GN. Intestinal metaplasia of the stomach. A status report. Cancer 1994;74:556–564.

42. Goldman H, Ming SC. Fine structure of intestinal metaplasia and adenocarcinoma of the human stomach. Lab Invest 1968; 18:203.

43. Stockton M, McCall I. Comparative electron microscopic features of normal, intermediate and metaplastic pyloric epithelium. Histopathology 1983;7:859–871.

44. Planteydt HT, Willighagen RGJ. Enzyme histochemistry of the human stomach with special reference to intestinal metaplasia. J Pathol 1960;80:713–722.

45. Matsukura N, Suzuki K, Kawachi T, et al. Distribution of marker enzymes and mucin in intestinal metaplasia of the stomach and relation of complete and incomplete types of metaplasia to minute gastric cancer. J Natl Cancer Inst 1980;65:231–236.

46. Goldman H, Ming SC. Mucins in normal and metaplastic gastrointestinal epithelium: Histochemical distribution. Arch Pathol Lab Med 1968;85:580.

47. Gad A. A histochemical study of human alimentary tract mucosubstances in health and disease. II. Inflammatory conditions. Br J Cancer 1969;23:64.

48. Jass JR, Filipe MI. The mucin profiles of normal gastric mucosa, intestinal metaplasia and its variants and gastric carcinoma. Histochem J 1981;13:931–939.

49. Iida F, Murata F, Nagata T. Histochemical studies of mucosubstances in metaplastic epithelium of the stomach with special reference to the development of intestinal metaplasia. Histochemistry 1978;56:229–237.

50. Teglbjaerg PS, Nielson HO. "Small intestinal type" and "colonic type" intestinal metaplasia of the human stomach. Acta Pathol Microbiol Scand 1978(A);86:351.

51. Segura DI, Montero C. Histochemical characterization of different types of intestinal metaplasia in gastric mucosa. Cancer 1983;52: 498–503.

52. Rubin W, Ross LL, Jeffries GH, et al. Some physiologic properties of heterotopic intestinal epithelium. Lab Invest 1967;16:813.

53. Siurala M, Tarpila S. Absorptive function of intestinal metaplasia of the stomach. Scand J Gastroenterol 1968;3:75.

54. Bordi C, Ravazzola M. Endocrine cells in the intestinal metaplasia of gastric mucosa. Am J Pathol 1979;90:391–395.

55. Filipe MI, Potet F, Bogomoletz WV, et al. Incomplete sulphomucin-secreting intestinal metaplasia for gastric cancer. Preliminary data from a prospective study from three centres. Gut 1985;26: 1319–1326.

56. Morson BC. Carcinoma arising from areas of intestinal metaplasia in the gastric mucosa. Br J Cancer 1955;9:377–385.

57. Lauren P. The two histological main types of gastric carcinoma: Diffuse and so-called intestinal type carcinoma. An attempt at a histoclinical classification. Acta Pathol Microbiol Scand 1965;64: 31–49.

58. Ming SC, Goldman H, Freiman DG. Intestinal metaplasia and histogenesis of carcinoma in human stomach: Light and electron microscopic study. Cancer 1967;20:1418.

59. Jass JR, Filipe MI. A variant of intestinal metaplasia associated with gastric carcinoma: A histochemical study. Histopathology 1979;3: 191–199.

60. Sipponen P, Seppa"la" K, Varis K, Hjelt L, et al. Intestinal metaplasia with colonic-type sulphomucins in the gastric mucosa; its association with gastric carcinoma. Acta Pathol Microbiol Scand 1980;A88: 217–224.

61. Iida F, Kusama J. Gastric carcinoma and intestinal metaplasia. Significance of types of intestinal metaplasia upon development of gastric carcinoma. Cancer 1982;50:2854–2858.

62. Lei D-N, Yu J-Y. Types of mucosal metaplasia in relation to the histogenesis of gastric carcinoma. Arch Pathol Lab Med 1984;108: 220–224.

63. Turoni H, Lurie B, Chaimoff CH, et al. The diagnostic significance of sulfated acid mucin content in gastric intestinal metaplasia with early gastric cancer. Am J Gastroenterol 1986;81:343–345.

64. Huang C-B, Xu J, Huang J-F, et al. Sulphomucin colonic type intestinal metaplasia and carcinoma in the stomach. A histochemical study of 115 cases obtained by biopsy. Cancer 1986;57: 1370–1375.

65. Parl FF, Lev R, Thomas E, et al. Histologic and morphometric study of chronic gastritis in alcoholic patients. Hum Pathol 1979; 40:45.

66. Cheli R, Giacosa A, Molinari F. Chronic atrophic gastritis and duodenogastric reflux. Scand J Gastroenterol 1981;16 (Suppl. 67):125.

67. Emmanouilidis A, Nicolopoulou-Stamati P, Manousos O. The histologic pattern of bile gastritis. Gastrointest Endosc 1984;30: 179–182.

68. Myers BM, Smith JL, Graham DY. Effect of red pepper and black pepper on the stomach. Am J Gastroenterol 1987;82:211–214.

69. Steer HW. Ultrastructure of cell migration through the gastric epithelium and its relationship to bacteria. J Clin Pathol 1975;28:639–646.

70. Warren JR, Marshall BJ. Unidentified curved bacilli on gastric epithelium in active chronic gastritis. Lancet 1983;1:1273.

71. Jones DM, Lessells AM, Eldridge J. Campylobacter-like organisms in the gastric mucosa: Culture, histological and serological studies. J Clin Pathol 1984;37:1002.

72. Johnston BJ, Reed PI, Ali MH. Campylobacter-like organisms in duodenal and antral endoscopic biopsies: Relationship to inflammation. Gut 1986;27:1132–1137.

73. Taylor DE, Hargreaves JA, Lai-King NG, et al. Isolation and characterization of Campylobacter pyloridis from gastric biopsies. Am J Clin Pathol 1987;87:49–54.

74. Drumna B, Sherman P, Cutz E, et al. Association of Campylobacter pylori on the gastric mucosa with antral gastritis in children. N Engl J Med 1987;316:1557–1561.

75. Pettross CW, Appelman MD, Cohen H, et al. Prevalence of Campylobacter pylori and association with antral mucosal histology in subjects with and without upper gastrointestinal symptoms. Dig Dis Sci 1988;33:649–653.

76. Marshall BJ. Helicobacter pylori. Am J Gastroenterol 1994;89:S116–S128.

77. Leung KM, Hui PK, Chan WY, et al. Helicobacter pylori-related gastritis and gastric ulcer. A continuum of progressive epithelial degeneration. Am J Clin Pathol 1992;98:569–574.

78. Barbosa AJA, Queiroz DMR, Mender EN, et al. Immunocytochemical identification of Campylobacter pylori in gastritis and correlation with culture. Arch Pathol Lab Med 1988;112:523–525.

79. Rathbone BJ, Wyatt JI, Worsley BW, et al. Systemic and local antibody response to gastric Campylobacter pyloridis in non-ulcer dyspepsia. Gut 1986;27:642–647.

80. Fabre R, Sobhani I, Laurent-Puig P, et al. Polymerase chain reaction assay for the detection of Helicobacter pylori in gastric biopsy specimens: Comparison with culture, rapid urease test, and histopathological tests. Gut 1994;35:905–908.

81. Karttunen TJ, Genta RM, Yaffe B, et al. Detection of Helicobacter pylori in paraffin-embedded gastric biopsy specimens by in situ hybridization. Am J Clin Pathol 1996;106:305–311.

82. Graham DY, Klein PD, Evans DJ Jr, et al. Campylobacter pylori detected noninvasively by the ^{13}C-urea breath test. Lancet 1987;1:1174–1177.

83. Montgomery EA, Martin DF, Peura DA. Rapid diagnosis of Campylobacter pylori by Gram stain. Am J Clin Pathol 1988;90:606–609.

84. Nichols L, Sughayer M, DeGirolami PC, et al. Evaluation of diagnostic methods for Helicobacter pylori gastritis. Am J Clin Pathol 1991;95:769–773.

85. Rollason TP, Stone J, Rhodes JM. Spiral organisms in endoscopic biopsies of the human stomach. J Clin Pathol 1984;37:23–26.

86. Price AB, Levi J, Dolby JM, et al. Campylobacter pyloridis in peptic ulcer disease: Microbiology, pathology, and scanning electron microscopy. Gut 1985;26:1183–1188.

87. Chen XG, Correa P, Offerhaus J, et al. Ultrastructure of the gastric mucosa harboring Campylobacter-like organisms. Am J Clin Pathol 1986;86:575–582.

88. Caselli M, Aleotti A, Boldrini P, et al. Ultrastructural patterns of Helicobacter pylori. Gut 1993;34:1507–1509.

89. Dooley CP, Cohen H, Fitzgibbons PL, et al. Prevalence of Helicobacter pylori infection and histologic gastritis in asymptomatic persons. N Engl J Med 1989;321:1562–1566.

90. Rathbone BJ, Wyatt JI, Heatley RV. Campylobacter pyloridis—A new factor in peptic ulcer disease. Gut 1986;27:635–641.

91. Blaser MJ. Gastric Campylobacter-like organisms, gastritis, and peptic ulcer disease. Gastroenterology 1987;93:371–383.

92. NIH Consensus Conference. Helicobacter pylori in peptic ulcer disease. JAMA 1994;272:65–69.

93. Frierson HF, Caldwell SH, Marshall BJ. Duodenal biopsy findings for patients with non-ulcer dyspepsia with or without Campylobacter pylori gastritis. Mod Pathol 1990;3:271–276.

94. Noach LA, Rolf TM, Bosma NB, et al. Gastric metaplasia and Helicobacter pylori infection. Gut 1993;34:1510–1514.

95. Paull G, Yardley JH. Gastric and esophageal Campylobacter pylori in patients with Barrett's esophagus. Gastroenterology 1988;95:216–218.

96. Loffeld RJ, Ten Tije BJ, Arends JW. Prevalence and significance of Helicobacter pylori in patients with Barrett's esophagus. Am J Gastroenterol 1992;87:1598–1600.

97. Dye KR, Marshall BJ, Frierson HF, et al. Campylobacter pylori colonizing heterotopic gastric tissue in the rectum. Am J Clin Pathol 1990;3:144–147.

98. McNulty CAM, Gearty JC, Crump B, et al. Campylobacter pyloridis and associated gastritis. Investigator-blind, placebo-controlled trial of bismuth salicylate and erythromycin ethylsuccinate. Br Med J 1986;293:645.

99. Genta RM, Lew GM, Graham DY. Changes in the gastric mucosa following eradication of Helicobacter pylori. Mod Pathol 1993;6:281–289.

100. Sung JJY, Chung SCS, Ling TKW, et al. Antibacterial treatment of gastric ulcers associated with Helicobacter pylori. N Engl J Med 1995;332:139–142.

101. Graham DY, Alpert LC, Smith JL, et al. Iatrogenic Campylobacter pylori infection as a cause of epidemic achlorrhydria. Am J Gastroenterol 1988;83:974–980.

102. Morris A, Nicholson G. Ingestion of Campylobacter pyloridis causes gastritis and raised fasting gastric pH. Am J Gastroenterol 1987;82:192–199.

103. McNulty CAM, Dent JC, Curry A, et al. New spiral bacterium in gastric mucosa. J Clin Pathol 1989;42:585–591.

104. Morris A, Ali MR, Thomsen L, et al. Tightly spiral shaped bacteria in the human stomach: Another cause of active chronic gastritis? Gut 1990;31:139–143.

105. Heilman KL, Borchard F. Gastritis due to spiral-shaped bacteria other than Helicobacter pylori: Clinical, histological, and ultrastructural findings. Gut 1991;32:137–140.

106. Oliva MM, Lazenby AJ, Perman JA. Gastritis associated with Gastrospirillum hominis in children. Comparison with Helicobacter pylori and review of the literature. Mod Pathol 1993;6:513–515.

107. Mazzucchelli L, Wildersmith CH, Ruchti C, et al. Gastrospirillum hominis in asymptomatic, healthy individuals. Dig Dis Sci 1993;38:2087–2090.

108. Hilzenrat N, Lamoureux E, Weintrub I, et al. Helicobacter heilmanii-like spiral bacteria in gastric mucosal biopsies. Prevalence and clinical significance. Arch Pathol Lab Med 1995;119:1149–1153.

109. Debongnie JC, Donnay M, Mairesse J. Gastrospirillum hominis ("Helicobacter heilmanii"): A cause of gastritis, sometimes transient, better diagnosed by touch cytology? Am J Gastroenterol 1995;90:411–416.

110. Wyatt JI. Histopathology of gastroduodenal inflammation: The impact of Helicobacter pylori. Histopathology 1995;26:1–15.

111. Genta RM, Hamner HW, Graham DY. Gastric lymphoid follicles in Helicobacter pylori infection: Frequency, distribution, and response to triple therapy. Hum Pathol 1993;24:577–583.

112. Eidt S, Stolte M. Prevalence of lymphoid follicles and aggregates in Helicobacter pylori gastritis. J Clin Pathol 1993;46:832–836.

113. Stamp GWH, Palmer K, Misiewicz JJ. Antral hypertrophic gastritis: A rare cause of iron deficiency. J Clin Pathol 1985;38:390–392.

114. Genta RM, Gurer IE, Graham DY, et al. Adherence of Helicobacter pylori to areas of incomplete intestinal metaplasia in the gastric mucosa. Gastroenterology 1996;111:1206–1211.

115. Glass GBJ, Pitchumoni CS. Atrophic gastritis. Hum Pathol 1975;6:219.

116. Chisholm M. Immunology of gastritis. Clin Gastroenterol 1976;5:419.

117. Coghill NF, Doniach D, Roitt IM, et al. Autoantibodies in simple atrophic gastritis. Gut 1965;6:48.

118. Wright R, Whitehead R, Wangel AG, et al. Autoantibodies and microscopic appearance of gastric mucosa. Lancet 1966;1:618–621.

119. Doniach D, Roitt IM, Taylor KB. Autoimmune phenomena in pernicious anaemia. Serologic overlap with thyroiditis, thyrotoxicosis, and systemic lupus erythematosus. Br Med J 1963;1:1374.

120. Lillibridge CA, Brandborg LL, Rubin CE. Childhood pernicious anaemia. Gastrointestinal secretory histological and electron microscopic aspects. Gastroenterology 1967;52:792.

121. Irvine WJ, Cullen DR, Mawhinney H. Natural history of autoimmune achlorhydric atrophic gastritis. A 1–15 year follow-up study. Lancet 1974;2:482–485.

122. McGuigan JE, Trudeau WL. Serum gastrin concentrations in pernicious anaemia. N Engl J Med 1970;282:358–361.

123. Jeffries GH, Todd JE, Sleisenger MH. The effect of prednisolone on gastric mucosal histology, gastric secretion, and vitamin B12 absorption in patients with pernicious anemia. J Clin Invest 1966;45:803.

124. Cheli R, Santi L, Ciancamerla G, et al. A clinical and statistical follow-up study of atrophic gastritis. Am J Dig Dis 1973;18:1061–1066.

125. Siurala M, Lehtola J, Ihamaki T. Atrophic gastritis and its sequelae. Results of 19–23 years of follow-up examinations. Scand J Gastroenterol 1974;9:441–446.

126. Meshkinpour H, Orlando RA, Arguello JF, et al. Significance of endoscopically visible blood vessels as an index of atrophic gastritis. Am J Gastroenterol 1979;71:376.

127. Overholt BF, Jeffries GH. Hypertrophic hypersecretory protein-losing gastropathy. Gastroenterology 1970;58:80–87.

128. Meuwissen SGM, Ridwan BU, Hasper HJ, et al. Hypertrophic protein-losing gastropathy. A retrospective analysis of 40 cases in the Netherlands. Scand J Gastroenterol 1992;27 Suppl 194:1–80.

129. Lewin KJ, Dowling F, Wright JP, et al. Gastric morphology and serum gastrin levels in pernicious anemia. Gut 1976;17:551.

130. Rubin W. A fine structural characterization of the proliferated endocrine cells in atrophic gastric mucosa. Am J Pathol 1973;70:109.

131. Flejou JF, Bahame P, Smith AC, et al. Pernicious anemia and Campylobacter like organisms: Is the gastric antrum resistent to colonization? Gut 1989;30:60–64.

132. Scharschmidt BF. The natural history of hypertrophic gastropathy (Menetrier's disease). Am J Med 1977;63:644.

133. Simon L, Figus AI, Bajtai A. Chronic gastritis following resection of the stomach. Am J Gastroenterol 1973;60:477.

134. Sauktonen M, Sipponen P, Varis K, et al. Morphological and dynamic behavior of the gastric mucosa after partial gastrectomy with special reference to the gastroenterostomy area. Hepatogastroenterology 1980;27:48.

135. Bechi P, Amorosi A, Mazzanti R, et al. Gastric histology and fasting bile reflux after partial gastrectomy. Gastroenterology 1987;93:335–343.

136. Nogahata Y, Kawakita N, Azumi Y, et al. Etiological involvement of Helicobacter pylori in "reflux" gastritis after gastrectomy. Am J Gastroenterol 1996;91:2130–2134.

137. Hoare AM, Jones EL, Alexander-Williams J, et al. Symptomatic significance of gastric mucosal changes after surgery for peptic ulcer. Gut 1977;18:295.

138. Geboes K, Rutgeerts P, Broeckaert L, et al. Histologic appearances of endoscopic gastric mucosal biopsies 10–20 years after partial gastrectomy. Ann Surg 1980;192:179.

139. Pickford IR, Craven JL, Hall R, et al. Endoscopic examination of the gastric remnant 31–39 years after subtotal gastrectomy for peptic ulcer. Gut 1984;25:393–397.

140. Joffe N, Goldman H, Antonioli DA. Recurring hyperplastic gastric polyps following subtotal gastrectomy. AJR Am J Roentgenol 1978;130:301.

141. Stemmermann GN, Hayashi T. Hyperplastic polyps of the gastric mucosa adjacent to gastroenterostomy stomas. Am J Clin Pathol 1979;71:341.

142. Clarke AC, Lee SP, Nicholson GI. Gastritis varioliformis. Am J Gastroenterol 1977;68:599–602.

143. Lambert R, Andre C, Moulinier B, Bugnon B. Diffuse varioliform gastritis. Digestion 1978;17:159–167.

144. Green PHR, Gold RP, Marboe CC, et al. Chronic erosive gastritis: Clinical, diagnostic and pathological features in nine patients. Am J Gastroenterol 1982;77:543–547.

145. Elta GH, Fawaz KA, Dayal Y, et al. Chronic erosive gastritis—a recently recognized disorder. Dig Dis Sci 1983;28:7–12.

146. Haot J, Jouret A, Willette M, et al. Lymphocytic gastritis—prospective study of its relationship with varioliform gastritis. Gut 1990;31:282–285.

147. Wolber RA, Owen DA, Anderson FH, et al. Lymphocytic gastritis and giant gastric folds associated with gastrointestinal protein loss. Mod Pathol 1991;4:13–15.

148. Wolber R, Owen D, DelBuono L, et al. Lymphocytic gastritis in patients with celiac sprue or spruelike intestinal disease. Gastroenterology 1990;98:310–315.

149. Dixon MF, Wyatt JI, Burke DA, et al. Lymphocytic gastritis—Relationship to Campylobacter pylori infection. J Pathol 154:1988;125–132.

150. Niemela S, Karttunen T, Kerola T, et al. Ten year follow up study of lymphocytic gastritis: Further evidence on Helicobacter pylori as a cause of lymphocytic gastritis and corpus gastritis. J Clin Pathol 1995;48:1111–1116.

151. Vogelsang H, Oberhuber G, Wyatt J. Lymphocytic gastritis and gastric permeability in patients with celiac disease. Gastroenterology 1996;111:73–77.

152. Alsaigh N, Odze R, Goldman H, et al. Gastric and esophageal intraepithelial lymphocytes in pediatric celiac disease. Am J Surg Pathol 1996;20:865–870.

153. Kimura K. Gastric xanthelasma. Arch Pathol Lab Med 1969;87:110–117.

154. Drude RB, Balart LA, Herrington JP, et al. Gastric xanthoma: Histological similarity to signet ring cell carcinoma. J Clin Gastroenterol 1982;4:217–221.

155. Domellof L, Ericksson S, Helander HF, et al. Lipid islands in the gastric mucosa after resection for benign ulcer disease. Gastroenterology 1977;72:14.

156. Terruzzi V, Minoli G, Butti GC, et al. Gastric lipid islands in the gastric stump and in nonoperated stomach. Endoscopy 1980;2:58–62.

157. Kaiserling E, Heinle H, Itabe H, et al. Lipid islands in human gastric mucosa: Morphological and immunohistochemical findings. Gastroenterology 1996;110:369–374.

158. Ming SC, Goldman H. Gastric polyps: A histogenetic classification and its relation to carcinoma. Cancer 1965;18:721.

159. Tomasulo J. Gastric polyps: Histologic types and their relationship to gastric carcinoma. Cancer 1971;27:1346.

160. Marcial MA, Villafana M, Hernandez–Denton J, et al. Fundic gland polyps: Prevalence and clinicopathologic features. Am J Gastroenterol 1993;88:1711–1713.

161. Antonioli DA. Precursors of gastric carcinoma: A critical review with a brief description of early (curable) gastric cancer. Hum Pathol 1994;25:994–1005.

162. Elsborg L, Mosbech J. Pernicious anemia as a risk factor in gastric cancer. Acta Med Scand 1979;206:315.

163. Hansson L-E, Engstrand L, Nyren O, et al. Helicobacter pylori infection: Independent risk indicator of gastric adenocarcinoma. Gastroenterology 1993;105:1098–1103.

164. Tatsuta M, Iishi H, Okuda S, et al. The association of Helicobacter pylori with differentiated-type early gastric cancer. Cancer 1993;72:1841–1845.

165. Hu PJ, Mitchell HM, Li YY, et al. Association of Helicobacter pylori with gastric cancer and observations on the detection of this bacterium in gastric cancer cases. Am J Gastroenterol 1994;89:1806–1810.

166. Schrumpf E, Serck-Hanssen A, Stadaar J, et al. Mucosal changes in the gastric stump 20 to 25 years after partial gastrectomy. Lancet 1977;2:467.

167. Domellof L, Eriksson S, Janunger KG. Carcinoma and possible precancerous change of the gastric stump after Billroth II resection. Gastroenterology 1977;73:462.

168. Schuman BM, Waldbaum JR, Hitz SW. Carcinoma of the gastric remnant in a U.S. population. Gastrointest Endosc 1984;30:71–73.

169. Viste A, Opheim P, Thunald J, et al. Risk of carcinoma following gastric operations for benign disease. A historical cohort study of 3470 patients. Lancet 1986;2:502–505.

170. Pointner R, Schwab G, Konigsrainer A, et al. Early cases of the gastric remnant. Gut 1988;29:298–301.

171. Schafer LW, Larson DE, Melton J, et al. The risk of gastric carcinoma after surgical treatment for benign ulcer disease. A population-based study in Olmsted County, Minnesota. N Engl J Med 1983;309:1210–1213.

172. Sandler RS, Johnson MD, Holland KL. Risk of stomach cancer after gastric surgery for benign conditions. A case-control study. Dig Dis Sci 1984;29:703–708.

173. Ming SC, Bajtai A, Correa P, et al. Gastric dysplasia. Significance and pathologic criteria. Cancer 1984;54:1794–1801.
174. Lewin KJ, Appelman HD. Tumors of the esophagus and stomach. Atlas of tumor pathology, 3rd series, fascicle 18. Washington DC: Armed Forces Institute of Pathology, 1996.
175. Graem N, Fischer AB, Beck H. Dysplasia and carcinoma in the Billroth II resected stomach 27–35 years post-operatively. Acta Pathol Microbiol Scand 1984;92:185–188.
176. Offerhaus G, Volstadt J, Huibregtse K, et al. Endoscopic screening for malignancy in the gastric remnant: The clinical significance of dysplasia in gastric mucosa. J Clin Pathol 1984;37:748–754.
177. von Holstein CS, Hammar E, Eriksson S, et al. Clinical significance of dysplasia in gastric remnant biopsy specimens. Cancer 1993;72: 1532–1535.
178. Saraga E-P, Gardial D, Costa J. Gastric dysplasia. A histological follow-up study. Am J Surg Pathol 1987;11:788–796.
179. Morson BC, Sobin LH, Grundmann E, et al. Precancerous conditions and epithelial dysplasia of the stomach. J Clin Pathol 1980;33: 231–240.
180. del Corral MJM, Pardo-Mindon FJ, Razquin S, et al. Risk of cancer in patients with gastric dysplasia. Follow-up study of 67 patients. Cancer 1990;65:2078–2085.
181. de Dombal FT, Price AB, Thompson H, et al. The British Society of Gastroenterology early gastric cancer/dysplasia survey: An interim report. Gut 1990;31:115–120.
182. Bearzi I, Brancorsini D, Santinelli A, et al. Gastric dysplasia—A 10 year follow-up study. Pathol Res Pract 1994;190:61–68.
183. Rugge M, Farinati F, Baffa R, et al. Gastric epithelial dysplasia in the natural history of gastric cancer: A multicenter prospective follow-up study. Gastroenterology 1994;107:1288–1296.
184. Hirota T, Itabashi M, Suzuki K, et al. Clinicopathologic study of minute and small early gastric cancers. Pathol Annu 1980;15:1.
185. Green PHR, O'Toole KM, Weinberg LM, et al. Early gastric cancer. Gastroenterology 1981;81:247–256.
186. Polak JM, Hoffbrand AV, Reed PI, et al. Qualitative and quantitative studies of antral and fundic G cells in pernicious anemia. Scand J Gastroenterol 1973;8:361.
187. Harris AI, Greenberg H. Pernicious anemia and the development of carcinoid tumors of the stomach. JAMA 1978;239:1160.
188. Borch K, Renvall H, Ludberg G. Gastric endocrine cell hyperplasia and carcinoid tumors in pernicious anemia. Gastroenterology 1985; 88:638–648.
189. Muller J, Kirchner T, Muller-Hermelink HK. Gastric endocrine cell hyperplasia and carcinoid tumors in atrophic gastritis type A. Am J Surg Pathol 1987;11:909–917.
190. Itsuno M, Watanabe H, Iwafuchi M, et al. Multiple carcinoids and endocrine cell micronests in type A gastritis. Their morphology, histogenesis, and natural history. Cancer 1989;63: 881–890.
191. Thomas RM, Baybick JH, Elsayed AM, et al. Gastric carcinoids. An immunohistochemical and clinicopathologic study of 104 patients. Cancer 1994;73:2053–2058.
192. D'Adda T, Pilato FP, Sivelli R, et al. Gastric carcinoid tumor and its precursor lesions. Arch Pathol Lab Med 1994;118:658–663.
193. Hodges JR, Isaacson P, Wright R. Diffuse enterochromaffin-like (ECL) cell hyperplasia and multiple gastric carcinoids: A complication of pernicious anemia. Gut 1981;22:237–241.
194. Isaacson PG. Gastrointestinal lymphoma. Hum Pathol 1994;25: 1020–1029.
195. Parsonnet J, Hansen S, Rodriquez L, et al. Helicobacter pylori infection and gastric lymphoma. N Engl J Med 1994;330:1267–1271.
196. Wotherspoon AC, Doglioni C, Diss TC, et al. Regression of primary low-grade B-cell gastric lymphoma of mucosa-associated lymphoid tissue type after eradication of Helicobacter pylori. Lancet 1993;342: 575–578.
197. Citron B, Pincus I, Geokas M, et al. Chemical trauma of the esophagus and stomach. Surg Clin North Am 1968;48:1303.
198. Allen R, Thoshinsky M, Stallone R, et al. Corrosive injuries of the stomach. Arch Surg 1970;100:409.
199. Lowe JE, Graham DY, Bolsaubin EV Jr, et al. Corrosive injury to the stomach: The natural history and role of fiberoptic endoscopy. Am J Surg 1979;137:803–806.
200. Marks I, Bank S, Werbeloff M, et al. The natural history of corrosive gastritis. Am J Dig Dis 1963;8:509.
201. Sugawa C, Mullins RJ, Lucas CE, et al. The value of early endoscopy following caustic ingestion. Surg Gynecol Obstet 1981;153: 553–556.
202. Dworkin B, Wormser GP, Rosenthal WS, et al. Gastrointestinal manifestations of the acquired immunodeficiency syndrome: A review of 22 cases. Am J Gastroenterol 1985;80:774–778.
203. Wilderlite L, Trier JS, Blacklow NR, et al. Structure of the gastric mucosa in acute infectious nonbacterial gastroenteritis. Gastroenterology 1975;68:425.
204. Nash G, Ross J. Herpetic esophagitis: A common cause of esophageal ulceration. Hum Pathol 1974;5:339.
205. Howiler W, Goldberg HI. Gastroesophageal involvement in herpes simplex. Gastroenterology 1976;70:775.
206. Sperling HV, Reed WG. Herpetic gastritis. Am J Dig Dis 1977;22: 1034.
207. Campbell DA, Piercey JRA, Shnitka TK, et al. Cytomegalovirus-associated gastric ulcer. Gastroenterology 1977;72:533–535.
208. Andrade JS, Bambirra EA, Lima GF, et al. Gastric cytomegalic inclusion bodies diagnosed by histologic examination of endoscopic biopsies in patients with gastric ulcer. Am J Clin Pathol 1983;79: 493–496.
209. Hinnant KL, Rotterdam HZ, Bell ET, et al. Cytomegalovirus infection of the alimentary tract: A clinicopathological correlation. Am J Gastroenterol 1986;81:944–950.
210. Chetty R, Roskell DE. Cytomegalovirus infection in the gastrointestinal tract. J Clin Pathol 1994;47:968–972.
211. Franzin G, Muolo A, Griminelli T. Cytomegalovirus inclusions in the gastroduodenal mucosa of patients after renal transplantation. Gut 1981;22:698–701.
212. Strayer DS, Phillips GB, Barker KH, et al. Gastric cytomegalovirus infection in bone marrow transplant patients. Cancer 1981;48:1478–1483.
213. Palmer ED. The morphologic consequences of acute exogenous (staphylococcic) gastroenteritis on the gastric mucosa. Gastroenterology 1951;19:462–475.
214. Gonzalez-Crussi F, Hackett RL. Phlegmonous gastritis. Arch Surg 1966;93:990–995.
215. Nevin NC, Eakins D, Clarke SD, et al. Acute phlegmonous gastritis. Br J Surg 1969;56:268–270.
216. Miller AI, Smith M, Rogers AI. Phlegmonous gastritis. Gastroenterology 1975;68:231.
217. Nicholson BW, Maull KI, Scher LA. Phlegmonous gastritis: Clinical presentation and surgical management. South Med J 1980;73:875.
218. Gonzalez L, Schowengerdt C, Skinner H, et al. Emphysematous gastritis. Surg Gynecol Obstet 1963;116:79.
219. Binmoeller KF, Benner KG. Emphysematous gastritis secondary to gastric infarction. Am J Gastroenterol 1992;87:526–529.
220. Sud A, Lehl SS, Bhasin DK, et al. Emphysematous gastritis. Am J Gastroenterol 1996;91:604–605.
221. Palmer ED. Tuberculosis of the stomach and the stomach in tuberculosis: A review with particular reference to gross pathology and gastroscopic diagnosis. Am Rev Tuberc 1950;61:116–130.
222. Chazan R, Aitchison J. Gastric tuberculosis. Br Med J 1960;2:1288.
223. Misra RC, Agarwal SK, Prakash P, et al. Gastric tuberculosis. Endoscopy 1982;14:235–237.
224. Subei I, Attar B, Schmitt G, et al. Primary gastric tuberculosis: A case report and literature review. Am J Gastroenterol 1987;82: 769–772.
225. Rotterdam H. Contributions of gastrointestinal biopsy to an understanding of gastrointestinal disease. Am J Gastroenterol 1983;78: 140–148.
226. Berardi RS. Abdominal actinomycosis. Surg Gynecol Obstet 1979; 149:257.
227. Wilson E. Abdominal actinomycosis with special reference to the stomach. Br J Surg 1962;49:266.
228. Van Olmen G, Larmuseau MF, Geboes K, et al. Primary gastric actinomycosis: A case report and review of the literature. Am J Gastroenterol 1984;79:512–516.
229. Mitchell R, Bralow S. Acute erosive gastritis due to early syphilis. Ann Intern Med 1964;61:933.
230. Butz WC, Watts JC, Rosales-Quintana S, et al. Erosive gastritis

as a manifestation of secondary syphilis. Am J Clin Pathol 1975; 63:895.

231. Besses C, Sans-Sabrofen J, Badia X, et al. Ulceroinfiltrative syphilitic gastropathy: Silver stain diagnosis from biopsy specimen. Am J Gastroenterol 1987;82:773–774.

232. Reisman TN, Leverett FL, Hudson JR, et al. Syphilitic gastropathy. Am J Dig Dis 1975;20:588–593.

233. Beckman JW, Schuman BM. Antral gastritis and ulceration in a patient with secondary syphilis. Gastrointest Endosc 1986;32:353–356.

234. Fyfe B, Poppiti RJ Jr, Lubin J, et al. Gastric syphilis. Primary diagnosis by gastric biopsy: Report of four cases. Arch Pathol Lab Med 1993;117:820–823.

235. Atten MJ, Attar BM, Teopengco E, et al. Gastric syphilis: A disease with multiple manifestations. Am J Gastroenterol 1994;89:2227–2229.

236. Morin ME, Tan A. Diffuse enlargement of gastric folds as a manifestation of secondary syphilis. Am J Gastroenterol 1980;74:170–172.

237. Inagaki H, Kawai T, Miyata M, et al. Gastric syphilis: Polymerase chain reaction detection of treponemal DNA in pseudolymphomatous lesions. Hum Pathol 1996;27:761–765.

238. Smith JMB. Mycoses of the alimentary tract: Progress report. Gut 1969;10:1035.

239. Eras P, Goldstein MJ, Sherlock P. Candida infection of the gastrointestinal tract. Medicine 1972;51:367.

240. Katzenstein ALA, Maksen J. Candidal infection of gastric ulcers: Histology, incidence and clinical significance. Am J Clin Pathol 1979;71:137.

241. Peters M, Weiner J, Whelan G. Fungal infection associated with gastroduodenal ulceration: Endoscopic and pathologic appearances. Gastroenterology 1980;78:350.

242. Gotlieb-Jensen K, Andersen J. Occurrence of Candida in gastric ulcers. Significance for the healing process. Gastroenterology 1983;85:535–537.

243. Loffeld RJ, Loffeld BC, Arends JW, et al. Fungal colonization of gastric ulcers. Am J Gastroenterol 1988;83:730–733.

244. Nelson R, Bruni M, Goldstein M. Primary gastric candidiasis in uncompromised subjects. Gastrointest Endosc 1975;22:92.

245. Gillespie PE, Green PH, Barrett PJ, et al. Gastric candidiasis. Med J Aust 1978;1:228.

246. Minoli G, Terruzzi V, Rossini A. Gastroduodenal candidiasis occurring without underlying diseases (primary gastroduodenal candidiasis). Endoscopy 1979;1:18–22.

247. Scott BB, Jenkins D. Gastro-oesophageal candidiasis. Gut 1982;23:137–139.

248. Young JA, Elias E. Gastro-oesophageal candidiasis: Diagnosis by brush cytology. J Clin Pathol 1985;38:293–296.

249. Pinkerton H, Iverson L. Histoplasmosis: Three fatal cases with disseminated sarcoid–like lesions. Arch Intern Med 1952;90:456–467.

250. Nudelman H, Rakatansky H. Gastric histoplasmosis—a case report. JAMA 1966;195:44.

251. Fisher JR, Sanowski RA. Disseminated histoplasmosis producing hypertrophic gastric folds. Dig Dis Sci 1978;23:282.

252. Miller DP, Everett ED. Gastrointestinal histoplasmosis. J Clin Gastroenterol 1979;1:233.

253. Kahn LB. Gastric mucormycosis: A report of a case with a review of the literature. S Afr Med J 1963;37:1265–1269.

254. Deal WB, Johnson JE III. Gastric phycomycosis: Report of a case and review of the literature. Gastroenterology 1969;57:579.

255. Lawson H, Schmaman A. Gastric phycomycosis. Br J Surg 61:743, 1974.

256. Lyon DT, Schubert TT, Mantia AG, et al. Phycomycosis of the gastrointestinal tract. Am J Gastroenterol 1979;72:379–391.

257. Garone MA, Winston BJ, Lewin JH. Cryptosporidiosis of the stomach. Am J Gastroenterol 1986;81:465–470.

258. Forester G, Sidhom O, Nahass R, et al. AIDS-associated cryptosporidiosis with gastric stricture and a therapeutic response to Paromomycin. Am J Gastroenterol 1994;89:1096–1098.

259. Alpert L, Miller M, Alpert E, et al. Gastric toxoplasmosis in acquired immunodeficiency syndrome: Antemortem diagnosis with histopathologic characterization. Gastroenterology 1996;110:258–264.

260. Watt IA, McLean NR, Girdwood RWA, et al. Eosinophilic gastroenteritis associated with a larval anisakine nematode. Lancet 1979;2:893–894.

261. Hsiu J–G, Gomsey AJ, Ives CE, et al. Gastric anisakiasis: Report of a case with clinical, endoscopic, and histological findings. Am J Gastroenterol 1986;81:1185–1187.

262. Kakizoe S, Kakizoe H, Kakizoe K, et al. Endoscopic findings and clinical manifestation of gastric anisakiasis. Am J Gastroenterol 1995;90:761–763.

263. Scowden EB, Schaffner W, Stone WJ. Overwhelming strongyloidiasis. An unappreciated opportunistic infection. Medicine 1978;57:527.

264. Ainley CC, Clarke DG, Timothy AR, et al. Strongyloides stercoralis hyperinfection associated with cimetidine in an immunosuppressed patient: Diagnosis by endoscopic biopsy. Gut 1986;27:337–338.

265. Strickland GT. Gastrointestinal manifestations of schistosomiasis. Gut 1994;35:1334–1337.

266. Jacob GS, Al Nakib B, Al Ruwaih A. Ascariasis producing upper gastrointestinal hemorrhage. Endoscopy 1983;15:67.

267. Choudhuri G, Saha SS, Tandon RK. Gastric ascariasis. Am J Gastroenterol 1986;81:788–790.

268. Mallory GK, Weiss S. Hemorrhages from lacerations of the cardiac orifice of the stomach due to vomiting. Am J Med Sci 1929;178:506.

269. Knauer CM. Mallory-Weiss syndrome. Gastroenterology 1976;71:5.

270. Graham DY, Schwartz SJ. The spectrum of the Mallory-Weiss tear. Medicine 1978;57:307.

271. Harris JM, DiPalma JA. Clinical significance of Mallory-Weiss tears. Am J Gastroenterol 1993;88:2056–2058.

272. Levin E, Clayman CB, Palmer WL, et al. Observations on the value of gastric irradiation in the treatment of duodenal ulcer. Gastroenterology 1957;32:42.

273. Clayman CB, Palmer WL, Kirsner JB. Gastric irradiation in the treatment of peptic ulcer. Gastroenterology 1968;55:403.

274. Novak JM, Collins JT, Donowitz M, et al. Effects of radiation on the human gastrointestinal tract. J Clin Gastroenterol 1979;1:9.

275. Berthrong M, Fajardo LF. Radiation injury in surgical pathology. II. Alimentary tract. Am J Surg Pathol 1981;5:153.

276. Goldgraber MB, Rubin CE, Palmer WL, et al. The early gastric response to irradiation, a serial biopsy study. Gastroenterology 1954;27:1–20.

277. McIlrath DC, Hallenbeck GA. Review of gastric freezing. JAMA 1964;190:715.

278. Barner HB, Collins CH, Jones TI, et al. Morphology of human stomach after therapeutic freezing. Arch Surg 1965;90:358.

279. Perry GT, Dunphy JV, Fruin RC, et al. Gastric freezing for duodenal ulcer. A double blind study. Gastroenterology 1964;47:6.

280. Klein NC, Hargrove RL, Sleisenger MH, et al. Eosinophilic gastroenteritis. Medicine 1970;40:299.

281. Goldman H, Proujansky R. Allergic proctitis and gastroenteritis in children. Clinical and mucosal biopsy features in 53 cases. Am J Surg Pathol 1986;10:75–86.

282. Johnstone JM, Morson BC. Eosinophilic gastroenteritis. Histopathology 1978;2:335–348.

283. Katz AJ, Goldman H, Grand RJ. Gastric mucosal biopsy in eosinophilic (allergic) gastroenteritis. Gastroenterology 1977;73:705.

284. Snyder JD, Rosenblum N, Wershil B, et al. Pyloric stenosis and eosinophilic gastroenteritis in infants. J Ped Gastroenterol Nutr 1987;6:543–547.

285. Eras P, Beranbaum S. Gastric diverticula: Congenital and acquired. Am J Gastroenterol 1972;57:120.

286. Kadian RS, Rose JF, Mann NS. Gastric bezoars—spontaneous resolution. Am J Gastroenterol 1978;70:79–80.

287. Holloway W, Lee S, Nicholson G. The composition and dissolution of phytobezoars. Arch Pathol Lab Med 1980;104:159.

288. Goldstein HM, Cohen LE, Hagen RO, et al. Gastric bezoars: A frequent complication in the postoperative ulcer patient. Radiology 1973;107:341–344.

289. Force T, MacDonald D, Eade OE, et al. Ischemic gastritis and duodenitis. Dig Dis Sci 1980;25:307.

290. Cherry RD, Jabbari M, Goresky CA, et al. Chronic mesenteric vascular insufficiency with gastric ulceration. Gastroenterology 1986;91:1548–1552.

291. Burke AP, Sobin LH, Virmani R. Localized vasculitis of the gastrointestinal tract. Am J Surg Pathol 1995;19:338–349.

292. Taylor NS, Gueft B, Lebowich RJ. Atheromatous embolization: A cause of gastric ulcers and small bowel necrosis. Gastroenterology 1964;47:97.

293. Petras RE, Hart WR, Bukowski RM. Gastric epithelial atypia associated with hepatic arterial infusion chemotherapy. Its distinction from early gastric carcinoma. Cancer 1985;56:745–750.

294. Jewell LD, Fields AL, Murray CJW, et al. Erosive gastroduodenitis with marked epithelial atypia after hepatic infusion chemotherapy. Am J Gastroenterol 1985;80:421–424.

295. Doria MI Jr, Doris LK, Faintuch J, et al. Gastric mucosal injury after hepatic arterial infusion chemotherapy with floxuridine. A clinical and pathologic study. Cancer 1994;73:2042–2047.

296. Kwee WS, Wils JA, Schlangen J, et al. Gastric epithelial atypia complicating hepatic arterial infusion chemotherapy. Histopathology 1994;24:151–154.

297. Jabbari M, Cherry R, Lough JO, et al. Gastric antral vascular ectasia: The watermelon stomach. Gastroenterology 1984;87:1165–1170.

298. Kruger R, Ryan ME, Dickson KB, et al. Diffuse vascular ectasia of the gastric antrum. Am J Gastroenterol 1987;82:421–426.

299. Ma CK, Behrle KM, Rosenberg BF, et al. Gastric antral vascular ectasia: The watermelon stomach. Surg Pathol 1988;1:231–239.

300. Gouldesbrough DR, Pell ACH. Gastric antral vascular ectasia: A problem of recognition and diagnosis. Gut 1991;32:954–955.

301. Potamiano S, Carter CR, Anderson JR. Endoscopic laser treatment of diffuse gastric antral vascular ectasia. Gut 1994;35:461–463.

302. McCormack TT, Sims J, Eyre-Brook I, et al. Gastric lesions in portal hypertension: Inflammatory gastritis or congestive gastropathy? Gut 1985;26:1226–1232.

303. Tarnowski AS, Sarfeh IJ, Stochura J, et al. Microvascular abnormalities of the portal hypertensive gastric mucosa. Hepatology 1988;1488–1494.

304. D'Amico G, Montabano L, Traina M, et al. Natural history of congestive gastropathy in cirrhosis. Gastroenterology 1990;99:1558–1564.

305. Parikh SS, Desai SB, Prabhu SR, et al. Congestive gastropathy: Factors influencing development, endoscopic features, Helicobacter pylori infection, and microvessel changes. Am J Gastroenterol 1994;89:1036–1042.

306. Marmaduke DP, Greenson JK, Cunningham I, et al. Gastric vascular ectasia in patients undergoing bone marrow transplantation. Am J Clin Pathol 1994;102:194–198.

307. Sherman L, Shenoy SS, Satchidanand SK, et al. Arteriovenous malformation of the stomach. Am J Gastroenterol 1979;72:160–164.

308. Ona FV, Ahluwalia M. Endoscopic appearance of gastric angiodysplasia in hereditary hemorrhagic telangiectasia. Am J Gastroenterol 1980;3:148–149.

309. Gunnlaugsson O. Angiodysplasia of the stomach and duodenum. Gastrointest Endosc 1985;31:251–254.

310. Jules GL, Labitzke HG, Lamb R, et al. The pathogenesis of Dieulafoy's gastric erosion. Am J Gastroenterol 1984;79:195–200.

311. Van Zanten SJOV, Bartelsman JFWM, Schipper ME, et al. Recurrent massive haematemesis from Dieulafoy vascular malformations—a review of 101 cases. Gut 1986;27:213–222.

312. Miko TL, Thomazy VA. The caliber persistent artery of the stomach: A unifying approach to gastric aneurysm, Dieulafoy's lesion, and submucosal arterial malformation. Hum Pathol 1988;19:914–921.

313. Haggitt RC. Granulomatous diseases of the gastrointestinal tract. In: Iochim HL, ed. Pathology of granulomas. New York: Raven Press, 1983:257–305.

314. Shapiro JL, Goldblum JR, Petras RE. A clinicopathologic study of 42 patients with granulomatous gastritis. Is there really an "idiopathic" granulomatous gastritis? Am J Surg Pathol 1996;20:462–470.

315. Harned RK, Anderson JC, Owen DR. Suture granuloma of the stomach following splenectomy. Am J Gastroenterol 1979;72:302–305.

316. Morson BC, Dawson IMP. Gastrointestinal pathology, 2nd ed. London: Blackwell Scientific, 1979:113–114.

317. Rutgeerts P, Onette E, Vantrappen G, et al. Crohn's disease of the stomach and duodenum: A clinical study with emphasis on the value of endoscopy and endoscopic biopsies. Endoscopy 1980;12:288.

318. Korelitz BI, Waye JD, Kreuning J, et al. Crohn's disease in endoscopic biopsies of the gastric antrum and duodenum. Am J Gastroenterol 1981;76:103–109.

319. Pryse-Davies J. Gastro-duodenal Crohn's disease. J Clin Pathol 1964;17:90.

320. Fielding JF, Toye DKM, Beton DC, et al. Crohn's disease of the stomach and duodenum. Gut 1970;11:1001.

321. Haggitt RC, Meissner WA. Crohn's disease of the upper gastrointestinal tract. Am J Clin Pathol 1973;59:613–622.

322. Fahimi HD, Deren JJ, Gottlieb LS, et al. Isolated granulomatous gastritis. Gastroenterology 1963;45:161.

323. Khan MH, Lam R, Tamoney HJ. Isolated granulomatous gastritis. Am J Gastroenterol 1979;71:90.

324. Schinella RA, Ackert J. Isolated granulomatous disease of the stomach: Report of 3 cases presenting as incidental findings in gastrectomy specimens. Am J Gastroenterol 1979;72:30–35.

325. Brown KM, Kass M, Wilson R. Isolated granulomatous gastritis. Treatment with corticosteroids. J Clin Gastroenterol 1987;9:442–446.

326. Ectors EL, Dixon MF, Geboes KJ, et al. Granulomatous gastritis: A morphological and diagnostic approach. Histopathology 1993;23:55–61.

327. Littler ER, Gleibermann E. Gastritis cystica polyposa (gastric mucosal prolapse at gastroenterostomy site, with cystic and infiltrative epithelial hyperplasia). Cancer 1972;29:205.

328. Honore LH, Lewis AS, Ohara KE. Gastritic glandularis et cystica profunda—report of 3 cases with discussion of etiology and pathogenesis. Dig Dis Sci 1979;24:48–52.

329. Franzen G, Novelli P. Gastritis cystica profunda. Histopathology 1981;5:555–547.

330. Fonde EC, Rodning CB. Gastritis cystica profunda. Am J Gastroenterol 1986;81:459–464.

331. Qizilbash AH. Gastritis cystica and carcinoma arising in old gastrojejunostomy stomach. Can Med Assoc J 1975;112:1432–1433.

332. Bogomoletz WV, Potet F, Barge J, et al. Pathological features and mucin histochemistry of primary gastric stump carcinoma associated with gastritis cystica polyposa. A study of six cases. Am J Surg Pathol 1985;9:401–410.

333. Snover DC, Weisdorf SA, Vercolotti GM, et al. A histopathologic study of gastric and small intestinal graft-versus-host disease following allogeneic bone marrow transplantation. Hum Pathol 1985;16:387–392.

334. Ferrara JLM, Deeg HJ. Graft-versus-host disease. N Engl J Med 1991;324:667–674.

335. Brooks JJ, Enterline HT. Gastric pseudolymphoma. Its three subtypes and relation to lymphoma. Cancer 1983;51:476–486.

336. Franzin G, Musola R, Mencarelli R. Morphological changes of the gastroduodenal mucosa in regular dialysis uraemic patients. Histopathology 1982;6:429.

337. Musola R, Franzin G, Mora R, et al. Prevalence of gastroduodenal lesions in uremic patients undergoing dialysis and after renal transplantation. Gastrointest Endosc 1984;30:343–346.

338. Yamada M, Hatakeyama S, Tsukagoshi H. Gastrointestinal amyloid deposition in AL (primary or myeloma-associated) and AA (secondary) amyloidosis. Diagnostic value of a gastric biopsy. Hum Pathol 1985;16:1206–1211.

339. Rocken C, Saeger W, Linke RP. Gastrointestinal amyloid deposits in old age—report on 110 consecutive autopsical patients and 98 retrospective bioptic specimens. Pathol Res Pract 1994;190:641–649.

340. Calletti RB, Trainer TD. Collagenous gastritis. Gastroenterology 1989;97:1552–1555.

341. Goldman H, Antonioli DA. Mucosal biopsy of the esophagus, stomach, and proximal duodenum. Hum Pathol 1982;13:423–448.

342. Whitehead R. Mucosal biopsy of the gastrointestinal tract. 4th ed. Philadelphia: WB Saunders, 1990:41–157.

343. Rotterdam H. Stomach. In: Rotterdam H, Sheahan DG, Sommers SC, eds. Biopsy diagnosis of the digestive tract. 2nd ed. New York: Raven Press, 1993:62–255.

344. Fung WP, Papadimitriou JM, Matz LR. Endoscopic, histologic, and ultrastructural correlations in chronic gastritis. Am J Gastroenterol 1979;71:269–279.

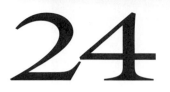

24 STRESS ULCER AND CHRONIC PEPTIC ULCER DISEASE

Harvey Goldman

Practically all causes of mucosal inflammation can lead to localized areas of destruction, and the sloughing of the necrotic mucosa results in the appearance of erosions or ulcers. An erosion represents a tissue deficit that is shallow and limited to the mucosa, whereas an ulcer crater extends into the submucosa or deeper parts of the gut wall. The focus of this chapter is on the disorders of acute stress-produced ulcers and of chronic peptic ulcer disease, both of which are dominantly located in the stomach and duodenum. Details of other inflammatory conditions of these areas that can develop secondary ulcers are provided in Chapters 11, 23, and 30.

STRESS ULCER

DEFINITION, ETIOLOGY, AND PATHOGENESIS

This condition is characterized by the appearance of acute erosions or ulcers of the stomach and duodenum in patients who are severely ill as a result of a variety of physical stresses, including trauma, burns, increased intracranial pressure, and sepsis (1–4). The lesions in burn cases are also called Curling ulcer (5–7) and those associated with cranial damage are termed Cushing ulcer (8, 9). The common pathogenetic factor is probably mucosal ischemia, related to overt shock or to the release and circulation of vasoconstrictive substances, and the reduced blood flow, together with the indigenous acid in the gastric lumen, accounts for the mucosal injury (1, 10).

Hyperacidity is noted only in those patients with increased intracranial pressure, owing to trauma or to a brain tumor, and is mediated by the vagus nerves because it can be suppressed by anticholinergic drugs. Most patients with stress ulcer have normal or reduced gastric acid, but the presence of some acid in the lumen is a prerequisite for the formation of the erosions and ulcers (11–13). The reduced mucosal blood flow can lead to damage of the surface and foveolar mucous cells, favoring the back diffusion of acid and the loss of cytoprotective substances, such as prostaglandins, and to a delay in renewal of these cells.

In numerous experimental models in animals, stress ulcers have been induced by restraint, exertion, burns, and traumatic or hemorrhagic shock (14–16). As in human subjects with this disease, the presence of gastric acid in the lumen is needed for the full development of the lesion, because the effect of the stress can be ameliorated or eliminated by the prior use of agents that inhibit or neutralize acid secretion. This effect on acid secretion is the basis for the prophylactic use of antacids and H2 blockers in high-risk patients, as discussed subsequently.

CLINICAL FEATURES

The dominant clinical findings relate to the underlying traumatic and septic conditions, and patients often present with signs of shock, respiratory or renal failure, and jaundice (2–4, 17, 18). With the appearance of the stress ulcers comes the added potential for gastrointestinal hemorrhage, which may prove life-threatening in these fragile patients (17–19). The bleeding varies in amount and typically has an abrupt onset without prior signs of gastric distress. Rarely, deep penetration or perforation of the ulcer leads to peritonitis. The clinical diagnosis of the stress ulcers is readily determined by gross endoscopic examination; the lesions usually are too superficial to be detected by ordinary radiographic studies.

Following the successful use of modern techniques to sustain patients with severe trauma and shock, an increase in the frequency of stress ulcers was observed in the surgical intensive care units, leading to significant hemorrhage in about 10% of cases (1, 3, 18). To combat this complication, the prophylactic use of antacids or other acid-neutralizing agents in high-risk patients became standard and resulted in a significant decline in the incidence of prominent hemorrhage and the overall mortality related to stress ulcer (20, 21). It was noted, however, that the sustained use of H2 blockers can promote the growth of coliform organisms and the development of pneumonia, particularly in patients receiving artificial ventilation for long periods, and these agents are no longer used routinely (22). At present, greater medical care has resulted in a lower incidence of stress ulcers, except for patients with coagulation problems or severe pneumonia (23).

The treatment of patients with established stress ulcers consists of correcting the underlying promoting condition, especially the shock, and of neutralizing the acid or inhibiting the gastric secretions (24, 25). The latter therapy also helps to deter the hemorrhage, because coagulation is optimal at a neutral pH and pepsins interfere with platelet agglutination. In patients with uncontrolled bleeding, angiographic injections of vasopressin, Gelfoam, or preformed clots are attempted. Surgical resection or devascularization may ultimately be required (4, 26, 27).

PATHOLOGY

GROSS FEATURES

The primary lesions noted in stressed patients are confined to the mucosa of the stomach and proximal duodenum (Fig. 24.1) and consist of a spectrum of alterations, ranging from patchy hemor-

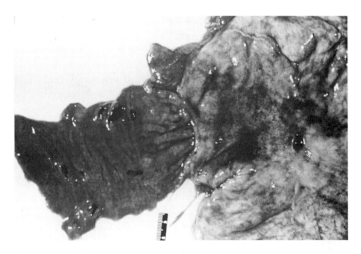

Figure 24.1 Acute stress ulcers. Multiple, small hemorrhagic ulcers are noted in the duodenum *(left)*, and a single ulcer together with diffuse mucosal congestion and hemorrhage in the gastric antral mucosa *(right)*.

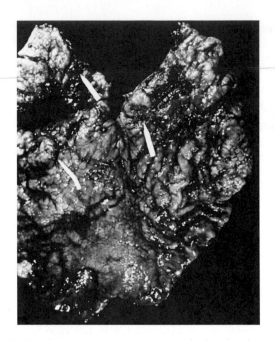

Figure 24.2 Gastrectomy specimen, with duodenal portion at the bottom. Multiple ulcers *(arrows)* are seen in the gastric corpus and a larger one in the upper right portion.

rhages to discrete erosions and ulcers (28). The ulcers may be single or multiple and most often are concentrated in the corpus and fundus of the stomach (Fig. 24.2), in contrast to the antral localization of chronic peptic ulcers and of the erosive cases of acute or chronic gastritis attributable to ethanol and drug exposure. The lesions typically are less than 1 cm in diameter and elliptical or circular, with sharply defined margins. Of interest, the early lesions noted in experimental models in animals, such as those related to restraint or exertion, often have a linear configuration, but this appearance is not characteristic of ulcer formation in humans. The ulcers usually are shallow and have a red base; rarely, findings may include a deeper penetration into the wall or a perforation with exudate on the peritoneal surface.

HISTOLOGIC FEATURES

Stress-induced erosions and ulcers are acute processes (17, 28). The earliest lesion, which is best visualized in experimental animals, consists of a localized area of hemorrhage and necrosis without inflammation that is limited to the mucosa and has the appearance of an acute ischemic infarction (Fig. 24.3) (16). Sloughing of the necrotic tissue follows, resulting in the ulcer crater and an acute inflammatory reaction, consisting of congested vessels and many neutrophils, in the adjacent intact mucosa and in the underlying submucosa (Fig. 24.4). The deeper parts of the wall are unaffected, unless there is a perforation. With healing, the eroded area is replaced by regenerating glands and the transient presence of a slight depression of the mucosal surface can result (Fig. 24.5) (17). Because the ulcer is superficial, there usually is no significant granulation tissue or fibrosis. Stress lesions typically heal without any sequelae and do not recur in the absence of the underlying stress condition. Ordinarily, no signs of chronic inflammation are seen in the ulcer or the surrounding mucosa.

DIFFERENTIAL DIAGNOSIS

The diagnosis of stress ulcer is promptly suggested by the appearance of upper gastrointestinal hemorrhage in a severely ill patient. Endoscopy is often performed for confirmation and to exclude other causes of bleeding; biopsy is not needed if the typical lesions are observed. Acute erosions and ulcers can be seen in the more severe cases of acute toxic gastritis owing to the use of ethanol or drugs and to bile reflux, but these lesions typically are confined to the antral region and usually are associated with more widespread mucosal hemorrhage or edema. Although some studies have included these examples of toxic or chemical gastritis in a broad list of stress conditions that can cause acute ulceration of the stomach and duodenum, this lumping should be avoided because the lesions seen in association with severe bodily injury have a different pathogenesis and generally more aggressive behavior. Chronic peptic ulcers are readily distinguished from acute stress ulcer by their limited localization to the antrum or the first part of the duodenum. They usually are single and reveal evidence of chronic inflammation and scarring in the ulcer and adjacent mucosa.

CHRONIC PEPTIC ULCER DISEASE

The following general sections address the features of peptic ulcer disease in the common sites of the antrum and duodenum. Characteristics of the disease in other locations of the gut are presented subsequently.

DEFINITIONS

A peptic ulcer is a localized ulcerating lesion of the gut, usually present in the stomach or the duodenum, that is attributable in part to the action of gastric acid and pepsin. In most conditions, however, gastric secretions are not the primary cause of the injury but rather are a necessary factor in its development. The term "acute

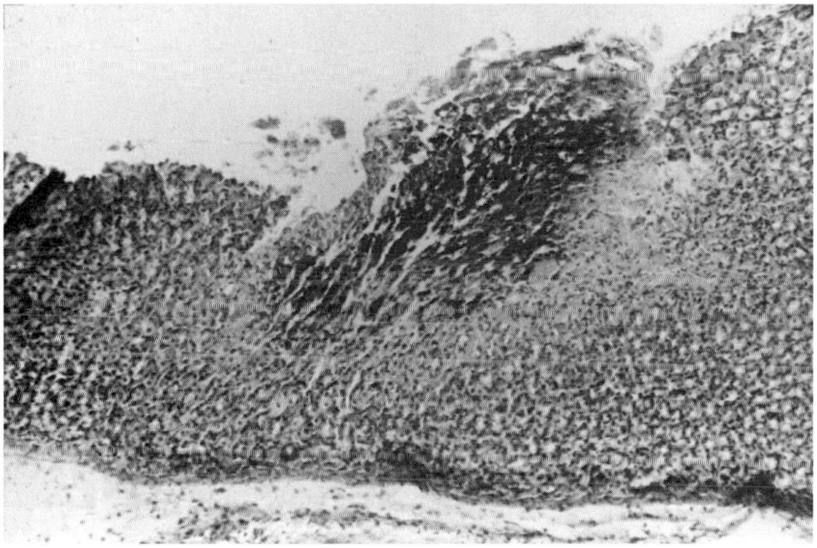

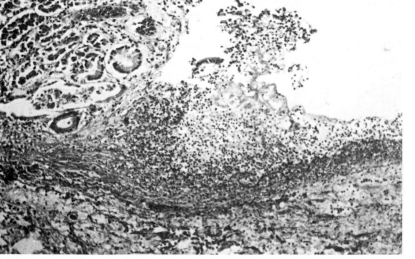

Figure 24.3 Gastric corpus mucosa from a rodent, following restraint-induced stress. The submucosa is at the bottom. A sharply localized area of hemorrhage and necrosis involves the superficial half of the mucosa (H & E, ×80).

Figure 24.4 Acute stress ulcer of the stomach, with some intact mucosa at top left. There is mucosal destruction with a marked neutrophilic reaction. The underlying submucosa (bottom) shows congestion and a slight inflammatory infiltrate but no fibrosis (H & E, ×100). Contrast with Figures 24.10 and 24.11 of chronic peptic ulcers.

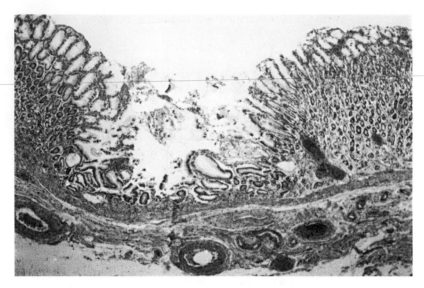

Figure 24.5 Healing stress ulcer of the stomach. Note mucosal loss and regenerative glands at the base of the mucosa. The underlying muscularis mucosae and submucosa *(bottom)* are intact without evidence of chronic features, such as fibrosis (H & E, ×80).

TABLE	
24.1	**Conditions Associated with Chronic Peptic Ulcers**

Promoting conditions
  Chronic pulmonary disease
  Chronic renal failure
  Hepatic cirrhosis
  Hyperparathyroidism
  Multiple endocrine neoplasia, type I
  Systemic mastocytosis
Precipitating factors
  Analgesics
  Anti-inflammatory drugs
  Ethanol and smoking
  Psychologic stress

peptic ulcer" is rarely used in an unqualified fashion because it embraces a variety of disorders of different etiologies, including acute stress lesions and ulcers caused by exposure to toxic chemicals and drugs (29) (see preceding section and Chapters 11 and 23).

Chronic peptic ulcer disease is a common disorder characterized by the recurrent appearance of ulcers that usually are solitary and most often are found in the antrum and in the first part of the duodenum (29, 30). Because the same etiologic factors are involved in the genesis of inflammatory lesions in these areas, principally H. pylori infection and hyperacidity, patients may encounter a spectrum of pathologic effects ranging from gastritis or duodenitis to overt ulceration (31–34).

EPIDEMIOLOGY

Chronic peptic ulcer disease is more common in whites (35) and in persons living in highly industrialized nations (36); it is estimated that more than 10 million people in the United States are affected.

Duodenal ulcer disease is about three times more common than gastric ulcer disease, but its incidence has shown a decline over the past two decades (37). Males are affected more often than females, with ratios of 4 : 1 or higher for duodenal ulcers and 1.5 to 2 : 1 for gastric ulcers. Duodenal ulcers affect persons of all ages, including children and young adults, whereas gastric ulcers are more frequently noted in patients over age 40. The disease is more common in persons who smoke cigarettes (38) but it is difficult to sort out this component from the general lifestyle of affected individuals (39, 40). The development of ulcers does not appear to have any constant relationship to dietary factors.

ETIOLOGY AND PATHOGENESIS
REVIEW OF NORMAL GASTRIC SECRETION

Hydrochloric acid is produced in the parietal (or oxyntic) cells and the class of pepsinogens in the chief cells that are located in the specialized glands of the fundic and corpus mucosa. The major physiologic stimuli for gastric secretion are the vagus nerves and the gastrin-producing endocrine cells (G cells) that are concentrated amidst the pyloric glands in the antral mucosa. The parietal cells also respond to other agents, such as histamine, and their function depends on an adequate mucosal blood supply. In the first or cerebral phase of gastric secretion, the vagi act both directly on the parietal cells and indirectly by stimulation of the G cells. The second or gastric phase is characterized by antral distention and greater stimulation of the gastrin cells. The final or intestinal phase depends on the release of other hormones, such as enterogastrone and somatostatin, that inhibit and curtail the gastric secretions. The pepsinogens are converted by the low pH to the active pepsins that are proteolytic enzymes. After the ingestion of a solid meal, the pyloric sphincter remains closed, and the major function of the stomach is the churning and physical disruption of the nutrients as well as the secretion of the gastric fluid; the pylorus opens in response to sensors in its mucosa when the solution becomes isotonic. The gastric acid is partially diluted by the alkaline secretions from the antral pyloric and duodenal Brunner glands and ultimately is neutralized by the biliary and pancreatic secretions in the small intestine (see Chapter 2 for further details).

GENERAL FACTORS

Factors involved in the etiology of chronic peptic ulcer disease have been investigated extensively, and the reader is referred to the reviews on this subject for more details (29, 30, 41, 42). The two most important factors are the amount of gastric acid (43) and the mucosal resistance (44, 45). In order for a peptic ulcer to develop, some gastric acid must be present but an increase in gastric secretions is only regularly seen in some cases of duodenal ulcers and in conditions with hypergastrinemia, such as the Zollinger-Ellison syndrome. Mucosal resistance depends on numerous components (44, 45), including adequate blood supply, normal renewal and differentiation of the surface epithelial cells, and the production of the mucous coat that covers the surface (46) and possibly of other protective agents, such as prostaglandins (13). A higher rate of peptic ulcers, especially of the duodenum, has been noted in persons with blood group type 0 and in those persons who do not secrete the blood substances into the gastrointestinal tract (47, 48).

An increase in duodenal ulcer incidence is also seen in first-degree relatives of patients, and a genetic basis is suggested by the higher frequency of concordance of ulcer disease in monozygotic than in dizygotic twins (49). Further support for a genetic predisposition comes from the observations of more ulcers in persons with an elevated level of serum pepsinogen type I (50) and possibly in individuals with the HLA-B5 and HLA-B12 phenotypes (51).

Psychologic factors have also been incriminated, because emotional stress can lead to vagal stimulation and an increase in the gastric secretion of acid and pepsin (39, 40, 52, 53). One has the image of the harassed executive popping pills to abort the ulcer symptoms. Such stresses apparently are not the primary cause of peptic ulcer disease, but they are promoting or precipitating factors. Other conditions that can facilitate the development of peptic ulcers are listed in Table 24.1 and include chronic pulmonary and renal diseases, hyperparathyroidism, hepatic cirrhosis, and systemic mastocytosis (54–58). In most of these disorders, gastric acid secretion is enhanced (see Chapter 19). A large variety of noxious chemicals and drugs, such as ethanol, salicylates, corticosteroids, indomethacin, and other nonsteroidal agents, can cause an acute gastritis or ulcer but also can activate a chronic peptic ulcer (59–66). These agents probably operate by further damaging the mucosa and reducing its resistance (see Chapter 11 for further details).

ROLE OF *HELICOBACTER PYLORI*

These bacteria are observed in the gastric antral mucosa in three quarters or more of patients with chronic peptic ulcer affecting either the stomach or the duodenum (67–70). In the duodenum, bacteria are found in areas of gastric mucous cell metaplasia. The organisms are also regularly seen in patients with chronic active gastritis involving the antrum who do not have ulcers (see Fig. 23.9). Consequently, it has been proposed that the bacteria may be the cause of both the gastritis and the reduced mucosal resistance that leads to ulcer formation in the stomach (71, 72). The relationship to duodenal ulcer is less clear, because less bacteria and inflammation are noted in this area and hyperacidity is often present. It remains possible that colonization is a secondary event or that organisms can add to the mucosal injury to promote the ulcer formation. It is noteworthy that healing of peptic ulcers of either the stomach or duodenum is usually facilitated by specific antimicrobial treatment and elimination of the bacteria (73), supporting the contention that the organisms are the principal cause of ulcer disease (see discussion of chronic antral gastritis in Chapter 23).

DUODENAL ULCER

Many patients with duodenal peptic ulcer have demonstrable hyperacidity, either fasting or after stimulation with a test meal, and it is thought that this hyperacidity is the dominant factor in the development of ulcer disease in this area (41–43). It is probable that the small intestinal epithelium is innately less resistant than the gastric mucosa to the effects of the acid and pepsin, which would explain the preferential localization of the ulcer in the mucosa that is just distal to the pyloris in the first part of the duodenum. This area is the first to be exposed to the acid-pepsin load, whereas tissue beyond this region benefits from neutralization by the biliary and pancreatic secretions. It has also been suggested that patients with duodenal ulcers have more rapid gastric emptying, which promotes the delivery of high acid concentrations into the duodenum (74). It is noteworthy that the site of peptic ulcers is similar in other situations; the recurrent stomal ulcer is typically in the jejunum just beyond the anastomosis, and ulcers that develop in association with gastric heterotopia (such as in a Meckel diverticulum) are also in the immediately adjacent small intestinal mucosa. In contrast, Zollinger-Ellison syndrome is associated with so much acid secretion that ulcers may be observed throughout the duodenum and even in the jejunum.

Some patients with duodenal ulcer disease have an associated peptic duodenitis, and the same etiologic factors may be involved in the initiation and precipitation of the two disorders. Concomitant inflammation and infection with H. pylori are noted in the gastric antrum in greater than 80% of cases of duodenal peptic ulcer (75). The organisms are only seen in the duodenum in association with gastric mucous cell metaplasia, which occurs following sustained inflammation of the mucosa (76). Accordingly, H. pylori is considered a likely factor in continued ulceration, which explains the beneficial response of most patients to antibiotic therapy.

GASTRIC ULCER

In gastric peptic ulcer, in contrast to duodenal disease, the relative importance of the two major factors of acid amount and mucosal resistance is reversed. Typically, the concentration of gastric acid is normal or reduced, and prior mucosal injury from other causes appears to be a prerequisite for the development of the gastric ulcer (77). Practically all patients have evidence of diffuse inflammation of the surrounding mucosa (78, 79), indicative of a chronic antral gastritis that is mainly caused by H. pylori infection (67–72); in some cases, gastritis may result from repeated exposure to toxic substances, including alcohol, drugs, and bile salts (59–65, 80–82). Typically, no increase in gastric secretion of acid and pepsin occurs. About 10% of patients have ulcers in both the antrum and the duodenum, and these patients more often demonstrate hyperacidity. Some individuals initially develop a duodenal ulcer with pyloric obstruction that leads to gastric antral distention, stimulation of the gastrin-producing cells, and increased acid production (83).

Unresolved issues are why only a small fraction of patients with chronic antral gastritis form ulcers and why the ulcers typically are solitary and recur in the same location. Many antral ulcers are located at the junction with the corpus mucosa, suggesting that this area may be exposed to a higher concentration of gastric secretions. Considering that patients with gastric ulcers are often older, one suggestion is that degenerative vascular disease of the local arteries may be an added factor in determining the occurrence and site of the lesion.

CLINICAL FEATURES

Patients with peptic ulcers typically experience episodes of epigastric burning pain that are related to times of acid secretion and to the absence of food in the stomach (84–86); i.e., pain usually occurs 1 to 2 hours after a meal or at night when the stomach has acid but is relatively empty of solid contents. Although the interval between eating and the appearance of pain may be shorter in cases of gastric ulcer compared to those of duodenal lesions, considerable overlap is noted. Some episodes are precipitated by the ingestion of a drug or an emotional crisis, but more often there is no special antecedent history. Other symptoms include occasional nausea, vomiting, and bleeding—manifestations that generally are present in more severe cases (see subsequent discussion of complications). The disease is characterized by periods of resolution or remission and of repeated recurrences or relapses, and patients usually are not completely cured. Milder "attacks" without overt ulceration are thought to result from underlying or associated mucosal inflammation, referred to as antral gastritis and peptic duodenitis.

The presence and particular location of the peptic ulcer are ordinarily determined by radiographic study. Endoscopic examination with biopsy and cytology are often added in the evaluation of gastric ulcers, particularly in older patients and when healing is slow, to distinguish the ulcer from a malignant tumor. Acid secretion, both basal and stimulated by histamine or pentagastrin, and serum gastrin levels also are determined in uncertain or unusual cases (43, 87, 88). The standard medical treatment of peptic ulcer disease involves the use of a large variety of antacid compounds, as well as antibiotics to eradicate H. pylori, H2-blocking agents, and other protective drugs. Resolution of the ulcer is monitored by radiographic and/or endoscopic procedures (89–91). The use of a bland diet may help to alleviate symptoms, but it does not by itself promote healing of the ulcer, and no evidence exists to support the use of medications in the prevention of recurrences. Surgical intervention is reserved for intractable disease and other complica-

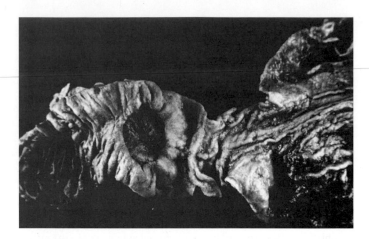

Figure 24.6 Segment of stomach *(right)* and duodenum reveals a large chronic peptic ulcer in the first portion of the duodenum. Note sharp demarcation of ulcer edges.

tions and for cases of persistent gastric ulcer that cannot be distinguished from malignancy (see subsequent discussion of complications).

PATHOLOGY

Despite the differences in the etiology and pathogenesis of peptic ulcers involving the stomach, duodenum and other locations, the morphologic features are the same (92–94).

LOCATION OF DISEASE

About 75% of chronic peptic ulcers occur in the pyloric region and the first portion of the duodenum and 20% in the gastric antrum (Table 24.2). Ulcers in the antrum are more often noted in the junctional area next to the corpus mucosa and along the lesser curvature, but they can involve any part (95–97). The fundic-corpus region of the stomach typically is spared, in contrast to tumors that can occur in this area. Other sites are the lower esophagus in patients with reflux esophagitis, recurrent stomal ulcers after gastric resection, ulcers that can occur in association with foci of gastric heterotopia, and more widespread lesions of the duodenum and jejunum in the Zollinger-Ellison syndrome (see discussion in the section concerning other conditions).

GROSS FEATURES

The ulcers of either the duodenum (Fig. 24.6) or the stomach (Figs. 24.7 and 24.8) are commonly single and vary from one to several centimeters in diameter. Uncommonly, gastric lesions can be 10 cm or larger and are referred to as giant ulcers (98, 99). Multiple ulcers, usually only two, are seen in about 10% of cases. These lesions usually are present in the stomach or one occurs in the stomach and one occurs in the duodenum (100, 101). The lesions are sharply demarcated and the mucosal edges have a regular contour. Although the margins appear flat on gross examination of specimens, a uniform elevation owing to edema is commonly appreciated by radiography and endoscopy. The surrounding mucosa, particularly

TABLE	
24.2	**Location of Chronic Peptic Ulcers**

Common disease	
First part of duodenum	(70–75%)
Gastric antrum	(20–25%)
Other conditions	
Distal esophagus in reflux esophagitis	
Jejunum in recurrent stomal ulcer following antral resection	
Distal duodenum and jejunum in patients with the Zollinger-Ellison syndrome	
Meckel diverticulum, ileum and rectum in cases of gastric heterotopia	

in cases of gastric ulcer, often has a granular appearance that reflects the presence of the associated diffuse mucosal inflammation. The serosal surface is either normal or shows adhesions or puckering in cases of deep ulcers. Ulcers that extend through the wall can penetrate a variety of neighboring structures, such as the pancreas, spleen, biliary tract, liver, and colon (102–106). The features of the other complications, including hemorrhage, perforation, and obstruction, are presented subsequently. With healing can come a prominence of the mucosal folds that radiate from the lesion (Fig. 24.9) (107), and the deeper ulcers that extend into the muscularis propria may cause a weakening of the wall, leading to the formation of a localized diverticulum.

HISTOLOGIC FEATURES

The histologic features of chronic peptic ulcers are entirely nonspecific and consist of those of the active disease, the reparative process, and scarring from previous episodes. The ulcers extend at least into the submucosa and often into the muscularis propria (Fig. 24.10). Active lesions demonstrate zones of necrosis, neutrophilic reaction, granulation tissue, and fibrosis that extend from the mucosal surface into the wall (Figs. 24.11 and 24.12). The surrounding intact mucosa of the gastric ulcers is always inflamed and reveals acute and chronic inflammatory cells and variable amounts of intestinal metaplasia (78, 79, 108). Numerous small bacteria, representing H. pylori, are present on the surface and in the lumina of the superficial gastric pits in most gastric cases (see Fig. 23.9) (67–70, 109). The effects of degeneration and regeneration seen in the gastric epithelium in the surface and foveolar region (Fig. 24.13) should not be confused with dysplasia; the distinction may be particularly difficult in the small and often distorted mucosal biopsy samples. The epithelial cell nuclei are enlarged and have a central nucleolus, but they typically are regular in size and shape and lack hyperchromatism.

The appearance of the mucosa around a duodenal ulcer is more variable. Usually, less inflammation is noted, and H. pylori, when observed, are present only in areas of gastric mucous cell metaplasia (75, 76). There is less concern about the regenerative epithelium in the duodenum because carcinoma does not ordinarily occur in this

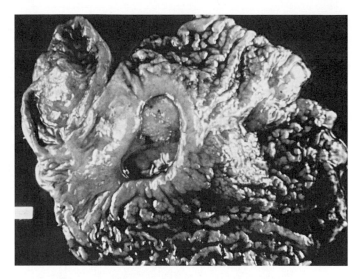

Figure 24.8   Segment of stomach with contiguous duodenum *(upper left)*. Note the large chronic peptic ulcer of the antrum. The rugae near the ulcer are irregular, but the ulcer edges appear uniform and sharply demarcated. The tissue at the ulcer base represents granulation tissue.

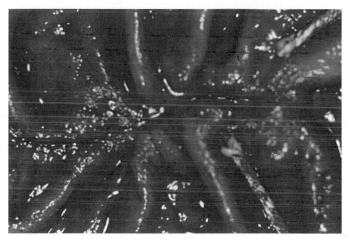

Figure 24.9   Healed chronic peptic ulcer of the stomach. Irregular and enlarged rugae appear to radiate from the ulcer lesion.

area and mucosal biopsies are not performed routinely. Other bacteria are frequently noted in the necrotic area of large ulcers of both the stomach and the duodenum, but they are thought to represent saprophytes that do not affect the lesion. Candida organisms are also seen occasionally (see Fig. 23.22), and they may contribute to the necrosis, resulting in a greater chance of perforation and an overall worse prognosis (110, 111). Other studies have failed to confirm these results, however, and the issue is not completely resolved (112, 113). Additional variable features include the presence of eroded vessels, giant cells, or poorly formed granulomas that probably represent a reaction to entrapped foreign material, and rarely the presence of abundant eosinophils without an apparent cause (see Fig. 12.2) (114). Furthermore, the number of antral G cells is increased in some cases of duodenal ulcer (115, 116) (see Chapter 15).

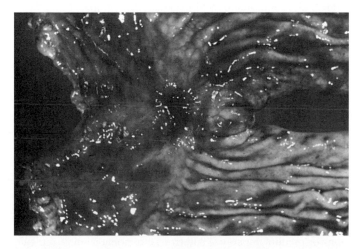

Figure 24.7   Segment of stomach with corpus at the right. There is a small chronic peptic ulcer of the gastric antrum at the junction with the corpus.

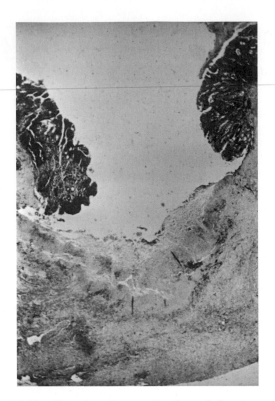

Figure 24.10 Chronic active peptic ulcer of the stomach. An ulcer crater extends into the submucosa and shows intact, inflamed mucosa at the edges. The ulcer base is composed of necrotic tissue and fibrosis, the latter serving as evidence of chronic disease (H & E, ×13). Contrast with Figure 24.4 of an acute stress ulcer.

With healing of the lesion, there is less necrosis, more abundant granulation tissue and fibrosis, and transient hyperplasia of the surface-foveolar mucous cells. The fibrosis replaces the normal structures of the submucosa and muscularis propria (see Fig. 24.11), and its amount relates to the overall size and depth of the lesion. The blood vessels at the bottom of the lesion often show patchy inflammation and fibrous thickening of the intima that are especially pronounced in the fibrotic areas. These changes are considered to be of a secondary nature.

EXAMINATION OF SURGICAL SPECIMEN

Gastric antral resection is performed in patients with chronic peptic ulcers of both the stomach and the duodenum, to either remove a gastric lesion or excise the area containing the gastrin-producing endocrine cells. The specimen is opened along the greater curvature, unless there is a lesion in this area, and measurements are obtained of the circumferences of the proximal and distal margins and of the lengths of the stomach along the lesser and greater curvatures. The distal end should be inspected to identify the pyloric sphincter; when normal, this structure appears as a thickened area of musculature with a slight elevation of the mucosal surface that then slopes sharply into the duodenum. Sections should be taken from any lesions observed, from random areas of the antrum to determine the presence and extent of any associated gastritis, and from the resection margins to confirm that the antrum has been completely excised. In particular, sections should be obtained to identify duodenal mucosa at the distal end and gastric corpus-type mucosa at the proximal end. These findings are then incorporated into the pathologic report.

DIFFERENTIAL DIAGNOSIS

GENERAL ASPECTS

The diagnosis of a chronic peptic ulcer is determined in most cases by the typical location of the lesion together with the characteristic clinical and radiographic features. The differential diagnosis includes a variety of inflammatory lesions associated with the development of ulcers in the stomach and duodenum. In most infections, the ulcers are multiple and relatively shallow, and the diagnosis is supplied by the characteristic histologic or culture findings. Ulcers can be caused directly by chemicals and drugs; aside from the history, a paucity of inflammation in the adjacent mucosa helps to identify these ulcers as acute lesions (117, 118). Crohn disease occasionally manifests with a large ulcer of the stomach or duodenum, and its distinction depends on finding other characteristic features, such as fissures and granulomas, or disease in other parts of the intestine.

DUODENAL ULCER

Carcinoma is rare in the duodenum and usually is located beyond the first portion, particularly in the region of the papilla of Vater. Stress ulcers are acute lesions that tend to be multiple and shallow, and they manifest in patients with severe bodily trauma or shock. Peptic ulcer and peptic duodenitis share the same etiology and clinical features, and their distinction is based simply on whether an ulcer can be grossly identified. As noted previously, these two conditions are parts of a spectrum of peptic disease of the duodenum and probably differ only in severity (see Chapter 30).

GASTRIC ULCER

The principal distinction to be made in a case of a gastric ulcer is between a benign peptic lesion and a malignant tumor (119–124) (usually an adenocarcinoma or malignant lymphoma). Carcinomas can occur in any part of the stomach, whereas chronic peptic ulcers are limited to the antral region. Although carcinomas occur less often at the lesser curvature where most peptic ulcers occur, overlap is considerable and investigation of any persistent ulcer of the stomach is required. Size alone is not a helpful criterion, because peptic ulcers can be large (98, 99), whereas early gastric carcinoma can be small and can mimic a benign ulcer in appearance (124–126). When an ulcerated lesion is estimated to be benign or malignant on the basis of gross radiographic or endoscopic examination, the impression is erroneous in over 25% of cases (Fig. 24.14). Accordingly, histologic study is mandatory, and it has been observed that taking at least four biopsy specimens, including one from the center of the lesion, together with brush cytology, should make the distinction in practically all cases (127–131). The detection of malignant lymphoma and its distinction from marked inflammation (or pseudolymphoma) and from carcinoma is more difficult, and resection may be needed to resolve the issue (see Chapters 17 and 27).

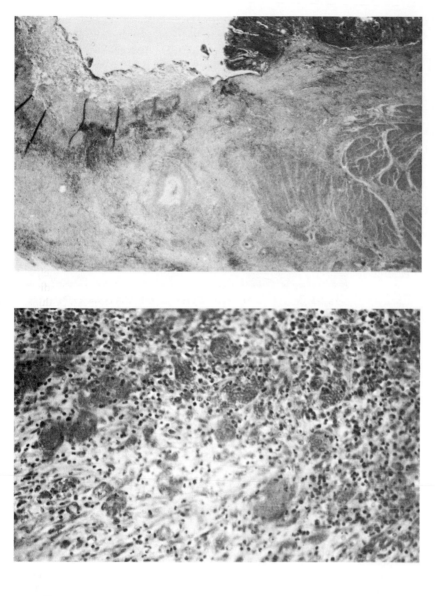

Figure 24.11 Chronic active peptic ulcer of the stomach. Ulceration and necrosis extend into the submucosa. Note extensive fibrosis of the underlying muscularis at lower left, a vessel in the center, and intact mucosa and muscularis propria at right (H & E, ×16).

Figure 24.12 Base of chronic active peptic ulcer reveals prominent granulation tissue (H & E, ×200).

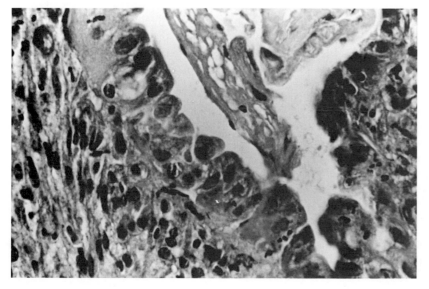

Figure 24.13 Edge of chronic active peptic ulcer of the stomach. There are signs of marked degeneration and regeneration of the surface and foveolar (pit) epithelia. Although enlarged, the epithelial nuclei tend to be regular in size and shape, and the cells have abundant cytoplasm (H & E, ×500). Contrast with the example of dysplastic epithelium seen in Figure 23.20. (Reproduced with permission from Goldman H, Antonioli DA. Mucosal biopsy of the esophagus, stomach, and proximal duodenum. Hum Pathol 1982;13:423–448.)

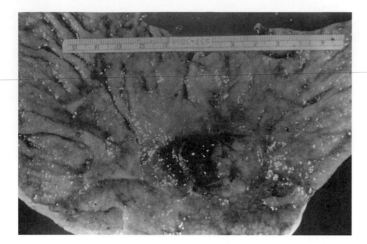

Figure 24.14 Segment of stomach with a large ulcer in the antrum that proved to be a carcinoma. Compare with Figures 24.7 and 24.8.

Erosions of the gastric antral mucosa can occur in association with acute toxic gastritis and chronic antral gastritis, and are readily distinguished by their multiple and shallow nature. Stress ulcers associated with severe bodily trauma or shock are often multiple and typically occur in the fundic-corpus region.

COMPLICATIONS

MEDICAL COMPLICATIONS

Common major complications directly related to peptic ulcer disease include hemorrhage, penetration into contiguous tissues, perforation, and obstruction (132) (Table 24.3). Although most patients experience some slight bleeding, massive hemorrhage requiring several units of blood replacement is observed at some time in the course of about 10% of cases (Fig. 24.15). This massive bleeding typically is associated with a deep ulcer and erosion of one or more large vessels (133, 134). When a relatively small ulcer is noted together with a single large bleeding artery, the possibility of a vascular malformation, such as Dieulafoy lesion of the stomach, should be considered; this malformation is more common in young adults and usually is located in the proximal stomach (135, 136).

A free perforation into the peritoneal cavity, seen in about 5 to 10% of hospitalized patients, results from the extension of an ulcer through the anterior wall of the stomach or duodenum (Fig. 24.16) (137, 138) and is associated with the presence of a purulent exudate on the serosal surface (Fig. 24.17). Patients typically present with signs of an "acute" abdomen and require immediate surgical intervention to avoid fatality. Extension of an ulcer through the posterior wall is commonly accompanied by penetration into the pancreas (102, 139) and, less often, into other neighboring organs, such as the spleen (Fig. 24.18), biliary tract, liver, and colon (103–106). Such lesions are noted in about 15% of patients with gastric ulcers and 25% of patients with duodenal lesions, leading to greater pain and signs of an acute pancreatitis or a fistula. Gastric outlet obstruction can result from either edema or fibrosis around an ulcer in the pyloric channel or duodenum (Fig. 24.19), and permanent effects are observed in about 5% of cases (140, 141).

SURGICAL COMPLICATIONS

Surgery is required for patients with chronic peptic ulcer who have intractable disease that has not responded to medical therapy; for any of the complications of uncontrolled hemorrhage, perforation, penetration, or fibrotic obstruction; and for lesions that cannot be adequately distinguished from malignancy (132, 142, 143). The three main types of operations are resection of a gastric lesion, correction of a particular complication (e.g., an omental patch over a site of perforation or a bypass gastrojejunostomy for pyloric obstruction), and a procedure to reduce gastric acid secretion. The latter, most often performed in patients with duodenal ulcer, consists, at least, of a vagotomy (truncal, selective, or highly selective aimed at just the innervation of the parietal cell area) together with a drainage procedure, such as a pyloroplasty. Alternatively, an

TABLE	
24.3	**Complications of Chronic Peptic Ulcer Disease**

Medical complications
  Intractable disease
  Hemorrhage
  Perforation
  Penetration into adjacent organs
  Obstruction
Surgical complications
  Recurrent stomal ulcer
  Retained antrum
  Postgastrectomy gastritis
  Dumping syndrome
  Afferent loop syndrome
Gastric adenocarcinoma
  Antrum related to associated chronic antral gastritis
  Proximal stomach (stump) following antral resection

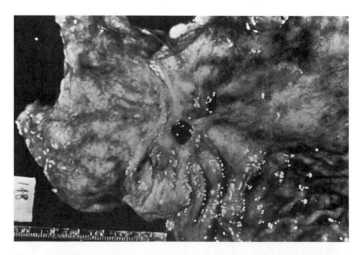

Figure 24.15 Segment of stomach with contiguous duodenum at left. Despite its relatively small size, this discrete chronic peptic ulcer of the lower antrum was the source of massive hemorrhage that necessitated performing surgical resection.

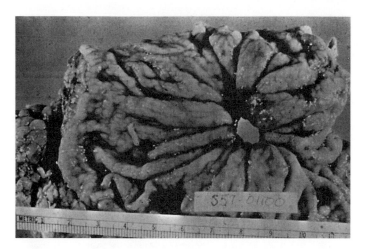

Figure 24.16 Segment of stomach with a transmural perforation of a chronic peptic ulcer. A portion of the ulcer can be seen next to the perforation. Rugae radiate from the lesion, a feature that is indicative of chronicity.

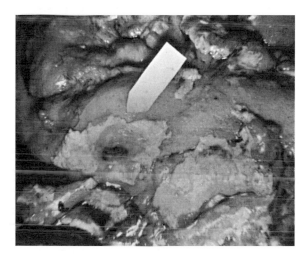

Figure 24.17 Peritoneal surface of the stomach. A perforated chronic peptic ulcer is surrounded by inflammatory exudate *(arrow)*.

antrectomy or large subtotal resection is performed to eliminate the gastrin-producing endocrine cells, and the proximal stomach is connected either to the duodenum (Billroth I) or to a loop of proximal jejunum (Billroth II).

More extensive surgical procedures with gastric resection generally are associated with less recurrence of ulcer disease but with a greater chance of other complications from the operation (144). Thus, recurrent ulcers are observed in about 10% of cases after a vagotomy but in only a few percent after a subtotal gastrectomy. The ulcers occur in the part of the small intestine, either the duodenum or the jejunum, that is immediately adjacent to the stomach (Fig. 24.20). Patients who have undergone gastric resection regularly develop gastritis of the residual stomach that is thought to result from the constant reflux of bile salts through the stoma. Reflux gastritis is productive of pain and mild bleeding in about 10% of cases (145) (see Chapter 23). Other complications of

gastric resection include the dumping syndrome (146) and a maldigestive disorder (147, 148). The former is caused by rapid passage of a hyperosmolar meal into the jejunum and results in pain and diarrhea. A mild degree of steatorrhea noted in most patients is probably the result of poor dilution and mixing of the meal with the biliary and pancreatic secretions; it usually is seen just in the chemical analysis of the stool and rarely produces symptoms. In the afferent loop syndrome, bacterial overgrowth in the static small bowel segment proximal to the stoma can lead to bile salt deconjugation, a greater amount of maldigestion, and clinically evident steatorrhea.

RELATION OF ULCER TO GASTRIC CARCINOMA

It was formerly thought that adenocarcinoma could develop in a benign peptic ulcer lesion as a late complication, but this appears to be a rare event (149, 150). Rather, peptic ulcer disease is invariably

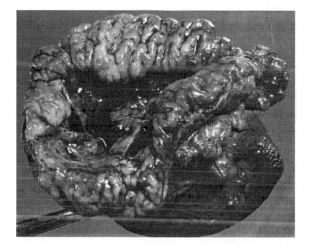

Figure 24.18 Large chronic peptic ulcer of the stomach that penetrated into the spleen (external surface of spleen at lower right).

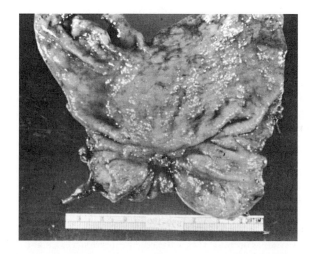

Figure 24.19 Segment of distal stomach shows a chronic active peptic ulcer and contraction of the pyloric region *(bottom)*.

associated with a more diffuse chronic gastritis in the surrounding antral mucosa, and it is the latter condition that has a greater frequency of cancer development. Thus, patients with chronic peptic ulcers of the stomach do have a slightly higher incidence of gastric carcinoma, but the tumors can occur in any part of the stomach and not preferentially in the area of the prior ulcer.

A similar situation exists in patients who have undergone an antral resection and gastroduodenostomy or gastrojejunostomy for the treatment of peptic ulcers of either the stomach or the duodenum. These patients regularly develop a chronic gastritis in the proximal stomach and experience an increased risk for the formation of adenomas, dysplasia, and adenocarcinoma (151–153) (see Chapters 23 and 27).

It should also be noted that some patients with gastric carcinoma present with a relatively small lesion and a secondary ulcer that can mimic the appearance of a benign ulcer (see Fig. 24.14) (124, 126). Indeed, medical therapy can result in partial or, rarely, complete healing of the ulcerated area, stressing the need for close observation and biopsy of any suspicious or unusual gastric ulcer lesion.

OTHER ULCER CONDITIONS

ESOPHAGUS

Ulcers as well as mucosal inflammation are frequent findings in patients with reflux esophagitis of the primary type or related to various motor disturbances, such as systemic sclerosis. Reflux disease is a common condition in which incompetence of the lower esophageal sphincter allows excess reflux and retention of acid and pepsin in the lower esophagus (see Chapter 20).

GASTRIC HETEROTOPIA

Foci of well-formed gastric fundic-corpus mucosa are observed in the many parts of the gut, including the upper esophagus, duodenum, rectum, Meckel diverticulum, and duplication cysts (154–158) (see Chapter 30). The cells of the specialized gastric glands in these ectopic lesions are functional and produce acid and pepsin, but whether or not an ulcer develops depends on other local factors. Thus, ulceration has only rarely been noted in the esophageal lesions (159), presumably because of rapid transit from this area, and has not been described in duodenal lesions where the abundant biliary and pancreatic secretions neutralize the acid.

In contrast, peptic ulcers can occur in areas of gastric heterotopia affecting the rectum (160, 161) or a Meckel diverticulum (162, 163), because these regions are relatively static, allowing time for the acid and pepsin to act. The ulcers typically occur in the area of intestine that is immediately adjacent to the ectopic gastric mucosa. In the Meckel lesion, the ulcer usually is in the diverticulum, but may be located in the contiguous ileum when there is diffuse heterotopia of the diverticular mucosa. The lesions can result in massive hemorrhage or in perforation of the diverticulum, and this condition is a major factor in the differential diagnosis in children with colonic bleeding or peritonitis. The original gastric foci can be obliterated by the secondary inflammation, as evidenced by its presence in only 50% of resected diverticula. Rectal involvement is rare, and patients typically have deep ulcers and complex fistulae that can penetrate into the perineum (see Chapter 30).

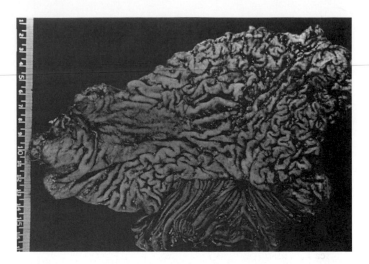

Figure 24.20 Segment of stomach *(top)* and jejunum connected by a side-to-side anastomosis following a Billroth II procedure. There is a small, recurrent, chronic peptic ulcer in the jejunum (lower) just next to the anastomosis.

STOMAL ULCERS

Stomal ulcers are recurrent lesions in patients who have undergone gastric resection for the treatment of peptic ulcer disease of either the stomach or the duodenum (164) (see previous discussion of surgical complications). The ulcers usually are small and are regularly located in the small intestine that is immediately contiguous to the residual stomach at the anastomosis, either in the duodenum after a Billroth I operation or in the jejunum following a Billroth II resection (see Fig. 24.20). Patients typically present with pain or bleeding (165). Radiographic and endoscopic studies are performed to distinguish recurrent peptic ulcer disease from the postgastrectomy type of gastritis and from other complications of the surgical procedure. Because ulcer recurrence after gastric resection is relatively uncommon, it is appropriate to search for a particular provocative condition, such as the ingestion of a toxic chemical or drug, a retained distal antrum, the Zollinger-Ellison syndrome, or an imperfectly constructed anastomosis.

RETAINED ANTRUM

This rare circumstance can occur in a patient who has undergone a Billroth II operation when a part of the distal antrum and pyloric sphincter is not excised. It is more likely to happen if a pyloric channel or duodenal ulcer with marked scarring results in the obliteration of the normal configuration of the pyloric sphincter. Because the retained portion of the antrum is a blind sac that is attached only to the duodenum and is not exposed to any acid formed in the proximal stomach, maximum stimulation of the antral G cells results in hypergastrinemia and recurrent stomal ulcers (166). A similar problem does not regularly develop if a part of the proximal antrum is retained, because this tissue is in contact with the gastric corpus and acid. Nevertheless, if too much antrum remains, the original operation can be ineffective. Therefore, it is important to examine the resection margins of any gastrectomy specimen, as noted previously. The diagnosis of a retained distal antrum is provided by serum gastrin and radiographic studies, and it is promptly corrected by surgical excision.

ZOLLINGER-ELLISON SYNDROME

This uncommon disorder probably accounts for less than 1% of cases of peptic ulcer disease. It is characterized by the presence of an autonomous source of gastrin leading to parietal cell hyperplasia, sustained hyperacidity, and multiple refractory ulcers of the stomach and small intestine (167–170). The syndrome is associated most often with a pancreatic islet cell tumor or "gastrinoma" (75 to 80% of cases), a diffuse islet cell hyperplasia (10%), or a tumor in the duodenal wall (5 to 10%) (171–173); rare sources include gastrinomas of the stomach, jejunum, liver, ovary, and parathyroid, and a diffuse G-cell hyperplasia in the gastric antrum. About 25% of pancreatic tumors are associated with the multiple endocrine neoplasm type I syndrome (174, 175), which includes pituitary chromophobe adenomas and parathyroid hyperplasia; about 66%

are malignant. The basal gastric acid level is regularly elevated and often approaches the stimulated level. The serum gastrin level is increased and is stimulated further by infusions of secretin and calcium (176, 177). These substances ordinarily suppress the gastrin level in persons without the syndrome.

The number of parietal cells may expand to three to five times normal, with extension of the parietal cells into the gastric pit region (Figs. 24.21 and 24.22). This situation usually results in gross enlargement of the gastric rugae, which can be appreciated radiographically and endoscopically (Fig. 24.23) (168, 169, 172). In contrast to ordinary peptic ulcer disease, the ulcers in Zollinger-Ellison syndrome more often are multiple (about 25% of cases) and occur in unusual sites, such as the distal duodenum (15%) and the jejunum (10%). Additional areas of inflammation and superficial erosions are often noted in the intervening small intestinal mucosa (178). Other consequences of the high gastric acid and fluid volume include the appearance of diarrhea and, occasionally, of steatorrhea resulting from the dilution and inactivation of the bile salts (178, 179).

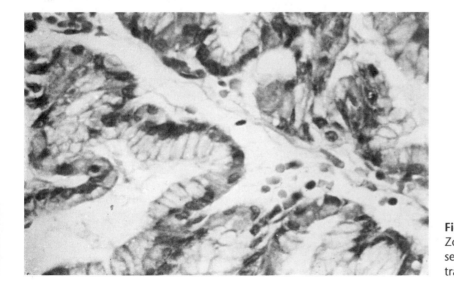

Figure 24.21   Gastric corpus mucosa in a case of Zollinger-Ellison syndrome. Significant hyperplasia of the parietal cells extends into the neck and foveolar region *(top)* (H & E, ×80).

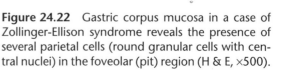

Figure 24.22   Gastric corpus mucosa in a case of Zollinger-Ellison syndrome reveals the presence of several parietal cells (round granular cells with central nuclei) in the foveolar (pit) region (H & E, ×500).

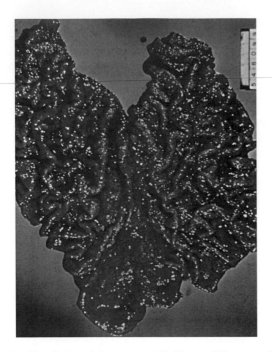

Figure 24.23 Stomach in a case of Zollinger-Ellison syndrome. Note the enlargement of the rugae.

The diagnosis of Zollinger-Ellison syndrome usually is apparent from the constellation of radiographic and chemical findings (170, 180). Elevation of the serum gastrin level is also seen in some patients with chronic fundic gastritis and pernicious anemia, a retained gastric antrum, and occasionally in patients with renal insufficiency or massive intestinal resection. Rugal hypertrophy may be a normal variant and is observed in individuals with Menetrier disease and tumors. Treatment consists of the removal of any benign tumors, which represent only a minority of cases, and is mainly directed at reducing the acid secretion by the use of H2-blocking drugs or, if needed, by gastrectomy (170, 181, 182). Even though patients often have a malignant tumor, these lesions usually are indolent and most of the morbidity and early fatality is related to the ulcers (see Chapters 15 and 25).

MUCOSAL BIOPSY

The general techniques and uses of endoscopy and biopsy are discussed in Chapter 3. These procedures are commonly used to help in the recognition of gastric and duodenal ulcers, to distinguish erosive gastritis or duodenitis and acute ulcers from chronic peptic ulcer disease, to monitor the clinical course after therapy, and to detect complications (34, 183–185). Endoscopy is generally more sensitive than radiography in the detection of small ulcers, especially if they are relatively shallow. Biopsy of an ulcer edge sometimes indicates that the lesion is acute, such as occurs after exposure to a drug (117, 118). A lack of inflammation is typical of most acute cases, whereas inflammation is always prominent in the mucosa next to a chronic peptic ulcer. The most important use of endoscopy is in distinguishing a benign peptic ulcer from a malignant tumor (127–131, 186, 187), either a carcinoma or a lymphoma in the stomach (see previous discussion of differential diagnosis).

REFERENCES

1. Skillman JJ, Silen W. Stress ulcers. Lancet 1972;2:1303.
2. Eiseman B, Heyman RL. Stress ulcers—a continuing challenge. N Engl J Med 1970;282:372.
3. Moody FG, Cheung LY, Simons MA, et al. Stress and the acute gastric mucosal lesion. Am J Dig Dis 1976;21:148.
4. Skillman JJ, Silen W. Stress ulceration in the acutely ill. Annu Rev Med 1976;27:9.
5. Pruitt BA, Foley FD, Moncrief JA. Curling's ulcer: Clinicopathologic study of 323 cases. Ann Surg 1970;172:523.
6. Czaja AJ, McAlhany JC, Pruitt BA. Acute gastroduodenal disease after thermal injury. An endoscopic evaluation of incidence and natural history. N Engl J Med 1974;291:925.
7. Pruitt BA, Goodwin CW. Stress ulcer disease in the burned patient. World J Surg 1981;5:209.
8. Cushing H. Peptic ulcers and the interbrain. Surg Gynecol Obstet 1932;55:1.
9. Kamada T, Fusamoto J, Kawano S, et al. Gastrointestinal bleeding following head injury: A clinical study of 433 cases. J Trauma 1977;17:44.
10. McClelland RN, Shires GT, Pager M. Gastric secretory and splanchnic blood flow in man following severe trauma and hemorrhagic shock. Am J Surg 1971;121:134.
11. Fischer RP, Jelense S, Fulton RL. The maintenance of gastric mucosal barrier during the early erosive gastritis component of stress ulceration. Surgery 1976;80:40.
12. Kivilaakso E, Silen W. Pathogenesis of experimental gastric-mucosal injury. N Engl J Med 1979;301:364–369.
13. Robert A. Cytoprotection by prostaglandins. Gastroenterology 1979;77:761.
14. Robert A, Kauffman GL. Stress ulcers, erosions and gastric mucosal injury. In: Sleisenger MH, Fordtran JS, eds. Gastrointestinal disease. 4th ed. Philadelphia: WB Saunders, 1989;772–792.
15. Brodie DA, Hanson HM. A study of the factors involved in the production of gastric ulcers by the restraint technique. Gastroenterology 1960;38:353.
16. Goldman H, Rosoff CB. Pathogenesis of acute gastric stress ulcer. Am J Pathol 1968;52:227.
17. Skillman JJ, Bushnell LS, Goldman H, et al. Respiratory failure, hypotension, sepsis and jaundice: A clinical syndrome associated with lethal hemorrhage from acute stress ulceration of the stomach. Am J Surg 1969;117:523.
18. Lucas CF. Stress ulceration: The clinical problem. World J Surg 1981;5:139.
19. Flowers RS, Kyle K, Hoerr SO. Post-operative hemorrhage from stress ulceration of the stomach and duodenum. Am J Surg 1970;119:632–639.
20. Menguy R. The prophylaxis of stress ulceration. N Engl J Med 1980;302:461.
21. Priebe HJ, Skillman JJ. Methods of prophylaxis in stress ulcer disease. World J Surg 1981;5:223.
22. Navab F, Steingrub J. Stress ulcer: Is routine prophylaxis necessary? Am J Gastroenterol 1995;90:708–712.
23. Cook DJ, Fuller HD, Guyatt GH, et al. Risk factors for gastrointestinal bleeding in critically ill patients. N Engl J Med 1994;330:377–381.
24. Simonian SJ, Curtis LE. Treatment of hemorrhagic gastritis by antacid. Ann Surg 1976;184:429.
25. Cheung LY. Treatment of established stress ulcer disease. World J Surg 1981;5:235.
26. Cody HS, Wichern WA. Choice of operation for acute gastric mucosal hemorrhage. Report of 36 cases and literature review. Am J Surg 1977;135:322.
27. Hubert JP, Kernan PD, Welch JS, et al. The surgical management of bleeding stress ulcers. Ann Surg 1980;191:672.
28. Lev R. "Stress" ulcers following war wounds in Vietnam: A morphologic and histochemical study. Lab Invest 1971;25:471.
29. Bynum TE, Hartsuck J, Jacobson ED. Gastric ulcer. Gastroenterology 1972;62:1052.
30. Grossman MI, Isenberg JI, Walsh JH, et al. Peptic diseases. Gastroenterology 1975;69:1071.

31. Owen DA. Gastritis and duodenitis. In: Appleman HD, ed. Pathology of the esophagus, stomach, and duodenum. London: Churchill Livingstone, 1984;37–77.

32. Yardley JH. Pathology of chronic gastritis and duodenitis. In: Goldman H, Appelman HD, Kaufman N, eds. Gastrointestinal pathology. Baltimore: Williams & Wilkins, 1990:69–143.

33. Appelman HD. Gastritis: Terminology, etiology, and clinicopathological correlations: Another biased view. Hum Pathol 1994;25: 1006–1019.

34. Goldman H. Gastrointestinal mucosal biopsy. New York: Churchill Livingstone, 1996:95–159.

35. Kurata JH, Haile BH. Racial difference in peptic ulcer disease: fact or myth. Gastroenterology 1982;83:166.

36. Langman MJS. Changing patterns in the epidemiology of peptic ulcer. Clin Gastroenterol 1973;2:219.

37. Mendeloff AI. What has been happening to duodenal ulcer? Gastroenterology 1974;67:1020.

38. Friedman GD, Siegelaub AB, Seltzer CC. Cigarettes, alcohol, coffee and peptic ulcer. N Engl J Med 1974;290:469.

39. Thomas J, Grieg M, Piper DW. Chronic gastric ulcer and life events. Gastroenterology 1980;78:905.

40. Piper DW, McIntosh JH, Ariotti DE, et al. Life events and chronic duodenal ulcer: A case control study. Gut 1981;22:1011.

41. Ippoliti A, Walsh J. Newer concept in the pathogenesis of peptic ulcer disease. Surg Clin North Am 1976;56:1479.

42. Szabo S. Biology of disease: Pathogenesis of duodenal ulcer disease. Lab Invest 1984;51:121–147.

43. Grossman MI. Abnormalities of acid secretion in patients with duodenal ulcers. Gastroenterology 1978;75:524.

44. Cooke AR. The role of the mucosal barrier in drug-induced gastric ulceration and erosions. Am J Dig Dis 1976;21:155.

45. Guth PH. Pathogenesis of gastric mucosal injury. Annu Rev Med 1982;33.183.

46. Pabst MA, Wachter C, Holzer P. Morphologic basis of the functional gastric acid barrier. Lab Invest 1996;74:78–85.

47. Daintree-Johnson H, Love AHG, Rogers NC, et al. Gastric ulcers, blood groups and acid secretion. Gut 1964,5:402.

48. Johnson HD. Gastric ulcer: Classification, blood group characteristics, secretion patterns and pathogenesis. Ann Surg 1965;162:996.

49. Eberhard G. The personality and peptic ulcer. Preliminary report of a twin study. Acta Psychiatr Scand 1968;203:131.

50. Rotter JI, Rimoin DL, Gursky JM, et al. HLA-B5 associated with duodenal ulcer. Gastroenterology 1977;73:438.

51. Ellis A, Woodrow JC. HLA and duodenal ulcer. Gut 1979;20:760.

52. Alp MH, Court JH, Grant AK. Personality pattern and emotional stress in the genesis of gastric ulcer. Gut 1970;11:773.

53. Feldman EJ, Elashoff JD, Samloff IM, et al. Psychologic stress and duodenal ulcer. N Engl J Med 1980;302:1206.

54. Langman MJS, Cooke AR. Gastric and duodenal ulcer and their associated diseases. Lancet 1976;1:680–683.

55. Archibald SD, Jirsch DW, Bear RA. A. Gastrointestinal complications of renal transplantation. 1. The upper gastrointestinal tract. Can Med Assoc J 1978;119:1291.

56. Kirsner JB. The parathyroids and peptic ulcer. Gastroenterology 1958;34:145.

57. Kirk AP, Dooley JS, Hunt RH. Peptic ulceration in patients with chronic liver disease. Dig Dis Sci 1980;25:756.

58. Amman RW, Vetter D, Deyhle P, et al. Gastrointestinal involvement in systemic mastocytosis. Gut 1976;17:107.

59. Laine L, Weinstein WM. Histology of alcoholic hemorrhgic "gastritis": A prospective evaluation. Gastroenterology 1988;94:1254–1262.

60. Levy M. Aspirin use in patients with major upper gastrointestinal bleeding and peptic ulcer disease. N Engl J Med 1974;290:1158.

61. Piper DW, McIntosh JH, Ariotti DE, et al. Analgesic ingestion and chronic peptic ulcer. Gastroenterology 1981;80:427.

62. Conn HO, Blitzer BL. Nonassociation of adrenocorticosteroid therapy and peptic ulcer. N Engl J Med 1976;294:473.

63. Pemberton RE, Strand LJ. A review of upper gastrointestinal effects of the newer nonsteroidal anti-inflammatory agents. Dig Dis Sci 1979;24:53–64.

64. Graham DY, Smith JL. Gastroduodenal complications of chronic NSAID therapy. Am J Gastroenterol 1988;83:1081–1084.

65. Allison MC, Howatson AG, Torrance CJ, et al. Gastrointestinal damage associated with the use of nonsteroidal anti-inflammatory drugs. N Engl J Med 1992;327:749–754.

66. Armstrong CP, Blower AL. Non-steroidal anti-inflammatory drugs and life threatening complications of peptic ulceration. Gut 1987; 28:527–532.

67. Price AB, Levi J, Dolby JM, et al. Campylobacter pyloridis in peptic ulcer disease: Microbiology, pathology, and scanning electron microscopy. Gut 1985;26:1183–1188.

68. Andersen LP, Holck S, Poolsen CO, et al. Campylobacter pyloridis in peptic ulcer disease. I. Gastric and duodenal infection caused by C. pyloridis: Histopathologic and microbiologic findings. Scand J Gastroenterol 1987;22:219–224.

69. Blaser MJ. Gastric Campylobacter-like organisms, gastritis, and peptic ulcer disease. Gastroenterology 1987;93:371–383.

70. Leung KM, Hui PK, Chan WY, et al. *Helicobacter pylori*-related gastritis and gastric ulcer. A continuum of progressive epithelial degeneration. Am J Clin Pathol 1992;98:569–574.

71. Rathbone BJ, Wyatt JI, Heatley RV. Campylobacter pyloridis - A new factor in peptic ulcer disease. Gut 1986;27:635–641.

72. NIH Consensus Conference. *Helicobacter pylori* in peptic ulcer disease. JAMA 1994;272:65–69.

73. Rauws EAJ, Tytgat GNJ. Cure of duodenal ulcer associated with eradication of *Helicobacter pylori*. Lancet 1990;335:1233–1235.

74. Lam SK, Isenberg JI, Grossman MI, et al. Rapid gastric emptying in duodenal ulcer patients. Dig Dis Sci 1982;27:598.

75. Louw JA, Falck V, Vanrensburg C, et al. Distribution of *Helicobacter pylori* colonization and associated gastric inflammatory changes. Difference between patients with duodenal and gastric ulcers. J Clin Pathol 1993;46:754–757.

76. Khulusi S, Badve S, Patel P, et al. Pathogenesis of gastric metaplasia of the human duodenum: Rule of *Helicobacter pylori*, gastric acid, and ulceration. Gastroenterology 1996;110:452–458.

77. Rhodes J. Etiology of gastric ulcer. Gastroenterology 1972;63;171.

78. Gear MWL, Truelove SC, Whitehead R. Gastric ulcer and gastritis. Gut 1971;12:639–645.

79. Trier JS. Morphology of the gastric mucosa in patients with ulcer disease. Am J Dig Dis 1976;21:138–140.

80. Fisher RS, Cohen S. Pyloric-sphincter dysfunction in patients with gastric ulcer. N Engl J Med 1973;288:273.

81. Rovelstad RA. The incompetent pyloric sphincter: Bile and mucosal ulceration. Am J Dig Dis 1976;21:105.

82. Thomas WEG. Duodeno-gastric reflux: A common factor in pathogenesis of gastric and duodenal ulcer. Lancet 1980;2:1166.

83. Dragstedt LR, Woodward ER. Gastric stasis: A cause of gastric ulcer. Scand J Gastroenterol 1970;5:243.

84. Smith FH, Jordan SM. Gastric ulcer: A study of 600 cases. Gastroenterology 1948;11:575.

85. Chapman ML. Peptic ulcer. A medical perspective. Med Clin North Am 1978;62:39.

86. Misiewicz JJ. Peptic ulceration and its correlation with symptoms. Clin Gastroenterol 1978;7:571.

87. Wesdorp RIC, Fisher JE. Plasma-gastrin and acid secretion in patients with peptic ulceration. Lancet 1974;2:857–860.

88. Walsh JH, Lam SK. Physiology and pathology of gastrin. Clin Gastroenterol 1980;9:567.

89. Peterson WL, Studevant RAL, Frankl HD, et al. Healing of duodenal ulcer with an antacid regimen. N Engl J Med 1977;297:341–345.

90. Isenberg JI, Peterson WL, Elashoff JD, et al. Healing of benign gastric ulcer with low-dose antacid or cimetidine: A double-blind, randomized, placebo-controlled trial. N Engl J Med 1983;308: 1319–1324.

91. Sung JJY, Chung SCS, Ling TKW, et al. Antibacterial treatment of gastric ulcers associated with *Helicobacter pylori*. N Engl J Med 1995;332:139–142.

92. Karsner HT. The pathology of peptic ulcer of the stomach. JAMA 1925;85:1376.

93. Magnus HA. The pathology of peptic ulceration. Postgrad Med J 1954;30:131.

94. Shimazu H, Koniski T, Yamogishi T, et al. A histopathological study on pyloric ulcer. Gastroenterol Jpn 1980;15:362.

95. Oi M, Oshida K, Sugimura S. The location of gastric ulcer. Gastroenterology 1959;36:45–56.

96. Kimura K. Chronological transition of the fundic-pyloric border determined by stepwise biopsy of the lesser and greater curvatures of the stomach. Gastroenterology 1972;63:584.

97. Thomas J, Greig M, McIntosh J, et al. The location of chronic gastric ulcer. Digestion 1980;20:79.

98. Jennings DA, Richardson JE. Giant lesser curve gastric ulcers. Lancet 1954;2:343.

99. Lumsden K, MacLarnon JC, Dawson J. Giant duodenal ulcer. Gut 1970;11:592.

100. Boyle JD. Multiple gastric ulcers. Gastroenterology 1971;61:628.

101. Bonnevie O. Gastric and duodenal ulcers in the same patients. Scand J Gastroenterol 1975;10:657.

102. Ross JR, Reaves LE. Syndrome of posterior penetrating-ulcer. Med Clin North Am 1966;50:461.

103. Joffe N, Antonioli DA. Penetration into spleen by benign gastric ulcer. Clin Radiol 1981;32:177.

104. Sarr MG, Shepard AJ, Zuidema GD. Choledochoduodenal fistula: An unusual complication of duodenal ulcer disease. Am J Surg 1981;141:736.

105. Guerrieri C, Waxman M. Hepatic tissue in gastroscopic biopsy: Evidence of hepatic penetration by peptic ulcer. Am J Gastroenterol 1987;82:890–893.

106. Cody JH, DiVincenti FC, Cowick DR, et al. Gastrocolic and gastrojejunocolic fistulae: Report of twelve cases and review of the literature. Ann Surg 1975;181:376.

107. Mori K, Shinya H, Wolff WI. Polypoid reparative mucosal proliferation at the site of a healed gastric ulcer; sequential gastrocopic, radiological and histological observations. Gastroenterology 1971;61:523.

108. Oohara T, Tohma H, Aono G, et al. Intestinal metaplasia of the regenerative epithelia in 549 gastric ulcers. Hum Pathol 1983;14:1066–1071.

109. Steer HW. The gastro-duodenal epithelium in peptic ulceration. J Pathol 1985;146:355–362.

110. Katzenstein ALA, Maksen J. Candidal infection of gastric ulcers: Histology, incidence and clinical significance. Am J Clin Pathol 1979;71:137.

111. Peters M, Weiner J, Whelan G. Fungal infection associated with gastroduodenal ulceration: Endoscopic and pathologic appearance. Gastroenterology 1980;78:350.

112. Gotlieb-Jensen K, Andersen J. Occurence of Candida in gastric ulcers. Significance for the healing process. Gastroenterology 1983;85:535–537.

113. Loffeld RJ, Loffeld BC, Arends JW, et al. Fungal colonization of gastric ulcers. Am J Gastroenterol 1988;83:730–733.

114. Scolapio JS, DeVault K, Wolfe JT. Eosinophilic gastroenteritis presenting as a giant gastric ulcer. Am J Gastroenterol 1996;91:804–805.

115. Ganguli PC. Antral gastrin-cell hyperplasia in peptic ulcer disease. Lancet 1974;1:583.

116. Takahashi T, Shimazu H, Yamagishi T, et al. G-cell populations in resected stomachs from gastric and duodenal ulcer patients. Gastroenterology 1980;78:498–504.

117. McDonald WC. Correlation of mucosal histology and aspirin intake in chronic gastric ulcer. Gastroenterology 1973;65:381.

118. Hamilton ST, Yardley JH. Endoscopic biopsy diagnosis of aspirin-associated chronic gastric ulcers. Gastroenterology 1980;78:1178.

119. Salupere VP. Gastric biopsy in peptic ulcer: A follow-up study. Scand J Gastroenterol 1969;4:537–543.

120. Gear MWL, Truelove SC, Williams DG, et al. Gastric cancer simulating benign gastric ulcer. Br J Surg 1969;56:739.

121. Montgomery RD, Richardson BP. Gastric ulcer and cancer. Q J Med 1975;44:591.

122. Dekker W, Tytgat GN. Diagnostic accuracy of fiberendoscopy in the detection of upper intestinal malignancy. A follow-up analysis. Gastroenterology 1977;73:710.

123. Mountford RA, Brown P, Salmon PR, et al. Gastric cancer detection in gastric ulcer disease. Gut 1980;21:9–17.

124. Podolsky I, Storms PR, Richardson CT, et al. Gastric adenocarcinoma masquerading endoscopically as benign gastric ulcer. A five-year experience. Dig Dis Sci 1988;33:1057–1063.

125. Hirota T, Itabashi N, Suzuki K, et al. Clinicopathologic study of minute and small early gastric cancer. Pathol Annu 1980;15:1.

126. Green PHR, O'Toole KM, Weinberg LM, et al. Early gastric cancer. Gastroenterology 1981;81:247.

127. Witzel L, Halter F, Gretillat PA, et al. Evaluation of specific value of endoscopic biopsies and brush cytology for malignancies of the esophagus and stomach. Gut 1976;27:375.

128. Halter F, Witzel L, Gretillat PA, et al. Diagnostic value of biopsy, guided lavage, and brush cytology in esophagogastroscopy. Am Dig Dis 1977;22:129–131.

129. Qizilbash AH, Casteli M, Kowalski MA, et al. Endoscopic brush cytology and biopsy in the diagnosis of cancer of the upper gastrointestinal tract. Acta Cytol 1980;24:313.

130. Graham DY, Schwartz JT, Cain GD et al. Prospective evaluation of biopsy number in the diagnosis of esophageal and gastric carcinoma. Gastroenterology 1982;82:228.

131. Marshall JB, Diaz-Arias AA, Barthel JS, et al. Prospective evaluation of optimal number of biopsy specimens and brush cytology in the diagnosis of cancer of the colorectum. Am J Gastroenterol 1993;88:1352–1354.

132. Graham DY. Complications of peptic ulcer disease and indications for surgery. In: Sleisenger MH, Fordtran JS, eds. Gastrointestinal disease. 4th ed. Philadelphia: WB Saunders, 1989:925–938.

133. Chinn AB, Weckesser EC. Acute hemorrhage from peptic ulceration; an analysis of 322 cases. Ann Intern Med 1951;34:339.

134. Cotten PB, Rosenberg MT, Waldram RPL. Early endoscopy of esophagus, stomach, and duodenal bulb in patients with hematemesis and melena. Br Med J 1973;2:1505.

135. Van Zanten SJOV, Bartelsman JFWM, Schipper ME, et al. Recurrent massive haematemesis from Dieulafoy vascular malformations—a review of 101 cases. Gut 1986;27:213–222.

136. Miko TL, Thomazy VA. The caliber persistent artery of the stomach: A unifying approach to gastric aneurysm, Dieulafoy's lesion, and submucosal arterial malformation. Hum Pathol 1988;19:914–921.

137. Rees JR, Thorlyarnasson B. Perforated gastric ulcer. Am J Surg 1973;126:93.

138. Sawyers JL, Herrington JL Jr, Mulherin JL, et al. Acute perforated duodenal ulcer. Arch Surg 1975;110:527.

139. Norris JR, Haubrich WS. The incidence and clinical features of penetration in peptic ulceration. JAMA 1961;178:386.

140. Kozell DD, Meyer KA. Obstructing gastroduodenal ulcer, symptoms and signs. Arch Surg 1964;89:491.

141. Kreel L, Ellis H. Pyloric stenosis in adults: A clinical and radiological study of 100 consecutive patients. Gut 1965;6:253.

142. Pheils MT, Mayday GB, Gillett DJ, et al. Surgery for benign gastric ulcer. Med J Aust 1970;1:56.

143. Scott JW, Sawyers JL, Gobbel WG Jr, et al. Definitive surgical treatment in duodenal ulcer disease. Curr Probl Surg 1968;10:3.

144. Price WE, Grizzle JE, Postlethwait RW, et al. Results of operation for duodenal ulcer. Surg Gynecol Obstet 1970;131:233.

145. Meshkinpour H, Marks JW, Schoenfield LJ, et al. Reflux gastritis syndrome: Mechanism of symptoms. Gastroenterology 1980;79:1283.

146. Tabaquchali S. The pathophysiological role of small intestinal flora. Scand J Gastroenterol 1970;(Suppl 6) 5:139.

147. Lundh G. Intestinal digestion and absorption after gastrectomy. Acta Chir Scand 1958;231:1.

148. Brooke-Cowden GL, Braasch JW, Gibb SO, et al. Postgastrectomy syndromes. Am J Surg 1976;131:464.

149. Ellis J, Kingston RD, Brookes VS, et al. Gastric carcinoma and previous peptic ulceration. Br J Surg 1979;66:117.

150. Papachriston DN, Agnanti N, Fortner JG. Gastric carcinoma after treatment of ulcer. Am J Surg 1980;139:193.

151. Domellof L, Erickson S, Janunger KG. Carcinoma and possible precancerous changes of the gastric stump after Billroth II resection. Gastroenterology 1977;73:462.

152. Offerhaus GJA, Stodt J, Huibregtse K, et al. The mucosa of the gastric remnant harboring malignancy. Histologic findings in the biopsy specimens of 504 asymptomatic patients 15 to 46 years after partial gastrectomy with emphasis on non malignant lesions. Cancer 1989;64:698–703.

153. Lundegardh G, Adami H-O, Helmich C, et al. Stomach cancer after partial gastrectomy for benign ulcer disease. N Engl J Med 1988;319:195–200.

154. Jabbori M, Goesky CA, Lough J, et al. The inlet patch: Heterotopic gastric mucosa in the upper esophagus. Gastroenterology 1985;89: 352–356.

155. Franzin G, Musola R, Negri A, et al. Heterotopic gastric (fundic) mucosa in the duodenum. Endoscopy 1982;14:166–167.

156. Wolff M. Heterotopic gastric epithelium in the rectum: A report of three new cases with a review of 87 cases of gastric heterotopia in the alimentary canal. Am J Clin Pathol 1971;55:604–616.

157. Seagram CG, Louch RE, Stephens CA, et al. Meckel's diverticulum: A 10-year review of 218 cases. Can J Surg 1968;11:369–373.

158. Bower RJ, Seiber WK, Kiesewetter WB. Alimentary tract duplications in children. Ann Surg 1978;188:669–674.

159. Truong LD, Stroebein JR, McKechnie JC. Gastric heterotopia of the proximal esophagus: A report of four cases detected by endoscopy and review of the literature. Am J Gastroenterol 1986;81:1162–1166.

160. Debas HT, Chaum H, Thomson FB, et al. Functioning heterotopic oxyntic mucosa in the rectum. Gastroenterol Clin Biol 1983; 7:39–42.

161. Kaloni BP, Vaezzadeh K, Sieber WK. Gastric heterotopia in rectum complicated by rectovesical fistula. Dig Dis Sci 1983;28: 378–380.

162. Case record of the Massachusetts General Hospital. N Engl J Med 1980;302:958–962.

163. Meguid M, Erakis AJ. Complications of Meckel's diverticulum in infants. Surg Gynecol Obstet 1974;139:541–544.

164. Printen KJ, Scott D, Mason EE. Stomal ulcers after gastric bypass. Arch Surg 1980;115:525.

165. Hunt PS, Dowling J, Korman M, et al. Bleeding stomal ulceration. Aust J Surg 1979;49:15.

166. Webster MW, Barnes EL, Stremple JF. Serum gastrin levels in the differential diagnosis of recurrent peptic ulceration due to retained gastric antrum. Am J Surg 1978;135:248.

167. Zollinger RM, Ellison EH. Primary ulcerations of jejunum associated with islet cell tumors of pancreas. Ann Surg 1955;142:709–728.

168. Ellison EH, Wilson SD. The Zollinger-Ellison syndrome: Reappraisal and evaluation of 260 registered cases. Ann Surg 1964;160:512.

169. Isenberg JI, Walsh JH, Grossman MI. Zollinger-Ellison syndrome. Gastroenterology 1973;65:140–165.

170. Wolfe MM, Jensen RT. Zollinger-Ellison syndrome. Current concepts in diagnosis and management. N Engl J Med 1987;317.1200–1209.

171. Greider MH, Rosai J, McGuigan JE. The human pancreatic islet cells and their tumors. II. Ulcerogenic and diarrheogenic tumors. Cancer 1974;33:1423.

172. Creutzfeldt W, Arnold R, Creutzfeldt C, et al. Pathomorphologic, biochemical and diagnostic aspects of gastrinomas (Zollinger-Ellison syndrome). Hum Pathol 1975;6:47.

173. Solcia E, Capella C, Buffa R, et al. Pathology of the Zollinger-Ellison syndrome. In: Fenoglio CM, ed. Progress in surgical pathology, volume 1. New York: Masson, 1980:119–133.

174. Ballard HS, Frame B, Hartsock RJ. Familial multiple endocrine adenoma-peptic ulcer complex. Medicine 1964;43:481.

175. Craven DE, Goodman AD, Carter JH. Familial multiple endocrine adenomatosis: Multiple endocrine neoplasia type I. Arch Intern Med 1972;129:567.

176. McGuigan JE, Wolfe MM. Secretin injection test in the diagnosis of gastrinoma. Gastroenterology 1980;79:1324.

177. DeVeney CW, DeVeney KS, Jaffe BM, et al. Use of calcium and secretin in the diagnosis of gastrinoma (Zollinger-Ellison syndrome). Ann Intern Med 1977;87:680.

178. Mansbach CM, Wilkins RM, Dobbins WO, et al. Intestinal mucosal function and structure in the steatorrhea of Zollinger-Ellison syndrome. Arch Intern Med 1968;121:487.

179. Shimoda SS, Saunder DR, Rubin CE. The Zollinger-Ellison syndrome with steatorrhea. Mechanisms of fat and vitamin B-12 malabsorption. Gastroenterology 1968;55:705.

180. Straus E, Yalow RS. Differential diagnosis in hyperchlorhydric hypergastrinemia. Gastroenterology 1974;66:867.

181. Bonfils S, Mignon M, Gratton H. Cimetidine treatment of acute and chronic Zollinger-Ellison syndrome. World J Surg 1979;3:597.

182. McCarthy DM. The place of surgery in the Zollinger Ellison syndrome. N Engl J Med 1980;302:1344.

183. Goldman H, Antonioli DA. Mucosal biopsy of the esophagus, stomach, and proximal duodenum. Hum Pathol 1982;13:423–448.

184. Whitehead R. Mucosal biopsy of the gastrointestinal tract. 4th ed. Philadelphia: WB Saunders, 1990:41–157.

185. Rotterdam H. Stomach. In: Rotterdam H, Sheahan DG, Sommers SC, eds. Biopsy diagnosis of the digestive tract. 2nd ed. New York: Raven Press, 1993:62–255.

186. Kobayashi S, Prolla JC, Kirsner JB. Brushing cytology of the esophagus and stomach under direct vision by fiberscopes. Acta Cytol 1970;14:223.

187. Hanson JT, Thorenson C, Morrissey JF. Brush cytology in the diagnosis of upper gastrointestinal malignancy. Gastrointest Endosc 1980,26:33.

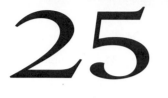

25 MUCOSAL HYPERTROPHY AND HYPERPLASIA OF THE STOMACH

Harvey Goldman

GENERAL ASPECTS

Localized or diffuse thickening or hypertrophy of the gastric mucosa can result from discrete hyperplasia of one or more of the epithelial elements of the mucosa or from inflammatory and tumor infiltrates. The epithelia that may be involved include the surface-foveolar (pit) mucous cells, the specialized parietal and chief cells of the corpus/fundus, the pyloric glands, and various combinations. The lesions can be focal, multifocal, or diffuse; the latter usually are concentrated in a particular region, such as the corpus (e.g., Zollinger-Ellison syndrome and Ménétrier disease) or antrum (most inflammatory lesions), or are present throughout the stomach (most tumors).

Depending on the location and extent of mucosal hypertrophy, the lesions are visualized as polyps, enlargement of the rugae, or some other deformity of the mucosal surface. Clinical features relate to the complications of polyps, the presence of hypersecretory states, or the effects of any underlying inflammatory or neoplastic disease. Most conditions that result in mucosal hypertrophy, such as gastritis, peptic ulcer disease, and gastric polyps, are discussed in Chapters 23, 24, and 26, respectively. The salient features of these disorders as well as the complete descriptions of other related conditions represent the focus of this chapter.

FOCAL MUCOSAL HYPERTROPHY OF THE STOMACH

The principal causes of focal or multifocal thickening of the gastric mucosa are polyps, the localized effects of inflammation

and repair, and the presence of heterotopic (ectopic) tissues (Table 25.1).

POLYPS

Gastric polyps (detailed in Chapter 26) include lesions that are inflammatory, hyperplastic (regenerative), hamartomatous, and neoplastic. Nonneoplastic polyps represent localized expansions of the mucosa and usually are composed of hyperplastic epithelial elements, mainly the surface-foveolar mucous cells and pyloric glands, together with varying amounts of edema, inflammatory cells, and proliferating stromal cells of the lamina propria (1, 2). Less common lesions are fundic gland polyps (3, 4), which contain specialized corpus epithelial cells with prominent cystic change, and benign lymphoid polyps that are localized areas of marked lymphoid hyperplasia (5). The polyps usually are single but can be multiple and exceptionally confluent in their appearance (see Fig. 23.14). Multiple gastric polyps of varying types are also encountered in the several polyposis syndromes, including familial adenomatous polyposis coli, generalized juvenile polyposis, the Peutz-Jeghers syndrome, and the Cronkhite-Canada syndrome (6–9).

INFLAMMATORY LESIONS

Commonly noted in the stomach are localized mucosal thickening related to inflammatory edema and regenerative tissue. These lesions are most often observed adjacent to ulcers and appear as a uniform elevation of the mucosa or as deformed folds (see Fig. 24.9). Mucosal biopsies are frequently performed to confirm the inflammatory nature of such areas and to exclude other more significant lesions, such as neoplasms.

TABLE 25.1	Causes of Focal Mucosal Hypertrophy of the Stomach

Polyps
   Inflammatory
   Hamartomatous
   Hyperplastic
   Neoplastic
Inflammatory lesions
   Edema
   Regeneration
Heterotopic tissues

HETEROTOPIC PANCREATIC TISSUE

Ectopic foci of mature pancreatic tissue may be observed in the stomach, more often in the distal portion, and in the duodenum (10–13). The gastric implants consist of the pancreatic elements alone or in combination with varying amounts of bile duct epithelia and smooth muscle. When the amount of muscle tissue is especially prominent, the lesions have also been termed adenomyomatous hamartoma and adenomyomas, but they are probably variants of the heterotopic process (14). The lesions usually are small and confined to the gastric wall, but they may enlarge and extend into the mucosal region (Fig 25.1). Endoscopic examination reveals as slightly raised, often umbilicated nodules (15), although biopsy samples are usually too superficial to detect the heterotopic glandular tissue. The umbilication represents the outlet of the exocrine duct (see Chapter 10).

The ectopic tissue should be distinguished from areas of pancreatic metaplasia, which consist of microscopic foci of pancreatic acinar tissue in the mucosa of patients with chronic gastritis (16) (see Fig. 23.4).

DIFFUSE MUCOSAL HYPERTROPHY OF THE STOMACH

The causes of a diffuse thickening or hypertrophy of the gastric mucosa, involving a major portion such as the corpus or antrum or the entire stomach, are listed in Table 25.2. It should be stressed that one of the principal causes, and perhaps the most common cause, of enlarged gastric folds or rugae is simply a variation of the normal size (17–19). Rugae are limited to the gastric fundus and corpus region and are composed of both mucosal and submucosal tissues. Their enlargement can be readily appreciated by radiographic and gross endoscopic examinations, and the diagnosis of a normal variation depends on noting that the rugae are simply enlarged but not deformed in any way and excluding any associated inflammation or hypersecretory state.

More significant causes of diffuse mucosal hypertrophy in the stomach include hyperplasia of the parietal cells (Zollinger-Ellison syndrome), of the surface-foveolar mucous cells (Ménétrier disease), or of some combination (other forms of hypertrophic

gastropathy) (14, 20). These disorders must be distinguished from a variety of inflammatory and neoplastic conditions that can also infiltrate and expand the mucosal region.

ZOLLINGER-ELLISON SYNDROME

This condition is detailed in Chapters 15 and 24, and is summarized briefly as follows.

DEFINITION, ETIOLOGY, AND PATHOGENESIS

The components of the syndrome include an autonomous source of gastrin, maximal stimulation and hyperplasia of the gastric parietal cells, and the presence of uncontrolled peptic ulcer disease and occasionally of maldigestion (21–23). Over 90% of cases are attributable to islet cell hyperplasia or tumors ("gastrinomas") of the pancreas, usually malignant but slowly growing (24, 25); other causes include tumors in the duodenal wall and rarely in the jejunum, and diffuse hyperplasia of antral G cells (26, 27).

CLINICAL FEATURES

Massive and continuous hypersecretion of gastric acid results in multiple erosions and ulcers of the stomach, all parts of the

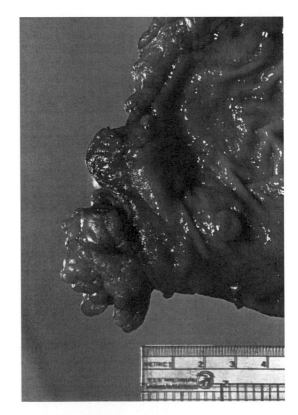

Figure 25.1 Heterotopic pancreatic tissue in the stomach. Lower part of the gastric antrum is shown, with the pylorus and rim of contiguous duodenum at the left. A localized, polypoid swelling *(bottom)* of the mucosa is attributable to the presence of the ectopic pancreatic tissue. The fine umbilication on the surface represents the outlet of a pancreatic duct. (Courtesy of Dr. Karoly Balogh, Deaconess Hospital, Boston, MA.)

TABLE	
25.2	**Causes of Diffuse Mucosal Hypertrophy of the Stomach**

Normal variation
Zollinger-Ellison syndrome
Menetrier disease
Hypertrophic, hypersecretory gastropathy
  (Other rare types)
Inflammatory disorders
  Tuberculosis, syphilis, and sarcoidosis
  Isolated granulomatous gastritis
  Allergic gastroenteritis
  Lymphocytic gastritis
  Gastritis cystica polyposa and profunda
Tumors
  Lymphoma
  Carcinoma

duodenum, and even the jejunum. Because of the great amount of acid and fluid produced, effects may include an inadequate dilution of the acid by the biliary secretions and inactivation of the primary bile salts, leading to diarrhea and maldigestion of fats. The diagnosis usually is secured by the detection of excess gastrin in the blood, made worse by calcium infusions, and by noting that the basal and stimulated acid outputs are equivalent (28). Treatment consists of removal of any resectable tumors and administration of H2-blocking agents; gastric resection is reserved for intractable cases (29).

PATHOLOGIC FEATURES

The gastric effects of the Zollinger-Ellison syndrome are described in Chapter 24 and include the presence of regularly enlarged rugae (see Fig. 24.23), the result of significant hyperplasia of the parietal cells in the fundus/corpus region (Fig 25.2; see Fig 24.21) (27). Many of the gastric glands are cystic owing to acid hypersecretion (Fig 25.3). The hyperplastic parietal cells are also noted in the foveolar region (see Fig. 24.22), which can be appreciated in endoscopic biopsy samples, but this feature is not specific for the syndrome (19). Although deeper aspiration-type mucosal biopsies can be performed in order to count and document the parietal cell hyperplasia, other functional studies are used more routinely for diagnosis. The corpus region shows no associated inflammation and no hyperplasia of the surface/foveolar mucous cells. Multiple mucosal erosions and ulcers, with acute and chronic inflammatory features, are observed within the antrum, all parts of the duodenum, and occasionally the jejunum. These features, together with the complications of peptic ulcer disease, are detailed in Chapter 24. Characteristics of those cases involving hyperplasia of the antral G cells are provided in Chapter 15.

DIAGNOSIS AND DIFFERENTIAL DIAGNOSIS

The diagnosis of Zollinger-Ellison syndrome is suspected in any patient with multiple or intractable peptic ulcer disease, and is confirmed by documentation of maximal acid production and

hypergastrinemia. Angiographic studies typically are needed to identify the presence and extent of the underlying tumor. The pathologic features in the gastric corpus are distinctive. Other causes of diffuse mucosal thickening in this area include Ménétrier disease, which reveals hyperplasia of the surface/foveolar mucous cells, lymphocytic (varioliform) gastritis showing significant inflammation, and infiltration by tumor. The rarer forms of hypertrophic gastropathy, described subsequently, may show hyperplasia of both the mucous cells and the specialized glands, and are not associated with a gastrinoma.

MÉNÉTRIER DISEASE

DEFINITION, ETIOLOGY, AND PATHOGENESIS

Ménétrier disease, originally described in 1888 (30), is a relatively rare disorder characterized by diffuse hyperplasia of the surface/foveolar mucous cells of the stomach (30–36); it usually is limited to the corpus/fundic region but may extend into the antrum (37). The etiology and pathogenesis are not known, although a frequent

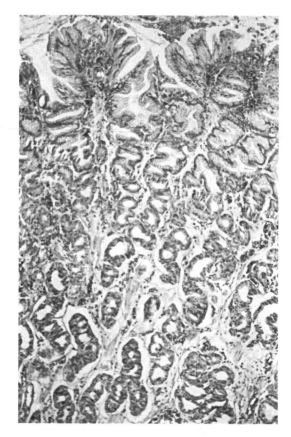

Figure 25.2 Gastric corpus mucosa in a case of Zollinger-Ellison syndrome, with surface at top. Expansion of the mucosa is due to hyperplasia of the parietal cells, which extend into the foveolar region. Most of the gastric glands are dilated, reflecting the increased secretion of the parietal cells. There is mild edema of the lamina propria but no significant increase in inflammatory cells (H & E, ×80).

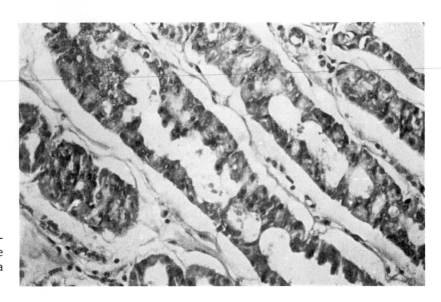

Figure 25.3 Gastric corpus glands in Zollinger-Ellison syndrome (same case as in Fig. 25.2). Note the dilation of the glands and edema of the lamina propria (H & E, ×200).

association with prior respiratory infections has been noted in cases in children. The disease is associated with normal or reduced gastric acid and with protein loss from the mucosa resulting in hypoalbuminemia (31, 38, 39). The reduction in gastric acid may be related to dilution by mucous secretions or to loss of the parietal cells secondary to expansion of the foveolar cells; this issue has not been decided.

A major problem in the understanding of Ménétrier disease relates to the poor or uncertain documentation of the essential features in many reported cases (20, 40, 41). The tendency has been to consider all cases with giant folds in the proximal stomach, usually with the exception of cases of Zollinger-Ellison, as potential examples of Ménétrier disease without further consideration of the histologic and functional features. This tendency has resulted in the inclusion of many cases that are probably examples of more ordinary chronic gastritis (42–44); indeed, the alleged association of carcinoma with Ménétrier disease may be related instead to this confusion with other cases of chronic gastritis. Definitive diagnosis of Ménétrier disease requires documentation of foveolar hyperplasia without significant inflammation, the lack of increased acid production, and the presence of protein loss from the mucosa (20).

CLINICAL FEATURES

Most adults with Ménétrier disease are 30 to 60 years of age, and 75% are men. Familial cases have been recorded rarely (45). Patients present with epigastric pain, weight loss, and diarrhea, and physical examination demonstrates evidence of peripheral edema in many cases. Further studies reveal enlargement of the gastric rugae, protein loss in the gut from the hyperplastic mucous cells, and hypoalbuminemia resulting in edema. Other causes of hypoalbuminemia such as renal diseases and other sources of the protein loss in the gut must be excluded. Medical treatment is mainly limited to albumin replacement and other maintenance of adequate nutrition. In some cases, the disease regresses spontaneously (46, 47), but when it persists in adult patients, surgical resection is often required to eliminate the lesion (48, 49).

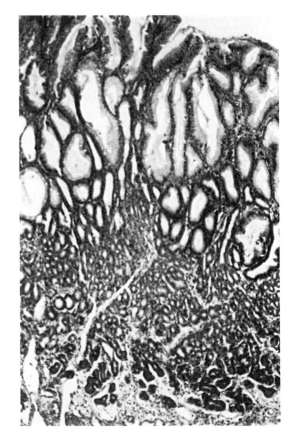

Figure 25.4 Gastric corpus mucosa in a patient with Ménétrier disease shows marked hyperplasia of the gastric foveolae (pits), with slight inflammation in the lamina propria, resulting in a thickening (hypertrophy) of the gastric mucosa. The normal corpus glands are at bottom. The foveolar region represents over 50% of the mucosal thickness in this sample; in the normal gastric body, the foveolae occupy only about 20% (H & E, ×13). (Courtesy of Dr. Donald Antonioli, Beth Israel Hospital, Boston, MA.)

PATHOLOGIC FEATURES

The essential pathologic feature is a pronounced hyperplasia of the foveolar (pit) mucous cells (14, 19, 20, 39, 44, 50, 51). The foveolae are greatly elongated, often tortuous, and cystic in appearance, and are composed mainly of mature mucous cells with little evidence of active regenerative cells or mitoses (Figs. 25.4 to 25.6). No ulcerations are evident, the amount of inflammatory cells in the epithelial layer and lamina propria typically is slight, and intestinal metaplasia is uncommon. The lesion is dominantly present in the corpus region, and the quantity of underlying parietal and chief cells is either normal or moderately reduced. Significant or complete loss of the specialized corpus glands, such as occurs in association with chronic atrophic gastritis, is not observed. The foveolar mucous cells can be accented with mucin stains, such as the periodic-acid Schiff (PAS) reaction, revealing intense staining throughout the cytoplasm (Fig. 25.7). In contrast, the neutral mucin granules typically are concentrated in the upper portions of the cells in the normal stomach.

At a gross level, the rugae are irregularly enlarged and often associated with polypoid areas, which are cystic and ooze mucus from the cut surface (Fig. 25.8). Mucosal biopsies allow ready identification of the foveolar hyperplasia and also exclude other causes of enlarged rugae, such as inflammatory lesions and tumors (19, 52, 53). Considering the limited size and amount of tissue obtained using mucosal biopsy, the sample may consist almost entirely of the hyperplastic foveolae, in contrast to a biopsy sample of normal or inflamed mucosa, which would contain a substantial component of the specialized glands (see Fig. 25.5); in such cases, the biopsy may offer the first suggestion that the patient has Ménétrier disease. No abnormalities of the rest of the gastric wall are evident, nor is there an association with other protein-losing disorders of the gut. Contrary to earlier reports, lesions usually show no signs of associated dysplasia or carcinoma.

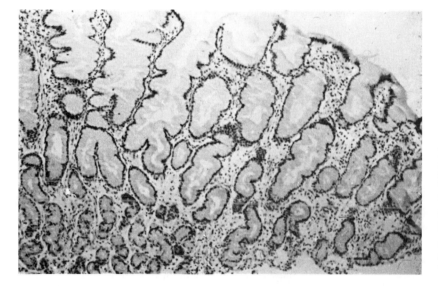

Figure 25.5 Gastric corpus mucosal biopsy sample in a case of Ménétrier disease shows marked hyperplasia of the foveolar mucous cells without significant inflammation. A small portion of the specialized glands is evident at lower left (H & E, ×80). (Reproduced with permission from Goldman H, Antonioli DA. Mucosal biopsy of the esophagus, stomach, and proximal duodenum. Hum Pathol 1982;13:423–448.)

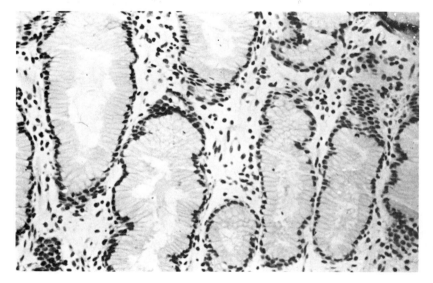

Figure 25.6 Gastric corpus mucosal biopsy in Ménétrier disease (same case as in Fig. 25.5). Hyperplastic and enlarged foveolar cells are filled with mucus in their cytoplasm. The nuclei are limited to the basal region of the cells and show no signs of active regeneration. Findings include mild edema and a small number of mononuclear inflammatory cells in the lamina propria but no inflammation in the epithelial layer (H & E, ×200).

DIAGNOSIS AND DIFFERENTIAL DIAGNOSIS

The diagnosis of definite cases of Ménétrier disease requires the demonstration of enlarged gastric rugae principally attributable to a hyperplasia of the foveolar mucous cells in the proximal part of the stomach that is not associated with significant inflammation; the absence of hyperplasia of other epithelial elements, such as parietal

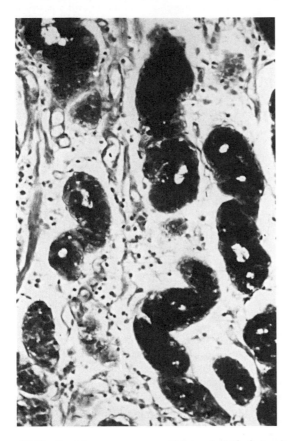

Figure 25.7   Gastric corpus mucosal biopsy in Ménétrier disease reveals intense staining for neutral mucin in the foveolar cells. Staining is evident in the entire cytoplasm, in contrast to normal foveolar cells, which show the mucin limited to the upper part of the cells (periodic acid-Schiff [PAS] reaction, ×100).

cells, and of excess acid production; and the presence of protein loss from the mucosa, leading to reduced serum albumin levels. In both the early and the healing phases of the disease, the morphologic features probably can exist without significant functional effects. Unfortunately, the clinical course in most cases of Ménétrier disease in adults is unpredictable.

Histologic confirmation is needed to verify the diagnosis and to exclude other causes of giant gastric folds in the proximal part of the stomach. Classic Zollinger-Ellison syndrome is associated with acid hypersecretion and no hyperplasia of the foveolar mucous cells or protein loss, and considerable inflammation is noted in cases of lymphocytic gastritis and other forms of chronic gastritis. Rarer types of hypertrophic gastropathy reveal hyperplasia of both the mucous cells and the specialized glands. Tumors such as large villous adenomas, carcinomas, and lymphomas can manifest with gross configurations that simulate enlarged mucosal folds and on occasion are associated with protein loss; these conditions are ultimately distinguished by histologic examination.

Problems can arise in the interpretation of small endoscopic biopsies. Because tissue specimens are limited in number and size, one must carefully correlate the histologic findings with the overall gross appearance of the mucosa and the functional features. Biopsies may reveal a localized area of foveolar hyperplasia that overlies a more ominous tumor lesion or that is a part of the healing phase of an inflammatory condition; the latter is more of a problem in the antrum, where most inflammatory disorders are concentrated. Such areas of foveolar hyperplasia usually are not composed entirely of mature mucous cells, as seen in Ménétrier disease. Typical findings include many mitoses and regenerating cells with enlarged nuclei and reduced cytoplasm. In selected cases, it may be advisable to perform the larger aspiration-type and snare biopsies, which permit evaluation of a greater depth of the mucosa and can help to exclude an underlying tumor (53).

RELATION TO CARCINOMA

In many isolated reports, authors have claimed that a link exists between Ménétrier disease and the development of carcinoma in adult patients, similar to that noted with chronic atrophic gastritis and pernicious anemia (32, 54). Documentation generally has been poor, however, and it is probable that most of these cases instead represent examples of the more common forms of chronic gastritis

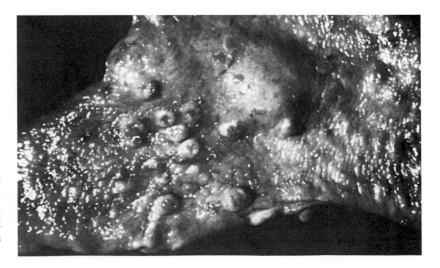

Figure 25.8   Stomach, in a case of Ménétrier disease; a portion of the antrum is at left. Note the irregular thickening of the corpus mucosa with numerous polypoid areas, extending to the junction with the antrum. The normal gastric rugae are not seen. (Courtesy of Dr. Karoly Balogh, Deaconess Hospital, Boston MA.)

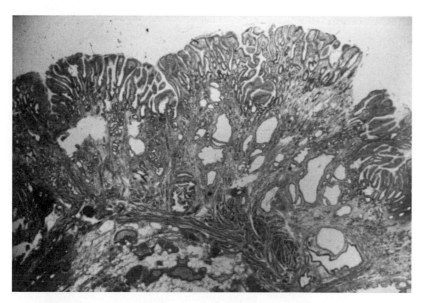

Figure 25.9 Gastric corpus mucosa in a case of gastritis cystica polyposa, with a small portion of submucosa at bottom. This condition developed in the proximal stomach remnant after subtotal resection of the distal stomach. Note the regeneration and hyperplasia of the gastric foveolae, some of which are cystic; considerable loss of the specialized corpus glands; and associated inflammation in the lamina propria (H & E, ×31).

or situations demonstrating newly developed inflammation and repair that is secondary to the tumor. This disclaimer is supported by the frequent presence of significant inflammation in the lesions and by the lack of a defined, long-term course before tumor development. The issue is not completely settled, but it seems unlikely that carcinoma is an important complication of Ménétrier disease (20).

CHILDHOOD CASES OF MÉNÉTRIER DISEASE

Although many children have an antecedent history of a respiratory infection and peripheral blood eosinophilia, the exact etiology and pathogenesis are not established. Compared to the clinical course in adults, Ménétrier disease in children is self-limited and regresses spontaneously after several weeks, surgical excision is not required (55–59). This disease neither recurs nor is it associated with carcinoma. The major differential diagnosis is allergic gastroenteritis, manifestations of which include enlarged gastric folds and protein loss (60). In the allergic condition, however, the lesion typically is in the gastric antrum, blood loss and anemia are often evident, and an increase of eosinophils is noted in biopsy tissue (see Chapter 12) (61).

OTHER TYPES OF HYPERTROPHIC, HYPERSECRETORY GASTROPATHY

These very rare disorders are characterized by variable hyperplasia of the foveolar mucous cells and the parietal cells (20). Their etiology and pathogenesis are not known. It is possible that some cases represent variants of Zollinger-Ellison syndrome and of Ménétrier disease.

CASES WITHOUT PROTEIN LOSS

Some cases have a focal and nodular thickening of the corpus mucosa that is due mainly to hyperplasia of parietal cells, acid hypersecretion, and multiple peptic ulcers of the gastric antrum and duodenum (62–64). Usually no significant hyperplasia of the surface/foveolar mucous cells is noted. The clinical and histologic features of the cases most closely resemble those in the Zollinger-Ellison syndrome, but affected patients lack a demonstrable source

of autonomous G cells and hypergastrinemia. Nevertheless, this condition may represent a milder form of the syndrome associated with a more focal hyperplasia of the parietal cell mass. Further studies are needed.

CASES WITH PROTEIN LOSS

In the few cases reported, findings included hyperplasia of the foveolar mucous cells and protein loss from the stomach. In contrast to typical Ménétrier disease, patients also demonstrate variable expansion of the parietal cells, acid hypersecretion, and development of peptic ulcers (65, 66).

INFLAMMATORY AND NEOPLASTIC CONDITIONS

INFLAMMATORY DISORDERS

A large variety of specific inflammatory conditions can be associated with gastric mucosal thickening, either localized or diffuse. These disorders mainly affect the antrum and include infections such as tuberculosis and syphilis, eosinophilic (allergic) gastroenteritis, isolated granulomatous gastritis, chronic granulomatous disease, and sarcoidosis (67–75). Mucosal hypertrophy can be dramatic, leading to pyloric obstruction and requiring biopsy to exclude tumors. Furthermore, any case of the more ordinary forms of chronic antral gastritis or chronic fundic gastritis can lead to the development of areas of polypoid or diffuse foveolar hyperplasia (76). These inflammatory disorders are typically distinguished from the syndromes described previously by the presence of significant inflammation.

Lymphocytic gastritis (also termed varioliform gastritis and chronic erosive gastritis) is associated with prominent mucosal hypertrophy of either the proximal part or the entire stomach (77–81). Characteristic findings include protein loss (82–84); heavy inflammatory infiltrate, particularly of lymphocytes in the epithelial layer; and alternating areas of erosions and mucosal thickening (see Fig 23.17). A significant degree of mucosal thickening is a common finding in gastritis cystica polyposa and gastritis cystica profunda (85–88); the former disorder is associated with cystic glands in the mucosa (Fig. 25.9), whereas in the latter, dilated glands are also found in the submucosa. These lesions may be diffuse or more localized, and they are especially prominent next to gastrojejunostomy stomas (see Fig. 23.27). The allergic disorders are described in Chapter 12 and the other inflammatory conditions of the stomach are discussed in Chapter 23.

TUMORS

Although most neoplasms of the stomach are solitary masses, they occasionally are more widespread and lead to diffuse mucosal thickening characterized by aberrant folds (89). These manifesta-

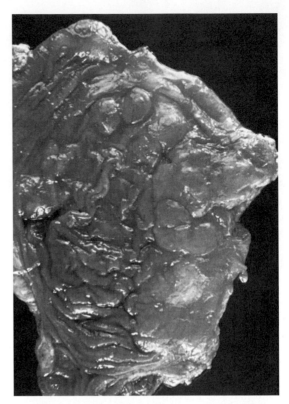

Figure 25.10   Stomach in a case of diffuse lymphoma, with antral region at the bottom. Pronounced thickening and deformity of the mucosal surface throughout the stomach are related to the tumor infiltration and associated edema. The normal gastric rugae are not seen.

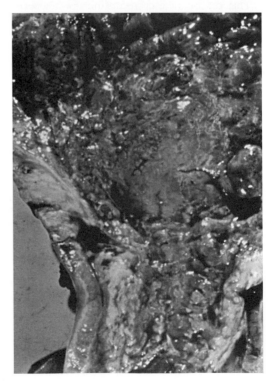

Figure 25.11   Stomach in a case of diffuse adenocarcinoma of the linitis plastica type, with antral region at bottom. In addition to the mural expansion, note the significant thickening of the mucosa and nodular irregularity of its surface. Some remnants of gastric rugae are seen at top.

tions are seen most often with lymphomas (Fig. 25.10), primary carcinomas of the linitis plastica type (Fig. 25.11), and, rarely, metastatic tumors (see Chapters 17 and 27).

REFERENCES

1. Ming SC, Goldman H. Gastric polyps: A histogenetic classification and its relation to carcinoma. Cancer 1965;18:721.
2. Tomasulo J. Gastric polyps: Histologic types and their relationship to gastric carcinoma. Cancer 1971;27:1346.
3. Lee RG, Burt RW. The histopathology of fundic gland polyps of the stomach. Am J Clin Pathol 1986;86:498–503.
4. Marcial MA, Villafana M, Hernandez-Denton J, et al. Fundic gland polyps: Prevalence and clinicopathologic features. Am J Gastroenterol 1993;88:1711–1713.
5. Ranchod M, Lewin KJ, Dorfman RF. Lymphoid hyperplasia of the gastro-intestinal tract: A study of 26 cases and review of the literature. Am J Surg Pathol 1978;2:383–400.
6. Watanabe H, Enjoji M, Yao T, et al. Gastric lesions in familial adenomatous polyposis coli: Their incidence and histological analysis. Hum Pathol 1978;9:269.
7. Sachatello CR, Pickren JW, Grace JT. Generalized juvenile gastro-intestinal polyposis. Gastroenterology 1970;58:669.
8. Williams GT, Bussey HJR, Morson BC. Hamartomatous polyps in Peutz-Jeghers syndrome. N Engl J Med 1978;299:101.
9. Burke AP, Sobin LH. The pathology of Cronkhite-Canada polyps. A comparison to juvenile polyposis. Am J Surg Pathol 1989;13:940–946.
10. Taylor AL. The epithelial heterotopias of the alimentary tract. J Pathol 1944;30:375–380.
11. Branch CD, Gross RE. Aberrant pancreatic tissue in GI tract. Surg Gynecol Obstet 1946;82:527.
12. Barbosa J de C, Dockerty MB, Waugh JM. Pancreatic heterotopia: Review of literature and report of 41 authenticated surgical cases, of which 25 were clinically significant. Surg Gynecol Obstet 1946;85:527–542.
13. Kaneda M, Yano T, Yamamoto T, et al. Ectopic pancreas on the stomach presenting as an inflammatory abdominal mass. Am J Gastroenterol 1989;84:663–666.
14. Ming SC. Tumors of the esophagus and stomach. In: Atlas of tumor pathology, 2nd series, fascicle 7. Washington DC: Armed Forces Institute of Pathology, 1973.
15. Caberwal D, Kogan SJ, Levitt SB. Ectopic pancreas presenting as an umbilical mass. J Pediatr Surg 1977;593–595.
16. Doglioni C, Laurino L, Dei Tos A, et al. Pancreatic (acinar) metaplasia of the gastric mucosa. Histology, ultrastructure, immunocytochemistry, and clinicopathologic correlations of 101 cases. Am J Surg Pathol 1993;17:1134–1143.
17. Reeder MM, Olmstead WW, Cooper PH. Large gastric folds, local or widespread. JAMA 1974;230:273.
18. Press AJ. Practical significance of gastric rugal folds. AJR Am J Roentgenol 1975;125:172.
19. Goldman H, Antonioli DA. Mucosal biopsy of the esophagus, stomach, and proximal duodenum. Hum Pathol 1982;13:423–448.
20. Appelman HD. Localized and extensive expansions of the gastric mucosa: Mucosal polyps and giant folds. In: Appelman HD, ed. Pathology of the esophagus, stomach, and duodenum. New York: Churchill Livingstone, 1984:79–119.
21. Zollinger RM, Ellison EH. Primary ulcerations of jejunum associated with islet cell tumors of pancreas. Ann Surg 1955;142:709–728.
22. Ellison EH, Wilson SD. The Zollinger-Ellison syndrome: Reappraisal and evaluation of 260 registered cases. Ann Surg 1964;160:512.
23. Isenberg JI, Walsh JH, Grossman MI. Zollinger-Ellison syndrome. Gastroenterology 1973;65:140–165.
24. Greider MH, Rosai J, McGuigan JE. The human pancreatic islet cells and their tumors. II. Ulcerogenic and diarrheogenic tumors. Cancer 1974;33:1423.
25. Creutzfeldt W, Arnold R, Creutzfeldt C, et al. Pathomorphologic, biochemical and diagnostic aspects of gastrinomas (Zollinger-Ellison syndrome). Hum Pathol 1975;6:47.
26. Gangul PC. Antral gastrin-cell hyperplasia in peptic ulcer disease. Lancet 1974;1:583.
27. Solcia E, Capella C, Buffa R, et al. Pathology of the Zollinger-Ellison syndrome. In: Fenoglio CM, Wolff M. Progress in surgical pathology, volume 1. New York: Masson, 1980:119–133.
28. Wolfe MM, Jensen RT. Zollinger-Ellison syndrome. Current concepts in diagnosis and management. N Engl J Med 1987;317:1200–1209.
29. McCarthy DM. The place of surgery in the Zollinger-Ellison syndrome. N Engl J Med 1980;302:1344.
30. Ménétrier P. Des polyadenomes gastriques et de leurs rapports avec le cancer de l'estomac. Arch Physiol Norm Pathol 1888;1:32–55, 236–262.
31. Chokas WV, Connor DH, Innes RC. Giant hypertrophy of the gastric mucosa, hypoproteinemia and edema (Ménétrier's disease). Am J Med 1959;27:125–131.
32. Scharschmidt BF. The natural history of hypertrophic gastropathy (Ménétrier's disease). Report of a case with 16 year follow-up and review of 120 cases from the literature. Am J Med 1977;63:644.
33. Davis JM, Gray GF, Thorbjarnarson B. Ménétrier's disease. A clinicopathologic study of six cases. Ann Surg 1977;185:456.
34. Fieber SS, Rickert RR. Hyperplastic gastropathy. Analysis of 50 selected cases from 1955–1980. Am J Gastroenterol 1981;76:321.
35. Komorowski RA, Caya JG. Hyperplastic gastropathy. Clinicopathologic correlation. Am J Surg Pathol 1991;15:577–585.
36. Meuwissen SGM, Ridwan BU, Hasper HJ, et al. Hypertrophic protein-losing gastropathy. A retrospective analysis of 40 cases in the Netherlands. Scand J Gastroenterol 1992;27 Suppl 194:1–80.
37. Olmsted WW, Cooper PH, Madewell JE. Involvement of the gastric antrum in Ménétrier's disease. AJR Am J Roentgenol 1976;76:524.
38. Smith RL, Powell DW. Prolonged treatment of Ménétrier's disease with an oral anticholinergic drug. Gastroenterology 1978;74:903.
39. Kelly DG, Miller LJ, Malagelada J-R, et al. Giant hypertrophic gastropathy (Ménétrier's disease): Pharmacologic effects on protein leakage and mucosal ultrastructure. Gastroenterology 1982;83:581–589.
40. Riegel N, DelVecchio A, Gillson VH. Ménétrier's disease. A case report and brief literature review. Am J Gastroenterol 1953;53:264.
41. Palmer ED. What Ménétrier really said. Gastrointest Endosc 1968;15:83.
42. Frank BW, Kern F Jr. Ménétrier's disease. Spontaneous metamorphosis of giant hypertrophy of the gastric mucosa to atrophic gastritis. Gastroenterology 1967;53:953.
43. Berenson MM, Sannella J, Freston JW. Ménétrier's disease. Serial morphological, secretory, and serological observations. Gastroenterology 1976;70:257.
44. Wolfsen HC, Carpenter HA, Talley NJ. Ménétrier's disease: A form of hypertrophic gastropathy or gastritis? Gastroenterology 1993;104:1310–1319.
45. Larsen B, Tarp V, Kristensen E. Familial giant hypertrophic gastritis (Ménétrier's disease). Gut 1987;28:1517–1521.
46. Lesser PB, Falchuk KR, Singer M, et al. Ménétrier's disease: Report of a case with transient and reversible findings. Gastroenterology 1975;68:1598–1601.
47. Walker FB IV. Spontaneous remission in hypertrophic gastropathy (Ménétrier's disease). South Med J 1981;74:1273.
48. Scott HW Jr, Shull HJ, Law DH IV, et al. Surgical management of Ménétrier's disease with protein-losing gastropathy. Ann Surg 1975;181:765.
49. Gold BM, Meyers MA. Progression of Ménétrier's disease with postoperative gastrojejunal intussusception. Gastroenterology 1977;73:583.
50. Kenney FD, Dockerty MB, Waugh JM. Giant hypertrophy of gastric mucosa. A clinical and pathological study. Cancer 1954;7:671.
51. Butz WC. Giant hypertrophic gastritis. A report of fourteen cases. Gastroenterology 1960;39:183.
52. Bjork JT, Geenen JE, Komorowski RA, et al. Ménétrier's disease diagnosed by electrosurgical snare biopsy. JAMA 1977;238:1755.
53. Komorowski RA, Caya JG, Geenen JE. The morphologic spectrum of large gastric folds: Utility of the snare biopsy. Gastrointest Endosc 1986;32:190–192.

54. Morson BC, Sobin LH, Grundmann E, et al. Precancerous conditions and epithelial dysplasia in the stomach. J Clin Pathol 1980;33:711–721.

55. Sandberg DH. Hypertrophic gastropathy (Ménétrier's disease) in childhood. J Pediatr 1971;78:866.

56. Chouraqui JP, Roy CC, Brochu P, et al. Ménétrier's disease in children: Report of a patient and review of sixteen other cases. Gastroenterology 1981;80:1042.

57. Stillman AE, Sieber O, Manthei U, et al. Transient protein-losing enteropathy and enlarged gastric rugae in childhood. Am J Dis Child 1981;135:29.

58. Kraut JR, Powell R, Hruby MA, et al. Ménétrier's disease in childhood: Report of two cases and a review of the literature. J Pediatr Surg 1981;16:707–711.

59. Baker A, Volberg F, Summer T, et al. Childhood Ménétrier's disease: Four new cases and discussion of the literature. Gastrointest Radiol 1986;11:131–134.

60. Teele RL, Katz AJ, Goldman H, et al. The radiographic features of eosinophilic gastroenteritis (allergic gastroenteropathy) of childhood. Am J Radiol 1979;132:575.

61. Goldman H, Proujansky R. Allergic proctitis and gastroenteritis in children: Clinical and mucosal biopsy features in 53 cases. Am J Surg Pathol 1986;10:75–86.

62. Schindler R. On hypertrophic glandular gastritis, hypertrophic gastropathy, and parietal cell mass. Gastroenterology 1963;45:77.

63. Stempien SJ, Dagradi AE, Reingold IM, et al. Hypertrophic hypersecretory gastropathy: Analysis of 15 cases and a review of the pertinent literature. Am J Dig Dis 1964;9:471.

64. Tan DTD, Stempien SJ, Dagradi AE. The clinical spectrum of hypertrophic hypersecretory gastropathy. Report of 50 patients. Gastrointest Endosc 1971;18:69.

65. Brooks AM, Isenberg J, Goldstein H. Giant thickening of the gastric mucosa with acid hypersecretion and protein-losing gastropathy. Gastroenterology 1970;58:73.

66. Overholt BF, Jeffries GH. Hypertrophic, hypersecretory protein-losing gastropathy. Gastroenterology 1970;58:80.

67. Subei I, Attar B, Schmitt G, et al. Primary gastric tuberculosis: A case report and literature review. Am J Gastroenterol 1987;82:769–772.

68. Tromba JL, Inglese R, Rieders B, et al. Primary gastric tuberculosis presenting as pyloric outlet obstruction. Am J Gastroenterol 1991;86:1820–1822.

69. Morin ME, Tan A. Diffuse enlargement of gastric folds as a manifestation of secondary syphilis. Am J Gastroenterol 1980;74:170–172.

70. Atten MJ, Attar BM, Teopengco E, et al. Gastric syphilis: A disease with multiple manifestations. Am J Gastroenterol 1994;89:2227–2229.

71. Katz AJ, Goldman H, Grand RJ. Gastric mucosal biopsy in eosinophilic (allergic) gastroenteritis. Gastroenterology 1977;73:705.

72. Khan MH, Lam R, Tamoney HJ. Isolated granulomatous gastritis. Am J Gastroenterol 1979;71:90.

73. Ectors EL, Dixon MF, Geboes KJ, et al. Granulomatous gastritis: A morphological and diagnostic approach. Histopathology 1993;23:55–61.

74. Ament ME, Ochs HD. Gastrointestinal manifestations of chronic granulomatous disease. N Engl J Med 1973;288:382.

75. Chinitz MA, Brandt LJ, Frank MS, et al. Symptomatic sarcoidosis of the stomach. Dig Dis Sci 1985;30:682–688.

76. Stamp GWH, Palmer K, Misiewicz JJ. Antral hypertrophic gastritis: A rare cause of iron deficiency. J Clin Pathol 1985;38:390–392.

77. Clarke AC, Lee SP, Nicholson GI. Gastritis varioliformis. Am J Gastroenterol 1977;68:599–602.

78. Lambert R, Andre C, Moulinier B, et al. Diffuse varioliform gastritis. Digestion 1978;17:159–167.

79. Green PHR, Gold RP, Marboe CC, et al. Chronic erosive gastritis: Clinical, diagnostic and pathological features in nine patients. Am J Gastroenterol 1982;77:543–547.

80. Elta GH, Fawaz KA, Dayal Y, et al. Chronic erosive gastritis—a recently recognized disorder. Dig Dis Sci 1983;28:7–12.

81. Haot J, Jouret A, Willette M, et al. Lymphocytic gastritis—prospective study of its relationship with varioliform gastritis. Gut 1990;31:282–285.

82. Crampton JR, Hunter JO, Neale G, et al. Chronic lymphocytic gastritis and protein losing gastropathy. Gut Festschrift 1989;71–74.

83. Haot J, Bogomoletz WV, Jouret A, et al. Ménétrier's disease with lymphocytic gastritis: An unusual association with possible pathogenic implications. Hum Pathol 1991;22:379–386.

84. Wolber RA, Owen DA, Anderson FH, et al. Lymphocytic gastritis and giant gastric folds associated with gastrointestinal protein loss. Mod Pathol 1991;4:13–15.

85. Littler ER, Gleibermann E. Gastritis cystica polyposa (gastric mucosal prolapse at gastroenterostomy site, with cystic and infiltrative epithelial hyperplasia). Cancer 1972;29:205.

86. Honore LH, Lewis AS, Ohara KE. Gastritic glandularis et cystica profunda—report of 3 cases with discussion of etiology and pathogenesis. Dig Dis Sci 1979;24:48–52.

87. Franzen G, Novelli P. Gastritis cystica profunda. Histopathology 1981;5:535–547.

88. Fonde EC, Rodning CB. Gastritis cystica profunda. Am J Gastroenterol 1986;81:459–464.

89. Lewin KJ, Appelman HD. Tumors of the esophagus and stomach. Atlas of tumor pathology, 3rd series, fascicle 18. Washington DC: Armed Forces Institute of Pathology, 1996.

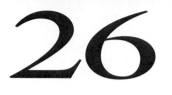

26

BENIGN EPITHELIAL POLYPS OF THE STOMACH

Si-Chun Ming

Polyps are nodular lesions that protrude above the mucosal surface of the stomach into the lumen. Such lesions can be neoplastic or nonneoplastic and imply no tissue or cellular composition. Their nature can be determined only by histologic examination. When the histologic composition is known, the term "polyp" is usually applied to a lesion with prominent epithelial components. The relative frequency of benign polypoid lesions is listed in Table 26.1 (1). Excluded from this table are the lesions caused by diffuse mucosal hyperplasia, which is discussed in Chapter 25.

The first report of a gastric polyp is said to be made by Amatus Lusitanus in 1557 (2). In 1761, Morgagni described a pedunculated polyp near the pylorus, and in 1835, Cruveilhier mentioned the possibility of the polyp causing obstruction or becoming malignant (3). Not until 1888, however, were the formation process and malignant transformation of the gastric polyp described and illustrated in detail by Ménétrier (4), who gave the name of polyadenomas to multiple polyps in the stomach, and classified them into two categories: polyadenomes polypeux (polypoid polyadenomas) and polyadenomes en nappe (cloth-like polyadenomas). The basic pathologic process was glandular hyperplasia, which in the former was localized in the form of sessile or pedunculated polyps, and in the latter formed large mucosal folds resembling ruffled cloth or cerebral convolutions. Ménétrier described two cases of carcinoma of the stomach with metastasis to the liver, one involving an ulcerated carcinoma accompanied by multiple polypoid polyadenomas and the other a diffusely infiltrating carcinoma associated with large mucosal folds. The latter condition of cloth-like polyadenomas is now known as Ménétrier disease (see Chapter 25 for details). The malignant potential of this rare condition is uncertain, although there are reports to this effect (5).

Ménétrier's polyadenomes polypeux are hyperplastic polyps that are not neoplastic, according to the current understanding of the disease. Ménétrier's case VI showed an ulcerated carcinoma in a stomach with multiple polyps. A similar case was reported by Mills (6). Both cases represent an association between polyp and carcinoma, not a developmental continuum. Yet some authors used the presence of a separate carcinoma as evidence for malignant potential of the polyp (7–9), and the reported incidence of carcinoma in the stomach with polyps was as high as 51% (8). Other authors reported malignant change in the polyp, with incidence rates varying from 0 to 29% (7, 10–13). These early reports are difficult to interpret because neither the histologic nature of the polyp nor the criteria for malignancy were always described. Some authors relied instead on the size and the number of the polyps as indicators of malignant potential. Predictably, the results varied greatly. The nature of the polyp and its malignant potential remain the main concerns regarding gastric polyps.

CLASSIFICATION OF EPITHELIAL POLYPS

The polyps can be classified as intraluminal and intramural types according to the location of the bulk of the lesion in relation to the wall of the stomach. Such a distinction is clinically relevant. The intraluminal polyp usually is a mucosal lesion, which may bleed if its surface is eroded, or obstruct if it is large and located near the orifices of the stomach. The intramural lesion usually is submucosal and is asymptomatic if small. When it is large, the covering mucosa may become ulcerated and bleed. A large intramural mass may also be

TABLE 26.1 Benign Polypoid Lesions of the Stomach in Order of Frequency

Type of Lesion	Total Number	Percent
Epithelial polyp	252	40.9
Leiomyoma	230	37.3
Inflammatory polyp	29	4.7
Heterotopic tissue	25	4.1
Lipoma	21	3.4
Neurogenic tumor	19	3.1
Vascular tumor	13	2.1
Eosinophilic granuloma	12	1.9
Fibroma	9	1.5
Miscellaneous lesions	6	1.0
Total	616	100.0

Modified from Ming SC. Tumors of the esophagus and stomach. In: Atlas of tumor pathology, second series, fascicle 7. Washington DC: Armed Forces Institute of Pathology. 1973:101.

obstructive if strategically located. Other symptoms typically are vague and infrequent, including epigastric discomfort, anorexia, and dyspepsia.

Ménétrier's classification of gastric polyps is based on the gross morphology. The first significant effort in the histologic classification of gastric polyps was made by Rieniets and Broders in 1945 and 1946 (14). In a series of publications, they divided gastric polyps into 18 different types in two basic forms. One form was called adenoma, made of hyperplastic glands and tubules, and the other form was called papillary adenoma. These forms correspond to the current terms of hyperplastic polyp and adenoma. Rieniets and Broders recognized the high incidence of malignant transformation in the papillary adenomas. Malignant change in such a lesion was reported as early as 1917 by Finney and Friedenwald (15). In 1951, Walk reviewed 51 reported and 2 new cases of villous tumors of the stomach (16). In a total of 67 tumors, malignancy was noted in 40 (60%). Additional case reports confirmed malignant change in villous adenomas of the stomach (17, 18).

By the early 1960s, it had become apparent that the significance of gastric polyps lay in their malignant potential, that the malignant potential is not uniform among the polyps, and that the polyps might be histologically heterogeneous. In 1965, Ming and Goldman recognized two basic forms of gastric polyps: one composed of normal-appearing cells lining elongated and hyperplastic foveolae and pyloric-type glands; the other containing glands made of atypical cells similar to those in a colonic adenoma (19). The former type was given the name of regenerative polyp, implying a reparative nature; the latter was called adenomatous polyp with the same pathologic implication as the adenomatous polyp of the colon. In addition to cytologic differences, these two types have different gross morphology and strikingly different malignant potential.

Since these basic concepts were recognized, some minor modifications have occurred. For instance, a more commonly used name for the regenerative polyp is hyperplastic polyp, as proposed by Tomasulo (20), although a reparative nature of the polyp remains most likely. Another modification is the recognition of a flat form of

adenoma in contrast to the papillovillous type (21). The flat adenoma was reported in Japan as a form of atypical epithelium (22) or borderline lesion (23). This lesion is relatively common in Japan but is rare in the United States. The third modification is the realization that stomach as well as other parts of the upper gastrointestinal tract are frequently affected in the genetically controlled polyposis syndromes, which primarily involve the colon. Gastric polyps are common in patients with Gardner syndrome or familial adenomatous polyposis (24) and juvenile polyposis (25). Similarly, the stomach is often involved in the nonhereditary Cronkhite-Canada syndrome (26).

The major subtypes of gastric polyps are listed in Table 26.2. The benign neoplastic polyps are adenomas composed of immature and dysplastic cells similar to those present in the colonic adenoma. On the basis of architectural pattern, the cytologic appearances of component cells, and the known biologic potentials, the adenomas are subdivided into flat type and papillary (villous) type. Rarely, dysplastic or adenomatous lesions are present in the hyperplastic polyp. Malignant epithelial tumors, namely carcinoma and carcinoid, may appear polypoid. Secondary metastatic tumors in the stomach may also take a polypoid form, although they are mostly submucosal. The nonneoplastic polyps are composed of disorganized epithelial structures but mostly normal-appearing cells, together with varying amounts of mesenchymal tissue. The most common subtype is the hyperplastic polyp, in which hyperplastic foveolae and pyloric-type glands are the dominant structures. Hamartomatous polyps are composed of tissues that are normal for

TABLE 26.2 Histologic Classification of Epithelial Gastric Polyps

I. Neoplastic polyp
  A. Benign: adenoma
    1. Flat (tubular) adenoma
    2. Papillary (villous) adenoma
  B. Malignant
    1. Primary polypoid carcinoma and carcinoid
    2. Secondary epithelial tumors
II. Nonneoplastic polyp
  A. Hyperplastic polyp
    1. Focal (polypoid) foveolar hyperplasia
    2. Hyperplastic (regenerative) polyp
    3. Hyperplastic polyp with dysplastic (adenomatous) lesion
  B. Hamartomatous polyp
    1. Peutz-Jeghers polyp
    2. Juvenile polyp
    3. Fundic gland polyp
  C. Inflammatory polyp
    1. Inflammatory pseudopolyp
    2. Inflammatory (retention) polyp
  D. Heterotopic polyp
    1. Ectopic pancreatic tissue
    2. Brunner gland hyperplasia
    3. Adenomyoma
  E. Nodular mucosal remnants

TABLE 26.3	Comparison of Classifications of Hyperplastic and Adenomatous Gastric Polyps					
Author (Reference)	**Nonneoplastic Polyp**			**Neoplastic Polyp**		
Ming (27)	- - - - - - - Hyperplastic (regenerative) polyp - - - - - - - -			- - - - - - - - - - - - - - - - - Adenoma - - - - - - - - - - - - - - - - -		
	Polypoid foveolar hyperplasia	- - - - - - Hyperplastic polyp - - - - - -		Adenomatous hyperplastic polyp	Flat adenoma	Papillary (villous) adenoma
Elster (28)	Focal foveolar hyperplasia	Hyperplasio-genous polyp	Adenoma with high differentiation		Borderline lesion, protruded	Adenoma with moderate differentiation
Koch (29)	Polypoid foveolar hyperplasia	Hyperplastic polyp	Hyperplastic adenomatous polyp	Adenomatous villous polyp		Villous polyp
Snover (30)	Foveolar hyperplasia	- - - - - - Hyperplastic polyp - - - - - -		Mixed adenomatous-hyperplastic polyp		Adenomatous villoglandular, villous polyp
Nakamura (31)	Type II polyp	- - - - - - - Type I polyp - - - - - - - - -			Type III polyp	Type IV polyp
Kozuka et al. (32)	- - - - - - - Hyperplastic (gastric type) polyp - - - - - - - -			Hyperplastic polyp with adenoma	Adenomatous (metaplastic) polyp	
Goldman and Appelman (33)	- - - - - - - Polyp without atypical hyperplasia - - - - - - -			- - - - - - - - - - - Polyp with atypical hyperplasia - - - - - - - - - - - -		

Not included: foveolar adenoma (30) and antral foveolar polyp (33). They do not have counterparts in other classifications.

the site, and often contain both epithelial and mesenchymal elements. The inflammatory polyps primarily consist of inflammatory tissue with a reduction of epithelial elements. The heterotopic polyps are choristomas containing tissues of neighboring organs and rarely misplaced tissues of the normal stomach. Lastly, the polyp may be composed of nodules of normal mucosa surrounded by atrophic tissue.

Other classifications of gastric polyps are compared in Table 26.3. The classification proposed by Elster (28), which is popular in Europe, introduces the concept of foveolar hyperplasia as a separate entity. Endoscopically, this lesion is small and sessile. It commonly arises in the region of a healing ulcer or erosion and in areas adjacent to carcinoma. In larger lesions, the hyperplastic foveolae expand and elongate toward the mucosal base where the glands proper remain mostly unchanged. Elster referred to this type of polyp as hyperplasiogenous polyp to indicate organ specificity and to distinguish it from the hyperplastic polyp of the colon. When the glands proper become hyperplastic and increased in number, the polyp takes on an adenomatous appearance. Elster considered this type of polyp a well-differentiated adenoma. Such a polyp has also been called hyperplastic adenomatous polyp (29, 34). All of these different forms are considered merely variants of hyperplastic polyp (21). Rarely, part of the hyperplastic polyp contains atypical glands identical to those in a true adenoma (35). Such a polyp is considered to have mixed adenomatous and nonneoplastic hyperplastic components and the adenomatous elements may be precancerous (27, 30, 35). Nakamura divided gastric polyps into four types (36): type I is an eroded sessile polyp with foveolar hyperplasia, type II corresponds to the usual hyperplastic polyp, type III is the flat adenoma, and type IV is the papillary adenoma.

In 1955, Morson stated that some gastric polyps were composed of intestinal-type epithelium (37). He noted that three of five such polyps had malignant change, whereas seven gastric-type polyps did not. A similar view was held by Kozuka et al., who divided gastric polyps also into gastric and metaplastic types (32). The metaplastic polyps are mostly adenomas and the gastric-type hyperplastic polyps (38). Malignant change was present in 42% of the former, less than 1% of the latter, and 10% of polyps with mixed epithelia. Goldman and Appelman classified gastric polyps according to the presence or absence of atypical hyperplasia (33). All polyps with malignant change had atypical hyperplasia. In addition, they described a form of antral polyp composed of compact foveolar cells that they called the antral foveolar polyp. Snover (30) described a similar lesion, called foveolar adenoma, although this lesion was located in the body of the stomach. Snover also documented seven polyps with mixed adenomatous and hyperplastic features.

Accurate histologic diagnosis of biopsy tissue is essential to establish a correct diagnosis and to render proper treatment. This requirement was dramatically illustrated by Niv and Bat, who reported that biopsy results demonstrated that nearly 50% of 99 polyps seen in 13,500 gastroscopies turned out to be either normal or inflammatory (39).

Interpretation of the biopsy also requires care. A mucosal or superficial biopsy of the polyp will not reveal the nature of a submucosally located intramural lesion. Even for the mucosal or intraluminal lesion, a superficial biopsy may not be diagnostic, because the histologic features of different types of lesions may be similar in focal areas. For instance, the hyperplastic, juvenile, and inflammatory polyps all have elongated and dilated foveolae and interstitial inflammation. A definite diagnosis may not be possible unless the entire lesion is examined. Seifert and Elster compared the diagnoses between biopsy specimens and excised tissues of the same polyps and noted that discrepancies were present in 53 of 75 polyps and significant inadequacy of the biopsy specimen was noted in 20 of these 53 polyps (40). Furthermore, an excisional biopsy is clearly necessary to evaluate possible malignant change within the polyp.

INCIDENCE OF GASTRIC POLYP

Gastric polyp is not common. Its incidence at autopsy and by radiologic survey is about 0.4 % (21). In a mass survey in Japan, gastric polyp was found in 0.23% of individuals (41). The incidence of gastric polyps found at endoscopy is higher (about 3 to 5%) (42–44). Whereas polyps used to account for 3.1% of all gastric tumors and 41% of benign tumors (1), the frequency has increased to about 90% of benign tumors in patients who have undergone biopsy (42). The incidence of gastric polyp is high in association with certain conditions: 22 to 37% in pernicious anemia (45, 46), 6% in chronic atrophic gastritis (47), and 4 to 20% in gastric stump after partial gastrectomy, depending on postresection duration (48, 49). Carcinoma often coexists with polyp formation in the same stomach (21, 50). Morson found polyps in 44% of consecutively resected carcinomatous stomachs (37). Gastric polyps are common in patients with familial adenomatous polyposis, 33% in one report (51) and 60% in another (52).

The types of polypoid lesions seen at the time of endoscopic biopsies vary in published reports. Of 244 lesions in 161 patients reported by Seifert and Elster (40), 54.1% were hyperplastic polyps, 21% inflammatory lesions, 10.6 % focal hyperplasia, 5.3% adenomas, 2% heterotopic lesions, 0.8% early carcinomas, and nonepithelial lesions in 7%. Single polyps were present in 140 patients and 2 to 3 polyps each in 15 patients. Four patients had 5 to 26 hyperplastic polyps each and two patients had Cronkhite-Canada syndrome with 5 and 10 polyps, respectively. In a report by Stolte et al. of 5515 gastric polyps from 4852 patients, 28.3% were hyperplastic polyps, 10% adenomas, carcinomas 7.2%, carcinoids 1.7%, Brunner gland heterotopia 1.2%, and inflammatory fibroid polyp 3.1% (53). The most common lesion in this group (47%) was glandular cyst of fundic glands. These cystic lesions are similar to fundic gland polyp which was found in 13% of gastric polyps reported by Snover (30).

In most reports, hyperplastic polyps account for 70 to 90% of epithelial gastric polyps (1, 30, 54). These polyps occur mostly in older individuals, with peaks in the sixth and seventh decades. Of 1353 patients reported by Kozuka, only 2 patients were in their second decade of life and 19 were in their third decade (38). Brooks reported intussusception of a hyperplastic polyp into the duodenum of an infant that caused obstruction and hematemesis (55). Hyperplastic polyp occurs about equally in women and men.

The frequency of adenoma among gastric polyps is about 7 to 10% (19, 30, 43, 54, 56, 57), although rates of incidence as high as 15.5 and 25% were reported by Stamm et al. (58) and Tomasulo (20). Among patients with familial adenomatous polyposis, gastric adenoma occurs in about 15% (51, 52). Affected individuals usually are in the early seventh decade of life (average age, 62.6 years) (59). The incidence of gastric adenoma increases with age, from only 0.1% in the third decade to 3.7% in the ninth decade (60). Men are affected more often than women (about 2:1 to 3:1). The preferred location is the distal portion of the stomach, particularly the antrum (19, 20, 22).

ADENOMA

HISTOGENESIS

Adenoma of the stomach resembles adenoma of the colon in its histologic appearance. It is composed of immature cells with varying degrees of dysplasia; tall columnar cells without specific markers predominate. Not uncommonly, however, a distinct, although often short and coarse, striated border is present on the luminal surface of the cells, indicating an intestinal character of the cells. Other intestinal features include goblet cells and Paneth cells. Argentaffin cells may also be present (19, 20, 61). The mucin in the adenoma is often acidic (62). The acid mucin is secreted by the intestines but not the normal stomach. Furthermore, the mucosa surrounding the adenoma often shows atrophic gastritis with prominent intestinal metaplasia, including the incomplete type (19, 29, 38). These features suggest a relationship between gastric adenoma and intestinal metaplasia, and the term metaplastic polyp or intestinal type adenoma has been applied to such an adenoma (32, 59). The adenomas showing mainly gastric-type cells and mucin secretion have been called gastric-type adenomas (59, 63). Gastric-type adenomas are rare; of 144 gastric adenomas reported by Hirota, only 4.2 % were gastric type, 93.7% intestinal type, and 2.1% mixed type (59).

PATHOLOGIC FEATURES AND SUBTYPES

The adenomas usually are solitary lesions. In a series of 75 cases described by Watanabe, single adenomas were seen in 50, two adenomas in 19, three adenomas in 5 and five adenomas in 1 patient (61). The lesions may arise anywhere in the stomach; about 50% are at the lesser curvature and only 5% are in the upper one third of the stomach (59).

The World Health Organization Histologic Typing divides the gastric adenomas into tubular, tubulovillous (papillotubular), and villous (papillary) types (64). These histologic patterns are reflected by two gross forms, namely flat and papillary. The flat adenoma is a tubular adenoma microscopically and the papillary adenoma shows tubulovillous and villous histologic features. They are schematically represented in Figure 26.1.

FLAT ADENOMA

Flat adenoma, recognized first by Nakamura (36), is the most common form of adenoma in the stomach, especially in Japan. Its gross appearance resembles that of early gastric carcinoma so that it has been classified accordingly (see Chapter 27). Most flat adenomas are slightly elevated lesions (type IIa-like) with an irregular but flat surface or that show varying degrees of nodularity (Fig. 26.2). Some adenomas have a smooth surface that is even with the surface of the surrounding mucosa (IIb-like lesion) (59, 60). A grossly depressed form (IIc-like lesion) has also been reported (65). The protruded adenomas (I-like) may be sessile (Is-like) or pedunculated (Ip-like). The respective frequencies of these types among 144 flat adenomas analyzed by Hirota and coworkers (59) were as follows: Is-like type, 8.3%; Ip-like type, 0.7%; IIa-like type, 68.8%; IIb-like type, 12.5%; IIc-like type, 5.5%; and combined IIa+IIc-like lesions, 4.2%. More than 80% of flat adenomas are less than 2 cm in diameter (average, 1 cm).

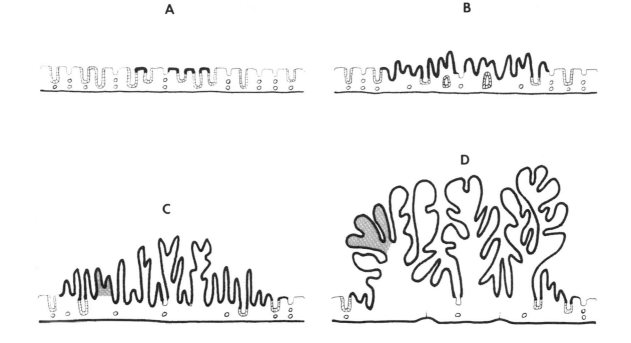

NORMAL GLAND, METAPLSTIC GLAND, ADENOMATOUS GLAND, MALIGNANT GLAND, MUSCULARIS MUCOSA.

Figure 26.1 Subtypes of gastric adenoma. **A.** Adenoma develops in the superficial epithelium, usually in a metaplastic mucosa. **B.** Flat (tubular) adenoma shows horizontal growth and occupies the upper layer of the mucosa. Nonneoplastic gastric tissue remains in the deep region. **C.** Villous or papillotubular adenoma shows vertical as well as horizontal growth with villous projections. **D.** Papillary adenoma shows a balanced horizontal and vertical growth. Deep crevices separate the adenoma into nodular partitions. Malignant change may occur in any area, more frequently in the elevated lesions. (Reprinted from Ming SC. Tumors of the esophagus and stomach, supplement. In: Atlas of tumor pathology, second series, fascicle 7. Washington DC: Armed Forces Institute of Pathology, 1984;S24–S32.)

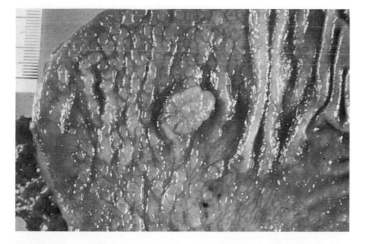

Figure 26.2 Flat adenoma, gross morphology. This IIa-like lesion is raised slightly above the mucosal surface. (Courtesy of Dr. T. Hirota, National Cancer Center Research Institute, Tokyo, Japan.)

The histologic features of flat adenoma are unique. Whereas the atypical cells in other adenomas, including those in the colon, extend through the entire thickness of the mucosa, the gastric flat adenoma, particularly the IIa-like type, usually occupies only the upper one third to one half of the gastric mucosa and maintains a two-layer structure (Figs. 26.3 and 26.4). The depressed adenomas usually occupy the entire thickness of the mucosa.

The cells in flat adenoma are slender and compact, and the rows of nuclei form a picket-fence appearance along the base of the cells (see Fig. 26.4). Pleomorphism and mitosis are not evident. Electron microscopy reveals sparse microvilli, reduced endoplasmic reticulum and mucin granules, and the presence of blebs on the apical surface (66). The deep glands are cytologically normal, although cystic dilatation and metaplastic changes are common. The dilatation of the deep glands is probably related to interruption of the excretory upper portion of the glands by the adenomatous tissue. The two-layer architecture and relative indolence of the immature epithelial cells are hallmarks distinguishing the flat adenoma from the papillary adenoma.

The possibility that flat adenoma is the earlier form of papillary adenoma has not been confirmed in follow-up studies. Most flat adenomas appear stationary. When Kamiya et al. monitored 85 lesions in 74 patients for 6 months to 12 years, only 8 showed gross changes: 4 became smaller and 4 grew larger (60); none disappeared. In spite of the lack of growth, the flat adenoma is clearly neoplastic, as evidenced by the cellular atypism and a relatively high incidence of malignant change (about 10%) within the lesion.

Because of the abnormal appearance of its constituent cells, flat adenoma had been called simply "atypical epithelium" (22) or "borderline lesion" (23). It is important to note, however, that flat adenoma and dysplasia are not synonymous, and these entities must

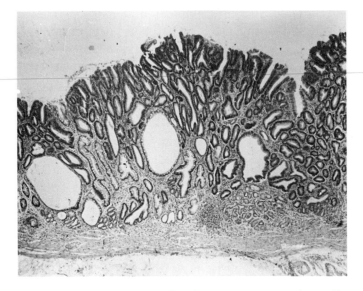

Figure 26.3 Flat adenoma, histologic appearance of a IIa-like lesion. The adenomatous tissue occupies the upper one half of the mucosa. The deep glands are focally dilated. The glands at left show intestinal metaplasia (×80).

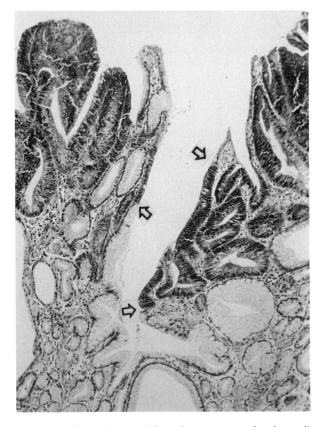

Figure 26.4 Flat adenoma. The adenomatous glands are lined by compact columnar cells. The slender nuclei are basally located. Transitions between the compact columnar cells of the adenoma and the neighboring normal foveolar cells *(arrows)* are abrupt (×120).

be distinguished. The flat adenoma is a grossly recognizable lesion characterized by relative uniformity in its composition of immature cells lining the branching and interrelated network of tubules (67). As a neoplasm, the adenoma is a sharply delimited lesion and, although noninvasive, nevertheless spreads horizontally within the confines of the epithelium, resulting in a sharp demarcation between the adenoma and the neighboring nonneoplastic epithelium (see Fig. 26.4). These features are common to all adenomas in the digestive tract. In contrast, the common dysplastic epithelium exhibits a reactive process in a labile state. The degree of dysplasia fluctuates from area to area and in various times. The change is gradual and the mucosa as a whole usually is atrophic, although the shortened glands proliferate actively. Details of dysplastic changes in the gastric mucosa is described in Chapter 27.

PAPILLARY (VILLOUS) ADENOMA

Papillary adenomas of the stomach are sessile or broad-based nodular lesions with a lobulated contour and deep crevices (Fig. 26.5). On radiologic examination, barium trapped in the crevices gives a soap-bubble appearance. These lesions are soft and velvety and freely mobile. Fixation to the deep tissue indicates carcinomatous change with invasion. The average size of papillary adenoma is 4 cm (16, 19), although lesions as large as 15 cm in greatest dimension have been reported (17). Papillary adenomas are located mostly in the antrum.

Histologically, the papillary or villous pattern is evident (Figs. 26.6 and 26.7). Columnar cells, some of which have striated borders (Fig. 26.8), predominate, but goblet cells (Fig. 26.9) and rarely Paneth cells are also seen. Sulfomucin as well as sialomucin are often present, although some authors report negative results for sulfomucin (68). Other findings include cells containing gastrin, somatostatin, and glicentin (69). In contrast to the relative unifor-

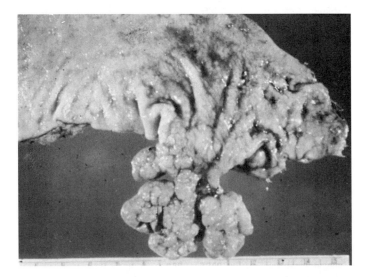

Figure 26.5 Papillary adenoma. The papillary nodules are partitioned by deep crevices. The base is broad and the adenomatous tissue extends to the adjacent mucosa. (Reprinted with permission from Ming SC. Tumors of the esophagus and stomach. In: Atlas of tumor pathology, second series, fascicle 7. Washington DC: Armed Forces Institute of Pathology, 1973: 124–143.)

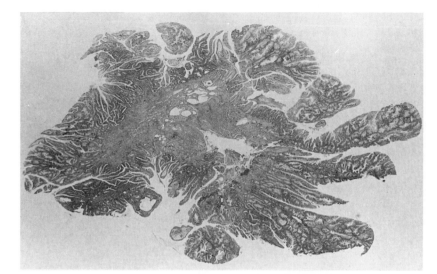

Figure 26.6   Papillary adenoma. This scanning histologic view of the adenoma in Figure 26.5 shows papillary lobulation of the lesion with focal areas of villous formation (×10). (Reprinted with permission from Ming SC. The classification and significance of gastric polyps. In: Yardley JH, Morson, BM, eds. The gastrointestinal tract. Baltimore: Williams & Wilkins, 1977:149–175.)

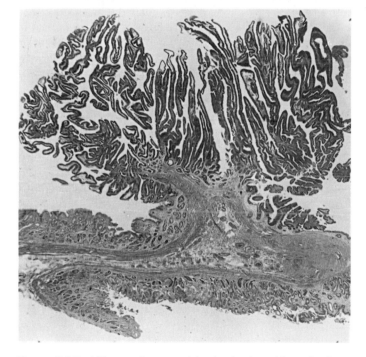

Figure 26.7   Villous adenoma, histologic view. Note the long slender villous fronds (×11).

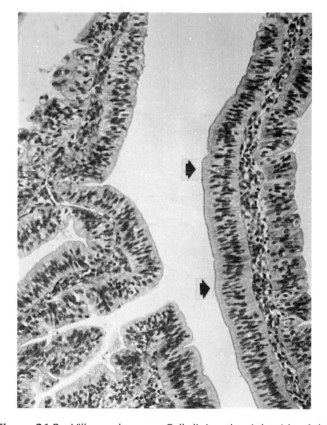

Figure 26.8   Villous adenoma. Cells lining the right side of the glandular crevice show a distinct striated border on their luminal surface *(arrows)*. Cells on the left of the crevice have a faintly stained and thinner apical border. The nuclei are pseudostratified and centrally seated. There is no mucous secretion (×300).

mity of cells in the flat adenoma, pleomorphism and mitoses are common in the papillary adenoma. The neoplastic cells end abruptly at the junction with the neighboring epithelium, which often exhibits prominent intestinal metaplasia (Fig. 26.10). Adenomas with malignant change are positive for carcinoembryonic antigen (68).

MOLECULAR STUDIES

Adenomas have a high rate of cell proliferation, as shown by positive immunohistochemical staining for Ki-67 in 28% of cells in ad-

enomas and an average apoptotic cell count of 26 per 1,000 cell (70). Studies of p53 expression in adenomatous lesions yielded mixed results. Some investigators found no overexpression of p53 (71, 72). Lauwers et al. (73) found p53 expression in adenomatous tissue in only 7 of 17 adenomas and in carcinomatous foci in only 3 others. Five adenomas with carcinoma or severe dysplasia were negative. Mutation of p53 was found in 30% of adenomas by Tohdo et al. (72) and 8% by Tamura et al. (74). The latter group also detected microsatellite instability in 8% of adenomas and

commented that these low rates suggested the rare occurrence of an adenoma-carcinoma sequence in gastric carcinogenesis. Semba et al., on the other hand, found microsatellite instability in 42% of gastric adenomas (75). In another study, APC gene mutation was present in 4 of 10 flat adenomas (76). Loss of heterozygosity of chromosome 9p was not detected in 10 adenomas investigated (77).

MALIGNANT TRANSFORMATION

Carcinomas may develop within the gastric polyps, particularly in adenomas, as well as outside the polyp. Reported frequencies of these events are summarized subsequently in Table 26.4. The frequency of malignant transformation in the adenoma ranges from 5 (65) to 76% (56), with an average of 31%. The flat adenomas have a lower incidence of malignant change. The incidence increases with the grade of dysplasia, the papillary pattern, and the size of the lesion (59). Independent carcinoma coexisting with adenoma in the same stomach is common. In a series of 121 cases described by Hirota et al., early carcinoma was present in 55 and advanced cancer in 29 cases (59). Only 1 of 29 patients reported by Laxen et al., however, had gastric cancer outside the adenoma (43).

In follow-up studies, Laxen et al. reported new polyps in 6 of 14 cases within 5 years (43) and carcinomas in 3 cases in 15 years (78). Sugano et al. noted no change of the "atypical epithelium" in a 2-year follow-up study (22). Kamiya et al. monitored 85 adenomas, mostly of the flat type, in 74 patients for 6 months to 12 years, and reported that carcinoma developed in 9 adenomas (60). These authors also noted gross change in size in 8 and a shift of the degree of dysplasia in 12. Tatsuta et al. (79) conducted a follow-up study (average of 15 months) in which 31 flat adenomas were tested for the expression of c-myc oncogene. Carcinoma developed in 5 of 11 adenomas positive for c-myc, but in none of 19 c-myc-negative adenomas.

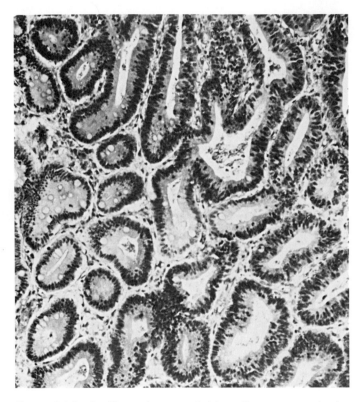

Figure 26.9   Papillary adenoma. Goblet cells are present in the differentiated glands. The less differentiated cells are markedly pseudostratified (×200).

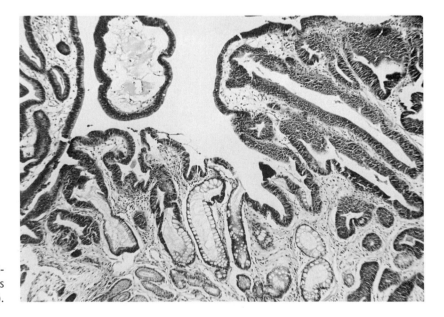

Figure 26.10   Papillary adenoma. The nonneoplastic mucosa below the adenomatous tissue shows intestinal metaplasia. Goblet cells are evident (×140).

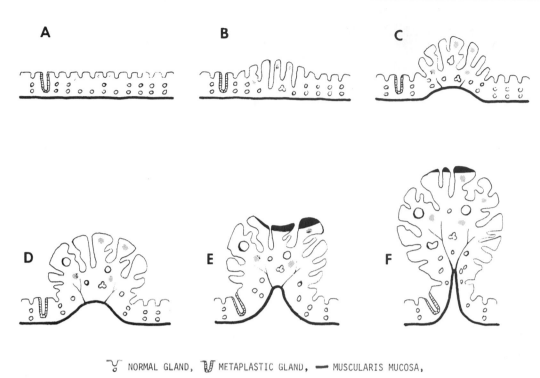

NORMAL GLAND, METAPLASTIC GLAND, ━ MUSCULARIS MUCOSA, ▪ ACUTE INFLAMMATION, ▨ CHRONIC INFLAMMATION.

Figure 26.11 Various forms of hyperplastic polyp. **A.** The mucosa in which the hyperplastic polyp arises usually show focal chronic inflammation and mild atrophy. Intestinal metaplasia is mild or absent. **B** and **C.** Polypoid foveolar hyperplasia resulting from elongation of the hyperplastic foveolae. **D.** Dome-shaped sessile polyp with branching and cystic foveolae and pyloric glands at base. **E.** Sessile polyp with erosion and acute inflammation at the top. **F.** Well-formed polyp with a short pedicle. (Reprinted from Ming SC. Tumors of the esophagus and stomach, supplement. In: Atlas of tumor pathology, second series, fascicle 7. Washington DC: Armed Forces Institute of Pathology, 1984;S24–S32.)

HYPERPLASTIC (REGENERATIVE) POLYP

Associated Conditions

The etiology of hyperplastic polyp is not known. It usually occurs in association with gastritis. Because *Helicobacter pylori* is a major cause of gastritis, its relation with hyperplastic polyp has been studied. In one report, H. pylori was present in 81% of stomachs with inflammatory polyps and 45 and 48% of cases with hyperplastic polyp or foveolar hyperplasia, respectively (80). The polyp cases also showed mucosal atrophy of the upper part of the stomach, the presence of antiparietal cell antibody, and an increased serum gastrin level, suggestive of autoimmune gastritis. In another report (81), H. pylori antibody was present in 84% of patients with hyperplastic polyps, 41% of controls, and 19% of patients with fundic gland polyp.

A genetic influence was shown in a report by Carneiro et al. (82) of a family with familial gastric polyposis and increased incidence of gastric cancer. When the authors examined gastric specimens from nine members of this family, five members had hyperplastic polyps; two had diffuse-type carcinoma, one of which originated in a hyperplastic polyp; two had foveolar hyperplasia; and three had atrophic gastritis with intestinal metaplasia. p53 was not detected in any of the specimens, but carcinoembryonic antigen was present in six and ras p21 in 8. H. pylori was present in all but two cancer cases. Hyperplastic polyps were reported in 3 of 4 patients with Cowden disease (83). The development of gastric polyps has been reported in patients receiving long-term omeprazole therapy. The type of polyps are variable, including hyperplastic polyp (84), fundic gland polyp (85), and glandular cyst (86).

Histogenesis and Subtypes

The hyperplastic polyp is composed, for the most part, of elongated and hyperplastic foveolae of the gastric glands. Expansion of the cell proliferation zone in the mucosa is an early event, as shown by bromodeoxyuridine labeling and immunohistochemical staining of proliferating cell nuclear antigen (87). Figure 26.11 illustrates various forms of the hyperplastic polyp. The hyperplasia usually occurs in chronically inflamed mucosa with a mild degree of atrophy (see Fig. 26.11A). The small polyps are sessile hemispheric lesions in the form of polypoid foveolar hyperplasia (see Fig. 26.11B and C). The number of foveolae does not appear to increase. These small lesions do not evolve into fully developed hyperplastic polyps (88). Further enlargement of the polyp (see Fig. 26.11D to F) appears to be the result of branching and dilatation of the hyperplastic foveolae. The newly formed foveolae are not connected with the deep glands, which are almost entirely of the pyloric type. In some cases, the deep

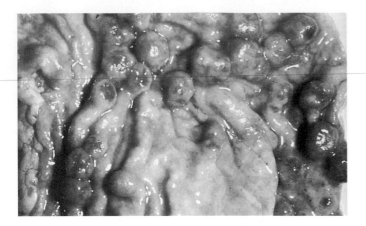

Figure 26.12 Hyperplastic polyp. Multiple polyps are relatively uniform in size, mostly about 1 cm in diameter. Several polyps had evidence of erosion at top. (See color plate.)

glands are increased in number. In general, they contribute little to the size of the polyp.

Secondary surface erosion is common (Figs. 26.11E, 26.12, and 26.13). In some cases, the erosion and acute inflammation destroy the glands and reduce their number. A reparative response to the erosion with secondary hyperplasia of the surrounding glands as suggested by Nakamura's type II polyp (31), is not common, although active regeneration with immature cells and presence of mitosis may accompany the erosion. A well-developed hyperplastic polyp is a distinct oval lesion (see Figs. 26.11F, 26.12, and 26.13). This scheme of the development of hyperplastic polyp proposes that the polyp is the result of excessive and apparently unchecked regenerative growth of the normal proliferative zone of the gastric epithelium, namely the deep foveolae and the neck region of the glands on a background of chronic gastritis.

The incidence of hyperplastic polyp is particularly high in the gastric remnant following partial gastrectomy. Polyp was present in 20% of patients whose stomach was resected more than 20 years previously (89). Koga found local hyperplastic changes in 66% of resected specimens of postgastrectomy stump (90). Enterogastric reflux is common in these patients, but its role in polyp formation is not certain. The immediate stimulus for the formation of the polyp has not been determined. Lastly, hyperplastic polyps may enlarge, shrink or disappear (43, 45, 60, 91). In most cases, the polyps remain stationary.

PATHOLOGIC FEATURES

Hyperplastic polyps generally are small and have a smooth domelike or olive-shaped appearance (see Figs. 26.12 and 26.13). Erosion may occur at the top. Most polyps are less than 1.5 cm in diameter (average size, 1 cm) (21), although polyps up to 12 cm in diameter have been reported (44). These large polyps may have a papillary appearance similar to that of a papillary adenoma (92). Most polyps are sessile, but some have a long pedicle. The number of patients with single or multiple polyps are nearly equal. Multiple polyps generally are uniform in shape and size. When the polyps number more than 50, the term "hyperplastic polyposis" is applied (42). Such cases are rare. Hyperplastic polyps are randomly distributed

with a slight prevalence in the antrum. In the body of the stomach, they typically sit on the rugal folds (34).

Histologically, the hyperplastic polyp is composed principally of dilated, elongated, and branching foveolae (see Figs. 26.13 and 26.14). The hyperplastic foveolae are lined by either normal appearing mucous cells or hypertrophic cells with abundant cytoplasm. The cells in some glands have eosinophilic cytoplasm, hyperchromatic nuclei and prominent nucleoli. The hyperplastic cells are crowded and intraglandular infolding is common (see Fig. 26.14). No pseudostratification occurs, however, and the nuclei remain basally located. Mitotic activities are rare except in the surface area, where active proliferation may be present in response to erosion and acute inflammation. Less than 25% of hyperplastic polyps have focal intestinal metaplasia, usually accompanied by metaplasia in the surrounding mucosa (38). The histologic appearance of cellular normalcy is reflected by DNA measurements showing a diploid pattern and the labeling index with ^{3}H-thymidine identical to that of the normal mucosa (93).

The deep glands are of pyloric type, even if the polyp is located in the fundic mucosa, apparently a result of pseudopyloric metaplasia. In small polyps, the number of these glands is the same as that in the surrounding mucosa. At this stage, the lesion is termed

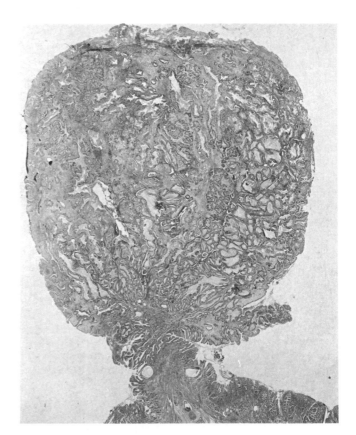

Figure 26.13 Hyperplastic polyp. This pedunculated polyp measured 2 cm in diameter. It is composed of closely packed hyperplastic foveolae, many of which are dilated and tortuous. Cystic glands are also present in the stalk and adjacent mucosa. (Reprinted from Ming SC. Tumors of the esophagus and stomach. In: Atlas of tumor pathology, second series, fascicle 7. Washington DC: Armed Forces Institute of Pathology, 1973:124–143.)

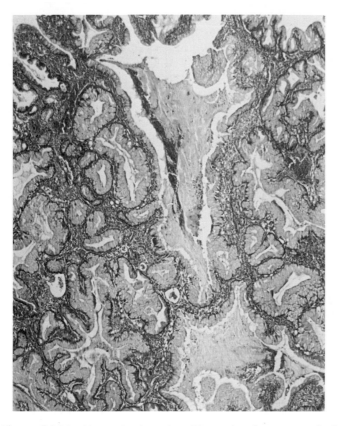

Figure 26.14   Hyperplastic polyp. The polyp is composed of many hyperplastic and dilated foveolae. The stroma is chronically inflamed and edematous (×140).

polypoid foveolar hyperplasia as a descriptor of the small mucosal elevation commonly seen endoscopically. In some clinics, this entity is the most common form of hyperplastic polyp (29). In the well-formed polyp, the number of pyloric glands varies. In some, the presence of many glands gives a superficial resemblance to an adenoma and the term "hyperplastic adenomatous polyp" is applied (28, 29). The morphology of the deep glands is normal, however, and no cellular atypia is noted (Fig. 26.15).

The lamina propria in the hyperplastic polyp shows varying degrees of chronic inflammation and edema, most prominent in the superficial region (see Fig. 26.14). Nodular collections of lymphocytes are common, occasionally with a germinal center. The surface area of the polyp may show erosion and acute inflammation accompanied by granulation tissue formation, prominent vascularity, and telangiectasia. In the loose connective stromal tissue, bundles of smooth muscle cells are often present, extending from their origin in the muscularis mucosae into the deep portions of the polyp (see Fig. 26.15). The muscle bundles are slender and taper off toward the upper portion of the polyp and usually do not reach the surface region.

Rarely dysplastic or adenomatous tissue is present in the hyperplastic polyp, admixed with hyperplastic foveolae (Fig. 26.16). The dysplastic immature cells may resemble either foveolar cells or metaplastic cells. Because the overall configuration and the majority of tissue in such a polyp are identical to those of hyperplastic polyp, the adenomatous change is considered to be a secondary process (27, 94), and the term "dysplastic (adenomatous) hyperplastic

polyp" has been applied (27). Snover gave the name of mixed adenomatous-hyperplastic polyp and placed it under the category of adenoma (30). He found 7 such lesions in 182 cases, one of which had in situ carcinoma in it. p53 is expressed only in the adenomatous foci, and not in the hyperplastic tissue (71, 73).

Another unusual anomaly associated with the hyperplastic polyp is the presence of globoid signet ring-like cells in the dilated foveolae (Fig. 26.17). These cells are large and secrete sialomucin. The nuclei are compressed against the cell membrane and are irregularly oriented. The significance of this change is not clear.

MALIGNANT POTENTIAL

None of the regenerative polyps studied by Ming and Goldman (19) showed cellular atypism or malignant transformation. Although it had since been generally accepted that the hyperplastic (regenerative) polyp had no malignant potential, there have been reports to the contrary (Table 26.4). The incidence of malignancy within the polyp is low, 1.0% of polyps and 1.7% of cases on average. Size of the polyp does not appear to be an important factor; carcinomas have been found in polyps smaller than 2 cm in size (51, 97, 98). In one case, the polyp measured 5 × 15 mm (51). Malignancy has not been reported in focal foveolar hyperplasia, however. In this regard, Stolte suggested that this small lesion should no longer be referred to as a gastric polyp (88).

The incidence of coexisting gastric carcinoma away from the polyp is higher than malignant change within the polyp, in an average of 13% of polyp-bearing patients (see Table 26.4). This observation emphasizes the importance of careful evaluation of the entire stomach when the polyp is present. In addition, Laxen et al. found 3 carcinomas in association with, but none within, the inflammatory polyps in 130 cases (43), indicating the unstable state of gastric mucosa in that clinical situation as well.

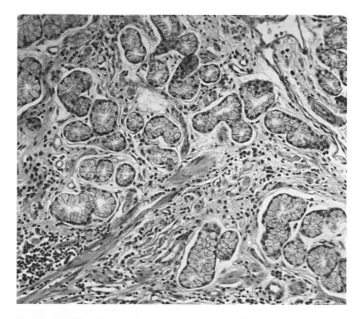

Figure 26.15   Hyperplastic polyp. Normal-appearing pyloric-type glands are separated by inflamed stromal tissue and thin bundles of muscle cells (×200).

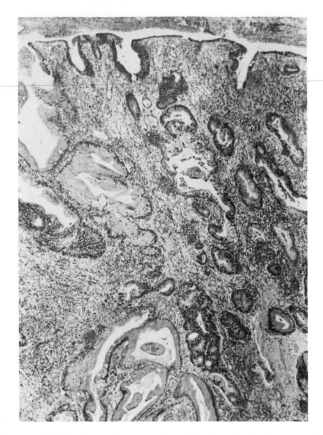

Figure 26.16 Hyperplastic polyp with dysplastic changes. Hyperplastic and dilated foveolae are shown at upper left and lower center. Other glands show varying degrees of dysplasia with hyperchromatic and pseudostratified cells (×80). (Courtesy of Dr. I. Kline, Lankenau Hospital, Philadelphia, PA.)

Follow-up studies of hyperplastic polyp have been reported. In a 15.5-year follow-up series involving 147 patients, Laxen reported that carcinoma developed in 3 cases outside the polyp and none in the polyp (78). Kawai et al. monitored 110 polyps up to 15 years and noted that carcinoma developed in one at 3 years (99). None of 974 polyps followed for 6 months to 11 years by Yamagata and Hisamichi developed carcinoma (100). In a study by Orlowska et al. (54), in which 131 polyps were monitored for an average of 2 years and 8 months, 2 developed carcinoma, 1 dysplasia, and 2 intestinal metaplasia. In addition, gastric carcinoma occurred outside the polyp in 2 of 58 patients under observation. So far, metastasis and death from malignant change in a hyperplastic polyp has not been reported.

The mechanism of malignant transformation in the hyperplastic polyp is unknown. Kozuka emphasized metaplastic change and reported a malignant incidence of 11% when metaplasia is present in contrast to 2% when it is absent (32). On the other hand, of 14 carcinomatous lesions among 421 hyperplastic polyps reported by Kushima and Hattori (95), 11 showed no metaplasia in the polyps. The importance of dysplastic or adenomatous change in the polyp (Fig. 26.18), as stressed by Ming (21, 35), is supported by the following observations. Snover reported malignant change in 1 of 7 mixed adenomatous-hyperplastic polyps in contrast to 1 in 127 hyperplastic polyps (30). The malignant polyp reported by Ghazi

et al. was in the adenomatous area of a 6-cm polyp (44). Dysplastic changes in the polyp have also been noted (29, 94, 101). Hattori (101) found dysplasia in 11 of 67 polyps, 9 in gastric epithelium, and 2 in intestinalized epithelium. Carcinomas were present in 3 of these polyps. Two carcinomas were of gastric type and one of intestinal type. The high frequency of involvement of gastric-type cells may be expected because they are the dominant cells in the hyperplastic polyp. Laxen et al. (43) noticed the increasing average age of patients with different types of polyps: 58 years for patients with inflammatory polyp, 60 years for foveolar hyperplasia, 64 years for hyperplastic polyp, and 72 years for adenomas, suggesting a chronologic order for the development of these lesions. Kozuka proposed a histogenetic sequence, from gastritis to carcinoma through stages of hyperplastic polyp and adenoma (38).

HAMARTOMATOUS POLYP

The hamartomatous polyps are tumor-like nodules composed of tissues normally present in the location, usually in a disorganized arrangement. Because the stomach consists of many different types of cells, the composition of hamartomatous polyps is not uniform. They occur most commonly in association with the hereditary gastrointestinal polyposis syndromes, namely Peutz-Jeghers syndrome, Gardner syndrome and related familial adenomatous polyposis, and juvenile polyposis. The genetic aspects of these conditions are discussed in Chapter 7. In these syndromes, the polyps are located more commonly and in larger numbers in the intestines than in the stomach. The morphology and characteristics of the intestinal polyps are described in Chapter 33.

It is noteworthy that gastric and intestinal polyps in the same disease may be of different types. For instance, whereas the intestinal polyps in Gardner syndrome and familial polyposis coli are mostly adenomas, the most common form of gastric polyp in these syndromes is hamartomatous, involving mainly the fundic mucosa. Although the polyps in Peutz-Jeghers syndrome and juvenile

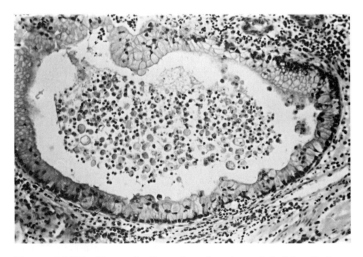

Figure 26.17 Hyperplastic polyp showing globoid cells in a dilated foveola. These oval cells are bulging with acidic mucin and the nuclei are compressed against the cell membrane as in the signet-ring cells. Some cells are free in the lumen, admixed with inflammatory cells (×200).

TABLE 26.4		Reported Frequency of Malignant Change in Coexisting Carcinoma Outside the Gastric Polyp at the Time of Diagnosis of the Polyp			
Reference		Malignant Change in Polyp		Coexisting Carcinoma Outside Polyp	
No.	Year	Adenoma	Hyperplastic Polyp	Adenoma	Hyperplastic Polyp
21[a]	1946–	41% (150/362)[b]	2.0% (4/204)[b]	48% (52/108)[b]	—
	1972	19% (11/57)[c]	1.0% (3/293)[c]	42% (52/123)[c]	22% (46/208)[c]
57[d]	1977–	30% (120/406)[b]	0.7% (20/2845)[b]	—	—
	1988	32% (14/44)[c]	2.2% (8/367)[a]	54% (89/165)[c]	7.4% (24/325)[c]
95	1993	—	3.3% (14/421)[b]	—	—
79	1994	16% (5/31)[b]	—	—	—
96	1995	—	1.7% (4/236)[b]	—	—
54	1995	10% (6/60)[b]	2.1% (10/483)[b]	13% (4/30)[b]	7.1% (19/265)[b]
97	1996	—	1.8% (4/112)[b]	—	—
98	1996	25% (1/4)[b]	9.7% (3/31)[b]	—	—
Subtotal	1993–	13% (12/95)[b]	2.6% (32/1252)[b]	13% (4/30)[b]	7.1% (19/265)[b]
	1996				
TOTAL		31% (284/903)[b]	1.0% (31/3526)[b]	48% (52/108)[b]	7.1% (19/265)[b]
		25% (25/101)[c]	1.7% (11/660)[c]	49% (141/288)[c]	13% (70/533)[c]

[a]Includes review of nine reports.

[b]Number of polyps.

[c]Number of cases.

[d]Includes 12 reports.

polyposis are both hamartomatous, they have different histologic characteristics. Lastly, the hamartomatous polyps may be seen in patients without other characteristics of these syndromes.

PEUTZ-JEGHERS SYNDROME

The polyps in the Peutz-Jeghers syndrome are prototypes of the hamartomatous polyp. They occur most commonly in the small intestines; gastric polyps are present in 25 to 49% of patients (102–104). Most of these lesions are less than 1 cm in diameter, and rarely are large enough to cause symptoms. Microscopically, the polyps show prominent foveolar hyperplasia and a varying amount of deep glands, the type of which corresponds to the location of the polyp (Fig. 26.19). Smooth muscle bundles of variable thickness extend from muscularis mucosae into the polyp, occasionally up to the surface area. Irregularity of muscle thickness may also be present in the media of blood vessels. All cells appear normal, and there is no inflammation in the lamina propria. These features distinguish the hamartomatous nature of the Peutz-Jeghers polyp from other types of gastric polyp.

Some patients with Peutz-Jeghers syndrome have only pigmentation or only polyposis (102, 105). Conversely, hamartomatous polyps of Peutz-Jeghers type without pigmentation or familial history have also been reported (106, 107). In two such cases reported by Katz et al., polyps measured 5 × 11 and 4 × 6 cm, respectively, causing obstruction and bleeding (107).

The possibility of malignant change in the Peutz-Jeghers polyp is a controversial issue. Reid recognized malignant change in 2 to 3%

of cases (108). The carcinoma, as the polyp, occurs more commonly in the intestines (103), but its location in the stomach and duodenum is disproportionately high (108). In most cases, the carcinoma is large and the polyps are small. Actual demonstration of carcinoma in the polyp is rarely accomplished (109, 110). The carcinoma develops in the adenomatous or dysplastic area of the polyp or coexisting independent adenoma (110). Cochet reported dysplastic changes in the polyp in association with a gastric carcinoma in a son and a duodenal carcinoma in his mother (111).

Peutz-Jeghers syndrome manifests early and the diagnosis is made in the first three decades of life. Patients with carcinoma are also in the early age as compared to cancer patients in the general population. Dodds et al. reported an average age of 27 years for patients with gastric carcinoma, 38 years for duodenal carcinoma, and 41 years for colonic carcinoma (103).

JUVENILE POLYPOSIS SYNDROME

Juvenile polyps are characterized grossly by a smooth surface and histologically by many dilated glands filled with mucus and an inflamed stroma (112). Because this type of polyp occurs mostly in children, it has been called juvenile polyp. This term has become a pathologic entity and is applied to any polyp with similar histologic features irrespective of the age of the patient at the time of diagnosis.

The cause of isolated juvenile polyp is unknown. Some pathologists favor inflammation as an etiologic factor, in view of the presence of many inflammatory cells and retention of mucus in the dilated glands. Thus, juvenile polyps had also been called inflam-

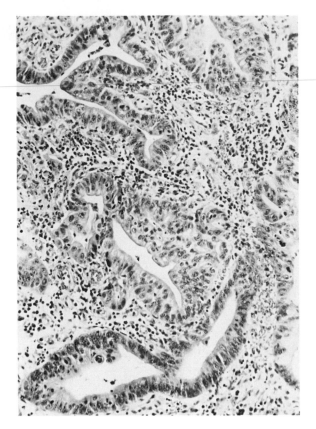

Figure 26.18 Carcinomatous lesion in the hyperplastic polyp with dysplastic changes shown in Figure 26.16 (×200). (Courtesy of Dr. I. Kline, Lankenau Hospital, Philadelphia, PA.)

matory or retention polyps. Morson, on the other hand, noting the similarity between the stromal tissue in the polyp and the lamina propria of normal colon, considered juvenile polyps as hamartomatous lesions (113). The detection of juvenile polyposis in infancy (114, 115) and the hyperplastic changes without retention cyst or inflammation in the early lesions (116) favor the theory of a hamartomatous nature of the juvenile polyp, at least in patients with hereditary syndromes.

Juvenile polyps exist in four situations (Table 26.5). The most common presentation is the presence of isolated polyps in the rectum or colon of the children (112). In juvenile polyposis coli, numerous polyps arise in the colon and a few in the small intestines (117). Generalized juvenile gastrointestinal polyposis affects the entire digestive tract, and the stomach is involved in about 15% (25, 114–116). This condition occurs at all ages. A positive family history is noted in 20 to 50% of cases (118, 119). The infantile type has a recessive genetic pattern of transmission, whereas the type involving older persons has dominant genetic transmission (115). As the patient grows older, the number of new polyps decreases (120). There have also been cases in which polyposis is limited to the stomach (121, 122). These syndromes may be related. Hofting et al. reported a family with prominent stomach involvement (123). Three members in the first generation died of gastric carcinoma and one of colon cancer. Three members of the second generation had extensive juvenile polyposis of the stomach and another one had both colon and stomach carcinomas. An example of gastric lesions

is shown in Figure 26.20. This patient had numerous small and one large juvenile polyps in the stomach and many juvenile polyps and an adenoma in the colon.

The juvenile polyp in the stomach is composed of hyperplastic foveolae and edematous stroma with inflammatory cells (Fig. 26.21). This composition resembles closely the common hyperplastic polyp of the stomach. Another type of polyp that requires differentiation is the inflammatory polyp with retention cysts associated with Cronkhite-Canada syndrome. The distinction between these three types of polyps is difficult. Definitive diagnosis requires the knowledge of the clinical background of the patient, such as the age, the symptoms, and the distribution and number of the polyps.

Carcinomas develop occasionally in patients with juvenile polyposis (in 17% in one report [118]), as well as in family members who do not have this type of polyp (124). Most carcinomas are found in the colon and a few occur in the stomach. Carcinomas in the colon may develop independently in adenomas that occur either coincidentally or as a secondary change within the juvenile polyp (25, 116, 125). In the stomach, carcinoma develops in the dysplastic juvenile polyp (116, 126). Figure 26.22 shows carcinomatous tissue in the dysplastic area of a large lobulated juvenile polyp in the stomach shown in Figure 26.20.

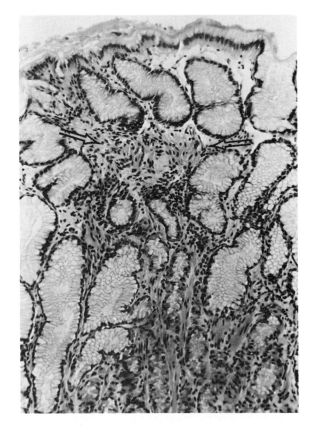

Figure 26.19 Peutz-Jeghers polyp. The foveolae are hyperplastic, but the fundic glands are normal. Both are separated by thin bundles of muscle cells, some of which are near the mucosal surface (arrows). There is no inflammation (×200). (Reprinted with permission from Ming SC. The classification and significance of gastric polyps. In: Yardley JH, Morson, BM, eds. The gastrointestinal tract. Baltimore: Williams & Wilkins, 1977:149–175.)

TABLE 26.5	Subtypes of Juvenile Polyps	
Types (Reference)	Location of Polyps	Familial History
Solitary juvenile polyp (112)	Colorectum	Absent
Juvenile polyposis coli (117)	Colorectum, few in small bowel	Present
Generalized juvenile gastrointestinal polyposis (114)	Stomach to rectum	Present in 20–50%
Familial juvenile polyposis of stomach (121)	Stomach	Present

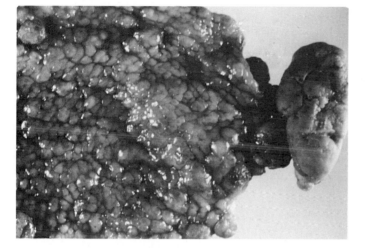

Figure 26.20 Juvenile gastrointestinal polyposis. The stomach mucosa was studded with numerous small polyps of uniform size, except for one large polyp shown at right. The polyps were composed of dilated foveolae and edematous stroma with chronic inflammation. The large polyp measured 5 × 3 × 2 cm and had focal malignant change, shown in Figure 26.22. The patient had numerous juvenile polyps and one adenoma in the colon that was resected 4 years prior to the gastrectomy. The patient demonstrated neither ectodermal changes nor a positive familial history of polyposis. (Courtesy of Dr. Arthur Aufdeheide, St. Luke's Hospital, Duluth, MN.)

FUNDIC GLAND POLYP

Fundic gland polyp, also known as fundic gland hyperplasia (30) and glandular cysts (53, 127), occurs in the oxyntic mucosa of the stomach. It was first described in detail by Watanabe et al. in 6 of 22 patients with familial polyposis coli (24), appearing as numerous sessile polyps less than 5 mm in diameter. Subsequently, fundic gland polyps have been found in patients with Gardner syndrome (128, 129) as well as polyposis coli patients (130–132). These lesions are composed of fundic glands lined with increasing numbers of normal appearing parietal and chief cells. Many glands are cystically dilated, tortuous, or budding (42, 133), hence the term "glandular cyst" (127). In one report, muscle cells were also present in a single polyp (134). Histochemical studies reveal that fundic gland polyps secrete O-acylated sialic acid (125), glucagon, and glicentin (135), which normally are present only in the fetal stomach. Histologically, however, the constituent cells of the polyp appear normal. Furthermore, the polyp may regress and disappear (30, 127–129, 132, 135, 136), suggesting that these lesions may not be hamartomatous. The stomach in familial polyposis coli patients may also contain adenoma, carcinoma, or carcinoid (23, 137–139).

Fundic gland polyps also arise in persons without colonic polyposis (30, 106, 127), probably even more commonly than in polyposis patients (127). Tsuchikame et al. reported three related patients with fundic gland polyposis in the stomach, but no polyps in the duodenum or colon (140). Eidt and Stolte (127) reviewed 1500 cases, of which 596 patients were examined for colonic lesions. Familial adenomatosis coli or Gardner syndrome was present in only 21 cases, simple adenomas in 66, adenocarcinomas in 21, and other types of polyps in 50. The remaining 438 patients had normal clinical findings in the colon. In a report by Stolte et al. (53), glandular cysts were the most common gastric lesion, accounting for 47% of 5515 gastric polyps examined. In a report by Marcial et al. (141), the prevalence rate of fundic gland polyp in gastroscopic examination was 0.8%; patients ranged in age from 27 to 82 years (average, 53 years); women were affected more often than men (5:1); each patient had an average of four polyps (range of 1 to 11); and the average size of the polyp was 2.3 +/- 1.2 mm.

FOVEOLAR POLYP

In 1972, Goldman and Appelman described 11 antral foveolar polyps in 8 patients (33). The polyps were composed of tightly packed, arborized foveolae lined by normal-appearing tall mucous cells that contained only neutral glycoprotein. The stroma was delicate and no inflammation was noted. About 33% of the polyps had mild metaplasia and about 25% were larger than 2 cm. Carcinoma of the stomach and colon was present in one case each. Snover (30) described an 8-cm polyp of this type found in the body of the stomach and called it a foveolar adenoma. This type of polyp, probably hamartomatous, can be readily distinguished from hyperplastic polyp and polypoid foveolar hyperplasia by the lack of stromal inflammation and cystic dilatation.

INFLAMMATORY POLYP

Inflammatory polyps accounted for one third of gastric polyps in the series reported by Laxen et al. (43). None of the polyps showed malignant change, but gastric carcinoma outside the polyps was present in 3 of 130 cases.

Inflammatory polyps are heterogeneous and encompass several entities. A polyp made of inflammatory granulation tissue can be properly called inflammatory pseudopolyp because glandular tissue is either lost or absent. A special form of inflammatory polyp, known as inflammatory fibroid polyp, occurs most commonly in the stomach and constitutes 3.1% of gastric polyps (53) (see Chapter 18). Another example of an inflammatory polyp of interest is the eosinophilic granuloma, which is discussed in Chapter 23.

An inflammatory polyp with prominent cystic glands may be called retention polyp because the dilated glands are filled with retained mucus. Such a polyp is rare in the stomach. The retention polyp resembles the hyperplastic polyp on one hand and the juvenile polyp on the other. The differentiation is difficult on the basis of histologic findings alone. Characteristics of the retention polyp are the edematous and inflamed stroma, the much dilated foveolae, and the absence of deep glands proper.

The polyps associated with the Cronkhite-Canada syndrome are of this type. This syndrome is characterized by diffuse gastrointestinal polyposis and ectodermal changes. Polyps are common in the stomach of patients with this syndrome. In one case, the patient had polyposis in the stomach and duodenum, but not in the colon (26). The gastric polyps are 0.5 to 1.5 cm in diameter, and are either long and finger-like (142) or resemble hydatid mole (26, 143). In two reported cases, carcinoma was found in the stomach (144), but not within the polyp. Additional information on Cronkhite-Canada syndrome is presented in Chapter 33.

HETEROTOPIC POLYP

Misplaced gastric glands may present as a polypoid mass (145). The glands may also be found in the submucosa (146). More commonly, heterotopic polyps are made of tissues from the neighboring pancreas and duodenum. They account for 4% of polypoid lesions in the stomach (see Table 26.1).

HETEROTOPIC PANCREATIC TISSUE

The heterotopic pancreas occurs in the intestines as well as in the stomach. Among 543 cases reviewed by Busard and Walters in which heterotopic pancreatic tissue was found, 276 involved the intestine, 149 the stomach, and 30 a Meckel diverticulum (147). Lai et al. reported a case of heterotopic pancreas in a duplicated stomach (148). The prepyloric region is a favored site in the stomach (149). In a case reported by DeBord et al., the patient had two lesions, one in the antrum and the other at the esophagogastric junction (150). Many patients are children (42, 115). The average age of adult patients was 45 years (53).

Heterotopic pancreas is primarily a submucosal, nipple-like lesion that has a dimpled center corresponding to the excretory duct. Clinical symptoms correlate with the size of the lesion and the

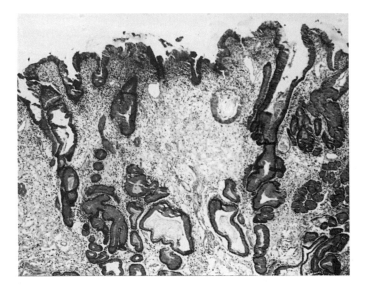

Figure 26.21 Juvenile gastrointestinal polyposis. Photomicrograph of one of the small polyps shown in Figure 26.20. Note the dilated glands and edematous and inflamed stroma (×80). (Courtesy of Dr. Arthur Aufdeheide, St. Luke's Hospital, Duluth, MN.)

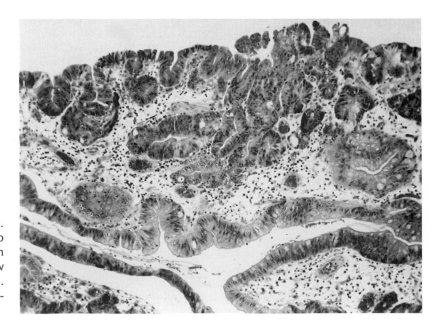

Figure 26.22 Juvenile gastrointestinal polyposis. Photomicrograph of the large gastric juvenile polyp in Figure 26.20. A focus of carcinoma is shown in the surface region. The glands beneath it show intestinal metaplasia and dysplastic changes (×300). (Courtesy of Dr. Arthur Aufdeheide, St. Luke's Hospital, Duluth, MN.)

extent of mucosal involvement (151). Ulceration and bleeding are common manifestations. Rarely, heterotopic pancreatic tissue resembles a malignant lesion (152), although actual malignant change is rare (153, 154). Histologically, the heterotopic tissue is composed mainly of exocrine glands and ducts; islet cells are present in varying amounts (155). San Juan et al. described a case of Zollinger-Ellison syndrome associated with a non-beta islet cell tumor in the heterotopic pancreas (156).

Brunner Gland Polyp (Hyperplasia)

Polypoid lesions made of Brunner glands have been called adenomas because of tightly packed glands. In reality, only hyperplasia is present and the glands are normal. The lesion occurs mainly in the duodenum and only rarely in the stomach, always in the prepyloric region (157, 158), where it may be obstructive. It accounts for 1.2% of gastric polyps (53). Whether Brunner gland polyp is a hamartoma or simple hyperplasia is not clear, although its stationary appearance favors the former.

Adenomyoma

A rare gastric lesion related to heterotopic tissues is known as adenomyoma or adenomyosis, which is composed of a mixture of ducts lined by columnar cells and bundles of smooth muscle in a haphazard arrangement (159–161). Pancreatic tissue and Brunner glands are often present. Most of the lesions are less than 2 cm and some are as large as 5 cm in diameter. In one case, excessive mucus secretion caused pseudomyxoma peritonei (152).

References

1. Ming SC. Tumors of the Esophagus and Stomach. In Atlas of Tumor Pathology, Second Series, Fascicle 7. Armed Forces of Pathology. Washington, DC 1973:99–101.
2. Marshak RH, Feldman F. Gastric polyps. Am J Dig Dis 1965;10:909–935.
3. Spriggs EI. Polyps of the stomach and polypoid gastritis. Q J Med, New Series 1943;12:1–60.
4. Ménétrier P. Des polyadenomes gastriques et de leurs rapport avec le cancer de l'estomac. Arch Physiol Norm Pathol 1888;1:32–55, 236–262.
5. Williams SM, Harned RK, Settles RH. Adenocarcinoma of the stomach in association with Menetrier's disease. Gastrointest Radiol 1978;3:387–390.
6. Mills GP. Multiple polypi of the stomach (gastritis polyposa): With the report of a case. Br J Surg 1922;10:226–231.
7. Eklof O. Benign tumours of the stomach and duodenum. A clinical and roentgenographic study with special reference to adenomatous polyps and the relation to malignancy. Acta Chir Scand Suppl 1962;291:1–57.
8. Lawrence JC. Gastrointestinal polyps: Statistical study of malignancy incidence. Am J Surg 1936;31:499–505.
9. Pearl FL, Brunn H. Multiple gastric polyposis; a supplementary report of 41 cases, including 3 personal cases. Surg Gynecol Obstet 1943;76:257–281.
10. Plachta A, Speer FD. Gastric polyps and their relationship to carcinoma of the stomach. Review of literature and report of 65 cases. Am J Gastroenterol 1957;28:160–175.
11. Berg JM. Histological aspects of the relation between gastric adenomatous polyps and gastric cancer. Cancer 1958;11:1149–1155.
12. Rosato F, Noto JA. Gastric polyps. Am J Surg 1966;111:647–650.
13. McNeer G, Joly DJ, Berg JW. The significance of adenomatous polyps. In: McNeer G, Pack GT, eds. Neoplasm of the stomach. Philadelphia: JB Lippincott, 1967:56–80.
14. Rieniets JH, Broders AC. Gastric adenomas. A pathologic study. West J Surg Obstet Gynecol 1945;53:163–170; 1946;54:21–39.
15. Finney JMT, Friedenwald J. Gastric polyposis. Am J Med Sci 1917;154:683–689.
16. Walk L. Villous tumors of the stomach. Clinical review and report of 2 cases. Arch Intern Med 1951;87:560–569.
17. Meltzer AD, Ostrum BJ, Isard HJ. Villous tumors of the stomach and duodenum. Radiology 1966;87:511–513.
18. Ross RJ. Villous adenoma of the stomach. J Am Med Assoc 1966;195:583–584.
19. Ming SC, Goldman H. Gastric polyps: A histogenetic classification and its relation to carcinoma. Cancer 1965;18:721–726.
20. Tomasulo J. Gastric polyps; histologic types and their relationship to gastric carcinoma. Cancer 1971;27:1346–1355.
21. Ming SC. The classification and significance of gastric polyps. In: Yardley JH, Morson BM, eds. The gastrointestinal tract. Baltimore: Williams & Wilkins, 1977:149–175.
22. Sugano H, Nakamura K, Takagi K. An atypical epithelium of the stomach. A clinicopathological entity. Gann Monogr Cancer Res 1971;11:257–269.
23. Nagayo T. Histological diagnosis of biopsied gastric mucosa with special reference to that of borderline lesions. Gann Monogr Cancer Res 1971;11:245–256.
24. Watanabe H, Enjoji M, Yao T, et al. Gastric lesions in familial adenomatosis coli. Their incidence and histological analysis. Hum Pathol 1978;9:269–283.
25. Beacham DH, Shields HM, Raffensperger EC, et al. Juvenile and adenomatous gastrointestinal polyposis. Am J Dig Dis 1978;23:1137–1143.
26. Kindblom LG, Angervall L, Santesson B, et al. Cronkhite-Canada syndrome. Case report. Cancer 1977;39:2651–2657.
27. Ming SC. Malignant potential of epithelial polyps of the stomach. In: Ming SC, ed. Precursors of gastric cancer. Praeger, Philadelphia. 1984:219–231.
28. Elster K. Histologic classification of gastric polyps. Curr Top Pathol 65:77–93.
29. Koch HK, Lesch R, Cremer M, et al. Polyp and polypoid foveolar hyperplasia in gastric biopsy specimens and their precancerous prevalence. Front Gastrointest Res 1979;4:183–191.
30. Snover DC. Benign epithelial polyps of the stomach. Pathol Annu 1985;20:303–329.
31. Nakamura T, Nakano G. Histopathological classification and malignant change in gastric polyps. J Clin Pathol 1985;38:754–764.
32. Kozuka S, Masamoto K, Suzuki S, et al. Histogenetic types and size of polypoid lesion of the stomach, with special reference to cancerous changes. Gann 1977;68:267–274.
33. Goldman DS, Appelman HD. Gastric mucosal polyps. Am J Clin Pathol 1972;58:434–444.
34. Ming SC. Tumors of the esophagus and stomach. In: Atlas of tumor pathology, second series, fascicle 7. Washington DC: Armed Forces of Pathology, 1973;124–143.
35. Ming SC. Tumors of the esophagus and stomach, supplement. In: Atlas of tumor pathology, second series, fascicle 7. Washington DC: Armed Forces of Pathology, 1985:S24–S32.
36. Nakamura T. Nakamura type III gastric polyp: History of the study. Proc 1st International Gastric Cancer congress. Bologna, Italy: Monduzzi Editore, 1995:209–212.
37. Morson BC. Gastric polyps composed of intestinal epithelium. Br J Cancer 1955;9:550–557.
38. Kozuka S. Gastric polyps. In: Filipe MI, Jass JR, eds. Gastric carcinoma. London: Churchill Livingstone, 1986;132–151.
39. Niv Y, Bat L. Gastric polyps-a clinical study. Isr J Med Sci 1985;21:841–844.
40. Seifert E, Elster K. Gastric polypectomy. Am J Gastroenterol 1975;63:451–456.
41. Ueno K, Oshiba S, Yamagata S, et al. Histo-clinical classification and follow–up study of gastric polyp. Tohoku J Exp Med 1976;118 (Suppl): 23–38.
42. Rosch W. Epidemiology, pathogenesis, diagnosis, treatment of benign gastric tumours. Front Gastrointest Res 1980;6:167–184.
43. Laxen F, Sipponen P, Ihamaki T, et al. Gastric polyps; their morphological and endoscopical characteristics and relation to gastric carcinoma. Acta Pathol Microbiol Scand (A) 1982;90:221–228.

44. Ghazi A, Ferstenberg H, Shinya H. Endoscopic gastroduodenal polypectomy. Ann Surg 1984;200:175–180.
45. Elsborg L, Andersen D, Myhere–Jensen O, et al. Gastric mucosal polyps in pernicious anaemia. Scand J Gastroenterol 1977;12:49–52.
46. Stockbrugger RW, Menon GG, Beilby JO, et al. Gastroscopic screening in 80 patients with pernicious anaemia. Gut 1983;24: 1141–1147.
47. Siurala M. Gastritis, its fate and sequelae. Ann Clin Res 1981;13: 111–113.
48. Janunger K, Domellof L. Gastric polyps and precancerous mucosal changes after partial gastrectomy. Acta Chir Scand 1978;144: 293–298.
49. Ovaska JT, Ekfors TO, Havia TV, et al. Endoscopic follow–up after resection for gastric or duodenal ulcer. Acta Chir Scand 1986;152: 289–295.
50. Seifert E, Gail K, Weismuller J. Gastric polypectomy. Long–term results (survey of 23 centres in Germany). Endoscopy 1983; 15:8–11.
51. Marcello PW, Asbun HJ, Veidenheimer MC, et al. Gastroduodenal polyps in familial adenomatous polyposis. Surg Endosc 1996;10: 418–421.
52. Goedde TA, Rodriguez–Bigas MA, Herrera L, et al. Gastroduodenal polyps in familial adenomatous polyposis. Surg Oncol 1992;1: 357–361.
53. Stolte M, Sticht T, Eidt S, et al. Frequency, location, and age and sex distribution of various types of gastric polyp. Endoscopy 1994;26: 659-665.
54. Orlowska J, Jarosz D, Pachlewski J, et al. Malignant transformation of benign epithelial gastric polyps. Am J Gastroenterol 1995;90: 2152–2159.
55. Brooks GS, Frost ES, Wesselhoeft C. Prolapsed hyperplastic gastric polyp causing gastric outlet obstruction, hypergastrinemia, and hematemesis in an infant. J Pediatr Surg 1992;27:1537–1538.
56. Nagayo T. Histogenesis and precursors of human gastric cancer. New York: Springer, 1986:103–111.
57. Ming SC. Epithelial polyps of the stomach. In: Ming SC, Goldman H, eds. Pathology of the gastrointestinal tract. Philadelphia: WB Saunders, 1992:547–569.
58. Stamm B, Sulser H, Stahlberger–Bucher R. Pathology of gastric mucosa polyps. Schweiz Med Wochenschr 1985;115:1120–1127.
59. Hirota T, Okada T, Itabashi M, et al. Histogenesis of human gastric cancer—with special reference to the significance of adenoma as a precancerous lesion. In: Ming SC, ed. Precursors of gastric cancer. Philadelphia: Praeger, 1984:233–252.
60. Kamiya T, Morishita T, Asakura H, et al. Long term follow–up on gastric adenoma and its relation to gastric protruded carcinoma. Cancer 1982;50:2493–2503.
61. Watanabe H. Argentaffin cells in adenoma of the stomach. Cancer 1972;30:1267–1274.
62. Jass JR, Filipe MI. Sulphomucins and precancerous lesions of the human stomach. Histopathology 1980;4:271–279.
63. Kushima R, Muller W, Stolte M, et al. Differential p53 protein expression in stomach adenomas of gastric and intestinal phenotypes: Possible sequences of p53 alteration in stomach carcinogenesis. Virchows Arch 1996;428:223–227.
64. Watanabe H, Jass JR, Sobin LH. WHO histological typing of oesophageal and gastric tumours. 2nd ed. New York: Springer, 1990:19–20.
65. Nakamura K, Sagakuchi H, Enjoji M. Depressed adenoma of the stomach. Cancer 1988;62:2197–2202.
66. Riemann JF, Schmidt H, Hermanek P. On the ultrastructure of the gastric "borderline lesion". J Cancer Res Clin Oncol 1983;105: 285–291.
67. Takahashi T, Iwama N. Atypical glands in gastric adenoma. Three–dimensional architecture compared with carcinomatous and metaplastic glands. Virchows Arch [A] 1984;403:135–148.
68. Inaba S, Tanaka T, Okanoue T, et al. Villous tumor of the stomach associated with adenocarcinomas—a histochemical study of mucosubstances. Jpn J Clin Oncol 1984;14:691–698.
69. Ito H, Yokozaki H, Hata J, et al. Glicentin–containing cells in intestinal metaplasia, adenoma and carcinoma of the stomach. Virchows Arch [A] 1984;404:17–29.
70. Okuyama S, Yokota K, Yuki M. Cell proliferation and cell death (apoptosis) in epithelial tumors of the stomach—analysis of tumor tissues by the endoscopic mucosal resection. [Japanese] Nippon Shokakibyo Gakkai Zasshi 1995;92:130–139.
71. Kitayama Y, Sugimura H, Tanaka M, et al. Expression of p53 and flow cytometric DNA analysis of isolated neoplastic glands of the stomach: An application of the gland isolation method. Virchows Arch 1995; 426:557–562.
72. Tohdo H, Yokozaki H, Haruma K, et al. p53 gene mutations in gastric adenomas. Virchows Arch [B] 1993;63:191–195.
73. Lauwers GY, Wahl SJ, Melamed J, et al. p53 expression in precancerous gastric lesions: an immunohistochemical study of PAb 1801 monoclonal antibody on adenomatous and hyperplastic gastric polyps. Am J Gastroenterol 1993;88:1916–1919.
74. Tamura G, Sakata K, Maesawa C, et al. Microsatellite alterations in adenoma and differentiated adenocarcinoma of the stomach. Cancer Res 1995;426:57-562.
75. Semba S, Yokozaki H, Yamamoto S, et al. Microsatellite instability in precancerous lesions and adenocarcinomas of the stomach. Cancer 1996;77(Suppl):1620–1627.
76. Nakatsuru S, Yanagisawa A, Furukawa Y, et al. Somatic mutations of the APC gene in precancerous lesion of the stomach. Hum Mol Genet 1993;2:1463–1465.
77. Sakata K, Tamura G, Maesawa C, et al. Loss of heterozygosity on the short arm of chromosome 9 without p16 gene mutation in gastric carcinomas. Jpn J Cancer Res 1995;86:333–335.
78. Laxen F. Gastric carcinoma and pernicious anaemia in long–term endoscopic follow–up of subjects with gastric polyps. Scand J Gastroenterol 1984;19:535–540.
79. Tatsuta M, Iishi H, Baba M, et al. Expression of c–myc mRNA as an aid in histologic differentiation of adenoma from well differentiated adenocarcinoma in the stomach. Cancer 1994;73:1795–1799.
80. Varis O, Laxen F, Valle J. Helicobacter pylori infection and fasting serum gastrin levels in a series of endoscopically diagnosed gastric polyps. APMIS 1994;102:759–764.
81. Bonilla Palacios JJ, Miyazaki Y, Kanayuma S, et al. Serum gastrin, pepsinogens, parietal cell and Helicobacter pylori antibodies in patients with gastric polyps. Acta Gastroenterol Latinoam 1994; 24:77–82.
82. Carneiro F, David L, Seruca R, et al. Hyperplastic polyposis and diffuse carcinoma of the stomach. A study of a family. Cancer 1993;72:323–329.
83. Hizawa K, Iida M, Matsumoto T, et al. Gastrointestinal manifestations of Cowden's disease. Report of four cases. J Clin Gastroenterol 1994;18:13–18.
84. Tanaka J, Fujimoto K, Iwakiri R, et al. Hyperplastic polyps following treatment of acute gastric ulcers. Intern Med 1994;33:366–368.
85. Graham JR. Omeprazole and gastric polyposis in humans. Gastroenterology 1993;104:1584.
86. Stolte M, Bethke B, Seifert E, et al. Observation of gastric glandular cysts in the corpus mucosa of the stomach under omeprazole treatment. Z Gastroenterol 1995;33:146–149.
87. Mitsufuji S, Tsuchihashi Y, Kodama T. Histogenesis of hyperplastic polyps of the stomach in terms of cellular proliferation. J Gastroenterol 1994;29:559–568.
88. Stolte M, Bethke B, Sticht T, et al. Differentiation of focal foveolar hyperplasia from hyperplastic polyps in gastric biopsy material. Pathol Res Pract 1995;191:1198–1202.
89. Stemmermann GN, Hayashi T. Hyperplastic polyps of the gastric mucosa adjacent to gastroenterostomy stomas. Am J Clin Pathol 1979;71:341–345.
90. Koga S, Watanabe H, Enjoji M. Stomal polypoid hypertrophic gastritis: A polypoid gastric lesion at gastroenterostomy site. Cancer 1979;43:647–657.
91. Tsukamoto Y, Nishitani H, Oshiumi Y, et al. Spontaneous disappearance of gastric polyps: Report of four cases. AJR Am J Roentgenol 1977;129:893–897.
92. Mukada T, Kashiwagura J, Itasaka K, et al. Giant hyperplasiogenous polyp of the stomach simulating malignant polyp. Tohoku J Exp Med 1984;142:125–130.
93. Petrova AS, Subrichina GN, Tschistjakova OV, et al. Flow cytometry, cytomorphology, histology and autoradiography in human gastric hyperplastic polyps and the surrounding mucosa. Oncology 1982; 39:308–313.

94. Daibo M, Itabashi M, Hirota T. Malignant transformation of gastric hyperplastic polyps. Am J Gastroenterol 1987;82:1016–1025.

95. Kushima R, Hattori T. Histogenesis and characteristics of gastric–type adenocarcinomas in the stomach. J Cancer Res Clin Oncol 1993;120:103–111.

96. Hizawa K, Fuchigami T, Iida M, et al. Possible neoplastic transformation within gastric hyperplastic polyp. Application of endoscopic polypectomy. Surg Endosc 1995;9:714–718.

97. Zea–Iriarte WL, Sekine I, Itsuno M, et al. Carcinoma in gastric hyperplastic polyps. A phenotypic study. Dig Dis Sci 1996;41:377–386.

98. Ginsberg GG, Al–Kawas FH, Fleischer DE, et al. Gastric polyps: Relationship of size and histology to cancer risk. Am J Gastroenterol 1996;91:714–717.

99. Kawai K, Kizu M, Miyaoka T. Epidemiology and pathogenesis of gastric cancer. Front Gastrointest Res 1980;6:71–86.

100. Yamagata S, Hisamichi S. Precancerous lesions of the stomach. World J Surg 1979;3:671–673.

101. Hattori T. Morphological range of hyperplastic polyps and carcinomas arising in hyperplastic polyps of the stomach. J Clin Pathol 1985;38:622–630.

102. Bartholomew LG, Moore CE, Dahlin DC, et al. Intestinal polyposis associated with mucocutaneous pigmentation. Surg Gynecol Obstet 1962;115:1–11.

103. Dodds WJ, Schulte WJ, Hensley GT, et al. Peutz–Jeghers syndrome and gastrointestinal malignancy. AJR Am J Roentgenol 1972;115:374–377.

104. Utsunomiya J, Gocho H, Miyanaga T, et al. Peutz–Jeghers syndrome. Its natural course and management. Johns Hopkins Med J 1975;136:71–82.

105. Erbe RW. Inherited gastrointestinal polyposis syndromes. N Engl J Med 1976;294:1101–1104.

106. Tatsuta M, Okuda S, Tamura H, et al. Gastric hamartomatous polyps in the absence of familial polyposis coli. Cancer 1980;45:818–823.

107. Katz LB, Tenembaum MM, Kreel I. Gastric hamartomatous polyps in the absence of familial polyposis: Report of two cases. Mt Sinai J Med 1982;49:426–429.

108. Reid JD. Intestinal carcinoma in the Peutz–Jeghers syndrome. J Am Med Assoc 1974;229:833–834.

109. Perzin KH, Bridge MF. Adenomatous and carcinomatous changes in hamartomatous polyps of the small intestine (Peutz–Jeghers syndrome): Report of a case and review of the literature. Cancer 1982;49:971–983.

110. Hizawa K, Iida M, Matsumoto T, et al. Neoplastic transformation arising in Peutz–Jeghers polyposis. Dis Colon Rectum 1993;36:953–957.

111. Cochet B, Carrol J, Desbeillets L, et al. Peutz–Jeghers syndrome associated with gastrointestinal carcinoma. Gut 20:169–175.

112. Roth SI, Helwig EB. Juvenile polyps of the colon and rectum. Cancer 1963;16:468–479.

113. Morson BC. Some peculiarities in the histology of intestinal polyps. Dis Colon Rectum 1962;5:337–344.

114. Sachatello CR, Pickren JW, Grace JT Jr. Generalized juvenile gastrointestinal polyposis. A hereditary syndrome. Gastroenterology 1979;58:699–708.

115. Sachatello CR, Griffin WO Jr. Hereditary polypoid diseases of the gastrointestinal tract. A working classification. Am J Surg 1975;129:198–203.

116. Goodman ZD, Yardley JH, Milligan FD. Pathogenesis of colonic polyps in multiple juvenile polyposis: Report of a case associated with gastric polyps and carcinoma of the rectum. Cancer 1979;43:1906–1913.

117. Veale AMO, McCall I, Bussey HJR, et al. Juvenile polyposis coli. J Med Genet 1966;3:5–16.

118. Hofting I, Pott G, Stolte M. The syndrome of juvenile polyposis. Leber Magen Darm 1993;23:107–108, 111–112.

119. Desai DC, Neale KF, Talbot IC, et al. Juvenile polyposis. Br J Surg 1995;82:14–17.

120. Ray JE, Heald RJ. Growing up with juvenile gastrointestinal polyposis. Report of a case. Dis Colon Rectum 1971;14:368–380.

121. Watanabe A, Nagashima H, Motoi M, et al. Familial juvenile polyposis of the stomach. Gastroenterology 1979;77:148–151.

122. Dos Santos JG, de Magalhaes J. Familial gastric polyposis. A new entity. J Genet Hum 1980;28:293–297.

123. Hofting I, Pott G, Schrameyer B, et al. Familial juvenile polyposis with predominant stomach involvement. [German] Z Gastroenterol 1993;31:480–483.

124. Stemper TJ, Kent TH, Summers RW. Juvenile polyposis and gastrointestinal carcinoma. A study of a kindred. Ann Intern Med 1975;83:639–646.

125. Grigioni WF, Alampi G, Martinelli G, et al. Atypical juvenile polyposis. Histopathology 1981;5:361–376.

126. Sassatelli R, Bertoni G, Serra L, et al. Generalized juvenile polyposis with mixed pattern and gastric cancer. Gastroenterology 1993;104:910–915.

127. Eidt S, Stolte M. Gastric glandular cysts – Investigations into their genesis and relationship to colorectal epithelial tumors. Z Gastroenterol 1989;27:212–217.

128. Burt RW, Berenson MM, Lee RG, et al. Upper gastrointestinal polyps in Gardner's syndrome. Gastroenterology 1984;86:295–301.

129. Tonelli F, Nardi F, Bechi P, et al. Extracolonic polyps in familial polyposis coli and Gardner's syndrome. Dis Colon Rectum 1985;28:664–668.

130. Weill–Bousson M, Fischer D, Reyd P, et al. Complex recto–colic adenomatous and hamartomatous polyposis with hyperplastic gastric polyps in a 13–year–old girl. Gastroenterol Clin Biol 1984;8:621–626.

131. Bulow S, Lauritsen KB, Johansen A, et al. Gastroduodenal polyps in familial polyposis coli. Dis Colon Rectum 1985;28:90–93.

132. Nishiura M, Hirota T, Itabashi M, et al. A clinical and histopathological study of gastric polyps in familial polyposis coli. Am J Gastroenterol 1984;79:98–103.

133. Lee RG, Burt RW. The histopathology of fundic gland polyps of the stomach. Am J Clin Pathol 1986;86:498–503.

134. Hanada M, Takami M, Hirata K, et al. Hyperplastic fundic gland polyp of the stomach. Acta Pathol Jap 1983;33:1269–1277.

135. Hara M, Tsutsumi Y, Watanabe K, et al. Solitary gastric polyps in the fundic gland area. A histochemical study. Acta Pathol Jpn 1985;35:831–840.

136. Iida M, Yao T, Watanabe H, et al. Spontaneous disappearance of fundic gland polyposis: Report of three cases. Gastroenterology 1980;79:725–728.

137. Jarvinen H, Nyberg M, Peltokallio P. Upper gastrointestinal tract polyps in familial adenomatosis. Gut 1983;24:333–339.

138. Shemesh E, Bat L. A prospective evaluation of the upper gastrointestinal tract and periampullary region in patients with Gardner syndrome. Am J Gastroenterol 1985;80:825–827.

139. Coffey RJ Jr, Knight CD Jr, Van Heerden JA, et al. Gastric adenocarcinoma complicating Gardner's syndrome in a North American Woman. Gastroenterology 1985;88(Pt 1):1263–1266.

140. Tsuchikame N, Ishimaru Y, Ohshima S, et al. Three familial cases of fundic gland polyposis without polyposis coli. Virchows Arch (A) 1993;422:337–340.

141. Marcial MA, Villafana M, Hernandez–Denton J, et al. Fundic gland polyps: Prevalence and clinicopathologic features. Am J Gastroenterol 1993;88:1711–1713.

142. Jarnum S, Jenson H. Diffuse gastrointestinal polyposis with ectodermal changes. A case with severe malabsorption and enteric loss of plasma proteins and electrolytes. Gastroenterology 1966;50:107–118.

143. Manousos O, Webster CU. Diffuse gastrointestinal polyposis with ectodermal changes. Gut 1966;7:375–379.

144. Sagara K, Fujiyama S, Kamuro Y, et al. Cronkhite–Canada syndrome associated with gastric cancer: Report of a case. Gastroenterol Jpn 1983;18:260–266.

145. Hou W, Haruma K, Sumii K, et al. Solitary pedunculated polypoid gastric gland heterotopia. Gastroenterol Jpn 1993;28:415–419.

146. Kamata Y, Kurotaki H, Onodera T, et al. An unusual heterotopia of pyloric glands of the stomach with inverted downgrowth. Acta Pathol Jpn 1993;43:192–197.

147. Busard JM, Walters W. Heterotopic pancreatic tissue. Arch Surg 1950;60:674–682.

148. Lai EC, Tompkins RK. Heterotopic pancreas. Review of a 26 year experience. Am J Surg 1986;151:697–700.

149. Yamagiwa H, Ishihara A, Sekoguchi T, et al. Heterotopic pancreas in surgically resected stomach. Gastroenterol Jpn 1977;12:380–386.

150. Debord JR, Majarakis JD, Nyhus LM. An unusual case of heterotopic pancreas of the stomach. Am J Surg 1981;141:269–273.

151. Armstrong CP, King PM, Dixon JM, et al. The clinical significance of heterotopic pancreas in the gastrointestinal tract. Br J Surg 1981;68:384–387.

152. Beccaria A, Beccaria E, Oliaro A, et al. Aberrant pancreas in gastric site. Minerva Med 1977;68:1441–1446.

153. Goldfarb WB, Bennett D, Monafo W. Carcinoma in heterotopic gastric pancreas. Ann Surg 1963;158:56–58.

154. Hickman DM, Frey CF, Carson JW. Adenocarcinoma arising in gastric heterotopic pancreas. West J Med 1981;135:57–62.

155. Tomita T, Kanabe S. Islet tissue in the heterotopic pancreas. Arch Pathol Lab Med 1983;107:469–472.

156. San Juan F, Treiger M, Silvestre W, et al. Zollinger–Ellison syndrome. Presentation of a case of non–beta–cell adenoma in a heterotopic pancreas with duodeno–jejunal peptic ulceration. Hospital (Rio de J) 1965;67:1148–1160.

157. Williams AW, Michie W. Adenomatosis of the stomach of Brunner gland type. Br J Surg 1957;45:259–263.

158. Johnson CD, Bynum TE. Brunner gland heterotopia presenting as gastric antral polyps. Gastrointest Endosc 1976;22:210–211.

159. Goldberg HI, Margulis AR. Adenomyoma of the stomach. AJR Am J Roentgenol 1966;96:382–387.

160. Stewart TW Jr, Mills LR. Adenomyoma of the stomach. South Med J 1984;77:1337–1338.

161. Ng WC, Yeoh SC, Joseph VT, et al. Adenomyoma of the pylorus presenting as intestinal obstruction with pseudomyxoma peritonei – a case report. Ann Acad Med Singapore 1981;10:562–565.

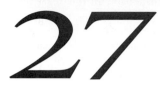

MALIGNANT EPITHELIAL TUMORS OF THE STOMACH

Si-Chun Ming and Teruyuki Hirota

Gastric cancer is a leading cause of cancer death in the world, in spite of a trend of decreasing incidence in most countries. The United States has the lowest incidence, where the estimated number of new cases of gastric cancer in 1997 is 22,400 (1). The estimated death from gastric cancer is 14,000, which is 2.5% of all cancer deaths, 11% of those of the digestive system and 17.1% of those of the gastrointestinal tract.

The stomach is a complex organ, particularly in its epithelial components. Its mucosa may be divided into three parts by the

functional anatomic features: cardia, fundus-body, and pyloric portions. Each part is made of specific glands, called, respectively, cardiac, fundic, and pyloric glands. The cardiac and pyloric glands are basically similar, composed of mucous columnar cells. The fundic glands contain chief and parietal cells. Details of structure and function of these glands are discussed in Chapter 2. In the presence of prolonged inflammation, irrespective of etiologic agents, the epithelium often shows metaplasia (see subsequent discussion of precancerous conditions as well as Chapter 23).

Carcinomas may develop in either metaplastic or nonmetaplastic epithelium. Thus, carcinomas of the stomach have complex and heterogeneous cell populations.

FREQUENCY AND CELL TYPES OF GASTRIC TUMORS

Many tumors of different tissue origin can occur in the stomach. The gastric tumors, like those in the other parts of the gastrointestinal tract, are dominated by tumors of epithelial origin. Among the epithelial tumors, the majority are malignant (2) (Table 27.1). This situation is distinctly different from that of the colon, in which the most frequent epithelial tumor is benign, but is analogous to that of other foregut-derived organs, the esophagus and the lung. This phenomenon probably has some etiologic implication. Whereas organ specificity is a possibility, the nature of carcinogenic exposure is also a likely factor, as suggested by the experimental models for gastric carcinogenesis. Use of these models shows that the most effective carcinogens used for stomach experiments are direct-acting (see section concerning experimental gastric carcinogenesis), whereas procarcinogens requiring metabolic activation are equally effective in colonic carcinogenesis (3).

The benign epithelial tumors of stomach, namely adenomas and polyps, are discussed in Chapter 26. Whereas nonneoplastic polyps are composed primarily of foveolar mucous cells of the normal stomach, adenomas often are composed of intestinal-type cells. Adenomas composed of gastric cells are rare (4). Intestinal features are also common in the carcinomas. In contrast to the adenomas, however, many carcinomas contain gastric-type cells, as well as endocrine cells and, less commonly, squamous cells (5). Thus, the composition of carcinomas of the stomach reflects the complexity of cell types seen in the normal and the metaplastic stomachs. They have more different types of cells than any other tumor in the body.

TABLE 27.1	Relative Frequency of Tumors of the Stomach	
Tumor Type	No. of Cases	Percent
Malignant tumors	4199	93.0
Carcinoma	3970	87.9
Lymphoma	136	3.0
Leiomyosarcoma	77	1.7
Carcinoid	11	0.3
Others	5	0.1
Benign tumors	315	7.0
Polyp	140	3.1
Leiomyoma	92	2.0
Inflammatory lesions	30	0.7
Heterotopic pancreas	20	0.4
Others	33	0.8

Modified from Ming SC. Tumors of the esophagus and stomach. In: Atlas of tumor pathology, second series, fascicle 7. Washington DC: Armed Forces Institute of Pathology, 1973;82.

The next most frequent tumor in the stomach after carcinoma is the smooth muscle cell tumor (see Chapter 18), in which the tumor is more often benign than malignant. In this regard, the stomach is the primary site for the epithelioid form of muscle cell tumor, which is intermediate in its behavior between leiomyoma and leiomyosarcoma. Muscle cell tumors, being submucosal, ordinarily are clinically silent until they are large enough to cause pressure symptoms or become ulcerated and bleed. The frequency rate shown in Table 27.1 is that of symptomatic tumors. The incidence increased to as high as 50% of all stomachs examined when an effort was made to search for small lesions (6). The third most frequent tumor in the stomach is lymphoma. This occurrence of lymphoma is interesting because the stomach, unlike the intestines, is not a principal lymphoid organ. The mucosal stroma is devoid of lymphocytic cells in the fetal and neonatal stomachs. With increasing age, however, lymphocytes and plasma cells become constant and are invariably present in the stomach of adults. Lymphomas of the stomach are discussed in detail in Chapter 17.

ADENOCARCINOMA

Carcinoma is the most important and the most common tumor of the stomach (see Table 27.1). Most gastric carcinomas are adenocarcinomas. Thus, adenocarcinoma is the main focus of concern when dealing with gastric cancers.

EPIDEMIOLOGY

GEOGRAPHIC DISTRIBUTION

The mortality rate associated with gastric carcinoma has a wide geographic variation (Fig. 27.1) (7). Rates also vary considerably within the same country. Results of epidemiologic studies comparing high-risk with low-risk regions give some insight into possible etiologic factors for gastric carcinoma. Additional information has been obtained by time-trend studies, which showed a steady decline in the mortality rate in most countries (8). The decline for the white male population in the United States has been most striking (1) (Fig. 27.2). Between 1973 and 1992, the incidence of gastric cancer in the United States decreased by 25.7% and the mortality rate decreased by 34.5% (9).

The causes of geographic variation and the decline in incidence are unknown. In epidemiologic studies, however, investigators noted that the intestinal type of carcinoma by Lauren classification (see subsequent section on histologic classifications) was more prevalent in the high-risk regions than the low-risk regions (9), and that its decline in incidence accounts for the decline of gastric cancer incidence in general (10). Other authors, however, did not confirm such findings (11).

AGE, SEX, AND RACIAL DISTRIBUTION

Gastric carcinomas, including early cancers, occur mainly in the elderly (Fig. 27.3) (9); infiltrative carcinoma tends to occur more often in younger patients. The male-to-female ratio is about 2 to 1 (see Figs. 27.1 and 27.3). The ratio is higher in expanding and intestinal-type carcinomas than in infiltrative and diffuse-type carcinomas (12, 13). In the United States, the lifetime risk of diagnosis

Age-Standardized Death Rates for Stomach Cancer per 100,000 Population

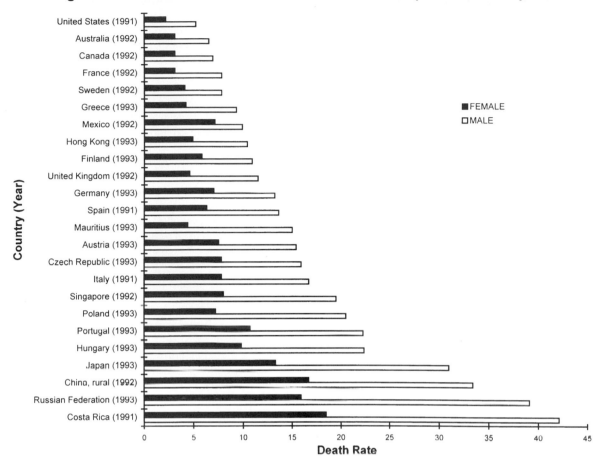

Figure 27.1   Mortality rates for gastric cancer in various countries. (Data from World Health Organization. 1994 World health statistics Annual. Geneva: World Health Organization, 1995;B396–B407.)

of gastric cancer is 1.24% for males and 0.79% for females, and the lifetime risk of dying from gastric cancer is 0.84% for males and 0.54% for females (9). In about 2% of cases, gastric carcinoma occurs in individuals 35 years of age and younger, with a reversed male-to-female ratio of 1:2.9 (14). Tumors in young patients are often diffusely infiltrating and large, and the prognosis is poor (14, 15). Bloss et al. (16) reported that of 37 young patients with gastric tumors, 28 had linitis plastica or poorly differentiated carcinoma, and only 2 of 37 patients survived 5 years.

The overall age and sex distribution of patients with early gastric carcinoma are similar to those of gastric cancer in general. Specific variations for early gastric cancer are noted in the following aspects. The number of patients 60 years of age and older has increased slightly since the early 1970s (17). Female predominance is noted until the fourth decade. Males predominate in the 40s and 50s, and a peak is reached in the 60s for both males and females (18).

In the United States, the incidence rate of gastric carcinoma in the black population is about twice that of the white population (11.2 versus 6.3 in 1992) (9). The male-to-female ratio is the same for both groups. The mortality rate in blacks is also twice that of the whites (6.7 versus 3.1). The survival rates are similar in both populations. The causes of the differences in the incidence and mortality between the populations have not been identified.

ETIOLOGIC FACTORS

The etiology of gastric carcinoma is unknown. Some systemic and local risk factors have been identified, however; the latter are described as precursor lesions in the following discussion.

The incidence of gastric carcinoma is known to be higher in individuals with blood type A, a family history of gastric cancer (19), or pernicious anemia (20). These findings suggest some weak genetic influence (see discussion of genetic factors in the development of gastric cancer in Chapter 7). The most important factors appear to be environmental, as shown by migrant studies. When people moved from the high-risk region to the low-risk region, the incidence of gastric carcinoma decreased (21, 22). The decrease is more pronounced in the second than in the first generation (23, 24), suggesting the lasting effect of carcinogenic exposure in early life. Such carcinogenic exposure is also indicated by the prevalence of chronic atrophic gastritis and intestinal metaplasia in the younger population living in the high-risk area relative to those in the low-risk area (25). A related factor is the low socioeconomic status of the high-risk population (8). Similarly, the higher incidence of gastric cancer in rural China than in urban regions (7) also supports the role of environmental factors.

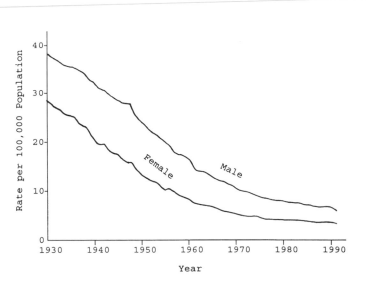

Figure 27.2   Decline of gastric cancer death rate in the United States by sex. (Data from Parker SL, Tong T, Bolden S, et al. Cancer statistics, 1997. CA Cancer J Clin 1997;47:5–27.)

DIET

Among the environmental factors, diet is the most important (8, 26), which has been credited with the decline of gastric cancer mortality (25–27). Foods that are starchy, pickled, smoked, and salted are risky, whereas fresh fruit, vegetables, beta-carotene, and vitamins C and E are beneficial (8, 26, 28). The importance of salt was emphasized by several investigators (26–28) and denied by others (29, 30). Experiments with rats showed that salt caused gastric mucosal damage, which then enhanced cell proliferation and carcinogen-induced carcinogenesis (31).

Soybean products are commonly eaten in Asia, where the incidence of gastric carcinoma is high. Soybean sauce mixed with sodium nitrite in vitro was found to be mutagenic, although the concentration of sodium nitrite necessary for the reaction was above the physiologic state in the human (32). On the other hand, soybean paste (miso), soybean curd (tofu), and soya milk inhibited nitrosamine formation from sodium nitrite in vitro (33). Other possible risk factors include asbestos (34–36) and radiation (37). The effect of alcohol and tobacco intake on the development of gastric cancer is uncertain (38).

CARCINOGENS

The carcinogens responsible for human gastric cancer have not been identified, but they are suspected to be N-nitroso compounds. Because atrophic gastritis is commonly associated with gastric

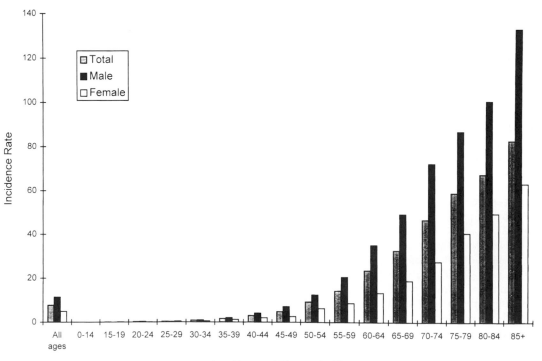

Figure 27.3   Incidence rates of gastric cancer in the United States by age and sex. (Data from Kosary CL, Ries LAG, Miller BA, et al. SEER cancer statistics review, 1973–1992: Tables and graphs. Bethesda: National Cancer Institute. NIH Publ. No. 96-2789, 1996.)

cancer, a hypothesis for the in vivo formation of these compounds has been proposed as follows: atrophic gastritis causes the decrease of the acidity of gastric juice, making possible the overgrowth of bacteria that convert nitrates to nitrites and catalyze in vivo N-nitrosation (8, 39). Several lines of evidence support this hypothesis. In Colombia, nitrate content in the well water and urinary nitrate excretion in the population are higher in the high-risk area than in the low-risk area (25). Saliva is another source of nitrate and nitrite, the amounts of which appear to be variable (40). The gastric juice pH, which increases in association with chronic atrophic gastritis, is positively related to the level of nitrite and nitrate-reducing bacteria and the concentration of N-nitroso compounds in the juice (41, 42). The gastric juice in high-risk patients is mutagenic (43). The carcinogenic nitroso compounds so formed are probably nitrosamides (40). Their formation can be blocked by vitamins C and E (8, 44).

HELICOBACTER PYLORI

Since its discovery in 1983 (45), *Helicobacter pylori* (HP) has been associated first with gastritis and peptic ulcer diseases (45, 46) and then with gastric cancer. Serologic studies for HP revealed that the risk for gastric cancer was three times higher in patients with HP than in those without it (47). H. pylori gastritis is a long-standing disease that may lead to atrophic gastritis (48) and intestinal metaplasia, which is a precancerous condition for intestinal-type gastric carcinoma through the stage of dysplasia. Thus, a sequence of events may be envisioned: H. pylori infection → acute gastritis → chronic gastritis → atrophic gastritis → intestinal metaplasia → dysplasia → carcinoma.

The first half of the sequence, i.e., infection leading to atrophic gastritis, has been elucidated. H. pylori has a unique affinity for gastric epithelium, primarily the surface and foveolar mucous cells, and its acid environment. In the duodenum, HP affects the areas with gastric metaplasia (49). It does not inhabit the intestinal epithelium, including the areas of intestinal metaplasia in the stomach, except the incomplete type (50). The organism and its products, including ammonia (51), injure the affected cells, causing acute gastritis with prominent neutrophils and stimulating cell proliferation. Chronic gastritis is associated with pronounced lymphocytic accumulation with lymphoid follicle formation (52). Gastric lymphoma may develop in some patients (53). The accompanying immunologic reaction (51) may contribute to exacerbated gastritis. Persistent injury eventually results in mucosal atrophy with hyperproliferative epithelium and intestinal metaplasia. Some reports (54, 55) of finding higher HP positivity in patients with intestinal-type gastric carcinoma than in those with diffuse-type carcinoma have not been confirmed by other authors (56, 57). Eradication of HP reduces the severity of atrophic gastritis and proliferative activity of the epithelium and inhibits intestinal metaplasia (58).

The mechanism of tissue changes in the latter half of the carcinogenic sequence, i.e., atrophic gastritis to dysplasia to carcinoma, has not been delineated. Evidence is derived from epidemiologic studies. HP gastritis is a common world-wide disease. The difference in incidence between high-risk and low-risk countries for gastritis is small. In any case, the majority of people with HP infection do not develop gastric cancer. The incidence of HP gastritis is about 80 to 90% in patients with duodenal ulcer, which

is not associated with gastric cancer. Furthermore, the ranges of odds ratios for gastric cancer in HP-infected individuals in high- and low-risk countries are not widely different, 0.6 to 4.2 in high-risk countries and 0.9 to 2.7 in low-risk countries (59).

In developing countries, the incidence of HP infection is high in children, and atrophic gastritis is common in young adults (48, 51). These observations lead to the suggestion that prolonged infection since childhood may be the basis for high gastric cancer incidence in these countries. In recent years, older persons are increasingly affected and there is a general decline in the infection rate (51). These changes may explain the trend in many countries of decreasing incidence of gastric cancer, particularly of the intestinal type (48).

The long latency period between the onset of initial HP infection and the appearance of gastric cancer indicates the cumulative effects of many factors. Prolonged HP infection results in atrophic gastritis and decreased acid secretion. The altered micro-environment, together with other risk factors just mentioned, allows colonization of other bacteria that may catalyze N-nitrosation to form carcinogens in the stomach. In addition, HP blocks gastric secretion of ascorbic acid, allowing carcinogens to exert their effect on the gastric epithelium (59).

At the late stage, the role of HP in carcinogenesis is no longer essential. In fact, the number of organisms is decreased because of mucosal atrophy and metaplasia. Eradication of the infection does not reverse the dysplastic epithelium (60), although it reduced the development of carcinoma in one study (61). Thus, HP is a precancerous agent, but it is not a carcinogen and its role in gastric carcinogenesis may be overrated (59).

Additional findings relevant to HP-initiated carcinogenesis have been reported. Vollmers et al. (62) isolated two monoclonal antibodies from patients with gastric carcinoma and HP gastritis. The antibodies cross-reacted with extracts of both HP and carcinoma cells. Furthermore, the antibodies showed stimulating and growth-enhancing effects on tumor cells in vitro. Strain differences among the bacteria have also been found. About 60% of HP possess the cagA gene. Infection with cagA-positive HP causes more severe gastritis and epithelial damage and higher risk of developing gastric carcinoma than infection with cagA-negative HP (63). A study in China, however, did not reveal a relation between cagA protein and gastric cancer (64).

To bring HP into focus in the evaluation of gastric diseases, a "Sydney system" for the classification of gastritis has been established (48). In this classification, the histologic diagnosis of gastritis requires a statement on the status of HP in the specimen. Other components of the diagnosis deal with the etiology, topographic extent of the disease, and graded assessment of morphologic changes. Such practices have been used routinely in the United States. In view of the frequent occurrence of the infection, the use of special stains to demonstrate the organism may be included in the routine examination of stomach specimens.

EPSTEIN-BARR VIRUS

Epstein-Barr virus (EBV) is the only other infectious agent that plays a role in the development of gastric carcinoma. The involved carcinoma is often undifferentiated and has prominent lymphoid stroma, so-called lymphoepithelioma-like carcinoma (65). Using in situ hybridization and polymerase chain reaction techniques, EBV was detected in over 80% of carcinomas with lymphoid stroma and 9% of ordinary adenocarcinomas (66). In another report (67), EBV was found in 70 of 1000 gastric carcinomas, including 8 of 9 (89%) of lymphoepithelioma-like carcinomas, 5.7% of poorly differentiated, and 6.8% of better differentiated adenocarcinomas. EBV was found in tumor cells but not in the lymphoid stroma or the normal epithelium. Thus, EBV appears to be involved in gastric carcinogenesis, although only a portion of the tumors are lymphoepithelioma-like. EBV infects the gastric epithelial cell through EBV-carrying lymphocytes (68), although the lymphocytes within the tumor might be responding to the tumor (67).

PRECURSORS

Since 1929, when Hurst (69) recognized chronic atrophic gastritis, peptic ulcer, adenoma, and polyps as precursors of gastric carcinoma, intestinal metaplasia, hyperplastic gastropathy, and gastric remnants after partial gastrectomy have also been associated with increased incidence of gastric cancer. The precancerous potential of these conditions is recognized primarily by clinical association with gastric cancer, whereas the pathologic lesions from which the carcinoma arises had largely been unknown until 1970s, when dysplasia of the epithelial cells was recognized as the fundamental premalignant lesion in all of these conditions.

The precursors of gastric carcinoma have been separated into two major categories: precancerous conditions and precancerous lesions (70). The precancerous conditions are clinical conditions in which the risk of gastric carcinoma is increased. The majority of patients with these conditions do not develop carcinoma. The precancerous lesions are pathologic changes from which the carcinoma eventually evolves. It is believed that the development of gastric carcinoma in precancerous conditions is preceded by the occurrence of a precancerous lesion. The incidence of early gastric carcinoma arising in various precancerous conditions in Japan is shown in Figure 27.4.

PRECANCEROUS CONDITIONS

Epithelial Polyps

Epithelial polyps are classified into five major categories: hyperplastic polyp, adenoma, hamartomatous polyp, inflammatory polyp, and heterotopic polyp. Inflammatory polyps have no malignant potential. Hyperplastic polyp and adenoma were the source of great confusion in the past with regard to their malignant potential. It is now generally accepted that the adenoma is a true neoplasm, and carcinoma develops in it in about 40% of cases. On the other hand, the hyperplastic polyp is probably the result of excessive regeneration after inflammation, and carcinomatous change occurs in only about 2% or less of cases. When carcinoma does develop in the hyperplastic polyp, it involves the dysplastic glands. Carcinoma rarely develops in the hamartomatous polyp and heterotopic pancreatic tissue. (See detailed discussion of malignant change in gastric polyps in Chapter 26.)

Chronic Atrophic Gastritis

A common condition, chronic atrophic gastritis (see Chapter 23 and previous discussion of its relation with H. pylori) is the most important among precursor lesions. Chronic atrophic gastritis was the precursor of 94.8% of early gastric cancer in Japan

— 1900 Cases —	N.C.C.H., Tokyo ~ April 1988		
Precancerous Lesion		No. of Cases	%
Hyperplastic polyp	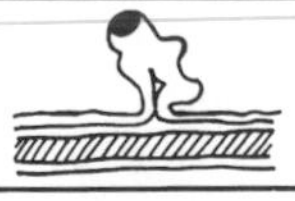	10	0.53
Adenoma	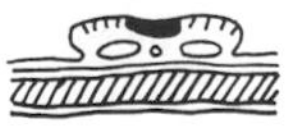	47	2.47
Chronic ulcer	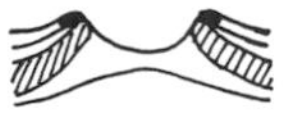	13	0.68
Atrophic gastritis	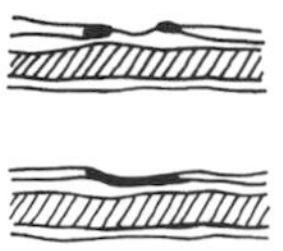	1802	94.84
Verrucous gastritis	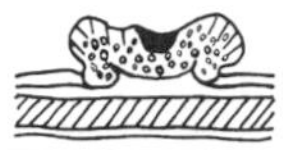	26	1.37
Stomach remnant	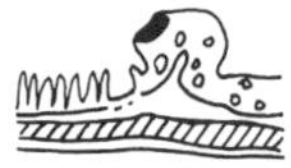	2	0.11
Aberrant pancreas	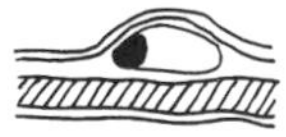	0	0
Total		1900	100 %

Figure 27.4 Incidence of early gastric cancer arising in various precancerous lesions at National Cancer Center Hospital, Tokyo. *Solid black areas* represent carcinomatous lesions.

(see Fig. 27.4). Its incidence increases with the advance of age and is seen mainly in older individuals. In high-risk areas for gastric cancer, however, this condition is common in young people as well (25). On the basis of epidemiologic data, Correa (71) proposed that chronic gastritis has three patterns, probably caused by separate etiologic factors: autoimmune type, involving acid-secreting fundic mucosa; hypersecretory type, involving the pyloric mucosa; and environmental type, involving multiple areas at random but more prominently at the fundopyloric junctional zone. Cancer develops more frequently in the first and the last types (72). The relative risk of developing gastric carcinoma in patients with severe chronic atrophic gastritis in the Finnish population was 18.1 in the antrum and 4.6 in the body of the stomach (72).

Atrophic gastric mucosa often shows intestinal metaplasia, but the extent of metaplasia varies greatly. With or without intestinal metaplasia, increased proliferative activity in the mucosa results in the presence of relatively immature cells in the glands (73). In metaplastic areas, cell proliferation is more evident in the lower portion of the glands; in nonmetaplastic mucosa, the superficial and foveolar cells are affected. As discussed previously, hypochlorhydria secondary to mucosal atrophy creates an altered environment in the stomach in which N-nitrosation may occur, initiating the carcinogenic events.

Intestinal Metaplasia

The surface and foveolae of the normal gastric mucosa are lined by a continuous layer of columnar mucous cells secreting neutral glycoproteins, whereas the goblet cells of the intestines are interspersed by absorptive cells and secrete acidic mucins, which are mainly sialomucins in the small intestines and sulfomucins in the colon. The sialomucins can be further separated into N- and O-acetylated types. The types of mucin are easily identified by simple staining procedures, such as periodic acid-Schiff reaction (PAS) for all mucoproteins, alcian blue for acidic mucins (74), periodate-borohydrite/potassium hydroxide/PAS for O-acetylated sialomucin (75), and high iron diamine for sulfomucin (76). The absorptive cells in the small intestine have well-formed microvilli that carry alkaline phosphatase and digestive enzymes, such as disaccharidases and peptidases, some of which can be demonstrated in the gross specimen (77). The absorptive cells in the colon, on the other hand, have only short and sparse microvilli lacking many enzymes. In intestinal metaplasia, the gastric mucosa is transformed into an intestinal-type mucosa with complex and heterogeneous features.

Intestinal metaplasia begins in the neck region, which is the proliferative zone of the normal gastric gland, and usually first appears at the antral-corpus junction (78). Based on the cell types and their functional features, intestinal metaplasia is divided into complete and incomplete types and several subtypes (79–81). Their composition is summarized in Table 27.2. In complete metaplasia, the gastric mucosa assumes the appearance of small intestinal mucosa but without villi (Fig. 27.5). The glands are lined by absorptive, goblet, Paneth, and endocrine cells. Early ultrastructural and histochemical studies confirm that these cells are identical to those of the small intestine (82). In the incompletely developed metaplasia, instead of absorptive cells, the columnar cells between the goblet cells resemble the mucous cells of the foveolae (82) (Fig. 27.6). The mucus in the goblet cells contains sialomucin, sulfomucin, or both (79). The mucus in the columnar cells of incompletely metaplastic glands may be neutral mucoproteins, sialomucin, or sulfomucin (Figs. 27.7 and 27.8).

Jass and Filipe (83) also divided intestinal metaplasia into complete (Type I) and incomplete (Type II) types, based on the presence of absorptive cells in the former and mucus-secreting columnar cells in the latter. The incomplete type was further

TABLE					
27.2	**Major Differences Among Subtypes of Intestinal Metaplasia**				

| | Complete Type | | Incomplete Type | | |
Feature	Small Intestinal	Colonic	Gastric	Small Intestinal	Colonic
Goblet cells	+	+	+	+	+
Mucous columnar cells	−	−	+	+	+
Paneth cells	+	−	−	−	−
Striated borders	+	±	−	−	−
Mucoproteins[a]	Sialomucin	Sulfomucin	Neutral	Sialomucin	Sulfomucin
Surface enzymes	+	±	−	−	−

+, present; −, absent.

[a]Mucoprotein indicated is in the goblet cells in the complete type and in the columnar cells in the incomplete type of metaplasia.

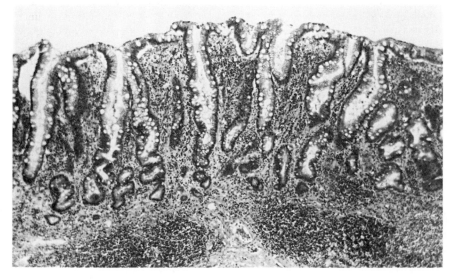

Figure 27.5 Complete type of intestinal metaplasia showing intestinal type crypts lined with goblet cells and absorptive cells. Severe chronic gastritis with lymphocytic infiltrates extends into the submucosa (×55).

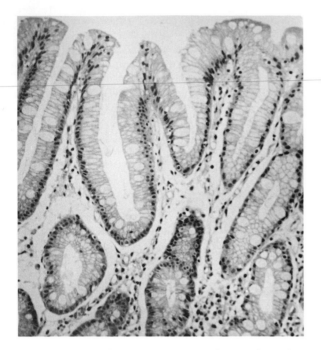

Figure 27.6 Incomplete type of intestinal metaplasia showing glands lined with goblet cells and mucous columnar cells. The latter resemble normal foveolar cells, but may secrete acidic intestinal mucins instead of neutral mucoproteins (×120).

divided into A and B subtypes: nonsulfated mucin in A and sulfated mucin in B. These types were subsequently renamed Types I, II, and III (84).

The precancerous nature of intestinal metaplasia is suggested by the observation that carcinoma often occurs in the area of intestinal metaplasia (Fig. 27.9), and that the risk of gastric cancer is proportional to the extent of metaplasia (85). Furthermore, positive immunohistochemical staining for carcinoembryonic antigen (CEA) has been found in the colonic type of metaplastic glands, but not in the small intestinal type of glands (86). The sulfomucin-secreting and the colonic types of metaplasia were said to be related to the intestinal or expanding type of gastric carcinoma by association (12, 87). In a study from India, however, Suvarna and Sasidharan (88) reported the absence of Type III metaplasia in cancerous stomachs, and follow-up studies of Type III metaplasia did not show an increased risk of gastric carcinoma (89, 90). In laboratory animals, intestinal metaplasia has been produced experimentally by treatments with carcinogens (91) and radiation (92), but its relationship with carcinoma has been inconsistent and it is not a required precancerous lesion (92). Thus, the Type III and colonic intestinal metaplasia may be a paracancerous rather than a precancerous lesion (93). In any case, the complete small intestinal-type metaplasia is so common that its precancerous potential is probably negligible.

Chronic Gastric Ulcer

Chronic gastric ulcers had been considered a precancerous lesion; e.g., in early reports from Japan, about 70% of cancer patients were said to have a pre-existing ulcer (94). The importance of chronic ulcer as a precancerous lesion has since been downgraded. At the National Cancer Center Hospital in Tokyo, chronic ulcer was considered a precursor of early gastric carcinoma in only 0.68% of cases (see Fig. 27.4). The incidence of deeply ulcerated (Type III) early gastric cancer in Japan has decreased steadily, and cases fulfilling the criteria of ulcer-cancer have virtually disappeared (18). In the meantime, Sakita et al. (95) reported that the malignant ulcer might heal, significantly in 18 to 25% of cases, thus invalidating the long-held view that an ulcer that heals is benign and that a carcinoma found in a healing ulcer has originated in a benign ulcer. Conversely, carcinomas have been found in about 2% of stomachs resected for clinically benign ulcer (96).

Farinati et al. (97) found 10 carcinomas in 144 ulcers on follow-up endoscopic biopsies, 9 within 1 year. In view of the slow growth of early gastric cancer, the relatively short history of the ulcer in such reports indicates that the carcinomas predated the ulcer. A 5-year study (98) revealed that none of 78 ulcer patients developed carcinoma. In another report of patients followed for nine or more years, the incidence was 2.2% (99).

Pathologically, the ulcer-associated carcinomas have a higher incidence of infiltrative type cancer than in the nonulcerated carcinomas (74, 100) (Fig. 27.10). Experimentally, chronically ulcerated gastric mucosa is more susceptible to experimental carcinogenic stimulation than the nonulcerated mucosa (101). More importantly, the malignant ulcer is often misdiagnosed as benign (102), emphasizing the need to obtain multiple endoscopic biopsy specimens from the ulcer margins to achieve a correct diagnosis.

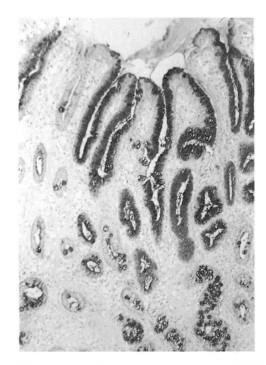

Figure 27.7 The tissue is stained with periodic acid-Schiff (PAS) reagent and alcian blue (AB) at pH 2.5. The goblet cells in metaplastic glands contain acidic mucin which is stained by AB and shown as blue. The normal foveolar cells *(at right)* contain neutral mucus and are stained red with PAS only. The columnar cells in incomplete metaplasia shown in the upper center contain both types of mucin and are stained by both PAS and AB (×200). (See color plate.)

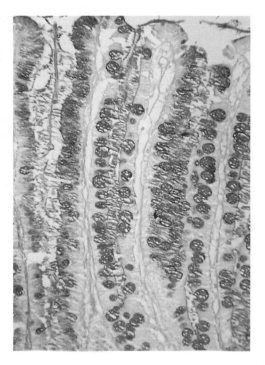

Figure 27.8 The gastric mucosa shows both complete and incomplete intestinal metaplasia. The tissue is stained with high iron diamine (HID) for sulfomucin in brown and alcian blue (AB) at pH 2.5 for sialomucin in blue. The mucin in goblet cells are mostly blue, a few on right both blue and brown. The mucin in mucous columnar cells are brown (×200). (See color plate.)

Gastric Remnants

A high incidence of carcinoma in the gastric remnants of partial gastrectomy has been reported in about 4000 cases (103). The incidence varied from 0 to 7.8%, mostly about 2% (104, 105). The incidence at autopsy was 11.3% in one series (106) and only 0.2% in another series (107). The latter was one fifth of the expected rate. The ratio of observed and expected cases in various reports varied from 0.34 to 2.21 (103). The variation is apparently related in part to the time factor. The incidence increases as the postoperative period lengthens (103, 108). This factor is in turn influenced by the age of the patient at the time of gastrectomy; younger patients had a longer interval between gastrectomy and diagnosis of carcinoma (104). The type of gastrectomy procedure and the nature of preoperative disease are not factors, although in most reports, the procedure was the Billroth II operation for duodenal ulcer.

Carcinoma usually develops more than 10 years after the initial gastrectomy. The tumor is often located at the stoma, but may also arise elsewhere in the stomach. The types of carcinoma are about equally divided between the intestinal and diffuse types (109). The gastric remnants commonly show gastritis, cystic glands, intestinal metaplasia, and dysplasia (78, 104, 110). Polyps may also occur, mostly of the hyperplastic type. The degree of dysplasia generally is mild and may regress (104, 111). Severe dysplasia probably plays an important role in the carcinogenesis, and its progression toward carcinoma has been reported (112).

The lack of sphincteric function at the gastroenterostomy stoma with consequent reflux of intestinal contents into the stomach has been cited as a cause of mucosal abnormalities and malignant changes in the stomach (105, 113). This conclusion is supported by the finding that the severity of intestinal metaplasia and dysplasia in the stomach stump correlates with the gastric pH (114). H. pylori is not an important factor (103). Experimentally, gastrojejunostomy increases the number of chemically induced cancer in the rat stomach (107). Denervation increased tumor yield in postgastrectomy remnants of stomach in carcinogen-treated rats (115).

Hyperplastic Gastropathy

Gastric mucosa may become thickened in association with a variety of conditions (see Chapter 25). When the mucosal hypertrophy is related to epithelial hyperplasia, it usually falls into three categories (116): glandular hyperplasia with hyperacidity, as in Zollinger-Ellison syndrome; mucous cell hyperplasia with protein loss, as in Ménétrier disease; and hyperplasia of mixed type, which often is asymptomatic. In the last situation, there is an increase of all glandular elements, which appear normal. Carcinoma is sometimes present in such a stomach. Patients tend to be young and female (116), and the carcinoma is often diffusely infiltrative. It has been postulated that fundic mucosal hyperplasia may be caused by endocrine substances secreted by the tumor cells (117).

The stomach in Zollinger-Ellison syndrome is not known to have increased incidence of carcinoma. Ménétrier disease is associated with hyperplasia of mucus-secreting foveolar cells, whereas the

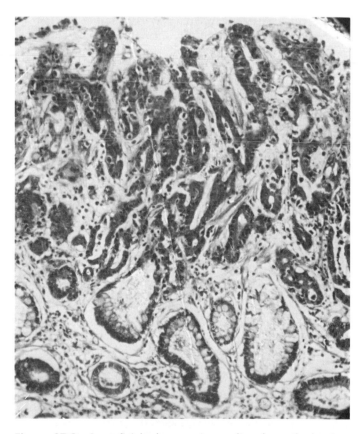

Figure 27.9 Superficial adenocarcinoma lies above the benign metaplastic glands (×150).

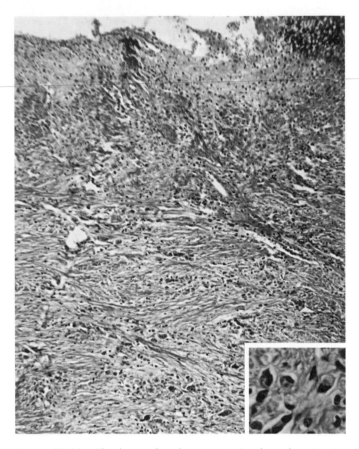

Figure 27.10   The base of a chronic peptic ulcer showing in-filtration of individual tumor cells (infiltrative type of carcinoma) in the scar tissue (×90). *Inset:* undifferentiated and signet ring cells in the fibrous tissue (×300).

deep glands are normal or more commonly atrophic. Carcinoma may develop in such a stomach, as first described by Ménétrier (118). Martin and coworkers collected 214 cases of the rare Ménétrier disease in the literature and found the frequency of malignant change to be 5 to 10% (78, 110, 119). In the case reported by Wood et al. (120), the carcinoma was located in grossly unremarkable antrum, whereas the mucosa of the body and fundus of the stomach were grossly hypertrophic. In a personally examined case, an early carcinoma was found in a small atrophic area in otherwise hyperplastic mucosa.

Other Conditions

Intramucosal cysts may be present in the normal appearing gastric mucosa away from a carcinoma. The incidence and the number of the cysts are higher in high-risk than in low-risk countries (121). The cystic glands are of gastric type when associated with diffuse carcinoma and of intestinal type when associated with intestinal-type cancer (122). Submucosal cystic glands also may accompany carcinoma, particularly underneath the early carcinoma (123, 124) (Fig. 27.11). Lastly, carcinoma may complicate gastric schistoso-miasis, as reported from China (125).

The diverse precancerous conditions share one basic histo-logic feature: increased proliferative activity of epithelial cells.

Reactive hyperplasia (Fig. 27.12) is evident in active chronic gastritis, margins of gastric ulcers, metaplastic epithelium, gastric remnants, and adenomas. Conditions with a low incidence of cancer risk, such as Ménétrier disease and hyperplastic polyps, show low epithelial proliferation. Thus, active epithelial hyperplasia may be considered the initial tissue alteration in the process of carcinogenesis.

PRECANCEROUS LESION: EPITHELIAL DYSPLASIA

Only a small percentage of patients who have one of the conditions just discussed develop gastric carcinoma. The only precursor lesion in which adenocarcinoma occurs with certainty is adenoma, and adenomas are composed of dysplastic cells. Epithelial dysplasia also plays an important role in the malignant change of other precan-cerous conditions. Thus, dysplasia has become the target of many investigations.

Broadly defined, dysplasia simply means abnormal growth, and the term has been applied to many conditions that have no relation to malignancy. In pathology and cytology, however, the term has become synonymous with premalignancy. As a precancerous lesion, dysplasia can be defined as an abnormal state of the tissue charac-terized by pronounced cellular and structural alterations and showing a propensity to malignant transformation (126). In the stomach, dysplasia can occur in the metaplastic as well as the nonmetaplastic gland (127).

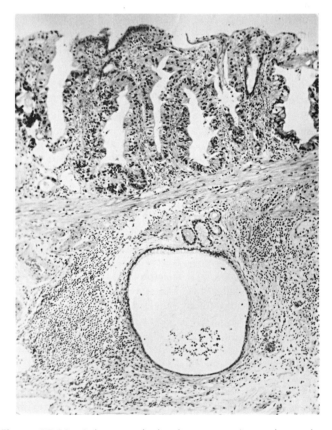

Figure 27.11   Submucosal glands, one cystic, underneath an intramucosal adenocarcinoma (×120).

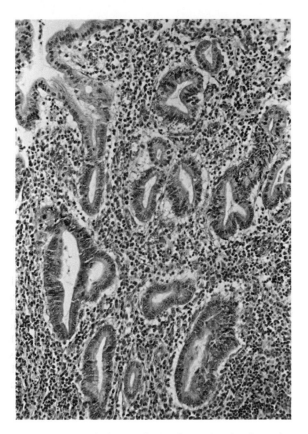

Figure 27.12 Simple hyperplasia of gastric glands at the margin of a chronic ulcer. The epithelial cells are immature and slightly pseudostratified. Intracellular mucin is reduced. The nuclei remain basally located. The lamina propria is heavily infiltrated by chronic inflammatory cells (×180).

Studies of gastric dysplasia include DNA and morphometric measurements, cell kinetic and molecular studies, and search for marker substances. The dysplastic cells have increased DNA and, when severe, polyploidy and occasionally aneuploidy (128, 129). The nuclear area is enlarged (130) and the cell cycle is lengthened, but the cell life span is shortened (128). Carcinoembryonic antigen and p21 ras are present in dysplastic cells (131, 132). The tumor suppressor gene p53 is overexpressed or mutated in 15 to 60% of cases (133, 134). The apoptosis inhibitor bcl-2 gene is also overexpressed (135). These studies indicate that in extreme cases, the dysplastic cells resemble malignant cells, and may in fact be malignant already.

For the clinical evaluation, light microscopic examination remains the most useful tool. Using this method, several grading systems have been reported (126). Morson et al. used the descriptive terms of mild, moderate, and severe (70). Cuello et al. (136) classified dysplasia into hyperplastic and adenomatous types, both of which were applied to the metaplastic mucosa. Similar classification was given by Jass (137): Type I was applied to adenomatous lesions and Type II to incompletely metaplastic and nonadenomatous mucosa.

The fundamental histologic feature of dysplasia is excessive cell proliferation resulting in an increased number of immature cells. Thus, dysplasia overlaps reparative regeneration on one end of the spectrum and carcinoma on the other end. For practical usage, the altered gastric epithelia may be classified in order of increasing abnormality (126).

Severe (Atypical) Hyperplasia (Figs. 27.13 and 27.14)

The immature cells vary slightly in size and shape and are pseudostratified. Normal maturation is still evident at the mucosal surface, which may be elevated because of the increased number of cells. This condition, seen at the ulcer border, in chronic atrophic gastritis, and occasionally in the hyperplastic polyp, is intermediate between simple hyperplasia and dysplasia and has also been classified as mild dysplasia or indefinite dysplasia. The term "atypical hyperplasia" is chosen because there is no clear evidence that this change is premalignant. Generally, the condition progresses to a higher degree of abnormality before malignant change occurs.

Dysplasia (Figs. 27.15 and 27.16)

The term "dysplasia" is applied to clearly abnormal glands. Cells show pleomorphism, variation in size and shape, increased nucleus-cytoplasm ratio, and poor cellular differentiation. Pseudostratification, nucleoli, and mitosis are common, but giant nuclei and abnormal mitosis are absent. The glands may show architectural derangements with budding, branching, and crowding. Dysplasia may be qualified as moderate and severe or low and high grade as in the colon.

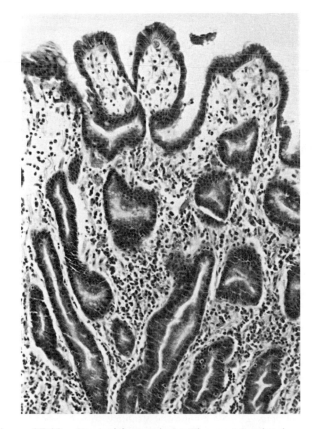

Figure 27.13 Atypical hyperplasia. The gastric glands are irregular. The cells are immature and there are mitotic figures. The stroma shows chronic inflammation (×150).

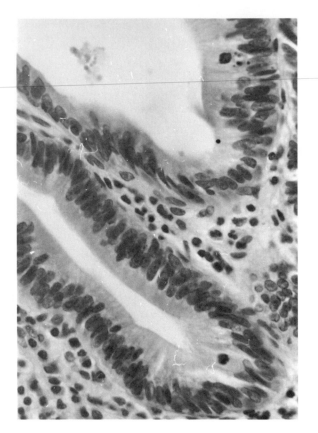

Figure 27.14 Atypical hyperplasia showing no mucus secretion and mild nuclear pseudostratification. The basally located nuclei are crowded but uniform in size and shape. There are no nucleoli. Mitoses are present (×480).

Because dysplasia is typically present in the adenoma, these two lesions must be differentiated. The distinction is important because the adenoma is a localized neoplasm that does not regress and is treated by excision. Dysplasia is a multifocal lesion and may regress. The differentiating features in favor of adenoma are: a circumscribed and grossly visible lesion, minimal inflammation in the stroma, and relatively uniform cellular features. The interface between adenoma and adjacent epithelium is abrupt. The dysplastic lesion is detectable only microscopically and shows gradations of abnormalities (see detailed discussion of differences between adenoma and dysplasia in Chapter 26).

Possible Cancer (Fig. 27.17)

This term is applied to a lesion with abnormalities so severe that it is difficult to decide whether it is dysplasia or carcinoma in situ. The most disturbing feature usually is the prominent pleomorphism. The tendency to put this lesion in the category of severe dysplasia clouds its true nature. This term should be used only as a temporary measure in favor of a definitive diagnosis as soon as possible after repeat biopsy. The key feature of malignancy is evidence of stromal invasion (Fig. 27.18). Unlike the stratified squamous epithelium and adenomas of the digestive tract, carcinoma in situ alone is a rare finding in the stomach. It usually is accompanied by invasive lesions in the neighboring tissue. Thus, a search for stromal invasion will

help to clarify a doubtful lesion. Alternatively, molecular studies may be helpful. The presence of aneuploidy and oncogenes favors the malignant nature of the lesion.

Evidence of the precancerous nature of dysplastic gastric epithelium has been found in two aspects: high grade of dysplasia is more common in cancerous than in benign stomachs (127) and carcinoma may develop in the dysplastic epithelium. Follow-up studies of dysplasia have been performed. A summary of 10 reports (138–147) is given in Table 27.3. Progression of dysplasia to higher grades and development of carcinoma occur more frequently in areas of severe dysplasia. Carcinoma occurs only infrequently in mild dysplasia, whereas the epithelium regresses to normal in 60% of cases. It is noteworthy that even severe dysplasia may regress. This phenomenon clearly distinguishes the nonneoplastic nature of dysplasia.

The majority of carcinomas have been found within 1 year of the diagnosis of dysplasia, suggesting that carcinoma was already present at the time of diagnosis of dysplasia. In view of these data, gastric dysplasia may be considered paracancerous rather than precancerous. Long-term studies are still needed to clarify the precancerous nature of gastric dysplasia.

In terms of management, the question of gastrectomy has been raised. Some investigators think dysplastic tissue is neoplastic (131) and should be treated by gastrectomy, as it is practiced for similar lesions in the colon. The circumstances surrounding gastric dysplasia are somewhat different from those in the colon, however, where dysplasia occurs almost exclusively in association with long-standing

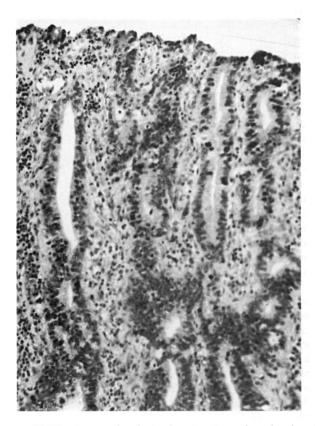

Figure 27.15 Severe dysplasia showing irregular glands with prominent nuclear stratification. The cells are short and slightly pleomorphic. There is no mucus secretion (×150).

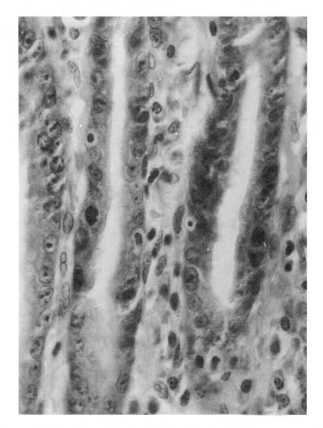

Figure 27.16 Severely dysplastic glands with immature cells. The cells are cuboidal and devoid of mucus secretion. The nuclei are large and slightly pleomorphic. The nucleoli are prominent. Mitosis is present (×480).

inflammatory bowel disease, the treatment of which includes colectomy even in the absence of dysplastic lesions. In the stomach, the dysplastic changes are multifocal with unpredictable location. These lesions are asymptomatic and may regress. A conservative approach to gastric dysplasia with follow-up examinations is appropriate in most cases (148). More importantly, efforts must be made to search for a coexisting carcinoma, a frequent concomitant, particularly if the dysplasia is severe or high grade. Diligent search in relatively short intervals may reveal a malignant focus only weeks or months later. Surgical resection is clearly indicated in such cases. Because most carcinomas so discovered are early lesions, they are highly curable (140, 143, 149). If no carcinoma is present, regular follow-up should continue for patients with high-grade dysplasia.

Dysplasia is closely associated with expanding or intestinal-type cancer (127, 137), but it does not play a prominent role in the development of the infiltrative or diffuse type of gastric cancer. The precancerous lesion of the latter remains uncertain. Some authors indicate, however, that infiltrative carcinoma may arise from the neck mucous cells (149a) or cells with globoid dysplasia. In globoid dysplasia, the foveolar cells take on a globoid appearance because their cytoplasm is engorged with excessive amounts of acidic mucin (128, 150). The eccentric nuclei are compressed and the cells resemble signet-ring cancer cells (Fig. 27.19). The presence of acid mucin indicates that it is a form of incomplete intestinal metaplasia. The polarity of the cells is lost and their nuclei are abnormally located. Globoid dysplasia may be seen in hyperplastic polyps.

EXPERIMENTAL GASTRIC CARCINOGENESIS

Adenocarcinoma of the stomach has been induced by radiation and a variety of carcinogens. Since the late 1960s, when Sugimura (151) used N-methyl-N'-nitro-N-nitrosoguanidine (MNNG) to produce adenomas, adenocarcinomas, and other tumors in the gastrointestinal tract in rats, MNNG has become the standard model for gastric carcinogenesis, mostly in rats. The susceptibility to MNNG is genetically controlled. Wistar and ACI rats are susceptible, but Buffalo rats and mice are resistant (151). The induced carcinoma resembles human gastric carcinoma. It is mostly well differentiated in rats (151), and signet-ring cells are common in dogs (152). Electron microscopy revealed both gastric and intestinal types of cells, as well as squamous cells (153). The tumors do not have pepsinogen 1 and the mucosal level of Pg 1 reduces dramatically in the precancerous period (154). The ethyl (ENNG) and propyl (PNNG) derivatives of MNNG are less tumorigenic. PNNG has been used in rats (155), ENNG is commonly used in dogs (151). A lower dose of ENNG in dogs produces mainly signet-ring cell carcinomas (Fig. 27.20), whereas a higher dose induces glandular adenocarcinomas (156). The induced signet-ring cell carcinoma may remain intramucosal for several years (157).

The MNNG-induced adenocarcinomas develop through the stages of superficial erosion, atrophy, and increasing degrees of dysplasia (158). Intestinal metaplasia, generally of the complete type, is common in rats, but the frequency varies (92). Change of

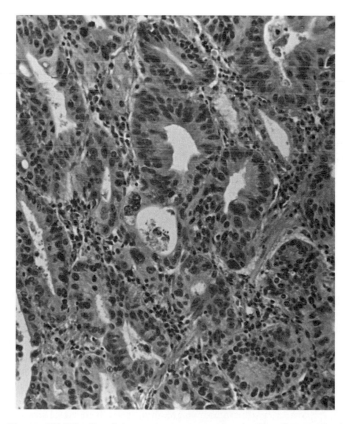

Figure 27.17 Possibly carcinomatous glands showing marked pseudostratification, moderate pleomorphism and no mucus secretion. The glands are crowded but there is no stromal invasion. Definite carcinoma is present in adjacent area (×200).

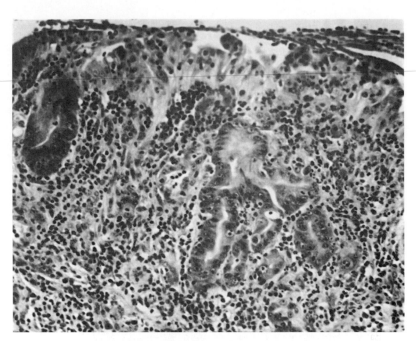

Figure 27.18 Small focus of superficial carcinoma with stromal invasion in an area of dysplasia (×120).

mucin secretion to acidic type occurs before the morphologic changes of metaplasia occur (159). In the dog and the monkey, intestinal metaplasia is rare or absent (160). On the other hand, PNNG induces metaplasia more frequently than carcinoma (155). Intestinal metaplasia appears to be an unimportant precancerous lesion in experimental gastric carcinogenesis.

NATURAL HISTORY OF GASTRIC ADENOCARCINOMA

The development and subsequent course of gastric adenocarcinoma go through several stages. The etiology of human gastric cancer is unknown, and whether the precancerous conditions are integral to the carcinogenic process or merely change the susceptibility of the tissue to carcinogenesis has not been determined. It has been postulated that carcinogenic exposure in high-risk regions probably occurs during early life, and carcinoma develops after a long latent period, in either metaplastic or gastric epithelium. In many but not all instances, dysplasia appears to be an intermediate step before carcinogenesis.

Histologic examination of early gastric carcinoma, particularly minute lesions, allows evaluation of the background mucosa from which the early cancerous lesion arises. Such studies have revealed that the glandular differentiated carcinoma was associated with intestinal metaplasia, whereas the nonglandular carcinomas arose from the gastric mucosa (161). Using serial-step sections, Hattori (162) noted that carcinoma, metaplasia, and dysplasia all began at the neck region of the glands, where regeneration of the epithelium normally occurred. Similar cellular origin from the gland neck was demonstrated for the signet-ring cell carcinoma by Grundmann (149a).

Because gastric carcinomas are often at an advanced stage at the time of diagnosis, it may be assumed that they are fast growing tumors. Actually, cell proliferation is slower in gastric cancer than in normal gastric mucosa, the cell cycle time being three times longer in the tumor (163). On the other hand, the mean cell life span is

TABLE 27.3	Summary of Gastric Epithelial Dysplasia Follow-Up Studies (1989–1994) in Percentages					
Dysplasia	Mild		Moderate		Severe	
Regression	36–74	(60)	27–87	(50)	0–60	(20)
Stationary	15–43	(20)	20–40	(25)	3–43	(20)
Progression	19–21	(20)	4–40	(25)	31–86	(60)
Carcinoma	0–7	(2)	4–36	(20)	31–80	(60)

Numbers in parentheses are average percents. Follow-up duration: 1 month to 5 years. From 50% to 80% of carcinomas were found within 1 year after biopsy diagnosis of dysplasia. From 39% to 80% of carcinomas were early. Percentages obtained from references 138–147.

shortened from 8 to 20 days in the normal mucosa to 1 day in the carcinoma (128). Combination of these two phenomena results in a slow rate of growth of the gastric carcinoma. From 1 to 4 years pass before the tumor is clinically recognized as an early carcinoma (164), which also grows slowly, with a doubling time of 2 to 3 years, and may remain superficial for as long as 14 to 21 years (164, 165). Advanced gastric carcinomas grow faster, with an average doubling time of 2 to 10 months, and that of the metastatic tumor is 0.6 to 2 months (164). Increasing DNA polyploidy and aneuploidy as the tumor advances and metastasizes (166) are indicative of progressive mutation of the tumor.

Gastric carcinomas have different modes of growth; some grow in a cohesive fashion and form large masses, whereas others invade by individual cells. These variations in the invasion pattern manifest early and persist throughout the course. Thus, growth patterns are intrinsic biologic characteristics of the cancer cells. The metastasis may be by either venous or lymphatic routes, resulting in different organ involvement and variations in the clinical courses and curability of the cancer. The terminal outcome, involving many factors, varies from patient to patient (see subsequent discussion of prognosis).

EARLY GASTRIC CARCINOMA AS A CLINICOPATHOLOGIC ENTITY

Japan has one of the highest rates of gastric carcinoma in the world. Because this malignancy accounts for the highest cancer mortality in Japan in both sexes, great efforts were placed on early diagnosis and treatment. As a result, many early gastric carcinomas have been detected, greatly improving the overall cure rate.

Verse was credited with the first description of early cancer of the stomach as an entity. In 1903, he reported seven cases of Schleimhautcarcinome with carcinoma involving the mucosa and submucosa (167). Subsequently, such a tumor has been reported variously as carcinoma in situ (168), superficial spreading type (169), and superficial carcinoma (170, 171). Not until 1962, however, when its macroscopic classification was presented by the Japan Gastroenterological Endoscopy Society (172), was the concept of early gastric cancer (EGC) firmly established.

Early gastric cancer is defined as a primary carcinoma of the stomach with carcinomatous infiltration limited to the mucosa and submucosa (Fig. 27.21), regardless of the presence or absence of lymph node metastases (173). "Early" indicates the possibility of complete surgical resection and does not imply a time dimension. Lymph node metastasis was found in 9% cases of EGC. Adequate regional lymphadenectomy has resulted in a 5-year survival rate higher than 95%.

From its opening in 1962 to December of 1991, the National Cancer Center Hospital (NCCH) in Tokyo has been the site for

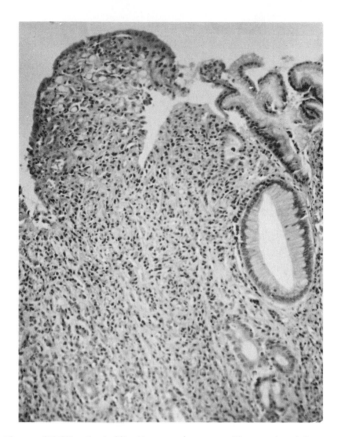

Figure 27.20 An infiltrative carcinoma without gland formation was induced in a dog with ENNG. There are neither intestinal metaplasia nor dysplasia in the adjacent mucosa (×120). (Courtesy of Dr. Rui-nien Wang, Professor of Pathology, Shanghai Second Medical University, China.)

surgical treatment of 6439 cases of gastric cancer. Early gastric cancer was found in 2400 (37%). The percentage of early cases among the surgically treated gastric cancers has steadily increased through subsequent years, so now, more than 50% of cases are in early stage, with a corresponding increase in the overall survival rate of gastric cancer. In Europe and the United States, the percentage of early cancer remains low. A study by the American College of Surgeons reported an incidence of 18% with a 5-year survival rate of 50% (174).

PATHOLOGY OF GASTRIC ADENOCARCINOMA

LOCATION

In the Japanese classification (173), the stomach is divided into the upper (C for corpus), middle (M), and lower (A for antrum) thirds along the long axis; and into the anterior and posterior walls, greater and lesser curvatures, and the whole circumference along the transverse axis. At NCCH, early cancer occurs most frequently in the M region (55.5%) and along the lesser curvature (47.8%), and least frequently in the C region (11.6%) and along the greater curvature (8.9%) (26). Among surgically treated patients in the Japan Registry, including advanced cases, cancer occurrence in the A region was the highest (44.6%), followed by the M (39.3%) and C (16.1%)

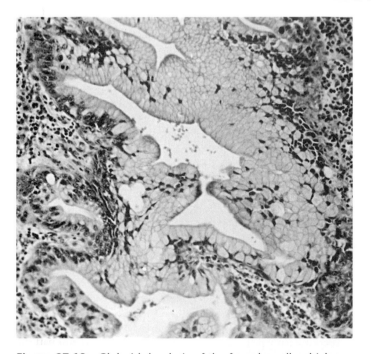

Figure 27.19 Globoid dysplasia of the foveolar cells which are distended by a large globule of mucus compressing the nuclei to the cell membrane. The polarity is lost and the cells are haphazardly oriented (×200).

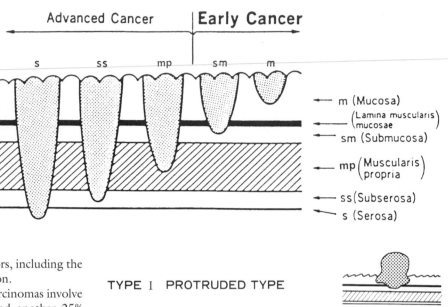

Figure 27.21 Definition of early and advanced gastric cancers according to the level of cancerous invasion in the gastric wall.

regions. These data probably reflect multiple factors, including the rate of detection and feasibility of surgical resection.

In the United States, about 50% of gastric carcinomas involve the pyloric mucosa, 25% the fundic mucosa, and another 25% both areas (12, 116). The number of carcinomas in the upper stomach has increased (175); currently, about 30% of tumors are found in the cardia.

SIZE

The size of gastric carcinoma at the time of diagnosis varies. Most EGCs are 2 to 5 cm in diameter. The more frequent detection of smaller lesions reflects the progress in diagnostic methods. At NCCH, 15% EGC were less than 1.1 cm in diameter and 29% were between 1.1 and 2 cm. The small cancer (less than 10 mm in diameter) and particularly the minute cancer (less than 5 mm in diameter) are important, not only in their potential for total curability, but also in their contribution to the understanding of premalignant lesions (176). Type IIb flat lesions constitute 58.3% of tumors less than 5 mm in diameter and 0% of tumors larger than 5 mm (177). These findings indicate that as the tumor grows larger, the originally flat lesion becomes either protruding or depressed or ulcerated. The advanced gastric carcinomas are larger; close to 50% of tumors are 6 cm or more in diameter and one seventh are larger than 10 cm (116).

GROSS MORPHOLOGY AND CLASSIFICATION

Grossly, adenocarcinomas of the stomach can be divided, according to a modified Borrmann classification (178), into five types (116):

1. Superficial carcinoma (Type 0 carcinoma, early carcinoma).
2. Polypoid carcinoma (Borrmann Type 1 carcinoma)
3. Fungating carcinoma (Borrmann Type 2 carcinoma)
4. Ulcerated carcinoma (Borrmann Type 3 carcinoma)
5. Diffusely infiltrative carcinoma (Borrmann Type 4 carcinoma, linitis plastica carcinoma)

The relative frequency of these types in our materials are 6% for the superficial, 7% polypoid, 25% ulcerated, 36% fungating, and 26% diffuse (12).

Type 0 carcinoma was not in Borrmann's original classification. It is applied by the Japanese Research Society for Gastric Cancer

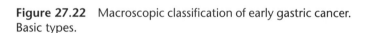

Figure 27.22 Macroscopic classification of early gastric cancer. Basic types.

(JRSGC) to early gastric cancers and includes all subtypes established by the Japanese Endoscopy Society (179). Because these tumors may persist for years and may metastasize, the descriptive term "superficial carcinoma" is more appropriate than the term of early carcinoma, although EGC is now a well-accepted term.

Early (Superficial) Gastric Carcinoma

MACROSCOPIC CLASSIFICATION   The macroscopic classification of early gastric cancer (EGC) is shown in Figure 27.22. The frequency of various types is listed in Table 27.4.

Type I tumor is a nodular lesion that often shows an irregular surface with crevices between the papillary projections (Fig. 27.23).

Type II lesions are further subdivided into Type IIa (superficial elevated type) with a slight elevation of the lesion approximately twice the thickness of mucosa to 5 mm (Fig. 27.24), Type IIb (superficial flat type) with the level of the lesion approximately the same as the surrounding mucosa, and Type IIc (superficial depressed type) with a shallow depression.

Type IIc cancer is the most frequent and most important lesion in clinical diagnosis (see Table 27.4). In this type, the erosive surface of the carcinoma is slightly lower than the surrounding mucosa and varies in size (Figs. 27.25 and 27.26). The tips of the mucosal folds converging at the Type IIc lesion show characteristic narrowing with indentation and an abrupt border. The depressed surface of the Type IIc lesion is characterized as follows: (*a*) Unlike the surrounding mucosa, it is flattened, occasionally accompanied by granular changes of various sizes; (*b*) within the depressed area, ulcer scar or open ulcer may be present, and these changes may be shallow; (*c*) the glistening surface disappears; and (*d*) color tone changes.

TABLE 27.4	Frequency of Macroscopic Types of Early Gastric Carcinoma at National Cancer Center Hospital in Tokyo		

Macroscopic Types	No. of Lesions	Percent
A. Predominantly protruded or elevated type	619	23.0
I	160	6.0
IIa	227	8.4
IIa + IIc	232	8.6
B. Flat type	80	3.0
IIb	80	3.0
C. Predominantly depressed or excavated type	1976	74.0
IIc	1659	62.1
IIc + III	174	6.5
IIc + IIa	72	2.7
III	15	0.6
III + IIc	56	2.1
Total	2675	100.0

Data represent findings from 2400 cases collected from May 1962 to December 1991.

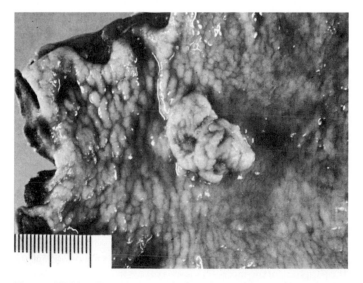

Figure 27.23 Type I protruded early gastric carcinoma. The tumor is papillary, with focal infiltration into submucosa.

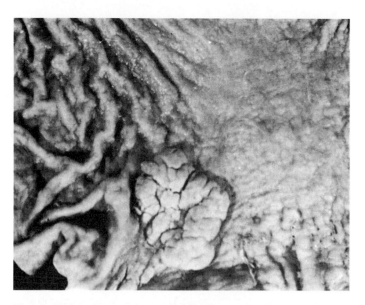

Figure 27.24 Type IIa superficially elevated early gastric carcinoma (Courtesy of Dr. Ying-Chang Zhang, Professor of Pathology, China Medical University, China.)

Type III cancer shows a deep ulcer-like excavation surrounded by a narrow rim of carcinomatous tissue along the ulcer border. This lesion may resemble a benign ulcer. Pure Type III lesion is rare, with a frequency rate of less than 1%.

Secondary ulceration was found in 65.4% of EGC, and more frequently in patients younger than age 65 years than in elderly patients. Formation of an ulcer scar is the main cause of the convergence of mucosal folds toward the carcinoma. It was commonly associated with submucosal invasion in Type IIc carcinoma measuring less than 3 cm, but not in larger lesions. The frequency of ulceration and/or ulcer scar decreased from 93.5% in 1962 to 71.9% in 1983 (180).

The combined type of EGC shows the coexistence of two or more macroscopic types in a single lesion (Fig. 27.27). In general, the type occupying the larger area is written first, regardless of the histogenesis. For example, when ulceration beyond the muscularis mucosa is found within a Type IIc lesion and the ulcer is smaller than the depressed region, this lesion is called Type IIc-Type III (Fig. 27.28). When elevation and excavation coexist, the lesion may be called Type IIa + Type IIc or Type IIc + Type IIa (Fig. 27.29). These designations make little difference as to the rate of lymph node metastases or prognosis, according to our statistical data.

Early gastric carcinomas have been classified by Inokuchi, Kodama, and colleagues according to size and growth patterns revealed on the cross section (181, 182). The tumors larger than 4 cm in diameter were classified as superficial spreading (Super type, 44.9%). Tumors less than 4 cm in diameter and showing no or slight submucosal invasion were classified as small mucosal type (36.5%). The small tumors with wide submucosal involvement were classified as penetrating type (Pen type, 17.4%). The mixed type tumors (1.2%) were larger than 4 cm in diameter and have submucosal involvement. The Pen type tumors were subdivided into A and B types, showing expanding and infiltrative form of submucosal growth, respectively. This observation is important because Pen A tumors were mostly elevated and had higher rates of lymphatic and

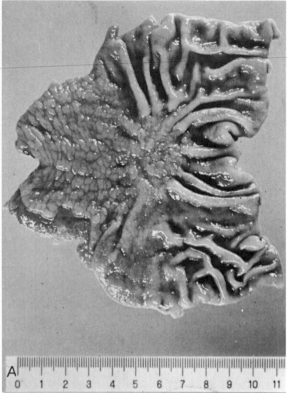

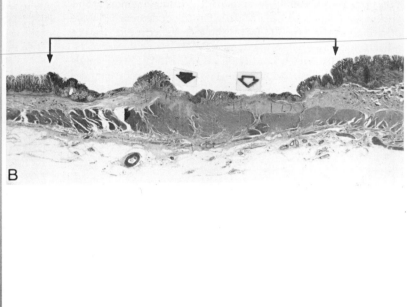

Figure 27.25 Type IIc superficially depressed early gastric carcinoma. **A.** Gross morphology. **B.** Scanning view of the microscopic morphology. Both open ulcer *(open arrow)* and scar tissue *(close arrow)* are present in the submucosa. The line marks the extent of the tumor.

hematogenous metastasis and worse prognosis than other types (182). Pen B tumors tended to have peritoneal recurrences. DNA measurements showed high ploidy of Pen A tumors and low ploidy of other tumors (182).

PREVALENCE AND CHRONOLOGIC CHANGES OF MACROSCOPIC TYPES The prevalence of macroscopic types of EGC varies somewhat among institutions. In the Japanese national statistics, Type IIc was seen most frequently (33.8%), followed by Type IIc + Type III (23.4%), Type I (9.7%), Type IIa (9%), and Type IIa + Type IIc (6.5%). In our data, IIc was most frequent (60.5%) and IIb was 3.3% (see Table 27.4). In contrast, among cases studied by Johansen (183), 13.3% of the tumors were of IIb type.

The distribution of macroscopic type has changed during the past 30 years. Initially, the depressed type accounted for 68.0%, with a recent increase to 75.3%. The frequency of elevated type is decreasing. Among the depressed types, the relatively shallow Type IIc lesion has become predominant. Type III lesions virtually disappeared after 1974 (17).

Advanced Gastric Carcinoma

The polypoid carcinoma (Fig. 27.30) is a broad-based, nodular tumor without gross ulceration. The fungating carcinoma (Fig. 27.31) is also a nodular tumor, but it has a large ulcer at the dome. The bottom of ulcer crater rests on the tumor mass and is above the level of the stomach wall. The ulcerated carcinoma (Figs. 27.32 and 27.33) is an excavated tumor, with a penetrating ulcer base and inconspicuous or only slightly elevated tumor mass at the periphery of the ulcer. This lesion differs from the Type III early carcinoma by the presence of tumor cells at the base as well as the margins of the ulcer. When the tumor tissue is scanty, the lesion may resemble a benign ulcer. In most instances, careful inspection allows

Figure 27.26 Minute type IIc early gastric carcinoma. **A.** Gross morphology. **B.** Scanning view of microscopic morphology. *Arrow* denotes the depressed cancer. The tumor is poorly differentiated.

the observer to distinguish a malignant ulcer from a benign ulcer without difficulty (Table 27.5). When the gross evidence for malignancy is absent, it is important that sections for microscopic examination include all ulcer margins. For endoscopic diagnosis, multiple biopsies may be necessary to avoid misdiagnosis.

The diffusely infiltrative carcinoma (Fig. 27.34) infiltrates through the stomach wall without forming a mass or becoming

COMBINED TYPE

IIa + IIc

IIc + IIa

IIb + IIc

IIc + III

III + IIc

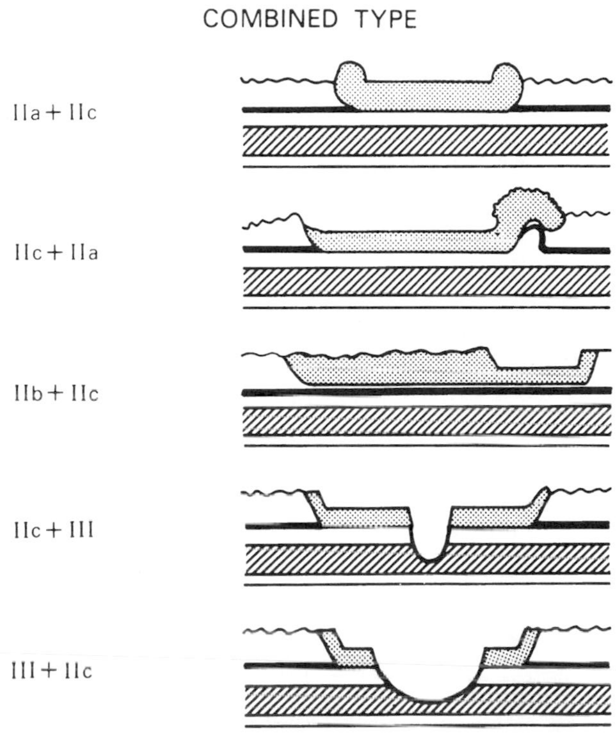

Figure 27.27 Macroscopic classification. Combined types. (Reprinted with permission from Hirota T, Ming SC, Itabashi M. Pathology of early gastric cancer. In: Nishi M, Ichikawa H, Nakajima T, et al., eds. Gastric cancer. Tokyo: Springer, 1993; 66–87.)

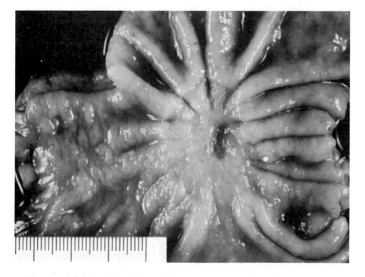

Figure 27.28 Combined Type IIc + III early gastric cancer.

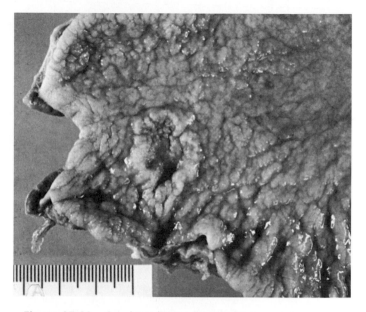

Figure 27.29 Combined Type IIa + IIc early gastric cancer.

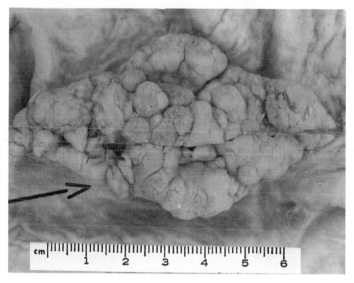

Figure 27.30 Polypoid carcinoma. Lesion is lobulated but not ulcerated. (Reprinted with permission from Ming SC. Tumors of the esophagus and stomach. In: Atlas of tumor pathology, second series, fascicle 7. Washington DC: Armed Forces Institute of Pathology, 1973:144–206.)

deeply ulcerated. It may involve the whole or a portion of the stomach. The thickened and stiff gastric wall is the reason that the term "linitis plastica" is used to describe this type of tumor. The tumor commonly is accompanied by prominent fibrosis and therefore is also called scirrhous carcinoma.

HISTOLOGIC COMPOSITION AND CLASSIFICATION

Histologic Composition

EPITHELIAL ELEMENTS The histologic features of gastric adenocarcinoma are complex. Many types of cells have been identified in the gastric carcinoma. Mucous cells are common. In glandular carci-

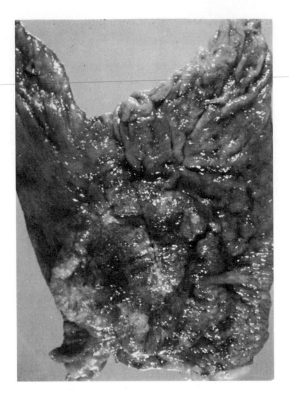

Figure 27.31 Fungating carcinoma in the antrum of the stomach. The tumor is raised and a large ulcer is on the surface.

noma, the majority are goblet cells (Fig. 27.35), which secrete intestinal acidic mucins (74, 116, 184, 185). In the diffusely infiltrative carcinoma, most signet-ring cells are also goblet cells (184). The others, however, secrete only neutral glycoprotein, thus resembling the foveolar or pyloric gland cells (184, 186). The gastric-type mucous cells are rare in glandular carcinoma. Intracellular cysts occasionally are present in the tumor cells (187). These cysts contain mucous granules and are lined by microvilli. The amount of mucus varies. The mucus is contained within the glandular structures in most cases. Excessive mucus may escape into the stroma.

The nonmucous tumor cells are mostly immature absorptive cells, with a distinct striated border (Fig. 27.36) made of well-formed microvilli (79, 184) and containing digestive enzymes (188). Additional cell types include pyloric gland cells (5, 184), endocrine cells (117, 189, 190), Paneth cells (191, 192), parietal cells (193, 194, 195), pepsinogen-secreting cells (196), chief cells, and squamous cells (5). Hepatoid cells have also been reported (197, 198). The argyrophil cells are sometimes abundant in solid carcinomas (199) and in diffusely infiltrating carcinoma (190). Solid carcinomas, which constitute about 6% of gastric carcinomas, are composed of sheets or masses of poorly differentiated or undifferentiated cells. Murayama et al. (199) examined 20 such tumors under the electron microscope and found mucous cells in 12 cases, neurosecretory cells in 5 cases, and both types of cells in 3 cases.

STROMAL ELEMENTS The stroma of many gastric carcinomas has distinctive features. Lymphocytic infiltration is prominent in some solid undifferentiated carcinomas (12). The latter type of lesion has

been associated with Epstein-Barr virus and given the names of lymphoepithelioma-like carcinoma (65) and carcinoma with lymphoid stroma (65–68, 200, 201) (Fig. 27.37).

The amount of fibrous stromal tissue varies. Tumors with little desmoplastic reaction form solid epithelial masses, usually showing poor gland or acinar formation; these lesions are called medullary carcinomas. Fibrosis is prominent in the infiltrative carcinomas (12, 202) (Fig. 27.38). The term "scirrhous carcinoma" is applied to such a tumor. The fibrous tissue is grossly evident. Procollagen I has been demonstrated in such tumors and in some cell lines but not in medullary carcinomas (203, 204). Furthermore, transforming growth factor from tumor cells may stimulate both tumor cells and fibroblasts to produce collagen (204).

The histologic composition of gastric carcinoma varies from case to case and from area to area within a case. As a result, several histologic classifications have been proposed, each with specific purposes.

World Health Organization (WHO) Classification

The World Health Organization classifies the gastric carcinomas into 10 types (205) (Table 27.6). The tubular adenocarcinomas are most common. This classification is highly reproducible (206) and

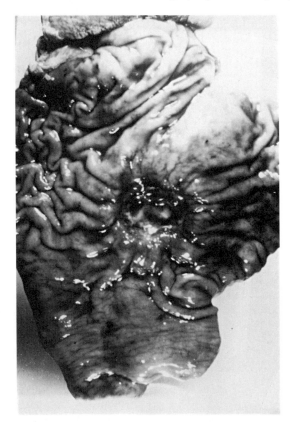

Figure 27.32 Ulcerated carcinoma in the distal portion of the body of the stomach. The ulcer base is shaggy and hemorrhagic. Mucosal folds are present at the ulcer margin except the distal region, where the mucosa slopes into the ulcer base. (Reprinted with permission from Ming SC. Tumors of the esophagus and stomach. In: Atlas of tumor pathology, second series, fascicle 7. Washington DC: Armed Forces Institute of Pathology, 1973: 144–206.)

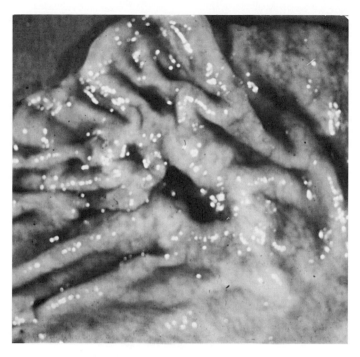

Figure 27.33 Ulcerated carcinoma. The deep ulcer is surrounded by a slightly raised wall. Microscopically, the tumor is a signet-ring cell carcinoma.

TABLE 27.5	Differentiation Between Benign Peptic Ulcer and Malignant Ulcer (Ulcerated Carcinoma without Forming Mass)	
	Benign Ulcer	Ulcerated Cancer
Ulcer border	Sharp	Fuzzy
Ulcer size	Small	Variable
Ulcer base	Clean, pearly	Necrotic, hemorrhagic
Tissue at base	Pale, rubbery	Granular, gritty
Ulcer depth	Muscularis or beyond	Variable
Mucosa around ulcer	Soft and mobile	Firm and fixed
	Congested, swollen	Pale, solid
Location	Antrum	Antrum and others
	Lesser curvature	
Perforation or massive bleeding	Relatively common	Uncommon
Age of patient	Middle age	Old

the terms are familiar to all pathologists. It is useful for routine pathologic diagnosis of gastric carcinoma, However, the histologic pattern of gastric carcinoma often varies, so the diagnosis is based on the dominant pattern and is accurate only for the materials examined.

The majority of gastric carcinomas are made of epithelial cells normally present in the stomach and intestines. These tumors are ordinary adenocarcinomas, and are discussed in the following section. (Those tumors containing cells of other organs are presented in separate discussions.) The structure of adenocarcinomas of the stomach generally takes two forms: one shows prominent cohesive gland formation, and the other shows individual or small groups of tumor cells forming no glands or incomplete glands or acini.

Papillary and tubular adenocarcinomas are glandular tumors. In the papillary tumor there are prominent intraglandular foldings and projections with cuboidal to high columnar carcinoma cells

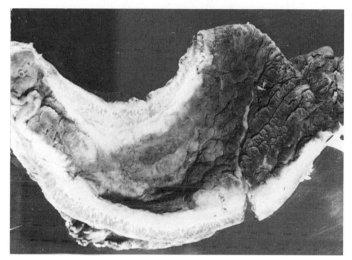

Figure 27.34 Diffusely infiltrative carcinoma (linitis plastica). The tumor involves the entire stomach. White scirrhous tumor tissue infiltrates the whole thickness of the gastric wall. (Reprinted with permission from Ming SC. Tumors of the esophagus and stomach. In: Atlas of tumor pathology, second series, fascicle 7. Washington DC: Armed Forces Institute of Pathology, 1973: 144–206.)

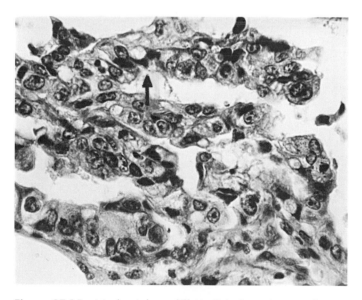

Figure 27.35 Moderately differentiated adenocarcinoma showing the presence of goblet cells, one of which is marked by an arrow (×480).

lining the narrow bands of interstitial tissue in an arborizing pattern (Fig. 27.39). In the tubular adenocarcinoma, the glands form branching tubules. The lumen of these tubules varies in size and may be cystic (Fig. 27.40). In both types, most tumor cells are absorptive type, with scattered goblet cells. The nuclei are nearly round or irregular, with abundant coarse chromatin pattern. Grossly, they usually form polypoid or fungating masses with a well-defined border.

Signet-ring cell carcinoma is so named because of the shape of the tumor cells, which are distended by abundant intracytoplasmic mucus compressing the crescentic nuclei against the cell wall (Fig. 27.41). The tumor characteristically infiltrates by individual cells. No or scanty gland formation is observed, although small alveolar or cordlike arrangement may be present. Signet-ring cell carcinoma is a prototype of diffusely infiltrative carcinoma.

All differentiated gastric adenocarcinomas secrete mucus, which is primarily intracellular and intraglandular. Excessive amounts of mucus may rupture the cells and glands and form mucus pools in the stroma, which may be grossly visible. When the mucus occupies more than 50% of tumor mass, the term "mucinous adenocarcinoma" is applied. Tumors with lesser amount of mucin are called adenocarcinoma with prominent mucinous components. The mucinous carcinoma is also called mucoid or colloid carcinoma. About 10% of the gastric carcinomas are of this type (207). Floating in the mucus pool are fragmented tumor gland or individual signet ring cells (see Fig. 27.41). The mucinous carcinoma is therefore a variant of either the glandular carcinoma or the signet-ring cell carcinoma.

The gastric adenocarcinomas are further graded as well-differentiated, moderately differentiated, or poorly differentiated. The undifferentiated carcinoma, showing total lack of glandular or cellular differentiation, is classified as a separate entity. The degrees of differentiation are judged at two levels: architectural and cellular. At the architectural level, a well-differentiated carcinoma is made of well-formed glands (see Figs. 27.36 and 27.40). Papillary projections may be present in the dilated glandular spaces. In the moderately differentiated type, the glandular structures are irregular, complex, or incomplete (see Fig. 27.35). The tumor cells may aggregate to form ribbons or masses (Fig. 27.42). A poorly

differentiated carcinoma has no or ill-formed glands (Fig. 27.43) or may represent only individually scattered tumor cells (Fig. 27.44). At the cellular level, a well-differentiated carcinoma is composed of mature functioning cells, such as absorptive cells with striated borders (see Fig. 27.36) and mucus-secreting goblet cells (see Fig. 27.35) or signet-ring cells (see Fig. 27.41). A poorly differentiated carcinoma has primitive nonfunctioning cells (see Figs. 27.37

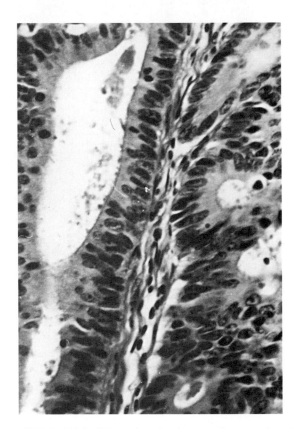

Figure 27.36 Well-differentiated adenocarcinoma showing a striated border on the luminal surface of the tumor cells (×375).

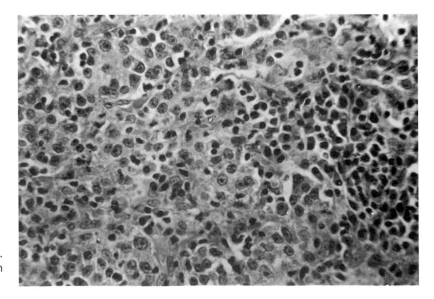

Figure 27.37 Carcinoma with lymphoid stroma. Many lymphocytes and few plasma cells mingle with undifferentiated carcinoma cells (×150).

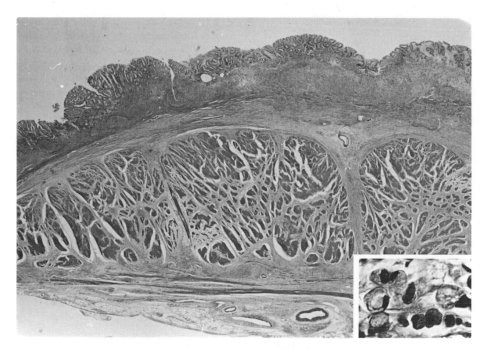

Figure 27.38 Infiltrative carcinoma showing diffuse infiltration of tumor cells and desmoplastic tissue throughout the gastric wall. The mucosa shows no intestinal metaplasia or dysplasia (×15). The tumor is a signet-ring cell carcinoma (*inset,* ×480).

TABLE	
27.6	**World Health Organization Histologic Typing of Malignant Epithelial Tumors of the Stomach**

Adenocarcinoma
  Papillary adenocarcinoma
  Tubular adenocarcinoma
  Mucinous adenocarcinoma
  Signet-ring cell carcinoma
Adenosquamous carcinoma
Squamous cell carcinoma
Small cell carcinoma
Undifferentiated carcinoma
Others

tubular adenocarcinoma. Special types of carcinomas include adenosquamous carcinoma, squamous cell carcinoma, carcinoid, and other tumors. In addition to tumor typing, the Japanese histologic classification includes the status of lymphatic and venous penetration; tissue level of tumor invasion; cancer-stroma relation; pattern of tumor growth; lymph node, hepatic, and peritoneal metastasis; as well as clinical and operative features.

At NCCH in Tokyo, papillary adenocarcinoma and tubular adenocarcinoma accounted for 43.7% of gastric carcinomas and poorly differentiated adenocarcinomas and signet-ring cell carcinomas accounted for 56.3%. Signet-ring cell carcinoma accounts for 29.6% of early cancer and 22.7% of advanced cancer. The frequency of poorly differentiated adenocarcinoma, on the other hand, was 11.7% in cases of early cancers, and 29.5% in those involving advanced cancer. Mucinous adenocarcinoma is rare and accounts for only 0.8% of early gastric cancer and 5.2% of advanced gastric cancer.

and 27.44). These two levels of differentiation may not go together. In practice, glandular formation is often used to judge the degree of differentiation of an adenocarcinoma. Thus, the signet-ring cell carcinoma may be considered a poorly differentiated tumor, because it does not form glands, even though the cells are well differentiated.

Japanese Classification

The Japanese histologic classification, which is similar to but more detailed and comprehensive than the WHO classification (see Table 27.6), facilitates staging of the cancer and overall evaluation of the patient's status. It has two major categories: common type and special type (173). The common type includes papillary, tubular, mucinous adenocarcinomas and signet-ring cell carcinoma. In addition, poorly differentiated adenocarcinoma is a separate subtype and is subdivided into solid and nonsolid types. The well- and moderately differentiated adenocarcinomas are subtypes of

Lauren Classification

Lauren (13) divided gastric carcinomas into two types: intestinal and diffuse, with a relative frequency of 53% and 33%, respectively. The remaining 14% of carcinomas did not fit into these patterns and were unclassified. The intestinal-type carcinoma was so named because it has features resembling a differentiated colonic carcinoma (see Figs. 27.35, 27.36, and 27.40). The diffuse type is characterized by diffuse infiltration of tumor cells individually or in small nests (see Figs. 27.38 and 27.44). Thus, the tumor types are decided by two different criteria. The intestinal type is characterized by its histologic morphology, and the diffuse type is characterized by its biologic behavior. They are not entirely compatible. Signet-ring cell carcinoma occurs also in the intestine, but it is not classified as intestinal-type carcinoma in the stomach.

The Lauren classification has been modified to include three subtypes: intestinal, diffuse, and mixed types. Their respective frequencies in a survey by the American College of Surgeons (174)

Clinically, the intestinal-type carcinoma is more common in older male patients, whereas the diffuse carcinoma is more common in younger female patients. The Lauren classification has been used in many epidemiologic studies (10, 21, 23). The intestinal-type carcinoma is prevalent in high-risk countries (21). The decline in gastric cancer incidence in many countries has been attributed by some investigators (10) to a decline in the incidence of intestinal-type carcinoma.

Ming Classification

This classification is based on the patterns of tumor growth and invasiveness, which are pathologic manifestations of tumor biology. Accordingly, the gastric carcinomas are divided into expanding and infiltrative types (12). The expanding carcinoma grows by expansion into cohesive nodules or masses, with sharply defined periphery compressing the neighboring tissue (Fig. 27.45; see also Fig. 27.42). The infiltrative carcinoma shows infiltration by individual cells (see Figs. 27.38 and 27.44) or small glands (Fig. 27.46). The relative frequencies of these type of gastric carcinomas are 67% and 33%, respectively. The difference in growth pattern is related to cell adhesion molecules, such as E-cadherin, which is largely preserved in the expanding carcinoma and lost in the infiltrative carcinoma (209). Both types of carcinoma show varying degrees of cell maturation and differentiation. Large glands, however, are present only in the expanding type. Under the electron microscope, the tumor cells in expanding carcinoma show well-developed desmosomes, which usually are absent in the infiltrative carcinoma even when the cells are in close contact (210). Lymphocytic infiltration is heavy in the expanding carcinoma, and desmoplastic response is prominent in the infiltrative carcinoma. The expanding carcinoma is often associated with chronic atrophic gastritis, prominent intestinal metaplasia, and dysplasia. These changes are either mild or absent in the stomach with infiltrative carcinoma.

The designation of infiltrative carcinoma is based on the infiltrative pattern of the entire tumor and not just the periphery

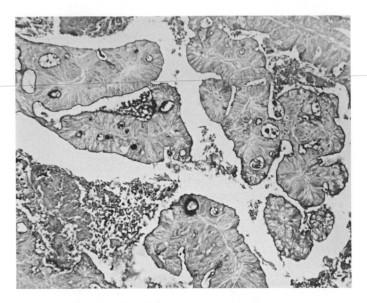

Figure 27.39 Papillary fronds in a large cystic area of a carcinoma. The tissue is stained with periodic acid-Schiff method, which shows black mucus in the tumor tissue and on the surface of the fronds (×120).

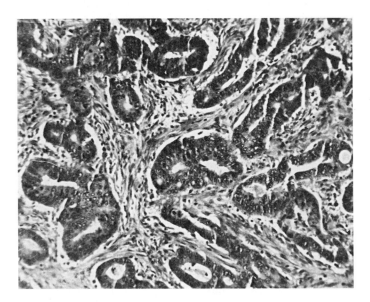

Figure 27.40 Adenocarcinoma showing irregular branching glands lined by pseudostratified tumor cells. Scattered lymphocytes are present in the scanty fibrous stroma (×120).

were 31%, 55%, and 5% (208). The mixed type tumors are treated as diffuse types in clinicopathologic evaluations.

This classification is reasonably reproducible (206). In spite of apparent histologic differences, however, electron microscopy and mucin histochemistry have revealed characteristics of intestinal cells, such as well-developed microvilli and acidic mucin, in both intestinal and diffuse types (184, 185). On the other hand, only the intestinal-type carcinoma is associated with chronic atrophic gastritis, severe intestinal metaplasia, and dysplasia in the neighboring mucosa.

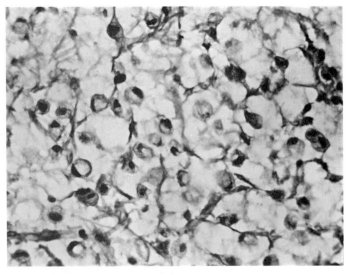

Figure 27.41 Signet-ring cell carcinoma cells with eccentric flattened nuclei and large globules of intracytoplasmic mucin in a mucinous stroma (×300).

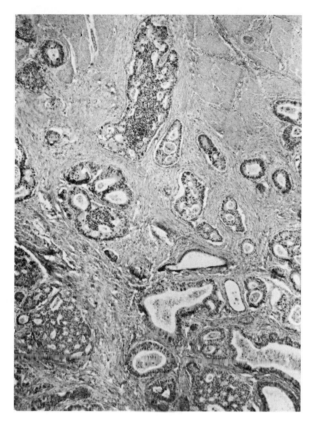

Figure 27.42 Expanding type adenocarcinoma showing glandular tumor tissue forming tubules and masses (×65).

of the tumor. As tumor growth progresses, the periphery of an expanding carcinoma may become less defined and show focal points of deep infiltration. Such a limited focal feature is insufficient to classify the tumor as infiltrative type. Instead, such a tumor may be qualified as an expanding carcinoma with focal infiltrative features, indicating a potential for diffuse infiltration.

The microscopic patterns of tumor growth are reflected in the gross appearances of the tumor. The expanding carcinoma shows sharply demarcated tumor mass (see Fig. 27.45), whereas the infiltrative carcinoma has indistinct tumor boundaries and does not form gross masses (see Fig. 27.34). These features correlate well with the gross morphology of the tumor (12, 211): the expanding carcinomas are polypoid or fungating and the infiltrative carcinomas are diffusely infiltrative. The ulcerated carcinomas are equally divided between the two types. Thus, this classification can be adopted for clinical usage and image analysis and at the time of surgical exploration.

Because the Ming classification is based on the growth pattern of the tumor, it imparts an important prognostic value. The survival rate of patients with expanding carcinoma has been found to be better than that in patients with infiltrative carcinoma (12, 210, 212, 213).

The Ming and Lauren classifications have some similarities. Intestinal-type carcinomas are mostly expanding carcinomas and the diffuse type carcinomas are infiltrative carcinomas. The solid carcinoma, unclassified in the Lauren classification, is an expanding carcinoma. Conversely, an intestinal-type tumor that is composed of

small glands and infiltrated diffusely without mass formation is an infiltrative-type carcinoma.

Other Classifications

In Japan, Nakamura (213) simply divided the gastric cancers into differentiated and undifferentiated types, using gland formation as the indicator for differentiation. The undifferentiated carcinomas include the poorly differentiated adenocarcinomas, signet-ring cell carcinomas, and mucinous carcinomas. Thus, the undifferentiated tumor in this classification is very different from the undifferentiated carcinoma in WHO histologic typing. This classification is used frequently in Japan, particularly in research pursuits.

In other classifications, Jass (214) separated gastric carcinomas into gastric and intestinal types based on a point system for various

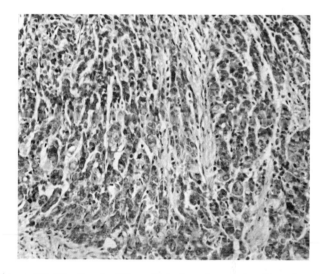

Figure 27.43 Poorly differentiated carcinoma in a Type IIc early gastric carcinoma shown in Figure 27.25.

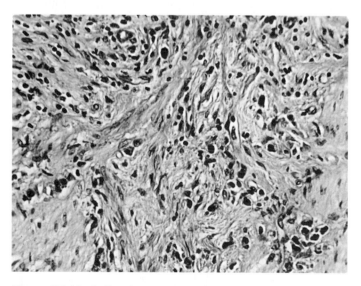

Figure 27.44 Infiltrative type carcinoma showing individual largely undifferentiated tumor cells between fascicles of muscle cells. A few cells have mucous globule in the cytoplasm (×200).

histologic features. Mulligan (215) divided gastric carcinomas into mucus cell (46.7%), pylorocardiac gland cell (29.7%), and intestinal cell types (23.6%). Goseki et al. classified gastric carcinoma into four groups based on the degree of tubular differentiation and amount of intracytoplasmic mucus (216): group I (40.0%): tubular differentiation well, mucus poor; group II (3.5%): tubular differentiation well, mucus rich; group III (20.0%): tubular differentiation poor, mucus poor; group IV (36.5%): tubular differentiation poor, mucus rich. Group I patients had a high frequency of liver metastasis, whereas group IV patients had more lymph node metastasis, peritoneal dissemination, and direct invasion of adjacent organs. Group III patients had intermediate findings.

Variants of Adenocarcinoma

Gastric adenocarcinomas are capable of differentiating into many types of cells that may or may not be indigenous to the normal stomach. Different types of cells are often present in the same tumor.

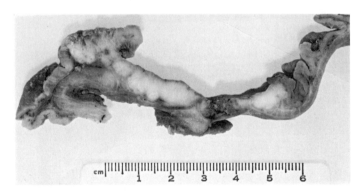

Figure 27.45 Cross-section of an expanding carcinoma showing the circumscribed tumor tissue involving the muscular layer. (Reprinted with permission from Ming SC. Tumors of the esophagus and stomach. In: Atlas of tumor pathology, second series, fascicle 7. Washington DC: Armed Forces Institute of Pathology, 1973:144–206.)

Occasionally, a specific cell type dominates and presents as a unique clinicopathologic entity. Such variant tumors include parietal cell carcinoma, Paneth cell carcinoma, hepatoid carcinoma, and mixed carcinoid-carcinoma.

Parietal cell carcinoma was first described by Capella et al. (193). The parietal cells in the tumor, which may vary in number (194), form poorly cohesive sheets resembling lymphoma (195). The identity of the cells is determined using electron microscopy. The patient profile is that of an old male with no specific symptoms.

Paneth cell carcinoma (192) is very rare. Only 4 cases have been reported. The cells are identified by electron microscopy and by the demonstration of lysozyme in the cells. No unusual clinical or gross morphologic features are found.

Hepatoid carcinoma and mixed carcinoid-carcinoma are described in subsequent sections.

MOLECULAR BIOLOGY AND MARKER SUBSTANCES

Many substances, including cancer-associated antigens, oncogenes, and other cell regulatory genes and proteins participate in the development of gastric carcinoma. The development of monoclonal antibodies against these substances allows direct pathologic study of the tumor tissue by immunohistochemical techniques. Advancement in molecular technology, such as the polymerase chain reaction and flow cytometry, further expands the scope of investigation. The application of these techniques in gastrointestinal cancer is presented in detail in Chapters 5, 7, and 8. Cell proliferation and kinetics of gastric carcinoma are discussed in Chapter 9.

Because gastric carcinomas are composed of gastric as well as intestinal cells, many types of mucins (74, 75, 83, 217), enzymes (190, 196, 211, 213, 218, 219), and hormones (190, 220, 221) related to these cells have been found in the carcinoma. The neutral mucus, being specific for the gastric mucous cells, is useful in identifying the gastric origin of secondary tumors (222).

The carcinoembryonic antigen (CEA), a commonly tested oncofetal antigen, has been demonstrated in gastric tumors as well as in the dysplastic and metaplastic tissue (86, 223, 224). The serum

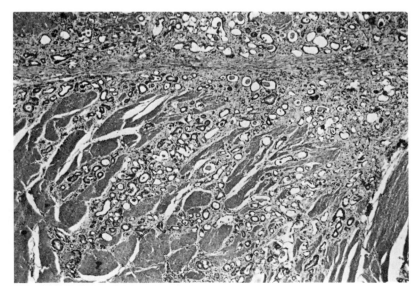

Figure 27.46 Infiltrative carcinoma showing infiltration of muscularis propria by individual small glands (×50).

levels of CEA and CA19-9 have been used to evaluate clinical courses (225–227). Another possible application of tumor markers is for screening a high-risk population. Serum levels of pepsinogen I and II have been used in screening (228). Fetal sulfoglycoprotein antigen was used in a mass survey (229). Positive results were obtained in about 9% of persons tested, of whom only 1% had carcinoma.

Gastric carcinomas have been studied for their DNA content and ploidy patterns. In general, 60 to 70% of gastric carcinomas are aneuploid (230, 231), more frequent in the glandular tumors, whereas the nonglandular infiltrative carcinomas are mostly diploid, particularly in the early stage. It has been noted that the intramucosally located signet-ring cells are nearly always diploid and the aneuploid cell population is found only focally in the deeply invasive portions of the tumor (230, 232). This finding correlates well with the slow rate of growth at the early stage of such tumors in both men and animals (157, 164). The polyploid and aneuploid carcinomas have high cell-proliferation activity and positive expression of epidermal growth factor receptor (233). They show deeper invasion, more lymph node metastases, and worse prognosis than diploid tumors and tumors with homogeneous ploidy (166, 230, 231, 234, 235). The ploidy patterns in the primary and recurrent tumors are consistent (236). The poor prognosis of the infiltrating carcinoma may be related to their invasiveness and frequent peritoneal metastasis, in spite of their low ploidy. Genetic alterations are different between the well-differentiated glandular carcinomas and the nonglandular infiltrative carcinomas (237): the former show alterations in c-erbB-2, bcl-2, cyclin E, APC, DCC; the latter show amplification of K-sam and mutation or loss of cadherin.

Several oncogenes, including K-sam, c-met, c-erbB-2, ras, and c-myc, have been demonstrated in gastric carcinoma (237–240). Expression and mutation of tumor suppressor gene p53 occur early in the intestinal and expansive types of tumors and late in the diffuse tumors, but no type difference is noted in advanced carcinomas (78, 241–243). Genome instability in gastric carcinomas has been shown to involve microsatellites on chromosomes 3p, 5q (APC and MCC loci), and 17p (p53 loci) with repair errors or loss of heterozygosity (244–246), but not on loci seen in hereditary nonpolyposis colorectal cancers (247). Such tumors tend to be advanced and poorly differentiated (244, 248). The expression of bcl-2 gene, known to suppress programmed cell death, has been detected in intestinal-type cancer, as well as in areas of intestinal metaplasia and dysplastic tissue (249). Many other genes, growth factors and their receptors, and cell proliferation regulators have been studied. The results are well summarized by Tahara and other authors (237–239, 243), who indicate that genetic instability, telomerase activity, p53 mutation, and CD44 abnormality are present in the early stage of gastric oncogenesis and oncogene activation and overexpression of growth factors are involved in cancer progression (237).

PROGRESSION OF GASTRIC CARCINOMA

LOCAL SPREAD

Gastric carcinomas break through the basement membrane and invade the lamina propria early in the course (250); the stage of in situ carcinoma is rarely observed (251). From the lamina propria, the tumor cells infiltrate along the blood vessels through muscularis mucosae into the submucosa, in which the cells proliferate to form balloon-like expansion (252). As the tumor penetrates the serosa, it may involve the neighboring organ or seed the peritoneal lining; the latter is more common in nonglandular than glandular carcinomas (253). A tumor of the upper part of the stomach may extend directly into the esophagus. At the pyloric end, involvement of the duodenum is usually subserosal and only rarely does the tumor extend into the submucosa or mucosa.

METASTASIS

Lymphatic permeation may occur in the deep mucosa (254, 255), and lymph node metastases have been reported in 0 to 17% of intramucosal carcinomas and 13 to 30% of submucosal carcinomas in Japan (256, 285). The corresponding ranges in Europe were 1.5 to 7% and 4 to 12.3%, respectively (285). At NCCH, lymph node metastases were seen in 2.1% of patients with mucosal tumors and in 13.9% of patients with submucosal invasion. The rate of lymph node metastasis for early cancer was related to the size (257), growth pattern (182), and ulceration of the primary tumor. The metastasis from mucosal cancer was limited to the primary regional nodes, but submucosal cancers may spread to the secondary or tertiary nodes (258). With deeper tumor invasion comes an increase in the incidence of lymph node involvement.

Blood vessel invasion begins in the submucosa (250). By these vascular channels, the tumor cells spread to distant organs. Liver and lung are most frequently involved. Hematogenous spread to the ovary occurs more frequently in signet-ring cell carcinoma than in glandular carcinoma. Such an ovarian tumor is known as Krukenberg tumor. The stomach is the site of the primary tumor in 70% of cases (259).

RECURRENCE AFTER RESECTION

The rate of recurrence of early gastric cancer 5 years postoperatively is around 3% in patients with intramucosal carcinoma and 8 to 9% in those with submucosal carcinoma. The recurrence rates 10 years postoperatively may be as high as 10 to 22% in patients with submucosal carcinoma and 8 to 14% in those with intramucosal tumor. Early recurrence generally occurs in cases with submucosal cancer, whereas late recurrence is common in those with mucosal tumor. Papillary and differentiated adenocarcinomas frequently show hepatic metastases, whereas other types of carcinoma more often lead to local recurrence, including peritoneal seeding of cancer cells. The study by the American College of Surgeons (174) cited a recurrence rate of 38.9%. The level of CEA was elevated in 50% of patients with recurrence.

TNM STAGING

The American Joint Committee on Cancer (AJCC) and UICC (Union Internationale Contre le Cancer, International Union Against Cancer) developed a TNM staging system (260) based on the depth of tumor invasion (T), the extent of lymph node involvement (N), and the presence of distant metastasis (M). This system has been revised periodically so that the stages would correlate closely with the survival rate. The AJCC system and definitions of the terms published in 1992 (208) are summarized in Table 27.7. It should be noted that pure in situ gastric carcinoma is rare and stage 0 patients have not been listed in the reported series of cases. The data are further specified as cTNM if clinically obtained or pTNM if pathologically verified. A report by the American College of Surgeons on 6742 patients with histologically confirmed gastric adenocarcinoma revealed that 17.1% of patients had stage I carcinoma, 16.9% stage II, 35.5% stage III, and 30.5% stage IV. (174). The stage of tumor is directly related to the outcome of the disease.

The UICC TNM system has also undergone several revisions (261–263) (see Table 27.7). In addition to the TNM categories just listed, a residual tumor (R) classification is required to indicate postoperative status of the tumor. The R0 status implies resection for cure. R0 may be further divided into R0a for negative tests for tumor markers and R0b for elevated or rising marker levels within 4 months of a R0 operation.

In view of the prognostic significance of the number of tumor-positive lymph nodes and of the ratio between the number of metastatic lymph nodes and that of total lymph nodes examined (263–266), the N0 status requires pathologic confirmation of

---

TABLE 27.7 TNM Staging of Gastric Carcinoma According to AJCC and UICC

Stage grouping
  Stage 0: Tis N0 M0
  Stage IA: T1 N0 M0
       IB: T1 N1 M0; or T2 N0 M0
  Stage II: T1 N2 M0; or T2 N1 M0; or T3 N0 M0
  Stage IIIA: T2 N2 M0; or T3 N1 M0; or T4 N0 M0
       IIIB: T3 N2 M0; or T4 N1 M0
  Stage IV: T4 N2 M0; or any T any N M1
Definitions and additional subdivisions
  Tis—In situ tumor
  T1—T1a: Tumor invades lamina propria
       T1b: Tumor invades submucosa
  T2—T2a: Tumor invades muscularis propria
       T2b: Tumor invades subserosa
  T3—Tumor penetrates serosa without invading adjacent structures
  T4—Tumor invades adjacent structures
  N0—No lymph node metastasis
  N1—Involved node within 3 cm of primary tumor
  N2—Involved nodes more than 3 cm from primary tumor
       For either N1 or N2: a: involving 1–3 nodes, b: involving 4–6 nodes, c: involving 7 or more nodes
  M0—No distant metastasis
  M1—M1a: metastasis to distant nodes
       M1b: metastasis to viscera
       M1c: metastasis to peritoneum or pleura
  R0—No residual tumor
  R1—Microscopic residual tumor present
  R2—Gross residual tumor present

Data from Beahrs OH, Henson DE, Hunter RVP, et al., eds. Manual for staging of cancer. 4th ed. Philadelphia: JB Lippincott, 1992:63–67; Hermanek P, Sobin LH, eds. UICC: TNM classification of malignant tumours. 4th ed. 2nd rev. Berlin: Springer, 1992; Hermanek P, Henson DE, Hutter RVP, et al., eds. UICC: TNM supplement 1993—a commentary on uniform use. Berlin: Springer, 1992; Hermanek P, Wittekind C. News of TNM and its use for classification of gastric cancer. World J Surg 1995;19:491–495.

---

negative nodes among a minimum of 15 nodes examined in an extended gastrectomy specimen.

In the Japanese classification of gastric cancer, the presence of hepatic (H) and peritoneal (P) metastasis is also taken into account in the staging of gastric cancer. The N categories are designated N1 to N4 according to the four location groups of lymph nodes listed by the Japanese Research Society for Gastric Cancer (173).

PROGNOSTIC FACTORS

The most important prognostic factor for gastric carcinoma is the TNM stage of the tumor at the time of diagnosis or resection. The report by the American College of Surgeons (174) showed that the overall 5-year survival rate for U.S. patients was 14%, and disease-specific survival rate was 26%. The survival rate for stage I patients was 50%, stage IA 59%, stage IB 44%, stage II 29%, stage III 13%, stage IIIa 15%, stage IIB 9%, and stage IV 3%. The survival rate for R0 patients was 35%, R1 patients 13%, and R2 patients 3%. The reported overall 5-year survival rate was 37% in Germany (264), 47% in Korea (267), and 72% in Japan (268). The higher survival rates in these countries may be related to a high percentage of stage I carcinomas (50% in Japan and 17% in the United States) and extensive surgical dissection (268). Among the stage-related factors, lymph node involvement is the most important factor among surgically treated patients. Extended lymphadenectomy results in improved survival.

The biologic behavior of the tumor, as manifested in its growth patterns, influences the prognosis (12, 212, 269, 270). The survival rate of the expanding carcinoma is better than that of the infiltrative carcinoma, independent of other features of the tumor (211, 271, 272). Similarly, the prognosis of intestinal-type carcinoma is better than that of diffuse carcinoma (13, 212, 263, 271), in part related to lymphatic involvement (211, 272). Prognosis is influenced by the extent of serosal and peritoneal involvement (273, 274), which is common in the infiltrative carcinoma (274). Furthermore, the percentage of signet-ring cells in the tumor is inversely related to the survival rate (275). Heavy infiltration of lymphocytes and Langerhans cells in the tumor stroma is a favorable prognostic sign (276, 277). Also favorable is the presence of parietal cells (194, 195, 278), endocrine cells (220), or oncogene c-myc product p62 (279). Unfavorable indicators are the overexpression of epidermal growth factor and its receptor (280, 281), c-erbB-2 (282, 283), p53 (284–286), CEA (287), HCG (288), lysozyme (289), estrogen receptor (290), and aneuploidy of the tumor cells (230, 231, 233, 234, 291). Reduction or loss of E-cadherin, a tumor invasion suppressor, is seen in tumors with a low rate of survival (292). Prognosis is poor for tumors of the upper stomach or entire stomach (173, 234, 263), but other locations have no effect on outcome. Factors with questionable effects include the grade of tumor differentiation (174, 268, 293), the size of the tumor (268, 269, 294), and Goseki's classification (295, 296). Factors that appear to have little significance include the gender, age, and race of patients, the duration of symptoms, and WHO histologic type of the tumor (269, 293).

CLINICOPATHOLOGIC CORRELATION
CLINICAL PRESENTATIONS AND DIAGNOSIS

The stomach is a voluminous organ. Its large chamber allows the tumor to grow to a large size before its effects become clinically evident. Obstruction is neither an early nor a common manifestation of the gastric tumors, unless they occur at the portal of entry or exit. The symptoms are usually nonspecific and vague. Epigastric discomfort and dyspepsia are common, resulting in part from tumor-associated conditions, such as gastritis. Ulcerated lesions may bleed and cause anemia. Occult blood in the stool is common, but massive bleeding is rare (297). Anemia may be associated with gastritis. Weight loss is seen in patients with advanced malignant tumors and is the common finding (298). Unusual presentations include free perforation of the stomach (299), hypoglycemia (300), granulocytosis (301), pneumatosis cystoides (302), thrombocytopenic purpura and immune complex disease (303), microangiopathy (304), and hepatic failure owing to intrasinusoidal metastasis (305). The duration of symptoms generally is less than 1 year, although the tumor is large and advanced at the time of diagnosis.

These clinical manifestations are not specific and the diagnosis often depends on direct visualization of the lesion by either radiologic imaging or endoscopic studies, which have an accuracy rate of nearly 90%. The rate of correct diagnosis reaches 97% when both methods are applied (306).

Even with such examinations, the nature of the lesion may not be determined until a histologic examination is performed. Biopsy may be problematic. According to the authors of one study, the major reasons for false-negative diagnosis after biopsy are inadequate number of biopsy specimens (less than 7) and misdiagnosis by the pathologists when the number of positive biopsy samples was three or less (307). Conversely, a false-positive diagnosis may be given because of misinterpretation of abnormal but benign cells in the specimen (308).

Difficulties in diagnosis may be encountered in specific situations. For instance, an early Type IIb gastric carcinoma may be grossly invisible, and an ulcerated carcinoma may be indistinguishable from a benign ulcer. For such lesions and for follow-up examination of patients with severe dysplasia, a liberal number of biopsy specimens may be required to achieve a high rate of correct diagnoses. Another helpful procedure is the cytologic examination (309), which can also be fruitful for screening and follow-up studies. (See Chapters 3 and 4 for detailed discussions of endoscopic and cytologic studies, respectively.)

The differential diagnosis of primary gastric tumors mainly involves the distinction between primary lymphoma of the stomach and solid undifferentiated gastric carcinoma of expanding type. Features favoring carcinoma include pleomorphism of tumor cells; circumscription of tumor nodules; the presence of markers for epithelial tumors such as mucin, cytokeratin, and CEA; desmoplastic response in the stroma; the polyclonal and heterogeneous nature of lymphoid cells; and precancerous lesions in the adjacent mucosa.

The primary nature of a gastric carcinoma usually is evident. Occasionally, it must be differentiated from a metastatic tumor. Metastatic tumors in the stomach are rare. They usually are small and submucosal, covered by intact mucosa. When a pancreatic or esophageal adenocarcinoma extends into the stomach, the differentiation against the primary tumor may be difficult and at times impossible. Identification is based primarily on the location of the bulk of the tumor and the presence of precursor lesions in the surrounding mucosa.

TREATMENT AND END RESULTS

Surgical resection of the tumor remains the treatment of choice. In the United States, many cases are diagnosed in the advanced stage,

and resection was performed in about 55% of cases (174). Curable resection is possible in only 30 to 60% of resected cases (174, 175). The end results of treatment are poor: overall 5-year survival rate is around 14% and that in patients with curable resection is about 30% (174, 310). Only 3% of the patients who did not undergo resection survived 4 years (311). In Germany (284) and Japan (268), curable resection was performed on 71.5 and 76.6% of patients, respectively, and the 5-year survival rate of these patients was 47.8 and 87.5%, respectively. The better survival rates in these countries than in the United States is related to extensive surgical dissection (312).

The 5- and 10-year survival rates after resection for early cancer without lymph node metastasis is 94 to 100% (313–315). The 5-year survival rates for EGC with N1 and N2 status are 67% and 42%, respectively (314). In recent years, EGC less than 1 cm in diameter and without node metastasis have been treated endoscopically, primarily by snare resection, followed by surgical resection or endoscopic laser therapy if residual tumor is present. Hiki reported complete disappearance of 43 tumors so treated (314). He also reported that endoscopic laser therapy alone showed a high rate of residual tumor if the lesion was 4 cm in diameter or larger. The residual lesions disappeared after repeated therapy. Post-therapy biopsy was emphasized.

For advanced cancer, postoperative adjuvant chemotherapy and radiotherapy have shown few beneficial effects (316–320). On the other hand, preoperative neoadjuvant chemotherapy for locally advanced cancer may cause remission and render unresectable tumors resectable in 40 to 60% of cases (317, 320). Kim used postoperative immunochemotherapy to enhance patients' immune response, followed by a multidrug chemotherapy regimen for stage III patients. The 5-year survival rate of treated patients was 45%, whereas that of patients treated with surgery alone was 24% (314). It is hopeful that new treatment methods may be developed to control advanced lesions (320).

ADENOCARCINOMA OF THE ESOPHAGOGASTRIC JUNCTION AND GASTRIC CARDIA

Adenocarcinoma of the esophagogastric junction (EGJ) is defined as a tumor with the center located within 2 cm of the anatomic EGJ. The distal one half of this region encompasses the gastric cardia. A similar proposal was made by Misumi and colleagues (321) and Siewert et al. (322), who used 1 cm above the EGJ as the upper limit for the tumor. A tumor located above the EGJ is an esophageal adenocarcinoma (EAC), and that below the EGJ is a cardiac adenocarcinoma (CAC). In the presence of Barrett epithelium, however, the squamocolumnar junction is no longer a marker for EGJ. Furthermore, the tumor may have destroyed or altered the appearance of the EGJ. The basis for deciding the origin of the tumor in such cases is circumstantial, relying on factors such as the appearance of the surrounding tissues and the presence of specific constituent structures of the respective organs. Clearly, these features are not applicable to a biopsy specimen. In some cases, the incompletely intestinalized epithelium, if present, is a reasonably reliable clue to the esophageal origin of the tumor tissue.

Adenocarcinomas of the EGJ and esophagus share many clinical features, including age at presentation, male predominance, symptom complexes related to hiatal hernia and reflux esophagitis, and a history of smoking and drinking (323–327). Thus, EAC and

CAC at the EGJ may be considered a single entity. In terms of full understanding and management of the case, these tumors should be separated. For instance, it is best to examine the extent and location of Barrett epithelium in patients with EAC and the degree and extent of intestinal metaplasia in the stomach of patients with CAC.

The incidence of adenocarcinoma at the EGJ has increased (328). At Temple University Hospital, the percentage of cardiac carcinoma among gastric carcinomas increased from 16% for 1976 to 1980 to 25% for 1991 to 1995. Antonioli and Goldman (329) reported an increase in the incidence of cardiac carcinoma in Boston from 0 to 27% of all gastric carcinomas. They also noted, however, an increase in the number of signet-ring cell carcinomas, a decreased male-to-female ratio, and an increase in the age of patients. Similar observations were made in the United Kingdom (330).

Most early cardiac carcinomas are elevated (331). Of 500 advanced carcinomas analyzed in China (332) 16% were fungating, 36.4% ulcerated with raised margins, 28% ulcerated infiltrative, and 19.2% diffusely infiltrative. Histologically, most tumors are well differentiated and about one tenth are mucinous. In our cases, 10% were signet-ring cell carcinomas. In contrast, among carcinomas of the distal stomach, 28% were signet ring type, and 8% of the tumors had well-differentiated glands resembling hyperplastic cardiac glands (332).

The cardiac carcinomas often invade the esophagus (57% of cases in one study) (333). The prognosis is poor (173, 294, 324). The overall postresection survival rate is 19.2% at 5 years and 8.5% at 10 years (332). The survival rate is lower in patients with esophageal involvement than in those without involvement of the esophagus (333). Aneuploidy has been found in 61 to 96% of adenocarcinomas of the EGJ, more frequently in tumors with infiltrative growth (234, 335). Aneuploid carcinomas were in late stages, had more lymph node metastasis, and were associated with short disease-free intervals after surgery.

SQUAMOUS CELL CARCINOMA, ADENOSQUAMOUS CARCINOMA, AND MUCOEPIDERMOID CARCINOMA

Squamous cells have been identified by electron microscopy in human gastric adenocarcinomas as well as in experimentally induced carcinomas in rats (5, 336), although they rarely are sufficiently prominent to justify the diagnosis of adenosquamous carcinoma. Pure squamous cell carcinoma is even rarer. Mori et al. (337) found 16 adenosquamous carcinomas (0.3%) and 4 squamous cell carcinomas (0.08%) among 5000 resected gastric carcinomas. The incidences of adenosquamous carcinoma reported by other authors were about 0.2 to 0.5% (338–340). In 1995, Volpe et al. reported that only 22 cases of pure squamous cell carcinoma had been reported (341).

The tumors may occur anywhere in the stomach; more than 50% arise in the antrum. One pure squamous cell carcinoma occurred in a gastric stump (342). Most tumors are large and ulcerated. Diffusely infiltrative lesions are rare. Histologically, the adenosquamous carcinomas are composed of elements of adenocarcinoma and squamous cells, separately or intermingled (Fig. 27.47). The glandular components have features of intestinal-type carcinoma and the adjacent mucosa shows evidence of gastritis and colonic type of intestinal metaplasia (343). Of 28 cases of adenocarcinoma studied by Mori et al. (344), 16 were differentiated and 12 were undifferentiated. The squamous cell carcinomas are moderately differentiated with keratinization and pearl formation. Reexamination with multiple sections allowed Mori et al. to find minute areas of adenocarcinoma in three of four tumors originally diagnosed as pure squamous cell carcinoma (337). The biologic behavior of these tumors in terms of their gross forms, depth of invasion, and mode of vascular permeation corresponded with that of similar adenocarcinomas without squamous differentiation.

Histogenesis of these tumors is uncertain, but the following possibilities have been suggested: invasion or metastasis from carcinomas in the neighboring organs, particularly the esophagus; squamous differentiation from totipotential stem cells; squamous metaplasia of adenocarcinoma; and malignant change of preexisting squamous mucosa, which may be ectopic or metaplastic.

Invasion of esophageal squamous carcinoma into the gastric cardia usually can be determined by the gross appearance, and the metastatic lesion is submucosal, often from a midesophageal tumor (345). Uncommonly, a large cardiac tumor may represent a metastasis from a small esophageal tumor (346). Some tumors are accompanied by benign squamous epithelium in the gastric mucosa, suggesting that the tumor originated from the preexisting squamous cells, either metaplastic (340) or heterotopic (347). In most cases, no benign squamous mucosa is present. In these cases, it is difficult to assess whether the squamous cells in the tumor are metaplastic cells of adenocarcinoma or are derived from totipotential stem cells. The presence of both tonofilaments and mucous granules in the same cell (348) support either view.

Clinically, men are affected more often than women (male-to-female ratio, 2.5:1 (340, 341, 343, 344). Patients range in age from 29 to 88 years (340), and many are under the age of 40 years (343, 344). The symptoms and sign are the same as for other gastric cancers. The prognosis is poor (344, 349).

Mucoepidermoid carcinoma is another tumor that contains both glandular and squamous cells. Szogi (350) found 21 cases in the literature and reported another case, postulating the origin of this lesion from ectopic pancreatic tissue. Hayashi et al. (351) reported another case and described tumor cells in continuity with ectopic submucosal glands.

HEPATOID ADENOCARCINOMA

Hepatoid adenocarcinoma contains a mixture of histologically recognizable features of hepatocellular carcinoma and adenocarcinoma (197, 198, 352, 353). The hepatoid cells are capable of secreting albumin, α-fetoprotein (AFP), α-1-antitrypsin, α-1-antichymotrypsin, and, occasionally, bile (197, 352). The serum level of AFP is often increased (352). Most tumors are fungating, but they may be ulcerated. Metastasis to the liver is common, and prognosis is poor (197, 353, 354). AFP has also been found in carcinomas without hepatoid cells. Nagai et al. (353) found 28 hepatoid tumors among 7200 gastric carcinomas and 22 adenocarcinomas that were AFP-positive but had no hepatoid cells. Of the hepatoid tumors, 15 were AFP-positive and 13 were AFP-negative. Irrespective of AFP status, the 5-year survival rate for these cases was 11.9%. The survival rate for AFP-positive adenocarcinomas is 38.2%. One patient had primary hepatoid carcinoma of the stomach

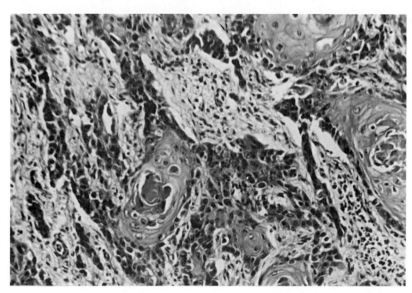

Figure 27.47 Adenosquamous carcinoma showing squamous cells with keratinizing pearls admixed with poorly differentiated tubular adenocarcinoma (×200).

with liver metastases and a primary hepatocellular carcinoma of the liver associated with hepatitis C infection (355). The gastric tumor was AFP-positive, but the primary tumor of the liver was AFP-negative.

TERATOMA, CHORIOCARCINOMA, AND YOLK SAC CARCINOMA

Teratomas and choriocarcinomas are rare in the stomach. Teratoma was first described in 1922 by Eusterman and Senty (356), who reported two cases of dermoid cysts in the stomach; one weighed 1000 g in an 8-year-old boy and the other measured 6 cm in the greatest dimension in a 31-year-old man. By 1981, Cairo et al. (357) reviewed 51 cases, with only 2 in female patients. The majority of gastric teratomas occurred in infants, some in utero (358). They accounted for 1% of teratomas in boys, but only 6 cases involved tumors in female infants (359). The tumor manifests as an abdominal mass, sometimes bleeding and occasionally causing obstruction. Pathologically, teratomas are large and may project either into the stomach or outward into the abdominal cavity. Tissues of all three germ layers are present, including teeth (357). Teratomas are benign and curable by resection (360).

Choriocarcinomas, the highly malignant tumors with poor prognosis, are characterized by the presence of syncytial and cytotrophoblasts that secrete human chorionic gonadotropin (HCG) (361–364). The serum level of HCG may be elevated and serves as a marker for prognosis (364). Immunohistochemical studies reveal that both α- and β-subunits of HCG are secreted by the tumor (365), and that the secretion is more abundant in the syncytial than in the cytotrophoblasts (362, 366). Human placental lactogen and pregnancy-specific glycoprotein have also been found in the cytotrophoblasts (363). Clinically, a male patient may manifest gynecomastia (367). It should be noted that HCG is commonly present in gastric adenocarcinoma cells. Among 124 carcinomas analyzed by Fukayama et al. (365), HCG-α was present in 39, HCG-β in 63, and both subunits in 26 tumors—α-subunits

in papillary and tubular tumors and normal gastric epithelium, and β-subunits in microtubular and mucocellular tumors and, rarely, normal cells. In four tumors, both units were present synchronously.

Choriocarcinoma often occurs together with adenocarcinoma. Of 47 cases analyzed by Garcia and Ghall (366), 28 had both adenocarcinoma and choriocarcinoma in the primary tumor; 13 had only choriocarcinoma and 6 only adenocarcinoma in the stomach and choriocarcinoma in the metastasis. In one case, only a focus of intramucosal carcinoma was found. In another report, choriocarcinoma coexisted with hepatoid carcinoma in the same tumor (368). In yet another case, yolk sac tumor with positive α-antitrypsin was found in the same tumor (366). Yolk sac carcinoma is rarely found in the stomach. Only two other cases have been reported (369), one together with adenocarcinoma components, and the other demonstrating positive AFP and gastrin immunostaining.

CARCINOID, CARCINOID-ADENOCARCINOMA, AND SMALL CELL CARCINOMA

The stomach is a common location for carcinoid, accounting for 10 to 30% of all such lesions (370). They arise mainly from the enterochromaffin-like cell located in the upper portion of the stomach, under the influence of hypergastrinemia (370). Thus, they are associated with chronic atrophic gastritis or Zollinger-Ellison syndrome with multiple endocrine neoplasia type 1. The lesions are multiple, small, and benign. In sporadic cases, these lesions have different cell types and are large and aggressive (371).

Rarely, carcinoid-carcinoma occurs in the stomach. In such tumors, the carcinoid cells are near diploid and carcinoma cell aneuploid (372). They are either combination tumors with admixed endocrine and exocrine cells, or composite tumors with separate groups of cell types. The endocrine cells secrete a variety of hormones (373). In one case, the tumor secreted parathyroid hormone-related protein causing hypercalcemia (374). In one report, a carcinoid-carcinoma was accompanied by multiple separate carcinoids in the fundic mucosa in a woman with nonantral gastric atrophy (375). (See Chapter 15 for detailed information about these tumors.)

Small cell carcinomas rarely occur in the stomach. Only eight cases have been reported up to 1990 (376). In one case, the tumor was early, with three independent foci of adenocarcinomas in the same stomach (377). These tumors manifest as an ulcerated mass and are composed of small cells with hyperchromatic nuclei and scanty cytoplasm (Fig. 27.48), similar to those seen in the small cell carcinoma of the lung. Foci of adenocarcinoma or squamous cell differentiation were present in one half of reported tumors (378, 379). The tumor cells contain neurosecretory granules and show positive reactions for chromogranin and nonspecific enolase and negative reactions for carcinoembryonic antigen and epithelial

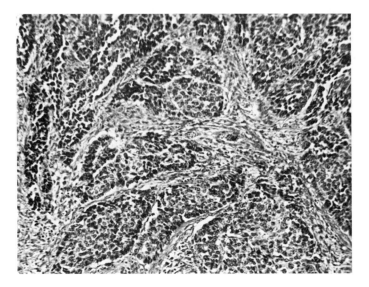

Figure 27.48   Small cell carcinoma showing groups of small tumor cells with dark nuclei and scanty cytoplasm (×120).

membrane antigen (376). The prognosis is poor (380). Most patients died within 1 year of diagnosis.

CARCINOSARCOMA

Carcinosarcoma of the stomach is composed in part of adenocarcinoma and in part of spindle-cell sarcoma in varying degrees of intermingling and admixture (Fig. 27.49). When two tumor components are in contact only at the interface, the tumor is a collision tumor formed by two separate tumors. In a composite tumor, two elements are largely separate but mixed irregularly in some portions, probably the result of separate growth from different cell lines within the same tumor. A combination tumor has evenly mixed components, suggesting differentiation of the same cell line along separate pathways. Of 24 cases of carcinosarcoma of the stomach analyzed by Tanimura and Furuta (381), 9 were thought to be collision tumors, 7 combination tumors, 6 composite tumors, and 2 of uncertain type.

By immunohistochemical study (382), the epithelial tumor cells showed positive reaction for cytokeratin, carcinoembryonic antigen, and epithelial membrane antigen. The spindle tumor cells were positive for vimentin, desmin, and, focally, cytokeratin as well. Thus, the sarcomatous tissue probably derived from the carcinoma cells; the term "sarcomatoid carcinoma" has been applied. The tumor reported by Kumagai et al. (383) was mostly sarcomatous, with teratomatous areas in addition to papillary adenocarcinoma. The sarcomatous tissue may show cartilaginous (384) or smooth muscle (385) differentiation.

UNDIFFERENTIATED CARCINOMA

Undifferentiated carcinoma in the WHO classification lacks any specific evidence of differentiation, structurally or functionally. This tumor is not equal to the "undifferentiated" carcinoma in the

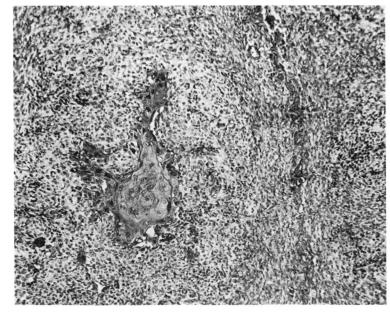

Figure 27.49   Carcinosarcoma showing a patch of squamous cells surrounded by sarcomatous tissue. (Reprinted with permission from Ming SC. Tumors of the esophagus and stomach. In: Atlas of tumor pathology, second series, fascicle 7. Washington DC: Armed Forces Institute of Pathology, 1973:144–206.)

Japanese classification; the latter term is applied to any tumor without good glandular or tubular structures and includes the poorly differentiated as well as some of the differentiated carcinomas, such as signet-ring cell carcinoma.

A subset of undifferentiated carcinomas show prominent lymphocytic infiltration in and around solid carcinoma nodules. They have been called carcinomas with lymphoid stroma or lymphoepithelioma-like carcinomas (65, 200), and are thought to be related to EBV (see previous section concerning Epstein-Barr virus). These tumors have been found in 3.8 to 7.2% of gastric carcinomas (200, 201). Within these tumors, T lymphocytes were in and around tumor cell nests, but B cells were clustered in lymphoid follicles outside the tumor mass. Such tumors occur predominantly in males and are located mainly in the upper part of the stomach (201, 386). Grossly, they manifest no special features. In one report, 50% of the tumors were early lesions (201). The advanced tumors are ulcerated (387). More than 80% of these tumors are EBV positive (65, 67, 386). The prognosis is better than that for ordinary adenocarcinoma of the stomach (388).

MULTIPLE PRIMARY CARCINOMAS

Multiple primary adenocarcinomas have been found in 5 to 21% of resected stomachs (183, 389, 390). The incidence of multiplicity is 8.4% among EGC and 4.7% among advanced cancers (391). Multiple early carcinomas were found in 8.3% of 500 gastric cancer cases at NCCH in Tokyo. Two lesions were present in 77% of the cases, 3 lesions in 20%, and 4 or more lesions in 3%. In patients 65 years of age and older, the rate of multiple tumors was 13%, twice that of the group younger than age 65 years. Kodera et al. (392) found multiple gastric carcinoma in 160 of 2790 surgical patients (5.7%). The diagnosis was made preoperatively in 50% of the cases. Of 126 patients with multiple gastric cancers, only one developed another carcinoma in the remnant stomach. The background gastric mucosa frequently revealed extensive intestinal metaplasia. It was suggested that the large early carcinomas might be formed by the collision of multiple small lesions (390). The presence of coexisting small early carcinoma in the cancerous stomach is often overlooked during routine endoscopy. Accuracy of diagnosis can be improved with the use of congo red-methylene blue test during the examination (393).

From 2 to 7% of patients with gastric carcinoma have malignant lesions in other organs, synchronously in about one third to one half of cases (394–396). One half to one third of the lesions were in other segments of the digestive tract, most commonly the colorectum. Ikeda et al. (397) found 13 patients with both gastric and colonic carcinomas among 447 gastric (2.9%) and 199 colorectal (6.5%) cancer patients. It is not clear, however, whether or not the incidence of second tumor is higher than that in the general population (394, 398).

SECONDARY AND METASTATIC TUMORS

Tumors of neighboring organs, such as esophagus, pancreas, and transverse colon, may extend directly into the stomach. Metastasis to the stomach is uncommon; evidence was found at autopsy in about 0.2% of cases (399). The majority of these tumors were carcinomas. The primary site of the tumors was the lung in about 50% of cases (400). The other relatively common primary sites were pancreas, esophagus, colon, breast, and melanomas of the skin. The metastatic lesions in the stomach are mainly submucosal. The large tumors may become polypoid with an ulcerated crater, causing bleeding, pain, or obstruction (400).

Metastasis from esophageal carcinoma to the gastric cardia was found in 5.6% of cases, mainly by intramural spread (401). The incidence of metastasis to the gastrointestinal tract from breast carcinoma is 8 to 15% (399), sometimes resulting in diffuse thickening of the gastric wall as in linitis plastica (402, 403). The metastatic lesion in the stomach from cutaneous melanoma may become ulcerated and cause massive bleeding (404, 405).

REFERENCES

1. Parker SL, Tong T, Bolden S, et al. Cancer statistics, 1997. CA Cancer J Clin 1997;47:5–27.
2. Ming SC. Tumors of the esophagus and stomach. In: Atlas of tumor pathology, second series, fascicle 7. Washington DC: Armed Forces Institute of Pathology, 1973;82.
3. Ming SC, Yu PL. Histogenesis of experimental colonic carcinoma. In: Rozen P, Reich CB, Winawer SJ, eds. Large bowel cancer: Policy, prevention, research and treatment. Front Gastrointest Res 1991;18:200–224.
4. Hirota T, Okada T, Itabashi M, et al. Histogenesis of human gastric cancer—with special reference to the significance of adenoma as a precancerous lesion In: Ming SC, ed. Precursors of gastric cancer. New York: Praeger, 1984;233–252.
5. Sasano N, Nakamura K, Arai M, et al. Ultrastructural cell patterns in human gastric carcinoma compared with non neoplastic gastric mucosa—histogenetic analysis of carcinoma by mucin histochemistry. J Natl Cancer Inst 1969;43:783–802.
6. Meissner WA. Leiomyoma of the stomach. Arch Pathol Lab Med 1944;38:207–209.
7. World Health Organization. 1994 World health statistics Annual. Geneva: World Health Organization, 1995;B396–B407.
8. Neugut AI, Hayek M, Howe G. Epidemiology of gastric cancer. Semin Oncol 1995;23:281–291.
9. Kosary CL, Ries LAG, Miller BA, et al. SEER cancer statistics review, 1973–1992: Tables and graphs. Bethesda: National Cancer Institute. NIH Publ. No. 96-2789, 1996.
10. Munoz N, Asvall J. Time trends of intestinal and diffuse types of gastric cancer in Norway. Int J Cancer 1971;8:144–157.
11. Whitehead R, Skinner JM, Heenan PJ. Incidence of carcinoma of stomach and tumor type. Br J Cancer 1974;30:370–372.
12. Ming SC. Gastric carcinoma: A pathobiological classification. Cancer 1977;39:2475–2485.
13. Lauren P. The two histological main types of gastric carcinoma. Diffuse and so-called intestinal type carcinoma. An attempt at histoclinical classification. Acta Pathol Microbiol Scand 1965;64:31–49.
14. Tso PL, Bringaze WL 3rd, Dauterive AH, et al. Gastric carcinoma in the young. Cancer 1987;59:1362–1365.
15. Grabiec J, Owen DA. Carcinoma of the stomach in young persons. Cancer 1985;56:388–396.
16. Bloss RS, Miller TA, Copeland EM III. Carcinoma of the stomach in the young adult. Surg Gynecol Obstet 1986;150:883–886.
17. Hirota T, Itabashi M, Daibo M, et al. Chronological changes in the morphological features of early gastric cancer, especially recent changes in macroscopic findings. Jpn J Clin Oncol 1984;14:181–199.
18. Hirota T, Ming SC, Itabashi M. Pathology of early gastric cancer. In: Nishi M, Ichikawa H, Nakajima T, et al., eds. Gastric cancer. Tokyo: Springer, 1993;66–87.

19. La Vecchia C, Negri E, Francheschi S, et al. Family history and the risk of stomach cancer and colorectal cancer. Cancer 1992;70:50–55.

20. Hsing A, Hansson L, McLaughlin J, et al. Pernicious anemia and subsequent cancer: A population based cohort study. Cancer 1993; 71:745–750.

21. Correa P, Haenszel W, Tannenbaum S. Epidemiology of gastric carcinoma. Review and future prospects. Natl Cancer Inst Monogr 1982;62:129–134.

22. Nomura A, Grove JS, Stemmerimann GN, et al. A prospective study of stomach cancer and its relation to diet, cigarettes, and alcohol consumption. Cancer Res 1990;50:627–631.

23. McMichael AJ, McCall MG, Hartshorne JM, et al. Patterns of gastro-intestinal cancer in European migrants to Australia: The role of dietary change. Int J Cancer 1980;25:431–437.

24. Locke, FB, King H. Cancer mortality risk among Japanese in the United States. J Natl Cancer Inst 1980;65:1149–1156.

25. Cuello C, Correa P, Haenszel W, et al. Gastric cancer in Colombia. I. Cancer risk and suspect environmental agents. J Natl Cancer Inst 1976;57:1015–1020.

26. Aoki K. Epidemiology of stomach cancer. In: Nishi M, Ichikawa H, Nakajima T, et al., eds. Gastric cancer. Tokyo: Springer, 1993:2–15.

27. Tominaga S. Decreasing trend of stomach cancer in Japan. Jpn J Cancer Res 1987;78:1–10.

28. Weisburger JH, Horn CL. Human and laboratory studies on the causes and prevention of gastrointestinal cancer. Scand J Gastroenterol Suppl 1985;104:15–26.

29. Lu JB, Qin YM. Correlation between high salt intake and mortality rates for oesophageal and gastric cancers in Hunan Province, China. Int J Epidemiol 1987;16:171–176.

30. Kono S, Ikeda M, Ogata M. Salt and geographical mortality of gastric cancer and stroke in Japan. J Epidemiol Community Health 1983; 37:43–46.

31. Charnley G, Tannebaum SR. Flow cytometric analysis of the effect of sodium chloride on gastric cancer risk in the rat. Cancer Res 1985;45:5608–5616.

32. Nagahara A, Ohshita K, Nasuno S. Relation of nitrite concentration to mutagen formation in soy sauce. Food Chem Toxicol 1986;24: 13–15.

33. Kurechi T, Kikugawa K, Fukuda S, et al. Inhibition of N-nitrosamine formation by soya products. Food Cosmet Toxicol 1981;19: 425–428.

34. Hirayama T. Relationship of soybean paste soup intake to gastric cancer risk. Nutr Cancer 1982;3:223–233.

35. Enterline PE, Hartley J, Henderson V. Asbestos and cancer: A cohort followed up to death. Br J Ind Med 1987;44:396–401.

36. Kogan FM, Vanchugova NN, Frasch VN. Possibility of inducing glandular stomach cancer in rats exposed to asbestos. Br J Ind Med 1987;44:682–686.

37. Hansson LE, Baron J, Nyren O, et al. Tobacco, alcohol and the risk of gastric cancer. A population-based case-control study in Sweden. Int J Cancer 1994;57:26–31.

38. Jedrychowski W, Boeing H, Wahrendorf J, et al. Vodka consumption, tobacco smoking and risk of gastric cancer in Poland. Int J Epidemiol 1993;22:606–613.

39. Leach SA, Thompson M, Hill M. Bacterially catalysed N-nitrosation reactions and their relative importance in the human stomach. Carcinogenesis 1987;8:1907–1912.

40. Mirvish SS. The etiology of gastric cancer. Intragastric nitrosamide formation and other theories. J Natl Cancer Inst 1983;71: 629–647.

41. Reed PI, Smith PLR, Haines K, et al. Gastric juice N-nitrosamines in health and gastroduodenal disease. Lancet 1981;2:550–552.

42. Schlag P, Bockler R, Peter M. Nitrite and nitrosamines in gastric juice: Risk factors for gastric cancer? Scand J Gastroenterol 1982; 17:145–150.

43. Morris DL, Youngs D, Muscroft TJ, et al. Mutagenicity in gastric juice. Gut 1984;25:723–727.

44. Mirvish SS. Effects of vitamins C and E on N–nitroso compound formation, carcinogenesis and cancer. Cancer 1986;58(Suppl): 1842–1850.

45. Warren JR, Marshall BJ. Unidentified curved bacilli on gastric epithelium in active chronic gastritis. Lancet 1983;1:1273–1275.

46. Marshall BJ, Warren JR. Unidentified curved bacilli in the stomach of patients with gastritis and peptic ulceration. Lancet 1984;1:1311–1315.

47. Hansson L-E, Engstrand L, Nyren O, et al. Helicobacter pylori infection: Independent risk indicator of gastric adenocarcinoma. Gastroenterology 1993;105:1098–1103.

48. Sipponen P. Helicobacter pylori: A cohort phenomenon. Am J Surg Pathol 1995;19(Suppl 1):S30–S36.

49. Noach LA, Rolf TM, Bosma NB, et al. Gastric metaplasia and Helicobacter pylori infection. Gut 1993;34:1510–1514.

50. Genta RM, Gurer IE, Graham DY, et al. Adherence of Helicobacter pylori to areas of incomplete intestinal metaplasia in the gastric mucosa. Gastroenterology 1996;111:1206–1211.

51. Graham DY, Go MF. Helicobacter pylori: Current status. Gastroenterology 1993;105:279–282.

52. Eidt S, Stolte M. Prevalence of lymphoid follicles and aggregates in Helicobacter pylori gastritis in antral and body mucosa. J Clin Pathol 1993;46:832–835.

53. Eidt S, Stolte M, Fischer R. Helicobacter pylori gastritis and primary gastric non-Hodgkin's lymphomas. J Clin Pathol 1994;47:436–439.

54. Endo S, Ohkusa T, Saito Y, et al. Detection of Helicobacter pylori infection in early stage gastric cancer. A comparison between intestinal- and diffuse-type gastric adenocarcinomas. Cancer 1995; 75:2203–2208.

55. Parsonnett J, Vandersteen D, Goates J, et al: Helicobacter pylori infection in intestinal and diffuse type gastric adenocarcinoma. J Natl Cancer Inst 1991;83:640–642.

56. Wee A, Kang JY. The M. Helicobacter pylori and gastric cancer: Correlation with gastritis, intestinal metaplasia and tumor histology. Gut 1993;33:1029–1032.

57. Clarkson KS, West KP. Gastric cancer and Helicobacter pylori infection. J Clin Pathol 1993;46:997–999.

58. Cahill RJ, Xia H, Kilgallen, et al. Effect of eradication of Helicobacter pylori infection on gastric epithelial cell proliferation. Dig Dis Sci 1995;40:1627–1631.

59. Crespi M, Citarda F. Helicobacter pylori and gastric cancer: An overrated risk? Scand J Gastroenterol 1996;31:1041–1046.

60. Borody TJ, Clark IW, Andrews P, et al. Eradication of Helicobacter pylori may not reverse severe gastric dysplasia. Am J Gastroenterol 1995;90:498–499.

61. Uemura N, Mukai T, Okamoto S, et al. Helicobacter pylori eradication inhibits the growth of intestinal type of gastric cancer in initial stage (abstract). Gastroenterology 1996;110:A83.

62. Vollmers HP, Dammrich J, Ribbert H, et al. Human monoclonal antibodies from stomach carcinoma patients react with Helicobacter pylori and stimulate stomach cancer cells in vitro. Cancer 1994;74: 1525–1532.

63. Blaser MJ, Perez-Perez GI, Kleanthous H, et al. Infection with Helicobacter pylori strains possessing CagA is associated with an increased risk of developing adenocarcinoma of the stomach. Cancer Res 1995;55:2111–2115.

64. Mitchell HM, Hazell SL, Li YY, et al. Serological response to specific Helicobacter pylori antigens: Antibody against CagA antigen is not predictive of gastric cancer in a developing country. Am J Gastroenterol 1996;91:1785–1788.

65. Shibata D, Tokunaga M, Uemura Y, et al. Association of Epstein-Barr virus with undifferentiated gastric carcinomas with intense lymphoid infiltration. Lymphoepithelioma-like carcinoma. Am J Pathol 1991; 139:469–474.

66. Nakamura S, Ueki T, Yao T, et al. Epstein-Barr virus in gastric carcinoma with lymphoid stroma. Special reference to its detection by the polymerase chain reaction and in situ hybridization in 99 tumors, including a morphologic analysis. Cancer 1994;73: 2239–2249.

67. Imai S, Koizumi S, Sugiura M, et al. Gastric carcinoma: Monoclonal epithelial malignant cells expressing Epstein-Barr virus latent infection protein. Proc Natl Acad Sci USA 1994;91:9131–9135.

68. Fukayama M, Hayashi Y, Iwasaki Y, et al. Epstein-Barr virus-associated gastric carcinoma and Epstein-Barr infection of the stomach. Lab Invest 1994;71:73–81.

69. Hurst AF. Precursors of carcinoma of the stomach. Lancet 1929;2: 1023–1028.

70. Morson BC, Sobin LH, Grundmann E, et al. Precancerous conditions and epithelial dysplasia in the stomach. J Clin Pathol 1980;33: 711–721.

71. Correa P. Chronic gastritis as a cancer precursor. Scand J Gastroenterol Suppl 1985;104:131–136.

72. Sipponen P, Kekki M, Haapakoski J, et al. Gastric cancer risk in chronic atrophic gastritis: Statistical calculation of cross-sectional data. Int J Cancer 1985;35:173–177.

73. Lipkin M, Correa P, Mikol YB, et al. Proliferative and antigenic modifications in human epithelial cells in chronic atrophic gastritis. J Natl Cancer Inst 1985;75:613–619.

74. Goldman H, Ming SC. Mucins in normal and neoplastic gastrointestinal epithelium. Histochemical distribution. Arch Pathol Lab Med 1968;85:580–586.

75. Teglbjaerg PS, Nielson HO. "Small intestinal type" and "colonic type" intestinal metaplasia of the human stomach and their relationship to the histogenetic types of gastric adenocarcinoma. Acta Pathol Microbiol Scand 1978;86A:351–355.

76. Spicer SS. Diamine methods for differentiating mucosubtances histochemically. J Histochem 1965;13:211–234.

77. Stemmermann GN, Hyashi T. Intestinal metaplasia of the gastric mucosa, a gross and microscopic study of its distribution in various disease states. J Natl Cancer Inst 1968;41:627–634.

78. Fenoglio-Preiser CM, Noffsinger AE, Belli J, et al. Pathologic and phenotypic features of gastric cancer. Semin Oncol 1995;23: 292–306.

79. Goldman H, Ming SC. Fine structure of intestinal metaplasia and adenocarcinoma of the human stomach. Lab Invest 1968;18: 203–210.

80. Ming SC. Intestinal metaplasia: Its heterogeneous nature and significance. In: Ming SC, ed. Precursors of gastric cancer. Philadelphia: Praeger, 1984;219–231.

81. Matsukura N, Suzuki K, Kawachi T, et al. Distribution of marker enzymes and mucin in intestinal metaplasia in human stomach and relation of complete and incomplete types of intestinal metaplasia to minute gastric carcinomas. J Natl Cancer Inst 1980;65: 231–240.

82. Segura DI, Montero C. Histochemical characterization of different types of intestinal metaplasia in gastric mucosa. Cancer 1983;82: 498–503.

83. Jass JR, Filipe MI. The mucin profile of normal gastric mucosa, intestinal metaplasia and its variants and gastric carcinoma. Histochem J 1981;13:931–939.

84. Filipe MI, Potet F, Bogomoletz WV, et al. Incomplete sulphomucin secreting intestinal metaplasia for gastric cancer. Preliminary data from a prospective study from three centres. Gut 1985;26:1319–1326.

85. Stemmermann GN. Intestinal metaplasia of the stomach. A status report. Cancer 1994;74:556–564.

86. Nielsen K, Teglbjaerg PS. On the occurrence of carcinoembryonic antigen (CEA) in different types of intestinal metaplasia of the human stomach. Tumour Biol 1984;5:313–320.

87. Hirota T, Okada T, Itabashi M, et al. Significance of intestinal metaplasia as a precancerous condition of the stomach. In: Ming SC, ed. Precursors of gastric cancer. Philadelphia: Praeger, 1984; 179–193.

88. Suvarna N, Sasidharan VP. Histopathological and histogenetic study of carcinoma of stomach in a high risk area. Indian J Cancer 1995;32:36–42.

89. Ectors N, Dixon MF. The prognostic value of sulphomucin positive intestinal metaplasia in the development of gastric cancer. Histopathology 1986;10:1271–1277.

90. Ramesar KC, Sanders DS, Hopwood D. Limited value of type III intestinal metaplasia in predicting risk of gastric carcinoma. J Clin Pathol 1987;40:1287–1290.

91. Tatematsu M, Furihata C, Katsuyama T, et al. Independent induction of intestinal metaplasia and gastric cancer in rats treated with N-methyl-N'-nitro-N-nitrosoguanidine. Cancer Res 1983;43:1335–1341.

92. Watanabe H, Ito A. Relationship between gastric tumorigenesis and intestinal metaplasia in rats given X-radiation and/or N-methyl-N'-nitro-N-nitrosoguanidine. J Natl Cancer Inst 1986;76:865–870.

93. Hattori T. Development of adenocarcinomas in the stomach. Cancer 1986;57:1528–1534.

94. Sano R. Pathological analysis of 300 cases of early gastric cancer with special reference to cancer associated with ulcer. Gann Monogr Cancer Res 1971;11:81–89.

95. Sakita T, Oguro Y, Takasu S, et al. Observations on the healing of ulcerations in early gastric cancer; the life cycle of the malignant ulcer. Gastroenterology 1971;60:835–844.

96. Haukland HH, Johnson JA, Eide JT. Carcinoma diagnosed in excised gastric ulcers. Acta Chir Scand 1981;147:439–443.

97. Farinati F, Cardin F, Di Mario F, et al. Early and advanced gastric cancer during follow-up of apparently benign gastric ulcer: Significance of the presence of epithelial dysplasia. J Surg Oncol 1987;36: 263–267.

98. Rollag A, Jacobsen CD. Gastric ulcer and risk of cancer. A five year follow-up study. Acta Med Scand 1984;216:105–109.

99. Kawai K, Kizu M, Miyaoka T. Epidemiology and pathogenesis of gastric cancer. Front Gastrointest Res 1980;6:71–86.

100. Hirota T, Itabashi M, Suzuki K, et al. Clinical study of minute and small early gastric cancer. Histogenesis of gastric cancer. Pathol Annu 1980;15:1–19.

101. Takahashi M, Shirai T, Gukushima S, et al. Effects of fundic ulcers induced by iodoacetamide on development of gastric tumors in rats treated with N-methyl-N'-nitro-N-nitrosoguinidine. Gann 1975;67: 47–54.

102. O'Brien MJ, Burakoff R, Robbins EA, et al. Early gastric cancer. Clinicopathologic study. Am J Med 1985;78:195–202.

103. Domellof L. Remnant stomach and gastric cancer. In: Nishi M, Ichikawa H, Nakajima T, et al., eds. Gastric cancer. Tokyo: Springer, 1993;168–183.

104. Gad A. Carcinoma of the resected stomach. In: Ming SC, ed. Precursors of gastric cancer. Philadelphia: Praeger, 1984;287–313.

105. Schafer LW, Larson DE, Melton J III, et al. The risk of gastric carcinoma after surgical treatment of benign ulcer diseases. N Engl J Med 1983;309:1210–1213.

106. Dittrich S, Theuring F. Das Karzinom im operierten Magen - eine autoptische Studie. Zentralbl Allg Pathol 1985;130:211–216.

107. Tokudome S, Kono S, Ikeda M, et al. A prospective study on primary gastric stump cancer following partial gastrectomy for benign gastroduodenal diseases. Cancer Res 1984;44:2208–2212.

108. Graem N, Fischer AB, Beck H. Dysplasia and carcinoma in the Billroth II resected stomach 27, 35 years post operatively. Acta Pathol Microbiol Immunol Scand (A) 1984;92:185–188.

109. Hammar E. The localization of precancerous changes and carcinoma after previous gastric operation for benign condition. Acta Pathol Microbiol Scand (A) 1976;84:495–507.

110. Antonioli DA. Precursors of gastric carcinoma: A critical review with a brief description of early (curable) gastric cancer. Hum Pathol 1994;25:994–1005.

111. Schrumpf E, Serck-Hanssen A, Stadaas J, et al. Mucosal changes in the gastric stump, 20–25 years after partial gastrectomy. Lancet 1977;2:467–469.

112. Offerhaus GJ, Huibregtse K, de Boer J, et al. The operated stomach: A premalignant condition? A prospective endoscopic follow-up study. Scand J Gastroenterol 1984;19:521–524.

113. Miwa K, Hattori T, Miyazaki I. Duodenogastric reflux and foregut carcinogenesis. Cancer 1995;75(Suppl):1426–1432.

114. Watt PC, Sloan JM, Spencer A, et al. Histology of the postoperative stomach before and after diversion of bile. Br Med J 1983;287:1410–1412.

115. Kaminishi M, Shimizu N, Yamaguchi H, et al. Different carcinogenesis in the gastric remnant after gastrectomy for gastric cancer. Cancer 1996;77(Suppl):1646–1653.

116. Ming SC. Tumors of the esophagus and stomach. In: Atlas of tumor pathology, second series, fascicle 7. Washington DC: Armed Forces Institute of Pathology, 1973:144–206.

117. Stamm B, Saremaslani P. Coincidence of fundic glandular hyperplasia and carcinoma of the stomach. Cancer 1989;63:354–359.

118. Ménétrier P. Des polyadenomas gastriques et de leurs rapports avec le cancer de l'estomac. Arch Physiol Norm Path 1888;1: 32–55.

119. Martin ED. Frequency and evolution of precancerous and dysplastic

lesions in the stomach. Excerpta Med Int Congr Ser 1981;555: 225–230.

120. Wood MG, Bates C, Brown RC, et al. Intramucosal carcinoma of the gastric antrum complicating Ménétrier's disease. J Clin Pathol 1983;36:1071–1075.

121. Rubio CA, Kato Y, Sugano H, et al. The intramucosal cysts of the stomach. VII. A pathway of gastric carcinogenesis? J Surg Oncol 1986;32:214–219.

122. Zhu FG, Deng XJ, Cheng NJ. Intramucosal cysts in gastric mucosa adjacent to carcinoma and peptic ulcer: A histochemical study. Histopathology 1987;11:631–638.

123. Pillay I, Petrelli M. Diffuse cystic glandular malformation of the stomach associated with adenocarcinoma. Cancer 1976;38: 915–920.

124. Iwanaga T, Koyama H, Takahashi Y, et al. Diffuse submucosal cysts and carcinoma of the stomach. Cancer 1975;36:606–614.

125. Zhou XX. Relationship between gastric schistosomiasis and gastric cancer, chronic gastric ulcer and chronic gastritis: Pathological analysis of 79 cases (in Chinese). Chung hua Ping Li Hsueh Tsa Chih 1986;15:62–64.

126. Ming SC, Bajtai A, Correa P, et al. Gastric dysplasia. Significance and pathologic criteria. Cancer 1984;54:1794–1801.

127. Ming SC. Dysplasia of gastric epithelium. Front Gastrointest Res 1979;4:164–172.

128. Oehlert W. Preneoplastic lesions of the stomach. In: Ming SC, ed. Precursors of gastric cancer. New York: Praeger, 1984;73–82.

129. Macartney JC, Camplejohn RS. DNA flow cytometry of histological material from dysplastic lesions of human gastric mucosa. J Pathol 1986;150:113–118.

130. Jarvis LR, Whitehead R. Morphometric analysis of gastric dysplasia. J Pathol 1985;147:133–138.

131. Jass JR, Strudley I, Faludy J. Histochemistry of epithelial metaplasia and dysplasia in human stomach and colorectum. Scand J Gastroenterol Suppl 1984;104:109–130.

132. Li J, Zhao A, Lu Y, et al. Expression of p185erbB2 and p21ras in carcinoma, dysplasia, and intestinal metaplasia of the stomach: An immunohistochemical and in situ hybridizaton study. Semin Surg Oncol 1994;10:95–99.

133. Brito MJ, Williams GT, Thompson H, et al. Expression of p53 in early (T1) gastric carcinoma and precancerous adjacent mucosa. Gut 1994;35:1697–1700.

134. Shiao Y-H, Rugge M, Correa P, et al. p53 alteration in gastric precancerous lesions. Am J Pathol 1994;144:511–517.

135. Lauwers GY, Scott GV, Hendricks J. Immunohistochemical evidence of aberrant bcl-2 protein expression in gastric epithelial dysplasia. Cancer 1994;73:2900–2904.

136. Cuello C, Correa P, Zarama G, et al. Histopathology of gastric dysplasia. Correlations with gastric juice chemistry. Am J Surg Pathol 1979;3:491–500.

137. Jass JR. A classification of gastric dysplasia. Histopathology 1983;7: 181–193.

138. Farinati F, Rugge M, DiMario F, et al. Early and advanced gastric cancer in the follow-up of moderate and severe gastric dysplasia patients. A prospective study. Endoscopy 1993;25:261–264.

139. DiGregorio C, Morandi P, Fante R, et al. Gastric dysplasia. A follow-up study. Am J Gastroenterol 1993;88:1714–1719.

140. Von Holstein CS, Hammar E, Eriksson S, et al. Clinical significance of dysplasia in gastric remnant biopsy specimens. Cancer 1993;72: 1532–1535.

141. Rugge M, Farinati F, Baffa R, et al. Gastric epithelial dysplasia in the natural history of gastric cancer: A multicenter prospective follow-up study. Gastroenterology 1994;107:1288–1296.

142. Rugge M, Farinati F, DiMario F, et al. Gastric epithelial dysplasia: A prospective multicenter follow-up study from the interdisciplinary group on gastric epithelial dysplasia. Hum Pathol 1991;22:1008–1022.

143. del Corral MJC, Pardo-Mindan FJ, Razquin S, et al. Risk of cancer in patients with gastric dysplasia. Follow-up study of 67 patients. Cancer 1990;65:2078–2085.

144. Burke AP, Sobin LH, Shekitka KM, et al. Dysplasia of the stomach and Barrett esophagus: A follow-up study. Mod Pathol 1991;4:336–341.

145. Thompson H, Price A, Williams GT, et al. The British Society of Gastroenterology Early Gastric Cancer/Dysplasia study. An interim

report. In: Ming SC. Significance of epithelial dysplasia in the esophagus and stomach. Endoscopy 1989;21(Suppl):38–45.

146. Koch HK, Oehlert M, Oehlert W. An evaluation of gastric dysplasia in the years 1986 and 1987. In: Ming SC. Significance of epithelial dysplasia in the esophagus and stomach. Endoscopy 1989;21(Suppl): 38–45.

147. Zampi G, Amorosi A, Bianchi S. Gastric dysplasia: Precancerous or paracancerous lesion? In: Ming SC. Significance of epithelial dysplasia in the esophagus and stomach. Endoscopy 1989;21(Suppl):38–45.

148. Andersson AP, Lauritsen KB, West F, et al. Dysplasia in gastric mucosa: Prognostic significance. Acta Chir Scand 1987;153:29–31.

149. Ming SC. Significance of epithelial dysplasia in the esophagus and stomach. Endoscopy 1989;21:38S–49S.

149a. Grundmann E, Schlake W. Histology of possible precancerous stage in stomach, In: Herfarth CH, Schlag P, eds. Gastric Cancer. Berlin: Springer-Verlag, 1979:72-82.

150. Borchard F. Precancerous conditions and lesions of the stomach. In: Rugge M, Arslan-Pagnini C, DiMario F, eds. Carcinoma gastrico e lesioni precancerose dello stomaco. Milano: Edizioni Unicopi, 1986; 175–210.

151. Sugimura T. Experimental gastric cancer. In: Nishi M, Ichikawa H, Nakajima T, et al., eds. Gastric cancer. Tokyo: Springer, 1993:28–39.

152. Saito T, Sasaki O, Tamada R, et al. Sequential studies of development of gastric carcinoma in dogs induced by N-methyl-N'-nitro-N-nitrosoguanidine. Cancer 1978;42:1246–1254.

153. Kobori O, Gedigk P, Totovic V. Adenomatous changes and adenocarcinoma of glandular stomach in Wistar rats induced by N-methyl-N'-nitro-N-nitrosoguanidine. An electron microscopic and histochemical study. Virchows Arch [A] 1977;373:37–54.

154. Tatematsu M, Furihata C, Katsuyama T, et al. Immunohistochemical demonstration of pyloric gland-type cells with low-pepsinogen isozyme 1 in preneoplastic and neoplastic tissues of rat stomachs treated with N-methyl-N'-nitro-N-nitrosoguanidine. J Natl Cancer Inst 1987;78:771–777.

155. Wang CX, Williams GM. Comparison of stomach cancer induced in rats by N-methyl-N'-nitro-N-nitrosoguanidine or N-propyl-N'-nitro-N-nitrosoguanidine. Cancer Lett 1987;34:173–185.

156. Sunagawa M, Takeshita K, Nakajima A, et al. Duration of ENNG administration and its effect on histological differentiation of experimental gastric cancer. Br J Cancer 1985;52:771–779.

157. Szentirmay Z, Ohgaki H, Maruyama K, et al. Early gastric cancer induced by N-ethyl-N'-nitro-N-nitrosoguanidine in a Cynomolgus monkey six years after initial dignosis of the lesion. Jpn J Cancer Res 1990;81:6–9.

158. Kunze E, Schauer A, Eder M, et al. Early sequential lesions during development of experimental gastric cancer with special reference to dysplasias. J Cancer Res Clin Oncol 1979;95:247–264.

159. Tsiftsis D, Jass JR, Filipe MI, et al. Altered patterns of mucin secretion in precancerous lesions induced in the glandular part of the stomach by the carcinogen N-methyl-N'-nitro-N-nitroguanidine. Invest Cell Pathol 1980;3:399–408.

160. Fujita S. Natural history of human gastric carcinoma in terms of their genesis and progression. Asian Med J 1983;26:787–805.

161. Nakamura K. Histogenesis of the gastric carcinoma and its clinicopathological significance. In: Nishi M, Ichikawa H, Nakajima T, et al. eds. Gastric cancer. Tokyo: Springer, 1993;112–132.

162. Hattori T. Development of adenocarcinoma in the stomach. Cancer 1986;57:1528–1534.

163. Clarkson B, Ota T, Okhita T, et al. Kinetics of proliferation of cancer cells in neoplastic effusions in man. Cancer 1965;18:1189–1213.

164. Fujita S. Natural history of human gastric carcinoma in terms of their genesis and progression. Asian Med J 1983;26:787–805.

165. Tsukuma H, Mishima T, Oshima A. Prospective study of "early" gastric cancer. Int J Cancer 1983;31:421–426.

166. Korenaga D, Okamura T, Saito A, et al. DNA ploidy is closely linked to tumor invasion, lymph node metastasis, and prognosis in clinical gastric cancer. Cancer 1988;62:309–313.

167. Verse M. Die Histogenese der Schleimhautcarcinome. Leipzig, 1903.

168. Mallory TB. Carcinoma in situ of the stomach and its bearing on the histogenesis of malignant ulcers. Arch Pathol Lab Med 1948;30: 348–362.

169. Stout AP. Superficial spreading type of carcinoma of the stomach. Arch Surg 1942;44:651–657.

170. Konjetzny GE. The superficial cancer of the gastric mucosa. Am J Dig Dis 1953;20:91–96.
171. Ming SC. Classification of gastric carcinoma. In: Filipe MI, Jass JR, eds. Gastric carcinoma. London: Churchill Livingstone, 1986;197–216.
172. Japanese Research Society for Gastric Cancer. The general rules for the gastric cancer study in surgery and pathology. Jpn J Surg 1981;11:127–145.
173. Japanese Research Society for Gastric Cancer. Japanese classification of gastric cancer. Tokyo: Kanehara, 1995.
174. Wanebo HJ, Kennedy BJ, Chmiel J, et al. Cancer of the stomach. A patient care study by the American College of Surgeons. Ann Surg 1993;218:583–592.
175. Meyers WC, Damiano RJ Jr, Rotolo FS, et al. Adenocarcinoma of the stomach. Changing patterns over the last 4 decades. Ann Surg 1987;205:1–8.
176. Hirota T, Itabashi M, Suzuki K, et al. Clinical study of minute and small early gastric cancer. Histogenesis of gastric cancer. Pathol Annu 1980;15:1–19.
177. Kurihara M, Keiichi K, Shirakabe H. Diagnosis of small early gastric cancer by X-ray, endoscopy and biopsy. Cancer Dect Prev 1981;4:377–383.
178. Borrmann R. Geshwelste des Magens und Duodenums. In: Henke F, Lubarsch O, eds. Handbuch der Spezieller Pathologischen Anatomie und Histologie. Berlin: Springer, 1926;4:865.
179. Japanese Research Society for Gastric Cancer. The general rules for the gastric cancer study in surgery and pathology. Jpn J Surg 1981;11:127–145.
180. Hirota T, Itabashi M, Daibo M, et al. Chronological changes in the morphological features of early gastric cancer, especially recent changes in macroscopic findings. Jpn J Clin Oncol 1984;14:181–199.
181. Kodama Y, Inokuchi K, Soejima K, et al. Growth patterns and prognosis in early gastric carcinoma. Superficially spreading and penetrating growth types. Cancer 1983;51:320–326.
182. Inukuchi K, Sugimachi K. Growth patterns of gastric cancer. In: Nishi M, Ichikawa H, Nakajima T, et al., eds. Gastric cancer. Tokyo: Springer, 1993;88–101.
183. Johansen A. Early gastric cancer. Bispebjerg Hospital, Copenhagen, Denmark, 1981.
184. Fiocca R, Villani L, Tenti P, et al. Characterization of four main cell types in gastric cancer: Foveolar, mucopeptic, intestinal columnar and goblet cells. An histologic, histochemical and ultrastructural study of "early" and "advanced" tumours. Path Res Pract 1987;182:308–325.
185. Nevalainen TJ, Jarvi OH. Ultrastructure of intestinal and diffuse carcinoma. J Pathol 1977;122:129–136.
186. Sugihara H, Hattori T, Fukuda M, et al. Cell proliferation and differentiation in intramucosal and advanced signet ring cell carcinomas of the human stomach. Virchows Arch [A] 1987;411:117–127.
187. Nevalainen TJ, Jarvi OH. Intracellular cysts in gastric carcinoma. Acta Pathol Microbiol Scand (A) 1976;84:517–522.
188. Kobori O, Oota K. Mucous substance and enzyme histochemistry of non-neoplastic and neoplastic gastric epithelium in man. Acta Pathol Jap 1974;24:119–1304.
189. Soga J, Tazawa K, Aizawa O, et al. Argentaffin cell adenocarcinoma of the stomach: An atypical carcinoid? Cancer 1971;28:999–1003.
190. Tahara E, Ito H, Nakagami K, et al. Scirrhous argyrophil cell carcinoma of the stomach with multiple production of polypeptide hormones, amine, CEA, lysozyme, and HCG. Cancer 1982;49:1904–1915.
191. Capella C, Cornaggia M, Usellini L, et al. Neoplastic cells containing lysozyme in gastric carcinomas. Pathology 1984;16:87–92.
192. Kazzaz BA, Eulderink F. Paneth cell-rich carcinoma of the stomach. Histopathology 1989;15:303–305.
193. Capella C, Frigerio B, Cornaggia M, et al. Gastric parietal cell carcinoma a newly recognized entity: Light microscopic and ultrastructural features. Histopathology 1984;8:813–824.
194. Byrne D, Holley MP, Cuschieri A. Parietal cell carcinoma of the stomach: Association with long-term survival after curative resection. Br J Cancer 1988;58:85–87.
195. Robey-Cafferty SS, Ro JY, McKee EG. Gastric parietal cell carcinoma with an unusual, lymphoma-like histologic appearance: Report of a case. Mod Pathol 1989;2:536–540.
196. Stemmermann GN, Samloff IM, Hayashi T. Pepsinogens I and II in carcinoma of the stomach: An immunohistochemical study. Appl Pathol 1985;3:159–163.
197. Ishikura H, Kirimoto K, Shamoto M, et al. Hepatoid adenocarcinomas of the stomach. An analysis of seven cases. Cancer 1986;58:119–126.
198. Matias-Guiu X, Guix M. Hepatoid gastric adenocarcinoma. Pathol Res Pract 1989;185:397–400.
199. Murayama H, Imai T, Kikuchi M. Solid carcinomas of the stomach. A combined histochemical, light and electron microscopic study. Cancer 1983;51:1673–1681.
200. Lertprasertsuke N, Tsutsumi Y. Gastric carcinoma with lymphoid stroma. Analysis using mucin histochemistry and immunohistochemistry. Virchows Arch [A] 1989;414:231–241.
201. Moritani S, Kushima R, Sugihara H, et al. Phenotypic characteristics of Epstein-Barr virus-associated gastric carcinomas. J Cancer Res Clin Oncol 1996;122:750–756.
202. Nagai Y, Sunada H, Sano J, et al. Biochemical and immunohistochemical studies on the scirrhous carcinoma of human stomach. Ann NY Acad Sci 1985;460:321–332.
203. Niitsu Y, Ito N, Kohda K, et al. Immunohistochemical identification of type I procollagen in tumour cells of scirrhous adenocarcinoma of the stomach. Br J Cancer 1988;57:79–82.
204. Yoshida K, Yokozaki H, Nimoto M, et al. Expression of TGF-β and procollagen type I and type III in human gastric carcinomas. Int J Cancer 1989;44:394–398.
205. Watanabe H, Jass JR, Sabin LH. Histological typing of oesophageal and gastric tumours. World Health Organization international histological classification of tumours. Berlin: Springer, 1989;20–26.
206. Arslan Pagnini C, Rugge M. Gastric cancer: Problems in histological diagnosis. Histopathology 1982;6:391–398.
207. Blander WL, Needham PRG, Morgan AD. Indolent mucoid carcinoma of stomach. J Clin Pathol 1974;27:536–541.
208. Beahrs OH, Henson DE, Hunter RVP, et al., eds. Manual for staging of cancer. 4th ed. Philadelphia: JB Lippincott, 1992;63–67.
209. Wang R-N, Cai J-C, Jiang C-Y, et al. Role of cell adhesion molecules in determining glandular differentiation and growth pattern of gastric carcinoma. Cell Vision 1995;2:120–125.
210. Ming SC. Tumors of the esophagus and stomach. Supplement. In: Atlas of tumor pathology, second series, fascicle 7. Washington DC: Armed Forces Institute of Pathology, 1985;533–554.
211. Ribeiro MM, Sarmento JA, Simoes S, et al. Prognostic significance of Lauren and Ming classifications and other pathologic parameters in gastric carcinoma. Cancer 1981;47:780–784.
212. Daves K Sr, Hale J, Kessimian N, et al. Histological classification of gastric adenocarcinoma. Lab Invest 1988;58:22A.
213. Nakamura K. Histogenesis of the gastric cancer and its clinical application. Ibaraki, Japan: Tsukura International Center, 1983.
214. Jass JR. Role of intestinal metaphasia in the histogenesis of gastric carcinoma. J Clin Pathol 1980;33:801–810.
215. Mulligan RM. Histogenesis and biological behavior of gastric carcinoma. Pathol Annu 1972;7:349–415.
216. Goseki N, Takizawa T, Koike M. Differences in the mode of extension of gastric cancer classified by histological type: New histological classification of gastric carcinoma. Gut 1992;33:606–612.
217. Filipe MI, Barbatis C, Sandey A, et al. Expression of intestinal mucin antigens in the gastric epithelium and its relationship with malignancy. Hum Pathol 1988;19:19–26.
218. Osborn M, Mazzoleni G, Santini D, et al. Villin, intestinal brush border hydrolases and keratin polypeptides in intestinal metaplasia and gastric cancer; an immunohistologic study emphasizing the different degrees of intestinal and gastric differentiation in signet ring cell carcinomas. Virchows Arch [A] 1988:303–312.
219. Fiocca R, Cornaggia M, Villani L, et al. Expression of pepsinogen II in gastric cancer. Its relationship to local invasion and lymph node metastasis. Cancer 1988;61:956–962.
220. Radi MJ, Fenoglio-Preiser CM, Bartow SA, et al. Gastric carcinoma in the young: A clinicopathological and immunohistochemical study. Am J Gastroenterol 1986;81:747–756.

221. Ito H, Hata J, Oda N, et al. Serotonin in tubular adenomas, adenocarcinomas and endocrine tumours of the stomach. An immunohistochemical study. Virchows Arch [A] 1986;410:239–245.

222. Cook HC. Neutral mucin content of gastric carcinomas as a diagnostic aid in the identification of secondary deposits. Histopathology 1982;6:591–599.

223. Skinner JM, Whitehead R. Tumor markers in carcinoma and in premalignant states of the stomach in humans. Eur J Cancer Clin Oncol 1982;180:227–235.

224. Wurster K, Rapp W. Histological and immunohistological studies on gastric mucosa. 1. The presence of CEA in dysplastic surface epithelium. Pathol Res Pract 1979;164:270–281.

225. Posner MR, Mayer RJ. The use of serologic tumor markers in gastrointestinal malignancies. Hematol Oncol Clin North Am 1994; 3:533–553.

226. Maehara Y, Kusumoto T, Takahashi I, et al. Predictive value of preoperative carcinoembryonic antigen levels of the prognosis of patients with well-differentiated gastric cancer. Oncology 1994;51: 234–237.

227. Janssen CW Jr, Orjasaeter H. Carcinoembryonic antigen in patients with gastric carcinoma. Eur J Surg Oncol 1986;12:19–23.

228. Miki M, Ichinose M, Ishikawa KB, et al. Clinical application of serum pepsinogen I and II levels for mass screening to detect gastric cancer. Jpn J Cancer Res 1993;84:1086–1090.

229. Hakkinen IPT, Heinonen R, Inberg MV, et al. Clinicopathological study of gastric cancers and precancerous states detected by fetal sulfoglycoprotein antigen screening. Cancer Res 1980;40:4308–4312.

230. Hattori T. DNA ploidy pattern and cell kinetics. In: Nishi M, Ichikawa H, Nakajima T, et al., eds. Gastric cancer. Tokyo: Springer, 1993:184–195.

231. Rugge M, Sonego F, Panozzo M, et al. Pathology and ploidy in the prognosis of gastric cancer with no extranodal metastasis. Cancer 1994;73:1127–1133.

232. Sugihara H, Hattori T, Fugita S, et al. Regional ploidy variations in signet ring cell carcinomas of the stomach. Cancer 1990;65: 122–129.

233. Yonemura Y, Sugiyama K, Fugimura T, et al. Correlation of DNA ploidy and proliferative activity in human gastric cancer. Cancer 1988;62:1497–1502.

234. Schneeberger AL, Finley RJ, Troster M, et al. The prognostic significance of tumor ploidy and pathology in adenocarcinoma of the esophagogastric junction. Cancer 1990;65:1206–1210.

235. Wyatt JI, Quirke P, Ward DC, et al. Comparison of histopathological and flow cytometric parameters in prediction of prognosis in gastric cancer. J Pathol 1989;158:195–201.

236. Korenaga D, Haraguchi M, Okamura T, et al. Consistency of DNA ploidy between primary and recurrent gastric carcinomas. Cancer Res 1986;46:1544–1546.

237. Tahara E, Semba S, Tahara H. Molecular biological observations in gastric cancer. Semin Oncol 1995;23:307–315.

238. Katoh M, Terada M. Oncogenes and tumor suppressor genes. In: Nishi M, Ichikawa H, Nakajima T, et al., eds. Gastric cancer. Tokyo: Springer, 1993:196–208.

239. Wright PA, Quirke P, Attanoos R, et al. Molecular pathology of gastric carcinoma: Progress and prospects. Hum Pathol 1992;23: 848–859.

240. Czerniak B, Herz F, Gorczyca W, et al. Expression of ras oncogene p21 protein in early gastric carcinoma and adjacent gastric epithelia. Cancer 1989;64:1467–1473.

241. Brito MJ, Williams GT, Thompson H, et al. Expression of p53 in early (T1) gastric carcinoma and precancerous adjacent mucosa. Gut 1994;35:1697–1700.

242. Fukunaga M, Monden T, Nakanishi H, et al. Immunohistochemical study of p53 in gastric carcinoma. Am J Clin Pathol 1994;101: 177–180.

243. Stemmermann G, Heffelfinger SC, Noffsinger A, et al. The molecular biology of esophageal and gastric cancer and their precursors: Oncogenes, tumor suppressor genes, and growth factors. Hum Pathol 1994;25:968–981.

244. Chong J-M, Fukayama M, Hayashi Y, et al. Microsatellite instability in the progression of gastric carcinoma. Cancer Res 1994;54:4595–4597.

245. Rhyu M-G, Park W-S, Meltzer SJ. Microsatellite instability occurs frequently in human gastric carcinoma. Oncogene 1994; 9:29–32.

246. Tamura G, Sakata K, Maesawa C, et al. Microsatellite alterations in adenoma and differentiated adenocarcinoma of the stomach. Cancer Res 1995;55:1933–1936.

247. Akiyama Y, Nakasaki H, Nihei Z, et al. Frequent microsatellite instabilities and analyses of the related genes in familial gastric cancers. Jpn J Cancer Res 1996; 87:595–601.

248. Han H-J, Yanagisawa A, Kato Y, et al. Genetic instability in pancreatic cancer and poorly differentiated type of gastric cancer. Cancer Res 1993;53:5087–5089.

249. Lauwers GY, Scott GV, Karpeh MS. Immunohistochemical evaluation of bcl-2 protein expression in gastric adenocarcinomas. Cancer 1995;75:2209–2213.

250. Schade RKO. The borderline between benign and malignant lesions in the stomach. In: Grundmann E, Grunze H, Witte S, eds. Early gastric cancer: Current status of diagnosis. Berlin: Springer, 1974: 45–53.

251. Kraus B, Cain H. Is there a carcinoma in-situ of gastric mucosa? Pathol Res Pract 1979;164:342–355.

252. Sakuma A, Ouchi A, Sugawara T, et al. Histologic infiltrating pattern of gastric microcarcinoma by means of serial sections. Cancer 1985;55:1087–1092.

253. Esaki Y, Hirayama R, Hirokawa K. A comparison of patterns of metastasis in gastric cancer by histologic type and age. Cancer 1990;65:2086–2090.

254. Lehnert T, Erlandson RA, Decosse JJ. Lymph and blood capillaries of the human gastric mucosa. A morphologic basis for metastasis in early gastric carcinoma. Gastroenterology 1989;89:939–950.

255. Bogomoletz WV. Early gastric cancer. Am J Surg Pathol 1984;8: 381–391.

256. Korenaga D, Haraguchi M, Tsujitani S, et al. Clinicopathological features of mucosal carcinoma of the stomach with lymph node metastasis in eleven patients. Br J Surg 1986;73:431–433.

257. Fukutomi H, Sakite T. Analysis of early gastric cancer cases collected from major hospitals and institutes in Japan. Jpn J Clin Oncol 1984;14:169–179.

258. Murakami T. Early cancer of the stomach. World J Surg 1979;3: 685–692.

259. Yakushiji M, Tazaki T, Nishimura H, et al. Krukenberg tumors of the ovary: A clinicopathologic analysis of 112 cases. Nippon Sanka Fujinka Gakkai Zasshi 1987;39:479–485.

260. Kennedy BJ. Staging of gastric cancer. In: Nishi M, Ichikawa H, Nakajima T, et al., eds. Gastric cancer. Tokyo: Springer, 1993; 102–111.

261. Hermanek P, Sobin LH, eds. UICC: TNM classification of malignant tumours. 4th ed. 2nd rev. Berlin: Springer, 1992.

262. Hermanek P, Henson DE, Hutter RVP, et al., eds. UICC: TNM supplement 1993—a commentary on uniform use. Berlin: Springer, 1992.

263. Hermanek P, Wittekind C. News of TNM and its use for classification of gastric cancer. World J Surg 1995;19:491–495.

264. Roder JD, Bher K, Siewert JR, et al. Prognostic factors in gastric carcinoma. Results of the German Gastric Carcinoma Study 1992. Cancer 1993;72:2089–2097.

265. Aurello P, Ramacciato G, Barillari P, et al. Prognostic value of the number of regional lymph nodes involved in gastric cancer: N1 or N2 a, b, c new staging. In: Siewert JR, Roder JD, eds. Progress in gastric cancer research 1997. Bologna: Monduzzi Editore, 1997; 219–222.

266. Juvan R, Repse S, Omejc M, et al. Prognostic value of lymph node metastasis ratio in gastric cancer. In: Siewert JR, Roder JD, eds. Progress in gastric cancer research 1997. Bologna: Monduzzi Editore, 1997;223–228.

267. Kim J-P. Results of surgery on 6589 gastric cancer patients indicating immunochemosurgery as being the best modality treatment for advanced gastric cancer. In: Nishi M, Ichikawa H, Nakajima T, et al., eds. Gastric cancer. Tokyo: Springer, 1993:358–377.

268. Kinoshita T, Maruyama K, Sasako M, et al. Treatment results of gastric cancer patients: Japanese experience. In: Nishi M, Ichikawa H, Nakajima T, et al., eds. Gastric cancer. Tokyo: Springer, 1993: 319–330.

269. Okada M, Kojima S, Murakami M, et al. Human gastric carcinoma: Prognosis in relation to macroscopic and microscopic features of the primary tumor. J Natl Cancer Inst 1983;71:275–279.

270. Haraguchi M, Okamura T, Sugimachi K. Accurate prognostic value of morphovolumetric analysis of advanced carcinoma of the stomach. Surg Gynecol Obstet 1987;164:335–339.

271. Cimerman M, Repse S, Jelenc F, et al. Comparison of Lauren's, Ming's and WHO histological classifications of gastric cancer as a prognostic factor for operated patients. Int Surg 1994;79:27–32.

272. Arslan Pagnini C, Rugge M. Advanced gastric carcinoma and prognosis. Virchows Arch [A] 1985;406:213–222.

273. Kaibara N, Iitsuka Y, Kimura A, et al. Relationship between area of serosal invasion and prognosis in patients with gastric carcinoma. Cancer 1987;60:136–139.

274. Baba H, Korenaga D, Haraguchi M, et al. Width of serosal invasion and prognosis in advanced human gastric cancer with special reference to the mode tumor invasion. Cancer 1989;64:2482–2486.

275. Santini D, Bazzocchi F, Mazzoleni G, et al. Signet-ring cells in advanced gastric cancer. A clinical, pathological and histochemical study. Acta Pathol Microbiol Immunol Scand (A) 1987;95:225–231.

276. Okamura T, Kodama Y, Kamegawa T, et al. Gastric carcinoma with lymphoid stroma: Correlation to reactive hyperplasia in regional lymph nodes and prognosis. Jpn J Surg 1983;13:177–183.

277. Tsujitani S, Furukawa T, Tamada R, et al. Langerhans cells and prognosis in patients with gastric carcinoma. Cancer 1987;59:501–505.

278. Gaffney EF. Favourable prognosis in gastric carcinoma with parietal cell differentiation. Histopathology 1987;11:217–218.

279. Yamamoto T, Yasui W, Ochiai A, et al. Immunohistochemical detection of c-myc oncogene product in human gastric carcinomas: Expression in tumor cells and stromal cells. Jpn J Cancer Res 1987;78:1169–1174.

280. Tahara E, Sumiyoshi H, Hata J, et al. Human epidermal growth factor in gastric carcinoma as a biologic marker of high malignancy. Jpn J Cancer Res 1986;77:145–152.

281. Sakai K, Mori S, Kawamoto T, et al. Expression of epidermal growth factor receptors on human gastric epithelia and gastric carcinomas. J Natl Cancer Inst 1986;77:1047–1052.

282. Uchino S, Tsuda H, Maruyama K, et al. Overexpression of c-erbB-2 protein in gastric cancer: Its correlation with long-term survival of patients. Cancer 1993;72:3179–3184.

283. Mizutani T, Onda M, Tokunaga A, et al. Relationship of C-erbB-2 protein expression and gene amplification to invasion and metastasis in human gastric cancer. Cancer 1993;72:2083–2088.

284. Joypaul BU, Hopwood D, Newman EL, et al. The prognostic significance of the accumulation of p53 tumor-suppressor gene protein in gastric adenocarcinoma. Br J Cancer 1994;69:943–946.

285. Kakeji Y, Korenaga D, Tsujitani S, et al. Gastric cancer with p53 overexpression has high potential for metastasizing to lymph nodes. Br J Cancer 1993;67:589–593.

286. Lim BHG, Soong R, Grieu F, et al. p53 accumulation and mutation are prognostic indicators of poor survival in human gastric carcinoma. Int J Cancer 1996;69:200–204.

287. Kojima O, Ikeda E, Uehara Y, et al. Correlation between carcinoembryonic antigen in gastric cancer tissue and survival of patients with gastric cancer. Gann 1984;75:230–236.

288. Ito H, Tahara E. Human chorionic gonadotropin in human gastric carcinoma. A retrospective immunohistochemical study. Acta Pathol Jpn 1983;33:287–296.

289. Tahara E, Ito H, Shimamoto F, et al. Lysozyme in human gastric carcinoma: A retrospective immunohistochemical study. Histopathology 1982;6:409–421.

290. Yokozaki H, Takekura N, Takanashi A, et al. Estrogen receptors in gastric adenocarcinoma: A retrospective immunohistochemical analysis. Virchows Arch [A] 1988;413:297–302.

291. Johnson H Jr, Belluco C, Masood S, et al. The value of flow cytometric analysis in patients with gastric cancer. Arch Surg 1993;128:314–317.

292. Gabbert HE, Mueller W, Schneiders A, et al. Prognostic value of E-cadherin expression in 413 gastric carcinomas. Int J Cancer 1996;69:184–189.

293. Hermanek P. Prognostic factors in stomach cancer surgery. Eur J Surg Oncol 1986;12:241–246.

294. Sjostedt S, Pieper R. Gastric cancer. Factors influencing long term survival and postoperative mortality. Acta Chir Scand (Suppl) 1986;530:25–29.

295. Martin IG, Dixon MF, Sue-ling H, et al. Goseki histological grading of gastric cancer is an important predictor of outcome. Gut 1994;35:758–763.

296. Guglielmi A, DeManzoni G, Verlato G, et al. Is the Goseki histological grading of gastric cancer a new prognostic factor? In: Siewert JR, Roder JD, eds. Progress in gastric cancer research 1997. Bologna: Monduzzi Editore, 1997;181–186.

297. Allum WH, Brearley S, Wheatley KE, et al. Acute haemorrhage from gastric malignancy. Br J Surg 1990;77:19–20.

298. Fuchs CS, Mayer RJ. Gastric carcinoma. N Engl J Med 1995;333:32–41.

299. Wilson TS. Free perforation in malignancies of the stomach. Can J Surg 1966;9:357–364.

300. Macdougall IC, Fleming S, Frier BM. Hypoglycaemic coma associated with gastric carcinoma. Postgrad Med J 1986;62:761–764.

301. Obara T, Ito Y, Kodama T, et al. A case of gastric carcinoma associated with excessive granulocytosis. Production of a colony-stimulating factor by the tumor. Cancer 1885;56:782–788.

302. Bhathal PS, Brown RW, Doyle TC, et al. Pneumatosis cystoides gastrica associated with adenocarcinoma of the stomach. Acta Cytol 1985;29:147–150.

303. Zimmerman SE, Smith FP, Phillips TM, et al. Gastric carcinoma and thrombotic thrombocytopenic purpura: Association with plasma immune complex concentrations. Br Med J (Clin Res) 1982;284:1432–1434.

304. Hugh A, Beris P. Eleven cases of neoplastic microangiopathy. Nouv Rev Fr Hematol 1989;31:223–230.

305. Sawabe M, Ohashi I, Kitagawa T. Diffuse intrasinusoidal metastasis of gastric carcinoma to the liver leading to fulminating hepatic failure. A case report. Cancer 1990;65:169–173.

306. Barentsz JO, Rosenbusch GR, Strijk SP, et al. Radiologic examination in gastric cancer. A retrospective study of 188 patients. Acta Radiol (Diagn) 1986;27:547–552.

307. Vyberg M, Hougen HP, Tonnesen K. Diagnostic accuracy of endoscopic gastrobiopsy in carcinoma of the stomach. A histopathological review of 101 cases. Acta Pathol Microbiol Immunol Scand (A) 1983;91:483–487.

308. Isaacson P. Biopsy appearances easily mistaken for malignancy in gastrointestinal endoscopy. Histopathology 1982;6:377–389.

309. Au FC, Koprowska I, Berger A, et al. The role of cytology in the diagnosis of carcinoma of the stomach. Surg Gynecol Obstet 1980;151:601–603.

310. Shiu MH, Karpeh M Jr, Brennan MF. End results of surgical treatment of gastric adenocarcinoma: American experience. In: Nishi M, Ichikawa H, Nakajima T, et al., eds. Gastric cancer. Tokyo: Springer, 1993;331–340.

311. Curtis RE, Kennedy BJ, Myers MH, et al. Evaluation of AJC stomach cancer staging using the SEER population. Semin Oncol 1985;12:21–31.

312. Noguchi Y, Imada T, Matsumoto A, et al. Radical surgery for gastric cancer. Cancer 1989;64:2053–2062.

313. Habu H, Takeshita K, Sunagawa M, et al. Prognostic factors of early gastric cancer—results of long-term follow-up and analysis of recurrent cases. Jpn J Surg 1987;17:248–255.

314. Hiki Y. Endoscopic treatment of early gastric cancer. In: Nishi M, Ichikawa H, Nakajima T, et al., eds. Gastric cancer. Tokyo: Springer, 1993;392–403.

315. Yamazaki H, Oshima A, Murakami R, et al. A long-term follow-up study of patients with gastric cancer detected by mass screening. Cancer 1989;63:613–617.

316. Nakajima T. Adjuvant and neoadjuvant chemotherapy in gastric cancer: A review. In: Nishi M, Ichikawa H, Nakajima T, et al., eds. Gastric cancer. Tokyo: Springer, 1993;404–414.

317. Preusser P, Wilke H. New systemic chemotherapy. In: Nishi M, Ichikawa H, Nakajima T, et al., eds. Gastric cancer. Tokyo: Springer, 1993;415–424.

318. Kelsen DP. Adjuvant and neoadjuvant therapy for gastric cancer. Semin Oncol 1996;23:379–389.

319. Wils J. The treatment of advanced gastric cancer. Semin Oncol 1996;23:397–406.

320. Minksy BD. The role of radiation therapy in gastric cancer. Semin Oncol 1996;23:390–396.

321. Misumi A, Murakami A, Harada K, et al. Definition of carcinoma of the gastric cardia. Langenbecks Arch Chir 1989;374:221–226.

322. Siewert JR, Holscher AH, Becker K, et al. Kardiakarzinom: Versuch einer therapeutisch relevanten Klassifikation. Chirurg 1987;58: 25–34.

323. Wang HH, Antonioli DA, Goldman H. Comparative features of esophageal and gastric adenocarcinomas: Recent changes in type and frequency. Hum Pathol 1986;17:482–487.

324. Schumpelick V, Dreuw B, Ophoff K, et al. Adenokarzinom des osophagogastralen Uberganges: Assoziation mit Barrett-Osophagus und gastroosophagealer Refluxkrankheit-Chirurgische Ergebnisse bei 122 Patienten. Leber Magen Darm 1996;26:75–76, 79–80, 83–86.

325. Kalish RJ, Clancy PE, Orringer MB, et al. Clinical, epidemiologic, and morphologic comparison between adenocarcinoma arising in Barrett's esophageal mucosa and in the gastric cardia. Gastroenterology 1984;86:461–467.

326. Duhaylongsod FG, Wolfe WG. Barrett's esophagus and adenocarcinoma of the esophagus and gastroesophageal junction. J Thorac Cardiovas Surg 1991;102:36–41.

327. Brown LM, Silverman DT, Pottern LM, et al. Adenocarcinoma of the esophagus and esophagogastric junction in white men in the United States: Alcohol, tobacco, and socioeconomic factors. Cancer Causes Control 1994;5:333–340.

328. Locke GR 3rd, Talley NJ, Carpenter HA, et al. Changes in the site- and histology-specific incidence of gastric cancer during a 50-year period. Gastroenterology 1995;109:1750–1756.

329. Antonioli DA, Goldman H. Changes in the location and type of gastric adenocarcinoma. Cancer 1982;50:775–781.

330. Allum WH, Powell DJ, McConkey CC, et al. Gastric cancer: A 25-year review. Br J Surg 1989;76:535–540.

331. Mori M, Kitagawa S, Iida M, et al. Early carcinoma of the gastric cardia. A clinicopathologic study of 21 cases. Cancer 1987;59:1758–1766.

332. Li L, Pan GL. Pathology of the gastric cardia. In: Huang GJ, Wu YK, eds. Carcinoma of the esophagus and gastric cardia. Berlin: Springer, 1984:117–155.

333. Okamura T, Tsujitani S, Marin P, et al. Adenocarcinoma in the upper third part of the stomach. Surg Gynecol Obstet 1987;165: 247–250.

334. Nakane Y, Okamura S, Boku T, et al. Prognostic differences of adenocarcinoma arising from the cardia and the upper third of the stomach. Am Surg 1993;59:423–429.

335. Sarbia M, Molsberger G, Willers R, et al. The prognostic significance of DNA ploidy in adenocarcinomas of the esophagogastric junction. J Cancer Res Clin Oncol 1996;122:186–188.

336. Uchida Y, Roessner A, Schlake W, et al. Development of tumors in the glandular stomach of rats after oral administration of carcinogens. II. Different cell types in antral carcinoma as revealed by electron microscopy. Z Krebsforsch 1976;87:213–228.

337. Mori M, Iwashita A, Enjoji M. Squamous cell carcinoma of the stomach: Report of three cases. Am J Gastroenterol 1986;81: 339–342.

338. Toyota N, Minagi S, Takeuchi T, et al. Adenosquamous carcinoma of the stomach associated with separate early gastric cancer (type IIc). J Gastroenterol 1996;31:105–108.

339. Sato N, Wada K, Kobayashi K, et al. A case of primary adenosquamous carcinoma of the stomach associated with gastric polyposis (in Japanese). Gan No Rinsho 1984;30:292–295.

340. Callery CD, Sanders MM, Pratt S, et al. Squamous cell carcinoma of the stomach: A study of four patients with comments on histogenesis. J Surg Oncol 1985;29:166–172.

341. Volpe CM, Hameer HR, Masetti P, et al. Squamous cell carcinoma of the stomach. Am Surg 1995;61:1076–1078.

342. Ruck P, Wehrmann M, Campbell M, et al. Squamous cell carcinoma of the gastric stump. A case report and review of the literature. Am J Surg Pathol 1989;13:317–324.

343. Mingazzini PL, Barsotti P, Malchiodi-Albedi F. Adenosquamous carcinoma of the stomach: Histological, histochemical and ultrastructural observations. Histopathology 1983;7:433–443.

344. Mori M, Iwashita A, Enjoji M. Adenosquamous carcinoma of the stomach. A clinicopathologic analysis of 28 cases. Cancer 1986;57: 333–339.

345. Saito T, Iizuka T, Kato H, et al. Esophageal carcinoma metastatic to the stomach. A clinicopathologic study of 35 cases. Cancer 1985;56: 2235–2241.

346. Talerman A, Woo-Ming MO. The origin of squamous cell carcinoma of the gastric cardia. Cancer 1968;22:1226–1232.

347. Won OH, Farman J, Krishnan MN, et al. Squamous cell carcinoma of the stomach. Am J Gastroenterol 1978;69:594–598.

348. Mori M, Fukuda T, Enjoji M. Adenosquamous carcinoma of the stomach. Histogenetic and ultrastructural studies. Gastroenterology 1987;92:1078–1082.

349. Lissens P, Peperstraete L, Mulier K, et al. Primary pure squamous cell carcinoma of the antrum of the stomach: A case report. Acta Chir Belg 1995;95(Suppl):184–186.

350. Szogi S. Muco-epidermoid carcinoma of the stomach. Acta Pathol Microbiol Scand 1959;46:37–42.

351. Hayashi I, Muto Y, Fujii Y, et al. Mucoepidermoid carcinoma of the stomach. J Surg Oncol 1987;34:94–99.

352. Ishikura H, Aizawa M. Hepatoid adenocarcinoma of the stomach. Lab Invest 1987;56:33A.

353. Nagai E, Ueyama T, Yao T, et al. Hepatoid adenocarcinoma of the stomach. A clinicopathologic and immunohistochemical analysis. Cancer 1993;72:1827–1835.

354. deLorimier A, Park F, Aranha GV, et al. Hepatoid carcinoma of the stomach. Cancer 1993;71:293–296.

355. Morinaga S, Takahashi Y. Primary hepatocellular carcinoma and hepatoid adenocarcinoma of the stomach with liver metastasis: An unusual association. Jpn J Clin Oncol 1996;26:258–263.

356. Eusterman GB, Senty EG. Benign tumors of the stomach, report of 27 cases. Surg Gynecol Obstet 1922;34:5–15.

357. Cairo MS, Grosfeld JL, Weetman RM. Gastric teratoma: Unusual cause for bleeding of the upper gastrointestinal tract in the newborn. Pediatrics 1981;67:721–724.

358. Nmadu PT, Mabogunje OA, Lawrie JH. Gastric teratoma: A case report. Ann Trop Paediatr 1993;13:291–292.

359. Gengler JS, Ashcraft KW, Slattery P. Gastric teratoma: The sixth reported case in a female infant. J Pediatr Surg 1995;30:889–890.

360. Haley T, Dimler M, Hollier P. Gastric teratoma with gastrointestinal bleeding. J Pediatr Surg 1986;21:949–950.

361. Imai Y, Kawabe T, Takahashi M, et al. A case of primary gastric choriocarcinoma and a review of the Japanese literature. J Gastroenterol 1994;29:642–646.

362. Mori H, Soeda O, Kamano T, et al. Choriocarcinomatous change with immunocytochemically HCG-positive cells in the gastric carcinoma of the males. Virchows Arch [A] 1982;396:141–153.

363. Ramponi A, Angeli G, Arceci F, et al. Gastric choriocarcinoma; an immunohistochemical study. Pathol Res Pract 1986;181:390–396.

364. Saigo PE, Brigati DJ, Sternberg SS, et al. Primary gastric choriocarcinoma. An immunohistological study. Am J Surg Pathol 1981;5: 333–342.

365. Fukayama M, Hayashi Y, Koike M. Human chorionic gonadotropin in gastric carcinoma. An immunohistochemical study suggesting independent regulation of subunits. Virchows Arch [A] 1987;411: 205–212.

366. Garcia RL, Ghali VS. Gastric choriocarcinoma and yolk sac tumor in a man: Observations about its possible origin. Hum Pathol 1985;16: 955–958.

367. Regan JF, Kremin JH. Chorioepithelioma of the stomach. Am J Surg 1960;100:224–233.

368. Motoyama T, Aizawa K, Fujiwara Y, et al. Coexistence of choriocarcinoma and hepatoid adenocarcinoma in the stomach. Pathol Int 194;44:716–721.

369. Zamecnik M, Patrikova J, Gomolcak P. Yolk sac carcinoma of the stomach with gastrin positivity. Hum Pathol 1993;24:927–928.

370. Gilligan CJ, Lawton GP, Tang LH, et al. Gastric carcinoid tumors: The biology and therapy of an enigmatic and controversial lesion. Am J Gastroenterol 1995;90:338–352.

371. Rappel S, Altendorf-Hofmann A, Stolte M. Prognosis of gastric carcinoid tumours. Digestion 1995;56:455–462.

372. Nagaoka S, Toyoshima H, Bandoh T, et al. Composite carcinoid-adenocarcinoma tumor of the stomach: Report of a case. Surg Today 1996;26:184–188.

373. Tahara E. Endocrine tumors of the gastrointestinal tract: Classification, function and biological behavior. In: Watanabe S, Wolff M, Sommers SC, eds. Digestive disease pathology. vol. 1. Philadelphia: Field & Wood, 1988;121–147.

374. Sugishita K, Tanno M, Kijima M, et al. Malignant hypercalcemia due to gastric endocrine cell carcinoma. Intern Med 1995;34: 104–107.

375. Caruso ML, Pilato FP, D'Adda T, et al. Composite carcinoid-adenocarcinoma of the stomach associated with multiple gastric carcinoids and nonantral gastric atrophy. Cancer 1989;64:1534–1539.

376. Hussein AM, Otrakji CL, Hussein BT. Small cell carcinoma of the stomach. Case report and review of the literature. Dig Dis Sci 1990;35:513–518.

377. Fukuda T, Ohnishi Y, Nishimaki T, et al. Early gastric cancer of the small cell type. Am J Gastroenterol 1988;83:1176–1179.

378. Shibuya H, Azumi N, Abe F. Gastric small-cell undifferentiated carcinoma with adeno and squamous cell components. Acta Pathol Jpn 1985;35:473–480.

379. Lo Re G, Canzonieri V, Veronesi A, et al. Extrapulmonary small cell carcinoma: A single institution experience and review of the literature. Ann Oncol 1994;5:909–913.

380. Masuyama K, Oonishi Y, Sawataishi M, et al. A case of small cell carcinoma of the stomach with multiple liver metastases. [Japanese] Gan To Kagaku Ryoho 1994;21:2338–2340.

381. Tanimura H, Furuta M. Carcinosarcoma of the stomach. Am J Surg 1967;113:702–709.

382. Robey-Cafferty SS, Grignon DJ, Ro JY, et al. Sarcomatoid carcinoma of the stomach. A report of three cases with immunohistochemical and ultrastructural observations. Cancer 1990;65:1601–1606.

383. Kumagai K, Kawai K, Kusano H, et al. A case of so-called carcinosarcoma of the stomach (in Japanese). Gan No Rinsho 1984;30: 1931–1936.

384. Minamoto T, Okada Y, Nakanishi I, et al. So called gastric carcinosarcoma—a case of chondrosarcomatous undifferentiated in the metastatic foci (in Japanese). Gan No Rinsho 1984;30:1321–1326.

385. Dundas SA, Slater DN, Wagner BE, et al. Gastric adenocarcinoleiomyosarcoma: A light, electron microscopic and immunohistological study. Histopathology 1988;13:347–350.

386. Tokunaga M, Land CE, Uemura Y, et al. Epstein-Barr virus in gastric carcinoma. Am J Pathol 1993;143:1250–1254.

387. Adachi Y, Yoh R, Konishi J, et al. Epstein-Barr virus-associated gastric carcinoma (review). J Clin Gastroenterol 1996;23:207–310.

388. Matsunou H, Konishi F, Hori H, et al. Characteristics of Epstein-Barr virus-associated gastric carcinoma with lymphoid stroma in Japan. Cancer 1996;77:1998–2004.

389. Honmyo U, Misumi A, Murakami A, et al. Clinicopathological analysis of synchronous multiple gastric carcinoma. Eur J Surg Oncol 1989;15:316–321.

390. Esaki Y, Hirokawa K, Yamashiro M. Multiple gastric cancers in the aged with special reference to intramucosal cancers. Cancer 1987;59: 560–565.

391. Marrano D, Viti G, Grigioni W, et al. Synchronous and metachronous cancer of the stomach. Eur J Surg Oncol 1987;13:493–498.

392. Kodera Y, Yamamura Y, Torii A, et al. Incidence, diagnosis and significance of multiple gastric cancer. Br J Surg 1995;82:1540–1543.

393. Iishi H, Tatsuta M, Okuda S. Diagnosis of simultaneous multiple gastric cancers by the endoscopic Congo red-methylene blue test. Endoscopy 1988;20:78–82.

394. Yoshino K, Asanuma F, Hanatani Y, et al. Multiple primary cancers in the stomach and another organ: Frequency and the effects on prognosis. Jpn J Clin Oncol 1985;15(Suppl 1):183–190.

395. Kasakura Y, Fujii M, Mochizuki M, et al. Clinical study on double cancer and triple cancer in the stomach and other organs. In: Siewert JR, Roder JD, eds. Progress in gastric cancer research 1997. Bologna: Monduzzi Editore, 1997;57–62.

396. Akehira K, Nakane Y, Iiyama H, et al. Second malignancies after gastrectomy for cancer. In: Siewert JR, Roder JD, eds. Progress in gastric cancer research 1997. Bologna: Monduzzi Editore, 1997; 63–66.

397. Ikeda Y, Mori M, Kajiyama K, et al. Multiple primary gastric and colorectal cancer in Japan. Int Surg 1995;80:37–40.

398. Lynge E, Jensen OM, Carstensen B. Second cancer following cancer of the digestive system in Denmark, 1943–80. Natl Cancer Inst Monogr 1985;68:277–308.

399. Ming SC. Tumors of the esophagus and stomach. In: Atlas of tumor pathology, second series, fascicle 7. Washington DC: Armed Forces Institute of Pathology, 1973;253–255.

400. Green LK. Hematogenous metastases to the stomach. A review of 67 cases. Cancer 1990;65:1596–1600.

401. Maeta M, Koga S, Shimizu N, et al. Clinicopathologic study of esophageal cancer associated with simultaneous metastatic lesions in the stomach. J Surg Oncol 1988;38:143–146.

402. Choi SH, Sheehan FR, Pickren JW. Metastatic involvement of the stomach by breast cancer. Cancer 1964;17:791–797.

403. Walker Q, Bilous M, Tiver KW, et al. Breast cancer metastases masquerading as primary gastric carcinoma. Aust NZ J Surg 1986; 56:395–398.

404. Gutman M, Klausner JM, Inbar M, et al. Surgical approach to malignant melanoma in the gastrointestinal tract. J Surg Oncol 1987;36:17–20.

405. Klausner JM, Skornick Y, Lelcuk S, et al. Acute complications of metastatic melanoma to the gastrointestinal tract. Br J Surg 1982; 69:195–196.

PART V

SMALL INTESTINE, COLON, AND RECTUM

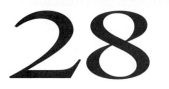

28 INFECTIOUS DISORDERS OF THE INTESTINES

Gerald D. Abrams

THE GASTROINTESTINAL TRACT AS AN ECOSYSTEM

THE NORMAL MICROBIAL FLORA

The gastrointestinal tract, in addition to being a complex apparatus for the digestion and absorption of nutrients, is actually a vast interface between the host and the environment. In approaching the infectious disorders of the intestine, it is therefore essential to view the subject with an ecologic perspective, recognizing the true relationship between the gastrointestinal mucosa and its surroundings.

Beginning at the moment of birth and throughout the life of the individual, the gastrointestinal tract is exposed to a continual stream of living microbial agents, and is quite literally "infected." From early infancy, a huge microbial population comes to inhabit the tract, from one end to the other. The microbial strains that associate in this fashion with the healthy host constitute the normal flora.

This complex microbial population, which reaches concentrations of 10^{12} cells per milliliter of intestinal content, is of reasonably predictable composition, given the fact that only a fraction of the microbial species encountered in the environment can survive and establish themselves in the particular conditions afforded by the gut (1). Moreover, the distribution of various species within the gastrointestinal tract is predictable, because the physicochemical microenvironment of one level of the tract differs from that of the others (with respect to pH, oxidation-reduction potential, nutrient concentrations, and the like), and a different set of microbial strains is adapted to each set of conditions. Finally, even at a given level of the gastrointestinal tract, there may be a predictable ordering of the flora, with some strains associating closely with or even adhering to the mucosal surface and others living within the luminal contents (2). In the normal host, all available "niches" are thus occupied, and the various microbial strains of flora in each location interact with one another and with the host.

The inevitable infection of the gastrointestinal tract with this normal flora does not produce disease and, in fact, even contributes to the physiologic well-being of the individual. The flora is a large, metabolically active mass, normally responsible for the biotransformation of many substances, both exogenous and endogenous, within the lumen (3). The normal luminal environment itself is actually the reflection of this metabolic activity, and even certain enzymes normally active within the lumen are known to be of microbial origin (4). The normal transit time of intestinal contents through the tract reflects a significant influence of the flora on peristaltic activity (5).

In the same fashion, even the normal histologic features of the gastrointestinal mucosa are shaped by the flora (Fig. 28.1). Comparison of germ-free animal hosts with those harboring a conventional flora has shown that the customarily observed cellularity of the lamina propria is largely a reaction to the flora, and that the normal histology of the gut-associated lymphoid tissues in general is likewise a response to the flora (6). The rate of epithelial cell renewal in the mucosa of normal or conventional animals is significantly faster than that of animals without the usual microbial load, and the mucosal content of certain enzymes is also influenced by the normal microbial presence (6, 7). Microflora also can modulate the endocrine cells of the gastrointestinal mucosa (8). Thus, the gastrointestinal tract normally "infected" by its resident flora is, in a general biologic sense, an ecosystem in which many complex interlocking equilibria are established and maintained within fairly narrow limits under ordinary conditions.

The conditions that are considered infectious disorders of the intestines can be comprehended in this perspective as significant perturbations of the ecosystem resulting from either invasion of exogenous agents capable of gaining a foothold among the normal residents or a change in the balance of endogenous strains and their relationship to one another and to the host.

STABILIZING FACTORS IN THE GASTROINTESTINAL ECOSYSTEM

Certain features of the normal gastrointestinal ecosystem, including both host and microbial factors, act in concert to maintain

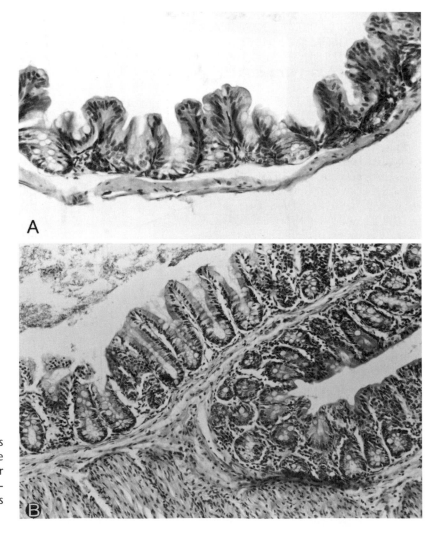

Figure 28.1   Large intestine of the germ-free (**A**), as compared with the conventional (**B**), mouse. The impact of the indigenous, normal flora in the latter animal is evident from differences in mucosal architecture and expansion of the lamina propria to its "normal" state as a response to the flora.

equilibrium and the status quo and to make it difficult for exogenous microbial stains to invade and successfully colonize the host. These stabilizing influences can be viewed as mucosal defense mechanisms.

GASTRIC ACIDITY

One factor that acts as an important initial defense mechanism, by diminishing the microbial load impinging on the small and large intestine, is the strongly acid pH of the normal stomach. Many microbial strains ingested from the environment are promptly killed on exposure to a pH of less than 4.0 (9). This microbicidal effect of acid has been clearly shown not only in vitro by direct test, but also in vivo by a number of observations. The variety of microbial strains that can be cultured from samples of gastric juice has been found to be much greater in patients with achlorhydria (pH ranging between 6.8 and 8.4) than in patients with acid gastric juice (pH between 1.3 and 3.4) (10). Furthermore, in a controlled experimental setting, the size of the dose of certain pathogens required to establish infection is significantly reduced if challenge occurs simultaneously with neutralization of gastric acidity (11). Finally, certain infections of the gastrointestinal tract have been found with greater frequency in postgastrectomy patients and in individuals who are achlorhydric for other reasons (12, 13).

INTESTINAL FACTORS

Those organisms that remain viable as they pass through the stomach generally are prevented from colonizing the small intestine by a set of defenses of a different sort. The major factor at this second level is the speedy propulsion of contents to the colon. Even in the absence of any significant microbicidal activity of the sort encountered in the stomach, simple mechanical flushing of the entering organisms prevents buildup of the intraluminal microbial population (14). It is primarily for this reason that microbial counts characteristically remain low in the small intestine. This mechanical defense of the small intestine is undoubtedly assisted by the constant production of mucus, which coats the mucosal surface and tends to minimize the chance that organisms can contact and perhaps adhere to the mucosa.

The importance of intestinal motility in mucosal defense is highlighted by certain observations in situations of impaired motility. For instance, studies show that an efficient means of ensuring the establishment of active infection after experimental challenge is the pharmacologic inhibition of peristalsis with opiates (15). Similarly, it has been observed that the clinical manifestations of shigellosis may actually be prolonged by antimotility drugs (16). Observations such as these argue strongly against the widespread use of antimotility preparations in the treatment of infectious diarrheal disease. Other intestinal factors that may play a role in stabilizing the gastrointestinal tract include antibiotic properties of the pancreatic juice and bile, lysozyme, and the normally brisk renewal of the lining of the tract (13).

MUCOSAL IMMUNE SYSTEM

An important additional factor, working in concert with the mechanisms just described, is the mucosal immune system (see Chapter 6). One major immunologic protection mechanism is mediated by secretory IgA, which inhibits microbial adherence to the epithelial lining of the gut, thus assuring rapid expulsion of microbes by mechanical means (17). The importance of antibody- and cell-mediated defenses in the intestine has been vividly underscored in recent years by the patterns of illness seen in immunocompromised patients, particularly those with acquired immunodeficiency syndrome (AIDS) (see Chapter 16). These patients frequently are overwhelmed by environmental microbes that are so unlikely to colonize normal subjects that we are generally unaware of their presence in our surroundings.

COLONIZATION RESISTANCE OF NORMAL FLORA

In the lower gastrointestinal tract, a very different set of conditions exists. At the colonic level, there is neither a strongly acid intraluminal pH nor a rapid defensive expulsion of contents. Rather, the major defensive mechanism is one of microbial ecology. This effect has been variously designated as "colonization resistance," "bacterial interference," or "bacterial antagonism," and is the direct result of a massive normal flora. The potential invaders that retain their viability on their way through the stomach and small intestine enter the colon in relatively small numbers and immediately confront a dense, established, resident flora.

The ability of this flora to inhibit the growth of invaders appears to be a reflection of competition for limited nutrients and/or the effect of metabolic inhibitors produced by the flora (18). Suppression of the resident flora is a well-recognized means of manipulating this ecologic defense experimentally. Furthermore, epidemiologic studies of certain *Salmonella* infections in the community have implicated the use of antibiotics as a risk factor in the development of infection, possibly reflecting lowered colonization resistance resulting from a disturbance in the normal flora (19, 20).

PERTURBATIONS OF THE GASTROINTESTINAL ECOSYSTEM

Viewing the gastrointestinal tract from an ecologic perspective is important because much of the infectious disease encountered in the gut is in reality not simply the result of an unlucky encounter with a passing pathogen. Actually, it is a reflection of some perturbation of the mucosal ecosystem, broadly defined. A microbial strain that functions as a colonizing pathogen in one situation may be handled as a transient visitor or even trivial symbiont in another situation with different conditions prevailing in the ecosystem. In fact, given sufficient disturbance of the gastrointestinal ecosystem, even components of the normal flora assume the role of pathogens.

CONTAMINATED SMALL BOWEL SYNDROME

An excellent example of the normal flora becoming pathogenic is the so-called contaminated small bowel syndrome, in which a large microbial population, especially the anaerobes normally inhabiting the colon, come to colonize the upper intestine (21). This situation can occur when the continuous unidirectional peristaltic cleansing of the small intestine is hampered, such as in association with various strictures and obstructions or after surgical construction of loops and bypasses. Such colonization may also accompany continuous microbial seeding of the small intestine, as in the presence of hypochlorhydria, enterocolic fistulas, or multiple, stagnant, small-intestinal diverticula. Because the normal characteristics of the tract reflect certain host-microbe equilibria, it stands to reason that such

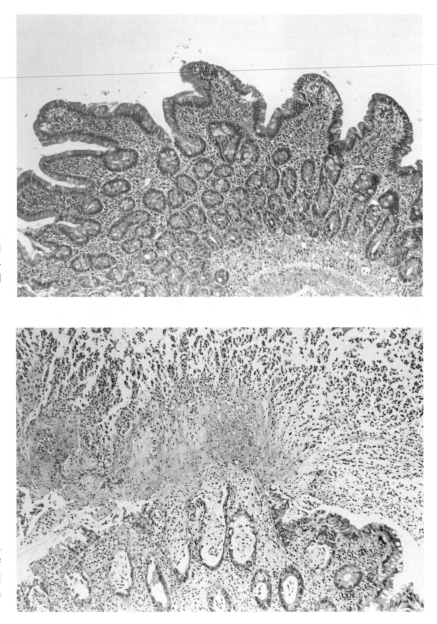

Figure 28.2 Mucosa of contaminated small bowel. Even the normal (colonic) flora in an abnormal setting is capable of altering host tissues, as evidenced by expansion of the lamina propria and architectural distortion.

Figure 28.3 Antibiotic-associated pseudomembranous colitis, type II lesion. A "mushroom" of exudate is adherent to the superficially damaged mucosal surface. Deeper portions of the mucosa survive.

a dramatic change in the habitat of the flora will alter these equilibria. In the contaminated small bowel syndrome, the results of these changes include steatorrhea owing to altered bile salt metabolism, macrocytic anemia reflecting microbial interaction with vitamin B_{12}, malabsorption of various nutrients, and even morphologic evidence of mucosal damage (Fig. 28.2). Somewhat analogous conditions may be noted in association with another sort of ecologic aberration in which subjects are exposed chronically to a grossly polluted environment that affords essentially continuous exposure to exogenous fecal contamination (21).

CLOSTRIDIUM DIFFICILE INFECTION AND PSEUDOMEMBRANOUS COLITIS

A far more important example of an ecologic perturbation is the recent emergence of *Clostridium difficile* in the role of intestinal pathogen. This organism is harbored by some healthy asymptomatic subjects, presumably in small numbers held in check by ecologic defenses. Many other individuals ordinarily are resistant to the organism, even though it is frequently present in the environment. *C. difficile* is an especially common environmental contaminant in hospitals and nursing facilities (22). When the normal intestinal flora is altered sufficiently, usually by antibiotic therapy, colonization resistance decreases and *C. difficile* is able to flourish, colonize the gut lumen, and produce an array of toxins (23). Two of these toxins have been well characterized: toxin A, which is both cytotoxic and enterotoxic, and toxin B, a potent cytotoxin that is principally responsible for changes noted in diagnostic toxin assays (24).

Proliferation of *C. difficile* can be associated with a variety of conditions, including pseudomembranous colitis and antibiotic-associated diarrhea. Although the histologic lesions of pseudomembranous colitis have been reproduced by exposure of the mucosa to cell-free, toxin-containing filtrates (25), the range of variation in the clinical expression of *C. difficile* infection, from asymptomatic carriage to fulminant colitis, has not been explained completely. Presumably, such variable expression is related to quantitative variations in bacillary proliferation and/or toxin production. *C. difficile* is thought to be responsible for a significant proportion of cases of antibiotic-associated diarrhea (without colitis), and for almost all cases of pseudomembranous colitis (22).

The morphologic lesion characteristically associated with *C. difficile* is pseudomembranous colitis, typified in type II lesions by groups of superficially damaged crypts covered by a mushrooming cloud of fibrinopurulent exudate, epithelial debris, and admixed mucus (Fig. 28.3). Alternation of affected areas with more normal areas produces the characteristic gross appearance (Fig. 28.4). Price and Davies stated that the diagnosis of pseudomembranous colitis

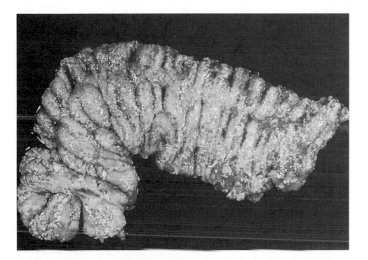

Figure 28.4 Antibiotic-associated pseudomembranous colitis, gross appearance. The yellow patches, which become confluent in some areas, represent adherent plaques of exudate corresponding to that shown in Figure 28.3. Transmural inflammation and developing megacolon led to colonic resection in this case. (See color plate.)

can also be made on finding a more limited lesion, which they designated a type I lesion, type II being the classic pseudomembranous lesion (26). The type I lesion consists of a focus of epithelial damage on the intercryptal surface or "summit," associated with a small cluster of leukocytes (Fig. 28.5). At the other extreme, *C. difficile* infection may produce full-thickness mucosal necrosis, which these authors described as a type III lesion.

Infection with *C. difficile* can produce a wide range of mucosal appearances. In one published study of biopsy material from patients with proven *C. difficile* infection, some individuals had no lesion, or only congestion and edema, some had a nonspecific colitis, and slightly more than 50% had the classic pseudomembranous lesion (27).

Our experience has been similar and has emphasized the importance of recognizing subtle variants of the early type I lesion. Conversely, we have seen transmural colonic inflammation in *C. difficile* infection (see Fig. 28.4), and other authors have described cases involving massive mural edema and toxic megacolon necessitating colonic resection (28, 29).

Although antibiotic therapy is the usual factor behind the ecologic perturbation that leads to *C. difficile* infection, this organism occasionally colonizes in patients without prior antibiotic exposure, has been associated with antineoplastic chemotherapy, and has been found in association with symptomatic flares of chronic inflammatory bowel disease (23, 30, 31).

NEUTROPENIC ENTEROCOLITIS

A third example of ecologic perturbation of the gastrointestinal tract leading to disease is the syndrome of necrotizing enterocolitis encountered in patients with malignancies, especially leukemia. This condition, variously termed "agranulocytic or neutropenic colitis," "typhlitis," and "ileocecal syndrome," is generally seen in patients receiving aggressive chemotherapy (32). In this clinical situation, the ecologic disturbance is complex, involving the host as well as possibly the flora. The lesions of neutropenic enterocolitis center about the terminal ileum and right colon and consist of patchy areas of transmural edema, necrosis, and microbial (bacterial and fungal)

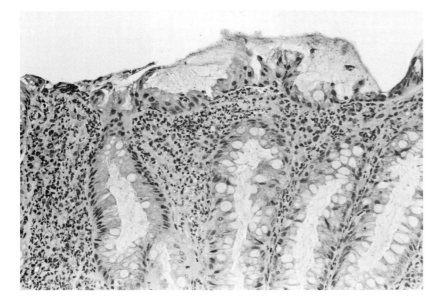

Figure 28.5 Antibiotic-associated pseudomembranous colitis, type I lesion. At the "summits" between crypts are small collections of neutrophils associated with tufts of damaged surface epithelium.

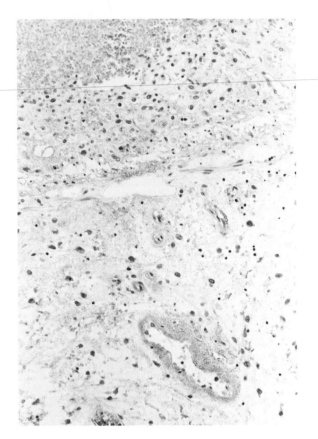

Figure 28.6   Neutropenic enterocolitis, showing *Candida* over-growth in the mucosa *(upper left)* and diffuse bacterial spread into the submucosa, lending a fuzzy character to the edematous tissue, evident especially around the blood vessel near the lower margin of the field. Note the paucity of cellular response.

invasion, with minimal cellular response (Fig. 28.6). These gastrointestinal lesions frequently are associated with positive blood cultures, most often with recovery of intestinal organisms. On the host side of the ecosystem, the critical pathogenetic factors are thought to include neutropenia and damage to the integrity of the mucosa, both related to chemotherapy. Given these alterations, microbial invasion could be a secondary phenomenon. These patients, however, generally have also been exposed to antibiotics, and it has been suggested that under these conditions, *Clostridium septicum* may be favored in a manner analogous to *C. difficile* in antibiotic-associated colitis. In neutropenic enterocolitis, however, the Clostridium appear actually to invade the wall (33).

A final related example of microecologic disturbance associated with significant disease is the observation that the combination of neutropenia and *C. difficile* infection may lead to polymicrobial bacteremia. This phenomenon may reflect entry of organisms from the bowel lumen through areas of clostridial mucosal damage (34).

EXOGENOUS INFECTION

VIRULENCE FACTORS

In the examples thus far discussed, infections have been secondary to a significant derangement of one or more elements of the digestive ecosystem. Under ordinary circumstances, this ecosystem has an impressive degree of stability and resistance to exogenous agents because of the defensive mechanisms intrinsic to it. Even so, there is a significant worldwide incidence of infection with enteric pathogens, reflecting not only unfavorable environmental conditions but also the development in some microbial species (i.e., the "pathogens") of mechanisms enabling them to overcome gastrointestinal defenses. The microbial attributes responsible for this ability to override host defenses are viewed as virulence factors, many of which have been mapped to microbial plasmids and chromosomes. It has been noted that the virulence factors of a microbe may be as important as its species in determining its status as a pathogen (35). *Escherichia coli* provides an excellent illustration of this principle. Various strains of this organism can produce disease through a wide variety of mechanisms, including enterotoxigenic, enteropathogenic, enteroinvasive, and enterohemorrhagic. Molecular aspects of microbial virulence factors are discussed in Chapter 8.

Descriptively, these virulence factors involve several general mechanisms: mucosal adhesion, tissue invasion, and microbial toxins.

MUCOSAL ADHESION

One set of virulence factors endows certain microbes with the ability to resist being swept rapidly through the gut. If peristaltic elimination can be avoided, colonization may then occur. This resistance to expulsion is accomplished by actual microbial adhesion to the surface of the intestine effected by ligand-receptor interaction between microbial surface structures and the host epithelial cell membrane. These microbial factors, termed "adhesins," reside on fimbriae or pili projecting from the microbial surface, as in the case of certain *E. coli*, or can be associated with surface structures other than fimbrial proteins, as in the case of *Vibrio cholerae* (36, 37). Antibody directed against these adhesins effectively prevents colonization and, thereby, production of disease. Certain organisms such as the cholera *Vibrio* are also equipped to supplement their adhesive properties with additional virulence factors conferring the ability to penetrate quickly through the layer of mucus protecting the mucosa and reach the epithelial surface. These ancillary factors include motility, chemotactic responsiveness, and mucinase production (38, 39).

TISSUE INVASION

A second set of virulence factors endows certain agents (e.g., *Shigella, Salmonella, Yersinia, Campylobacter*) with the ability to invade the mucosa after initial colonization. The first step in invasion involves entry into epithelial cells, apparently accomplished by a microbe-stimulated endocytosis on the part of the host cell (40). The M cells of follicle-associated epithelium may be preferentially involved in this process (41). Some organisms, such as *Salmonella*, are transported within phagosomes in the epithelial cell to be discharged into the lamina propria. Others organisms, such as *Shigella*, apparently spread laterally into other epithelial cells. In order to establish disease, the entering organisms must also be capable of intracellular multiplication, an attribute mediated by yet another set of virulence factors. The attributes of some organisms permit survival only in the lamina propria, whereas other agents are able to spread to regional lymph nodes or even systemically.

MICROBIAL TOXINS

Toxins, which are damaging substances produced by microbial agents, constitute yet another class of virulence factors. The two major groups of toxins of enteropathogens are enterotoxins and cytotoxins. Enterotoxins, without killing the epithelial cells or producing a significant histologic lesion, sharply alter cellular transport of electrolytes and water, producing a net secretion of water that may overwhelm the absorptive capacities of the colon, producing diarrhea (42). Cytotoxins injure and kill cells and are therefore associated with histologic lesions of the mucosa.

Despite a precise definition of the pathogenic role of toxins in some of the enterotoxigenic secretory diarrheas, such as cholera, the details of pathogenesis have not been as clearly elaborated with respect to most invasive pathogens. For these agents, toxin production alone is insufficient and must be accompanied by invasion of the mucosa. Furthermore, diarrhea in these latter cases cannot be explained simply as a result of anatomic mucosal disruption. There is some evidence for a role of activated inflammatory mediators in some invasive infection (43, 44). These mediators may stimulate intestinal secretion by acting on both enterocytes and enteric nerves (45). Toxins may also act as virulence factors by altering the intestinal environment in a way that directly favors the microbial agent (e.g., release of some essential nutrient from the affected mucosa) (46). Less directly, it can be argued that toxins augment microbial spread in the environment through the provocation of diarrhea.

PATTERNS OF HOST-MICROBE INTERACTION

Because various microbial strains are endowed with different sets of virulence factors, it follows that these agents should manifest a variety of patterns of interaction with the host. Levine proposed the following classification of enteric pathogens that is based on their relative degrees of invasiveness (37).

MUCOSAL ADHESION OF ORGANISMS WITH ENTEROTOXIN PRODUCTION

In the infections of this class, the mucosa is not invaded and no histopathologic lesion is discernible. Organisms first attach to and colonize the mucosal surface of the small intestine and then elaborate and release enterotoxin, which leads to secretory diarrhea. Cholera, the classic example of this class of disease, involves enterotoxic activation of the adenylate cyclase system of the epithelium and secretion of large quantities of water with a histologically intact mucosa (37, 46, 47). Simultaneously, water absorption in the colon is suppressed (48). Enterotoxigenic E. coli organisms also exemplify this class of infection, producing infant diarrhea and traveler's diarrhea, especially in developing countries.

MUCOSAL ADHESION OF ORGANISMS WITH MICROVILLOUS DAMAGE

The best example of this type of infection is infant diarrhea associated with enteropathogenic E. coli. In this condition, microbial adherence is followed not by true cellular invasion, but by significant injury to microvilli. This ultrastructural cellular damage, together with the effects of the toxin, may produce the diarrhea (49).

MUCOSAL INVASION OF ORGANISMS WITH INTRACELLULAR PROLIFERATION

Shigella infections with invasion of the epithelial cells of the distal small intestine and colon typify this class. Bacteria tend to remain localized in epithelial cells, with some spread into the lamina propria. Cell damage leads to the inflammation, hemorrhage, and ulceration associated with signs and symptoms of dysentery. Varying degrees of watery diarrhea may also be seen in individuals with shigellosis. The pathogenic role of Shigella-associated toxin, which is cytotoxic, neurotoxic, and enterotoxic, is not entirely clear (50). Fluid secretion may be related in part to increased concentration of prostaglandins associated with inflammation (43). A similar pattern of disease is also seen in the dysenteric syndrome produced by enteroinvasive E. coli.

MUCOSAL INVASION OF ORGANISMS WITH PROLIFERATION IN LAMINA PROPRIA AND REGIONAL LYMPH NODES

This class of infection includes diseases related to nontyphoid Salmonella species, Yersinia, and Campylobacter. Although toxins have been associated with these organisms, details of pathogenesis are incompletely understood.

MUCOSAL TRANSLOCATION OF ORGANISMS WITH SYSTEMIC SPREAD

Salmonella typhi and Salmonella paratyphi are examples of agents that, through their virulence factors, are able to survive the inflammatory response in the lamina propria, spread into the regional lymph nodes, and ultimately spread to the circulation. Survival within macrophages of the nonimmune host appears to be a key factor (37).

HEMORRHAGIC COLITIS

Another pattern of host-microbe interaction that does not conform precisely to those just listed is exemplified by the hemorrhagic colitis caused by strains of E. coli that produce toxins cytopathic for HeLa and Vero cells. These toxins are similar or identical to Shiga toxins. E. coli 0157:H7 is the most prominent of several verotoxin-producing strains. These "enterohemorrhagic" E. coli organisms, transmitted in food (especially poorly cooked hamburger) or water, cause a generally nonfebrile illness characterized by abdominal cramps and first watery and then bloody diarrhea. The organisms are noninvasive, but the mucosa can nonetheless be damaged significantly, either by direct contact or through the effect of the cytotoxins. Lesions are nonspecific and can resemble those of acute self-limited (infectious) colitis described subsequently, but they can also have the pattern of ischemic injury or even pseudomembranous colitis (51, 52). Although the colitis most often is self-limited, the hemolytic uremic syndrome or thrombotic thrombocytopenic purpura may be a complication (53).

PATHOLOGY OF INTESTINAL INFECTIONS

GENERAL CONSIDERATIONS

Given the multiple types of microbial agents that can infect the digestive tract, their differing degrees of invasiveness, and the variety of their virulence factors, it is difficult to characterize the pathology of intestinal infections succinctly.

At one extreme, some infectious agents may be associated with dramatic or even lethal physiologic derangements but produce no significant pathologic lesion. In cholera, the classic example of this sort of disease, enterotoxin production by the *Vibrio* organisms colonizing the gut triggers a massive secretion of water, but without an accompanying enteritis. The recognition of this important principle is a relatively recent event historically, correcting a misconception that originated in the time of Virchow. Observations at autopsy, confounded by inevitable autolytic changes in the intestinal mucosa, had led to the concept that the diarrhea of cholera was the result of mucosal denudement. Many years later, biopsy results showed that the mucosa was actually intact during the active stages of disease (54). A corollary to this principle is that even in those diseases associated with a significant histopathologic lesion, all clinically observed derangements are not necessarily correlated with that particular lesion.

At the opposite extreme, some enteric infections are associated with a characteristic or even pathognomonic histopathologic appearance. Such is the case with certain viral infections (e.g., cytomegalovirus), wherein cytopathologic changes are virtually diagnostic, as well as for those infectious agents (e.g., protozoans, helminths, and certain fungi) that can be recognized readily in tissue sections.

For most enteric infections encountered by the pathologist, however, the recognition of a particular histopathologic lesion does not in itself allow a specific etiologic diagnosis. Many diverse infections are associated with the same spectrum of mucosal changes, including damage to the surface and/or crypt epithelium, regenerative alterations in epithelial cell renewal patterns, altered mucin secretion, hyperemia and edema of the lamina propria, and leukocytic infiltration of varying degree. Only when these changes are correlated with microbial, immunologic, and clinical information is it possible to make a specific diagnosis.

ACUTE SELF-LIMITED ENTEROCOLITIS

An issue of crucial practical importance for the pathologist is distinguishing between mucosal lesions of the sort produced by various microbial agents and those of idiopathic bowel disease, such as chronic ulcerative colitis or Crohn's disease. Patients presenting with bloody diarrhea of sudden onset may have an acute infectious enterocolitis or may be suffering the first clinical manifestations of idiopathic inflammatory bowel disease. In the former, the disease is usually short-lived and even self-limited, whereas in the latter, a protracted chronic course can be expected. Although stool cultures would appear to be the obvious way to make the distinction, it is estimated that enteric pathogens are recovered in only 50% of cases of self-limited colitis. Therefore, biopsy assumes a role of great importance.

Kumar and colleagues delineated the histopathologic features that are helpful in making this distinction (55). They studied a group of patients with "acute self-limited colitis" (ASLC), defined as a first episode of bloody diarrhea, accompanied by a sigmoidoscopic appearance consistent with inflammatory bowel disease, a rapid clinical resolution (usually within 2 weeks), and normal clinical follow-up examinations. Their study group included patients from whom *Campylobacter, Salmonella, Shigella,* and *Yersinia* were recovered; in 57.5% of their patient population, no "pathogen" was recovered. The most important characteristic changes in sigmoidoscopic biopsy samples were seen within the first 4 days after the onset of clinical disease. These changes included mucosal edema; superficial ulcers with a neutrophilic surface exudate; cryptitis, crypt ulcers, and crypt abscesses; diminution in the amount of intracellular mucin; and increased cellularity of the lamina propria, with neutrophils and lesser numbers of lymphocytes, plasma cells, and eosinophils (Fig. 28.7). During the next several days, the edema was variable; regenerative epithelial changes appeared; active crypt

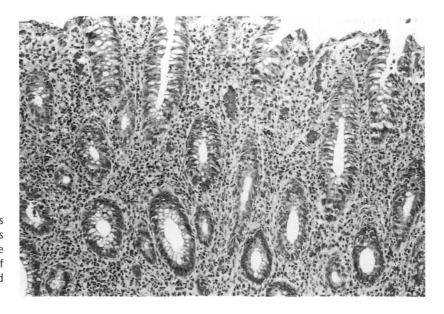

Figure 28.7 Acute self-limited colitis. Goblet cells are partly depleted of mucin, and the mucosa is diffusely inflamed, with a neutrophilic infiltrate in the epithelium. The appearance differs from that of ulcerative colitis in the lack of basal plasmacytosis and of significant crypt distortion.

lesions became more focal; and neutrophils were less prominent in the lamina propria. In the later stages of resolution, at the latter part of the second week, mucosal edema had disappeared; active crypt lesions had resolved, leaving some persistent features of regeneration; a slight increase in lamina propria cellularity was noted; and some biopsies were essentially normal. At none of these stages was there evidence of significant crypt distortion (abnormal shapes, branching, loss of parallelism) or plasmacytosis in the lower one fifth of the mucosa. The absence of crypt distortion and basal plasmacytosis was the most useful criterion in separating a self-limited colitis from a chronic colitis.

In a follow-up study, patients with ASLC were compared with ulcerative colitis patients, and the differential diagnostic validity of these features was confirmed (56). The resolving phase of ASLC, however, with its residual focal cryptitis, may be confused with Crohn's disease, and appropriate clinical follow-up is required. The utility of biopsy and distinguishing between ASLC and idiopathic inflammatory bowel disease has been independently confirmed (57). Results of other studies have indicated, however, that almost one third of patients presenting with acute diarrhea and histologic findings of ASLC may eventually develop idiopathic chronic inflammatory bowel disease (58), and that interobserver disagreement limits the discriminant value of histologic analysis (59). Thus, it appears that although histopathologic interpretation is of significant value in many cases, it must be considered in the context of other laboratory data, clinical findings, and results of imaging studies.

EXCLUSION OF NONINFECTIOUS CAUSES

An important factor to consider in the interpretation of biopsy material is the effect of agents used to prepare the bowel for endoscopic examination, because these effects may include mild "colitic" changes (see Chapters 3 and 11 for additional information.) Hypertonic phosphate enemas can produce damage and/or detachment of surface epithelium, partial depletion of cellular mucin, and edema of the lamina propria (60). Bisacodyl has been associated with similar changes, as well as with deeper crypt damage and occasional neutrophilic accumulation (61). Finally, it should be noted that a mucosal colitis (with crypt abscesses, epithelial cell degeneration, regenerative changes, inflammatory infiltrates, and lymphoid hyperplasia) has been seen in excluded segments of colon after diversion of the fecal stream (see Chapter 30). This colitic lesion does not appear to be related to known intestinal "pathogens," is reversible with correction of the diversion, and seems to respond to topical application of short-chain fatty acids that are absent from the excluded segment (62, 63).

VIRAL INFECTIONS
VIRAL GASTROENTERITIS

Acute viral gastroenteritis is an exceedingly common ailment in many parts of the world that is responsible for abundant, generally self-limited morbidity, and occasional mortality. Although multiple viral agents may be responsible for these frequent infections, the rotaviruses, Norwalk virus, and enteric adenoviruses are recognized as etiologically most important in nonbacterial acute gastroenteritis (64). These infections are characterized by invasion of mature enterocytes of the small intestine (65). Mucosal injury leads to shortening of villi and lengthening of crypts, with heightened

mitotic activity and cellular infiltration of the lamina propria (66). The diarrhea associated with these infections represents a net secretion of water by the intestine. In the case of rotavirus enteritis, evidence suggests that the functional abnormalities are related not to direct damage of enterocytes, but to altered differentiation of epithelial cells as cell renewal patterns change (65). Although the histopathologic lesions associated with these infections have been characterized in limited biopsy studies, diagnosis is most often circumstantial or immunologic.

OTHER VIRAL LESIONS

Although less common than the gastroenteritides just described, certain other viral lesions are encountered by the pathologist in surgical material. Lesions associated with these viruses can be identified by demonstration of characteristic cytopathic changes. Immunoperoxidase techniques can be applied to show specific antigen in these lesions.

Herpesvirus Infection

Herpes simplex virus is an important cause of proctitis in homosexual males having anal receptive intercourse (67). Signs and symptoms include anorectal pain, tenesmus, constipation, difficulty in urinating, sacral paresthesias, and inguinal adenopathy. Physical examination may reveal perianal vesicular lesions, and sigmoidoscopic findings include mucosal friability and distal rectal ulcers or vesicles. Histopathologic findings in herpetic proctitis may be largely nonspecific, with crypt abscesses and increased numbers of neutrophils in the lamina propria. Some patients also manifest other more characteristic findings, including perivascular lymphocytic cuffing in the submucosa, intranuclear inclusions, and multinucleated giant cells with "ground-glass" nuclei in the submucosa.

Cytomegalovirus Infection

Cytomegalovirus infection of the digestive tract is an increasingly frequent clinical finding because of its common occurrence in patients with AIDS and in iatrogenically immunosuppressed transplant patients (68, 69). The infection can also be seen in immunocompetent subjects, as a complicating feature of ulcerative colitis (70–72). In the intestinal tract, cytomegalovirus has been associated with a variety of lesions, including hemorrhage, ulceration, and perforation, but the role of the virus in initiating the mucosal damage is not clear. Some evidence suggests that the virus is simply an opportunist that colonizes established lesions, whereas other data point to a primary role. Another suggestion is that cytomegalovirus preferentially infects rapidly proliferating granulation tissue, perhaps aggravating various primary injuries (73). Some authors have claimed that such cytomegalovirus infection may lead to worsening or intractability of underlying ulcerative colitis, whereas others have considered the infection without effect on the course of the colitis (71, 74).

In most instances, the cytomegalovirus associated with ulcerative lesions seems to have a special affinity for cells in and around small vessels (Fig. 28.8) but is rarely found in epithelial cells. Infected cells are significantly enlarged, with an increase in both nuclear and cytoplasmic volume. The typical virocyte has a large, basophilic to amphophilic intranuclear inclusion surrounded by a

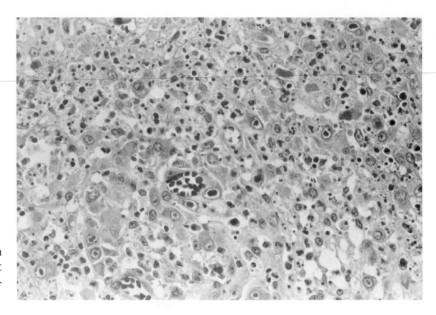

Figure 28.8 Granulation tissue in the colon of a patient with ulcerative colitis. The cytopathologic features of cytomegalovirus infection, centered especially around small vessels are evident.

zone of nuclear clearing. Somewhat granular inclusion material of similar tinctorial character may be seen in the cytoplasm as well.

Adenovirus Infection

Although adenovirus gastroenteritis is common in pediatric populations, pathologic material is rarely seen in the usual, uncomplicated clinical setting. It has been noted, however, that a significant association exists between adenovirus infection and ileocecal intussusception (75, 76). In such cases, characteristic intranuclear inclusions are seen in the epithelial cells of terminal ileum and/or appendix (Fig. 28.9), frequently associated with lymphoid hyperplasia.

CHLAMYDIAL INFECTIONS

Chlamydiae, well recognized as etiologic agents of ocular, respiratory, and genital infections, are increasingly being documented as a cause of disease in the distal large intestine. Certain subtypes of the species *Chlamydia trachomatis* are known to produce a spectrum of infection, ranging from trachoma and inclusion conjunctivitis to salpingitis and nongonococcal urethritis; others subtypes are associated with lymphogranuloma venereum (LGV). Both LGV and non-LGV immunotypes infect the large bowel (77). Anorectal LGV is a recognized secondary complication of genital LGV, especially in women (78). Primary chlamydial bowel infection, however, is recognized most often in homosexual males and can involve non-LGV as well as LGV immunotypes of *C. trachomatis*. Definitive diagnosis of chlamydial proctitis is based on isolation of the agent from the rectum or serologic evidence of its presence.

LGV strains appear to be associated with more severe disease than non-LGV stains (77). Some patients with proven infection are essentially asymptomatic; at the opposite extreme, patients present with significant pain, bleeding, and discharge of exudate. Endoscopically, findings range from mild erythema and friability to severe mucosal disruption with ulceration and formation of fistulas. The histologic appearance of chlamydial infection is similarly variable. Some cases show only nonspecific changes of mild ASLC; others can

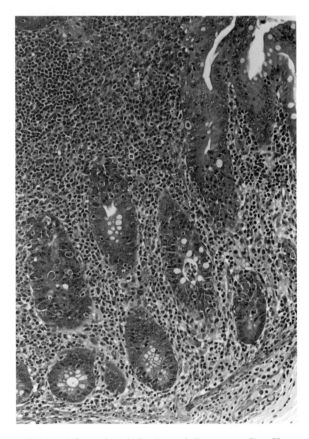

Figure 28.9 Adenovirus infection of the appendix. Characteristic inclusions in crypt epithelium are seen at far left and at far right.

easily be confused with chronic inflammatory bowel disease. In proctocolitis produced by LGV strains of *C. trachomatis*, biopsy specimens with chronic, focally granulomatous mucosal lesions can be indistinguishable from those of Crohn's disease, and this differential diagnosis must be kept in mind. A detailed autopsy study of the bowel in patients with clinically recognized genital LGV suggests that the lesions of LGV, as contrasted with those of Crohn's colitis, are rarely seen proximal to the midportion of the descending colon (78).

BACTERIAL INFECTIONS

Bacteria of many different types infect the human digestive tract and produce various combinations of gastroenteritis and/or enterocolitis. As outlined previously, the pathogenesis and pathophysiology of these infections are complex and involve colonization of the small and large intestines in varying combination. Clinical manifestations of these diseases may involve simple diarrhea related to enterotoxin-induced alterations in mucosal water absorption and secretion, dysentery owing to the invasive and destructive action of the bacteria, or a combination of the two. Specific diagnosis of bacterial infections generally involves cultural or serologic identification of the etiologic agent, because clinical syndromes tend to overlap and pathologic features are most often nonspecific. Practical aspects of laboratory diagnosis have been reviewed (79).

SALMONELLOSIS AND SHIGELLOSIS

The "classic" bacterial pathogens of the intestinal tract are *Salmonella* organisms, typically agents of "food poisoning," and *Shigella* organisms of various species, often associated with epidemics of bacillary dysentery. These organisms can actually produce a range of signs and symptoms, from watery diarrhea to full-blown dysentery, with fever, abdominal pain, and bloody diarrhea. These agents are thought to colonize both the small intestine and the large intestine, but the detailed pathologic features of the small intestine have not been as well studied as has the appearance of the large intestine, especially the rectum. Findings from a colonoscopic study of shigellosis indicate that the rectosigmoid is the most frequently and most severely affected level of the colon, and that there are lesser degrees of proximal extension during the course of the disease (80). In fatal cases, pancolitis is common (81). The endoscopic appearance of *Salmonella* and *Shigella* colitis can vary from relatively mild mucosal inflammation with hyperemia and contact bleeding to a raggedly eroded surface. Biopsy studies in both salmonellosis and shigellosis cases have shown the proctocolitis is characterized by nondistortive, relatively superficial changes detailed previously as those of ASLC (82, 83)(Fig. 28.10). These histopathologic characteristics do not permit the designation of a specific etiologic agent without collateral microbiologic or serologic data, but do generally allow the distinction between "acute infectious colitis" and chronic inflammatory bowel disease, such as ulcerative colitis. A study from West Bengal demonstrated, to the contrary, that lesions of shigellosis may mimic the crypt distortion of ulcerative colitis (84). Similar observations in a study from Bangladesh have been reported (81). These contradictory findings may be a reflection of the particular characteristics and environment of those study populations.

CAMPYLOBACTER ENTEROCOLITIS

Since 1977, when effective and practical means of culture became available, members of the genus *Campylobacter*, especially *C. jejuni*, have emerged as important intestinal pathogens (85, 86). These organisms are widespread in mammals and birds and can survive well in the environment. Thus, sources of human infection include food, milk, water, and animal contact. The infection tends to involve young patients with no particular predisposing factors. The clinical features of *Campylobacter* infection do not allow it to be distinguished from other enteric infections without culture. Like many other enteric infections, the disease is usually self-limited. At one extreme, some patients have a mild diarrheal disease suggestive of viral gastroenteritis; at the other, signs and symptoms of a severe colitic illness with grossly bloody stools may closely mimic ulcerative colitis. The colonoscopic appearance likewise may be confused with that of ulcerative colitis, with mucosal congestion and edema, friability, and granularity.

Campylobacter infection apparently involves the small intestine as well as the colon, but the disease in the small intestine has not been as well characterized by biopsy study. Some evidence suggests that *C. jejuni* produce an enterotoxin leading to a secretory diarrhea of

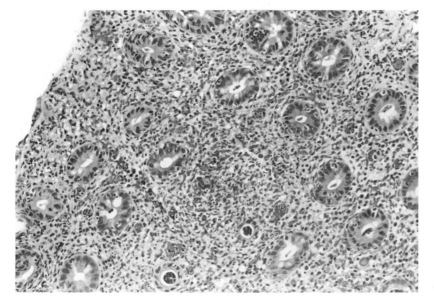

Figure 28.10 *Salmonella* colitis. The neutrophilic infiltrate, acute cryptitis, and the lack of significant crypt distortion are characteristic of acute infectious colitis or so-called acute self-limited colitis. Compare with Figure 28.7.

the sort seen in cholera (85). Other evidence demonstrates that the organisms are invasive in the manner of *Shigella* and *Salmonella,* usually within the bowel wall but occasionally extending parenterally.

The biopsy appearance of *Campylobacter* colitis has been well characterized, and it does not differ from that associated with other enteric agents, such as *Salmonella* or *Shigella,* i.e., with a range of appearances from mild mucosal edema and increased cellularity of the lamina propria to a full-blown picture of acute ASLC (87, 88)(Fig. 28.11). Because of the clinical mimicry of ulcerative colitis by *Campylobacter* infection, the importance of distinguishing between the two entities is clear. Because a significant proportion of truly infected patients may appear "negative" on the basis of culture results, biopsy assumes great practical significance and has been shown to be an effective means of making this important distinction (56).

Another important aspect of this disease is the fact that *C. jejuni* infection often precedes the development of Guillain-Barré syndrome (89).

YERSINIA ENTEROCOLITIS

Another group of enteric bacterial infections recognized with increased frequency are those involving members of the genus *Yersinia*—aerobic, gram-negative organisms formerly classified in the genus *Pasteurella* (90, 91). Infection with these organisms has been traced to contaminated food, animal contact, and even person-to-person transmission. Infants, children, and young adults are affected most often. The most common manifestations of *Yersinia* infection are those of a self-limited enterocolitis with abdominal pain, diarrhea, fever, and bloody stools. In a significant number of patients, particularly older children and adults, signs and symptoms are suggestive of right lower quadrant disease, closely mimicking appendicitis. In a small number of patients, yersinial septicemia may ensue.

Yersinial lesions are recognized most often in material obtained at laparotomy for presumed appendicitis. The usual gross features in such cases are those of a striking mesenteric lymphadenopathy, often a normal-appearing appendix, and evidence of inflammation of the terminal ileum and proximal colon, with thickening and edema of the bowel wall, prominence of Peyer's patches, and scattered mucosal ulcers. The findings may be suggestive of Crohn's disease or even tuberculosis. In *Y. enterocolitica* infections, the characteristic microscopic feature is lymphofollicular hyperplasia with microabscesses in the mesenteric lymph nodes and bowel wall. In the ileum, colon, and appendix, mucosal ulcers of various sizes are surfaced by fibrinopurulent exudate and sometimes associated with clusters of gram-negative bacteria. Characteristically, the small aphthous ulcers are situated over hyperplastic lymphoid follicles (Fig. 28.12) (92). Similar changes have been described in association with *Y. pseudotuberculosis,* but with a distinct granulomatous component surrounding the microabscesses in lymphoid tissue (93). In addition to the lesions recognized in the ileocecal area, colorectal endoscopy has revealed more widespread colitic lesions, including aphthous ulcers (90).

TUBERCULOSIS

Mycobacteria of various types occasionally are encountered as a cause of intestinal disease. *Mycobacterium tuberculosis,* long recognized as an etiologic agent of enteric disease, remains an important pathogen in developing countries but is less common in the western world. *Mycobacterium avium,* on the other hand, has emerged as a "new" infectious agent in immunocompromised hosts (see Chapter 16).

Tubercle bacilli apparently are capable of penetrating the intestinal mucosa after being swallowed. At one time, bovine strains of *M. tuberculosis* were important in this regard, but bovine tuberculosis has been virtually eliminated in economically developed countries. Most gastrointestinal tuberculosis in much of the world now represents infection with human strains, presumably with a pulmonary route of initial entry. Older studies (94) showing the greater incidence of intestinal tuberculosis in patients with more advanced pulmonary tuberculosis with cavitation suggest swallowing of infected sputum as an initiating event. Increasingly, however,

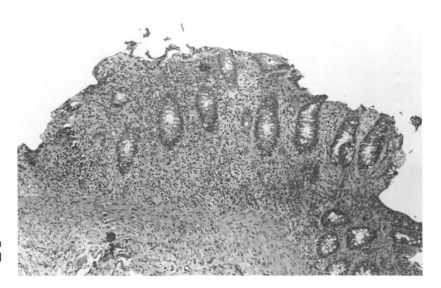

Figure 28.11 *Campylobacter* colitis. This infection is characterized by the pattern of acute self-limited colitis.

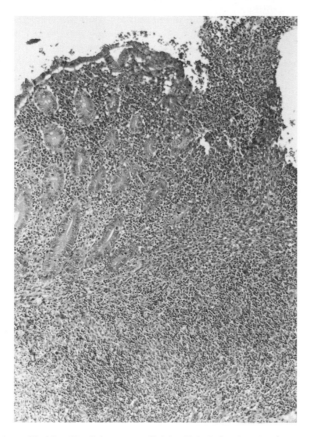

Figure 28.12 *Yersinia* appendicitis. This infection is characterized by aphthous ulcers *(top)* overlying hyperplastic lymphoid follicles, and microabscesses in regional nodes.

it has become apparent that at the time of clinical presentation of the enteric tuberculous lesion, affected individuals may have no radiographic evidence of pulmonary infection.

The signs and symptoms associated with enteric tuberculosis are highly variable, given the fact that various levels of the small and large bowel may be involved and that perforation, hemorrhage, obstruction, and fistula formation may all occur. Enteric tuberculosis has manifested as mechanical small-bowel obstruction, apparent appendicitis, and even segmental colonic stricture (95). Abdominal pain is a universal finding, as is the demonstration of abnormality on contrast-enhanced radiographic studies. Reflecting the fact that the ileocecal region is by far the most common site of intestinal tuberculosis, the presence of a right lower quadrant mass is a common sign (96).

Intestinal tuberculosis is grossly characterized by an inflammatory mass in the affected segment of gut, usually with secondary mesenteric lymphadenopathy. Lesions exhibit various combinations of mucosal ulceration, classically transverse, and inflammatory thickening of the wall. Grossly, as well as radiographically, the features of enteric tuberculosis and Crohn's disease may be virtually identical. Microscopically, intestinal lesions of tuberculosis are similar to tuberculous lesions elsewhere in the body, with necrotizing granulomata as their hallmark. The granulomata tend to be more florid than those of Crohn's disease, and caseation is found in the larger granulomata (Fig. 28.13). Even when necrosis is not especially prominent in the intramural lesions, the associated lymph

nodes usually show caseation (94). As in any tuberculous lesions, acid-fast bacilli are variably demonstrable histologically with appropriate stains.

ACTINOMYCOSIS

Actinomycosis is another infection with one of the "higher bacteria" (i.e., organisms related to *Streptomyces, Mycobacterium,* and *Nocardia*) that may be encountered in the bowel. *Actinomyces israelii* is the usual etiologic agent of human actinomycosis, other species of the genus being found only occasionally (97). The organism is a normal commensal inhabitant of the digestive tract, especially in the oropharyngeal region. Actinomycosis apparently results from the introduction of the organism from the lumen into the tissues in the course of some other disease of after accidental or surgical trauma. A synergistic role by other microbes occasionally demonstrated in actinomycotic lesions has been suggested, but the evidence is not conclusive. Abdominal actinomycosis accounts for one fifth to one third of cases, the majority being cervicofacial and thoracic (98). Many cases of abdominal actinomycosis have been reported to follow appendectomy, cholecystectomy, or operations to treat diverticular disease, trauma, or neoplasm. The clinical manifestations are extremely variable but generally consist of inflammation with draining abscesses.

The typical gross lesions of actinomycosis associated with the gut, as elsewhere in the body, are abscesses with tough, fibrous walls

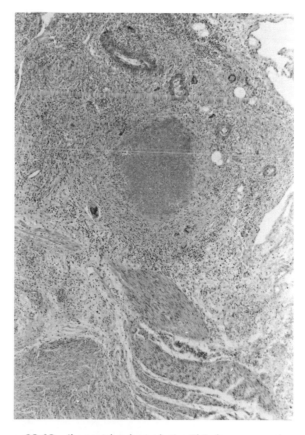

Figure 28.13 Ileocecal tuberculosis. This large granuloma in the submucosa, unlike those of Crohn's disease, shows central caseation.

enclosing loculi filled with yellow to white pus, often associated with sinus tracts. Although, classically, "sulfur granules" are described in the exudate, these granules are not always evident grossly. Microscopically, the typical actinomycotic lesion is an abscess, often multiloculated, with a surrounding zone of vascular granulation tissue and scar. Large, foamy macrophages surround the suppurative centers of the lesions, with scattered lymphocytes and plasma cells in the granulation tissue (98). The feature that is histologically diagnostic of the infection (cultural verification is often difficult) is the grain or granule found floating in the pus. In preparations stained with hematoxylin and eosin, the granules are spherical to ovoid masses averaging approximately 300 μm in diameter with lightly basophilic to amphophilic central regions and a peripheral fringe of radiating eosinophilic clubs (Fig. 28.14). Organisms per se cannot be resolved well in routine preparations. In Brown-Brenn-stained sections, gram-positive, slender, branching, beaded bacilli can be demonstrated, tangled in the center of the granules, more parallel in their arrangement at the periphery in relation to the clubs. Differential diagnosis includes nocardiosis, staphylococcal botryomycosis, and fungal infections, all of which may involve granular clusters of organisms. *Nocardia* tends to form loose masses without clubs and, unlike *Actinomyces*, is acid-fast. Staphylococci and fungi can be distinguished by their morphologic characteristics.

INTESTINAL SPIROCHETOSIS

So-called intestinal spirochetosis should be mentioned, although its inclusion with the intestinal infections is somewhat debatable. The morphologic features of spirochetal colonization of the colon were first specifically delineated in 1967, although the presence of spirochetes in gut flora had long been known (99). This study revealed a 9% incidence of spirochetosis in consecutive biopsy specimens. The dense population of spirochetes is readily recognized by light microscopy (Fig. 28.15) and by electron microscopy appears regularly oriented among the microvilli of epithelial cells (Fig. 28.16). In many published studies, the incidence of colorectal or appendiceal spirochetosis ranges between 1 and 10%, and evidence suggests that the organisms are nonpathogenic (100, 101). In some instances, however, spirochetosis has been associated with symptoms, with resolution of the symptoms and disappearance of the spirochetes after antimicrobial therapy (102, 103). Spirochetosis has also been found to have a higher incidence in "pseudo-appendicitis" (i.e., cases in which the appendix was removed because of symptoms of appendicitis and found to be not inflamed) than in appendices removed incidentally through other procedures (104). Spirochetosis has also been found with significantly greater frequency in homosexual male subjects, although the significance of this finding is as yet obscure (105).

GONORRHEA AND SYPHILIS

In addition to the various bacteria listed in the preceding discussion, others not ordinarily thought of as intestinal pathogens can be found infecting the gut. Because most of these do not have unique symptoms or produce pathognomonic morphologic changes, diagnosis generally depends on demonstrating the specific organisms or serologic evidence of their presence. In particular, sexually transmitted agents of many sorts, including *Neisseria gonorrhoeae* and *Treponema pallidum* are frequent findings in homosexual males with symptomatic anorectal disease (106).

In a series of men with culture-proven rectal gonorrhea but without concomitant gastrointestinal infections, many had no anorectal symptoms, and in 84%, the rectal mucosa appeared normal by proctoscopic examination; a few had signs of distal proctitis. Histologically, only 42% of these men showed any abnormality, most often an increase in lymphocytes and plasma cells in the lamina propria. Only a few subjects had an acute inflammatory infiltrate in the mucosa (107). In another study of 89 homosexual men with intestinal symptoms, less than one half had histologic abnormalities on biopsy (108). No sigmoidoscopic appearance or histologic pattern was specific for any infection. Acute inflammatory changes were the most common histologic abnormalities. Chronic inflammatory changes (including increased chronic inflammatory cells in the submucosa, granulomas, and lymphoid follicles) were uncommon but were significantly associated with syphilis, herpes simplex virus, and *C. trachomatis*. The authors concluded that when histologic features of idiopathic inflammatory bowel disease are found in a homosexual man, syphilis and chlamydial infection in

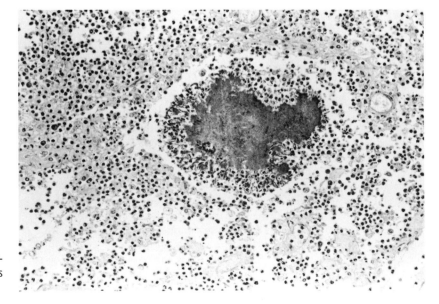

Figure 28.14   Actinomycosis. This infection is characterized by the presence of "granules" within areas of suppuration.

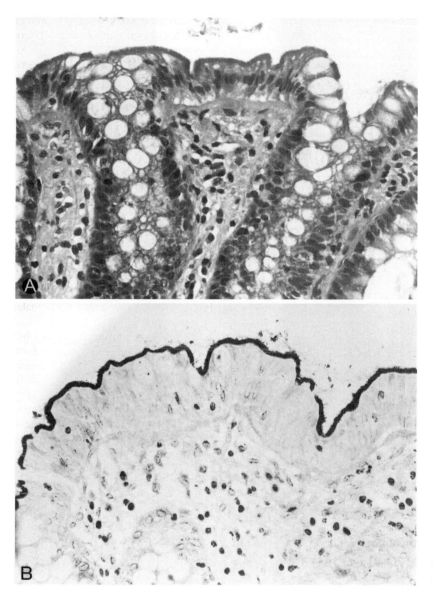

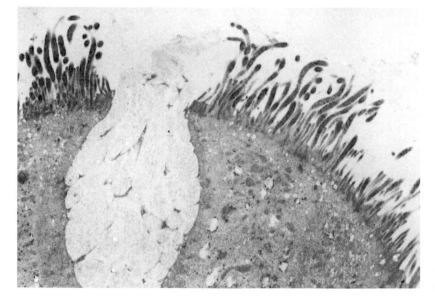

Figure 28.15   Colonic spirochetosis. **A.** Routine preparation shows "accentuation" of the luminal border of epithelial cells. **B.** With Warthin-Starry (or Churukian-Schenk) silver stain, an oriented layer of bacteria is visible.

Figure 28.16   Colonic spirochetosis. Electron micrography reveals spirochetes oriented longitudinally among microvilli.

particular need to be ruled out carefully before a diagnosis of idiopathic inflammatory bowel disease is entertained (108).

FUNGAL INFECTIONS

CANDIDIASIS, MUCORMYCOSIS, AND ASPERGILLOSIS

Mycotic infections of the gut usually are encountered as secondary phenomena in debilitated patients, especially those with leukemia or lymphoma; those with other diseases associated with immunologic impairment; and those who have been treated with cytotoxic agents, steroids, and antibiotics. Candidiasis and mucormycosis (Fig. 28.17) appear to be the most important of the opportunistic infections, but *Aspergillus* infection has also been reported (109). Although any level of the tract may be involved, infections with *Candida* species are more likely to be found in the mouth, esophagus, and stomach; lesions of mucormycosis show a predilection for the stomach and colon (110, 111). The organisms

ordinarily are recognized in profusion in the lesions, which vary from areas of superficial erosion to foci of transmural hemorrhage and necrosis.

HISTOPLASMOSIS

The digestive tract is occasionally involved as part of a primary mycotic infection, i.e., in individuals who are not first overtly debilitated by some other disease. Infection with *Histoplasma capsulatum*, found in many parts of the world but endemic in the eastern central United States, usually is acquired by inhalation of spores from organisms residing in the soil. Although histoplasmosis is most often a benign, asymptomatic pulmonary infection, disseminated infection develops in some affected individuals (112). Autopsy studies indicate that approximately 75% of patients with disseminated histoplasmosis have lesions in the small intestine, colon, or liver. The ileum is involved most frequently, followed closely by the colon, with occasional lesions in the appendix or at

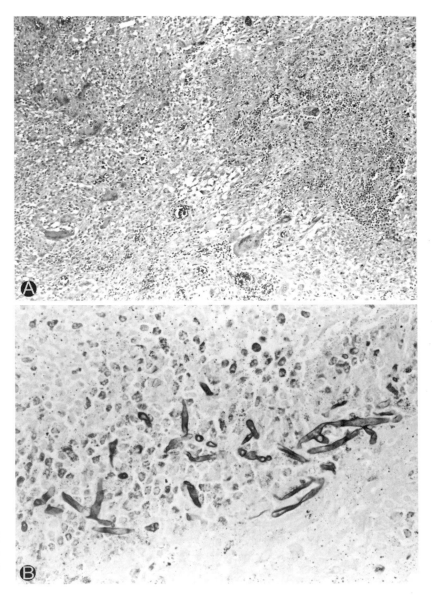

Figure 28.17 Colonic mucormycosis. An area of necrotizing, suppurative, and granulomatous inflammation in the wall (**A**) is seen with the methenamine silver stain (**B**) to be mycotic.

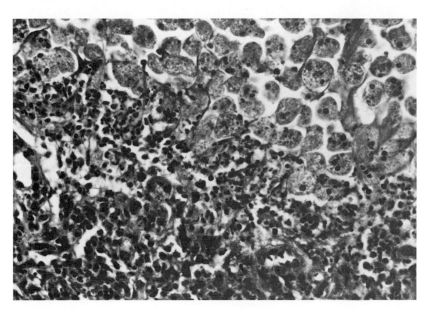

Figure 28.18 Amebiasis. Features of the mucosal inflammatory process in the lower part of this field are nonspecific. Diagnosis rests on recognition of amebae in the surface exudate, in profusion at the top of this field.

various other levels of the digestive tract. These gastrointestinal lesions are evident clinically in only a minority of cases. In these few patients, the fungal lesions may mimic carcinoma, lymphoma, tuberculosis, or idiopathic inflammatory bowel disease; pain and diarrhea are the most frequent complaints. Although it seems probable that intestinal lesions reflect spread of organisms from the lung, the possibility of an enteric portal of primary entry cannot be excluded in all cases. The intestinal lesions are ulcerative and granulomatous, with presumptive diagnosis resting on demonstration of budding yeast forms in the lesions and definitive diagnosis made possible by culture of the organism (113).

PROTOZOAN INFECTION

AMEBIASIS

Infection with *Entamoeba histolytica* is prevalent in much of the world and is sometimes endemic in developing countries. Amebiasis has also been recognized recently as a particular problem in homosexual males (106). The possibility of confusion clinically and endoscopically with ulcerative colitis and with Crohn's disease makes recognition of this infection important.

The amebae are ingested as cysts from the environment; after excystation, the trophozoites colonize the large intestine. This process is facilitated by an association between the amebae and bacteria resident in the gut. As is true for many other enteric organisms, specific adherence of the *E. histolytica* to mucosal lining cells is a critical step in pathogenesis. The organisms are then capable of invading the bowel wall and destroying host tissue, a process apparently mediated by proteolytic enzymes, cell-free cytotoxins, and a process of contact-dependent cytolysis (114).

On the basis of autopsy study, the primary target of amebic attack appears to be the cecum and ascending colon, with subsequent spread to other locations. The usual lesions in the gut are ulcerative, but exuberant inflammation and formation of granulation tissue produce an ameboma, which may simulate a neoplasm. Complications of amebiasis include direct extension to perineal skin, intestinal perforation, and parenteral dissemination through blood vessels and lymphatics (115).

In a detailed rectal biopsy study, Prathap and Gilman (116) recognized the following types of amebic lesions:

1. A nonspecific lesion characterized by mucosal hyperemia, edema, patchy mucin depletion, and focal neutrophilic infiltration. At best, few amebae are seen in surface exudate.
2. A mucopenic depression in the mucosa, produced by depletion of epithelial mucin, with focal surface erosion. Amebae are present immediately adjacent to the area of superficial lysis of epithelium.
3. An early invasive lesion with superficial ulceration and amebae present in the tissue.
4. A late invasive lesion with deep ulceration, the classic flask-shaped ulcer. Amebae are present in the exudate, which is not especially cellular.
5. A granulating ulcer with a nonspecific appearance and no amebae.

In general, the diagnosis is suggested only when the amebae happen to be visualized in the biopsy specimen (Fig. 28.18), and strands of mucus associated with the mucosa therefore deserve careful scrutiny. In a sigmoidoscopic biopsy study involving patients with documented amebic colitis, Pittman and Hennigar (117) stressed that a diffuse nonspecific inflammatory response was characteristic, and that amebae might be absent from a significant proportion of biopsies. Conversely, many accounts suggest that amebae often evoke little or no inflammatory response. Conceivably, amebae may differ in this regard, or possibly a brisk inflammatory response reflects secondary infection. Chances for making the diagnosis of amebiasis are best, in any event, if the organisms are sought in fresh stool or exudate obtained at the time of endoscopy.

GIARDIASIS

Giardia lamblia is another protozoan found worldwide that is often a cause of infectious diarrhea (118). Water containing the cyst forms of the organism appears to be the major source of infection. After ingestion, excystation begins in the stomach, and the small intestine is then colonized by the trophozoites. The organisms attach to the microvillous border of enterocytes by adhesive disks, and they can often be seen in biopsy specimens as arched or sickle-shaped forms attached to the microvillous border (Fig. 28.19).

Clinically, giardiasis varies from an asymptomatic infection to a severe diarrheal illness that may become chronic, with malabsorption and weight loss (119). This disease has a particular association with various hypogammaglobulinemic disorders. Biopsy of the upper small intestine yields a spectrum of nonspecific changes; in many infected patients, biopsy tissue has a normal histologic appearance (120). The degree of enterocyte damage varies; findings include shortening of the villi, expansion of lamina propria, and an increase in epithelial mitotic activity. In the extreme, the histologic picture may resemble that of sprue. More severe structural abnormalities tend to be found in immunodeficient patients. The pathogenesis of the disease is not completely understood, but it may involve enzymatic alterations associated with direct damage to enterocytes, loss of surface area associated with atrophy of the villi, altered turnover of epithelial cells, and release of prostaglandin from macrophages (118). Diagnosis depends on demonstration of the organisms in duodenal jejunal biopsy specimens, aspirates of duodenal fluid, or stool specimens.

COCCIDIOSIS

Protozoans of the subclass Coccidia, long recognized in infection of other animal species, have also been implicated in human infection. These infections may be zoonotic or transmitted person-to-person and are associated with variable syndromes of diarrhea and malabsorption (121, 122). Organisms of the genus *Isospora* and the genus *Cryptosporidium* have been identified in human hosts, the former as intracytoplasmic parasites within enterocytes of the small intestine and the latter closely associated with the microvillous border of enterocytes, possibly within host cell membrane (123). *Isospora* infection has been identified as a rare cause of intractable diarrhea and malabsorption (124).

Cryptosporidiosis, only recently identified as a significant problem in humans, manifests as an opportunistic infection in immunocompromised patients, especially those with AIDS, but also infects immunocompetent subjects. One massive outbreak was traced to an urban water supply (125). The diarrheal disease in immunocompetent individuals tends to be of short duration,

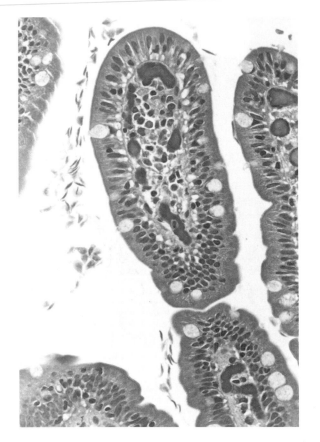

Figure 28.19 Giardiasis. Numerous organisms are seen along the villous surface (separation is an artifact), in profile, as crescent or sickle shapes, or occasionally *en face*, as at lower left.

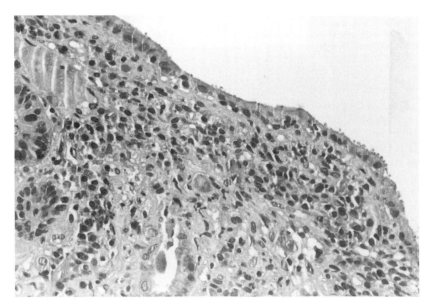

Figure 28.20 Cryptosporidiosis. The organisms have the appearance of tiny spheres along the microvillus border.

whereas in the immunocompromised population, it often is intractable, persisting to the death of the subject. The small bowel seems to be the main site of colonization, but in immunocompromised subjects, organisms may be seen from pharynx to rectum. Infection

of the small intestine may be accompanied by abnormalities in crypt architecture and variable inflammation in the lamina propria. The organisms are seen as tiny basophilic spheres seemingly attached to the microvillous border (Fig. 28.20). Diagnosis can be confirmed not only by biopsy but also by examination of fecal concentrates (126).

HELMINTHIC INFECTION

The human gut can be infected by a wide variety of helminthic parasites. Descriptions of these parasites are beyond the scope of this discussion, and the reader is referred to detailed presentations in standard references (127). Two infections, however, warrant specific mention: schistosomiasis and strongyloidiasis. Schistosomiasis, a serious disease in many parts of the world, may be associated with significant lesions of the bowel. Adult *Schistosoma japonicum* and *Schistosoma mansoni* live in the mesenteric circulation, and the large numbers of ova produced by the parasites pass through the bowel wall. The granulomatous inflammatory reaction elicited by the ova may lead to polypoid and ulcerative gross lesions of the distal large bowel reminiscent of Crohn's disease or even of neoplasia (128). The continuing mucosal proliferative changes in chronic schistosomiasis may be associated with the development of colonic carcinoma in a manner analogous to that in ulcerative colitis (129). Accurate diagnosis of colonic schistosomiasis rests on recognition of the ova. The inflammatory reaction to the ova varies with time, ranging from diffuse and cellular to granulomatous to fibrotic (Fig. 28.21).

Strongyloidiasis is important not only because the infection is widespread, affecting on the order of 100 million people, but also because of unique host-parasite relationships in this infection. Strongyloidiasis can be maintained for many years in a given subject by a process of autoinfection, with conversion to an overwhelming hyperinfection should the subject become immunocompromised (130). The parasites can be seen in relation to the intestinal mucosa (Fig. 28.22) and can also produce a transmural eosinophilic-granulomatous lesion associated with invasive larvae (131).

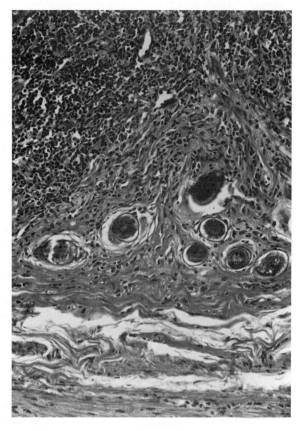

Figure 28.21 Schistosomiasis. Diagnosis rests on recognition of ova, surrounded by an inflammatory reaction, which is often granulomatous (giant cells around ova at left).

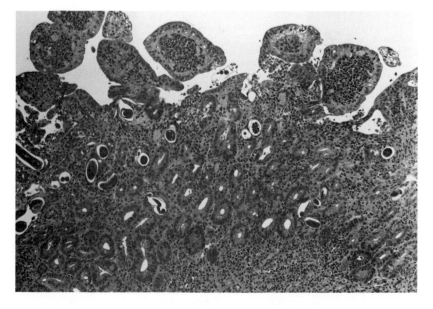

Figure 28.22 Hyperinfection of small intestine with *Strongyloides*. Numerous worms are obvious in the distorted, inflamed mucosa.

REFERENCES

1. Simon G, Gorbach SL. Intestinal flora in health and disease. Gastroenterology 1984;86:174–193.
2. Savage DC. Overview of the association of microbes with epithelial surfaces. Microecol Ther 1984;14:169–182.
3. Drasar BS, Hill MS. The metabolic activities of gut bacteria. In: Drasar BS, Hill MS. Human intestinal flora. New York: Academic Press, 1974;51–168.
4. Prizont R, Konigsberg N. Identification of bacterial glycosidases in rat cecal contents. Dig Dis Sci 1981;26:773–777.
5. Abrams GD, Bishop JE. Effect of the normal microbial flora on gastrointestinal motility. Proc Soc Exp Biol Med 1967;126:301–304.
6. Abrams GD, Bauer H, Sprinz H. Influence of the normal flora on mucosal morphology and cellular renewal in the ileum: A comparison of germfree and conventional mice. Lab Invest 1963;12:355–364.
7. Yolton DP, Stanley C, Savage DC. Influence of the indigenous gastrointestinal microbial flora on duodenal alkaline phosphatase activity in mice. Infect Immun 1971;3:768–773.
8. Uribe A, Alam M, Johansson O, et al. Microflora modulates endocrine cells in the gastrointestinal mucosa of the rat. Gastroenterology 1994;107:1259–1269.
9. Gianella RA, Broitman SA, Zamcheck N. The gastric barrier to microorganisms in man: In vivo and in vitro studies. Gut 1972;13:251–256.
10. Borriello SP, Reed PJ, Dolby JM, et al. Microbial and metabolic profile of achlorhydric stomach: Comparison of pernicious anemia and hypogammaglobulinaemia. J Clin Pathol 1985;38:946–953.
11. Hornick RB, Music SI, Wenzel R, et al. The Broad Street pump revisited: Response of volunteers to ingested cholera vibrios. Bull NY Acad Med 1971;47:1181–1191.
12. Gianella RA, Broitman SA, Zamcheck N. Influence of gastric acidity on bacterial and parasitic enteric infections. Ann Intern Med 1973;78:271–276.
13. Sarker SA, Gyr K. Non-immunological defence mechanisms of the gut. Gut 1992;33:987–993.
14. Dixon JMS. The fate of bacteria in the small intestine. J Pathol Bacteriol 1960;79:131–140.
15. Formal SB, Abrams GD, Schneider H, et al. Experimental Shigella infections. VI. Role of the small intestine in an experimental infection in guinea pigs. J Bacteriol 1963;85:119–125.
16. Dupont HL, Hornick RB. Adverse effect of lomotil therapy in Shigellosis. JAMA 1973;226:1525–1528.
17. Abraham SN, Beachey EH. Host defenses against adhesion of bacteria to mucosal surfaces. In: Gallin JI, Fauci AS, eds. Advances in host defense mechanisms 4. New York: Raven Press, 1985;63–88.
18. Freter R. Interdependence of mechanisms that control bacterial colonization of the large intestine. Microecol Ther 1984;14:89–96.
19. Holmberg SD, Osterholm MT, Senger KA, et al. Drug-resistant *Salmonella* from animals fed antimicrobials. N Engl J Med 1984;311:617–622.
20. Spika JS, Waterman SH, Soo Hoo GW, et al. Chloramphenicol-resistant *Salmonella newport* traced through hamburger to dairy farms. N Engl J Med 1987;316:565–570.
21. Gracey M. The contaminated small bowel syndrome: Pathogenesis, diagnosis and treatment. Am J Clin Nutr 1979;32:234–243.
22. Kelly CP, Pothoulakis C, LaMont JT. *Clostridium difficile* colitis. N Engl J Med 1994;330:257–262.
23. Trnka YM, LaMont JT. *Clostridium difficile* colitis. Adv Intern Med 1984;29:85–107.
24. Bartlett JG, Laughon B. *Clostridium difficile* toxins. Microecol Ther 1984;14:35–42.
25. Abrams GD, Allo M, Rifkin GD, et al. Mucosal damage mediated by clostridial toxin in experimental clindamycin-associated colitis. Gut 1980;21:493–499.
26. Price AB, Davies DR. Pseudomembranous colitis. J Clin Pathol 1977;30:1–12.
27. Rocca JM, Pieterse AD, Rowland R, et al. *Clostridium difficile* colitis. Aust NZ J Med 1984;14:606–610.
28. Cone JB, Wetzel W. Toxic megacolon secondary to pseudomembranous colitis. Dis Colon Rectum 1982;25:478–482.
29. Schnett S, Antonioli A, Goldman H. Massive mural edema in severe pseudomembranous colitis. Arch Pathol Lab Med 1983;107:211–213.
30. Cudmore M, Silva J, Fekety R. Clostridial enterocolitis produced by antineoplastic agents in hamsters and humans. Curr Chem Infect Dis 1980;2:1460–1461.
31. Trnka YM, LaMont JT. Association of *Clostridium difficile* toxin with symptomatic relapse of chronic inflammatory bowel disease. Gastroenterology 1981;80:693–696.
32. Steinberg D, Gold J, Brodin A. Necrotizing enterocolitis in leukemia. Arch Intern Med 1973;131:538–544.
33. King A, Rampling A, Wight DGD, et al. Neutropenic enterocolitis due to *Clostridium septicum* infection. J Clin Pathol 1984;37:335–343.
34. Rampling A, Warren RE, Bevan PC, et al. *Clostridium difficile* in hematological malignancy. J Clin Pathol 1985;38:445–451.
35. Guerrant RL, Bobak DA. Bacterial and protozoal gastroenteritis. N Engl J Med 1991;325:327–340.
36. Klemm P. Fimbrial adhesins of *Escherichia coli*. Rev Infect Dis 1985;7:321–340.
37. Levine MM, Kaper JB, Black RE, et al. New knowledge on pathogenesis of bacterial infections as applied to vaccine development. Microbiol Rev 1983;47:510–550.
38. Freter R, O'Brien PCM. Role of chemotaxis in the association of motile bacteria with intestinal mucosa: In vivo studies. Infect Immun 1981;34:234–240.
39. Burnet FM. The mucinase of *Virio cholerae*. Aust J Exp Med Sci 1948;26:71–80.
40. Formal SB, Hale TL, Sansonetti PJ. Invasive enteric pathogens. Rev Infect Dis (Suppl 4) 1983;5:S702–S707.
41. Grutzkau A, Hanski C, Hahn H, et al. Involvement of M cells in the bacterial invasion of Peyer's patches: A common mechanism shared by *Yersinia enterocolitica* and other enteroinvasive bacteria. Gut 1990;31:1011–1015.
42. Gianella RA. Pathogenesis of acute diarrheal disorders. Annu Rev Med 1981;32:341–357.
43. Gots RE, Formal SB, Gianella RA. Indomethacin inhibition of *Salmonella typhimurium, Shigella flexneri* and *Vibrio cholerae* mediated rabbit ileal secretion. J Infect Dis 1974:130:280–284.
44. Rask-Madsen J. Eicosanoids and their role in the pathogenesis of diarrheal diseases. Clin Gastroenterol 1986;15:546–566.
45. Powell DW. New paradigms for the pathophysiology of infectious diarrhea. Gastroenterology 1994;106:1705–1707.
46. Mekalanos JJ. Cholera toxin: Genetic analysis, regulation and role in pathogenesis. Curr Top Microbiol Immunol 1985;118:97–118.
47. Rabbani GH. Cholera. Clin Gastroenterol 1986;3:507–528.
48. Speelman P, Butler T, Kabir I, et al. Colonic dysfunction during cholera infection. Gastroenterology 1986;91:164–170.
49. Ulshen MH, Rollo JL. Pathogenesis of *Escherichia coli* gastroenteritis in man: Another mechanism. N Engl J Med 1980;302:99–101.
50. O'Brien AD, Marques LRM, Newland JW, et al. Shiga and Shiga-like toxins. Microecol Ther 1984;14:25–30.
51. Griffin PM, Olmstead LC, Petras RE. Escherichia coli 0157:H7-associated colitis. A clinical and histological study of 11 cases. Gastroenterology 1990;99:142–149.
52. Kelly J, Oryshak A, Wenetsek M, et al. The colonic pathology of *Escherichia coli* 0157:H7 infection. Am J Surg Pathol 1990;14:87–93.
53. Boyce TG, Swerdlow DL, Griffin PM. *Escherichia coli* 0157:H7 and the hemolytic uremic syndrome. N Engl J Med 1995;333:364–368.
54. Gangarosa EG, Beisel WR, Benyajati C, et al. The nature of the gastrointestinal lesion in Asiatic cholera and its relation to pathogenesis: A biopsy study. Am J Trop Med Hyg 1960;9:125–135.
55. Kumar NB, Nostrant TT, Appelman HD. The histopathologic spectrum of acute self-limited colitis (acute infectious-type colitis). Am J Surg Pathol 1982;6:523–529.
56. Nontrant TT, Kumar NB, Appelman HD. Histopathology differentiates acute self-limited colitis from ulcerative colitis. Gastroenterology 1987;92:318–328.
57. Surawicz CM, Haggitt RC, Husseman M, et al. Mucosal biopsy diagnosis of colitis: Acute self-limited colitis and idiopathic inflammatory bowel disease. Gastroenterology 1994;107:755–763.

58. Therkildsen MH, Jensen BN, Teglbjaerg PS, et al. The final outcome of patients presenting with their first episode of acute diarrheoea and an inflamed rectal mucosa with preserved crypt architecture. Scand J Gastroenterol 1989;24:158–164.

59. Allison MC, Hamilton-Dutoit SJ, Dhillon AP, et al. The value of rectal biopsy in distinguishing self-limited colitis from early inflammatory bowel disease. Q J Med 1987;65:985–995.

60. Leriche M, Devroede G, Sanchez G, et al. Changes in the rectal mucosa induced by hypertonic enemas. Dis Colon Rectum 1978;21:227–236.

61. Meisel JL, Bergman D, Graney D, et al. Human rectal mucosa: Proctoscopic and morphological changes caused by laxatives. Gastroenterology 1977;72:1274–1279.

62. Glotzer DJ, Glick ME, Goldman H. Proctitis and colitis following diversion of the fecal stream. Gastroenterology 1981;80:438–441.

63. Harig JM, Soergel KH, Komorowski RA, et al. Treatment of diversion colitis with short-chain-fatty acid irrigation. N Engl J Med 1989;320:23–28.

64. Blacklow NR, Greeberg HB. Viral gastroenteritis. N Engl J Med 1991;325:252–264.

65. Davidson GP. Viral diarrhoea. Clin Gastroenterol 1986;15:39–53.

66. Schreiber DS, Blacklow NR, Trier JS. The mucosal lesion of the proximal small intestine in acute infectious nonbacterial gastroenteritis. N Engl Med 1973;288:1318–1323.

67. Goodell SE, Quinn TC, Mkrtichian E, et al. Herpes simplex proctitis in homosexual men. N Eng J Med 1983;308:868–871.

68. Bodey GP, Fainstein V. Infections of the gastrointestinal tract in the immunocompromised patient. Annu Rev Med 1986;37:271–281.

69. Foucar E, Mukai D, Foucar K, et al. Colon ulceration in lethal cytomegalovirus infection. Am J Clin Pathol 1981;76:788–801.

70. Keren DF, Milligan FD, Strandberg JD, et al. Intercurrent cytomegalovirus colitis in a patient with ulcerative colitis. Johns Hopkins Med J 1975;136:178–182.

71. Cooper HS, Raffansperger EC, Jonas L, et al. Cytomegalovirus inclusions in patients with ulcerative colitis requiring colonic resection. Gastoenterology 1977;72:1253–1256.

72. Chetty R, Roskell DE. Cytomegalovirus infection in the gastrointestinal tract. J Clin Pathol 1994;47:968–972.

73. Goodman ZD, Boitnot JK, Yardley JH. Perforation of the colon associated with cytomegalovirus infection. Dig Dis Sci 1979;24:376–380.

74. Eyre-Brook IA, Dundas S. Incidence and clinical significance of colonic cytomegalovirus infection in idiopathic inflammatory bowel disease requiring colectomy. Gut 1986;27:1419–1425.

75. Yunis EJ, Atchison RW, Michaels RH, et al. Adenovirus and ileocecal intussusception. Lab Invest 1975;33:347–351.

76. Montgomery EA, Popek EJ. Intussusception, adenovirus, and children: A brief reaffirmation. Hum Pathol 1994;25:169–174.

77. Quinn TC, Goodell SE, Mkrtichian E, et al. *Chlamydia trachomatis* proctitis. N Engl J Med 1981;305:195–200.

78. dela Monte SM, Hutchins GM. Follicular proctocolitis and neuromatous hyperplasia with lymphogranuloma venereum. Hum Pathol 1985;16:1025–1032.

79. Nolte FS. Practical considerations in the laboratory diagnosis of bacterial enteric infections. Am J Clin Pathol 1994;101(Suppl 1):S14–S17.

80. Speelman P, Kabir I, Islam M. Distribution and spread of colonic lesions in shigellosis: A colonscopic study. J Infect Dis 1984;150:899–903.

81. Islam MM, Azad AK, Bardhan PK, et al. Pathology of shigellosis and its complications. Histopathology 1994;24:65–71.

82. Day DW, Mandal BK, Morson BC. The rectal biopsy appearances in Salmonella colitis. Histopathology 1978;2:117–131.

83. McGovern VJ, Slavutin LJ. Pathology of Salmonella colitis. Am J Surg Pathol 1979;3:483–490.

84. Anand BS, Malhorta V, Bhattacharya SK, et al. Rectal histology in acute bacillary dysentery. Gastroenterology 1986;90:654–660.

85. Walker RI, Caldwell MB, Lee EC, et al. Pathophysiology of Campylobacter enteritis. Microbiol Rev 1986;50:81–94.

86. Blaser MJ, Reller LB. Campylobacter enteritis. N Engl J Med 1981;305:1444–1452.

87. Price AB, Jewkes J, Sanderson PJ. Acute diarrhea: Campylobacter colitis and the role of rectal biopsy. J Clin Pathol 1979;32:990–997.

88. Colgan T, Lambert JR, Newman A, et al. *Campylobacter jejuni* enterocolitis. Arch Pathol Lab Med 1980;104:571–574.

89. Rees JH, Soudain SE, Gregson NA, et al. *Campylobacter jejuni* infection and Guillain-Barré syndrome. N Engl J Med 1995;333:1374–1379.

90. Vantrappen G, Agg HO, Panette E, et al. Yersinia enteritis and enterocolitis: Gastroenterological aspects. Gastroenterology 1977;72:220–227.

91. Simmonds SD, Noble MA, Freeman JH. Gastrointestinal features of culture-positive *Yersinia enterocolitica* infection. Gastroenterology 1987;92:112–117.

92. Gleason TH, Patterson SD. The pathology of *Yersinia enterocolitica* ileocolitis. Am J Surg Pathol 1982;6:347–355.

93. El-Maraghi NRH, Mair NS. The histopathology of enteric infection with *Yersinia pseudotuberculosis*. Am J Clin Pathol 1979;71:631–639.

94. Abrams JS, Holden WD. Tuberculosis of the gastrointestinal tract. Arch Surg 1964;84:282–293.

95. Breiter JR, Hajjar JJ. Segmental tuberculosis of the colon diagnosed by colonscopy. Am J Gastroenterol 1981;76:369–373.

96. Palmer KR, Patil DH, Basran GS, et al. Abdominal tuberculosis in urban Britain—a common disease. Gut 1985;26:1296–1305.

97. Bennhoff DF. Actinomycosis: Diagnostic and therapeutic considerations and a review of 32 cases. Laryngoscope 1981;94:1198–1217.

98. Brown JR. Human actinomycosis: A study of 181 subjects. Hum Pathol 1973;4:319–330.

99. Harland WA, Lee FD. Intestinal spirochetosis. Br Med J 1967;3:718–719.

100. Henrik-Nielsen R, Orholm M, Pederson JO, et al. Colorectal spirochetosis: Clinical significance of the infestation. Gastroenterology 1983;85:62–67.

101. Lee FD, Kraszewski A, Gordon J, et al. Intestinal spirochaetosis. Gut 1971;12:126–133.

102. Burns DG, Hayes MM. Rectal spirochetosis: Symptomatic response to metronidazole and mebendazole. S Afr Med J 1985;68:335–336.

103. Gebbers JO, Ferguson DJP, Mason C, et al. Spirochaetosis of the human rectum associated with an intraepithelial mast cell and IgE plasma cell response. Gut 1987;81:588–593.

104. Henrik-Nielson R, Lundbeck FA, Stubbe-Teglbjaerg P, et al. Intestinal spirochetosis of the vermiform appendix. Gastroenterology 1985;88:971–977.

105. Ruane PJ, Nakata MM, Reinhardt JF, et al. Spirochete-like organisms in the human gastrointestinal tract. Rev Infect Dis 1989;11:184–196.

106. Quinn TC, Corey L, Chaffee RG, et al. The etiology of anorectal infections in homosexual men. Am J Med 1981;71:395–406.

107. McMillan A, McNeillage G, Gilmour IIM, et al. Histology of rectal gonorrhoea in men, with a note on anorectal infection with *Neisseria meningitidis*. J Clin Pathol 1983;36:511–514.

108. Surawicz CM, Goodell SE, Quinn TC, et al. Spectrum of rectal biopsy abnormalities in homosexual men with intestinal symptoms. Gastroenterology 1986;91:651–659.

109. Prescott RJ, Harris M, Banerjee SS. Fungal infections of the small and large intestine. J Clin Pathol 1992;45:806–811.

110. Smith JMB. Mycoses of the alimentary tract. Gut 1969;10:1035–1040.

111. Eras P, Goldstein MJ, Sherlock P. Candida infection of the gastrointestinal tract. Medicine 1972;51:367–379.

112. Goodwin RA, Loyd JE, DesPrez RM. Histoplasmosis in normal hosts. Medicine 1981;60:231–266.

113. Miller DP, Everett ED. Gastrointestinal histoplasmosis. J Clin Gastroenterol 1979;1:233–236.

114. Ravdin J. Pathogenesis of disease caused by *Entamoeba histolytica*: Studies of adherence, secreted toxins, and contact-dependent cytolysis. Rev Infect Dis 1986;8:247–260.

115. Brandt H, Perez Tamayo R. Pathology of human amebiasis. Hum Pathol 1970;1:351–385.

116. Prathap K, Gilman R. The histopathology of acute intestinal amebiasis. Am J Pathol 1970;60:229–245.

117. Pittman FE, Hennigar GR. Sigmoidoscopic and colonic mucosal biopsy findings in amebic colitis. Arch Pathol Lab Med 1974;97:155–158.

118. Smith PD. Pathophysiology and immunology of giardiasis. Annu Rev Med 1985;36:295–307.

119. Hartong WA, Gourley WK, Arvanitakis C. Giardiasis: Clinical spectrum and functional—structural abnormalities of the small intestinal mucosa. Gastroenterology 1979;77:61–69.

120. Oberhuber G, Stolte M. Giardiasis: Analysis of histological changes in biopsy specimens of 80 patients. J Clin Pathol 1990;43:641–643.

121. Navin TR, Juranek DD. Cryptosporidiosis: Clinical, epidemiologic, and parasitologic review. Rev Infect Dis 1984;6:313–327.

122. Casemore DP, Sands RL, Curry A. Cryptosporidium species. A "new" human pathogen. J Clin Pathol 1985;38:1321–1336.

123. Bird RG, Smith MD. Cryptosporidiosis in man: Parasite life cycle and fine structural pathology. J Pathol 1980;132:217–233.

124. Liebman WM, Thaler MM, DeLorimer A, et al. Intractable diarrhea of infancy due to intestinal coccidiosis. Gastroenterology 1980;78:579–584.

125. MacKenzie WR, Hoxie NJ, Proctor ME, et al. A massive outbreak of cryptosporidium infection transmitted through the public water supply. N Engl J Med 1994;331:161–167.

126. Casemore DP, Armstrong M, Sands RL. Laboratory diagnosis of cryptosporidiosis. J Clin Pathol 1985;38:1337–1341.

127. Marcial-Rojas RA, ed. Pathology of protozoal and helminthic infections. Baltimore: Williams & Wilkins, 1971.

128. Dimmette RM, Sproat HF. Rectosigmoid polyps in schistosomiasis. Am J Trop Med Hyg 1955;4:1057–1067.

129. Chen MC, Chuang CY, Chang FY, et al. Evolution of colorectal cancer in schistosomiasis. Cancer 1980;46:1661–1675.

130. DeVault GA, King JW, Rohr MS, et al. Opportunistic infections with *Strongyloides stercoralis* in renal transplantation. Rev Infect Dis 1990;12:653–671.

131. Gutierrez Y, Bhatia P, Barbadawala ST, et al. *Strongyloides stercoralis* eosinophilic granulomatous enterocolitis. Am J Surg Pathol 1996;20:603–612.

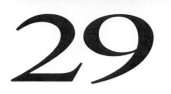

ULCERATIVE COLITIS AND CROHN'S DISEASE

Harvey Goldman

Two common disorders affecting the intestinal tract, particularly in persons from the more developed countries, are ulcerative colitis and Crohn's disease (1–3). They are often referred to under the common term of inflammatory bowel disease, or IBD. Since many other intestinal diseases with known etiologies also have an inflammatory basis, it has been suggested that ulcerative colitis and Crohn's disease should more appropriately be linked under the title of idiopathic inflammatory bowel disease, but this latter term is not as widely used.

The precise etiology and pathogenesis of ulcerative colitis and Crohn's disease are unknown, and they share many common features (4, 5). Accordingly, the diagnostic separation of these two disorders depends at all times on a consideration of the combined clinical, distributional, macroscopic, and histological characteristics (5–8). In this regard, the results obtained from radiographic and gross endoscopic examinations are vital for the accurate determination of the location of the disease and of other gross features prior to the pathologic study of the resected intestinal specimen. In this chapter, the two conditions are presented separately, followed by a section detailing the comparative features. A final section describes the uses and interpretations of endoscopic biopsies in these disorders.

ULCERATIVE COLITIS

GENERAL ASPECTS

DEFINITION

Ulcerative colitis is a chronic inflammatory disorder of unknown etiology that involves exclusively the large intestine and appendix. It is the most common cause of chronic colitis in the United States. Since the rectum is invariably affected, the disease has also been termed ulcerative proctocolitis. It was originally suspected that it may have an infectious etiology because of similarities in the inflammatory reaction, but a constant agent has never been established. The study by Warren and Sommers in 1949 provided a detailed account of the pathologic features (9); although these investigators initially thought that ulcerative colitis might be caused by a vasculitis, this was not confirmed.

DIAGNOSTIC CRITERIA

Before the diagnosis of ulcerative colitis can be considered, all other possible causes of inflammatory disease must be excluded, including infections, ischemic disease, known immune and toxic disorders,

TABLE	
29.1	**Diagnostic Features of Ulcerative Colitis**

Absence of known etiology.

Rectum always involved.

Colonic disease in majority of cases. When present, it is always diffuse and there are no skip areas except in the right colon.

Appendix may be affected, but there is no involvement of other parts of the gut.

Inflammation and ulceration is usually limited to the mucosa and submucosa. Involvement of deeper parts of bowel wall is seen in one-third of surgical resections, and in toxic megacolon.

Absence of discrete inflammatory sinus tracts, fissures, and fistulae. Must distinguish from multiple "cracks" in wall that may be seen in cases with toxic megacolon.

Absence of well formed, sarcoid-type granulomas. Must distinguish from granulomas due to ruptured crypts or foreign bodies.

and mechanical effects. Since there is no pathognomonic feature, the diagnosis of ulcerative colitis depends on a combination of clinical, distributional, and structural characteristics (Table 29.1). There is constant involvement of the rectum, variable extension of the disease to the more proximal portions of the colon in a diffuse fashion, and limitation of the disorder to the large intestine and appendix (1–3, 5, 9). The dominant inflammatory effect, at least in the initial stages, is in the mucosa, and the inflammatory reaction is essentially nonspecific. Compared to Crohn's disease and some infections of the colon, there is usually less inflammation in the deeper portions of the bowel wall. In addition, there are no skip areas (except in the right colon), discrete inflammatory sinus tracts, or granulomas.

EPIDEMIOLOGY

The disease may affect persons of all ages, including children and older adults, with a major peak in the third decade (10–12). A second, smaller peak has been suggested for the sixth–seventh decades, but it is uncertain whether this apparent peak is not confounded by the presence of other disorders in elderly persons such as ischemic disease (13). There is a slight preponderance of females, and ulcerative colitis is decidedly more common in persons from Western developed countries, in the White population, and in Jewish people. The overall incidence in areas where the disease is more common is approximately 5 to 6 per 100,000 persons. About 1 to 2% of the cases are familial. It has been noted that persons who smoke cigarettes are less likely to develop ulcerative colitis, and treatment with transdermal nicotine patches has been tried with variable results (14, 15). Also observed is that prior appendectomy has a protective effect; this was seen in 1 of 74 (0.6%) patients with ulcerative colitis compared to 41 of 161 (25%) persons without the disease (16).

ETIOLOGY AND PATHOGENESIS

The cause and pathogenesis of ulcerative colitis are not known (4). An infectious etiology was once considered because of the similarity of the inflammatory reaction to that seen in some human intestinal

infections and animal models. Furthermore, some of the relapses may be associated with or actually precipitated by secondary infections, such as those due to *Salmonella* and *Clostridium difficile*. However, the inflammatory reaction has proven to be completely nonspecific, there is no response to antimicrobial drugs except in the special case of secondary infections, and a constant infectious agent has not been identified as the primary cause of the colitis. There is also no evidence of a vasculitis or a reaction to known toxins. Although stressful situations may induce diarrhea, in general, and may be a precipitating factor for a relapse in a patient with ulcerative colitis, there is as yet no solid evidence to support this as having a primary role in the etiology of the disease.

Animal models of chronic colitis, both naturally occurring and experimentally induced, have been used to evaluate the pathologic features and particularly the development of neoplasia (17, 18). Although helpful in describing the sequential changes noted in the tumor formation, their relation to human colitis is not established.

It is currently believed that immune mechanisms are the probable cause of ulcerative colitis. As evidence supporting this theory, some of the patients have other disorders of a probable immunologic basis such as rheumatoid arthritis, there is a common presence of serum auto-antibodies including those directed to elements of the colonic mucosa, and the disease usually responds to corticosteroids and other immunosuppressive therapy. However, most of these features could be of a secondary or nonspecific nature, and the actual immunologic event responsible for the colitis is not established. A subset of patients, mainly cases involving the rectum, has been identified in whom there is a high concentration of IgE-bearing plasma cells in the lamina propria and a beneficial response to antihistamine medications (19, 20). It was suggested that these cases might be due to an immediate hypersensitivity type of allergic reaction, but it is unclear how they relate to the overall condition of ulcerative colitis.

CLINICAL FEATURES

In ulcerative colitis there is usually an abrupt onset, and major symptoms include crampy abdominal pain, tenesmus, mucous discharge in milder cases, diarrhea, and bleeding (21, 22). Laboratory tests reveal, in the severe cases, leukocytosis, anemia, hypokalemia, and hypoproteinemia. An increased serum level of antineutrophil cytoplasmic antibodies, particularly of the perinuclear type (p-ANCA), has been noted in patients with ulcerative colitis (23). This appears to be a secondary effect, and the levels tend to correlate with the degree of activity of the colitis but not with the development of pouchitis (24, 25). The presence of proctitis or proctocolitis is established by radiographic and/or sigmoidoscopic examinations. As noted previously, other known causes of colonic inflammation must be excluded before the diagnosis of ulcerative colitis can be made. It may be difficult to distinguish an initial episode of ulcerative colitis from a case of acute self-limited colitis. Mucosal biopsy may be especially helpful at this time in the detection or confirmation of the colitis, and in the determination of whether it is in the acute or chronic stage (26–28).

About 90% of the patients present with disease that is confined to the rectum and sigmoid colon, but over 50% eventually progress to develop more extensive colitis. The disease is characterized by periods of remission (inactive or quiescent colitis) and relapses (active colitis), and the recurrences may be associated with proximal extension of the colitis. The presence of proctitis appears to accentuate the development of perianal complications, including fissures and abscesses, which occur in about 15% of the patients (see Chapter 36 on Diseases of the Anal Region). Medical therapy includes mainly sulfasalazine derivatives, such as 5-aminosalicylate, and corticosteroids, administered by rectum or orally, with antibiotics used for secondary infections. Surgery is reserved for intractable disease and complications, and requires a complete proctocolectomy that is performed in one or two stages. The surgery is associated with the creation of a permanent ileostomy of the standard or continent type or, most commonly, with the formation of an ileal reservoir and ileoanal anastomosis. It is essential that the complete rectal mucosa be removed because of the concern for the late development of carcinoma in this area (29, 30). The overall mortality for ulcerative colitis is very low, with deaths mainly related to perforated megacolon, to septic complications of surgery or immunosuppressive therapy, and to carcinoma.

PATHOLOGY

The pathologic features of ulcerative colitis are similar in all age groups, including young children and elderly patients (31, 32).

DISTRIBUTION OF DISEASE

There is always involvement of the rectum and a variable extension of the disease upward in a diffuse fashion into the colon (1–3, 33). The disease remains limited to the rectum (ulcerative proctitis) in approximately 5 to 10% of the cases, proceeds at time of recurrence to involve the sigmoid and descending colon (left-sided colitis) in about 35% of the cases, and extends to the proximal transverse colon or beyond (extensive colitis) in over 50% of patients (Fig. 29.1). When the colitis involves the entire colon, it is also referred to as universal colitis or pan-colitis (Fig. 29.2). In surgical specimens, a

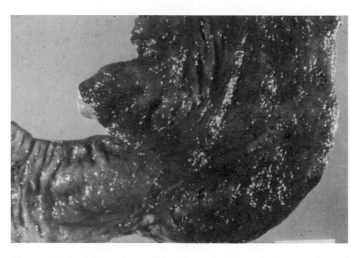

Figure 29.2   Ulcerative colitis. There is diffuse inflammation of the mucosa in the right colon including the cecum that stops abruptly at the ileocecal valve. The ileum *(left)* is slightly dilated but not ulcerated.

disproportionate number of cases with extensive involvement are seen, since these tend to be derived from patients with more severe and complicated disease.

There are no skip areas of normal colon amidst the inflamed segment of colon. Occasionally, there is an uneven degree of inflammation and repair resulting in areas that grossly simulate a skip region, but histological examination of such areas confirms the presence of diffuse colitis (34). Also, patients with severe colitis associated with colonic dilation who have a normal right colon may develop a localized area of colitis in the cecum, probably due to the effect of higher pressure in this region. Appendiceal involvement is usually associated with universal colitis but may occur in the face of relative sparing of the right side of the colon (35, 36). The lesion in the appendix is typically diffuse and limited to the superficial layers, in contrast to the transmural acute inflammation noted in an ordinary case of acute suppurative appendicitis (see Chapter 35, Disorders of the Vermiform Appendix).

The terminal portion of the ileum, usually limited to the distal-most 10 cm, may be dilated, particularly in cases with universal colitis (Fig. 29.2). It is thought that this results from regurgitation of colonic secretions through a dilated, relatively incompetent ileocecal valve, and this has been termed "backwash ileitis." It should be stressed, however, that there is no ulceration of the ileal mucosa; at most, there may be a patchy increase in inflammatory cells within the lamina propria together with the dilation. Accordingly, there is no evidence to support the conjecture that the ileum is involved with the same process that is damaging the colonic mucosa. There are also no ulcerative lesions of any other portion of the small intestine or upper gastrointestinal tract in cases of ulcerative colitis—i.e., the disease, true to its name, is limited to the colon and rectum. When a destructive lesion is found in some other portion of the gut, an alternative explanation must be sought.

In the cases limited to the rectum, referred to as ulcerative proctitis, the symptoms are characteristically less severe, there are fewer complications, and surgical excision is rarely needed (22). The pathologic features of ulcerative proctitis, as determined by study of mucosal biopsies, are otherwise similar to those of ulcerative colitis.

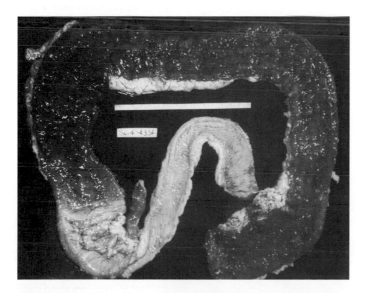

Figure 29.1   Ulcerative colitis. Subtotal colectomy specimen, showing diffuse involvement with hemorrhagic mucosa from the distal resection margin *(bottom right)* to the lower part of the ascending colon. The more proximal part of the colon and cecum, the appendix, and the ileal segment are normal.

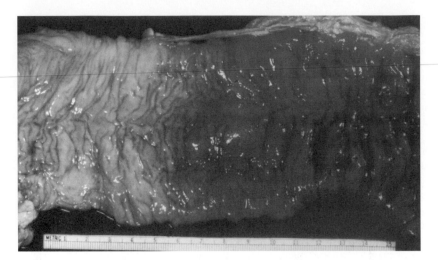

Figure 29.3 Segment of colon in ulcerative colitis, revealing a sharp demarcation between the inflamed, hemorrhagic mucosa *(right)* and the normal mucosa *(left)*.

GROSS FEATURES

Many of the early changes are best appreciated in vivo at the gross endoscopic examination (37, 38). The lesion begins with a diffuse erythema and patchy hemorrhage of the mucosa, and proceeds to a stage of friability and overt ulceration. The disease involves the rectum and colon in a continuous fashion, and there is usually a relatively sharp demarcation between the inflamed mucosa at the proximal end of the lesion and the adjacent normal colon (Fig. 29.3). More advanced lesions show extensive undermining of the intact but inflamed mucosa by the ulcerations resulting in the formation of mucosal bridges (Fig. 29.4). The ulcers tend to be superficial, usually limited to the mucosa or upper submucosa, and there are typically no gross abnormalities of the underlying muscularis propria or serosa. In about one-third of surgically resected specimens, which presumably represent the more severe cases, ulcers are found to extend into the muscularis propria. This is associated with focal inflammation of the serosa, but the change is usually not grossly conspicuous. There are no discrete inflammatory sinus tracts or fistulas in uncomplicated cases of ulcerative colitis.

With time and intermittent repair of the colitis, there is the variable formation of inflammatory polyps which are also termed pseudopolyps (39). These inflammatory polyps result in part from a persistence of intact mucosa that is relatively raised next to an ulcerated area, but also from the intense inflammation and repair that is present in that mucosa (Fig. 29.5). The presence of such polyps is a good indicator of chronic colitis, but it is not specific for ulcerative colitis since they may be seen in other causes of chronic inflammation such as in Crohn's disease of the colon and in ischemic colitis (40). The polyps vary considerably in their amount, size, and distribution. There may be only a few scattered inflammatory polyps or a veritable sea of such lesions over a large portion of the colon (Fig. 29.6). Most inflammatory pseudopolyps are sessile or have a short stalk, and they exhibit a relatively smooth surface, in contrast

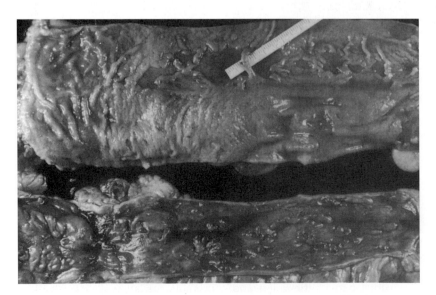

Figure 29.4 Ulcerative colitis. There is extensive ulceration and the presence of mucosal bridges. The bowel wall is not thickened.

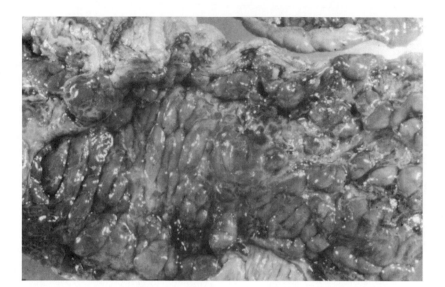

Figure 29.5   Ulcerative colitis, showing an admixture of ulceration and inflammatory pseudopolyps.

to the more convoluted or frankly papillary surface contour of adenomas. Occasionally, an inflammatory polyp may be very large and localized (giant pseudopolyp) and mimic the appearance of a polypoid neoplasm (41, 42). Close inspection of such polyps reveals that they are composed of anastomosing strands of mucosa, as can be readily demonstrated by passing a probe through the various channels and arches of the lesion (Fig. 29.7); a neoplasm, in contrast, is composed of a more solid mass and has a continuous attachment at its base with the mucosa. The polyps may also persist after the cessation of the ulcerating and inflammatory phase of active colitis. This appears to be due to the formation of a fibromuscular core in the polyp, analogous to the development of fibroepithelial polyps in other tissues. The overlying mucosa in such polyps may lose all signs of active inflammation, and superficial mucosal biopsies may fail to appreciate their nature. These persistent polyps frequently have a villous or finger-like configu-

ration and have also been called filiform polyps (43). Lesions in the rectum may develop a covering of squamous metaplasia and have an opaque surface.

The inactive or quiescent phase of ulcerative colitis is characterized grossly by the absence of ulcers and the occasional persistence of inflammatory pseudopolyps. There is usually a simplification of the haustral markings, and severe cases show a relatively flat mucosal surface. By endoscopic examination, there may be enhanced vascular markings due to the greater visualization of the submucosal vessels through an atrophic mucosa. Upon recurrence and progression of the disease, there may be an uneven degree of inflammation. In most patients, the worst disease remains in the distal colon and rectum, but some show more prominent disease in the proximal front of the colon. More severe cases of active ulcerative colitis may be associated with pronounced dilation of the lumen and thinning of the bowel wall, and late lesions include a

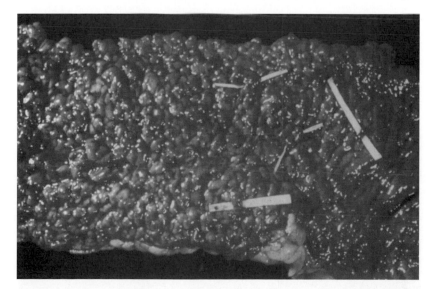

Figure 29.6   Ulcerative colitis. The mucosal surface is altered by the presence of a massive number of small inflammatory pseudopolyps.

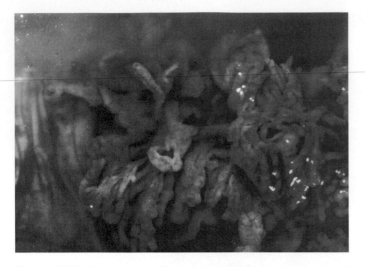

Figure 29.7   Single large inflammatory pseudopolyp in a case of chronic ulcerative colitis. The polyp is composed of numerous, fine mucosal bridges.

shortening of the colon and fibrous stricture formation. These are discussed in the section on Complications.

HISTOLOGICAL FEATURES

The microscopic features noted in ulcerative colitis are essentially nonspecific (1–3, 5–9, 34, 44–46). Indeed, it is often impossible to distinguish the initial stage of ulcerative colitis from other causes of acute colitis, particularly in the examination of small mucosal biopsies. With progression of the disease, however, the mucosa undergoes a series of architectural and inflammatory changes that serve to identify the lesion as a chronic disorder (27, 28). In the initial acute phase, there is marked infiltration of the mucosa with neutrophils together with signs of degeneration of the surface and crypt epithelia (Fig. 29.8). The neutrophils are present both in the

lamina propria and in the damaged epithelial layer. The injury to the crypt ranges from the simple presence of neutrophils in the epithelium, to focal denudation of the epithelial cells, and finally to complete destruction of the crypt surrounding a pool of luminal neutrophils (crypt abscess). The term cryptitis may be applied to the full variety of inflammatory changes affecting the crypts (45, 46). Also present are features of prominent regeneration of the epithelial cells, including elongation and pallisading of the nuclei, with central enlarged nucleoli, and numerous mitoses.

Mucosal erosions and superficial ulcerations, usually limited to the upper submucosa, develop in the more severe cases and are typically associated with inflammatory pseudopolyps in the adjacent mucosa (Figs. 29.9 and 29.10). In nonulcerated areas, the normal architecture of relatively straight and parallel crypts with minimal branching may remain in an acute case of ulcerative colitis (26). Giant cells, representing multinucleated macrophages, may be present in the mucosa that is actively inflamed and eroded, and these are thought to result from a nonspecific reaction to luminal contents. Occasionally seen are poorly formed granulomas surrounding a ruptured crypt (Fig. 29.11), and multiple sections may be required to identify the crypt injury as the source of the lesion (47). Well formed sarcoid-type granulomas that are unassociated with necrosis or foreign material are not seen in ulcerative colitis.

Complete regeneration and restoration of the mucosa to normal is observed following most cases of acute self-limited colitis, such as those due to acute infections. In contrast, when a patient with ulcerative colitis attains a remission, there usually are persistent and characteristic alterations in the mucosa present that serve to identify the disorder as a chronic colitis (Table 29.2). Some of these features have been observed as early as three weeks after the onset of ulcerative colitis. The major mucosal changes are an abnormal architecture characterized by extensive budding and branching of the crypts (Fig. 29.12), an atrophy of the crypts as evidenced by their shortening and diffuse separation from the muscularis mucosae (Fig. 29.13), and a villous-like transformation of the mucosal surface (28). Also commonly present are an overall increase in mononuclear inflammatory cells and eosinophils in the lamina propria (48–50), the presence of small lymphoid nodules and

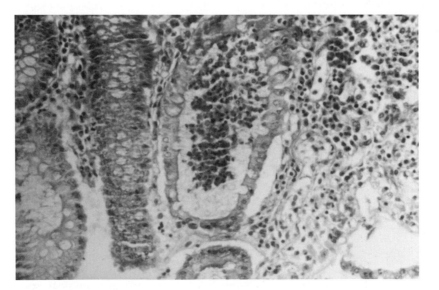

Figure 29.8   Colonic mucosa in an active case of ulcerative colitis, showing acute cryptitis with a crypt abscess. H & E, ×100.

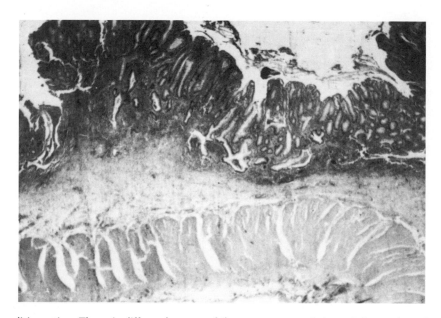

Figure 29.9 Ulcerative colitis, active. There is diffuse damage of the mucosa, consisting of alternating ulcers and inflamed mucosa. The inflammation extends into the upper submucosa, but the deeper parts of the wall, including the muscularis propria and serosa (*at the bottom*), are usually normal. H & E, ×20.

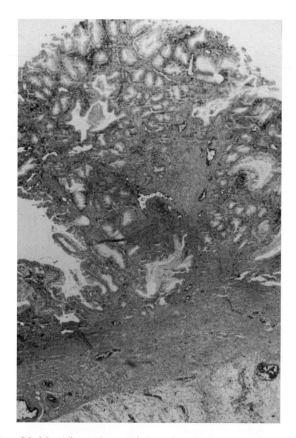

Figure 29.10 Ulcerative colitis, showing an inflammatory pseudopolyp. The polyp is composed of regenerating glands and inflamed mucosa. H & E, ×60.

increased plasma cells at the base of the mucosa separating the crypts and the muscularis mucosae (27) (Fig. 29.14), and the appearance of Paneth cell metaplasia in the crypt epithelium (46, 51) (Fig. 29.15). It should be remembered that Paneth cells are normally indigenous to the cecum and proximal ascending colon and that their presence, therefore, can only be considered abnormal if seen in the mid and distal portions of the colon. It has been estimated that at least one of these features of chronic colitis can be found in almost 80% of initial mucosal biopsies in cases of ulcerative colitis (26). In contrast, they are never present in a case of acute self-limited colitis. By immunocytochemical staining, the increase in plasma cells is seen to affect all classes including the IgG, IgM, and IgA types (52). Some cases of ulcerative proctitis show a preferential increase in IgE-type plasma cells and are thought to have an allergic component (19, 20) (see Chapter 12).

Also noted in chronic colitis to a variable degree are a hyperplasia of the crypt endocrine cells (53), columnar cells with mucin limited to the luminal aspect that resemble the mucous cells of gastric pits, rare patches of pyloric glandular metaplasia, foci of squamous metaplasia in distal lesions, the incorporation of adipose tissue in the mucosa probably resulting from prior ulceration, and fibrosis of the base of the lamina propria in longstanding cases. It is important to distinguish artifactual spaces in the lamina propria, referred to as pseudolipomatosis and commonly present in distorted biopsies, from true adipose tissue in the mucosa (54); the latter is usually associated with disruption of the muscularis mucosae. Although these various features of chronic colitis are commonly seen, they may not be appreciated in small biopsy samples in all cases. Furthermore, the mucosa more often appears normal during a remission if the patient has been treated with steroid enemas (55).

During a relapse, noted are both the changes of chronic colitis and the inflammatory and degenerative effects of the active disease. Considering the duration of the disease and the histological features in the mucosa, cases of ulcerative colitis can be categorized into

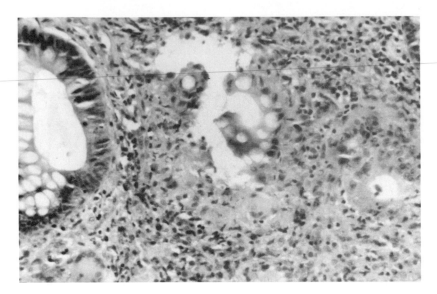

Figure 29.11   Colonic mucosa in active ulcerative colitis, revealing a poorly formed granulomatous reaction to a ruptured crypt. H & E, ×400.

three groups: acute colitis for the initial episode, chronic inactive colitis at time of remission, and chronic active colitis during relapses.

The primary and dominant injury in ulcerative colitis is at the level of the mucosa, and the disease has also been called mucosal colitis to distinguish it from the transmural colitis seen in most cases of Crohn's disease. When the mucosa is completely destroyed, there is sloughing of the necrotic tissue and formation of ulcers. The ulcers are usually superficial and limited to the upper submucosa (Fig. 29.9), but they may in severe cases extend to the muscularis propria, as noted in about one-third of surgical resections. A nonspecific acute inflammatory response, consisting of edema and neutrophils, surrounds the ulcers. This inflammation is usually confined to the submucosa but may extend through the wall when there is deeper ulceration. Other alterations in the submucosa are nonspecific and include congestion, presence of mononuclear inflammatory cells (plasma cells, lymphocytes, and macrophages)

with occasional lymphoid nodules, and slight lymphatic dilatation. Underlying areas of prior ulceration, the muscularis mucosae may be either thinned-out and disrupted or show focal areas of hypertrophy. In long-standing cases, there may be focal areas of fibrosis and neural proliferation in the submucosa, but this change is rarely as prominent as that seen in Crohn's disease. The muscularis propria and serosa are usually normal or show, at most, a patchy acute and chronic inflammation in cases with deep ulcers. There are no discrete inflammatory fissures extending into the muscularis.

In some patients requiring surgery, an initial subtotal colectomy is performed and the rectum is temporarily left in situ as a mucous fistula. The rectal mucosa continues to show the effects of chronic colitis and intermittent changes of active disease. Occasional cases reveal marked hyperplasia of lymphoid nodules within the mucosa and submucosa, and this has been referred to as follicular proctitis; it is possible that this change reflects a reaction to substances in the static segment of rectum. This alteration may also be seen, but usually to a lesser degree, in cases with an intact colon.

PATHOLOGIC DIAGNOSIS

Lacking any specific markers, the diagnosis of ulcerative colitis is essentially one of exclusion. Other causes of acute and chronic colitis of known etiology must be ruled out by appropriate clinical and laboratory studies. The diagnosis of ulcerative colitis (Table 29.1) is established by the demonstration of all of the following features: (1) absence of a known or presumed etiology; (2) rectal involvement and variable degree of colonic and appendiceal disease, which is always diffuse (i.e., has no skip areas, except in the right colon); (3) no involvement of other portions of the gut; (4) absence of discrete inflammatory sinus tracts extending into the wall; and (5) relatively nonspecific inflammatory reaction, largely confined to the mucosa and submucosa, without the presence of well formed sarcoid-type granulomas. After the first few weeks, most cases also reveal characteristic changes in the mucosa that signify a chronic colitis.

TABLE 29.2	Histologic Features of Chronic Colitis

Common Features:	More Variable Features:
Abnormal mucosal architecture characterized by prominent branching of crypts	Endocrine cell hyperplasia
	Pyloric gland metaplasia
	Squamous metaplasia
Atrophy of crypts	Fibrosis of lamina propria
Villiform surface	
Increase of mononuclear inflammatory cells and eosinophils in lamina propria	
Presence of lymphoid nodules and increased plasma cells at base of lamina propria	
Paneth cell metaplasia	

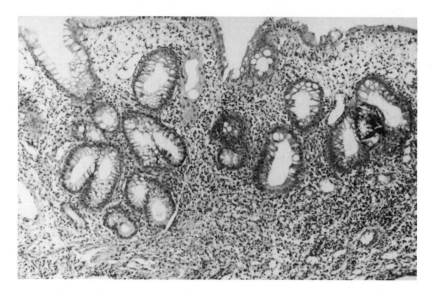

Figure 29.12   Colonic mucosa in chronic ulcerative colitis. There is a prominent architectural alteration due to multiple branching and slight shortening of the crypts. H & E, ×60. (Reprinted with permission from Goldman H, Antonioli DA. Mucosal biopsy of the rectum, colon and distal ileum. Hum Pathol 1982;13:981-1012.)

DIFFERENTIAL DIAGNOSIS

Acute infections of the colon can usually be distinguished from ulcerative colitis in the very early stages because they more often exhibit focal lesions (46, 56, 57). In some infections, such as those due to *Campylobacter* and *Chlamydia* agents, granulomas may also be present (26, 47, 58). The later stage of infections is commonly associated with a more diffuse colitis, and only the demonstration of the microorganism, typically by culture of the stool or its examination for ova, serves to distinguish it from an acute case of ulcerative colitis (59–63). Furthermore, some infections, including those due

to *Shigella* and *Chlamydia* organisms, may persist and develop features of a chronic colitis, but this event is uncommon and the histologic alterations are usually not as prominent as that seen in ulcerative colitis. Pseudomembranous colitis, typically due to *C. difficile*, reveals characteristic, small, sharply demarcated, yellow to white patches on the mucosa, and histology shows a relatively normal mucosa next to the inflamed areas (64–66). Amebic colitis due to *Entamoeba histolytica* can cause an acute and chronic colitis with diffuse lesions that is identical to ulcerative colitis (67, 68). There may be extensive ulcerations, and the diagnosis is established by the identification of the characteristic ova in the stool or in smears

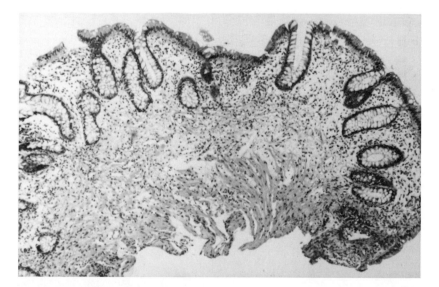

Figure 29.13   Colonic mucosa in chronic ulcerative colitis. Example of inactive phase showing crypt atrophy. The crypts are fewer in number and markedly shortened, as evidenced by the increased space between their bases and the muscularis mucosae *(at bottom)*. H & E, ×60. (Reprinted with permission from Goldman H, Antonioli DA. Mucosal biopsy of the rectum, colon and distal ileum. Hum Pathol 1982;13:981-1012.)

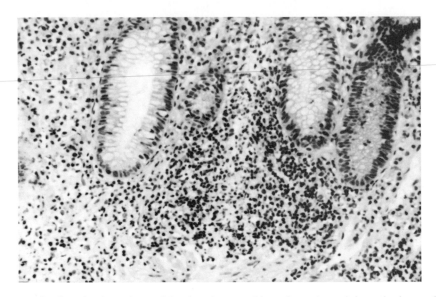

Figure 29.14   Colonic mucosa in chronic ulcerative colitis, showing small lymphocytic nodule at the base of the mucosa between the crypts and the muscularis mucosae. H & E, ×250.

obtained by direct imprints of the lesion. See Chapter 28 on Infectious Disorders of the Intestines for further details.

Cases of ischemic colitis are more common in older patients, and there is a tendency for segmental involvement with frequent sparing of the rectum; microscopy reveals extensive necrosis which is more often concentrated in the superficial half of the mucosa (69, 70). There also may be prominent hemorrhage and hemosiderin deposits in cases of ischemic colitis, but this is not a distinguishing feature as it may be seen in any case of colitis with prominent bleeding. Less common causes of colitis that can simulate ulcerative colitis include reactions to drugs and the effects of vasculitis (71, 72). These tend to be milder and more focal but may exceptionally present with a fulminant colitis; their distinction is dependent on the history and the presence of associated con-

ditions such as lupus erythematosus. The major differential diagnosis of ulcerative colitis, particularly in the chronic phase, is Crohn's disease (1, 2, 5–8, 46, 73). Most cases can be readily distinguished by a consideration not only of the histological features but also of the gross and distributional characteristics. Thus, the diagnosis of Crohn's disease is manifested by the presence of some combination of focal lesions in the colon and other parts of the gut, the development of mural sinus tracts, and the appearance of granulomas.

COMPLICATIONS

Clinical problems resulting from severe episodes of ulcerative colitis include anemia from repeated hemorrhages, hypovolemia and

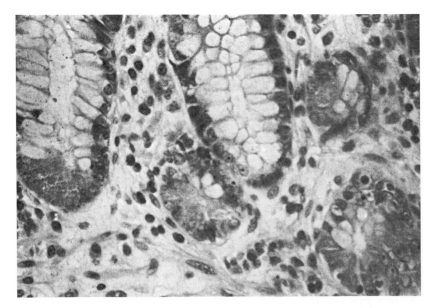

Figure 29.15   Colonic mucosa in chronic ulcerative colitis, revealing Paneth cell metaplasia in the bottom of the crypts. H & E, ×250.

hypokalemia due in part from the inflammation but mostly from reduced absorption, and hypoproteinemia resulting from oozing of protein from the mucosal ulcerations.

TOXIC MEGACOLON

A severe episode of active colitis, either in the acute phase or at a recurrence, can result in extreme outpouring of fluid and hemorrhage into the colonic lumen. This leads to progressive dilation of the lumen, pressure-induced extension of the necrosis and thinning of the bowel wall, and ultimately to perforation if this complication is not checked. The patients are very sick and exhibit high fever and prominent leukocytosis; the lesion is best monitored by serial abdominal radiographs, and surgery becomes indicated if there is progression of the bowel dilation over a period of 3 to 5 days. Inspection of the bowel wall reveals thinning due to ischemic-type necrosis with prominent vascular congestion and focal cracks or fissures in the most inflamed areas (Fig. 29.16). These fissures must be distinguished from the discrete sinus tracts that occur in an otherwise normal or thickened bowel wall in Crohn's disease (34). Perforation of the colon in a case of toxic megacolon results in a generalized peritonitis and an overall poor prognosis.

SECONDARY INFECTIONS

Some of the relapses seen in ulcerative colitis are due to the development of secondary infections rather than to recrudescence of the primary disease. This may be caused by any of the ordinary pathogens (74, 75), but more commonly noted are infections due to *Salmonella* and *C. difficile* (76, 77). Rare cases due to protozoa such as *Balantidium* have also been recorded (78). It is important to recognize this possibility at time or relapse and to perform the appropriate stool culture and toxin assays, because the cases respond preferentially to specific antimicrobial therapy. The pathologic features of these infections are identical to that seen in ordinary recurrent ulcerative colitis; specifically, the pseudomembranes associated with *C. difficile* disease in non-colitis patients are not present in cases complicating ulcerative colitis. Occasionally, in patients receiving high doses of corticosteroids or other immunosuppressive therapy, opportunistic infections due mainly to herpes simplex and cytomegalovirus occur (79, 80). These tend to be associated with very severe cases and may promote increased necrosis and perforation. Exceptionally, there is spread of the opportunistic infection to internal organs, and death can result from generalized sepsis or massive hepatic necrosis. In such cases, one should look for the characteristic inclusions of the viruses, and this search can be abetted by specific immunocytochemical stains.

COLITIS CYSTICA

In cases with extensive ulceration, there may be the downgrowth and persistence of dilated colonic glands into the submucosa and occasionally the muscularis propria, and this is called colitis cystica profunda (81). The lesions may also be associated with inflammatory pseudopolyps, and the overall mass may be confused with an adenocarcinoma. The distinction is made by noting that the misplaced glands are either normal or show at most the effects of inflammation, and there is no dysplasia of the epithelium. Although there have been many descriptions of colitis cystica, it appears that the prominent polypoid form is very uncommon. Other benign conditions in ulcerative colitis that reveal spaces or nodules in the submucosa include pneumatosis intestinalis which is due to the growth of gas-forming bacteria in areas of acute or active colitis, and clusters of macrophages containing barium, so-called "barium granuloma" (see Chapter 30 for further details).

POSTSURGICAL ILEAL ABNORMALITIES

Since ulcerative colitis is a disease that is limited to the rectum and colon, it is expected that total proctocolectomy will be curative.

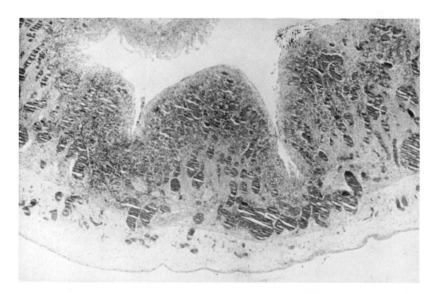

Figure 29.16 Colonic wall in a case of severe ulcerative colitis. There is deep ulceration, and the underlying muscularis propria shows marked congestion, granulation tissue, and superficial cracks in the tissue. H & E, ×20.

Nevertheless, a small proportion of the patients develop problems with the ileum, associated either with an ileostomy or an ileal reservoir following an ileal-anal anastomosis (8, 82–84). Up to 5% of patients who have had a regular ileostomy require one or more revisions of this structure, due mainly to a tight stoma, mucosal prolapse, or local sepsis. The resected ileum is frequently normal or shows just mucosal atrophy characterized by an increase in mononuclear inflammatory cells in the lamina propria together with a variable degree of villous shortening (85–88). Occasionally noted is a complete loss of villi and transformation to a colonic-type mucosa with sulfomucins in the goblet mucous cells (89). Other abnormalities that may be present include hemorrhagic necrosis in cases of prolapse, focal ulceration, and sinus tracts. These changes are usually confined to the stoma and distal 5 cm of the ileostomy segment. Exceptionally, prominent granulomas may be encountered at an ileostomy stoma and in the adjacent skin, due to suture reaction or to the insertion of foreign objects in the opening.

Some patients develop what has been termed prestomal ileitis, characterized by the presence of focal and shallow ulcers in a longer segment of ileum proximal to the stoma (90). The involved ileal segment is either of normal caliber or dilated, in contrast to the stenosis that is commonly seen in cases of recurrent Crohn's disease of the ileum. It is thought that prestomal ileitis might be due to a relative obstruction and formation of stasis-type ulcers. Histologic study of the ulcers shows nonspecific inflammation, and there are no mural fissures or granulomas. The incidence of abnormalities affecting continent-type ileostomies is much higher, with some estimates of 40 to 50%, and they are due largely to vascular compromise and obstruction (91, 92). This is ordinarily corrected by conversion to a standard ileostomy.

POUCHITIS

In an effort to retain the anal sphincter in patients with ulcerative colitis who require a colectomy, there has been a recent increase in operations involving an ileoanal anastomosis with creation of an ileal reservoir, particularly in younger patients. About 25% of these patients develop superficial ulcerations of the ileal mucosa, termed "pouchitis," which are due mainly to stasis or to secondary infections from various microbial agents, and they typically respond to antibiotic therapy with few recurrences. The ileum in the reservoir shows a mild to moderate degree of mucosal atrophy, together with focal erosions or ulcers and a nonspecific acute inflammatory reaction (93–95). Occasional lesions reveal a prominent inflammatory membrane, pseudopolyps, or mucosal prolapse (96).

Noted in fewer than 5% of cases are multiple episodes of pouchitis and the development of chronic alterations of the ileal mucosa (97). The later lesions show greater villous atrophy and branching of the crypts, an increase in mononuclear inflammatory cells, and the presence of colonic-type mucins and antigens (84, 98–100). The mucosa may ultimately take on the characteristics of the colonic type, and it has been suggested that further inflammation in this tissue represents recurrence of the chronic ulcerative colitis (101). As an additional consequence, the pouch mucosa may be at later risk for the appearance of dysplasia and carcinoma (102–105).

In situations in which disease appears in an ileostomy area or an ileal reservoir, particularly in cases with ulceration, concern may arise that the original diagnosis of ulcerative colitis was an error and that the patient instead has Crohn's disease (106). It may prove useful, in such instances, to review the clinical findings and the pathologic features of the prior colectomy specimen. Stringent criteria are required in assessing the ileal lesions. Features sought to support the diagnosis of Crohn's disease in the ileum include transmural inflammation with fibrosis and stricture formation, and the presence of inflammatory sinus tracts or granulomas away from the area of the stoma or anastomosis (87) (see section on Crohn's Disease for further details).

EXTRA-INTESTINAL MANIFESTATIONS

In about one-third of the patients with ulcerative colitis, a variety of inflammatory conditions affecting other organ systems may occur at some time during the course of the disease (107). These include uveitis, joint abnormalities in the form of polyarthritis or ankylosing spondylitis, and the skin diseases of erythema nodosum and pyoderma gangrenosum. The conditions are much more common in patients with extensive colitis than in those with left-sided colitis or proctitis (108). It is thought that these manifestations are due to effects of circulating immune complexes, induced by antigens that are derived from the gut lumen or the damaged colonic mucosa. In support of this notion, all of these conditions disappear when the patient has a total colectomy. Alterations are also commonly seen in the liver, consisting of fatty change from poor nutrition or high dose corticosteroid therapy, and the appearance of focal infiltration of mononuclear inflammatory cells in the portal triads (chronic pericholangitis) most likely representing a nonspecific reaction to toxic substances that are absorbed from the inflamed colon.

A less frequent effect noted in the liver and biliary tract in cases of ulcerative colitis is sclerosing cholangitis, characterized by the development of progressive fibrosis that encircles the large extrahepatic and intrahepatic bile ducts as well as the ductules in the portal tracts. This results in a characteristic beaded appearance of the large bile ducts that is best visualized by radiographic study, and in obstruction of the ductal system. The liver may show the added features of obstructive injury in the form of prominent bile stasis and acute cholangiolitis. The etiology of sclerosing cholangitis is unknown and, unlike the other extra-intestinal manifestations seen in ulcerative colitis, this lesion does not regress after the performance of a total colectomy (109). Patients with sclerosing cholangitis have a further problem in that there is an increased incidence of bile duct adenocarcinoma (110). The tumors may affect any part of the intrahepatic and extrahepatic ducts, typically present as advanced lesions with progression of the stenosis and obstruction, and are rarely amenable to surgical resection. Primary sclerosing cholangitis is a rare disorder. Since most cases are associated instead with chronic inflammatory bowel disease, either ulcerative colitis or Crohn's disease, these latter conditions should be considered in any patient with the appearance of sclerosing cholangitis or stenotic bile duct carcinoma.

DYSPLASIA AND CARCINOMA
INCIDENCE AND RISK FACTORS

Patients with ulcerative colitis have an increased incidence of colonic adenocarcinoma (111–113). The two major risk factors are the extent and the duration of the colitis (114–116). It has been estimated that cases of extensive colitis (i.e., disease extending to at

TABLE 29.3	Carcinoma in Ulcerative Colitis	
Extensive colitis[a]		15%
10 years	1%	
15 years	4.5%	
20 years	13%	
30 years	34%	
Left-sided colitis		5%

Table modified from Greenstein AJ, Sachar DB, Smith H, et al. Cancer in universal and left-sided ulcerative colitis: factors determining risk. Gastroenterology 1979;99:290–294.

[a]Colitis extending to at least the hepatic flexure.

least the hepatic flexure) have an overall incidence of tumor development of about 15% whereas the rate in those with left-sided colitis is about 5% (Table 29.3). The incidence clearly increases with respect to time, with a 1 to 2% annual rise in tumors after 10 years of extensive disease. Although the risk of tumor occurrence is least in the first decade, this is the period when most patients have not yet had a colectomy for other indications, and it appears that about 20% of the tumors arise at this time, particularly after 5 years of disease (117). It has also been suggested that the frequency of dysplasia complicating ulcerative colitis may be greater in older patients, independent of the overall duration of disease (118). The degree of cancer risk is variable, however, and probably depends on the geographic location and the particular group of patients studied (119). There is no independent relation of tumor development to the age of onset of the colitis, to the activity or severity of the disease, to the type of medical therapy, or to the sex, race, or ethnic background of the patients. Recent reports indicate that cases of ulcerative colitis with sclerosing cholangitis have a greater tendency for the development of dysplasia and carcinoma in the colon (120, 121).

There are claims that the incidences of leukemia and colonic lymphomas are increased in patients with ulcerative colitis (122–124), but this is not a major problem. Also recorded have been increases of bile duct carcinoma (110), of colonic carcinoid tumors (125), and possibly of uterine and vaginal cancers (126). Most of the carcinoid tumors appear as microscopic lesions and are detected as incidental findings during the process of routine endoscopy and biopsy (127, 128); it is not clear whether prompt excision or simple follow-up is needed in these cases. There are rare reports of lymphoepithelial carcinoma (129) and malignant melanoma (130) of the colon as well as the development of an appendiceal carcinoma (131).

It has been noted that there may be an increased chance of primary adenocarcinoma occurring in ileostomy sites, typically seen 20 or more years after colectomy for ulcerative colitis (132–134). Carcinomas have also been detected in ileoanal reservoirs, but this may be related in part to inadvertently retained rectal mucosa (103, 104). There is no enhanced frequency of other tumors of the colon or of other portions of the gastrointestinal tract.

CARCINOMA

There are approximately 1000 new cases of carcinoma complicating chronic inflammatory bowel disease in the United States each year,

accounting for about 1% of all new colonic adenocarcinomas (135). When compared with the noncolitic population, tumors in ulcerative colitis arise in younger patients, with an average age that is about 10 years less, and they are more frequently multiple (113, 136, 137). They are also distributed more diffusely throughout the colon and do not show the strong predilection for the rectosigmoid area; indeed, recent studies suggest that there are an increasing number of cases in the right portion of the colon (138). The tumors tend to be restricted to areas of prior inflammation, and they may also develop in rectal stumps following a subtotal colectomy (29, 30).

The majority of symptomatic cases present with stenotic lesions, and the usual adenoma-carcinoma sequence of a patient without colitis is not seen. A comparison of tumors with and without colitis at equivalent stages of growth reveals a similar behavior (136, 139). Nevertheless, because it may be exceedingly difficult to distinguish stenosing tumors from the effects of the underlying colitis, most cases of carcinoma complicating ulcerative colitis in symptomatic patients appear at an advanced stage and the prognosis is generally poor. The advanced tumors vary in size, with lesions extending over several centimeters, and they frequently are circumferential (Fig. 29.17). The adjacent mucosa is often raised and may represent areas of residual dysplasia. The overall spread of the carcinomas is similar to that seen in patients without colitis, and there is invasion into and through the bowel wall to the peritoneum, and metastases to regional lymph nodes and liver. The earlier

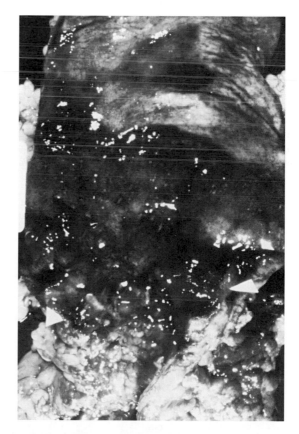

Figure 29.17 Adenocarcinoma of the colon, in a case of chronic ulcerative colitis. The carcinoma is located in the stenotic portion (*at bottom*) and the adjacent mucosa is slightly raised due to associated dysplasia.

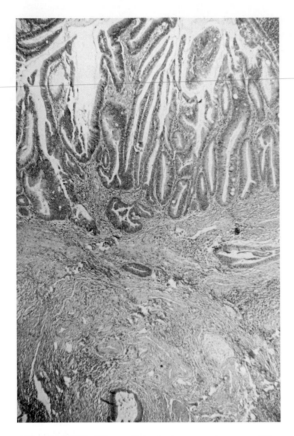

Figure 29.18   Well-differentiated adenocarcinoma of the colon, complicating chronic ulcerative colitis. The carcinomatous glands are well formed and their nature is revealed only by the invasion into the submucosa and muscularis propria. The overlying mucosa *(top)* shows the dysplastic glands. H & E, ×20.

carcinomas, which are presently being detected with greater frequency because of the use of surveillance programs, tend to be smaller and appear as more discrete, slightly raised or polypoid lesions (140). These early tumors are associated with prominent

dysplasia in the mucosa and usually show less invasion by the carcinoma. The remaining colonic mucosa shows signs of chronic colitis, which is usually in the inactive stage, and may reveal other foci of gross or microscopic dysplasia alone or together with other carcinomas.

Histological examination of the adenocarcinomas in ulcerative colitis reveals variable gland formation, and a high proportion, in the order of 35 to 40%, are very well differentiated or of the mucinous type (141, 142) (Fig. 29.18). Indeed, it may be difficult to appreciate the carcinoma in mucosal biopsies because the samples may be too superficial to detect the invasion. All other histological forms are encountered, including poorly differentiated carcinoma, signet ring cell type, and tumors mixed with neuroendocrine cells (adenocarcinoid tumors) (143, 144). There is no relation between the degree of differentiation of the carcinomas and their behavior.

A clinical suspicion of carcinoma complicating ulcerative colitis is raised if there develops obstructive signs, bleeding, or weight loss that cannot be explained by the underlying inflammatory disease. The tumors are localized by radiographic and endoscopic studies, and a specific diagnosis is obtained by directed mucosal biopsy. The level of serum carcinoembryonic antigen has not proven to be of value, because it may vary considerably as a result of active colitis and its repair. Because of the common presence and occasional large size of inflammatory pseudopolyps, it was once thought that these lesions might be a precursor to the carcinoma, but this view is no longer accepted. Indeed, it is rare for an inflammatory polyp to be the site for even the presence of dysplasia.

DYSPLASIA

Dysplasia represents a neoplastic transformation of the colonic epithelium and serves as a marker that a patient with ulcerative colitis either already has or is particularly prone to the development of carcinoma (145). Synonyms for colonic dysplasia include precancer, precarcinoma, and adenomatous epithelium. Early studies of carcinoma in ulcerative colitis noted the presence of such dysplasia at the edge of many tumors (146), and Morson and Pang in 1967 demonstrated that this could be detected in mucosal biopsies that were obtained from sites away from the overt tumor (147).

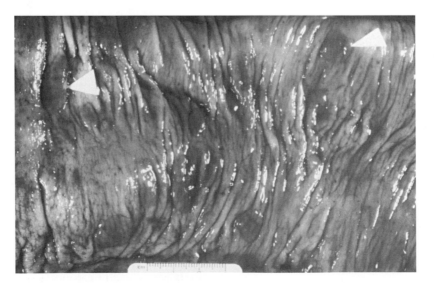

Figure 29.19   Colon segment in a case of inactive ulcerative colitis. There are several small plaques *(arrows)* in the mucosa which revealed epithelial dysplasia on histologic examination (see Figure 29.32).

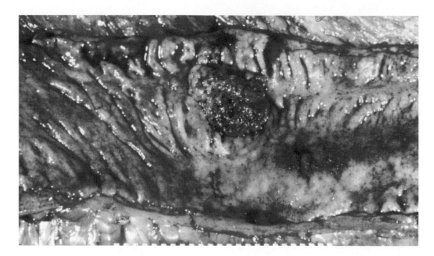

Figure 29.20   Polypoid lesion of dysplasia in ulcerative colitis.

Subsequent investigations showed that about 90% of cases of ulcerative colitis with carcinoma contain foci of dysplasia, either adjacent to or remote from the gross cancer (136, 148–158). The dysplasia, like the carcinoma, may be present in any portion of the colon, and only about 65% of the lesions are detected if the inspection is limited to the left-side of the colon (138, 159). It may be observed as a microscopic alteration in the flat atrophic mucosa or, when severe, is associated with a gross lesion (referred to as dysplasia-associated mass lesion or DALM) (160). The gross areas of dysplasia vary in size from a few millimeters to several centimeters in diameter, and they are typically sessile and slightly raised lesions with a prominent velvety or villous-like surface pattern (148) (Figs. 29.19 and 29.20). Ordinary inflammatory polyps (pseudopolyps), in contrast, tend to have a smoother or rounded surface contour. Signs of carcinoma within a gross dysplastic lesion include the presence of ulceration, induration, or stenosis. However, many of the carcinomas lack these surface changes and are revealed only by detection of invasion into the colonic wall, particularly in early and well differentiated tumors (Fig. 29.18). It has been estimated that the appearance of dysplasia, particularly in the flat mucosa, may precede the development of overt carcinoma by as long as 7 years (150). On the other hand, in grossly evident lesions, the dysplasia may be the first sign of an underlying invasive tumor. Dysplasia is less often found in cases of carcinoma that occur in areas of prior strictures or fistulae (161).

The histological diagnosis of dysplasia in cases of ulcerative colitis is often difficult because of the persistent inflammatory and reparative effects of the underlying disease. The latter features cause complex branching of the crypts and other architectural changes that may be confused with a neoplastic proliferation, especially in cases that also show regenerative effects in the epithelium. It is essential, therefore, to be aware of the full range of inflammatory changes that may affect the mucosa in cases of chronic ulcerative colitis before the diagnosis of dysplasia can be made with certainty (45, 46). To assist in this distinction, a standardized classification of colonic dysplasia with uniform nomenclature and criteria has been provided (145) (Table 29.4). This was primarily designed for the interpretation of mucosal biopsy samples but can be applied to the general examination of the mucosa. Tissues are rated in this classification as Negative, Indefinite, or Positive for dysplasia on the basis of a combination of histological and cytological characteristics. The Negative category includes tissues that are normal or show the expected effects of inactive or active colitis (see section of Histological Features under Pathology). There is rarely any difficulty in evaluating tissues with inactive colitis; these may show irregular branching and shortening of the crypts, but the epithelial cells have a normal or slightly regenerative appearance without prominence of the nuclei (Fig. 29.21).

The greatest caution must be applied in the examination of specimens with active colitis to avoid the overdiagnosis of dysplasia (Fig. 29.22). The features should not be compared with the normal mucosa, but rather the changes of chronic colitis should serve as the baseline. Because of the severe confounding effects of active inflammation, the examination of ulcerated areas or ordinary pseudopolyps should be avoided; rather, samples should be taken from the flat, more atrophic appearing regions or from villous-like lesions. Active colitis is associated with greater regeneration, and some crypts may show prominent elongation and pallisading of the nuclei (Fig. 29.23). Also present are numerous mitoses and occasional "dystrophic" goblet cells with mucin displaced to the basal portion of the cell (Fig. 29.24). However, there is no, or just minimal, hyperchromatism or pleomorphism. Although the nuclear changes may be similar to that seen in low grade dysplasia, the inflammatory nature is usually evident because of the associated neutrophilic infiltration of the crypts and lamina propria.

TABLE 29.4	Classification of Dysplasia in Chronic Colitis	
Negative for Dysplasia	Indefinite for Dysplasia	Positive for Dysplasia
Normal mucosa	Probably negative	Low grade dysplasia
Inactive (quiescent)	(inflammatory)	High grade dysplasia
colitis	Probably positive	
Active colitis	(dysplastic)	

Table modified from Riddell RH, Goldman HG, Ransohoff, et al. Dysplasia in inflammatory bowel disease: standardized classification with provisional clinical applications. Hum Pathol 1983;14:931–968.

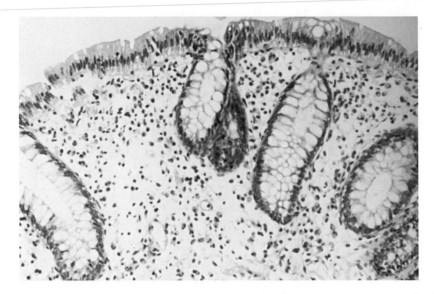

Figure 29.21   Colonic mucosa in ulcerative colitis, rated as negative for dysplasia. There is crypt atrophy but no cytologic atypism. H & E, ×100.

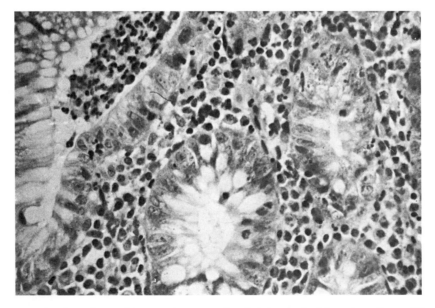

Figure 29.22   Colonic mucosa in ulcerative colitis, rated as negative for dysplasia. There is active colitis with crypt abscesses and increased inflammation in the lamina propria. Some of the epithelial cells contain elongated nuclei without hyperchromasia. H & E, ×250. (Reprinted with permission from Goldman H, Antonioli DA. Mucosal biopsy of the rectum, colon and distal ileum. Hum Pathol 1982;13:981-1012.)

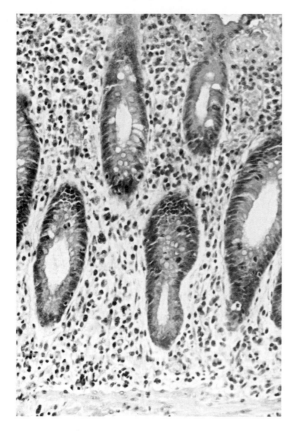

Figure 29.23   Colonic mucosa in ulcerative colitis, rated as negative for dysplasia. There is prominent regeneration of the crypts with reduction in the cytoplasmic mucin. The epithelial cell nuclei are slightly enlarged but uniform (in size and cellular location) and are not hyperchromatic. H & E, ×100.

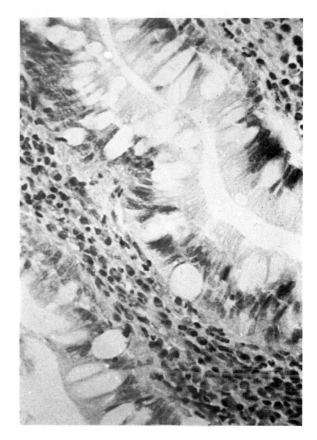

Figure 29.24   Colonic mucosa containing dystrophic goblet mucous cells, rated as negative for dysplasia. The dystrophic goblet cells are characterized by the presence of cytoplasmic mucin in the basal rather than the normal luminal position of the cell. Although dystrophic goblet cells are more often seen in dysplasia, there is no nuclear atypism in this example. H & E, ×250.

The category of Indefinite for dysplasia is employed when the mucosal changes appear to exceed that usually seen in active colitis but the features are insufficient for an unequivocal diagnosis of dysplasia. It is often used when signs of active disease are less conspicuous in the mucosa sampled (Fig. 29.25) or when there is the appearance of unusual forms of inflammation or growth. The latter include the degenerative effects in the surface cells overlying lymphoid nodules in cases of follicular proctitis or colitis

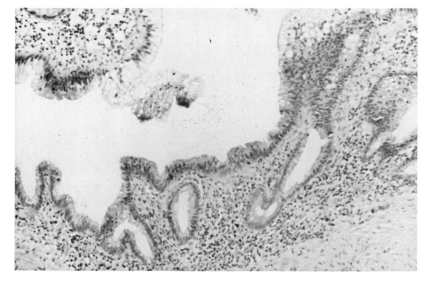

Figure 29.25   Colonic mucosa in ulcerative colitis, rated as indefinite for dysplasia. The surface epithelium (center) shows loss of mucin and enlarged palisading nuclei suspicious of dysplasia. However, the affected region is depressed and it is more likely that this represents active regeneration of a previously ulcerated area. H & E, ×100.

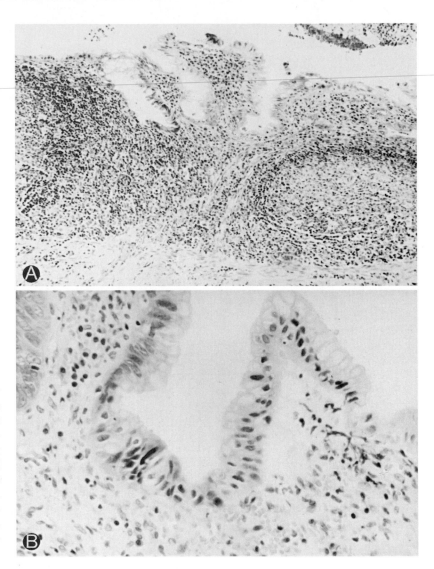

Figure 29.26   (A) Colonic mucosa with follicular inflammation in ulcerative colitis, rated as indefinite for dysplasia. There are numerous lymphoid nodules in the mucosa and the overlying epithelium is attenuated. H & E, ×100. **(B)** Closer view of the colonic mucosa, showing atypical cells in the surface and upper crypt epithelia. Such cells are often seen in cases with follicular inflammation and usually regress. H & E, ×400. (Reprinted with permission from Goldman H, Antonioli DA. Mucosal biopsy of the rectum, colon and distal ileum. Hum Pathol 1982;13:981-1012.)

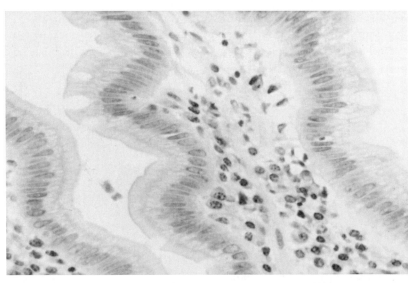

Figure 29.27   Colonic mucosa with incomplete maturation of the crypts, rated as indefinite for dysplasia. The mucin is reduced and limited to the luminal portion of the cells, and the nuclei are generally enlarged. Such changes can occur in regeneration but have also been noted next to overt dysplastic lesions. H & E, ×400.

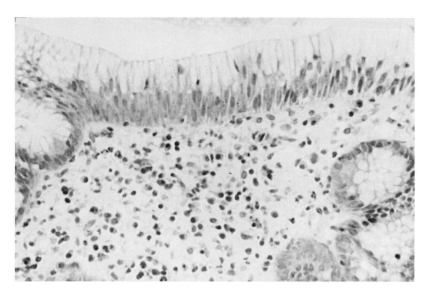

Figure 29.28 Colonic mucosal biopsy in ulcerative colitis, rated as positive for low grade (or mild) dysplasia. There is a prominent elongation and stratification of the nuclei in the surface epithelial cells in the absence of acute inflammation. The nuclei occupy the basal half of the epithelial cells, and there is no hyperchromasia. H & E, ×400. (Reprinted with permission from Goldman H. Dysplasia and carcinoma in inflammatory bowel disease. In: Rachmilewitz D, ed. Inflammatory Bowel Diseases. The Hague: Martinus Nijhoff Publishers, 1982;3:27–40.)

(Fig. 29.26), a hyperplastic-type growth with prominent papillary, infoldings similar to that seen in hyperplastic polyps, and the appearance of incomplete maturation of the crypts with uniformly enlarged nuclei (Fig. 29.27). In all of these instances, the assessment is primarily based on the quality of the nuclei. Uncertainties in diagnosis may also be due to technical factors, including mainly the effects of fixatives, and to reactions to toxic enema solutions. Whenever possible, the rating of Indefinite should be further qualified as probably negative (inflammatory) or probably positive (dysplastic) because of the implications for further management, as described in the section on Clinical Applications.

A two tier system is used for the rating of colonic dysplasia, consisting of low grade and high grade degrees, to match the potential clinical options of further biopsy or colectomy. Low grade

dysplasia reveals no architectural changes in excess of that seen in chronic colitis and a mild to moderate degree of cytologic atypism of the epithelial cells in the absence of any significant active inflammation (Fig. 29.28). There is elongation and stratification of the nuclei which tend to occupy about half of the cell height. The cells are otherwise fairly regular and show only focal and modest hyperchromatism. High grade dysplasia, in contrast, shows some combination of: stratified nuclei that extend beyond the midpoint of the cells (Fig. 29.29); glandular proliferation that is more than expected in chronic colitis; greater number of dystrophic goblet cells; and more prominent hyperchromatism and pleomorphism (Fig. 29.30) There may also be many mitoses, but these are also seen in ordinary regeneration. Carcinoma in situ, characterized by severe epithelial changes and a cribriform glandular arrangement, is

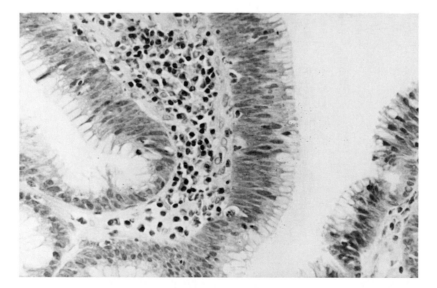

Figure 29.29   Colonic mucosal biopsy of raised mucosal lesion in ulcerative colitis, rated as positive for high grade (or moderate) dysplasia. Compared to Figure 29.28, the glands are more irregular, the nuclear stratification is more prominent, and the nuclei extend into the luminal half of the cells. H & E, ×400. (Reprinted with permission from Goldman H. Dysplasia and carcinoma in inflammatory bowel disease. In: Rachmilewitz D, ed. Inflammatory Bowel Diseases. The Hague: Martinus Nijhoff Publishers, 1982;3:27–40.)

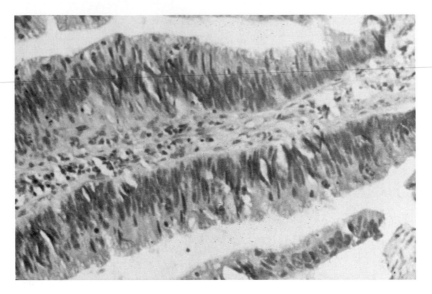

Figure 29.30 Colonic mucosal biopsy of raised mucosal lesion in ulcerative colitis (same case as Figure 29.17), rated as positive for high grade (or severe) dysplasia. There was a villiform surface, and the epithelial cell nuclei show considerable pleomorphism and hyperchromasia. H & E, ×400.

not considered a separate entity but rather is included in the diagnostic term of high grade dysplasia because the clinical implication is the same (Fig. 29.31). In any case of dysplasia, one should also look for infiltrating carcinoma, either limited to the lamina propria and muscularis mucosae (intramucosal carcinoma), or extending into the submucosa or beyond (invasive carcinoma). In this regard, many of the carcinomas are well differentiated and only identified by the feature of invasion.

The dysplasia is usually most prominent in the crypt bases when associated with a gross mass (Fig. 29.32), whereas it tends to be concentrated on the surface of flat atrophic mucosa (Fig. 29.28); in all instances, the degree of dysplasia, whether low or high grade, is rated by the worst area. Inflammatory polyps (pseudopolyps) may show considerable glandular proliferation, but it is rare for dysplasia to develop in such lesions. One problem that is seen in older patients is how to distinguish a polypoid area of dysplasia from an incidental development of an adenoma (Table 29.5). Isolated adenomas tend to be pedunculated and appear in areas of the colon that are otherwise normal, whereas the dysplastic lesions are more typically sessile and located in a region of chronic colitis (162). Furthermore,

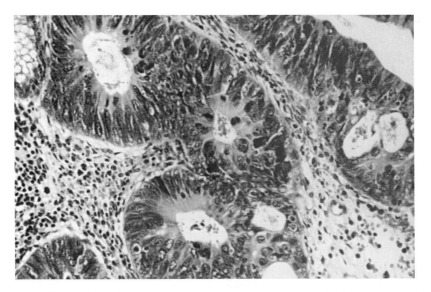

Figure 29.31 Colonic mucosa in ulcerative colitis, rated as positive for high grade dysplasia. There is marked nuclear atypicality and cribriform glands without invasion into the lamina propria. Such features have also been called adenocarcinoma in situ but fit within the category of high grade dysplasia. H & E, ×250. (Reprinted with permission from Goldman H. Dysplasia and carcinoma in inflammatory bowel disease. In: Rachmilewitz D, ed. Inflammatory Bowel Diseases. The Hague: Martinus Nijhoff Publishers, 1982;3:27–40.)

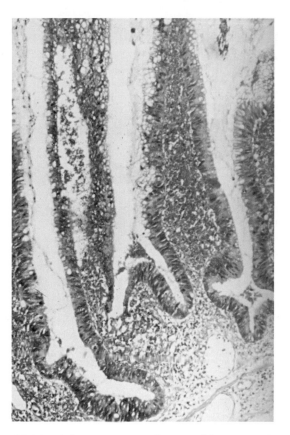

Figure 29.32 Colonic mucosa of a raised lesion in ulcerative colitis (same case as Figure 29.19), showing a villiform surface. The dysplastic cells are concentrated in the basal portion of the crypts, whereas the cells at the surface appear mature. H & E, ×100.

the neoplastic growth is limited to the head of an adenoma and spares the stalk mucosa; in contrast, the dysplasia often extends to involve parts of the stalk, if present, and the adjacent colonic mucosa. If there is major doubt, a conservative polypectomy might be initially favored in an older patient with a stalked polyp.

OTHER STUDIES

Other, unsuccessful, methods that have been tested to diagnose dysplasia have included immunocytochemical stains for carcinoembryonic antigen and secretory component (163). A reduction in sulfomucins and an increase in sialomucins has been noted in many cases of dysplasia (164), but this alteration is also seen in most of the negative cases and may be a nonspecific reaction of the colonic mucosa in inflammatory states. Similarly, the colonic mucosa in cancer cases reveals a reduction in the large intestine-type mucous antigens and the appearance of small intestine-type antigens (165). An increase in abnormal glycoconjugates, identified by lectin-binding studies, was also observed in patients who subsequently developed dysplasia (166).

The application of scanning electron microscopy with quantitative analyses has revealed reductions in the density and size of the surface cells and their microvilli in dysplastic lesions (167, 168). The microvillar changes, particularly a reduction in their density and

thickness, appear to be fairly specific and may help to distinguish dysplasia from inflammatory effects in cases that require repeat biopsy because of uncertainties in the diagnosis. The identification of aneuploidal cells by DNA flow cytometry has been noted in about 50% of the cases of dysplasia, and this method may also prove useful in problem cases (169–173).

Further investigations of colonic dysplasia revealed increased staining and abnormal cytoplasmic localization of sucrase-isomaltase (174). This enzyme is ordinarily localized to the absorptive cells of the normal small intestine; it is present in the normal fetal colon but disappears in the adult colon. There is also enhanced reaction of cell cycle markers such as Ki-67 and topoisomerase in the dysplastic cells with extension of the staining from the lower half of the crypt in the normal colon to the surface of the neoplastic lesions (175, 176). Many other molecular alterations have been detected in colonic dysplasia, including the early appearance of mutations in $p53$, loss of heterozygosity for many other gene products, and microsatellite instability (177–184). See Chapter 5 on special studies and Chapter 8 on Molecular Biology for further details.

CLINICAL APPLICATIONS

Considering the statistical data, it has been recommended that patients with extensive ulcerative colitis lasting more than 10 years should have a prophylactic colectomy, but this has not been accepted by most patients. An effort to detect early carcinoma by periodic radiographic and endoscopic studies has proved difficult because of the flat and stenosing character of most tumors, which are similar to the inflammatory effects of the underlying colitis. Furthermore, many of the carcinomas are well differentiated and not easily appreciated in mucosal biopsy. It is currently recommended that patients with extensive ulcerative colitis lasting more than 8 to 10 years should have periodic colonoscopic examinations to look for dysplasia and to determine which cases should have a colectomy (117, 145, 150, 157). From past cumulative studies of all patients with ulcerative colitis, including those seen for the first time and those with symptoms, it appeared that if high grade dysplasia was identified in an endoscopic biopsy, there was about one chance in three that the patient had an occult carcinoma of the colon and some of these were deeply invasive (159). More recent investigations have revealed that this chance of carcinoma is much less, even if the dysplasia is derived from a gross lesion, in patients who are asymptomatic and seen as part of a surveillance program. Accordingly, the primary aim of the surveillance program is to detect significant dysplasia and to prevent the appearance of carcinoma.

Raised velvety lesions should be sought for biopsy at endoscopy, and overtly inflamed areas and ordinary pseudopolyps should

TABLE 29.5	Isolated Adenoma versus Polypoid Dysplasia of the Colon	
	Adenoma	Dysplasia
Adjacent mucosa	Normal	Chronic colitis
Presence of stalk	Common	Rare
Location of dysplastic epithelium	Polyp head only	Polyp head, stalk, and adjacent mucosa

be avoided (145). In the absence of a gross lesion, which is the usual case, multiple (8 to 12) random biopsies should be obtained from the flat mucosa in all parts of the colon. The biopsies are rated by light microscopy as negative, indefinite or positive for dysplasia, and all positive cases should be confirmed by additional examiners or repeat study. If the biopsies are taken from the flat mucosa, regular surveillance can be continued if they are rated as negative or indefinite–probably negative, earlier repeat biopsy should be done if rated as other indefinite or as low grade dysplasia, and colectomy is considered if the confirmed diagnosis is high grade dysplasia. These actions are slightly modified if the biopsies are taken from a gross lesion, with repeat biopsy for any indefinite lesion and consideration of colectomy for both low and high grade dysplasia. Further accumulation of data from prospective studies is needed to determine whether these recommendations will prove valid in the prevention of carcinoma in patients with ulcerative colitis (185–187).

CROHN'S DISEASE

GENERAL ASPECTS

DEFINITION AND TERMINOLOGY

Crohn's disease is a chronic inflammatory disorder of unknown etiology that may affect any portion of the alimentary tract. The disease is characterized by the frequent presence of transmural inflammation, strictures, fistulas, and granulomas (1–3). It most commonly involves the small intestine, particularly the distal ileum, and the colon. Because of the tendency for there to be a segmental distribution, the disease has also been termed regional enteritis (or ileitis), regional enterocolitis, and segmental or regional colitis. Since predominant involvement of the colon was at one time considered to be uncertain, another old term for the disease in that area was granulomatous colitis (5, 6). The entity was firmly established and separated from other known inflammatory disorders, such as infections, by Crohn in 1932 who described involvement of the terminal ileum (188). Several reports over the ensuing 5 years illustrated disease in other portions of the small intestine, colon, and upper gastrointestinal tract. However, there remained a tendency to ascribe idiopathic inflammatory disease that affected mainly the colon to ulcerative colitis until 1960, when studies by Lockhart-Mummery and others reestablished that Crohn's disease could affect the colon (189). The spelling of the eponym has been a persistent challenge, as aptly documented in a published letter (190).

DIAGNOSTIC CRITERIA

Before the diagnosis of Crohn's disease can be considered, other known causes of inflammation of the gut must be excluded by relevant laboratory tests, and by radiographic and endoscopic procedures. The principal disorders to be distinguished include infections, ischemic disease, and diverticulitis. Furthermore, when the disease is confined to or predominantly affects the colon, the differential includes ulcerative colitis (5–7). The diagnosis of Crohn's disease is best accomplished by using a combination of distributional, gross, and microscopic features, including the presence of skip or segmental disease, sinus tracts and fistulas, and

TABLE 29.6	Diagnostic Features of Crohn's Disease

Absence of known etiology.

Common involvement of distal small intestine and/or colon. Disease tends to have a focal or segmental distribution, and rectum is often spared.

May affect all other parts of the gut, including the oral cavity, esophagus, stomach, proximal small intestine, appendix, and anal region.

Characterized by ulceration and inflammation extending deep into the bowel wall and by early fibrous stricture formation.

Presence of discrete inflammatory sinus tracts, fissures, or fistulae in two-thirds of cases. Must distinguish from multiple "cracks" in wall that may been seen in cases with toxic megacolon.

Presence of well formed, sarcoid-type granulomas in one-half of the cases. Must distinguish from granulomas due to ruptured crypts or foreign bodies.

NOTE: All of the features may not be present in an individual case.

granulomatous inflammation (Table 29.6). Further details are provided in the section on Pathologic Diagnosis.

EPIDEMIOLOGY

Crohn's disease has many epidemiologic features in common with ulcerative colitis (10, 191). Thus, it is more common in the Western developed countries, and it is about two to five times more frequent in the White population and two to three times in Jewish people. The annual incidence in countries where the disease is more often seen is about 1 to 3 per 100,000, and there is a familial history in 3 to 11% of reported series. The disease has a peak incidence in the third decade but may affect all age groups, including children and elderly persons, and there is no definite gender predilection. It was formerly thought that Crohn's disease was much less common than ulcerative colitis, by a factor of 1/5 to 1/7, but this was due to the misplacement of many cases of colonic Crohn's disease into the ulcerative colitis category. Overall, ulcerative colitis is slightly more frequent, whereas studies of surgical specimens reveal more cases of Crohn's disease since they more often require operations.

ETIOLOGY AND PATHOGENESIS

The cause and evolution of Crohn's disease are not known. Considering the character of the inflammatory reaction, with the presence of prominent lymphoid nodules and occasional granulomas, a chronic infection has long been suspected. Transfer studies in animals employing ultrafiltrates of disease tissue have implicated viruses and cell-wall–defective bacteria, but a consistent agent has not been identified (192, 193). Other investigations have noted the appearance of bacteria with an antigenic profile resembling *Mycobacterium paratuberculosis* (194) and granulomas containing antigens of the Measles virus (195). However, these observations have not been confirmed in other studies (196–198). An immunologic mechanism has also been considered because of the frequent presence of allergic and other immune disorders in the patients and by the beneficial response to immunosuppressive therapy (4, 199). There have been extensive investigations of the immune cells, and it has been suggested that Crohn's disease is due to an altered T cell response to various antigens including infectious agents. Other theories have included vascular disease (200), lymphatic obstruction, and emotional stress, but there is no firm data to support their roles in the primary etiology of the disease.

The earliest lesion, well seen by scanning electron microscopy, appears to be a tiny erosion of the surface overlying normal mucosal lymphoid tissue (201). These coalesce to form small aphthous ulcers and eventually more diffuse ulceration of the mucosa. With progression of the disease, there is marked hyperplasia of the lymphoid tissue which extends through the wall, fibrosis and muscular hypertrophy leading to strictures, and discrete inflammatory sinus tracts that pierce the wall. Granulomas are also present in about 50% of the cases. The mechanisms responsible for this advancement of the disease are not known.

CLINICAL FEATURES

The clinical findings are variable and depend on the particular distribution of the disease (202). Most patients have involvement of the ileum and present with fever, crampy abdominal pain from obstruction, and watery diarrhea due mainly to the toxic effects of unabsorbed bile salts on the colonic mucosa. An acute attack, seen in about 20% of the cases, may simulate a case of acute appendicitis. More marked small intestinal disease is characterized by the appearance of abdominal masses and sepsis due to localized perforations; sinus tracts and fistulae which may extend to other viscera and the skin; and malabsorption due to various factors, including reduced bile salt reabsorption from the diseased or bypassed ileum, bacterial proliferation states and, least often, extensive mucosal loss in the jejunum. The nutritional deficit can be a special problem in preadolescents since it may interfere with the normal maturation and cause a stunting of growth (203). When there is prominent colonic disease, the clinical features are similar to that seen in cases of ulcerative colitis and include the acute onset of purulent diarrhea and rectal bleeding. Perianal disease in the form of fistulae and abscesses is seen in about 20 to 25% of all cases and is the presenting feature in about 5% of the patients. Exceptionally, the disease may affect the upper gastrointestinal tract and reveals focal ulceration of the oral cavity, or lesions that mimic reflux esophagitis and chronic peptic ulcer disease.

Medical therapy consists of nutritional support, various anti-inflammatory and immunosuppressive agents including corticosteroids and 6-mercaptopurine, and antibiotics for secondary infections and perforations. The disease is characterized by frequent periods of relapses and remissions, and there is often extension and worsening of the lesions at time of recurrence. Surgery is commonly required for the various complications and intractable disease in the intestines, and an attempt is made to limit this to conservative resections of the bowel (204, 205); there is a strong likelihood of postoperative recurrences which is independent of the amount of normal tissue removed (206, 207). The distribution of the disease permits in most cases a segmental resection and anastomosis of the bowel, with an expected recurrence rate of about 5% per year. The recurrent disease tends to appear in the same site, either the small intestine or the colon, as the original lesion, usually next to the anastomosis (207, 208). When surgery is needed for severe colonic disease with rectal involvement, a total colectomy is required. Despite the tendency for repeated relapses and for the need of multiple resections, it is rare for the patients to become nutritional cripples (8, 209), and the overall mortality from Crohn's disease and its complications is only about twice that of the general population (210).

PATHOLOGY

There have been several detailed studies of the pathology of Crohn's disease affecting the small intestine and the colon (1, 2, 211–213). The pathologic features are generally similar in patients of all age groups, including children and elderly patients (31, 214).

DISTRIBUTION OF DISEASE

Any part of the alimentary tract may be affected in Crohn's disease. At the microscopic and ultrastructural level there is often evidence, in the form of patchy inflammation, axonal degeneration, or granulomas, of widespread lesions in the mucosa and submucosa throughout the gut (201, 215–220). These features may serve as a marker that the patient has Crohn's disease, but do not predict that a clinically significant gross lesion will develop in that particular region. At the onset of the disease, there is gross involvement of the small intestine alone in about 45%, the small bowel and colon in 35%, and the colon alone in 15% of patients. When there is involvement of both the small and large intestines, it is frequently dominant in one or the other area. As the disease progresses, the lesions tend to remain in their original tissues, and only a small proportion of the cases later extend between the small and large bowel. Most of the cases with small intestinal disease affect the terminal portion of the ileum, and this frequently, but not invariably, extends to the ileocecal valve region (Fig. 29.33). In about 5 to 10% of the small intestinal cases there is eventually involvement, either by direct extension or over skip areas, to the proximal ileum and jejunum.

The pattern of colonic disease is highly variable (1–3, 189). More commonly noted are a predominantly right-sided colitis or segmental disease of the colon with a normal rectum (Fig. 29.34). About 50% of the colonic cases reveal proctitis and this may be associated with continuous disease of the left colon, simulating ulcerative colitis. Intrinsic involvement of the appendix is frequent in patients with small intestinal disease and less often noted in those with mainly colonic lesions. Perianal disease is noted in about 25% of the cases with either small intestinal or colonic disease.

Cases of Crohn's disease have a propensity for the development of sinus tracts and fistulae that frequently extend to other parts of the intestinal tract. It is important to distinguish these secondary openings from intrinsic disease in that region, as this information may be needed in the planning of surgical resections. A small proportion of cases reveal gross lesions in the upper part of the gut, including the oral cavity, esophagus, stomach, and proximal duodenum. These lesions are usually seen in conjunction with gross disease of the small or large intestine, but exceptionally they may be the presenting feature of Crohn's disease. There have been several reports that purport to show the presence of primary Crohn's disease in tissues outside of the alimentary tract, including the skin, musculoskeletal system, lung, gall bladder, and genital region (221–230). In the absence of a histological marker for Crohn's

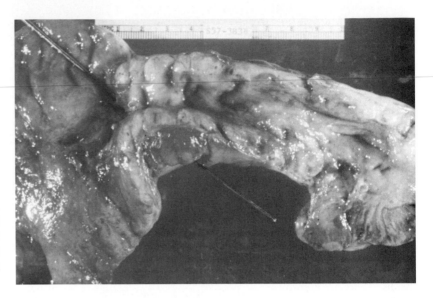

Figure 29.33 Crohn's disease of the terminal ileum, characterized by stenosis, mucosal ulceration, marked mural thickening, and a transmural sinus tract *(identified by probe)*. The lesion appears to stop at the ileocecal valve, and the contiguous cecum *(left)* is not overtly involved.

disease, however, there remains the possibility that these nonintestinal lesions are of a nonspecific or secondary nature.

GROSS FEATURES OF INTESTINAL DISEASE

The earliest grossly evident lesion in Crohn's disease is a small sharply demarcated ulcer of the mucosa (Fig. 29.35), referred to as an aphthous ulcer, and is well visualized at endoscopic examination (231, 232). They may also be seen away from the major site of the disease, and this offers evidence that the lesions of Crohn's disease are often segmental and widespread. The aphthous ulcers are often

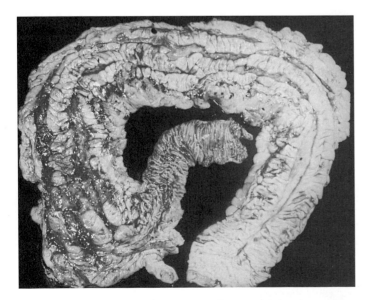

Figure 29.34 Crohn's disease, involving mainly the colon. There are prominent longitudinal ulcers extending from the cecum *(lower left)* to the descending colon, but the more distal part of the colon and rectum were normal. Compared to Figure 29.33, there is no stenosis and the wall is not thickened. The disease also crosses the ileocecal valve and extends into the terminal ileum for a short distance.

multiple, and vary in size from 1 to 2 mm up to 1 cm in greatest diameter. The intervening mucosa is either edematous or normal in appearance. Radiographic studies reveal in some cases a nodule or "hump" of edema and inflammatory tissue around the ulcers (233). These small lesions may eventually coalesce to form more diffuse ulceration of the intestinal mucosa.

The larger ulcers extend over a variable length of intestine, and they may be separated by patches or segments of normal mucosa, resulting in a cobblestone-like appearance in the affected areas. There is a tendency for the ulcers to occupy the deep part of the submucosa, and about 65% of the cases are further associated with the presence of fine inflammatory fissures or sinus tracts that extend well into the muscularis propria (234) (Fig. 29.36). These tracts are best seen by making multiple longitudinal cuts into the specimen and inspecting the bowel wall on profile. They must be distinguished from the multiple short cracks in the tissue that accompany the severe dilation and secondary ischemic necrosis of the bowel wall in any case of severe colitis (34) (see Fig. 29.16). Further extension of the sinus tracts through the bowel wall leads to localized perforation and external abscess formation (Fig. 29.33). The containment of the inflammatory process and the abscesses to a limited region is a characteristic feature of Crohn's disease. Free perforation of the gut with the development of generalized peritonitis can occur but is much less common than in cases of ulcerative colitis (235). The sinus tracts and external inflammatory reaction may further adhere to other tissues and promote the development of fistulous communications. The gross fistulas are observed at some time during the course of the disease in about 35% of the cases, and may connect the previously diseased area with other parts of the bowel and anal canal, the urinary bladder, vagina, and skin of the abdomen and perineal regions. Concomitant with the burrowing ulcers and deep inflammation, there is commonly a marked submucosal fibrosis which leads to early and progressive stricture formation (236). The muscularis propria may undergo considerable hypertrophy, and the adjacent fat tends to wrap itself around the external surface and to obscure most of the serosal surface (Fig. 29.37); this has been referred to as "creeping fat." There are also prominent peritoneal adhesions which often bind together and distort adjacent segments of bowel, particularly of the small intestine.

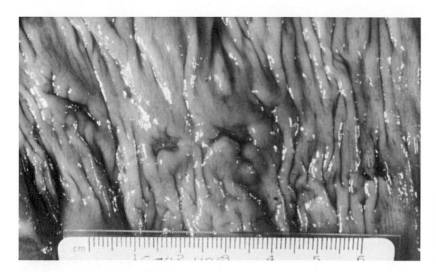

Figure 29.35 Crohn's disease of the colon, showing an early lesion of multiple small aphthous ulcers. The mucosa next to the ulcers is slightly raised due to inflammation, but the rest of the mucosa appears normal.

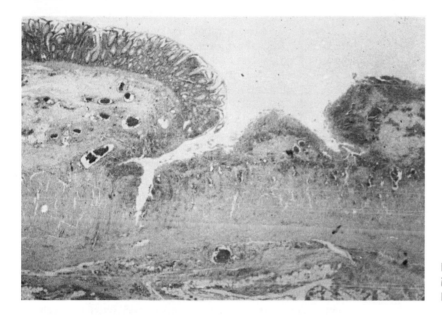

Figure 29.36 Crohn's disease of the colon, revealing a superficial fissure into the muscularis propria. H & E, ×20.

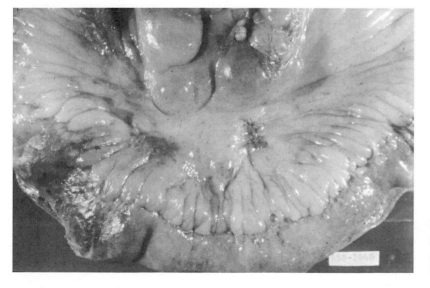

Figure 29.37 Crohn's disease of the small intestine, demonstrating serosal inflammation, creeping fat *(left)*, and enlargement of the mesenteric lymph nodes *(top)*.

The gross features of Crohn's disease vary to some degree in the different regions. Disease of the small intestine, especially the terminal ileum, is much more commonly characterized by marked stenosis, muscular hypertrophy, encircling adipose tissue, and fistula formation (Fig. 29.33). Abscesses may surround nearby structures such as the appendix and uterine adnexa, and the sinus tracts frequently undermine the adjacent cecal mucosa. Colonic disease usually has less prominent thickening of the bowel wall, and frequently noted are longitudinal ulcers that overlie the region of the taeni coli (Fig. 29.34). About 20% of the colonic cases are characterized by more superficial ulceration (237) and the presence of numerous inflammatory pseudopolyps (238), similar to that seen in ulcerative colitis; the diagnosis of Crohn's disease in these cases depends on the demonstration of definite skip areas or coexisting ileal disease (5). The absence of prominent muscular thickening and of serosal inflammation in many cases probably contributed to the underdiagnosis of Crohn's disease of the colon in the past. Longitudinal sinus tracts may result from multiple fissures piercing through the colon wall, and these tracts may extend for a considerable distance. Similar lesions are seen in diverticular disease, and the distinction from Crohn's disease often requires histological examination (see Differential Diagnosis). Indeed, the colon may be affected concurrently by both disorders.

In the examination of a surgically resected specimen, it is important to determine the exact location and extent of the disease and to decide whether the resection margins are affected or not. Only the presence of gross ulceration, usually in the form of the small aphthous lesions, at a margin is a strong indicator that the disease will progress and clinically recur (205, 207, 239). The appearance of various histological abnormalities such as increased inflammatory cells or granulomas in the absence of mucosal necrosis at the margin does not affect the clinical course. Accordingly, at time of operating room consultation, the gross extent of the disease should be relied upon, and frozen sections used only for doubtful cases to confirm the presence of an ulcer at a margin. Indeed, considerable errors are noted when depending on the finding of other features in the frozen sections.

HISTOLOGICAL FEATURES OF INTESTINAL DISEASE

The early lesion of the aphthous ulcer reveals relatively superficial necrosis that is usually limited to the mucosa and upper submucosa, and the inflammatory reaction at the edge of the ulcer is nonspecific (201, 240). There is prominent edema and neutrophilic infiltration in the initial stage, and this is followed by the appearance of granulation tissue and mononuclear inflammatory cells. There are often no granulomas or proliferation of lymphoid nodules in these early lesions. The mucosa between the ulcers is intact and lacks any features of active or of chronic colitis.

The histologic features of the larger and advanced lesions in Crohn's disease are more striking and characteristic (Table 29.7). These include a relatively sharp demarcation between the edge of the ulcer and the adjacent normal mucosa (Fig. 29.38); a marked proliferation of small lymphoid nodules that is often most pronounced in the submucosa but may involve any layer from the mucosa to the serosa (Fig. 29.39); prominent dilatation of the lymphatics which is best seen in the submucosa (Fig. 29.40); considerable expansion of the submucosa by fibrosis which is often associated with marked proliferation of neural elements (Figs. 29.39 and 29.41); variable hypertrophy of the muscularis propria; and foci of inflammation in the muscle and serosa (Fig. 29.38). The larger

TABLE 29.7	Histologic Features of Crohn's Disease

Focal (segmental) ulceration
Proliferation of lymphoid nodules
Dilation of submucosal lymphatics
Submucosal fibrosis
Neuronal hyperplasia
Hypertrophy of muscularis propria
Serosal inflammation
Inflammatory sinus tracts that extend into or through the muscularis propria
Sarcoid-type granulomas

NOTE: The frequency of the features varies with the location of the disease (see Text).

ulcers have a variable depth but frequently extend into the lower submucosa or reach the muscularis propria. The lining of the sinus tracts and fistulae is composed of acute and chronic inflammatory cells with varying degrees of granulation tissue and fibrosis (Fig. 29.42); they may contain scattered foreign body type giant cells, but well formed granulomas are not typically found in these tracts. Vascular alterations are also commonly seen in the chronic cases and consist of intimal fibrous thickening, thrombosis, and old occlusions affecting the medium-sized arteries and veins (241). Occasionally noted is a focal inflammation of the media but this is not associated with prominent necrosis of the vessel wall. The vascular changes are typically located in the outer part of the wall and in the mesentery, and are most often observed in cases with deep ulcerations. These changes are thought to represent a secondary phenomenon, and there is no conclusive evidence to support a vasculitic etiology in Crohn's disease.

Variations in the histological features are noted in the different regions, especially during the reparative phase. Crohn's disease of the small intestine reveals a more constant and greater degree of submucosal fibrosis, neural proliferation, and muscular hypertrophy. The regenerated mucosa is simplified with a reduction or absence of villi, and frequently noted are a hyperplasia of the Paneth cells causing the cells to be higher in the crypts, and a pyloric glandular metaplasia which is typically concentrated at the base of the glands (Fig. 29.43). The intact mucosa often shows numerous slightly raised nodules, and these are usually due to lymphoid tissue or to florid pyloric gland metaplasia (242).

In Crohn's disease of the colon, the submucosal and muscular features are often less pronounced, with a normal muscle thickness noted in over 50% of patients. Indeed, when prominent muscular hypertrophy is seen in a case of Crohn's disease of the colon but is not associated with deep ulcers or fissures, the possible presence of concomitant diverticular disease of the colon must be considered. In about 20% of the colonic cases, the ulcers are relatively shallow and limited to the mucosa or upper submucosa. In contrast to ulcerative colitis, however, there is usually present some inflammation in the muscle and serosa even in areas of superficial ulceration (Fig. 29.38). This observation supports the notion that the presence of marked and often transmural inflammation with strong predominance of lymphoid nodules in Crohn's disease is an independent phenomena and not directly related to the degree of ulceration. The histological

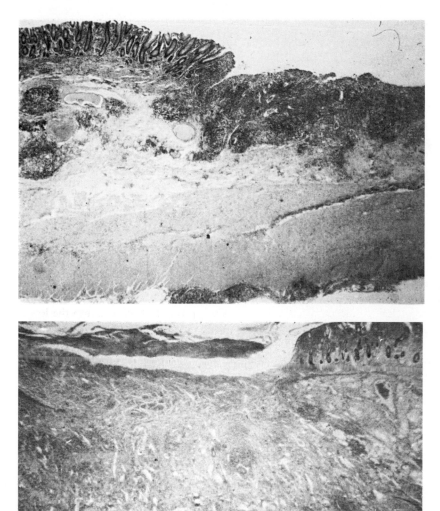

Figure 29.38   Crohn's disease of the colon, revealing a relatively sharp demarcation between the ulcerated area and adjacent intact mucosa *(top left)* and prominent serosal inflammation in the absence of deep ulceration. H & E, ×20.

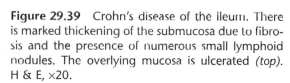

Figure 29.39   Crohn's disease of the ileum. There is marked thickening of the submucosa due to fibrosis and the presence of numerous small lymphoid nodules. The overlying mucosa is ulcerated *(top)*. H & E, ×20.

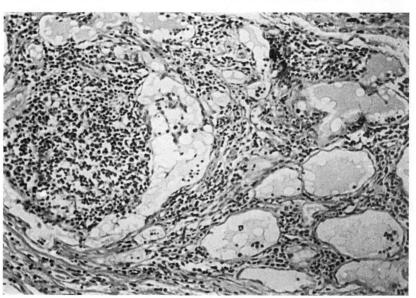

Figure 29.40   Crohn's disease of the small intestine, showing marked lymphatic dilation and lymphoid nodules in the submucosa. H & E, ×100.

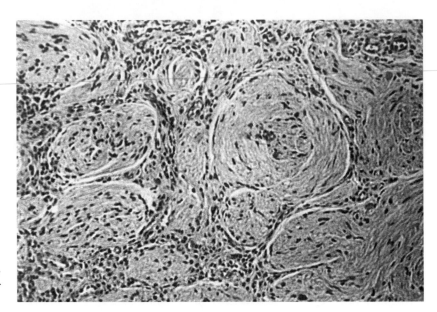

Figure 29.41 Crohn's disease of the small intestine, revealing prominent neural proliferation in the submucosa. H & E, ×100.

characteristics of chronic colitis that are so prominent in the mucosa of cases of ulcerative colitis may also be seen in Crohn's disease, but they tend to exhibit a patchy distribution and to be separated by areas of completely normal mucosa. The mucosal features of chronic colitis include complex branching or atrophy of the crypts, a marked increase of mononuclear inflammatory cells and eosinophils in the lamina propria, a villiform surface, and the presence of Paneth cell metaplasia (see section on Pathology of Ulcerative Colitis for further details). Many of the colonic cases of Crohn's disease also contain inflammatory pseudopolyps which are identical in size, configuration, and other characteristics to those seen in ulcerative colitis (238).

One of the hallmark histological features of Crohn's disease is the presence of granulomas (243–245). However, these are noted in only 50% of the cases, and there are no clinical or morphological differences between the cases with and without granulomas. It has been suggested that granulomas are more commonly noted in younger patients, that they are seen earlier in the course of the disease, and that their presence might have prognostic significance, but none of these proposals has been substantiated (246). The mechanism responsible for the development of granulomas is not known, and there is no explanation for why in many of the cases of Crohn's disease granulomas do not form. The granulomas may be observed in any portion of the bowel wall, from the mucosa to the serosa, and are also noted in the regional lymph nodes in about 5 to 10% of the cases. One study using an injection technique suggested that the granulomas within the bowel wall are preferentially located in close contact to the mural arteries (195), but this has been disputed (247). The granulomas typically appear as discrete nodules of compact macrophages with giant cells, and there is a variable admixture with other inflammatory cells such as lymphocytes and eosinophils (Fig. 29.44). Necrosis is usually not present, and the granulomas most resemble those seen in sarcoidosis (47). Exceptionally, granulomas in the serosa may exhibit extensive necrosis, and it is probable that this is a consequence of adjacent sinus tracts and abscesses, or represents a reaction to foreign material including suture, vegetable matter, talc, and starch. Some of the granulomas are less well formed and consist of just a small aggregate of macrophages; these are usually observed in the mucosa and referred to as microgranulomas (248). Before considering a granuloma as a supportive feature for the diagnosis of Crohn's disease, it is important to exclude lesions due to a reaction to ruptured crypts (see Fig. 29.11) or to foreign material, especially in the perianal region.

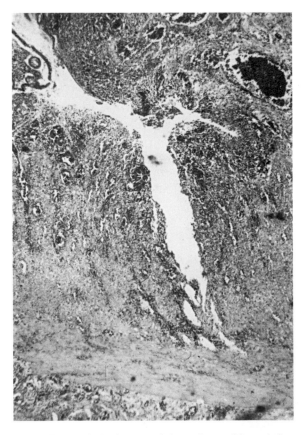

Figure 29.42 Crohn's disease of the colon, with an inflammatory sinus tract extending through the muscularis propria to the serosa. The tract is lined with nonspecific inflammatory cells and granulation tissue. H & E, ×60.

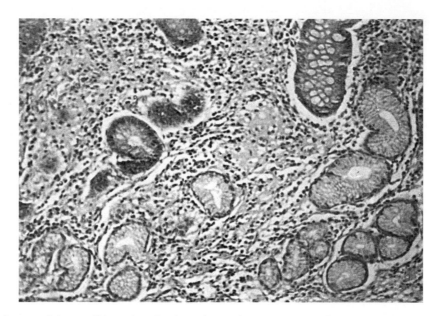

Figure 29.43   Crohn's disease of the small intestine. Section of granular mucosa revealing prominent pyloric gland metaplasia in the basal portion. The cells of the pyloric glands are mature, are distended with mucus of the neutral type, and have flattened basal nuclei. H & E, ×100.

The granulomas may appear in the inflamed and ulcerated areas but are more frequently noted in the otherwise normal mucosa. Overall, the presence of granulomas is not considered a sign of active disease but rather may serve as a marker that the patient has Crohn's disease. Thus, granulomas may be seen in the mucosa of both the upper and lower gastrointestinal tract far removed from the grossly evident disease, and biopsies of such accessible areas can be helpful in making the diagnosis in uncertain cases (215, 216). In this regard, it may be difficult to distinguish by radiographic study some cases of

Crohn's disease of the small intestine from other disorders such as malignant lymphoma, and endoscopic examination and random biopsies of the colon can be employed to look for microscopic evidence of colitis or granulomas (249). In the colon, the incidence of granulomas appears to relate to the presence and extent of grossly evident areas of disease. Thus, granulomas are seen in random biopsies of the rectum in about 5% of cases with gross lesions limited to the small intestine, 10 to 15% of those with right-sided colonic lesions, and 25% of patients with left-sided involvement. It has also

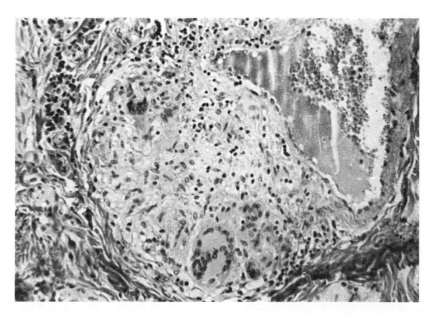

Figure 29.44   Well formed granuloma, located in the intestinal submucosa, in a case of Crohn's disease. The granuloma is composed primarily of enlarged macrophages and giant cells. Other inflammatory cells, especially plasma cells and eosinophils, are often admixed at the edge, but there is no necrosis. H & E, ×100.

been demonstrated that granulomas can be detected with increased frequency by the examination of en-face sections of the intestinal mucosa (250).

PATHOLOGIC DIAGNOSIS OF INTESTINAL DISEASE

Before considering the diagnosis of Crohn's disease, all other known inflammatory disorders of the gut must be excluded. Furthermore, when Crohn's disease affects the colon, it must be distinguished from chronic ulcerative colitis. The diagnosis of Crohn's disease, and its separation from ulcerative colitis, depends on the demonstration of any one or more of the following features (Table 29.7): (1) involvement of the small intestine or the upper part of the alimentary tract; (2) segmental disease of the colon, including a normal rectum or the presence of other skip areas; (3) appearance of fissures–sinus tracts or fistulae that are not a secondary result of severe acute colitis; and (4) presence of well formed, sarcoid-type granulomas. More than one of these features is usually present, but it should be emphasized that the diagnosis of Crohn's disease does not require the finding of all of them in an individual case. Overall, the appearance of focal or segmental disease is the most frequent feature and seen in about 90% of cases, microscopic fissures in about 65%, gross sinus tracts in about 35%, and granulomas in 50% of the cases. Other common findings in Crohn's disease include stricture formation due to submucosal fibrosis, transmural inflammation, and prominent perianal disease, but none of these is specific.

DIFFERENTIAL DIAGNOSIS OF INTESTINAL DISEASE

SMALL INTESTINE

About 20% of the cases of Crohn's disease affecting the terminal ileum have an abrupt onset and may mimic primary inflammation of the appendix or uterine adnexal structures. If an operation is performed for a case of suspected acute appendicitis, it is usually recommended that the appendix be removed to avoid future confusion with Crohn's disease, provided the appendix is not in direct contiguity with the intestinal lesion. The principal disorders that must be distinguished from Crohn's disease of the small intestine are lymphoma, ischemic disease, and chronic granulomatous infections with a predilection for the ileocecal area including those due to tuberculosis, *Yersinia*, *Histoplasma*, and *Anisakiasis*. The similarity with lymphoma is largely at a clinical or radiographic level, and the tumor usually forms a mass that extends into the lumen and is readily identified by its characteristic histology. Exceptionally, ischemic disease may be localized to the terminal ileum and mimic Crohn's disease (251).

Cases of intestinal tuberculosis are rare in the United States but may totally resemble Crohn's disease at a gross level (252). They tend to have stenosing lesions of the terminal ileum and the contiguous cecum, transmural inflammation, and occasional sinus tracts. The granulomas, however, including those in the bowel wall as well as in the mesentery, show prominent caseous necrosis, and the specific diagnosis is provided by special stains and cultures. Because of the large number and coalescence of the granulomas, tuberculosis may be suspected grossly by the presence of numerous tiny nodules on the serosal and free peritoneal surfaces. Histoplasmosis may show disease in the ileocecal area or patchy involvement of the colon, and the diagnosis depends on the finding of caseous

necrosis and specific stains and cultures (253, 254). Anisakiasis is a helminthic infection due to the ingestion of raw fish containing the nematode eggs and is more prevalent in countries where this is a common practice (255). It results in a destructive lesion of the small intestine with prominent sinus tracts; there is an intense eosinophilic reaction, and the worm is identified in the inflamed areas. Yersinial infections, due to *Yersinia pseudotuberculosis* and *Yersinia enterocolitica*, cause an acute and chronic inflammatory lesion of the terminal ileum (256, 257). They may be associated with pronounced lymphoid hyperplasia and contain characteristic microabscesses and granulomas that may have spotty necrosis. Although the organism may be identified in the tissues by immunocytochemical stains, the diagnosis is usually obtained by specific culture. See Chapter 28 on Infectious Disorders of the Intestines for further details.

COLON

The differential diagnosis of Crohn's disease of the colon is dependent on the particular distribution of the cases. Examples of right-sided colitis must be distinguished from certain infections including tuberculosis and amebiasis. Infection due to *E. histolyticum* may reveal more widespread colonic lesions, resembling ulcerative colitis, or be concentrated in the cecal region (67, 68). There are characteristic discrete ulcers which often penetrate deeply into the wall and show undermining of the adjacent heaped-up mucosa. Abundant organisms are present on the surface and in the submucosa of the ulcerated areas, and these can be readily identified with conventional stains or the periodic acid–Schiff (PAS) reaction. When Crohn's disease of the colon presents with segmental disease, the differential includes ischemic colitis, diverticular disease, and neoplasms. Chronic ischemic disease may be associated with patchy ulceration, stricture formation from submucosal fibrosis, and inflammatory pseudopolyps (69, 70). Distinguishing features include a tendency for the ulcers to be relatively shallow, the appearance of much less chronic inflammation without prominent lymphoid nodules, and the absence of discrete inflammatory sinus tracts and fistulae in the cases of ischemic colitis (see Chapter 14 on Vascular Diseases).

Diverticular disease of the colon, particularly when complicated by rupture and peridiverticulitis, may share clinical and radiographic features with Crohn's disease (258, 259). The lesions may be segmental and associated with complex transmural and pericolic tracts and abscesses, and hypertrophy of the muscularis propria is often present (260, 261). The discriminating features of diverticular disease (Table 29.8) include the lesser degree of intrinsic colitis which can be assessed by endoscopic examination (262), the frequent presence of colonic mucosa in the inner lining of the diverticula, the occurrence of muscular hypertrophy that is not associated with inflammatory fissures, and the appearance of loosely formed granulomas or just a collection of giant cells containing foreign material that are limited to the pericolic tissue (see Chapter 32 on Diverticular Diseases of Colon). Since Crohn's disease and colonic diverticulosis are each fairly common disorders, there are cases in which both disorders are present. A neoplasm must be considered in cases of Crohn's disease with a large pseudopolyp, a progressive stricture, and sinus or fistulous tracts that are unassociated with prominent mucosal disease. In cases of Crohn's disease with mainly left-sided or diffuse colitis, the differential includes

TABLE 29.8	Crohn's Disease versus Diverticular Disease of the Colon	
	CDC	DDC
Intrinsic colitis	Present	Absent or mild
Lining of mural sinus tracts	By inflammatory tissue only	In part, by colonic mucosa
Granulomas	Well formed, sarcoid-type in all parts of bowel wall	Loose, foreign body-type only in pericolic tissue

CDC-Crohn's disease of colon

DDC-Diverticular disease of colon

other common colonic infections and ulcerative colitis, and this is discussed in the section on Differential Diagnosis of Ulcerative Colitis.

DISEASE OF OTHER PARTS OF THE ALIMENTARY TRACT

Crohn's disease may also affect all other portions of the gut, including the oral cavity, esophagus, stomach and proximal duodenum, appendix, and anal region. The presence in these other locations is usually seen in conjunction with disease of the small or large intestines, but it may exceptionally be the initial or dominant site. The diagnosis is based on the finding of the characteristic pathologic features and is abetted by the demonstration of the disease in the more common regions.

ORAL CAVITY

Lesions of the mucosa of the oral cavity develop in about 5 to 10% of patients with Crohn's disease (263–265). They are usually in the form of multiple, small, non-healing aphthous ulcers which must be distinguished from those due to the more common viral and other infections. Biopsies reveal granulomatous inflammation, and the ulcers are typically superficial and uncommonly associated with nodular inflammation and sinus tracts. Less often noted is inflammation of the gingiva and lips. Granulomatous lesions have also been observed rarely in the salivary glands, where they may cause rupture of the ducts and localized mucocele formation (266).

ESOPHAGUS

This is the least commonly affected area, and primary Crohn's disease in this site is extremely rare (267–269). The lesions may present with multiple superficial aphthous ulcers, or there may develop a more diffuse disease with stenosis and sinus tracts (see Chapter 20 on Esophagitis for further details).

STOMACH AND PROXIMAL DUODENUM

In cases of Crohn's disease affecting the intestines, random biopsies of the gastric and proximal duodenal mucosa reveal patchy inflammation or granulomas in about 25% to 50% of the patients (215, 216) (Fig. 29.45). This does not signify, however, the presence or subsequent development of clinically significant gross lesions in this area. Ulcerated lesions of the stomach and contiguous duodenum are observed in about 5% of patients with Crohn's disease (Fig. 29.46), and this is almost always seen together with involvement of the distal small intestine (270–272). The lesions usually cause a diffuse erosion of the gastric antral and/or duodenal mucosa and resemble peptic inflammation; biopsy examination may reveal extensive necrosis over a large area and occasional granulomas to support the diagnosis of Crohn's disease. Some cases have a more localized and deeper ulcer, and the distinction from chronic peptic ulcer usually depends on the radiographic demonstration of an odd location, multiple lesions, or sinus tracts (273). Furthermore, the stomach and duodenum may be secondarily involved by fistulae that extend from active disease of the small intestine or colon. In these instances, the mucosa and wall immediately adjacent to the fistulae show inflammation, but there is no evidence of intrinsic disease in the stomach or duodenum (see Chapter 23 on Gastritis and Chapter 31 on Malabsorptive Disorders for further details).

APPENDIX

The appendix is commonly involved in cases of Crohn's disease affecting the intestines, and it may be the initial specimen examined because of the performance of an appendectomy in an unsuspected case of Crohn's disease (274–276). Intrinsic disease is characterized by the presence of patchy or diffuse mucosal ulceration, marked mural thickening with numerous lymphoid nodules in all layers,

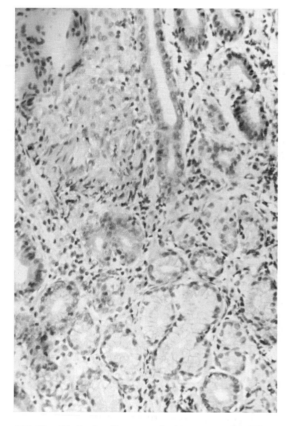

Figure 29.45 Crohn's disease of the stomach. The gastric mucosa reveals slight inflammation and irregularity of the glands and a granuloma *(upper left)*. H & E, ×100.

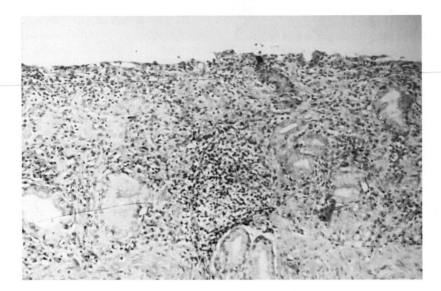

Figure 29.46   Crohn's disease of the duodenum, showing ulceration and inflammation of the mucosa *(top)*. H & E, ×40.

occasional sinus tracts, and scattered granulomas. The major disorders to be distinguished are persistent inflammation following a previous appendiceal rupture, and helminthic infections. In addition, the appendix may be secondarily involved and simply encased by an abscess or adhesions resulting from the rupture of an adjacent area of diseased intestine. The inflammation in such cases, typically of a nonspecific character, is limited to the peri-appendiceal and serosal regions, and the mucosa and wall of the appendix are of normal caliber and show no intrinsic signs of inflammation (see Chapter 35 on Disorders of the Appendix for further details).

ANAL REGION

Lesions in the anal and perianal region are seen in about 20 to 25% of patients with Crohn's disease of the small or large intestines (277–279). It starts in this location in up to 5% of the cases and may precede the development of overt intestinal disease by 2 to 3 years. The lesions are characterized by the appearance of multiple and complex fissures and perianal abscesses. Fistulae frequently extend to the perineal skin and to other adjacent organs. The contiguous rectum may show signs of proctitis or be completely normal. Biopsy samples of the anal area show marked but nonspecific acute and chronic inflammation with granulation tissue and fibrosis and frequent multinucleated giant cells. Granulomas are also often present, particularly in the anal skin, but most of these are loosely formed and appear to be of the foreign body type. Since granulomas of this nature are also frequently seen in patients with perianal disease that is not associated with Crohn's disease, it is unsafe to use this feature for the diagnosis. Rather, it is recommended that additional biopsies be obtained from the rectal mucosa, even if it appears grossly normal, to look for evidence of proctitis or granulomas (see Chapter 36 on Disorders of the Anal Region for further details).

COMPLICATIONS

Clinical problems may result from fluid and electrolyte losses, anemia from repeated hemorrhages which is more prevalent with

disease of the colon, and malabsorption in cases involving the small intestine. Most of the cases of malabsorption are due to decreased bile salts from a reduction in their reabsorption in the distal ileum. This occurs after about 100 cm of terminal ileum is lost due to mucosal disease, bypass from fistulae, or by surgical resections. Disease of the more proximal small intestine and bacterial proliferation states due to stenoses and fistulae also contribute to the malabsorption. Additional complications of Crohn's disease include: intestinal obstruction, most common in the terminal ileum and at sites of anastomosis, due to stenosis from fibrotic strictures and to extensive peritoneal adhesions; secondary sepsis that results from the localized bowel perforations and peri-intestinal abscesses; and fistulous communication with adjacent tissues and organs. The fistulae may connect with and cause secondary inflammation in the abdominal and perineal skin, other segments of the gut, the urinary bladder, and the genital region particularly the vagina. Secondary amyloidosis may also uncommonly develop, as a consequence of the longstanding inflammatory condition. Most of the other complications, including those principally affecting the colon and the extraintestinal manifestations, are similar to those seen in ulcerative colitis. Their details are in the section on Complications under Ulcerative Colitis, and they are briefly summarized here.

TOXIC MEGACOLON

This is less common than in ulcerative colitis, presumably because of the tendency for cases of Crohn's disease to develop considerable fibrosis that walls off the inflammatory lesions. It occurs in cases with extensive colitis and is due to a great production of fluid and blood in the lumen which leads by increased pressure to a dilation of the lumen and thinning of the bowel wall. Further complications include an ischemic-type necrosis of the wall and perforation into the free peritoneal cavity.

SECONDARY INFECTIONS

Aside from the septic complication of the fistulae and abscess, secondary infections may also occur at the level of the mucosal lesions. Some of the relapses may be due to infectious agents such as *C. difficile* and respond best to specific antimicrobial therapy (74–77). In addition, opportunistic infections such as those due to herpes and cytomegalovirus may develop in patients receiving high doses of anti-inflammatory and immunosuppressive medicines, and these may lead to greater necrosis and the threat of systemic spread of the infection (79, 80).

COLITIS AND ENTERITIS CYSTICA

In areas of mucosal regeneration, some of the glandular tissue may extend through breaks in the muscularis mucosae and be misplaced in the submucosa (280–282). The submucosal glands are often dilated and there may be an overlying inflammatory polyp. The lesions are usually small and just an incidental finding. Larger lesions may be confused grossly with carcinoma but readily distinguished by the mature nature of the epithelium. See Chapter 30 for further details.

POSTSURGICAL ILEAL AND COLONIC ABNORMALITIES

Following surgery, the ileum just proximal to an anastomosis or an ileostomy stoma frequently shows some degree of mucosal atrophy, and this is possibly due to stasis or to the exposure of the mucosa to an increased number of bacteria (85–88). The features noted include some shortening of the villous height and associated crypt hyperplasia, an increase in the number of goblet mucous cells in the villi, a hyperplasia of the Paneth cells with extension of the cells to upper part of the crypts, and greater lymphoid nodules and patchy infiltrates of mononuclear inflammatory cells in the lamina propria. There is, however, no evidence of active ileitis in the form of erosion or neutrophilic infiltration in this atrophic mucosa, and the changes have no clinical significance.

Whenever an ulcerated lesion is noted in the ileum following surgery, the immediate concern is whether this represents recurrent Crohn's disease (83, 106, 283). It should be remembered, however, that other ileal abnormalities may occur, as evidenced by their presence in patients who have had a colectomy for ulcerative colitis or for familial polyposis (8, 82). Thus, less specific alterations are seen in about 5% of patients who have an ileostomy and include hemorrhagic necrosis from mucosal prolapse, suture abscesses, and ulcers and occasional sinus tracts in the distal few centimeters and stoma that are due to mechanical effects or localized sepsis. Uncommonly, a longer segment of ileum may reveal focal ulcerations, termed prestomal ileitis, which is thought to be due to a tight stoma (90). In all of these situations, the problem is ordinarily corrected by a revision of the ileostomy. Similar changes are less frequently noted in the ileum just proximal to an anastomosis; these tend to be milder and usually do not require corrective surgery.

More prominent inflammation and erosions can develop in ileal reservoirs, called pouchitis (84, 93–95), in patients with ulcerative colitis who have had a total colectomy and ileoanal anastomosis. The presence of this ileitis can lead to questions concerning the original diagnosis of the colitis, and this subject is discussed in the section on Complications of Ulcerative Colitis. Because of the propensity of Crohn's disease to involve the small intestine, the Koch-type continent ileostomy and ileoanal reservoir procedures are not performed in these patients.

Recurrent Crohn's disease of the ileum proximal to a stoma or an anastomosis has a variable appearance (87). Milder cases may show just focal ulcerations, and it may be impossible to distinguish them from the nonspecific ileal alterations unless there is granulomatous inflammation in the ulcerated areas. The finding of random granulomas in the intact mucosa cannot by itself be considered as conclusive evidence that the patient has recurrent Crohn's disease, since such isolated granulomas may be seen in patients without active disease. Furthermore, granulomas are seen in only 50% of cases of Crohn's disease, and, interestingly, they are found in recurrences only if granulomas were evident in the primarily resected disease. Advanced lesions show more certain features, in the form of sinus tracts away from the stoma or anastomosis and prominent stenosis that may extend over a long segment of the ileum. About 35% of ilea resected for recurrent disease lack characteristic features and the diagnosis is determined by the subsequent clinical course.

The lesions of recurrent Crohn's disease following surgery tend to appear in the same region, whether the small intestine or colon, where there was the primary disease (207). Thus, if the previous intestinal resection contained Crohn's disease in the colon, the recurrent disease is also apt to be in the colon just distal to the anastomosis. Indeed, a patient with recurrent Crohn's disease of the colon is more likely to eventually require a total colectomy than one with primarily small bowel disease. There is usually no diagnostic difficulty in assessing the colonic lesions, because nonspecific mechanical changes such as those described above in the ileum do not apparently affect the colon that is immediately distal to the anastomosis. In patients who have had an ileocolic resection and temporary ileostomy, however, the bypassed segment of distal colon and rectum can develop mild nonspecific inflammatory changes in the mucosa. This condition has been termed diversion-related colitis and is thought to be due to stasis in the excluded segment (284, 285); the lesion completely regresses after continuity of the bowel is restored by an anastomosis (see Chapter 30 for further details).

EXTRAINTESTINAL MANIFESTATIONS

Several inflammatory conditions that are possibly due to the effects of circulating immune complexes are seen in 25 to 30% of patients with Crohn's disease (107, 277). These are similar to those seen in ulcerative colitis and include uveitis, polyarthritis and ankylosing spondylitis, and the skin lesions of erythema nodosum and pyoderma gangrenosum. The lesions tend to regress following surgical extirpation of the intestinal disease but may reappear at time of recurrent disease. Hepatic and biliary abnormalities include fatty change of the liver from nutritional deficiency, chronic pericholangitis, sclerosing cholangitis which further promotes the development of bile duct carcinoma, and an increased incidence of gallstones; granulomas may also be found in the portal tracts in a few percent of the cases. In addition, renal calculi are commonly noted in patients with active small bowel disease, and hydronephrosis may occur due to extrinsic compression of a ureter from an adjacent abscess.

DYSPLASIA AND CARCINOMA

The major description of these conditions is provided in the section on Dysplasia and Carcinoma under Ulcerative Colitis, and only the salient points relating to Crohn's disease are presented here.

INCIDENCE AND RISK FACTORS

An increased incidence of adenocarcinoma of both the small intestine and colon is seen in patients with long-standing Crohn's disease, although it is not as great as that observed in cases of ulcerative colitis (286–289). It has been estimated that patients with chronic disease of the small intestine have a 20-fold increase in carcinoma of that area and that the overall incidence for tumor development in the colon is about 3%. The tumor formation is directly related to the duration of disease, with the major rise noted after 15 to 20 years. The development of carcinoma complicating Crohn's disease may be greater in patients who had their onset of inflammatory disease before age 30 (290). Compared to ulcerative colitis, there is a lower incidence of and longer interval before the appearance of carcinoma of the colon in Crohn's disease. This may be due to there being less colonic tissue at risk, because the lesions tend to be more focal and earlier surgery is done for other indications in Crohn's disease (291).

There is also an increase of squamous cell carcinomas of the anal region and of adenocarcinomas in perianal fistulae in cases of Crohn's disease, related to the greater degree of chronic disease in these areas (292–294). Aside from the occurrence of bile duct carcinomas complicating sclerosing cholangitis and a possible slight increase in intestinal lymphomas, there is no evidence of an enhanced frequency of other tumors affecting the intestines and upper part of the gut (110, 126).

CARCINOMA

Compared to the normal population, the carcinomas occur in younger patients by an average of 10 years, are more often multiple, and tend to be more evenly distributed in the intestines at sites of Crohn's disease (295–301). At an earlier time, bypass of a diseased segment of small intestine was favored over primary resection, and it was later noted that almost 40% of the carcinomas developed in these excluded segments. Most of the cases present at an advanced stage with stenosis and evidence of deep invasion. Tumors may also arise in fistulous tracts (294). Since stricture and fistula formations are common characteristics of Crohn's disease, it is extremely difficult to detect the development of a superimposed carcinoma at an early stage. Occasionally, an early carcinoma is detected, more often in the colon, and these are usually associated with dysplasia; they appear as smaller, more circumscribed and flat lesions (302).

The histological characteristics of the adenocarcinomas are the same as that seen in ulcerative colitis, with over 30% of the cases of the well differentiated and mucinous types. This factor adds to the difficulty of the pre-operative diagnosis of carcinoma, even if the tumors are in the colon and accessible to endoscopic biopsy.

DYSPLASIA

As in cases of ulcerative colitis, epithelial dysplasia can often be identified in the marginal mucosa of carcinomas of both the small intestine and colon in Crohn's disease (297, 298, 302–304). This dysplasia can also be occasionally found in the mucosa away from the carcinoma, but its utility in early diagnosis is limited to the colon where the mucosa can be surveyed by endoscopic examination (305). The histological features of dysplasia are identical to that seen in ulcerative colitis, and the same classification can be employed, with the following categories: Negative for dysplasia, including

normal, inactive and active inflammatory disease; Indefinite for dysplasia which is further rated, if possible, as probably negative or probably positive; and Positive for dysplasia, including low grade and high grade degrees (145). A full description is provided in the section under Ulcerative Colitis.

CLINICAL APPLICATIONS

Since there are fewer cases than in ulcerative colitis, it has been debated whether a surveillance program to detect dysplasia in Crohn's disease is warranted (291). Part of the reason stems from the fact that there are relatively few cases of chronic disease of the colon in which most or all of the colon has not been surgically removed for other indications. Nevertheless, in cases of long-standing Crohn's disease of the intact colon with relatively diffuse lesions (i.e., those resembling ulcerative colitis), the risk for dysplasia and carcinoma remains high and surveillance probably should be performed (289, 300). It has also been suggested that regions with persistent strictures and fistulas should be excised, because these may be preferred sites for tumor formation.

COMPARATIVE FEATURES

Since the precise etiology of ulcerative colitis and Crohn's disease is unknown and they share several clinical and morphological features, it has been long suspected that the two conditions might be variants of the same common disorder. Both are chronic inflammatory conditions that appear to have an immunologic basis, are often precipitated by stressful situations, and they respond to equivalent anti-inflammatory and immunosuppressive drugs. There are a common set of extraintestinal manifestations, and the incidence of dysplasia and carcinoma is increased in both conditions. Major differences in the distributional and structural characteristics and in the overall behavior are noted, however, that justify the current separation of the two diseases. There are also dissimilarities in the immunologic studies, with T cell alterations more typical of Crohn's disease. Until the exact etiology is established, the issue of whether cases of idiopathic inflammatory bowel disease represent one or two diseases, or even more, will remain in doubt. For the present, we tentatively accept the division into the two disorders. There are rare cases in which both patterns appear to be present, with the colon showing features of ulcerative colitis and the ileum those of Crohn's disease (306). Again, lacking any truly specific markers, it is impossible to ascertain whether these patients have both conditions or just Crohn's disease with a variable pattern in different regions of the intestine.

PATHOLOGIC AND DIAGNOSTIC FEATURES

It should be stressed at the outset that before the diagnosis of either ulcerative colitis or Crohn's disease can be made, other known causes of inflammatory conditions must be excluded. This is not always possible at the start of the disease, and the definitive diagnosis may depend on the response to therapy and the subsequent clinical course. The diagnosis of Crohn's disease becomes evident when the disease dominantly affects the small intestine or the upper part of the gut. In contrast, considerable difficulty may be encountered in separating the two diseases in the colon.

TABLE 29.9	Ulcerative Colitis versus Crohn's Disease of the Colon	

Discriminating Features		
	UC	CDC
Rectal involvement	100% (diffuse)	50% (usually focal)
Colonic disease	Always diffuse	Focal in 90%
Level of inflammation	Limited to mucosa and submucosa in 67%	Extends to muscularis propria and serosa in 80%
Mural sinus tracts	Absent	About 67%
Fistulae	Absent	About 33%
Granulomas	Absent	About 50%

UC-Ulcerative colitis

CDC-Crohn's disease of colon

DISCRIMINATING FEATURES IN COLONIC DISEASE

The information obtained from all modalities, including the results of radiographic and endoscopic examinations, are usually needed to distinguish ulcerative colitis and Crohn's disease of the colon, particularly in cases that have not yet had a surgical resection. Mucosal biopsy study may be especially helpful in determining the presence or absence of a grossly suspected skip area and in the detection of granulomas (44, 46, 244, 307–315). The separation is best made by considering the combined distributional, gross, and histological features (Table 29.9). Ulcerative colitis is characterized by constant involvement of the rectum, a variable extent of disease of the colon which is always diffuse (except in the right colon), the absence of ulcerating lesions of the ileum, **AND** the lack of discrete inflammatory sinus tracts or sarcoid-type granulomas. Crohn's disease, in contrast, is distinguished by the identification of an atypical distribution (in the form of a normal rectum, other skip areas of disease in the colon, or ulcerating lesions of the ileum), the presence of discrete inflammatory sinus tracts or fistulae, **OR** the appearance of well-formed granulomas. Difficulty may arise in a case of severe active ulcerative colitis, when multiple cracks or superficial fissures can appear in the bowel wall as a result of the increased intraluminal pressure (Fig. 29.16), and these must be distinguished from the more isolated and longer sinus tracts (Figs. 29.36 and 29.42) of Crohn's disease (34). Some cases of ulcerative colitis during the reparative phase reveal an uneven degree of residual inflammation resulting in the gross appearance of a skip area, but histological examination confirms the presence of diffuse disease. Also, nonspecific granulomas reacting to ruptured crypts or foreign material are occasionally seen in ulcerative colitis (Fig. 29.11) and must be discounted (47).

SHARED FEATURES IN COLONIC DISEASE

There are many other morphological features that may be present in both ulcerative colitis and Crohn's disease of the colon, although they may be more frequent or prominent in one or the other disorder (5, 7, 312, 316). Thus, inflammatory pseudopolyps tend to be more extensive in ulcerative colitis, whereas stenosis is more frequent and appears earlier in Crohn's disease. Crypt abscesses, mononuclear inflammatory cells, eosinophils, and microscopic features of chronic colitis are common in both disorders. Cases of Crohn's disease show a greater frequency and degree of lymphoid nodular hyperplasia, fibrosis, neural and muscular proliferation, and serosal inflammation (Figs. 29.38 to 29.41). The notion that ulcerative colitis takes the form of a mucosal colitis and Crohn's disease a transmural colitis is at best an idealization, and the reverse may be seen in both conditions (8, 237).

INDETERMINATE COLITIS

In about 10 to 15% of cases of idiopathic inflammatory bowel disease, there is either insufficient data or the presence of prominent overlapping features that interfere with the clear distinction between ulcerative colitis and Crohn's disease of the colon, and these cases have been called indeterminate colitis (34, 317). Most of the difficulties arise in patients who have not had an intestinal resection and in whom the exact distribution of the disease has not yet been adequately defined by complete radiographic and endoscopic studies. In some instances, the term appears to be misused because of the failure to consider the combined information provided by the various diagnostic procedures. For example, a rectal mucosal biopsy may reveal a chronic active inflammation without granulomas suggesting ulcerative colitis, whereas the radiographic examination may show segmental disease and/or sinus tracts in the colon; in such instances, it should be recognized that the results of the radiographic study are more specific and that the patient has Crohn's disease despite the limited findings of the rectal biopsy.

In the examination of surgical specimens, the diagnosis of indeterminate colitis is often applied to cases that grossly resemble ulcerative colitis, with diffuse involvement of the rectum and colon, but have one or more of the following added features: (1) cracks or superficial fissures in the bowel wall in regions of severe disease that may be difficult to distinguish from discrete inflammatory sinus tracts; (2) one or a few small isolated ulcers appearing like aphthous lesions, that are proximal to the main site of the colonic disease; and (3) poorly formed granulomas that are usually related to ruptured crypts or reactions to foreign material. It is probable that most of these cases represent ulcerative colitis; in these instances, the diagnosis of Crohn's disease would depend on the finding of characteristic lesions in the proximal colon or ileum. Some cases of idiopathic inflammatory bowel disease have been called indeterminate because of the unwillingness of the observer to completely accept segmental disease in the colon as a proven and solitary criterion of Crohn's disease. Thus, one may encounter descriptions of ulcerative colitis with a normal rectum and segmental ulcerative colitis, or, as a compromise, they may be called indeterminate colitis. Assuming that the spared areas of mucosa are confirmed to be completely normal by histological examination, these cases should more appropriately be diagnosed as Crohn's disease, because ileal recurrences have been documented in such patients.

It is the author's impression that the category of indeterminate colitis has been overused. It may be employed as a tentative or provisional term in cases that do not have complete information about the distribution of the lesions, with the understanding that the more specific diagnosis of either ulcerative colitis or Crohn's disease will eventually be forthcoming (34). Even in these instances, however, it might be sufficient to classify the cases as chronic idiopathic colitis, thus avoiding the addition of a new term, and to simply await further data before making the particular diagnosis. If one considers the combined information provided by the radiographic and endoscopic procedures as well as the results of biopsy and specimen examinations, the great majority of cases can be readily separated into ulcerative colitis or Crohn's disease. Indeterminate colitis is best regarded as a descriptive term, and it should not be used to indicate a separate and distinct disease entity.

CLINICAL COURSE

The major reason for attempting to distinguish ulcerative colitis and Crohn's disease is because of the differences in the clinical behavior of the two conditions (5, 83). Recurrences are essentially limited to the colon and rectum in ulcerative colitis, and the disease can be ultimately controlled, if necessary, by a total colectomy. In contrast, the majority of cases with Crohn's disease have their major effects in the small intestine which cannot be completely eliminated; thus, there is a high incidence of recurrent disease in the residual intestine following surgical resections, resulting in greater functional problems (206, 207).

Some of the cases of Crohn's disease are characterized by dominant or exclusive involvement of the colon, and their clinical course may be initially similar to that of ulcerative colitis. Compared to ulcerative colitis, patients with Crohn's disease of the colon less often develop toxic megacolon but more frequently require earlier surgery for complications such as strictures and fistulas, and they are at risk for the occurrence and progression of disease in the small intestine. Because Crohn's disease frequently spares the rectum and the distal colon, segmental resections of the colon or of the ileum and colon with preservation of intestinal continuity is often possible. In patients who have an ileostomy, revisions for various mechanical, vascular, and septic problems may be required in both conditions; overall, the revision rate is greater in cases of Crohn's disease because of the added complication of recurrent disease.

The types and frequency of extraintestinal manifestations involving the eyes, joints, skin, liver, and biliary tract are similar in the two disorders, whereas renal calculi are mainly seen in Crohn's disease (107). Dysplasia and carcinoma can occur in both conditions but is decidedly more common in cases of extensive ulcerative colitis.

MUCOSAL BIOPSY

The general information pertaining to endoscopic procedures and biopsies is provided in Chapter 3. Presented here are the particular uses and interpretations of mucosal biopsies as they relate to cases of ulcerative colitis and Crohn's disease, with special reference to biopsies of the rectum, colon, and ileum. Consonant with the development of flexible colonoscopes and with the overall increase in endoscopic procedures, the examination of the colon is being performed more often in cases of inflammatory bowel disease and there is now greater reliance on the microscopic findings than in previous years (26–28, 44–46, 231, 307–315).

RECTAL AND COLONIC BIOPSY

There are several reasons for performing endoscopy and obtaining mucosal biopsies of the rectum and colon in inflammatory bowel disease (Table 29.10), and it is important that the particular

TABLE 29.10	Rectocolonic Mucosal Biopsy in Inflammatory Bowel Disease

Uses

Detection or exclusion of other colonic diseases
Identification or confirmation of colitis
Separation of acute and chronic colitis
Distinction between ulcerative and Crohn's colitis
Determination of extent and severity of disease
Detection of dysplasia and carcinoma

indication be conveyed by the clinician and that there be a relevant response by the pathologist to the questions posed (45, 46, 312, 316).

OTHER CAUSES

In some instances, the biopsy is obtained to detect or to exclude other inflammatory conditions that may have a fairly distinctive or specific histology. Thus, the biopsy may reveal the characteristic pseudomembrane in antibiotic-associated colitis, the bland hemorrhagic necrosis in early ischemic disease, and the particular microorganisms or their typical effects in fungal, protozoal, and some viral infections. Endoscopy may also assist in the distinction of diverticular disease of the colon from Crohn's colitis by showing the absence or only minor changes of intrinsic mucosal disease.

IDENTIFICATION OF COLITIS

There are times when the results of the radiographic and gross endoscopic examinations are equivocal and it is uncertain whether the patient has colitis. Some of the endoscopic features observed such as edema and erythema may be a consequence of the preparatory enemas or of the mechanical effects of the procedure itself (312, 318, 319). Biopsy is often obtained, in these situations, to establish, confirm, or exclude the presence of an inflammatory disease. Even if the gross appearance is normal, it is probably good practice to secure a biopsy since there may still be evidence of colitis at a microscopic level. Conversely, biopsy might also be considered in cases with flagrant signs of colitis to obtain an objective confirmation and permanent record, in the form of the histologic slide, of the existence of colitis. In this regard, provided taking biopsies from deeply ulcerated areas which may have an underlying thin wall is avoided, the chance of complications appears to be very low (320).

ACUTE VERSUS CHRONIC COLITIS

Once a definite diagnosis of proctitis or colitis is made in a case with a relatively abrupt onset, the question usually arises as to whether it is an example of an acute self-limited colitis or of the early phase of a chronic colitis. Stool cultures will identify the common pathogens, but there remain cases of acute colitis without a clear etiology. Biopsy study can assist in this distinction and often provides definite evidence that the patient has a chronic disorder (26–28). Major and common signs of chronic colitis that are noted in the mucosa include prominent branching or atrophy of the crypts, Paneth cell metaplasia, a villiform surface, and a marked increase of eosinophils and mononuclear inflammatory cells in the lamina propria with the appearance of lymphoid nodules and increased plasma cells just above the muscularis mucosae (Figs. 29.12 to 29.15). One or more of these features is seen in almost 80% of the cases of chronic colitis, as early as three weeks after the onset of the disease, whereas they are never seen in patients with acute self-limited colitis. Furthermore, if the results of the initial biopsy are not discriminatory, a repeat biopsy should be considered at a time that the patient is well. The mucosa will revert to normal if the case was one of acute self-limited colitis, while the mucosal alterations will usually progress and become evident in the chronic cases.

ULCERATIVE VERSUS CROHN'S COLITIS

Having established that the patient has a chronic colitis and that it is of the idiopathic type, biopsy examination is often of assistance in deciding whether the case is ulcerative colitis or Crohn's disease of the colon (44–46, 308, 311, 312, 316). Certain features that are characteristic of Crohn's disease such as deep fissures and transmural inflammation cannot be detected in the superficial biopsies. The possible appearances that can be observed in the mucosal biopsies include a normal mucosa, a diffuse colitis (Fig. 29.47), a focal colitis meaning that part of the biopsy is completely normal or shows just a slight lengthening of the crypts (Fig. 29.48), and the presence of sarcoid-type granulomas that may occur in the otherwise normal or in the inflamed mucosa (Fig. 29.49). The finding in the biopsies of a normal mucosa to confirm rectal sparing or other skip areas, of a focal colitis or of granulomas offers evidence for the diagnosis of Crohn's disease, since these features are not seen in ulcerative colitis. Only the demonstration of diffuse colitis in the biopsy would be consistent with ulcerative colitis; since this pattern may also be identified amidst an area of Crohn's disease, however, the specific diagnosis in such cases must depend on further data. At the time of initial biopsy in a patient with colitis, the differential diagnosis is usually broader and the finding of a biopsy pattern other than diffuse colitis serves simply to exclude ulcerative colitis. In these cases, showing a focal colitis and/or granulomas in the biopsy, the major differential includes certain infections as well as Crohn's disease.

EXTENT AND SEVERITY OF DISEASE

Whichever the particular type of idiopathic colitis is present, endoscopy and mucosal biopsy offer the most sensitive tools for the determination of the extent and the severity of the lesions, for monitoring the response of the disease to therapy, and for the detection of recurrences (321). Prior to surgery for Crohn's disease of the distal ileum, colonoscopy is often performed to accurately determine the presence and extent of any colonic involvement; this information is needed to decide on the amount of colon that should be resected. The determination is based primarily on the degree of gross disease found, because microscopic lesions alone do not necessarily presage the early development of clinically significant colitis. In particular, isolated granulomas in an otherwise normal mucosa are simply a marker that the patient has Crohn's disease, and they are not an indicator of impending colitis in the region where they are noted. At the preoperative colonoscopy, biopsies are usually obtained of suspected lesions to confirm the appearance of an ulceration. Another important indication for the performance of colonoscopic examination is in patients with long-standing ulcerative colitis in whom radiographic studies have identified only left-sided disease. Since the incidence of carcinoma is probably greater in cases with extensive ulcerative colitis than in those with only distal disease, the procedure is done to determine the true extent of the disease and to decide whether a surveillance program for the detection of dysplasia should be started. In this regard, although the radiographic and even the gross endoscopic appearances of the colonic mucosa may be normal, evidence of chronic colitis can be more sensitively detected by histologic examination. In all of these situations, it should be emphasized that the information sought is not the particular diagnosis, whether ulcerative or

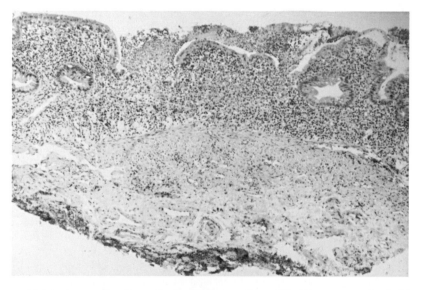

Figure 29.47   Colonic mucosal biopsy, revealing the pattern of diffuse active colitis. The mucosa *(top)* of the entire sample is inflamed. H & E, ×40. (Reprinted with permission from Goldman H, Antonioli DA. Mucosal biopsy of the rectum, colon and distal ileum. Hum Pathol 1982;13:981-1012.)

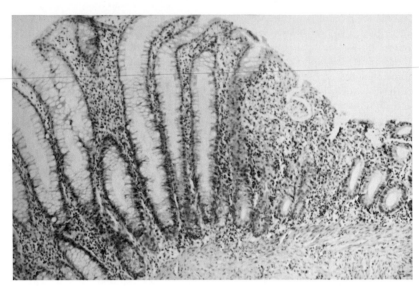

Figure 29.48 Colonic mucosal biopsy, demonstrating the pattern of a focal active colitis. Ulceration is noted on the right, whereas the crypts on the left are intact, noninflamed, and show only slight elongation. H & E, ×100. (Reprinted with permission from Goldman H, Antonioli DA. Mucosal biopsy of the rectum, colon and distal ileum. Hum Pathol 1982;13: 981-1012.)

Crohn's colitis, which is already known, but rather the extent or severity of the disease. Accordingly, the pathologic report should attempt to address these specific issues.

NEOPLASIA

Mucosal biopsies are also obtained from large or other unusual polypoid lesions, from strictures, and from the flat atrophic mucosa as part of a surveillance program to look for dysplasia and carcinoma. This subject is presented in the sections on Dysplasia and Carcinoma under Ulcerative Colitis and under Crohn's disease.

ILEAL BIOPSY

Examination of the intact terminal ileum is limited usually by the inability of the endoscopist to pass the colonoscope through the ileocecal valve (322, 323). Even when biopsies are taken from the valve region, they are more often from the colonic side. There have been a few studies in which a more concerted and successful effort

has been made to obtain samples from the terminal ileum, and useful information has been obtained in about 29% of the cases (324). Features observed include those of typical Crohn's disease or of other causes of ileitis such as infections and ischemic disease; in many instances, the identification of a normal mucosa helps to exclude Crohn's disease from consideration in the patients. In the assessment of the distal ileum, the histological features of the normal mucosa of this region must be appreciated. Compared to the mucosa of the jejunum, there is usually an increased number of goblet mucous cells in the villi and a greater prominence of lymphoid tissue with mature lymphoid follicles (Peyer's patches) in the mucosa and submucosa of the ileum.

Following surgical resections, mucosal biopsy may be obtained from the ileum proximal to a stoma or an anastomosis with the colon or anal region. As a consequence of the surgical procedure itself, the ileal mucosa often reveals some degree of atrophy in the form of variable shortening of the villi and reactive crypt hyperplasia, more goblet mucous cells in the villous region, appearance of Paneth cells higher in the crypts, and increased mononuclear inflammatory cells

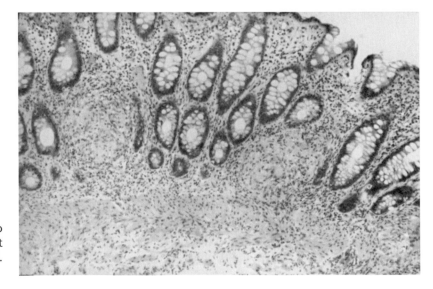

Figure 29.49 Colonic mucosal biopsy, showing two well formed granulomas in the basal portion. The rest of the mucosa including the crypts appear normal. H & E, ×100.

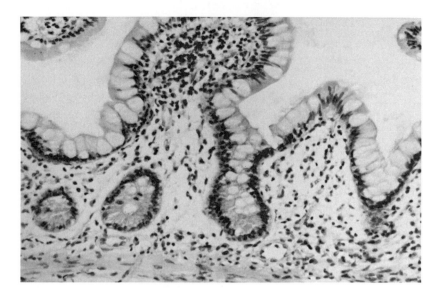

Figure 29.50   Ileal mucosal biopsy. There is a mild atrophy, characterized by a slight shortening of the villi and an increased number of goblet mucous cells over the villous surface. More marked cases show greater villous shortening, crypt hyperplasia and proliferation of Paneth cells. H & E, ×100.

(macrophages, lymphocytes and plasma cells) in the lamina propria (85–88) (Fig. 29.50). These histological features are usually unassociated with any gross changes, and they have no functional or clinical significance. Accordingly, they must be discounted before the diagnosis of ileitis can be considered. The major features sought to define a case of active ileitis (84, 93–95) are: (1) destructive lesions ranging from erosion of the surface epithelium to overt ulceration (Fig. 29.51), (2) the presence of neutrophils in the surface or crypt epithelia (cryptitis and crypt abscesses) and in the lamina propria; and (3) the appearance of granulomas in cases of

Crohn's disease. It is important to remember that in patients with ulcerative colitis who have had a total colectomy, the mucosa proximal to an ileostomy stoma may reveal ileitis that is due to various mechanical, vascular, and septic causes (82, 88, 90). Similar alterations can occur in the ilea proximal to a stoma or an anastomosis in cases of Crohn's disease, and these must be distinguished from recurrent disease in such patients (87, 325). The details of this subject are presented in the sections on Postsurgical Ileal Abnormalities and Pouchitis under Ulcerative Colitis and under Crohn's Disease.

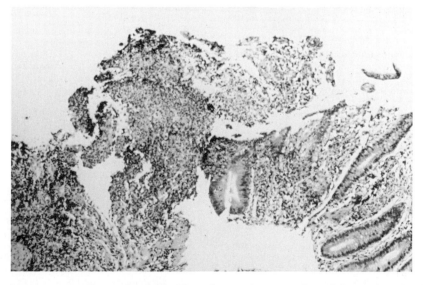

Figure 29.51   Ileal mucosal biopsy, revealing active ileitis. There is prominent erosion of the surface *(top)* and acute inflammation. H & E, ×100.

REFERENCES

1. Mottet NK. Histopathologic spectrum of regional enteritis and ulcerative colitis. Philadelphia: WB Saunders Co, 1971.
2. Price AB, Morson BC. Inflammatory bowel disease: the surgical pathology of Crohn's disease and ulcerative colitis. Hum Pathol 1975;6:7–29.
3. Hamilton SR. Diagnosis and comparison of ulcerative colitis and Crohn's disease involving the colon. In: Norris HT, ed. Pathology of the colon, small intestine, and anus. New York: Churchill Livingstone, 1983:1–19.
4. Sachar DB, Auslander MD, Walfish JS. Aetiological theories of inflammatory bowel disease. Clin Gastroenterol 1980;9:231–257.
5. Glotzer DJ, Gardner RC, Goldman H, et al. Comparative features and course of ulcerative and granulomatous colitis. N Engl J Med 1970;282:582–589.
6. Schachter H, Goldstein MJ, Rappaport H, et al. Ulcerative and "granulomatous" colitis: validity of differential diagnostic criteria. A study of 100 patients treated by total colectomy. Ann Intern Med 1970;72:841–851.
7. Cook MG, Dixon MF. An analysis of the reliability of detection and diagnostic value of various pathological features in Crohn's disease and ulcerative colitis. Gut 1973;14:255–262.
8. Fawaz KA, Glotzer DJ, Goldman H, et al. Ulcerative colitis and Crohn's disease of the colon: a comparison of the long-term postoperative courses. Gastroenterology 1976;71:372–378.
9. Warren S, Sommers SC. Pathogenesis of ulcerative colitis. Am J Pathol 1949;25:657–679.
10. Garland CF, Lilienfeld AM, Medeloff AI, et al. Incidence rates of ulcerative colitis and Crohn's disease in fifteen areas of the United States. Gastroenterology 1981;81:1115–1124.
11. Monsen U, Brostrum O, Nordenvall B, et al. Prevalence of inflammatory bowel disease among relatives of patients with ulcerative colitis. Scand J Gastroenterol 1987;22:214–218.
12. Mayberry JF. Some aspects of the epidemiology of ulcerative colitis. Gut 1985;26:968–974.
13. Brandt L, Boley S, Goldberg L, et al. Colitis in the elderly. A reappraisal. Am J Gastroenterol 1981;76:239–245.
14. Pullen R, Rhodes J, Ganesh S, et al. Transdermal nicotine for active ulcerative colitis. N Engl J Med 1994;330:811–815.
15. Thomas GAO, Rhodes J, Mani V, et al. Transdermal nicotine as maintenance therapy for ulcerative colitis. N Engl J Med 1995;332:988–992.
16. Rutgeerts P, D'Haens G, Hiele M, et al. Appendectomy protects against ulcerative colitis. Gastroenterology 1994;106:1251–1253.
17. Warren BF, Watkins PE. Animal models of inflammatory bowel disease. J Pathol 1994;172:313–316.
18. Elson CO, Sartor RB, Tennyson GS, Riddell RH. Experimental models of inflammatory bowel disease. Gastroenterology 1995;109:1344–1367.
19. Rosekrans PCM, Meijer CJLM, VanDerWal AM, et al. Allergic proctitis, a clinical and immunopathological entity. Gut 1980;21:1017–1023.
20. Murdock DL, Piris J. Immunoglobulin E in nonspecific proctitis and ulcerative colitis. Studies with a monoclonal antibody. Digestion 1983;25:201–204.
21. Edwards FC, Truelove SC. The course and prognosis of ulcerative colitis. Gut 1963;4:299–315.
22. Sparberg M, Fennessey J, Kirsner JB. Ulcerative proctitis and mild ulcerative colitis: a study of 220 patients. Medicine (Baltimore) 1966;45:391–412.
23. Ridman BU, Dolman KM, von Blomberg BME, et al. Neutrophil cytoplasmic antibodies (p-ANCA) in ulcerative colitis. J Clin Pathol 1994;47:253–257.
24. Lee JCW, Lennard-Jones JE, Cambridge G. Antineutrophil antibodies in familial inflammatory bowel disease. Gastroenterology 1995;108:428–433.
25. Esteve M, Mallolas J, Klaassen J, et al. Antineutrophil cytoplasmic antibodies in sera from colectomised ulcerative colitis patients and its relation to the presence of pouchitis. Gut 1996;38:894–898.
26. Surawicz CM, Belic L. Rectal biopsy helps to distinguish acute self-limited colitis from idiopathic inflammatory bowel disease. Gastroenterology 1984;86:104–113.
27. Nostrant TT, Kumar NB, Appelman HD. Histopathology differentiates acute self-limited colitis from ulcerative colitis. Gastroenterology 1987;92:313–328.
28. Surawicz CM, Haggitt RC, Husseman M, McFarland LV. Mucosal biopsy diagnosis of colitis: acute self-limited colitis and idiopathic inflammatory bowel disease. Gastroenterology 1994;107:755–763.
29. Johnson WR, McDermott FT, Hughes ESR, et al. The risk of rectal carcinoma following colectomy in ulcerative colitis. Dis Colon Rectum 1983;26:44–46.
30. Filipe MI, Edwards MR, Ehsanullah M. A prospective study of dysplasia and carcinoma in the rectal biopsies and rectal stump of eight patients following anastomosis in ulcerative colitis. Histopathology 1985;9:1139–1153.
31. Chong SKF, Blackshaw AJ, Boyle S, et al. Histologic diagnosis of chronic inflammatory bowel disease in childhood. Gut 1985;26:55–59.
32. Zimmerman J, Gavish D, Rachmilewitz D. Early and late onset ulcerative colitis: distinct clinical features. J Clin Gastroenterol 1985;7:492–498.
33. Lumb G. Pathology of ulcerative colitis. Gastroenterology 1961;40:290–298.
34. Price AB. Overlap in the spectrum of non specific inflammatory bowel disease—colitis indeterminate. J Clin Pathol 1978;31:567–577.
35. Groisman GM, George J, Harpaz N. Ulcerative appendicitis in universal and nonuniversal ulcerative colitis. Modern Pathol 1994;7:322–325.
36. Kroft SH, Stryker SJ, Rao MS. Appendiceal involvement as a skip lesion in ulcerative colitis. Modern Pathol 1994;7:912–914.
37. Powell-Tuch J, Day DW, Buchell NA, et al. Correlations between defined sigmoidoscopic appearances and other measures of disease activity in ulcerative colitis. Dig Dis Sci 1982;27:533–537.
38. Holdstock G, DuBoulay CE, Smith CL. Survey of the use of colonoscopy in inflammatory bowel disease. Dig Dis Sci 1984;29:731–734.
39. Teague RH, Read AE. Polyposis in ulcerative colitis. Gut 1975;16:792–795.
40. Levine DS, Surawicz CM, Spencer GD, et al. Inflammatory polyposis two years after ischemic colon injury. Dig Dis Sci 1986;31:1159–1167.
41. Hinrichs HR, Goldman H. Localized giant pseudopolyposis of the colon. JAMA 1968;205:248–249.
42. Kelly JK, Langevin JM, Price LM, et al. Giant and symptomatic inflammatory polyps of the colon in idiopathic inflammatory bowel disease. Am J Surg Pathol 1986;10:420–428.
43. Brozna JP, Fisher RL, Barwick KW. Filiform polyposis. An unusual complication of inflammatory bowel disease. J Clin Gastroenterol 1985;7:451–458.
44. Morson BC. Rectal biopsy in inflammatory bowel disease. N Engl J Med 1972;287:1337–1339.
45. Yardley JH, Donowitz M. Colo-rectal biopsy in inflammatory bowel disease. In: Yardley JH, Morson BC, Abell MR, eds. The gastrointestinal tract. Baltimore: Williams & Wilkins, 1977:50–94.
46. Goldman H. Interpretation of large intestinal mucosal biopsies. Hum Pathol 1994;25:1150–1159.
47. Haggitt RC. Granulomatous diseases of the gastrointestinal tract. In: Ioachim HL, ed. Pathology of granulomas. New York: Raven Press, 1983.
48. Sommers SC, Korelitz BI. Mucosal cell counts in ulcerative and granulomatous colitis. Am J Clin Pathol 1975;63:359–365.
49. Sarin SK, Malkotra V, Gupta SS, et al. Significance of eosinophil and mast cell counts in rectal mucosa in ulcerative colitis. A prospective controlled study. Dig Dis Sci 1987;32:363–367.
50. Bischoff SC, Wedemeyer J, Herrmann A, et al. Quantitative assessment of intestinal eosinophils and mast cells in inflammatory bowel disease. Histopathology 1996;28:1–13.
51. Symonds DA. Paneth cell metaplasia in diseases of the colon and rectum. Arch Pathol 1974;97:343–347.
52. Scott BB, Goodall A, Stephenson P, Jenkins D. Rectal mucosal plasma cells in inflammatory bowel disease. Gut 1983;24:519–524.
53. Skinner JM, Whitehead R, Piris J. Argentaffin cells in ulcerative colitis. Gut 1971;12:636–638.

54. Snover DC, Sandstad J, Hutton S. Mucosal pseudolipomatosis of the colon. Am J Clin Pathol 1985;84:575–580.

55. Odze R, Antonioli D, Peppercorn M, Goldman H. Effect of topical 5-aminosalicylic acid (5-ASA) therapy on rectal mucosal biopsy morphology in chronic ulcerative colitis. Am J Surg Pathol 1993;17: 869–875.

56. Dickinson RJ, Gilmour HM, McClelland DBL. Rectal biopsy in patients presenting to an infectious disease unit with diarrhoeal disease. Gut 1979;20:141–148.

57. Jewkes J, Larson HE, Price AB, et al. Etiology of acute diarrhea in adults. Gut 1981;22:388–392.

58. Quinn TC, Goodell SE, Mhrtichian PAC, et al. Chlamydia trachomatis proctitis. N Engl J Med 1981;305:195–200.

59. Islam MM, Azad AK, Bardhan PK, et al. Pathology of shigellosis and its complications. Histopathology 1994;24:65–71.

60. Day DW, Mandal BK, Morson BC. The rectal biopsy appearances in salmonella colitis. Histopathology 1978;2:117–131.

61. McGovern VJ, Slarutin LJ. Pathology of salmonella colitis. Am J Surg Pathol 1979;3:483–490.

62. Price AB, Jewkes J, Sanderson PJ. Acute diarrhea: campylobacter colitis and the role of rectal biopsy. J Clin Pathol 1979;32: 990–997.

63. Van Spreeuwel JP, Duursma GC, Meijer CJLM, et al. Campylobacter colitis: histological, immunohistochemical and ultrastructural findings. Gut 1985;26:945–951.

64. Price AB, Davies DR. Pseudomembranous colitis. J Clin Pathol 1977;30:1–12.

65. Bartlett JG. Antibiotic-associated colitis. Clin Gastroenterol 1979;8: 783–801.

66. Kelly CP, Pothoulakis C, LaMont JT. Clostridium difficile colitis. N Engl J Med 1994;330:257–262.

67. Pittman FE, Hennigar GR. Sigmoidoscopic and colonic mucosal biopsy findings in amebic colitis. Arch Pathol 1974;97:145–158.

68. Gonzalez-Ruiz A, Haque R, Aguirre A, et al. Value of microscopy in the diagnosis of dysentery associated with invasive Entamoeba histolytica. J Clin Pathol 1994;47:236–240.

69. Whitehead R. The pathology of ischemia of the intestines. Pathol Annu 1976;11:1–52.

70. Norris HT. Reexamination of the spectrum of ischemic bowel disease. In: Norris HT, ed. Pathology of the colon, small intestine, and anus. New York: Churchill Livingstone, 1983:109–120.

71. Atherton LD, Leib ES, Kaye MD. Toxic megacolon associated with methotrexate therapy. Gastroenterology 1984;86:1583–1588.

72. Burke AP, Sobin LH, Virmani R. Localized vasculitis of the gastrointestinal tract. Am J Surg Pathol 1995;19:338–349.

73. Hellstrom HR, Fisher ER. Estimation of mucosal mucin as an aid in the differentiation of Crohn's disease of the colon and chronic ulcerative colitis. Am J Clin Pathol 1967;48:259–268.

74. Lambert JR, Karmali MA, Newman A. Campylobacter enterocolitis. Ann Intern Med 1979;91:929–930.

75. Gebhard RL, Greenberg HB, Singh N, et al. Acute viral enteritis and exacerbation of inflammatory bowel disease. Gastroenterology 1982; 83:1207–1209.

76. Lindemann RJ, Weinstein L, Levitan R, Patterson JF. Ulcerative colitis and intestinal Salmonellosis. Am J Med Sci 1967;254: 855–861.

77. Trnka YM, LaMont JT. Association of *Clostridium difficile* toxin with symptomatic relapse of chronic inflammatory bowel disease. Gastroenterology 1981;80:393–396.

78. Kamberoglou D, Savva S, Adraskelos N, et al. Balantidiosis complicating a case of ulcerative colitis. Am J Gastroenterol 1990;85: 765–766.

79. Cooper IIS, Roffensperger EC, Jonal L. Cytomegalovirus inclusions in patients with ulcerative colitis and toxic dilatation requiring colonic resection. Gastroenterology 1977;72:1253–1256.

80. Sidi S, Gragam JH, Razvi SA, Banks PA. Cytomegalovirus infection of the colon associated with ulcerative colitis. Arch Surg 1979;114: 857–859.

81. Magidson JG, Lewin KC. Diffuse colitis cystica profunda. Report of a case. Am J Surg Pathol 1981;5:393–399.

82. Turnbull RB Jr, Weakley FL, Farmer RG. Ileitis after colectomy and ileostomy for nonspecific ulcerative colitis. Dis Colon Rectum 1964; 7:427–435.

83. Steinberg DM, Allan RN, Brooke BN, et al. Sequelae of colectomy and ileostomy: comparison between Crohn's colitis and ulcerative colitis. Gastroenterology 1975;68:33–39.

84. Knober H, Ligumchy M, Ohon E, et al. Pouch ileitis — recurrence of the inflammatory bowel disease in the ileal reservoir. Am J Gastroenterol 1986;81:199–220.

85. Bechi P, Romagnoli P, Cortesini C. Ileal mucosal morphology after total colectomy in man. Histopathology 1981;5:667–678.

86. Go PM, Lens J, Bosmon FT. Mucosal alterations in the reservoir of patients with Kock's continent ileostomy. Scand J Gastroenterol 1987;2:1076–1080.

87. Bull DM, Peppercorn MA, Glotzer DJ, et al. Crohn's disease of the colon (clinical conference). Gastroenterology 1979;76:607–621.

88. Hallak A, Baratz M, Santo M, et al. Ileitis after colectomy for ulcerative colitis or carcinoma. Gut 1994;35:373–376.

89. Berman JJ, Ullah A. Colonic metaplasia of ileostomies. Biological significance for ulcerative colitis patients following total colectomy. Am J Surg Pathol 1989;13:955–960.

90. Knill-Jones RP, Morson BC, Williams R. Prestomal ileitis: clinical and pathological findings in five cases. Q J Med 1970;63:287–297.

91. Cranley B. The Koch reservoir ileostomy: a review of its development, problems, and role in modern surgical practice. Br J Surg 1983;70: 94–99.

92. Svaninger G, Nordgren S, Oresland T, Hulten L. Incidence and characteristics of pouchitis in the Koch continent ileostomy and the pelvic pouch. Scand J Gastroenterol 1993;28:695–701.

93. Madden MV, Farthing MJG, Nicholls RJ. Inflammation in ileal reservoirs: "pouchitis". Gut 1990;31:247–249.

94. Apel R, Cohen Z, Andrews CW Jr, et al. Prospective evaluation of early morphological changes in pelvic ileal pouches. Gastroenterology 1994;107:435–443.

95. Sandborn WJ. Pouchitis following ileal pouch—anal anastomosis: definition, pathogenesis, and treatment. Gastroenterology 1994; 107:1856–1860.

96. Blazeby JM, Durdey P, Warren BF. Polypoid mucosal prolapse in a pelvic ileal reservoir. Gut 1994;35:1668–1669.

97. Carraro PS, Talbot IC, Nicholls RJ. Long-term appraisal of the histological appearances of the ileal reservoir mucosa after restorative proctocolectomy for ulcerative colitis. Gut 1994;35:1721–1727.

98. Salemans JM, Nogengast FM, Lubbers EJ, Kuijper SJ. Postoperative and long-term results of ileal pouch anal anastomosis for ulcerative colitis and familial polyposis coli. Dig Dis Sci 1992;37:1882–1889.

99. Santos MC, Thompson JS. Late complications of the ileal pouch—anal anastomosis. Am J Gastroenterol 1993;88:3–10.

100. Campbell AP, Merrett MN, Kettlewell M, et al. Expression of colonic antigens by goblet and columnar epithelial cells in ileal pouch mucosa: their association with inflammatory change and faecal stasis. J Clin Pathol 1994;47:834–839.

101. Luukkonen P, Jarvinen H, Tanskanen M, Kahri A. Pouchitis—recurrence of the inflammatory bowel disease? Gut 1994;35: 243–246.

102. Veress B, Reinholt FP, Lindquist K, et al. Long-term histomorphological surveillance of the pelvic ileal pouch: dysplasia develops in a subgroup of patients. Gastroenterology 1995;109:1090–1097.

103. Taylor BA, Wolff BG, Dozois RR, et al. Ileal pouch—anal anastomosis for chronic ulcerative colitis and familial polyposis coli complicated by adenocarcinoma. Dis Colon Rectum 1988;31:358–362.

104. Stern H, Wolfisch S, Mullen B. Cancer in an ileoanal reservoir: a new late complication? Gut 1990;31:473–475.

105. Attanoos R, Billings PJ, Hughes LE, Williams GT. Ileostomy polyps, adenomas, and adenocarcinomas. Gut 1995;37:840–844.

106. Subramani K, Harpaz N, Bilotta C, et al. Refractory proctitis: does it reflect underlying Crohn's disease? Gut 1993;34:1539–1542.

107. Greenstein AJ, Janowitz HD, Sachar DB. The extra-intestinal complications of Crohn's disease and ulcerative colitis: a study of 700 patients. Medicine (Baltimore) 1976;55:401–412.

108. Monsen V, Sorstad J, Hellers G, Johansson C. Extracolonic diagnoses in ulcerative colitis: an epidemiological study. Am J Gastroenterol 1990;85:711–716.

109. Cangemi JR, Wisner RH, Beaver SJ, et al. Effect of proctocolectomy for chronic ulcerative colitis on the natural history of primary sclerosing cholangitis. Gastroenterology 1989;96:790–794.

110. Wee A, Ludwig J, Coffey RJ, et al. Hepatobiliary carcinoma associated with primary sclerosing cholangitis and chronic ulcerative colitis. Hum Pathol 1985;16:719–726.

111. Goldgraber MC, Humphreys EM, Kirsner JB, Palmer WL. Carcinoma and ulcerative colitis: a clinical-pathologic study. II. Statistical analysis. Gastroenterology 1958;34:840–846.

112. Devroede GJ, Taylor WF, Sauer WG, et al. Cancer risk and life expectancy of children with ulcerative colitis. N Engl J Med 1971; 285:17–21.

113. Lennard-Jones JE, Morson BC, Ritchie JK, et al. Cancer in colitis: assessment of the individual risk by clinical and histological criteria. Gastroenterology 1977;73:1280–1289.

114. Greenstein AJ, Sachar DB, Smith H, et al. Cancer in universal and left-sided ulcerative colitis: factors determining risk. Gastroenterology 1979;99:290–294.

115. Pinczowski D, Ekbom A, Baron J, et al. Risk factors for colorectal cancer in patients with ulcerative colitis: a case-control study. Gastroenterology 1994;107:117–120.

116. Bansal P, Sonnenberg A. Risk factors of colorectal cancer in inflammatory bowel disease. Am J Gastroenterol 1996;91:44–48.

117. Nugent FW, Haggitt RC, Colcher H, et al. Malignant potential of chronic ulcerative colitis. Preliminary report. Gastroenterology 1979;76:1–5.

118. Biasco G, Grandi G, Paganelli GM, et al. Colorectal cancer in patients with ulcerative colitis. A prospective cohort study in Italy. Cancer 1995;75:2045–2050.

119. Gyde SN, Prior P, Allan RN, et al. Colorectal cancer in ulcerative colitis: a cohort study of primary referrals from three centers. Gut 1988;29:206–217.

120. Brentnall TA, Haggitt RC, Rabinovitch PS. Alimentary tract. Risk and natural history of colonic neoplasia in patients with primary sclerosing cholangitis and ulcerative colitis. Gastroenterology 1996; 110:331–338.

121. Loftus EV, Sandborn WJ, Tremaine WJ, et al. Risk of colorectal neoplasia in patients with primary sclerosing cholangitis. Gastroenterology 1996;110:432–440.

122. Hanauer SB, Wong KK, Frank PH, et al. Acute leukemia following inflammatory bowel disease. Dig Dis Sci 1982;27:545–548.

123. Greenstein AJ, Mullin GE, Strauchen JA, et al. Lymphoma in inflammatory bowel disease. Cancer 1992;69:1119–1123.

124. Robert ME, Kuo FC, Longtine JA, et al. Diffuse colonic mantle cell lymphoma in a patient with presumed ulcerative colitis. Detection of a precursor monoclonal lymphoid population using polymerase chain reaction and immunohistochemistry. Am J Surg Pathol 1996;20: 1024–1031.

125. Owen DA, Hwang WS, Thorlakson RH, Walli E. Malignant carcinoid tumor complicating chronic ulcerative colitis. Am J Clin Pathol 1981;76:333–338.

126. Mir-Madjlessi SH, Farmer RG, Easley KA, Beck GJ. Colorectal and extracolonic malignancy in ulcerative colitis. Cancer 1986;58:1569–1574.

127. Haidor A, Dixon MF. Solitary microcarcinoid ulcerative colitis. Histopathology 1992;21:487–488.

128. McNeely B, Owen DA, Pezim M. Multiple microcarcinoids arising in chronic ulcerative colitis. Am J Clin Pathol 1992;98:112–116.

129. Palazzo JP, Mittal KR. Lymphoepithelioma-like carcinoma of the rectum in a patient with ulcerative colitis. Am J Gastroenterol 1996;91:398–399.

130. Greenstein AJ, Sackar DB, Shafir M, et al. Malignant melanoma in inflammatory bowel disease. Am J Gastroenterol 1992;87:317–320.

131. Odze RD, Medline P, Cohen Z. Adenocarcinoma arising in an appendix involved with chronic ulcerative colitis. Am J Gastroenterol 1994;89:1905–1907.

132. Carter D, Choi H, Otterson M, Telford GL. Primary adenocarcinoma of the ileostomy after colectomy for ulcerative colitis. Dig Dis Sci 1988;33:509–512.

133. Suarez V, Alexander-Williams J, O'Connor HJ, et al. Carcinoma developing in ileostomies after 25 or more years. Gastroenterology 1988;95:205–208.

134. Johnson JA, Talton DS, Poole GV. Adenocarcinoma of a Brooke ileostomy for adenomatous polyposis coli. Am J Gastroenterol 1993;88:1122–1124.

135. Riddell RH. Dysplasia in inflammatory bowel disease. Clin Gastroenterol 1980;9:439–458.

136. Cook MG, Goligher JD. Carcinoma and epithelial dysplasia complicating ulcerative colitis. Gastroenterology 1975;68:1127–1136.

137. Greenstein AJ, Sachar DB, Smith H, et al. Patterns of neoplasia in Crohn's disease and ulcerative colitis. Cancer 1980;46:403–407.

138. Vatn MH, Elgjo K, Bergan A. Distribution of dysplasia in ulcerative colitis. Scand J Gastroenterol 1984;19:893–895.

139. Gyde SN, Prior P, Thompson H, et al. Survival of patients with colorectal cancer complicating ulcerative colitis. Gut 1984;25: 228–231.

140. Butt JH, Konishi F, Morson BC, et al. Macroscopic lesions in dysplasia and carcinoma complicating ulcerative colitis. Dig Dis Sci 1983;28:18–26.

141. Symonds DA, Vickery AL. Mucinous carcinoma of the colon and rectum. Cancer 1976;37:1891–1900.

142. Goldman H. Dysplasia and carcinoma in inflammatory bowel disease. In: Rachmilewitz D, ed. Inflammatory bowel diseases. The Hague: Martinus Nijhoff Publishers, 1982:27–40.

143. Riddell RH. The precarcinomatous lesion of ulcerative colitis. In: Yardley JH, Morson BC, Abell MR, eds. The gastrointestinal tract. Baltimore: Williams & Wilkins Co, 1977:109–123.

144. Lyss AP, Thompson JJ, Glick JH. Adenocarcinoid tumor of the colon arising in pre-existing ulcerative colitis. Cancer 1981;48:833–839.

145. Riddell RH, Goldman HG, Ransohoff DF, et al. Dysplasia in inflammatory bowel disease: standardized classification with provisional clinical applications. Hum Pathol 1983;14:931–968.

146. Dawson IMP, Pryse-Davies J. The development of carcinoma of the large intestine in ulcerative colitis. Br J Surg 1959;47:113.

147. Morson BC, Pang LSC. Rectal biopsy as an aid to cancer control in ulcerative colitis. Gut 1967;8:423–434.

148. Yardley JH, Keren DF. "Precancer" lesions in ulcerative colitis. A retrospective study of rectal biopsy and colectomy specimens. Cancer 1974;34:835–844.

149. Kewenter J, Hulten L, Ahren C. The occurrence of severe epithelial dysplasia and its bearing on the treatment of long-standing ulcerative colitis. Ann Surg 1982;195:209–212.

150. Lennard-Jones JE, Ritchie JK, Morson BC, Williams CB. Cancer surveillance in ulcerative colitis. Experience over 15 years. Lancet 1983;2:149–152.

151. Nugent FW, Haggett RC, Gilpin PA. Cancer surveillance in ulcerative colitis. Gastroenterology 1991;100:1241–1248.

152. Rosenstock E, Farmer RG, Petras R, et al. Surveillance for colonic carcinoma in ulcerative colitis. Gastroenterology 1985;89:1342–1346.

153. Fochios SE, Sommers SC, Korelitz BI: Sigmoidoscopy and biopsy in surveillance for cancer in ulcerative colitis. J Clin Gastroenterol 1986;8:249–254.

154. Brostrom O, Lofberg R, Ost A, Reichard H. Cancer surveillance of patients with long-standing ulcerative colitis: a clinical, endoscopical, and histological study. Gut 1987;27:1408–1413.

155. Manning AP, Bulgin OR, Dixon MF, Axon ATR. Screening by colonoscopy for colonic epithelial dysplasia in inflammatory bowel disease. Gut 1987;28:1489–1494.

156. Bernstein CN, Shanahan F, Weinstein WM. Are we telling patients the truth about surveillance colonoscopy in ulcerative colitis? Lancet 1994;343:71–74.

157. Connell WR, Lennard-Jones JE, Williams CB, et al. Factors affecting the outcome of endoscopic surveillance for cancer in ulcerative colitis. Gastroenterology 1994;107:934–944.

158. Pascal RR. Dysplasia and early carcinoma in inflammatory bowel disease and colorectal adenomas. Hum Pathol 1994;25:1160–1171.

159. Dobbins WO, Stock M, Ginsberg AL. Early detection and prevention of carcinoma of the colon in patients with ulcerative colitis. Cancer 1977;40:2542–2548.

160. Blackstone MO, Riddell RH, Rogers RHG, et al. Dysplasia-associated lesion or mass (DALM) detected by colonoscopy in long-standing ulcerative colitis. An indication for colectomy. Gastroenterology 1981;80:366–374.

161. Reiser JR, Waye JD, Janowitz HD, Harpaz N. Adenocarcinoma in strictures of ulcerative colitis without antecedent dysplasia by colonoscopy. Am J Gastroenterol 1994;89:119–122.

162. Odze R, Krauss M, Antonioli D. Clinicopathologic evaluation of adenomas and polypoid dysplastic lesions in chronic ulcerative colitis [Abstract]. Modern Pathol 1996;9:63A.

163. Isaacson P. Tissue demonstration of carcinoembryonic antigen (CEA) in ulcerative colitis. Gut 1976;17:561–567.

164. Ehsanullah M, Morgan MN, Filipe MI, Gazzard B. Sialomucins in the assessment of dysplasia and cancer risk patients with ulcerative colitis treated with colectomy and ileo-rectal anastomosis. Histopathology 1985;9:223–235.

165. Itzkowitz SH, Young E, Dubois D, et al. Sialosyl-Tn antigen is prevalent and precedes dysplasia in ulcerative colitis: a retrospective case-control study. Gastroenterology 1996;110:694–704.

166. Boland CR, Lance P, Levin B, Riddell RH, Kim YS. Abnormal goblet cell glycoconjugates in rectal biopsies associated with an increased risk of neoplasia in patients with ulcerative colitis: early results of a prospective study. Gut 1984;25:1364–1371.

167. Shields HM, Bates ML, Goldman H, et al. Scanning electron microscopic appearance of chronic ulcerative colitis with and without dysplasia. Gastroenterology 1985;89:62–72.

168. Shields HM, Best CJ, Goldman H. Use of scanning electron microscopy with morphometric analyses in the distinction of dysplasia from inflammatory changes in ulcerative colitis. Surg Pathol 1988;1:183–192.

169. Fozard JBJ, Quirke P, Dixon MF, et al. DNA aneuploidy in ulcerative colitis. Gut 1987;27:1414–1418.

170. Cuvelier CA, Morson BC, Roels HJ. The DNA content in cancer and dysplasia in chronic ulcerative colitis. Histopathology 1987;11:927–929.

171. Melville DM, Jass JR, Shepherd NA, et al. Dysplasia and deoxyribonucleic acid aneuploidy in the assessment of precancerous changes in chronic ulcerative colitis. Observer variation and correlations. Gastroenterology 1988;95:668–675.

172. Lofberg R, Caspersson T, Tribukait B, Ost A. Comparative DNA analyses in long-standing ulcerative colitis with aneuploidy. Gut 1989;30:1731–1736.

173. Rubin CE, Haggitt RC, Burmer GC, et al. DNA aneuploidy in colonic biopsies predicts future development of dysplasia in ulcerative colitis. Gastroenterology 1992;103:1611–1620.

174. Andrews CW, O'Hara CJ, Goldman H, et al. Sucrase-isomaltase expression in chronic ulcerative colitis and dysplasia. Hum Pathol 1992;23:774–779.

175. Noffsinger AE, Miller MA, Cost MV, Fenoglio-Preiser CM. The pattern of cell proliferation in neoplastic and non-neoplastic lesions of ulcerative colitis. Cancer 1996;78:2307–2312.

176. Fogt F, Nikulasson ST, Holden JA, et al. Topoisomerase II alpha expression in normal, inflammatory and neoplastic conditions of the gastric and colonic mucosa. Modern Pathol 1997;in press.

177. Brentnall TA, Crispin DA, Rabinovitch PS, et al. Mutations in the p53 gene: an early marker of neoplastic progression in ulcerative colitis. Gastroenterology 1994;107:369–378.

178. Harpaz N, Peck AL, Yin J, et al. p53 protein expression in ulcerative colitis-associated colorectal dysplasia and carcinoma. Hum Pathol 1994;25:1069–1074.

179. Chaubert P, Benhattar J, Saraga E, Costa J. K-ras mutations and p53 alterations in neoplastic and non-neoplastic lesions associated with long-standing ulcerative colitis. Am J Pathol 1994;144:767–775.

180. Redston MS, Papadopoulos N, Caldas C, et al. Common occurrence of APC and K-ras gene mutations in the spectrum of colitis-associated neoplasias. Gastroenterology 1995;108:383–392.

181. Chang M, Tsuchiya K, Batchelor RG, et al. Deletion mapping of chromosome 8p in colorectal carcinoma and dysplasia arising in ulcerative colitis, prostatic carcinoma, and malignant fibrous histiocytomas. Am J Pathol 1994;144:1–6.

182. Cartwright CA, Coad CA, Egbert BM. Elevated c-src tyrosine kinase activity in premalignant epithelia of ulcerative colitis. J Clin Invest 1994;93:509–515.

183. Fogt F, Vortmeyer AO, Goldman H, et al. Loss of heterozygosity in the development of dysplasia and carcinoma in ulcerative colitis: a genetic characterization [abstract]. Modern Pathol 1997;in press.

184. Kern SE, Redston M, Seymour AB, et al. Molecular genetic profiles of colitis-associated neoplasms. Gastroenterology 1994;107:420–428.

185. Collins RH Jr, Feldman M, Fordtram JS. Colon cancer, dysplasia, and surveillance in patients with ulcerative colitis. A critical review. N Engl J Med 1987;316:1654–1658.

186. Fozard JBJ, Dixon MF: Colonoscopic surveillance in ulcerative colitis—dysplasia through the looking glass. Gut 1989;30:285–292.

187. Choi PM, Nugent FW, Schoetz DJ, et al. Colonoscopic surveillance reduces mortality from colorectal cancer in ulcerative colitis. Gastroenterology 1993;105:418–424.

188. Crohn BB, Ginzburg L, Oppenheimer GD. Regional ileitis: a pathologic and clinical entity. JAMA 1932;99:1323–1329.

189. Lockhart-Mummery HE, Morson BC. Crohn's disease (regional enteritis) of the large intestine and its distinction from ulcerative colitis. Gut 1960;1:87–105.

190. Yardley JH: Crohnology [letter]. Gastroenterology 1984;87:744.

191. Mayberry JF, Rhodes J. Epidemiologic aspects of Crohn's disease: a review of the literature. Gut 1984;25:886–899.

192. Gitnick GL, Arthus MH, Shibata I. Cultivation of viral agents from Crohn's disease. A new sensitive system. Lancet 1976;2:215–221.

193. Parent K, Mitchell P. Cell wall-defective variants of pseudomonas-like (group Va) bacteria in Crohn's disease. Gastroenterology 1978;75:368–372.

194. Fidler HM, Thurrell W, Johnson NMcI, Rook GAW, et al. Specific detection of Mycobacterium paratuberculosis DNA associated with granulomatous tissue in Crohn's disease. Gut 1994;35:506–510.

195. Wakefield AJ, Ekbom A, Dhillon AP, et al. Crohn's disease: pathogenesis and persistent measles virus infection. Gastroenterology 1995;108:911–916.

196. Frank TS, Cook SM. Analysis of paraffin sections of Crohn's disease for Mycobacterium paratuberculosis using polymerase chain reaction. Modern Pathol 1996;9:32–35.

197. Haga Y, Funakoshi O, Kuroe K, et al. Absence of measles viral genomic sequence in intestinal tissues from Crohn's disease by nested polymerase chain reaction. Gut 1996;38:211–215.

198. Liu Y, Van Kruiningen HJ, West AB, et al. Immunocytochemical evidence of Listeria, Escherichia coli, and Streptococcus antigens in Crohn's disease. Gastroenterology 1995;108:1396–1404.

199. Keren DF. Immunopathogenesis of inflammatory bowel disease. In: Norris HT, ed. Pathology of the colon, small intestine, and anus. New York: Churchill Livingstone, 1983:61–76.

200. Wakefield GJ, Sawyerr AM, Dohllon AP, et al. Pathogenesis of Crohn's disease. Multifocal gastrointestinal infarction. Lancet 1989;2:1057–1062.

201. Rickert RR, Carter HW. The "early" ulcerative lesion of Crohn's disease: correlative light and scanning electron microscopic studies. J Clin Gastroenterol 1980;2:11–19.

202. Farmer RJ, Hawk WA, Turnbull RB Jr. Clinical patterns in Crohn's disease: a statistical study of 615 cases. Gastroenterology 1975;68:627–635.

203. Homer DR, Grand RJ, Colodny AH. Growth, course, and prognosis after surgery for Crohn's disease in children and adolescents. Pediatrics 1977;59:717–725.

204. Farmer RG, Hawk WA, Turnbull RB Jr. Indications for surgery in Crohn's disease. Analysis of 500 cases. Gastroenterology 1976;71:245–250.

205. Pennington L, Hamilton SR, Bayless TR, et al. Surgical management of Crohn's disease: influence of disease at margin of resection. Ann Surg 1980;192:311–318.

206. Greenstein AJ, Sachar DB, Pasternack BS, Janowitz HD. Reoperation and recurrence in Crohn's colitis and ileocolitis. Crude and cumulative rates. N Engl J Med 1975;293:685–690.

207. Trnka YM, Glotzer DJ, Kasdon EJ, et al. The long-term outcome of restorative operation in Crohn's disease: influence of location, prognostic factors, and surgical guidelines. Ann Surg 1982;196:345–355.

208. Rutgeerts P, Geboes K, Vantrappen G, et al. Natural history of Crohn's disease at the ileocolonic anastomosis after curative surgery. Gut 1984;25:665–672.

209. Nugent FW, Veidenheimer MC, Meissner WA, Haggitt RC. Prognosis after colonic resection for Crohn's disease of the colon. Gastroenterology 1973;65:398–402.

210. Prior P, Gyde S, Cooke WT, et al. Mortality in Crohn's disease. Gastroenterology 1981;80:307–312.

211. Warren S, Sommers SC. Cicatrizing enteritis (regional ileitis) as a pathologic entity: analysis of 120 cases. Am J Pathol 1948;24:475–501.

212. Rappaport H, Burgoyne FH, Smetana HP. Pathology of regional enteritis. Milit Surg 1951;109:463–502.

213. Geboes K. Morphological aspects of Crohn's disease. Maldegem: Druk Van Hoetenberghe, 1984.

214. Shapiro PA, Peppercorn MA, Antonioli DA, et al. Crohn's disease in the elderly. Am J Gastroenterol 1981;76:132–137.

215. Korelitz BI, Waye JD, Kreuning J, et al. Crohn's disease in endoscopic biopsies of the gastric antrum and duodenum. Am J Gastroenterol 1981;76:103–109.

216. Alcantara M, Rodriguez R, Potenciano JLM, et al. Endoscopic and bioptic findings in the upper gastrointestinal tract in patients with Crohn's disease. Endoscopy 1993;25:282–286.

217. Dunne WT, Cooke WT, Allan RN. Enzymatic and morphometric evidence for Crohn's disease as a diffuse lesion of the gastrointestinal tract. Gut 1977;18:290–294.

218. Dvorak AM, Osage JE, Monahan RA, et al. Crohn's disease: transmission electron microscopic studies. III. Target tissues: proliferation and injury to smooth muscle and the autonomic nervous system. Hum Pathol 1980;11:620–635.

219. Steinhoff MM, Kodner JJ, De Schryver-Kecskemeti K. Axonal degeneration/necrosis: a possible ultrastructural marker for Crohn's disease. Modern Pathol 1988;1:182–187.

220. Nagel E, Bartels M, Pichlmayr R. Scanning electron-microscopic lesions in Crohn's disease: relevance for the interpretation of postoperative recurrence. Gastroenterology 1995;108:376–382.

221. Sutphen JL, Cooper PH, Machel SE, Nelson DL. Metastatic cutaneous Crohn's disease. Gastroenterology 1984;86:941–944.

222. Attanoos RL, Appleton MAC, Hughes LE, et al. Granulomatous hidradenitis suppurativa and cutaneous Crohn's disease. Histopathology 1993;23:111–115.

223. Marotta PJ, Reynolds RPE. Metastatic Crohn's disease. Am J Gastroenterol 1996;91:373–375.

224. Nugent FW, Glaser D, Fernandez-Herlihy L. Crohn's disease associated with granulomatous bone disease. N Engl J Med 1976;294:262–263.

225. Bayless TM, Stevens MB. Granulomatous synovitis and Crohn's disease. N Engl J Med 1976;294:903.

226. Menard DB, Haddad H, Blain JG, et al. Granulomatous myositis and myopathy associated with Crohn's colitis. N Engl J Med 1976;295:818–819.

227. Lemann M, Messing B, D'Agay F, Modigliani R. Crohn's disease with respiratory tract involvement. Gut 1987;28:1669–1672.

228. McClure J, Banerjee SS, Schofield PS. Crohn's disease of the gallbladder. J Clin Pathol 1984;37:516–518.

229. Schulman D, Beck LS, Roberts IM, Schwartz AM. Crohn's disease of the vulva. Am J Gastroenterol 1987;82:1328–1330.

230. Slaney G, Muller S, Clay J, et al. Crohn's disease involving the penis. Gut 1986;27:329–333.

231. Geboes K, Vantrappen G. The value of colonoscopy in the diagnosis of Crohn's disease. Gastrointest Endosc 1975;2:18–23.

232. Watier A, Devroede G, Perey B, et al. Small erythematous mucosal plaques: an endoscopic sign of Crohn's disease. Gut 1980;21:835–839.

233. Joffe N, Antonioli DA, Bettman M, Goldman H. Focal granulomatous (Crohn's) colitis: radiological-pathological correlation. Gastrointest Radiol 1978;3:73–80.

234. Kelly JK, Siu TO. The strictures, sinus, and fissures of Crohn's disease. J Clin Gastroenterol 1986;8:594–598.

235. Greenstein AJ, Mann DA, Sachar DB, Aufses AH Jr. Free perforation in Crohn's disease. I. A survey of 99 cases. Am J Gastroenterol 1985;80:682–689.

236. Kelly JK, Sutherland LR. The chronological sequence in the pathology of Crohn's disease. J Clin Gastroenterol 1988;10:28–33.

237. McQuillon AC, Appelman HD. Superficial Crohn's disease: a study of 10 patients. Surg Pathol 1989;2:231–239.

238. Kahn E, Daum F. Pseudopolyps of the small intestine in Crohn's disease. Hum Pathol 1984;15:84–86.

239. Klein O, Colombel J-F, Lescut D, et al. Remaining small bowel endoscopic lesions at surgery have no influence on early anastomotic recurrences in Crohn's disease. Am J Gastroenterol 1995;90:1949–1952.

240. Dourmashkin RR, Davies H, Wells C, et al. Epithelial patchy necrosis in Crohn's disease. Hum Pathol 1983;14:643–648.

241. Geller SA, Cohen A. Arterial inflammatory-cell infiltrates in Crohn's disease. Arch Pathol Lab Med 1983;107:473–475.

242. Ming SC, Simon M, Tandar BN. Gross gastric metaplasia of ileum after regional enteritis. Gastroenterology 1963;44:63–68.

243. Chambers TJ, Morson BC. The granuloma in Crohn's disease. Gut 1979;20:269–274.

244. Surawicz CM, Meisel JL, Ylvisaker T, et al. Rectal biopsy in the diagnosis of Crohn's disease: value of multiple biopsies and serial sectioning. Gastroenterology 1981;80:66–71.

245. Kuramoto S, Oohara T, Ihara O, et al. Granulomas of the gut in Crohn's disease. A step sectioning study. Dis Colon Rectum 1987;30:6–11.

246. Wolfson DM, Sachar DB, Cohen A, et al: Granulomas do not affect postoperative recurrence rates in Crohn's disease. Gastroenterology 1982;83:405–409.

247. Matson AP, Van Kruiningen HJ, West AB, et al. The relationship of granulomas to blood vessels in intestinal Crohn's disease. Modern Pathol 1995;8:680–685.

248. Rotterdam H, Korelitz BI, Sommers SC. Microgranulomas in grossly normal rectal mucosa in Crohn's disease. Am J Clin Pathol 1977;67:550–554.

249. Hyams JS, Goldman H, Katz AJ. Differentiating small bowel Crohn's disease from lymphoma: role of rectal biopsy. Gastroenterology 1980;79:340–343.

250. Hamilton SR, Bussey HJR, Morson BC. En face histopathologic technique for examining colonic mucosa of resection specimens. Am J Clin Pathol 1982;78:514–517.

251. Brophy CM, Frederick WG, Schlessel R, Barwick KW. Focal segmental ischemia of the terminal ileum mimicking Crohn's disease. J Clin Gastroenterol 1988;10:343–347.

252. Singh V, Kumar P, Kamal J, et al. Clinicocolonoscopic profile of colonic tuberculosis. Am J Gastroenterol 1991;91:565–568.

253. Miller DP, Everett ED. Gastrointestinal histoplasmosis. J Clin Gastroenterol 1979;1:233–236.

254. Cimponeriu D, LoPresti P, Lavelanet M, et al. Gastrointestinal histoplasmosis in HIV infection: two cases of colonic pseudocancer and review of the literature. Am J Gastroenterol 1994;89:129–131.

255. Pinkus GS, Coolidge C, Little MD. Intestinal anisakiasis. First case report from North America. Am J Med 1975;59:114–120.

256. El-Maraghi NRH, Mair NS. The histopathology of enteric infection with *Yersinia pseudotuberculosis*. Am J Clin Pathol 1979;71:631–639.

257. Gleason TH, Patterson SD. The pathology of *Yersinia enterocolitica* ileocolitis. Am J Surg Pathol 1982;6:347–355.

258. Ming SC, Fleischner FG. Diverticulitis of the sigmoid colon: reappraisal of the pathology and pathogenesis. Surgery 1965;58:627–633.

259. Morson BC. Pathology of the diverticular disease of the colon. Clin Gastroenterol 1975;4:37–52.

260. Meyers MA, Alonso DR, Morson BC, et al. Pathogenesis of diverticulitis complicating granulomatous colitis. Gastroenterology 1978;74:24–31.

261. Marshak RH, Lindner AE, Maklansky D. Paracolic fistulous tracts in diverticulitis and granulomatous colitis. JAMA 1980;243:1943–1946.

262. Makapugay LM, Dean PJ. Diverticular disease-associated chronic colitis. Am J Surg Pathol 1996;20:94–102.

263. Bishop RP, Brewster AC, Antonioli DA. Crohn's disease of the mouth. Gastroenterology 1972;62:302–306.

264. Basu MK, Asquith P, Thompson RA, et al. Oral manifestations of Crohn's disease. Gut 1975;16:249–254.

265. Scully C, Cochran KM, Russell RI, et al. Crohn's disease of the mouth: an indicator of intestinal involvement. Gut 1982;23:198–201.

266. Schnitt SJ, Antonioli DA, Jaffe B, Peppercorn MA. Granulomatous inflammation of minor salivary gland ducts. A new oral manifestation of Crohn's disease. Hum Pathol 1987;18:405–407.

267. Li Volsi VA, Jaretzki A. Granulomatous esophagitis: a case of Crohn's disease limited to the esophagus. Gastroenterology 1973;64:313.

268. Geboes K, Janssen J, Rutgeerts P, Van Trappen G. Crohn's disease of the esophagus. J Clin Gastroenterol 1986;8:31–37.

269. Taskin V, von Sohsten R, Singh B, et al. Crohn's disease of the esophagus. Am J Gastroenterol 1995;90:1000–1001.

270. Fielding JF, Toye DKM, Beton DC, et al. Crohn's disease of the stomach and duodenum. Gut 1970;11:1001–1006.

271. Nugent FW, Richmond M, Park SK. Crohn's disease of the duodenum. Gut 1977;18:115–120.

272. Schuffler MD, Chaffee RE. Small intestinal biopsy in a patient with Crohn's disease of the duodenum (The spectrum of abnormal findings in the absence of granulomas). Gastroenterology 1979;76:1009–1014.

273. Marshak RH, Maklansky D, Kurzban JD, Lindner AE. Crohn's disease of the stomach and duodenum. Am J Gastroenterol 1982;77:340–341.

274. Ewen SWB, Anderson J, Galloway JMD, et al. Crohn's disease initially confined to the appendix. Gastroenterology 1971;60:853–857.

275. Ariel I, Vinograd I, Hershlag A, et al. Crohn's disease isolated to the appendix: truths and fallacies. Hum Pathol 1986;17:1116–1121.

276. Huang JC, Appelman HD. Another look at chronic appendicitis resembling Crohn's disease. Mod Pathol 1996;10:975–981.

277. Rankin GB, Watts HD, Melnyk CS, Kelley ML Jr. National Cooperative Crohn's Disease Study: extraintestinal manifestations and perianal Crohn's. Gastroenterology 1979;77:914–920.

278. Alexander-Williams J, Bachman P. Perianal Crohn's. World J Surg 1980;4:203.

279. Lockhart-Mummery HE. Anal lesions in Crohn's disease. Br J Surg 1985;72:S95–S96.

280. Aftalion B, Lipper S. Enteritis cystica profunda associated with Crohn's disease. Arch Pathol Lab Med 1984;108:532–533.

281. Saul SH, Wong LK, Zinsser KR. Enteritis cystica profunda: association with Crohn's disease. Hum Pathol 1986;17:600–603.

282. Alexis J, Lubin J, Wallach M: Enteritis cystica profunda in a patient with Crohn's disease. Arch Pathol Lab Med 1989;113:947–949.

283. Sachar DB, Wolfson DM, Greenstein AJ, et al. Risk factors for postoperative recurrence of Crohn's disease. Gastroenterology 1983;85:917–921.

284. Glotzer DJ, Glick ME, Goldman H. Proctitis and colitis following diversion of the fecal stream. Gastroenterology 1981;80:438–441.

285. Korelitz BI, Cheskin LJ, Sohn N, Sommers SC. Proctitis after fecal diversion in Crohn's disease and its elimination with reanastomosis: implications for surgical management. Report of four cases. Gastroenterology 1984;87:710–713.

286. Weedon DD, Shorter RG, Ilstrup DM, et al. Crohn's disease and cancer. N Engl J Med 1973;289:1099–1103.

287. Lightdale CJ, Sternberg SS, Posner G, et al. Carcinoma complicating Crohn's disease. Am J Med 1975;59:262–268.

288. Lashner BA. Risk factors for small bowel cancer in Crohn's disease. Dig Dis Sci 1992;37:1179–1184.

289. Gillen CD, Walmsley RS, Prior P, et al. Ulcerative colitis and Crohn's disease: a comparison of the colorectal cancer risk in extensive colitis. Gut 1994;35:1590–1592.

290. Gillen CD, Andrews HA, Prior P, Allan RN. Crohn's disease and colorectal cancer. Gut 1994;35:651–655.

291. Glotzer DJ. The risk of cancer in Crohn's disease [editorial]. Gastroenterology 1985;89:438–441.

292. Connell WR, Sheffield JP, Kamm MA, et al. Lower gastrointestinal malignancy in Crohn's disease. Gut 1994;35:347–352.

293. Nikias G, Eisner T, Katz S, et al. Crohn's disease and colorectal carcinoma: rectal cancer complicating long-standing active perianal disease. Am J Gastroenterol 1995;90:216–219.

294. Chaikhouni A, Requeyra FI, Stevens JR. Adenocarcinoma in perineal fistulas of Crohn's disease. Dis Colon Rectum 1981;24:639–643.

295. Thompson EM, Clayden G, Price AB. Cancer in Crohn's disease—an "occult" malignancy. Histopathology 1983;7:365–376.

296. Collier PE, Turowski P, Diamond DL. Small intestinal adenocarcinoma complicating regional enteritis. Cancer 1985;55:516–521.

297. Hamilton SR. Colorectal carcinoma in patients with Crohn's disease. Gastroenterology 1985;89:398–407.

298. Petras RE, Mir-Madjlessi SH, Farmer RG. Crohn's disease and intestinal carcinoma. A report of 11 cases with emphasis on associated epithelial dysplasia. Gastroenterology 1987;93:1307–1314.

299. Senay E, Sachar DB, Keohane M, Greenstein AJ. Small bowel carcinoma in Crohn's disease. Distinguishing features and risk factors. Cancer 1989;63:360–363.

300. Choi PM, Zelig MP. Similarity of colorectal cancer in Crohn's disease and ulcerative colitis: implications for carcinogenesis and prevention. Gut 1994;35:950–954.

301. Bernstein D, Rogers A. Malignancy in Crohn's disease. Am J Gastroenterol 1996;91:434–440.

302. Cuvelier C, Bekaert E, DePother C, et al. Crohn's disease with adenocarcinoma and dysplasia. Macroscopical, histological, and immunohistochemical aspects of two cases. Am J Surg Pathol 1989;13:187–196.

303. Craft CF, Mendelsohn G, Cooper HS, et al. Colonic "precancer" in Crohn's disease. Gastroenterology 1981;80:578–584.

304. Simpson S, Traube J, Riddell RH. The histologic appearance of dysplasia (precarcinomatous change) in Crohn's disease of the small and large intestine. Gastroenterology 1981;81:492–501.

305. Warren R, Barwick KW. Crohn's colitis with carcinoma and dysplasia. Report of a case and review of 100 small and large bowel resections for Crohn's disease to detect incidence of dysplasia. Am J Surg Pathol 1983;7:151–159.

306. White CL, Hamilton SR, Diamond MP, Cameron JL. Crohn's disease and ulcerative colitis in the same patient. Gut 1983;24:857–862.

307. Hill RB, Kent TH, Hansen RN. Clinical usefulness of rectal biopsy in Crohn's disease. Gastroenterology 1979;77:938–944.

308. Iliffe GD, Owen DA. Rectal biopsy in Crohn's disease. Dig Dis Sci 1981;26:321–324.

309. Surawicz CM. Serial sectioning of a portion of a rectal biopsy detects more focal abnormalities. A prospective study of patients with inflammatory bowel disease. Dig Dis Sci 1982;27:434–436.

310. Goldman H, Antonioli DA. Mucosal biopsy of the rectum, colon, and distal ileum. Hum Pathol 1982;13:981–1012.

311. Malatjalian DA. Pathology of inflammatory bowel disease in colorectal mucosal biopsies. Dig Dis Sci 1987;32:5S–15S.

312. Goldman H. Colonic mucosal biopsy in inflammatory bowel disease. Surg Pathol 1991;4:3–24.

313. Rotterdam H, Sheahan DG, Sommers SC, eds. Biopsy diagnosis of the digestive tract, 2nd ed. New York: Raven Press, 1993.

314. Goldman H. Gastrointestinal mucosal biopsy. New York: Churchill Livingstone, 1996.

315. Whitehead R. Mucosal biopsy of the gastrointestinal tract, 5th ed. Philadelphia: WB Saunders, 1996.

316. Haggitt RC. Differential diagnosis of colitis. In: Goldman H, Appelman HD, Kaufman N, eds. Gastrointestinal pathology. Baltimore: Williams & Wilkins, 1990;325–355.

317. Lee KS, Medline A, Shockey S. Indeterminate colitis in the spectrum of inflammatory bowel disease. Arch Pathol Lab Med 1979;103:173–176.

318. Meisel JL, Bergman D, Graney D, et al. Human rectal mucosa: proctoscopic and morphological changes caused by laxatives. Gastroenterology 1977;72:1274–1279.

319. Levine DS, Haggitt RC. Normal histology of the colon. Am J Surg Pathol 1989;13:966–984.

320. Shahmis M, Schuman BM. Complications of fiberoptic endoscopy. Gastrointest Endosc 1960;26:86–91.

321. Korelitz BI, Sommers SC. Responses to drug therapy in ulcerative colitis. Am J Dig Dis 1976;21:441–447.

322. Goldin E, Rachmilewitz D. Ileoscopic diagnosis of terminal ileitis. Gastrointest Endosc 1984;30:11–14.

323. Coremans G, Rutgeerts P, Geboes K, et al. The value of ileoscopy with biopsy in the diagnosis of intestinal Crohn's disease. Gastrointest Endosc 1984;30:167–172.

324. Borsch G, Schmidt G. Endoscopy of the terminal ileum. Diagnostic yield in 400 consecutive specimens. Dis Colon Rectum 1985;28:499–501.

325. Goldblatt MS, Corman ML, Haggitt RC, et al. Ileostomy complications requiring revision: Lahey Clinic experience, 1964–1973. Dis Colon Rectum 1977;20:209–214.

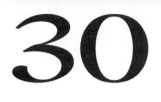

There are numerous conditions that are characterized by the presence of inflammatory lesions in the small and large intestines (1) (Table 30.1). The most common disorders are those due to infections and the idiopathic diseases of ulcerative colitis and Crohn's disease. Inflammatory lesions may occur and become the dominant finding during the course of many other diseases, including allergic and other immune disorders, radiation and chemical injuries, motor and mechanical disturbances, ischemic disease, and various metabolic conditions. Since all of these lesions affect the mucosa, considerable information has been acquired by the study of mucosal biopsies of the various segments of the intestinal tract (2–11).

The present chapter presents those inflammatory diseases and tumor-like lesions of the small and large intestines that are not completely covered in other parts of the book. Lesions primarily involving the jejunum are detailed in Chapter 31 on Malabsorptive Disorders, and other inflammatory conditions that can affect multiple organs of the alimentary tract are included in Chapter 19 on Systemic and Miscellaneous Disorders. Necrotizing enterocolitis

is described in Chapter 14 on Vascular Diseases, and obstructive colitis in Chapter 13 on Motor and Mechanical Disorders.

DUODENITIS

PEPTIC DUODENITIS

DEFINITION

Peptic duodenitis is an acute and chronic inflammatory disorder of the duodenal mucosa that is largely due to the toxic effect of excess gastric acid, and possibly abetted by activated gastric proteolytic enzymes and bacteria (12, 13). It is a highly prevalent condition which, in the acute form, probably affects all persons at some time, and it is estimated that 5 to 10% of the population in Western developed countries have prolonged or chronic disease. The condition is thought to be a part of the spectrum of peptic ulcer disease in which the patients have the characteristic symptoms and mucosal

TABLE	
30.1	**Inflammatory Diseases of the Intestines**

Idiopathic Inflammatory Bowel Disease
   Ulcerative Colitis
   Crohn's Disease
Infections
Ischemic Bowel Disease and Vasculitis
Motor and Mechanical Diseases
Radiation and Chemical Injuries
Allergic and Other Immune Disorders
Miscellaneous Conditions
   Peptic Duodenitis and Ulcer
   Bypass Enteritis and Diversion Colitis
   Collagenous Colitis and Lymphocytic Colitis
   Enteritis and Colitis Cystica Profunda
   Stercoral and Nonspecific Ulcers

inflammation, but lack overt ulceration (14–16). Furthermore, there are many cases in which the inflammation is minimal and difficult to identify, yet the patients respond to specific antacid therapy.

ETIOLOGY AND PATHOGENESIS

The cause of peptic duodenitis is believed to be the same as that of peptic ulcer disease of the duodenum. Most patients have increased gastric acid secretion either at the basal level or, more commonly, after stimulation by a test meal, histamine, or pentagastrin. The acid acts on the mucosa of the proximal duodenum, which is not protected by the neutralizing effect of the biliary secretions, and causes damage of the surface epithelium (17). Whether the injury is directly due to the erosive action of the acid and enzymes or is mediated by vasoconstrictive effects on the small vessels in the lamina propria is not established. In either event, the inflammation that follows is of a secondary or reactive nature. Some cases of peptic duodenitis progress to the development of discrete ulcers, or the duodenitis may appear and persist after the healing of an ulcer. This supports the notion that peptic duodenitis is a variant and milder form of peptic ulcer disease.

It has been recently noted that about 67 to 75% of patients with peptic ulcer disease of the duodenum contain *Helicobacter pylori* in the gastric antral mucosa, and supplemental treatment with antibiotics may speed recovery and help to prevent recurrences of the ulcer (18, 19). Possible mechanisms by which the bacteria facilitate the development or persistence of the duodenitis include added stimulation of gastric acid secretion and secondary damage to the duodenal mucosa. Of interest, they are not seen in the mucosa of the normal or acutely inflamed duodenum but are frequently present when there is gastric mucous cell metaplasia in cases of chronic duodenitis (20, 21). The organisms are located on the surface adjacent to the gastric-type mucous cells, and they are best visualized with silver and Giemsa stains. See Chapter 23 on Gastritis and Chapter 24 on Peptic Ulcer Disorders for further details.

CLINICAL FEATURES

The clinical aspects of peptic duodenitis are essentially the same as those of duodenal peptic ulcer disease, and the condition often follows a chronic course with repeated recurrences (12). The most common symptom is a burning, midepigastric pain that appears when the stomach is relatively empty, at about 1 to 2 hours after eating or during the night. Severe cases may reveal more persistent pain, episodes of nausea and vomiting, and evidence of bleeding. Medical therapy is mainly intended to buffer the gastric acid by the use of frequent small meals, antacids, and H2 blockers. As noted, antibiotics may be added if *H. pylori* is present. There is also the avoidance of stressful situations and of the ingestion of any substances that may precipitate or promote acid-peptic injury such as ethanol, aspirin, and other medications. Surgical procedures to reduce gastric acid secretion are infrequent but may be needed in severe cases with erosions and bleeding.

GROSS PATHOLOGY

The lesion of peptic duodenitis primarily affects the mucosa, and the inflammation extends at most into the upper part of the submucosa, sparing the deeper portions of the bowel wall. Since surgical resections of the inflamed duodenum are not performed, the information on the pathology of duodenitis is mainly derived from endoscopic examination and the histologic study of mucosal biopsy specimens. The lesion is typically limited to the first portion of the duodenum, except in cases with extreme acid production such as is seen in the Zollinger-Ellison syndrome where the inflammation may extend throughout the organ. Early gross features of duodenitis include edema, erythema, and patchy hemorrhages of the mucosa, and severe cases reveal friability and superficial erosions (14, 22–24). Based on the dominant appearance of the lesions, the cases have been categorized as hemorrhagic or erosive duodenitis, but these terms simply denote a more severe form of the disease and do not imply any differences in their development (25).

MICROSCOPIC PATHOLOGY

There have been a large number of histologic studies of the mucosa in peptic duodenitis (15, 16, 26–28). The interpretation is made difficult because of the relatively distorted appearance of the normal duodenal mucosa when compared with that of the jejunum (2, 4, 13, 26, 29). The villi of the normal duodenum are not as straight and frequently show slight shortening which is due in part to the presence of variable amounts of Brunner glands in the mucosa (Fig. 30.1). In addition, the first part of the duodenum is normally exposed to large quantities of unbuffered gastric acid and is, therefore, the site of what might be called physiologic peptic injury. These features are often seen in biopsies of patients who are shown to have other disorders and in the rims of duodena attached to gastrectomy specimens. Accordingly, these changes must be discounted before one can consider the diagnosis of clinically significant acid-peptic injury.

More certain histologic features of acute or active duodenitis include evidence of degeneration of the surface epithelium, and the presence of neutrophils and a variable increase of mononuclear inflammatory cells in the lamina propria and in the epithelial layer (Fig. 30.2). Milder cases show some shortening of the villi with the inflammation limited to this region. The more severe cases are associated with greater blunting and occasional loss of the villi, extension of the epithelial damage and inflammation to the crypts, focal hemorrhages in the lamina propria, and superficial erosions. The lesions may be diffuse, which is more common, or show a patchy distribution. There may also be acute inflammation in the upper submucosa in the marked cases, but the muscularis propria is normal. The healing phase of duodenitis is characterized by the transient persistence of shortened villi, crypt hyperplasia which is best visualized in areas with few Brunner glands, remaining foci of increased mononuclear inflammatory cells in the lamina propria, increased intraepithelial lymphocytes, and a reduction or absence of neutrophils.

As a result of repeated episodes of peptic injury, features of chronic duodenitis appear in the mucosa, and these include a retention of the changes noted in the healing phase, a hyperplasia of the Brunner glands (30), and a gastric mucous cell metaplasia over the surface of the villi (28, 31, 32). The proliferation of the Brunner glands is often diffuse, resulting in the greater distortion of the villi and crypts, or it may produce a localized nodule (Fig. 30.3). Such nodules may become grossly evident and have been called in the past Brunner gland "adenomas"; there is, however, no cytologic atypism to indicate a neoplasm and it is more appropriate to refer to them as hyperplastic nodules to signify their reparative nature. The gastric mucous cells in the metaplastic areas are of the surface/foveolar type, and they typically appear as a continuous layer of cells that is concentrated at the top or over the upper one-third of the villous surface (Fig. 30.4). The character of the gastric mucous cells is easily recognized in standard H & E preparations and can be accentuated by the use of differential mucin stains. Whereas the intestinal goblet mucous cells have a distended shape and contain acid mucins which stain with alcian blue, the gastric surface-type mucous cells are relatively thin and have mucous granules that are restricted to the luminal end of the cytoplasm and that stain intensely with the periodic acid-Schiff (PAS) reaction for neutral glycoproteins. As noted previously, *H. pylori* may be seen in the areas of gastric mucous cell metaplasia. Some reports favor the interpretation that the appearance of the gastric mucous cell metaplasia is primarily a consequence of the acid (33), and others that it is more closely

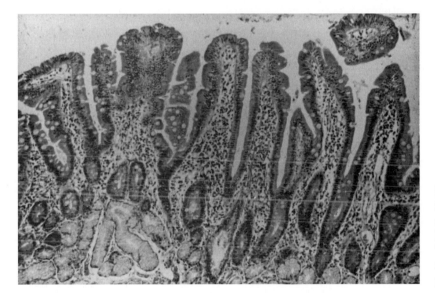

Figure 30.1 Normal duodenal mucosa. Compared to the normal jejunum, the duodenal villi are slightly shortened and irregular, due in part to the nests of Brunner glands at the base of the mucosa *(bottom)*. There is a moderate amount of inflammatory cells, mainly of the mononuclear types, in the lamina propria, and the epithelial cells are intact. H & E, ×120.

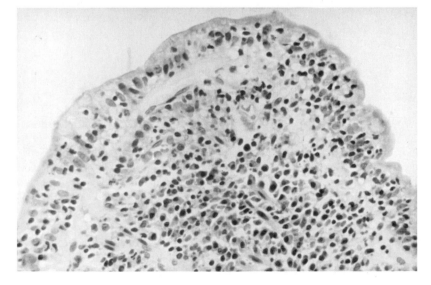

Figure 30.2 Duodenal mucosa in a case of active peptic duodenitis. The villus is blunted and widened, and the surface epithelial cells are markedly shortened and infiltrated with inflammatory cells. There is also an increase of inflammatory cells, including neutrophils as well as mononuclear cells, in the lamina propria. H & E, ×400.

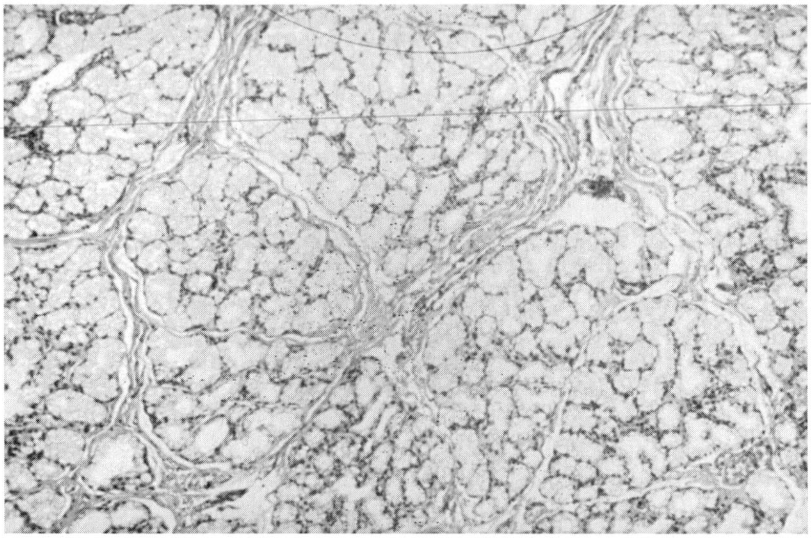

Figure 30.3 Nodule of Brunner gland hyperplasia in a case of chronic peptic duodenitis. There is a marked amount of mature Brunner glands without any nuclear atypicality. H & E, ×100.

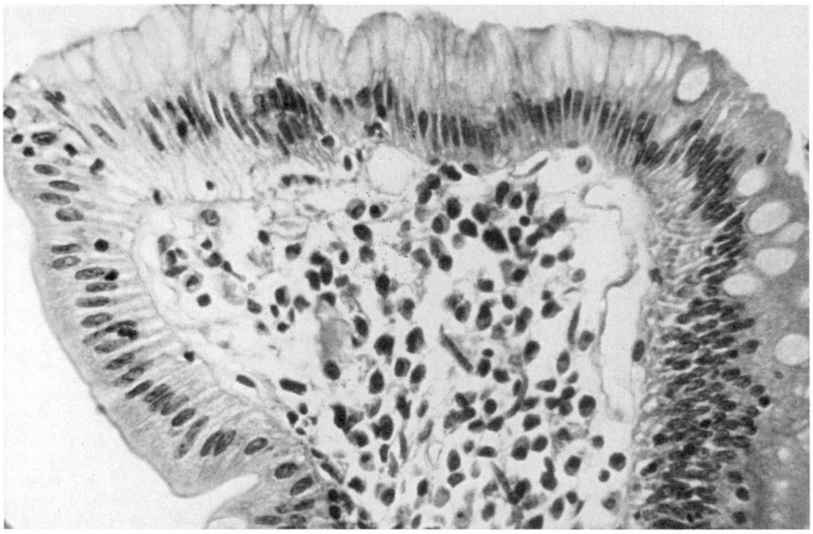

Figure 30.4 Duodenal mucosa in a case of chronic peptic duodenitis, showing gastric surface mucous cell metaplasia on the top of the villus. The gastric mucous cells are columnar and the cytoplasmic mucin is concentrated in the luminal portion of the cells. H & E, ×400.

related to the presence of *H. pylori* (34). The mere presence of mononuclear inflammatory cells in the lamina propria, even if they appear slightly increased in amount, in the absence of other features does not constitute evidence of chronic duodenitis, since these cells may be seen in the intestinal mucosa of normal persons.

COMPLICATIONS

In long-standing cases of duodenitis, the mucosal surface may be irregularly raised. This has been termed nodular duodenitis (35). Some of these cases are due to hyperplasia of the Brunner glands, but most are the result of marked proliferation of lymphoid tissue in the mucosa and upper submucosa. Since the lesion of a peptic duodenitis is largely confined to the mucosa, complications of the sort that are seen in diseases with deeper lesions, such as fibrous stricture, sinus tracts, and perforation, are not encountered. Despite the persistence of the inflammation over many years, there is apparently no increase in the incidence of carcinoma, lymphoma, or other tumors in this condition. Patients with peptic duodenitis are more prone to develop acid-peptic disease of other organs, mainly the stomach and the esophagus, presumably because excess gastric acid production may also be a contributing factor in the genesis of the lesions in the other areas.

DIAGNOSIS

The diagnosis of peptic duodenitis is mainly based on the clinical features, including the characteristic pain and response to antacid therapy in a patient who does not have a demonstrable ulcer (12). Radiographic study is commonly performed to exclude the presence of a peptic ulcer; findings are usually normal, or they may reveal edema and, in late cases, a nodular appearance of the mucosa due to hyperplasia of the Brunner glands or lymphoid nodules. Endoscopic examination with mucosal biopsy is added in many cases to identify or document the presence of inflammation, to determine the exact site of the injury (whether the esophagus, stomach, or duodenum), to exclude other causes, and to monitor the disease after therapy. Overall, there is a relatively poor correlation between the gross and microscopic features in the milder cases of duodenitis (22, 23). The gross features of early and mild disease, such as edema and erythema of the mucosa, may be difficult to distinguish from the traumatic effects of the endoscopic procedure. Conversely, there may be microscopic evidence of active duodenitis in cases with a normal gross appearance. The histologic interpretation of duodenitis must be conservative, since it is usually impossible to separate the various architectural and traumatic effects from the changes of early disease. Accordingly, the clinical diagnosis of active duodenitis is usually dependent on the characteristic symptomatology and on the presence of either a compatible gross or microscopic appearance.

DIFFERENTIAL DIAGNOSIS

The pathologic features noted in peptic duodenitis are entirely nonspecific, and the diagnosis depends on the finding of disease restricted to the proximal duodenum and on the exclusion of other causes. Equivalent inflammation may be seen in many other disorders, including radiation, chemical, and drug reactions, and ischemic disease, and the separation from these requires the relevant clinical information. Infections may be associated with prominent mucosal inflammation and are distinguished by the identification of the organism or viral inclusions, either in the tissue or by appropriate cultures. In allergic disease affecting the duodenum, the lesions are usually patchy and occasionally noted are large clusters of eosinophils in the lamina propria. The duodenum is ordinarily involved in celiac disease with active lesions showing marked or complete villous atrophy together with prominent crypt hyperplasia, but neutrophilic infiltration is usually minimal or absent. Crohn's disease may occasionally involve the duodenum, and severe lesions reveal greater destruction with a tendency for deep ulceration; the disease may be present in any portion of the duodenum, and granulomas are noted in many of the cases. The gross appearance of nodular duodenitis can raise the suspicion of a tumor, and biopsy examination is usually required to make the distinction.

OTHER TYPES OF DUODENITIS

Many other inflammatory conditions can affect the duodenum (Table 30.2). The detailed information about these disorders is provided in other chapters, and only some of the salient points that relate to disease in the duodenum are presented here.

TABLE	
30.2	**Inflammatory Diseases of the Duodenum**

Peptic Duodenitis and Chronic Peptic Ulcer
Acute Stress Ulcer
Infections
   Post gastric surgery
   Opportunistic
Radiation, Drug, and Toxic Injuries
Vasculitis
Crohn's Disease
Celiac Disease
Allergic Disease

INFECTIONS

The common viral and bacterial infections of the intestines do not usually involve the duodenum, possibly due to the antagonistic effects of acid and other toxic substances in this area (36). It has been noted, however, that some peptic ulcers reveal a localized overgrowth of bacteria and fungi, and these may be associated with greater severity and with delay in healing (37, 38). Following a Billroth II operation, the afferent loop leading to the gastrojejunostomy may become stagnant and favor the development of bacterial proliferation in the lumen (4, 39). The functional problems that ensue are largely due to the effects of bacteria on the bile salts and to the utilization of vitamins, while the mucosa may be normal or show a variable degree of inflammation which is usually mild and patchy.

The duodenum is a common site for infection in cases of the acquired immunodeficiency syndrome (AIDS) and other immune disorders, and both biopsies and aspirates are frequently obtained from this area (40, 41). Included are direct invasion by the HIV virus (42), and opportunistic infections due to cytomegalovirus (43, 44), fungi (45), *Giardia* (46–48), *Isospora* (49–51), *Cryptosporidia* (52–59), *Microsporidia* (60–62), *Cyclospora* (63), *Toxoplasma* (64), and *Leishmania* (65), and their distinctive structures can be readily visualized in the tissues. The amount of mucosal destruction and inflammatory reaction is highly variable in these infections, as a result of the marked immunosuppression, ranging from minimal alterations to overt ulceration. The lesions are typically confined to the mucosa and submucosa. Infection with *Mycobacterium avium* complex is also most commonly seen in the AIDS patients (66, 67). The mucosa typically shows clusters of foamy macrophages or poorly formed granulomas but occasionally may be completely normal in appearance on H&E sections; the specific diagnosis is provided by the acid fast stain which reveals abundant organisms both in the macrophages and in the intervening lamina propria (Fig. 30.5). The organisms also react with other stains including the periodic acid-Schiff (PAS), which has led to confusion with Whipple's disease in the past.

A variety of helminthic infections (68–70), identified by the specific ova, and foci of Whipple's disease (71) have also been observed in the duodenum. The overall identification of duodenal infections, particularly of the opportunistic types, has increased in recent years, and this is mainly attributable to the greater performance of endoscopy and mucosal biopsy of this area. See Chapter 28 on Infectious Disorders of the Intestines and Chapter 31 on Malabsorptive Disorders for further details.

PHYSICAL AND CHEMICAL INJURIES

The duodenum may be damaged by radiation which is usually applied for tumors in adjacent tissues (72). The acute changes include prominent edema and hemorrhage of the mucosa and submucosa, followed by ulceration and marked inflammatory reaction. Obstruction may result from the inflammatory edema or fibrous stricture formation. Chronic effects include persistence of the ulcers which may penetrate the deeper parts of the bowel wall, fibrosis and sinus tract formation, and progressive thickening of the small vessels leading to secondary ischemic effects. Histologic examination may reveal enlarged and atypical mesenchymal cells in the inflamed and fibrotic areas, and the diagnosis is based on the

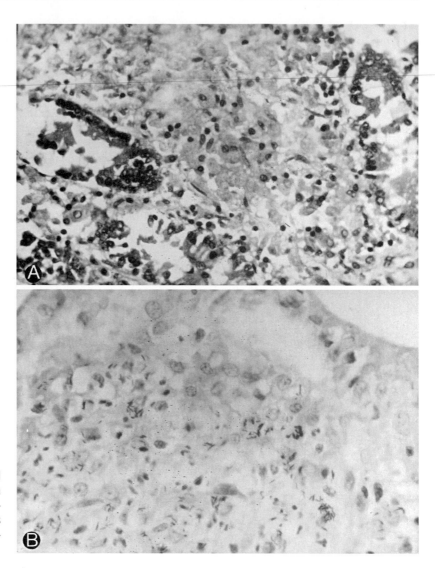

Figure 30.5 Duodenal mucosa in a case of acquired immunodeficiency syndrome. **(A)** *(top)*. There is a sheet of vacuolated macrophages in the lamina propria *(center)*. H & E, ×400. **(B)** *(bottom)*. Numerous acid-fast bacilli are in the lamina propria. Ziehl-Neelsen stain, ×400.

clinical history and the finding of compatible pathologic features. Mucosal biopsy of ulcerated areas is often obtained to exclude the presence of tumor or opportunistic infections.

Various chemicals, such as ethanol (73) and medications (74–76), acting as direct toxins or mediated by immunologic injury, can also damage the duodenum. There has been increasing use of nonsteroidal anti-inflammatory drugs (NSAIDs), and these can cause a variety of lesions in the small and large intestines (77, 78). Included are foci of inflammation, ulcers, strictures, and diaphragms composed of fibromuscular tissue. In addition, the duodenal epithelium may reveal marked atypism following infusion chemotherapy for hepatic tumors (79, 80). After the toxic substances are discontinued, there is usually prompt healing, but some cases, possibly due to secondary infections, show persistence and progression of the lesions. See Chapter 11 on Physical and Chemical Disorders for further details.

VASCULAR DISEASE

Because of the extensive vascular collaterals encircling the duodenum, ischemic disease due to thrombotic occlusion of vessels or to low blood flow is rarely observed. In an effort to stop or reduce a massive hemorrhage from a peptic ulcer, vasoconstrictive agents and preformed clots or gelfoam have been inserted into the mesenteric vessels at time of angiography, and this sometimes results in extensive ischemic damage of the duodenal mucosa and wall (81). Vasculitis (82–84) and atheromatous emboli (85) may affect any part of the intestine, including the duodenum, and may lead to focal infarction and ulceration of the overlying tissues. See Chapter 14 on Vascular Disease for details.

CROHN'S DISEASE

In cases of Crohn's disease affecting the ileum and colon, microscopic abnormalities are commonly noted in the duodenal mucosa, consisting of focal cryptitis and/or granulomas (86–89). Such changes are seen in random sections of the mucosa in 25 to 50% of cases, and in about 80% if serial sections are obtained, but their presence is not associated with any functional problems. Gross lesions, indicating clinically significant disease, are much less commonly observed and reveal prominent mucosal necrosis and ulceration that may affect any part of the duodenum (90) (see Fig. 29.46

in Chapter 29). The pathologic features are similar to those seen in the distal intestine and include the tendency for deep ulceration, fibrous stricture and sinus tract formation, muscular hypertrophy, and transmural inflammation. Distinguishing Crohn's disease from peptic duodenitis and duodenal peptic ulcer is readily accomplished by noting the more diffuse distribution of the lesions in the duodenum and by the presence of sinus tracts and granulomas. Separation of Crohn's disease from other necrotizing lesions of the duodenum such as severe infections is often dependent on finding associated lesions in the more characteristic sites of the distal ileum and colon. See Chapter 29 on Ulcerative Colitis and Crohn's Disease for details.

CELIAC DISEASE

The duodenum is invariably involved in cases of celiac disease, which is also termed nontropical sprue and gluten-sensitive enteropathy (91, 92). The lesion is identical to that described in the jejunum and consists of a diffuse and uniform injury in the mucosa, with the deeper parts of the bowel wall uninvolved (4, 93–95). Major histologic features include a marked shortening ("atrophy") or absence of the villi, reactive crypt hyperplasia which is proportional to the degree of villous damage, evidence of degeneration of the surface epithelial cells with increased intraepithelial lymphocytes, and a prominent infiltrate of mononuclear inflammatory cells (mostly plasma cells and lymphocytes) in the lamina propria. Neutrophils may be present but are usually not conspicuous. The healing phase is characterized by the reappearance of the normal tall surface epithelial cells with well formed brush borders, a decline in the inflammation, a slow reformation of the villi, and persistence of the crypt hyperplasia until the villi are completely normal (96). Since the histologic features are nonspecific in nature and can be seen in many other conditions, including peptic disease, infections, and allergic conditions, the diagnosis of celiac disease depends on the response to a gluten free diet; in children, a gluten challenge is also often required after the patient is well to effectively exclude the other causes of enteritis (97). It has recently been demonstrated that the effects of gluten can be seen in the rectal and gastric mucosae, and biopsy of these areas following dietary challenge may also prove useful (98, 99).

With the greater use of endoscopy, mucosal biopsy of the duodenum is being increasingly used as a screening test for celiac disease (5, 11). If the duodenal biopsy is normal or shows only minimal changes in a patient with suspected celiac disease, that disorder is effectively excluded because of the expected involvement of the duodenum in all active cases. Conversely, the finding of duodenal disease on biopsy, particularly if there is not complete villous loss, could be the result of the much more common disorder of peptic duodenitis; in such cases, a jejunal mucosal biopsy would then be needed. See Chapter 31 on Malabsorptive Disorders for details.

ALLERGIC DISEASE

The proximal small intestine, including the duodenum, is one of the preferential sites for involvement by allergic disease (100). The lesions may be isolated to the small intestine but are more often associated with disease affecting other parts of the upper tract, including the esophagus and the stomach (101–103). A specific causative food substance such as milk protein (104, 105) or soy (106, 107) protein is identified in many of the patients with small bowel disease, whereas other cases (termed allergic or eosinophilic gastroenteritis) are related to multiple allergens (103, 108). Severe cases reveal prominent mucosal edema which can be appreciated by radiographic and endoscopic examinations (109). In most cases, however, the lesions are detected by microscopic study of the duodenum or jejunum which reveals a variable shortening of the villi together with a patchy infiltrate of eosinophils in the lamina propria and adjacent epithelia (4, 103–107, 110). The inflammation may extend into the upper submucosa, but the deeper parts of the bowel wall are unaffected. Since the lesions are so focal, multiple biopsy samples of the duodenum and jejunum may be required to establish the diagnosis (111). In this regard, it has been observed that the gastric antrum is more constantly and severely involved, and biopsy of this region should also be obtained in cases of suspected allergic disease (102). See Chapter 12 on Allergic Disorders for further details.

OTHER IMMUNE DISORDERS

The proximal small intestine is often involved in the various primary and acquired immunodeficiency diseases, leading to alterations of the mucosa (112, 113). Abnormalities that are identified in duodenal and jejunal mucosal biopsies include the appearance of a focal or diffuse enteritis, a variable reduction of plasma cells in the lamina propria, and the presence of opportunistic microorganisms. In transient hypogammaglobulinemia of infants, the mucosa is usually normal, but about 25% of the cases show signs of an active or healing enteritis in mucosal biopsies (114). The small intestinal mucosa is one of the target tissues in graft-versus-host reactions, and the lesions observed range from a patchy enteritis (115) to extensive ulceration (116). See Chapters 6, 16, and 31 for details on the immune-mediated disorders.

STRESS ULCERS OF THE DUODENUM

This subject is covered in Chapter 24.

MISCELLANEOUS INFLAMMATORY DISORDERS OF THE SMALL INTESTINE

ULCERATIVE JEJUNOILEITIS

DEFINITION AND ETIOLOGY

Ulcerative jejunoileitis is a rare condition of uncertain etiology, characterized by the appearance of multiple and persistent ulcers of the jejunum and ileum (117–119). The disorder was originally delineated and separated from Crohn's disease by noting the absence of mural thickening and of granulomas and that lesions did not develop in the colon. The existence of ulcerative jejunoileitis as a distinct entity has been subsequently questioned, however, and it has been suggested that it may represent an uncommon complication of long-standing celiac disease and of cases of refractory sprue in which ulcers can develop (120, 121).

PATHOLOGY

The ulcers vary in size, are usually sharply demarcated, and are concentrated in the jejunum and proximal ileum. The intervening mucosa appears grossly intact, and there are no diffuse alterations of the bowel wall. The inflammatory reaction surrounding the ulcers is entirely nonspecific, and there are no granulomas or sinus tracts. In support of the notion that ulcerative jejunoileitis may simply be a complication of celiac disease, the mucosa of the nonulcerated areas frequently reveals some degree of villous shortening, crypt hyperplasia, and increased mononuclear inflammatory cells in the lamina propria (120–122).

DIFFERENTIAL DIAGNOSIS

The disorder must be distinguished from other conditions that are associated with multiple small intestinal ulcerations. These conditions are mainly infections, as shown by cultures, and Crohn's disease, shown by the presence of mural thickening, sinus tracts, granulomas, and colonic lesions. As noted, the separation of ulcerative jejunoileitis from the ulcerated phase of celiac disease or of refractory sprue is probably a moot point (92, 123). In addition, the appearance of ulcers in a case of celiac disease may signal the development of the complication of malignant lymphoma. It may be exceedingly difficult to appreciate the tumor grossly because of the absence of a discrete mass, and mucosal biopsies may be too superficial to detect the tumor which is usually concentrated in the intestinal wall and the mesentery. The diagnosis of lymphoma, which is most often of the T-cell type (124), usually requires a full thickness sample at operation. See Chapter 31 on Malabsorptive Disorders for further details.

BYPASS ENTERITIS

DEFINITION, ETIOLOGY, AND CLINICAL FEATURES

Bypass of long segments of the jejunum and of the ileum were formerly performed in patients with extreme obesity, and subsequent examinations of these excluded segments often revealed inflammatory changes in the mucosa (125). Although the mucosal alterations are usually mild and not associated with prominent clinical problems related to the intestine, it is possible that drainage of toxic substances from the inflamed areas contribute to the portal tract lesions of the liver that are frequently noted in these patients (126). Exceptionally, a more pronounced degree of enteritis has been observed (127). The mucosal inflammation seen in the excluded tissues is probably a consequence of stasis, but a specific microbiologic agent or other toxic substance has not been determined. The intestinal lesions typically disappear when the bypass is eliminated and normal luminal flow is restored in the gut segment. A temporary bypass or diverting ileostomy may be performed for other inflammatory conditions of the small intestine to allow time for some healing and localization to occur prior to resection, and it is important to recognize, in all of these situations, that newly developed inflammatory charges may simply be the effect of stasis rather than extension of the primary disease. Such information might prove important in determining the extent of any planned surgical resections or in decisions to restore intestinal continuity.

PATHOLOGY

The changes noted in the excluded intestinal segments are mainly limited to the mucosa and are of a nonspecific nature (125, 126). There often are an increased number of hypertrophied lymphoid nodules and an overall increase of mononuclear inflammatory cells in the lamina propria, which may result in a slight granularity of the mucosal surface. Changes of active enteritis are less frequent and range from focal areas of cryptitis and villous atrophy to overt erosions and ulcers (127). Neutrophils predominate in the active lesions, and the presence of granulomas has only rarely been noted (128). In some patients, particularly in those who have had a longstanding bypass for a chronic enteritis such as Crohn's disease, there may develop a marked contraction of the bowel with the lumen narrowed to 1 to 2 cm in diameter; there is often an associated hypertrophy of the muscularis propria (129), but this may reflect the underlying condition of chronic enteritis.

ENTERITIS CYSTICA PROFUNDA

DEFINITION, ETIOLOGY, AND CLINICAL FEATURES

Enteritis cystica profunda is an uncommon condition of the small intestine, characterized by the extension of mature or regenerative epithelium through the muscularis mucosae into the submucosa and occasionally the deeper parts of the bowel wall (130, 131). The lesion is seen most commonly in chronic inflammatory disorders such as Crohn's disease (132, 133) and in association with the hamartomatous polyps of the Peutz-Jeghers syndrome (134, 135). It is thought to result from disruptions of the muscularis mucosae that permit the proliferating mucosal tissue to extend past the natural barrier into the underlying tissues. The clinical features are usually dominated by the underlying disease, and the enteritis cystica lesion is typically an incidental finding. Exceptionally, when the lesion is large, the features of an expanded or polypoid mucosa together with presence of glands in the wall may simulate a neoplasm, and this can be an important consideration because the primary diseases are prone to the development of carcinomas. Similar lesions are observed in other parts of the gut and are termed by their specific location as gastritis cystica profunda and colitis cystica profunda.

PATHOLOGY

The lesions may rarely be isolated but are more often multiple and observed as a complication of a chronic inflammatory or polypoid condition. They vary in size and location, with the majority detected in the ileum, and most are grossly obscured by the underlying disease. Larger lesions reveal cystic spaces or a mucinous appearance of the wall and mimic a neoplastic mass but are readily distinguished by microscopic examination. There is an irregular proliferation of glands, many of which are cystic, and the lesion is usually limited to the submucosa; more pronounced cases show further extension of the glands into the muscularis propria and rarely to the serosa. The epithelium lining the glands and cystic spaces is usually completely mature, with small basal-oriented nuclei and abundant mucus-filled cytoplasm, or it may show the features of inflamed or regenerating cells. Associated with the misplaced glands are variable amounts of lamina propria which help to identify the nature of the lesion. There is typically no inflammatory reaction around the misplaced glands, unless there is rupture of the cysts and extravasation of mucus which may evoke a mild proliferation of macrophages. Mucinous carcinomas, in contrast, show some degree of atypism of the epithelial nuclei (in the form of elongated and pallisading nuclei, hyperchromasia, and pleomorphism) and often the presence of a loose connective tissue stroma (so-called tumor stroma) between the glands and the indigenous tissues. The appearance of the overlying mucosa reflects the primary disease, revealing inflammation and pseudopolyps in Crohn's disease and other chronic forms of enteritis or the characteristic features of the hamartomatous polyps.

OTHER ULCERS OF THE SMALL INTESTINE

Multiple ulcers are seen in the major diffuse inflammatory conditions of the small intestine (Table 30.1), including infections (see Chapter 28) and Crohn's disease (Chapter 29), and as a complication of some cases of celiac disease (Chapter 31). In addition, ulcers can occur as a result of radiation and chemical injuries (Chapter 11), stasis and mechanical obstruction (Chapter 13), vasculitis and ischemic disease (Chapter 14), graft-versus-host disease and other immunologic conditions (Chapter 16), and various systemic disorders (Chapter 19). In the Zollinger-Ellison syndrome, multiple ulcers are occasionally noted in the distal duodenum and proximal jejunum and are due to the sustained, marked elevations in gastric acid secretion (see Chapter 24). Ulcerated lesions of the ileum are also noted in many patients with the Behçet's syndrome, described in the section on Miscellaneous Disorders of the Colon.

NONSPECIFIC ULCER OF THE SMALL INTESTINE

This category embraces cases in which ulcers of unknown or uncertain etiology involve the jejunum and/or the ileum (136–138). It is clearly a mixed group and includes cases with single or multiple lesions which may be acute or associated with fibrous stricture formation. The ulcers may affect either sex and all age groups, with a tendency for lesions of the jejunum to be more common in children and those of the ileum to occur in adult patients (136). Overall, about 75% of the cases involve the ileum, but deep ulcers and perforation are more frequent in the jejunum. The major presenting symptoms are those of intestinal obstruction, bleeding, and perforation, and surgery is often required for these complications and to establish the diagnosis. The pathologic features are nonspecific, revealing ulcers of variable size and depth, acute and chronic inflammatory cells, and the formation of prominent granulation tissue and fibrosis which can extend deep into the wall and cause marked stenosis. There are no sinus tracts or granulomas, and the mucosa and bowel wall adjacent to or between the ulcers is typically normal. The diagnosis of a case of nonspecific ulcer(s) of the small intestine depends on the identification by radiographic study or operative findings of ulcerated or stenotic lesions and on the exclusion of all other possible causes. In particular, ulcers due to less common infections such as the *Yersinia* agents (139, 140), to drug effects from enteric-coated potassium (141–143), gold (144, 145), NSAIDs (77, 78), digitalis and oral contraceptive pills (74, 146), and to ischemic lesions resulting from constricting fibrous bands in the serosa and adjacent mesentery may often present without a clear history, and these conditions should be considered in the differential diagnosis.

MISCELLANEOUS INFLAMMATORY DISORDERS OF THE COLON

LYMPHOCYTIC (MICROSCOPIC) COLITIS

DEFINITION AND ETIOLOGY

The term microscopic colitis was applied by Bo-Linn et al. in 1985 to a group of patients with recurrent secretory diarrhea of unknown etiology, and in whom morphologic investigations revealed only histologic alterations that were limited to the colonic mucosa (147). The condition was initially identified in patients with cases of suspected Crohn's disease who lacked and did not develop the characteristic features of that disease after a long follow-up period (148). Considering the disparity between the functional problem and the microscopic features, it is highly unlikely that the structural change is a cause of the diarrhea; rather, the histologic findings serve as a potential marker of the disease and also to exclude other causes of chronic inflammatory bowel disease. It is also possible that the microscopic changes are a simple consequence of the diarrhea and potential colonic stagnation or that they represent a nonspecific response to a primary etiologic agent. The use of the term "microscopic colitis" is not ideal, because it is often employed as a descriptive phrase in other inflammatory conditions. A recent study of a larger series of cases noted the constant presence of an increased number of lymphocytes in the surface epithelial layer, and the term of lymphocytic colitis was proposed as a preferred name for this condition (149). The appearance of the increased intraepithelial lymphocytes is similar to that observed in chronic erosive (lymphocytic) gastritis (see Chapter 23) and in celiac disease (Chapter 31), but there is no established connection among these three disorders.

CLINICAL FEATURES

This is an uncommon condition, and the described cases have been mainly in middle-aged and older women (150, 151). Unlike collagenous colitis, however, cases have been noted in men and in younger patients as well. All patients present with persistent, watery diarrhea, and functional studies have revealed reduced colonic absorption of water due to a decrease in the active and passive absorptions of sodium and chloride (148). Of interest, a decrease in water absorption in the small intestine has also been noted in some of the cases, but this has not been associated with any structural abnormalities in the jejunal mucosa. Rarely noted is the association of medications with the onset of the lymphocytic colitis (152). There are no radiographic or gross endoscopic alterations, and stool cultures are normal. Other investigators have noted the appearance of anemia, hypokalemia, and hypoproteinemia in cases referred to as microscopic colitis, but it is not at all clear whether these represent the same condition as that with watery diarrhea alone (153). The diarrhea tends to persist, and some cases respond to anti-inflammatory drugs with improvement of the symptoms and the colonic biopsy features.

PATHOLOGY

There are no gross alterations, and histologic examination of the small intestinal mucosa is normal. Based on studies of mucosal biopsies of the colon, the constant abnormality is an increase of lymphocytes within the surface epithelium, without any erosions or thickening of the underlying collagen layer (149). Variable features include the presence of neutrophils and increased eosinophils and mononuclear cells in the lamina propria in the absence of cryptitis (150, 151, 154). The inflammatory reaction is entirely nonspecific, and granulomas or a prominence of lymphoid nodules are not observed. The histologic features, even in patients with recurrent or chronic disease, resemble most a mild acute colitis except for the presence of the increased mononuclear inflammatory cells in the surface layer. The more characteristic findings of chronic colitis (155), such as complex branching or atrophy of the crypts, a villiform surface, and Paneth cell metaplasia, have not been described (see section on Ulcerative Colitis in Chapter 29).

DIFFERENTIAL DIAGNOSIS

The diagnosis of lymphocytic colitis depends on the exclusion of other causes of recurrent or chronic colitis and secretory diarrhea, and on the finding of patchy inflammation that is restricted to the colonic mucosa. Mild cases of acute colitis due to infections, known toxic substances, vascular diseases, and immunologic disorders are separated by stool cultures, relevant clinical information, and the limited duration of the disease. A diffuse colitis and gross alterations are seen in ulcerative colitis, and Crohn's disease of the colon ultimately reveals ulceration, mural inflammation, and often granulomas. In cases in which the secretory diarrhea is the dominant or sole feature, other diagnostic considerations would include celiac disease, which is identified by the typical alterations in the small bowel mucosa and by the absence of colitis, and functional endocrine tumors which lack structural alterations. Fully developed cases of collagenous colitis show a characteristic thickening of the basement membrane in the colonic mucosa and typically lack signs of acute inflammation and rectal bleeding.

COLLAGENOUS COLITIS
DEFINITION AND ETIOLOGY

First described by Lindstrom in 1976 (156), collagenous colitis is an uncommon condition characterized by prolonged episodes of watery diarrhea and the presence of marked thickening of the collagen layer beneath the surface epithelial cells of the colonic mucosa (151, 154, 157–164). The cause of this disorder is not known, but it has been suggested that the collagenous band may interfere with the normal reabsorption of water by the colonic mucosa resulting in the diarrhea (156). Alternatively, both the diarrhea and the structural change may be the consequences of a common etiologic event. In studies of serial mucosal biopsies, there is a general correlation between the degrees of the diarrhea and thickened membrane, but also the observation that the diarrhea may be the initial feature (160, 165). It is currently thought that one or more toxic substances, as yet not identified, can cause this condition and that the colonic mucosa reveals a patchy inflammation together with the gradual development of the collagenous band (163). There are rare cases of collagenous colitis that have abnormalities of other tissues, including atrophy of the small intestinal mucosa (166, 167)

and pulmonary fibrosis (168), but it is not clear whether this association is real, or just coincidental.

CLINICAL FEATURES

The exact incidence of collagenous colitis is not known, but it has been noted recently with increasing frequency. The disorder occurs predominantly in middle-aged and older women, and cases typically present with the gradual onset of watery diarrhea and abdominal crampy pain. There are rare reports suggesting that the collagenous colitis is precipitated by NSAIDs (169), but this has not been confirmed by others (170). The diarrhea often progresses, or remits and recurs (171), and has a variable duration of up to several years, but it eventually subsides in most cases (158, 170). Radiographic and stool culture examinations are normal, and the diagnosis was overlooked in the past because the colonic mucosa appears normal at endoscopic study and biopsy was not obtained. The patients have frequently been tagged as having the irritable bowel syndrome or a psychosomatic disorder, and are often relieved once the diagnosis of collagenous colitis is established by colonic mucosal biopsy. Most cases respond to treatment with anti-inflammatory drugs (172).

PATHOLOGY

There are no gross abnormalities, and the histologic lesion is limited to the mucosa of the large intestine; the abnormality is more commonly noted and usually more severe in the colon than in the rectum (163, 164, 173). In the fully developed lesion, there is marked thickening of the basement membrane region by collagen deposition, ranging from 15 to 65 μm in width, immediately beneath the surface epithelial cells (Fig. 30.6). In contrast, the thickness of the basement membrane in the colonic mucosa of normal persons is typically less than 5 to 6 μm (174). The lesion at this stage is usually diffuse within the biopsy and easily appreciated by H & E staining, and it can be accentuated by the use of Trichrome stains for connective tissues. Ultrastructural studies have demonstrated that the basement lamina of the epithelial cells is of normal dimension and appearance and that the thickening is due solely to the deposition of mature type I and type III collagens in the subjacent tissue (159). Amyloid stains are negative, and no other proteins including immune complexes have been identified by immunocytochemical stains in the abnormal area (175). The thickened band is limited to the surface area and does not extend down to involve the basement membrane region of the underlying crypts. Other histologic features in cases of collagenous colitis include a patchy increase of mononuclear inflammatory cells in the superficial part of the lamina propria and in the surface epithelial layer (149); less commonly observed are tiny foci of epithelial degeneration, small numbers of neutrophils, and Paneth cell metaplasia (170). There are no granulomas or other signs of chronic colitis such as complex branching and atrophy of the crypts, or a villiform surface (155).

Serial biopsy examinations have been performed in some patients who eventually developed the classic lesion of collagenous colitis, and these have permitted a delineation of the earlier phase of the lesion (160, 165). The earliest biopsies, obtained just days or a few weeks after the onset of the symptoms, are often nonspecific, revealing just patchy areas of increased inflammation and occasional surface erosion but no collagen deposition. Samples taken even after several weeks of disease may show variable persistence of the

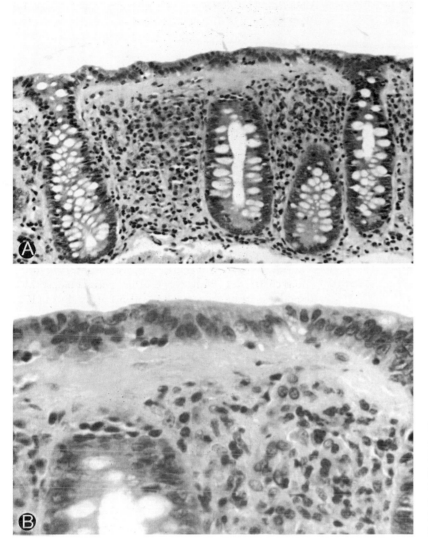

Figure 30.6 Colonic mucosa in collagenous colitis. **(A)** *(top).* There is a marked thickening of the collagen layer that is limited to the region just beneath the surface epithelium. The crypts are normal. H & E, ×100. **(B)** *(bottom).* Closer view, showing the thickened collagen layer and increased mononuclear inflammatory cells in the surface epithelial layer. H & E, ×400.

inflammation and a definite but focal and usually slight collagen increase in the superficial basement membrane area (Fig. 30.7). At this stage, the diagnosis of collagenous colitis can be suspected but not made with certainty, because equivalent degrees of collagen deposition can be seen in other forms of colitis, notably in radiation damage, ischemic disease, ulcerative colitis, and Crohn's disease (164, 174, 176). The later and more diagnostic biopsies contain the fully developed and diffuse lesions. Recovery from the condition is associated with elimination of the collagenous band and return of the mucosa to a completely normal appearance, but the condition may recur (163, 171).

DIFFERENTIAL DIAGNOSIS

The diagnosis of collagenous colitis is established by finding the characteristic lesion in the mucosa of a patient with a pure secretory form of diarrhea. It should be remembered that the lesion may be less obvious or absent in the rectum, and therefore, biopsies should be obtained higher up from the colon if the disease is suspected. Cases of acute and chronic colitis, including infections and the idiopathic forms of ulcerative colitis and Crohn's disease of the

colon, typically present with purulent and bloody diarrhea and reveal ulcerations or other gross abnormalities of the colon. A patchy thickening of the basement membrane by collagen beneath the surface epithelial cells is occasionally seen in cases of ischemic, radiation, and ulcerative colitis, but the collagen band is usually less than 10 μm in thickness and the distinction from collagenous colitis is apparent from the presence of other features (164, 174). It is of interest that the identical collagenous thickening of the surface basement membrane is noted in many cases of hyperplastic polyps of the colon (159). This should cause no confusion with the diagnosis of collagenous colitis since the clinical setting is entirely different, but the presence of the fibrous band may help to identify the particular type of polyp when the lesion is small and tangentially sectioned.

Other disorders that may be manifested by a secretory diarrhea include celiac disease and Crohn's disease of the small intestine, which are readily distinguished by lesions in that area of the gut, and functional endocrine tumors which show no structural changes. Cases of lymphocytic colitis may present with prominent watery diarrhea, but they often have other signs of an active colitis such as bleeding and foci of acute inflammation in the mucosa and lack the

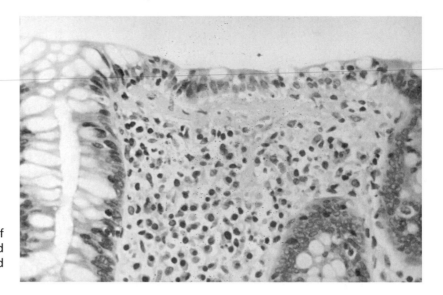

Figure 30.7 Colonic mucosa in an earlier case of collagenous colitis. The thickened collagen band beneath the surface epithelium is less prominent and more patchy in distribution. H & E, ×250.

collagenous band (147, 149). Probably the biggest problem in the diagnosis of collagenous colitis has been the failure to consider the possibility in an otherwise healthy patient who complains simply of watery diarrhea. Since there are no gross abnormalities evident upon radiographic and endoscopic examinations, the diagnosis can only be secured by biopsy of the colon, preferably above the rectal area.

DIVERSION-RELATED COLITIS

DEFINITION AND ETIOLOGY

Following a diverting ileostomy or colostomy, inflammatory changes of a nonspecific nature often appear in the mucosa of the excluded colonic segment that is distal to the stoma (177–185). The gross features observed at endoscopy may mimic a mild case of ulcerative colitis, but the condition also occurs in patients without an antecedent history of inflammatory bowel disease, and lesions are not observed in the gut proximal to the stoma. Furthermore, the inflammatory changes completely resolve after intestinal continuity is restored. It is thought that the disorder results from the effects of stagnation in the excluded segment, but a specific microbiologic agent or other toxic substance has not been identified.

CLINICAL FEATURES

There have been no detailed prospective studies of this disorder, and its frequency and time of onset after the diverting procedure are not known. It has been observed following ileostomy or, more often, colostomy at all sites for various conditions, including diverticular disease, motor disturbances, drug reactions, antibiotic-associated colitis, and Crohn's disease (177, 178, 183). Most patients are asymptomatic, and the lesion is only detected at time of endoscopy that might be performed in advance of a planned reanastomosis of the intestine. Some patients, particularly in cases with a long duration, develop a mucous discharge, diarrhea, and rectal bleeding (179–182). Amelioration of symptoms and histologic improvement have been observed following rectal irrigation with short chain fatty acids (186). The condition can persist for many months to years and does not appear to completely resolve until the intestine is reconnected permitting normal fecal flow. In the past, the finding of such inflammatory changes has resulted in delays in reanastomosis or even in resection of involved areas because of uncertainty in the diagnosis or significance of the lesion (177, 181). This is of particular importance in cases with known Crohn's disease who have had a temporary diverting procedure, and the dilemma arises as to whether the mucosal changes in the excluded segment are related to the surgery or represent evidence of persistent or recurrent Crohn's disease (178). Since the lesions due to diversion are typically most prominent in the rectum, at stake is the decision of either to connect the bowel to the inflamed area or to resect the rectum and leave the patient with a permanent enterostomy. In the absence of certain signs of Crohn's disease such as extensive granulomatous inflammation and sinus tracts in the rectum of such cases, it is probably worthwhile to explain the situation to the patient and to perform an anastomotic procedure. Ultimately, the determination of whether a patient had diversion-related colitis rests on its complete resolution following elimination of the stoma and reconnection of the intestine.

PATHOLOGY

The lesions are limited to the mucosal layer and are often confined to or most severe in the distal colon and rectum. The gross appearance, as observed at endoscopic examination, typically reveals some combination of erythema, granularity, and mild friability, and discrete aphthous-type ulcers have been noted in the more prolonged cases (179, 182, 183, 187). The changes may be very similar to those seen in idiopathic inflammatory bowel disease, but the distinction can be readily made by microscopic study of mucosal biopsies. Since the lesions are often patchy, the mucosa may be completely normal or show just a prominence of lymphoid nodules (188). Signs of active colitis or proctitis are observed in most cases and include the focal presence of acute cryptitis and degeneration of surface epithelial cells with neutrophils in the adjacent lamina propria (Figs. 30.8 and 30.9). The ulcers that sometimes develop have a nonspecific inflammatory reaction. There may also be regenerative signs in the crypts and foci of increased mononuclear inflammatory cells, and rarely observed are features of chronic colitis such as branching or atrophy of the crypts (182, 183, 189). Loose granulomas of the foreign body-type may uncommonly be found in the anorectal region in long-standing cases, and pneumatosis has been noted in cases with large ulcers (190). The inflammatory changes are generally restricted to the mucosa, and the deeper parts of the bowel wall are uninvolved. In particular, prominent submucosal fibrosis and mural sinus tracts have not been observed. After reanastomosis and recovery from the condition, the mucosa reverts to normal and there are no sequelae seen in biopsy samples.

DIFFERENTIAL DIAGNOSIS

The diagnosis of diversion-related colitis is tentatively suspected by the finding of nonspecific, mild inflammatory changes in the mucosa of an excluded colonic and rectal segment, and secured by reversion of the mucosa to normal after intestinal continuity is restored. The differential diagnosis would include any of the several conditions

that may complicate a surgical procedure. Ordinary infections are excluded by stool cultures and ischemic disease by the absence of the typical features of hemorrhagic necrosis and extensive ulceration; furthermore, ischemic lesions are much less common in the rectum and tend not to persist at such a mild level of injury. Antibiotic-associated colitis is characterized by the frequent presence of small pseudomembranes on the mucosal surface and by the positive assay for *C. difficile* in the stool (191). In ulcerative colitis, there is usually a prior history of the disease, and the lesions are invariably diffuse and frequently associated with histologic features of chronic colitis. As noted in the section on Clinical Features, the distinction between diversion colitis and extension of Crohn's disease in a patient with overt gross lesions in the ileum or proximal colon may be a particular challenge, since both conditions may reveal microscopic patches of inflammation and aphthous ulcers. In such cases, the definite diagnosis of Crohn's disease affecting the distal colon and rectum would require the finding of characteristic features such as prominent submucosal fibrosis, sinus tracts, transmural inflammation, or granulomas excluding those of the foreign body-type.

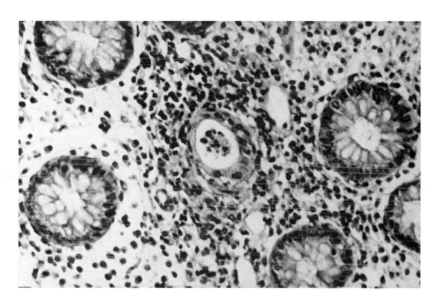

Figure 30.8   Rectal mucosa in a case of diversion-related colitis. There is a focal crypt abscess *(center)* amidst an otherwise normal mucosa. H & E, ×400.

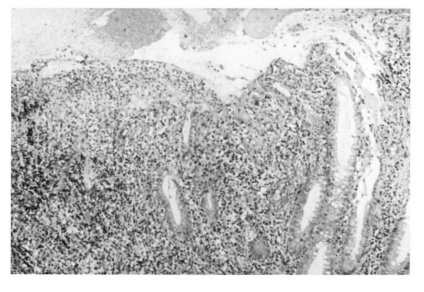

Figure 30.9   Rectal mucosa in diversion-related colitis, showing a more advanced lesion, characterized by superficial ulceration and greater inflammation. H & E, ×100.

ACUTE SELF-LIMITED COLITIS

This is not a specific disease entity but rather a descriptive term that is applied to cases of acute colitis and proctitis that ultimately recover and leave no traces of injury in the mucosa (155, 192). Although an infectious agent or toxic substance is often identified, the particular cause is not established in about 25% to 33% of the cases. The major importance of this category, particularly of those cases without an apparent etiology, is in the distinction from early or acute cases of idiopathic inflammatory bowel disease. Both groups may have an abrupt onset of colitis and identical radiographic and gross endoscopic appearances. Mucosal biopsy can be of considerable assistance in sorting out these disorders. Changes of chronic colitis are frequently seen in cases of ulcerative colitis and Crohn's disease, and include an altered architecture by complex branching and atrophy of the crypts, a villiform surface, Paneth cell metaplasia, a marked increase of mononuclear inflammatory cells in the lamina propria, and the interposition of numerous plasma cells and small lymphoid nodules between the crypt bases and the muscularis mucosae. In contrast, none of these histologic features is observed in cases of acute self-limited colitis. In the acute stage, there is evidence of cryptitis and a marked infiltrate of neutrophils which are concentrated in the superficial half of the mucosa, but the crypts remain relatively straight and there is no prominence of mononuclear inflammatory cells. Upon recovery, there is complete restoration of the mucosa to normal in cases of acute self-limited colitis, whereas the changes of chronic colitis persist in the great majority of cases of ulcerative colitis.

COLITIS CYSTICA PROFUNDA

DEFINITION AND ETIOLOGY

This denotes a condition in which mature colonic epithelium extends through the muscularis mucosae into the submucosa or deeper parts of the intestinal wall (193–196). It is most commonly observed as an isolated lesion in the late stages of the solitary rectal ulcer syndrome which is described in a separate section. Multiple small lesions are less often seen as a consequence of a chronic inflammatory condition of the colon such as ulcerative colitis, Crohn's disease, radiation colitis, and colonic schistosomiasis (197–200); rare cases have been observed in an apparently normal colon (201, 202). In the inflammatory disorders, it is believed that the colitis cystica forms as a result of an ulceration with destruction of the muscularis mucosae and subsequent regeneration of the mucosal glands that extend through the gap into the underlying tissues of the bowel wall. Considering the high frequency of ulceration in such disorders, however, it is not clear why colitis cystica is not more commonly seen, suggesting that additional factors may be involved in its genesis. Equivalent lesions are seen in the stomach and small intestine and referred to respectively as gastritis cystica profunda and as enteritis cystica profunda.

CLINICAL FEATURES

Colitis cystica is usually a small and incidental histologic finding, and the clinical course is determined by the underlying inflammatory disease. Exceptionally, there may be a larger lesion associated with a polypoid mucosa or deep extension into the wall, and

the appearance may grossly resemble a tumor (202). This circumstance takes on special significance since the underlying inflammatory conditions are particularly prone to the development of adenocarcinoma.

PATHOLOGY

Gross alterations may be observed in the larger lesions and include a raised or polypoid mucosa and a mucinous appearance of the wall. The histologic features are distinctive and reveal the presence of cystically dilated colonic glands within the submucosa and occasionally into the deeper parts of the intestinal wall. The epithelial cells lining the glands are usually normal or hyperplastic, containing basal nuclei and abundant cytoplasm, or they may show signs of regeneration. There is no dysplasia of the epithelium, and the stromal tissue around the misplaced glands is typically composed of the lamina propria.

DIFFERENTIAL DIAGNOSIS

The diagnosis of colitis cystica profunda is based on the finding of colonic glands with mature or regenerative epithelium beneath the mucosal layer. In the normal colonic mucosa, there are numerous lymphoid follicles which frequently extend into the uppermost portion of the submucosa. The muscularis mucosae is interrupted at these points, and small portions of the crypt bases are often present in the superficial submucosa in such areas. This appearance may cause some difficulty, particularly in tangential or peripheral microscopic sections that do not reveal the complete lymphoid follicle, but it can be readily separated from colitis cystica by knowing of its existence and by noting that the glands are collapsed rather than cystic and that they are invariably associated with lymphoid tissue. The most important distinction of colitis cystica is with adenocarcinoma which can also develop as a complication of chronic colitis. In this regard, well-differentiated or mucinous carcinomas are often encountered in these inflammatory diseases. The diagnosis of carcinoma is dependent on finding some degree of dysplasia of the epithelial cells and on the frequent presence of inflammation and a loose stroma between the neoplastic glands and the normal tissues. Some cases of hyperplastic polyps (203, 204) and adenomas (205) of the colon reveal misplacement of the glands into the submucosa, but these lesions can be easily recognized by noting the characteristic features of the mucosal component and of the dysplastic epithelium.

SOLITARY RECTAL ULCER SYNDROME

DEFINITION AND ETIOLOGY

This condition is characterized by the presence of ulcers or polypoid inflammatory lesions in the rectum and is often associated with mucosal prolapse (206–217). It is thought to be due to a malfunction of the internal anal sphincter or of the overall rectal musculature resulting in chronic straining upon defecation and the development of rectal prolapse and mucosal erosions (209, 210, 216, 218). Following repeated episodes, there is often exuberant repair leading to the formation of a polyp and to the extension of glands into the submucosa. The term "syndrome" has been applied to this condition, because the initial ulcerative phase may be either not identified or associated with multiple lesions. Considering the variability of the early features and of the manometric studies as well as the frequent dominance of the polypoid stage, it has also been suggested that the condition might be due to a hamartomatous process (207). Other names that have been proffered to describe the various features include localized colitis (or proctitis) cystica profunda in cases with submucosal involvement (206, 214), inflammatory cloacogenic polyp in those with a prominent mass (219–221), and mucosal prolapse syndrome (213) to depict the full range of changes associated with rectal prolapse.

CLINICAL FEATURES

Although the solitary rectal ulcer syndrome was once considered to be rare, it is now being encountered with increased frequency and it is probable that the condition has been greatly overlooked in the past (215). In this regard, the clinical diagnosis is often delayed and is suspected in only about 33% of the cases, and its initial recognition is usually provided by morphologic study. The lesion is more common in women, and the peak incidence is in the third and fourth decades. Major symptoms include straining on defecation, constipation, anorectal or abdominal pain, rectal bleeding, and a mucous discharge (212, 218, 222, 223). Rectal prolapse is identified in about 80% of the cases, and recognition of the mucosal lesions often requires that the patient strain down at time of proctoscopic examination (210). There is no definitive medical therapy and attempts of local surgical resection are usually not successful (212). The disorder typically persists or recurs and only a minority of cases completely resolve. Treatment is typically limited to the use of laxatives and the assurance to the patient that a more serious condition is not present.

PATHOLOGY

About 85% of the lesions are noted on the anterior wall of the rectum, and they are located up to 18 cm above the anal verge with most occurring in the distal 3 to 5 cm (209, 212, 215). The early lesion is typically a single small and shallow ulcer, ranging up to 1 cm in diameter, which is relatively well-demarcated and often associated with erythema and slight elevation of the adjacent mucosa. Larger ulcers up to 6 cm have been uncommonly observed. Multiple ulcers are infrequently seen, whereas the initial ulcerated lesion may be absent in about 33% of the cases (218), possibly because the patient is not evaluated at the early stage of the disease. Histologic examination reveals necrosis that is often limited to the superficial half of the mucosa together with acute inflammation and prominent hemorrhage in the adjacent mucosa. In addition, there is a characteristic fibromuscular hyperplasia in the lamina propria, which is best visualized by examination of the adjacent nonulcerated mucosa. Accordingly, biopsy samples should be selected from the edges of the ulcer to permit its detection.

The older lesions are associated with the development of a polypoid mass in the majority of the cases. The polyps vary in size, ranging up to 3 or 4 cm in diameter, are typically sessile, and have either a smooth surface or a papillary contour resembling an adenoma. There may be patches of superficial necrosis but there is usually no discrete ulceration at this stage. The polyps are composed of regenerating glands with variable reduction of mucus and a faint serrated appearance, similar to that seen in hyperplastic polyps, and they are distinguished by the presence of a marked fibromuscular proliferation in the lamina propria (224) (Fig. 30.10). The larger polyps are often associated with a villiform surface (Fig. 30.11) and

occasionally reveal focal loss of the muscularis mucosae and extension of cystic colonic glands into the submucosa (Fig. 30.12), representing a localized form of colitis cystica profunda (206). There is no dysplasia of the epithelium, and the misplaced glands are not associated with any inflammation or newly-formed stroma (Fig. 30.13). Other features of mucosal prolapse may be observed in the adjacent mucosa, including foci of hemorrhagic necrosis and patchy inflammation (213). The submucosal ganglia and nerves appear to be normal, and there are no abnormalities of the muscularis propria.

DIFFERENTIAL DIAGNOSIS

The diagnosis of the solitary rectal ulcer syndrome depends on the findings of the characteristic fibromuscular hyperplasia in the lamina propria at the edge of an ulcer or in a polyp and of the absence of any epithelial dysplasia. Rectal ulcers may be seen in many other common inflammatory conditions, including infections, ischemic injury, ulcerative colitis, and Crohn's disease, but the lesions in these disorders are more often multiple or diffuse and diarrhea is a prominent feature. Localized ulcers can also occur as a result of stasis, pressure necrosis from a stercoral lesion, and various generalized diseases, and they are separated by the non-specific nature of the histologic features or by the clinical information. The most important distinction of the lesions in the later stages is with other polyps and with adenocarcinoma of the rectum. It may be very difficult to separate the polyps of the solitary ulcer syndrome from inflammatory and juvenile-type polyps on the basis of the histologic features alone, and one must rely on the clinical findings in such cases. Hyperplastic polyps are typically small and barely raised, and they lack necrosis, inflammation, and the fibromuscular proliferation in the lamina propria. Adenomas, with or without misplaced epithelium, and carcinomas are readily distinguished by the presence of dysplasia of the epithelium; furthermore, there is often prominent inflammation and a loose connective tissue stroma around the submucosal glands in cases of invasive carcinoma.

EFFECTS OF LAXATIVES AND ENEMAS

MELANOSIS COLI

This is a common asymptomatic condition that is characterized by the prominent presence of a lipofuscin-type pigment in the macrophages of the lamina propria of the large bowel (225–229). Since the pigment is not melanin, it has been suggested that the condition might be termed instead pseudomelanosis coli. It is thought to be due mainly to the continued use of anthracene-containing laxatives which include cascara sagrada, senna, aloe, rhubarb, and frangula. The condition is more commonly noted in adult females which may simply reflect the rate of laxative usage. Estimates of its frequency range from 5% in endoscopic studies to 10% in autopsy surveys, and it has been determined that it takes from 4 to 12 months for the lesion to grossly appear and an equivalent time for its regression after the cessation of the laxative use. There are no clinical problems that are directly related to the pigment deposition. The lesion involves all parts of the rectum, colon, and appendix but tends to spare the regions of the mucosa occupied by lymphoid nodules, polyps, and carcinomas. When the deposition is very marked, the mucosa may be grossly dark brown

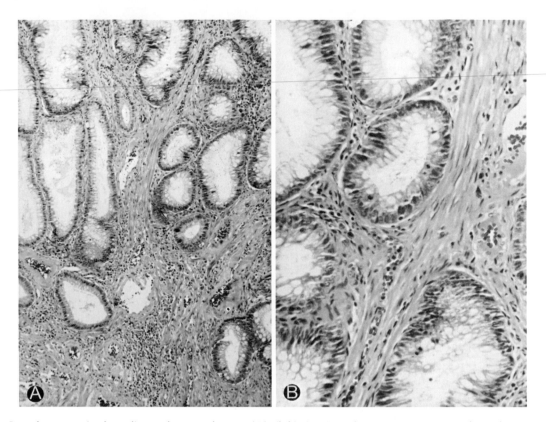

Figure 30.10 Rectal mucosa in the solitary ulcer syndrome. **(A)** *(left)*. Section of mucosa next to an ulcer, showing the prominent fibromuscular stroma and the serrated appearance of the glands. H & E, ×100. **(B)** *(right)*. Closer view of the mucosa revealing the fibromuscular hyperplasia in the lamina propria. H & E, ×400.

(Fig. 30.14), and the appearance must be distinguished from old hemorrhages and necrosis which would show a loss of the normal mucosal luster. Histologic study reveals that the brown, finely granular pigment is within macrophages (Fig. 30.15) and that it has the tinctorial characteristics of a lipofuscin based on positive staining with fat stains and the periodic acid-Schiff reaction. Similar pigment deposition may be seen in various storage diseases and in chronic granulomatous disease (see Chapter 19), but the macrophages in these disorders tend to be larger and arranged in clusters or nodules. The storage diseases also show pigment in other mesenchymal cells and in nerves. Scattered macrophages containing lesser amounts of lipofuscin are occasionally seen in the mucosa of normal persons, and the distinction from melanosis coli is a matter of degree (230).

Patches of pseudomelanin deposition have also been noted in the duodenal mucosa at endoscopic examination (231–233), particularly in patients with chronic renal failure (234). The pigment appears to be an iron derivative and may be due to episodes of mucosal hemorrhage in these patients (235, 236). There does not appear to be any relationship to laxative use or to the colonic condition.

CATHARTIC COLON

This is an uncommon disorder that can result from the extensive and long-term use of laxatives leading to the development of a dilated and hypotonic colon (237, 238). It is more common in

women and usually requires over 15 years of laxative use before its formation. The laxatives employed have been of all sorts including anthracene compounds, resins, and irritant oils. The patients typically present with chronic constipation and abdominal pain, and there are no signs of fever, diarrhea, or bleeding. It is thought that the cause is a toxic effect on the nerves and plexuses leading to secondary muscle damage in the bowel wall (239). The effects typically begin in the region of the ileocecal valve and right colon and progress with time to the distal portion, showing a dilated and tubular-appearing bowel with loss of the haustral markings and a dried-out mucosal surface (240, 241). Histologic features include the variable presence of mucosal and crypt atrophy, a thickening of the muscularis mucosae, and a vacuolization of the ganglion cells. Melanosis coli may also be present but is an independent effect of some of the laxatives. The cathartic colon must be distinguished from other causes of colonic dilation such as pseudo-obstruction disorders (242), and this is accomplished by the history and the lack of lesions in other parts of the gut (see Chapter 13 on Motor and Mechanical Disorders).

LAXATIVE ABUSE SYNDROME

This is due to the excessive and surreptitious use of laxatives leading to the appearance of unexplained chronic diarrhea and loss of protein and potassium (243, 244). It must be suspected when thorough gross and microscopic evaluation of the intestines fails to reveal any pathologic lesions.

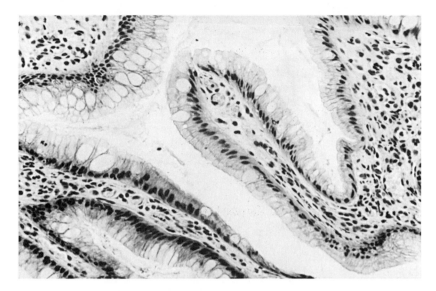

Figure 30.11   Rectal polyp in an advanced case of the solitary ulcer syndrome. The surface has a prominent villous configuration but there is no nuclear atypicality. H & E, ×400.

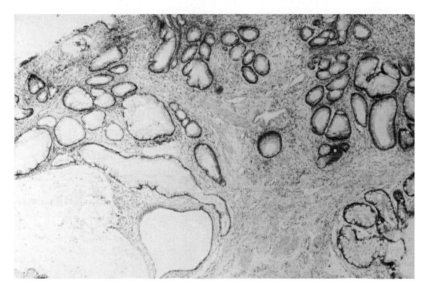

Figure 30.12   Rectal polyp in the solitary ulcer syndrome. The glands are irregular and extend into the submucosa *(lower left)*, representing a localized form of colitis cystica profunda. H & E, ×60.

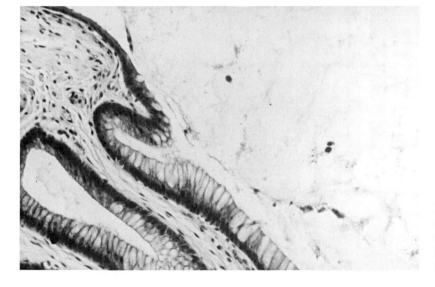

Figure 30.13   Rectal polyp in the solitary ulcer syndrome. Section of the submucosa, revealing the misplaced glands with mature cells and adjacent lamina propria type of stroma. There is no cellular atypicality. H & E, ×400.

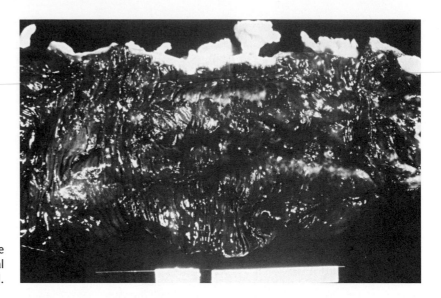

Figure 30.14 Melanosis coli. Mucosal surface of the colon, showing the dark brown color. The haustral folds are intact and the mucosa is otherwise normal.

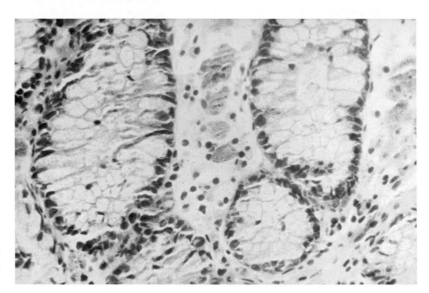

Figure 30.15 Colonic mucosa in melanosis coli. There are clumps of macrophages in the lamina propria, containing the finely granular and refractile lipofuscin material. The crypts are normal and there is no increase of other inflammatory cells. H & E, ×400.

EFFECTS OF ENEMAS

Saline enemas and other mild solutions used in the preparation of patients for colonoscopy often cause an edema of the lamina propria but no damage of the epithelium (8, 245, 246). More alterations are commonly noted with enemas containing Fleet Phospho-Soda (CB Fleet Co, Lynchburg, VA), bisacodyl, hydrogen peroxide, and other hypertonic solutions (246–249); the changes include a flattening and sloughing of the surface epithelium, a decrease in the staining of the upper crypt epithelial cells, a depletion of the goblet cell mucus, and the occasional presence of neutrophils in the lamina propria (Fig. 30.16). There are usually no symptoms from these enemas, but the histologic features may resemble those seen in a mild case of acute colitis or proctitis and must be discounted in the assessment of a mucosal biopsy. The enema changes typically resolve within a week.

Greater injury has been noted in the intestines following the use of enema or oral preparations that contain Kayexalate (sodium polystyrene sulfonate)-sorbitol solution (Sanofi Winthrop Pharma-ceuticals, NY) (250, 251). There is ischemic necrosis of the bowel that may be limited to the mucosa or extend into the wall leading to potential perforation, and the Kayexalate crystals can be seen in mucosal biopsy samples. A much more severe form of colitis has been observed with enemas using a soap solution, characterized by mucosal necrosis and greater inflammation leading to diarrhea and rectal bleeding (252, 253). The lesion is usually confined to the mucosa but may exceptionally extend deeper into the bowel wall (254, 255). Because of the frequency of these effects as well as the uncertain need of such irritating solutions, soap enemas are no longer recommended.

OTHER ULCERS OF THE COLON

Ulceration of the mucosa is a feature of many intrinsic colonic diseases, and the lesions tend to be multiple or diffuse and are associated with inflammatory changes in the intervening mucosa (Table 30.1). The present section deals with those ulcers that are localized and have a relatively nonspecific histologic appearance.

BEHÇET'S DISEASE

This is an uncommon disorder characterized by the presence of small aphthous ulcers of the oral cavity and the external genital region together with uveitis or iriditis (256, 257). It is thought to be an immune disorder, possibly mediated by a vasculitis, and lesions have also been noted in the skin, joints, and neuromuscular system. The gastrointestinal tract is involved in about 50% of the cases, and the ulcers tend to be concentrated in the distal ileum and proximal colon (258–261). The lesions are small and cause slight undermining of the adjacent mucosa; although most are superficial, they can exceptionally extend into the wall and cause perforation. The inflammatory reaction around the ulcers is nonspecific, and a vasculitis has not been well documented in the intestinal lesions. Based on the distribution of the disease in the intestine and the appearance of the aphthous ulcers, the syndrome may resemble early stage Crohn's disease but is readily separated by the lack of progression to larger ulcerated and strictured lesions, of sinus tracts, and of granulomas. Multiple, small shallow ulcers have also been noted in the esophagus (262–264) and in the stomach and duodenum (265, 266) in some cases of Behçet's disease.

STERCORAL ULCERS

These are most common in the distal colon and rectum and are due mainly to fecal impactions resulting in pressure-induced necrosis of the mucosal surface (267). They are analogous to the decubitus ulcers that occur in other surfaces such as the skin. The patients typically present with severe constipation, abdominal or rectal pain, and bleeding, and the clinical diagnosis is usually apparent. The ulcers may be single or multiple, vary in size from a few millimeters to several centimeters in diameter, and usually display sharply defined edges with congestion of the adjacent mucosa. They are most often confined to the submucosa, but deeper lesions and perforation may occur (268–270). The histologic features are fairly distinctive in the early lesions, revealing an ischemic-type injury characterized by extensive necrosis, marked congestion and patchy

hemorrhage, entrapped fecal material, and little inflammation. Chronic ulcers show the effects of repair and secondary infection, including neutrophilic reaction, variable fibrosis, and the appearance of giant cells and poorly formed granulomas in response to the fecal matter. Mucosal biopsy may be obtained in large lesions to exclude other inflammatory causes of ulceration and neoplasms.

NONSPECIFIC ULCERS OF THE COLON

Isolated ulcers of unknown or uncertain etiology spontaneously appear in all parts of the colon (271–276). Before considering this category, it is essential that ulcers due to the various intrinsic and secondary colonic diseases be excluded. In particular, localized ulcers of the rectum are usually part of the solitary rectal ulcer syndrome and are distinguished by their characteristic clinical and histologic features (206–215), as described in the previous section. Localized ulcers of the colon and rectum have also been noted in patients with radiation injury (72), with reactions to ergotamine suppositories (277, 278), contraceptive pills (279, 280) and other drugs (74–78, 281), and with atheromatous emboli (85, 282) and vasculitis (83, 84, 283). A predilection for cecal lesions occurs in cases of renal failure (284, 285), agranulocytosis (286–288), and of colonic obstruction (289). Rare cases have been recorded as a result of cocaine ingestion (290, 291) and of retained cleansing solutions in endoscopes (292).

The nonspecific ulcers of the colon have been noted most commonly in the cecum and proximal ascending portion, followed by the sigmoid colon, and appear to be least frequent in the transverse and descending parts. They may be seen in all age groups and typically present with bleeding from right-sided lesions and hemorrhage or obstruction from sigmoid cases. The lesions are identified by radiographic and endoscopic examination, and the diagnosis is obtained by noting the nonspecific nature on biopsy study and by the exclusion of other known causes of colonic ulceration.

Detailed pathologic studies have concentrated on the cecal ulcers, revealing that they are typically located on the antimesenteric border and that they vary in size and depth (273). The ulcers may be up to several centimeters in diameter, and deep penetration of the

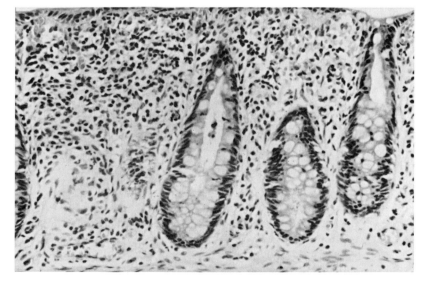

Figure 30.16 Rectal mucosa in a mild case of enema-induced colitis. There is a flattening of the surface epithelium, a slight pallor of the superficial mucosa, and the presence of rare neutrophils. H & E, ×100. Reproduced, with permission, from Goldman H, Antonioli DA. Mucosal biopsy of the rectum, colon and distal ileum. Hum Pathol 1982;13:981–1012.

intestinal wall and perforation have been described. The histologic features are essentially nonspecific, showing acute and chronic inflammation, prominent granulation tissue, variable fibrosis, and fibrin thrombi in small vessels. It has been considered that the ulcer might be a consequence of inflammation and effacement of a localized diverticulum of the cecum (293), and this might apply in the younger patients in whom such limited diverticula away from the mesenteric border are more commonly observed. In older patients, an ischemic process has been postulated, based in part on its greater probability in this age group, but also on the histologic character of the lesion (274). In this regard, the lesion of vascular ectasia (or angiodysplasia) is known to occur in the cecum of older patients and is thought to be the result of chronic constipation leading to increased transmural pressure in this area (294). Although these vascular cases usually present with massive hemorrhage and inconspicuous mucosal lesions, it is possible that they might be a nidus for secondary injury and the development of some of the cecal ulcers.

SECONDARY ULCERS OF THE COLON

Colonic ulcers can occur in other conditions that may affect the entire alimentary tract, and these are presented in detail in other parts of the book, including radiation and chemical injury (Chapter 11), motor and mechanical disorders (Chapter 13), vasculitis and other vascular diseases (Chapter 14), graft-versus-host reaction (295, 296) and other immunologic injuries (Chapter 16), and uremia (285), chronic granulomatous disease (297, 298), and other systemic disorders (Chapter 19).

IRRITABLE BOWEL SYNDROME

This is a common condition in which the patients present with intermittent crampy abdominal pain and watery or mucus-filled diarrhea, and the symptoms are often precipitated by stressful situations (299, 300). It has long been suspected that this is a functional disorder, but recent manometric studies have suggested the possibility of a motor disturbance. There are no gross or microscopic alterations. Endoscopy and mucosal biopsy are often obtained to exclude some form of enteritis or colitis. As noted previously, some of these patients are found to have collagenous or lymphocytic colitis.

OTHER TUMOR-LIKE LESIONS OF THE INTESTINES

PNEUMATOSIS INTESTINALIS

DEFINITION AND ETIOLOGY

This is a relatively common disorder characterized by the presence of air or other gas-filled cysts in the intestinal wall (301–305). Other names for this condition are pneumatosis cystoides intestinalis to honor the prominent cysts that may be present, and pneumatosis coli when the lesion is limited to the colon. It may involve the small or the large intestine, and there appear to be two major forms of the disease. The more common type often appears as an asymptomatic radiographic abnormality of the small intestine, and it is seen in patients with pulmonary emphysema or an obstructing peptic ulcer

of the gastric pylorus (306). In these situations, it is believed that air under high pressure escapes from a ruptured pulmonary bleb or through a penetrating posterior ulcer and passes through the retroperitoneum and along the adventitia of the mesenteric vessels to reach the bowel wall where it is deposited. The other type, which is seen more often in the colon, is thought to be the consequence of mucosal disease resulting in the penetration of luminal gases or gas-forming bacteria into the mucosa and underlying tissues (303–305, 307). Pneumatosis has been observed in a wide variety of inflammatory conditions affecting the small intestine and colon, including infections, necrotizing enterocolitis, ischemic disease, ulcerative colitis, Crohn's disease, and mechanical obstruction. It may also be seen following trauma to the mucosa as a result of an endoscopic procedure (304, 308). Other theories of the genesis of pneumatosis suggest that there is a primary chemical injury of the mucosal and submucosal tissues (309) or that the gas is mainly contained within the mural lymphatics (310).

CLINICAL FEATURES

The disease may affect all age groups, including infants and children, and is more common in males, possibly reflecting their higher incidence of pulmonary disease and peptic ulcers. Most of the cases related to pulmonary disease or to pyloric obstruction are asymptomatic and the lesion is typically an incidental radiographic finding (306). Symptoms are more often present in the cases of pneumatosis that are associated with intestinal disease and reflect the underlying enteritis or colitis. Uncommonly, the lesion may be localized and large resembling a polypoid mass on radiographic and endoscopic examination or there may be signs of intestinal obstruction (307). The finding of pneumatosis in a patient with a clinically evident inflammatory or ischemic condition is often an ominous sign because it tends to correlate with cases that have greater necrosis. The pneumatosis may persist after the initiating event has subsided or it may regress after a variable period of time. Therapy is mainly directed at the underlying disease and treatment is not required for the pneumatosis lesion.

PATHOLOGY

The lesions are more common in the small intestine than the colon, and may involve any part of the bowel wall but are particularly prominent in the looser submucosal and subserosal layers (303–305). There is a marked expansion of the submucosa by the gas-filled cystic spaces, which range from a few millimeters to several centimeters in diameter, imparting a honeycomb or spongelike appearance. The mucosa is usually elevated over the cysts, and localized lesions may look like a broad-based polyp (Fig. 30.17). Less pronounced changes are noted in the subserosal area, and the muscularis propria is often spared except for the region around the piercing vessels in its superficial portion. The histologic features differ somewhat in the two major types of pneumatosis, particularly in the character of the inflammatory reaction. Both reveal cystic spaces of variable size that are lined mainly by flattened cells. It has long been debated whether these might be endothelial cells in support of the theory that the gas is contained within dilated lymphatics (310), but most believe that the lining is composed of indigenous mesenchymal cells that are compressed by the gas. There may be small foci of inflammation in the adjacent tissues in both types of pneumatosis, and cases related to mucosal disease often

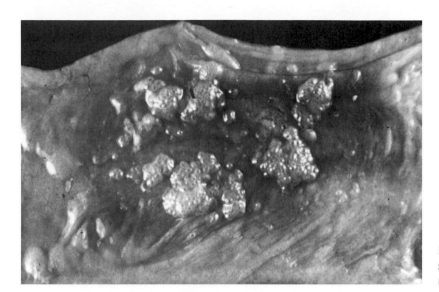

Figure 30.17 Pneumatosis coli. Mucosal surface showing an irregularly polypoid lesion composed of numerous gas-filled cysts.

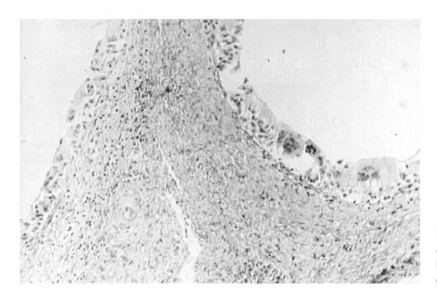

Figure 30.18 Colonic wall in a case of pneumatosis coli. There is a large gas-filled cyst *(upper right)*, lined by inflammatory tissue and a few multinucleated giant cells. H & E, ×100.

show more prominent proliferation of macrophages and giant cells at the edge of the cystic spaces (303) (Fig. 30.18). It is thought that this might represent a reaction to luminal products, although bacteria and fecal matter are not ordinarily found in the spaces. The mucosa frequently reveals inflammation, dilatation, and rupture of crypts, as well as microcysts with giant cells in the lamina propria (309, 311), and these features together with the cysts in the upper submucosa can be readily detected in biopsy samples (6, 312) (Fig. 30.19).

DIFFERENTIAL DIAGNOSIS

The diagnosis of pneumatosis intestinalis is easily accomplished by the demonstration of gas-filled spaces in the bowel wall. This is ordinarily done by radiographic and gross examinations and may be abetted by mucosal biopsy of lesions that protrude into the lumen. It is important that the intestine, particularly the mucosa, be carefully inspected to look for evidence of inflammatory or ischemic lesions, since the clinical course is largely dependent on the presence

and extent of any primary intestinal disease. The postmortem formation of gas gangrene, due to invasion and proliferation of gas forming bacteria such as *Clostridium welchii*, can also produce the appearance of large gaseous cysts in the intestinal wall. This can be readily distinguished from pneumatosis by histologic examination, which reveals extensive autolysis of the tissues in the absence of an inflammatory reaction together with the finding of many large bacterial rods. In patients with severe neutropenia, a necrotizing colitis that is mainly due to virulent streptococci can occur, and irregular spaces are often seen in the intestinal wall upon microscopic examination (286–288). There are typically no gross cystic lesions, however, and the specific diagnosis is provided by the finding of many bacteria in the wall and by cultures of the stool and tissues.

Other conditions that may need to be distinguished from pneumatosis intestinalis because of the presence of irregular or cystic spaces include areas of fat necrosis, foreign body reactions to other fatty substances that are dissolved during the tissue preparation (such as an oleogranuloma), enteritis or colitis cystica profunda, and

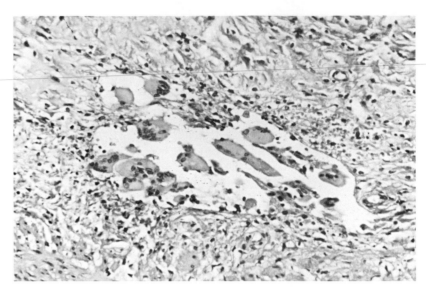

Figure 30.19   Colonic biopsy in a case of pneumatosis coli, revealing slit-like spaces lined by inflammatory giant cells in the submucosa. H & E, ×400. Reproduced, with permission, from Goldman H, Antonioli DA. Mucosal biopsy of the rectum, colon and distal ileum. Hum Pathol 1982;13:981–1012.

a lymphangioma. Areas of fat necrosis, which can be seen in any inflammatory disorder affecting the submucosa, are characterized by the appearance of small spaces and a marked inflammatory reaction with many foamy lipid-filled macrophages and fibrosis. A similar inflammatory reaction is noted in oleogranulomas, and these lesions are typically solitary and confined to the rectal area. In enteritis and colitis cystica profunda, the cysts are filled with mucus and lined by tall columnar epithelial cells. Lymphangiomas are usually solitary and more often circumscribed, and they may reveal lymph fluid within the cystic spaces and an attenuated, incomplete muscular wall.

ENDOMETRIOSIS

DEFINITION AND ETIOLOGY

This is a common condition characterized by the presence of ectopic endometrial tissue. It is most often encountered in the uterine wall, the pelvic adnexa and soft tissues, and in the peritoneum, and it may rarely be found in regional lymph nodes and in distant sites such as the lungs and pleura. Gastrointestinal involvement is noted in about 33% of the cases, and the most common location is in the distal colon and rectum (313–316). There are two major theories regarding the development of endometriosis. It has been suggested that endometrial tissue may extrude through the Fallopian tubes at time of normal menstruation, and this would explain the concentration of the lesions in the pelvic tissues and on the peritoneal surface. Alternatively, it is known that the celomic epithelium is capable of pleuripotential differentiation and is the probable source of tumors of Mullerian origin affecting the uterine adnexa, and this hypothesis would allow for the finding of endometriosis in all regions, including areas that are remote from the uterus. In either situation, the ectopic endometrial tissue can respond to the cyclic hormonal stimulation resulting in hemorrhage, fibrosis, and pressure effects in the affected tissues.

CLINICAL FEATURES

The disorder is typically seen in women during their reproductive years, with a peak incidence of severe symptoms in the fourth decade, and it declines or abates during pregnancy and after menopause. In most cases affecting the intestinal tract, the lesions are at a microscopic level and not productive of clinical problems from this area. Symptoms referable to involvement of the distal colon and rectum include constipation, abdominal or rectal pain, and occasional diarrhea which may be cyclic. Rectal bleeding is only rarely observed presumably because the lesions do not often extend into the mucosal layer (317–319). Obstruction is less common and is usually seen with larger lesions in the sigmoid colon and ileum, and this results from an intraluminal mass or stricture (313, 318), an intussusception (320), or serosal fibrosis and peritoneal adhesions. Such masses, which are composed mainly of fibrosis and hypertrophied smooth muscle, may persist in older patients and simulate a neoplasm. The presence of endometriosis in the appendix can also be associated with prominent bleeding and with an intussusception (321, 322). Patients with intestinal endometriosis may present with prominent symptoms but lack any findings on radiographic and endoscopic examinations, and they are often initially thought to have the irritable bowel syndrome or a functional complaint. Furthermore, even when gross lesions of intestinal endometriosis are detected by such studies, their exact nature is not revealed and the clinical diagnosis is typically dependent on the finding of compatible features of the disease in other more common locations. Treatment is identical to that for endometriosis in general and includes hormones and analgesics, and surgery may be required for the cases with obstruction, a mass of undetermined nature, or a rare perforation (323).

PATHOLOGY

Estimates of involvement of the gastrointestinal tract by endometriosis have ranged up to 34% (313–315, 320). Of these cases, lesions have been noted in the sigmoid colon and rectum in over 80%, the appendix in 5 to 10%, the cecum in 4%, and the small intestine, usually the distal ileum, in about 7%. Rare examples have also been noted in the proximal small intestine and in a Meckel's diverticulum. The endometriosis is most commonly present in the serosal surface and in the muscularis propria, and it may extend into the submucosa but only rarely into the mucosa. Lesions range in size from microscopic foci to several centimeters in diameter, and the smaller implants are soft and red due to the dominant presence of the endometrial tissue and hemorrhage. In contrast, most of the mass of the large lesions is composed of fibrous and muscle tissue imparting a pale and hard appearance. The gross features of endometriosis are also somewhat dependent on its location in the bowel wall. Lesions concentrated in the serosa are often associated with prominent fibrosis which may extend into the mesentery or mesocolon, whereas those embedded in the muscularis propria typically evoke a hypertrophy of the smooth muscle which may simulate a tumor of the intestinal wall. Least frequent is the appearance of a polypoid mass in the submucosa and mucosa (317–319).

Histologic examination reveals the characteristic endometrial tissue with glands and stroma, foci of fresh and old hemorrhage with inflammation and hemosiderin deposits, and variable fibrosis and smooth muscular hypertrophy (Fig. 30.20). In the larger lesions that are usually dominated by the presence of fibrous and muscular tissues, multiple histologic sections may be required to identify the endometriotic foci (Fig. 30.21). The major complication is intestinal obstruction which is most often at the level of the sigmoid colon (313) or the terminal ileum (314), and this results usually from a constricting lesion of the bowel wall or peritoneal fibrous adhesions. Obstruction due to a polypoid mass or its intussusception, major hemorrhage into the gut lumen, and perforation of the bowel wall are rarely seen (320, 323). Endoscopic examination and mucosal biopsy are mainly used to exclude other diseases and exceptionally

may detect the endometriosis when it involves the mucosa or upper submucosa (317) (Fig. 30.22). Rare cases of adenocarcinoma arising in endometriotic tissue within the colon have been reported (324), and these must be distinguished from the spread of a primary uterine tumor.

DIFFERENTIAL DIAGNOSIS

The diagnosis of endometriosis is dependent on the histologic finding of the typical glands and stroma of the ectopic tissue in the wall of the intestine. As noted, the residual foci of the endometriotic tissue may be sparse in the larger lesions, particularly in those affecting the muscularis propria, and it may be necessary to examine multiple tissue sections. Furthermore, repeated hemorrhages may result in considerable distortion and even loss of the stromal component, but the finding of the glands together with a surrounding fibromuscular proliferation should alert one to the possibility of endometriosis. The disease must be distinguished from other conditions that may be associated with an intestinal stricture, including mainly: ischemic disease, which usually affects older persons and has prominent bleeding; Crohn's disease, by the presence of greater diarrhea and the characteristic lesions of sinus tracts and granulomas; and adenocarcinoma of the colon, by the finding of dysplastic features in the glandular epithelium. Difficulties may arise in the assessment of mucosal biopsies containing endometriosis if there has been distortion or loss of the stroma component, but there should still be no atypism of the

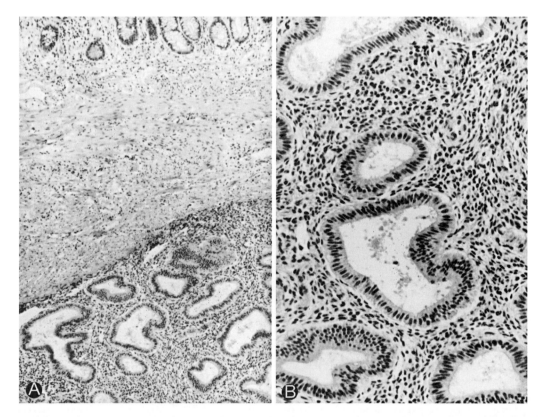

Figure 30.20   **(A)** *(left)*. Endometriosis of the ileum, with mucosal surface at top. There is a large nodule of endometriotic tissue in the intestinal wall *(bottom)*. H & E, ×60. **(B)** *(right)*. Closer view of the endometriotic tissue showing the characteristic glands and stroma. H & E, ×250.

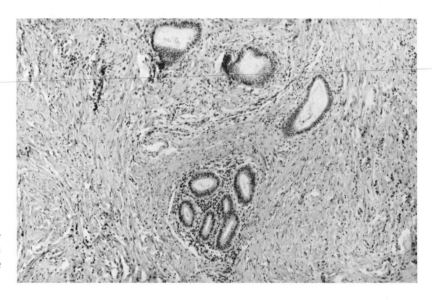

Figure 30.21 Endometriosis of the rectosigmoid colon. There is a small focus of endometriotic tissue in the muscle layer together with a proliferation of the smooth muscle tissue. H & E, ×60.

glands. In cases of endometriosis that are mainly in the muscularis propria, the associated muscular hypertrophy can mimic the appearance of a leiomyoma. The smooth muscle tumors tend to be well circumscribed, whereas endometriosis is more often circumferential or has ill-defined margins. The separation is provided by histologic examination of multiple sections to look for foci of ectopic tissue. The appearance of mural lesions, particularly in the distal ileum and appendix, with surrounding fibrosis that may extend into the contiguous mesentery, can also be caused by carcinoid tumors, and the distinction from endometriosis is readily made by the histologic finding of the typical neuroendocrine cells.

GASTRIC HETEROTOPIA

DEFINITION AND ETIOLOGY

This is a relatively common condition characterized by the presence of mature gastric fundic-corpus–type mucosa in ectopic locations throughout the alimentary tract (325, 326). The lesions are most commonly observed in the upper esophagus (327–331), proximal duodenum (332–334), and rectum (335–338), possibly because these are sites that are commonly inspected by endoscopic examinations. Nodules have also been noted in the jejunum (339), in Meckel's diverticulum (340–342), and in enteric and colonic duplication cysts (343, 344), whereas they are rarely seen in the normal distal ileum and proximal colon. The lesions are thought to arise from congenital rests, and this concept is supported by the appearance of fully developed gastric corpus mucosa, by the more common occurrence in children and young adults, by the frequent association with other anomalies of the intestinal tract, and by the absence of an underlying inflammatory condition in the affected tissues.

Such heterotopias in the intestines must be distinguished from the more common process of gastric metaplasia, which typically consists of the appearance of gastric pyloric glands (2, 4, 8) or surface-foveolar–type of mucous cells (31–33), and which develops as a consequence of chronic inflammatory disorders such as peptic duodenitis, celiac disease, Crohn's disease, and ulcerative colitis.

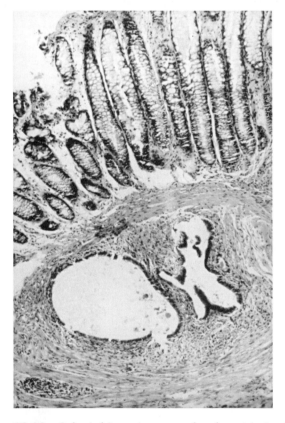

Figure 30.22 Colonic biopsy in a case of endometriosis, showing a small focus of endometrial glands in the submucosa. There is no cytologic atypicality. H & E, ×60.

Similarly, gastric heterotopia of the esophagus must be separated from Barrett's esophagus which occurs in patients with chronic esophagitis. The ectopic gastric tissue in typically confined to the upper esophagus and is composed of mature corpus tissue, whereas the Barrett lesion is located in the distal portion and shows a mixture of gastric and intestinal mucous cells (11).

CLINICAL FEATURES

Gastric heterotopia of the intestines may be seen in either sex and in all age groups, but the symptomatic cases appear to be more common in children. Most cases are asymptomatic and are observed as incidental findings during endoscopic examination of the duodenum (332) or as part of the pathologic study of excised diverticula and cysts (342–344). The specialized glandular cells are functional and secrete acid and proteolytic enzymes (328, 335), but the occurrence of peptic injury is mainly related to the location of the lesions. Thus, ulceration of the adjacent unprotected mucosa is often observed when gastric heterotopia involves relatively stagnant areas such as the rectum (336–338), congenital diverticula, and duplication cysts (342), whereas peptic injury is rarely seen in cases affecting the duodenum, possibly because of the prompt dilution of the acid by biliary secretions in this area. Lesions of the duodenum typically present with a small solitary nodule at endoscopy, and the diagnosis is readily established by biopsy study. It is important to separate gastric heterotopia, which may be seen in any part of the duodenum, from the changes of peptic duodenitis, which are concentrated in the first portion, because there is no relation between these two conditions. Exceptionally, there may be larger heterotopic nodules in the duodenum or jejunum and these can bleed or be the source for an intussusception (339). The esophageal cases are usually asymptomatic but may exceptionally develop ulceration and stricture (330).

Patients with lesions of the rectum and of developmental diverticula and cysts more often present with painless rectal bleeding, and the diagnosis is commonly made by a technetium scan. In the rectal cases, the luminal pH is typically less than 4 and vital stains such as Congo Red can be applied to detect the parietal cells (335). The cases with ulceration are prone to deep penetration of the wall and perforation, and fistulas may develop in the rectal lesions (337). Surgical excision is ordinarily required for these symptomatic cases.

PATHOLOGY

The primary lesion of gastric heterotopia is essentially the same in whatever part of the intestinal tract that it is located. It consists of a fairly well circumscribed nodule of variable size, with most less than 1 cm in diameter, that is typically sessile and slightly raised, and that has a smooth surface contour. The lesions are usually single, but multiple nodules and simultaneous involvement of different parts of the tract (e.g., both the esophagus and the duodenum) are occasionally noted. The histologic features are distinctive, revealing completely normal gastric corpus-fundic mucosa in most cases (Fig. 30.23). The flat surface and short foveolae (or pits) are lined by a continuous layer of tall columnar cells with mucous granules, which stain strongly with the periodic acid-Schiff reaction, concentrated in the luminal portions of the cytoplasm. Of interest, *Helicobacter pylori* may be noted next to the gastric mucous cells (345, 346). Most of the mucosa is occupied by the specialized glands which are closely packed and contain abundant parietal and

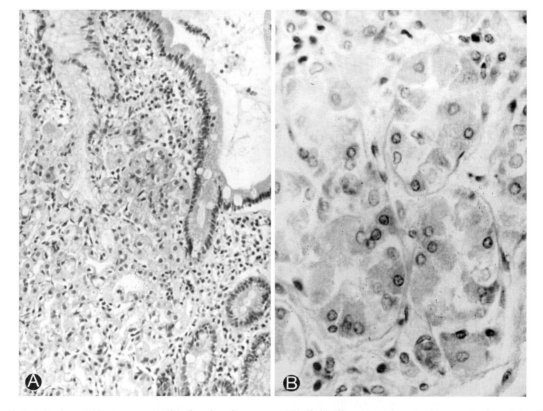

Figure 30.23 Heterotopic gastric mucosa in the duodenal mucosa. **(A)** *(left)*. There is a sharply demarcated nodule of normal gastric corpus-fundic type mucosa in the left portion, consisting of surface-foveolar mucous cells at the top and the specialized glands at the bottom. A small area of normal duodenal mucosa is at the right, and there is no inflammatory reaction. H & E, ×60. **(B)** *(right)*. Closer view of the specialized corpus glands showing both normal parietal and chief cells. There is no inflammation. H & E, ×400.

chief cells, and the margins of the lesions are sharply separated from the adjacent intestinal mucosa. The gastric tissue in the Meckel's diverticulum may show the changes of reflux gastritis due to action of the adjacent intestinal secretions, similar to what is noted in the stomach following reflux of duodenal material (347). Observed are edema and fibromuscular hyperplasia of the lamina propria together with variable hyperplasia of the gastric pits.

The duodenal cases are rarely associated with ulceration, and the finding of inflammation should alert one to the possible presence of a coexisting but unrelated duodenitis. Larger lesions of the small intestine are rare, and these can become inflamed or cause obstruction by an intussusception (339). In addition, cases of adenocarcinoma thought to arise in areas of gastric heterotopia involving the esophagus, jejunum, and a Meckel's diverticulum have been described (348–350).

In the gastric heterotopia involving the rectum and developmental cysts and diverticula, the ulcerations that occur are typically located in the intestinal mucosa that is immediately adjacent to the ectopic tissue (340, 342), since this area is unprotected and receives the highest concentration of gastric acid. This is analogous to the selective appearance of peptic injury in the first part of the duodenum or on the jejunal side of a gastrojejunostomy stoma. The ulcers vary in size and they are often deep, leading to free perforation or to the development of localized fistulae, with the latter more commonly observed in the rectal cases (337). It is also likely that the chance of perforation is enhanced in the cases involving diverticula and cysts by the pressure effects of inflammation and secondary ischemic damage in these relatively contained structures. The inflammation around the ulcerated areas may extend into the heterotopic nodules resulting in damage and loss of some or all of the ectopic tissue. In this regard, gastric heterotopic tissue is noted in only about 50% of the cases of ruptured Meckel's diverticulum (341), and it is possible that some of these cases may have lost the identifiable ectopic tissue rather than representing examples of simple mechanical perforation.

DIFFERENTIAL DIAGNOSIS

The diagnosis of gastric heterotopia depends simply on the histologic identification of normal gastric corpus-fundic mucosa in any other part of the alimentary tract. At a microscopic level, it must be distinguished from gastric metaplasia which is a frequent finding in many chronic inflammatory conditions of the esophagus and intestinal tract. The metaplasia typically consists of a proliferation of pyloric glands (2, 4, 11) and a more variable presence of the surface-foveolar–type of mucous cells. Scattered parietal and chief cells or small clusters of these cells may uncommonly be present, particularly in cases affecting the esophagus, but the appearance of a completely normal gastric corpus is not seen in the metaplastic process. In cases of Barrett's esophagus, the gastric metaplasia is admixed with intestine-type mucous cells and distal samples may show some parietal and chief cells; the presence of a normal gastric fundus in this area is typically indicative of a hiatal hernia. Furthermore, gastric heterotopia is usually in the cervical part of the esophagus (327), whereas the changes of Barrett's esophagus start in and are concentrated in the distal portion. Chronic peptic duodenitis often reveals a partial transformation of the epithelial cells overlying the villi into those of the gastric surface-type (31–33), and similar changes together with patches of pyloric glands have

been noted in long-standing cases of celiac disease. Pyloric gland metaplasia is also a common finding in Crohn's disease, particularly of the small intestine, where it appears as patches of mature glands at the base of the inflamed mucosa. Gastric heterotopia of the duodenum frequently presents with small nodules, and the gross differential includes mainly Brunner gland hyperplasia and lymphoid hyperplasia in this area.

FOREIGN BODY REACTIONS

This subject is presented in part in the section on Foreign Bodies in Chapter 13 on Motor and Mechanical Disorders, and in the section on Granulomatous Disorders in Chapter 19 on Systemic and Miscellaneous Disorders, and the present section concentrates on those conditions that have their major or exclusive effects in the intestinal tract.

Foreign objects that are ingested or that are introduced through the rectum or a stoma can cause clinical problems by laceration of the mucosal surface and by obstruction of the lumen. The inflammatory reaction, in such cases, is often nonspecific but may reveal focal granulomas, and the intensity is largely determined by the degree of trauma to the intestinal wall. The foreign body may lodge in an area of preexisting intestinal disease, and the combination may be responsible for the onset of symptoms. Perforation and fibrous stricture can develop, and surgery is often required for these complications and for the removal of objects that are not spontaneously passed in the feces.

Localized granulomatous reactions in the intestinal mucosa and wall can occur in response to a wide assortment of foreign substances (Table 30.3). These include: mucin that has escaped from ruptured crypts in cases of enteritis or colitis, or from tissues that have been traumatized by prior biopsy or a surgical procedure; fecal matter at the sites of bowel perforations and, less commonly, in the wall of sinus tracts; and suture material that is part of a healing process or in a stitch abscess (351) (Fig. 30.24). The nature of the foreign substance can be readily identified in standard histologic sections in all of these situations, and there are usually no clinical problems that can be attributed to the granulomas alone. Reactions to talc (352–354) or to starch (355, 356) that was introduced during prior surgery have been most often noted on the peritoneal surface where they may be the cause of an exudative peritonitis, and the character of the substance is defined by its birefringent appearance. In any of these circumstances, if the foreign body nature of the granuloma is not evident, it may be necessary to consider other causes of granulomatous inflammation of the intestines, principally infections and Crohn's disease.

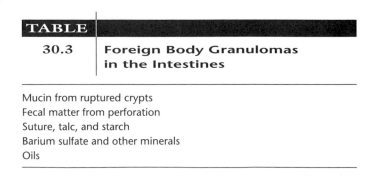

TABLE	
30.3	**Foreign Body Granulomas in the Intestines**

Mucin from ruptured crypts
Fecal matter from perforation
Suture, talc, and starch
Barium sulfate and other minerals
Oils

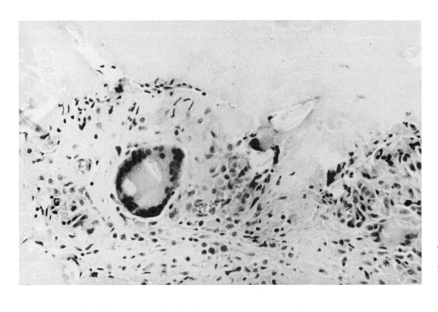

Figure 30.24 Suture reaction in the colonic wall. There are many multinucleated inflammatory giant cells that contain and surround the suture material. H & E, ×250.

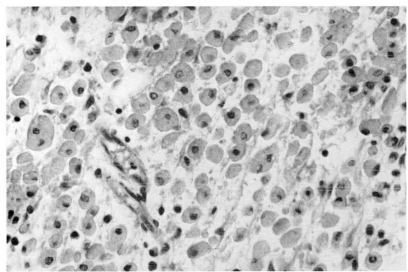

Figure 30.25 Barium granuloma in the colonic submucosa. There is a mass of macrophages containing the fine brown, refractile barium sulfate material. Otherwise, there is very little inflammatory reaction. H & E, ×400.

BARIUM GRANULOMA

This is a nodule of barium sulfate and reactive macrophages that is most commonly seen in the submucosa of the rectum (357, 358). It results from the passage of barium through the mucosal layer at time of radiographic study, and its occurrence is facilitated by prior endoscopic or biopsy examination and by the presence of preexisting mucosal disease (359). Most lesions are small incidental findings, whereas patients with larger nodules typically present with rectal pain and constipation. The granulomas vary in size, ranging up to 10 cm in diameter, are usually concentrated in the submucosa as a fairly well circumscribed mass, and may contain pale green crystals of barium sulfate upon gross inspection. The larger lesions may also show a central umbilication or small ulcer on the mucosal aspect, and the barium sulfate may extrude into the perirectal tissues (360). The histologic appearance is fairly distinctive, revealing a mass of macrophages that contain the barium sulfate granules, which have a faint brownish color on H & E stained slides and are refractile but not birefringent (361) (Fig. 30.25). There may be an

occasional giant cell but well formed, discrete granulomas of the sarcoid type are not seen. Since the barium sulfate is an inert substance, there are no other signs of inflammation unless the nodule has occurred in an area of prior disease. Most of the lesions eventually regress, and surgical excision is usually not required. Barium granulomas are less commonly seen in other parts of the intestine and are typically revealed as incidental findings on histologic examination (359).

OIL GRANULOMA

This is an uncommon condition that represents an inflammatory reaction to exogenous oily substances, and it has also been called an oleogranuloma (351, 362–365). The lesions are located in the rectum and are due to the introduction of a lubricant in this area or of an oil-based medium at time of local sclerosis of hemorrhoidal varices (362, 365). As is noted in other tissues in the body, the strongest inflammatory reactions are caused by mineral oil. Most

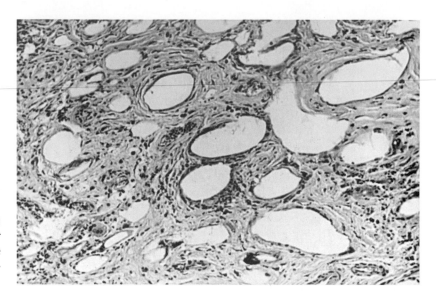

Figure 30.26 Oil granuloma (oleogranuloma) in the rectal submucosa. There are many ovoid clear spaces due to the extraction of the lipid in the tissue preparation, together with a prominent inflammatory and fibrotic reaction. H & E, ×100.

cases are observed as a small incidental finding during a rectal examination, or the patient may present with pain, constipation, and occasional bleeding. It is usually a single well circumscribed nodule, ranging up to a few centimeters in diameter, and it is concentrated in the submucosa but may show focal extension into the mucosa and muscularis propria. The histologic features are characteristic, revealing irregular spaces that are surrounded by macrophages and prominent fibrosis (Fig. 30.26). Giant cells containing lipid are sparse and well formed granulomas of the sarcoid type are not observed. Some cases, possibly representing an earlier stage or a reaction to more toxic oils, show a greater amount of acute and chronic inflammatory cells including eosinophils (351). The spaces result from the extraction of the lipid during the slide preparation, and their nature can be confirmed by fat stains performed on frozen sections, although this is typically not needed for the diagnosis. The lesions appear as a solitary mass or, uncommonly, as a stricture in the rectum resembling a neoplasm (363), and biopsy and surgery may be required to establish the diagnosis and to relieve any obstruction.

Oil granulomas must be distinguished from other rectal lesions that reveal cystic changes in the submucosa. Areas of fat necrosis are usually associated with less fibrosis and reveal a greater prominence of foamy macrophages due to the deposition of the triglycerides within the cells in the form of fine droplets, and there is often other evidence of a proctitis. The lesions of pneumatosis intestinalis typically show very little inflammation and fibrosis and are more diffuse. In the solitary rectal ulcer syndrome involving the submucosa, the cystic spaces are filled with mucus and lined by tall columnar epithelial cells.

REFERENCES

1. Owen DA, Kelly JK. Inflammatory diseases of the gastrointestinal tract. Modern Pathol 1995;8:97–108.
2. Goldman H, Antonioli DA. Mucosal biopsy of the esophagus, stomach and proximal duodenum. Hum Pathol 1982;13:423–448.
3. Chang MH, Wang TH, Hsu JY, et al. Endoscopic examination of the upper gastrointestinal tract in infancy. Gastrointest Endosc 1983;29:15–17.
4. Perera DR, Weinstein WM, Rubin CE. Small intestinal biopsy. Hum Pathol 1975;6:157–217.
5. Scott BB, Jenkins D. Endoscopic small intestinal biopsy. Gastrointest Endosc 1981;27:162–167.
6. Goldman H, Antonioli DA. Mucosal biopsy of the rectum, colon and distal ileum. Hum Pathol 1982;13:981–1012.
7. Yardley JH, Donovitz M. Colo-rectal biopsy in inflammatory bowel disease. In: Yardley JH, Morson BC, Abell MR, eds. The gastrointestinal tract. Baltimore: Williams & Wilkins, 1977:50–94.
8. Goldman H. Interpretation of large intestinal mucosal biopsies. Hum Pathol 1994;25:1150–1159.
9. Rotterdam H, Sheahan DG, Sommers SC, eds. Biopsy diagnosis of the digestive tract, 2nd ed. New York: Raven Press, 1993.
10. Whitehead R. Mucosal biopsy of the gastrointestinal tract, 5th ed. Philadelphia: WB Saunders, 1996.
11. Goldman H. Gastrointestinal mucosal biopsy. New York: Churchill Livingstone, 1996.
12. Jaffe SN, Lee FD, Blumgart LH. Duodenitis. Clin Gastroenterol 1978;7:635.
13. Owen DA. Gastritis and duodenitis. In: Appelman HD, ed. Pathology of the esophagus, stomach, and duodenum. New York: Churchill Livingstone, 1984:37–77.
14. McCallum RW, Singh D, Wollman J. Endoscopic and histologic correlations of the duodenal bulb: the spectrum of duodenitis. Arch Pathol Lab Med 1979;103:169–172.
15. Greenlaw R, Sheahan DG, DeLuca V, et al. Gastroduodenitis: a broader concept of peptic ulcer disease. Dig Dis Sci 1980;25:660.
16. Hasan M, Sirius W, Ferguson A. Duodenal mucosal architecture in non-specific and ulcer-associated duodenitis. Gut 1981;22:637–641.
17. Steer HW. Surface morphology of the gastroduodenal mucosa in duodenal ulceration. Gut 1984;25:1203–1210.
18. Hazell SL, Hennessy WB, Brody TJ, et al. Campylobacter pyloridis gastritis II: distribution of bacteria and associated inflammation in the gastroduodenal environment. Am J Gastroenterol 1987;82:297–301.
19. Wyatt JI. Histopathology of gastroduodenal inflammation: the impact of Helicobacter pylori. Histopathology 1995;26:1–15.
20. Frierson HF, Caldwell SH, Marshall BJ. Duodenal biopsy findings for patients with non-ulcer dyspepsia with or without Campylobacter pylori gastritis. Modern Pathol 1990;3:271–276.
21. Shabib SM, Cutz E, Drumm B, Sherman PM. Association of gastric metaplasia and duodenitis with Helicobacter pylori infection in children. Am J Clin Pathol 1994;102:188–191.
22. Paoluzi P, Pallone F, Palazzesi P, et al. Frequency and extent of bulbar duodenitis in duodenal ulcer, endoscopic and histological study. Endoscopy 1982;14:193–195.

23. Odeida G, Forni M, Farina L, et al. Duodenitis in children: clinical, endoscopic and pathological aspects. Gastrointest Endosc 1987;33: 366–369.

24. Shousha S, Spiller RC, Parkins RA. The endoscopically abnormal duodenum in patients with dyspepsia: biopsy findings in 60 cases. Histopathology 1983;7:23–34.

25. Weinstein WM. The diagnosis and classification of gastritis and duodenitis. J Clin Gastroenterol 1981;3(Suppl 2):7–16.

26. Jenkins D, Goodall A, Gille FR, Scott BB. Defining duodenitis: quantitative histological study of mucosal responses and their correlations. J Clin Pathol 1985;38:1119–1126.

27. Earlam RJ, Amerigo J, Kakavoulis T, Pollock DJ. Histological appearances of oesophagus, antrum and duodenum and their correlation with symptoms in patients with duodenal ulcer. Gut 1985; 26:95–100.

28. Yardley JH. Pathology of chronic gastritis and duodenitis. In: Goldman H, Appelman HD, Kaufman N, eds. Gastrointestinal Pathology. Baltimore: Williams & Wilkins, 1990:69–143.

29. Kreunig J, Bosman FT, Kuiper G, et al. Gastric and duodenal mucosa in healthy individuals. J Clin Pathol 1978;31:69–77.

30. Franzin G, Musola R, Ghidini O, et al. Nodular hyperplasia of Brunner's glands. Gastrointest Endosc 1985;31:374–378.

31. James AH. Gastric epithelium in the duodenum. Gut 1964;5: 285–294.

32. Shousha S, Parkins RA, Bille TB. Chronic duodenitis with gastric metaplasia: electron microscopic study including comparison with normal. Histopathology 1983;7:873–885.

33. Noach LA, Rold TM, Bosma NB, et al. Gastric metaplasia and Helicobacter pylori infection. Gut 1993;34:1510–1514.

34. Khulusi S, Badve S, Patel P, et al. Pathogenesis of gastric metaplasia of the human duodenum: role of Helicobacter pylori, gastric acid, and ulceration. Gastroenterology 1996;110:452–458.

35. Triadafilopoulos G. Clinical and pathologic features of the nodular duodenum. Am J Gastroenterol 1993;88:1058–1064.

36. Giannella RA, Broitman SA, Zamcheck N. Influence of gastric acidity on bacterial and parasitic enteric infections. Ann Intern Med 1973; 78:271–276.

37. Peters M, Weiner J, Whelan G. Fungal infection associated with gastroduodenal ulceration: endoscopic and pathologic appearances. Gastroenterology 1980;78:350–354.

38. Thomas E, Reddy KR. Non-healing duodenal ulceration due to candida. J Clin Gastroenterol 1983;5:55–58.

39. King CE, Toskes PP. Small intestine bacterial overgrowth. Gastroenterology 1979;76:1035–1055.

40. Rotterdam H, Tsang P. Gastrointestinal disease in the immunocompromised patient. Hum Pathol 1994;25:1123–1140.

41. Bown JW, Savides TJ, Mathews C, et al. Diagnostic yield of duodenal biopsy and aspirate in AIDS-associated diarrhea. Am J Gastroenterol 1996;91:2289–2292.

42. Ehrenpreis ED, Patterson BK, Brainer JA, et al. Histopathologic findings of duodenal biopsy specimens in HIV-infected patients with and without diarrhea and malabsorption. Am J Clin Pathol 1992;97:21–28.

43. Hinnant KL, Rotterdam HZ, Bell ET, Tapper ML. Cytomegalovirus infection of the alimentary tract: a clinicopathological correlation. Am J Gastroenterology 1986;81:944–950.

44. Chetty R, Roskell DE. Cytomegalovirus infection in the gastrointestinal tract. J Clin Pathol 1994;47:968–972.

45. Eras P, Goldstein MJ, Sherlock P. Candida infection of the gastrointestinal tract. Medicine 1972;51:367–379.

46. Ament ME, Rubin CE. Relation of giardiasis to abnormal intestinal structure and function in gastrointestinal immunodeficiency syndromes. Gastroenterology 1972;62:216–226.

47. Sun T. The diagnosis of giardiasis. Am J Surg Pathol 1980;4: 265–271.

48. Marshall JB, Kelley DH, Vogele K. Giardiasis: diagnosis by endoscopic brush cytology of the duodenum. Am J Gastroenterol 1984; 79:517–519.

49. Trier JS, Moxey PC, Schimmel EM. Chronic intestinal coccidiosis in man: intestinal morphology and response to treatment. Gastroenterology 1974;66:923.

50. DeHovitz JA, Pape JN, Boncy M, Johnson WD Jr. Clinical manifestations and therapy of Isospora belli infection in patients with the acquired immunodeficiency syndrome. N Engl J Med 1986; 315:87–90.

51. Marcial-Seoane MA, Serrano-Olmo J. Intestinal infection with Isospora belli. PRHSJ 1995;14:137–140.

52. Nime FA, Burek JD, Page DL, et al. Acute enterocolitis in a human being infected with the protozoan Cryptosporidium. Gastroenterology 1976;70:592–598.

53. Current WL, Reese NC, Ernst JV, et al. Human cryptosporidiosis in immunocompetent and immunodeficient persons. Studies of an outbreak and experimental transmission. N Engl J Med 1983;308: 1252–1257.

54. Guarda LA, Stein SA, Cleary KA, Ordonez NG. Human cryptosporidiosis in the acquired immune deficiency syndrome. Arch Pathol Lab Med 1983;107:562–566.

55. Lefkowitch JH, Krumholz S, Feng Chen KC, et al. Cryptosporidiosis of the human small intestine: a light and electron microscopic study. Hum Pathol 1984;15:746–752.

56. Isaacs D, Hunt GH, Phillips AD, et al. Cryptosporidiosis in immunocompetent children. J Clin Pathol 1985;38:76–81.

57. Wolfson JS, Richter JM, Waldron MA, et al. Cryptosporidiosis in immunocompetent patients. N Engl J Med 1985;312: 1278–1282.

58. Genta RM, Chappell CL, White AC, et al. Duodenal morphology and intensity of infection in AIDS-related intestinal cryptosporidiosis. Gastroenterology 1993;105:1769–1775.

59. Papp JP Jr, DeYoung BR, Fromkes JJ. Endoscopic appearance of cryptosporidial duodenitis. Am J Gastroenterol 1996;91: 2235–2236.

60. Simon D, Brandt LJ. Diarrhea in patients with the acquired immunodeficiency syndrome. Gastroenterology 1993;105: 1238–1242.

61. Shadduck JA, Orenstein JM. Comparative pathology of microsporidiosis. Arch Pathol Lab Med 1993;117:1215–1219.

62. Schwartz DA, Sobottka I, Leitch GJ, et al. Pathology of microsporidiosis. Emerging parasitic infections in patients with acquired immunodeficiency syndrome. Arch Pathol Lab Med 1996; 120:173–188.

63. Sun T, Ilardi CF, Asnis D, et al. Light and electron microscopic identification of cyclospora species in the small intestine. Evidence of the presence of asexual life cycle in human host. Am J Clin Pathol 1996;105:216–220.

64. Bonacini M, Kanel G, Alamy M. Duodenal and hepatic toxoplasmosis in a patient with HIV infection: review of the literature. Am J Gastroenterol 1996;91:1838–1840.

65. Zimmer G, Guillou L, Gauthier T, et al. Digestive leishmaniasis in acquired immunodeficiency syndrome: a light and electron microscopic study of two cases. Mod Pathol 1996;10:966–969.

66. Roth RI, Owen RZ, Keren DF, Volberding PA. Intestinal infection with Mycobacterium avium in acquired immune deficiency syndrome (AIDS). Histological and clinical comparison with Whipple's disease. Dig Dis Sci 1985;30:497–504.

67. Dworkin B, Wormser GP, Rosenthal WS, et al. Gastrointestinal manifestations of the acquired immunodeficiency syndrome: a review of 22 cases. Am J Gastroenterol 1985;80:774–778.

68. Witham RR, Mosser RS. An unusual presentation of schistosomiasis duodenitis. Gastroenterology 1979;77:1316.

69. Thatcher BS, Fleischer D, Rankin GB, Petras R. Duodenal schistosomiasis diagnosed by endoscopic biopsy of an isolated polyp. Am J Gastroenterol 1984;79:927–929.

70. Bone MF, Chesner LM, Oliver R, Asquith P. Endoscopic appearances of duodenitis due to strongyloidiasis. Gastrointest Endosc 1982;28: 190–191.

71. Volpicelli NA, Salyer WR, Milligan FD, et al. The endoscopic appearance of the duodenum in Whipple's disease. Johns Hopkins Med J 1976;138:19–23.

72. Berthrong M, Fajardo LF. Radiation injury in surgical pathology. Part II. Alimentary Tract. Am J Surg Pathol 1981;5:153–178.

73. Millan MS, Morris GP, Beck IT, et al. Villous damage induced by suction biopsy and by acute ethanol intake in normal human small intestine. Dig Dis Sci 1980;25:513–525.

74. Riddell RH. The gastrointestinal tract. In: Riddell RH, ed. Pathology of drug-induced and toxic diseases. New York: Churchill Livingstone, 1982:515–606.

75. Lee FD. Drug-related pathological lesions of the intestinal tract. Histopathology 1994;25:303–308.

76. Cunningham D, Morgan RJ, Mills PR, et al. Functional and structural changes of the human proximal small intestine after cytotoxic therapy. J Clin Pathol 1985;38:265–270.

77. Allison MC, Howatson AG, Torrance CJ, et al. Gastrointestinal damage associated with the use of non-steroidal anti-inflammatory drugs. N Engl J Med 1992;327:749–754.

78. Bjornason I, Hayllar J, Macpherson AJ, Russell AS. Side effects of non-steroidal anti-inflammatory drugs on the small and large intestine in humans. Gastroenterology 1993;104:1832–1847.

79. Jewell LD, Fields AL, Murray CJW, Thomson ABR. Erosive gastroduodenitis with marked epithelial atypia after hepatic infusion chemotherapy. Am J Gastroenterol 1985;80:421–424.

80. Schuger L, Peretz T, Goldin E, et al. Duodenal epithelial atypia. A specific complication of hepatic arterial infusion chemotherapy. Cancer 1988;61:663–666.

81. Shapiro N, Brandt L, Sproyregan S, et al. Duodenal infarction after therapeutic gel-foam embolization of bleeding duodenal ulcer. Gastroenterology 1981;80:176–180.

82. Shepherd HA, Patal C, Bamforth J, Isaacson P. Upper gastrointestinal endoscopy in systemic vasculitis presenting as an acute abdomen. Endoscopy 1983;15:307–311.

83. Camilleri M, Pusey CD, Chadwick VS, Rees AJ. Gastrointestinal manifestations of systemic vasculitis. Quart J Med 1983;206: 141–149.

84. Burke AP, Sobin LH, Virmani R. Localized vasculitis of the gastrointestinal tract. Am J Surg Pathol 1995;19:338–349.

85. Holly DC, Zachary PE. Cholesterol embolization leading to small and large bowel infarction. Am J Gastroenterol 1995;2075–2076.

86. Rutgeerts P, Onette E, Vantrappen G, et al. Crohn's disease of the stomach and duodenum: a clinical study with emphasis on the value of endoscopy and endoscopic biopsies. Endoscopy 1980;12:288.

87. Korelitz BI, Waye JD, Kreuning J, et al. Crohn's disease in endoscopic biopsies of the gastric antrum and duodenum. Am J Gastroenterol 1981;76:103–109.

88. Tanaka M, Kimura K, Sakai H, et al. Long-term follow-up for minute gastroduodenal lesions in Crohn's disease. Gastrointest Endosc 1986;32:206–209.

89. Alcantara M, Rodriguez R, Potenciano JLM, et al. Endoscopic and bioptic findings in the upper gastrointestinal tract in patients with Crohn's disease. Endoscopy 1993;25:282–286.

90. Frandsen PJ, Jarnum S, Malmstrom J. Crohn's disease of the duodenum. Scand J Gastroenterol 1980;15:683–688.

91. Falchuk ZM. Update on gluten-sensitive enteropathy. Am J Med 1979;67:50.

92. Collin P, Reunala T, Pukkala E, et al. Coeliac disease—associated disorders and survival. Gut 1994;1215–1218.

93. Yardley JH, Bayless TM, Norton JH. et al. Celiac disease: a study of the jejunal epithelium before and after a gluten-free diet. N Engl J Med 1962;267:1173–1179.

94. Schenk EA, Samloff IM, Klipstein FA. Morphologic characteristics of jejunal biopsy in celiac disease and tropical sprue. Am J Pathol 1965;47:765–781.

95. Variend S, Phillips AD, Walker-Smith JA. The small intestinal mucosal biopsy in childhood. Perspect Pediatr Pathol 1984;1:57–78.

96. Kluge F, Koch HK, Grosse-Wilde H, et al. Follow-up of treated adult celiac disease: clinical and morphological studies. Hepato-Gastroenterol 1982;29:17–23.

97. Bramble MG, Zucolato S, Wright NA, Record CC. Acute gluten challenge in treated adult coeliac disease: a morphometric and enzymatic study. Gut 1985;26:159–174.

98. Loft DE, Marsh MN, Crowe PT. Rectal gluten challenge and diagnosis of coeliac disease. Lancet 1990;335:1293–1295.

99. Alsaigh N, Odze R, Goldman H, et al. Gastric and esophageal intraepithelial lymphocytes in pediatric celiac disease. Am J Surg Pathol 1996;20:865–870.

100. Grybowski JD. Gastrointestinal milk allergy in infants. Pediatrics 1967;40:354–360.

101. Dobbins JW, Sheahan DG, Behar J. Eosinophilic gastroenteritis with esophageal involvement. Gastroenterology 1977;72:1312–1316.

102. Katz AJ, Goldman H, Grand RJ. Gastric mucosal biopsy in eosinophilic (allergic) gastroenteritis. Gastroenterology 1977;73:705–709.

103. Goldman H, Proujansky R. Allergic proctitis and gastroenteritis in children. Clinical and mucosal biopsy features in 53 cases. Am J Surg Pathol 1986;10:75–86.

104. Shiner M, Ballard J, Brook CGD, et al. Intestinal biopsy in the diagnosis of cow's milk protein intolerance without acute symptoms. Lancet 1975;2:1060–1063.

105. Walker-Smith JA, Harrison M, Kilby A, et al. Cow's milk-sensitive enteropathy. Arch Dis Child 1978;53:375–380.

106. Ament M, Rubin CE. Soy protein—another cause of the flat intestinal lesion. Gastroenterology 1972;62:227–234.

107. Perkkio M, Savilahti E, Kuitunen P. Morphometric and immunohistochemical study of jejunal biopsies from children with intestinal soy allergy. Fin Eur J Pediatr 1981;137:63–69.

108. Klein NC, Hargrove RL, Sleisenger MH, et al. Eosinophilic gastroenteritis. Medicine 1970;40:299–319.

109. Teele RL, Katz AJ, Goldman H, et al. Radiographic features of eosinophilic gastroenteritis (allergic gastroenteropathy) of childhood. Am J Radiol 1979;132:575–580.

110. Rosekrans PCM, Meijer CJLM, Cornelisse CJ, et al. Use of morphometry and immunohistochemistry of small intestinal biopsy specimens in the diagnosis of food allergy. J Clin Pathol 1980;33: 125–130.

111. Leinbach GE, Rubin CE. Eosinophilic gastroenteritis: a simple reaction to food allergies? Gastroenterology 1970;59:874–889.

112. Ament ME, Ochs HD, Davis SD: Structure and function of the gastrointestinal tract in primary immunodeficiency syndromes: a study of 39 patients. Medicine 1973;52:227–248.

113. Washington K, Stenzel TT, Buckley RH, Gottfried MR. Gastrointestinal pathology in patients with common variable immunodeficiency and X-linked agammaglobulinemia. Am J Surg Pathol 1996;20: 1240–1252.

114. Perlmutter PH, Leichtner AM, Goldman H, Winter HS. Chronic diarrhea associated with hypogammaglobulinemia and enteropathy in infants and children. Dig Dis Sci 1985;30:1149–1155.

115. Snover DC, Weisdorf SA, Vercolotti GM, et al. A histopathologic study of gastric and small intestinal graft-versus-host disease following allogeneic bone marrow transplantation. Hum Pathol 1985;16: 387–392.

116. Spencer GD, Shulman HM, Mayerson D, et al. Diffuse intestinal ulceration after marrow transplantation: a clinicopathologic study of 13 patients. Hum Pathol 1986;17:621–633.

117. Jeffries GH, Steinberg H, Sleisenger MH. Chronic ulcerative (nongranulomatous) jejunitis. Am J Med 1968;44:47–59.

118. Modigliani R, Poitras P, Galian A, et al. Chronic non-specific ulcerative duodenojejunoileitis: report of four cases. Gut 1979;20: 318–328.

119. Ruan EA, Komorowski RA, Hogan WJ, Soergel KH. Nongranulomatous chronic idiopathic enterocolitis: clinicopathologic profile and response to corticosteroids. Gastroenterology 1996;111:629–637.

120. Isaacson P, Wright DH. Malignant histiocytosis of the intestine. Its relationship to malabsorption and ulcerative jejunitis. Hum Pathol 1978;9:661–677.

121. Baer AN, Bayless TM, Yardley JH. Intestinal ulceration and malabsorption syndromes. Gastroenterology 1980;79:754–765.

122. Robertson DAF, Dixon MF, Scott BB, et al. Small intestinal ulceration: diagnostic difficulties in relation to coeliac disease. Gut 1983;24:565–574.

123. Bayless TM, Kapelowitz RF, Shelley WM, et al. Intestinal ulceration—a complication of celiac disease. N Engl J Med 1967; 276:996–1002.

124. Isaacson PG. Gastrointestinal lymphoma. Hum Pathol 1994;25: 1020–1029.

125. Passaro E Jr, Drenick E, Wilson SE. Bypass enteritis: a new complication of jejunoileal bypass for obesity. Am J Surg 1976;131: 169–174.

126. Drenick EJ, Ament ME, Finegold SM, et al. Bypass enteropathy: intestinal and systemic manifestations following small bowel bypass. JAMA 1976;236:269–272.

127. Francis WW, Iannuccilli E. Acute fulminating transmural ileocolitis after small bowel bypass for morbid obesity. Am J Surg 1978;135: 524–528.

128. Causey JQ. Granulomatous colitis and ileitis complicating jejunoileal bypass. Arch Intern Med 1978;138:1727.

129. Morson BC, Dawson IMP. Gastrointestinal pathology, 2nd ed. London: Blackwell Scientific Publishers, 1979:565.

130. Baillie EE, Abell MR. Enteritis cystica polyposa. Am J Clin Pathol 1970;54:643–649.

131. Kyriakos M, Condon SC. Enteritis cystica profunda. Am J Clin Pathol 1978;69:77–85.

132. Aftalion B, Lipper S. Enteritis cystica profunda associated with Crohn's disease. Arch Pathol Lab Med 1984;108:532–533.

133. Saul SH, Wong LK, Zinsser KR. Enteritis cystica profunda: association with Crohn's disease. Hum Pathol 1986;17:600–603.

134. Bolwell JS, James PD. Peutz-Jeghers syndrome with pseudoinvasion of hamartomatous polyp and multiple epithelial neoplasms. Histopathology 1979;3:39–50.

135. Shepherd NA, Bussey HJR, Jass JR. Epithelial misplacement in Peutz-Jeghers polyps. A diagnostic pitfall. Am J Surg Pathol 1987;11:743–749.

136. Boydstan JS Jr, Gaffey TA, Bartholomew LG. Clinicopathologic study of non-specific ulcers of the small intestine. Dig Dis Sci 1981;26:911–916.

137. Wayte DM, Helwig EB. Small bowel ulceration—iatrogenic or multifactorial origin? Am J Clin Pathol 1968;49:26–40.

138. Wilson IH, Cooley NV, Luibel FJ. Non-specific stenosing small bowel ulcers. Am J Gastroenterol 1968;50:449–455.

139. Bradford WD, Noce PS, Gutman LT, et al. Pathologic features of enteric infection with *Yersinia enterocolitica*. Arch Pathol 1974;98:17–22.

140. El-Maraghi NRH, Mair NS. The histopathology of enteric infection with *Yersinia pseudotuberculosis*. Am J Clin Pathol 1979;71:631–639.

141. Lawrason FD, Alpert E, Mohr FL, McMahon FG. Ulcerative-obstructive lesions of the small intestine. JAMA 1965;191:641–644.

142. Weiss SM, Rutenberg HL, Paskin DL, Zaren HA. Gut lesions due to slow-release KCl tablets. N Engl J Med 1977;246:111.

143. Barloon T, Moore SA, Mitros FA. A case of stenotic obstruction of the jejunum secondary to slow-release potassium. Am J Gastroenterol 1986;81:192–194.

144. Jackson CW, Haboubi NY, Whorwell PJ, Schofield PF. Gold-induced enterocolitis. Gut 1986;27:452–456.

145. Geltner D, Sternfeld M, Becker SA, Kori M. Gold-induced ileitis. J Clin Gastroenterol 1986;8:184–186.

146. Deana DG, Dean PJ. Reversible ischemic colitis in young women. Association with oral contraceptive use. Am J Surg Pathol 1995;19:454–462.

147. Bo-Linn GW, Vendrell DD, Lee E, Fordtran JS. An evaluation of the significance of microscopic colitis in patients with chronic diarrhea. J Clin Invest 1985;75:1559–1569.

148. Read NW, Krejs GJ, Read MG, et al. Chronic diarrhea of unknown origin. Gastroenterology 1980;78:264–271.

149. Lazenby AJ, Yardley JH, Giardiello FM, et al. Lymphocytic ("microscopic") colitis: a comparative histopathologic study with particular reference to collagenous colitis. Hum Pathol 1989;20:18–28.

150. Veress B, Lofberg R, Bergman L. Microscopic colitis syndrome. Gut 1995;36:880–886.

151. Jawhari A, Talbot IC. Microscopic, lymphocytic and collagenous colitis. Histopathology 1996;29:101–110.

152. Beaugerie L, Luboinski J, Brousse N, et al. Drug induced lymphocytic colitis. Gut 1994;35:426–428.

153. Kingham JGC, Levinson DA, Ball JA, Dawson AM. Microscopic colitis—a cause of chronic watery diarrhea. Br Med J 1982;285:1601–1604.

154. Saul SH. The watery diarrhea-colitis syndrome. A review of collagenous and microscopic/lymphocytic colitis. Int J Surg Pathol 1993;1:65–82.

155. Surawicz CM, Haggitt RC, Husseman M, McFarland LV. Mucosal biopsy diagnosis of colitis: acute self-limited colitis and idiopathic inflammatory bowel disease. Gastroenterology 1994;107:755–763.

156. Lindstrom CG. "Collagenous colitis" with watery diarrhea—a new entity? Pathol Eur 1976;11:87–89.

157. Bogomoletz WV, Adnet JJ, Birembaut P, et al. Collagenous colitis: an unrecognized entity. Gut 1980;21:164–168.

158. Pieterse AS, Hecker R, Rowland R. Collagenous colitis: a distinctive and potentially reversible disorder. J Clin Pathol 1982;35:338–340.

159. Flejou JF, Grimaud JA, Molas G. Collagenous colitis. Ultrastructural study and collagen immunotyping of four cases. Arch Pathol Lab Med 1984;198:977–982.

160. Teglbjaerg PS, Tharpen EH, Jensen HH. Development of collagenous colitis in sequential biopsy specimens. Gastroenterology 1984;87:703–709.

161. Kingham JGC, Levison DA, Morson BC, Dawson AM. Collagenous colitis. Gut 1986;27:550–557.

162. Hwang WS, Kelley JK, Shaffer EA, Hershfield NB. Collagenous colitis: a disease of pencryptal fibroblastic sheath. J Pathol 1986;149:33–40.

163. Jesserun J, Yardley JH, Giardiello FM, et al. Chronic colitis with thickening of the subepithelial collagen layer (collagenous colitis). Histopathologic findings in 15 patients. Hum Pathol 1987;18:839–848.

164. Wang HH, Owings DV, Antonioli DA, Goldman H. Increased subepithelial collagen deposition is not specific for collagenous colitis. Modern Pathol 1988;1:329–335.

165. Carpenter HA, Tremaine WJ, Batts KP, et al. Sequential histologic evaluations in collagenous colitis. Dig Dis Sci 1993;37:1903–1909.

166. Hamilton I, Sander S, Hopwood D, Bouchier IAD. Collagenous colitis associated with small intestinal villous atrophy. Gut 1986;27:1394–1398.

167. Eckstein RP, Dowsett JF, Riley JW. Collagenous enterocolitis: a case of collagenous colitis with involvement of the small intestine. Am J Gastroenterol 1988;83:767–771.

168. Wiener MD. Collagenous colitis and pulmonary fibrosis. Manifestations of a single disease? J Clin Gastroenterol 1986;8:677–680.

169. Riddell RH, Tonaka M, Mazzoleni G. Non-steroidal anti-inflammatory drugs as a possible cause of collagenous colitis: a case-control study. Gut 1992;33:683–686.

170. Goff JS, Barnett JL, Pelke T, Appelman HD. Collagenous colitis: histopathology and clinical course. Am J Gastroenterol 1997;92:57–60.

171. Palmer KR, Berry H, Wheeler PJ, et al. Collagenous colitis—a relapsing and remitting disease. Gut 1986;27:578–580.

172. Zins BJ, Sandborn WJ, Tremaine WJ. Collagenous and lymphocytic colitis: subject review and therapeutic alternatives. Am J Gastroenterol 1995;90:1394–1400.

173. Tanaka M, Mazzoleni G, Riddell RH. Distribution of collagenous colitis: utility of flexible sigmoidoscopy. Gut 1992;33:65–70.

174. Gledhill A, Cole FM. Significance of basement membrane thickening in the human colon. Gut 1984;25:1085–1088.

175. Mosnier J F, Larvol L, Barge J, et al. Lymphocytic and collagenous colitis: an immunohistochemical study. Am J Gastroenterol 1996;91:709–713.

176. Gardiner GW, Goldberg R, Currie D, Murray D. Colonic carcinoma associated with an abnormal collagen table. Cancer 1984;54:2973–2977.

177. Glotzer DJ, Glick ME, Goldman H. Proctitis and colitis following diversion of the fecal stream. Gastroenterology 1981;80:438–441.

178. Korelitz BI, Cheskin LJ, Sohn N, Sommers SC. Proctitis after fecal diversion in Crohn's disease and its elimination with reanastomosis: implication for surgical management. Report of four cases. Gastroenterology 1984;87:710–713.

179. Lush LB, Reichen J, Levine JS. Aphthous ulceration in diversion colitis. Clinical applications. Gastroenterology 1984;87:1171–1173.

180. Ona FV, Bogar JN. Rectal bleeding due to diversion colitis. Am J Gastroenterol 1985;80:40–41.

181. Murray FE, O'Brien MJ, Birkett DH, et al. Diversion colitis. Pathologic findings in a resected sigmoid colon and rectum. Gastroenterology 1987;93:1404–1408.

182. Ma CK, Gottlieb C, Haas PA. Diversion colitis: a clinicopathologic study of 21 cases. Hum Pathol 1990;21:429–436.

183. Komorowski RA. Histologic spectrum of diversion colitis. Am J Surg Pathol 1990;14:548–554.

184. Geraghty JM, Talbot IC. Diversion colitis: histological features in the colon and rectum after defunctioning colostomy. Gut 1991;32:1020–1023.

185. Warren BF, Shepherd NA, Bartolo DCC, Bradfield JWB. Pathology of the defunctioned rectum in ulcerative colitis. Gut 1993;34:514–516.

186. Harig JM, Soergel KH, Komorowski RA, Wood CM. Treatment of diversion colitis with short chain-fatty acid irrigation. N Engl J Med 1989;320:23–28.
187. Geraghty JM, Charles AK. Aphthoid ulceration in diversion colitis. Histopathology 1994;24:395–397.
188. Yeong ML, Bethwaite PB, Prasad J, Isbister WH. Lymphoid follicular hyperplasia—a distinctive feature of diversion colitis. Histopathology 1991;19:55–61.
189. Roe AM, Warren BF, Brodribb AJM, Brown C. Diversion colitis and involution of the defunctioned anorectum. Gut 1993;34:382–385.
190. Lu ES, Lin T, Harms BL, et al. A severe case of diversion colitis with large ulcerations. Am J Gastroenterol 1995;90:1508–1510.
191. Price AB, Davies DR. Pseudomembranous colitis. J Clin Pathol 1977;30:1–12.
192. Nostrant TT, Kumar NB, Appelman HD. Histopathology differentiates acute self-limited colitis from ulcerative colitis. Gastroenterology 1987;92:318–328.
193. Goodall HB, Sinclair ISR. Colitis cystica profunda. J Pathol Bacteriol 1957;73:33–42.
194. Epstein SE, Ascari WQ, Ablow RC, et al. Colitis cystica profunda. Am J Clin Pathol 1966;45:186–201.
195. Herman AH, Nabseth DC. Colitis cystica profunda: localized, segmental, and diffuse. Arch Surg 1973;106:337.
196. Martin JK Jr, Culp CE, Werland LH. Colitis cystica profunda. Dis Colon Rectum 1980;23:488.
197. Dyson JD. Herniation of mucosal epithelium into the submucosa in chronic ulcerative colitis. J Clin Pathol 1975;28:189.
198. Clark RM. Microdiverticula and submucosal epithelial elements in ulcerative and granulomatous diseases of the ileum and colon. Can Med Assoc J 1970;103:24.
199. Gardiner GW, McAuliffe N, Murray D. Colitis cystica profunda occurring in a radiation-induced colonic stricture. Hum Pathol 1984;15:295–298.
200. Ng WK, Chan KW. Postirradiation colitis cystica profunda. Case report and literature review. Arch Pathol Lab Med 1995;119:1170–1173.
201. Magidson JG, Lewin KJ. Diffuse colitis cystica profunda. Report of a case. Am J Surg Pathol 1981;5:393.
202. Bentley E, Chandrasoma P, Cohen H, et al. Colitis cystica profunda: presenting with complete intestinal obstruction and recurrence. Gastroenterology 1985;89:1157–1161.
203. Sobin LH. Inverted hyperplastic polyps of the colon. Am J Surg Pathol 1985;9:265–272.
204. Shepherd NA. Inverted hyperplastic polyposis of the colon. J Clin Pathol 1993;46:56–60.
205. Muto T, Bussey HJR, Morson BC. Pseudo-carcinomatous invasion in adenomatous polyps of the colon and rectum. J Clin Pathol 1973;26:25–31.
206. Wayte DM, Helwig EB. Colitis cystica profunda. Am J Clin Pathol 1966;48:159–169.
207. Allen MS. Hamartomatous inverted polyps of the rectum. Cancer 1966;19:257.
208. Madigan MR, Morson BC. Solitary ulcer of the rectum. Gut 1969;10:871–881.
209. Rutter K, Riddell RH. The solitary ulcer syndrome of the rectum. Clin Gastroenterol 1975;4:505–530.
210. Schweiger M, Williams JA. Solitary ulcer syndrome of the rectum—its association with occult rectal prolapse. Lancet 1977;2:170–171.
211. Franzin G, Dina R, Scarpa A, Fratton A. The evolution of the solitary ulcer of the rectum. An endoscopic and histopathological study. Endoscopy 1982;14:131–134.
212. Ford MJ, Anderson JR, Gilmour HM, et al. Clinical spectrum of "solitary ulcer" of the rectum. Gastroenterology 1983;84:1533–1540.
213. DuBoulay CE, Fairbrother J, Isaacson PG. Mucosal prolapse syndrome—a unifying concept for solitary ulcer syndrome and related disorders. J Clin Pathol 1983;36:1264–1268.
214. Stuart M. Proctitis cystica profunda. Incidence, etiology and treatment. Dis Colon Rectum 1984;27:153–156.
215. Saul SH, Sollenberger LC. Solitary rectal ulcer syndrome. Its clinical and pathological underdiagnosis. Am J Surg Pathol 1985;9:411–421.
216. Levine DS. Solitary rectal ulcer syndrome. Are "solitary" rectal ulcer syndrome and "localized" colitis cystica profunda analogous syndromes caused by rectal prolapse? Gastroenterology 1987;92:243–253.
217. Kang YS, Kamm MA, Engel AF, Talbot IC. Pathology of the rectal wall in solitary rectal ulcer syndrome and complete rectal prolapse. Gut 1996;38:587–590.
218. Keighley MR, Shouler P. Clinical and manometric features of the solitary rectal ulcer syndrome. Dis Colon Rectum 1984;27:507–512.
219. Lobert PF, Appelman HP. Inflammatory cloacogenic polyp—a unique inflammatory lesion of the anal transitional zone. Am J Surg Pathol 1981;5:761–766.
220. Saul SH. Inflammatory cloacogenic polyp: relationship to solitary rectal ulcer syndrome/mucosal prolapse and other bowel disorders. Hum Pathol 1987;18:1120–1125.
221. Levey JM, Banner B, Darrah J, et al. Inflammatory cloacogenic polyp: three cases and literature review. Am J Gastroenterol 1994;89:438–441.
222. Niv Y, Bat L. Solitary rectal ulcer syndrome—clinical, endoscopic, and histological spectrum. Am J Gastroenterol 1986;81:486–491.
223. Tjandra JJ, Fazio VW, Church JM, et al. Clinical concepts of solitary rectal ulcer. Dis Colon Rectum 1992;25:227–234.
224. Levine DS, Surawicz CM, Ajer T, et al. Diffuse excess mucosal collagen in rectal biopsies facilitates differential diagnosis of solitary rectal ulcer syndrome from other inflammatory bowel diseases. Dig Dis Sci 1988;33:1345–1352.
225. Bockus HL, Willard JH, Bank J. Melanosis coli: the etiologic significance of the anthracene laxatives: a report of 41 cases. JAMA 1933;101:1–6.
226. Wittoesch JH, Jackman RJ, MacDonald JR. Melanosis coli: general review and study of 887 cases. Dis Colon Rectum 1958;1:172–180.
227. Steer HW, Colin-Jones DG. Melanosis coli: studies of the toxic effects of irritant purgatives. J Pathol 1975;115:199.
228. Walker NI, Smith MM, Smithers BM. Ultrastructure of human melanosis coli with reference to its pathogenesis. Pathology 1993;25:120–124.
229. Ghadially FN, Walley VM. Melanoses of the gastrointestinal tract. Histopathology 1994;25:197–207.
230. Levine DS, Haggitt RC. Normal histology of the colon. Am J Surg Pathol 1989;13:966–984.
231. Cowen ML, Humphries TJ. Pseudomelanosis of the duodenum. Gastrointest Endosc 1980;26:107–108.
232. Sharp JR, Insalaco SJ, Johnson LF. "Melanosis" of the duodenum associated with a gastric ulcer and folic acid deficiency. Gastroenterology 1980;78:366–369.
233. Yamare H, Norris M, Gillier C. Pseudomelanosis duodeni: a clinicopathologic entity. Gastrointest Endosc 1985;31:83–86.
234. Gupta TP, Weinstock JV. Duodenal pseudomelanosis associated with chronic renal failure. Gastrointest Endosc 1986;32:358–360.
235. Kang JY, Wu AYT, Chia JLS, et al. Clinical and ultrastructural studies in duodenal pseudomelanosis. Gut 1987;28:1673–1681.
236. Ghadially FN, Walley VM. Pigments of the gastrointestinal tract: a comparison of light microscopic and electron microscopic findings. Ultrastruct Pathol 1995;19:213–220.
237. Smith B. Pathology of cathartic colon. Proc Roy Soc Med 1972;65:288.
238. Urso FP, Urso MJ, Lee CH. The cathartic colon: pathological findings and radiological/pathological correlation. Radiology 1975;116:557–559.
239. Smith B. Pathologic changes in the colon produced by anthraquinone purgatives. Dis Colon Rectum 1973;16:455–458.
240. Heilbrun N, Bernstein C. Roentgen abnormalities of the large and small intestine associated with prolonged cathartic ingestion. Radiology 1955;65:549–556.
241. Ziter FMH Jr. Cathartic colon. NY State J Med 1967;67:546–549.
242. Anuras S, Shirazi SS. Colonic pseudoobstruction. Am J Gastroenterol 1984;79:525–532.
243. Heizer WD, Warshaw AL, Walkman TA. Protein-losing gastroenteropathy and malabsorption associated with factitious diarrhea. Ann Intern Med 1968;839–852.
244. Oster JR, Materson BJ, Rogers AI. Laxative abuse syndrome. Am J Gastroenterol 1980;74:451–458.

245. Pockros PJ, Foroozan P. Golytely lavage versus standard colonoscopy preparation. Effect on normal colonic mucosal histology. Gastroenterology 1985;88:845–848.

246. Meisel JL, Bergman D, Graney D, et al. Human rectal mucosa: proctoscopic and morphological changes caused by laxatives. Gastroenterology 1977;72:1274–1279.

247. Leriche M, Devroede G, Sanchez G, et al. Changes in the rectal mucosa induced by hypertonic enemas. Dis Colon Rectum 1978;21:227–236.

248. Meyer CT, Brand M, DeLuca VA, Spriro HM. Hydrogen peroxide colitis: a report of three patients. J Clin Gastroenterol 1981;3:31–35.

249. Hardin RD, Tedesco FJ. Colitis after Hibiclens enema. J Clin Gastroenterol 1986;8:572–575.

250. Scott TR, Graham SM, Schweitzer EJ, Bartlett ST. Colonic necrosis following sodium polystyrene sulfonate (Kayexalate)-sorbitol enema in a renal transplant patient. Dis Colon Rectum 1993;36:607–609.

251. Rashid A, Hamilton SR. Necrosis of the gastrointestinal tract in uremic patients as a result of sodium polystyrene sulfonate (Kayexalate) in sorbitol. Am J Surg Pathol 1997;21:60–69.

252. Barker CS. Acute colitis resulting from soapsuds enema. Can Med Assoc J 1945;52:285–286.

253. Pike BF, Phillippi PJ, Lawson EH. Soap colitis. N Engl J Med 1971;285:217–218.

254. Bendit M. Gangrene of the rectum as a complication of an enema. Br Med J 1945;1:664.

255. Segal I, Tim LO, Hamilton DG, et al. Ritual-enema–induced colitis. Dis Colon Rectum 1979;22:195–199.

256. Chajek T, Fainaru M. Behcet's disease: report of 41 cases and a review of the literature. Medicine 1975;54:179–196.

257. Lakhanpal S, Tani K, Lie JT, et al. Pathologic features of Behcet's syndrome. A review of Japanese autopsy registry data. Hum Pathol 1985;16:790–795.

258. Smith GE, Kime LR, Pitcher JL. The colitis of Behcet's disease. A separate entity? Colonoscopic findings and literature review. Dig Dis Sci 1973;18:987–1000.

259. Baba S, Maruta M, Ando K, et al. Intestinal Behcet's disease. Report of five cases. Dis Colon Rectum 1976;19:428–440.

260. Lee RG. The colitis of Behcet's syndrome. Am J Surg Pathol 1986;10:888–893.

261. Masugi J, Matsui T, Fujimori T, Maeda S. A case of Behcet's disease with multiple longitudinal ulcers all over the colon. Am J Gastroenterol 1994;89:778–780.

262. Mori S, Yoshihira A, Kawamura H, et al. Esophageal involvement in Behcet's disease. Am J Gastroenterol 1983;78:548–553.

263. Yashiro K, Nagasako K, Hasegawa K, et al. Esophageal lesions in intestinal Behcet's disease. Endoscopy 1986;18:57–60.

264. Anti M, Marra G, Rapaccini GL, et al. Esophageal involvement in Behcet's syndrome. J Clin Gastroenterol 1986;8:514–519.

265. Good AE, Mutchnick MG, Weatherbee L. Duodenal ulcer, hepatic abscess, and fatal hemobilia with Behcet's syndrome: a case report. Am J Gastroenterol 1982;77:905–909.

266. Satake K, Yada K, Ikehara T, et al. Pyloric stenosis: an unusual complication of Behcet's disease. Am J Gastroenterol 1986;81:816–818.

267. Grinvalsky HT, Bowerman CI. Stercoraceous ulcers of the colon. Relatively neglected medical and surgical problem. JAMA 1959;171:1941–1946.

268. Milliser RV, Greenberg SR, Neiman BH. Exsanguinating stercoral ulceration. Am J Dig Dis 1970;15:485–488.

269. Liedberg G. Stercoraceous perforations of the colon. Acta Clin Scand 1969;135:552.

270. Gekas P, Schuster MM. Stercoral perforation of the colon: case report and review of the literature. Gastroenterology 1981;80:1054–1058.

271. Yates LN, Clausen EG. Simple nonspecific ulcers of the sigmoid colon. Arch Surg 1960;81:535–541.

272. Smithwick W, Anderson RP, Ballinger WF. Nonspecific ulcer of the colon. Arch Surg 1968;97:133–138.

273. Benninger GW, Honig LJ, Fein HD. Nonspecific ulceration of the cecum. Am J Gastroenterol 1971;55:594–601.

274. Corry RJ, Bartlett NK, Cohen RB. Erosions of the cecum: a cause of massive hemorrhage. Am J Surg 1970;119:106–110.

275. Mahoney TJ, Bubrick MP, Hitchcock CR. Nonspecific ulcers of the colon. Dis Colon Rectum 1978;21:623–626.

276. Shah NC, Ostrov AH, Cavallero JB, Rodgers JB. Benign ulcers of the colon. Gastrointest Endosc 1986;32:102–104.

277. Wormann B, Hochter W, Seib H-J, Ottenjann R. Ergotamine-induced colitis. Endoscopy 1985;17:165–166.

278. Eckardt VF, Kanzler G, Remmele W. Anorectal ergotism: another cause of solitary rectal ulcers. Gastroenterology 1986;91:1123–1127.

279. Bernardino ME, Lawson TL. Discrete colonic ulcers associated with oral contraceptives. Dig Dis Sci 1976;21:503–506.

280. Tedesco FJ, Volpicelli NA, Moore FS. Estrogen- and progesterone-associated colitis: a disorder with clinical and endoscopic features mimicking Crohn's colitis. Gastrointest Endosc 1982;28:247–249.

281. Stamm C, Burkhalter E, Pearce W, et al. Benign colonic ulcers associated with nonsteroidal anti-inflammatory drug ingestion. Am J Gastroenterol 1994;89:2230–2233.

282. Moolenaar W, Lamers CBHW. Cholesterol crystal embolization to the alimentary tract. Gut 1996;38:196–200.

283. Tribe CR, Scott DGI, Bacon PA. Rectal biopsy in the diagnosis of systemic vasculitis. J Clin Pathol 1981;34:843–850.

284. Sutherland DER, Chan FY, Foucar E, et al. The bleeding cecal ulcer in transplant patients. Surgery 1979;86:386–398.

285. Huded F, Posner GL, Tick R. Nonspecific ulcer of the colon in a chronic hemodialysis patient. Am J Gastroenterol 1982;77:913–916.

286. Dosik GM, Luna M, Valdovieso M, et al. Necrotizing colitis in patients with cancer. Am J Med 1979;67:646–656.

287. Kies MS, Luedke DW, Boyd JF, McCue MJ. Neutropenic enterocolitis. Cancer 1979;43:730–734.

288. Wade DS, Nava HR, Douglas HO Jr. Neutropenic enterocolitis. Clinical diagnosis and treatment. Cancer 1992;69:17–23.

289. Levine TS, Price AB. Obstructive enterocolitis: a clinico-pathological discussion. Histopathology 1994;25:57–64.

290. Nalbundian H, Sketh N, Dietrich R, et al. Intestinal ischemia caused by cocaine ingestion. Report of two cases. Surgery 1985;97:374–376.

291. Brown DN, Rosenholtz MJ, Marshall JB. Ischemic colitis related to cocaine abuse. Am J Gastroenterol 1994;89:1558–1561.

292. Jonas G, Mahoney A, Murray J, Gertler S. Chemical colitis due to endoscopic cleansing solutions: a mimic of pseudomembranous colitis. Gastroenterology 1988;95:1403–1408.

293. Williams KL. Acute solitary ulcers and acute diverticulitis of the cecum and ascending colon. Br J Surg 1960;47:351–358.

294. Mitsudo SM, Boley SJ, Brandt LJ, et al. Vascular ectasias of the right colon in the elderly: a distinct pathologic entity. Hum Pathol 1979;10:585–600.

295. Sale GE, Shulman HM, McDonald JB, et al. Gastrointestinal graft-versus-host disease in man: a clinicopathologic study of the rectal biopsy. Am J Surg Pathol 1979;3:291.

296. Gallucci BB, Sale GE, McDonald GB, et al. The fine structure of human rectal epithelium in acute graft-versus-host disease. Am J Surg Pathol 1982;6:293–305.

297. Ament ME, Ochs HD. Gastrointestinal manifestations of chronic granulomatous disease. N Engl J Med 1973;288:382–387.

298. Werlin SL, Chusid MJ, Caya J, et al. Colitis in chronic granulomatous disease. Gastroenterology 1982;82:328–331.

299. Lennard-Jones JE. Functional gastrointestinal disorders. N Engl J Med 1983;308:431–435.

300. Lynn RB, Friedman RS. Irritable bowel syndrome. N Engl J Med 1993;329:1940–1945.

301. Hughes DTD, Gordon KCD, Swann JC, Bolt GL. Pneumatosis cystoides intestinalis. Gut 1966;7:553–557.

302. Ecker JA, Williams RG, Clay KL. Pneumatosis cystoides intestinalis—bullous emphysema of the intestine. A review of the literature. Am J Gastroenterol 1971;56:125–136.

303. Yale CE, Balish E. Pneumatosis cystoides intestinalis. Dis Colon Rectum 1976;19:107–111.

304. Galondiuk S, Fazio VW. Pneumatosis cystoides intestinalis: a review of the literature. Dis Colon Rectum 1986;29:358–363.

305. Heng Y, Schuffler MD, Haggitt RC, et al. Pneumatosis intestinalis: a review. Am J Gastroenterol 1995;90:1747–1758.

306. Keyting WS, McCarver RR, Kovarik JL, et al. Pneumatosis intestinalis: a new concept. Radiology 1961;76:733.

307. Smith BH, Welter LH. Pneumatosis intestinalis. Am J Clin Pathol 1967;48:455–465.

308. Heer M, Altorfer J, Pirovino M, Schmid M. Pneumatosis cystoides coli: a rare complication of colonoscopy. Endoscopy 1983;15:119–120.

309. Pieterse AS, Leong AS, Rowland R. The mucosal changes and pathogenesis of pneumatosis cystoides intestinalis. Hum Pathol 1985;16:683–688.

310. Haboubi NY, Honan BP, Hasleton PS, et al. Pneumatosis coli: a case report with ultrastructural study. Histopathology 1984;8:145–155.

311. Suarez V, Chesner IM, Price AB, Newman J. Pneumatosis cystoides intestinalis. Histological mucosal changes mimicking inflammatory bowel disease. Arch Pathol Lab Med 1989;113:898–901.

312. Pemberton HW, Smith WG, Holman CB. Pneumatosis cystoides intestinalis diagnosed sigmoidoscopically. Am J Surg 1957;94:472–477.

313. Jenkinson EL, Brown WH. Endometriosis—a study of 117 cases with special reference to constricting lesions of the rectum and sigmoid colon. JAMA 1943;122:349–354.

314. Boles RS, Hodes PJ. Endometriosis of the small and large intestine. Gastroenterology 1958;34:367.

315. Spjut HJ, Perkins DE. Endometriosis of the sigmoid colon and rectum. A roentgenographic and pathologic study. Am J Roentgenol 1959;82:1070–1075.

316. Parr NJ, Murphy C, Holt S, et al. Endometriosis and the gut. Gut 1988;29:1112–1115.

317. Caccese WJ, McKinley MJ, Bronzo RL, Bronson R. Endoscopic confirmation of colonic endometriosis. Gastrointest Endosc 1984;30:191–193.

318. Bashist B, Forde KA, McCaffrey RM. Polypoid endometrioma of the rectosigmoid. Gastrointest Radiol 1983;8:85–88.

319. Langlois NEI, Park KGM, Keenan RA. Mucosal changes in the large bowel with endometriosis: a possible cause of misdiagnosis of colitis? Hum Pathol 1994;25:1030–1034.

320. Aronchuck CA, Brooks FP, Dyson WL, et al. Ileocecal endometriosis presenting with abdominal pain and gastrointestinal bleeding. Dig Dis Sci 1983;28:566–572.

321. Shome GP, Nagaraju M, Munis A, Wiese D. Appendiceal endometriosis presenting as massive lower intestinal hemorrhage. Am J Gastroenterol 1995;90:1881–1883.

322. Panzer S, Pitt HA, Wallach EE, et al. Intussusception of the appendix due to endometriosis. Am J Gastroenterol 1995;90:1892–1893.

323. Ledley GS, Shenk IM, Heit HA. Sigmoid colon perforation due to endometriosis not associated with pregnancy. Am J Gastroenterol 1988;83:1424–1426.

324. Amano S, Yamada N. Endometrioid carcinoma arising from endometriosis of the sigmoid colon: a case report. Hum Pathol 1981;12:845–849.

325. Wolff M. Heterotopic gastric epithelium in the rectum: a report of three new cases with a review of 87 cases of gastric heterotopia in the alimentary canal. Am J Clin Pathol 1971;55:604–616.

326. Yokoyama I, Kozuka S, Ito K, et al. Gastric gland metaplasia in the small and large intestine. Gut 1977;18:214–218.

327. Jabbori M, Goresky CA, Lough J, et al. The inlet patch: heterotopic gastric mucosa in the upper esophagus. Gastroenterology 1985;89:352–356.

328. Shah KK, DeRidder PH, Shah KK. Ectopic gastric mucosa in proximal esophagus. Its clinical significance and hormonal profile. J Clin Gastroenterol 1986;8:509–513.

329. Truong LD, Stroebein JR, McKechnie JC. Gastric heterotopia of the proximal esophagus: a report of four cases detected by endoscopy and review of the literature. Am J Gastroenterol 1986;81:1162–1166.

330. Steadman C, Kerlin P, Teague C, Stephenson P. High esophageal stricture: a complication of "inlet patch" mucosa. Gastroenterology 1988;94:521–524.

331. Borkan-Manesh F, Fornum JB. Incidence of heterotopic gastric mucosa in the upper oesophagus. Gut 1991;32:968–972.

332. Franzin G, Musola R, Negri A, et al. Heterotopic gastric (fundic) mucosa in the duodenum. Endoscopy 1982;14:166–167.

333. Spiller RC, Shousha S, Barrison IG. Heterotopic gastric tissue in the duodenum. A report of eight cases. Dig Dis Sci 1982;27:880–883.

334. Vizcarrondo FJ, Wang T-Y, Brady PG. Heterotopic gastric mucosa: presentation as a rugose duodenal mass. Gastrointest Endosc 1983;29:107–111.

335. Debas HT, Chaun H, Thomson FB, et al. Functioning heterotopic oxyntic mucosa in the rectum. Gastroenterology 1980;79:1300–1302.

336. Pistoia MA, Guadagni S, Tisiano D, et al. Ulcerated ectopic gastric mucosa of the rectum. Gastrointest Endosc 1987;33:41–43.

337. Kaloni BP, Vaezzadeh K, Sieber WK. Gastric heterotopia in rectum complicated by rectovesical fistula. Dig Dis Sci 1983;28:378–380.

338. Schwarzenberg SJ, Whitington PF. Rectal gastric mucosa heterotopia as a cause of hematochezia in an infant. Dig Dis Sci 1983;28:470–472.

339. Galligan ML, Uhlich T, Lewin KJ. Heterotopic gastric mucosa in the jejunum causing intussusception. Arch Pathol Lab Med 1983;107:335–336.

340. Seagram CG, Louch RE, Stephens CA, Wentworth P. Meckel's diverticulum: a 10-year review of 218 cases. Can J Surg 1968;11:369–373.

341. Meguid M, Erakis AJ. Complications of Meckel's diverticulum in infants. Surg Gynecol Obstet 1974;139:541–544.

342. Case Records of the Massachusetts General Hospital. N Engl J Med 1980;302:958–962.

343. Gross RE, Holcomb GW Jr, Farber S. Duplications of the alimentary tract. Pediatrics 1952;9:449–467.

344. Bower RJ, Sieber WK, Kiesewetter WB. Alimentary tract duplications in children. Ann Surg 1978;188:669–674.

345. Dye KR, Marshall BJ, Frierson HF, et al. Campylobacter pylori colonizing heterotopic gastric tissue in the rectum. Am J Clin Pathol 1990;93:144–147.

346. Flejou JF, Potet F, Molas G, et al. Campylobacter-like organisms in heterotopic gastric mucosa of the upper oesophagus. J Clin Pathol 1990;43:961.

347. Cserni G. Gastric pathology in Meckel's diverticulum. Review of cases resected between 1965 and 1995. Am J Clin Pathol 1996;106:782–785.

348. Sperling RM, Grendell JH. Adenocarcinoma arising in an inlet patch of the esophagus. Am J Gastroenterol 1995;90:150–152.

349. Caruso ML, Marzullo F. Jejunal adenocarcinoma in congenital heterotopic gastric mucosa. J Clin Gastroenterol 1988;10:92–94.

350. Kusumoto H, Yoshitake H, Mochida K, et al. Adenocarcinoma in Meckel's diverticulum: report of a case and review of 30 cases in the English and Japanese literature. Am J Gastroenterol 1992;87:910–913.

351. Haggitt RC. Granulomatous diseases of the gastrointestinal tract. In: Ioachim HL, ed. Pathology of granulomas. New York: Raven Press, 1983:257–305.

352. Lichtman AL, McDonald JR, Dixon CF, Mann FC. Talc granuloma. Surg Gynecol Obstet 1946;83:531–546.

353. Eiseman B, Seelig MG, Wormach NA. Talcum powder granuloma: a frequent and serious postoperative complication. Ann Surg 1947;126:820–832.

354. Anani PA, Ribaux C, Gardiol D. Unusual intestinal talcosis. Am J Surg Pathol 1987;11:890–894.

355. Humphrey SR, Cameron AJ, Harrison EG Jr. Acute granulomatous peritonitis due to starch glove powder. Gastroenterology 1972;63:1062–1065.

356. Nissim F, Ashkenazy M, Borenstein R, Czernobilsky B. Tuberculoid corn starch granulomas with caseous necrosis. A diagnostic challenge. Arch Pathol Lab Med 1981;105:86–88.

357. Carney JA, Stephens DH. Intramural barium (barium granuloma) of colon and rectum. Gastroenterology 1973;65:316.

358. Lewis JW, Kerstein MD, Koss N. Barium granuloma of the rectum: an uncommon complication of barium enema. Ann Surg 1980;81:418–423.

359. McKee PH, Cameron CHS. Barium granuloma of the transverse colon. Postgrad Med J 1968;54:698–702.

360. Phelps JE, Sanowski RA, Kozarek RA. Intramural extravasation of barium simulating carcinoma of the rectum. Dis Colon Rectum 1981;24:388.

361. Levison DA, Crocker PR, Smith A. Varied light and scanning electron

microscopic appearance of barium sulphate in smears and histologic sections. J Clin Pathol 1984;37:481–487.

362. Susnow DA. Oleogranulomas of the rectum: following rectal instal-lation of petrolatum or ointments containing petrolatum. Am J Surg 1952;83:496–499.

363. Hernandez V, Hernandez IA, Berthrong M. Oleogranuloma simulating carcinoma of the rectum. Dis Colon Rectum 1967;10: 205–209.

364. Greaney MG, Jackson PR. Oleogranuloma of the rectum produced by Lasonil ointment. Br Med J 1977;2:997–998.

365. Mazier WP, Sun KM, Robertson WG. Oil-induced granuloma (oleoma) of the rectum. Dis Colon Rectum 1978;21:292–294.

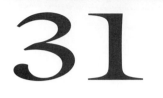

CHAPTER

31 MALABSORPTIVE DISORDERS

John H. Yardley

INTRODUCTION

This chapter deals with those chronic conditions that can lead to abnormal absorption of nutrient substances from the small intestine. The classification of these conditions is given in Table 31.1. Major attention is given to disorders such as celiac disease and Whipple's disease for which malabsorption is a cen-tral feature of their clinical presentation. Clinicopathologic corre-lation is included to enhance general comprehension of patho-logic changes and because it is often essential for full and correct pathologic interpretation. Diseases that can be associated with malabsorption, but which are discussed more fully elsewhere in the book (e.g., infections and Crohn's disease), are considered only briefly.

TABLE

31.1 | Classification of Disorders of Malabsorption

Diseases Associated with Normal Mucosal Histology
  Pancreatic insufficiency
  Bile salt insufficiency
  Postgastrectomy
  Short bowel syndrome
  Alcoholism
  Inborn disaccharidase deficiencies
    Adult-type lactase deficiency (hypolactasia)
    Other disaccharidase deficiencies
Diseases Associated with Nonspecific Mucosal Inflammatory Lesions
  Peptic duodenitis and jejunitis (Chapter 30)
  Celiac disease (Gluten-induced enteropathy)
  Celiac-related conditions
    Refractory celiac disease
    Refractory sprue (some cases)
    Collagenous sprue
    Dermatitis herpetiformis
  Celiac-like reactions to agents other than gluten
    Soy milk, MER–29 (triparanol)
  Lymphocytic enterocolitis (Chapter 30)
  Tropical sprue
  Stasis (blind-loop) syndrome
    Various motor and mechanical disturbances
  Deficiency states
    Protein deficiency
    Zinc deficiency and acrodermatitis enteropathica
    Iron deficiency
  Unclassified nonspecific inflammatory lesions
Infection-Associated Mucosal Lesions
  Viral infections (Chapters 16 and 28)
  Bacterial infections
    Mycobacterium avium intracellulare (Chapter 16)
    Whipple's disease
    Various other agents (Chapter 28)
  Fungus infections
    Moniliasis (Chapters 16 and 28)
    Histoplasmosis (Chapter 28)
  Protozoan parasites
    Giardiasis (Chapter 28)
    Cryptosporidiosis (Chapter 16)
    Microsporidiosis
    Coccidiosis *(Isospora)* (Chapter 28)

  Metazoan parasites
    Ascariasis (with protein deficiency)
    Hookworm
    Strongyloidiasis
    Capillariasis
Mucosal Lesions Associated with Altered Immune Response
  AIDS-associated diseases
    AIDS enteropathy (idiopathic)
    Opportunistic infections (Chapter 16)
  Autoimmune enteropathy
  Chronic granulomatous disease (Chapters 16 and 19)
  Graft-vs-host disease (Chapters 6 and 16)
  Immune deficiency states (Chapter 16)
Miscellaneous Diseases Associated with Characteristic Mucosal Lesions
  Abetalipoproteinemia (Chapter 19)
  Amyloidosis (Chapter 19)
  Crohn's disease (Chapter 29)
  Drug-associated lesions (Chapter 11)
  Eosinophilic gastroenteritis (Chapter 12)
  Histiocytosis X (Chapter 19)
  Lipid storage disease (Chapter 19)
  Lymphangiectasis
    Primary
    Secondary (Chapter 19)
  Lymphomas (Chapter 17)
  Mastocytosis
  Microvillous inclusion disease
  Radiation changes (Chapter 11)
  Waldenström's macroglobulinemia

Note: Chapter numbers in parentheses refer to the place where the listed disorder is discussed. All others are covered in this chapter.

Useful monographs and reviews covering malabsorption and associated pathologic changes are included in the reference list (1–5).

BIOPSIES—SPECIAL CONSIDERATIONS

Pathologic study of malabsorptive disorders depends almost entirely on duodenal and small intestinal biopsy. Prior to availability of fiberoptic endoscopy, most biopsies of the small intestine were obtained by using a fluoroscopically guided capsule device. Capsule biopsy, which can be performed anywhere in the small intestine, is now largely supplanted by endoscopically guided biopsy of the duodenum. Although endoscopic biopsy is usually adequate for diagnosis of such conditions as celiac disease (6), the presence of peptic duodenitis (or just the possibility of its presence) frequently confounds interpretation of inflammatory and degenerative changes, especially for biopsies taken from the duodenal bulb. (For additional discussion of this problem see the discussion under celiac disease). Furthermore, the proximal and distal small intestine are not necessarily involved to comparable degrees in all conditions. Thus "blind" biopsy from the jejunum and beyond by means of a capsule device or a "jejunoscope" is still needed at times for adequate study of some of the diseases and lesions described in this chapter.

The small intestinal mucosa is often not uniformly involved in malabsorption-associated conditions, a fact that should always be kept in mind, especially when examining biopsies obtained blindly via a capsule instrument. For instance, celiac disease alters the mucosa diffusely and all capsule biopsies taken from the same level of the small intestine can be expected to have a similar appearance, whereas biopsies from patients with segmental and focal disorders (e.g., Crohn's disease, dermatitis herpetiformis, Whipple's disease, and lymphoma) have an unpredictable degree of involvement. In addition, even with endoscopically guided biopsy, a specimen may not necessarily come from the intended biopsy site, since the operator does not always have full control over location of the forceps at the moment when tissue is obtained.

Two special procedures which can at times be of value for studying small intestinal biopsies in malabsorptive disorders are: (1) macroscopic examination and photography of specimens, and (2) study of smears prepared from the biopsy specimen. Direct macroscopic study is most often done to identify changes in the configuration of villi. It is also helpful for correlating endoscopic and histological findings, and for immediate verification that small intestinal mucosa was obtained, and for making preliminary assessment of mucosal architecture. An ordinary dissecting microscope, or even a strong hand lens, can provide useful observations. Correct lighting of the specimen, with the light source set in the near horizontal plane, is needed for good visualization and for photography of villi and other surface features (7).

Stained smears obtained from a biopsy specimen by dabbing it against a clean glass slide are useful for examining luminal contents for detached cells or microorganisms. They can be especially helpful for assessing cytologic characteristics and for detecting *Giardia lamblia* and other protozoan parasites.

CLINICOPATHOLOGIC CONSIDERATIONS

When used alone, the term *malabsorption* broadly describes dysfunction in the uptake of *any* substance by the small intestine. By this definition, malabsorption occurs in a wide range of disorders having varied clinical presentations. For instance, in pancreatic insufficiency the clinical picture is often dominated by abnormal lipid absorption, whereas the defect in adult lactase deficiency is malabsorption of lactose. The term *malabsorption syndrome* pertains more narrowly to a constellation of clinical findings that includes chronic diarrhea, steatorrhea, and variable secondary changes such as weight loss and evidence of vitamin deficiencies. The term *sprue* is an older generic term for diseases that are associated with steatorrhea, weight loss, deficiency states, etc., and thus is a synonym for malabsorption syndrome.

When considering biopsy findings in patients with malabsorption, it is often useful to consider whether the malabsorption has come about because of abnormalities of intraluminal digestion, abnormalities of uptake of nutrients by the mucosa, or some combination of the two.

Abnormalities of digestion (maldigestion) chiefly result from derangements in intraluminal breakdown of foodstuffs and can occur with:

(a) Inadequate mixing and time for interaction of enzymes and food, as in altered motility, with short bowel, and after gastrectomy.
(b) Bile salt deficiency.
(c) Pancreatic insufficiency.
(d) Deficiency of a specific digestive enzyme, lactase deficiency being the commonest example.

In general, the mucosa will show little or no abnormality when the principal cause of malabsorption is maldigestion.

Abnormalities of uptake occur when ability of the mucosa to absorb foodstuff is reduced either because of mucosal injury, as in celiac disease, or functionally as in ileal bypass, and in altered motility.

PROTEIN LOSING ENTEROPATHY

Protein losing enteropathy (PLE) condition occurs when serum proteins, especially albumin, leak across the mucosal barrier in excessive amounts and are lost in the fecal stream, or are resorbed as breakdown products after digestion. Since patients with PLE can develop severe hypoalbuminemia, peripheral edema is often the presenting manifestation. Additionally, PLE can be "primary," i.e., develop as a *de novo* condition in patients who demonstrate only widespread intestinal lymphangiectasia (see below under Miscellaneous Diseases Associated with Characteristic Mucosal Lesions), or it can be "secondary" (see Chapter 19), resulting from mucosal injury, as in celiac disease, or because of lymphatic obstruction as in constrictive pericarditis or Whipple's disease. Thus PLE is an important accompanying manifestation in some patients with malabsorption.

DISEASES ASSOCIATED WITH NORMAL MUCOSAL HISTOLOGY

Normal mucosal histology (Fig. 31.1) is most often seen in conditions where the malabsorption has resulted chiefly from intraluminal maldigestion (Table 31.1). Examples are patients with *chronic pancreatic insufficiency* or *intraluminal bile salt deficiency* (8, 9). These patients characteristically show elevated stool fat because of resulting fat maldigestion (10), whereas they have normal *d*-xylose uptake because their mucosa is unaffected. Normal histology can also be seen in patients with *rapid transit* of foodstuff through the small intestine, with a resulting reduction in total mucosal surface and inadequate mixing of foodstuff and digestive enzymes. Examples are *postgastrectomy* patients and patients who have a *short bowel*. Again, the mucosa in these individuals will be normal or show insufficient alterations to account for the malabsorption. *Alcoholism* presents a special problem, particularly for the "binge drinker" who may, through a combination of incompletely understood factors, show malabsorption of a variety of substances even though by light microscopy the mucosa is normal when alcohol alone is administered (11, 12). On the other hand, chronic alcoholics often have dietary deficiencies which may be crucial to the resulting mucosal changes, as was shown in those patients with associated folate deficiency (12). Pancreatic insufficiency secondary to alcoholism may also play a role (13).

Patients with *primary disaccharidase deficiency* represent another class of patients in whom a normal-looking intestinal mucosa accompanies a highly specific form of maldigestion-malabsorption. A large percentage of the world's population develops lactase deficiency (hypolactasia) on reaching adolescence or adulthood, especially persons of oriental and black ethnic origin. The lactose splitting enzyme is concentrated in the brush border of the small intestinal absorptive cells (14). Individuals with adult-type hypolactasia are unable to convert adequate amounts of lactose into its constituent monosaccharides, glucose and galactose, an essential step before its absorption can occur. When lactose remains in the intestinal lumen, the patient experiences symptoms of *milk intolerance* (abdominal cramps, bloating, flatulence, and diarrhea) as a result of osmotic retention of water in the lumen and bacterial action on the lactose that reaches the colon, with resulting production of gas and irritant substances, especially lactic acid (15).

Mucosal biopsies obtained from patients with adult-type hypolactasia look entirely normal in a conventional slide (Fig. 31.1) even though these biopsies demonstrate the hypolactasia by chemical analysis, and by enzymatic stain they show total absence or greatly reduced and mosaic distribution of lactase (16, 17) (Fig. 31.2). Other types of primary disaccharidase deficiency (e.g. sucrase and maltase deficiencies) are rare, and are present from birth; the intestinal mucosa also appears microscopically normal in these patients even though the clinical consequences may be severe. *Secondary lactase deficiency* can occur in patients with extensive damage to absorptive epithelium (e.g., in celiac disease).

From a practical standpoint, the important idea is that clinically significant forms of malabsorption can occur in the absence of visible mucosal alterations. It should also be stressed that a normal-looking biopsy can be encountered if the biopsy instrument happens to be positioned away from relevant focal disease (e.g., in lymphoma).

DISEASES PRIMARILY SHOWING NONSPECIFIC INFLAMMATION AND MUCOSAL ALTERATIONS

Malabsorptive disorders in this group show variable degrees of mucosal inflammatory changes, none of which are diagnostic or even characteristic by themselves. Inflammatory changes can vary as to severity, predominant cell types, and location.

Celiac disease is the major entity in this group of diseases among patients in developed Western countries (18) (Table 31.1).

CELIAC DISEASE

Synonyms for celiac disease, some no longer appropriate, are "nontropical sprue," "idiopathic sprue," "idiopathic steatorrhea," "celiac sprue," and "gluten-induced enteropathy." Excellent reviews of this subject are available and should be consulted for detailed descriptions of clinical and pathophysiologic observations (18–20).

ETIOLOGY AND PATHOGENESIS

Etiology of Celiac Disease

The central finding in celiac disease is an unusual sensitivity of the small intestinal mucosa to *gluten*, the major protein constituent of wheat flour and to a lesser degree, to gluten-related proteins in rye, oats, and barley (21–24). The relevant protein constituent in gluten

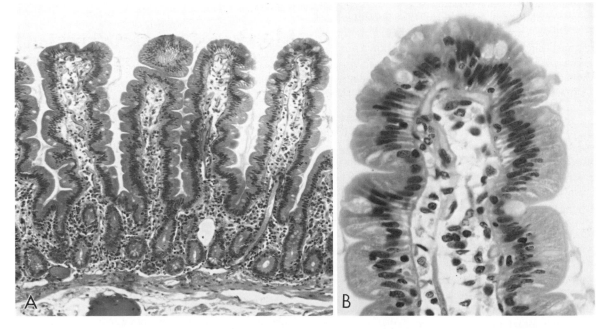

Figure 31.1 **(A)** Jejunal biopsy. Normal appearing small intestinal mucosa (adult-type lactase deficiency (hypolactasia). Villi are narrow, have a ruffled outline, and a villus to crypt ratio of almost 3:1 (×125). **(B)** Villus tip showing tall columnar epithelium with intact brush border. There are only scattered intraepithelial lymphocytes and mononuclear cells in the lamina propria (×450).

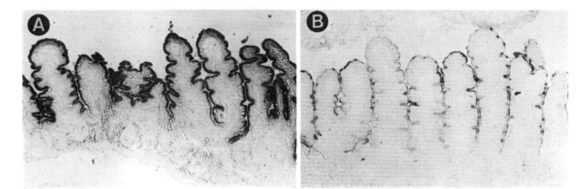

Figure 31.2 Human mucosal lactase demonstrated by enzymohistochemistry. **(A)** Adult subject with high lactase activity. All villi show uniform staining of enterocyte brush borders. **(B)** Subject with adult-type hypolactasia. Activity is present in only a few enterocytes over each villus; other enterocytes are weakly stained or unstained, giving a mosaic staining pattern. Note that crypt cells are negative in both specimens. (Reproduced with permission from Maiuri L, Rossi M, Raia V, et al. Surface staining on the villus of lactase protein and lactase activity in adult-type hypolactasia. Gastroenterology 1993;105:708–714.)

has been further identified as the alcohol-soluble fraction *gliadin*, and symptom-provoking subfractions of crude gliadin, termed α-gliadins, has also been identified, which in turn show other active subcomponents, including A-gliadin. Most patients who adhere closely to a *gluten free diet* show both clinical remission and eventual restoration of normal or near normal mucosal histology. Although by no means fully established, the underlying mechanism of mucosal injury in celiac patients is widely considered to be autoimmune.

Findings in serial biopsies of the small intestine before and at various intervals after gluten withdrawal have shown a clear relation between the mucosal findings and exposure to dietary gluten (25–28). The central feature is epithelial injury during gluten exposure that disappears on gluten withdrawal and reappears after reinstituting dietary gluten (27, 28). Parallel functional studies demonstrating impaired epithelial transport of lipid in active celiac disease, with recovery on a gluten free diet, have also emphasized the central role of epithelial damage in celiac disease (26).

It is useful to consider the typical response to a gluten free diet in full-blown celiac disease in three stages (Table 31.2). At each stage the pathologist must anticipate a different set of findings, and definitive assessment without knowledge of the patient's dietary status should not be attempted.

Pathogenesis of Celiac Disease

The mechanisms by which gluten injures the absorptive epithelium in celiac disease are not fully established, but current knowledge fits well with a combined genetic, environmental, and autoimmune pathogenesis.

GENETIC FACTORS There is much evidence favoring genetic factors. There is often familial occurrence, including occult jejunal lesions in asymptomatic relatives that is equivalent to latent celiac disease (29–31). Also, monozygotic twins show a high frequency of concordance for celiac disease (32). In one family study evidence of the disorder was found in 11% of first degree relatives of patients examined (29), while other investigators noted that 8.7% were affected (30). Furthermore, striking associations are found between celiac disease and class II major histocompatibility genes in the HLA-D region, especially DR3, DR7, DQw2, and a 4 kD restric-

TABLE	
31.2	**Celiac Disease**

Cardinal Features Under Varied Conditions of Gluten Exposure

BEFORE GLUTEN-FREE DIET (FULL EXPOSURE TO GLUTEN)
- Malabsorption syndrome.
- *Flat* jejunal biopsy (*Absent* or severely blunted villi) with:
   Surface epithelium, thinned, injured.
   Intraepithelial lymphocytes increased at surface.
   Chronic inflammation increased in lamina propria.
   Crypt mitoses increased; crypts elongated.
GLUTEN-FREE DIET–SHORT TERM (1 WK.–3 MOS.)
- Marked clinical improvement.
- Diminished surface epithelial injury.
- Reduced number of intraepithelial lymphocytes.
- Villi return partially.
GLUTEN-FREE DIET–LONG TERM (GREATER THAN 3 MOS.)
- Villi gradually become fully normal.
- Mitotic hyperactivity gradually subsides.
- Chronic inflammation much diminished.
GLUTEN RESTORED TO DIET
- Rapid return of all lesions and malabsorption findings.
- Early increase in intraepithelial lymphocytes and injury to epithelium over villi.

tion fragment in the DP subregion (33–35), while Marsh et al. demonstrated increased intraepithelial lymphocytes in first degree relatives of patients with celiac disease, especially in relatives of HLA DR3 phenotype (36). A close association exists, too, between celiac disease and the class I HLA-B8 haplotype that is thought to reflect strong linkage disequilibrium with HLA-DR3 (35). Thus the available data strongly support a multigenic, HLA-associated susceptibility to celiac disease (35).

The term *latent celiac disease* is applied to persons who are asymptomatic for malabsorption but who nevertheless show evidence of gluten sensitivity. These individuals are often first degree relatives of persons with known celiac disease. Latent celiac disease can be accompanied by small bowel mucosal changes, and it is important for pathologists to be aware that the changes can fall anywhere along a spectrum of severity. In some persons with latent celiac disease the mucosal lesion approaches that seen in the full-blown symptomatic disorder while at the other extreme there may be normal looking mucosa. Common denominators among these patients can be elevated antigliadin antibody production and intestinal surface epithelial lymphocytosis (37–39). Detection of increased IgA and IgM antigliadin antibodies in intestinal secretions may be especially relevant as well (37, 38).

The importance of genetic factors in celiac disease is further confirmed by the close connection between celiac disease and dermatitis herpetiformis (see below) and by the heightened association between celiac disease and other autoimmune diseases (e.g., Type I diabetes mellitus and pernicious anemia) thereby additionally demonstrating genetically determined susceptibility (40–42). See Chapter 7 for further details.

IMMUNOLOGIC FACTORS   The prominent lymphocytic and plasma cell infiltrates suggest the fundamental importance of immune response in celiac disease. But in addition, elegant in vitro (organ culture) techniques used by Falchuk and colleagues demonstrated that not only gluten, but also an endogenous mediator present only in actively affected intestine is needed to cause injury (18). The local (intramucosal) immune system—either humoral,

cellular, or both—is the best candidate as "endogenous mediator." The favorable response by celiac patients to corticosteroids both in vivo (43) and in vitro (44) adds further weight to a role for immunity.

Elevated circulating antibodies to gluten and its fractions have long been noted, but celiac patients also often show parallel increases in antibodies to unrelated foodstuffs such as casein (45, 46). Increased IgA antibodies to gluten and its products are found, too, in persons with other forms of intestinal disease, and antigliadin antibodies (usually IgG) were sometimes detected in normal individuals (47–49). Thus it is possible that there is only nonspecific immune response to gluten, as well as to other foodstuffs, which result when the damaged mucosa absorbs undigested peptides. Furthermore, since celiac patients can have selective IgA deficiency (up to ten times or more expected frequency [50]), it is hard to see how IgA antibodies could be an essential causative factor. Nonetheless, there is strong correlation between the level of circulating IgA antigliadins and both clinical and histologic status of the celiac disease (47–49), and IgA antigliadin-producing mucosal lymphocytes are increased in active celiac disease (51).

Along with the antibodies against gluten and its fractions, celiac patients with active disease often show circulating IgA antibodies against reticulin (52), a feature that it shares with dermatitis herpetiformis. These findings, along with antigliadin antibodies (see above) are the bases of valuable screening tests for celiac disease. Furthermore, a 90 kD gliadin-binding glycoprotein is found in the intestine and skin of normal individuals. It is noteworthy that both

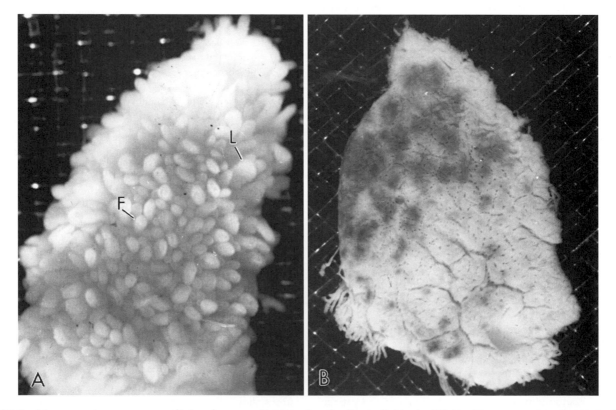

Figure 31.3   Macroscopic appearance of jejunal mucosa in normal and celiac individuals. **(A)** Healthy person showing typical normal pattern of predominantly finger-like *(F)* and scattered leaf-shaped *(L)* villi (×13). **(B)** Active (untreated) Celiac disease. No villi are detected. Numerous crypt openings are evident *(arrows)*. Dark splotches are artefactual hemorrhage, probably induced during suction biopsy (×13).

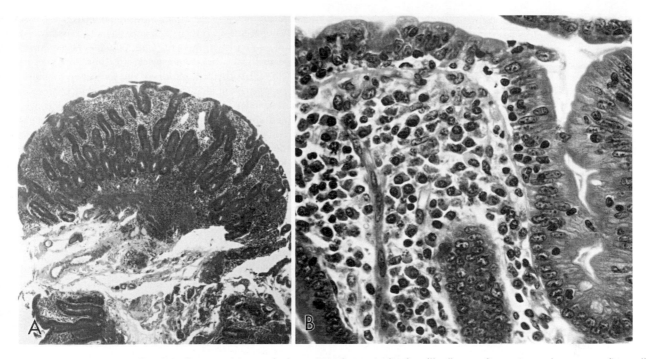

Figure 31.4   Active (untreated) celiac disease—histopathology. **(A)** The typical colon-like flat configuration at low power fits well with the macroscopic appearance seen in Figure 31.3B (×50). **(B)** Same specimen, detail of surface and upper crypt epithelium. The surface epithelium appears thinned, damaged, and "pseudostratified" and is infiltrated by lymphocytes (small dark nuclei). It has also detached from the basement membrane (to which the biopsy procedure probably contributed). The deeper crypt epithelium is much less affected. The lamina propria contains predominately plasma cells and lymphocytes (×430).

observations are consistent with autoantibody production. The incidence of other autoantibodies (antinuclear, antiparietal cell, antithyroid, etc.) has been described as high in adults, although celiac children seldom show them (42).

There are also observations which point to a role for cellular immunity in celiac disease: a striking correlation has been noted between exposure to gluten and the number of intraepithelial lymphocytes. These lymphocytes, which are predominantly cytotoxic/suppressor T cells, diminished in number on gluten withdrawal and reappeared in as little as two hours when gluten was restored to the diet (27, 53, 54). A similar response occurred in the rectum and was suggested as a diagnostic test for celiac disease (55–57). It is reasonable to postulate that these intraepithelial lymphocytes, in concert with gluten, actually lead to epithelial damage through release of injurious mediator substances. In other studies T cells from celiac patients demonstrated enhanced migration inhibition when exposed in vitro to an active gluten fraction (58, 59). Investigations using an A-gliadin-derived peptide which was homologous to a peptide derived from type 12 adenovirus (see below) gave similar results (60, 61).

Kagnoff and colleagues have provided highly provocative evidence that individuals who develop celiac disease are first "primed" to become susceptible by initial exposure to a specific viral agent—type 12 adenovirus (Ad12) (62). A central observation is that the Ad12 virus contains a protein that shares homology with α-gliadin (63). In addition, the authors demonstrated that celiac patients show a high frequency of circulating antibodies to the Ad12 virus (62). It is their general hypothesis that the viral protein may play a role in the pathogenesis of celiac disease, "perhaps by virtue

of immunologic cross-reactivity between determinants shared by the viral protein and α-gliadin" (19).

The concept of a preceding infectious component in the genesis of celiac disease is highly attractive from a clinicopathologic standpoint. It helps account for individual variations in findings, especially as demonstrated by celiac disease in identical twins. While some identical twin pairs have shown similar clinical presentations (29, 32, 64), in others the celiac-related findings were dissimilar, with absence of clinical and pathologic changes in the second twin (65, 66), or with the second twin developing symptoms at a later time (67), or with marked discrepancy in severity between twins (68). In another report a second twin manifested dermatitis herpetiformis instead of celiac disease (69).

PATHOLOGY

A jejunal biopsy specimen from a patient with active, untreated celiac disease is strikingly abnormal. Villi are completely absent, as shown both macroscopically (Fig. 31.3B) and histologically (Fig. 31.4A). Indeed, the absence of villi can be so complete that the first impression is that one is examining a biopsy of colon rather than jejunum. The loss of villi is often referred to as "villous atrophy," but the term, along with its various degrees—partial and subtotal—are misnomers since the villi are not "atrophic" in the literal sense. The mucosal flattening seems to result from remolding of the mucosa by a combination of increased inflammation, surface epithelial injury, and altered epithelial turnover. Overall mucosal thickness is not significantly altered in celiac

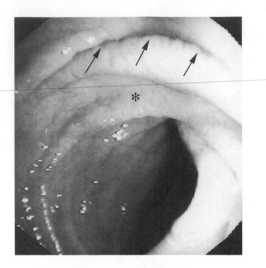

Figure 31.5 Endoscopically visualized counterpart to mucosal "atrophy" in untreated celiac disease, seen here as a striking "scalloped" appearance along the edge of a valvula connivente *(arrows)*. The same changes have a mosaic pattern when seen face-on *(*)*. (Endoscopic picture kindly provided by Dr. William Ravich.) (See color plate).

restoration of healthy-looking columnar cells with well-formed brush borders (i.e., return of microvilli) and possibly a reduction in intraepithelial lymphocytes (Fig. 31.7B). These improvements can occur in as little as one week after initiating the gluten-free diet (25). That this restoration of the surface epithelium accounts well for the patient's rapid improvement is evident from the return of intracellular enzymes by histochemical tests as well as the regained ability to transport lipid contained in a test meal (74). There may be reduction in epithelial mitoses by actual count (25), but the elevated mitotic levels typically persist long after gluten withdrawal. Since the heightened epithelial turnover is a response to injury, persistent elevation of epithelial mitoses may reflect continued presence of gluten in the diet, since wheat products are ubiquitous, and total avoidance of gluten is difficult even with rigorous compliance.

There is progressive morphological improvement with continued adherence to the gluten-free diet. Although the time required for return of villi varies from patient to patient, all who respond clinically will show at least some return of villi after about three months. This is accompanied by a gradual reduction in chronic inflammation and diminution of epithelial mitoses. After one to two years on a strict diet the villus to crypt ratio may be near normal (Fig. 31.8A), as will the appearance of the epithelium covering the

disease (70), and epithelium lining the upper ends of the lengthened ("hyperplastic") crypts in celiac disease have the histochemical characteristics of villus epithelium (71).

The mucosal "atrophy" seen macroscopically and histologically is also detectable endoscopically, thereby providing a valuable early clue to the correct diagnosis. The most striking endoscopic changes in active celiac disease are a scalloped appearance to the valvulae conniventes (72) (Fig. 31.5), and loss of mucosal folds (valves of Kerckring) in the distal duodenum (73).

Comparison of the surface and crypt epithelia in active celiac disease demonstrates that the surface epithelium shows strikingly greater evidence of damage (25) (Fig. 31.4B). Surface epithelium often appears cuboidal rather than columnar, the cytoplasm looks condensed and eosinophilic, the brush border is absent or thinned, the epithelial nuclei are scattered rather than basally placed ("pseudostratification") and numerous lymphocytes are intercalated between the surface cells.

Histochemical and electron microscopic study of the surface epithelium have confirmed their damaged state (26, 71, 74–76). The crypt epithelium shows little or no evidence of damage or inflammation, but there is typically a moderate to marked increase in mitotic figures (25) (Fig. 31.6). Goblet and Paneth cells are normal in appearance though they may be reduced in numbers. The inflammatory response in the lamina propria is predominantly mononuclear, with numerous plasma cells, except for those few individuals who also have immune deficiency.

Response to a gluten-free diet is clinically and morphologically dramatic in the patient with previously untreated celiac disease. Patients may report an improved sense of well-being within a few days, and in the ensuing days and weeks, there is rapid improvement with diminution of malabsorption findings and rapid weight gain (25). Rebiopsy of the jejunum soon after beginning the gluten free diet (Table 31.2) reveals little or no return of villi or reduction in chronic inflammation (Fig. 31.7). There is, however, evidence of improvement in the surface epithelium with

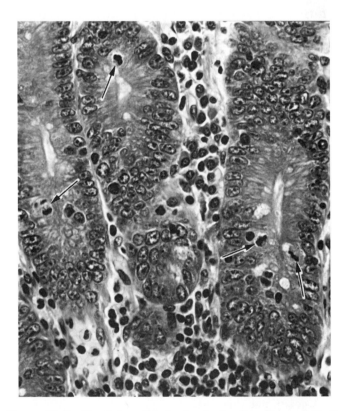

Figure 31.6 Crypts in active (untreated) celiac disease. Mitotic figures *(arrows)* are increased in numbers and some are located in the upper crypts *(top of figure)*, findings that indicate heightened epithelial proliferation. (A normal jejunal biopsy typically demonstrates only 1 mitotic figure per 2 to 3 crypts, most of which are located in the lower halves of the crypts.) Increased chronic inflammation consisting predominantly of plasma cells and lymphocytes is also noted here (×430).

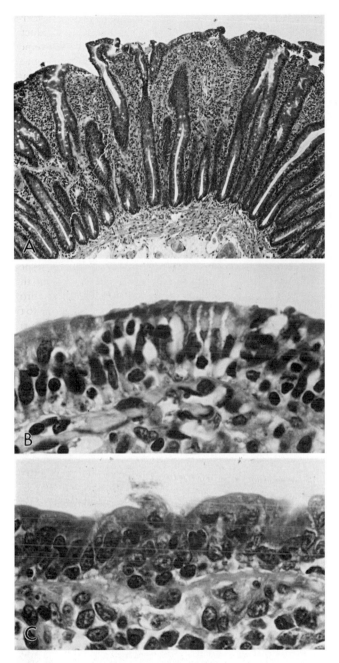

Figure 31.7 Celiac disease 3 weeks after instituting a gluten-free diet. **(A)** The surface epithelium has a faintly wavy outline which suggests incipient return of villi (×90). **(B)** At higher magnification the surface epithelium looks somewhat columnar and taller and the nuclei are more basally located as compared to the biopsy shown in 31.7C (×675). **(C)** For comparison, surface epithelium from the untreated celiac disease patient shown in Figure 31.4 (×675).

villi (Fig. 31.8B). On the other hand even limited exposure to gluten seems to cause some continuing inflammation, villus blunting, and epithelial injury.

Patients who have undergone long-term treatment with a gluten-free diet usually retain their sensitivity to gluten, and this has been confirmed for both the small intestine (27, 77) and rectum (55, 56). Furthermore, the histologic response of the mucosa in treated patients who are re-exposed to gluten gives additional insight into the nature of the response. The time required for reappearance of histologic changes can vary from 2 hours to 6 days (27, 54). Initially, intraepithelial lymphocytes are increased and the epithelium over the upper part of the villus is damaged; a rapid and specific intraepithelial lymphocytic response has also been seen in the rectum on re-exposure to gluten (55, 56). These observations fit well with the hypothesis that the surface epithelium in these patients is sensitive to gluten and that intraepithelial lymphocytes play a key role in the injurious response (see below). Of interest, these lymphocytes are chiefly T cells of the gamma/delta type (78). With continued exposure to gluten, there is overall increase in chronic inflammation, and if gluten ingestion continues, the full-blown syndrome returns.

DIFFERENTIAL DIAGNOSIS AND DIAGNOSTIC PITFALLS

Changes in the jejunal mucosa in celiac disease are so highly characteristic, especially in full-blown active disease with a flat small intestinal biopsy, that one usually does not fail to consider the diagnosis. On the other hand, one should never make the diagnosis of celiac disease solely on the basis of histologic findings since it is possible to have a flat small intestinal biopsy in a variety of other entities (Table 31.3). Furthermore, the range of diagnostic possibilities becomes very large, encompassing most of the disorders described in this section, when intermediate degrees of villus shortening and blunting ("partial villous atrophy") and mucosal inflammation are considered.

Differential Diagnosis

It is curious and potentially important to our understanding of pathogenetic mechanisms in celiac disease that, with minor exceptions, gluten remains the only noninfectious agent to have been established as a specific cause of severe chronic, mucosal injury and resulting malabsorption of the type seen in celiac disease. Isolated cases have been encountered in which soy protein, used as a milk substitute in infants, has caused celiac-like lesions (79). The mucosa showed chronic inflammation and flattening, and there was recovery after soy protein withdrawal. Only a few additional cases of this nature have been reported.

Patients given the drug triparanol (MER-29), on occasion developed a strikingly celiac-like mucosal lesion with loss of villi, chronic inflammation, etc. Withdrawal of the drug led to recovery from malabsorption and disappearance of the mucosal lesion (80).

Neomycin is another drug that is associated with nonspecific inflammation and blunting of villi (81), but it is less of a mimic of celiac disease than are the lesions associated with soy protein and triparanol. The neomycin lesion is said to be dose-related and to regress when the drug is discontinued.

Diagnostic Pitfalls

Depending on the patient's dietary status, plus individual variation, the pathologist must be alert to the wide spectrum of findings that can be seen in small intestinal biopsies from celiac patients. Difficulties for pathologists are compounded when they are asked to

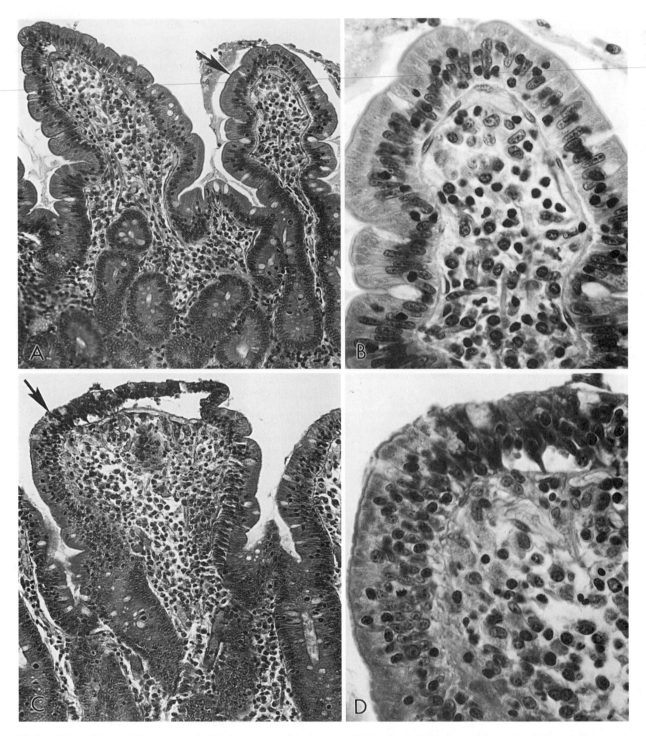

Figure 31.8   Celiac disease. Effects on intestinal mucosa of long-term gluten-free diet followed by restoration of dietary gluten. All frames are of biopsies from the same patient made two years after initiating a gluten-free diet. **(A)** Before administering gluten villi are somewhat short but otherwise normal looking. Lamina proprial and intraepithelial chronic inflammation are about normal in amount. The surface epithelium is columnar and has a prominent brush border. A close-up view of the villus indicated *(arrow)* is shown in B (×200). **(B)** The villus indicated by the arrow in A (×575). **(C)** Intestinal mucosa six days after re-instituting dietary gluten. The villi appear bulbous and shortened, chronic inflammation has increased, and numerous lymphocytes are now seen in the epithelium. Also, the surface epithelium is strikingly condensed and shows detachment from the basement membrane. An expanded view of the area indicated *(arrow)* is shown in D (×200). **(D)** Area indicated by the arrow in C (×575). (B, C, and D are reproduced with permission from Bayless TM, Rubin S, Topping T, Yardley JH, Hendrix TR. Morphologic and functional effects of gluten feeding on jejunal mucosa and celiac disease. In: Booth CC, Dowling RH, eds. Coeliac disease. Edinburgh: Churchill-Livingstone, 1970:76–89.)

TABLE 31.3	Malabsorptive Disorders for Which Biopsies Can Resemble Untreated Celiac Disease[a]

Disorder/Agent	Comments
Dermatitis herpetiformis	Focal or patchy lesions
Autoimmune enteropathy[b,c]	Other autoimmune features
Lymphocytic enterocolitis[d]	
Lymphoma	See Chapter 17
Microvillous inclusion disease[e]	Infants; inborn abnormality
Peptic disease	Chiefly duod. bulb (except Zollinger-Ellison Syndrome)
Soy protein[f]	Probably soy allergy
Triparanol (MER–29)[g]	Historical interest only; drug removed from market
Tropical sprue	Unusual for mucosa to be completely flat

[a]Disorders that can demonstrate a flat or nearly flat mucosa. Other features of celiac disease (thinned surface epithelium, intraepithelial lymphocytes, chronic inflammation, increased mitoses, etc.) may not be present.

[b]Unsworth DJ, Walker-Smith JA. Autoimmunity in diarrhoeal disease. J Pediatr Gastroenterol Nutr 1985;4:375–380.

[c]Cuenod B, Brousse N, Goulet O, et al. Classification of intractable diarrhea in infancy using clinical and immunohistological criteria. Gastroenterology 1990;99:1037–1043.

[d]Dubois RN, Lazenby AJ, Yardley JH, et al. Lymphocytic entero-colitis in patients with 'refractory' sprue. JAMA 1989;262:935–937.

[e]Cutz E, Rhoads JM, Drumm B, et al. Microvillus inclusion disease: an inherited defect of brush-border assembly and differentiation. New Engl J Med 1989;320:646–651.

[f]Ament ME, Rubin CE. Soy protein—another cause of the flat intestinal lesion. Gastroenterology 1972;62:227–234.

[g]McPherson JR, Shorter RG. Intestinal lesions associated with triparanol. A clinical and experimental study. Am J Dig Dis 1965;10:1024–1033.

assess duodenal or jejunal mucosa for possible celiac disease in patients who have already been placed on a gluten-free diet without a pretreatment biopsy, or in those who may not be fully compliant with their diet, or when the dietary history is incomplete.

The biopsy site along the small intestine can profoundly affect pathologic findings. To a degree that varies widely between patients, the severity of the lesion diminishes distally in active celiac disease, as does the total length of intestine involved. Thus a typical flat biopsy can be obtained occasionally from an asymptomatic person if most of their small intestine is still functioning normally. The reduced severity distally is presumed to result from progressive proteolysis and hence dilution of intact gluten as it moves down the intestine.

Another pitfall for the pathologist is overreliance on biopsies obtained from the proximal duodenum. This can cause either overdiagnosis or underdiagnosis of celiac disease, especially for biopsies that are obtained from the duodenal bulb (Fig. 31.9). On the one hand, severe peptic duodenitis, with or without associated peptic ulcer, occasionally causes a biopsy to appear flat and heavily inflamed, thereby mimicking the changes of celiac disease. On the

other hand, proximal duodenal biopsies from celiac patients who also have peptic duodenitis with marked replacement of absorptive cells by gastric mucous cells can show an intact villus architecture (Fig. 31.9B). Presumably the gastric metaplasia provides localized protection against the injurious effects of gluten.

SEROLOGIC TESTS FOR CELIAC DISEASE

Demonstration of circulating antibodies to gliadin, reticulin, or endomysium (reticulin that lines primate smooth muscle) (82) are now of proven usefulness as a noninvasive screening test, in early diagnosis, and for monitoring response to treatment in celiac disease (83). Correlation between "villous atrophy" and elevated antireticulin or antiendomysium levels was 90 to 100% in some hands, and in adults and older children may be present in the absence of mucosal abnormality (37). Antiendomysial testing is probably superior to antigliadin, but variation between laboratories is to be expected.

MALIGNANCY IN CELIAC DISEASE

There is no doubt that malignancy occurs at significantly higher than expected frequency in celiac patients (84–86). Primary non-Hodgkins lymphoma of the small intestine is the most commonly seen tumor (see Chapter 17), accounting for about 50% of all malignant conditions found in celiac patients (84, 85). The lymphomas that arise in celiac disease are mostly derived from mucosal T cells ("enteropathy-associated T-cell lymphoma"), probably those that migrate into the epithelial layer (87, 88). Furthermore, the T-cell subset characteristics of the lymphoma are similar to those that predominate in celiac disease (see above under Pathogenesis of celiac disease), thereby additionally supporting a direct relationship between the lymphoma and the celiac disease (89). Recently, it was shown that the same clonal gene rearrangements seen in enteropathy-associated T-cell lymphoma could be demonstrated in reactive T cell populations from adjacent nontumorous mucosa (90).

Adenocarcinoma of the small intestine, carcinoma of the esophagus, and carcinoma of the mouth and pharynx are the principal other malignancies that arise with greater than expected frequency in celiac disease (84–86). Swinson et al. found 19 instances of small intestinal adenocarcinoma, compared with 0.23 cases expected, among 119 nonlymphomatous malignancies in their registry (85). Those tumors occur predominantly in the jejunum and duodenum. One patient with celiac disease demonstrated villous adenoma, a likely precursor of carcinoma, and others have been seen with multiple adenocarcinomas (91–93). Conventional squamous esophageal and oropharyngeal tumors are also increased in celiac disease patients; Holmes et al. found the relative risk for those lesions to be 12.3 (P<.01) and 9.7 (P<.01) respectively (86). There is no obvious explanation for the increased squamous lesions, but vitamin A deficiency associated with the malabsorption syndrome has been suggested (85).

Holmes et al. observed a significantly reduced risk of malignancy among patients who adhered closely to a gluten-free diet for five or more years. While nonlymphomatous malignancy has been seen at numerous other sites in celiac patients (e.g., pancreas, stomach, colon, bladder, breast, and brain), with the possible

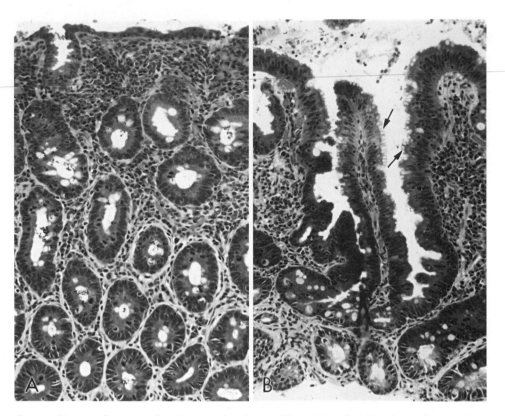

Figure 31.9   Celiac disease. Biopsies from two locations in duodenum illustrating that the diagnosis may be overlooked if only the duodenal bulb is biopsied. **(A)** Biopsy from second portion of duodenum demonstrating typical flat biopsy of Celiac disease (×180). **(B)** Biopsy of bulb obtained at same time as A. Findings are consistent with peptic duodenitis with inflammation and distorted villi demonstrating gastric mucous cells metaplasia *(arrows)* (×180). (Reproduced with permission from Yardley, JH. Pathology of chronic gastritis and duodenitis. In: Goldman H, Appelman HD, Kaufmann N, eds. Gastrointestinal pathology. USCAP Monograph in Pathology 31. Baltimore: Williams & Wilkins, 1990:49–143.)

exception of testis (*P*<.001) in one report (85), malignancy has have not been described in excess numbers in other locations.

CELIAC-RELATED CONDITIONS

REFRACTORY CELIAC DISEASE AND REFRACTORY SPRUE

Most persons with celiac disease remain well on a gluten-free diet for many years, but some patients later develop recurrent symptoms despite close adherence to the diet. This loss of previously shown responsiveness to the gluten-free diet I prefer to term *refractory celiac disease* although it is called, by other authors, generically, *refractory sprue* (94) (Fig. 31.10). There are also some patients with malabsorption and a typical flat biopsy who do not respond to gluten withdrawal even when their illness is first diagnosed (Fig. 31.11). It is to the condition afflicting these individuals that I prefer to restrict the term *refractory sprue* (synonyms: unclassified sprue, atypical sprue) since their intestinal lesion is of uncertain or unknown etiology, although some of these patients could in fact have demonstrated underlying celiac disease (95).

Both refractory celiac disease and refractory sprue can be accompanied by ulcerations in the small intestine (Fig. 31.12). The ulcerations can cause bleeding, perforation, or stricture (94–96). They can be small and superficial or large and extend to the muscularis propria. The ulcers may be accompanied by pyloric

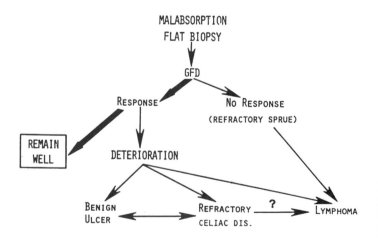

Figure 31.10   Celiac disease. Summary of possible clinical courses. Most patients who are found to have a flat biopsy and who subsequently adhere to a gluten-free diet (GFD) improve and remain well *(thick arrows)*. A few patients with malabsorption and flat biopsies, however, fail to respond to the diet from the outset (Refractory Sprue) while others relapse after an initial satisfactory response (Refractory Celiac Disease). Other possible outcomes are shown in the lower portion of the diagram.

metaplasia or ectopic gastric mucosa (97), but those features are typically lacking and the pathogenesis of the ulcers is not known. Patients in full remission from their celiac disease as a result of treatment with either a gluten-free diet or corticosteroids can also develop ulcers (95, 96). Presence of ulcers in refractory celiac disease or refractory sprue should always lead to a high index of suspicion of celiac-associated intestinal lymphoma.

Some ulcer-associated cases, especially those with refractory sprue, have been categorized in the past as "chronic ulcerative (nongranulomatous) jejunoileitis" (98). This is felt, however, to be a misleading term which should be avoided since it gives the impression that a distinct entity is described while failing to focus attention on the underlying malabsorptive disorder.

Active (acute) inflammation is seen only rarely in celiac patients who respond well to gluten withdrawal. Thus a biopsy specimen showing acute inflammation, with or without demonstrated ulceration (which could be nearby), should always cause suspicion that the individual may have ulcers and possibly refractory sprue or refractory celiac disease. The patient may also have an infectious or other condition unrelated to celiac disease.

Lymphoma can present clinically as refractory celiac disease or refractory sprue and should be included in the differential diagnosis for unexplained or recrudescent malabsorption (Fig. 31.10). Furthermore, in addition to the inherent sampling problem, early histologic changes in celiac disease-associated malignant lymphoma may be subtle and all but impossible to recognize, being noted only as scattered atypical lymphoid (often "histiocytic") cells that tend to infiltrate crypt epithelium. Lymphoma accompanying ulceration is also easily overlooked (95, 99).

In some patients with refractory celiac disease the poor response to a gluten-free diet may be related to associated hyperacidity that leads to additional mucosal injury (100). Biopsies from the duodenum in these patients will show peptic duodenitis combined with changes of celiac disease. The Brunner gland enlargement associated with the peptic disease leads to a nodular appearance in the duodenum that at times is seen radiologically as a bubbly appearance to the barium column ("bubbly bulb") (Fig. 31.13) (100). The importance of hyperacidity in genesis of the lesion was supported by favorable response in some patients to combined treatment with a gluten-free diet and H_2 blocking drugs (100).

Cavitation of mesenteric lymph nodes and *hyposplenism* are two additional findings that are especially prone to occur in refractory celiac disease (97, 101). Cavitated mesenteric nodes are readily detected either as a palpable abdominal mass or by CT radiologically (Fig. 31.14) (102). The nodes tend to concentrate in the jejunal mesentery; individual nodes can measure 5 cm or more. Lymphoma is frequently suspected in these individuals, but is an infrequent association (97). The cavitated nodes demonstrate a large central "pseudocystic" cavity from which fluid may gush on sectioning; histologically the cavitary space contains hyaline material and is surrounded by fibrosis and an outer rim of surviving lymphoid tissue. These patients also typically show hyposplenism clinically (presence of Howell-Jolly bodies and target cells in circulating erythrocytes) and have an atrophic spleen. The two findings are presumably associated in some way, although their pathogenesis is otherwise unknown. Some degree of hyposplenism is also common in celiac disease when cavitated mesenteric nodes are not detected (103). Studies of its possible relationship to malignant disease (104) and to autoimmune phenomena (103) have been negative.

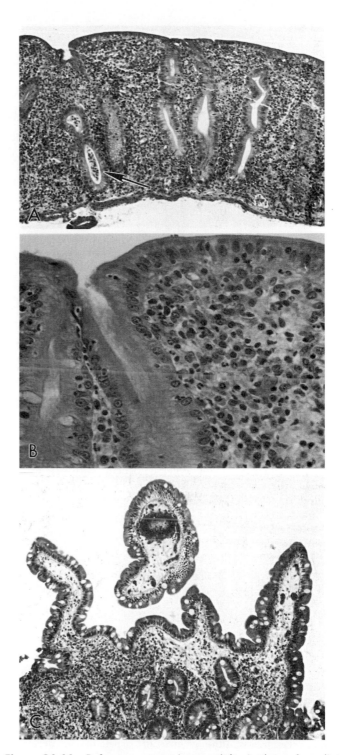

Figure 31.11 Refractory sprue in an adult. A gluten-free diet was ineffective, but the patient's malabsorption improved dramatically on corticosteroids. **(A)** Initial flat biopsy with intense inflammation, including gland abscess *(arrow)* (×90). **(B)** Detail of specimen shown in A; the surface epithelium appears thinned and regenerating. Acute and chronic inflammation are present in the lamina propria, but the paucity of intraepithelial lymphocytes is in striking contrast to the typical findings in untreated celiac disease (×340). **(C)** Restoration of villi seen after corticosteroid therapy (×90).

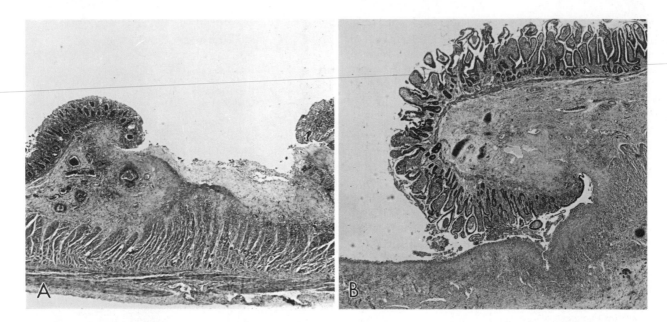

Figure 31.12   Ulceration in refractory sprue and refractory celiac disease. **(A)** Ulcer in patient with malabsorption who never responded to a gluten-free diet and thus was an example of refractory sprue (×18). **(B)** Ulcer in another patient who had longstanding celiac disease who responded well to a gluten-free diet but then later developed multiple small intestinal ulcers. Note the tall villi in adjacent mucosa, indicating recovery from gluten withdrawal (×18). (Reproduced with permission from Baer AN, Bayless TM, Yardley JH. Intestinal ulceration and malabsorption syndromes. Gastroenterology 1980;79:754–765.)

COLLAGENOUS SPRUE

A curious and uncommon subset of patients with flat mucosal biopsies are those with so called *collagenous sprue* (105). In this condition the flattened mucosa shows intense scarring in the lamina propria. Others have found some degree of subepithelial collagen deposition in about one-third of their patients with untreated celiac disease, and the collagen diminished on a gluten-free diet (106). The clinical presentation in collagenous sprue is comparable to other instances of refractory celiac disease and refractory sprue, and the condition is now generally viewed as a variant form of celiac disease (107, 108).

DERMATITIS HERPETIFORMIS

Most patients with *dermatitis herpetiformis* have an associated derangement in their intestinal mucosa which closely resembles that seen in active celiac disease (40, 109–111). However, in dermatitis herpetiformis the mucosal lesion varies markedly in severity from patient to patient; also, its distribution in the intestine is less uniform than in celiac disease. Although up to 20% of patients with dermatitis herpetiformis show abnormal laboratory tests for malabsorption, only about 4% of the patients have intestinal symptoms (40).

It was believed initially that dermatitis herpetiformis was not related to celiac disease or to gluten sensitivity. Subsequent experience, however, showed that individuals with dermatitis herpetiformis also have a high frequency of the same histocompatibility antigens (e.g., HLA-B8 and HLA-DR3) as celiac patients, and that both the intestinal and skin lesions in dermatitis herpetiformis can be improved by adherence to a gluten-free diet. Reinstitution of dietary gluten in dermatitis herpetiformis leads to worsening of skin and gastrointestinal lesions with increase in IgA and IgM containing plasma cells (112).

While the skin and intestinal lesions are histopathologically dissimilar, dermatitis herpetiformis patients almost always demonstrate deposition of IgA in the skin at the basement membrane, and this may be related to intestinal involvement (40). The full pathogenesis of dermatitis herpetiformis and the nature of its relationship to celiac disease remain to be clarified. See Chapter 19 for further details.

CELIAC-LIKE AND CELIAC-RELATED CONDITIONS ELSEWHERE IN THE GASTROINTESTINAL TRACT

Lymphocytic infiltration into the epithelium comparable to that seen in celiac disease is a prominent feature in lymphocytic gastritis (Chapter 23) and in lymphocytic and collagenous colitis (Chapter 30). In fact, collagenous colitis resembles and took its name from collagenous sprue (113).

While these various forms of gastritis and colitis that share features with celiac disease most often occur as freestanding clinical entities in patients who give no historic or other evidence of celiac disease, lymphocytic gastritis and lymphocytic and collagenous colitis are sometimes seen in celiac patients. Among a group of celiac-type patients for whom gastric biopsy were available, lymphocytic gastritis was noted in 45% (114). In one investigation lymphocytic colitis was found in 11% of celiac patients (115) while in another a much higher frequency (31%) was noted (116). Celiac disease has also been reported in at least three patients with collagenous colitis (117–119).

Small intestinal inflammatory changes which resemble celiac disease, but which are refractory to gluten withdrawal, can also be found in patients with lymphocytic ("microscopic") or collagenous colitis (42, 115, 118, 120). The accompanying small intestinal lesion has consisted only of chronic inflammation and villus blunting in some patients while in others there was collagenous change. Still other patients with small intestinal changes resembling celiac disease, but who had never responded to a gluten-free diet (and hence had "refractory sprue"), have also demonstrated lymphocytic infiltration of colonic epithelium. One such group of patients was said to have *lymphocytic enterocolitis* (115).

Occurrence of celiac-like and celiac-related findings outside the small intestine has obvious significance from the standpoint of differential diagnosis. It is also of theoretical interest since autoim-

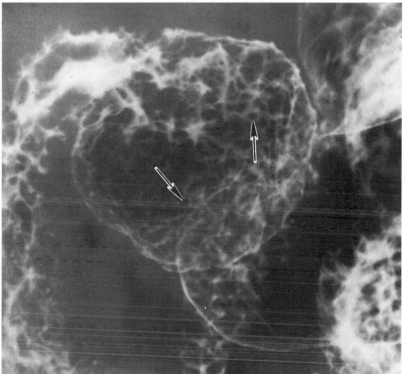

Figure 31.13 Refractory celiac disease showing "bubbly bulb." (The patient became unresponsive to a gluten-free diet after undergoing initial remission.) Contrast material outlines the radiolucent nodules that are believed to represent enlarged Brunner's glands accompanying flattened mucosa of Celiac disease. (Reproduced with permission from Jones B, Bayless TM, Hamilton SR, Yardley JH. "Bubbly" duodenal bulb in celiac disease: radiologic-pathologic correlation. Am J Roentgenol 1984;142:119–122.)

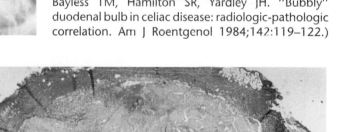

Figure 31.14 Cavitated mesenteric nodes in refractory celiac disease. **(A)** CT scan showing greatly enlarged, cavitated node demonstrating fat-fluid levels *(arrows)*. **(B)** Histologic section of a cavitated node containing hyaline material *(H)* and a separate region containing abundant lipid. The largely destroyed lymph node has a thick fibrous capsule. (Reproduced with permission from Rubesin SE, Herlinger H, Saul SH, Grumbach K, Laufer I, Levine MS. Adult celiac disease and its complications. Radiographics 1989;9:1045–1066.)

mune phenomena that are similar and/or related to celiac disease may be involved in other lymphocytic and collagenous inflammatory conditions that occur outside the small intestine (121).

TROPICAL SPRUE (POSTINFECTIVE TROPICAL MALABSORPTION)

Numerous definitions for tropical sprue have been proposed over the years, many with varying emphasis on particular findings. For all-encompassing conciseness, however, it is hard to improve upon the definition provided by Baker and Mathan (122): "Intestinal malabsorption of unknown etiology, occurring among residents in, or visitors to, the tropics."

There are several noteworthy points about tropical sprue. One, the malabsorption is *chronic* and is typically accompanied by various nutritional deficiencies with folate deficiency a usual hallmark. However, the deficiencies are secondary and do not, as was believed at one time, seem to be a primary etiologic factor. Two, tropical sprue occurs only in certain areas, chiefly the West Indies (especially Puerto Rico, Haiti, and the Dominican Republic), portions of Central America and the northern countries of South America, the Indian subcontinent, south China, Southeast Asia, and central and south Africa. Three, adults are affected much more commonly than children. Expatriates such as military personnel who immigrate to endemic areas are often afflicted, but their illness tends to be more acute and they are less likely to present with severe folate and/or Vitamin B12 deficiency and anemia. And four, the disorder is found in endemic and epidemic forms. Under both circumstances the patients' findings suggest an infectious etiology, including a frequent history of onset following an episode of an acute and presumably infectious diarrheal illness.

ETIOLOGY AND PATHOGENESIS

The etiology of tropical sprue is unknown, and, indeed, there may be no single inciting agent. It is widely postulated, however, that tropical sprue begins with an episode of infectious diarrhea from a bacterial, parasitic, or viral organism (123, 124). This is believed to be followed by residual and persistent damage to the mucosa, including absorptive cells. In addition, there is bacterial overgrowth by enterotoxigenic organisms (most commonly *E. coli*, and *Haemophilus*) which may be important in sustaining the disease (125). Thus broad spectrum antibiotics are of major importance in treatment of tropical sprue (126, 127). The reason for the chronic bacterial overgrowth is poorly understood, but excess production of enteroglucagon with resulting reduced motility and stasis, thereby favoring heavy colonization, has been suggested (123). At the same time it should be stressed that the bacteria that colonize the intestine in tropical sprue are not predominantly of the anaerobic, bile salt depleting variety found in the *stasis syndrome* (see below) (128–130).

Because it is a major site of folate and Vitamin B12 absorption, damage to ileal mucosa leads to malabsorption of those vitamins with resulting deficiencies, especially of folate (131). Individuals who are already malnourished are especially vulnerable. At the same time there is evidence that folate and Vitamin B12 deficiency can each *cause* derangements in intestinal mucosal structure and func-

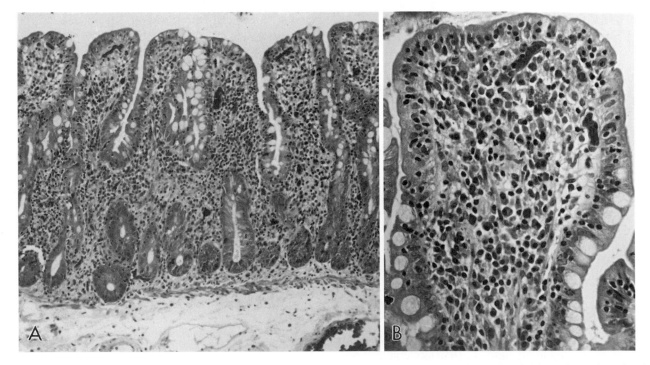

Figure 31.15 Moderately severe tropical sprue. **(A)** The villi are blunted and shortened and the crypts elongated. On the other hand, there is not the *complete* absence of villi commonly seen in Celiac disease. There is overall increased chronic inflammation involving the lamina propria and epithelium (×120). **(B)** The epithelium and lamina propria are infiltrated by lymphocytes and other mononuclears. The epithelium is cuboidal and somewhat stratified (×250).

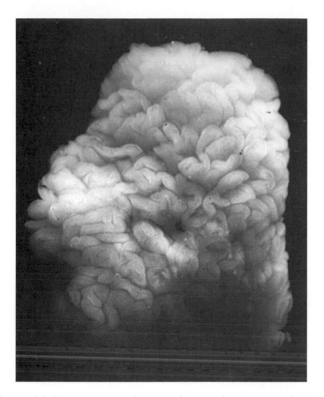

Figure 31.16 Macroscopic view of tropical sprue-type changes in jejunal mucosa. (Alcoholic patient with malabsorption and folate deficiency comparable to that seen in tropical sprue.) Ridges and large leaves have replaced the predominantly finger architecture of normal small intestine (compare with Figure 31.3A). While architectural shift of this type is characteristic of tropical sprue, it is a finding in many other conditions that demonstrate chronic inflammation with blunting and shortening of villi.

tion (12, 132). Thus the vitamin deficiencies, once in place in tropical sprue, are able to further enhance the intestinal mucosal damage and lead to megaloblastic anemia and other associated clinical findings (131). Further support for the concept of direct damage by deficiency of the two vitamins is found in the favorable response to treatment with folic acid and/or Vitamin B12 alone. Epithelial mitotic figures tend to reappear, nuclear size diminishes, and villi become more normal (133). Ethyl alcohol, either ingested by the patient or produced locally by resident bacteria, may also be an important cofactor in mucosal damage.

PATHOLOGY

Histologically, the most common pattern in small intestinal biopsies in tropical sprue is blunting and shortening of villi without total absence (Fig. 31.15). This appearance matches well with findings in the dissecting microscope of altered villus architecture with a shift towards leaves and ridges instead of tubular villi (Fig. 31.16). There is chronic inflammation with increased lymphocytes, plasma cells, and eosinophils and the surface epithelium is usually cuboidal and somewhat pseudostratified (Fig. 31.15B). Intraepithelial lymphocyte infiltration also occurs, most prominently in the upper crypt and crypt-villus interzones (134). The lymphocytic infiltration

appears *after* onset of epithelial derangement, suggesting that cell-mediated immune response in the epithelium in tropical sprue is secondary (134), unlike celiac disease where lymphocyte infiltration precedes or is concurrent with epithelial injury due to gluten.

Total absence of villi comparable to that seen in celiac disease is only rarely noted in tropical sprue. Marsh et al. (134) stated: "Biopsies of proximal jejunum in over 1500 South Indian patients with tropical sprue have not revealed any with the "flat" mucosa characteristic of untreated celiac sprue." On the other hand, unlike celiac disease, overall mucosal thinning occurs in more severely affected persons with tropical sprue, and thus it can be said that a true mucosal and villus atrophy can be seen (70, 135).

In the severest forms of untreated tropical sprue, the crypt epithelium shows reduced mitoses and nuclear enlargement (Fig. 31.17) (136). Another noteworthy feature of the mucosal changes in tropical sprue is their *variability* both from patient to patient and from area to area in the small intestine of single individuals; this can be especially apparent under the dissecting microscope (70, 135). Despite the variability, severity of the mucosal alterations tend to correlate with severity of the clinical symptoms and laboratory findings (137).

Although epithelial changes are usually less prominent in tropical sprue than in celiac disease, there is good evidence that they contribute importantly to the malabsorption. Schenk et al. demonstrated diminished epithelial ATPase activity (70) and increased numbers of lipid droplets are seen in the surface epithelium, in the basement membrane, and in the lamina propria (70, 138). The

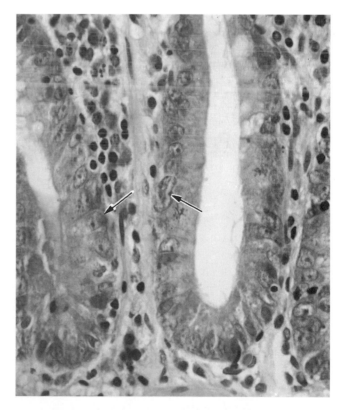

Figure 31.17 Tropical sprue. Lower crypts showing enlarged, pale nuclei. In addition, epithelial mitotic figures were sparse in this specimen, another characteristic feature of more severe tropical sprue (×550).

subepithelial region also often shows increased collagen, and, by electron microscopy, finely granular and sometimes fibrillar material of unknown nature and significance. Similar material is occasionally seen in asymptomatic persons from the same part of the world, and in other conditions affecting the small bowel, including celiac disease (138).

Presence of mild to severe gastritis in about one-half of a group of patients with tropical sprue led to the suggestion that the stomach is a possible additional site of disease (139). However, there has been no confirmation of these findings. Furthermore, the available photomicrographs (139) show a nonspecific chronic gastritis comparable to that which is now recognized to be due to *Helicobacter pylori*. There is no evidence that deficiency of intrinsic factor plays a role in the Vitamin B12 deficiency sometimes seen in tropical sprue. Instead, the deficiency is thought to result from consumption of the vitamin by intraluminal bacteria combined with ileal malabsorption.

Rare comments about histopathology of the colorectum suggest only that it appeared normal. Impaired absorption of water and electrolytes from the colorectum has, however, been described in tropical sprue (140), and the mucosa showed low levels of sodium-potassium ATPase (141). These abnormalities in the colorectum could contribute to the diarrhea. Findings in both the stomach and colorectum in tropical sprue probably deserve further investigation.

CLINICOPATHOLOGIC CORRELATION

Occurrence of histologic changes of the type seen in tropical sprue do not always correlate well with clinical and laboratory findings of malabsorption. Jejunal biopsies from symptom-free individuals living in areas where tropical sprue is endemic often show some blunting of villi and inflammatory changes that are qualitatively and at times quantitatively comparable to those seen in patients with demonstrated malabsorption. While there are undoubtedly many variables such as malnutrition, the patient's microflora, and nature of inciting agents that determine the final clinical and pathologic picture, in all likelihood *distribution* of the lesion is a factor in the discrepancy between pathologic changes and clinical findings, too. In its earlier and milder stages the mucosal changes in tropical sprue diminish distally, but in chronic and advanced disease the ileum and jejunum typically are affected histologically to a similar degree (142).

DIFFERENTIAL DIAGNOSIS

Because of the nonspecific character of the histopathologic changes, the importance of a maximal effort to exclude the many other possible causes of villus blunting and inflammatory changes (Table 31.1) before arriving at a diagnosis of tropical sprue cannot be overstressed. It is especially important to rule out malabsorption-associated syndromes due to known infectious causes (e.g., *Giardia lamblia*, *Strongyloides stercoralis*, or *Capillaria phillipinensis*). Obviously demonstration of clinical features such as folate and/or Vitamin B12 deficiency and a history of residence in the appropriate area of the world are also crucial.

STASIS (BLIND-LOOP) SYNDROME

The stasis syndrome is characterized by stagnation of intestinal contents, with secondary proliferation of colonic type bacteria occurring in a patient who has an underlying small intestinal disorder that has led to delayed or altered movement of its contents. There is accompanying malabsorption of fat and, at times, of Vitamin B12, carbohydrates, and other substances. Synonyms are blind-loop syndrome, stagnant loop syndrome, and bacterial overgrowth syndrome.

Conditions associated with the stasis syndrome include primary motor disturbances (see Chapter 13) and mechanical abnormalities resulting from a gastrointestinal disease or following surgical alterations (Table 31.4). It occurs in the small subset of *scleroderma* patients who develop saccular dilatations and diverticula of the small intestine secondary to degeneration of the muscularis propria. In patients with *pseudo-obstruction* there is dysmotility (143) and, at times, diverticulum formation due to nerve or muscle degeneration from an inherited defect. Bacterial overgrowth in even a single diverticulum in the duodenum can lead to malabsorption (130). Patients with *diabetes mellitus* occasionally show motility disturbances as a result of peripheral neuropathy. Among various mechanical disturbances, stasis syndrome can be seen with spontaneous strictures and fistulae (as in Crohn's disease) or in a surgically isolated segment of intestine (blind loop). An enteroenterostomy can functionally become an isolated segment, and in gastro-jejunocolic fistulae bacteria are constantly fed from the colon into the proximal small intestine. Stasis syndrome has also been described occasionally in elderly patients who lacked demonstrable underlying disease (144, 145).

PATHOGENESIS

The role of bacterial overgrowth in stasis syndrome has been studied extensively and is considered a main factor in its pathogenesis (Fig. 31.18) (130, 146). At first the major focus centered on the effects of anaerobic bacteria on conjugated bile salts, compounds that are important to solubilization of fat into absorbable micelles.

TABLE	
31.4	**Diseases and Conditions Associated With the Stasis (Blind-loop) Syndrome**

Motor Disturbances
  Scleroderma
  Pseudo-obstruction
  Diabetes mellitus
  Amyloidosis
  Thyroid
Structural Abnormalities
  Diverticula of small intestine
  Strictures and narrowings
    Crohn's disease
    Tuberculosis
    Adhesions
  Surgically isolated segments
    Self-filling "pouches"
    Afferent limb in gastro-jejunostomy
  Entero-enterostomy
  Gastro-jejuno-colic fistula

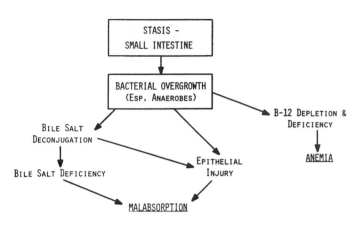

Figure 31.18 Stasis (blind-loop) syndrome. Summary of pathogenetic factors leading to malabsorption and (in some patients) anemia.

Anaerobic bacteria are not normally found in the small intestine, but typically occur in large numbers in patients with stasis syndrome. Certain of the anaerobic bacteria (*Bacteroides* and several others) can deconjugate bile salt to free bile acids. Free bile acids are ineffective as fat solubilizers, and fat malabsorption is felt to result from reduced availability of the conjugated bile salt. On the other hand, an association between fat solubilization and amounts of conjugated and free bile acids is not always demonstrated (147).

The absorptive epithelium is also altered in stasis syndrome, and this could have as much or more importance than effects of changes in luminal bile salts and bile acids on micelle formation. Ultrastructural studies in patients (147) and in experimental animals (148) have shown epithelial damage and evidence of abnormal epithelial fat transport. Defective absorption and reduced brush border and other epithelial enzymes have been noted, too (148–150). The cause of the epithelial injury is unclear, but presence of unconjugated bile acids and bacterial metabolic products are suggested factors.

Depletion of nutrients by the luminal bacteria is an important factor in the Vitamin B12 deficiency that these patients often show. Nutrient depletion by bacteria may also cause other deficiencies, as suggested by the loss of administered d-xylose that occurs from bacterial action.

Definitive correction of mechanical conditions causing stasis syndrome such as blind loop is typically curative (151). Furthermore, significant improvement in malabsorption is usually seen after reduction in intestinal flora from antibiotic treatment, thus confirming the importance of bacterial overgrowth (146, 152).

PATHOLOGY

Descriptions of the underlying disorders that can lead to stasis syndrome are covered in other chapters. Obviously, a mucosal biopsy will not serve to demonstrate changes in deep musculature or nerves or to identify gross mechanical disturbances that have led to stasis syndrome.

The light microscopic changes in small intestinal biopsies from patients with stasis syndrome are easily summarized: they are nonspecific in character, variable in severity (Fig. 31.19), and do not necessarily correlate with clinical findings (147). Although moderate and even severe changes may be noted, many biopsies show few if any abnormalities, and the changes are usually limited to chronic inflammation with some villus blunting and reduction in villus to crypt ratio (147). Vesicles may be seen in the absorptive epithelium, especially over the villus tips; they probably reflect "hang-up" of absorbed lipid by damaged cells. The mucosal changes are often patchy in distribution and severity, and multiple biopsies may be needed to demonstrate them. On occasion a smear prepared from the jejunal biopsy will show numerous bacteria in the mucus overlying the epithelium, but because of possible saliva-associated organisms, their presence must be interpreted cautiously.

Experience with the markedly deranged mucosa of celiac disease during the early period after invention of the biopsy capsule was probably responsible for widespread initial failure to appreciate the potential importance in bacterial overgrowth conditions of relatively inconspicuous changes seen in villus epithelium by light microscopy (153). The ultrastructural, enzymic, and functional changes in absorptive epithelium described above under Pathogenesis do not always correlate closely with alterations seen by light microscopy, being typically more frequently observed and more prominent. This is a point to be kept in mind when evaluating biopsies from these patients.

DEFICIENCY STATES

In addition to the numerous deficiency states that *result* from malabsorption, some deficiency states can *cause* malabsorption by damaging the small intestinal mucosa. The direct effects of folate and Vitamin B12 deficiency on the small intestine are discussed in the section on tropical sprue (under Etiology and Pathogenesis).

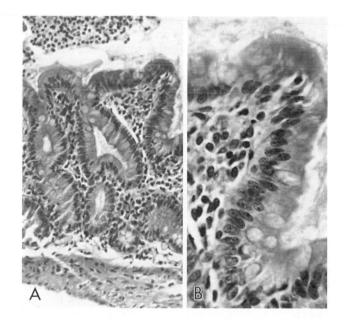

Figure 31.19 Jejunal biopsy from patient with gastro-colic fistula (post-Billroth II), which led to a stasis syndrome. **(A)** The mucosa shows blunting and shortening of villi and increased chronic inflammation. **(B)** The epithelium does not appear especially damaged or inflamed, in keeping with the frequent poor correlation between pathologic changes and clinical findings in this condition (×675).

Protein deficiency (or "protein-calorie malnutrition" when total calorie intake is also inadequate), iron deficiency, and zinc deficiency have been shown to cause mucosal alterations of themselves and will be considered here. There are undoubtedly other deficiency states, too, whose relationships to malabsorption have gone unrecognized or are less well defined.

PROTEIN DEFICIENCY

It is known from experimental studies that protein deficiency can lead to alterations in the small intestine with overall mucosal and muscle layer thinning, blunting of villi, epithelial thinning, and increased chronic inflammation (predominantly lymphocytes and plasma cells) (Fig. 31.20) (154, 155). There is frequently malabsorption, although not necessarily with steatorrhea or diarrhea; associated infection can lead to enhancement of histologic and clinical changes (155). However, the effects of protein deficiency are variable. Rats placed on a low protein diet for 22 weeks developed reduction in some epithelial enzymes such as acid phosphatase and succinic dehydrogenase, but epithelial ultrastructure remained normal (156). On the other hand, only 3 weeks on a no protein diet were required for rats to develop ultrastructural changes in absorptive epithelium (154).

While it is difficult to verify the impact on the human intestine of isolated protein deficiency, changes comparable to those produced experimentally have been reported in humans subjected to chronic protein malnutrition (157–161). Klipstein et al. have summarized the difficulties of distinguishing between protein-calorie malnutrition, tropical sprue, superimposed infection, and other unknown factors in producing intestinal changes and malabsorption in Haitian patients (162). Those authors considered patients who demonstrated both diarrhea and megaloblastic anemia to have tropical sprue while those who showed reduced serum albumin without megaloblastic anemia, with or without diarrhea, were considered to have protein deficiency. Mucosal changes were more severe in those with tropical sprue, but lesser degrees of villus blunting, chronic inflammation, etc. were seen in both protein deficient and asymptomatic patients.

In other studies, conducted in a tropical area where superimposed parasitic infection was common, it was found that treatment of protein calorie malnutrition in children led to improvement in mucosal thickness, epithelial cell height, and brush border thickness (163). However, when there was also chronic diarrhea (cause not specified) the epithelium showed greater inflammatory infiltrate. Control patients without past or present malnutrition showed minimal epithelial inflammatory infiltrate, but nonetheless demonstrated macroscopic changes in villus architecture with blunting and ridge formation. Furthermore, inflammatory cells in the lamina propria were comparable in number and type for protein-calorie malnourished children before and after recovery and for controls (163). These studies emphasize that in the real world "pure" malnutrition rarely if ever exists, and that multiple associated factors are the rule and usually always include undefined acute and chronic infections.

IRON DEFICIENCY

Malabsorption associated with nonspecific mucosal abnormalities, including blunted villi and chronic inflammation, can occur in dietary iron-deficiency anemia, and the abnormalities are corrected by adequate iron intake (164). It is noteworthy that the malabsorp-

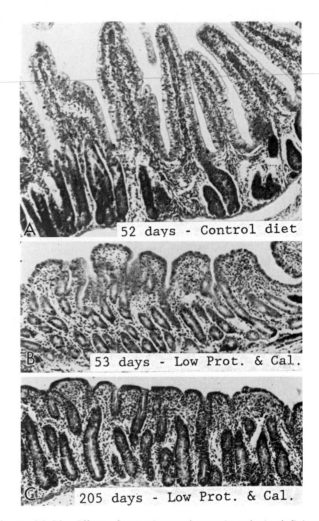

Figure 31.20   Effect of experimental protein-calorie deficiency on jejunum in 3 week old pigs. **(A)** Normal appearing jejunum after 52 days on a balanced commercial diet. **(B)** Increased lymphocyte infiltration and blunting of villi after 53 days on reduced protein and calories. **(C)** Severe changes produced after 205 days on slightly higher protein and calorie deficient diet. Note similarity of crypt depth in all three specimens. (Reproduced with permission from Platt BS, Heard CRC, Stewart RJC. The effects of protein-calorie deficiency on the gastrointestinal tract. In: Munro HN, ed. The role of the gastrointestinal tract in protein metabolism. Philadelphia: FA Davis, 1964:227–237.)

tion associated with iron-deficiency anemia in children may include impaired iron absorption, so that parenteral iron repletion may be needed for these patients (165). The mechanism by which iron deficiency causes gastrointestinal abnormalities is incompletely understood, but cellular enzymes are reduced in the mucosa of iron-deficient patients, including iron-dependent enzymes such as cytochrome oxidase.

ZINC DEFICIENCY AND ACRODERMATITIS ENTEROPATHICA

Zinc is an essential component of a number of metalloenzymes that participate in a variety of metabolic processes, including carbohydrate, lipid, protein, and nucleic acid synthesis (166). Zinc deficiency can arise in a variety of clinical settings through diminished intake, competitive binding by certain foodstuffs, increased demand by the body, or increased excretion, and it can be accompanied by a wide range of clinical manifestations (166).

Zinc deficiency is the underlying cause of acrodermatitis enteropathica, an inherited autosomal recessive disease in children. In addition to severe skin changes, the patient has diarrhea and malabsorption, and if left untreated the condition can lead to death. On the other hand, administration of zinc sulfate brings about rapid, complete remission. A similar syndrome can also occur at any age when zinc-free intravenous solutions are used for total parenteral alimentation over a prolonged (longer than 1 month) period (167–169).

Purely dietary zinc deficiency may also play an important causative role in duration and severity of diarrheal illnesses among infants and young children. In a recent study from India oral zinc supplementation led to clinically important reductions in the duration and severity of diarrhea in infants and young children with acute infectious diarrhea (170).

The exact abnormality in zinc transport and/or metabolism in acrodermatitis enteropathica is not understood, but it has been suggested that the patients have a defective intestinal oligopeptidase that serves in normal persons to eliminate a zinc-chelating oligopeptide (171). As a result, zinc remains bound to the oligopeptide and thus is unavailable for absorption. Symptoms of acrodermatitis enteropathica typically appear soon after weaning, perhaps because normal human milk provides the necessary enzyme. A smaller subset of patients with acrodermatitis enteropathica do not show reduced serum zinc, yet respond to zinc administration (172).

Studies of the small intestine in acrodermatitis enteropathica have given variable results. Three untreated patients investigated by Kelly et al. showed "loss of villous architecture with flattening of villi, which in some areas was as severe as that seen in coeliac disease" (173). The surface epithelium was cuboidal and increased chronic inflammation was seen in the lamina propria and epithelium. Some improvement occurred after treatment with human milk and diiodohydroxyquinoline (an older therapy for acrodermatitis enteropathica). Normal mucosal architecture was totally restored after six months of zinc administration. In another study, conducted before the importance of zinc was recognized, numerous proximal small bowel biopsies showed *patchy* moderate to severe mucosal abnormalities with thinning, flattening, focal crypt necrosis, and reduction in crypts; rectal biopsies were also abnormal (174).

Other investigators have described normal or minimally abnormal intestinal mucosa by light microscopy in acrodermatitis enteropathica (175, 176). The discrepancies between these observations and the severe changes cited above are not readily explained, but possible differences in the degree and duration of zinc deficiency needed to produce skin versus intestinal lesions could be a factor. It is known that clinical manifestations can vary according to the severity of the zinc deficiency (166). Another possible factor is the treatment other than zinc supplementation that was sometimes used.

Bohane et al. noted rod-like, spherical, and fibrillar inclusions in Paneth cells in small intestinal biopsy specimens from patients with acrodermatitis enteropathica, even though the specimens were normal by dissecting and light microscopy (176). The Paneth cells became normal after zinc replacement. Similar changes in Paneth cells were described in experimental zinc deficiency in rats (177).

Ultrastructural abnormalities in Paneth cells were used to support a diagnosis of acrodermatitis enteropathica in a patient whose serum zinc levels were normal (172). Other authors, however, have felt that the Paneth cell findings are not specific for zinc deficiency, occurring also in malnutrition from a variety of other causes (178).

UNCLASSIFIED NONSPECIFIC INFLAMMATORY LESIONS

It is important to recognize that in the final analysis a significant proportion of small intestinal biopsies from patients with malabsorption will show nonspecific chronic inflammation, villus blunting, and other changes that are not accounted for by any known or identifiable causative factor or aspect of the patient's clinical history. Absence of known causation is especially true for biopsies from patients who live in or have lived in tropical and developing countries, but can also occur elsewhere. Many such idiopathic cases could be infectious, but it is usually not possible to verify this in individual patients. Also, more than one factor may be operative, including multiple deficiency states and infections. It is preferable, therefore, for the pathologist to take a conservative stance and to consider such cases to be "unclassified."

INFECTION-ASSOCIATED MUCOSAL LESIONS

In this section some general points about infection-associated malabsorption will be mentioned, while the infections that bear a special relation to chronic malabsorption such as Whipple's disease will be covered in detail. Discussions of additional gastrointestinal infections are found in Chapters 16 and 28.

VIRAL INFECTIONS

Only nonspecific histopathologic changes (e.g., epithelial damage, villus blunting, and chronic inflammation) are found in most known viral infections of the small intestine. Pathologists are, therefore, usually unable to detect viral infection from conventional histologic material alone (179). Nevertheless, it is important, if only from the standpoint of differential diagnosis, that they be aware that virally-induced lesions in the small intestine can (1) be limited to that portion of the gastrointestinal tract, and (2) be associated with significant clinical findings, including malabsorption.

It is also important to realize that many types of viruses have been implicated as causes or potential causes of gastroenteritis (Table 31.5) and that the list will undoubtedly grow. Furthermore, while viral infections of the gastrointestinal tract are largely associated with acute gastroenteritis from which the patient soon recovers, it is entirely possible that some viruses will be shown to be associated with chronic disease in the small intestine. Viruses may also play an indirect but essential role in chronic malabsorptive disease, as is hypothesized for type 12 adenovirus and celiac disease (61).

BACTERIAL INFECTIONS
WHIPPLE'S DISEASE

This rare chronic infectious disease is the principal bacterial infection that has a strong association with chronic malabsorption. Its histopathologic characteristic is accumulation of periodic acid-Schiff (PAS) positive macrophages in the lamina propria and in other organs (180, 181). Complete reviews of this topic, including historical overviews, can be found in references (182, 183).

Etiology and Pathogenesis

The causative agent is a small (1.0 to 1.5 μm) rod-shaped bacterium, *Tropheryma whippelii*, a so far uncultured organism that was recently identified by polymerase chain reaction (PCR) techniques on a 16S ribosomal RNA-derived nucleotide-sequence that is unique to *T. whippelii*. The findings have also been subjected to phylogenetic analysis to identify the organism as a form of actinomycete (180, 181). Although Whipple himself described bacteria in the tissues of his 1907 case and remarked on their possible causative significance (184), for many years the disorder was nevertheless viewed as a possible lipid storage problem and then later, following discovery of the PAS-positive macrophages, as a possible polysaccharide storage

disorder. The bacterial causation of Whipple's disease was only (re)discovered with the advent of ultrastructural techniques (185, 186). The Whipple bacillus occurs both extracellularly and within PAS-positive granules in the macrophages. The macrophage granules are phagosomes that result from bacterial phagocytosis and digestion (see below under Pathology).

Malabsorption in Whipple's disease occurs mainly because nutrient movement via the lamina propria and mesenteric lymphatic drainage system is impeded by masses of PAS-positive macrophages. As a result, lipid accumulation in the mucosa of the small intestine and in mesenteric lymph nodes is a prominent feature and led Whipple to call the disorder "intestinal lipodystrophy" (184).

The possibility that individuals who develop Whipple's disease have a host-related, and perhaps genetically determined susceptibility to infection by *T. whippelii* has been examined by several investigators. Such studies are hampered by the rarity of the condition and the need to study both the active and treated infection as optimal controls. A recent study, however, suggests that patients with Whipple's disease may have innate defects in their cell mediated immunity (187).

Pathology

A small intestinal biopsy from full-blown, untreated Whipple's disease has a characteristic appearance, and the diagnosis can be suspected even from ordinary H & E stained sections. The villi often have a rounded and somewhat blunted appearance. Extracellular lipid collections are frequently seen in the lamina propria and lymphatic channels. Grossly, the process of chylous obstruction can lead to a spectacular appearance with multiple white spots on the mucosa due to underlying accumulation of chyle in the lymphatics and lamina propria (Fig. 31.21).

Histologically, the diagnostic *sine qua non* of Whipple's disease is the presence in the lamina propria of numerous macrophages showing pink, foamy cytoplasm (Figs. 31.22A and 31.22B). Other inflammatory cell types are reduced in number,

TABLE	
31.5	**Virus Infections of the Small Intestine**

Major Causes of Enteritis:[a]
   Norwalk-like viruses
   Rotaviruses
Other Known or Possible Causes of Enteritis:
   Enteric adenoviruses
   Astroviruses
   Caliciviruses
   Minirotaviruses
   Cytomegaloviruses[a]

[a]See Chapters 16 and 28 for additional information

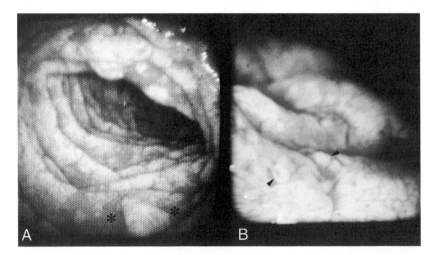

Figure 31.21   Whipple's disease—endoscopy. **(A)** Low power endoscopic view of the second duodenum. Thickened folds seem to be coated with granular, whitish material in patchy distribution. Reddish areas *(*)* represent more normal mucosa. **(B)** Close-up view demonstrating swollen villi *(arrowheads)* from whitish areas of A. Histologically, these villi were distended by chyle and bacteria-filled macrophages, as shown in Figure 31.22. (Reproduced with permission from Volpicelli NA, Salyer WR, Milligan FD, Bayless TM, Yardley JH. The endoscopic appearance of the duodenum in Whipple's disease. Johns Hopkins Med J 1976;138:19–23.) (See color plate).

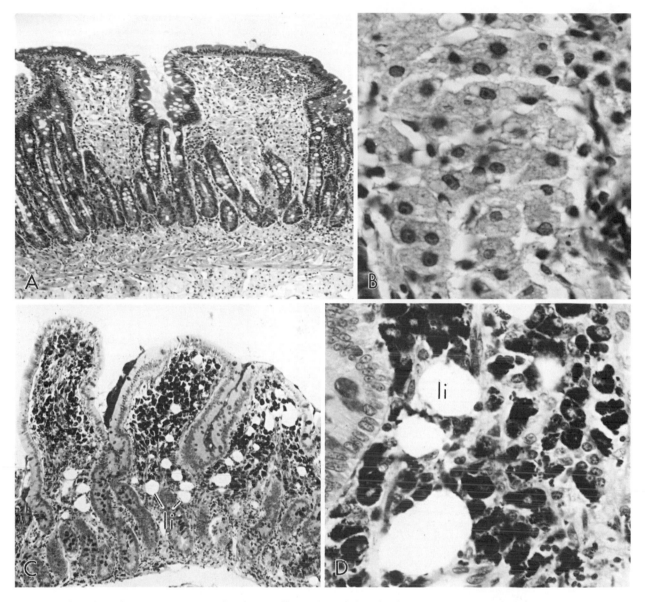

Figure 31.22 Whipple's disease—histopathology. **(A)** Blunted and fused villi containing foamy-looking macrophages (×90). **(B)** Detail of foamy macrophages occupying lamina propria (×675). **(C)** Periodic acid-Schiff (PAS) stain of another case demonstrating intensely PAS-positive *(dark)* macrophage contents. Extracellular lipid droplets *(li)* are also present as a result of chyle stasis (×100). **(D)** The foamy macrophages are crammed with granular PAS-positive material. Lipid droplets are designated *(li)* (×510).

while collections of neutrophils are observed on occasion. A PAS stain demonstrates that the foamy-looking cytoplasm of the H & E-stained macrophages is in fact stuffed with PAS-positive granules (Figs. 31.22C and 31.22D). At times it is also possible to discern very small, rod-shaped PAS-positive and Gram-positive objects in the extracellular space that are consistent with the causative organisms.

By electron microscopy, the rod-shaped bacteria are seen both extracellularly and in the macrophages (Fig. 31.23A). The macrophage granules are membrane-bound phagosomes that show a variable content. Some granules contain intact bacteria, while in others the bacteria are degenerating, and in still others the granules contain no recognizable bacteria, showing only a membranous-looking material in irregularly patterned parallel ar-

rays (Fig. 31.23C). The intracellular granules begin, therefore, as phagosomes containing the bacteria. These ingested bacteria then undergo degeneration, becoming less and less recognizable in the granules until only the membranous elements remain. These ultrastructural findings support the conclusion that the bacteria proliferate in the extracellular space, followed by phagocytosis by macrophages, which then are unable to completely dispose of them. Ultrastructural studies have shown that the bacteria have an outer membrane of uncertain nature and an underlying cell wall with dimensions that are consistent with a Gram-positive species. The cell wall also includes an inner membrane that accounts for the residual PAS-positive membranous material in the macrophage granules after degradation of other bacterial components (188). Rod-shaped intracellular bacteria are also found

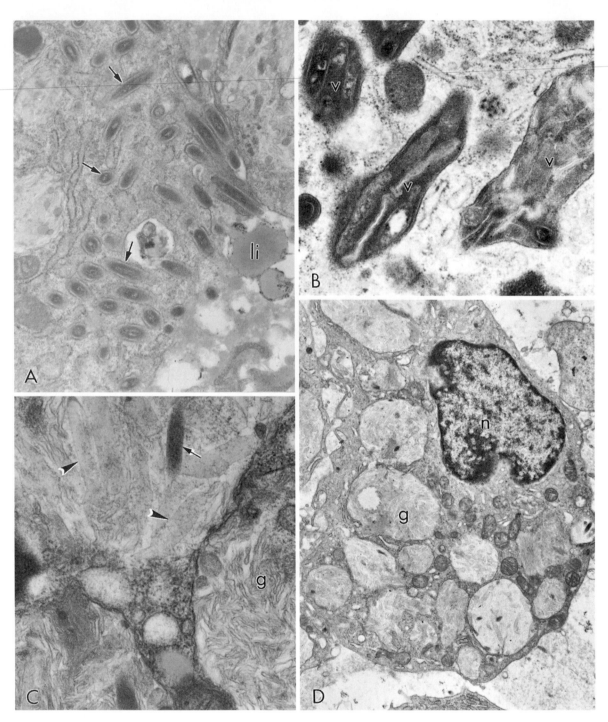

Figure 31.23 Whipple's disease—ultrastructural findings in lamina propria. **(A)** Bacilli *(arrows)* are located in the cytoplasm of a macrophage, presumably soon after ingestion. Dark (osmiophilic) extracellular lipid droplets *(li)* are also evident (×15,400). **(B)** Phagocytic vacuoles *(v)* in macrophages, each containing outlines of organisms undergoing digestion (×27,500). **(C)** Transformation of phagocytic vacuoles into mature granules containing occasional residual bacilli *(arrow)* and ghost-like outlines of bacilli *(arrowheads)*. Another granule *(g)* demonstrates typical end-stage membranous inclusions (×28,400). **(D)** Overview of "mature" Whipple macrophage; the nucleus *(n)* and a granule *(g)* are identified (×7,300).

in other cell types in Whipple's disease. These include epithelium, fibroblasts, endothelium, leukocytes, lymphocytes, mast cells, and smooth muscle cells. Taken together, these observations suggest that the causative agent is primarily an intracellular pathogen (189).

Extragastrointestinal Manifestations

Although Whipple's disease almost always includes involvement of the small intestine and presence of malabsorption, it is in fact a systemic illness (190) that commonly affects other organs, especially the heart, brain and eyes (191), joints, and R-E system. At the same time, a few well-studied patients, especially those with Whipple's disease of the central nervous system, have been reported in whom PAS-positive macrophage infiltration of the small intestine was not seen (192, 193). With expanded use of more sensitive molecular diagnosis, recognition of such cases should become more common (see below under Diagnosis). Pathologists and gastroenterologists need to be aware of these possibilities when asked to examine the GI tract in patients with suspected non-GI lesions of Whipple's disease (e.g., in the brain).

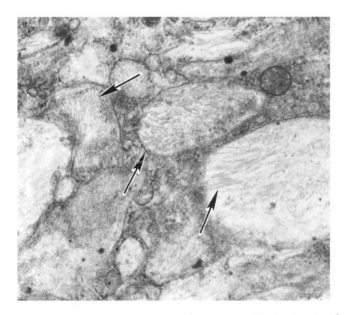

Figure 31.24 Post-treatment findings in Whipple's disease. A few residual macrophages showing pale PAS positive granularity were noted following antibiotic treatment. As seen here, by electron microscopy these macrophages demonstrate intracyto-plasmic membrane-bound bundles of fibrillar material. Bacteria and granules containing residual membranous material like that shown in Figure 31.23C are no longer detected. ×37,800.

Diagnosis

Jejunal biopsy is for now still the optimal method for diagnosis and verification of Whipple's disease (194), although its diagnosis can be *suggested* by endoscopic recognition of enlarged, lipid-choked villi. This feature also identifies optimal sites for biopsy detection (195). There are, however, potential pitfalls and limitations to be avoided in biopsy diagnosis of Whipple's disease. In the small intestine, these include: (1) Sampling errors because of patchy distribution of the lesion or restriction of PAS-positive macrophages to the submucosa (196). (2) Treatment of Whipple's disease with antibiotics can markedly reduce the number of PAS positive macrophages. Furthermore, after prolonged treatment the residual macrophages may no longer show bacteria and by electron micros-copy the granules may instead contain a characteristic posttreatment fibrillary material (Fig. 31.24). (3) The pathologist must also be wary of a false positive diagnosis: normal intestinal mucosa can occasionally show PAS-positive granule-containing macrophages, although the granules may be small and otherwise atypical for Whipple's disease (Table 31.6). *Mycobacterium avium/intracellu-lare* infection in an AIDS patient presenting with diarrhea and malabsorption is another potential source of error; a positive acid fast stain will distinguish the lesion from Whipple's disease (197). (See Chapter 16 under AIDS for additional information about *Mycobacterium avium/intracellulare.*)

It is possible that Whipple's disease can at least theoretically be suspected or diagnosed based on demonstration of PAS-positive macrophages in many tissues other than small intestine such as rectum (198), stomach, liver, lymph nodes, spleen, tonsil, brain, heart, etc. However, because PAS-positive inclusions seen in mac-rophages in those tissues in most cases have resulted from conditions other than Whipple's disease (Table 31.6), it is strongly advised that suspected Whipple's disease in those other locations be interpreted cautiously and that whenever possible its presence be verified by electron microscopy to demonstrate the characteristic macrophagic granules containing organisms and/or membranous material.

In the future, availability of the new molecular techniques for confirming Whipple's disease should make a major contribution to its diagnosis and offer an alternative to electron microscopy for questionable cases. Use of polymerase chain reaction (PCR) meth-ods to demonstrate infection with *T. whippelii* organisms has already

			Typical Staining		
Organ	Mimicking Cell(s)	PAS	Alcian Blue[a]	AFB	Other
Small Intestine	Macrophages: nongranular or granular (lipofuscin by EM)	+	−	−	
	Mycobacterium avium/intracellulare in AIDS	+	−	+	
Lymph Nodes and Liver	Macrophages: Nongranular or granular (often lipofuscin by EM)	+	−	−	
Stomach	Macrophage as above	+	−	−	Cytokeratin +
	Carcinoma (signet ring)	+	+	−	
Colorectum	Muciphages	+	+	−	

TABLE 31.6 PAS Positive Cells in Various Organs That Can Mimic Macrophages of Whipple's Disease

[a]Alcian blue at pH 2.5.

led to diagnosis of the disorder in intestinal biopsy specimens that did not show the histopathologic findings of Whipple's disease, and in vitreous fluid from the eye (199). In addition, it is now known that the infection can be diagnosed in peripheral blood by means of molecular methodology and, as a result of that observation, it was demonstrated that blood smears from two patients with Whipple's disease can show erythrocytes with numerous adherent rod-shaped bacteria consistent with the Whipple's bacilli (200).

FUNGAL INFECTION

Fungus infections of the alimentary tract are discussed in Chapters 16 and 28. They are not a significant cause of malabsorption. However, *Monilia* and *Histoplasma* are rarely mentioned as infectious agents in the small intestine, and will be briefly discussed.

MONILIASIS

Ten hospitalized patients with severe noncolitic, secretory diarrhea due to overwhelming infection by monilial (candidal) organisms have been described (201). Most were elderly individuals being treated with multiple antibiotics or chemotherapeutic agents. We have seen severe moniliasis in an immunodeficient patient under treatment for leukemia. There was monilial esophagitis and marked destruction of villi over the entire length of the small bowel. The stomach was largely spared, presumably because of low pH. Histo-

logically, the small intestine revealed a heavy superficial coating of yeast and pseudohyphae. The underlying villi had undergone necrosis and acute inflammation. The patient experienced cholera-like watery diarrhea, presumably because of diminished absorptive capacity combined with secretion from intact crypts.

HISTOPLASMOSIS

Although *Histoplasma capsulatum* is capable of infecting all parts of the gastrointestinal tract from the mouth to the anus, with the ileum being most frequently involved, it is an extremely rare cause of malabsorption (202). In the single case report of that association in the world's literature, there was disseminated histoplasmosis and the patient presented with watery diarrhea of explosive onset along with laboratory evidence of malabsorption (202). *H. capsulatum* was grown from a small bowel biopsy. Histologically, the biopsy showed blunted villi and a heavy mononuclear infiltration. Organisms were seen in the mononuclear cells in the intestine as well as in liver, breast, and skin.

PROTOZOAN PARASITOSIS

A general discussion of parasitic disease and malabsorption has been published (195). A recent review of the "new" gastrointestinal spore-forming protozoal pathogens (*Cryptosporidia, Microsporidia, Isospora*, and *Cyclospora*) is also available (203).

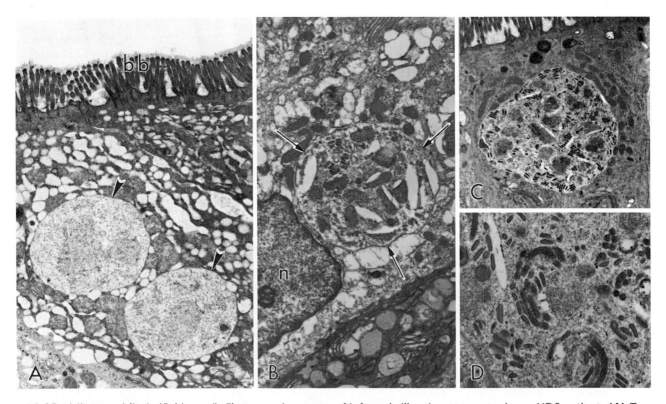

Figure 31.25 Microsporidiosis (*E. bieneusi*). Electron microscopy of infected villus tip enterocytes in an AIDS patient. **(A)** Two pale, early plasmodia *(arrowheads)* are seen just beneath the brush border *(bb)*. The enterocyte epithelium is vacuolated—evidence of cellular injury (×8,400). **(B)** Plasmodium *(outlined by arrows)* undergoing sporogeny; nuclear material has divided into separate darker clumps. Note the characteristic open clefts in the organism and the typical concave deformity in the adjacent enterocyte nucleus *(n)* (×7,200). **(C)** Multiple polar filaments have appeared in this organism during sporogeny (×6,200). **(D)** Detail of polar filaments during their formation (×18,200). (Electron micrographs kindly provided by Dr. Joel Greenson and Dr. Audrey Lazenby.)

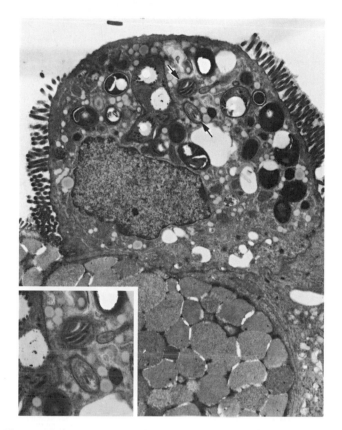

Figure 31.26 Microsporidiosis (*E. bieneusi*) (AIDS patient). An enterocyte that contains multiple mature spores is extruding from the villus tip. Adjacent goblet cell is seen below. Coiled polar filaments are visible inside two of the spores *(arrows)* (×6,300). *Inset*: Close-up of spores with their tightly coiled polar filaments (×17,250). (Electron micrograph kindly provided by Dr Joel Greenson.)

The principal protozoan infections that can cause malabsorption are giardiasis, coccidiosis, cryptosporidiosis, and microsporidiosis. Pathologists should be able to recognize these protozoan organisms in small intestinal biopsies, and it is worthwhile to develop the habit of searching for them in intestinal biopsies from all patients with unexplained diarrhea and/or malabsorption. There is also some evidence to suggest that malaria may also be associated with malabsorption, perhaps because of effects on the microcirculation (204). Giardiasis and coccidiosis are covered in Chapter 28, and cryptosporidiosis is considered in Chapter 16. Microsporidiosis is increasingly recognized as a common cause of diarrhea and malabsorption in AIDS patients (205), and is discussed here.

MICROSPORIDIOSIS

Although long known to occur in arthropods and fish, infections due to organisms of the phylum *Microspora* were only rarely described in warm blooded animals, including man, until recently (205). They are obligate intracellular parasites whose life cycle has both proliferative and spore-producing phases (206). The defining feature of these organisms is presence in each spore of a coiled *polar filament* that is used to transmit the infection to a host cell by injecting it with the spore contents. Intestinal microsporidiosis in

humans is largely due to a newly described agent—*Enterocytozoon bieneusi* (207), although infection with another microsporidian *Septata (Encephalitozoon) intestinalis* is also described (208, 209). Correct diagnosis with respect to the latter could be important to patient treatment because of superior response by *S. intestinalis* to the drug albendazole.

E. bieneusi is the apparent causative agent in a sizable proportion of AIDS patients who develop chronic diarrhea. Orenstein et al. found *E. bieneusi* in small intestinal epithelium from 20 of 67 AIDS patients who had chronic diarrhea and no other pathogen demonstrable by either light microscopy or by microbiological techniques (210). Similarly, other investigators found microsporidia in five of eleven AIDS patients with diarrhea (211). *E. bieneusi* were present much more consistently in jejunal than in duodenal biopsies (210).

Electron microscopy is the most reliable method for detecting the infection, and is required for species identification (205, 211, 212). The plasmodial (meront) form of the organism always occurs in the supranuclear cytoplasm of villus epithelium, especially at the villus tips (Fig. 31.25B). The plasmodia have an average diameter of about 5 μm; a characteristic feature is the presence of one or more empty clefts or slits in the organism. The spores can be observed in various stages of development, beginning with appearance of polar filaments, and when mature measure about 1.0 μm × 1.5 μm (Figs. 31.25C, 31.25D and 31.26).

Light microscopic study of methylene blue-Azure II stained "thick" (ca 1 μm) sections from plastic embedded tissue is almost as reliable as electron microscopy for demonstrating microsporidial plasmodia and spores (Fig. 31.27) (210). In these preparations the plasmodia are paler than the surrounding cytoplasm whereas the

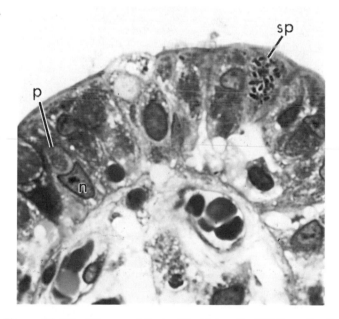

Figure 31.27 Microsporidiosis (*E. bieneusi*) (AIDS patient). 1 μm plastic section of a villus tip demonstrating a plasmodium *(p)* containing faintly visible open clefts. The adjacent enterocyte nucleus *(n)* appears indented by the organism. Dark staining spores *(sp)* are seen elsewhere. Clumps of dark, amorphous material in other enterocytes are of uncertain significance. Methylene blue–Azure II stain (×1,225).

spores are dense. Another approach that could prove to be both simple and reliable for detecting microsporidia is the use of Giemsa stained dried smears prepared from small intestinal biopsies or stool (212, 213); duodenal fluid can also be efficacious (214).

Detection of microsporidial organisms in H & E stained paraffin sections is possible and should be attempted, although it is considerably more difficult and less dependable than electron microscopy or methylene blue-Azure II stained "thick" sections. Optimal results with conventional histologic material require thin sections of well-preserved and uniformly stained tissue (210). The plasmodial form, which is basophilic in H & E stained sections, is especially difficult to demonstrate since it is not only small, but its staining is often only slightly darker than the surrounding epithelial cytoplasm. The organisms are typically most numerous in degenerating and sloughing epithelium at the villus tips (Fig. 31.28A). Associated intraepithelial spores may also be seen in H & E stained paraffin sections as very small refractile bodies (210). The spores are, however, Gram positive and thus at times easily identified in paraffin sections with use of bacterial stains (e.g., Brown and Brenn) (215) (Fig. 31.28B). Unfortunately, the spores may be sparse or even absent (212).

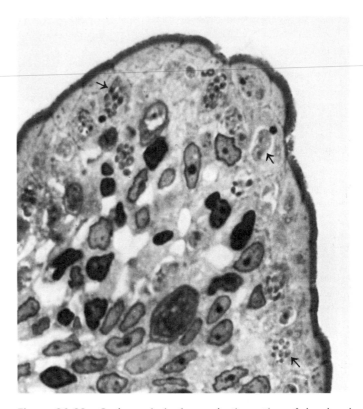

Figure 31.29 Cyclosporiasis. 1 μm plastic section of duodenal biopsy showing many cyclospora organisms *(arrows)* in enterocytic cytoplasm. A single large organism in a vacuole represents a trophozoite, whereas clusters of small organisms are mature and immature schizonts. Toluidine blue stain (×1450). (Reproduced with permission from Sun T, Ilardi CF, Asnis D, et al. Light and electron microscopic identification of Cyclospora species in the small intestine. Evidence of the presence of asexual life cycle in human host. Am J Clin Pathol 1996;105:216–220.)

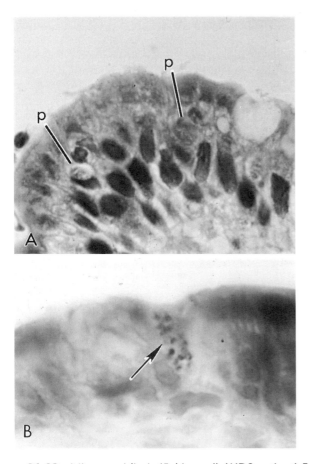

Figure 31.28 Microsporidiosis (*E. bieneusi*) (AIDS patient) Formalin fixed, paraffin embedded tissue. **(A)** Hematoxylin and eosin-stain. Plasmodia *(p)* are visible, one with indentation of the subjacent nucleus (×1225). **(B)** Brown and Brenn stain. Gram positive staining of spores (×1850).

Histologically, the mucosa in patients with microsporidiosis shows blunting and shortening of villi, chronic inflammation with numerous lymphocytes and plasma cells in the lamina propria, and increased intraepithelial lymphocytes (210, 211). Small intestinal microsporidiosis has so far been limited to patients with AIDS, and it should be noted that the mucosal changes are also consistent with that condition alone (see below on AIDS).

Laboratory diagnosis of microsporidiosis on stool or duodenal aspirate is a useful alternative to endoscopic biopsy (216, 217).

CYCLOSPORIASIS

Etiology and Pathogenesis

The causative agent in cyclosporiasis is *Cyclospora cayetanensis* (218), the only species in the genus known to infect humans. Other terms that have been used for the organism are cyanobacter-like body (219), coccidia-like body (220), and coccidian-like body (221). It is the most recently identified of several intracellular spore forming protozoans known to infect human beings, the others being *Cryptosporidia*, *Microsporidia*, and *Isospora* (203). Recent molecular phylogenetic studies suggest that *Cyclospora* is closely related to *Eimeria* (222), a class of coccidial protozoan considered primarily an infectious agent of nonhuman species. The cyclosporal infection in humans is centered in the small intestinal epithelium. The life cycle and transmission of the disease are not fully worked out. For a good general review and summary see Brennan et al. (223).

Clinical Findings

Cyclosporiasis typically presents as acute watery diarrhea. There can be associated nausea, vomiting, and abdominal pain, and the acute phase usually turns into a chronic, and often relapsing, illness that can last for six weeks or more in adults (220). There can be weight loss and associated malabsorption (220). Both immunocompetent and immunocompromised individuals (e.g., those with AIDS) are affected, with the disease tending to be more persistent in the latter. Children can have a shorter illness than adults. The disease is typically self-limited although good response to trimethoprim-sulfamethoxazole is described.

Epidemiology

Cyclosporiasis is most prevalent in developing countries; however, occasional clustered and sporadic cases are seen in Western countries, including the United States and Canada (224–226), especially among travelers to areas where cyclosporiasis is endemic but also in nontravelers. Fecally contaminated food (imported raspberries in one noteworthy study in the United States [226]) and unpurified water are thought to be the chief sources of transmission (225).

Pathology

The pathologic findings center on the small intestine where mucosa shows chronic and acute inflammation with prominent plasma cells in the lamina propria and variable blunting and shortening of villi. Increased intraepithelial lymphocytosis can be a noteworthy feature, too.

The oocysts that occur in stool specimens are sometimes also demonstrable in duodenal aspirate (220). Some authors have observed intracytoplasmic parasites in formalin fixed, paraffin embedded duodenal epithelium. In a recent report it was shown that intraepithelial *Cyclospora* could be well demonstrated in routine paraffin sections, by using 5 μm thick sections and prolonged exposure to hematoxylin without eosin or other counterstain (227). However, for detailed, reliable demonstration of the organisms in small intestine use of plastic embedded 1 μm stained sections (Fig. 31.29) or electron microscopy (Fig. 31.30) is recommended (219, 228, 229). In this way sporozoites, trophozoites, schizonts, merozoites, and possibly sexual (229) forms have been identified. As with *Microsporidia*, enterocytes that cover the upper villi and villous tips are the ones chiefly affected by *Cyclospora*. It is also noteworthy that even with heavy infection only the small intestinal epithelium is invaded; cells in the lamina propria and submucosa of the small intestine are not involved. The colorectum is completely spared (227).

Diagnosis

The primary means for clinical diagnosis of cyclosporiasis is detection of the spherical oocysts in stool. The oocysts are 8 to 10 μm in diameter and show a variable degree of acid fast staining from deep red to nonstaining (Fig. 31.31). The oocysts can also be recognized

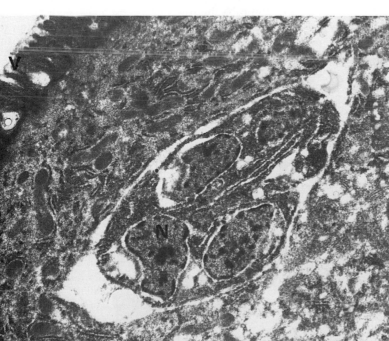

Figure 31.30 Cyclosporiasis. Electron micrograph of an immature schizont at a stage with four nuclei *(N)* in the cytoplasm of an absorptive cell. The brush border with its microvilli is seen *(V)* (×23,400). (Reproduced with permission from Sun T, Ilardi CF, Asnis D, et al. Light and electron microscopic identification of Cyclospora species in the small intestine. Evidence of the presence of asexual life cycle in human host. Am J Clin Pathol 1996;105:216–220.)

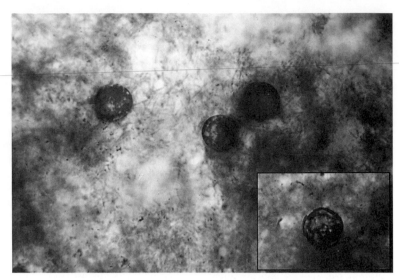

Figure 31.31 Cyclosporiasis. Cyclosporal oocysts seen in an acid fast stain of stool specimen from an actively infected individual. This technique provides the principal means for diagnosis of cyclosporiasis. Note the granular character of the intracellular staining and associated unstained vacuoles. *Inset*: Example of a much paler staining oocyst from elsewhere in the same stool preparation, to illustrate typical variability of acid fast staining; there may be no uptake of stain whatsoever by some oocysts. (Case material kindly provided by Mr. Tom Spahr.) (See color plate.)

by their autofluorescence under ultraviolet stimulation. It is important that the cyclosporal oocysts not be confused with the structurally similar but smaller (4 to 5 μm diameter) oocysts of *Cryptosporidia*.

METAZOAN PARASITOSIS

Nematodes (round worms) and cestodes (tapeworms) are the principal metazoan parasites that infect the small intestine. Most are largely asymptomatic, or cause minimal discomfort. The larger nematodes and cestodes do rarely cause obstructive symptoms. Also, intestinal tapeworms (especially *Diphyllobothrium latum*) can be associated with secondary Vitamin B12 deficiency (204), and hookworm infection can lead to iron deficiency anemia and be accompanied by hypoproteinemia if the worm burden is large (230). In general, however, visible changes in the mucosa and associated malabsorption are not found in metazoan parasite infections. The exceptions are possibly ascariasis, strongyloidiasis, Capillariasis, and schistosomiasis (especially *Schistosoma japonicum* since the egg-laying female resides in the superior mesenteric artery [204]; see Chapter 28).

ASCARIASIS

Infection with *Ascaris lumbricoides* is frequent in economically deprived individuals living under poor sanitary conditions in tropical and subtropical areas. Although *Ascaris* sometimes causes obstruction to hollow viscera, the large (up to 35 cm) organism lives free in the lumen and is not known to cause mucosal injury or inflammation or to lead to malabsorption by direct means. However, its potential importance in small bowel function when malnutrition is also present was shown in one investigation in which malabsorption was noted in children having both a large *Ascaris* burden and poor protein intake (231). Steatorrhea and d-xylose absorption improved after *Ascaris* organisms were eradicated even though the children continued their low protein intake. Unfortunately, jejunal biopsies could not be done in that study and the exact role of the *Ascaris* in the malabsorption was not examined further.

STRONGYLOIDIASIS

The causative agent is *Strongyloides stercoralis*. It, like Capillariasis and schistosomiasis, differs from the other intestinal worm infections in that the organism resides in the mucosa so that mucosal alterations may be present and the diagnosis can be made from an intestinal biopsy. *Strongyloides* occurs in tropical and temperate areas throughout the world, but is most common in warm, moist climates where in some instances (e.g., Brazil) up to 85% of the population may be infected (232). It also is endemic in warmer areas of the United States, and can be found in individuals who have traveled to heavily infected regions such as Southeast Asia.

The mature female remains in the crypts indefinitely (e.g., 30 years or longer), typically in the duodenum, where eggs are produced, probably by parthenogenesis. Eggs embryonate into larvae in the crypt epithelium. The larvae usually then escape into the bowel lumen and pass harmlessly out of the host with the stool. If, however, the host is subjected to generalized debilitation as from tumor, or becomes malnourished, or if there is supervening immunosuppression or other immunodeficiency state, including AIDS, the patient can develop an *internal autoinfection* or *hyperinfection* with *Strongyloides* larvae (233). In this condition larvae reinvade the host instead of passing only into the stool. This leads to widespread vascular dissemination and a resulting severe systemic illness. There may be malabsorption and hypoproteinemia and rarely, associated urinary, cardiac, or CNS symptoms. Eosinophilia, which is common in the mild cases, will frequently disappear during hyperinfection. Early diagnosis of hyperinfection is critical since it is potentially lethal.

Unexplained bacteremia due to enteric organisms associated with hyperinfection in strongyloidiasis has been described (233). It is believed that the larvae carry bacteria into the host either by surface adherence or in the larval intestine. Gram-negative bacillary meningitis can be a prominent aspect of the illness.

Diagnosis of strongyloidiasis is most frequently based on demonstration of larvae in the stool (Fig. 31.32) (234). A fresh specimen is required, since a stool specimen which contains hookworm eggs that is allowed to stand at room temperature can hatch the hookworm larvae, and these closely resemble *Strongyloides* larvae. Also, *Strongyloides* larvae can, if stored, mature into distinctive types of free-living filariform larvae or adults. As an additional test, the larval forms of various worm species are distinguishable by their characteristic tracks in soft agar (235). Strongyloidiasis can also be diagnosed from duodenal aspirate.

The appearance of *Strongyloides* in small intestinal biopsies is characteristic: eggs may be seen in crypt epithelium (Fig. 31.33A) and some of the eggs will be embryonating. There can also be larvae, and more rarely, adult worms. The adult female is recognized by its larger size and presence of reproductive tubes. Thus all stages of the *Strongyloides* organism can be noted in the crypts, with hatching larvae seen escaping from the mucosa (Fig. 31.33B).

Reactive changes in the mucosa are nonspecific. However, tissue eosinophilia may be striking, and there is usually chronic inflammation and some blunting of villi. Thus even when it is not possible to see the organisms, heavy concentrations of eosinophils

suggest the diagnosis which is in turn verified by stool examination (Fig. 31.32). Hyperinfection may be associated with large numbers of larvae in the mucosa, along with erosions and migrating larvae in deeper structures (Fig. 31.34). The colon can be involved in hyperinfection (232), too, so that it is also possible to make the diagnosis from a colonic or rectal biopsy.

CAPILLARIASIS

The causative agent is a nematode *Capillaria phillipinensis* (236, 237). Capillariasis has been described only since 1964. Most patients reside in the Philippines, although cases have been noted more recently in Taiwan, Southeast Asia, and the Middle East (238, 239). Thus, while Capillariasis is confined to a relatively small region of the world, it may be spreading, and the high mobility of modern society could eventually lead to much wider dissemination.

Patients are believed to acquire the infection by eating fish whose flesh contains larvae; birds may also be an important vector (240). It is uncertain whether ingestion of nematode eggs can infect human beings directly. Autoinfection is believed to occur in the human host with resulting huge numbers of worms. Intestinal Capillariasis can be epidemic. In its chronic form the symptoms resemble tropical sprue; emaciation can be severe and lead to death (237).

The infection is centered primarily in the jejunum and ileum, although the duodenum is sometimes involved (241). The nematodes are found burrowing into crypts of the small intestine with both adults and larvae being noted side-by-side (236). The adult worms are small and slender, measuring about 2.5 to 4 mm long by 20 to 50 μm in width (236). Eggs and embryonating eggs are observed developing internally in adult female worms. The anterior ends of the infecting worms reach into the lamina propria, and the

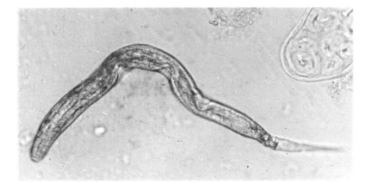

Figure 31.32   Strongyloidiasis. Rhabditiform larva in stool. The stool examination was crucial to this patient's diagnosis, a mucosal biopsy showing only nonspecific inflammation with prominent eosinophils and villus blunting.

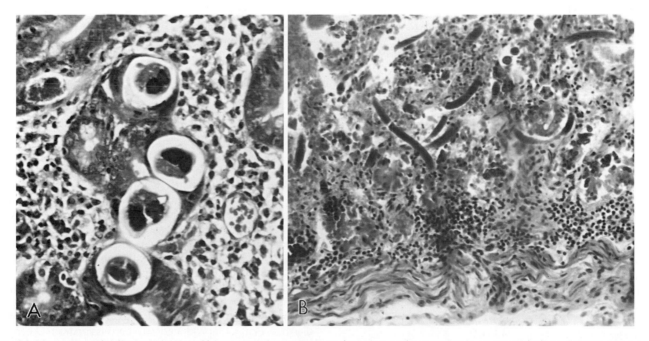

Figure 31.33   Strongyloidiasis. **(A)** Jejunal biopsy specimen. Eggs undergoing embryonation in crypt epithelium (×210). **(B)** Jejunum at autopsy showing heavy *S. stercoralis* infection. Numerous rhabditiform larvae are moving from the mucosa towards the lumen (×340).

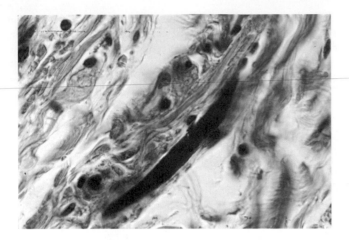

Figure 31.34 Strongyloidiasis. Internal autoinfection. A reinvasive larva is seen in the submucosa in the autopsy specimen shown in Figure 31.33B (×540).

mucosa shows chronic inflammation with blunting and shortening of villi. Adult worms are occasionally found in the liver (236, 241).

A major differential point for the pathologist is to distinguish between Capillariasis and strongyloidiasis. A key feature in making the distinction is to note the location of embryonating eggs; they occur only inside the female adults in Capillariasis (236), in contrast to their presence in crypt epithelium in strongyloidiasis.

MUCOSAL LESIONS ASSOCIATED WITH ALTERED IMMUNE RESPONSE

The possibility that altered immunity may underlie a patient's intestinal dysfunction should be routinely considered when examining a small bowel biopsy. Presence of a viral, bacterial, fungal, or parasitic agent should suggest that there may be an abnormal immune response, especially in those infections that are typical for AIDS. Common variable immune deficiency should be considered whenever giardiasis is noted. It should also be remembered that malnutrition, treatment with corticosteroids, cytotoxic agents, or other immunosuppressants, and presence of protein losing enteropathy can all lead to reduction in both humoral and cellular immune response.

Entities associated with alterations in immune response are largely covered elsewhere in this volume. Most primary and secondary immunodeficiency states are described in Chapter 16; graft-vs-host disease is considered there and additionally in Chapter 6. Eosinophilic gastroenteritis is reviewed in Chapter 12 along with other allergic conditions. Kagnoff has provided an excellent general discussion of altered immune states in gastrointestinal disease (242).

Two specialized aspects of altered immunity in the small intestine that are associated with malabsorption will be considered here: idiopathic AIDS enteropathy and autoimmune enteropathy.

IDIOPATHIC AIDS ENTEROPATHY

Chronic diarrhea, often with malabsorption and weight loss, is an important finding in AIDS (243, 244), representing a major complaint in about half of all AIDS patients (211, 243). In

approximately 50% of such cases the diarrheal/malabsorption syndrome results from secondary infection in the small intestine and/or colorectum (245, 246) (see Chapter 16 and see above for microsporidiosis). Altered gastrointestinal immunity with diminished mucosal CD4+ (helper) cells and increased CD8+ (cytotoxic/suppressor) cells correlate well with the AIDS patient's enhanced vulnerability to infection (247). However, no secondary infectious agents can be demonstrated in the intestine of many AIDS patients with diarrhea even after all available methods have been used. This condition is here termed *idiopathic AIDS enteropathy*.

Mucosal biopsies from patients with idiopathic AIDS enteropathy have shown by morphometry decreased villus to crypt ratios (Fig. 31.35) because of villus atrophy and crypt elongation. In addition, however, the architectural changes were also found in AIDS patients without diarrhea as compared with normal controls (*P*<.0001) (211). Furthermore, AIDS patients without diarrhea, and those with diarrhea whether demonstrating an enteropathogen or not, all showed comparable frequencies of epithelial mitoses. Thus the altered villus and crypt architecture and the patients' epithelial proliferative activity were independent of the presence

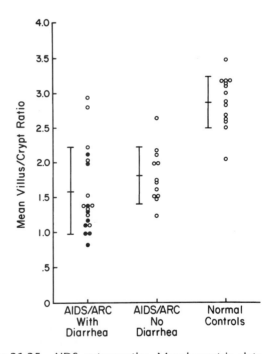

Figure 31.35 AIDS enteropathy. Morphometric data for duodenal mucosa in patients with AIDS or ARC (AIDS Related Complex) and chronic diarrhea, in other patients with AIDS or ARC but without diarrhea, and for healthy controls. Open circles: no pathogens identified. Closed circles: occult enteropathogens present (chiefly *Mycobacterium avium-intracellulare* and microsporidia). The villus to crypt ratios were reduced for patients with AIDS or ARC irrespective of whether or not diarrhea was present (*P*>.001). For patients with AIDS, diarrhea, and an enteropathogen as compared to patients with AIDS and diarrhea without infections, *P*=.06, and as compared to AIDS without diarrhea, *P*<.03. (Reproduced with permission from Greenson JK, Belitsos PC, Yardley JH, Bartlett JG. AIDS enteropathy-occult enteric infections and duodenal mucosal alterations in chronic diarrhea. Ann Inter Med 1991;114:366–372.)

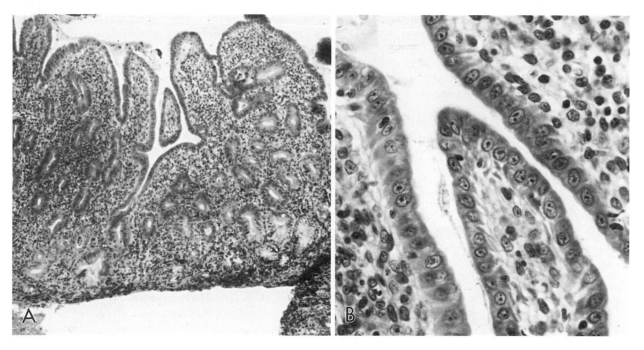

Figure 31.36 Autoimmune enteropathy in an infant who demonstrated severe malabsorption and autoimmune phenomena involving several systems. **(A)** Villi are markedly rounded and shortened and there is intense inflammation, chiefly chronic (×100). **(B)** The villi are covered with regenerating epithelium that, however, shows a striking *absence* of lymphocytic infiltration (×510).

of diarrhea or demonstrable enteric infection in advanced HIV infection.

Possible causes of idiopathic AIDS enteropathy include undetected secondary infection, direct effect of the HIV agent or its products on the intestine, and indirect effects of immunodeficiency or other immune dysregulation.

The role played in the mucosal morphometric changes by HIV is unclear. The virus has been described by some investigators in epithelial cells, leading them to postulate that the virus itself is responsible for idiopathic AIDS enteropathy (248, 249), but others failed to confirm those findings and noted HIV only in monocytes of the lamina propria (250, 251). The relatively sporadically seen HIV could in fact be a chance occurrence without direct bearing on the mucosal alterations.

The effects of HIV virus on T cells might also explain the villus atrophy and crypt hyperplasia seen in HIV-infected patients. Similar striking villus atrophy and crypt hyperplasia were noted in fetal small bowel explants when T cells were activated with pokeweed mitogens or anti-CD3 monoclonal antibody (252, 253). Comparable findings were also observed after rejection of mouse small intestine allografts and in graft-versus-host disease of the intestine following bone marrow transplantation (254). Thus it is conceivable that alterations in mucosal T cells in AIDS somehow lead to down regulation of small bowel epithelial proliferation and maturation with resulting alterations in mucosal architecture. Additional support for this hypothesis is suggested by the marked decrease in duodenal brush border lactase activity that was noted in HIV-infected patients (255).

AUTOIMMUNE ENTEROPATHY

The term encompasses a group of pediatric patients, usually infants, who have watery diarrhea, derangement of the intestinal mucosa

with inflammation and loss of villi, and evidence of circulating autoantibodies against intestinal epithelium (42, 256, 257). The patients characteristically have multiple other autoimmune reactions such as type I diabetes and hemolytic anemia, and demonstrate other organ-specific or nonspecific autoantibodies. The disease is typically severe and intractable, requiring intravenous feeding; favorable response to immunosuppressive agents may be noted (258). These patients represent a distinctive subset among young patients, most of whom are infants, who have unexplained intractable diarrhea (257, 259).

A small intestinal biopsy in autoimmune enteropathy typically appears flat, with near total loss of villi (Fig. 31.36A). Chronic inflammation is increased in the lamina propria, whereas there is only limited if any increase in intraepithelial lymphocytes, an important distinguishing feature from celiac disease (Fig. 31.36B). Acute inflammation may also be seen. Severity of the lesion is proportional to titer of circulating antienterocyte antibodies (257). There is evidence of epithelial damage to both villus and crypt epithelium (256), and presence of crypt necrosis has been regarded as an especially poor prognostic sign (259). It has recently been emphasized that these patients frequently also show colitis, which in some patients is severe and may resemble ulcerative colitis (260).

The etiology of autoimmune enteropathy is unknown. However, there is frequent mention of a similar disorder in siblings and of the presence of other autoimmune and allergic disorders in other relatives (257, 259). Also, in some patients the illness had begun as an acute diarrheal episode that coincided with a similar acute illness in other family members in at least one instance (256). Furthermore, it is noteworthy that the illness is *not* present at birth and that the antienterocyte antibodies have been noted to appear *after* the illness began (256). These findings suggest that a combination of one or more extrinsic agents and inherited factors are operative, and that while autoimmunity is unlikely to be the primary mechanism of epithelial injury, it probably does play an important secondary pathogenetic role. Cuenod et al. noted that activated T cells, as indicated by presence of interleukin-2-receptor bearing cells, were markedly increased in number in their patients and have suggested that this might account for the villous atrophy (259). They and others have also noted enhancement of epithelial HLA-DR antigens, with especially prominent involvement of crypts in those patients with high antiepithelial antibody titers (261). It is of special interest that treatment with cyclosporine has led to dramatic and prolonged clinical and histologic improvement with restoration of villi (258).

MISCELLANEOUS DISEASES ASSOCIATED WITH CHARACTERISTIC MUCOSAL LESIONS

This section encompasses an otherwise diverse collection of disorders all of which have in common the presence of one or more characteristic features that allow them to be definitively recognized or strongly suspected solely from a mucosal biopsy. Most of the listed entities are described in other chapters (see Table 31.1 for locations). Mastocytosis, microvillous inclusion disease, primary lymphangiectasia, and Waldenström's macroglobulinemia will be discussed here.

MASTOCYTOSIS

This condition is characterized by abnormal accumulation of mast cells in various tissues, accompanied by symptoms which result from excessive release of vasoactive and possibly other substances by the mast cells, especially histamine. Mastocytosis presents most commonly during childhood as a localized disease manifested as a pigmented rash *(urticaria pigmentosa)*, although the disorder can first appear during adulthood, too. Pruritis and dermatographia are the principal manifestations. About 10% of all patients with urticaria pigmentosa also have, or later develop, *systemic mastocytosis* with increased mast cells in other organs—most frequently bone marrow, lymph nodes, liver, and spleen (262). Systemic mastocytosis in the absence of skin lesions is usually viewed as rare, although at least one group found no skin involvement in 44% of their patients (262). Major clinical findings in systemic mastocytosis are episodic headache, flushing, weakness, abdominal pain, and diarrhea. Cherner et al. found that among 16 consecutive patients with systemic mastocytosis nine had either duodenal ulcer or duodenitis and five showed impaired absorption from the small intestine, although it was usually mild (263a). More severe malabsorption is an infrequent but well recognized finding in systemic mastocytosis (264–272).

For the pathologist to deal effectively with mastocytosis it is crucial that he know the techniques required to demonstrate mast cells, including aspects that are peculiar to the gastrointestinal tract. Special stains such as Giemsa and toluidine blue are needed to reveal the characteristic mast cell granules and their metachromasia. Mast cells *cannot* be distinguished from other mononuclear cell types in H & E stained sections. Furthermore, after releasing their granule contents in response to immunological or other stimulation, mast cells become undetectable even by special stains, and electron microscopy is then required for their identification. As was shown

for rats and mice (273, 274), and more recently for human beings (274a, 275), at least two types of mast cells are recognizable. The more widespread and common type occurs in dermis and connective tissue in many organs, including intestinal submucosa and muscularis. This type, termed a connective tissue mast cell (CTMC), is well shown by an appropriate stain such as toluidine blue after fixation in buffered or other ordinary formalin solutions. On the other hand, the mast cells found in the lamina propria of the intestinal mucosa are predominantly of a different type, and are termed mucosal mast cells (MMC). MMC are poorly demonstrated after conventional types of formalin fixation, requiring especially chosen fixatives (see below). Pulmonary mast cells have similar properties.

Strobel et al. found that whereas only a few mast cells could be seen in the lamina propria after buffered formalin, formol-sublimate, or saline-formol fixation, a four-fold to six-fold increase in visible mast cells was observed with Carnoy's fixative. Other fixatives tested, including basic lead acetate, formalin-acetic acid, Baker's (formalin-calcium chloride), and Bouin's, gave intermediate results (and in descending order) (274a). Similarly, formalin-acetic acid was found by Ruitenberg et al. to be much more effective than standard 10% formalin for demonstrating MMC (275). Later quantitative studies have shown that formaldehyde treatment can block cationic dye binding to granules in most MMC, suggesting that this is a special property of the particular glycosoaminoglycan composition of proteoglycan core in MMC (263). Submucosal mast cells, in keeping with the predominance of CTMC in that location, show a less pronounced relationship to type of fixation.

There are other features of human MMC that distinguish them from CTMC. These are smaller in size, with fewer and smaller granules which tend to be located in peripheral cytoplasm, differences in the content of their granules (137, 275), and different reactivities to monoclonal antibodies against tryptase and chymase (276). A possible additional mast cell type occurs under the crypt epithelium in humans (275). These findings are in keeping with the constantly expanding evidence of morphologic, cytochemical, and functional heterogeneity of mast cells generally (277).

Gross and microscopic changes have often been described in the intestine in systemic mastocytosis with severe malabsorption. The wall may appear thickened (266, 278), and several authors have reported mucosal nodularity (262, 267). One group of investigators saw "exudative duodenitis" (271). Ammann et al. have suggested that the mucosal changes can result from exposure to extrinsic substances, observing by endoscopy that "papular edema" and hyperemia appeared after a provocation test using a peptone or polymyxin containing solution (268).

Histologically, villus shortening ("atrophy"), edema, and increased mucosal lymphocytes and plasma cells are typically described; most authors also have stated that eosinophils are prominent (264, 266–271). Braverman et al. saw short clubbed villi and absence and destruction of some crypts (271) leading to an initial diagnosis of celiac disease.

In contrast to the architectural and nonspecific inflammatory changes that are consistently described in the intestinal mucosa in systemic mastocytosis with malabsorption, there is inconsistency between authors in regard to the number of mucosal mast cells. Only normal or unimpressive numbers were described in the lamina propria in several reports (264, 266, 268, 270), e.g., 3 to 4 mast cells per high powered field (usually defined as with 40× objective and 10× eyepiece) (270). On the other hand, other investigators found definite increases (265, 267, 271, 272, 278) with values for mast cells per high powered field ranging between 7 to 10 (272) and 50 to 100 (271). In addition, degranulated mast cells and abnormal mast cells with irregular and double nuclei have been reported by electron microscopy (271).

The variability in observed numbers of lamina propria mast cells in mastocytosis could occur in several ways, including *true* variation in numbers between patients, or variable numbers at different times in the same patient, or only an *apparent* lack of increase that results from granule depletion that in turn leads to reduced ability to detect their presence. However, before the nature of variation in number of lamina propria mast cells found in mastocytosis can be determined with certainty, it is obviously essential to consider the type of fixation used. In fact, of the authors mentioned above who describe malabsorption in mastocytosis by light microscopy, only two (265, 271) have provided information about fixation. And if it is assumed that ordinary formalin was the fixative used in the many of the reported cases, it is very possible, in view of the cited studies on the effects of fixation (274a, 275), that many if not all of the cases described as showing normal numbers of lamina propria mast cells in mastocytosis would have shown an increase if Carnoy's, formalin-acetic acid, or other more appropriate fixation technique had been used (Fig. 31.37). This conclusion is supported by the observation of Braverman et al. that whereas mast cells were not increased in formalin fixed intestine, an estimated 50 to 100 per high powered field were seen after fixation in Bouin's solution (271).

Among authors who mention the status of *submucosal* mast cells in mastocytosis, several describe an increase (265–267), and this was seen in one case (266) even when no increase was noted in lamina propria mast cells. Such an observation would fit with the fact that the submucosa largely contains CTMC, which are not affected adversely by ordinary formalin fixation.

It is not clear how the increase in mast cells comes about in systemic mastocytosis, or how it can sometimes lead to malabsorption and to altered mucosal architecture. It is generally agreed, however, that local increase in mast cells occurs in humans during a variety of acute and chronic inflammatory responses, during certain immune responses, and in fibrotic reactions. It is also known from experiments in rats that the intestinal mast cell population undergoes marked expansion following infection with a parasite, *Nippostrongylus brasiliensis* (279), and that such expansion appears to be under T cell control (274). Furthermore, a 30-fold increase in intestinal mast cells occurred in nude mice after interleukin-3 injections (280). Although in vitro studies did not confirm a similar relationship of mast cell proliferation to IL-3 in humans (281), observations of this type are consistent with the hypothesis that abnormal regulation of mast cell proliferation is of central importance in mastocytosis.

MICROVILLOUS INCLUSION DISEASE

This is an autosomally inherited recessive condition in newborns, presenting as severe, intractable diarrhea with steatorrhea (282, 283). The diarrhea does not abate on total parenteral alimentation. Absorptive tests and transepithelial electrolyte fluxes in microvillous inclusion disease have indicated sugar malabsorption and profound net secretion of fluid and electrolytes (282, 284). Few if any of the infants live beyond the eighteenth month of life.

By endoscopy, atrophic folds may be seen in the duodenum. Small intestinal biopsies show markedly blunted or absent villi and a thin surface epithelium resembling that seen in celiac disease, except that intraepithelial lymphocytes are not increased (Fig. 31.38).

Electron microscopy is definitive, consistently demonstrating striking and highly characteristic ultrastructural abnormalities in the surface enterocytes (283). The microvilli at the apical border are shortened, disorganized, and in places are greatly reduced in number or even absent. At the same time, many enterocytes demonstrate large, pathognomonic microvillous inclusions just below the surface and in the apical cytoplasm. These inclusions consist of an apparently circularized fragment of complete microvillous border that are bounded externally by a terminal web (Fig. 31.39). There is also evidence of autophagocytosis with various other lysosome-like vesicular inclusions that sometimes contain microvilli.

The possibility has been raised that MVID is part of a spectrum of microvillous disorders. A condition termed *microvillus dystrophy* is described in three patients (including two siblings of consanguineous parents) in whom surface microvilli were haphazardly formed or absent and accompanied by cytoplasmic vesicles but no true microvillous inclusions (285).

It has been suggested for MVID that there are abnormalities in assembly of the microvilli at the apical surface of the enterocytes (283). Goblet cells, Paneth cells, and endocrine cells are not affected. Similar changes have been noted in surface epithelium

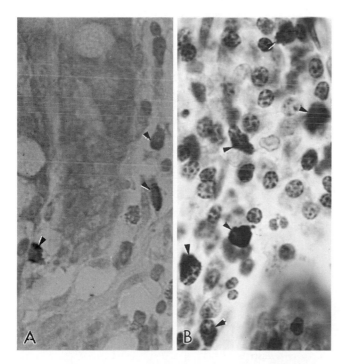

Figure 31.37 Mucosal mast cells. Relation of mast cell demonstration to type of fixative used for separate portions of small intestine from the same patient. **(A)** 10% buffered formalin. A typical field showing no more than three widely scattered, small-sized mast cells *(arrowheads)* containing a limited number of granules. **(B)** Carnoy's. A greater concentration of mast cells *(arrowheads)*, each containing a large number of intracellular granules, is evident after using Carnoy's fixation. (Differences in background staining are an unrelated feature.) Toluidine blue stain (×875).

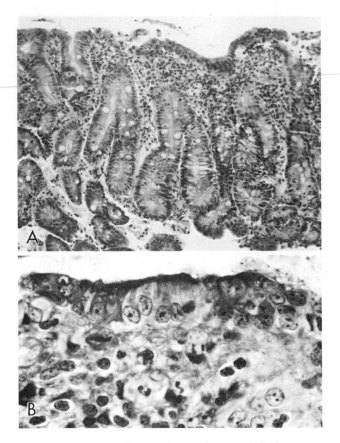

Figure 31.38 Microvillous inclusion disease. **(A)** Flat mucosa. Hematoxylin and eosin stain (×120). **(B)** Disorganized appearance of surface epithelium which shows prominent apical PAS-positive layer but lacks a clearly defined brush border. Periodic acid-Schiff stain (×675).

in the colon, rectum, and gallbladder (283, 284). The crypt enterocytes show well-preserved brush borders although the cells are said to demonstrate increased numbers of vesicular bodies (283).

While transmission electron microscopy is the diagnostic *sine qua non*, microvillous inclusion disease can also be strongly suspected from conventional histologic preparations (Fig. 31.38B). The brush border in places can be so thin as to be barely visible after PAS staining. In addition, the absorptive cells show prominent PAS positive droplets in their upper cytoplasm. Staining for alkaline phosphatase, which is normally found in the brush border, also stains the vesicles, thereby adding further specificity to light microscopic study (286). More recently, immunostaining for carcinoembryonic antigen (CEA), which is also present in brush border, has been described as a useful technique for demonstrating MVID by light microscopy (287).

PRIMARY INTESTINAL LYMPHANGIECTASIA

Patients with this condition present with PLE (see Introduction), hypoproteinemia, and peripheral edema (288–290). Diarrhea and steatorrhea are often noted, and reductions in serum globulins and peripheral lymphocytes with associated immunological disorders may be found (291). Presence of dilated lymphatics in the mucosa of the small intestine is the cardinal finding in intestinal lymphangiectasia, and the only apparent cause is "disturbance of the lymphatic system" (288). The condition develops mainly as a sporadic disorder in children and young adults, although familial occurrence is described. The patient and other family members may also show evidence of abnormal lymphatic drainage in one or more extremities (primary or idiopathic lymphedema), and there may be chylous ascites (288, 292). In a study of 52 patients with primary lymphedema, 12 (22%) were found to have significant PLE (293). Isolated instances of intestinal blood loss in patients with lymphangiectasia are described (294, 295).

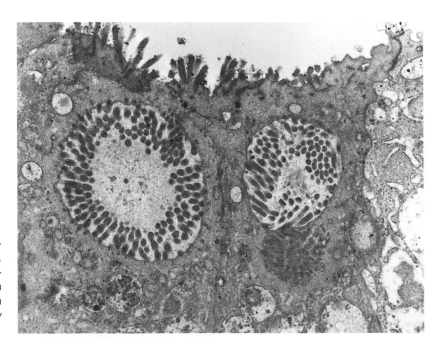

Figure 31.39 Microvillous inclusion disease. Electron micrograph of an abnormal surface enterocyte. Characteristic intracytoplasmic inclusions with apparent internalized microvilli are present beneath a markedly attenuated and abnormal intact brush border (×14,750). (Picture kindly provided by Dr. Joy Young-Ramsaran and Dr. Jean Olson.)

Grossly (or endoscopically), the mucosa shows white spots, white villi, and overlying chyle-like substance (296). The lesions are focal and may require multiple biopsies or serial sections to demonstrate their presence (290, 297). The reader is reminded that similar gross findings are present in Whipple's disease (Fig. 31.21) and in macroglobulinemia with intestinal involvement (see section on Waldenström's macroglobuinemia below) (195, 298).

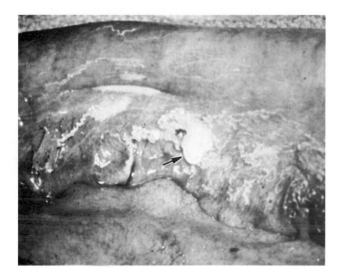

Figure 31.40 Primary lymphangiectasia. External appearance of small intestine at laparotomy showing tortuous, dilated lymphatic vessels filled with chyle. A large drop of chyle has formed where a vessel was nicked *(arrow)*.

In some persons the subserosal intestinal and mesenteric lymphatics have shown evidence of chylous distention indicative of more distal obstruction (Fig. 31.40). The cause of this condition is unclear. However, Waldman et al. demonstrated mesenteric lymphatic obstruction associated with thickening and fragmentation of the elastica interna and luminal fibrosis in four of five patients for whom specimens were available; mesenteric lymph nodes were also fibrotic (288). It was not clear whether the changes were congenital or acquired.

Histologically, the dilated mucosal lymphatics are seen typically in the villi just under the epithelium (Fig. 31.41), but can occur throughout the lamina propria and in the submucosa. The lymphatic endothelium is usually well-outlined, and protein and scattered foamy macrophages may be present in the lumen and lamina propria. Mild to moderate blunting of villi and slight chronic inflammation are sometimes described (290), and generalized edema of the lamina propria, presumably secondary to hypoproteinemia, may be seen. Intraepithelial lymphocytes were noted to be reduced whereas plasma cells were present in normal numbers (299). Ultrastructural studies have shown increases in collagen, basal lamina, and supporting cells around the dilated lymphatics along with prominent intracellular fibrils in the lymphatic endothelium (294). Additionally, large lipid droplets were observed at the base of the absorptive cells, and chylomicrons were seen in the extracellular spaces and lymphatic lumina (294, 296).

The luminal protein loss probably occurs through a combination of leakage through the epithelium and rupture of the lymphangiectatic lesions with release of chyle. The steatorrhea seen in primary intestinal lymphangiectasia appears to result from enteric loss of fat rather than malabsorption (300).

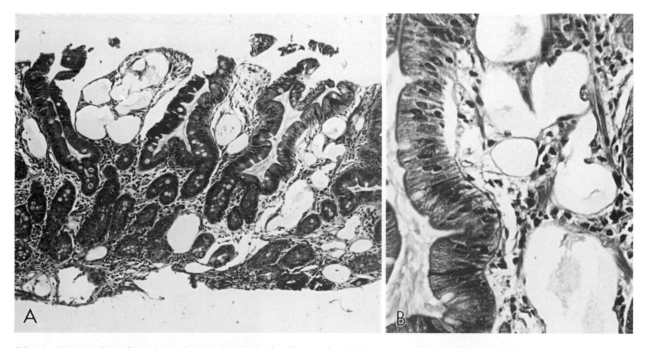

Figure 31.41 Primary lymphangiectasia in a patient with edema of multiple extremities. **(A)** Greatly dilated, tortuous central lacteals are present in villi and deep parts of an otherwise unremarkable looking mucosa. (Detachment of surface epithelium is artefactual.) (×105). **(B)** The multiple lymphatic channels are lined by an intact endothelial layer (×340).

It should be stressed that lymphangiectasia may be found incidentally during endoscopy or in an isolated biopsy of the small intestine in the absence of any clinical evidence of PLE or hypoproteinemia. In addition, Patel and DeRidder described patients with "functional lymphangiectasia" in whom the changes were not associated with PLE, appeared to be transient, and required no follow-up (301).

WALDENSTRÖM'S MACROGLOBULINEMIA

Intestinal involvement in Waldenström's macroglobulinemia is a rare complication of that disorder. These patients present with diarrhea, malabsorption, and PLE along with typical findings of a monoclonal IgM spike by serum immunoelectrophoresis, and neoplastic plasmacytoid cells in the bone marrow.

Grossly, myriads of small, whitish nodules comparable to those seen in primary lymphangiectasia and in Whipple's disease carpet an edematous, thickened, small intestinal mucosa (Fig. 31.42) (298, 302). The mesenteric nodes are enlarged and contain pale cheesy material, as can the dilated lymphatics that may be seen draining into them (302). Involvement of the stomach or colon has not been described.

Deposition of large amounts of eosinophilic, amorphous-looking proteinaceous material that is located in the mucosal lymphatics and lamina propria is the principal histologic finding in the intestine (Fig. 31.43). By electron microscopy the material is also seen between epithelial cells. The proteinaceous material is PAS positive and congo red negative (302–304). It also stains immunohistochemically for monoclonal IgM, thereby demonstrating its identity with the circulating monoclonal macroglobulin (298, 305, 306). Lipid droplets can be found extracellularly, sometimes admixed with the macroglobulin (305). In addition, there are lipid-containing, largely PAS-negative foam cells, but very little evidence of intracellular protein deposits are noted by either light or electron microscopy. The proteinaceous material involving the regional lymph nodes has the same characteristics as that in the intestine.

Neoplastic cellular infiltration is seen much less commonly than macroglobulin deposition as the cause of intestinal symptoms in

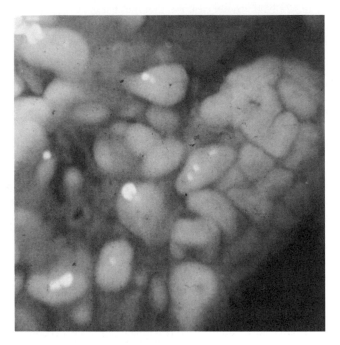

Figure 31.42 Waldenström's macroglobulinemia. Macroscopic view of intestinal mucosa. Swollen villi appear as multiple whitish nodules.

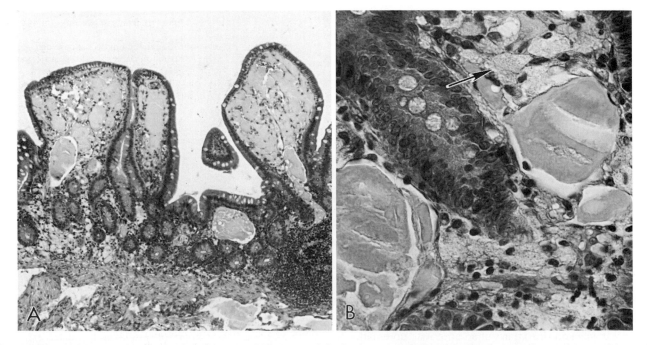

Figure 31.43 Waldenström's macroglobulinemia. **(A)** Macroglobulin has accumulated in the lymphatics and interstitium of the lamina propria, thereby creating the nodules seen in Figure 31.42 (×90). **(B)** Macroglobulin accumulations in lymphatics. Numerous foamy macrophages are present in the interstitium *(arrow)* (×400). (Case kindly provided by Dr. Geoffrey Mendelssohn.)

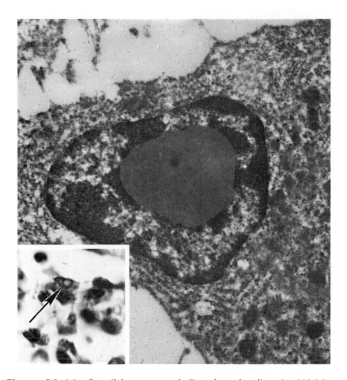

Figure 31.44 Possible mucosal Dutcher bodies in Waldenström's macroglobulinemia. Electron micrograph demonstrating an amorphous intranuclear inclusion consistent with accumulated macroglobulin in a lymphoplasmacytoid cell. ×18,700. *Inset*: Light micrograph of mucosal Dutcher body-like inclusion *(arrow)* H & E (×900). (Reproduced with permission from Bedine MS, Yardley JH, Elliott HL, Banwell JG, Hendrix TR. Intestinal Involvement in Waldenström's macroglobulinemia. Gastroenterology 1973;65:308–315.)

patients with Waldenström's macroglobulinemia (283). Furthermore, the mononuclear cellular infiltrate that is associated with massive intestinal macroglobulin deposition is usually considered benign. Nevertheless, in some cases of macroglobulin deposition several authors have described accompanying plasmacytoid lymphocytes, atypical plasma cells, and Dutcher bodies (intranuclear globulin deposits) (Fig. 31.44) (302–304). Those observations suggest that neoplastic infiltration in the mucosa may at times be involved in local deposition of macroglobulin (303). In all likelihood, however, deposition of circulating macroglobulins *per se*, with secondary lymphatic obstruction, is the most probable underlying mechanism of the mucosal disease and malabsorption. This conclusion is supported by the demonstration of accompanying massive macroglobulin deposition in mesenteric lymph nodes in most if not all patients, and by the dramatic regression of thickened mucosa and enlarged lymph nodes that can be seen after circulating macroglobulins are reduced therapeutically by means of plasmaphoresis (298, 307).

ACKNOWLEDGMENTS

The collaboration and cooperation of my many clinical colleagues in studies of malabsorption over the years is gratefully acknowledged. Special thanks go to Dr. Thomas R. Hendrix and Dr. Theodore M. Bayless; they first introduced me to the subject of malabsorption and contributed much to my understanding of it. I also want to express my gratitude to my wife, Eritha, for the outstanding help she provided in the preparation and assembly of this manuscript.

Except when otherwise indicated, original photomicrographs were prepared by Raymond E. Lund, RBP, FBPA.

REFERENCES

1. Riley SA, Turnberg LA. Maldigestion and malabsorption. In: Sleisenger MH, Fordtran JS, eds. Gastrointestinal disease, 5th ed. Philadelphia: WB Saunders, 1993:1009–1027.
2. Dobbins WO III. Small bowel biopsy in malabsorptive states. In: Norris HT, ed. Pathology of the colon, small intestine and anus. New York: Churchill Livingstone, 1983:121–167.
3. Lewin KJ, Riddell RH, Weinstein WM. Gastrointestinal pathology and its clinical implications. New York: Igaku-Shoin, 1992:750–800.
4. Goldman H. Gastrointestinal mucosal biopsy. New York: Churchill Livingstone, 1996:221–343.
5. Shiner M. Ultrastructure of the small intestinal mucosa. Normal and disease related appearances. New York: Springer-Verlag, 1983.
6. Holdstock G, Eade DE, Isaacson P, Smith CL. Endoscopic duodenal biopsy in coeliac disease and duodenitis. Scand J Gastroenterol 1979;14:717.
7. Brackenbury W, Stewart JS. Macroscopic appearances of mucosal biopsies from the small intestine. Med Biol Illustr 1963;13: 220–227.
8. Atkinson M, Nordin BEC, Sheshock S. Malabsorption and bone disease in prolonged obstructive jaundice. Quart J Med 1956;25: 299–312.
9. Marin GA, Clark ML, Senior JR. Studies of malabsorption occurring in patients with Laennec's cirrhosis. Gastroenterology 1969;56: 727–736.
10. Bo-Linn GW, Fordtran JS. Fecal fat concentration in patients with steatorrhea. Gastroenterology 1984;87:319–322.
11. Rubin E, Ryback BJ, Lindenbaum J, et al. Ultrastructural changes in the small intestine induced by ethanol. Gastroenterology 1972;63: 801–814.
12. Hermos JA, Adams WH, Liu Yong K, et al. Mucosa of the small intestine in folate-deficient alcoholics. Ann Intern Med 1972;76: 957–965.
13. Mezey E. Intestinal function in chronic alcoholism. Ann NY Acad Sci 1975;252:215–227.
14. Auricchio S. Genetically determined disaccharidase deficiencies. In: Walker WA, Durie PR, Hamilton JR, et al., eds. Pediatric gastrointestinal disease. Philadelphia & Toronto: Decker, 1991:647.
15. Bayless TM, Christopher NL. Disaccharidase deficiency. Amer J Clin Nutr 1969;22:181–190.
16. Maiuri L, Raia V, Potter J, et al. Mosaic pattern of lactase expression villous enterocytes in human adult-type hypolactasia. Gastroenterology 1991;100:359–369.
17. Maiuri L, Rossi M, Raia V, et al. Surface staining on the villus of lactase protein and lactase activity in adult-type hypolactasia. Gastroenterology 1993;105:708–714.
18. Walker-Smith JA, Guandalini S, Schmitz J, et al. Revised criteria for diagnosis of coeliac disease. Arch Dis Child 1990;65:909–911.
19. Kagnoff MF. Immunopathogenesis of celiac disease. Immunol Invest 1989;18:499–508.
20. Trier JS. Celiac sprue. In: Sleisenger MH, Fordtran JS, eds. Gastrointestinal disease, 5th ed. Philadelphia: WB Saunders, 1993: 1078–1105.
21. Dicke WK. Coeliac disease: investigation of harmful effects of certain types of cereal on patients with coeliac disease [Doctoral thesis], English summary. Utrecht, Netherlands: University of Utrecht, 1950:106–116.
22. Dicke WK, Weijers HA, v.d.Kamer JH. Coeliac disease. II. The presence in wheat of a factor having a deleterious effect in cases of coeliac disease. Acta Paediatrica 1953;42:34–42.
23. Rubin CE, Brandborg LL, Phelps PC, Taylor HC Jr. Studies of celiac disease. I. Apparent identical and specific nature of duodenal and proximal jejunal lesion in celiac disease and idiopathic sprue. Gastroenterology 1960;38:28–49.

24. Sleisenger MH, Rynbergen HJ, Pert JH, Almy TP. Treatment of non-tropical sprue: wheat-, rye-, and oat-free diet. J Am Dietet A 1957;33:1137–1140.

25. Yardley JH, Bayless TM, Norton JH, Hendrix TR. Celiac disease: a study of the jejunal epithelium before and after a gluten-free diet. New Engl J Med 1962;267:1173–1179.

26. Samloff IM, Davis JS, Schenk EA. A clinical and histochemical study of gluten-free diet. Gastroenterology 1965;48:155–172.

27. Bayless TM, Rubin S, Topping T, et al. Morphologic and functional effects of gluten feeding on jejunal mucosa and celiac disease. In: Booth CC, Dowling RH, eds. Coeliac disease. Edinburgh: Churchill-Livingstone, 1970:76–89.

28. McNicholl B, Egan-Mitchell B, Stevens F, et al. Mucosal recovery in treated childhood celiac disease (gluten-sensitive enteropathy). J Pediatr 1976;89:418–424.

29. MacDonald WC, Dobbins WO, Rubin CE. Studies on the familial nature of celiac sprue using biopsy of the small intestine. New Engl J Med 1965;272:448–455.

30. Auricchio S, Mazzacca G, Tosi R, et al. Coeliac disease as a family condition: identification of asymptomatic coeliac patients within family groups. Gastroenterol Internat 1988;1:25–31.

31. Troncone R, Greco L, Mayer M, et al. Latent and potential coeliac disease. Acta Paediatrica 1996;412(Suppl):10–14.

32. Khuffash FA, Barakat MH, Majeed HA, et al. Coeliac disease in monozygotic twin girls. Synchronous presentation. Gut 1984;25:1009–1012.

33. Mearin ML, Biemond I, Peña AS, et al. HLA-DR phenotypes in Spanish coeliac children: their contribution to the understanding of the genetics of the disease. Gut 1983;24:532–537.

34. Niven MJ, Caffrey C, Sachs JA, et al. Susceptibility to coeliac disease involves genes in HLA-DP region. Lancet 1987;2:805.

35. Kagnoff MF. Understanding the molecular basis of coeliac disease. Gut 1990;31:497–499.

36. Marsh MN, Bjarnason I, Shaw J, et al. Studies of intestinal lymphoid tissue. XIV-HLA status, mucosal morphology, permeability, and epithelial lymphocyte populations in first degree relatives of patients with coeliac disease. Gut 1991;31:32–36.

37. Arranz E, Ferguson A. Intestinal antibody pattern in celiac disease: occurrence in patients with normal jejunal biopsy histology. Gastroenterology 1993;104:1263–1272.

38. Marsh MN. Gluten sensitivity and latency: can patterns of intestinal antibody secretion define the 'silent majority'? Gastroenterology 1993;104:1150–1153.

39. Catassi C, Ratsch I-M, Fabianai E, et al. Coeliac disease in the year 2000: exploring the iceberg. Lancet 1994;343:200–203.

40. Katz SI, Hall RP III, Lawley TJ, Strober W. Dermatitis herpetiformis: the skin and the gut. Ann Intern Med 1980;93:857–874.

41. Mulder CJJ, Tytgat GNJ. Coeliac disease and related disorders. Netherlands J Med 1987;31:286–299.

42. Unsworth DJ, Walker-Smith JA. Autoimmunity in diarrhoeal disease. J Pediatr Gastroenterol Nutr 1985;4:375–380.

43. Wall AJ, Douglas AP, Booth CC, Pearse AGE. Response of the jejunal mucosa in adult coeliac disease to oral prednisolone. Gut 1970;11:7–14.

44. Katz AJ, Falchuk ZM, Strober W, Schwachman H. Gluten-sensitive enteropathy. Inhibition by cortisol of the effect of gluten protein in vitro. N Engl J Med 1976;295:131–136.

45. Ferguson A, Carswell F. Precipitins to dietary proteins in serum and upper intestinal secretions of coeliac children. Brit Med J 1972;1:75–77.

46. Kendrick KG, Walker-Smith AJ. Immunoglobulins and dietary protein antibodies in childhood coeliac disease. Gut 1970;11:635–640.

47. Lindberg T, Nilsson LA, Borulf S, et al. Serum IgA and IgG gliadin antibodies and small intestinal mucosal damage in children. J Pediatr Gastroenterol Nutr 1985;4:917–922.

48. Juto P, Fredrikzon B, Hernell O. Gliadin-specific serum immunoglobulins A, E, G, and M in childhood: relation to small intestinal mucosal morphology. J Pediatr Gastroenterol Nutr 1985;4:723–729.

49. Stahlberg MR, Savilahti E, Viander M. Antibodies to gliadin by ELISA as a screening test for childhood celiac disease. J Pediatr Gastroenterol Nutr 1986;5:726–729.

50. Collin P, Maki M, Keyrilainen O, et al. Selective IgA deficiency and coeliac disease. Scand J Gastroenterol 1992;27:367–371.

51. Lycke N, Kilander A, Nilsson L-A, et al. Production of antibodies to gliadin in intestinal mucosa of patients with coeliac disease: a study at the single cell level. Gut 1989;30:72–77.

52. Unsworth DJ, Leonard NL, Fry L. Antireticulin and antigliadin antibodies in dermatitis herpetiformis and celiac disease. In: Beutner EH, Chorzelski TC, Kumar V, eds. Immunopathology of the skin, 3rd ed. New York: John Wiley & Sons, 1987:455–470.

53. Ferguson A, Murray D. Quantitation of intraepithelial lymphocytes in human jejunum. Gut 1971;12:988–994.

54. Freedman AR, Macartney JC, Nelufer JM, Ciclitira PJ. Timing of infiltration of T lymphocytes induced by gluten into the small intestine in coeliac disease. J Clin Pathol 1987;40:741–745.

55. Austin LL, Dobbins WO. Studies of the rectal mucosa in coeliac sprue: the intraepithelial lymphocyte. Gut 1988;29:200–205.

56. Loft DE, Marsh MN, Crowe PT. Rectal gluten challenge and diagnosis of coeliac disease. Lancet 1990;335:1293–1295.

57. Loft DE, Marsh MN, Sandle GI, et al. Studies of intestinal lymphoid tissue. XII. Epithelial lymphocyte and mucosal responses to rectal gluten challenge in celiac sprue. Gastroenterology 1989;97:29–37.

58. Corazza GR, Sarchielli P, Londei M, et al. Gluten specific suppressor T cell dysfunction in coeliac disease. Gut 1986;27:392–398.

59. Guan R, Rawcliffe PM, Priddle JD, Jewell DP. Cellular hypersensitivity to gluten derived peptides in coeliac disease. Gut 1987;28:426–434.

60. Karagiannis JA, Priddle JD, Jewell DP. Cell-mediated immunity to a synthetic gliadin peptide resembling a sequence from adenovirus 12. Lancet 1987;1:884–886.

61. Mantzaris GJ, Karagiannis JA, Priddle JD, Jewell DP. Cellular hypersensitivity to a synthetic dodecapeptide derived from adenovirus 12 which resembles a sequence of A-gliadin in patients with coeliac disease. Gut 1990;31:668–673.

62. Kagnoff MF, Paterson YJ, Kumar PJ, et al. Evidence for the role of a human intestinal adenovirus in the pathogenesis of coeliac disease. Gut 1987;28:995–1001.

63. Kagnoff MF, Austin RK, Hubert JJ, Kasarda DD. Possible role for human adenovirus in the pathogenesis of celiac disease. J Exp Med 1984;160:1544–1557.

64. Penna FJ, Mota JA, Roquete ML, et al. Coeliac disease in identical twins. Arch Dis Child 1979;54:395–397.

65. Hoffman HN, Wollaeger EE, Greenberg E. Discordance for nontropical sprue (adult coeliac disease) in a monozygotic twin pair. Gastroenterology 1966;51:36–42.

66. Walker-Smith JA. Discordance of childhood celiac disease in monozygotic twins. Gut 1973;14:374–375.

67. Salazar-de-Sousa J, Ramos-de-Almeida JM, Monteiro MV, Magalhaes-Ramalho P. Late onset coeliac disease in the monozygotic twin of a coeliac child. Acta Paediatr Scand 1987;76:172–174.

68. Lee FI, Prior J, Murray SM. Celiac disease in monozygous twin boys. Asynchronous presentation. Dig Dis Sci 1982;27:1137–1140.

69. Jepsen LV, Ullman S. Dermatitis herpetiformis and gluten-sensitive enteropathy in monozygotic twins. Acta Derm Venereol (Stockh) 1980;60:353–355.

70. Schenk EA, Samloff IM, Klipstein FA. Morphologic characteristics of jejunal biopsy in celiac disease and tropical sprue. Am J Pathol 1965;47:765–781.

71. Padykula HA. Recent functional interpretations of intestinal morphology. Fed Proc 1962;21:873–879.

72. Jabbari M, Wild G, Goresky CA, et al. Scalloped valvulae conniventes: an endoscopic marker of celiac sprue. Gastroenterology 1988;95:1518–1522.

73. Brocchi E, Corazza G, Caletti G, et al. Endoscopic demonstration of loss of duodenal folds in the diagnosis of celiac disease. New Engl J Med 1988;319:741–744.

74. Schenk EA, Samloff IM. Clinical and morphologic changes following gluten administration to patients with treated celiac disease. Am J Pathol 1968;52:579–593.

75. Zetterqvist H, Hendrix TR. A preliminary note on an ultrastructural abnormality of intestinal epithelium in adult celiac disease (nontropical sprue) which is reversed by a gluten free diet. Bull Johns Hopkins Hosp 1960;106:240–249.

76. Rubin W, Ross LL, Sleisenger MH, Wesser E. An electron microscopic study of adult celiac disease. Lab Invest 1966;15:1720–1747.

77. Rubin CE, Brandborg LL, Flick AL, et al. Studies of celiac sprue. 3. The effect of repeated wheat instillation into the proximal ileum of patients on a gluten free diet. Gastroenterology 1968;54:793.

78. Arranz E, Bode J, Kingstone K, Ferguson A. Intestinal antibody pattern of coeliac disease: association with gamma/delta T cell receptor expression by intraepithelial lymphocytes, and other indices of potential coeliac disease. Gut 1994;35:476–482.

79. Ament ME, Rubin CE. Soy protein—another cause of the flat intestinal lesion. Gastroenterology 1972;62:227–234.

80. McPherson JR, Shorter RG. Intestinal lesions associated with triparanol. A clinical and experimental study. Am J Dig Dis 1965;10:1024–1033.

81. Rogers AI, Vloedman DA, Bloom EC, Kalser MH. Neomycin-induced steatorrhea. JAMA 1966;197:185–190.

82. Chorzelski TP, Beutner EH, Sulej J, et al. IgA anti-endomysium antibody: A new immunological marker of dermatitis herpetiformis and coeliac disease. Br J Dermatol 1984;111:395–402.

83. Diagnosis of celiac disease [Editorial]. Lancet 1991;337:590.

84. Cooper BT, Holmes GK, Ferguson R, Cooke WT. Celiac disease and malignancy. Medicine 1980;59:249–261.

85. Swinson CM, Slavin G, Coles EC, Booth CC. Coeliac disease and malignancy. Lancet 1983;1:111–115.

86. Holmes GK, Prior P, Lane MR, et al. Malignancy in coeliac disease—effect of a gluten free diet. Gut 1989;30:333–338.

87. Isaacson PG, O'Connor NTJ, Spencer J, et al. Malignant histiocytosis of the intestine: a T-cell lymphoma. Lancet 1985;2:688–691.

88. Spencer J, Cerf-Bensussan N, Jarry A, et al. Enteropathy-associated T cell lymphoma (malignant histiocytosis of the intestine) is recognized by a monoclonal antibody (HML-1) that defines a membrane molecule on human mucosal lymphocytes. Am J Pathol 1988;132:1–5.

89. Spencer J, MacDonald TT, Diss TC, et al. Changes in intraepithelial lymphocyte subpopulations in coeliac disease and enteropathy associated T cell lymphoma (malignant histiocytosis of the intestine). Gut 1989;30:339–346.

90. Murray A, Cuevas EC, Jones DB, Wright DH. Study of the immunohistochemistry and T cell clonality of enteropathy-associated T cell lymphoma. Am J Pathol 1995;146:509–519.

91. Fishman MJ, Jeejeebhoy KN, Gopinath N, et al. Small intestinal villous adenoma and celiac disease. Am J Gastroenterol 1990;85. 748–751.

92. Dannenberg A, Godwin T, Rayburn J, et al. Multifocal adenocarcinoma of the proximal small intestine in a patient with celiac sprue. J Clin Gastroenterol 1989;11:73–76.

93. Straker RJ, Gunasekaran S, Brady PG. Adenocarcinoma of the jejunum in association with celiac sprue. J Clin Gastroenterol 1989;11:320–323.

94. Trier JS, Falchuk ZM, Carey MC, Schreiber DS. Celiac sprue and refractory sprue (clinical conference). Gastroenterology 1978;75:307–316.

95. Baer AN, Bayless TM, Yardley JH. Intestinal ulceration and malabsorption syndromes. Gastroenterology 1980;79:754–765.

96. Bayless TM, Kapelowitz RF, Shelley WM, et al. Intestinal ulceration—a complication of celiac disease. New Engl J Med 1967;276:996–1002.

97. Freeman HJ, Chiu BK. Small bowel malignant lymphoma complicating celiac sprue and the mesenteric lymph node cavitation syndrome. Gastroenterology 1986;90:2008–2012.

98. Jeffries GH, Steinberg H, Sleisenger MH. Chronic ulcerative (non-granulomatous) jejunitis. Am J Med 1968;44:47–59.

99. Robertson DA, Dixon MF, Scott BB, et al. Small intestinal ulceration: diagnostic difficulties in relation to coeliac disease. Gut 1983;24:565–574.

100. Jones B, Bayless TM, Hamilton SR, Yardley JH. "Bubbly" duodenal bulb in celiac disease: radiologic-pathologic correlation. Am J Roentgenol 1984;142:119–122.

101. Matuchansky C, Colin R, Hemet J, et al. Cavitation of mesenteric lymph nodes, splenic atrophy, and a flat small intestinal mucosa. Gastroenterology 1984;87:606–614.

102. Rubesin SE, Herlinger H, Saul SH, et al. Adult celiac disease and its complications. Radiographics 1989;9:1045–1066.

103. O'Grady JG, Stevens FM, Harding B, et al. Hyposplenism and gluten-sensitive enteropathy. Natural history, incidence, and relation-

ship to diet and small bowel morphology. Gastroenterology 1984;87:1326–1331.

104. O'Grady JG, Stevens FM, McCarthy CF. Celiac disease: does hyposplenism predispose to the development of malignant disease? Am J Gastroenterol 1985;80:27–29.

105. Weinstein WM, Saunders DR, Tytgat GN, Rubin CE. Collagenous sprue—an unrecognized type of malabsorption. New Engl J Med 1970;283:1297–1301.

106. Bossart R, Henry K, Booth CC, Doe WF. Subepithelial collagen in intestinal malabsorption. Gut 1975;16:18–22.

107. Holdstock DJ, Oleesky S. Successful treatment of collagenous sprue with combination of prednisolone and gluten-free diet. Postgrad Med J 1973;49:664–667.

108. Guller R, Anabitarte M, Mayer M. Kollagensprue und ulzerierende Jejunoileitis bei einem Patienten mit gluteninduzierter Enteropathie. Schweiz Med Wochenschr 1986;116:1343–1349.

109. Marks J, Shuster S, Watson AJ. Small bowel changes in dermatitis herpetiformis. Lancet 1966;2:1280–1282.

110. Shuster S, Watson AJ, Marks J. Coeliac syndrome in dermatitis herpetiformis. Lancet 1968;1:1101–1106.

111. Gebhard RL, Falchuk ZH, Katz SI, et al. Dermatitis herpetiformis. Immunologic concomitants of small intestinal disease and relationship to histocompatibility antigens HL-A8. J Clin Invest 1974;54:98–103.

112. Kosnai I, Karpati S, Savilahti E, et al. Gluten challenge in children with dermatitis herpetiformis: a clinical, morphological and immunohistological study. Gut 1986;27:1464–1470.

113. Lindstrom CG. "Collagenous colitis" with watery diarrhea. A new entity? Pathologia Europ 1976;11:87–89.

114. Wolber R, Owen D, DelBuono L, et al. Lymphocytic gastritis in patients with celiac sprue of spruelike intestinal disease. Gastroenterology 1990;98:310–315.

115. Dubois RN, Lazenby AJ, Yardley JH, et al. Lymphocytic enterocolitis in patients with 'refractory' sprue. JAMA 1989;262:935–937.

116. Wolber R, Owen D, Freeman H. Colonic lymphocytosis in patients with celiac sprue. Hum Pathol 1990;21:1092–1096.

117. O'Mahony S, Nawroz IM, Ferguson A. Coeliac disease and collagenous colitis. Postgrad Med J 1990;66:238–241.

118. Hamilton I, Sanders S, Hopwood D, Bouchier IA. Collagenous colitis associated with small intestinal villous atrophy. Gut 1986;27:1394–1398.

119. Breen EG, Farren C, Connolly CE, McCarthy CF. Collagenous colitis and coeliac disease. Gut 1987;28:364.

120. Eckstein RP, Dowsett JF, Riley JW. Collagenous enterocolitis: a case of collagenous colitis with involvement of the small intestine. Am J Gastroenterol 1988;83:767–771.

121. Yardley JH, Lazenby AJ, Giardiello FM, Bayless TM. Collagenous, "microscopic," lymphocytic, and other gentler and more subtle forms of colitis. Hum Pathol 1990;21:1089–1091.

122. Baker SJ, Mathan VI. Syndrome of tropical sprue in South India. Am J Clin Nutr 1968;21:984–993.

123. Cook GC. Aetiology and pathogenesis of postinfective tropical malabsorption (tropical sprue). Lancet 1984;1:721–723.

124. Cook GC. Postinfective malabsorption (including tropical sprue). In: Bouchier AD, Alan RN, Hodgson JF, Deighley MRB, eds. Gastroenterology. Clinical practice and science. Philadelphia: WB Saunders, 1993:522–537.

125. Klipstein FA, Holdeman LV, Corcino JJ, Moore WEC. Enterotoxigenic intestinal bacteria in tropical sprue. Ann Intern Med 1973;79:632–641.

126. Guerra R, Wheby MS, Bayless TM. Long-term antibiotic therapy in tropical sprue. Ann Intern Med 1965;63:619–634.

127. Rickles FR, Klipstein FA, Tomasini J, et al. Long-term follow-up of antibiotic-treated tropical sprue. Ann Intern Med 1972;76:203–210.

128. Gorbach SL, Banwell JG, Mitra R, et al. Bacterial contamination of the upper small bowel in tropical sprue. Lancet 1969;1:74–77.

129. Cassells JS, Banwell JG, Gorbach SL, et al. Tropical sprue and malnutrition in West Bengal. IV. Bile salt deconjugation in tropical sprue. Am J Clin Nutr 1970;23:1579–1581.

130. Simon GL, Gorbach SL. Intestinal microflora. Med Clin North Am 1982;66:557–574.

131. Klipstein FA. Folate in tropical sprue. Brit J Haematol 1972;23(Suppl):119–133.

132. Foroozan P, Trier JS. Mucosa of the small intestine in pernicious anemia. New Engl J Med 1967;277:553–559.
133. Hendrix TR. Interpretation of intestinal biopsies. Gastroenterology 1968;54:976–978.
134. Marsh MN, Mathan M, Mathan VI. Studies of intestinal lymphoid tissue. VII. The secondary nature of lymphoid cell "activation" in the jejunal lesion of tropical sprue. Am J Pathol 1983;112:302–312.
135. Swanson VL, Thomassen RW. Pathology of the jejunal mucosa in tropical sprue. Am J Pathol 1965;46:511–581.
136. Swanson VL, Wheby MS, Bayless TM. Morphologic effects of folic acid and vitamin B-12 on the jejunal lesion of tropical sprue. Am J Pathol 1966;49:167–191.
137. Sheey TW, Legeters LJ, Wallace DK. Tropical jejunitis in Americans serving in Vietnam. Am J Clin Nutr 1968;21:1013-1022.
138. Brunser O, Eidelman S, Klipstein FA. Intestinal morphology of rural Haitians. A comparison between overt tropical sprue and asymptomatic subjects. Gastroenterology 1970;58:655–668.
139. Vaish SK, Sampathkumar J, Jacob R, Baker SJ. The stomach in tropical sprue. Gut 1965;6:458–465.
140. Ramakrishna BS, Mathan VI. Role of bacterial toxins, bile acids, and free fatty acids in colonic malabsorption in tropical sprue. Dig Dis Sci 1987;32:500–505.
141. Ramakrishna BS, Mathan VI. Absorption of water and sodium and activity of adenosine triphosphatases in the rectal mucosa in tropical sprue. Gut 1988;29:665–668.
142. Wheby MS, Swanson VL, Bayless TM. Comparison of ileal and jejunal biopsies in tropical sprue. Am J Clin Nutr 1971;24:117–123.
143. Goyal RK, Compton CC, Ferrucci JT. Case records of the Massachusetts General Hospital. Weekly clinicopathological exercises. Case 25-1990. A 63-year-old man with recurrent diarrhea. N Engl J Med 1990;322:1796–1806.
144. McEvoy A, Dutton J, James OFW. Bacterial contamination of the small intestine is an important cause of occult malabsorption in the elderly. Br Med J 1983;287:789–793.
145. Roberts SH, James O, Jarvis EH. Bacterial overgrowth syndrome without "blind loop": a cause for malnutrition in the elderly. Lancet 1977;2:1193–1195.
146. King CE, Toskes PP. Small intestine bacterial overgrowth. Gastroenterology 1979;76:1035–1055.
147. Ament ME, Shimoda SS, Saunders DP, Rubin CE. Pathogenesis of steatorrhea in three cases of small intestinal stasis syndrome. Gastroenterology 1972;63:728–747.
148. Toskes PP, Giannella RA, Jervis HR, et al. Small intestinal mucosal injury in the experimental blind loop syndrome. Light- and electron-microscopic and histochemical studies. Gastroenterology 1975;68:193–203.
149. Giannella RA, Rout WR, Toskes PP. Jejunal brush border injury and impaired sugar and amino acid uptake in the blind-loop syndrome. Gastroenterology 1974;67:965–974.
150. Riepe SP, Goldstein J, Alpers DH. Effect of secreted *Bacteroides* proteases on human intestinal brush border hydrolases. J Clin Invest 1980;66:314–322.
151. Drenick EJ, Roslyn JJ. Cure of arthritis-dermatitis syndrome due to intestinal bypass by resection of nonfunctional segment of blind loop. Dig Dis Sci 1990;35:656–660.
152. Kahn IJ, Jeffries GH, Sleisenger MH. Malabsorption in intestinal scleroderma. Correction by antibiotics. New Engl J Med 1966;274:1339–1344.
153. Paulley JW. Gut damage in human blind-loop syndrome. Gastroenterology 1981;81:195.
154. Takano J. Intestinal changes in protein-deficient rats. Exp Mol Pathol 1964;3:224–231.
155. Platt BS, Heard CRC, Stewart RJC. The effects of protein-calorie deficiency on the gastrointestinal tract. In: Munro HN, ed. The role of the gastrointestinal tract in protein metabolism. Philadelphia: FA Davis, 1964:227–237.
156. Tandon BN, Newberne PM, Young VR. A histochemical study of enzyme changes and ultrastructure of the jejunal mucosa in protein-depleted rats. J Nutr 1969;99:519–530.
157. Herskovic T. The effect of protein malnutrition on the small intestine. Am J Clin Nutr 1969;22:300–304.
158. James WPT. Intestinal absorption in protein caloric malnutrition. Lancet 1968;1:333–335.
159. Mayoral LG, Bolanos O, Lotero H, Duque E. Enteropathy in adult protein malnutrition: a review of the Cali experience. Am J Clin Nutr 1975;28:894–900.
160. Duque E, Bolanos O, Lotero H, Mayoral LG. Enteropathy in adult protein malnutrition: light microscopic findings. Am J Clin Nutr 1975;28:901–913.
161. Duque E, Lotero H, Bolanos O, Mayoral LG. Enteropathy in adult protein malnutrition: ultrastructural findings. Am J Clin Nutr 1975;28:914–924.
162. Klipstein FA, Samloff IM, Smarth G, Schenk E. Malabsorption and malnutrition in rural Haiti. Am J Clin Nutr 1968;21:1042–1052.
163. Schneider RE, Viteri FE. Morphological aspects of the duodenojejunal mucosa in protein-calorie malnourished children and during recovery. Am J Clin Nutr 1972;25:1092–1102.
164. Naiman JL, Oski FA, Diamond LK, et al. The gastrointestinal effects of iron-deficiency anemia. Pediatrics 1964;33:83–99.
165. Gross SJ, Stuart MJ, Swender PT, Oski FA. Malabsorption of iron in children with iron deficiency. J Pediatr 1976;88:795–799.
166. Prasad AS. The role of zinc in gastrointestinal and liver disease. Clinics Gastroenterol 1983;12:713–741.
167. Kay RG, Tasman-Jones C, Pybus J, et al. A syndrome of acute zinc deficiency during total parenteral alimentation in man. Ann Surg 1976;183:331–340.
168. Brazin SA, Johnson WT, Abramson LJ. The acrodermatitis enteropathica-like syndrome. Arch Dermatol 1979;115:597–599.
169. Strobel CT, Byrne WJ, Abramovits W, et al. A zinc-deficiency dermatitis in patients on total parenteral nutrition. Int J Dermatol 1978;17:575–581.
170. Sazawal S, Black RE, Bhan MK, et al. Zinc supplementation in young children with acute diarrhea in India. N Engl J Med 1995;333:839–844.
171. Walling A, Householder M, Walling A. Acrodermatitis enteropathica. Am Fam Physician 1989;39:151–154.
172. Mack D, Koletzko B, Cunnane S, et al. Acrodermatitis enteropathica with normal serum zinc levels: diagnostic value of small bowel biopsy and essential fatty acid determination. Gut 1989;30:1426–1429.
173. Kelly R, Davidson GP, Townley RRW, Campbell PE. Reversible intestinal mucosal abnormality in acrodermatitis enteropathica. Arch Dis Child 1976;51:219–222.
174. Ament ME, Broviac J. Acrodermatitis enteropathica (AE)—demonstration of small and large intestinal mucosal lesions: failure of hyperalimentation, Intralipid, and Diodoquin to reverse the intestinal lesions and generalized malabsorption syndromes [Abstract]. Gastroenterology 1973;64:A-9/692.
175. Braun OH, Heilmann K, Pauli W, et al. Acrodermatitis enteropathica: recent findings concerning clinical features, pathogenesis, diagnosis and therapy. Europ J Pediat 1976;121:247–261.
176. Bohane TD, Hamilton JR, Gall DG. Acrodermatitis enteropathica, zinc and the Paneth cell. A case report with family studies. Gastroenterology 1977;73:587–592.
177. Elmes ME, Jones JG. Ultrastructural changes in the small intestine of zinc deficient rats. J Pathol 1980;130:37–43.
178. Kobayashi Y, Suzuki H, Konno T, et al. Ultrastructural alterations of Paneth cells in infants associated with gastrointestinal symptoms. Tohoku J Exp Med 1983;139:225–230.
179. Blacklow NR, Cukor G. Viral gastroenteritis. New Engl J Med 1981;304:397–406.
180. Wilson KH, Blitchington R, Frothingham R, Wilson JA. Phylogeny of the Whipple's-disease-associated bacterium. Lancet 1991;338:474–475.
181. Relman DA, Schmidt TM, MacDermott RP, Falkow S. Identification of the uncultured bacillus of Whipple's disease. New Engl J Med 1992;327:293–301.
182. Keren DF. Whipple's disease: a review emphasizing immunology and microbiology. Crit Rev Clin Lab Sci 1981;14:75–108.
183. Dobbins WO III. Whipple's disease. Springfield, Ill.: Charles C Thomas, 1987.
184. Whipple GH. A hitherto undescribed disease characterized anatomically by deposits of fat and fatty acids in the intestinal and mesenteric lymphatic tissue. Bull Johns Hopkins Hosp 1907;18:382–391.
185. Chears WC, Ashworth CT. Electron microscopic study of intestinal mucosa in Whipple's disease: demonstration of encapsulated bacilliform bodies in the lesion. Gastroenterology 1961;41:129–138.

186. Yardley JH, Hendrix TR. Combined electron and light microscopy in Whipple's disease: demonstration of "bacillary bodies" in the intestine. Bull Johns Hopkins Hosp 1961;109:80–95.

187. Marth T, Roux M, von Herbay A, et al. Persistent reduction of complement receptor 3 alpha-chain expressing mononuclear blood cells and transient inhibitory serum factors in Whipple's disease. Clin Immunol Immunopathol 1994;72:217–226.

188. Silva MT, Macedo PM, Moura Nunes JF. Ultrastructure of bacilli and the bacillary origin of the macrophagic inclusions in Whipple's disease. J Gen Microbiol 1985;131:1001–1013.

189. Dobbins WO 3d, Kawanishi H. Bacillary characteristics in Whipple's disease: an electron microscopic study. Gastroenterology 1981;80:1468–1475.

190. Sieracki JC, Fine G. Whipple's disease—observations on systemic involvement. Arch Pathol 1959;67:81–93.

191. Knox DL, Bayless TM, Pittman FE. Neurologic disease in patients with Whipple's disease. Medicine 1976;55:467–476.

192. Radvany J, Rosales RK. Whipple's disease confined to the brain: a case studied clinically and pathologically. J Neurol Neurosurg Psychiatry 1977;40:901–909.

193. Knox DL, Green WR, Troncoso JC, et al. Cerebro-ocular Whipple's disease: a 62 year odyssey from death to diagnosis. Neurology 1995;45:617–625.

194. Dobbins WO III. The diagnosis of Whipple's disease [Editorial]. New Engl J Med 1995;332:390–392.

195. Volpicelli NA, Salyer WR, Milligan FD, et al. The endoscopic appearance of the duodenum in Whipple's disease. Johns Hopkins Med J 1976;138:19–23.

196. Kuhajda FP, Belitsos NJ, Keren DF, Hutchins GM. A submucosal variant of Whipple's disease. Gastroenterology 1982;82:46–50.

197. Roth RI, Owen RL, Keren DF, Volberding PA. Intestinal infection with Mycobacterium avium in acquired immune deficiency syndrome (AIDS). Histological and clinical comparison with Whipple's disease. Dig Dis Sci 1985;30:497–504.

198. Gonzalez-Licea AG, Yardley JH. Whipple's disease in the rectum. Light and electron microscopic findings. Am J Path 1968;52:1191–1206.

199. Rickman LS, Freeman WR, Green WRG, et al. Brief report: uveitis caused by Tropheryma whippelii (Whipple's bacillus). New Engl J Med 1995;332:363–366.

200. Lowsky R, Archer GL, Fyles G, et al. Brief report: diagnosis of Whipple's disease by molecular analysis of peripheral blood. New Engl J Med 1994;331:1343–1346.

201. Gupta TP, Ehrinpreis MN. Candida-associated diarrhea in hospitalized patients. Gastroenterology 1990;98:780–785.

202. Orchard JL, Luparello F, Brunskill D. Malabsorption syndrome occurring in the course of disseminated histoplasmosis: case report and review of gastrointestinal histoplasmosis. Am J Med 1979;66:331–336.

203. Goodgame RW. Understanding intestinal spore-forming protozoa: cryptosporidia, microsporidia, isospora, and cyclospora. Ann Intern Med 1996;124:429–441.

204. Brasitus TA. Parasites and malabsorption. Clin Gastroenterol 1983;12:495–510.

205. Cali A, Owen RL. Microsporidiosis. In: Balows A, ed. Laboratory diagnosis of infectious disease: principles and practices. New York: Springer-Verlag, 1988;1:929–950.

206. Cali A, Owen RL. Intracellular development of Enterocytozoon, a unique microsporidian found in the intestine of AIDS patients. J Protozool 1990;37:145–155.

207. Desportes I, LeCharpentier Y, Galian A, et al. Occurrence of a new microsporidian Enterocytozoon bieneusi n. g., n. sp., in the enterocytes of a human patient with AIDS. J Protozool 1985;32:250–254.

208. Orenstein JM, Tenner M, Cali A, Kotler DP. A microsporidian previously undescribed in humans, infecting enterocytes and macrophages, and associated with diarrhea in an acquired immunodeficiency syndrome patient. Hum Pathol 1992;23:722–728.

209. Hartskeerl RA, Van Gool T, Schuitema AR, et al. Genetic and immunological characterization of the microsporidian Septata intestinalis Cali, Kotler and Orenstein, 1993: reclassification to Encephalitozoon intestinalis. Parasitology 1995;110(Pt 3):277–285.

210. Orenstein JM, Chiang J, Steinberg W, et al. Intestinal microsporidiosis as a cause of diarrhea in human immunodeficiency virus-infected patients. Hum Pathol 1990;21:475–481.

211. Greenson JK, Belitsos PC, Yardley JH, Bartlett JG. AIDS enteropathy—occult enteric infections and duodenal mucosal alterations in chronic diarrhea. Ann Intern Med 1991;114:366–372.

212. Rijpstra AC, Canning EU, Ketel RJV, et al. Use of light microscopy to diagnose small intestinal microsporidiosis in patients with AIDS. J Infect Dis 1988;157:827–831.

213. van Gool T, Hollister WS, Schattenkerk JE, et al. Diagnosis of Enterocytozoon bieneusi microsporidiosis in AIDS patients by recovery of spores from faeces. Lancet 1990;336:267–268.

214. Orenstein JM, Zierdt W, Zierdt C, Kotler DP. Identification of spores of enterocytozoon-bieneusi in stool and duodenal fluid from AIDS patients. Lancet 1990;336:1127–1128.

215. Lucas SB, Papadaki L, Conlon C, et al. Diagnosis of intestinal microsporidiosis in patients with AIDS. J Clin Pathol 1989;42:885–890.

216. Conteas CN, Sowerby T, Berlin GW, et al. Fluorescence techniques for diagnosing intestinal microsporidiosis in stool, enteric fluid, and biopsy specimens from acquired immunodeficiency syndrome patients with chronic diarrhea. Arch Pathol Lab Med 1996;120:847–853.

217. Weber R, Bryan RT, Owen RL, et al. Improved light-microscopical detection of microsporidia spores in stool and duodenal aspirates. New Engl J Med 1992;326:161–166.

218. Ortega YR, Sterling CR, Gilman RH, et al. Cyclospora species—a new protozoan pathogen of humans. N Engl J Med 1993;328:1308–1312.

219. Bendall RP, Lucas S, Moody A, et al. Diarrhoea associated with cyanobacterium like bodies: a new coccidian enteritis of man [Review]. Lancet 1993;341:590–592.

220. Connor BA, Shlim DR, Scholes JV, et al. Pathologic changes in the small bowel in nine patients with diarrhea associated with a coccidia-like body. Ann Intern Med 1993;119:377–382.

221. Hoge CW, Shlim DR, Rajah R, et al. Epidemiology of diarrhoeal illness associated with coccidian-like organism among travellers and foreign residents in Nepal. Lancet 1993;341:1175–1179.

222. Relman DA, Schmidt TM, Gajadhar A, et al. Molecular phylogenetic analysis of Cyclospora, the human intestinal pathogen, suggests that it is closely related to Eimeria species. J Infect Dis 1996;173:440–445.

223. Brennan MK, Macpherson DW, Palmer J, Keystone JS. Cyclosporiasis—a new cause of diarrhea. Can Med Assoc J 1996;155:1293–1296.

224. Ooi WW, Zimmerman SK, Needham CA. Cyclospora species as a gastrointestinal pathogen in immunocompetent hosts. J Clin Microbiol 1995;33:1267.

225. Huang P, Weber JT, Sosin DM, et al. The first reported outbreak of diarrheal illness associated with Cyclospora in the United States. Ann Intern Med 1995;123:409–414.

226. Update: outbreaks of Cyclospora cayetanensis infection—United States and Canada, 1996. Morb Mortal Wkly Rep 1996;45:611–612.

227. Van Nhieu JT, Nin F, Fleuryfeith J, et al. Identification of intracellular stages of Cyclospora species by light microscopy of thick sections using hematoxylin. Human Pathol 1996;27:1107–1109.

228. Sun T, Ilardi CF, Asnis D, et al. Light and electron microscopic identification of Cyclospora species in the small intestine. Evidence of the presence of asexual life cycle in human host. Am J Clin Pathol 1996;105:216–220.

229. Deluol A-M, Teilhac MF, Poirot J-L, et al. Cyclospora sp: life cycle studies in patient by electron microscopy. J Eukaryot Microbiol 1996;43:128S–129S.

230. Saraya AK, Tandon BN. Hookworm anaemia and intestinal malabsorption associated with hookworm infestation. Prog Drug Res 1975;19:108–118.

231. Tripathy K, Gonzalez F, Lotero H, Bolanos O. Effects of Ascaris infection on human nutrition. Am J Trop Med Hyg 1970;20:212–218.

232. Meyers WM, Connor DH, Neafie RC. Strongyloidiasis. In: Binford CH, Connor DH, ed. Pathology of tropical and extraordinary diseases. Washington, D.C.: Armed Forces Institute of Pathology, 1976:428–432.

233. Scowden EB, Schaffner W, Stone WJ. Overwhelming strongyloidi-

asis. An unappreciated opportunistic infection. Medicine 1978;57:527–544.

234. Milder JE, Walzer PD, Kilgore G, et al. Clinical features of *Strongyloides stercoralis* infection in an endemic area of the United States. Gastroenterology 1981;80:1481–1488.

235. Arakaki T, Iwanaga M, Kinjo F, et al. Efficacy of agar-plate culture in detection of Strongyloides stercoralis infection. J Parasitol 1990;76:425–428.

236. Neafie RC, Connor DH, Cross JH. Capillariasis (intestinal and hepatic). In: Binford CH, Connor DH, eds. Pathology of tropical and extraordinary diseases. Washington, D.C.: Armed Forces Institute of Pathology, 1976:402–408.

237. Intestinal capillariasis: a new disease of man [Editorial]. Lancet 1973;1:587–588.

238. Chen CY, Hsieh WC, Lin JT, Liu MC. Intestinal capillariasis: report of a case. Taiwan I Hsueh Hui Tsa Chih 1989;88:617–620.

239. Youssef FG, Mikhail EM, Mansour NS. Intestinal capillariasis in Egypt: a case report. Am J Trop Med Hyg 1989;40:195–196.

240. Cross JH, Basaca-Sevilla V. Experimental transmission of Capillaria phillipinensis to birds. Trans R Soc Trop Med Hyg 1983;77:511–514.

241. Fresh JW, Cross JH, Reyes V, et al. Necropsy findings in intestinal capillariasis. Am J Trop Med Hyg 1972;21:169–173.

242. Kagnoff MF. Immunology and inflammation of the gastrointestinal tract. In: Sleisenger MH, Fordtran JS, eds. Gastrointestinal disease, 5th ed. Philadelphia: WB Saunders, 1993:45–86.

243. Bartelsman JFWM, Sars PRA, Tytgat GNJ. Gastrointestinal complications in patients with acquired immunodeficiency syndrome. Scand J Gastroenterol 1989;24(Suppl 171):112–117.

244. HIV-associated enteropathy [Editorial]. Lancet 1989;2:777–778.

245. Laughon BE, Druckman DA, Vernon A, et al. Prevalence of enteric pathogens in homosexual men with and without acquired immunodeficiency syndrome. Gastroenterology 1988;94:984–993.

246. Rodgers VD, Fassett R, Kagnoff MF. Abnormalities in intestinal mucosal T cells in homosexual populations including those with the lymphadenopathy syndrome and acquired immunodeficiency syndrome. Gastroenterology 1986;90:552–558.

247. Rodgers VD, Kagnoff MF. Abnormalities of the intestinal immune system in AIDS. Gastroenterol Clin North Am 1988;17:487–494.

248. Nelson JA, Wiley CA, Reynolds-Kohler C, et al. Human immunodeficiency virus detected in bowel epithelium from patients with gastrointestinal symptoms. Lancet 1988;1:259–262.

249. Mathijs JM, Hing M, Grierson J, et al. HIV infection of rectal mucosa [Letter]. Lancet 1988;1:1111.

250. Fox CH, Kotler D, Tierney A, et al. Detection of HIV-1 RNA in the lamina propria of patients with AIDS and gastrointestinal disease. J Infect Dis 1989;159:467–471.

251. Jarry A, Cortez A, Rene E, et al. Infected cells and immune cells in the gastrointestinal tract of AIDS patients. An immunohistochemical study of 127 cases. Histopathology 1990;16:133–140.

252. Ferreira RD, Forsyth LE, Richman PI, et al. Changes in the rate of crypt epithelial cell proliferation and mucosal morphology induced by a T-cell-mediated response in human small intestine. Gastroenterology 1990;98:1255–1263.

253. MacDonald TT, Spencer J. Evidence that activated mucosal T cells play a role in the pathogenesis of enteropathy in human small intestine. J Exp Med 1988;167:1341–1349.

254. MacDonald TT, Ferguson A. Hypersensitivity reactions in the small intestine. 3. The effects of allograft rejection and of graft-versus-host reaction on epithelial cell kinetics. Cell Tissue Kinet 1977;10:301–312.

255. Ullrich R, Zeitz M, Heise W, et al. Small intestinal structure and function in patients infected with human immunodeficiency virus (HIV): evidence for HIV-induced enteropathy. Ann Intern Med 1989;111:15–21.

256. Unsworth J, Hutchins P, Mitchell J, et al. Flat small intestinal mucosa and autoantibodies against the gut epithelium. J Pediatr Gastroenterol Nutr 1982;1:503–513.

257. Mirakian R, Richardson A, Milla PJ, et al. Protracted diarrhoea of infancy: evidence in support of an autoimmune variant. Br Med J 1986;293:1132–1136.

258. Seldman EG, Localle F, Russo P, et al. Successful treatment of autoimmune enteropathy with cyclosporine. J Pediatr 1990;117:929–932.

259. Cuenod B, Brousse N, Goulet O, et al. Classification of intractable diarrhea in infancy using clinical and immunohistological criteria. Gastroenterology 1990;99:1037–1043.

260. Hill SM, Milla PJ, Bottazzo GF, Mirakian R. Autoimmune enteropathy and colitis: is there a generalised autoimmune gut disorder? Gut 1991;32:36–42.

261. Mirakian R, Hill S, Richardson A, et al. HLA product expression and lymphocyte subpopulations in jejunum biopsies of children with idiopathic protracted diarrhoea and enterocyte autoantibodies. J Autoimmun 1988;1:263–277.

262. Webb TA, Li CY, Yam LT. Systemic mast cell disease: a clinical and hematopathologic study of 26 cases. Cancer 1982;49:927–938.

263. Enerbäck L, Pipkorn U, Aldenborg F, Wingren U. Mast cell heterogeneity in man: properties and function of human mucosal mast cells. In: Galli SJ, Austen FK, eds. Mast cell and basophil differentiation and function in health and disease. New York: Raven Press, 1989:27–37.

263a. Cherner JA, Jensen RT, Dubois A, et al. Gastrointestinal dysfunction in systemic mastocytosis. A prospective study. Gastroenterology 1988;95:657–667.

264. Bank S, Marks IN. Malabsorption in systemic mast cell disease. Gastroenterology 1963;45:535–549.

265. Jarnum S, Zachariae H. Mastocytosis (urticaria pigmentosa) of skin, stomach, and gut with malabsorption. Gut 1967;8:64–68.

266. Broitman SA, McCray RS, May JC, et al. Mastocytosis and intestinal malabsorption. Am J Med 1970;48:382–389.

267. Dantzig PI. Tetany, malabsorption, and mastocytosis. Arch Intern Med 1975;135:1514–1518.

268. Ammann RW, Vetter D, Deyhle P, et al. Gastrointestinal involvement in systemic mastocytosis. Gut 1976;17:107–112.

269. Fishman RS, Fleming CR, Li CY. Systemic mastocytosis with review of gastrointestinal manifestations. Mayo Clin Proc 1979;54:51–54.

270. Bredfeldt JE, O'Laughlin JC, Durham JB, Blessing LD. Malabsorption and gastric hyperacidity in systemic mastocytosis. Am J Gastroenterol 1980;74:133–137.

271. Braverman DZ, Dollberg L, Shiner M. Clinical, histological, and electron microscopic study of mast cell disease of the small bowel. Am J Gastroenterol 1985;80:30–37.

272. Reisberg IR, Oyakawa S. Mastocytosis with malabsorption, myelofibrosis, and massive ascites. Am J Gastroenterol 1987;82:54–60.

273. Enerbäck L. Mast cells in rat gastrointestinal mucosa. I. Effects of fixation. Acta Pathol Microbiol Scand 1966;66:289–302.

274. Befus AD, Pearce FL, Gauldie J, et al. Isolation and characteristics of mast cells from the lamina propria of the small bowel. In: Pepys J, Edwards AM, eds. Baltimore: University Park Press, 1979:702–709.

274a. Strobel S, Miller HRP, Ferguson A. Human intestinal mucosal mast cells: evaluation of fixation and staining techniques. J Clin Pathol 1981;34:851–858.

275. Ruitenberg EJ, Gustowska L, Elgersma A, Ruitenberg HM. Effect of fixation on the light microscopical visualization of mast cells in the mucosa and connective tissue of the human duodenum. Int Arch Allergy Appl Immunol 1982;67:233–238.

276. Irani AM, Bradford TR, Kepley CL, et al. Detection of MCT and MCTC types of human mast cells by immunohistochemistry using new monoclonal anti-tryptase and anti-chymase antibodies. J Histochem Cytochem 1989;37:1509–1515.

277. Barrett KE, Metcalfe DD. Mast cell heterogeneity: evidence and implications. J Clin Immunol 1984;4:253–261.

278. Scott BB, Hardy GJ, Losowsky MS. Involvement of the small intestine in systemic mast cell disease. Gut 1975;16:918–924.

279. Befus AD, Denburg J, Bienenstock J. Mechanisms of intestinal mastocytosis. In: Pepys J, Edwards AM, eds. The mast cell: its role in health and disease. Baltimore: University Park Press, 1979:115–122.

280. Abe T, Ochiai H, Minamishima Y, Nawa Y. Induction of intestinal mastocytosis in nude mice by repeated injection of interleukin-3. Int Arch Allergy Appl Immunol 1988;86:356–358.

281. Saito H, Hatake K, Dvorak AM, et al. Selective differentiation and proliferation of hematopoietic cells induced by recombinant human interleukins. Proc Natl Acad Sci USA 1988;85:2288–2292.

282. Davidson GP, Cutz E, Hamilton JR, Gall DG. Familial enteropathy: a syndrome of protracted diarrhea from birth, failure to thrive, and hypoplastic villus atrophy. Gastroenterology 1978;75:783–790.

283. Cutz E, Rhoads JM, Drumm B, et al. Microvillus inclusion disease: an inherited defect of brush-border assembly and differentiation. New Engl J Med 1989;320:646–651.

284. Rhoads JM, Vogler RC, Lacey SR, et al. Microvillus inclusion disease. In vitro jejunal electrolyte transport. Gastroenterology 1991;100: 811–817.

285. Raafat F, Green NJ, Nathavitharana KA, Booth IW. Intestinal microvillous dystrophy: a variant of microvillous inclusion disease or a new entity? Hum Pathol 1994;25:1243–1248.

286. Lake BD. Microvillus inclusion disease: specific diagnostic features shown by alkaline phosphatase histochemistry. J Clin Pathol 1988; 41:880–882.

287. Groisman GM, Ben-Izhak O, Schwersenz A, et al. The value of polyclonal carcinoembryonic antigen immunostaining in the diagnosis of microvillous inclusion disease. Hum Pathol 1993;24:1232–1237.

288. Waldman TA, Steinfeld JL, Dutcher TF, et al. The role of gastrointestinal system in "idiopathic hypoproteinemia." Gastroenterology 1961;41:197–207.

289. Waldmann TA. Protein-losing enteropathy. Gastroenterology 1966; 50:422–443.

290. Abramowsky C, Hupertz V, Kilbridge P, Czinn S. Intestinal lymphangiectasia in children: a study of upper gastrointestinal endoscopic biopsies. Pediatr Pathol 1989;9:289–297.

291. Strober W, Wochner RD, Carbone PP, Waldman TA. Intestinal lymphangiectasia: a protein-losing enteropathy with hypogammaglobulinemia, lymphocytopenia and impaired homograft rejection. J Clin Invest 1967;46:1643–1656.

292. Pomerantz M, Waldman TA. Systemic lymphatic abnormalities associated with gastrointestinal protein loss secondary to intestinal lymphangiectasia. Gastroenterology 1963;45:703–711.

293. Eustace PW, Gaunt JI, Croft DN. Incidence of protein-losing enteropathy in primary lymphoedema using chromium-51 chloride technique. BMJ 1975;4:737.

294. Dobbins WO III. Electron microscopic study of the intestinal mucosa in intestinal lymphangiectasia. Gastroenterology 1966;51: 1004–1017.

295. Perisic VN, Kokai G. Bleeding from duodenal lymphangiectasia. Arch Dis Child 1991;66:153–154.

296. Asakura H, Miur S, Morishita T, et al. Endoscopic and histopathological study on primary and secondary intestinal lymphangiectasia. Dig Dis Sci 1981;26:312–320.

297. Hart MH, Vanderhoof JA, Antonson DL. Failure of blind small bowel biopsy in the diagnosis of intestinal lymphangiectasia. J Pediatr Gastroenterol Nutr 1987;6:803–805.

298. Harris M, Burton IE, Scarffe JH. Macroglobulinemia and intestinal lymphangiectasia: a rare association. J Clin Pathol 1983; 36:30–36.

299. Myszor MF, Davidson A, Hodgson HJF. The local mucosal immune system in intestinal lymphangiectasia. J Clin Lab Immunol 1988; 26:1–3.

300. Mistilis SP, Skyring AP, Stephen DD. Intestinal lymphangiectasia. Mechanism of enteric loss of plasma protein and fat. Lancet 1965; 1:77–80.

301. Patel AS, DeRidder PH. Endoscopic appearance and significance of functional lymphangiectasia of the duodenal mucosa. Gastrointest Endosc 1990;36:376–378.

302. Cabrera A, de la Pava S, Pickren JW. Intestinal localization of Waldenstrom's disease. Arch Intern Med 1964;114:399–407.

303. Bedine MS, Yardley JH, Elliott HL, et al. Intestinal involvement in Waldenstrom's macroglobulinemia. Gastroenterology 1973;65: 308–315.

304. Brandt LJ, Davidoff A, Bernstein LH, et al. Small intestinal involvement in Waldenstrom's macroglobulinemia. Case report and review of the literature. Dig Dis Sci 1981;26:174–180.

305. Pruzanski W, Warren RE, Goldie JH, Katz A. Malabsorption syndrome with infiltration of the intestinal wall extracellular monoclonal macroglobulin. Am J Med 1973;54:811–818.

306. Amrein PC, Compton CC. Case records of the Massachusetts General Hospital. Weekly clinicopathological exercises. Case 3-1990. A 66-year-old woman with Waldenstrom's macroglobulinemia, diarrhea, anemia, and persistent gastrointestinal bleeding. N Engl J Med 1990;322:183–192.

307. Aspelin P, Adielsson G, Dimitrov N, et al. Abdominal computed tomography in macroglobulinemia (Waldenstrom's disease). Acta Radiologica 1989;30:197–200.

32 DIVERTICULAR DISEASE OF THE COLON

Si-Chun Ming

A diverticulum of the gastrointestinal tract is a blind pouch leading off the gut. Its mucosa, including muscularis mucosae, is in continuance with that of the organ from which it arises, and it communicates with the main lumen of the gut. The diverticulum may partially or completely penetrate the muscularis propria so that the apex of diverticulum is covered only by the mesenteric tissue or the serosa. These features distinguish the diverticulum from a duplication of the alimentary tract, which is most commonly a noncommunicating cystic structure containing a full or partial layer of muscularis propria. The duplications are discussed in detail in Chapter 10.

The presence of diverticula is termed diverticulosis. In the majority of cases, the diverticulum is asymptomatic. Therefore, diverticulosis in the clinical sense may be considered an incidental phenomenon and not a disease. In many cases, however, the diverticulum may become inflamed, bleed, obstruct, and perforate to cause extramural abscess, fistula, and diffuse sepsis. The term diverticular disease encompasses the variable clinical spectrum of manifestations, particularly diverticulitis and its complications.

The diverticular disease of the colon is discussed in detail in this chapter. Those of the upper gastrointestinal tract are presented briefly. Additional information is presented in Chapter 10 on congenital diverticula, Chapter 20 on esophageal diverticula, Chapter 13 on small intestinal diverticula associated with muscular or neural diseases, Chapter 35 on appendiceal diverticula and, in brief passages, in various chapters on inflammatory and neoplastic disorders.

CLASSIFICATION OF DIVERTICULA

The diverticula have been classified in several ways (Table 32.1). Basically, the diverticula can be divided into two groups: true and false. A true diverticulum is a wide-mouthed pouch lined by a wall identical to that of the adjacent normal colon, including a full complement of muscular layer. It occurs most commonly as a single lesion in the cecum and ascending colon. The congenital diverticulum is usually a true diverticulum. The false diverticulum (pseudodiverticulum) does not have a full muscularis propria. The acquired diverticulum is usually a pseudodiverticulum.

The diverticula have also been classified by the mechanisms of their formation into pulsion and traction types. The pulsion diverticulum is the result of increased intraluminal pressure pushing the mucosa through a weak point in the muscularis propria. It is therefore a pseudodiverticulum. The traction diverticulum is caused by scar tissue outside the gut pulling a portion of gut wall outward to form a sac. The traction diverticulum has a full thickness muscular layer.

TABLE	
32.1	**Classification of Diverticulum of the Digestive Tract**

I. Anatomic Classification
   A. True diverticulum
      Diverticular wall containing full muscularis propria
   B. False (pseudo) diverticulum
      Diverticular wall lacking all or part of muscularis propria
II. Developmental Classification
   A. Congenital diverticulum
      True or false diverticulum, mostly true
   B. Acquired diverticulum
      True or false diverticulum, mostly false
III. Classification by Location
IV. Clinical Classification
   A. Symptomatic diverticular disease
   B. Asymptomatic diverticular disease

DIVERTICULOSIS OF THE UPPER GASTROINTESTINAL TRACT

Diverticula can occur in any segment of the gastrointestinal tract. The most common and most serious ones are found in the colon, in about 10 to 66% of barium enema examinations, and are more common in the Western countries (1). Diverticula of the upper gastrointestinal tract are less frequent. Among 20,000 barium examinations, Wheeler found diverticula of the esophagus in 0.15%, of the stomach in 0.1%, and of the duodenum in 5.1% (2).

In the esophagus, the diverticula are found at the pharyngoesophageal junction, just above the diaphragm and the midthorax, with a frequency ratio of approximately 7:1:2 (2). The diverticulum at midthoracic esophagus is usually a traction diverticulum caused by tuberculous lymphadenitis at the level of bifurcation of trachea. With marked decline of tuberculosis, the incidence of traction diverticulum has virtually disappeared. The diverticula at either end of the esophagus are of the pulsion type. A congenital diverticulum at this location in the infant, on the other hand, has a muscular wall. The pharyngoesophageal diverticulum, also known as Zenker's diverticulum, is invariably located at the posterior wall between the oblique fibers of inferior constrictor and the crossing fibers of cricopharyngeus muscle (3).

The epiphrenic diverticula occur just above the diaphragm and are often associated with conditions causing functional or structural obstruction of the distal esophagus, such as hiatus hernia (4), diffuse esophageal spasm, and achalasia (5). In one report, the diverticulum occurred in a boy with Ehlers-Danlos syndrome (6).

Clinically, the pulsion diverticula occur in the middle or later years of life and more frequently in males than females. Many patients are asymptomatic. Symptoms are related to obstruction, inflammation, and hemorrhage (7). Carcinoma develops in about 0.3% of Zenker's diverticulum (8).

The diverticula discussed above are usually single, large, and project beyond the esophageal wall. In diffuse intramural esophageal diverticulosis (also called pseudodiverticulosis), there are many small diverticula within the wall, and these are more numerous in the upper esophagus (9–11). They were thought to be dilated ducts of the esophageal glands lined with metaplastic squamous cells.

Diverticula of the stomach occur in the posterior wall near cardia in 75% of the cases, and in the prepyloric region in 15% (12, 13). The former ones may be congenital or acquired (13, 14). They are often asymptomatic, but may become ulcerated and bleed (14, 15). The prepyloric diverticula are usually acquired, probably related to peptic ulcer. Rarely, the diverticula are intramural (16). Additional information on gastric diverticula is given in Chapter 23.

Diverticula of the small intestine occur most frequently in the duodenum. They are rare in the jejunum and ileum, appearing in about 0.1% of barium examinations (17). They may be congenital or acquired. Meckel's diverticulum is the prototype of a congenital type (see Chapter 10). It has been found in 0.3% to 2% of the autopsies (17, 18). There is a slight male predominance in the symptomatic patients. In the adult, it is located at the antimesenteric border of the ileum, 80 to 90 cm above the ileocecal valve, measuring up to 12 cm in length (17). The mucosa is composed mostly of the small intestinal type of tissue, but heterotopic mucosa of other parts of the gastrointestinal tract, and pancreatic tissue, may be present (19). The oxyntic gastric mucosa is associated with peptic ulceration, often in the adjacent ileum, and may cause obstruction by kinking or volvulus. The presence of fecalith may induce acute inflammation (20). One case of Meckel's diverticulitis was reported in a neonatal infant (21). Rarely, neoplasms, epithelial or mesenchymal in origin, may arise in Meckel's diverticulum (22–24) (see Chapter 34). The incidence of complications in Meckel's diverticulum has been estimated at 87 per 100,000 cases, with a lifetime risk of 6.4% (21).

Diverticula of the duodenum have been found in 1 to 6% of radiologic examinations, with an average of 1.7%, and in an average of 8.6% of autopsies (17). They were discovered in 13.4% of patients examined with endoscopic retrograde cholangiopancreatography. They are mostly single, projecting out at the medial aspect of the second portion of duodenum in the periampullary region. In about 33% of the cases they are located in the third and fourth portions of duodenum (25). Most patients are asymptomatic, but some diverticula may cause dysfunction of sphincter of Oddi (26) and increased intrabiliary pressure (27), causing obstructive jaundice. Hemorrhage, perforation, and acute pancreatitis may also occur (28, 29). Rarely, fecalith may form in the diverticulum causing obstruction of the distal gut (30). The rare congenital duodenal diverticula may be extramural or intramural (31). The intraluminal diverticulum is a pocket created by a membrane made of mucosa on both sides (32). There is often a small opening on the membrane allowing communication between the diverticulum and the duodenal lumen. The membrane may be excised endoscopically or surgically (33).

Diverticula of the jejunum and ileum, other than Meckel's diverticulum, are mostly acquired (34), possibly due to defects in the muscular coat or nerve plexus (see Chapter 13). Jejunal diverticula occur in 0.07 to 2.0% of the population (35). They are usually multiple and typically occur at the mesenteric border where blood vessels enter the intestinal wall (36). The diverticula may cause hemorrhage, inflammation, perforation, and obstruction (36, 37) requiring surgical management in 10% of cases (34). Complications of the abdominal wall and hepatic abscesses were reported (38, 39). Malabsorption syndrome, particularly Vitamin

B_{12} deficiency leading to macrocytic anemia, may occur, due to overgrowth of bacteria in the diverticula (36) (see Chapter 31).

EPIDEMIOLOGY OF DIVERTICULAR DISEASE OF THE COLON

Accounts of historical events related to the description of colonic diverticula and their clinical consequences were given by Painter and Burkitt (1). Cruveilhier (40) was credited for giving the first detailed description of diverticula of colon in 1849. In 1899 Graser (41) related the herniation of diverticulum to the point of vascular entrance into the colon wall. In 1904, Beer (42) believed that fecal masses in the diverticula caused diverticulitis, progressing to perforation and fistula. Thus the concept of diverticular disease of colon took shape around the turn of the 20th century. However, the condition was uncommon and its importance as a clinical problem was not generally appreciated, until the advent of radiology demonstrating the prevalence of colonic diverticula in the general population (1). Radiologic studies and autopsy data showed that the incidence had increased dramatically in the Western countries, coinciding with the change of life style and eating habits, from a high-residue diet containing plenty of cereal fiber to a low-residue diet deficient in dietary fiber.

The influence of westernization in dietary habits on the incidence of colonic diverticula is shown clearly by the geographic distribution of the disease. In the recent reports the incidence has increased in the urbanized Africans (43) and Indians (44) to over 2%. The incidence in Japan increased from 3.9 to 9.0% in 1970s up to 8.4 to 23.3% in 1984 (45, 46). In Hong Kong the rate was 5% in 1985 (47). In Singapore, however, colonic diverticula were found in 20% of barium examinations (48). The rate among Arabs in Israel increased by seven-fold to 9.5% (49). While the sigmoid colon is affected in 90% of cases in the Western countries, 75% of diverticula, mostly of congenital type, were found in the cecum and ascending colon in the Asians (45–48, 50). Another difference is in the sex distribution: while nearly equal between the sexes in the Westerners, there is a 3:2 male predominance in the Asians (45).

ETIOLOGY AND PATHOGENESIS OF DIVERTICULAR DISEASE OF COLON

Two factors determine the development of acquired colonic diverticula: (1) a higher intraluminal pressure of the gut than the ambient peritoneal pressure, and (2) a weak point in the intestinal wall where herniation of the mucosa occurs. The effects of these factors on the diverticula of upper gastrointestinal tract are briefly mentioned above. The situation is more complicated in the colon. The muscularis propria, which generates the intraluminal pressure by contraction and maintains the integrity of the intestinal wall, has a unique anatomic arrangement in that the longitudinal muscle is gathered into three equidistant bands: one mesenteric taenia at the attachment of mesocolon to colon and two antimesenteric taeniae on the opposing free wall. The blood vessels in the mesentery pass over the mesenteric taenia to enter the circular muscle coat between the mesenteric taenia and each antimesenteric taenia, corresponding to the usual location of diverticula (Fig. 32.1).

DEFECTS IN THE COLONIC WALL

The occurrence of diverticula at the point of vascular penetration, which serves as a weak point in the colonic wall, was recognized by Graser in 1899 (41). The relationship was confirmed by Noer in specimens studied after injection of latex into the vessels (51). He and others (52) recognized, however, that the relationship between vessels and diverticula was inconstant (Fig. 32.2). The contribution of a weakened point in the colonic wall to the development of diverticulum is demonstrated in scleroderma. In this condition, diverticula occur at areas where the muscular layer is replaced by fibrous tissue (53). Since the fibrotic area is relatively broad, the opening of the diverticulum is wide. On the other hand, the opening of a usual diverticulum is small and its neck is surrounded by circular muscle (Fig. 32.3). Scleroderma has also been associated with rectal diverticulum which is usually single and asymptomatic (54). The association of colonic diverticula with Marfan's (55) and Ehlers Danlos syndromes (56), diseases with defects in collagen formation, suggests a possible defect in collagen tissue in diverticulosis. Electron microscopy of the submucosal collagen of the colon revealed that the fibrils become smaller and more compact with aging and these features were more pronounced in colons with diverticula (57). Elastic fibers in the muscular taenia have also been shown to change with aging (58). There is a 200% increase of elastin between normal appearing muscle cells causing shortening of taeniae, which is a significant contributing factor in the development

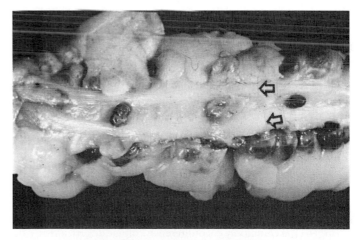

Figure 32.1   A colon at postmortem showing many diverticula along the wall between the antimesenteric taeniae *(arrows)* and mesenteric taenia, which is not seen because it lies on the other side of the colon and is covered by adipose tissue. The diverticula are dark in color, more prominently visible in the lower row, because of feces within. Only three diverticula are between the antimesenteric taeniae. The taeniae are prominent in this specimen because of increased thickness. Reproduced with permission from Fleischner FG, Ming SC, Henken EM. Revised concepts on diverticular disease of the colon. 1. Diverticulosis: emphasis on tissue derangement and its relation to the irritable colon syndrome. Radiology 1964;83:859–872.

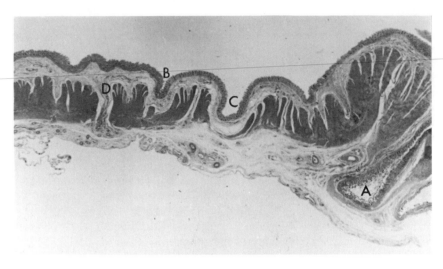

Figure 32.2 The colon was sectioned longitudinally. It shows a well developed diverticulum *(A)* in an area of thickened tunica muscularis. An artery runs alongside the diverticular wall. A beginning *(B)* and a partially developed diverticulum *(C)* burrow into tunica muscularis between the fascicles of circular muscle. No large blood vessels are seen in these areas. In another area *(D)*, penetrating vessels are present, but without diverticulum. The relationship between the site of diverticulum and vascular distribution is inconstant depending, in part, on the sampling of the tissue (×7).

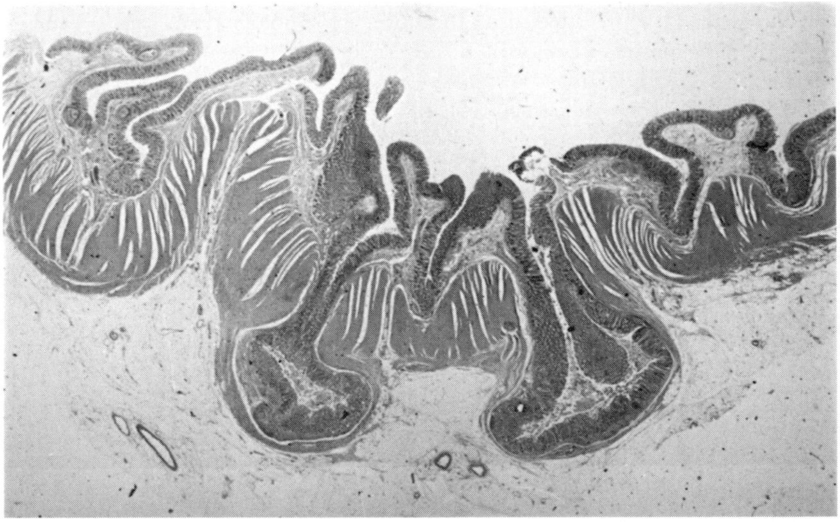

Figure 32.3 The longitudinal section of a resected colon showing two well developed diverticula and a beginning one *(right margin)*. The patient had a documented episode of perforation of a diverticulum 6 months earlier. The section shows only mild peridiverticular fibrosis. The mucosa in the diverticula are flask shaped. Their necks are narrow and surrounded by circular muscle. The colon was shortened and the mucosa was thrown into many redundant folds (×7). Reproduced with permission from Ming SC, Fleischner FG. Diverticulitis of the sigmoid colon: reappraisal of the pathology and pathogenesis. Surgery 1965;58: 627–633.

of colonic diverticula. There is also a decrease in the tensile strength and elasticity of colon wall with age (59).

ABNORMALITIES OF THE MUSCULAR LAYER

The radiologic observation of a deformed colon, particularly the sigmoid, variously described as a saw-tooth pattern (56), serrated pattern (60), contracted haustral pattern (60), and prediverticular shape (61), is commonly encountered in colonic diverticulosis. The last term was given since the abnormality was also seen in colons without diverticula, presumably a precursor of diverticulosis. These terms describe the shortened and distorted appearance of the sigmoid, with prominent saccules separated by thick folds of colonic wall (52). The cause of the deformity was thought to be inflammation and fibrosis. However, pathologic examination of surgically resected as well as postmortem specimens revealed that inflammation and fibrosis were absent or mild in many cases (52, 62). Instead, the deformity is caused by shortened longitudinal taeniae which become thick and hard with a cartilage-like consistency. Shortening of the taeniae causes the sigmoid colon to take a concertina-like appearance with bunched-up folds made of redundant mucosa and circular muscle layer (Figs. 32.4 and 32.5). The folds narrow the lumen, causing obstruction in some cases and subsequent dilatation of colon proximal to it. Removal of the shortened taeniae restores the colon to the normal length and contour (52). It was in these taeniae that Whitney and Morson found elastosis (58). Elastosis is the probable cause of muscle shortening, not spasm, as suggested by the contracted appearance of the muscle, since the muscle changes are not related to the motility of the colon (59).

The circular muscle is divided into small bands, the fasciculi (52, 62), between which the penetrating blood vessels reside (Fig. 32.2). It is not as markedly affected as the longitudinal taeniae. In the markedly contracted colon, the circular muscle is thickened, but the individual fibers do not appear hypertrophic.

The contracted state of the colon and the shortened taeniae suggest that the colon is in a state of spasm. The abdominal pain and constipation experienced by patients with spastic colon or irritable bowel syndrome are also major complaints of patients with colonic diverticular disease. It was therefore postulated that spastic colon was related to diverticulosis (52). The development of colonic diverticulosis in two infants with total colonic aganglionosis has been explained on the basis of spasm (63). Muscle relaxants may alleviate the symptoms in patients with diverticula (64). Recent studies, however, indicate that irritable bowel syndrome and diverticular disease may not be related (65, 66), since they show different frequency of myoelectric activity. Clinically, patients with diverticular disease usually are old and have a short history of symptoms, whereas patients with irritable bowel syndrome are young and usually have a long history of symptoms. The intraluminal pressure is increased in diverticular disease but not in irritable bowel syndrome (67).

INTRALUMINAL PRESSURE

The intraluminal pressure has been found to be increased in the sigmoid colon with diverticula (68, 69). The pressure recordings from adjacent areas of the colon show that the waves are independent of each other, implying that the pressure generated in one area does not always transmit to the adjacent areas (70). Painter et al. showed that in diverticulosis there was increased segmentation of colonic activity (71). The segmented colon was seen as a series of "little bladders" with obstruction at both ends by the contracting rings. The increased pressure generated by muscular contraction within the segment forced herniation of mucosa through the wall to form a diverticulum (1). This sequence of events implies the muscle contraction as the cause of both segmentation and mucosal herniation. Subsequent studies by others, however, showed no relation between increased motility and diverticulosis, although the high pressure activity was related to the colicky pain experienced by patients with diverticular disease (72). Furthermore, patients with asymptomatic diverticulosis have normal motility activity in the colon (73).

DIETARY FIBER

Epidemiologic data suggest that colonic diverticulosis is related to deficient fiber consumption (1). A four year follow-up study

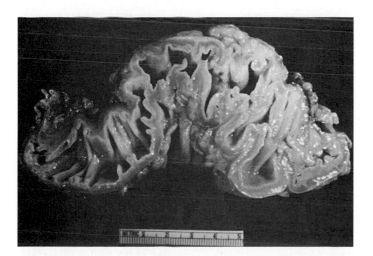

Figure 32.4   The longitudinal cut surface of a markedly contracted sigmoid colon, resected because of obstruction. The colon is markedly contracted and the lumen is narrowed by folds of thick muscle and redundant mucosa. A few diverticula (not shown) were present. Reproduced with permission from Ming SC, Fleischner FG. Diverticulitis of the sigmoid colon: reappraisal of the pathology and pathogenesis. Surgery 1965;58:627–633.

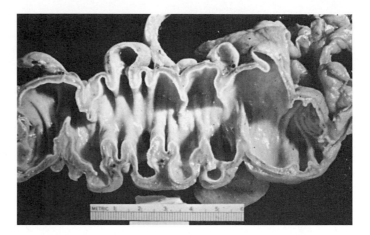

Figure 32.5   The longitudinally hemisectioned postmortem colon was fixed in a distended state by perfusing the lumen with formalin. Diverticula are present in the corrugated segment.

revealed that low dietary fiber, primarily fruit and vegetable fibers, increased the incidence of symptomatic diverticular disease as compared to a high fiber diet, and that a high fat and red meat diet augments the effects of fibers (74). Painter and Burkitt (75) postulated that a fiber-rich diet would increase the volume of feces, therefore the diameter of the colon. A wider colon would have lower pressure and less segmentation than a narrower colon, hence less diverticulosis. The low incidence of colonic diverticula in the Africans was also related to the observation that the food residue stayed in the African's gut for a shorter period allowing less time for absorption of water than the Westerner's. Therefore, the feces in the latter was drier and generated higher intraluminal pressure, thereby favoring the development of diverticula. This hypothesis was supported by the observation of Gear (76) that diverticulosis was three times more frequent in nonvegetarians than vegetarians. However, a recent report from India showed that most patients with colonic diverticulosis in India were vegetarians (50). Furthermore, Eastwood et al. (77) found no difference in the stool weight, transit time, and intraluminal pressure between individuals with and without diverticulosis.

Supplementary bran fiber absorbs water and increases the volume and moisture of the stool, thus reducing the intraluminal pressure. It has been used to treat diverticular disease. Hyland (78) treated 75 patients with acute complications of diverticular disease with high fiber diet, and 90% of them remained symptom free for a period of 5 to 7 years.

OTHER FACTORS

Genetic influence has been implicated in a report of severe sigmoid diverticulitis in a pair of identical twins in their third decade of life (79), and in another report on colonic diverticula in three siblings in Nigeria where the incidence of the disease is low (80). These occurrences, however, are very rare.

Flynn et al. reported the possible effect of fecal bile acid (81). Both fecal lithocholic and deoxycholic acids were lower in patients with colonic diverticula than in controls. Significant positive correlation was found between lithocholic acid concentration and 12 to 18 cycles per minute myoelectric activity, and between deoxycholic acid concentration and 9 cycles per minute activity. It was suggested that in diverticulosis there was increased absorption of bile acids causing alteration of myoelectric activity.

In summary, the formation of colonic diverticula follows the following sequence of events: biophysical alterations in the colonic wall of the aged person results in a reduction of tensile strength of the tissue and contraction and shortening of taeniae, particularly in the sigmoid. These changes in turn cause exaggerated haustration and redundant mucosal folds narrowing the lumen. A low-fiber diet produces small dry fecal mass and generates an increase in intraluminal pressure. Elevated pressure in a narrowed segment of the colon forces herniation of mucosa through the weak point of the colonic wall to form diverticula.

PATHOLOGY OF DIVERTICULAR DISEASE OF THE COLON

The etiologic factors discussed above contribute significantly to the morphologic appearance of diverticula of the colon, as well as to the clinical presentation and the natural course of the disease.

HANDLING OF GROSS SPECIMENS

The colon may be fixed in formalin before opening. In order to keep the diverticula distended, the colon should be filled with formalin under slight pressure and then immersed in a pail of formalin overnight. This treatment is suitable for a postmortem colon or a resected specimen which is not deformed by muscle abnormality or inflammatory process. Fixation will harden the tissue and make it difficult to identify all the diverticula and to pin-point the bleeding or perforated lesion. For such purposes it is better to examine the fresh specimen in detail, identify the diverticula by probing, fill them with cotton balls to maintain the shape, and mark the diseased foci. Only then fix the specimen in formalin for later sectioning for microscopic examination.

GROSS FEATURES OF DIVERTICULOSIS

The diverticula appear as dark green or brown, round or oval nodules of 0.5 to 1 cm in diameter, arranged in a longitudinal row along the lateral borders of the mesenteric taenia (Fig. 32.1). The color is that of the feces showing through the thin wall of the diverticula. If the diverticulum is empty and collapsed, it will not be readily recognized on external examination of the bowel. Viewed from the mucosal aspect, the openings of diverticula are depressed dimples, 3 to 5 mm in diameter, from which fecal materials can be pressed out. The presence of diverticula can be confirmed by probing. Occasionally, the diverticulum inverts back into the lumen of the colon and appears as a wrinkled polyp. It can be pushed back into its seat. In cases of suspected bleeding from a diverticulum, it is important to probe each diverticulum for the presence of blood in order to identify the source of bleeding. An angiograph may help to localize the bleeding vessel.

The gross features may be modified by the status of tunica muscularis, the number of diverticula, and the amount of pericolic adipose tissue. Prominent mucosal folds in a shortened, accordion-like colon, caused by either contraction of the taeniae or the presence of numerous diverticula, may obscure the openings of diverticula. In this situation, removal of the mucosa will expose the openings and greatly facilitate the localization of diverticula (Fig. 32.6). Externally, an excessive amount of mesocolic fat may cover up the diverticula. It is not unusual that the fat-covered diverticula may appear as appendices epiploicae.

HISTOLOGIC FEATURES OF DIVERTICULOSIS

The vast majority of diverticula of the colon are pseudodiverticula. They are shaped like a flask. The neck is surrounded by circular muscle, and the wall consists of mucosa, muscularis mucosae, submucosa, and, in some cases, a thin layer of longitudinal muscle (Figs. 32.3 and 32.7). The mucosa may appear normal or thinner than normal. The mucosa around the ostia of diverticula may show increased infiltration of lymphocytes and plasma cells (82). At or near the apex of diverticulum, lymphoid nodules are often present. The lumen usually contains amorphous fecal material. The muscularis mucosae is thinner than that of the adjacent colon. When muscularis propria does not cover the apex, the submucosa of the diverticulum merges with the subserosal or mesocolic adipose tissue, within which small and medium sized blood vessels may be present. Occasionally, the diverticulum penetrates partially into the circular muscle layer, compressing on the outer muscle fibers (Fig. 32.2). Such early diverticulum probably corresponds to the transient diverticulum seen radiologically in 4.1% of patients with diverticula (83).

CLASSIFICATION OF DIVERTICULAR DISEASES OF THE COLON

Based on the gross and microscopic findings, the diverticular disease of the colon can be classified as listed in Table 32.2. The specific pathologic characteristics of each category are described below.

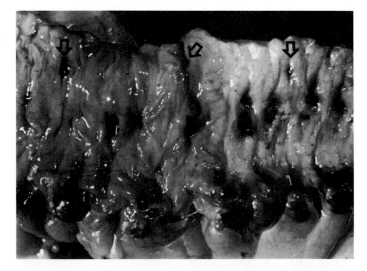

Figure 32.6 The luminal aspect of the colon shown in Fig. 32.1. The colon was opened just above the lower row of diverticula shown in Fig. 32.1. The upper row of diverticula is now in the middle of the colon and the openings of three diverticula between the antimesenteric taeniae in the upper row *(arrows).* The redundant mucosa was stripped off. The openings of diverticula with fecal materials within are clearly shown.

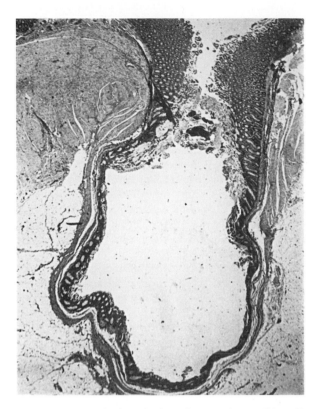

Figure 32.7 A simple diverticulum shows a thin wall lined by an atrophic mucosa, partial muscularis mucosae, and a thin layer of longitudinal muscle (×21).

PREDIVERTICULAR STATE

The colon in a prediverticular state is marked by the prominent muscle abnormalities described above, but without diverticula (68). The disease affects principally the sigmoid colon. Externally the involved segment appears narrow, thickened, and shortened, with the taeniae thick and rigid. Between the taeniae the colon wall shows sacculation, with bulging segments alternating with circular depressions. On opening of the lumen, the depressions correspond to bunched up muscle forming circular folds separating the contracted haustral sacs (Fig. 32.4). When the thick taeniae are trimmed off, the colon segment can be lengthened and the sacculation disappears. This state is, therefore, created by the contraction of taeniae coli. The circular muscle is thickened only at a later stage. It is in this corrugated segment of colon that there is an increased intraluminal pressure resulting in the development of diverticula in the contracted haustral sacs. This sequence of events has been demonstrated by follow-up radiologic examinations through many years (52, 68). The chronology of these changes depicts the contracted colon as a prediverticular state.

SIMPLE DIVERTICULOSIS

In this condition, simple diverticula, described above in the section on histologic features, are scattered along a colon of normal caliber and contour (Fig. 32.8). The haustra are regularly spaced and have a smooth mucosal surface. The taeniae and circular muscle are normal.

SIMPLE MASSED DIVERTICULOSIS

This term is applied by Fleischner et al. (52) to the colon with numerous simple diverticula. It involves primarily the left colon. The colon is shortened because a large portion of the mucosa is consumed by diverticula. The colonic wall is wrinkled and shrunk. The resultant folds are close to each other and uniform in appearance. The taeniae and circular muscle are normal.

DIVERTICULOSIS WITH MUSCLE ABNORMALITY (SPASTIC COLON DIVERTICULOSIS)

In this condition the thickened and shortened taeniae cause the colon to assume the shape of a concertina and force the develop-

TABLE 32.2	Pathologic Classification of Colonic Diverticular Disease

I. Prediverticular state
    Elastosis of muscularis with contraction and shortening of taeniae
    Mainly sigmoid involvement
II. Simple diverticulosis
    Multiple pseudodiverticula without muscle abnormality
    Random location; all colon involvement possible
III. Simple massed diverticulosis
    Numerous pseudodiverticula without muscle abnormality
    Diffuse distribution with shortening of colon
IV. Diverticulosis with muscle abnormality (spastic colon diverticulosis)
    Contracted and thick taeniae coli
    Exaggerated haustral sacculation with redundant mucosal folds
    Thick colon wall and narrow lumen
    Many or few pseudodiverticula
    Prominent sigmoid involvement
V. Giant diverticulum
VI. Diverticulitis
    A. Uncomplicated diverticulitis
    B. Complicated diverticulitis

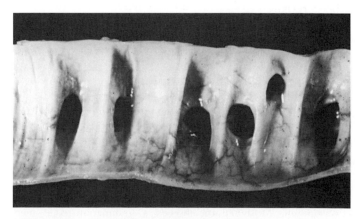

Figure 32.8 The hemisectioned strip of a colon with simple diverticulosis showing openings of diverticula in the haustral sacs. The wall of the colon is not thickened or deformed.

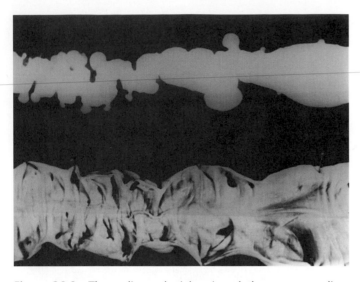

Figure 32.9 The radiograph *(above)* and the corresponding segment of a postmortem colon *(below)* showing diverticula in the narrowed and corrugated area, but not in the smooth area at right.

ment of diverticulum at the weak points of the muscular coat of the colon. The significance of muscle abnormality was emphasized also by Morson (62). We were so impressed by the contracted taeniae in sigmoid diverticulosis that the condition was termed spastic colon diverticulosis implying a relationship with the spastic colon syndrome (52). Although this relationship appears uncertain in view of different clinical and myoelectric features between them, as discussed in the section on Pathogenesis, the contracted state of the colon remains a significant factor in the development of this type of diverticulosis. The diverticula occur in the corrugated segment, usually close to the lateral borders of the thickened mesenteric taenia (Figs. 32.9 to 32.11). The thickness of circular muscle is variable, shown best in the longitudinal section (Fig. 32.12). This type of diverticulosis is limited to the left colon, particularly the sigmoid which is normally narrower and has thicker muscular tissue than the right colon. The effects of volume and consistency of the feces as related to dietary fiber intake are probably strongest in this region.

GIANT DIVERTICULUM

Giant diverticula are large sacs measuring 6 to 27 cm in diameter (84). Radiologically, they appear as persistent radiolucent "balloons" (85) or air filled cysts (86). In spite of their size, they are often missed in the initial radiologic examination (87). Fifty-two cases had been reported up to 1984 (88), occurring mostly in the sigmoid, and occasionally in the transverse, colon (89). McNutt et al. (90) described three types: (1) gradually enlarged pseudodiverticulum which contained muscularis mucosae in the wall, but the mucosal lining was usually replaced by granulation tissue; (2) focal perforation of diverticulum leading to abscess formation with intermittent communication with the colon lumen resulting in a large pseudocyst filled with gas from the infection; and (3) a true diverticulum. Most reports showed a granulation-tissue–lined cavity which can be an infected diverticulum or a pseudocyst. Communication with colonic lumen is present in 60% of cases (90).

The lesion may perforate into the peritoneal cavity (90). In one case carcinoma was found in the diverticulum (91).

DIVERTICULITIS AND COMPLICATIONS

Diverticulosis becomes a clinical entity when one or more diverticula are inflamed or the patient suffers abdominal pain, changes of bowel habits, or symptoms and signs of intra-abdominal infection. These symptoms occur in about 4 to 5% of all patients with diverticulosis. Diverticulitis develops in 10 to 20% of persons with diagnosed diverticulosis (84, 92), more frequently in patients under 40 years of age (93). Twenty-five to 50% of the patients are hospitalized and 15 to 30% of the hospitalized patients are operated on (94). Not all of the operated patients have pathologically confirmed diverticulitis, however. In our own materials, 26% of surgical specimens resected for diverticulitis showed no inflammation but muscular distortion, 8% of specimens had localized inflammation limited to the diverticular wall, and 66% of specimens had severe peridiverticulitis, secondary to focal perforation of the diverticula (95).

Pure acute diverticulitis, with inflammation limited to the diverticular wall (Fig. 32.13) is uncommon in the resected specimens. It was found usually at or near the apex of a diverticulum. The involved area is small, only a few millimeters in size. The mucosa is destroyed and replaced by acute inflammatory exudate. The muscularis mucosa is similarly affected. In some cases, the inflammation involves the submucosa and adjacent peridiverticular tissue. In three of seven such cases, there was erosion and rupture of small arteries in the involved submucosa, resulting in massive rectal bleeding requiring surgical resection of the colon (95). The bleeding vessel was found only after every diverticulum in the specimen was examined microscopically.

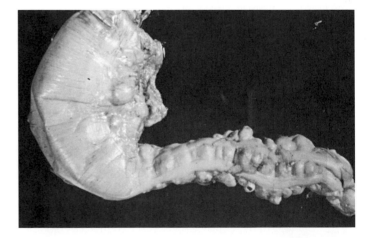

Figure 32.10 Many diverticula in the narrowed portion of the colon at right where the taeniae are thickened and the intervening colonic wall is contracted. There are many circular depressions corresponding to invaginating circular folds. The segment proximal to it is dilated and the taeniae are inconspicuous. Reproduced with permission from Fleischner FG, Ming SC, Henken EM. Revised concepts on diverticular disease of the colon. 1. Diverticulosis: emphasis on tissue derangement and its relation to the irritable colon syndrome. Radiology 1964;83:859–872.

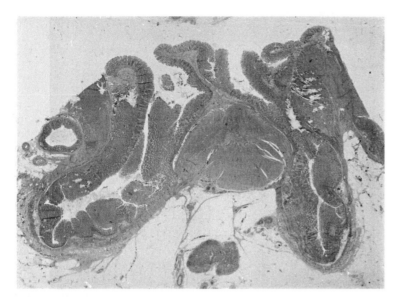

Figure 32.11   The cross section of a contracted segment of colon showing two well-formed diverticula, separated by the thickened antimesenteric taenia. Redundant mucosal folds project into the lumen (×7).

Minute foci of acute diverticulitis are probably quite common, but seldom documented, because they are not grossly visible and they may not cause symptoms. These small lesions may be readily healed, leaving no trace of inflammation or only slight fibrosis in the peridiverticular region, which is commonly seen in the surgical specimens.

Clinically manifest diverticulitis is in fact no longer pure diverticulitis, but complications of focal perforation (Fig. 32.14) resulting in severe pericolitis (Fig. 32.15), pericolic (Fig. 32.16) or pelvic abscess, fistula formation involving pelvic organs, or free perforation to the peritoneum causing purulent or fecal peritonitis (72, 95, 96). Histologic evidence of perforation of the diverticulum includes foreign body granulomas containing food particles, fecal matter, or barium sulfate crystals (Fig. 32.17). Such stigmas of perforation were present in 60% of resected specimens (95). Radiologic evidence of perforation, such as extravasation of barium sulfate and free air in the peritoneal cavity, are readily demonstrated in the acute cases (96). Occasionally, two or more diverticula are perforated giving rise to the formation of intercommunicating or dissecting abscesses along the pericolic tissue (96) and double tracking of barium in radiologic examination (97). A small perforation may heal, leaving a defect in the diverticular wall accompanied by peridiverticular inflammation (Fig. 32.18).

Marked pericolitis and abscess formation create an indurated mass (Figs. 32.14 and 32.15) which may compress and obstruct the bowel. Obstruction is encountered in 5 to 10% of complicated diverticula. The thickened wall may be erroneously interpreted as neoplastic. The accuracy of radiologic differentiation between diverticular mass and carcinoma is only 50%, while the accuracy of diagnosing diverticula is 92% (98).

The abscesses may rupture into other organs or the peritoneal cavity, producing fistula tracts involving other organs in 2.4% to 20% of cases (99, 100). Among these cases colovesical fistula is most frequent, in 65% of patients, colovaginal fistula in 25%, coloenteric fistula in 6.5%, colouterine fistula in 3%, and colocutaneous fistula in 1% (99). In one report, 35.6% of patients with diverticular disease had urinary tract symptoms and 3.6% of patients had colovesical fistula (101). These patients may have pneumaturia (102). Uncommon sites of fistula formation include the hip joint (103, 104),

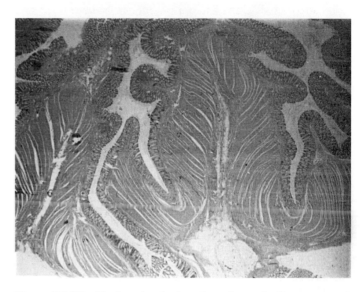

Figure 32.12   The longitudinal section of a markedly contracted sigmoid colon showing thick circular muscle, prominent mucosal folds, and three diverticula (×21).

perineum, scrotum, buttock, thigh, lower extremity, mediastinum, neck (103, 105–107), fallopian tube (108), and ureter (109). Sigmoid-appendiceal fistula have also been reported (110, 111).

Free perforation is also common. Among 105 patients with diverticular sepsis operated on by Lambert et al. (112), 73 had free peritonitis, 40 with communicating perforation and 33 with non-communicating perforation. Intestinal obstruction was present in 9 patients and localized abscess or mass in 23 patients. In another report, 32 of 93 operated patients had free perforation, obstruction in 14 and abscess in 11 (113). The mortality rate within 30 days was 10.8%. Rarely, a fistula perforates into portal veins, causing pneumopylephlebitis, thrombopylephlebitis, and liver abscess (114–117). Septic phlebitis of the inferior mesenteric vein was also reported (118). Patients on steroid therapy for other diseases may develop perforation of colonic diverticula (119, 120).

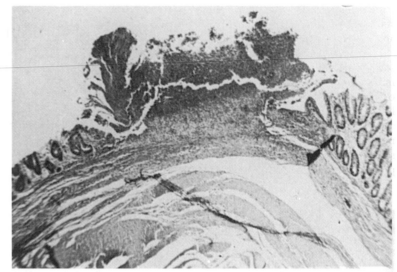

Figure 32.13 Acute diverticulitis with necrosis and inflammation involving the mucosa, muscularis mucosae, and adjacent submucosa (×35). Reproduced with permission from Ming SC, Fleischner FG. Diverticulitis of the sigmoid colon: reappraisal of the pathology and pathogenesis. Surgery 1965;58:627–633.

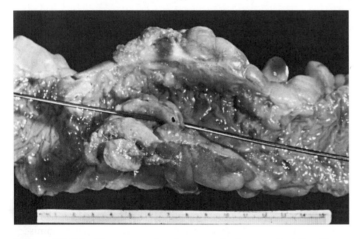

Figure 32.14 The opened colon, surgically resected for diverticulitis, showing a perforated diverticulum (with the probe through it) and a pericolic inflammatory mass compressing on the lumen.

Hinchey et al. (121) classified the perforated diverticulitis cases into 4 stages. A modified staging, including other inflammatory conditions, is listed in Table 32.3.

DIVERTICULA OF THE RIGHT COLON AND CECUM

The above accounts deal primarily with diverticula disease of the left colon, particularly the sigmoid. The diverticula of the right colon are different in several aspects.

1. Geographic Distribution: In Western countries colonic diverticula are found most frequently in the sigmoid (122). The right colon and cecum was involved in only 1 to 5% of cases (123). In Asians, diverticula occur more frequently in the right colon (46, 48, 50). Of 979 cases of colonic diverticulosis reported by Kubo (45), 76% were in the right colon.

2. Type of Diverticula: Diverticula of the left colon are nearly all of the false type, while those in the right colon may be true or false. The false diverticula of the right colon resemble those of the left colon, being multiple and associated with high intraluminal pressure and abnormal motility (124). They are accompanied by diverticula in the distal colon. The true diverticula are usually single or few, and located mostly in the cecum. The relative proportion of true diverticula varied in different reports. In one report, 90% of diverticula were of true type (125), but in another report, only 2 of 16 diverticula were true (126).

3. Age of the Patients: Diverticula of the colon in general increase in frequency with age. The average age of patients was 63 years (127). The average age of patients with diverticula of right colon was under 40 years (125, 128).

Cecal diverticulitis is rare, estimated to constitute only 0.1% of all diverticular disease cases (129). The congenital diverticulum is usually located on the anterior wall of the cecum close to the ileocecal valve (100). Acute cecal diverticulitis is misdiagnosed as acute appendicitis in the majority of cases (125, 128, 130). The inflammatory mass may also be mistaken as a malignant tumor (131, 132), even at operation. Free perforation occurs only rarely (133). The diverticulitis may be complicated by acute pylephlebitis and liver abscesses (134).

CLINICOPATHOLOGIC CORRELATION

CLINICAL FEATURES

Diverticular disease of the colon is a disease of the aged, with its incidence increasing progressively with age. According to Parks (94), two-thirds of patients at age 85 had diverticula by barium enema examination. Similar findings were noted by Rodkey and Welch (127). Among patients with colonic diverticula, only 0.6% were under the age of 30 and 4.8% under the age of 40 (94). These observations coincide with the age related decline in tensile strength and elasticity of colonic wall (59) and changes in the muscle of the colon (58). There is an equal sex distribution. Some reports showing a slightly higher incidence of diverticular disease in females are unexplained (94).

Symptoms of abdominal pain, and radiologic and sigmoidoscopic appearance of a narrowed and deformed colon segment could indicate either the prediverticular state with muscle abnormalities or pericolic inflammation. Pure diverticulitis with inflammation limited to the diverticular wall may be common, but is largely asymptomatic. Computerized tomography (CT) gives better diagnostic results than contrast enema for the extent of inflammatory sequelae and extracolic abnormalities (135, 136). Sonography provides an additional diagnostic advantage in selected cases (137).

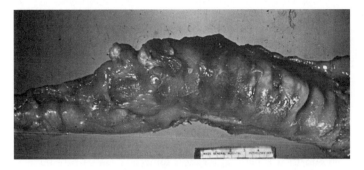

Figure 32.15 The external view of a surgical specimen showing markedly thickened pericolic tissue due to severe inflammation.

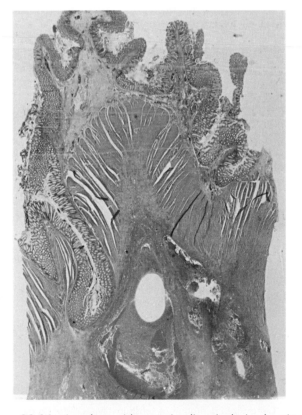

Figure 32.16 A colon with spastic diverticulosis showing a pericolic abscess with gas bubbles (empty spaces) secondary to perforation of a diverticulum (×10).

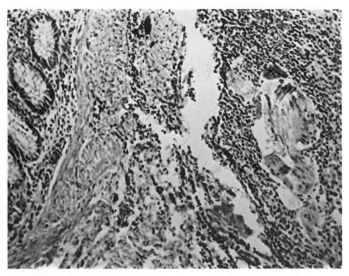

Figure 32.17 A colonic diverticulum showing severe chronic inflammation and a foreign body granuloma containing vegetable fibers (×150).

Diverticular disease of the colon may develop serious complications requiring surgical intervention. Orebaugh (138) reported that recurrent diverticulitis was the most common indication for operation, in 35% of cases, hemorrhage in 25%, perforation in 22%, suspicion of carcinoma in 17%, obstruction in 16%, and fistula in 10%. These add up to more than 100% because of the presence of more than one complication in 25% of cases. In a report by Alexander et al. (139), 14% of 673 patients with diverticular disease had operations. Of 93 operated cases, the indications for operation were abscess in 35, bleeding in 18, perforation in 10, obstruction in 10, fistula in 5, recurrent symptoms in 7, and suspicion of cancer in 8. The problem is particularly grave in immunocompromised patients, who respond poorly to medical treatment and usually require operation (140). Patients younger than 50 years developed more severe complications but were operated on less frequently than older patients (93, 141–143).

Some patients developed extraintestinal manifestations. There have been reports of patients with arthritis and pyoderma gangrenosum which resolved after resection of the involved colon (144, 145). One patient developed retroperitoneal fibrosis (146).

COMPLICATED DIVERTICULITIS WITH PERFORATION

Limited diverticulitis becomes critical when it is complicated by perforation, pericolic abscess, and fistulous tract formation involving other organs. For proper management of patients suffering from these complications, the staging system by Hinchey et al. (121), which categorizes patients according to the extent of extracolic infection has been useful. A modified staging system is listed in Table 32.3. Of 116 patients treated by Auguste et al. (147) 21% were in Stage 1, 35% in Stage 2, 35% in Stage 3, and 9% in Stage 4. Primary resection with anastomosis is preferred for limited diverticulitis, but a two or three stage operation may be necessary for advanced Stage diseases (148). The primary resection has lower mortality, shorter hospital stay, and shorter disability duration than

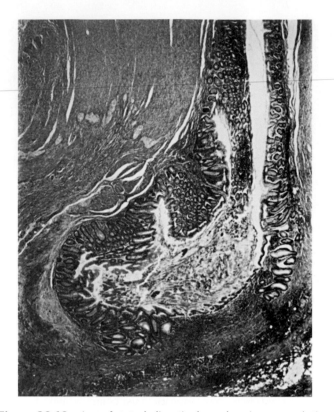

Figure 32.18 A perforated diverticulum showing granulation tissue and regenerating surface epithelium at the site of perforation and severe chronic pericolitis (×30). Reproduced with permission from Ming SC, Fleischner FG. Diverticulitis of the sigmoid colon: reappraisal of the pathology and pathogenesis. Surgery 1965;58:627–633.

the staged resection (147). A recurrence of diverticulitis had been reported in 30 to 40% of patients (94). There have been improvements in the results of surgical management of septic complications of diverticulitis in recent years in spite of the increased number of risk patients (149). For Stage 1 diverticulitis, laparoscopic resection has been shown to be beneficial (150).

HEMORRHAGE

Rectal hemorrhage occurs in 10 to 30% of patients with diverticular disease, severely in 3 to 5% (84). The bleeding stops spontaneously in 80% of cases, but recurs in 20 to 25% of cases. It had been stated that the source of bleeding was in the right colon in up to 70% of cases (84, 151), "even if diverticula are seen only in the sigmoid colon" (151). This view is clearly exaggerated, since this incidence equals or exceeds the incidence of right-sided colonic diverticula. The diverticula are found more often in the right than left colon in Japan. Bleeding occurred in only 3.9% of 1124 Japanese patients reported on by Kubo et al. (152), mostly in old patients with multiple diverticula in the left colon.

Another frequently stated belief, that most of the bleeding diverticulum is not inflamed, also requires qualification. Minor bleeding from granulation tissue is common in diverticulitis. Massive bleeding, on the other hand, is the result of erosion of an artery. Such a thick walled vessel will not bleed without injury. The damaged artery is difficult to identify because it is usually not accompanied by overt, grossly evident inflammation to mark its location. It may be found only after meticulous search in the pathologic specimen. When it is found, it is in an area of active inflammation (Fig. 32.19). In our materials, the bleeding artery was identified in three resected colons only when every diverticulum was subjected to microscopic examination (95). Meyers (153) noted the consistent finding of arterial changes in the diverticula, including eccentric intimal thickening, thinning of media, and duplication of internal elastic lamina. These changes are commonly seen in an area of chronic inflammation. They are nonspecific, but indicate past or continuing tissue injury. These arteries are not the source of bleeding in most instances.

Tedesco (154) noted that 20% of distal intestinal bleeding occurred in patients with diverticular disease, but in 40% of these patients, the bleeding source was other than the diverticulum. In the left colon, polyps, neoplasms, and other inflammatory conditions may coexist with diverticula and be the source of bleeding. In the right colon, angiodysplasia (also called arteriovenous malformation and vascular ectasia) is a recognized major source of colonic bleeding in older persons (155–157). This condition is discussed in Chapter 14. The abnormal vessels are mostly dilated veins and capillaries located primarily in the submucosa and, in some cases, also in the mucosa. These vessels bleed easily because the walls are thin and their superficial location subjects them to easy trauma. Compression by the tunica muscularis on the veins has been postulated as a possible cause of this condition in the colon (155). They often coexist with diverticula (158, 159). In some cases it may be difficult to determine the source of bleeding between these two conditions. If bleeding recurs in such a patient, an elective right hemicolectomy has been suggested (159).

The location of a bleeding vessel in diverticular disease can be identified by angiography and radionuclide scintigraphy (84). These techniques make it possible to surgically resect only the involved segment of colon. They also help the pathologist to limit the search for the responsible vessel to a likely area.

OBSTRUCTION

Obstruction in diverticular disease of the colon can be due to muscle thickening and mucosal folds in the prediverticular state and uncomplicated diverticulosis. In diverticulitis, a large inflammatory mass, often with abscess within, may compressed on the lumen,

TABLE	
32.3	**Pathologic Stages of Colonic Diverticulitis According to the Extent of Inflammation**

Stage 0: Diverticulitis confined to diverticular wall
Stage 1: Localized pericolitis and pericolic abscess confined to peridiverticular tissue
Stage 2: Perforated diverticulitis with abscess and fistula involving contiguous organs or tissues
Stage 3: Generalized peritonitis or sepsis involving distant organs
Stage 4: Fecal peritonitis

Modified from Hinchey EJ, et al. Adv Surg 1978;12:85.

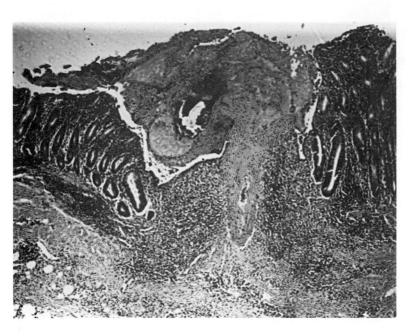

Figure 32.19 A bleeding diverticulum showing a thrombus covering a partially necrotic artery in an area of severe inflammation (×70).

sometimes circumferentially (96). Obstruction is noted in about 10% of cases (138, 139). It is an important indication for surgical intervention, partly because an obstructive lesion may mimic carcinoma.

COEXISTING COLONIC CONDITIONS

CARCINOMA

There is no evidence that diverticular disease predisposes the colon to malignant transformation. However, the development of colonic carcinoma is related to dietary fiber deficiency (see Chapter 34 for details) as is the development of diverticular disease of the colon. It may be expected, therefore, that there will be an increased incidence of one condition when the other is present. In fact, the incidences of carcinoma in colons with diverticula and vice versa are the same as in the control population: about 6 to 10% by colonoscopy in the former situation (160–162) and 39% by barium enema in the latter situation (163). The incidence of adenoma in the colon with diverticulosis was 27%, the same as the controls in one report (161) and twice more than the controls in another report (160). However, rare cases of carcinoma developing in a diverticulum have been reported (163–165). In one case, a mucinous carcinoid was found in a rectosigmoid diverticulum (166). The carcinoma may invade a coexisting diverticulum (95). More importantly, it is often difficult to differentiate an inflammatory mass from a carcinoma, even during operation. In this situation, perioperative fine needle aspiration biopsy has been found helpful (167).

INFLAMMATORY BOWEL DISEASES

Ulcerative colitis has a bimodal mode of development. The old age group may have coexisting diverticula, although these occurrences are uncommon. Jalan (168) found 23 such cases in 399 ulcerative colitis patients. The typical mucosal lesions of ulcerative colitis is readily recognized. Crohn's disease of colon is more commonly associated with diverticular disease (100). It is more difficult to differentiate them radiologically because both conditions are seg-

mental, have thickened colon wall and pericolic inflammation, and may have fistula. Marshak (169) outlined the major radiologic differences between them, which are applicable also to pathologic examination. Mainly, the diverticular disease involves a shorter segment, has shorter fistulous tract, and a more localized lesion than similar changes in Crohn's disease. Anal lesions, commonly seen in Crohn's disease, are absent in diverticular disease.

ISCHEMIC COLON DISEASE

The ischemic changes of the colon are characterized by coagulative necrosis of the mucosa and marked submucosal edema in the acute phase and cicatrical stricture in the chronic cases (see Chapter 14 for details). The splenic flexure of the colon is the favored site for ischemic changes. These lesions may superimpose on the diverticular disease.

ASSOCIATED EXTRACOLIC CONDITIONS

The patients with diverticular disease of the colon may have an increased incidence of other conditions. Saint's triad of colonic diverticulosis, hiatus hernia, and gallstones has been periodically reported. Burkitt and Walker considered the triad to be manifestations of fiber deficiency (170). Scaggion et al. (171) found 7 cases among 684 patients by barium examination. Eighty-six additional patients had two of the triad. In another report cholelithiasis was present in 45% of patients with, and in 22% of patients without, colonic diverticula (172). Other reported conditions, in addition to those mentioned in the section on Etiology, included polycystic disease of the kidney (173), ischemic heart disease (174), intra-abdominal panniculitis (175), and varicose veins (176). There were also reports of diverticulitis developing in patients in chronic renal failure (177), following cardiac or other surgical procedures (178, 179), in immunosuppressed heart transplant recipients, and patients on high dose cortisone treatment (180). Complicated diverticular disease is reportedly an important cause of death in rheumatoid arthritis patients (181).

REFERENCES

1. Painter NS, Burkitt DP. Diverticular disease of the colon: a deficiency disease of Western civilization. Br Med J 1971;2:450–454.
2. Wheeler D. Diverticula of foregut. Radiology 1947;49:476–482.
3. Lahey FH. Pharyngoesophageal diverticulum. Its management and complications. Ann Surg 1946;134:617–652.
4. Gage-Whote L. Incidence of Zenker's diverticulum with hiatus hernia. Laryngoscope 1988;98:526–530.
5. Rasmussen PC, Jensen BS, Winther A. Oesophageal achalasia combined with epiphrenic diverticulum. A case report. Scand J Thorac Cardiovas Surg 1988;22:81–82.
6. Toyohara T, Kaneko T, Araki H, et al. Giant epiphrenic diverticulum in a boy with Ehlers-Danlos syndrome. Ped Radiol 1989;19:437.
7. Hendren WG, Anderson T, Miller JI. Massive bleeding in a Zenker's diverticulum. South Med J 1990;83:362.
8. Zitsch RP, O'Brien CJ, Maddox WA. Pharyngoesophageal diverticulum complicated by squamous cell carcinoma. Head Neck Surg 1987;9:290–294.
9. Watarai N, Kataoka M, Taniwaki S, Masaoka A. A rare type of intramural esophageal diverticulosis. Am J Gastroenterol 1990;85:733–736.
10. Umlas J, Sakhuja R. The pathology of esophageal intramural pseudodiverticulosis. Am J Clin Pathol 1976;65:314–320.
11. Medeiros LJ, Doos WG, Balogh K. Esophageal intramural pseudodiverticulosis: a report of two cases with analysis of similar, less extensive changes in "normal" autopsy esophagi. Hum Pathol 1988;19:928–931.
12. Eells RW, Simril WA. Gastric diverticula: Report of thirty-one cases. Am J Roentgenol 1952;68:8–14.
13. Eras P, Beranbaum SL. Gastric diverticula: Congenital and acquired. Am J Gastroenterol 1972;57:120–132.
14. Benhamou PH, Lenaerts C, Carnarelli JP, et al. Diverticulum of the stomach in children. Apropos of a case of congenital diverticulum. Ann Ped 1989;36:467–478.
15. Gibbons CP, Harvey L. An ulcerated gastric diverticulum—A rare cause of haematemesis and melaena. Postgrad Med J 1984;60:693–695.
16. Cockrell CH, Cho SR, Messmer JM, et al. Intramural gastric diverticula: a report of three cases. Brit J Radiol 1984;57:285–288.
17. Localio A, Stahl WM. Diverticular disease of the alimentary tract Part II: The esophagus, stomach, duodenum and small intestine. Curr Probl Surg 1968;5:1–47.
18. Mackey WC, Dineen P. A fifty year experience with Meckel's diverticulum. Surg Gynecol Obstet 1983;156:56–64.
19. Artigas V, Calabuig R, Badia F, et al. Meckel's diverticulum: value of ectopic tissue. Am J Surg 1986;151:631–634.
20. Spence LD, Moran V. Meckel's diverticulitis secondary to an enterolith. Eur J Radiol 1995;21:92–93.
21. Cullen JJ, Kelly KA, Moir CR, et al. Surgical management of Meckel's diverticulum. An epidemiologic, population-based study. Ann Surg 1994;220:564–568.
22. Moyana TN. Carcinoid tumors arising from Meckel's diverticulum. A clinical, morphologic, and immunohistochemical study. Am J Clin Pathol 1989;91:52–56.
23. Niv Y, Abu-Avid S, Kopelman C, Oren M. Torsion of leiomyosarcoma of Meckel's diverticulum. Am J Gastroenterol 1986;81:228–291.
24. Bloch T, Tejada E, Brodhecker C. Malignant melanoma in Meckel's diverticulum. Am J Clin Pathol 1986;86:231–234.
25. Landor JH, Fulkerson CC. Duodenal diverticula. Arch Surg 1966;93:182–188.
26. Miyazaki S, Sakamoto T, Miyata M, et al. Function of the sphincter of Oddi in patients with juxtapapillary duodenal diverticula: evaluation by intraoperative biliary manometry under a duodenal pressure load. World J Surg 1995;19:307–312.
27. Nagakawa T, Kanno M, Ueno K, et al. Intrabiliary pressure measurement by duodenal pressure loading for the evaluation of duodenal parapapillary diverticulum. Hepatogastroenterology 1996;43:1129–1134.
28. Juler JL, List JW, Stemmer EA, Connolly JE. Duodenal diverticulitis. Arch Surg 1969;99:572–578.
29. Uomo G, Manes G, Ragozzino A, et al. Periampullary extraluminal duodenal diverticula and acute pancreatitis: an underestimated etiological association. Am J Gastroenterol 1996;91:1186–1188.
30. Chuang JH, Chan HM, Huang YS, et al. Enterolith ileus as a complication of duodenal diverticulosis—one case report and review of the literature. Kao Hsiung I Hsueh Ko Hsueh Tsa Chih 1993;9:488–493.
31. Abdel-Hafiz AA, Birkett DH, Ahmed MS. Congenital duodenal diverticula: a report of three cases and a review of the literature. Surgery 1988;104:74–78.
32. Soreide JA, Seime S, Soreide O. Intraluminal duodenal diverticulum: case report and update of the literature 1975–1986. Am J Gastroenterol 1988;83:988–991.
33. Adams DB. Management of the intraluminal duodenal diverticulum: endoscopy or duodenotomy? Am J Surg 1986;151:524–526.
34. Graupe F, Rassek D, Schwenk W, Stock W. Divertikulitis des Jejunums als seltene Ursache für eine akute gastrointestinale Blutung—Diagnostik und Therapie. Leber Magen Darm 1995;25:279–281.
35. Albu E, Parikh V, Alankar S, Gerst PH. Perforated solitary jejunal diverticulum. South Med J 1995;88:575–576.
36. Meagher AP, Porter AJ, Rowland R, et al. Jejunal diverticulosis. Aust N Z J Surg 1993;63:360–366.
37. Chendrasekhar A, Timberlake GA. Perforated jejunal diverticula: an analysis of reported cases. Am Surg 1995;61:984–988.
38. Alvarez OA, Mejia A, Ostrower VS, Lee M. Jejunal diverticulitis manifesting with abdominal wall abscess. Am J Gastroenterol 1995;90:2060–2062.
39. Posthuma EF, Bieger R, Kuypers TJ. A rare cause of a hepatic abscess: diverticulitis of the ileum. Neth J Med 1993;42:69–72.
40. Cruveilhier J. Traite d'Anatomie Pathologique Générale. Paris: Baillière 1849;592.
41. Graser E. Das falsche darm divitkel. Arch Klin Chir 1899;59:638.
42. Beer E. Some pathological and clinical aspects of acquired (false) diverticula of the intestine. Am J Med Sci 1904;128:135.
43. Segal I, Solomon A, Hunt JA. Emergence of diverticular disease in the urban South African black. Gastroenterology 1977;72:215–219.
44. Kochhar R, Goenka MK, Nagi B, et al. The emergence of colonic diverticulosis in urbanised Indians. A report of 23 cases. Trop Geograph Med 1989;41:254–256.
45. Kubo A, Ishiwata J, Maeda Y, et al. Clinical studies on diverticular disease of the colon. Jap J Med 1983;22:185–189.
46. Munakata A, Nakaji S, Takami H, et al. Epidemiological evaluation of colonic diverticulosis and dietary fiber in Japan. Tohoku J Exper Med 1993;171:145–151.
47. Coode PE, Chan KW, Chan YT. Polyps and diverticula of the large intestine: a necropsy survey in Hong Kong. Gut 1985;26:1045–1048.
48. Chia JG, Wilde CC, Ngoi SS, et al. Trends of diverticular disease of the large bowel in a newly developed country. Dis Colon Rectum 1991;34:498–501.
49. Levy N, Stermer E, Simon J. The changing epidemiology of diverticular disease in Israel. Dis Colon Rectum 1985;28:416–418.
50. Goenka MK, Nagi B, Kochhar R, et al. Colonic diverticulosis in India: the changing scene. Indian J Gastroenterol 1994;13:86–88.
51. Noer RJ. Hemorrhage as a complication of diverticulitis. Ann Surg 1955;141:674–685.
52. Fleischner FG, Ming SC, Henken EM. Revised concepts on diverticular disease of the colon. 1. Diverticulosis: emphasis on tissue derangement and its relation to the irritable colon syndrome. Radiology 1964;83:859–872.
53. Heinz ER, Steinberg AJ, Sackner MA. Roentgenographic and pathologic aspects of intestinal scleroderma. Ann Intern Med 1983;59:822–826.
54. Plavsic BM, Raider L, Drnovsek VH, Kogutt MS. Association of rectal diverticula and scleroderma. Acta Radiol 1995;36:96–99.
55. Mielke JE, Becker KL, Gross JB. Diverticulitis of the colon in a young man with Marfan's syndrome. Gastroenterology 1965;48:379–382.
56. Cook JM. Spontaneous perforation of the colon: report of two cases in a family exhibiting Marfan stigmata. Ohio Med J 1968;64:73.
57. Thomson HJ, Busuttil A, Eastwood MA, et al. Submucosal collagen changes in the normal colon and in diverticular disease. Int J Colorect Dis 1987;2:208–213.

58. Whiteway J, Morson BC. Elastosis in diverticular disease of the sigmoid colon. Gut 1985;26:258–266.

59. Watters DA, Smith AN. Strength of the colon wall in diverticular disease. Br J Surg 1990;77:257–259.

60. Shanks SC, Kerley P. A textbook of X-ray diagnosis. 3rd ed. Philadelphia: WB Saunders, 1959:426.

61. Spriggs EI, Marxer OA. Multiple diverticula of the colon. Lancet 1927;1:1067–1074.

62. Morson BC. Pathology of diverticular disease of the colon. Clin Gastroenterol 1975;4:37–52.

63. Ivanoev K, Fork T, Hagerstrand J, et al. Diverticulosis in total colonic aganglionosis. Acta Radiol Diag 1985;26:447–451.

64. Srivastava GS, Smith AN, Painter NS. Sterculia, bulk-forming agent with smooth-muscle relaxant, versus bran in diverticular disease. Br Med J 1976;1:315–318.

65. Almy TP, Howell, DA. Diverticular disease of the colon. N Engl J Med 1980;302:324–331.

66. Snape WJ Jr, Carlson GM, Cohen S. Colonic myoelectric activity in the irritable bowel syndrome. Gastroenterology 1976;70:326–330.

67. Trotman IF, Misiewicz JJ. Sigmoid motility in diverticular disease and the irritable bowel syndrome. Gut 1988;29:218–222.

68. Arfwidsson S. Pathogenesis of multiple diverticula of the sigmoid colon in diverticular disease. Acta Chi Scand Suppl 1964;342:11–26.

69. Ritsema GH, Thijn CJ, Smout AJ. Motility of the sigmoid in irritable bowel syndrome and colonic diverticulosis. Ned Tijdschrift Geneeskd 1990;134:1398–1401.

70. Connell AM. Applied physiology of the colon: factors relevant to diverticular disease. Clin Gastroenterol 1975;4:23–36.

71. Painter NS, Truelove SC, Ardan GM, Tuckery M. Segmentation and the localization of intraluminal pressures in the human colon, with special reference to the pathogenesis of colonic diverticula. Gastroenterology 1965;49:169–177.

72. Weinreich J, Andersen D. Intraluminal pressure in the sigmoid colon. II. Patients with sigmoid diverticula and related conditions. Scand J Gastroenterol 1976;11:581–586.

73. Howell DA, Crow HC, Almy TP, Ramsey WH. A controlled double-blind study of sigmoid motility using psyllium mucilloid in diverticular disease (DD). Gastroenterology 1978;74:1046.

74. Aldoori WH, Giovannucci EL, Rimm EB, et al. A prospective study of diet and the risk of symptomatic diverticular disease in men. Am J Clin Nutr 1994;60:757–764.

75. Painter, NS Burkitt, DP. Diverticular disease of the colon, a 20th century problem. Clin Gastroenterol 1975;4:3–21.

76. Gear JSS, Ware A, Furdson P, et al. Symptomless diverticular disease and intake of dietary fibre. Lancet 1979;1:511–514.

77. Eastwood MA, Smith AN, Brydon WG, Pritchard J. Colonic function in patients with diverticular disease. Lancet 1978;1:1181–1182.

78. Hyland JM, Talyor I. Does a high fibre diet prevent the complications of diverticular disease? Br J Surg 1989;67:77–79.

79. Frieden JH, Morgenstern L. Sigmoid diverticulitis in identical twins. Dig Dis Sci 1985;30:182–183.

80. Omojala MF, Mangete E. Diverticulosis of the colon in three Nigerian siblings. Trop Geograph Med 1988;40:54–57.

81. Flynn M, Hyland J, Hammond P, et al. Faecal bile acid excretion in diverticular disease. Br J Surg 1980;67:629–632.

82. Goldstein NS, Ahmad E. Histology of the mucosa in sigmoid colon specimens with diverticular disease: observations for the interpretation of sigmoid colonoscopic biopsy specimens. Am J Clin Pathol 1997;107:438–444.

83. Rawlinson J, Brunton FJ. Transient diverticula of the colon. Br J Radiol 1989;62:27–30.

84. Noitove A, Almy TP. Diverticular disease of the colon. In: Sleisenger MH, Fordtran JS, eds. Gastrointestinal Disease. Pathophysiology, Diagnosis, Management. 4th ed. Philadelphia: WB Saunders, 1989:1419–1434.

85. Rosenberg RF, Naidich JB. Plain film recognition of giant colonic diverticulum. Am J Gastroenterol 1981;76:59–69.

86. Van Niekerk AJ, Fourie PA. Giant colonic diverticulum—a radiological diagnostic problem. A case report. South Afr Med J 1989;75:447–448.

87. D'Almeida MJ, McQuiston JH. Giant sigmoid diverticulum. J Am Osteopath Assoc 1996;96:309–313.

88. Ellerbroek CJ, Lu CC. Unusual manifestations of giant colonic diverticulum. Dis Colon Rectum 1984;27:545–547.

89. Lepeyrie H, Balmes P, Loizon P, Delhoume JY. Giant diverticulum of the transverse colon. J Chir 1988;125:717–720.

90. McNutt R, Schmitt D, Schulte W. Giant colonic diverticula—three distinct entities. Report of a case. Dis Colon Rectum 1988;31:624–628.

91. Kricun R, Stasik JJ, Reither RD, Dex WJ. Giant colonic diverticulum. Am J Roentgenol 1980;135:507–512.

92. Freeman SR, McNally PR. Diverticulitis. Med Clin North Am 1993;177:1149–1167.

93. Ambrosetti P, Robert JH, Witzig JA, et al. Acute left colonic diverticulitis in young patients. J Am Coll Surg 1994;179:156–160.

94. Parks, TG. Natural history of diverticular disease of the colon. Clin Gastroenterol 1975;4:53–69.

95. Ming SC, Fleischner FG. Diverticulitis of the sigmoid colon: reappraisal of the pathology and pathogenesis. Surgery 1965;58:627–633.

96. Fleischner FG, Ming SC. Revised concept on diverticular disease of the colon. 2. So-called diverticulitis: diverticular sigmoiditis and perisigmoiditis, diverticular abscess, fistula, frank peritonitis. Radiology 1965;84:599–609.

97. Ferrucci JT, Ragsdale BD, Barrett PJ, et al. Double tracking in the sigmoid colon. Radiology 1976;120:307–312.

98. Schnyder P, Moss AA, Thoeni RF, Margulis AR. A double-blind study of radiologic accuracy in diverticulosis, diverticulitis and carcinoma of the sigmoid colon. J Clin Gastroenterol 1979;1:55–66.

99. Woods RJ, Lavery IC, Fazio VW, et al. Internal fistulas in diverticular disease. Dis Colon Rectum 1988;31:591–596.

100. Small WP, Smith AN. Fistula and conditions associated with diverticular disease of the colon. Clin Gastroenterol 1975;4:171–199.

101. Hafner CD, Ponka LJ, Brush BE. Genitourinary manifestations of diverticulitis of the colon. A study of 500 cases. JAMA 1962;179:76–78.

102. Benchimol D, Lagautriere F, Richelme H. Fistules sigmoido-vesicales d'origine diverticulaire. Ann Urol (Paris) 1995;29:26–30.

103. Ravo B, Khan SA, Ger R, et al. Unusual extraperitoneal presentations of diverticulitis. Am J Gastroenterol 1985;80:346–351.

104. McCrea ES, Wagner E. Femoral osteomyelitis secondary to diverticulitis. J Canad Assoc Radiol 1981;32:181–182.

105. Hur T, Chen Y, Shu GH, et al. Spontaneous cervical subcutaneous and mediastinal emphysema secondary to occult sigmoid diverticulitis. Eur Respir J 1995;8:2188–2190.

106. Gerber GS, Guss SP, Pielet RW. Fournier's gangrene secondary to intra-abdominal processes. Urology 1994;44:779–782.

107. Rothenbuehler JM, Oertli D, Harder F. Extraperitoneal manifestation of perforated diverticulitis. Dig Dis Sci. 1993;38:1985–1988.

108. Hain JM, Sherick DG, Cleary RK. Salpingocolonic fistula secondary to diverticulitis. Am Surg 1996;62:984–986.

109. Cirocco WC, Priolo SR, Golub RW. Spontaneous ureterocolic fistula: a rare complication of colonic diverticular disease. Am Surg 1994;60:832–835.

110. Libson E, Bloom RA, Verstandig A, et al. Sigmoid-appendiceal fistula in diverticular disease. Diag Imag Clin Med 1984;53:262–264.

111. van Hillo M, Fazio VW, Lavery IC. Sigmoidoappendiceal fistula—an unusual complication of diverticulitis. Report of a case. Dis Colon Rectum 1984;27:618–620.

112. Lambert ME, Knox RA, Schofield PF, Hancock BD. Management of the septic complications of diverticular disease. Br J Surg 1986;73:567–579.

113. Berry AR, Turner WH, Mortensen NJ, Kettlewell MG. Emergency surgery for complicated diverticular disease. A five-year experience. Dis Colon Rectum 1989;32:849–854.

114. Jensen JA, Tsang D, Minnis JF, et al. Pneumopylephlebitis and intramesocolic diverticular perforation. Am J Surg 1985;150:284–287.

115. Sonnenshein MA, Cone LA, Alexander RM. Diverticulitis with colovenous fistula and portal venous gas. Report of two cases. J Clin Gastroenterol 1986;8:195–198.

116. Burgard G, Cuilleron M, Cuilleret J. Une complication exceptionnelle de la sigmoidite diverticulaire perforee: l'aeroportie avec abces miliaires du foie. J Chir (Paris) 1993;130:237–239.

117. Duffy FJ Jr, Millan MT, Schoetz DJ Jr, Larsen CR. Suppurative pylephlebitis and pylethrombosis: the role of anticoagulation. Am Surg 1995;61:1041–1044.

118. Lee L, Kang YS, Astromoff N. Septic thrombophlebitis of the inferior mesenteric vein associated with diverticulitis CT diagnosis. Clin Imaging 1996;20:115–117.

119. Arsura EL. Corticosteroid-association perforation of colonic diverticula. Arch Intern Med 1990;150:1337–1338.

120. Weiner HL, Rezai AR, Cooper PR. Sigmoid diverticular perforation in neurosurgical patients receiving high-dose corticosteroids. Neurosurgery 1993;33:40–43.

121. Hinchey EJ, Schaal PG, Richards GK. Treatment of perforated diverticular disease of the colon. Adv Surg 1978;12:85–109.

122. Richter S, v.d. Linde J, Dominok GW. Diverticular disease. Pathology and clinical aspects based on 368 autopsy cases. Zentralbl Chir 1991;116:991–998.

123. Haubrich WS. Diverticula and diverticular disease of the colon. In: Berk JE, Haubrich WS, Kalser MH, et al. eds. Bockus Gastroenterology. 4th ed. Philadelphia: WB Saunders, 1985:2445–2473.

124. Sugihara K, Muto T, Morioka Y: Motility study in the right sided diverticular disease of the colon. Gut 1983;24:1130–1134.

125. Gharaibeh KI, Shami SK, Al-Qudah MS, et al. True caecal diverticulitis. Int Surg 1995;80:218–222.

126. Pieterse AS, Rowland R, Miliauskas JR, Hoffmann DC. Right-sided diverticular disease of the colon: a morphological analysis of 16 cases. Aust N Z J Surg 1986;56:471–475.

127. Rodkey GV, Welch CE. Diverticulitis of the colon: evolution in concept and therapy. Surg Clin North Am 1965;45:1231–1243.

128. Sardi A, Gokli A, Singer JA. Diverticular disease of the cecum and ascending colon. A review of 881 cases. Am Surgeon 1987;53:41–45.

129. Leichtling JJ. Acute cecal diverticulitis. Gastroenterology 1955;29:453–460.

130. Harada RN, Whelan TJ Jr. Surgical management of cecal diverticulitis. Am J Surg 1993;166:666–669.

131. Fischer MG, Farkas AM. Diverticulitis of the cecum and ascending colon. Dis Colon Rectum 1984;27:454–458.

132. Luoma A, Nagy AG. Cecal diverticulitis. Canad J Surg 1989;32:283–286.

133. Mittal VK, Cortez JA, Olson AM. Solitary perforated diverticulum of the ascending colon: report of two cases. J Dis Colon Rectum 1981;24:47–49.

134. Perez-Cruet MJ, Grable E, Drapkin MS, et al. Pylephlebitis associated with diverticulitis. South Med J 1993;86:578–580.

135. Cho KC, Morehouse HT, Alterman DD, Thornhill BA. Sigmoid diverticulitis: diagnostic role of CT—comparison with barium enema studies. Radiology 1990;176:111–115.

136. Birnbaum BA, Balthazar EJ. CT of appendicitis and diverticulitis. Radiol Clin North Am 1994;32:885–898.

137. Yacoe ME, Jeffrey RB Jr. Sonography of appendicitis and diverticulitis. Radiol Clin North Am 1994;32:899–912.

138. Orebaugh JE, Macris JA, Lee JF. Surgical treatment of diverticular disease of the colon. Am Surgeon 1978;44:712–715.

139. Alexander J, Karl RC, Skinner DB. Results of changing trends in the surgical management of complications of diverticular disease. Surgery 1983;94:683–690.

140. Perkins JD, Shield CF 3d, Chang FC, Farha GJ. Acute diverticulitis. Comparison of treatment in immunocompromised and nonimmunocompromised patients. Am J Surg 1984;148:745–748.

141. Freischlag J, Bennion RS, Thompson JE Jr. Complications of diverticular disease of the colon in young people. Dis Colon Rectum 1986;29:639–643.

142. Schauer PR, Ramos R, Ghiatas AA, Sirinek KR. Virulent diverticular disease in young obese men. Am J Surg 1992;164:443–446.

143. Vignati PV. Welch JP. Cohen JL. Long-term management of diverticulitis in young patients. Dis Colon Rectum 1995;38:627–629.

144. Klein S, Mayer L, Present DH, et al. Extraintestinal manifestations in patients with diverticulitis. Ann Intern Med 1988;108:700–702.

145. Kurgansky D, Foxwell MM Jr. Pyoderma gangrenosum as a cutaneous manifestation of diverticular disease. South Med J 1993;86:581–584.

146. Harbrecht PJ, Ahmad W, Fry DE, Amin M. Occult diverticulitis, a cause of retroperitoneal fibrosis. Dis Colon Rectum 1980;23:255–257.

147. Auguste L, Borrero E, Wise L. Surgical management of perforated colonic diverticulitis. Arch Surg 1985;120:450–452.

148. Pemberton JH, Armstrong DN, Dietzen CD. Diverticulitis. In: Yamada T, Alpers DH, Owyang C, Powell DW, Silverstein FE. eds. Textbook of gastroenterology. Philadelphia: JB Lippincott, 1995:1876–1890.

149. Khan AL, Ah-See AK, Crofts TJ, et al. Surgical management of the septic complications of diverticular disease. Ann R Coll Surg Engl 1995;77:16–20.

150. Sher ME, Agachan F, Bortul M, et al. Laparoscopic surgery for diverticulitis. Surg Endosc 1997;11:264–267.

151. Hughes LE. Complications of diverticular disease: inflammation, obstruction and hemorrhage. Clin Gastroenterol 1975;4:147–170.

152. Kubo A, Kagaya T, Nakagawa H. Studies on complications of diverticular disease of the colon. Jap J Med 1985;24:39–43.

153. Meyers MA, Alonso DR, Baer JW. Pathogenesis of massively bleeding colonic diverticulosis: new observations. Am J Roentgenol 1976;127:901–908.

154. Tedesco FJ, Waye JD, Raskin JB, et al. Colonoscopic evaluation of rectal bleeding; a study of 304 patients. Ann Intern Med 1978;89:907–909.

155. Boley SJ, Brandt LJ: Vascular ectasias of the colon—1986. Dig Dis Sci 1986;31(Suppl):26S–42S.

156. Santos JCM Jr, Aprilli F, Guimaraes AS, Rocha JJ. Angiodysplasia of the colon: endoscopic diagnosis and treatment. Br J Surg 1988;75:256–258.

157. Roberts PL, Schoetz DJ Jr, Coller JA. Vascular ectasia. Diagnosis and treatment by colonoscopy. Am Surg 1988;54:56–59.

158. Trendell-Smith NJ, Warren BF, Sheffield EA, Durdey P. An unusual case of colonic angiodysplasia. J Clin Pathol 1995;48:272–275.

159. Reinus JF, Brandt LJ. Vascular ectasias and diverticulosis. Common causes of lower intestinal bleeding. Gastroenterol Clin North Am 1994;23:1–20.

160. Morini S, de Angelis P, Manurita L, Colavolpe V. Association of colonic diverticula with adenomas and carcinomas. A colonoscopic experience. Dis Colon Rectum 1988;31:793–796.

161. Boulos PB, Cowin AP, Karamanolis DG, Clark CG. Diverticula, neoplasia, or both? Early detection of carcinoma in sigmoid diverticular disease. Ann Surg 1985;202:607–609.

162. De Masi E, Bertolotti A, Fegiz GF. The importance of endoscopy in the diagnosis of neoplasms associated with diverticular disease of the colon, and its effect on surgical treatment. Ital J Surg Sci 1984;14:195–199.

163. Hines JR, Gordon RT. Adenocarcinoma arising in a diverticular abscess of the colon: report of a case. Dis Colon Rectum 1975;18:49–51.

164. McCraw RC, Wilson SM, Brown FM, Gardner WA. Adenocarcinoma arising in a sigmoid diverticulum: report of a case. Dis Colon Rectum 1975;19:553–556.

165. Cohn KH, Weimar JA, Fani K, DeSoto-LaPaix F. Adenocarcinoma arising within a colonic diverticulum: report of two cases and review of the literature. Surgery 1993;113:223–226.

166. Hernandez FJ, Fernandez BB. Mucus-secreting carcinoid tumor in a colonic diverticulum: report of a case. Dis Colon Rectum 1976;19:63–67.

167. Axelsson CK, Francis D. Preoperative fine-needle aspiration biopsy: an aid to differential diagnosis between diverticular disease and colonic cancer? A preliminary report. Dis Colon Rectum. 1978;21:319–321.

168. Jalan KN, Walker RJ, Prescot RJ, et al. Fecal stasis and diverticular disease in ulcerative colitis. Gut 1970;11:688–696.

169. Marshak RH. Granulomatous colitis in association with diverticula. N Engl J Med 1970;283:1080–1084.

170. Burkitt DP, Walker AR. Saint's triad: confirmation and explanation. South Afr Med J 1976;50:2136–2138.

171. Scaggion G, Poletti G, Riggo S. Saint's triad: statistico-epidemiological research and case contribution. Minn Med 1987;78:1183–1187.

172. Capron JP, Piperaud R, Dupas J-L, et al. Evidence for an association between cholelithiasis and diverticular disease of the colon. Dig Dis Sci 1981;26:523–527.

173. Scheff RT, Zuckerman G, Harter H, et al. Diverticular disease in patients with chronic renal failure due to polycystic kidney disease. Ann Intern Med 1980;92:202–204.

174. Foster KJ, Holdstock G, Whorwell PJ, et al. Prevalence of diverticular disease of the colon in patients with ischaemic heart disease. Gut 1978;19:1054–1056.

175. Bak M. Nodular intra-abdominal panniculitis: an accompaniment of colorectal carcinoma and diverticular disease. Histopathology 1996; 29:21–27.

176. Brodribb AJ, Humphreys DM. Diverticular disease: three studies. Part I—Relation to other disorders and fibre intake. Br Med J 1976;1:424–425.

177. Galbraith P, Bagg MN, Schabel SI, Rajagopalan PR. Diverticular complications of renal failure. Gastrointest Radiol 1990;15:259–262.

178. Burton NA, Albus RA, Graeber GM, Lough FC. Acute diverticulitis following cardiac surgery. Chest 1986;89:756–757.

179. Badia-Perez JM, Valverde-Sintas J, Franch-Arcas G, et al. Acute postoperative diverticulitis. Int J Colorect Dis 1989;4:141–143.

180. Detry O, Defraigne JO, Meurisse M, et al. Acute diverticulitis in heart transplant recipients. Transpl Int 1996;9:376–379.

181. Myllykangas-Luosujarvi R. Diverticulosis—a primary cause of life-threatening complications in rheumatoid arthritis. Clin Exp Rheumatol 1995;13:79–82.

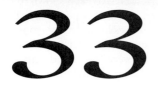
33 BENIGN EPITHELIAL POLYPS OF THE INTESTINES

Harry S. Cooper

The term polyp is a clinical term for a gross description of any circumscribed "tumor" that projects above the surrounding normal mucosa. The term polyp should not be used as a histologic diagnosis. Polyps may be neoplastic, inflammatory, hyperplastic, or hamartomatous in nature (Table 33.1); only through histologic examination can one be certain of their nature and clinical signifi-

cance. Solitary polyps (regardless of their histologic features) are much more common in the large intestine and rectum than in the small intestine; accordingly, most of this chapter will be devoted to lesions of the large intestine and rectum. However, in polyposis syndromes, involvement of the small intestine by these polyps is common.

TABLE 33.1	Classification of Solitary and Multiple Intestinal Polyps

Neoplastic Polyps
  Adenoma—tubular, tubulovillous, villous, flat, serrated
Nonneoplastic Polyps
  Hyperplastic (metaplastic) polyp
  Juvenile polyp
  Peutz-Jegher's
  Inflammatory polyp—Inflammatory fibroid, inflammatory (Nos),
    inflammatory cap, inflammatory myoglandular, diverticular,
    intestinal pyogenic, granulation tissue polyposis, atheroemboli
  Lymphoid polyp

NONNEOPLASTIC POLYPS

HYPERPLASTIC POLYPS

Hyperplastic (or metaplastic) polyps are small (most are less than 5 mm in size), convex elevations limited to the colon and rectum. They are commonly seen in the sigmoid colon and rectums of individuals 40 years of age or greater (1–7) and are considered nonneoplastic in nature (8).

SIZE, SITE DISTRIBUTION, INCIDENCE AND EPIDEMIOLOGY

In the older literature, it was stated that the vast majority of polyps of the colon and rectum less than 5 mm in size were hyperplastic polyps. In autopsy material Arthur noted that 80% of rectal polyps less than 5 mm in size were hyperplastic polyps (1). Similarly, Lane et al. (9), in a study of 2136 colorectal polyps (1581 adenomas and 555 hyperplastic polyps) in symptomatic adults, noted that 90% of lesions less than 3 mm in size were hyperplastic polyps. However, recent data from biopsy material have challenged this. Estrada and Spjut (10) reported that, of lesions 5 mm or less, 43.5% and 56.5% were hyperplastic polyps and adenomas, respectively. Waye et al. (11) found that among polyps 6 mm or less in size, 61% were adenomas and 20% were hyperplastic polyps.

Some studies have reported that small distal polyps (sigmoid colon and rectum) are more likely to be hyperplastic polyps rather than adenomas (3, 11) while others have reported just the opposite (4, 5, 12).

The incidence of hyperplastic polyps increases with the age of the population, and is uncommon below the age of 40 years (1, 7). In autopsy studies of adults more than 40 years of age in populations with Western lifestyles the incidence of hyperplastic polyps varies from 13 to 75% (1, 7). In biopsy studies the incidence has been reported as varying from 2 to 26% (sigmoid colon and rectum) (2, 4–6), and 10.3 to 30% for the entire colon and rectum (3, 4, 6). The incidence of hyperplastic polyps varies depending upon the geographic population studied. Epidemiologic studies indicate that the incidence of hyperplastic polyps parallels that of large-bowel adenomas and cancers. Studies from Western countries, where there is a high incidence of adenomas and cancers, have reported the incidence of hyperplastic polyps to be as high as 85%; in underdeveloped countries, where the incidence of adenomas and cancers is

low, the incidence of hyperplastic polyps may be as low as 2 to 3% (13). However, not all population studies report similar findings (14, 15). Dietary and other lifestyle factors have been shown to be associated with hyperplastic polyps in the United States. The health professionals follow-up study and the nurses health study reported that, by multivariate analysis, consumption of greater than 30 g of alcohol a day and cigarette smoking were associated with an increased risk of hyperplastic polyps, while a high intake of folate was associated with a decreased risk of hyperplastic polyps. Consumption of animal fat suggested an increased risk, but was attenuated in full multivariate analysis (16). Depending on the study, the male to female ratio varies from unity to 4:1 (1, 13, 17).

ETIOLOGY, CELL KINETICS, AND PATHOGENESIS

To date the etiology of hyperplastic polyps is unknown. Franzin et al. (18) believe that hyperplastic polyps may be of inflammatory or ischemic origin. Araki et al. (19) believe that chronic inflammation has some etiologic role. Cell kinetic studies (20, 21) have shown that hyperplastic polyps are nonneoplastic in nature and that the mode of cell renewal is the same as in the normal mucosa, but with a longer turnover time, a delayed migration from crypt to surface, and a slower exfoliation (i.e., hypermature epithelium). An immunohistochemical study of antigens related to cell differentiation supports the concept of earlier maturation along the crypt axis (hypermaturation) (22). Araki et al. present data which support the concept that hyperplastic polyps originate from a single abnormal crypt within a small region of the mucosa. Polyps grow by fission of abnormal crypts and fusion of polycentrically originated "polyps" (19).

CLINICAL ASPECTS

Hyperplastic polyps, because of their small size, rarely produce symptoms referable to the gastrointestinal tract. However, there have been reports of patients with large or multiple hyperplastic polyps that were responsible for GI symptoms (17, 23–27).

Recently there has been controversy about the clinical significance of hyperplastic polyps found on sigmoidoscopy and the presence or association of proximal colonic adenomas. Some investigators (2, 6, 12, 28) believe that the presence of hyperplastic polyps in the distal colon and rectum are markers for the presence of proximal adenomas which would then require a full colonoscopic exam. However, others present, just as convincingly, data to the contrary (3–5). A position paper by the American College of Gastroenterology states that a hyperplastic polyp found during proctosigmoidoscopy is not an indication for colonoscopy (29).

The close association of hyperplastic polyps with colon and rectal cancers and populations with a high prevalence of colorectal cancer has led many to consider hyperplastic polyps as markers for neoplasia. Studies by Risio et al. (30) of the epithelial proliferation labeling index in "normal mucosa" of patients with and without hyperplastic polyps, in conjunction with autopsy studies by Jass et al. (7) and Eide et al. (31), have led to the hypothesis that hyperplastic polyps may be markers of the action of environmental factors that interact in the initiation/mutagenesis phase of colorectal neoplasia.

There have been reports of patients who have so-called hyperplastic polyposis (17, 24, 26, 27, 32), in which the number of polyps ranges from "numerous" to hundreds. In these cases there was no reported familial incidence and there was a marked male predominance. Recently, Torlakovic and Snover (33) have raised the question as to whether some of the reported cases of hyperplastic polyposis are instead cases of the so called serrated adenomatous polyposis. In most of the reported cases of hyperplastic polyposis (17, 24, 26, 32) the illustrations are not sufficient to distinguish hyperplastic polyposis from serrated adenomatous polyposis. However, the case of Bengoecher et al. (27) most likely represents serrated adenomatous polyposis. Burt and Samowitz in their personal experience have seen cases of both hyperplastic polyposis and serrated adenomatous polyposis (34). Two cases of inverted hyperplastic polyposis have been reported (35). Both were middle aged males with concurrent colonic adenocarcinoma. The number of inverted polyps were 18 and 12, and they were present in the proximal ascending colons.

PATHOLOGY

On gross examination, hyperplastic polyps appear as small sessile rounded excrescences that are the same color or paler than the surrounding mucosa. They often sit on the mucosal folds and may be flattened or convex in nature (Fig. 33.1). Occasionally, hyperplastic polyps may be pedunculated with a well-developed stalk. The vast majority of hyperplastic polyps range from 3 to 6 mm in size. However, in large series of hyperplastic polyps approximately 1 to 4% of polyps are greater than 1 cm in size (17, 18). On microscopic examination, hyperplastic polyps have a serrated or saw-toothed appearance similar to that seen in a secretory endometrium. The serrated appearance is due to the extensive papillary enfolding of epithelial cells. In most series columnar cells predominate over goblet cells (1, 8, 18), although it has been claimed that goblet cells predominate in earlier lesions (1). The columnar cells take on a bright eosinophilic appearance often with a distinct brush border. The nuclei of both goblet cells and columnar cells are basally located, show no atypia, are ovoid to round, usually uniformly dark, and occasionally small nucleoli can be seen (Fig. 33.2). These nuclear features are important in differentiating a hyperplastic polyp from a serrated adenoma and from traditional adenomas. In well-oriented material the basal portion of the crypt shows an increased mitotic rate compared with the mitotic rate of the normal surrounding mucosa; however, mitoses are never located in the upper third of the crypt or surface epithelium. The nuclei in the basal

portion of the crypts are characteristically more crowded and hyperchromatic; however, this should not be misinterpreted as adenomatous change. Arthur has claimed that in the earlier lesions, there is simply a dilatation of the superficial parts of the glands, whereas in "older" lesions, full-thickness involvement of the crypt is seen (1). Often the specimen is less well oriented and is cut tangentially, in which case the crypts take on a star-shaped appearance (Fig. 33.3). Often one can appreciate a disordered muscularis mucosae, with muscle fibers radiating toward the surface. This disordered muscularis mucosa may account for pseudoinvasion of epithelium into the submucosa mimicking invasive cancer. Sobin (36) has described an inverted hyperplastic polyp with an endophytic growth pattern and complex epithelial growth pattern that may penetrate the muscularis mucosae and mimic cancer. These are more frequent in women and the right side of the colon. These lesions occasionally may overlay lymphoid nodules. In the classic hyperplastic polyp Paneth cells may also occasionally be present. In hyperplastic polyps there is widening or exaggeration of the collagen table beneath the surface epithelium (9). This is in contrast to classic and serrated adenomas, in which there is thinning of this subepithelial basement membrane table. Regarding large hyperplastic polyps (larger than 1 cm), Williams et al. (17) note that at low power they may take on the appearance of villous or tubulovillous adenomas. Franzin et al. (18) noted clear cut adenoma admixed with three of seven large hyperplastic polyps. In light of the recent characterization of serrated adenomas, one must query whether these lesions represent large hyperplastic polyps or serrated adenomas. The photos in these articles and other reported large hyperplastic polyps do not allow this distinction to be made. In the authors personal experience, cases which in the past I had considered as large hyperplastic polyps on re-review I now believe are the so called serrated adenomas.

Adenomatous foci admixed with hyperplastic polyps are known to occur (Fig. 33.4). The St. Mark's group found hyperplastic foci in 0.6% of adenomas (17). Franzin et al. found that 9.6% of adenomas had hyperplastic foci and five of seven hyperplastic polyps greater than 1 cm in size had adenomatous foci (18). Estrada and Spjut (10) reported 13% of hyperplastic polyps to have foci of adenomatous epithelium. However, this high incidence might be due to overinterpretation of the crowded hyperchromatic basally placed nuclei of hyperplastic polyps as adenomatous. These lesions are better considered admixed hyperplastic adenomatous polyps so as to avoid confusion from the term mixed hyperplastic adenomatous polyp (serrated adenoma). One must also be cautioned that small adenomas, when viewed at lower power magnification, may take on the appearance of a hyperplastic polyp; however, on more careful inspection they are truly adenomas. Goldman et al. (37) noted that 36% of villous adenomas less than 2 cm in size had foci of hyperplastic polyps whereas only 5% of villous adenomas greater than 2 cm had foci of hyperplastic polyps. While uncommon, there are reported cases of adenocarcinoma arising within hyperplastic polyps (18, 23, 32). In these cases the hyperplastic polyps were large. Hyperplastic epithelium has also been noted in 20 to 85% of juvenile polyps, Peutz-Jeghers polyps, and inflammatory polyps (18).

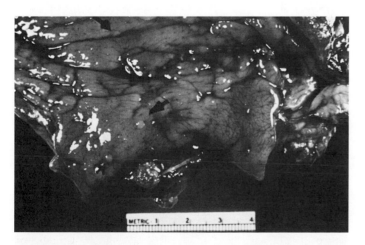

Figure 33.1   Gross appearance of hyperplastic polyps *(arrows).* The polyps are small and convex and appear to be of the same color as the surrounding mucosa.

SPECIAL STUDIES

Hyperplastic polyps have been shown to express K-ras mutations in 22% of cases studied while 0% of cases express APC mutations (38).

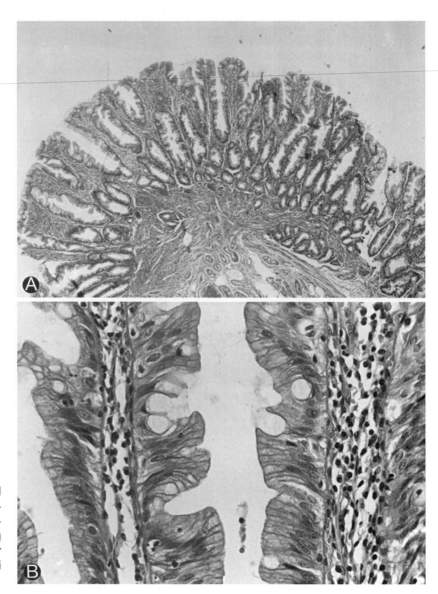

Figure 33.2   Hyperplastic polyp. **(A)** Well oriented specimen, showing a serrated, or papillary, enfolding of epithelium. The muscularis mucosa is distorted and splayed. **(B)** High power view showing serrated epithelium with an admixture of columnar and goblet cells. No mitoses are noted and the nuclei are bland in nature.

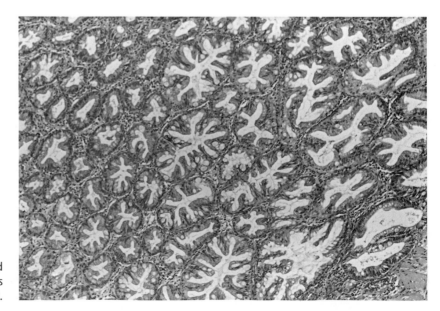

Figure 33.3   Low power view of a poorly oriented hyperplastic polyp. One can identify the lesion as such by the star-shaped appearance of the glands.

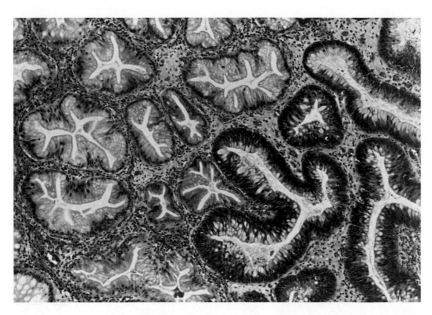

Figure 33.4 Hyperplastic polyp with focal adenomatous changes. The adenoma is on the right and the hyperplastic polyp is on the left. At this magnification the nuclear differences are obvious.

The data regarding expression of bcl-2 protein in hyperplastic polyps have been conflicting. Fioritio et al. (39) and Stern et al. (40) report that hyperplastic polyps fail to express bcl-2 protein. On the other hand Bosari et al. (41) and Bronner et al. (42) both report expression of bcl-2 protein in hyperplastic polyps in a pattern similar to the normal colon (i.e., limited to the proliferative zone). Hyperplastic polyps do not express $p53$ protein when studied with the Pab 1801 antibody (43). Torlakovic and Snover (33) using antibodies DO7 and Pab 1801 found $p53$ protein expression in two of ten hyperplastic polyps. However, these two cases also showed anomalous expression for blood group antigens Le[a] and Le[b] and peanut lectin. Other markers of epithelial cell differentiation or neoplastic association such as lectins and blood group antigens have been studied in hyperplastic polyps. For the most part, hyperplastic polyps express these markers in patterns more similar to normal mucosa than neoplastic mucosa, however, exceptions are noted where hyperplastic polyps express these markers in a pattern associated with neoplasia (22, 44–48).

SERRATED ADENOMA

Longacre et al. described the entity of mixed hyperplastic adenomatous polyps, which they believe represents an adenoma (so-called serrated adenoma), rather than a hyperplastic polyp (49). These findings have been corroborated by Torlakovic et al. (33). The entity of mixed hyperplastic adenomatous polyps and/or serrated adenoma will be discussed under hyperplastic polyps because of the morphologic similarity and confusion with hyperplastic polyps. For the rest of this discussion, I will use the term serrated adenoma rather than mixed hyperplastic adenomatous polyp.

CLINICAL ASPECTS

The serrated adenoma is uncommon, noted in 101 of 18,000 polyps (0.5%). They are most commonly found in the rectosigmoid colon. They range in size from 0.2 cm to 7.5 cm, 60% are 0.1 to 0.6 cm in size, and 21% are greater than 1.0 cm in size. In traditional hyperplastic polyps 93% are smaller than 0.5 cm and only 1 to 4% are larger than 1.0 cm. Sixty five percent of serrated adenomas are sessile

and 35% are pedunculated. Twenty four percent of serrated adenomas had foci of traditional adenoma and 10% had foci of intramucosal cancer (49). It is becoming more clear that many of the lesions in the past that were diagnosed as large hyperplastic polyps are probably serrated adenomas.

PATHOLOGY

At low power one sees a serrated pattern similar to that of traditional hyperplastic polyps. However, on closer scrutiny a serrated adenoma shows a more complicated branching. The cytoplasm may be very eosinophilic. Serrated adenomas tend to have elongated crypts with dilatation of the crypts (greater at the bases). Also present are horizontally oriented crypts running just above the muscularis mucosae often with goblet cells at the base of the crypt. The most dilated crypts tend to have an increased content of goblet cells mucous collecting in the crypts and surface mucosa. Generally, the serrated adenoma appears more villiform or complexly branched than does a traditional hyperplastic polyp. Probably the most discriminating feature is that of the nuclei. The nuclei of serrated adenomas are considered somewhat between that of a hyperplastic polyp and traditional adenoma (more atypia than a hyperplastic polyp but atypia that falls short of traditional adenomas). In traditional hyperplastic polyps the nuclei are ovoid or round, dark with occasional faint nucleoli, and basally placed with minimal pseudostratification. In the serrated adenoma, the nuclei are larger, ovoid and rounded, with focal elongation and pseudostratification. They can be hyperchromatic with chromatin clumping or nuclear membrane irregularities, or vesicular with "prominent" nucleoli (Fig. 33.5). Mitoses may occasionally be seen in the upper crypt and surface of serrated adenomas. Serrated adenomas lack the subepithelial thickened collagen layer seen in traditional hyperplastic polyps (33, 49). Torlakovic and Snover (33) list the following as a way of differentiating serrated adenomas from hyperplastic polyps. Compared to hyperplastic polyps, serrated adenomas will have:

1. Dilatation of the crypt that is most prominent at the base.
2. Presence of horizontally oriented crypts (just above the muscularis mucosae).

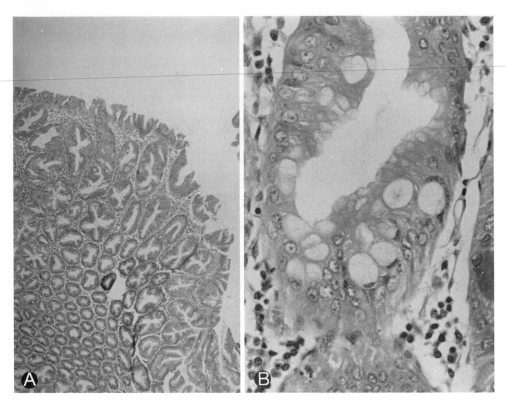

Figure 33.5   (A) Low power view of serrated adenoma. Note infolding of glands similar to classic hyperplastic polyp. **(B)** High power view. Please note nuclei are rounded with prominent nucleoli. Compare this to nuclear changes in Figure 33.2B.

3. Large areas without endocrine cells on H & E and Cherukian Shenk.
4. Nuclear atypia, including basally oriented oval or round nuclei that are enlarged with prominent nucleoli.
5. Focal mucous overproduction (resembling mucinous cystadenoma of appendix).
6. Proliferation zone frequently moved from the base of the crypt to middle or upper part of the crypt with presence of numerous goblet cells in base of crypt.
7. Frequent or focal eosinophilia of cytoplasm.

Figure 33.6 clearly shows the difference between a hyperplastic polyp, a serrated adenoma, and villous adenoma with serrated features.

Torlakovic and Snover (33) have also reported six cases of serrated adenomatous polyposis. Five of the six cases were male (similar to reported for hyperplastic polyposis), four had cancers in the colon, and two had associated adenomas. In four cases the polyps were described as more than 100 and in two cases more than 50 in number. The polyps were often sessile and large, 0.5 to 4.0 cm in size. They were not limited to any specific portion of the bowel.

PEUTZ-JEGHERS POLYP

The Peutz-Jeghers polyp is a nonneoplastic hamartomatous polyp that occurs in the stomach, small intestine, and colon. One usually associates the Peutz-Jeghers polyp with the syndrome of intestinal polyposis and mucocutaneous pigmentation. However, it has been noted that these Peutz-Jeghers polyps may occur as solitary lesions

in patients without the syndrome. In fact, it appears that those solitary polyps may be found as commonly as in patients with the syndrome (50–52).

ETIOLOGY

Peutz-Jeghers polyps are true hamartomas. There is a genetic etiology in those people with the syndrome (see section on Polyposis).

CLINICAL ASPECTS

These will be discussed under the section on Polyposis.

PATHOLOGY

On gross examination these polyps may be sessile or pedunculated and may vary in size, some being quite large (3.5 cm or more). The Peutz-Jeghers polyps are derived from intestinal glandular epithelium together with stroma that includes a branching muscular framework from the muscularis mucosa. Both the epithelial and the smooth muscle components give the Peutz-Jeghers polyp its characteristic appearance. Its arborescent arrangement should enable the pathologist to make the diagnosis at low-power magnification. The epithelium resembles the normal epithelium from the area of the gastrointestinal tract from which it comes. In the small intestine the epithelium consists of both absorptive columnar cells and goblet cells (Fig. 33.7). In the colon the glands often show extensive branching with predominantly hypertrophied goblet cells (Fig. 33.8). A normal distribution of endocrine cells is present. It is not uncommon to see areas of hyperplastic epithelium

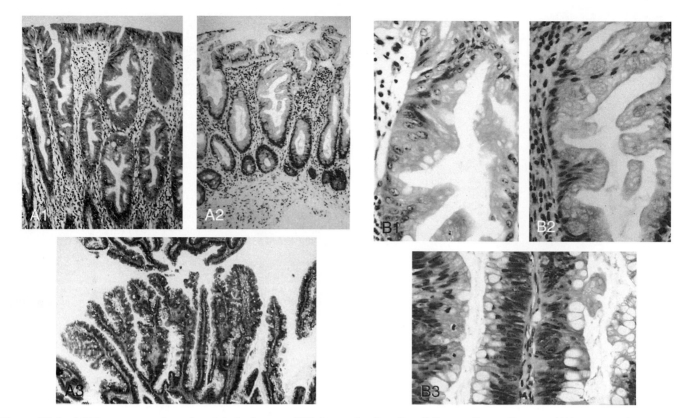

Figure 33.6   (A) Low power view of serrated adenoma *(A1)*, hyperplastic polyp *(A2)* and villous adenoma *(A3)*. Note: At lower power all have serrated appearance. **(B)** High power view of **A** differentiates the three lesions. Please note characteristic nuclear changes. Serrated adenoma *(B1)* with nuclei showing prominent nucleoli, hyperplastic polyp *(B2)* with ovoid hyperchromatic nuclei and no nucleoli, and villous adenoma *(B3)* with characteristic hyperchromatic, elongated and stratified nuclei. (See color plate.)

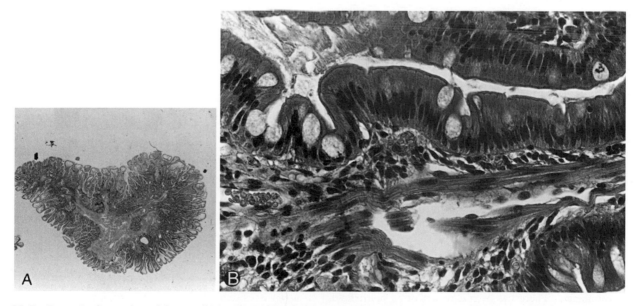

Figure 33.7   Peutz-Jegher polyp of the small intestine. **(A)** Whole mount view. **(B)** Higher power view showing normal absorptive and goblet cells. Smooth muscle fibers are extending through the core of the villous.

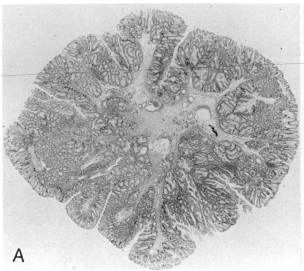

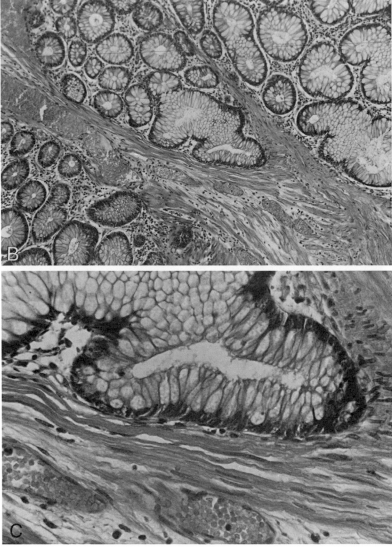

Figure 33.8 Peutz-Jegher polyp of the colon. **(A)** Whole mount view showing the branching and tortuosity of glands. **(B)** Medium power view, showing branching smooth muscle fibers circling and separating glands. **(C)** High power view showing benign goblet cells with adjacent smooth muscle fibers.

within these polyps. The epithelium in these polyps is non-neoplastic in nature; however, there have been reports of dysplastic adenomatous changes and adenocarcinomas arising within Peutz-Jeghers polyps of the small intestine and of the colon (53–67) (The malignant potential of Peutz-Jeghers polyps will be discussed further under the section on Polyposis). Occasionally one may see pseudoinvasion of the epithelium (herniation of mucosa) similar to that noted in adenomas, but this should not be taken as evidence of malignancy (Fig. 33.9). Bolwell and James reported a case of ileal Peutz-Jeghers polyps that appeared grossly to form a tumor mass and infiltrate to the serosa (68). On microscopic examination this proved to be herniation (pseudoinvasion of the mucosa with cystic formation that had extruded into the muscularis propria and serosa). Shepherd et al. (69) have reported that pseudoinvasion or epithelial misplacement is present in 10% of small-intestinal Peutz-Jeghers polyps but is extremely uncommon in the large intestine. There has been a report of an epithelioid leiomyosarcoma arising in a Peutz-Jeghers polyp that had metastasized to the liver (70).

INFLAMMATORY FIBROID POLYP

GENERAL ASPECTS

Inflammatory fibroid polyps are benign tumor masses that occur in the stomach, and the small and large intestines. These uncommon lesions occur at all ages and have a worldwide distribution (71–73). Their cause is unknown, and they are not associated with any known syndromes; however, they have been reported in ileal pouches or the terminal ileum in patients with ulcerative colitis (74) and Crohn's disease (71, 75). Other terms used to describe these lesions are eosinophilic granuloma, submucosal fibroma, hemangiopericytoma, inflammatory pseudotumor, and fibroma (71–73).

CLINICAL ASPECTS

Inflammatory fibroid polyps can occur at any age (range, 3 to 80 years). The symptoms, in decreasing order of incidence, are episodic abdominal pain, vomiting, blood in the stool, diarrhea, constipation, abdominal distention, and weight loss; they may cause intussusception. The vast majority of the lesions are noted in the small intestine (mainly in the ileum); however, they can occur less commonly in the colon. Inflammatory fibroid polyps are benign, and surgical resection is curative.

PATHOLOGY

The pathology is similar whether the polyps arise in the small or the large intestine. They range in size from 1.5 to 13 cm (average, 3.0 to 4.0 cm). On gross examination most lesions are polypoid with a broad base. The bulk of the lesion resides in the submucosa; however, these polyps may infiltrate into the muscularis propria and serosa. On cut surface they tend to be tan, gray or yellow, and the overlying mucosa is often ulcerated/eroded. Microscopic examination reveals a "fibrocytic"-like lesion in a loose stroma with variable blood vessels and an inflammatory infiltrate. Around muscular walled blood vessels one finds a characteristic rarefaction (myxoid change) to the stroma. In some areas the lesions are myxoid with sparse connective tissue fibers. Various cell types are randomly distributed throughout the lesion. There are stellate and spindle-shaped fibroblasts with indistinct basophilic cytoplasm. Eosinophils, lymphocytes, plasma cells, macrophages, and mast cells are noted. Eosinophils ranged from few to dense aggregates. Cellular fields may show cells with mitotic figures with some lesions showing two mitoses per high-power fields. It is notoriously difficult to diagnose inflammatory fibroid polyps via small endoscopic biopsies, as all one usually sees is the granulation tissue from the eroded surface (Fig. 33.10).

This lesion must be distinguished from malignant mesenchymal tumors. In addition to its characteristic histology, the inflam-

matory fibroid polyp may penetrate the bowel wall with a pattern of dissection between the muscle fibers, causing a splaying or splitting of the muscle wall layer. In contrast, mesenchymal neoplasms infiltrate pushing aside the muscle wall layer (71). To date immunohistochemical studies have shown that these lesions are not neural in nature but probably are derived from myofibroblasts, histiocytes, or fibroblasts (71, 76). Also noted is heterogeneity of the immunohistochemical profile.

INFLAMMATORY PSEUDOPOLYP

INCIDENCE

Inflammatory pseudopolyps are noted in the colon and rectum. As their name suggests they are secondary to inflammatory disorders of the large intestine, such as ulcerative colitis and Crohn's disease. They may also be seen in amebiasis, schistosomiasis, ischemic colitis, at surgical anastomotic sites, and adjacent to ulcers. It has been noted that inflammatory polyps may be seen in 10 to 20% of patients with ulcerative colitis (77). In Africa, inflammatory polyps account for 25 to 30% of all colonic polyps (78, 79).

ETIOLOGY AND PATHOGENESIS

In ulcerative colitis and Crohn's disease, inflammatory pseudopolyps are primarily the result of ulceration and undermining of the adjacent intact mucosa. Because of this, the intact mucosa stands out and projects into the lumen. At times inflammatory pseudopolyps may become so extensive that they carpet a large portion of the intestinal surface. In Africa there is a high incidence of bacterial proctocolitis, which may be etiologic, as is the incidence of schistosomal infestation (78, 79).

PATHOLOGY

In ulcerative colitis or Crohn's disease these polyps are nothing more than raised tags of mucosa or submucosa (Fig. 33.11). In some polyps there is essentially no inflammation, and they consist simply of long fingers of normal mucosa. When inflammation is present they may consist of cystically dilated glands and an inflamed intervening stroma; there may also be changes of epithelial hyperplasia. Occasionally these inflammatory polyps may have bizarre stromal changes which may "mimic a sarcoma" (80, 81). The vast majority of patients reported with these changes have had inflammatory bowel disease. These lesions are usually solitary (75% of cases) and range from 1 to 6 cm, although the majority are less than 2 cm. Histologically one sees bizarre spindle, epithelioid, large ganglion-like or multinucleated cells in a fibroblastic granulation tissue stroma. Cells with prominent viral-like nucleoli may also be present. Mitoses are rare and atypical mitoses are absent. There is often a zonation effect of atypical bizarre cells and more characteristic benign spindle cells. However, this may not be apparent on a small biopsy. In distinguishing this from a malignant process one should take into consideration the pattern of zonation of bizarre cells, scanty mitoses, and lack of atypical mitoses, and also the majority of the lesions are solitary, small, and often associated with inflammatory bowel disease. Local excision of the entire lesion is curative (80, 81). Inflammatory polyps may closely resemble early juvenile polyps, which are believed by some to have an inflammatory

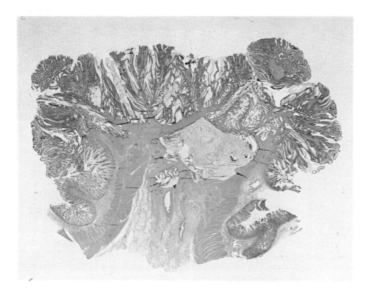

Figure 33.9 Low power view of Peutz-Jegher's polyp of the small intestine. At this power one can see mucinous cysts and herniated epithelium in the muscularis propria. This is not invasion, but entrapped or herniated mucosa (Reproduced with permission from Cooper HS. Intestinal neoplasms in diagnostic surgical pathology, Sternberg SS, ed. Raven Press).

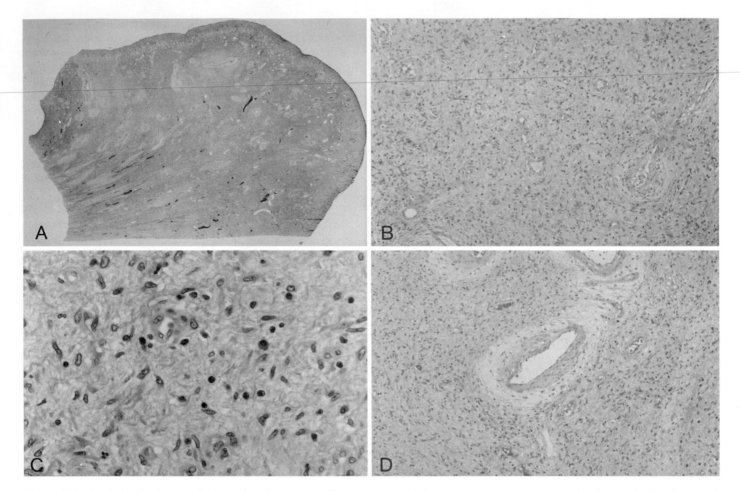

Figure 33.10 **(A)** Whole mount view of inflammatory fibroid polyp. At this power one can appreciate the eroded surface and vascularity. **(B)** Medium power view of polyp "stroma." **(C)** High power view showing loose connective tissue, bland fibrocytic spindle shaped cells, and occasional inflammatory cells. **(D)** Muscular walled blood vessel with characteristic surrounding rarefaction changes.

etiology. In young children with no history of inflammatory bowel disease and only a few polyps, care should be taken not to misdiagnose a small inflamed juvenile polyp as an inflammatory polyp.

The inflammatory polyps seen adjacent to ulcers, at surgical anastomotic sites, or in schistosomiasis tend to be small rounded nodules of granulation tissue with variable epithelial components (Fig. 33.12). With schistosomal polyps ova can often be seen.

INFLAMMATORY CAP POLYP

Inflammatory cap polyps are lesions that may be part of a spectrum of "inflammatory polyps" that have mucosal prolapse as their etiology. To date these lesions have been described only in the colon and limited to the rectosigmoid or distal colon. The majority of polyps have been described as sessile and vary in size from 0.5 to 2.0 cm. The polyps have been reported as being solitary or numerous (polyposis). Often these patients present with diarrhea and rectal bleeding. Some cases have been associated with ulcerative colitis or diverticular disease (82–85).

The histology is very similar to the spectrum of changes seen in the rectal prolapsed disorders. In general one sees an eroded

surface with a fibrinopurulent inflammatory cap. The body of the polyp shows acute and chronic inflammation, proliferation and splaying of the muscularis mucosae with fibromuscular obliteration of the lamina propria. The epithelial component is benign with hyperplastic changes, goblet cell hyperplasia, and tortuosity of glands.

INFLAMMATORY MYOGLANDULAR POLYP

This is a recently described entity which may have mucosal prolapse as its etiology. These polyps were initially described as limited to the colon (rectum, sigmoid, and descending colon) (86), however, they have also been described in the ileum causing intussusception (87).

These lesions are solitary, usually pedunculated but may also be sessile. They show a male predominance, and may present with hemorrhage. Grossly, they are spherical with a smooth surface showing erosions. On cross section one sees hyperplastic, branching and occasionally dilated glands within a background of smooth muscle fibers that have proliferated radially. The surface can be eroded with a fibrinous exudate. At low power, one is struck with the similarity of inflammatory myoglandular polyp to a juvenile polyp or a Peutz-Jeghers polyp. According to Nakamura et al. (86), juvenile polyps do not show the extent of smooth muscle proliferation as inflammatory myoglandular polyps. And Peutz-Jeghers polyps have an epithelial component that is "normal" and lacks erosions and surface granulation tissue.

DIVERTICULAR POLYP

These are polyps that arise in the background of diverticular disease and may have mucosal prolapse (at least in some part) as an etiology. Clinically these patients have symptomatology similar to that seen secondary to diverticular disease (88, 89). Endoscopically these lesions may show frank polypoid protuberances that can be confused grossly with an adenoma (88). In the study by Kelly (89) the polyps numbered from one to eleven per resection specimen and ranged in size from 0.5 to 3.0 cm. Grossly, the lesions were described as consisting of two types: (1) an "early minimal lesion" that consisted of swelling of the mucosal folds with brown stripped apices, and (2) an "advanced lesion" that was a large leaflike polyp with a broad base arising on mucosal folds. Histologically the minimal lesion showed mucosal and submucosal congestion, hemorrhage, and hemosiderin macrophages in the lamina propria and submucosa. The advanced lesions most distinctively resembled the changes seen in the mucosal prolapse disorders. There is mucosal edema, fibromuscular obliteration of the lamina propria, epithelial hyperplasia, crypt branching, crypt dilatation, and occasionally misplaced glands in the submucosa. Pseudosarcomatous changes in the stroma have been noted. Gross polyps may also be due to changes secondary to inverted diverticulum.

INTESTINAL PYOGENIC GRANULOMA

This entity was first reported in the English literature in 1995 by Yao (90) (there were two previous reported cases in the Japanese literature). Yao reported three cases—one in the colon, one in the ileum, and one on the jejunal side of a gastrojejunostomy. Clinically these patients had bleeding, anemia, and melena. Grossly, the lesions were polypoid and sessile, ranging from 0.7 to 2.5 cm in size and were described as dark brown or black, with a necrotic covering. Microscopically, two of the three cases involved the entire bowel wall thickness and the other was limited to the mucosa. All three cases were ulcerated. All cases showed a classic lobular arrangement of capillaries with a single layer of flattened or rounded endothelial cells. There was no papillary endothelial hyperplasia. There were sparse spindle cells and a delicate collagenous stroma. The stroma showed edema and inflammatory cells.

GRANULATION TISSUE POLYPOSIS

This is an uncommon polyposis disorder of "granulation tissue" proliferation associated with carcinoid tumors of the ileum (91). In the two reported cases, the polyps were limited to the segment of bowel with an infiltrating carcinoid tumor. These polyps are numerous (in the hundreds in one case), sessile, and up to 0.5 cm in size. They are nodular and pale brown in color. Microscopically they consist of nodules of granulation tissue (capillary, plasma cells, and lymphocytes) and smooth muscle cells, changes which are not unlike those seen in the mucosal prolapse disorders. Interestingly, the authors reviewed 55 random cases of ileal carcinoids and found two more cases with similar but less pronounced changes.

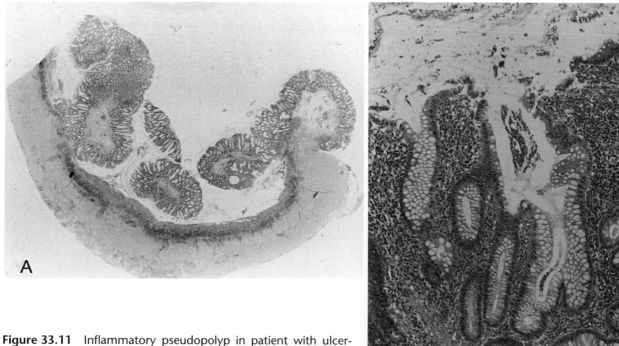

Figure 33.11 Inflammatory pseudopolyp in patient with ulcerative colitis. **(A)** Whole mount view. The polyps are due to residual mucosa adjacent to ulcerated epithelium. **(B)** Medium power view. The glands are distorted and leukocytes are noted in the lumen. The lamina propria has a dense chronic inflammatory infiltrate.

Figure 33.12 Colonic inflammatory pseudopolyp. **(A)** The surface is capped with granulation tissue and the basal glands are dilated and distorted. **(B)** Medium power view, showing distorted hypertrophic benign goblet cells. **(C)** High power view of the cap of granulation tissue.

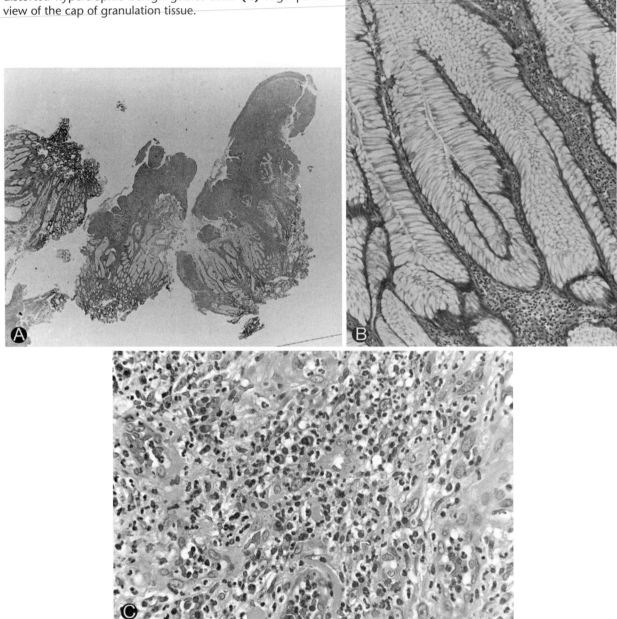

ATHEROEMBOLI ASSOCIATED INFLAMMATORY POLYPS

Chivelle et al. (92) reported a case of an individual with a two-year history of bloody diarrhea, abdominal pain, and atheroemboli associated inflammatory type polyps. These lesions consisted of broad-based polyps covered with a brown granular mucosa and occasional erosion, ranging in size from 0.3 to 1.9 cm. Microscopically these were essentially ischemic polypoid granulation tissue consisting of superficial erosion, granulation tissue, reactive epithe- lial cells, coagulative necrosis, hyperplasia of the muscularis muco- sae, and atheroemboli in the submucosal arterioles.

UNIFYING CONCEPT OF MUCOSAL PROLAPSE

The entities of inflammatory cap polyp(osis), inflammatory myo- glandular polyp, and diverticular polyp all have some histologic overlaps within the spectrum of mucosal prolapse. This has led some to consider that these lesions are all part of the same etiology and are not separate entities but may simply represent different stages of development on a temporal basis (83). On the other hand Nakamuro (86) feels strongly that the entity of inflammatory myoglandular polyp is distinctly different than inflammatory cap polyps and other mucosal prolapse related disorders.

JUVENILE POLYP

INCIDENCE AND EPIDEMIOLOGY

Juvenile polyps occur most commonly during the first two decades of life, but they are not uncommonly seen in adults. They are essentially limited to the colon and rectum, but the small intestine and stomach may be involved in cases of juvenile polyposis (see the section on Polyposis). In an autopsy study from the United States of patients younger than 21 years of age, the incidence of juvenile polyps was 1% (93). In Cali, Colombia, an autopsy study of children under 14 years of age reported an incidence of 3.1% (15). In Jordanians the calculated incidence is 1.6 per 100,000 of the total population and 2.8 per 100,000 in people under 10 years of age (94). In Nigeria, juvenile polyps are the most common type of polyp seen, representing from 53 to 60% of all polyps seen in surgically obtained material (78, 79). In these African studies the age distribution is similar to that seen in Western countries. The solitary juvenile polyp does not have an inherited (genetic) etiology.

ETIOLOGY AND PATHOGENESIS

Some authors believe that juvenile polyps are hamartomatous in nature (8), and others have proposed an inflammatory etiology (95, 96). Studies of patients with juvenile polyposis suggest that the initiating event is mucosal hyperplasia and the formation of small hyperplastic polyps. This is followed by inflammation and ulceration with sealing off of the surface, obstruction, and subsequent dilatation of crypts and the formation of a characteristic juvenile polyp (97–99). Subramony et al. (96), studying the random nonpolypoid and nodular mucosa of patients with juvenile polyposis, believe that the earliest event is a dense inflammatory infiltrate in the superficial upper third of the crypt prior to any epithelial changes.

CLINICAL ASPECTS

Juvenile polyps occur most commonly as solitary lesions (85 to 90% of the cases) localized mainly in the rectum. In the childhood and adult groups, rectal bleeding is the most common presenting symptom, occurring in approximately 80% of the patients. Abdominal cramps is also an associated symptom. In the childhood group, approximately 20% present with prolapse or protrusion of the polyp; in about 10% of children the polyp is first discovered when it has been spontaneously passed in the stool (autoamputation).

The solitary (nonpolyposis) juvenile polyp is a benign proliferation which rarely undergoes neoplastic change and is not associated with an increased risk for developing colorectal cancer (100). There have been four reports of adenomatous change within solitary juvenile polyps (94, 101–103) and two reported cases of adenocarcinoma arising in solitary juvenile polyps (94, 104). Another reported case involves a 17-year old female patient with two juvenile polyps and a concomitant villous adenoma with carcinoma in situ (105). The clinical manifestations and neoplastic changes associated with juvenile polyposis will be discussed under the section on Polyposis.

PATHOLOGY

On gross examination, juvenile polyps have a smooth, glistening surface and are of a reddish-tan to red color (Fig. 33.13). Cut section shows cystic spaces filled with grayish white or creamy yellow fluid. Most juvenile polyps are pedunculated, but occasionally they may be sessile.

In the "fully developed" juvenile polyp cystically dilated glands are seen in an inflamed stroma (Fig. 33.14). The glands, which are often tortuous, may be made up of well formed mucus-secreting cells. When the glands are filled with mucus the epithelial cells may be attenuated. Pink regenerative epithelium, similar to that in hyperplastic polyps, can be seen in 45% of the cases. When the cystically dilated glands rupture they incite an inflammatory reaction in the stroma. Occasionally areas of osseous metaplasia are present. The microscopic appearance of early juvenile polyps may be easily confused with that of inflammatory pseudopolyps, which appear as a cap of florid granulation tissue sitting on top of cystically dilated or hyperplastic crypts.

LYMPHOID POLYP

Lymphoid polyps occur mainly in the rectum and occasionally in the ileum. They occur in all age groups, but most commonly in the second through fifth decades of life. They may be found incidentally or may occasionally cause symptoms such as rectal bleeding, discomfort, or prolapse. Lymphoid polyps vary in size from a few millimeters up to 3 cm. Approximately 80% of polyps are sessile and 20% are pedunculated. The polyps are solitary in 80% of the cases, but occur in groups of two to six in the remaining 20%. Microscopically they consist of prominent lymphoid follicles with active germinal centers. These lymphoid aggregates are located mainly in the mucosa and the submucosa; however, they rarely may involve the muscularis propria. Local excision is curative, and recurrence is rare. Occasional spontaneous remission of these lesions has been noted (106, 107).

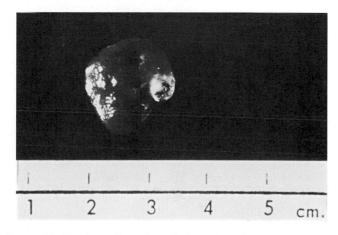

Figure 33.13 Juvenile polyp of the colon showing a smooth shiny surface. These polyps are of a tan, reddish color. In this instance, the point of transection by fulgeration can be appreciated.

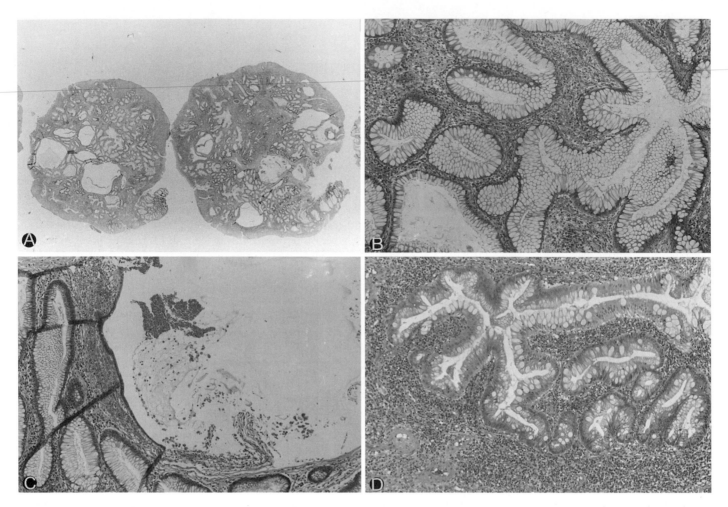

Figure 33.14 Juvenile polyp of the colon. **(A)** Whole mount section. There are cystically dilated glands interspersed with distorted branching glands. The intervening stroma is expanded. **(B)** Branching glands; the epithelium is totally benign. **(C)** Cystically dilated glands filled with mucin and polyps. **(D)** Focus of hyperplastic epithelium.

NEOPLASTIC POLYPS

ADENOMA

Adenomas are benign neoplastic polyps of the small and the large intestines and are classified pathologically (microscopically) as either tubular, tubulovillous, or villous. Classification of adenomas may also be based upon the gross appearance (e.g., flat adenoma). Adenomas are important clinically because they are premalignant lesions that have the potential for developing into cancer. Although this chapter describes polyps of both the small and the large intestines, the reader should be aware that adenomas are rare in the small intestine (except in hereditary polyposis syndrome) and quite common in the large intestine. The vast majority of what is discussed in this chapter relates to large intestinal adenomas. Small intestinal adenomas will only be briefly referred to.

INCIDENCE, EPIDEMIOLOGY, AND SITE DISTRIBUTION

The incidence or prevalence of colonic adenomas varies in different parts of the world. Autopsy studies indicate that colonic adenomas tend to be fairly common in Western cultures (as high as 60% in one autopsy study) (108) and rare in underdeveloped countries (as low as 5.5% in another autopsy study) (15). The incidence of adenomas generally parallels the incidence of cancer and the socioeconomic gradient, both of which are related to the Western lifestyle and diet. Race and country of origin, per se, do not have a role in the incidence of adenomas. Japanese and Africans who have migrated to Westernized societies take up the incidence of their new environment (13). All autopsy studies regardless of geographic location or incidence of colorectal cancer show an increased incidence of adenomas as the population ages, especially for the group 60 years of age and older (15, 108–110). In fact, in Cali, Colombia, the incidence of adenomas rises to 20% in the population over 65 years of age (15). Among asymptomatic individuals undergoing colonoscopy, the prevalence of adenomas has been reported as 39% (111). Among asymptomatic individuals undergoing sigmoidoscopy, the prevalence of individuals with distal adenomas is approximately 18% (4–6, 112). Adenomas usually appear singly, but may also be multiple (synchronous and metachronous). Two large colonoscopic studies from New York (113) and London (114) report an incidence of multiple adenomas (two or more) as 36% and 50%, respectively. The incidence of metachronous adenomas is approximately 30% in colonoscopic studies of patients with an adenoma (115, 116). Autopsy studies have shown multiple lesions in 2 to 16% of the population (15, 108–110), with the lower percentage being reported from underdeveloped countries. Regarding the incidence of histologic types of adenomas most autopsy studies report that of all adenomas, 95% are tubular, 2 to 4% are tubulovillous, and the remaining lesions are villous (15, 108–110, 117, 118). In colonoscopic material, however, the reported incidence of tubular adenomas is 65 to 85%; of tubulovillous adenomas, 8.2 to 27%; and of villous adenomas, 3 to 9% (113, 114, 119, 120). The distribution of colonic adenomas will vary, depending on whether data were obtained from autopsy or colonoscopic material. Most colonoscopic studies report that 75% of adenomas occur in the left colon with the great preponderance in the sigmoid colon (113, 114, 119). On the other hand, autopsy studies report an even distribution of adenomas throughout the entire length of the bowel (113, 114, 118). This discrepancy may be explained on the basis of size of the polyp. Most adenomas less than 1.0 cm in size tend to show an even distribution throughout the entire large intestine, whereas those greater than 1.0 cm tend to be located in the distal colon. It is easier to identify smaller lesions in careful autopsy studies than in colonoscopic studies. In fact, 88% of adenomas in autopsy material tend to be under 1.0 cm in size whereas only 48% of adenomas in colonoscopic material are under 1.0 cm in size.

ETIOLOGY

Carcinogenesis is a multistage process that includes inception (initiation) and growth (progression). Cannon-Albright et al. (112) comment that an underlying genetic susceptibility is present in the majority of persons with common adenomas and cancer and that environmental factors interact with genetic factors to determine which individuals develop adenomas or cancer. Hypotheses regarding the etiology of adenomas have accounted for both genetic and environmental factors. Hill et al. (121) have proposed that there is a recessive gene *(p)* that leads to the potential for development of adenomas. Thus persons who carry two *p* genes *(pp)* would have a tendency for development of adenomas. However, the development of an adenoma would be predicated solely on some environmental factor working on the *pp* population. Recent studies have confirmed the genetic susceptibility to developing sporadic adenomas. These studies have shown that patients with a first-degree relative with a history of colorectal cancer had twice the incidence of adenomas than those with no family history. These individuals also had a significantly greater incidence of high grade dysplasia and proximal location (111, 112, 122). Furthermore, other environmental factors act on the already formed adenoma to transform it into a cancer. As mentioned previously, those Japanese and Africans who have left their native lands and moved to new environments in the West have a much greater incidence of adenomas than do those who remain in their native environment (13). Other factors such as lifestyle and diet may also be important. Studies have reported adenomas to be associated with increased levels of dietary saturated fat, red meat, and decreased dietary consumption of cruciferous vegetables. A protective effect against the formation of adenomas has been associated with increased dietary fiber, Vitamin A, and vegetables. Cigarette smoking and alcohol consumption have also been implicated in the epidemiology of adenomas (123–126). See Chapter 7 for a detailed discussion of the genetics of adenomas.

CLINICAL ASPECTS

In patients with adenomas, the predominant symptom is rectal bleeding, followed by varying symptoms of altered bowel habits, abdominal pain, flatulence, and mucus discharge. However, today more and more patients have no symptoms but are discovered with the multiple screening techniques used in the over 40 years of age population (e.g., test for occult blood, barium enema, and colonoscopy).

POLYP CANCER SEQUENCE

The major clinical significance of adenomas is that they are precancerous lesions, i.e., adenomas may undergo change into carcinomas. This is true for both large-bowel adenomas and small-intestinal adenomas. The polyp cancer sequence discussed below relates to the large bowel only. Four major types of studies—epidemiologic, clinical, molecular, and morphologic (size, histologic type, and atypia)—are used. Many studies have shown that the incidence of adenomas parallels the incidence of large-bowel carcinoma (13-15). In general, those countries with low rates of colon cancer have low rates of adenomas. In populations where the incidence of colon cancer is low, intermediate, and high, the incidence of adenomas is 5.5%, 13 to 35%, and 50 to 60%, respectively (13-15). The relationship between sites of large-bowel cancer and the corresponding site distribution of large-bowel adenoma is also important in the polyp cancer sequence. Most colon cancers arise in the distal colon; however, autopsy studies report an even distribution of polyps throughout the large intestine, whereas colonoscopic studies report a predominance of adenomas to occur in the left side. However, such data must be considered in conjunction with other factors such as size and dysplasia as related to site. Smaller adenomas tend to be distributed evenly throughout the large intestine, whereas larger adenomas with high grade dysplasia tend to be located in the sigmoid colon (108, 109, 113, 114, 120), and size and high grade dysplasia play important roles in the malignant transformation of adenomas. The size of an adenoma is related to its malignant potential. Three major colonoscopic studies reported that carcinoma in situ was found in 5% of adenomas less than 1.0 cm, in 13% of adenomas from 1.0 to 1.9 cm, and in 18% of adenomas from 2.0 to 2.9 cm in size (113, 120). It also noted that invasive cancer was present in 0.5% of adenomas under 1.0 cm, in 5% of adenomas from 1.0 to 1.9 cm, and 10% of adenomas from 2.0 to 2.9 cm in size (113). Lesions larger than 1.0 cm in size (127, 128) tend to be located in the sigmoid colon, the region of the large intestine with the greatest incidence of cancer (109, 113, 114, 119).

The type of adenoma, or its growth pattern, has a role in its malignant potential. The incidence of carcinomatous change is higher in villous than in tubular adenomas while tubulovillous adenomas have an intermediate incidence (2 to 3% in tubular adenomas, 6 to 8% in tubulovillous adenomas, and 10 to 18% in villous adenomas) (113, 114, 119). When the size of the adenoma and its histologic type are considered, the incidence of invasive cancer in lesions smaller than 1.0 cm is 0.3% in tubular adenomas, 1.5% in tubulovillous adenomas, and 2.5% in villous adenomas; in lesions larger than 2.0 cm the incidence of invasive cancer is 6.5% in tubular adenomas, 11.4% in tubulovillous adenomas, and 17% in villous adenomas. These data show that although size is important in predicting malignant potential, villous adenomas of any size have

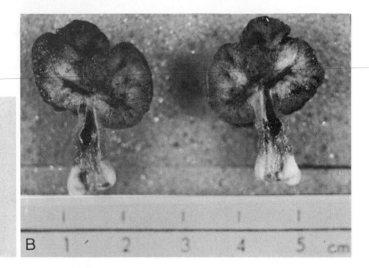

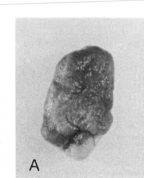

Figure 33.15 Adenoma of the colon. **(A)** Surface view of an adenoma with a short stalk. **(B)** Another adenoma with long stalk bisected after fixation. All important landmarks can be appreciated.

a greater propensity for malignant changes than do tubular adenomas. Similar studies by Morson support this (127).

High grade dysplasia (defined in the section on Pathology) is an important marker or determinant in the polyp cancer sequence. Colonoscopic studies have found that the sigmoid colon is the portion of the large intestine with the highest incidence of adenomas that show advanced high grade dysplasia (113, 114). This correlates with the major site for colon cancer. Autopsy studies show that the incidence of high grade dysplasia clearly parallels the incidence of carcinoma (14, 129). The incidences of invasive cancer in tubular adenomas, tubulovillous adenomas, and villous adenomas, with mild dysplasia present, was 2.0%, 13.9%, and 36.2%, respectively. Compare those values to 27%, 34%, and 50% in tubular adenomas, tubulovillous adenomas, and villous adenomas with high grade dysplasia (129). The size, degree of dysplasia, and histologic type can also be predictive of future cancer. Atkin et al. showed that patients with distal adenomas with a villous component larger than 1 cm in size, or high grade dysplasia, had an incidence of colon cancer 3.6 time higher than a control population. If adenomas were multiple, this increased to 6.0 times higher incidence (130).

Clinical studies also lend support for the adenoma cancer sequence. In a recent National Polyp Study, Winawer et al. found that by clearing the colon of adenomas (polypectomies) they were able to reduce the incidence of colorectal cancer by 90%, 88%, and 76% versus three control groups (131). A similar study of surveillance polypectomies in patients from families with purported hereditary nonpolyposis colon cancer showed a halving in the rate of colorectal cancer in at risk members of families with hereditary nonpolyposis colon cancer (132).

Molecular studies are also supportive of the adenoma cancer sequence. There has been an explosion of information regarding the molecular events from normal epithelium to early adenoma, advanced adenoma, and malignant (carcinomatous) changes in adenomas (133–135). These events have been sequenced as: (1) APC mutation; (2) hyperproliferative state; (3) early adenoma; (4) K-Ras mutation; (5) intermediate adenoma; (6) allelic loss of chromosome 18q (DCC); (7) late adenoma; (8) allelic loss of chromosome 17p (*p*53); (9) malignant change. See Chapter 8 for detailed discussion of molecular changes in adenoma cancer sequence.

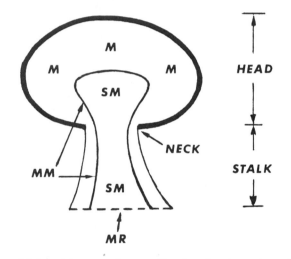

Figure 33.16 Diagram of normal landmarks of a pedunculated adenoma. mucosa (M), muscularis mucosae (MM), submucosa (SM), margin of resection (MR).

PATHOLOGY

For adequate evaluation of the pathology of an adenoma in the polypectomy specimen, particularly when a malignancy is suspected, it is important that the specimen be adequately fixed and grossly examined carefully so that the tissue is cut properly for optimal orientation. The gross lesion should be carefully examined for a stalk or pedicle. If a stalk or pedicle is short or absent, the site of transection can be identified by the diathermy mark, which is white or tan in color. The polyp should be transected longitudinally so that the slide shows all the landmarks in continuity (Fig. 33.15). The important histologic landmarks of an adenoma are: the head, the neck, transection margin, and the stalk (if pedunculated). The stalk consists of the nonneoplastic epithelium that makes up the pedicle of the adenoma. The point where the stalk meets the adenomatous epithelium is the neck, and the remainder of the polyp is the head. The point of transection or margin is the free edge of submucosa containing diathermy change (Fig. 33.16). The muscularis mucosae, another important landmark, separates the mucosa from the submucosa. These landmarks become important when reporting adenomas that contain invasive cancer.

SMALL-INTESTINAL ADENOMA

Adenomas of the small intestine are uncommon but are of either the tubular or the villous type. Grossly they are more commonly sessile. Microscopically they consist of papillary fronds with adenomatous epithelium, as in the colonic adenomas. Occasionally one may see adenomatous epithelium alternating with and adjacent to normal nonneoplastic villi. One may also see villi partially replaced by adenomatous epithelium. All degrees of dysplasia, including intramucosal in situ and invasive cancer, can occur (Fig. 33.17).

LARGE-INTESTINAL ADENOMA

Grossly, adenomas may be pedunculated (stalked), sessile, or flat. It has been generally taught that tubular adenomas were always pedunculated and that villous adenomas were characteristically sessile. However, tubular adenomas may be sessile and villous adenomas may be pedunculated. On gross examination tubular adenomas tend to be spherical and have a relatively smooth surface that is often divided into what appears to be "lobules," as a result of intercommunicating clefts in the head of the adenoma, while villous adenomas tend to have a papillary or shaggy-carpet–like appearance.

The adenoma is often darker or redder than the surrounding mucosa. A stalk may be present (Fig. 33.18). Villous adenomas tend to have a "shaggy" surface with obvious papillary fronds (Fig. 33.19). In autopsy material 88% of adenomas are smaller than

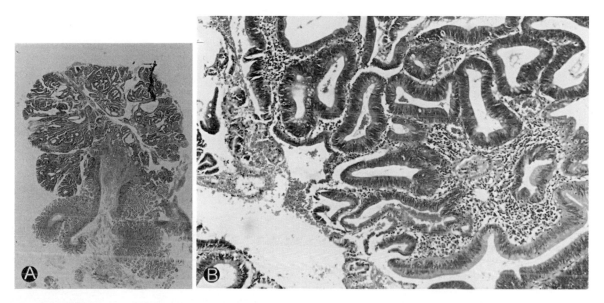

Figure 33.17 Small intestinal adenoma. **(A)** Whole mount view. **(B)** Microscopic view showing classic changes of adenoma with hyperchromatic and stratified nuclei.

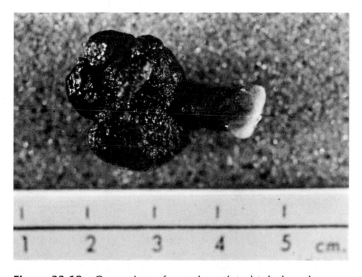

Figure 33.18 Gross view of a pedunculated tubular adenoma of the colon. The head of the polyp is dark (red), lobulated and fissured. A long stalk (pedicle) is obvious.

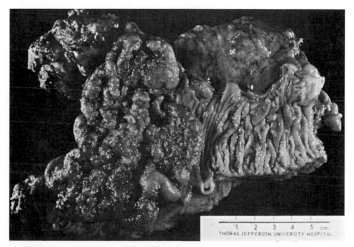

Figure 33.19 Gross photograph of a large villous adenoma. This lesion is spreading and sessile in nature.

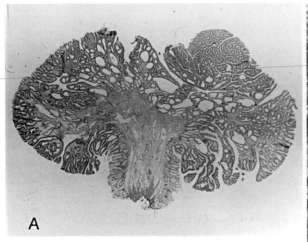

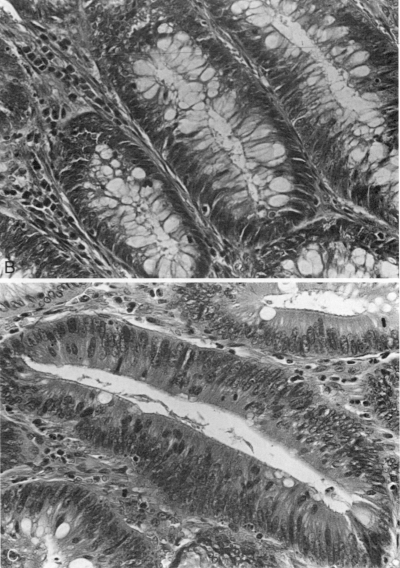

Figure 33.20 Tubular adenoma of the colon. **(A)** Whole mount view. At this magnification one can appreciate that the neoplastic glands are forming tubules. **(B)** High power view. Adenomatous epithelium with preserved mucus production (goblet cells) and intervening lamina propria is evident. **(C)** High power view. In this field there is marked decrease in mucus production.

1.0 cm (108, 109); in colonoscopy material 48% of adenomas are smaller than 1.0 cm, 35% are 1 to 2 cm in size, and 17% are larger than 2.0 cm (123). In general there is a correlation between the lesion's size and its histologic type. Regarding adenomas less than 1.0 cm in size, 91% are tubular adenomas, 7% are tubulovillous adenomas, and 2% are villous adenomas. However, of lesions greater than 2.0 cm in size, 48% are tubular adenomas, 38% are tubulovillous adenomas, 12% are villous adenomas, and 2% are polypoid carcinomas (119). Irrespective of type, all adenomas consist of neoplastic (adenomatous) epithelium. The overall growth pattern determines whether an adenoma qualifies as tubular, tubulovillous, or villous. In tubular adenomas there is a proliferation of adenomatous epithelium that forms tubules, which are usually separated from each other by normal lamina propria. In the usual tubular adenoma, the tubules are regular with little branching or tufting (changes that are seen with increasing degrees of dysplasia). The epithelial cells themselves show enlarged nuclei, which are hyperchromatic and elongated in shape; stratification of nuclei is common. Mucin may be absent or present, and can vary from well-formed goblets to small

apical mucin vacuoles. In general the loss of mucin production correlates with advanced degrees of dysplasia (Fig. 33.20). In villous adenomas, one sees similar epithelial changes; however, the overall configuration is that of a growth of fine fingerlets or villi that project perpendicularly from the muscularis mucosae to the outer tip of the adenoma (Fig. 33.21). Because many adenomas show mixed features of both tubules and villi, what determines the classification of a lesion as one or the other? Some authors say that if at least 80% of the lesion is either tubular or villous, then the lesion is classified as such, and all others are tubulovillous adenomas (114); others use a standard of at least 75% (113). The World Health Organization uses the 80% cutoff (136).

Adenomas by definition show dysplasia. The World Health Organization (136) and National Polyp Study (120) both use a classification of mild, moderate, and severe dysplasia, and/or a classification of low grade dysplasia (mild or moderate dysplasia) or high grade dysplasia (severe dysplasia). In today's practice of pathology the high grade-low grade system is most commonly used and is becoming the norm (120, 136, 137). The "usual" adenoma is considered to be of low grade dysplasia. The term high grade dysplasia is supplanting (replacing) the term carcinoma in situ which now with severe dysplasia falls into the category of high grade dysplasia. In high grade dysplasia one sees both architectural and cytologic changes. Architecturally the crypts show irregular branching or budding, or show a cribriform or back-to-back pattern. Cytologically the nuclei are greatly enlarged, ovoid or round, hyperchromatic, or vesicular with prominent nucleoli. Mitotic figures are prominent and some are abnormal. Areas of necrosis may be present and cytoplasmic mucin production may be absent or reduced (Figs. 33.22 and 33.23).

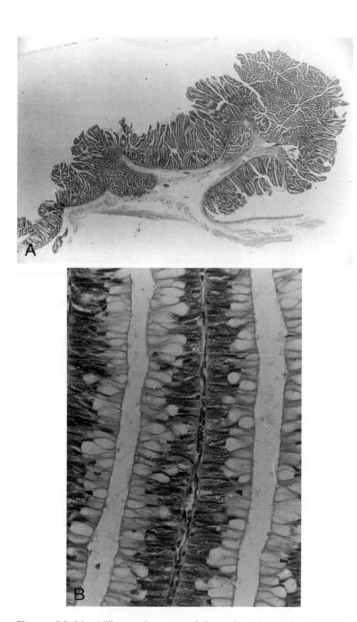

Figure 33.21 Villous adenoma of the colon. **(A)** Whole mount view. One can appreciate that the neoplastic epithelium is thrown up into villous projections. **(B)** High power view. The nuclei are stratified in a typical nature. In this instance, mucus production is preserved.

FLAT ADENOMA

In 1985 Muto et al. (138) reported on small (up to 1 cm) grossly flat polyps which showed a relatively high percentage of "malignancy" (severe dysplasia). Since this publication there have been numerous articles published on flat adenomas. The vast majority have been published by the Japanese and as of this writing controversy exists about these flat adenomas. Many investigators believe that these flat adenomas are precursors of small cancers that rapidly grow into deeply penetrating cancers, although some may grow into classic polypoid adenomas (139–141). Some believe that these aggressive adenomas are rare in Western societies (142).

In prospective colonoscopic screening studies, the incidence of flat adenoma has varied from 2.8% (143) to 24% (144). Other terms such as depressed adenomas can probably be equated with flat adenoma (139, 145). Grossly these lesions are usually less than 1 cm in size, have a reddish surface, and have a slight elevation. The surface is not dome shaped but rather flat and a central depression is occasionally seen. These lesions are difficult to detect endoscopically, however, with the use of dye spraying methods (chromoendoscopy) these lesions are more readily appreciated (144). Most articles report a male predominance of from 3:1 to 6:1 (138, 140, 146). The literature is conflicting as to site distribution, with some reporting no site predilection (143), others a right colon predilection (140). Reported studies indicate a family history of colorectal cancer in 10 to 20% of cases (144, 146, 147).

Adachi et al. (146) reported that 16% of cases had two or more flat adenomas while Wolber and Owen (147) reported that 50% of patients had two or more flat adenomas.

Histologically, the vast majority of lesions are reported as tubular adenomas (138, 144, 146, 147). At low power microscopy, the height of the flat adenoma is never greater than two times the height of the adjacent nonneoplastic mucosa. The central portion of the lesion shows full thickness dysplasia while the periphery of the lesion tends to show dysplastic glands at the surface of the crypt "sitting atop" nonneoplastic glands at the base of the crypt (Fig. 33.24). It is very important to remember that a flat adenoma is not defined solely by this "characteristic" histology but rather by its gross or endoscopic appearance. Samowitz et al. (148) have shown that among 127 sequentially accessioned adenomas, 25% showed the "classic" histologic features of flat adenoma "but none were grossly flat and none showed high grade dysplasia."

In the original article by Muto et al. (138) the reported incidence of high grade dysplasia was 40%. Wolber and Owen reported a 41% incidence of high grade dysplasia (147). However, subsequent studies of larger numbers have reported a lower incidence of high grade dysplasia ranging from 10 to 12% (143, 144, 146). In all studies the incidence of high grade dysplasia correlated directly with the size of the lesion. The incidence of high grade dysplasia in lesions less than 5 mm is less than 10% while the incidence of high grade dysplasia in lesions 1 cm in size has been 35 to 40%. If one compares the incidence of high grade dysplasia to classic polypoid adenomas under 1 cm in size, the incidence of high grade dysplasia in flat adenomas is much greater. The discrepancies of reported incidence of high grade dysplasia and so called small early invasive cancers could relate to differences in diagnostic criteria. Uno et al. (149) showed that among seven flat lesions one pathologist diagnosed five cases as flat depressed cancer and two cases as borderline cancer while another pathologist diagnosed one case as early flat depressed cancer and six cases as flat adenomas.

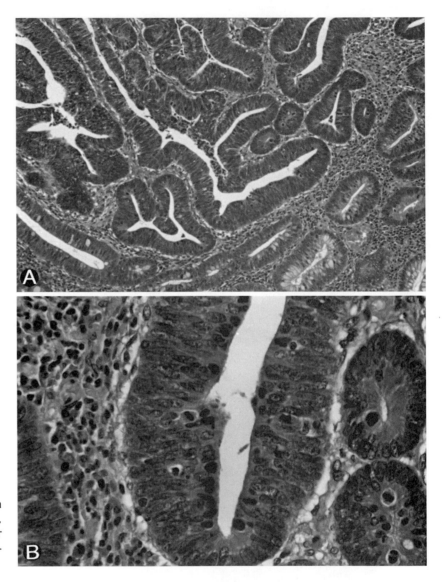

Figure 33.22 **(A)** Low power view of adenoma with high grade dysplasia. There is a branching, budding, or buckling of glands. **(B)** High power view showing nuclei proliferating to the gland lumen and loss of mucin.

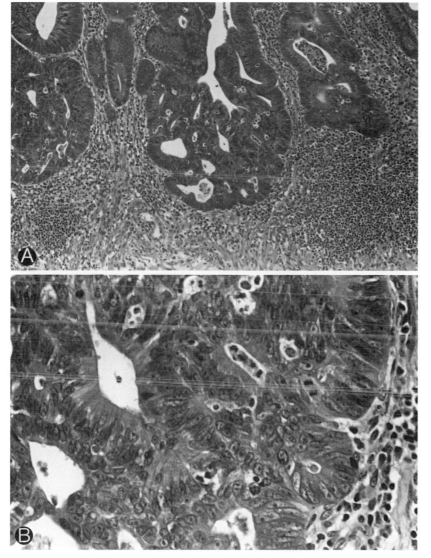

Figure 33.23 **(A)** Low power view of adenoma with high grade dysplasia. There is cribriforming or back to back glands. **(B)** High power view of **A**.

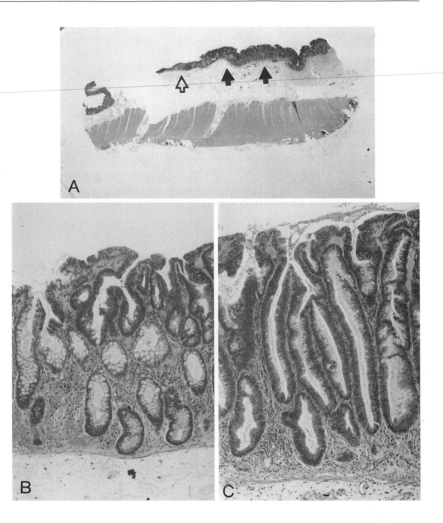

Figure 33.24 **(A)** Low power view of flat adenoma. The height of the adenoma *(closed arrow)* is not greater than twice the height of the nonneoplastic mucosa *(open arrow)*. **(B)** Periphery of adenoma, showing dysplastic (adenomatous) glands on the surface with nonneoplastic glands below. **(C)** Center of adenoma showing neoplastic (adenomatous) changes through the full thickness of the mucosa.

Therefore problems exist with interobserver variation and probably terminology. Minamoto et al. (140) emphasizes that there is a difference in definition of degrees of dysplasia and "carcinoma" between Japanese pathologists and Western pathologists. From reviewing illustrations of various articles, it would appear that in flat adenomas the diagnosis of high grade dysplasia is more often predicated on cytologic changes rather than architectural changes.

Flat adenomas have a significantly lower incidence of K-Ras codon 12 point mutations than do polypoid adenomas (23% versus 67%) (141, 150, 151).

ADENOMA IN HEREDITARY NONPOLYPOSIS COLON CANCER

Hereditary nonpolyposis colon cancer (HNPCC) is a genetic disorder with abnormalities on chromosomes 2p and 3p. This relates to mutations in the mismatch repair genes hMSH2, hMLH1, hPMS1, and hPMS2 (152). While this is not a polyposis disorder, it has been shown that adenomas are precursors of cancers and that screening and polypectomy in this group of patients will reduce the incidence of cancer (132). Most studies indicate that HNPCC patients do not have an increased number of adenomas compared to the general population (153, 154). However, it has been proposed

that adenomas in HNPCC patients have a greater predilection for malignant change (154, 155). Mecklin et al. (156) reported 23% of adenomas in HNPCC with cancer had high grade dysplasia versus 13% of controls. In an autopsy study, Jass and Stewart (157) reported that the adenomas from HNPCC patients with cancer had a significantly greater incidence of high grade dysplasia, villous configuration, and larger size compared to controls. In a colonoscopic study of patients at risk for HNPCC, Jass et al. (158) found a significantly higher incidence of high grade dysplasia and villous component compared to autopsy controls. However, the incidence of high grade dysplasia was not significantly higher than a surgical/sigmoidoscopy series from the St. Marks Hospital of London, England. In a prospective study of patients at risk for HNPCC, this increased prevalence of high grade dysplasia and villous growth has not been noted by Lynch et al. (159) who found only small tubular adenomas with no high grade dysplasia.

Microsatellite instability has been detected in the majority of adenomas from patients with HNPCC (160, 161) suggesting that the development of genomic instability is an early event. The number of altered microsatellite foci is smaller in completely benign adenomas than in adenomas with foci of cancer (162). However, in most studies to date, mutations in *p*53 are not found any more frequently in tumors with microsatellite instability than in those without it (163–165).

ADENOMA WITH CANCER

Both small-intestinal and large-intestinal adenomas are precancerous lesions. The incidence of high grade dysplasia (in situ cancer) arising in colonic adenomas is 12.3%, whereas the incidence of invasive cancer arising in colonic adenomas is about 5% (115). The term malignant polyp should be restricted to those adenomas (or polypoid carcinoma) in which there is true invasive cancer. The term invasive cancer should be used to describe only those lesions in which cancer has invaded beyond the muscularis mucosae into the submucosa. The lymphatics of the colon are closely associated with the muscularis mucosae, and only after the cancer has invaded into the submucosa does it have the biologic potential for metastasis. Cancer that is limited to the mucosa has been variously termed high grade dysplasia, in situ carcinoma, or intramucosal adenocarcinoma. However, none of these entities has the biological potential for metastases.

PATHOLOGY

High grade dysplasia (previously called in situ cancer) is diagnosed when there is "buckling," bridging, or cribriform growth of epithelial cells with accompanying cytologic atypia all within the confines of the basement membrane. Intramucosal cancer shows the same changes as high grade dysplasia; in addition, tumor cells invade into the mucosal stroma of the lamina propria and elicit an inflammatory or desmoplastic reaction (Fig. 33.25). In many adenomas the muscularis mucosae is quite irregular and appears splayed or splintered. This must be considered when a lesion with high grade dysplasia or intramucosal adenocarcinoma is examined, as the splayed muscularis mucosae may surround and envelope crypts, mimicking invasive cancer and possibly trapping the uninitiated observer into making an incorrect diagnosis of invasive cancer. Invasive cancer should be diagnosed only when tumor cells have invaded beyond the muscularis mucosae into the submucosa.

Figure 33.25   (A) Low power view of intramucosal adenocarcinoma. Note the cells invading into the lamina propria *(arrows)*. Compare this to high grade dysplasia (Figs. 33.22 and 33.23) where the neoplastic process remains confined within the basement membrane. **(B)** High power view showing cancer cells "invading" in the lamina propria.

The presence of an investment of "lamina propria" around epithelial glands is often helpful in differentiating entrapped epithelium from invasive cancer.

In the case of an adenoma with invasive cancer, the following parameters should be reported: (1) status of the resection margin, (2) histologic grade of the cancer, and (3) the presence or absence of lymphatic and or venous invasion by cancer (Figs. 33.26 through 33.30).

PATIENT MANAGEMENT IN LARGE-INTESTINAL MALIGNANT POLYPS

The pathologist plays an important role in the management of the patient with an endoscopically removed malignant colorectal polyp.

Among numerous reports of endoscopically removed malignant colorectal polyps, the incidence of adverse outcome (local and/or distant recurrence in polypectomy-only cases, or local residual disease and/or lymph node metastases in cases of surgical resection subsequent to polypectomy) is approximately 13% (166–179). However, there are certain histologic parameters which can predict which patients are more likely to have an adverse outcome and more likely need a definitive postpolypectomy surgical resection. In general, most investigators believe that if cancer is at or near the endoscopically transected margin, and/or grade III, and/or with lymphatic or venous invasion then a definitive surgical resection is recommended, while in the absence of all of these unfavorable histologic parameters, then endoscopic polypectomy most likely is adequate therapy (166–169, 172, 173, 175, 179). The

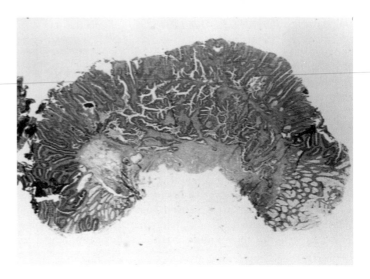

Figure 33.27   Short stalked adenoma of the colon with cancer invading the submucosa. The margin of resection is free of cancer.

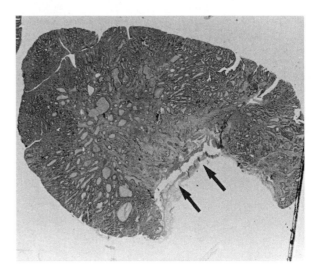

Figure 33.28   Sessile adenoma with invasive cancer extending to the transected margin of resection *(arrow)*.

incidence of adverse outcome in the presence of any unfavorable histologic parameter is approximately 20%. The incidence of adverse outcome in the absence of unfavorable histologic parameters as reviewed from the literature is 1.7% (179).

In a large interinstitutional study we found the incidence of adverse outcome to be 21.4% when tumor is at or near (within 1 mm) the margin, while the literature reports a 33% incidence (179). The margin of resection is the edge of submucosa that was transected. This usually has diathermy to help identify the margin. Tumor at the margin means tumor cells at the actual margin. The term negative margin is defined differently by various authors as: (1) not within the diathermy (166), (2) greater than one high power field from the diathermy (171), (3) greater than 1 mm from the margin (172), and (4) greater than 2 mm from the margin (180). In the literature the incidence of adverse outcome in the presence of

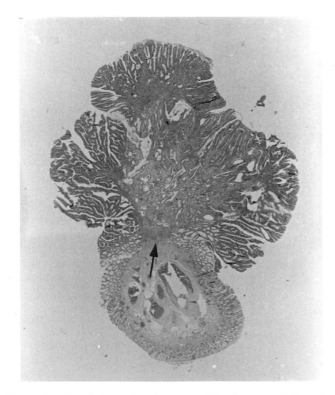

Figure 33.26   Pedunculated (long stalk) adenoma of the colon with invasive cancer limited to the head of the polyp and up to the neck *(arrow)*. The margin of resection is negative.

lymphatic invasion is 38.8% (167, 168, 171). All report cases with adverse outcome were associated with other unfavorable histology (lymphatic invasion and positive margin or grade III) while no cases with lymphatic invasion alone eventuated into an adverse outcome. Our data are contrary to this (179). We found that the incidence of adverse outcome in the presence of lymphatic invasion was 17.6% and that lymphatic invasion alone (in the absence of other unfavorable histology) was a significant indicator of adverse outcome. It should be noted that the detection of lymphatic invasion is very subjective and that the interobserver agreement was fair, moderate, or substantial for lymphatic invasion. Because of this variability, some investigators don't even attempt to report on the presence or absence of lymphatic invasion (181). In our study (179), we found venous invasion in 3.5% of cases (5 of 140) with two of the five having an adverse outcome, although both had other unfavorable histologic parameters. The literature is conflicting regarding venous invasion. Some feel that its presence is not significant (181) while others feel it is significant (174).

Nivatvongs et al. (182) reported that of the group with lymphatic/venous invasion (not separated out) 31% had lymph node metastases, but all of these with an adverse outcome were associated with other unfavorable histology (Haggitt level 4) (183).

The incidence of grade III cancer and adverse outcome is approximately 9% and 36% respectively (167–169, 171, 173, 177, 179, 182). These grade III cancers are usually associated with other unfavorable histology, further supporting their inherent aggressive biological nature.

In summary, endoscopic polypectomy usually is adequate therapy if: (1) the cancer is grade I or II, (2) the margin of resection is negative for cancer (more than 1 mm removed), and (3) there is no evidence of lymphatic or venous invasion. Subsequent surgical resection should probably be undertaken if: (1) the cancer is grade III, and/or (2) the cancer is at or near the margin of transection (within 1 mm), and/or (3) lymphatic and/or venous invasion is noted.

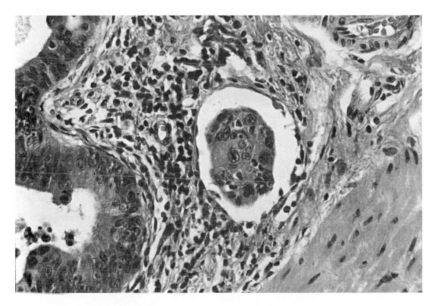

Figure 33.29   Malignant polyp with a tumor embolus in a lymphatic section.

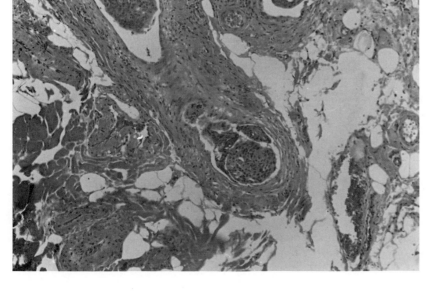

Figure 33.30   Malignant polyp with tumor emboli in muscular wall veins.

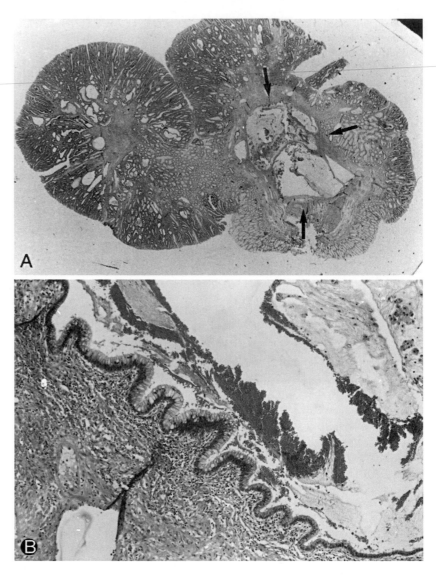

Figure 33.31   Colonic adenoma with pseudoinvasion. **(A)** Cystically dilated epithelial structures are present in the submucosa of the stalk *(arrows)*. **(B)** Medium power view of a pseudoinvasive submucosal gland. The gland is dilated and filled with blood and mucin. The lamina propria can be discerned surrounding this epithelial gland.

ADENOMA WITH PSEUDOINVASION

Pseudoinvasion occurs when the mucosa of the polyp has been "misplaced" into the submucosa, and hence mimics invasive carcinoma. Other terms used to describe this entity are epithelial misplacement and hamartomatous inverted polyps. It is important to recognize pseudoinvasion so that a misdiagnosis of invasive carcinoma and unnecessary surgery are avoided. In one retrospective study it was reported that 18 of 21 cases of pseudoinvasion were originally diagnosed as some form of cancer (184).

INCIDENCE AND ETIOLOGY

The incidence of pseudoinvasive adenomas in two large series of colonic lesions is 2.5 to 3.5% (119, 185). When one considers that 5% of adenomas will contain invasive cancer, the incidence of pseudoinvasion is not that uncommon. The male to female ratio is 3:1, and most of the polyps are located in the sigmoid colon and have long pedicles or stalks. The etiology probably has to do with rotation of the polyp's stalk and vascular compromise, which may act as a mechanical force that forces the mucosa to be misplaced and

herniated into the submucosa through defects in the muscularis mucosae (184, 185).

PATHOLOGY

The basic pathology is that of misplaced benign epithelial structures in the submucosa, in contrast to truly invasive cancer, in which the malignant epithelial glands themselves infiltrate into the submucosa and elicit a desmoplastic reaction. In pseudoinvasion the misplaced structures consist of both epithelium and surrounding lamina propria (Fig. 33.31). This may be somewhat analogous to adenomyosis in the uterus. These misplaced glands may be histologically normal epithelium or may show adenomatous changes, sometimes even with high grade dysplasia. The submucosal glands often show cystic dilatation with rupture, causing leakage of mucin into the stroma and secondary inflammation. Often the submucosa shows extensive deposits of hemosiderin. Careful examination of the actual polyp will reveal whether changes in the head of the lesion is cancerous or adenomatous. If the changes in the head are adenomatous, invasive cancer within an adenoma would be highly unlikely. Although many cases of pseudoinvasion are straightforward, there are some in which it is extremely difficult to differentiate pseudoinvasion from true invasive cancer.

POLYPOSIS SYNDROMES

A list of many polyposis syndromes is contained in Table 33.2.

FAMILIAL ADENOMATOSIS POLYPOSIS

Familial adenomatous polyposis (FAP) is an autosomal-dominant disorder in which the large intestine and rectum are carpeted with multiple adenomas (186–190). The number of adenomas ranged from hundreds to approximately 3000 (Fig. 33.32). The genetic defect is due to the chromosome allele loss 5q21, called the APC (adenomatous polyposis coli) gene. The coding region is 8.5 kb long and its protein product has a predicted molecular mass of 310 kd. The most common defects in APC are point mutations and microdeletions leading to truncated protein. The normal APC protein is localized to the cytoplasm and may be involved in cytoskeletal organization through its association with the catenins. The mutant or truncated protein could disrupt this normal process (190). No true case of FAP has fewer than 100 adenomas (see Attenuated FAP). Of interest there may be phenotypic variability in FAP patients even with the same genetic mutation. Giardiello et al. (191) studied patients from 11 unrelated families with identical 5-base–pair deletions at codon 1309. They noted phenotypic variability as polyp density varied from 3.8 to 13.1 polyps/cm^2. The distribution also varied, with some patients showing diffuse disease and others with relative sparing of the proximal colon. Besides having colonic polyps, most patients with FAP also have upper gastrointestinal polyps. A prospective upper GI screening of 102 asymptomatic FAP patients showed that 100 of 102 had microscopic pathology (often in the absence of macroscopic lesions). Ninety-four had adenomatous change in the duodenum, 44 had microscopic fundic gland polyps (stomach), and six had gastric adenomas (192). The incidence of FAP has been estimated

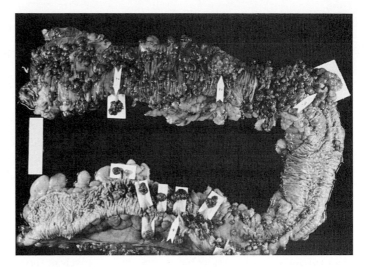

Figure 33.32 Gross specimen from patient with familial polyposis coli. Numerous adenomas of varying sizes can be appreciated.

to be 1 in 8000 births, 20% of which are the first instance in a family (a new mutation). The average age at detection in those patients who present with symptoms is 36.5 years. However, in those patients who are examined because of a family history of FAP, the average age at detection is 23.8 years. Adenomas usually do not appear before the age of 10; however, they have been reported rarely in younger children. Adenocarcinoma of the large intestine will develop in all patients who are left untreated. At the time of initial diagnosis, 67% of the probands will have colonic adenocarcinoma; however, only 7.5% of a screened group will have adenocarcinoma at initial examination (188). The average age at diagnosis of adenocarcinoma in the FAP group is 39 years, which is at least 25 years younger than the average age of diagnosis of adenocarcinoma in the general population. The lesions in FAP are adenomas, and they are histologically similar to those seen in the non-FAP patient. Samples of grossly normal mucosa can be examined, and microscopic adenomas consisting of only one or two glands may be found. Examination of the mucosa with a dissecting microscope shows that besides classic polypoid adenomas one can find flat/depressed adenomas (30% of adenomas). These flat/depressed adenomas make up 15% of all adenomas less than 1.5 mm in diameter, however, they were not found among adenomas larger than 2.0 mm in diameter. These findings suggest that some ordinary polypoid adenomas may originate from small flat/depressed adenomas (193). Kinetic studies using tritiated thymidine have shown that histologically normal epithelial cells will show DNA synthesis at all levels of the crypt in contradistinction to the lower two-thirds only seen in normal mucosa (194). Additional information on kinetic studies is presented in Chapter 9. Mucin studies have shown that 82% of the flat mucosa (nonadenomatous) of patients with FAP will show decreased staining for O-acylated sialomucins, findings noted also for colonic adenocarcinomas (195). Finally, one should be aware of the reports that patients with FAP may have benign lymphoid polyps of the terminal ileum (196), and that a member of an FAP family had multiple benign lymphoid polyps of the colon and ileum in the absence of any adenomas (197).

TABLE 33.2	**Polyposis Syndromes**

Familial Adenomatous Polyposis (FAP)
Gardner's Syndrome
Turcot's Syndrome
Attenuated FAP
Hereditary Flat Adenoma Syndrome
Muir Torre Syndrome
Juvenile Polyposis
Peutz-Jegher's Syndrome
Cronkhite-Canada Syndrome
Cowden's Disease
Intestinal Ganglioneuromatosis
Lymphoid Polyposis
Hereditary Mixed Polyposis Syndrome
Serrated Adenomatous Polyposis

GARDNER'S SYNDROME

Gardner's syndrome is an autosomal-dominant disorder that comprises the triad of intestinal polyposis, soft tissue abnormalities, and abnormalities of bone (186–190). Also noted is congenital hypertrophy of the retinal pigment epithelium consisting of single or multiple pigmented ovoid lesions occurring unilaterally or bilaterally and detected by routine fundoscopic examination. The genetic defect is identical to FAP, however, the biological basis for variable expression of extracolonic manifestations is unknown. Similarly to FAP, patients with Gardner's syndrome have upper gastrointestinal polyps (190). The intestinal polyps are adenomas as in FAP. Benign lymphoid polyposis of the ileum has been associated with this syndrome (198, 199). There is an increased incidence of adenocarcinoma of the pancreatic duodenal region. Cancers have also been reported in the thyroid gland and the adrenal gland. The soft tissue lesions are epidermal cysts, fibromas, lipomas, and desmoid tumors (occurring postoperatively or spontaneously). The bony lesions are osteomas and cortical thickening of the long bones and ribs. Dental abnormalities such as impacted teeth, supernumerary teeth, and dental cysts have been reported. At times, the soft tissue abnormalities may precede the intestinal manifestations by years. The colonic manifestations, numbers of adenomas, and the incidence of large-bowel cancer are as described for the FAP syndrome.

TURCOT'S SYNDROME

Turcot's syndrome was originally described in two siblings with polyposis coli who developed malignant brain tumors (187). This is a rare disorder which is probably an autosomal dominant disorder. The true frequency of Turcot's syndrome may be difficult to assess, as brain tumors are associated with a high mortality and may precede the detection of colonic polyps. To date, the association of Turcot's syndrome with the APC gene mutation is unclear (190). The lesions are adenomas, and the malignant potential may be the same as in FAP; however, patients may die of central nervous system lesions prior to the onset of intestinal carcinoma.

ATTENUATED FAP

This is a less severe form of polyposis with a low number of polyps (adenomas), usually less than 100, yet patients sustain a high risk for colorectal cancer. The cancers usually develop 15 years later than the classic FAP patient, but 10 years earlier than sporadic cancer (200). Leppert et al. (201) studied a large kindred (of 51 members) with a history of early onset colorectal cancers. Only two had more than 100 polyps while eight members had 2 to 40 polyps. These authors found linkage to the APC gene. The genetic defect in this disorder is linked to 5q21, similar to FAP (202). Four distinct mutations have been identified in a few families with attenuated FAP. These predict truncated proteins either by point mutations or frame shifts similar to mutations in APC, however, they differ in that the four mutated sites are very close to each other and are nearer the 5' end of the APC gene than any base substitutions or small deletions yet discovered in patients with classical APC (200).

HEREDITARY FLAT ADENOMA SYNDROME

Hereditary flat adenoma syndrome (HFAS) is presently thought to be a variant of FAP with the genetic defect linked to 5q21–22. Signs of HFAS in individuals are: (1) multiple colorectal adenomas, but usually fewer than 100, (2) the polyps tend to occur at a later age than in classic FAP, (3) the adenomas tend to show a proximal location, (4) the onset of colorectal cancer is later than in HNPCC and FAP, (5) these individuals have adenomas and cancers of the stomach and duodenum, and (6) fundic gland polyps of the stomach are also noted and in some patients fundic gland polyps may be present in the absence of colorectal adenomas (203, 204). The majority of the adenomas are of the flat type (see section on Flat Adenomas). However, Lynch et al. (203) report that in their experience, only 3 of 235 flat adenomas (1.2%) in the familial setting showed high grade dysplasia, which is much lower than reported in patients with sporadic flat adenoma (138, 143, 146, 147).

MUIR TORRE SYNDROME

The Muir Torre Syndrome was originally subclassified as a form of hereditary adenomatous polyposis (FAP) syndrome. The Muir Torre Syndrome is a rare autosomal dominant disorder with fewer than 100 adenomas, typically present in the proximal colon. This syndrome is associated with skin lesions such as basal cell carcinoma, sebaceous carcinoma, and squamous carcinoma. The genetics of this syndrome are unknown as of yet (190).

JUVENILE POLYPOSIS SYNDROME

The subject of juvenile polyposis is quite complex and confusing. This disorder represents a heterogeneous group: some patients have polyps limited to the colon, while others have polyps that involve the stomach and small bowel also; some cases are familial, others are not; and some patients have coexisting separate adenomas, whereas others have juvenile polyps with adenomatous changes (95–97, 205–213). Various authors have proposed the following definitions of juvenile polyposis: (1) juvenile polyps throughout the entire gastrointestinal tract; (2) any number of juvenile polyps in a patient with a family history; or (3) any patient with three or more, five or more, or ten or more juvenile polyps (depending upon author) (208, 211–213). In juvenile polyposis the number of polyps ranges from dozens to hundreds; however, they are not as numerous as in FAP. The reported distribution of juvenile polyps from the literature is colorectum 98%, stomach 13.6%, duodenum 2.3%, and jejunum and ileum 6.5% (211). In general, 20 to 50% of the patients have a familial or genetic history that probably indicates autosomal dominance inheritance. Extraintestinal congenital anomalies have been reported in 11 to 20% of both familial and nonfamilial cases (211). The various anomalies reported are malrotation of the gut, mesenteric lymphangioma, hypertelorism, amyotonia congenita, hydrocephalus, tetralogy of Fallot, coarctation of the aorta, thyroglossal duct cyst, and idiopathic hypertrophic subaortic stenosis. Most patients with the polyposis syndrome present in childhood and 15% present as adults (211). There is a rare form of juvenile polyposis of infancy with diarrhea, bleeding, protein losing enteropathy, alopecia, and clubbing of fingers and toes which is often fatal (211, 214). These cases clinically mimic the adult Cronkhite-Canada syndrome.

There is an increased risk for colon cancer in patients with juvenile polyposis. This increased risk is from 15 to 21% (211-213). Gastric cancers have also been reported (96, 215, 216).

The pathology of polyps in the polyposis syndrome shows a wider histopathologic spectrum than in the solitary lesions and has been characterized into typical and atypical juvenile polyps (212).

The typical polyps are grossly round and smooth and are histologically similar to solitary juvenile polyps. The atypical polyps have a characteristic gross appearance of a multilobulated mass (i.e., multiple closely packed juvenile polyps attached to a single stalk) or villiform. Histologically these lesions had relatively less lamina propria and more epithelium than is found in the more typical variety. They often adopt a villous or papillary configuration (212). In the St. Marks Study 81% were classified as typical polyps and 16% as atypical polyps (212). Adenomatous (dysplastic) changes are not infrequent. They have been noted in 46.7% of atypical polyps, and 9.0% of typical polyps (15% of all polyps) (212). Giardello et al. (213) reported either separate adenomas or adenomatous change in juvenile polyps in 31.5% of patients, the youngest patient was 3.0 years of age. Separate hyperplastic polyps can also be seen (212, 213).

PEUTZ-JEGHERS SYNDROME

The Peutz-Jeghers syndrome is an autosomal-dominant disorder of hamartomatous polyps associated with mucocutaneous pigmentation (186–190, 217). Polyps are located in the stomach and the small and large intestines. The number of polyps is usually counted in the dozens rather than in the hundreds, as in FAP. Most patients are diagnosed in their twenties, and the male to female ratio is 1:1. The clinical symptoms vary depending upon the location of the polyps. Most patients present with GI complaints, such as obstruction, abdominal pain, bloody stools, and anal extrusion (in decreasing order of frequency). Obstruction and abdominal pain are associated with small-intestinal polyps, and bloody stools and anal extrusion with large-intestinal and rectal polyps. Approximately 23% of cases are initially diagnosed because of changes in pigmentation, consisting of melanin deposition forming spots or freckles that usually appear in infancy or early childhood. Pigmentation occurs on the lips, buccal mucosa, eyelids, digits, and rarely the intestinal mucosa. The pigmentation in the lips is the most consistent finding, but this tends to fade with age. Also associated with the syndrome is the presence of sex cord tumors with annular tubules of the ovary (218), well-differentiated adenocarcinoma of the uterine cervix, and bilateral breast cancers (189) and feminizing sertoli cell tumors of the testis (190, 219).

A series of 222 Japanese patients with the Peutz-Jeghers syndrome reported the following distribution of polyps: 49% had gastric polyps, 64% had small-intestinal polyps, 53% had colonic polyps, and 32% had rectal polyps (58). In a series of 182 patients with the Peutz-Jeghers syndrome seen at the Mayo Clinic, 24% of the patients had gastric polyps, 96% had small-intestinal polyps, 26% had colonic polyps, and 24% had rectal polyps (220). In the Japanese study colonic polyps were twice as frequent as in the Mayo Clinic Study, but the Mayo Clinic reported a much higher frequency of small-intestinal polyps.

The pathologic features of these polyps are described earlier in this chapter. One major area of controversy has been whether there is a real association between this syndrome and malignancy. In the earlier literature it was claimed that malignant change in a Peutz-Jeghers polyp ran as high as 24% (221). This value was due to the erroneous interpretation of the admixed epithelial and mesenchymal elements and the presence of herniated mucosa as representing malignant change. Once the hamartomatous nature of this lesion was recognized, so was the fact that malignant change was uncommon. To date there have been well documented cases of adenomas and invasive cancers arising in Peutz-Jeghers polyps of both the small and large bowel, with some showing lymph node metastases (53–55, 60–65, 222). Hizawa et al. reported that 12.6% of Peutz-Jeghers polyps had foci of either adenoma or adenocarcinoma and of seven patients with the syndrome, three (43%) had adenomas (62). Adenomas may also occur separately and not be associated with the actual Peutz-Jeghers polyp. Reid has estimated that 2 to 3% of patients with the Peutz-Jeghers syndrome will develop a GI malignancy, mainly in the duodenal region (223). In a 1975 Japanese study of 222 histologically documented cases of Peutz-Jeghers syndrome, 15 (6.7%) had "early cancers" (three in the stomach, eight in the small intestine, and four in the intestine) and 11 (4.9%) had "advanced cancer" (three in the stomach, one in the small intestine, one in the small and the large intestines, and six in the large intestine) (58). However, the authors could document histologically malignant change in only two Peutz-Jeghers polyps. It is not known whether the cancers arose in Peutz-Jeghers polyps or in nonhamartomatous mucosa. More recent studies have shown a significant increase in both gastrointestinal and extragastrointestinal tumors in patients with the Peutz-Jeghers syndrome. Giardello et al. (66) reported an incidence of 48% malignancy in 31 patients with the syndrome. This was 18 times greater than what was expected in the general population (4 pancreatic, 2 breast, 2 stomach, 2 colon, 2 lung, 1 endometrial, 1 unspecified site, and 1 myeloma). Spiegelman et al. (67) found a 22% malignancy rate in 72 patients with the syndrome (9 gastrointestinal and 7 nongastrointestinal). Fifty percent of the GI cancers arose within an actual hamartomatous Peutz-Jeghers polyp. This incidence was 13 times greater than expected. Konishi et al. (65) in a review of the literature found a difference in site distributions of malignancies when comparing the Japanese reports with those from Western countries. Cancers of the stomach and small intestine were rare in Japan compared to the West. In Japan, cancers in the colon predominated while in the Western literature there was an equal distribution throughout the GI tract. This no doubt reflects the marked site difference incidences of Peutz-Jeghers polyps in Japan versus the West (58, 220).

CRONKHITE-CANADA SYNDROME

The Cronkhite-Canada syndrome (CCS) is a nonhereditary disorder of GI polyposis associated with alopecia, nail atrophy, and hyperpigmentation of the skin (224, 225). Cronkhite-Canada syndrome is noted worldwide, and unlike most cases of intestinal polyposis, the lesions first appear in late adult life, with approximately 80% of patients being 50 years or older at onset. The male to female ratio is close to 1:1. The clinical symptoms (in decreasing order of frequency) are diarrhea, weight loss, abdominal pain, anorexia, weakness, and hematochezia. The physical findings are nail changes (dystrophy, thinning, and splitting), hair loss, and pigmentary changes. Hair loss usually occurs rapidly over a period of weeks and has been noted in all parts of the body. It is of interest that regrowth of hair has been noted after therapy or during spontaneous remission. Pigmentary changes include hyperpigmentation (lentigo-like area) and white patchy vitiligo. Approximately 50% of the cases are fatal, usually secondary to cachexia and anemia. Supportive therapy may provide long term remission; in fact it has been reported that polyps may decrease in size or number (225). At present, surgery is recommended only for complications such as prolapse, bowel obstruction, or malignancy. Present data indicate that the potential risk for development of intestinal cancer is not great enough to indicate colectomy, although there have been

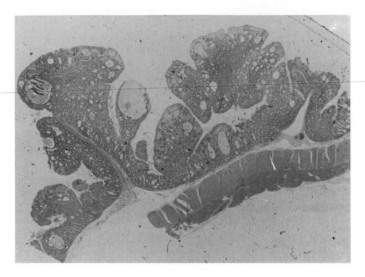

Figure 33.33   Whole mount view of Cronkhite-Canada polyps. The polypoid mucosa shows cystically dilated glands. Also note that the intervening flat mucosa has cystically dilated glands (courtesy of Dr. Klaus Lewin, University of California, Los Angeles, California).

several reported cases of colorectal cancer arising in conjunction with CCS (225–227).

The polyps of CCS are found in the stomach, small intestine, colon, and rectum and may be sessile or pedunculated. Histologically the polyps are identical to juvenile polyps. One sees tortuous glands that are cystically dilated and filled with inspissated mucus (Fig. 33.33). The lamina propria is edematous and inflamed. However, in CCS, the intervening nonpolypoid mucosa shows cystic dilatation of crypts and inflammation and edema in the lamina propria (Fig. 33.34). There have been reports of adenomatous changes in these polyps (226, 227).

COWDEN'S DISEASE

Cowden's disease is an uncommon autosomal-dominant disorder. In Cowden's disease one sees facial trichilemmomas, acral keratosis, and oral mucosal papillomas. This disorder is also associated with breast and thyroid cancer. Cowden's disease is mentioned under the polyposis syndromes because one can see numerous colonic and small-intestinal polyps. Some have described these as hamartomatous lesions (228), consisting of a mildly fibrotic, mildly disordered mucosa overlying a submucosa that displayed disorganization and splaying of smooth muscle fibers. These lesions show some similarities to the pathology seen in the solitary rectal ulcer syndrome. Other authors reported polyps that were described as inflammatory lesions, lipomas, and ganglioneuromas (229). There is no increased risk for gastrointestinal cancers in this disorder (190).

INTESTINAL GANGLIONEUROMATOSIS

Intestinal ganglioneuromatosis is a familial disorder that has been associated with the multiple endocrine neoplasia syndrome, type 2b, and with Recklinghausen's disease (230–233). There may be a diffuse proliferation of ganglioneuromatous elements, which at times may be polypoid. In some instances, the ganglioneuromatosis

has been found in association with juvenile polyposis and adenomas (232, 233).

LYMPHOID POLYPOSIS

Multiple benign lymphoid polyposis of the large bowel has been reported. Most cases occur in children (197, 234). Histologically similar to the solitary lymphoid polyps of the rectum, lymphoid polyposis consists of prominent active lymphoid nodules in the mucosa and submucosa (Fig. 33.35). The lesions are entirely benign and in some cases have been reported to disappear spontaneously. In one series there was a family history of lymphoid polyposis (234). In another report, a 12 year old boy with a family history of FAP was found to have multiple lymphoid polyps and no adenomas (197). In patients with family histories of polyps it is essential to determine the exact histologic nature of the lesions so that unnecessary surgery is not performed. Benign lymphoid polyposis of the terminal ileum has been reported in patients with Gardner's syndrome and FAP (198, 199).

HEREDITARY MIXED POLYPOSIS SYNDROME

This is an autosomal dominant disorder that has been mapped to chromosome 6q. Five types of polyps have been described in individuals with this disorder: tubular adenomas, villous adenomas, flat adenomas, hyperplastic polyps, and atypical juvenile polyps. Colorectal cancer is also seen in this disorder. This disorder might be

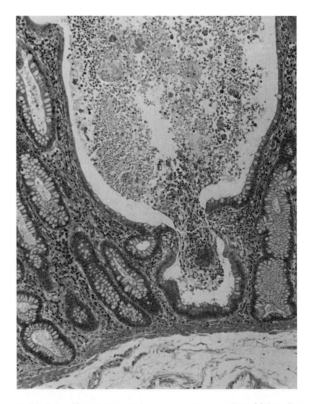

Figure 33.34   Flat intervening mucosa in Cronkhite-Canada syndrome. There is a dilated gland filled with mucus and leukocytes. The epithelium is benign (courtesy of Dr. Klaus Lewin, University of California, Los Angeles, California).

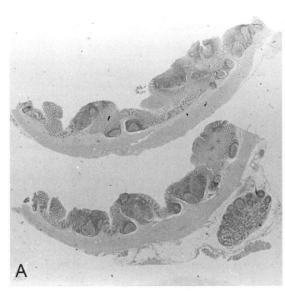

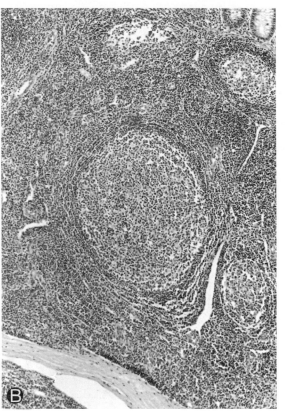

Figure 33.35 Lymphoid polyposis of the colon. **(A)** Whole mount view. One can appreciate that the polyps are due to prominent mucosal and submucosal lymphoid tissue. **(B)** Microscopic view showing lymphoid nodules with prominent germinal centers.

a variant of juvenile polyposis, however, in juvenile polyposis, adenomas are uncommon (2%) while in hereditary mixed polyposis the majority of polyps are adenomas. In hereditary mixed polyposis the number of polyps are fewer than seen in juvenile polyposis. Juvenile polyposis usually presents one decade earlier than hereditary mixed polyposis (235, 236).

REFERENCES

1. Arthur JF. Structure and significance of metaplastic nodules in the rectal mucosa. J Clin Pathol 1968;21:735–743.
2. Blue MG, Sivak MV, Achkar E, et al. Hyperplastic polyps seen at sigmoidoscopy are markers for additional adenomas seen at colonoscopy. Gastroenterology 1991;100:564–566.
3. Provenzale D, Garrett JW, Condon SE, Sandler RS. Risk for colon adenomas in patients with rectosigmoid hyperplastic polyps. Ann Intern Med 1990;113:760–763.
4. Rex DK, Smith JJ, Ulbright TM, Lehman GA. Distal colonic hyperplastic polyps do not predict proximal adenomas in asymptomatic average risk subjects. Gastroenterology 1992;102:317–319.
5. Brady PG, Straker RJ, McClave SA, et al. Are hyperplastic rectosigmoid polyps associated with an increased risk of proximal colonic neoplasms? Gastrointest Endosc 1993;39:481–485.
6. Foutch PG, Disario JA, Pardy K, et al. The sentinal hyperplastic polyp: a marker for synchronous neoplasia in the proximal colon. Am J Gastroenterol 1991;86:1482–1485.
7. Jass JR, Young PJ, Robinson EM. Predictors of presence, multiplicity, size and dysplasia of colorectal adenomas. A necropsy study in New Zealand. Gut 1992;33:1508–1514.
8. Morson BC: Some peculiarities in the histology of intestinal polyps. Dis Colon Rectum 1962;5:337–344.
9. Lane N, Kaplan H, Pascal RR. Minute adenomatous and hyperplastic polyps of the colon: divergent patterns of epithelial growth with specific associated mesenchymal changes; contrasting roles in the pathogenesis of carcinoma. Gastroenterology 1971;60:537–551.
10. Estrada RG, Spjut HJ. Hyperplastic polyps of the large bowel. Am J Surg Pathol 1980;4:127–133.
11. Waye JD, Lewis BS, Frankel A, Geller SA. Small colon polyps. Am J Gastroenterol 1988;83:899–906.
12. Pennazio M, Aragona A, Risio M, et al. Small rectosigmoid polyps as markers of proximal neoplasms. Dis Colon Rectum 1993;36:1121–1125.
13. Correa P. Epidemiology of polyps in cancer. In: Morson BC, ed. Pathogenesis of colorectal cancer. Philadelphia, WB Saunders, 1978:126–152.
14. Sato E, Oughi A, Sussano N, Ishidate T. Polyps and diverticulosis of the large bowel in autopsy populations of Akita Prefecture compared with Miyagi: high risk for colorectal cancer in Japan. Cancer 1976;37:1316–1321.
15. Correa P, Duque E, Cuello C. Haenszel W. Polyps of the colon and rectum in Cali, Colombia. Int J Cancer 1972;9:86–96.
16. Kearney J, Giovannucci E, Rimm EB, et al. Diet, alcohol, and smoking and the occurrence of hyperplastic polyps of the colon and rectum. Cancer Causes and Control 1995;6:45–56.
17. Williams GT, Arthur JF, Bussey HJR, Morson BC. Metaplastic polyps and polyposis of the colorectum. Histopathology 1980;4:155–170.
18. Franzin G, Zamboni G, Scarpa A, et al. Hyperplastic (metaplastic) polyps of the colon: a histological and histochemical study. Am J Surg Pathol 1984;8:687–698.
19. Araki K, Ogatat T, Kobayashi M, Yatani R. A morphological study of the histogenesis of human colorectal hyperplastic polyp. Gastroenterology 1995;109:1468–1474.
20. Hayoshi T, Yatani R, Apostal J, Stemmermann GN. Pathogenesis of hyperplastic polyps of the colon: a hypothesis based on ultrastructural and in vitro cell kinetics. Gastroenterology 1974;66:347–356.
21. Risio M, Coverlizza S, Ferrari A, et al. Immunohistochemical study of epithelial cell proliferation in hyperplastic polyps, adenomas, adenocarcinomas of the large bowel. Gastroenterology 1988;94:899–906.
22. Cooper HS, Marshall C. Ruggierio F, Steplewski Z. Hyperplastic polyps of the colon and rectum: an immunohistochemical study with monoclonal antibodies vs. blood group antigens (Sialosyl-Le^a, Le^a, Le^b, Le^x, Le^y, A, B, and H). Lab Invest 1987;57:421–428.

23. Cooper HS, Patchefsky AP, Marks G. Adenomatous and carcinomatous changes within hyperplastic colonic epithelium. Dis Colon Rectum 1979;22:152–156.

24. Sumner HW, Wasserman NF, McClain CJ. Giant hyperplastic polyposis of the colon. Dig Dis Sci 1981;26:58–89.

25. Whittle TS, Varner W, Brown FM. Giant hyperplastic polyp of the colon, simulating adenocarcinoma. Am J Gastroenterol 1978;69:105–107.

26. Warner AS, Glick ME, Fogt F. Multiple large hyperplastic polyps of the colon coincident with adenocarcinoma. Am J Gastroenterol 1994;89:123–125.

27. Bengoechea O, Martinez-Penula JM, Larrinaga B, et al. Hyperplastic polyposis of the colorectum and adenocarcinoma in a 24 year old man. Am J Surg Pathol 1987;11:323–327.

28. Achkar E, Carey W. Small polyps found during fiberoptic sigmoidoscopy in a symptomatic patient. Ann Intern Med 1988;109:800–803.

29. Bond JH. The Practice Parameters Committee of the American College of Gastroenterology. Polyp guideline: Diagnosis, treatment, and surveillance for patients with non-familial colorectal polyps. Ann Intern Med 1993;119:836–843.

30. Risio M, Arrigoni A, Pennazio M, et al. Mucosal cell proliferation in patients with hyperplastic colorectal polyps. Scand J Gastroenterol 1995;30:344–348.

31. Edei TJ. Prevalance and morphological features of adenomas of the large intestine in individuals with and without colorectal carcinoma. Histopathology 1986;10:111–118.

32. Teoh HH, Delahunt B, Isbister WH. Dysplastic and malignant areas in hyperplastic polyps of the intestine. Pathology 1989;21:138–142.

33. Torlakovic E, Snover DC. Serrated adenomatous polyposis in human. Gastroenterology 1996;110:748–755.

34. Burt RW, Samowitz WS. Serrated adenomatous polyposis: a new syndrome? Gastroenterology 1996;110:950–952.

35. Shepherd NA. Inverted hyperplastic polyposis of the colon. J Clin Pathol 1993;46:56–60.

36. Sobin LH. Inverted hyperplastic polyps of the colon. Am J Surg Pathol 1985;9:265–272.

37. Goldman H, Ming SC, Hickok DF. Nature and significance of hyperplastic polyps of the human colon. Arch Pathol 1970;89:349–354.

38. Jen J, Powell SM, Papadopoulus N, et al. Molecular determinants of dysplasia in colorectal lesions. Cancer Research 1994;54:5523–5526.

39. FIorito DE, Schwartz MR, Lechago J. Serrated adenomas: comparison with tubular/villous adenomas and hyperplastic polyps using p53, Bcl-2 and Ki-67. Lab Invest 1995;72:60a.

40. Stern RA, Greenson JK, Flint A. Evaluation of cell kinetics in hyperplastic using Mib-1 and image analysis and Nbcl-2. Lab Invest 1995;72:69a.

41. Bosari S, Moneghini L, Graziani D, et al. Bcl-2 oncoprotein in colorectal hyperplastic polyps, adenomas, and adenocarcinomas. Hum Pathol 1995;26:534–540.

42. Bronner MP, Culin C, Reed JC, Furth EE. The bcl-2 proto-oncogene and gastrointestinal epithelial tumor progression model. Am J Pathol 1995;146:20–26.

43. Purdie CA, O'Grady J, Piris J, et al. p53 expression in colorectal tumor. Am J Pathol 1991;138:807–813.

44. Jass JR, Filipe MI, Abbas S, et al. A morphologic and histochemical study of metaplastic polyps of the colorectum. Cancer 1984;53:510–515.

45. Cooper HS, Reuter VE. Peanut lectin binding sites in polyps of the colon and rectum: adenomas, hyperplastic polyps and adenomas with in situ carcinoma. Lab Invest 1983;49:655–661.

46. Boland CR, Montgomery CK, Kim YS. A cancer associated mucin alteration in benign colonic polyps. Gastroenterology 1982;82:664–672.

47. Cooper HS, Cox J, Patchefsky AS. Immunohistochemical study of blood group substances in polyps of the distal colon: expression of a fetal antigen. Am J Clin Pathol 1980;73:345–350.

48. Bara J, Languille O, Gendron MC, et al. Immunohistochemical study of precancerous mucus modification in human distal colonic polyps. Cancer Res 1983;43:3885–3891.

49. Longacre TA, Fenoglio-Preiser CM. Mixed hyperplastic adenomatous polyps/serrated adenomas. A distinct form of colorectal neoplasia. Am J Surg Pathol 1990;14:524–537.

50. Gibbs NM. Juvenile and Peutz-Jeghers polyps. In: Morson BC, ed. Pathogenesis of Colorectal Cancer. Philadelphia: WB Saunders, 1978:33–42.

51. Lewin KJ, Riddell RLT, Weinstein WM. Gastrointestinal pathology and its clinical implications. Igaku-Shoin 1992:1215.

52. Talbot IC, Price A. Biopsy pathology in colorectal disease. London: Chapman and Hall, 1987:254.

53. Perzin KH, Bridge MF. Adenomatous and carcinomatous change in hamartomatous polyps of the small intestine (Peutz-Jeghers syndrome): report of a case and review of the literature. Cancer 1982;49:971–983.

54. William JP, Knudsen A. Peutz-Jeghers syndrome with metastasizing duodenal carcinoma. Gut 1965;6:179–184.

55. Matuchanuky C. Babin P, Costrot S, et al. Peutz-Jeghers syndrome with metastasizing carcinoma arising from a jejunal hamartoma. Gastroenterology 1979;77:1311–1315.

56. Shibata HR, Phillips MJ. Peutz-Jeghers syndrome with jejunal and colonic adenocarcinoma. Can Med Assoc J 1970;103:285–287.

57. Cochet B, Carrel K, Desbaillets L, Widgren S. Peutz-Jeghers syndrome associated with gastrointestinal cancer. Gut 1979;20:169–175.

58. Utsunomiya J, Gocho H, Miyanga T, et al. Peutz-Jeghers syndrome: its natural course in management. Johns Hopkins Med J 1975;136:71–82.

59. Miller LJ, Bartholomew LG, Dozois RR, Dahlin DC. Adenocarcinoma of the rectum arising in a hamartomatous polyp in a patient with Peutz-Jeghers syndrome. Dig Dis Sci 1983;28:1047–1051.

60. Horn RC Jr, Payne WA, Fine G. The Peutz-Jeghers syndrome. Arch Pathol 1963;76:29–37.

61. Narita T, Eto T, Ito T. Peutz-Jeghers syndrome with adenomas and adenocarcinomas in colonic polyps. Am J Surg Pathol 1987;11:76–81.

62. Hizawa K, Iida M, Matsumoto T, et al. Neoplastic transformation arising in Peutz-Jeghers polyposis. Dis Colon Rectum 1993;36:953–957.

63. Hizawa K, Iida M, Matsumoto T, et al. Cancer in Peutz-Jeghers syndrome. Cancer 1993;72:277–281.

64. Foley TR, McGarrity TJ, Abt AB. Peutz-Jeghers syndrome, A clinicopathologic survey of the Harrisburg family with a 49 year follow-up. Gastroenterology 1988;95:1535–1540.

65. Konishi F, Wyse NE, Muto T, et al. Peutz-Jeghers polyposis associated with carcinoma of the digestive organs. Report of three cases and review of the literature. Dis Colon Rectum 1987;30:790–799.

66. Giardiello FM, Welsh SB, Hamilton SR, et al. Increased risk of cancer in the Peutz-Jeghers syndrome. N Engl J Med 1987;316:1511–1514.

67. Spigelman AD, Murday V, Phillips RKS. Cancer and Peutz-Jeghers syndrome. Gut 1989;30:1588–1590.

68. Bolwell JS, James PD. Peutz-Jeghers syndrome with pseudoinvasion of hamartomatous polyps and multiple epithelial neoplasms. Histopathology 1979;3:39–50.

69. Shepherd NA, Bussey HJR, Jass JR. Epithelial misplacement in Peutz-Jeghers polyps: a diagnostic pitfall. Am J Surg Pathol 1987;11:743–749.

70. Patterson MJ, Kernen JA. Epithelioid leiomyosarcoma originating in a hamartomatous polyp from a patient with Peutz-Jeghers syndrome. Gastroenterology 1985;88:1060–1064.

71. Shimer GR, Helwig EB. Inflammatory fibroid polyps of the intestine. Am J Clin Pathol 1984;81:708–714.

72. Benjamin SP, Hawk WA, Turnbull RB. Fibrous inflammatory polyps of the ileum and cecum: review of five cases with emphasis on differentiation from mesenchymal neoplasms. Cancer 1977;39:1300–1305.

73. LiVolsi VA, Perzin KH. Inflammatory pseudotumor (inflammatory fibrous polyp) of the small intestine, colon: a clinicopathological study. Am J Dig Dis 1975;20:325–336.

74. Tysk C, Schnurer LB, Wickbom G. Obstructing inflammatory fibroid polyp in pelvic ileal reservoir after restorative proctocolectomy in ulcerative colitis. Report of a case. Dis Colon Rectum 1994;37:1034–1037.

75. Williams GR, Jaffe S, Scott CA. Inflammatory fibroid polyp of the terminal ileum presenting in a patient with active Crohn's disease. Histopathology 1992;20:545–547.

76. Kolodziejczyk P, Yao T, Tsuneyoshi M. Inflammatory fibroid polyp of the stomach. Special reference to an immunohistochemical profile of 42 cases. Am J Surg Pathol 1993;17:1159–1168.

77. Price AB Benign lymphoid polyps and inflammatory polyps. In: Morson BC, ed. Pathogenesis of colorectal cancer. Philadelphia: WB Saunders, 1978:33–42.

78. Williams AO, Prince DL. Intestinal polyps in the Nigerian African. J Clin Pathol 1975;28:367–371.

79. Mabogunje OA, Subbuswamy SG, Lawrie JH. Rectal polyps in Zaria, Nigeria. Dis Colon Rectum 1978;21:474–479.

80. Shekitka KM, Helwig EB. Deceptive bizarre stromal cells in polyps and ulcers of the gastrointestinal tract. Cancer 1991;67:2111–2117.

81. Jessurun J, Paplanus SH, Nagle RB, et al. Pseudosarcomatous changes in inflammatory pseudopolyps of the colon. Arch Pathol Lab Med 1986;110:833–836.

82. Williams GT, Bussey HJR, Morson BC. Inflammatory cap polyps of the large intestine. Br J Surg 1985;72:S133.

83. Gehenot M, Colombel JF, Wolschies E, et al. Cap polyposis occurring in the post-operative course of pelvic surgery. Gut 1994;35:1670–1672.

84. Campbell AP, Cobb CA, Chapman RWG, et al. Cap polyposis—an unusual cause of diarrhea. Gut 1993;34:562–564.

85. Chetty R, Bhathal PS, Slavin JL. Prolapse induced inflammatory polyps of the colorectum and anal transitional zone. Histopathology 1993;23:63–67.

86. Nakamura SI, Kino I, Akagi T. Inflammatory myoglandular polyps of the colon and rectum. A clinical pathological study of 32 pedunculated polyps, distinct from other types of polyps. Am J Surg Pathol 1992;16:772–779.

87. Griffiths AP, Hopkinson JM, Dixon MF. Inflammatory myoglandular polyp causing ileal intussusception. Histopathology 1993;23:596–598.

88. Mathus-Veliegen EMH, Tytgat GNJ. A polyp simulating mucosal prolapse syndrome in (pre) diverticular disease. Endoscopy 1986,18:84–86.

89. Kelly JK. Polypoid prolapse in mucosal folds in diverticular disease. Am J Surg Pathol 1991;15:871–878.

90. Yao T, Nagai E, Utsunomiya T, Tsuneyoshi M. An intestinal counterpart of pyogenic granuloma of the skin A newly proposed entity. Am J Surg Pathol 1995;19:1054–1060.

91. Allibone RO, Hoffman J, Gooney JR, Helliwell TR. Granulation tissue polyposis associated with carcinoid tumors of the small intestine. Histopathology 1993;22:475–480.

92. Cheville JC, Mitros FA, Vanderzalm G, Platz CE. Atheroemboli associated polyps of the sigmoid colon. Am J Surg Pathol 1993;17:1054–1057.

93. Helwig EB. Adenomas of the large intestine in children. Am J Dis Child 1946;72:289–295.

94. Dajani YV, Kamal MF. Colorectal juvenile polyps: an epidemiological and histopathological study of 144 cases in Jordanians. Histopathology 1984;8:765–779.

95. Roth SI, Helwig EB. Juvenile polyps of the colon and rectum. Cancer 1963;16:468–479.

96. Subramony C, Scottconner CEH, Skelton D, Hall TJ. Familial juvenile polyposis. Study of the kindred: evolution of polyps in relationship to gastrointestinal carcinoma. Am J Clin Pathol 1994;102:91–97.

97. Goodman ZD, Yardley JH, Milligan FD. Pathogenesis of colonic polyps in multiple juvenile polyposis: report of a case associated with gastric polyps and carcinoma of the rectum. Cancer 1979;43:1906–1913.

98. Lipper S, Kahn LB, Sandler RS, Varma V. Multiple juvenile polyposis: the study of the pathogenesis of juvenile polyps and their relationship to colonic adenomas. Hum Pathol 1981;12:804–813.

99. Grigioni WF, Alampi G, Martinelli G, Piccaluga A. Atypical juvenile polyposis. Histopathology 1981;5:361–376.

100. Nugent KP, Talbot IC, Hodgson SV, Phillips RKS. Solitary juvenile polyps: not a marker for subsequent malignancy. Gastroenterology 1993;105:698–700.

101. Freeman CJ, Fechner RE. A solitary juvenile polyp with hyperplastic and adenomatous glands. Dig Dis Sci 1982;27:946–948.

102. Billingham RP, Bowman HE, Mackeigan JM. Solitary adenomas in juvenile patients. Dis Colon Rectum 1980;23:26–30.

103. Berg HK, Herrera L, Petrelli NJ, et al.. Mixed juvenile-adenomatous polyps of the rectum in an elderly patient. J Surg Oncol 1985;29:40–42.

104. Tung-Hua L, Min-Chang C. Hsien-Chiu LC, Chieh L. Malignant change of juvenile polyp of the colon: a case report. Chin Med J 1978;4:434–439.

105. Baptist SJ, Sabatini MT. Co-existing juvenile polyps in tubulovillous adenoma of colon with carcinoma in situ. Hum Pathol 1985;16:1061–1063.

106. Ranchod M, Lewin KJ, Dorfman RF. Lymphoid hyperplasia of the gastrointestinal tract: a study of 26 cases and review of the literature. Am J Surg Pathol 1978;2:383–400.

107. Corres JS, Wallace MH, Morson BC. Benign lymphomas of the rectum and anal canal: a study of 100 cases. J Pathol Bacteriol 1961;82:371–382.

108. Rickert RR, Auerbach O, Garfinkle L, et al. Adenomatous lesions of the large bowel and colon: an autopsy survey. Cancer 1979;43:1847–1857.

109. Williams AR, Baisoorya BAW, Day DW. Polyps and cancer of the large bowel: a necropsy study in Liverpool. Gut 1982;23:835–842.

110. Vatn MH, Stalsberg HH. The prevalence of polyps in the large intestine in Oslo: an autopsy study. Cancer 1982;49:819–825.

111. Bazzoli F, Fossi S, Sottili S, et al. The risk of adenomatous polyps in asymptomatic first degree relatives of persons with colon cancer. Gastroenterology 1995;109:783–788.

112. Cannon-Albright LA, Bishop T, Samowitz W, et al. Colonic polyps in an unselected population: prevalence, characteristics, and associations. Am J Gastroenterol 1994;89:827–831.

113. Shinya H, Wolff WI. Morphology, anatomic distribution and cancer potential of polyps: an analysis of 7000 polyps endoscopically removed. Ann Surg 1979;190:679–683.

114. Konishi F, Morson BC. Pathology of colorectal adenomas: a colonoscopic survey. J Clin Pathol 1982;35:830–841.

115. Neuget AI, Johnsen CM, Forde KA, Treat MR. Recurrence rates for colorectal polyps. Cancer 1985;55:1586–1589.

116. Winawer SJ, Zauber AG, O'Brien MJ, et al. Randomized comparison of surveillance intervals after colonoscopic removal of newly diagnosed endoscopic polyps. The National Polyp Workshop. N Eng J Med 1993;328:901–906.

117. Elde TJ, Stalsberg H. Polyps of the large intestine in Northern Norway. Cancer 1978;42:2839–2848.

118. Coode PE, Chan KW, Chan YT. Polyps and diverticuli of large intestine: a necroscopy study in Hong Kong. Gut 1985;26:1045–1048.

119. Gillespie PE, Chambers TJ, Chan KW, et al. Colonic adenomas: a colonoscopic survey. Gut 1979;20:240–245.

120. O'Brien MJ, Winawer SJ, Zauber AG, et al. The National Polyp Study Workgroup: patient and polyp characteristics associated with high grade dysplasia-colorectal adenomas. Gastroenterology 1990;98:371–379.

121. Hill MJ, Morson BC, Bussey HJR. Etiology of adenoma carcinoma sequence in large bowel. Lancet 1978;1:245–247.

122. Bonelli U, Martinez H, Conio M, et al. Family history of colorectal cancers a risk factor for benign and malignant tumors of the large bowel: a case controlled study. Int J Cancer 1988;41:513–517.

123. Nelson RL. Diet and adenomatous polyp risk. Sem Surg Oncol 1994;10:165–175.

124. Martinez ME, McPherson RS, Annegers JF, Levin B. Cigarette smoking and alcohol consumption as risk factors for colorectal adenomatous polyps. JNCI 1995;87:274–279.

125. Giovannucci E, Stampfer MJ, Colditz G, et al. Relationships of diet to risk of colorectal adenoma in men. JNCI 1992;84:91–98.

126. Neugut AI, Garbowski G, Lee WC, et al. Dietary risk factors for the incidence of recurrence of colorectal adenomatous polyps: a case control study. Ann Intern Med 1993;118:91–95.

127. Morson BC. A polyp sequence in the large bowel. Proc Soc Med 1974;67:451–457.

128. Day W, Morson BC. The adenoma-cancer sequence. In: Morson BC, ed. Pathogenesis of colorectal cancer. Philadelphia: WB Saunders, 1978:58–71.

129. Cuello C, Margio C, Correa P. Atypia in adenomas in three populations with different risks for large bowel cancer. Cali, Sao Paulo, and New Orleans. Natl Cancer Inst 1979;53:171–173 (monograph).

130. Atkin WS, Morson BC, Kuzick J. Long term risk of colorectal cancer after excision of rectosigmoid adenomas. N Engl J Med 1992;326:658–662.

131. Winawer SJ, Zauber AG, Ho MN, et al. Prevention of colorectal cancer by colonoscopic polypectomy. N Eng J Med 1993;329:1177–1181.

132. Jarven HJ, Mecklin JP, Sistonen P. Screening reduces colorectal cancer rate in families with hereditary non-polyposis colon cancer. Gastroenterology 1995;108:1405–1411.

133. Vogelstein B, Fearon ER, Hamilton SR, et al. Genetic alterations during colorectal tumor development. N Engl J Med 1988;319:525–532.

134. Fearon ER, Vogelstein B. A genetic model for colorectal tumorigenesis. Cell 1990;61:759–776.

135. Hamilton SR. The molecular genetics of colorectal neoplasia. Gastroenterology 1993;105:3–7.

136. Jass JR, Sobin LH. World Health Organization. International histological classification of tumors. Histological typing of intestinal tumors. 2nd ed. Berlin: Springer-Verlag, 1989.

137. Pascal RR. Dysplasia in early carcinoma in inflammatory bowel disease in colorectal adenomas. Human Pathol 1994;25:1160–1171.

138. Muto T, Kamiya J, Sawada T, et al. Small flat adenoma of the large bowel with special reference to its clinicopathological features. Dis Colon Rectum 1985;28:847–851.

139. Yao T, Tada S, Tsuneyoshi M. Colorectal counterpart of gastric depressed adenoma. A comparison with flat and polypoid adenomas with special reference to the development of pericryptal fibroblasts. Am J Surg Pathol 1994;18:559–568.

140. Minamoto T, Sawaguchi K, Ohta T, et al. Superficial type adenomas in adenocarcinomas of the colon and rectum: a comparative morphological study. Gastroenterology 1994;106:1436–1443.

141. Yamagata S, Muto T, Uchida Y, et al. Polypoid growth in K ras Codon 12 mutation in colorectal cancer. Cancer 1995;75:953–957.

142. Bond JH. Small flat adenomas appear to have little clinical importance in Western Countries. Gastrointest Endosc 1995;42:184–186.

143. Mitooka H, Fujimori T, Maeda S, Nagasako K. Minute flat neoplastic lesions of the colon detected by contrast chromoscopy using an indigo carmine capsule. Gastrointest Endosc 1995;41:453–459.

144. Jaramillo E, Watanabe EM, Slezak P, Rubio C. Flat neoplastic lesions of the colon and rectum detected by high resolution video endoscopy and chromoscopy. Gastrointest Endosc 1995;42:114–122.

145. Kubota O, Kino I. Depressed adenomas of the colon in familial adenomatous polyposis. Histology, immunohistochemical detection of proliferating cell nuclear antigen (PCNA), an analysis of the background mucosa. Am J Surg Pathol 1995;19:318–327.

146. Adachi M, Muto T, Okinaga K, Morioka Y. Clinicopathological features of the flat adenoma. Dis Colon Rectum 1991;34:981–986.

147. Wolber RA, Owen DA. Flat adenomas of the colon. Hum Pathol 1991;22:70–74.

148. Samowitz WS, Burt RL. The nonspecificity of histological findings reported for flat adenomas. Hum Pathol 1995;26:571–573.

149. Uno Y, Munakata A, Tanaka M. The discrepancy of histological diagnosis between flat adenomas. Gastrointest Endosc 1994;40:1–6.

150. Yamagata S, Muto T, Uchida Y, et al. Lower incidence of K-ras codon 12 mutation in flat colorectal adenomas than in polypoid adenomas. Jap J Cancer Res 1994;85:147–151.

151. Fujimori T, Satonaka K, Yamamura-Idei Y, et al. Noninvolvement of ras mutations in flat colorectal adenomas and carcinomas. Int J Cancer 1994;57:51–55.

152. Lynch HP, Smyrk KT. Colorectal cancer—survival advantage in hereditary nonpolyposis colorectal cancer. Gastroenterology 1996;110:943–954.

153. Mecklin JP, Jarvinen HJ. Clinical features of colorectal cancer in cancer family syndrome. Dis Colon Rectum 1986;29:160–164.

154. Smyrk TC. Colon cancer connections. Cancer syndrome meets molecular biology meets histopathology. Am J Pathol 1994;145:1–6.

155. Ahlquist DA. Aggressive polyps in hereditary nonpolyposis colorectal: targets for screening. Gastroenterology 1995;108:1590–1592.

156. Mecklin JP, Sipponen P, Jarvinen HJ. Histopathology of colorectal carcinomas and adenoma in cancer family syndrome. Dis Colon Rectum 1986;29:849–853.

157. Jass JR, Stewart SM. Evolution of hereditary nonpolyposis colorectal cancer. Gut 1992;33:783–786.

158. Jass JR, Smyrk TZ, Stewart SM, et al. Pathology of hereditary nonpolyposis colorectal cancer. Anticancer Research 1994;14:1631–1634.

159. Lynch HT, Smyrk TC, Watson P, et al. Genetics, natural history, tumor spectrum, and pathology of hereditary nonpolyposis colorectal cancer: an updated view. Gastroenterology 1993;104:1535–1549.

160. Aaltonen LA, Peltomaki P, Mecklin JP, et al. Replication errors in benign and malignant tumors from hereditary nonpolyposis colorectal cancer patients. Cancer Res 1994;54:1645–1648.

161. Shibata D, Peinado MA, Ionov Y, et al. Genomic instability in repeated sequences is an early somatic event in colorectal tumor genesis that after transformation. Nature Genet 1994;6:273–281.

162. Jacoby RF, Marshall DF, Kailas S, et al. Genetic instability with adenoma to carcinoma progression in hereditary nonpolyposis colon cancer. Gastroenterology 1995;109:73–82.

163. Aaltonen LA, Paltomaki P, Leach FS, et al. Clues to the pathogenesis of familial colorectal cancer. Science 1993;260:812–816.

164. Strickler JG, Zheng J, Shu Q, et al. p53 mutations in microsatellite instability in sporadic gastric cancer: when guardians fail. Cancer Res 1994;54:4750–4755.

165. Mirinov NM, Aguelonma M, Potapova GI, et al. Alterations of (CA) and DNA repeats in tumor suppression in human gastric cancer. Cancer Res 1994;54:41–44.

166. Morson BC, Whiteway JE, Jones EA, et al. Histopathology and prognosis of malignant colorectal polyps treated by endoscopic polypectomy. Gut 1984;25:437–444.

167. Cooper HS. Surgical pathology of endoscopically removed malignant polyps of the colon and rectum. Am J Surg Pathol 1983;7:613–623.

168. Cranley JP, Petras RE, Carey WD, et al. When is endoscopic polypectomy adequate therapy for colonic polyp containing invasive carcinoma? Gastroenterology 1986;91:419–427.

169. Kyzer S, Begin LR, Gordon PH, Mitmaker B. The care of patients with colorectal polyps that contain invasive adenocarcinoma. Endoscopic polypectomy or colectomy? Cancer 1992;70:2044–2050.

170. Christie JP. Polypectomy or colectomy? Management of 106 consecutive encountered colorectal polyps. Am Surg 1988;54:93–99.

171. Coverlizza S, Risio M, Ferrari A, et al. Colorectal adenomas containing invasive carcinoma. Pathological assessment of lymph node metastatic potential. Cancer 1989;64:1937–1947.

172. Richards WO, Webb WA, Morris SJ, et al. Patient management after endoscopic removal of the cancerous colon adenoma. Ann Surg 1987;205:665–672.

173. Williams CD, Geraghty JM. The malignant polyp—when to operate: St. Mark's experience. Can J Gastroenterol 1990;4:549–553.

174. Muller S, Chesner IM, Igan MA, et al. Significance of venous and lymphatic invasion in malignant polyps of the colon and rectum. Gut 1990;30:1385–1391.

175. Wolff WI, Shinya H. Definitive treatment of malignant polyps of the colon. Ann Surg 1975;185:516–525.

176. Shatney CH, Lober PH, Gilbertson V, Sosin H. Management of focally malignant pedunculated adenomatous colorectal polyps. Dis Colon Rectum 1976;19:334–341.

177. Nivatvongs S, Goldberg SM. Management of patients who have polyps containing invasive carcinoma removed via colonoscope. Dis Colon Rectum 1978;21:811.

178. Langer JC, Cohen Z, Taylor BR, et al. Management of patients with polyp containing malignancy removed by colonoscopic polypectomy. Dis Colon Rectum 1984;27:6–9.

179. Cooper HS, Deppisch LM, Gourley WK, et al. Endoscopically removed malignant colorectal polyps: clinical pathological correlations. Gastroenterology 1995;108:1657–1665.

180. Volk EE, Goldblum JR, Petras RE, et al. Management and outcome of patients with invasive carcinoma arising in colorectal polyps. Gastroenterology 1995;109:1801–1807.

181. Geraghty JM, Williams CB, Talbot IC. Malignant colorectal polyp: venous invasion and successful treatment by endoscopic polypectomy. Gut 1991;32:774–778.

182. Nivatvongs S, Rojanasakul A, Reiman HM, et al. The risk of lymph node metastasis in colorectal polyps with invasive adenocarcinoma. Dis Colon Rectum 1991;34:323–328.

183. Haggitt RC, Goltzbach RE, Soffer EE, Wribule D. Prognostic factors in colorectal carcinomas arising in adenomas: implications of lesions removed by endoscopic polypectomy. Gastroenterology 1985;89:328–336.
184. Greene FL. Epithelial misplacement in adenomatous polyps of the colon and rectum. Cancer 1974;33:206–217.
185. Muto T, Bussey HJR, Morson BC. Pseudocarcinomatous invasion in adenomatous polyps of the colon and rectum. J Clin Pathol 1973;26:25–31.
186. Erbe RW. Current concepts in genetics: inherited gastrointestinal-polyposis syndrome. N Engl J Med 1976;294:1101–1104.
187. Wennstrom J, Pierce ER, McKusick VA. Hereditary benign and malignant lesions of the large bowel. Cancer 1974;34:850–857.
188. Bussey HJR, Veale AMO, Morson BC. Genetics of gastrointestinal polyposis. Gastroenterology 1978;74:1325–1330.
189. Haggit RC, Reid BJ. Hereditary gastrointestinal polyposis syndromes. Am J Surg Pathol 1986;10:871–887.
190. Rustgi A. Hereditary gastrointestinal polyposis and nonpolyposis syndrome. N Engl J Med 1994;331:1694–1702.
191. Giardeillo FM, Krush AJ, Petersen GM, et al. Phenotypic variability of familial adenomatous polyposis in 11 unrelated families with identical APC gene mutation. Gastroenterology 1994;104:1542–1547.
192. Domizio P, Talbot IC, Spigelman D, et al. Upper gastrointestinal pathology in familial adenomatous polyposis: results from a prospective study of 102 patients. J Clin Pathol 1990;43:738–743.
193. Kobota O, Kino I. Minute adenomas of the depressed type in familial adenomatous polyposis of the colon. Cancer 1993;72:1159–1164.
194. Deschner EE, Lipkin M. Proliferative patterns in colonic mucosa in familial polyposis. Cancer 1975;35:413–418.
195. Muto T, Kamiya J, Sawada T, et al. Mucin abnormality of colon mucosa in patients with familial polyposis coli. Dis Colon Rectum 1985;28:147–148
196. Dorazio RA, Whelan TJ Jr. Lymphoid hyperplasia of the terminal ileum associated with familial polyposis coli. Ann Surg 1970;171:300–302.
197. Venkitachalam PS, Hirsch E, Elguezabal A, Littman L. Multiple lymphoid polyposis and familial polyposis of the colon: a genetic relationship. Dis Colon Rectum 1978;21:336–341.
198. Shaw EB Jr, Henningar GR. Intestinal lymphoid polyposis. Am J Clin Pathol 1974;61:417–422.
199. Thomford NR, Greenberger NJ. Lymphoid polyps of the ileum associated with Gardner's syndrome. Arch Surg 1968;96:289–291.
200. Spirio L, Olschwang S, Groden J, et al. Alleles of the APC gene: an attenuated form of familial polyposis. Cell 1993;75:951–957.
201. Leppert M, Burt R, Hughes JP, et al. Genetic analysis of an inherited predisposition to colonic colon cancer in a family with a variable number of adenomatous polyps. N Engl J Med 1990;322:904–908.
202. Spirio L, Otterud B, Stauffer D, et al. Linkage of a variant or attenuated form of adenomatous polyposis coli to the adenomatous polyposis coli (APC) locust. Am J Hum Genet 1992;51:92–100.
203. Lynch HT, Smyrk TC, Watson P, et al. Hereditary flat adenoma syndrome: a variant of familial adenomatous polyposis. Dis Colon Rectum 1992;35:411–421.
204. Lynch HT, Smyrk TC, Lanspa SJ, et al. Upper gastrointestinal manifestations in families with hereditary flat adenoma syndrome. Cancer 1993;71:2709–2714.
205. Veale AMO, McColl I, Bussey HJR, Morson BC. Juvenile polyposis coli. J Med Genet 1966;3:5–16.
206. Rozen P, Baratz M. Familial juvenile polyposis with associated colon cancer. Cancer 1982;49:1500–1503.
207. Jarvinen H, Franssila KO. Familial juvenile polyposis coli: increased risk of colorectal cancer. Gut 1984;25:792–800.
208. Sachatello CR, Pickren JW, Grace JT. Generalized juvenile gastrointestinal polyposis. Gastroenterology 1970;58:699–708.
209. Velcek FT, Coopersmith IS, Chen CK, et al. Familial juvenile adenomatosis polyposis. J Pediatr Surg 1976;11:781–787.
210. Restrepo C, Moreno J, Duque E, et al. Juvenile colonic polyposis in Colombia. Dis Colon Rectum 1978;29:600–612.

211. Desai DC, Neal KF, Talbot IC, et al. Juvenile polyposis. Br J Surg 1995;82:14–17.
212. Jass JR, Williams EB, Bussey HJR, Morson BC. Juvenile polyposis—a pre-cancerous condition. Histopathology 1988;13:619–630.
213. Giardiello FM, Hamilton SR, Kern SE, et al. Colorectal neoplasia in juvenile polyposis or juvenile polyps. Arch Dis Child 1991;66:971–975.
214. Scharf GM, Becker JHR, Laage NJ. Juvenile gastrointestinal polyposis or the infantile Cronkhite-Canada Syndrome. J Pediatr Surg 1986;21:953–954.
215. Sassatelli R, Bertoni G, Serra L, et al. Generalized juvenile polyposis with mixed pattern and gastric cancer. Gastroenterology 1993;104:910–915.
216. Stemper EJ, Kents TA, Summers RW. Juvenile polyposis and gastrointestinal carcinoma: a study of a kindred. Ann Intern Med 1975;183:639–646.
217. Jegher H, McKusick VA, Kat KH. General intestinal polyposis and melanin spots of oral mucosa, lips and digits. N Engl J Med 1949;241:993–1005, 1032–1036.
218. Scully RE. Sex cord tumor with annular tubules: a distinctive ovarian tumor of the Peutz-Jeghers syndrome. Cancer 1970;25:1107–1121.
219. Young S, Gooneratne S, Straus FH, et al. Feminizing Sertoli cell tumors in boys with Peutz-Jeghers syndrome. Am J Surg Pathol 1995;19:508.
220. Bartholomew LG, Dahlin DC, Waugh JGM. Intestinal polyposis associated with mucocutaneous melanin pigmentation (Peutz-Jegher's syndrome). Gastroenterology 1957;32:434–451.
221. Bailey D. Polyposis of the gastrointestinal tract: the Peutz-Jegher's syndrome. Br Med J 1957;2:433–438.
222. Hsu SD, Zaharopoulus PA, May JT, Costanzi JJ. Peutz-Jeghers syndrome with intestinal cancer: report of the association in one family. Cancer 1979;44:1527–1532.
223. Reid JD. Intestinal cancer in the Peutz-Jeghers syndrome. JAMA 1974;229:833–834.
224. Cronkhite LW, Canada WJ. Generalized gastrointestinal polyposis: an unusual syndrome of polyposis, pigmentation alopecia, and onychodystrophy. N Engl J Med 1955;252:1011–1015.
225. Daniel ES, Ludwig SL, Lew KJ, et al. The Cronkhite Canadian syndrome: an analysis of clinical and pathological features and therapy in 55 patients. Medicine 1982;61:293–309.
226. Katayama Y, Kimura M, Konn M. Cronkhite-Canada syndrome associated with rectal cancer and adenomatous changes in colonic polyps. Am J Surg Pathol 1985;9:65–71.
227. Nomomura A, Ohta G, Ihata T, et al. Cronkhite-Canada syndrome associated with sigmoid cancer. Acta Pathol Jap 1980;30:825–845.
228. Carlson GJ, Nivatvongs S, Snover DC. Colorectal polyps in Cowden's disease. Am J Surg Pathol 1984;8:763–770.
229. Weary PE, Gorlin RJ, Gentry WC Jr, et al. Multiple hamartoma syndrome: Cowden's disease. Arch Dermatol 1972;106:682–690.
230. Carney JA, Hayles AB. Alimentary tract manifestations of multiple endocrine neoplasia. Type II B. Mayo Clin Proc 1977;52:543–548.
231. Snover DC, Weigent CE, Sumncer HW. Diffuse mucosal ganglioneuromatosis of the colon associated with adenocarcinoma. Am J Clin Pathol 1981;75:225–229.
232. Weidner N, Flanders DJ, Mitros FA. Mucosal ganglioneuromatosis associated with multiple colonic polyps. Am J Surg Pathol 1984;8:779–786.
233. Mendelsohn G, Diamond MP. Familial ganglioneuromatosis polyposis of the large bowel: report of a family with associated juvenile polyposis. Am J Surg Pathol 1984;8:515–520.
234. Louw JH. Polypoid lesions of the large bowel in children with particular reference to benign lymphoid polyposis. J Pediatr Surg 1968;3:195–209.
235. Thomas HJW, Whitelaw SC, Cottrell SE, et al. Hereditary mixed polyposis syndrome: genetic mapping to chromosome 6q. Gastroenterology 1996;110:89.
236. Whitelaw S, Markie D, Murday V, et al. Hereditary mixed polyposis syndrome. A new disorder? Gut 1992(suppl);33:S56.

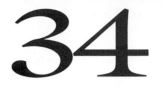

MALIGNANT EPITHELIAL TUMORS OF THE INTESTINES

Si-Chun Ming

MULTIPLE CARCINOMAS
SQUAMOUS CELL CARCINOMA AND ADENOSQUAMOUS CARCINOMA
ENDOCRINE CARCINOMA

COMPOSITE ADENOCARCINOMA AND CARCINOID AND ADENOCARCINOID
SMALL CELL CARCINOMA
OTHER RARE CARCINOMAS AND METASTATIC TUMORS

The small and large intestines have similar structural organizations and histologic components (details are described in Chapter 2). However, they exhibit a number of differences, primarily related to their different functions. The small intestine is principally an absorptive organ for nutrients. It has abundant absorptive cells with well developed microvilli which form a brush border recognizable under a light microscope. The large intestine contains few absorptive cells that do not have a distinct brush border. Goblet cells, on the other hand, are more abundant in the large than the small intestine. The endocrine cells secrete more products in the small than the large intestine. Similarly, lymphoid tissue is more abundant in the small than the large intestine. Tumors of the endocrine and lymphoid cells are presented in Chapters 15 and 17 respectively, and the mesenchymal tumors in Chapter 18. This chapter deals primarily with malignant epithelial tumors. The benign epithelial tumors, namely adenomas and polyps, are presented in Chapter 33.

INCIDENCE AND TYPES OF INTESTINAL CARCINOMA

A striking difference between the tumors of the small and large intestines is in the frequency of epithelial tumors. The average length of the small intestine is 7 m and that of the large intestine 1.5 m. Although the small intestine is much narrower than the large intestine, the presence of numerous circular mucosal folds (Kerckring's valves or plicae circularis) so greatly increases the mucosal surface in the small intestine that it makes up about 90% of the total surface area of the gastrointestinal tract. However, tumors of the small intestines are rare, constituting only 5 to 6% of all gastrointestinal tumors and 1 to 2% of all gastrointestinal cancers (1, 2). The estimated number of new cases of and deaths from gastrointestinal cancers in 1997 in the United States is

shown in Table 34.1 (3). The cancers of small intestine account for 2.2% of new cases and 0.9% of deaths from all cancers of the digestive system (3). On the other hand, cancers of the large intestine (colon and rectum) are much more common, accounting for 58.1% of new cases and 43.2% of deaths from all digestive system cancers (Table 34.1). The colorectal cancers caused 57,405 deaths in 1993, accounting for 10.8% of all cancer deaths in the United States (3).

The incidence, and mortality and survival rates from gastrointestinal cancers in the United States are shown in Table 34.2 (4). The incidence and mortality rates of the small intestinal cancers are lowest and those of the colorectal cancers highest. The rarity of small intestinal tumors is also seen in the hospital population, making up less than 0.1% of all admissions (5, 6). In one report on 17,070 autopsies, 93 patients (0.54%) had small intestinal tumors, 24% of which were malignant (7). Among the surgically treated symptomatic patients, 75% of small intestinal tumors were malignant.

Types of tumors and their distribution in the small intestine are listed in Table 34.3 (8–17). Among the benign tumors, only one-third are epithelial lesions. They are equally distributed among the segments of the small intestine. Although only 25 to 30 cm long, the duodenum has a disproportionately high number of adenomas and polyps. The mesenchymal tumors, both benign and malignant, occur more commonly in the jejunum and ileum. The angiomatous lesions are presented in Chapter 14. Among the malignant tumors of the small intestine, adenocarcinoma is the most common. About 80% of the carcinomas occur in the duodenum and jejunum. Carcinoid and lymphoma, on the other hand, occur most commonly in the ileum. Epithelial tumors dominate in the large intestine, accounting for 90 to 95% of both benign and malignant lesions. In contrast to the small intestine, adenomas and polyps of the large intestine are much more common than the carcinomas. The younger the patients, the more likely the tumors will be polyps.

TABLE 34.1	Estimated New Cases and Death for Gastrointestinal Cancer in the United States in 1997					
	New Cases			Deaths		
Cancer Site	Male	Female	Total	Male	Female	Total
All sites	785,800	596,600	1,382,400	294,000	265,900	560,000
Esophagus	9,400	3,100	12,500	8,700	2,800	11,500
Stomach	14,000	8,400	22,400	8,300	5,700	14,000
Small intestine	2,600	2,300	4,900	540	600	1,140
Colon	45,500	48,600	94,100	22,600	24,000	46,600
Rectum	20,900	16,200	37,100	4,400	3,900	8,300
All digestive system	120,000	105,900	225,900	67,440	59,630	127,070

Data source: Parker SL, Tong T, Bolden S, Wingo PA. Cancer statistics, 1997. CA 1997;47:5–27.

TABLE 34.2 Age-adjusted SEER Incidence and U.S. Mortality Rates per 100,000 Population in 1988-1992, and 5-year Relative Survival Rates (%) of Gastrointestinal Cancer in 1986-1991

Cancer Site	Incidence Rate			Mortality Rate			Survival Rate		
	Total	Male	Female	Total	Male	Female	Total	Male	Female
Esophagus	3.9	6.5	1.8	3.5	6.0	1.5	10.0	10.1	9.7
Stomach	7.7	11.4	4.9	4.7	6.8	3.1	20.0	17.2	24.9
Small intestine	1.2	1.5	1.0	0.3	0.4	0.3	51.2	49.7	52.8
Colon/rectum	47.7	58.2	40.0	18.7	23.1	15.6	61.0	61.6	60.4
Lung	58.6	81.7	41.5	49.6	74.4	31.4	13.4	12.1	15.4
Breast	60.1	0.9	109.6	15.2	0.2	27.1	83.2	83.9	83.2
Prostate	59.1	141.4	—	9.9	26.0	—	85.8	85.8	—

Data source: Kosary CL, Gloeckle-Ries LA, Miller BA, Hankey BF, Harras A, Edwards BK. SEER Cancer Statistics Review, 1973-1992. NIH publication 96-2789. Bethesda, MD: National Cancer Institute, 1996:152–180.

SEER (Surveillance, Epidemiology and End Results) program is a project of the National Cancer Institute.

TABLE 34.3 Frequency and Types of Tumors of the Small Intestine In Number and Percentage

Tumor Type	Total Cases[a]	Tumor Location Specified[b]			
		Duodenum	Jejunum	Ileum	Subtotal
Benign Total[c]	2859 (100.0)	531 (22.6)	759 (32.4)	1057 (45.0)	2347 (100.0)
Adenoma, polyp	795 (27.8)	230 (30.5)	265 (35.1)	259 (34.4)	754 (100.0)
Leiomyoma	803 (28.1)	123 (19.0)	275 (42.4)	250 (38.6)	648 (100.0)
Lipoma	494 (17.3)	100 (19.1)	196 (37.4)	228 (43.5)	524 (100.0)
Fibroma	192 (6.7)	8 (3.0)	130 (48.9)	128 (48.1)	266 (100.0)
Angioma	368 (12.9)	21 (7.5)	136 (48.6)	123 (43.9)	280 (100.0)
Nerve tumor	106 (3.7)	16 (14.7)	48 (44.0)	45 (41.3)	109 (100.0)
Miscellaneous	101 (3.5)	33 (43.4)	19 (25.0)	24 (31.6)	76 (100.0)
Malignant Total[d]	2446 (100.0)	375 (20.0)	560 (29.8)	945 (50.2)	1880 (100.0)
Carcinoma	855 (35.0)	267 (38.5)	290 (41.8)	137 (19.7)	694 (100.0)
Carcinoid	823 (33.6)	57 (9.3)	41 (6.7)	512 (83.8)	610 (100.0)
Sarcoma	268 (11.0)	38 (17.3)	88 (40.0)	94 (42.7)	220 (100.0)
Lymphoma	487 (19.9)	12 (3.5)	137 (39.5)	198 (57.0)	347 (100.0)
Miscellaneous	13 (0.5)	1 (11.1)	4 (44.4)	4 (44.5)	9 (100.0)

[a]Total number of cases in cited references irrespective of tumor location.

[b]Only reports listing tumor locations are included.

[c]For benign cases see: Wood DA. Tumors of the intestines. Atlas of Tumor Pathology, Fascicle 22. Washington, DC: Armed Forces Institute of Pathology, 1967. del Regato JA, Spjut HJ, Cox JD. Ackerman and del Regato's Cancer. Diagnosis, Treatment and Prognosis. 6th ed. St Louis: CV Mosby, 1985:512–530. Herbsman H, Wetstein L, Rosen V. Tumors of the small intestine. Curr Prob Surg 1980;17:121–184. Wilson JM, Melvin DB, Gray GF, et al. Benign small bowel tumor. Ann Surg 1975;181: 247–250. Mason GR. Tumors of the duodenum and small intestine. In: Sabiston DC Jr, ed. Textbook of Surgery. 13th ed. Philadelphia: WB Saunders, 1986:868–873. Braasch JW, Denbo HE. Tumors of the small intestine. Surg Clin N Am 1964;44:791–809.

[d]For malignant cases see: Darling RC, Welch CE. Tumors of the small intestine. New Engl J Med 1959;260:397–408. del Regato JA, Spjut HJ, Cox JD. Ackerman and del Regato's Cancer. Diagnosis, Treatment and Prognosis. 6th ed. St Louis: CV Mosby, 1985:512–530. Herbsman H, Wetstein L, Rosen V. Tumors of the small intestine. Curr Prob Surg 1980;17:121–184. Mason GR. Tumors of the duodenum and small intestine. In: Sabiston DC Jr, ed. Textbook of Surgery. 13th ed. Philadelphia: WB Saunders, 1986:868–873. Braasch JW, Denbo HE. Tumors of the small intestine. Surg Clin N Am 1964;44:791–809. Kelsey JR Jr. Small bowel tumors. In: Bockus HL, ed. Gastroenterology, 3rd ed. Philadelphia: WB Saunders, 1976:459–472. Barclay THC, Shapira DV. Malignant tumors of the small intestine. Cancer 1983;51:878–881. Wilson JM, Melvin DB, Gray DG, Thorbjarnason B. Primary malignancies of the small bowel: A report of 96 cases and reviews of the literature. Ann Surg 1974;180: 175–179. Williamson RCN, Welch CE, Malt RA. Adenocarcinoma and lymphoma of the small intestine. Distribution and etiologic associations. Ann Surg 1983;197: 172–178.

The constituent cells of the epithelial tumors, irrespective of their location in the intestine, are of the same lineage as the normal cells, mainly columnar absorptive cells, mucous cells, endocrine cells, and occasionally Paneth cells (18). Only rarely do cells of metaplastic or heterotopic origin play a role in the tumor development of the intestines. Two types of metaplasia or heterotopia may occur in the intestines: squamous metaplasia, and gastric metaplasia or heterotopia (see Chapter 30). Squamous metaplasia is rare and is seen mainly in the colon and rectum after tissue injury (19). It may also occur in an adenoma (20). Squamous cell carcinoma may develop from such metaplastic cells. Pure squamous cell carcinomas of the colon are rare (19, 21). Adenosquamous cell carcinoma is slightly more common (22). The squamous cells in the latter probably originate from the progenitor of the neoplastic cells rather than from a separate cell origin of metaplastic nature. Gastric metaplasia or heterotopia is common in the duodenum. The gastric cells are usually in association with duodenitis and consist primarily of surface and foveolar cells (23), and occasionally cells of fundic glands (24). Pyloric glands in the duodenal lesion are difficult to identify, because of the presence of Brunner glands. Polyps and adenomas in gastric metaplasia have been reported (23, 25). Gastric metaplasia with pyloric glands may be seen in the distal small intestine and colorectum, usually in association with chronic inflammatory bowel disease (26) and rarely as heterotopia (27). There was a case of jejunal adenocarcinoma in heterotopic gastric mucosa (28). Neoplastic change in the gastric tissue in the colorectum has not been reported.

ADENOCARCINOMA OF THE INTESTINES

GENERAL CONSIDERATIONS

Adenocarcinoma is the most important malignant tumor in the intestines. It is nearly fifty times more frequent in the large intestine than the small intestine (Table 34.2). The colorectal carcinoma ranks the third most common cause of cancer death in both men, after lung and prostate, and women, after lung and breast, in the United States (3). The probability of developing and dying of colorectal cancer in a life time is high (Table 34.4) (4). It is higher in the white than in the black population. Because of its high prevalence, colorectal carcinoma has attracted a great deal more attention and effort than the small intestinal cancer. Consequently, much more information is available concerning colorectal carcinoma.

The mucosa of the small and large intestines is exposed to a similar environment, namely a mixture of ingested substances and bodily secretions containing bile and metabolic products. In addition, there is a large number of bacteria, many of which are anaerobic. If the carcinogenic agents are exogenous and environmental in source as suspected, they are likely to be in this mixture, and the epithelium of both small and large intestines is exposed to them. It is, therefore, puzzling to see such a striking difference in the cancer incidence in the respective segments of the intestine. A number of possible factors have been postulated (1, 29, 30) and are listed below.

1. Rapid transit time of bowel contents in the small intestine may have reduced the contact time with carcinogens, whereas the solid feces in the large intestine remains for a much longer time.
2. The liquid content of the small intestine may dilute the carcinogens while absorption of water in the large intestine concentrates the carcinogens. Furthermore, liquid content may be less of an irritant and less injurious to the small intestinal mucosa than the solid and particulate fecal matter in the large intestine.
3. There is a much larger bacterial population with many anaerobes in the large intestine than the small intestine, which may convert bile salts and other procarcinogens into carcinogens (31).
4. The small intestine has higher enzyme activity than the large intestine to detoxify carcinogens. For instance, the benzpyrene hydroxylase in the small intestine may convert benzpyrene into less active metabolites (32).

TABLE 34.4	Lifetime Risk of Being Diagnosed with Cancer and Dying of Cancer by Race and Sex in Percentage. SEER Program 1990-1992					
	All Races		White		Black	
Lifetime Risk of	Males	Females	Males	Females	Males	Females
Developing Cancer						
Esophagus	0.71	0.26	0.66	0.25	1.26	0.99
Stomach	1.24	0.79	1.10	0.68	1.44	1.02
Colon/rectum	6.15	5.88	6.28	5.92	4.47	5.42
Dying of Cancer						
Esophagus	0.65	0.23	0.62	0.22	1.23	0.39
Stomach	0.84	0.54	0.75	0.48	1.04	0.65
Colon/rectum	2.59	2.57	2.65	2.60	2.04	2.60

Data source: Kosary CL, Gloeckle-Ries LA, Miller BA, Hankey BF, Harras A, Edwards BK. SEER Cancer Statistics Review, 1973–1992. NIH publication 96-2789. Bethesda, MD: National Cancer Institute, 1996:152–180.

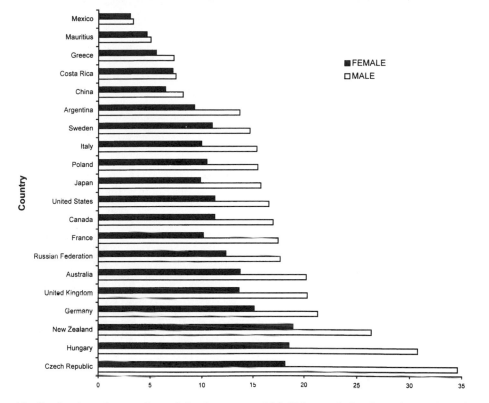

Figure 34.1 Geographic distribution of age-adjusted death rates per 100,000 population for colorectal carcinoma in 1990 to 1993. Data from Parker SL, Tong T, Bolden S, Wingo PA. Cancer statistics, 1997. CA 1997;47:5–27.

5. Rapid cell turnover in the small intestine may protect the mucosal cells by shedding. On the other hand, increased proliferation of mucosal cells may actually increase the malignant transformation (33) and the neoplastic cells do not shed but accumulate at the site of origin (34). Thus, the beneficial effect of rapid cell turnover may be limited to the initial stage of carcinogenesis.

6. The effective immune system in the small intestine with immunologically active lymphocytes may protect the tissue against oncogenic viruses (32), and the T lymphocytes against the cancer cells (35).

EPIDEMIOLOGY

Small Intestinal Carcinoma

The low incidence rate of small intestinal carcinoma seen in the United States (Tables 34.1 and 34.2) is also found in other countries (29). The incidence rate is higher in the developed Western countries than in the underdeveloped countries (29, 36) and parallels that of colon cancer (32). Within the United States, the incidence rate in Hawaiian whites is higher than in Hawaiian Japanese; the latter is higher than that in Japan (29). There is a slight male predominance (37). The incidence rate is higher in blacks than in whites (4). The survival rate of small intestinal cancer is lower than that of colorectal cancer, particularly in the male (Table 34.2). The

age of the patients ranges from 30 to 80, with a peak in the seventh decade (15, 38).

Large Intestinal Carcinoma

The incidence and mortality rates of large intestinal carcinoma vary greatly in different countries (Fig. 34.1), ranging from the low of 2.0 for males and 2.2 for females in Albania to the high of 34.6 for males in the Czech Republic and 18.9 for females in New Zealand (3). In general, the incidence rates are high in the European and North American countries and low in Asian, South American, and African countries. There is a male predominance in the high incidence regions (37). The sex difference is slight in the United States (Fig. 34.2). The incidence rates of the colon cancer is higher than that of the rectal cancer in the high incidence areas but the difference is small in the low incidence areas (39). Furthermore, the rectal cancer in the high risk regions is located more in the upper rectum and in the low risk regions more in the lower rectum (40).

The distribution of colorectal cancers among ethnic groups in the United States is shown in Table 34.5 (41). The incidence and mortality rates by sex and race are listed in Table 34.6 (4). The ratio between the incidence rate and the mortality rate of colorectal cancer in the United States is about 2.5. Between 1973 and 1992, there was an increase in the incidence rate of colon cancer, only slightly among the white male, but prominently in both sexes of the black race (Table 34.6). The incidence rate of rectal cancer had

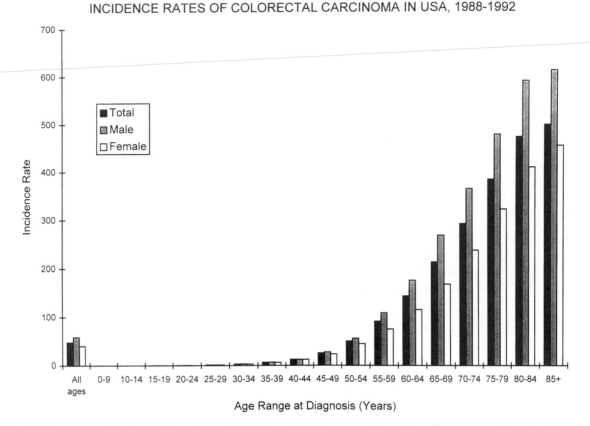

Figure 34.2   Incidence rates of colorectal carcinoma in 1988 to 1992 by sex and age. Data from Kosary CL, Gloeckle-Ries LA, Miller BA, Hankey BF, Harras A, Edwards BK. SEER Cancer Statistics Review, 1973–1992. NIH publication 96-2789. Bethesda, MD: National Cancer Institute, 1996:152–180.

increased only among the black male. The mortality rate of colorectal cancer during this period decreased in the white population but increased in the black male. A recent study in Detroit (42) revealed an increase in the incidence of carcinomas in the right colon, up to splenic flexure, in mid 1970s and early 1980s in African Americans. This increase is particularly evident for the late stage lesions in men and is associated with a decrease in survival rates.

Carcinomas of the colon and rectum are diseases of the elderly, with peak age in the 7th and 8th decades (Fig. 34.2). The mean age of the patients was 71.2 years for carcinoma of the right colon, 68.2 years for left colon cancer, and 65.6 years for rectal cancer (43). Colorectal carcinoma occurs rarely in the young. Only 3 to 6% of the patients were younger than 40 years (44–46). The symptoms in these patients are not different from those in the older patients (47). Some reports noted that the young patients had a high incidence of signet-ring cell and mucinous carcinomas (44, 46, 48–50) and poor prognosis (44, 45, 48–50). Other reports found a no worse survival rate in the young than in older patients (47, 51).

ETIOLOGY

The geographic, sex, and racial differences in the incidence rates of intestinal cancer appear to be caused by environmental rather then genetic factors as shown by migration studies. The incidence rates among migrants residing in the new country for a long time and

their next generations usually shift toward the prevailing rates of the local population (52–54). While racial genetics does not appear to be important, genetics does play a dominant role in the development of intestinal cancer in a number of hereditary diseases such as familial adenomatous polyposis and Gardner's and Lynch syndromes. In addition, alterations in gene expression have been demonstrated in the cancer cells. Table 34.7 lists possible risk factors of intestinal cancers. Detailed discussion of these findings is in the section on molecular and genetic alteration later in this chapter as well as in Chapters 7 and 8.

Carcinogens

The carcinogenic agents for human intestinal cancer have not been identified. There are, however, reliable animal models for the induction of intestinal carcinoma using chemical carcinogens. Two models in particular give information relevant to human intestinal carcinogenesis. One model involves the use of a strong direct-acting carcinogen, such as N-methyl-N′-nitro-N-nitrosoguanidine (MNNG), to induce the carcinoma at points of contact with the tissue (55). The other model uses chemicals which require metabolic activation before exerting the carcinogenic effect, such as analogues of cycasin and 1,2-dimethylhydrazine (DMH) (56, 57). Although MNNG is not organ-specific, DMH and related chemicals are strongly organotropic and cause intestinal tumors, mostly colonic, independent of route of administration. It is unlikely that exposure to a direct carcinogen is a major cause of human intestinal tumor. The indirect mechanism of carcinogenesis may be more applicable to the human situation. In addition to illustrating possible modes of carcinogenesis, the experimental models are used to evaluate suspected risk factors in the human by manipulating the dietary and other environmental conditions in the animals.

The sources of possible intestinal carcinogens may be environmental, occupational, diet-linked, or endogenous. The environmental agents include air pollutants such as sulfur dioxide in acid haze (58), hazardous chemical waste (59), automobile emissions (60), arsenic in well water (61), and asbestos (62). The importance of asbestos exposure has been disputed, however (63). A variety of occupations had an increased risk for colon cancer (64) including the petroleum product industry, printing machine operators, food manufacturing workers, and manufacturers of polypropylene (65). Food may be contaminated by carcinogens (66) or serve as substrate for endogenous carcinogen (67). Nitroso compounds have been found in the feces of persons with a diet high in protein and low in ascorbic acid and tocopherol (68). They may be formed in the stomach with chronic gastritis (69). Other endogenous substances which may be related to intestinal carcinogenesis include mutagenic agents, such as fecapentaenes, which are found in the human feces and thought to be produced by colonic microflora. They have been correlated with the incidences of colon cancer (70, 71) and polyps (72). However, no such relationship was found in a recent study (73). Mutagenic compounds have also been found in cooked meat (66, 74, 75). A study in New Zealand demonstrated DNA-damaging activity in fecal extract from persons on a mixed diet but none from Seventh-Day Adventists on an ovo-lacto-vegetarian diet (76).

Radiation as a possible carcinogenic agent is suspected when colonic carcinoma develops in patients who received radiation therapy to the pelvic region for various reasons, mostly for the treatment of gynecologic malignancy (77, 78). Jao et al. reviewed 76 cases of colon or anorectal cancer after pelvic radiation (77). The mean interval between radiation and cancer development was 15.2 years. About one-third of the tumors were mucinous adenocarcinomas. The 5-year survival rate was 48%. Carcinomas of the colon and rectum had also been reported in patients who received a single massive dose of radiation (79) and in atomic bomb survivors (80). The tissue surrounding the tumor may show reactive radiation effects which have been used as a marker for radiation-induced lesions.

Tubulovillous adenoma was induced in the duodenum of guinea fowls by intravenous injection of a virus strain pts-57 (81). A search for viral DNA for cytomegalovirus, Epstein-Barr virus, and human papillomavirus in biopsies of human colonic adenomas and adenocarcinomas has been negative (82).

Modifying Agents

Chemical carcinogenesis appears to be the most important cause of intestinal carcinoma. A variety of substances has been found to have a modifying effect on the process. The promoters include bile acids (83) and 3-ketosteroids (84). The inhibitors are generally antioxidants such as Vitamins C and E and selenium. Vitamins C and E reduce the level of fecal mitogens in the stool and inhibit the formation of nitrosamines, cell proliferation, and carcinogenesis (85). Supplementary administration of these vitamins for 2 years to patients who had colonic polyps removed showed them having a slightly lower recurrence rate than the control patients on placebo (86). Selenium reduces tumor formation in the colon in experimental animals (87), particularly in the right colon (88). The reported increase of cancer incidence in the right colon in Western countries has been attributed to selenium deficiency (89). Butylated hydroxytoluene, another antioxidant, reduces experimental colonic tumors in the male mice but not in the female (90).

Nonsteroidal anti-inflammatory drugs (NSAIDs), which include aspirin, indomethacin, proxicam, and sulindac, have been found to reduce the incidence and number of colorectal tumors in rodents induced by a variety of carcinogens such as DMH and azoxymethane (91, 92). In retrospective studies in the human, NSAIDs have been found to reduce the odds ratio for developing colon cancers (78, 93–95) and adenomas (96) by one-third to one-half. The inhibitory effect increased with the duration and dose of drug usage. Prospective studies showed less protective effect by aspirin (91). In one study, the protective effect was seen only in men younger than 65 years of age (97). A trial with sulindac on patients with familial adenomatous polyposis showed regression of polyps which regrew after the drug was discontinued (98). The mechanism of NSAID action has not been clarified. An NSAID reduces

TABLE	
34.5	**Percentage of Colon and Rectal Cancer in 1992 by Ethnicity, Site, and Stage**

	Colon Cancer	Rectal Cancer
Ethnicity		
Non-Hispanic White	85.1	85.7
Hispanic	2.2	2.8
African American	8.2	6.9
Native American	0.1	0.2
Asian	1.4	1.9
Unknown	3.0	2.6
Anatomic site		
Ascending/cecum	36.1	
Transverse	17.2	
Descending	6.9	
Sigmoid	33.4	
Multiple sites	1.2	
Unknown	5.2	
Rectosigmoid junction		32.6
Rectum		67.4
Stage		
0	6.9	6.3
I	18.1	23.4
II	23.8	19.0
III	19.4	20.3
IV	15.6	12.3
Unknown	16.2	18.7

Data source: Steele GD Jr, Jessup JM. Colorectal cancer. In: Steele GD Jr, Jessup JM, Winchester DP, Menck HR, Murphy GP, eds. National Cancer data base. Annual review of patient care, 1995. Atlanta: American Cancer Society, 1996;66–83.

TABLE
34.6

Age-adjusted SEER Incidence and U.S. Mortality Rates per 100,000 Population and 5-year Survival Rates in Percentage of Colorectal Cancer by Race and Sex and Their Percent Changes

Cancer Site	All Races		White		Black	
	Male	Female	Male	Female	Male	Female
Incidence Rate						
1988–1992						
Colorectum	58.2	40.0	58.1	39.6	61.0	46.3
Colon	40.0	29.7	40.0	29.4	46.5	36.6
Rectum	17.9	10.0	18.0	10.2	15.1	9.7
Percent change (1973 to 1992)						
Colorectum	3.8	−6.3	1.4	−8.2	40.4	15.9
Colon	11.1	−3.4	8.8	−5.8	42.2	30.6
Rectum	−9.7	−14.0	−12.4	−14.4	35.5	−20.4
Mortality Rate						
1988–1992						
Colorectum	23.1	15.6	22.9	15.3	28.1	20.4
Percent change (1973 to 1992)						
Colorectum	−11.3	−23.0	−13.5	−25.1	22.9	2.0
5-Year Survival Rate						
1986–1991						
Colorectum	61.6	60.4	62.5	61.0	51.1	53.6
Colon	62.7	60.8	63.7	61.4	51.3	53.6
Rectum	59.3	59.4	60.3	59.9	50.5	53.6
1974–1976						
Colorectum	48.6	50.3	49.0	50.5	41.2	47.2
Colon	49.4	50.7	49.7	50.8	43.9	46.6
Rectum	47.3	49.3	47.7	49.6	34.3	49.1
Percent change (1974–1976 to 1986–1991)						
Colorectum	26.7	20.1	27.5	20.8	24.0	13.6
Colon	26.9	19.9	28.2	20.9	16.9	15.0
Rectum	25.4	20.5	26.4	20.8	47.2	9.2

Data source: Kosary CL, Gloeckle-Ries LA, Miller BA, Hankey BF, Harras A, Edwards BK. SEER Cancer Statistics Review, 1973–1992. NIH publication 96-2789. Bethesda, MD: National Cancer Institute, 1996:152–180.

prostaglandin production by inhibiting the action of cyclooxygenase. Cyclooxygenase is increased in colon cancer cells (72, 99, 100). The action of prostaglandin on intestinal epithelium is not clear, however (101).

SYSTEMIC RISK FACTORS

Although precise etiologic agents for intestinal cancers are not known, many factors related to an increased risk of developing intestinal cancer, particularly colorectal cancer, have been identified. Some of these factors are systemic, affecting the body as a whole. Others are regional changes affecting the site of tumor formation. Thus the former factors are mainly metabolic in nature and the latter factors are tissue alterations preceding carcinogenesis, and are precancerous conditions.

The intestinal tract is exposed to many possible carcinogens, exogenous and endogenous, as discussed above. Since the likely possibility involves one or more carcinogenic agents requiring prior

metabolic activation before the carcinogenic effect is manifest, the tumors are often the result of complex interplay among a number of risk factors rather than the product of a single factor. In some instances, conflicting observations were made.

Genetic Factors

The genetic aspects of intestinal cancers are discussed in Chapter 7. In this section, only information related to pathologic features are presented. Genetic factors play a role in an estimated 20% of colorectal carcinomas (102). They have a primary role in several syndromes in which intestinal polyposis is the main or prominent component:

1. Familial adenomatous polyposis (FAP) and the related Gardner and Turcot syndromes. In addition to polyposis, Gardner syndrome manifests benign skin, soft tissue, and bone lesions (103).

2. Peutz-Jeghers syndrome in which, in addition to polyposis, there is mucocutaneous pigmentation (104).
3. Juvenile polyposis (105).

These syndromes are rare. Much more common are the hereditary nonpolyposis colorectal cancers (HNPCC) which account for about 5 to 15% of all colorectal cancers (106–108). Although these latter patients do not have polyposis, adenomas occur in a random fashion as in the general population in about one-third of the cases screened (102, 109). In addition, heredity plays a role in patients with discrete familial clustering of colonic polyps (110), with an estimated gene frequency of 19% (111).

TABLE	
34.7	**Risk Factors of Intestinal Carcinoma**

Carcinogenic Agents
  Chemical carcinogens
  Radiation
  Modifying agents
Systemic Risk Factors
  Genetic factors
  Cancer history
  Dietary factors
    High fat and meat intake
    Low intake of fiber, fruits, and vegetables
  Alcohol and tobacco
  Low physical activity and obesity
  Occupation
Intestinal Risk Factors
  Bile acids and sterols
  Intestinal bacterial flora
Associated Conditions
  Cholecystectomy
  Barrett's esophagus
  Gastrectomy and hypochlorhydria
Precancerous Conditions
  Benign epithelial polyps
    Adenomas and adenomatous polyposis
    Nonneoplastic polyps and polyposis
      Hyperplastic polyp
      Peutz-Jeghers syndrome
      Juvenile polyposis
  Intestinal diseases
    Ulcerative colitis and Crohn's disease
    Schistosomiasis
    Epithelial hyperplasia
Molecular and Genetic Alterations
Protective Factors
  High intake of dietary fibers, fruits, and vegetables
  Vitamins and antioxidants
  Folate and methionine
  Aspirin and nonsteroidal anti-inflammatory drugs
  Calcium
  High physical activity

Colorectal cancer can occur in all of these conditions, usually at a young age. In FAP, the mean age of polyposis patients is 16 years and the average age of cancer patients is 35. The incidence of carcinoma increases with age, and is 7% at 21 years of age, 50% by 39 years, and 90% by 45 years. These cases account for 1% of colorectal cancers (106, 107). Eventually, all polyposis patients develop colorectal cancer. The carcinoma develops from the adenoma and de novo carcinoma has not been seen in these cases (103). Carcinoma and adenoma can occur also in the stomach and small intestine, particularly the duodenum (112). Periampullary carcinoma is present in 10 to 12% of patients. A less severe form of FAP, called attenuated adenomatosis polyposis coli (AAPC), has been recognized recently (113). In AAPC the average number of colonic adenomas is 30. The manifestations of adenoma and carcinoma in AAPC are 10 years later than FAP on average. The carcinoma is present in the right colon in about 70% of cases. The polyps in the Peutz-Jeghers syndrome and familial juvenile polyposis are of nonneoplastic hamartomatous type. Carcinoma develops from the hamartomatous polyp or the associated adenoma (104, 114, 115). Recently, a family with a hereditary mixed polyposis syndrome was reported from St. Mark's hospital in England (116). The affected members of the family developed colonic polyps of different types including adenomas, hyperplastic polyps, atypical juvenile polyps, and polyps with mixed histology. The condition is inherited in autosomal dominant fashion. Of 71 patients with updated clinical information, 42 had colorectal cancer or polyps. Typically, fewer than 15 polyps were found in a patient. The cancers are distributed throughout the colon and rectum.

The HNPCC cases have been divided into two groups, named Lynch syndromes I and II (102, 117). The difference between these two syndromes is that familial aggregation of cancers in other organs, particularly the endometrial, ovarian, and pancreatic carcinomas, is present in Lynch syndrome II, but not in Lynch syndrome I. Lynch syndrome II is also known as cancer family syndrome (118, 119). The lifetime risk of developing colon cancer in HNPCC patients is 80% (120). The colorectal cancers in these cases have several characteristics (108, 119, 121). They are located mostly in the right colon (72%), and the mean age at diagnosis is 44.6 years. Multiple colorectal carcinomas are common, synchronous in 18% and metachronous in 24% of the cases. Histologically, mucinous and signet-ring cell carcinomas are more common than in the general population. The associated adenomas may be of flat type (102), which has a high rate of malignant change (122). Additional information on the polyposis syndromes is presented in Chapter 33, and the genetic aspects of these conditions are discussed in Chapter 7.

In addition to the genetics related to hereditary intestinal tumors, a change in the expression of many genes in the DNA is commonly involved in the carcinogenic process even though the tumor is not hereditary. A progressive series of steps in which tumor suppressor genes are deleted or mutated has been identified by biochemical and cytogenetic methods (123–125). These events are discussed in Chapters 7 and 8 and summarized in the section on molecular and genetic alterations later in this chapter.

Dietary Factors

Epidemiologic studies implicate diet as the major risk factor for colonic cancer. The marked regional variations in the incidence rates for colorectal carcinoma can be correlated with dietary habits. Experimental studies on animals fed with various modified diets support these views.

DIETARY FAT AND MEAT   It has been shown that the countries with high mortality rates from colorectal cancer had high fat and meat consumption (52, 126, 127). Dietary fat constituted 41.8% of total calories in the United States, a high risk country, and 12.2% in Japan, a low risk country (126). A similar positive correlation between incidence rates of large bowel cancer and consumption of animal fat, meat, and cholesterol, and inverse correlation with dietary fibers and Vitamins C and A were found in other studies (101, 128). The mortality rate of colorectal cancer is low among the Seventh-Day Adventists who consume less fat and cholesterol than their high risk compatriots (129). The types of fat or oil consumed are important factors (130). Saturated fat and red meat consumption are associated with increased incidence of colon cancer (131–134). However, experiments comparing the effects of saturated and unsaturated fat gave conflicting results (135, 136). The combination of high fat and low fiber in the diet gives a high yield of experimental colorectal tumors in rats (137). The mechanism of these effects is an increase in endogenous bile acids and fatty acids which promote colonic carcinogenesis (83). The meat protein enhances carcinogenesis by serving as substrate for possible carcinogenic substances and increasing bacterial growth (138).

TOTAL CALORIE INTAKE   High total calorie intake increases the risk for colon cancer (9, 134). Calorie restriction reduces colon tumor yield in rats even if the animals are on a high fat diet (139).

CHOLESTEROL AND FECAL STEROLS   High fat intake increases the fecal level of cholesterol and natural sterols, and the serum level of cholesterol and β-lipoprotein, which are associated with increased risk of colon cancer in man (140) and experimental animals (141). Reddy et al. found that the levels of fecal cholesterol and sterol excretion differed markedly in people with different dietary habits. In decreasing order are levels among Americans on a mixed diet, American vegetarians, Seventh-Day Adventists, Japanese, and Chinese (142); this order is in parallel with the incidence rates of colon cancer.

DIETARY FIBERS, FRUITS, AND VEGETABLES   High risk countries for colorectal cancer consume less vegetables, fruits, and fibers than the low risk countries (101, 128). Many antimutagenic and anticarcinogenic substances have been isolated from fruits and vegetables (143). In addition, they provide the protective effects of vitamins and fibers (131, 144). The negative effect of dietary fiber on colon cancer risk has been extensively studied. While most reports on humans show the protective effect of fiber against colon cancer, some reports show no effect (145). In animal experiments conflicting data have also been obtained, apparently related to the types of fibers used (146). In the human, insoluble and more fermentable fibers such as cellulose and bran are protective (131, 144). The mechanism of the modulating effects of fiber on colon carcinogenesis is complex and involves interactions between fiber and many substances in the gut. Insoluble fibers increases the bulk of the feces, dilutes the carcinogens and bile acids, and shortens the transit time (127). Carcinogens and bile acids can be bound to the fiber (147).

These effects reduce the exposure of colonic epithelium to the carcinogens and promoters. Fibers are fermented by the anaerobic organisms to produce short-chain fatty acids which increase the fecal acidity, stimulate the cell growth of colonic epithelium, and facilitate carcinogenesis (131, 145). In addition, the acid bowel contents may inhibit the metabolism of carcinogens and bile acids and reduce the carcinogenecity of these substances (148, 149).

VITAMINS AND CALCIUM   Vitamins C and E are antioxidants which may inhibit the formation of N-nitroso compounds, but their ability to reduce carcinogenesis is variable (134, 149–151). Vitamin A and related retinoids and beta-carotene are protective against esophageal carcinomas. Their role in colon carcinogenesis is equivocal (149, 152). The intake of dietary Vitamin D and calcium is inversely related to the incidence of colorectal cancer in a 19-year prospective study in man (153). Insoluble calcium soap formed with fatty acids or bile acids prevents mucosal damage and hyperplasia caused by these agents (154). Supplementary oral calcium has been shown to reduce the proliferative activity and promote differentiation of colon epithelial cells (155, 156). Calcium reduced colon tumors in experiments in rodents (85). Finally, folate reduces colon cancer risk while folate and methionine deficiency increases the risk (149, 157, 158). Vegetables and fruits are major sources of folate.

Alcohol and Tobacco

Alcohol and tobacco increase the risk for colonic cancer and adenoma (158–161). Heavy beer drinking has been associated with an increased incidence of rectal carcinoma (159, 162).

Hormones

Among hormones of the digestive tract, gastrin (163, 164) and intestinal active peptide (165) have been shown to promote colon cancer development, because of their effect on increased cell proliferation.

That sex hormones play a role in bowel cancer is suggested by the sex difference of tumor incidence: males are more affected than females (52, 166). Furthermore, the incidence was lower in women with previous pregnancies and who had never used estrogen supplements (167, 168). Oral contraceptive use increased the risk of rectal cancer but not colonic cancer in women (169). Estrogen and androgen receptors are present in the colonic tumors (170, 171). Injection of testosterone at birth increases DMH-induced tumors in both male and female mice, but more in the female. This is attributed to hyperestrogenization of the androgenized female (172). However, data on testosterone effect on tumor growth are contradictory (171, 173). Patients with acromegaly have an increased incidence of colon cancer and polyps (174, 175), probably because of the stimulation by insulin-like growth factors which are present in the tumor (176). Colonic cancer has been seen in patients with parathyroid adenoma (177), but the mechanism is not clear.

Cancer History

In genetic cancer syndromes, familial and personal history of previous bowel tumor is a characteristic feature. In the general population, 5 to 10% of persons have one first-degree relative with colon cancer. This incidence increases to 10 to 20% among colon cancer patients (178, 179). Persons who have one first-degree relative with colon cancer have a 3.5-fold increase of colon cancer risk (180), amounting to a 21% risk considering the lifetime risk of colon cancer in the general population is 6% (Table 34.4). The risk increases if the number of relatives with cancer is two or more and the age at time of diagnosis is 50 years or under (181, 182). Persons with a second-degree or third-degree relative with colon cancer have a 30 to 50% increase of risk (183). The incidence of colonic adenomas in first-degree relatives also increases the risk of colon cancer (184). One report (185) noted a high incidence of small bowel cancer in patients with prior large bowel cancer. There was also a slight increase in the relative incidence of cancer in extraintestinal organs, including bladder (in both sexes), breast, endometrium, ovary, and prostate (183, 185). There is no increased risk for the spouse of patients with colorectal cancer (186).

Social Status, Physical Activity, and Obesity

The incidence of colorectal carcinoma is higher in urban than in rural regions and more in the upper than lower socioeconomic class (52). The incidence is lower in Mormons and Seventh-Day Adventists than in other groups (75, 187). Life style and dietary habits are likely factors. Physical activity may also be a factor since it seems to reduce the mortality rate of colorectal cancer (188, 189). It also reduces the incidence of DMH-induced colon tumors (190). Risk for colon cancer is increased in obese persons, especially those with abdominal obesity (191). In such persons, there is an increase of serum insulin which may stimulate cell growth in the intestine.

Extraintestinal Conditions

CHOLECYSTECTOMY   There have been many reports on the relationship between prior cholecystectomy and subsequent development of colon cancer. Most reports indicated a positive relationship for both cancer (192–195) and adenoma (196, 197), but some reports showed no relationship (198, 199). The increased risk affects the right colon but not the left colon or rectum (192, 194) and women more than men (193, 194, 200). The colon carcinoma generally develops several years after cholecystectomy. The proposed mechanism is related to bile acid metabolism (192). After cholecystectomy, the enterohepatic circulation of bile salts is increased. This leads to increased secondary bile acids in the bowel by action of intestinal bacteria, and enhanced tumor production.

BARRETT'S ESOPHAGUS   There have been conflicting reports about the association of colonic neoplasms with Barrett's esophagus. In a review of published data (201), it was noted that the prevalence of colon cancer was 7.6% in patients with Barrett's esophagus and 1.6% in the control group. The risk was higher if the Barrett's esophagus was composed of metaplastic epithelium. On the other hand, no increase of colonic adenoma was found in patients with Barrett's esophagus (202, 203).

GASTRECTOMY AND HYPOCHLORHYDRIA   There is a two-fold increase of colorectal cancer after gastrectomy for gastroduodenal disease (204, 205). Hypochlorhydria and bile reflux causing increased levels of carcinogens and free secondary bile acids in the gastric remnant may be responsible for the increased risk of cancer in the colon and stomach (205). The same mechanism may be applied to the finding of a slight increase of colorectal cancer in patients with pernicious anemia (69).

INTESTINAL RISK FACTORS

Intestinal Contents

BILE ACIDS   Bile acids and their metabolites are involved in many ways in colorectal carcinogenesis as discussed above. The bile acid conjugates can be hydrolyzed by the intestinal anaerobes to free bile acids (31, 206), particularly the deoxycholic and lithocholic acids. Their fecal concentration is higher in colonic cancer patients than in adenoma patients (142). The free bile acid concentration in patients with small adenomas is the same as in normal persons, suggesting that the bile acids are involved in the growth but not the initiation of the adenomas (128).

Deoxycholic acid causes inflammation and necrosis followed by proliferation of colonic epithelium. These changes can be prevented by calcium which sequesters the bile acid (207). Lithocholic acid has an even more important role in promoting tumor growth since the lithocholic acid to deoxycholic acid ratio in the feces is highest in patients with colonic carcinoma, lowest in persons at low risk, and at an intermediate level in patients with adenomas (206). The free bile acids are potent inducers of chromosomal aneuploidy, whereas the conjugated bile acids are not (208).

INTESTINAL FLORA   Intestinal microorganisms, particularly the anaerobic *Clostridia*, play a crucial role in carcinogenesis of the gut (209). Enzymes produced by these bacteria, such as β-glucuronidase and hydroxylases, convert conjugated bile acids and procarcinogens to secondary bile acids and free active forms which may initiate or promote tumorigenesis (31, 133, 210). They ferment plant fibers to produce short-chain fatty acids and lower the pH of bowel contents, both of which influence the carcinogenic process (see the above section on dietary fibers). Germ-free animals produce much fewer intestinal tumors than conventional animals (211). Treatment of animals with antibiotics during the induction period reduces the cancer incidence (212).

FECAL CONTENTS   It is evident that the contents of fecal matter, whether exogenous or endogenous, are primary sources of carcinogens and substances which either promote or inhibit tumors. In one experiment, a segment of distal colon was bypassed by the fecal stream as a result of a surgical operation. Tumors were induced by DMH in the feces-filled segment and not in the empty bypassed segment (213). In another experiment, DMH administration did produce tumors in the isolated, defunctionalized, and cleansed segment of colon, although in fewer animals and in smaller numbers than in the reanastomosed intact colon (214). Since the isolated segment did not have contact with feces, the DMH probably reached the segment via the circulation and was converted to the active carcinogen by colonic cells.

Tissue Susceptibility

The colon is more susceptible to carcinogenic effects than the small intestine. In rats with surgical transposition of jejunum or cecum to distal colon or vice versa, administration of a carcinogen produced tumors in the colorectum of all animals, but tumors were absent or few in the transposed jejunum or cecum (215, 216).

PRECANCEROUS CONDITIONS

The precancerous conditions are intestinal diseases in which there is an increased risk of developing intestinal carcinoma. It is generally accepted that carcinomas do not develop from a totally normal cell. Instead, they develop from an altered cell which may appear normal in routine histologic examination but has altered functions so that it may express abnormal markers such as carcinoembryonic antigen (CEA). On the other hand, many premalignant cells are morphologically abnormal, showing hyperchromatism, pleomorphism, abnormal size and shape, loss of polarity, and frequent mitoses. Such cells are dysplastic and their propensity to malignancy is proportional to the degree of abnormality. Dysplastic cells are characteristic of adenomas and premalignant lesions of ulcerative colitis (217). It is the presence of such functionally or morphologically altered cells that marks the premalignant nature of the precancerous conditions.

Benign Epithelial Polyps

The pathologic features and malignant potential of intestinal polyps are presented in detail in Chapter 33. Only a brief account is given in this section.

ADENOMAS AND ADENOMATOSIS   The malignant potential of adenomas is proportional to the grades of dysplasia and the quantity of cell mass. When the individual adenoma is small, a large number of adenomas increases the malignant potential, as in FAP. When the lesion is small, but highly dysplastic, a high rate of malignant change is again evident, as in the flat adenomas (122, 218). The growth pattern is also a factor in that the presence of villous configuration, a sign of heightened vertical expansion, is a marker of high malignant potential (122, 217, 219, 220). These features in concert determine the outcome of an adenoma or the adenomatosis syndrome. A comparable relationship between adenoma and carcinoma is also present in the small intestine (221).

The process of carcinoma development in an adenoma is known as the adenoma-carcinoma sequence (222). The evolution of carcinoma from adenoma is usually histologically evident and the invasive carcinomas often contain a focus of remnant adenoma (223, 224) (Figs. 34.3 and 34.4). The incidence of carcinoma in untreated adenoma is 2.5% in 5 years, 8% in 10 years, and 24% in 20 years (225). Less than 10% of adenomas develop carcinoma in a lifetime (226). Polypectomy reduces the incidence of colon cancer. In the National Polyp Study of 1418 patients, only five carcinomas were found after a follow-up of 8401 patient-years, a reduction of 76 to 90% of the expected cancer incidence (227).

Many adenomas have markers of malignancy, including aberrant blood group antigens, oncofetal antigens such as CEA and CA19-9 (228), T antigens (229), and DNA aneuploidy (230). Recent investigations using molecular biology techniques have revealed a multi-step alteration in genes in the colonic carcinogenesis sequence (125, 231, 232), with changes in the adenoma as the initial step (see the section on molecular and genetic alterations later in this chapter). The question remains, however, whether all colorectal carcinomas, except those following long-standing inflammatory bowel disease, develop from a pre-existing adenoma. One

piece of evidence against this concept was the finding of small nonpolypoid carcinomas without a trace of adenomatous tissue (233, 234). Furthermore, experimental studies show that colonic carcinoma may develop without the adenoma stage (235, 236). The question of de novo carcinoma is further discussed in the section on histogenesis of the carcinoma.

NONNEOPLASTIC POLYPS AND POLYPOSIS

Hyperplastic Polyps   The hyperplastic polyps are small and generally considered to be innocuous lesions. However, a hyperplastic polyp may become adenomatous, and thus be indirectly involved in malignant change (237, 238). Furthermore, features of malignant change such as CEA and O-acylated sialomucin have been found in the hyperplastic polyps (239). Recently, some adenomas have been found to contain mixed hyperplastic and adenomatous features (240). About one-third of these lesions had significant dysplasia and 11% had intramucosal carcinoma.

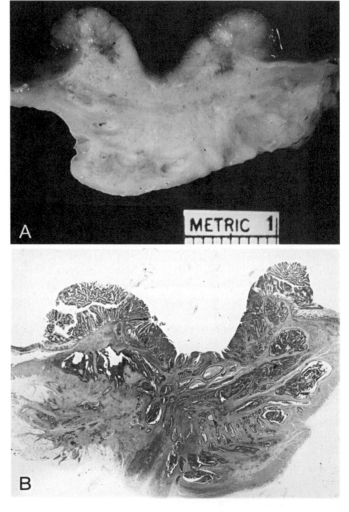

Figure 34.3   A small ulcerated adenocarcinoma of the colon, showing adenomatous tissue at the border of the invasive lesion. **(A)** Gross appearance of the cross sectional surface of the lesion. **(B)** Scanning view of the histologic section showing invasive carcinoma at the center and tubular adenoma at the periphery.

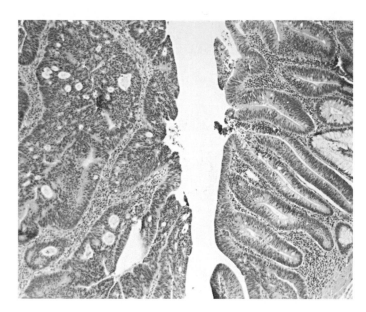

Figure 34.4 An area of adenocarcinoma *(left)* in a tubular adenoma *(right)* (×55).

Hamartomatous Polyposis   There are two kinds of hamartomatous polyps: polyps in the Peutz-Jeghers syndrome and polyps in juvenile polyposis. Both are composed of essentially normal epithelial cells and are not considered premalignant. However, intestinal cancers have been reported in both syndromes, mostly in the small intestines in the Peutz-Jeghers syndrome and in the colon in the juvenile polyposis syndrome. The carcinomas arise in the dysplastic or adenomatous lesions (104, 114, 115, 241) (Fig. 34.5).

Inflammatory and Other Bowel Disease

ULCERATIVE COLITIS AND CROHN'S DISEASE   Malignant and premalignant changes complicating ulcerative colitis and Crohn's disease are discussed in detail in Chapter 29. Only a brief account is given here.

The development of colonic carcinoma in patients with ulcerative colitis is related to the extent and the duration of colitis (242). The incidence rates of colorectal cancer in ulcerative colitis is 0.8% at 10 years of colitis, 5.5% at 20 years, and 13.5% at 30 years. The incidence rate is higher in patients who have sclerosing cholangitis (243). The wide geographic variation in the incidence of malignancy in ulcerative colitis (244) raises the possibility of a role for additional environmental factors (245). The colitis-associated carcinoma differs from the colonic carcinoma in the general population in its tendency to locate randomly in the colon, to be multiple, and to have an early onset (244). It originates from dysplastic tissue rather than adenoma (245, 246). The probability of cancer increases with the grades of dysplasia: 2% without dysplasia, 19% in low grade dysplasia, and 42% in high grade dysplasia (247). The survival rate of colitis-associated colorectal cancer is the same as that of ordinary colorectal carcinoma.

Carcinoma may arise in the affected segments of the intestine in patients with Crohn's disease. As in ulcerative colitis, the carcinoma arises from dysplastic tissue, and not from an adenoma (248, 249). The risk factors are long duration of the disease, and the presence of a fistula, stricture, and right-sided colon disease (250). The observed incidence of cancer of the small intestine in Crohn's

disease is 85.8 times that of the estimated rate of the general population (251). This high ratio is probably because of the low rate of carcinoma at this site in the general population.

An animal model of intestinal carcinoma associated with inflammatory lesions has been found in a species of marmoset (*Saguinus oedipus oedipus*, the cotton-top tamarin) (252). These carcinomas are multifocal, occurring in the colon as well as the small intestine. The model differs from human colitis-associated carcinoma in a number of ways, however. In the marmosets, most of the carcinomas are undifferentiated (253), the colitis is mild, and neither dysplasia nor adenoma are present.

SCHISTOSOMIASIS   Among the infectious diseases of the bowel in man, only infestation with *Schistosoma japonicum* is known to be complicated by colorectal carcinoma (254). The patients usually have a long history of diffuse involvement of the large intestine with pseudopolyps, disrupted muscularis mucosae, and ectopically regenerating glands. The carcinoma is often multicentric (255). Schistosomiasis is common in Egypt and is due to *Schistosoma mansoni* infection. This form of schistosomiasis is not associated with colon carcinoma or adenoma, although inflammatory polyps are common in the colon (256).

Epithelial Hyperplasia

Proliferating cells may be at risk for altered DNA replication when exposed to a carcinogen. Experimentally, adaptive hyperplasia of intestinal mucosa can be produced by jejunoileal resection, subtotal colectomy, enteric bypass, or pancreatobiliary diversion (257). Administration of carcinogen to these postoperative animals induces an increased number of intestinal tumors. A single dose of DMH induces multiple foci of atypia in the hyperplastic colon (258). In man, precancerous conditions usually have hyperplastic epithelium. Many of the risk factors in carcinogenesis are related to

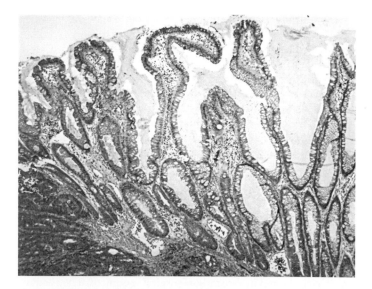

Figure 34.5 A focus of adenocarcinoma *(bottom)* in a Peutz-Jeghers polyp of the duodenum. Adenomatous lesion was present in other areas (×55).

cell proliferation (259). Tumor promoting agents such as fat, bile acids, and short-chain fatty acids increase cell proliferation, whereas a vegetarian diet decreases it.

HISTOGENESIS AND NATURAL HISTORY

Histogenesis

Adenocarcinomas of the intestines develop along two major pathways. Most commonly, they occur in the highly dysplastic or villous adenoma, and less commonly in the dysplastic epithelium of the flat intestinal mucosa following chronic inflammation of long duration. These events are discussed above in the section on precancerous conditions, as well as in Chapter 29 on ulcerative colitis and Crohn's disease, and Chapter 31 on benign intestinal polyps. The relatively recent recognition of small flat adenomas in the colon adds support to the adenoma-carcinoma pathway (122).

The fact that any residual adenoma might not be found by serial sectioning even in early carcinomas raises the possibility of de novo development of intestinal carcinoma (260). Such lesions have been reported by several investigators. Kjeldsberg and Altshuler (261) reported a case of carcinoma in situ of the colon without associated adenoma. Crawford (233) reported two minute colonic carcinomas measuring $0.3 \times 0.3 \times 0.1$ cm and 0.2×0.2 cm. The former was intramucosal and the latter had invaded the submucosa. Shimoda et al. (262) studied 178 early and 853 advanced carcinomas of the colorectum. Of the early carcinomas 146 (82%) were polypoid and 32 (18%) nonpolypoid. Adenomatous elements were found in 96% of pedunculated polypoid carcinomas and 86% of sessile polypoid carcinomas. The nonpolypoid early carcinomas ranged from 2 to 28 mm in size. Adenomatous tissue was absent in all. Among the advanced carcinomas, polypoid lesions were seen in 186 cases (22%), with residual adenoma in 40 lesions. The remaining advanced carcinomas were nonpolypoid. It was postulated that the carcinomas, which had not developed from adenoma, invaded early and grew rapidly to account for a high percentage of nonpolypoid carcinomas among the advanced cases. By colonoscopy, Kudo et al. (263) found 184 early carcinomas with submucosal invasion. Twenty of these tumors, all under 15 mm in size, were depressed and were considered to be de novo carcinomas.

Hyperplasia is commonly observed in the colonic mucosa adjacent to carcinoma, the so-called transitional mucosa, and occasionally in patchy areas remote from the carcinoma (264). The transitional mucosa is hyperplastic and thickened and the crypts are dilated and distorted (265, 266) (Fig. 34.6). Immature and intermediate cells are retained in the upper level of the crypts. The absorptive cells are often vesiculated and the microvilli are sparse (267). Similar changes can also be found in the mucosa adjacent to an adenoma (266, 268). The transitional mucosa shows affinity to concanavalin A (269), but there is no CEA (268). It is not clear whether these changes are precancerous or incidental.

In experimental colonic carcinogenesis in rodents, early microscopic changes involving one or multiple crypts are readily observed (270). These lesions, known as aberrant crypt foci (ACF), may be recognized grossly after the mucosal surface of the specimen is stained with methylene blue (271). The same method has been used endoscopically and in the study of surgical specimens. The aberrant crypts in the stained mucosa have stellar or elliptical luminal openings, while normal crypts have round openings (272, 273). The epithelium of aberrant crypts is thicker than normal and the

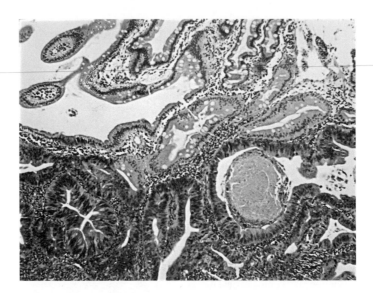

Figure 34.6 Transitional mucosa bordering an adenocarcinoma *(left lower corner)* of the colon, showing thickened mucosa containing dilated and hyperplastic glands (×32).

pericryptal region is widened. The average number of ACF in the colon per square centimeter was 20 in patients with FAP and 0.18 in inflammatory bowel disease (274). The microscopic appearance of the crypt epithelium in ACF may be hyperplastic, dysplastic, or adenomatous, but is rarely normal. Hyperplastic ACF are considered the earliest preneoplastic lesions. K-ras mutation at codon 12 is present in 58% of cases (275, 276). Carcinoembryonic antigen is present in 93%, and is related to the size of the ACF and the presence of dysplasia (277). Dysplastic ACF have mutations in the APC (adenomatous polyposis coli) gene (278).

Natural History

Colonic carcinomas are slow growing tumors. It was estimated that it would take 5 to 10 years for the normal colonic epithelium to become hyperplastic and then progress to an adenoma. The lesion would take an additional 3 to 5 years to become carcinoma and develop metastases (279). Cell kinetic studies (see Chapter 9) of tumor cells grown in vitro show that the cell cycle time is longer than that of normal crypt cells, with a lengthened S phase. Clinically, the mean doubling time of the tumor, i.e., the time for a tumor to double its diameter as measured by radiologic examinations, was 620 days, with a range of 111 to 3430 days in 20 colorectal carcinomas (280). This figure is undoubtedly influenced by the amount of necrosis in the tumor which may be as much as 90% of the tumor mass. It was estimated that it might take 6 to 8 years for a colonic carcinoma to reach the size of 6 cm (281). The mean doubling time of pulmonary metastasis was 109 days (282), and that of hepatic metastasis 50 to 95 days (283, 284).

MOLECULAR AND GENETIC ALTERATIONS

It has been long recognized that carcinogenesis is a multistep process. Pathologically, the process begins with increased cell proliferation resulting in epithelial hyperplasia, followed by increasing alterations of cells forming dysplasia or benign neoplasia, and ends in uncontrolled cancer growth. These changes are the results of altered DNA. The molecular and genetic basis of the alterations have been greatly illuminated in recent years since the pioneer work of Vogelstein and his colleagues (231, 232). Several genes and many other factors are involved. They are discussed in detail in Chapters 7 and 8. Briefly, the carcinogenic process in the colon begins with the loss of function of tumor suppressor genes APC and MCC (mutated in colorectal cancer) by allelic loss, mutation, or both in FAP and sporadic colorectal cancer (231, 232), and by alterations of DNA mismatch repair genes in HNPCC (285–287). These changes convert normal epithelium to adenoma. Additional changes in tumor suppressor genes DCC (deleted in colorectal cancer) and p53 and mutation of the oncogene K-ras cause the adenoma to progress and become malignant. The growth and invasion of the tumor is regulated by growth factors (288–291), cell cycle regulators (292, 293), and molecules related to angiogenesis, cell adhesion, apoptosis, and metastasis (294–301). Although these basic changes apply to colonic carcinogenesis in general, the sequence and timing of each event may differ in different clinical entities.

Familial Adenomatous Polyposis

Familial adenomatous polyposis is an autosomal dominant disease. The patients have germline deletion or mutation of the APC gene on chromosome 5q21. Adenomas develop at an early age. Following the adenoma-carcinoma sequence outlined above, some of the advanced adenomas convert to carcinoma. Similar genetic lesions are seen in Gardner syndrome (232) and Turcot syndrome (302).

Hereditary Nonpolyposis Colorectal Cancer

Hereditary nonpolyposis colorectal cancer is also an autosomal dominant disease. Although there is no polyposis, adenomas do exist in the colon in small numbers, and cancer can develop from the adenomas. However, HNPCC is not due to mutation or allelic loss of APC gene. In HNPCC, the initial genetic lesion causing colorectal carcinoma involves a germline mutation of genes in the DNA mismatch repair system (MRS). Defects in this system result in microsatellite instability or replication error (RER⁺) phenotype which is present in 86% of colon cancers and 57% of adenomas in HNPCC patients (286, 303). Four mutated genes have been identified in HNPCC: hMSH2, hMLH1, hPMS1, and hPMS2 (286, 304, 305). In addition, a mutation of G-T binding protein (GTBP), a homologue of the yeast *S. cerevisiae* MSH6 gene, was identified in a MRS-deficient colon cancer cell line (286). In families with Lynch syndrome II, excess endometrial and small intestinal carcinomas are associated with mutation of either the hMSH2 or hMLH1 genes, but excess risk for cancer of the urinary tract, stomach, and ovary is associated only with mutation of the hMSH2 gene (120).

Sporadic Colorectal Cancer

Sporadic colorectal cancers are not hereditary, although the risk increases if there is a family history of colon cancer. The sporadic colon carcinoma develops in the pre-existing adenoma, as in FAP. The genetic alterations are similar. The RER⁺ phenotype is found in 15% of sporadic cancers and 3% of adenomas (303). The ACF discussed earlier are the presumed precursors for sporadic colon cancer. Large ACF contain mutated K-ras oncogene in 58 to 85% of

lesions (275, 306), implicating early involvement of K-ras in the development of this lesion. The ACF may show microsatellite instability and mutations in APC (278, 307), but no p53 expression (276).

Colorectal Cancer in Ulcerative Colitis

Colorectal carcinomas develop in long-standing ulcerative colitis from dysplastic epithelium. Carcinoma was identified in 43% of colons with dysplasia associated lesions and masses, 42% in high grade dysplasia, 19% in low grade dysplasia, 9% in indefinite dysplasia, and 2% in negative for dysplasia (247). Molecular genetic studies of dysplastic and cancerous tissue revealed allelic loss in many chromosomes, including 5q (the location of APC) and 17p (the location of p53) (308). Mutation of the K-ras oncogene was detected in 44% of dysplastic tissue and 30% of carcinomas (309). Mutation of the p53 gene was present in 33% of low grade dysplasias, 63% of high grade dysplasias, and 85% of carcinomas. Loss of heterozygosity (LOH) of p53, Rb, MCC, and APC genes was detected in approximately 30% of the dysplastic or cancerous tissues (310). In another study, allelic loss of DCC was noted in 29%, p53 in 66%, Rb in 50%, NF1 in 14%, and APC/MCC region in 50% of samples (311). Microsatellite instability and mutation of the MSH2 gene were present in 26% and 27% of colitis-associated dysplasia and cancer, respectively (312, 313). These studies indicate a pattern of genetic alterations in colitis-associated neoplasia similar to that of sporadic colorectal cancer, although their histogenetic sequences are different. Additional information on molecular abnormalities in neoplastic lesions in inflammatory bowel disease is provided in Chapter 8.

EXPERIMENTAL CARCINOGENESIS

Experimental studies are useful in providing insight into the mechanisms of carcinogenesis. They can be used to evaluate risk factors by manipulating the experimental environment and to study the sequence of tissue changes in the target organ at planned time intervals. Colonic carcinomas have been produced by a variety of carcinogens in several species of rodents (55–57). A commonly used chemical is 1,2-dimethylhydrazine (DMH). 1,2-Dimethylhydrazine is a procarcinogen and is not mutagenic by itself. Animals exposed to DMH have tumors in the colon and, to a lesser degree, upper small intestine, regardless of the route of administration, whether given orally or injected subcutaneously or intraperitoneally. It is oxidized primarily in the liver to form azoxymethane (AOM), then N-hydroxylated to methylazoxymethanol (MAM) (57, 314, 315) which is secreted in the bile in conjugated form. The bacterial β-glucuronidase frees MAM in the intestinal lumen where it is metabolized to the active carcinogen (56). Both AOM and MAM have also been used to produce tumors. It is evident that this pathway to active carcinogen is subjected to modification by a variety of factors in the microenvironment of the intestinal tract. The DMH model is therefore commonly used to test the significance of risk factors. Another commonly used gastrointestinal carcinogen is N-methyl-N′-nitro-N-nitrosoguanidine (MNNG), a direct-acting carcinogen. It produces tumors in the stomach and upper small intestine when given in the drinking water (316), and colorectal tumors by intrarectal instillation (55).

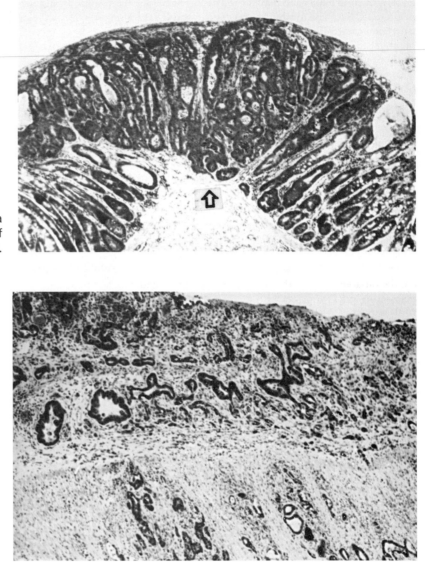

Figure 34.7 DMH-induced colonic adenoma in a mouse with a focus of adenocarcinoma at the center of base invading the muscularis mucosae *(arrow)* (×50).

Figure 34.8 Infiltrative adenocarcinoma of the colon from a MNNG treated mouse. There was no adenomatous tissue in the lesion (×50).

In either model, the initial change is an increase in cell proliferation with expansion of the proliferative compartment in the crypt before tumorigenesis (317). The DMH-induced tumors are adenomas and carcinomas. An adenoma-carcinoma sequence was noted in these tumors by some investigators (318, 319). Others found evidence for de novo origin of the carcinomas (214, 320). In our own experiments in mice (236), DMH produced two types of adenomas: the polypoid adenoma with a single-crypt origin and the flat adenoma with multiple-crypt origin. Carcinomas with superficial invasion arose in both of them (Fig. 34.7). Crypt hyperplasia was common in the preneoplastic stage but dysplasia was rare. In the MNNG treated mice, dysplasia was common. In addition to polypoid adenoma, deeply infiltrative carcinoma without adenomatous elements were also common (Fig. 34.8). Thus adenomas were produced in both models, but carcinomas differed in both origin and invasiveness. In another DMH experiment in rats, tumors appeared earlier and were in greater numbers in the distal colon than the proximal colon (321). The difference in tumor yield is probably related to the baseline proliferative state of different parts of the

colon: the untreated rats had longer crypt length and larger proliferative zone in the distal colon. It appears that the tissue origin of the intestinal carcinoma is related to the type and perhaps also the dose and the mode of action of the carcinogen, and that the latent period and tumor yield are influenced by the baseline proliferative state of the crypt cells.

For the study of genetic factors, a mouse model with an altered Apc gene has been developed. Apc is a mouse homologue of the human APC gene. The mutated gene was produced by ethylnitrosourea in B6 (C57BL/6J strain) mice (322, 323). The affected mice develop multiple intestinal adenomas and few adenocarcinomas, mostly in the small intestine. The mutated gene is called Min for multiple intestinal neoplasia. It also causes mammary adenocarcinoma and keratoacanthoma. The Min gene is located at the Apc locus on chromosome 18 (324). It is dominantly inherited. The number of intestinal tumors in the hybrid (AKRXB6 Min+) F1 mice reduces after backcross breeding to Min negative AKR mice, indicating the presence of a modifier gene in the AKR mice. The modifier, called Mom (modifier of Min) has been mapped on chromosome 4 (324). This model is useful for the study of the APC gene as well as its relationship to other genes or risk factors in colon carcinogenesis (325, 326).

PATHOLOGY

Although the gross and microscopic anatomy of the small and large intestines differ in many aspects, the pathologic features of adenocarcinoma are remarkably similar in these organs. All normally present cell types including columnar cells, goblet cells, less differentiated crypt cells, Paneth cells, and endocrine cells have been identified in the adenocarcinomas of both small and large intestines. Squamous cell differentiation has also been found in some tumors. Gross appearances of the carcinomas are also similar in the small and large intestines. On the other hand, the clinical presentations may vary regionally because of the relationship between the tumor and the neighboring organs. This relationship may affect the prognosis as well.

The common pathologic features are presented in this section and the variable clinicopathologic features are presented in the later sections on individual organs.

GROSS MORPHOLOGY AND CLASSIFICATION

Grossly, the intestinal adenocarcinomas take one of four forms: polypoid, fungating, ulcerative, or infiltrative.

Polypoid Type

In this type, the carcinoma forms an exophytic intraluminal mass without significant ulcerative defects (Fig. 34.9). It may have a nodular, lobulated, or papillary surface. The small ones may closely resemble adenomas and may be, in fact, an adenoma with carcinomatous focus. The large bulky ones are seen more commonly in the cecum and right colon than in the left colon or rectum. This type of carcinoma is likely to have arisen in an adenoma.

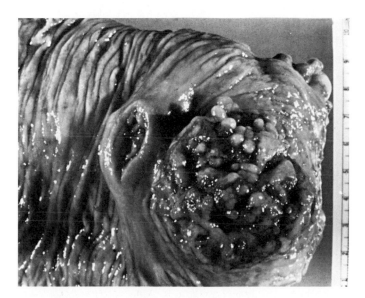

Figure 34.9 A polypoid carcinoma of cecum. The orifice of the ileum is shown *(left)*.

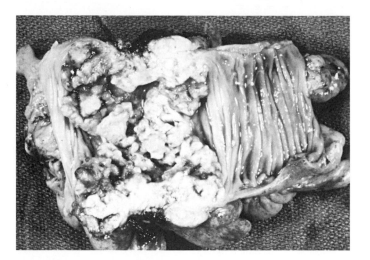

Figure 34.10 A fungating carcinoma of sigmoid colon, involving the entire circumference of the colon.

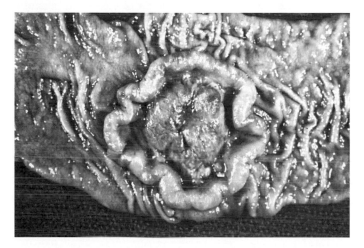

Figure 34.11 A fungating carcinoma of sigmoid colon, showing a raised rim of tumor tissue around a large ulceration.

Fungating Type

This type of carcinoma is basically a polypoid carcinoma with prominent ulceration (Fig. 34.10). The tumor often has a raised and rolled border in which residual adenomatous tissue may be present (Fig. 34.11). In some tumors, the ulceration destroys much of the tumor leaving only a small portion of exophytic lesion at the border of the tumor. The carcinomatous tissue, including the marginal region, is firm, whereas the residual adenomatous tissue is relatively soft and pliable. Careful inspection and palpation of the nonulcerated tumor margin can usually identify the adenomatous areas.

Ulcerative Type

This type of carcinoma invades deeply into the colonic wall, and the ulcerated surface is even with the normal mucosal surface or, more often, sinks below it (Fig. 34.12). The tumor margin is not raised and there is no grossly discernible adenomatous tissue. The carcinoma infiltrates and thickens the intestinal wall resulting in a discoid

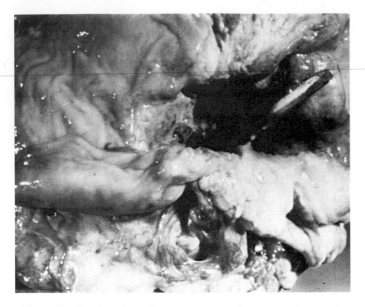

Figure 34.12 An ulcerative carcinoma of colon with a probe through the perforated ulcer crater.

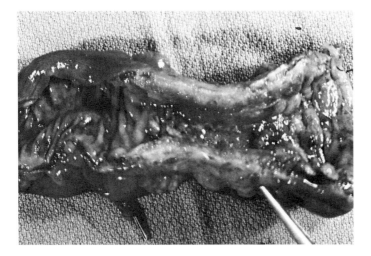

Figure 34.13 A diffusely infiltrative signet-ring cell carcinoma of the rectosigmoid, showing the uniformly thickened wall and shallow ulceration of the luminal surface. The tumor is circumferential and the lumen is narrowed.

or saucer-like appearance of the lesion. The ulcerative carcinoma is more commonly seen in the left colon than in the right colon. Shimoda et al. suggested that such nonpolypoid carcinomas arise de novo, without a pre-existing adenoma (262). However, it remains possible that the pre-existing adenoma may have been destroyed by either the carcinoma, the ulceration, or both.

Infiltrative Type

This type of carcinoma infiltrates the intestinal wall extensively and often circumferentially without forming a nodular mass (Fig. 34.13). Diffuse thickening of a long segment of the bowel

gives the lesion an appearance similar to the linitis plastica carcinoma of the stomach, and this term has been applied to these lesions (327, 328). In this regard, it should be kept in mind that a metastatic lesion from the linitis plastica type of gastric carcinoma may have the same appearance. On the cut surface, the carcinoma is pale gray or white. Its consistency is firm and gritty.

In the polypoid and fungating types, the periphery of the tumor tissue is sharply demarcated, at least focally. The periphery of infiltrative carcinoma, on the other hand, is indistinct. The border of an ulcerative carcinoma may have either appearance. The circum-

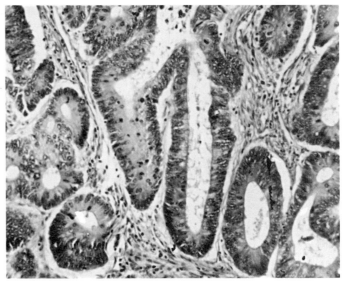

Figure 34.14 A well differentiated adenocarcinoma of the colon showing glands composed mainly of columnar cell, some of which contain small globules of mucus in the apical cytoplasm. Many mitotic figures are present (×150).

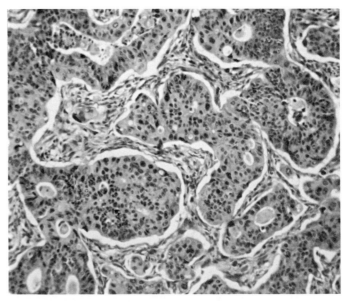

Figure 34.15 A moderately differentiated adenocarcinoma of colon with glandular formation in some areas (×180).

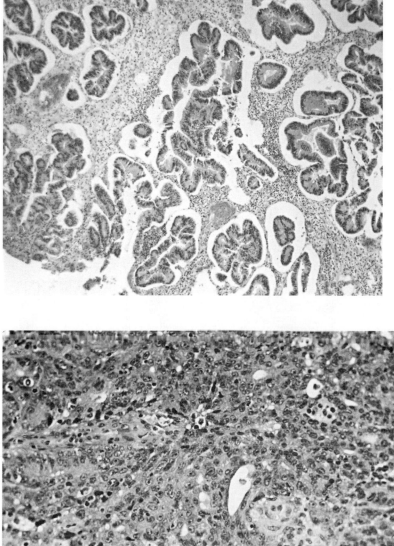

Figure 34.16   A papillary adenocarcinoma at the peri-ampullary region of duodenum (×50).

Figure 34.17   A poorly differentiated adenocarcinoma of the colon showing a compact sheet of tumor cells and a few small glandular spaces (×120).

ferential and obstructive lesions are also called stenosing or constrictive tumors.

The reported frequency of different types of carcinoma vary because of variations of the terms used. Shimoda et al. classified 20% of the carcinomas as polypoid and 80% nonpolypoid (262). Jackson and Beahrs noted that 65% of carcinomas were crater-like ulcerative lesions and 25% fungating tumors (329). Similar frequencies were found by Dionne (330).

HISTOLOGIC FEATURES AND CELL TYPES

Histologic Features

Intestinal adenocarcinomas are mostly well (25%) to moderately (60%) differentiated glandular tumors (331) (Figs. 34.14 and 34.15). Intraglandular papillary infoldings may be present in the well differentiated carcinomas (Fig. 34.16). Rare groups of neoplastic cells with few fenestrations may fill the glandular lumen (332). About 15% of the adenocarcinomas of the intestines are poorly differentiated or mostly undifferentiated. These tumors often grow expansively and form solid nodular masses (Fig. 34.17). In spite of the lack of gland formation, the cells in some tumors are not particularly pleomorphic or bizarre, and the prognosis is relatively good (333). The undifferentiated small cell carcinomas have been identified as endocrine tumors and carry a poor prognosis. They are described in a later section.

There are two main patterns of growth: expanding and infiltrative. The expanding growth pattern is characterized by nodular tumor aggregates made of large interconnecting glands (Fig. 34.18). In many tumors, the branching glands form a loosely intertwined network interposed by cellular fibrous tissue in which varying numbers of lymphocytic cells are present. The infiltrative

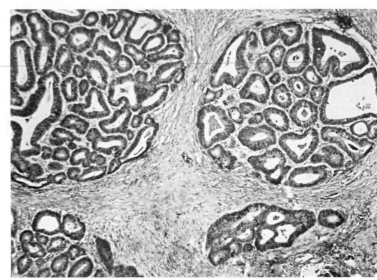

Figure 34.18 A well differentiated adenocarcinoma of colon showing expanding type of growth. Groups of glands form circumscribed nodules separated by fibrous stroma (×50).

growth pattern is characterized by narrow tubular glands with few bridging connections, invading the gut wall individually or in small groups (Fig. 34.19). The tubules are accompanied by relatively acellular collagenous tissue. Tumors with abundant fibrous stroma have been called scirrhous carcinomas which can be recognized grossly as firm fibrous tissue without discrete nodules. Some carcinomas have a mixed pattern of growth (Fig. 34.20), with the infiltrative tubules chiefly in the deeply invasive region, suggesting a change of biological behavior as the carcinoma advances. Diffuse infiltration by individual carcinoma cells, as commonly seen in the gastric carcinoma, is rare in the intestines. This pattern of invasion is characteristic of the signet-ring cell carcinoma, described below. Diffuse infiltration by undifferentiated individual cells is extremely rare.

Expanding carcinomas are usually polypoid or fungating in their gross presentation. Infiltrative carcinomas are ulcerative or infiltrative. The ulcerative carcinomas with slightly raised border often show mixed patterns of growth.

Cell Types

The majority of carcinoma cells are columnar cells with no, or only an ill-defined striated, border. Mucous cells are commonly present and the intraluminal secretion usually contains mucus, predominantly sulfomucin, mixed with lesser amounts of sialomucin. Neutral type mucoprotein is rarely present. Many mucous cells have only small globules of secretion (Fig. 34.14). Goblet cells are infrequent.

Endocrine cells, mostly argyrophilic and less frequently argentaffin, are commonly present. Iwafuchi et al. (334) found these cells in 18 of 24 small intestinal carcinomas, secreting serotonin and a variety of peptides. In the large intestine, endocrine cells have been found in 20 to 75% of the carcinomas (335, 336). They were found in 4% of mucinous and 5% of undifferentiated carcinomas of the rectum, and 52% of nonmucinous carcinomas of the colon (335). In most cases, the number of endocrine cells are small. In some cases, they are prominent enough to justify the name of neuroendocrine carcinoma or adenocarcinoid (337, 338). Additional information

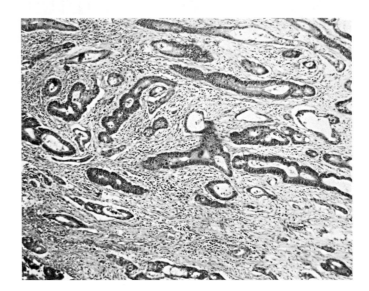

Figure 34.19 A well differentiated tubular adenocarcinoma showing infiltrative type of growth. Individual glands infiltrate the stroma in which many lymphocytes are present (×50).

on endocrine cell tumors is presented in Chapter 15. Neoplastic Paneth cells have also been identified in the adenocarcinomas of both the small intestine and colon (336, 339, 340). The endocrine and Paneth cells are normally derived from stem cells in the intestinal crypt, as are the columnar and goblet cells. The clonal origin of these cells in carcinoma is supported by the observation of differentiation into columnar, mucous, and endocrine cells from a single human rectal carcinoma cell in culture (341). In view of these findings, an intestinal adenocarcinoma with neoplastic endocrine and Paneth cells has been called crypt cell carcinoma (342) or stem cell carcinoma (343, 344). These tumors may also contain squamous cells (336). Tuft (caveolated) cells have been identified in two carcinoma cell lines (345). Neoplastic M and cup cells have not been described.

Ultrastructural and Morphometric Studies

Colonic carcinomas have been studied with electron microscopy (346, 347), showing varying degrees of cell differentiation. The mucin granules decrease with lower grade of differentiation. Conversely, the apical dense bodies, glycocalyceal bodies, cytoplasmic vesiculation, and desmosomes all increase. The microvilli are sparse and contain dense core microfilaments extending as long rootlets into a clear zone of apical cytoplasm. The long rootlets appear to be a marker for colonic adenocarcinoma (347). The nucleus of the carcinoma cells shows thin flat appendages which are connected with the main nucleus by lamellar bridges. These appendages were called nucleotesimals (348), thought to be related to an unusual form of amitotic division. Electron microscopy is instrumental in the identification of special cell types in the carcinoma, such as endocrine cells (342, 343). Morphometric studies of the carcinoma show expanded nuclear area, an increased nucleo-cytoplasmic ratio from the normal mean of 20.4 to the mean of 39.7 in the carcinomas, displacement of nuclear position in the cells, and variable nuclear size and shape (349, 350). There is no significant difference in these parameters between the primary carcinoma and the metastatic lesion (351).

VARIANTS OF ADENOCARCINOMA

Mucinous adenocarcinoma and signet-ring cell carcinomas are variants of adenocarcinoma with prominent mucus secretion. In the mucinous adenocarcinoma the mucus is primarily extracellular, while in the signet-ring cell carcinoma the mucus is intracellular (Figs. 34.21 and 34.22). Each has specific morphologic and biological characteristics to warrant a separate identify as noted in the World Health Organization Histological Typing of Intestinal Tumors (352). They occur more often in the younger patients and in patients with HNPCC and inflammatory bowel disease (46, 102, 108, 353–355).

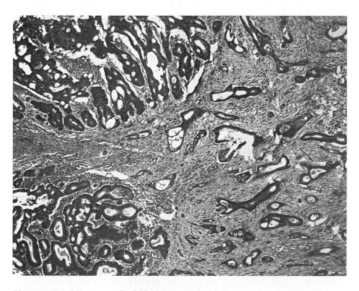

Figure 34.20   A well differentiated adenocarcinoma of the colon with mixed expanding and infiltrative types of growth (×32).

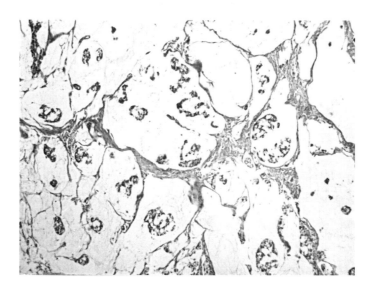

Figure 34.21   Mucinous adenocarcinoma of the colon. More than 80% of the tumor mass is occupied by mucus (×50).

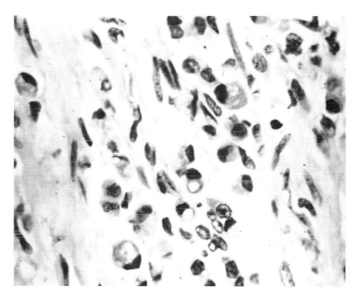

Figure 34.22   Signet-ring cell carcinoma of the colon showing single signet-ring shaped and undifferentiated carcinoma cells infiltrating the stroma (×480).

Mucinous Adenocarcinoma

In mucinous adenocarcinoma, abundant mucus forms pools in the connective tissue, surrounding the cancerous glands. The amount of mucus required to qualify the tumor as mucinous is 50% or more of the tumor mass (352, 353, 356). A minimum of 25% mucus is required for the tumor to be considered as having mucinous component (287, 357). With these criteria, 5 to 15% of colonic carcinomas are mucinous (353–355, 358) and an additional 5 to 6% of tumors have mucinous components (356, 357). The tumors with a large amount of mucus present a grossly gelatinous appearance and the term of mucoid or colloid carcinoma is applied. Most of the mucinous carcinomas appear to have originated from adenomas (358) and are composed of tubular structures. They are located more often in the right colon and rectum than other parts of the colon. There are differences in molecular alterations between mucinous and nonmucinous carcinomas. Mutation of p53 is less frequent, but mutation of K-ras and microsatellite instability are more frequent in the mucinous than nonmucinous carcinomas (355). Mucinous tumors are often in advanced stage when diagnosed, less resectable, and have poorer prognosis than the other carcinomas (354, 356, 358). Purtilo et al. reported a familial occurrence of mucinous colonic carcinoma in 13 members of a black family (359). The median age of the patients was 39 years. The transmission was of autosomal dominant trait.

Signet-Ring Cell Carcinoma

Signet-ring cell carcinoma occurs rarely in the intestines. Ojeda et al. in 1982 found only 52 reported cases in the English literature in a 50 year period (360). The reported incidences were 0.2 to 1% of carcinomas (361, 362), and 4% of mucinous carcinomas (363). It is characterized by tumor cells shaped like a signet-ring, with an eccentric crescent-shaped nucleus pushed by the intracytoplasmic mucus against the cell wall (Fig. 34.22). These cells infiltrate the gut wall individually or in small groups. Diffuse infiltration produces a linitis plastica type of gross appearance (328). The prognosis is poor, with only a few patients living more than one year after diagnosis (360, 364).

SPREAD OF ADENOCARCINOMA

Depending on the location of the carcinoma, deep penetration of the tumor may cause direct involvement of the neighboring organs or tissues. Tumor cells may seed the peritoneum, surgical wound, or areas of inflammation. Venous permeation usually results in metastasis in the liver via the portal system. Cells of the lower rectal carcinoma may enter the systemic venous circulation directly and be lodged in the lung.

The lymphatic spread of carcinoma differs between the small and large intestines. The small intestine has a rich lymphatic network in the mucosa. An intramucosal carcinoma, therefore, may be able to metastasize to the regional lymph node. The lymphatics of the colon reach only to the level of muscularis mucosae (365), so that only carcinomas with invasion into the submucosa or deeper layers may have lymphatic metastasis.

STAGING OF ADENOCARCINOMA

Intestinal adenocarcinomas have been divided into early and advanced cases, using the same definition applied to gastric cancers (262, 366). The early carcinomas are limited to the mucosa or submucosa and the advanced carcinomas have invaded the muscularis propria or deeper layers. The status of lymph node metastasis is not taken into consideration. Hermanek and Gall had 130 early cases, 3% of which had lymph node metastasis (367). The 10 year survival rate was 100% and a limited resection of the lesion was adequate in some cases.

A comprehensive staging system with specific reference to survival rate and prognosis was introduced by Dukes in 1932 (368). It was designed originally for rectal cancers but has now been applied to all intestinal cancers. Dukes classified the tumors into

three groups (Table 34.8): Group A with tumor within the rectal wall, up to but not through the muscularis propria; Group B with tumor penetrating through the rectal wall into the extramural tissue, but without lymph node metastasis; and Group C with metastasis to the regional lymph nodes. The five year survival rates for the respective groups were 93%, 65%, and 23% (369). With the recognition of additional factors, there have been several attempts to modify the grouping criteria. In 1949, Kirklin et al. divided Group A cases into A and B1 groups: A with carcinoma limited to the mucosa, and B1 with tumor extending into muscularis propria (370). The original Dukes' group B became B2. There was no significant difference between the survival rates of these two subgroups. This modification was adopted by Astler and Coller in 1954 (371) who introduced the subgroups of C1 and C2 for cases with lymph node metastasis. C1 patients had B1 primary tumor and C2 patients had B2 primary tumor. The respective 5-year survival rates were 100.0% for A, 66.6% for B1, 53.9% for B2, 42.8% for C1, and 22.4% for C2 patients. The differences between groups of B1, B2, and C1 were not great. Dukes also adopted C1 and C2 categories in 1949 and 1958 (372, 373): C1 for involvement of regional lymph nodes only, and C2 for positive nodes at the point of ligation of blood vessel at the time of surgical resection of the tumor. The latter nodes were called apical nodes, referring to their location in the surgical specimen. It was noted that the 5-year survival rate for C1 patients was 40.9% and for C2 patients 13.6% (373). Turnbull et al. introduced the category of group D for patients with metastasis in distant organs (374). In addition to the level of lymph node involvement, Dukes also recognized the importance of the number of involved nodes (373). Recent analyses indicate that metastasis to more than four lymph nodes imparts a poor prognosis (375, 376).

The American Joint Commission on Cancer (AJCC) has developed a staging system based on similar parameters: the extent of tumor invasion (T), the status of lymph node involvement (N), and distant metastasis (M). There are minor differences between tumors of the small and large intestines in the definition of T and N categories. The TNM staging system has undergone several modifications. The recent version (377) takes into consideration the number of involved lymph nodes. The AJCC staging (377) is compared with the Dukes' classification (373) and the modified classifications of Astler and Coller (371) and Turnbull et al. (374) in Table 34.8.

The pathologic features of intestinal tumors are complex. The staging systems discussed above encompass only a few of them. Other significant prognostic factors include the pattern of tumor growth, grade of tumor cell differentiation, and the density of lymphocytic infiltration in the tumor (378). Jass proposed a classification of colorectal carcinomas for prognostic prediction based on the evaluation of all the features using numeric indicators (378, 379). In practice, Dukes' method remains popular since it is simple and easy to use.

PATHOLOGIC EXAMINATION AND REPORT

Pathologic evaluation of the neoplasm serves multiple purposes: providing bases for clinical management of individual patients, documentation of the lesion for archival and follow-up studies, and research. To accomplish these, the specimens must be properly handled and carefully examined, to an extent depending on the nature of the specimens. There are three major sources of the specimens: endoscopic biopsy, excision biopsy, and major resection.

TABLE 34.8	Staging Method for Intestinal Carcinoma

AJCC TNM System			Dukes Classification	Astler-Coller & Turnbull Modification
0 : Tis	N0	M0	—	—
I : T1	N0	M0	A : intramural	A : mucosa
T2	N0	M0	A : intramural	B1 : muscularis propria
II : T3,4	N0	M0	B : extramural	B2 : extramural
III : T1–4	N1–3	M0	C1 : regional nodes	C1 : B1 + positive nodes
			C2 : apical nodes	C2 : B2 + positive nodes
IV : T1–4	N1–3	M1		D : dist. met.

Definition of TNM Categories by AJCC	
Small Intestine	Large Intestine

	Small Intestine	Large Intestine
T-Primary tumor		
T0	No evidence of tumor	No evidence of tumor
Tis	Carcinoma in situ	Carcinoma in situ or invading lamina propria
T1	Invading lamina propria or submucosa	Invading submucosa
T2	Invading muscularis propria	Invading muscularis propria
T3	Invading subserosa, mesentery, or retroperitoneum	Invading subserosa or pericolic tissue
T4	Through serosa or invading contiguous organs	Through serosa or invading contiguous organs
N-Regional node		
N0	No metastasis	No metastasis
N1	Metastasis to any number of nodes	1 to 3 positive nodes
N2	—	4 or more positive nodes
N3	—	Any positive node along a named vessel
M-Distant metastasis		
M0	No distant metastasis	No distant metastasis
M1	Distant metastasis	Distant metastasis

—: not applicable.

Data sources: AJCC—Beahrs OH, Henson DE, Hutter RVP, Kennedy BJ, eds. Manual for staging of cancer. 4th ed. Philadelphia: JB Lippincott, 1992:69–73. Dukes classification—Dukes CE, Bussey HJR. The spread of rectal cancer and its effect on prognosis. Br J Cancer 1958;12:309–320. Astler-Coller—Astler VB, Coller FA. The prognostic significance of direct extension of the carcinoma of the colon and rectum. Ann Surg 1954;139:846–851. Turnbull modification—Turnbull RB, Kyle K, Watson FR, et al. Cancer of the rectum: the influence of the no-touch isolation technique on survival rates. Ann Surg 1967;166:420–427

In order to preserve the tissue for microscopic examination, the specimen should be placed in a fixative, mainly neutralized formalin, as soon as possible. However, certain features, such as color, texture, and size, are best viewed when the specimen is fresh. Furthermore certain tests can only be done on fresh specimens such as cytogenetic analysis, enzyme histochemical stain, and molecular studies. In addition, procedures such as electron microscopy, require special fixatives. For these requirements, samples of fresh tissue must be obtained immediately.

Biopsy specimens are usually prefixed before arriving at the laboratory. Proper orientation of specimens is essential for obtaining a section perpendicular to the intestinal wall. A close clinician-pathologist liaison and cooperation is essential in this situation. This relationship is also important for the pathologist to receive detailed clinical information for proper evaluation of the case. The excised specimen may have been cut into several pieces. They may be prefixed or fresh. Identification of the source of each fragment and the nature of original whole lesion must be obtained.

The surgically resected segments of intestine should be kept intact until examination in the laboratory so that the relationship between the lesions and the organ is preserved. The specimen should be immediately examined for any abnormality on the exterior of the specimen. Then the intestine is opened longitudinally along the mesenteric border so that it can be laid flat. The mucosa is carefully inspected for any tumor, erosion, ulcer, or change of colon. Photographs are taken before the tissue is cut.

Certain features must be obtained when the tissue is fresh, such as the color, texture, consistency, size, and location of the lesion. Fixation will change these features and also shrink the tissue. One important feature to determine is the distance between the lesion and the resection margins of the specimen. Fixation will change the measurements. Samples for special studies requiring fresh tissue or special fixation should be obtained immediately. It is prudent to save samples in a low temperature freezer or liquid nitrogen for possible future studies. The lymph nodes should be located, measured, and examined for gross evidence of metastatic tumor. The number and location of the nodes must be established. The apical nodes and nodes at different locations should be separately labeled. The intestinal wall and attached mesentery or soft tissue are palpated to detect any tumor, thickening, or adhesion. The lesion itself should be examined for its location, size, shape, color, and consistency. The height of a protruding mass and the depth of the ulcerated region are measured. The depth of tumor invasion can best be seen on the cut surface, which will also reveal any areas of necrosis, hemorrhage, or fistula. The distance between the border of the tumor and the resection margin of the intestine must be measured. The specimen is examined again after fixation. Small polyps and changes in the mucosal patterns are more clearly shown after fixation. Methylene blue painting of the mucosa may enhance the appearance of these changes and is used to detect ACF.

Tissue sections for microscopic study should be prepared to show the whole picture of the lesion, including the extent of invasion, margins of the tumor, various compartments of the lesion, the nature of other lesions, any alteration of the flat mucosa, the histology of all lymph nodes, and the status of the resection margin of the intestine. The sections supply information for the histologic diagnosis of the tumor, grade of differentiation, extent of invasion, lymphatic and vascular permeation, and TNM stage of the tumor.

The pathology report should be detailed to list all the information including the results of any special study such as DNA ploidy, molecular alterations, and karyotypic analysis. The College of American Pathologists did a study of the pathologic information on colorectal carcinoma in the surgical pathology reports of 532 laboratories (380). Interinstitutional differences were noticeable. A comprehensive checklist was recommended for general use. The list includes pathologic classification of the tumor as well as TNM evaluations. A comparable checklist was proposed by the Association of Directors of Anatomic and Surgical Pathology (381).

SMALL INTESTINAL ADENOCARCINOMA

Carcinomas of the small intestine share many of the pathologic features and precursor conditions with colorectal cancers. The etiologic factors are presumably similar also. The epidemiologic data, however, show less geographic variation than that shown by carcinomas of other segments of the digestive tract.

PATHOLOGY

Location

Adenocarcinomas of the small intestine occur mostly in the upper segments, with about 40% each in the duodenum and jejunum (Table 34.3). In one report, carcinoma of the duodenum was nearly twice as common as that of the jejunum and ileum combined (221). Duodenal carcinomas occur in the periampullary region in 65% of cases, in the supraampullary region in 21%, and in the infraampullary region in 14% (8). Involvement of the duodenal bulb is rare (382). In the jejunum, the carcinomas are located mostly in the upper segment. In both the duodenum and the jejunum, adenocarcinoma is the most common malignant tumor. In the ileum, on the other hand, the most common tumor is carcinoid, and the distal segment is the favored site for carcinoma (13).

The location of adenocarcinoma is influenced by the precancerous conditions from which they arise. Seventy-five percent of carcinomas associated with Crohn's disease, for instance, occur in the ileum (383) which is the primary site for Crohn's disease. The jejunum is the site for carcinoma in Crohn's disease in 24% of cases. The duodenum is involved only rarely (384). These carcinomas develop from the dysplastic epithelium (385). In patients with FAP

or Gardner syndrome, carcinomas and adenomas often occur in the duodenum, particularly in the periampullary region (386, 387). In celiac disease and nontropical sprue, duodenal and jejunal carcinomas may occur (388, 389). Other sites of small intestinal carcinoma include Meckel's diverticulum (390), aberrant pancreas (391), ectopic gastric mucosa (28), ileostomy (392, 393), and possibly Brunner's gland (394).

Pathologic Features and Pattern of Spread

The adenocarcinomas of the proximal small intestine tend to be polypoid or fungating, possibly related to their origin in adenoma (Figs. 34.23 and 34.24), whereas those of the distal segment are often ulcerated and infiltrating. In about 80% of cases, the carcinoma is annular and constrictive (2). The carcinoma complicating Crohn's disease may not be grossly evident in one-half of the cases (383). Occasionally, they are multifocal.

Microscopically, most adenocarcinomas of the small intestine are well to moderately differentiated. Papillary (Fig. 34.16) and villous appearances are seen mainly in the polypoid tumors (395). About 20% of tumors are poorly differentiated (396). Most cells are columnar, with varying degrees of microvillar development (397). Mucous cells are commonly present, secreting both sialomucin and sulfomucin in most cases, although the adjacent normal mucosa secretes only the sialomucin (398). Argyrophilic cells are commonly found, especially in carcinomas of the ileum (334, 398). Paneth cells may be present also, occasionally in large numbers (399).

In most cases, the carcinoma is already deeply invasive at the time of diagnosis. Early carcinoma is rarely diagnosed, except as a focal lesion in an adenoma. Carcinomas of the ampullary region can invade the head of pancreas, pancreatic duct, or common bile duct. In such a situation, it may be difficult to decide the origin of the tumor. In an analysis of 233 periampullary tumors, Yamaguchi and Enjoji found 109 carcinomas of the ampulla of Vater, 19 of the duodenum, 38 of the distal bile duct, and 48 of the head of pancreas (400). In 12 cases, the origin of the carcinoma was not determined. In other regions, penetration of the tumor through serosa may cause peritoneal dissemination or adherence between the tumor and loops of adjacent intestine.

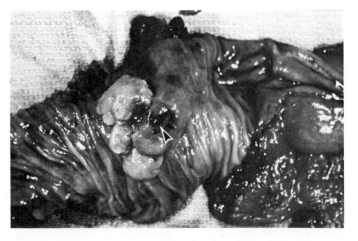

Figure 34.23 Carcinoma of the duodenum at the periampullary region. The orifice of the ampulla of Vater is indicated *(arrowhead)*.

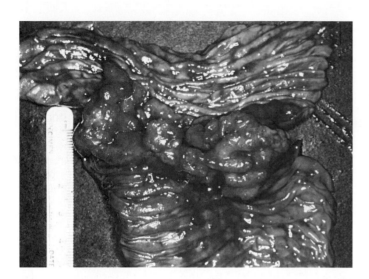

Figure 34.24 A circumferential polypoid carcinoma of the jejunum. The lumen above the tumor is dilated.

The small intestine is rich in lymphatics. Lymphatic permeation is common in the primary lesion. Carcinomas of the duodenum metastasize to the posterior pancreaticoduodenal lymph nodes, those of the jejunum and ileum to the mesenteric nodes, and those of the terminal ileum to the ileocolic and posterior cecal nodes. The carcinomas of the ampulla have lower rates of lymph node involvement, only 20 to 35% of cases (395). Venous invasion of carcinoma in all parts of the small intestine leads into the portal venous system and eventually the liver, from which the tumor spreads to the lung and other organs.

CLINICAL PRESENTATION

Adenocarcinomas of the small intestine occur mainly in the elderly with 86% of patients older than 50 years (30, 401). Since most carcinomas are annular, symptoms of intestinal obstruction are common and pain is the most frequent complaint (1, 30). Tumors of the upper intestine produce nausea and vomiting, whereas those in the distal small intestine cause abdominal distention and periumbilical pain. Weight loss is frequent (402). Acute abdominal emergency due to perforation of the tumor is uncommon (403). Bleeding is common, but usually occult and chronic. Acute massive bleeding is rare.

The periampullary carcinomas often cause obstruction of the common bile duct and jaundice. Of the cases reviewed by Yamaguchi et al. 111 were icteric and 31 nonicteric (404). The carcinomas in the icteric group were more advanced, less papillary, and showed less intraluminal and more periductal growth than those in the nonicteric group. The 10-year survival rates were 57% for the nonicteric patients and 23% for the icteric patients.

The primary choice of treatment is surgical resection of the carcinoma. The reported resectability rate was, on average, 72% for carcinomas of the duodenum, 76% for those of the jejunum, and 82% for those of the ileum (1). The 5-year survival rates of the resected cases were 20%, 17%, and 9% for the respective groups. The 5-year survival rate for all carcinomas of the small intestine was 51% and the mortality rate was 0.3 per 100,000 population (Table 34.2).

COLORECTAL ADENOCARCINOMA

PATHOLOGY

Location

Most colorectal adenocarcinomas are located in the sigmoid and rectum (Table 34.5). There has been an increase in the incidence of carcinomas in the proximal or right colon from the cecum to splenic flexure and a decrease in the incidence of carcinomas in the distal or left colon (405–407). The change is particularly evident within the same institution. Cady et al. reported that in a forty-year period, from 1940 to 1979, the percentage of carcinoma in the right colon at The Lahey Clinic in Boston increased from 7% to 22%, whereas that of the sigmoid and rectal carcinoma decreased from 80% to 62% (408). The report by Slater et al. showed an increase from 18.7% to 27.5% for right colon cancer and a decrease from 72.1% to 62.5% for left colon cancer (409). A similar change is found by comparing the frequencies of tumors in different segments of the colorectum. In 1967, Wood (8) reported that the frequency of carcinoma in cecum and ascending colon was only 10% and that in sigmoid and rectum 75%. In recent reports, the corresponding frequencies were about 25% and 60% respectively (331, 408).The shift of frequency to the right colon parallels a similar shift of the location of the adenomas and an increase in the age of the patients (410).

The location of colorectal carcinoma coincides with the location of precancerous conditions from which the cancer develops. In ulcerative colitis, the carcinoma is widely distributed. In Crohn's disease, the carcinoma is located more in the right colon than in the left colon (411). Carcinoma has also been reported in the rectal stump after colectomy for colitis (412). The location of colonic carcinoma is also affected by genetic factors. In Lynch syndromes, greater than 70% of the carcinomas occur in the right colon and only 25% in the sigmoid and rectum (102).

The carcinomas of the right and left colon differ in several aspects. The carcinomas in the left colon tend to occur more frequently in the male, have three times more concomitant adenomas, and are twice as likely to have adenomatous tissue in the tumor than those in the right colon. Carcinoid and mucinous components are more prominent in the carcinomas of the right colon.

Pathologic Features

Grossly, carcinomas of the right colon, particularly the cecum, tend to be polypoid and fungating (Fig. 34.9), whereas those of the left colon ulcerative (Fig. 34.12) as well as fungating (Figs. 34.10 and 34.11). Diffusely infiltrative (linitis plastica) type of carcinoma occur more often in the distal colon (Fig. 34.13). Circumferential involvement is more common in the left colon which is normally narrower than the right colon. The carcinomas complicating inflammatory bowel disease are often flat and may not be grossly evident (413).

Histologically, the colorectal carcinomas are mostly well to moderately differentiated. In a recent report (414), 39.4% of the tumors were well differentiated, 37.3% moderately differentiated, 14.1% poorly differentiated, and 9.2% mucinous. Endocrine and mucinous elements are more common in the tumors of the right than the left colon (413, 415). The carcinomas associated with Crohn's disease may be less differentiated than others (415).

Patterns of Spread

LOCAL SPREAD The mucosal origin of colorectal carcinoma causes the carcinomas to grow intraluminally, particularly in tumors arising in an adenoma. Intramural spread may be circumferential or longitudinal along the long axis of the bowel. The extent of intramural spread under an intact mucosa is an important concern at the time of surgical resection. Fortunately, in most cases, deep-seated lateral spread of the tumor is limited. A study by Lozorthes et al. on 119 rectal carcinomas (416) revealed that in 74% of cases, the extent of deep-seated carcinomatous tissue was the same as that seen grossly. In 21% of cases, the border of tumor spread was beyond the gross margin by less than 5 mm. In only 5% did the tumor extend for 5 to 15 mm beyond the gross margin. A similar observation was made by Madsen et al. (417) who concluded that 1.5 cm was an adequate distal margin. Kameda et al. noted that the intramural spread of the tumor was within 0.5 cm of the gross margin in a localized tumor and 2.1 cm in an infiltrative tumor, and that a lymph node with metastatic tumor was usually located within 1 cm of the margin of the primary lesion (418). They, therefore, recommended a resection margin of 2 cm for localized carcinomas and 3 cm for infiltrative carcinomas. The highly infiltrative signet-ring cell carcinoma is an exception to this rule. Rarely, perineural invasion may extend far beyond the gross tumor margin (417).

The carcinomas may invade directly into the neighboring tissue. A cecal carcinoma may extend into the lateral abdominal gutter and the abdominal wall. Carcinoma of the transverse colon may involve the stomach, pancreas, liver, gallbladder, and spleen. Carcinomas of the ascending and descending colons may involve the retroperitoneal tissue. Carcinomas of the sigmoid and rectum may involve the pelvic organs, urinary bladder in the males and vagina in the female. The anterior surface of the colon is covered by the peritoneum. The carcinoma may penetrate the serosa and seed the peritoneal surface. Fibrous adhesion forms when the carcinoma involves the adjacent loops of intestine, mesentery, or omentum.

LYMPHATIC SPREAD Lymphatic spread of the tumor to the regional lymph nodes usually occurs along the arteries. The first group of involved lymph nodes are in the pericolic or perirectal tissue. The ileocolic and middle colic lymphatic chains drain into the central nodes of the superior mesenteric artery. There may be aberrant lymphatics draining the lower rectum to nodes along the inferior mesenteric artery, skipping the nodes adjacent to the primary tumor (419). Retrograde lymph node metastasis may occur when the normal lymphatic flow is blocked by metastatic tumor (420). Lymph node metastasis is present in about 40 to 50% of colorectal carcinomas, mostly advanced (373, 421, 422). Lymph node metastasis is rare in early carcinomas. Of 178 early colorectal carcinomas studied by Shimoda et al., 32 of 146 polypoid carcinomas and 22 of 32 nonpolypoid carcinomas had submucosal involvement. Lymph node metastasis was present in only four cases, all nonpolypoid (262).

VENOUS SPREAD Venous invasion may occur in colorectal carcinomas and tumor cells have been found in both regional and peripheral venous blood (423). Mesenteric venous flow lodges the tumor cells in the liver which is the most frequent site of visceral metastasis. Another route for the tumor cells to reach the liver is via blood vessel invasion in the lymph node (424). From the liver, tumor cells advance to the lung and other organs. Metastasis to the lung alone may occur from carcinomas of the lower rectum which has a dual venous system: superior hemorrhoidal veins to the portal system and liver, and middle and inferior hemorrhoidal veins to the systemic circulation and lung. Occasionally, direct metastasis to the vertebra occurs by way of Batson's venous plexus (425).

METASTASIS The frequency of metastasis in the visceral organs at autopsy was reported by Berge et al. (426). The liver was involved in 75.7% of colonic carcinomas and 61.9% of rectal carcinomas. The corresponding percentages for metastasis in the lung were 47.7% and 64.2%. The higher percentage in rectal carcinoma is explained in the section on venous invasion above. Lymph node metastasis was present in 77.0% and 78.4% respectively. The other frequently involved organs included peritoneum (in 49.4% and 25.4% of respective cases), adrenal (13.8% and 18.7%), ovary (17.3% and 3.6%), bone (11.7% and 19.4%), pleura (11.3% and 12.7%), brain (6.3% and 8.2%), kidney (5.0% and 4.5%), skin (5.0% and 3%), and spleen (6.7% and 2.2%). Micrometastasis with few scattered cancer cells, as seen in bone marrow, is easily missed in routine microscopy, but may be detected by reverse-transcription polymerase chain reaction for keratin (427), or by immunohistochemical staining for cytoskeleton (428).

Metastasis to the ovary by signet-ring cell carcinoma produces Krukenburg tumors with bilateral enlargement of ovaries (429). In one report, metastasis of a cecal adenocarcinoma to the ovary caused excessive estrogen production and post-menopausal uterine bleeding (430). Other uncommon sites of metastasis include testis (431), jaw (432), nasopharynx (433), pelvic bone (434), and phalangeal bone (435). The metastatic lesion may become ossified (436).

IMPLANTATION Peritoneal seeding of carcinoma cells is relatively common, particularly in patients with the infiltrative type of carcinoma. Occasionally the tumor implant grows in the rectouterine (Douglas) or rectovesical pouch to form a palpable mass by rectal examination, known as Blumer's shelf. Implantation of tumor cells at the time of surgical operation may be responsible for tumor growth in surgical wounds (437) and at the anastomotic suture line (438, 439). Intraluminal seeding of exfoliated cancer cells may cause implantation in fistula in ano (440). The occurrence of some of the synchronous colonic carcinomas with identical DNA indices has been postulated to be on similar basis (441). Peritoneal seeding is the main cause of local recurrence of the tumor which occurs in about 10% of patients after resection of tumor for cure (442).

MARKER SUBSTANCES

Since the isolation of CEA in 1965 (443), many biochemical markers have been demonstrated in the colorectal carcinoma (444–447). The development of monoclonal antibody techniques and immunohistochemical methods further facilitated the investigation. Carcinoembryonic antigen is the prototype of a group of oncofetal antigens. It is a glycoprotein present in the fetal cells as well as some adult cells (448) and in increased amount in many malignant tumors. In the colorectum, it is associated with the striated border of the normal columnar cells and apical cell wall of the carcinoma cells. Intracytoplasmic presence is seen mainly in the mucus-secreting cells (449). Carcinoembryonic antigen is demonstrable also in the adenomas (444, 450), inflammatory bowel disease (450), and ACF (277). The serum level of CEA is related to the tumor mass. The upper limit of normal serum level is 5 ng/mL. Eighteen percent of patients with early colonic carcinoma had an elevated CEA serum level, while 83% of patients with advanced carcinoma had a high serum level (447). Although CEA is not specific enough for the diagnosis of colorectal carcinoma, its serum level, together with that of tumor associated glycoprotein TAG-72, has been used to monitor post-operative tumor recurrence (451, 452). Preoperative serum CEA level was found to be related to the stage of the carcinoma and the survival rate (445, 453, 454).

CA19-9 is an example of an antigen synthesized by cancer cells (444, 445, 455). It is related to blood group antigen Le^a and is present in up to 80% of colonic carcinomas and other benign lesions such as polyps and dysplastic cells. Elevated serum levels of CA19-9 are present in up to 50% of cancer patients. It is less sensitive but more specific than CEA for cancer diagnosis (456). Altered expressions of Lewis and ABH blood group antigens are often noted in the colorectal adenomas and carcinomas (444, 457–459). T antigen, a precursor for blood group M and N antigens, is demonstrated by binding with peanut agglutinin in nearly all colonic carcinomas (444). Other lectins have also been found to bind colonic carcinomas and polyps (460). Colon-specific antigen p (CSAp) is another glycoprotein found in the serum of patients with advanced colonic carcinomas (445, 461). Several cancer-related antigens recognize mucin-type glycoproteins, including M1 antigen and colon-ovarian tumor antigen (COTA) (462–464).

DNA contents of carcinoma cells have been studied by many investigators. Aneuploidy was found in 53% of colonic carcinomas, 27% of tubular adenomas, and 19% in ulcerative colitis (465). However, 68% of hereditary nonpolypoid carcinomas were found to be diploid (466). The polypoid carcinomas were aneuploid in 17%, while the crater-shaped carcinomas were aneuploid in 77% of cases (216). The ploidy of carcinoma has been correlated with CEA serum level (450), depth of tumor invasion (467), stage of tumor (468), and prognosis (468, 469). Some studies, however, did not find such relationships (470). In any case, the ploidy of the tumor is not as significant a prognostic factor as the morphologic features of the carcinoma (379). Using tritiated thymidine labeling or antibody Ki-67, more proliferating cells were found in carcinomas than in adenomas or normal mucosa (471, 472). However, the number of these cells in colonic carcinoma varied widely and there was no relation to any known parameter of prognostic significance (473).

SURVIVAL RATES AND PROGNOSIS

The latest available 5-year survival rates of colorectal cancer by race and sex in the SEER (Surveillance, Epidemiology, and End Results) program of the National Cancer Institute are listed in Table 34.6 (4). The rates in the 1986 to 1991 period were 20% higher than the corresponding rates in the 1974 to 1976 period. The improvement in survival rates is most pronounced for rectal cancer in black males and least pronounced for rectal cancer in black females. The survival rates by stage and location of the tumors from the National Cancer Data Base are listed in Table 34.9 (41). The survival rates were highest for Stage I carcinomas at 72%, and lowest for Stage IV tumors with distant metastasis at 7%.

The survival rates are influenced by many factors which are listed in Table 34.10. The College of American Pathologists classified them into four categories, according to the reported information regarding the extent of studies on them and their usage

TABLE 34.9	Relative 5-Year Survival Rates (%) of Colon Cancer and Rectal Cancer Diagnosed in 1986/87 by Site and Stage	
	Colon Cancer	Rectal Cancer
Anatomic Site		
Ascending/cecum	49	
Transverse	49	
Descending	54	
Sigmoid	55	
Multiple sites	47	
Unknown	51	
Rectosigmoid junction		50
Rectum		50
Stage		
All stages	51	50
I	72	72
II	63	57
III	45	41
IV	7	6

Data source: Steele GD Jr, Jessup JM. Colorectal cancer. In: Steele GD Jr, Jessup JM, Winchester DP, Menck HR, Murphy GP, eds. National Cancer data base. Annual review of patient care, 1995. Atlanta: American Cancer Society, 1996;66–83.

in clinical management of patients (474). Among the pathologic factors, the stage of tumor at the time of diagnosis or surgical operation is the most important. Patients with liver metastasis have a mean survival period of 4.5 months (101). However, small and solitary metastatic tumor in the liver or lung are resectable and potentially curable if there is no other residual tumor (442). Histologic type and growth pattern of the tumor are also important. The signet-ring cell tumor with a diffusely infiltrative pattern has poor prognosis (360, 364).

Serum CEA is often used to monitor the tumor status after surgical resection of the tumor. It provides a guideline for second exploration and resection for recurrent tumor. Twenty percent of these patients were cured by resection of recurrent tumor (442). TAG-72 has been used for similar purposes (452).

DNA ploidy of the tumor has been found to be an important prognostic factor. In a study on 363 postresection patients by Chapman et al. (475), 60% of colorectal cancers were aneuploid. The 5-year survival rate for diploid tumors was 76% and for aneuploid tumors 64%. There was no relation between ploidy and stage, histologic grade, or site of the tumor. Another report (476) also showed no relation between aneuploidy and distant metastasis or survival.

The nm23 gene is a metastasis suppressor gene. The expression of nm23 by immunohistochemical staining showed only marginal relationship with death of patients (477). A similar finding was obtained by Northern blot hybridization technique for nm23-H1 RNA (478). On the other hand, allelic loss or mutation of nm23 gene was found in four of eight tumors with distant metastasis and none of twelve tumors without metastasis (296). In another report (476), patients with allelic deletion of nm23 had three times the risk

TABLE	
34.10	**Prognostic Factors for Colorectal Carcinoma**

Pathologic factors
  Stage of carcinoma at time of diagnosis
  Extent of local invasion of carcinoma
  Lymph node metastasis
  Number of lymph nodes with metastasis
  Type of carcinoma
  Growth pattern of carcinoma
  Length of resection margin from tumor
  Grade of differentiation of carcinoma
  Vascular permeation by carcinoma
  Perineural invasion by carcinoma
  Serosal involvement by carcinoma
  Inflammatory reaction in carcinoma
  Location of carcinoma
  Size and shape of carcinoma
Molecular and genetic factors
  DNA ploidy of carcinoma
  Tumor suppressor genes
  Apoptosis inhibition gene
  Metastasis inhibition gene
Biologic markers
  Carcinoembryonic antigen serum level
  Tumor-associated antigens
  Mucin related markers

of developing distant metastasis than patients without nm23 deletion. However, an increased level of nm23 expression was related to large size and deep invasion of the tumor (477).

Apoptosis, the programmed cell death, is inhibited by the bcl-2 gene. Lack of bcl-2 expression in tumor cells by immunohistochemical stain is associated with larger tumors and lower rate of survival than bcl-2 positive tumors, although bcl-2 expression was not related to tumor stage (479). Overexpression of p53 was associated with a lower survival rate than p53 negative tumors in Stage III (480), but p53 expression did not show overall prognostic significance (481, 482). Tumors with K-ras mutation had worse prognosis than those without K-ras mutation (483). The expression of DCC, a tumor suppressor gene, is inversely related to the survival rates of Stage II and III tumors (484).

CLINICAL PRESENTATION

Symptoms and Signs

The symptoms and signs of colorectal carcinoma, in order of frequency, are abdominal pain or cramping (78%), change in bowel habits (67%), hematochezia (56%), weight loss (38%), anemia (24%), intestinal obstruction (11%), symptoms related to metastasis (7%), and palpable abdominal mass (485). There are regional variations in the frequency of these manifestations because of differences in the caliber of the bowel, the nature of feces, and the type of tumor. Fresh blood in the stool and a change of bowel habits are common in patients with carcinomas of the distal colon and rectum, whereas anemia, weight loss, and palpable mass are main manifestations of carcinomas of the proximal colon (486). Carcinoma of the rectum may involve pelvic organs and produce genitourinary symptoms.

Complications

Obstruction and perforation are the main complications, affecting 29% of colonic carcinomas and 7% of rectal carcinomas (487). Obstruction alone was present in 15% of cases and perforation with or without obstruction in 4%. Compared to noncomplicated cases, these patients were older, the tumors were less resectable, the surgical mortality was four times higher, and the overall 5-year survival rate was only one-half of that for noncomplicated cases (487, 488). Acute obstruction due to intussusception is relatively common in association with benign tumors of the intestine, but is only rarely reported in patients with carcinoma (489). Chronic obstruction is mostly due to circumferential infiltration of the tumor with napkin-ring shaped constriction. The perforated cases fared worse, with a 5-year survival rate of only 10% (490). In an analysis of 51 perforated cases among 1551 colorectal cancer cases (3.3%) (491), localized perforation with abscess formation was present in 31 (61%), and free perforation with generalized peritonitis in 20 (39%). Excluding 19 cases with Stage IV disease or postoperative death, the 5-year survival rate of the remaining 32 aggressively treated patients was 58%, similar to the overall survival rate of all patients.

The colorectal carcinomas are often ulcerated and bleed. The blood loss may be frank or occult. The ulcerated tumor may serve as a locus for infection which induces further necrosis of the tumor and contributes to perforation and fistula formation. The infection may spread to other organs. There have been reports of streptococcus bovis septicemia and endocarditis (492–494), clostridial septicemia and soft tissue gangrene (495), meningitis, and abscesses in various organs (492).

The lower urinary tract is affected in 38% of patients causing obstruction, gross hematuria, or neurogenic bladder (496). It is more commonly associated with recurrent than primary colorectal carcinoma. Other uncommon complications include coagulopathy in patients with metastasizing mucus-producing tumors (497), microangiopathic hemolytic anemia (498), dermatomyositis (499), extrahepatic obstructive jaundice (500), and nodular intra-abdominal panniculitis (501).

Associated Conditions

In addition to the common association of colorectal carcinoma with precancerous conditions listed in Table 34.7, colon carcinoma has been reported in patients with a variety of other conditions. Colonic diverticulosis is common in the Western countries and affects mostly the distal colon, as does the carcinoma. It is therefore not surprising to find that both conditions may coexist in a high percentage of cases in both men and women (502, 503). The carcinoma may fortuitously involve one or more diverticula. Patients with colorectal carcinoma were found to have hyperplastic gastric polyps in 18.7% and gastric adenomas in 3.5% (504). Appendicitis was present in 10 of 519 patients with cecal carcinoma (505). Coexisting carcinomas in other parts of the digestive tract include that of ampulla of Vater (506), gall bladder (507), appendix (507), and squamous cell carcinoma of the anus (508). Other reported coexisting tumors were astrocytoma in a 16 year old boy (509), extragenital malignant mixed mesodermal tumor (510), and mesenteric fibromatosis (511).

Screening, Diagnosis, and Treatment

Many patients with colorectal cancer do not have symptoms. Therefore, screening of asymptomatic patients over the age of 50 has been urged. Two main tests used are fecal occult blood test (FOBT) and endoscopy. A variety of tests for occult blood in the feces have been used. A 6-day test resulted in the detection of adenoma in 8.77 and carcinoma in 2.54 per 1000 tested persons (512). The detected carcinomas were in a relatively early stage in most of the cases (513, 514). Screening with proctosigmoidoscopy has only limited benefit (515). Colonoscopy is useful in screening high risk populations such as first-degree relatives of patients with familial traits. In one such study, adenoma was detected in 21% of 114 tested persons (516). In spite of the benefits of FOBT, the efficacy of FOBT has been debated (517). It is evident that FOBT is insensitive. It fails to detect many tumors and most bleeding lesions are not neoplastic. Although FOBT screening reduced colorectal cancer mortality, it did not influence the cancer incidence (518). Furthermore, false results of the test may indirectly harm the patient. To overcome some of the limitations, it has been suggested that the combination of FOBT and flexible sigmoidoscopy should be used for screening (519). However, sigmoidoscopy up to 60 cm level may miss one-third of the lesions (520). Colonoscopy is sensitive and specific. Rex et al. examined 209 asymptomatic patients with colonoscopy (521). An adenoma was found in 25% and carcinoma in 1% of patients. It has been estimated that colonoscopic polypectomy might reduce the risk for colorectal cancer by 76% to 90% (227). Screening colonoscopy with polypectomy reduced the risk for colorectal cancer in families with HNPCC by 62% (522). Endoscopic surveillance of patients with ulcerative colitis detected dysplasia in 8.5% (523).

The diagnosis of colorectal carcinoma in symptomatic patients requires increasingly sophisticated imaging techniques, endoscopic examination with biopsy (see Chapter 3), and cytological study (see Chapter 4). Magnetic resonance imaging (MRI) and immunoscintigraphy are also used (524). Local spread of carcinoma and lymph node metastasis can be detected by endoluminal ultrasonography with an accuracy rate of greater than 80%, much better than computerized tomography (CT) scan (525). CT and MRI are complementary in diagnosing complications (526). Endoscopy is indispensable in diagnosing the colorectal tumors. Total colonoscopy is necessary to detect synchronous lesions preoperatively and metachronous lesions postoperatively (527, 528). Endoscopic biopsy is accurate for diagnosis in 90% of cases and fine needle aspiration cytology is particularly useful for infiltrative type of growth with an accuracy rate of 97%, whereas brush cytology is accurate in 83% of cases (529). In terms of reliability of pathologic diagnosis on the resected specimens, routine histologic sections have been found to be quite adequate and representative (530, 531).

The colorectal carcinomas are treated primarily by surgical resection (532). The resectability of the tumor depends on the stage of the tumor when first diagnosed and the surgical techniques used. In general, 85% of colorectal carcinomas are resectable for cure, 10% are unresectable or resectable for palliation only, and 5% are inoperable (533). Endoscopic transrectal resection has been applied

to patients with poor operative risk or small tumors (534). This treatment is curative for only 5% of rectal cancers (532). Fifty percent of patients develop local, regional, or systemic recurrence of the tumor after curable resection of the primary lesion (532, 535). A surveillance program for early detection of recurrent disease in asymptomatic patients has not resulted in survival benefit, however. Adjuvant postoperative radiation has been used to control local recurrence and improve the survival rate (536, 537). Radiation has also been used to improve operability of rectal cancer (101, 538). Chemotherapy with 5-fluorouracil (5-FU) alone or in combination with interferon has been tried on advanced cancer patients with partial response (539). Combined use of 5-FU and levamisole, an immunostimulant, showed beneficial effects on postresection patients (540). Liver metastases have been treated surgically, with low operative mortality and an increased 5-year survival rate up to 43% (541, 542). Arterial infusion of 5-FU to the liver results in partial remission and prolongs the survival interval (543).

MULTIPLE CARCINOMAS

Adenocarcinomas of the colon and rectum are often multiple, occurring synchronously in 3 to 8% of patients, and metachronously in 2 to 3% of patients surviving the first carcinoma (101, 527, 544, 545). Synchronous carcinomas are diagnosed perioperatively in 2 to 3% of cases (546). The origin of synchronous carcinomas was investigated retrospectively by DNA ploidy of the tumors (441). In four cases, all tumors were diploid, and in three cases the tumors had identical aneuploid patterns, suggesting the possibility of monoclonal origin of the tumors. Synchronous carcinomas are more common in patients with familial polyposis (21%) (547), HNPCC (18%) (117), ulcerative colitis (18%) (547), and pelvic irradiation (548). In one report, each of a pair of monozygotic twins had three colonic carcinomas (549). In a study in Japan (550), 35% of synchronous carcinomas were all advanced, 59% a mix of advanced and early, and 6% all early. In 62% of cases, the synchronous carcinomas were in the sigmoid and rectum. In another study (551), 88% of synchronous carcinomas were in different segments of the colon. Sixty percent of these colons had adenomas. Patients with synchronous carcinomas had a higher incidence of metachronous cancer than those with single cancer at first diagnosis (552). The intervals between the first and second carcinoma varied, between 2 and 5 years in 40 to 50% of cases (527), but an interval longer than 20 years has been noted (549).

The preoperative diagnosis of synchronous carcinomas is achieved mainly by colonoscopy. The early lesions might be easily missed and correct preoperative diagnosis was made in only 42% of cases (553). In 24% of cases, the second carcinoma was discovered at operation, and in 34% incidentally in the resected specimen. Postoperative colonoscopy is mandatory for early diagnosis of metachronous carcinomas (553).

SQUAMOUS CELL CARCINOMA AND ADENOSQUAMOUS CARCINOMA

Occasional squamous cells are present in about 5% of colorectal adenocarcinomas. About one-half of such tumors were found in the rectum and sigmoid and 20% in the cecum (554). They are rare,

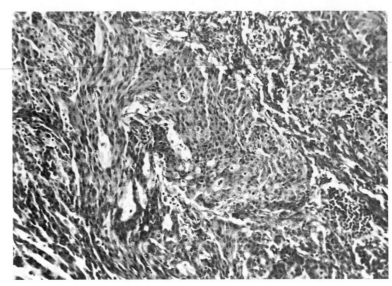

Figure 34.25   Adenosquamous carcinoma showing squamous component of the tumor (×120).

occurring in only 0.05% of adenocarcinomas (555). Squamous cell carcinoma of the colon was first reported in 1919 (556). By 1988, more than 60 cases were reported (557). The reported location of the tumor varied, more frequent in the right colon in some reports (558, 559), and more in the left colon in other reports (21). Occasional squamous cell carcinomas have glandular components and are called adenosquamous carcinoma (Fig. 34.25). The squamous cells in these tumors are identified by electron microscopy and immunohistochemistry (560, 561). In rare cases, hypercalcemia was present (562). The clinical presentation of squamous and adenosquamous carcinomas are similar to that of adenocarcinoma. There is no sex difference. Grossly, the tumors form fungating masses (19). They are aggressive tumors, and 5-year survival rates were reported to be 50% for Dukes' B, 33% for Dukes' C, and 0% for Dukes' D tumors (557). Squamous cell and adenosquamous carcinoma probably originate from crypt cells. The presence of carcinoid cells in an adenosquamous carcinoma supports this view (563). Colonic adenoma may have areas of squamous metaplasia (20) (Fig. 34.26) and squamous cell carcinoma may develop in such an adenoma (517). They may also arise from an area of squamous metaplasia in the flat mucosa (564). These tumors have also been reported in patients with ulcerative colitis (557, 565), and after radiation treatment to ovarian carcinoma (566). In one case, the squamous cell carcinoma developed in a duplication of the colon (567).

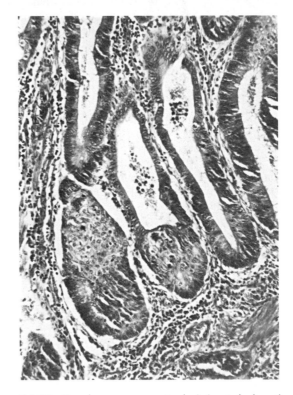

Figure 34.26   Focal squamous metaplasia in a tubular adenoma of the colon (×120).

ENDOCRINE CARCINOMA

Endocrine cells of the gut are of endodermal origin and differentiated from stem cells in the crypt. The crypt origin of these cells explains their presence in a wide range of intestinal neoplasms (334, 336, 342, 568), occasionally in conjunction with Paneth (337) or squamous cells (563, 568). In addition, there are tumors which are composed of both carcinoid and carcinoma or of carcinomatous cells with endocrine functions. These tumors are discussed in detail in Chapter 15. A brief discussion is given below.

COMPOSITE ADENOCARCINOMA AND CARCINOID, AND ADENOCARCINOID

In some of these tumors, carcinoid coexists with either adenoma or adenocarcinoma (Fig. 34.27) as composite tumors (569, 570). In other cases, the carcinoma and carcinoid cells intimately intermingle to form adenocarcinoid (571, 572). The latter, particularly the variant known as goblet cell carcinoid, occurs most frequently in the appendix (See Chapter 35).

SMALL CELL CARCINOMA

Small cell carcinomas of the intestines have been identified as an unusual form of endocrine carcinoma. They are histologically identical with the pulmonary eponym. The cells are uniformly small with a dense chromatin pattern and scanty cytoplasm (Fig. 34.28). Occasional glandular structures may be present (338). Some tumors appear to have developed in an adenoma. Of five cases reported by Mills et al., four were associated with villous or tubulovillous adenoma (573). Occasional cases have coexisting adenocarcinoma (574) (Fig. 34.29). Grossly, small cell carcinomas may be polypoid, fungating, or constrictive (573–575). Electron microscopic examination of the tumor reveals neurosecretory dense core granules of variable sizes, tonofilaments, and desmosomes (338, 575). Immu-

nohistochemical studies show positive reaction for medium and low molecular weight cytokeratin, epithelial membrane antigen, neuron-specific enolase, and neurofilaments (576). Small cell carcinomas are very aggressive, and even a small superficial tumor may have already metastasized to the lymph node (573). Of 20 colonic tumors reviewed by Redman (574), widespread metastasis was present in 85%. Nearly all patients died, mostly within a year (573). Radiation and chemotherapy may provide temporary remission (574, 575).

OTHER RARE CARCINOMAS AND METASTATIC TUMORS

Bak reported four cases of pleomorphic (giant cell) carcinoma, two in the small intestine and two in the colon (577). The tumors were

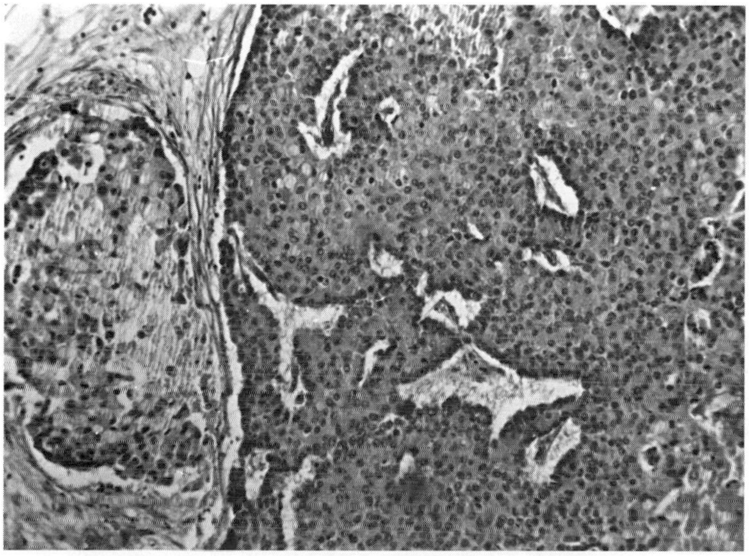

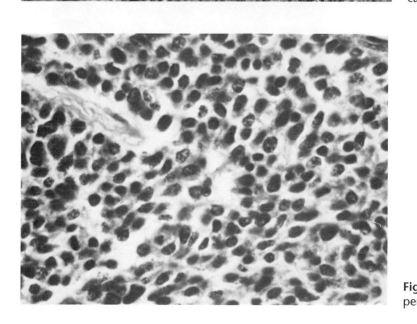

Figure 34.27   Composite adenocarcinoma and carcinoid of the colon, showing a small group of mucous carcinoma cells left to a patch of carcinoid cells. In other areas, the carcinoma is mostly tubular and infiltrative (×120).

Figure 34.28   Small cell carcinoma of colon showing hyperchromatic nuclei and scanty cytoplasm (×480).

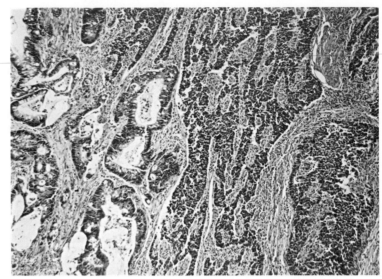

Figure 34.29   Small cell carcinoma *(right)* of the colon with a focus of adenocarcinoma *(left)*. A high magnification view of the small cell carcinoma is shown in Figure 34.28. Both elements were present in the metastatic lesion in the lymph node (×50).

composed of a mixture of giant, polygonal, and spindle cells. Dense core granules, keratin, vimentin, and neuron-specific enolase were present in the cells. There was early spread of the tumor and prognosis was poor. Jewel et al. reported four cases of colonic adenoma and carcinoma composed of uniform clear cells with abundant glycogen in the cytoplasm (578). Kubosawa et al. reported a case of choriocarcinoma, together with papillary adenocarcinoma, in the sigmoid colon of a 50 year old woman with high serum level of human chorionic gonadotropin (579). The metastatic lesions contained only choriocarcinoma. Robey-Cafferty et al. reported six cases of anaplastic sarcomatoid carcinoma in the jejunum and ileum (580). The tumors were large endophytic masses and composed of large cells with prominent nucleoli and spindle cells which by electron microscopy were shown to be epithelial cells. They took an aggressive course and five patients died within 40 months. Amano and Yamada reported an endometrioid carcinoma arising from endometriosis in the sigmoid (581). Rare carcinomas in the duplication of gastrointestinal tract have been reported (582).

Primary melanomas of the anus and anal canal may extend into the lower rectum (583). Primary melanoma of the rectum is rare (584). The diagnosis of primary melanoma of the small bowel is usually based on the lack of a known primary lesion elsewhere. Such cases are rare (585, 586). On the other hand, melanoma of the skin often metastasizes to the gut, particularly the small intestine (587, 588).

Carcinomas of other parts of the digestive tract may metastasize to the intestines. The linitis plastica type of gastric carcinoma may metastasize to the colon and cause segmental stricture which can be mistaken as a primary colonic lesion (589, 590). Metastatic colonic carcinoma may cause annular narrowing of the small intestine (591). Other tumors which metastasize relatively commonly to the intestines are carcinomas of the breast (592, 593) and lung (594, 595). The metastatic lesions in the intestine are usually submucosally located (Fig. 34.30) and small. The covering mucosa is intact. Occasionally, a polypoid lesion may lead to intussusception (596). The infiltrative lesions may cause obstruction and ulcerated lesions may bleed or perforate (594, 595).

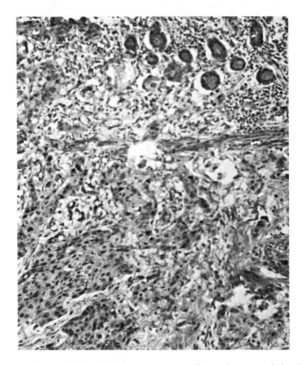

Figure 34.30   Metastatic squamous cell carcinoma of the lung in the submucosa and adjacent mucosa of jejunum (×120).

References

1. Sindelar WF. Cancer of the small intestine. In: De Vita VT, Hellman S, Rosenberg SA, eds. Cancer. Principle and Practice of Oncology. 2nd ed. Philadelphia: JB Lippincott, 1985:771–794.
2. Jaffe BM, McFadden D. Tumors of the small intestine. In: Moossa AR, Robson MC, Schimpff SC, eds. Comprehensive textbook of Oncology. Baltimore: Williams & Wilkins, 1986:1052–1062.
3. Parker SL, Tong T, Bolden S, Wingo PA. Cancer statistics, 1997. CA 1997;47:5–27.
4. Kosary CL, Gloeckle-Ries LA, Miller BA, et al. SEER Cancer

Statistics Review, 1973–1992. NIH publication 96-2789. Bethesda, MD: National Cancer Institute, 1996:152–180.

5. McPeak CJ. Malignant tumors of the small intestine. Am J Surg 1967;114:402–411.

6. Eckel JH. Primary tumors of the jejunum and ileum. Surgery 1948;23:467–475.

7. Darling RC, Welch CE. Tumors of the small intestine. New Engl J Med 1959;260:397–408.

8. Wood DA. Tumors of the intestines. Atlas of Tumor Pathology, Fascicle 22. Washington, DC: Armed Forces Institute of Pathology, 1967.

9. del Regato JA, Spjut HJ, Cox JD. Ackerman and del Regato's Cancer. Diagnosis, Treatment and Prognosis. 6th ed. St Louis: CV Mosby, 1985:512–530.

10. Herbsman H, Wetstein L, Rosen V. Tumors of the small intestine. Curr Prob Surg 1980;17:121–184.

11. Wilson JM, Melvin DB, Gray GF, et al. Benign small bowel tumor. Ann Surg 1975;181:247–250.

12. Mason GR. Tumors of the duodenum and small intestine. In: Sabiston DC Jr, ed. Textbook of Surgery. 13th ed. Philadelphia: WB Saunders, 1986:868–873.

13. Kelsey JR Jr. Small bowel tumors. In: Bockus HL, ed. Gastroenterology, 3rd ed. Philadelphia: WB Saunders, 1976:459–472.

14. Barclay THC, Shapira DV. Malignant tumors of the small intestine. Cancer 1983;51:878–881.

15. Wilson JM, Melvin DB, Gray GF, Thorbjarnarson B. Primary malignancies of the small bowel: A report of 96 cases and reviews of the literature. Ann Surg 1974;180:175–179.

16. Williamson RCN, Welch CE, Malt RA. Adenocarcinoma and lymphoma of the small intestine. Distribution and etiologic associations. Ann Surg 1983;197:172–178.

17. Braasch JW, Denbo HE. Tumors of the small intestine. Surg Clin N Am 1964;44:791–809.

18. Ho SB, Itzkowitz SH, Friera AM, et al. Cell lineage markers in premalignant and malignant colonic mucosa. Gastroenterology 1989;97:392–404.

19. Lafreniere R, Ketcham AS. Primary squamous carcinoma of the rectum. Report of a case and review of the literature. Dis Colon Rectum 1985;28:967–972.

20. Almagro UA, Pintar K, Zellmer RB. Squamous metaplasia in colorectal polyps. Cancer 1984;53:2679–2682.

21. Pigott JP, Williams GB. Primary squamous cell carcinoma of the colorectum: case report and literature review of a rare entity. J Surg Oncol 1987;35:117–119.

22. Griesser GH, Schumacher U, Elfeldt R, et al. Adenosquamous carcinoma of the ileum: report of a case and review of the literature. Virchows Arch (A) 1985;406:483–487.

23. Shousha S, Spiller RC, Parkins RA. The endoscopically abnormal duodena in patients with dyspepsia: biopsy findings in 60 cases. Histopathology 1983;7:23–34.

24. Tsadilas T. Duodenal polyp composed of ectopic gastric mucosa. Dig Dis Sci 1984;29:475–477.

25. Russin R, Krevsky B, Caroline DF, et al. Mixed hyperplastic and adenomatous polyp arising from ectopic gastric mucosa of the duodenum. Arch Pathol Lab Med 1986;110:556–558.

26. Ming SC, Simon M, Tandar BN. Gross gastric metaplasia of ileum after regional enteritis. Gastroenterology 1963;44:63–68.

27. Tayler AL. The epithelial heterotopias of the alimentary tract. J Pathol 1930;30:415–449.

28. Caruso ML, Marzullo F. Jejunal adenocarcinoma in congenital heterotopic gastric mucosa. J Clin Gastroenterol 1988;10.92–96.

29. Lightdale CJ, Koepsell TD, Sherlock P. Small intestine. In: Schottenfeld D, Fraumeni JF, eds. Cancer epidemiology and prevention. Philadelphia: WB Saunders, 1982:692–702.

30. Lance P. Tumors and other neoplastic diseases of the small bowel. In: Yamada T. ed. Textbook of gastroenterology. Philadelphia: JB Lippincott, 1995:1696–1713.

31. Roberton AM. Roles of endogenous substances and bacteria in colorectal cancer. Mutat Res 1993;290:71–78.

32. Lowenfels AB. Why are small bowel tumors so rare? Lancet 1973; 1:24–26.

33. Williamson RCN, Rainey JB. The relationship between intestinal

hyperplasia and carcinogenesis. Scand J Gastroenterol Suppl 1985; 104:57–76.

34. Lipkin M. Phase 1 and phase 2 proliferative lesions of colonic epithelial cells in diseases leading to colonic cancer. Cancer 1974;34: 878–888.

35. Calman KC. Why are small bowel tumors rare? An experimental model. Gut 1974;15:552–554.

36. WHO (World Health Organization). Cancer Incidence in Five Continents, Vol III. International Agency for Research on Cancer, Lyon, France. 1976.

37. Cutler SJ, Young JR Jr. Demographic patterns of cancer incidence in the United States. In: Fraumeni JR Jr, ed. Persons at high risk of cancer: an approach to cancer etiology and control. New York: Academic Press, 1975:307–342.

38. Sinar D. Small bowel neoplasms (other than carcinoid and lymphoma). In: Sleisenger MH, Fordtran JS, eds. Gastrointestinal disease. Physiology, diagnosis, management. 5th ed. Philadelphia: WB Saunders, 1993:1393–1401.

39. Schottenfeld D, Winawer SJ. Large intestine. In: Schottenfeld D, Fraumeni JF, eds. Cancer epidemiology and prevention. Philadelphia: WB Saunders, 1982:703–727.

40. Correa P. Comments on the epidemiology of large bowel cancer. Cancer Res 1975;35:3395–3397.

41. Steele GD Jr, Jessup JM. Colorectal cancer. In: Steele GD Jr, Jessup JM, Winchester DP, Menck HR, Murphy GP, eds. National cancer data base. Annual review of patient care, 1995. Atlanta: American Cancer Society, 1996;66–83.

42. Demers RY, Severson RK, Shottenfeld D, Lazar L. Incidence of colorectal carcinoma by anatomic subsite: an epidemiologic study of time trends and racial differences in the Detroit, Michigan area. Cancer 1997;79:441–447.

43. Fleshner P, Slater G, Aufses AH Jr. Age and sex distribution of patients with colorectal cancer. Dis Colon Rectum 1989;32:107 111.

44. Pitluk H, Poticha SM. Carcinoma of the colon and rectum in patients less than 40 years of age. Surg Gynecol Obstet 1983;157: 335–337.

45. Adkins RB Jr, DeLozier JB, McKnight WG, Waterhouse B. Carcinoma of the colon in patients 35 years of age and younger. Am Surgeon 1987;53:141–145.

46. Heys SD, O'Hanrahan TJ, Brittenden J, Eremin O. Colorectal cancer in young patients: a review of the literature. Eur J Surg Oncol 1994;20:225–231.

47. Beckman EN, Gathright JB, Ray JE. A potentially brighter prognosis for colon carcinoma in the third and fourth decades. Cancer 1984; 54:1478–1481.

48. VanVoorhis B, Cruikshank DP. Colon carcinoma complicating pregnancy. A report of two cases. J Reproductive Med 1989;34: 923–927.

49. Heydenrych JJ, Warren B. An unusual presentation of carcinoma of the colon in a child. A case report. S Afr Med J 1984;65:617–618.

50. Yamamoto T, Matsumoto K, Iriyama K. Colorectal cancer in a patient younger than 20 years of age: report of a case and a review of the Japanese literature. Surg Today 1996;26:810–813.

51. Sarma DP. Colorectal carcinoma in young adults: an autopsy study. J Surg Oncol 1987;35:52–54.

52. Correa P, Haenszel W. The epidemiology of large bowel cancer. Adv Cancer Res 1978;26:1–141.

53. King H, Locke FB. Cancer mortality among Chinese in the United States. J Natl Cancer Inst 1980;65:1141–1148.

54. Locke FB, King H. Cancer mortality risk among Japanese in the United States. J Natl Cancer Inst 1980;65:1149–1156.

55. So BT, Magadia NE, Wynder EL. Induction of carcinomas of the colon and rectum in rats by intrarectal instillation of N-methyl-N'-nitro-N-nitrosoguanidine. J Natl Cancer Inst 1973;50:927–932.

56. LaMont JT, O'Gorman TA. Experimental colon cancer. Gastroenterology 1978;75:1157–1169.

57. Pozharisski KM, Likhachev AJ, Klimashevski VF, Shaposhinikov JD. Experimental intestinal cancer research with special reference to human pathology. Adv Cancer Res 1979;30:165–237.

58. Gorham ED, Garland CF, Garland FC. Acid haze air pollution and breast and colon cancer mortality in 20 Canadian cities. Canad J Public Health 1989;80:96–100.

59. Griffith J, Duncan RC, Riggan WB, et al. Cancer mortality in the U.S. counties with hazardous waste sites and ground water pollution. Arch Environ Health 1989;44:69–74.

60. Ippen M, Fehr R, Krasemann EO. Cancer in residents of heavy traffic areas. Versicherungsmedizin 1989;41:39–42.

61. Chen CJ, Chuang YC, Lin TM, et al. Malignant neoplasms among residents of a blackfoot disease-endemic area in Taiwan: High-arsenic artesian well water and cancers. Cancer Res 1985;45:5895–5899.

62. Frumkin H, Berlin J. Asbestos exposure and gastrointestinal malignancy review and meta-analysis. Am J Ind Med 1988;14:79–95.

63. Edelman DA. Exposure to asbestos and the risk of gastrointestinal cancer: a reassessment. Br J Ind Med 1988;45:75–82.

64. Brownson RC, Zahm SH, Chang JC, et al. Occupational risk of colon cancer. An analysis by anatomic subsite. Am J Epidemiol 1989;130:675–678.

65. Acquavella JF, Douglass TS, Phillips SC. Evaluation of excess colorectal cancer incidence among workers involved in the manufacture of polypropylene. J Occup Med 1988;30:438–442.

66. Nagao M, Sugimura T. Carcinogenic factors in food with relevance to colon cancer development. Mutat Res 1993;290:43–51.

67. Habs M, Schmahl D. Carcinogenic substances in food. Inn Med 1979;6:237–249.

68. Bruce WR, Varghese AJ, Wang S, et al. The endogenous production of nitroso compounds in the colon and cancer at that site. Int Symp Princess Takamatsu Cancer Res Fund 1979:221–228.

69. Talley NJ, Chute CG, Larson DE, et al. Risk for colorectal adenocarcinoma in pernicious anemia. A population-based cohort study. Ann Intern Med 1989;111:738–742.

70. Ehrich M, Aswell JE, Van Tassell RL, et al. Mutagens in the feces of three South African populations at different levels of risk for colon cancer. Mutat Res 1979;64:231–240.

71. Bruch WR. Recent hypotheses for the origin of colon cancer. Cancer Res 1987;47:4237–4242.

72. Correa P, Paschal J, Pizzolato P, et al. Fecal mutagens and colorectal polyps: preliminary report of an autopsy study. In: Bruce WR, Correa P, Lipkin M, et al. eds. Gastrointestinal cancer: endogenous factors. Cold Spring Harbor, New York: Cold Spring Laboratory, 1981:119–123.

73. Schiffman MH, Van Tassell RL, Robinson A, et al. Case-control study of colorectal cancer and fecapentaene excretion. Cancer Res 1989;49:1322–1326.

74. Hatch FT, Felton JS, Stuermer DH, et al. Identification of mutagens from the cooking of food. Chem Mutagens 1984;9:111–164.

75. Sugimura T. Carcinogenicity of mutagenic heterocyclic amines formed during the cooking process. Mutat Res 1985;150:33–42.

76. Ferguson LR, Alley PG, Gribben BM. DNA-damaging activity in ethanol-soluble fractions of feces from New Zealand groups at varying risks of colorectal cancer. Nutr Cancer 1985;7:93–103.

77. Jao SW, Beart RW Jr, Reiman HM, et al. Colon and anorectal cancer after pelvic irradiation. Dis Colon Rectum 1987;30:953–958.

78. Gajraj H, Davies DR, Jackson BT. Synchronous small and large bowel cancer developing after pelvic irradiation. Gut 1988;29:126–128.

79. Rotmensch S, Avigad I, Soffer EE, et al. Carcinoma of the large bowel after a single massive dose of radiation in healthy teenagers. Cancer 1986;57:728–731.

80. Kato H. Radiation-induced cancer and its modifying factor among A-bomb survivors. Int Symp Princess Takamatsu Cancer Res Fund 1987;18:117–124.

81. Kirev TT, Toshkov IA, Mladenov ZM. Virus-induced duodenal adenomas in guinea fowls. J Natl Cancer Inst 1987;79:1117–1121.

82. Boguszakova L, Hirsch I, Brichacek B, et al. Absence of cytomegalovirus, Epstein-Barr virus, and papillomavirus DNA from adenoma and adenocarcinoma of the colon. Acta Virol J (Praha) 1988;32:303–308.

83. Suzuki K, Bruce WR. Increase by deoxycholic acid of the colonic nuclear damage induced by known carcinogens in C57B1/6J mice. J Natl Cancer Inst 1986;76:1129–1132.

84. Smith LL. Carcinogenic cholesterol products. In: Smith LL, ed. Cholesterol autoxidation. New York: Plenum Press, 1981:432–446.

85. Greenwald P, Kelloff GJ, Boone CW, McDonald SS. Genetic and cellular changes in colorectal cancer: proposed targets of chemopreventive agents. Cancer Epidemiol Biomarkers Prev 1995;4:691–702.

86. Mckeown-Eyssen G, Holloway C, Jazmaji V, et al. A randomized trial of vitamins C and E in the prevention of recurrence of colorectal polyps. Cancer Res 1988;48:4701–4705.

87. Temple NJ, Basu TK. Selenium and cabbage and colon carcinogenesis in mice. J Natl Cancer Inst 1987;79:1131–1134.

88. Soullier BK, Wilson PS, Nigro ND. Effect of selenium on azoxymethane-induced intestinal cancer in rats fed high fat diet. Cancer Lett 1981;12:343–348.

89. Nelson RL. Is the changing pattern of colorectal cancer caused by selenium deficiency? Dis Colon Rectum 1984;27:459–461.

90. Clapp NK, Bowels ND, Satterfield LC, et al. Selective protective effect of butylated hydroxytoulene against 1,2-dimethylhydrazine carcinogenesis in balb/c mice. J Natl Cancer Inst 1979;63:1081–1087.

91. DuBois RN, Giardiello FM, Smalley WE. Non-steroidal anti-inflammatory drugs, eicosanoids, and colorectal cancer prevention. Gastroenterol Clin North Am 1996;25:773–791.

92. Greenberg ER, Baron JA. Prospects for preventing colorectal cancer death. J Natl Cancer Inst 1993;85:1182–1184.

93. Greenberg ER, Baron JA. Aspirin and other nonsteroid anti-inflammatory drugs as cancer-preventive agents. IARC Sci Publ 1996;139:91–98.

94. Rosenberg L, Palmer JR, Zaube AG, et al. A hypothesis: nonsteroidal anti-inflammatory drugs reduce the incidence of large bowel cancer. J Natl Cancer Inst 1991;83:355–358.

95. Hill MJ, Aries BC. Faecal steroid composition and its relationship to cancer of the large bowel. J Pathol 1971;104:129–139.

96. Logan RF, Little J, Hawtin PG, et al. Effect of aspirin and non-steroidal anti-inflammatory drugs on colorectal adenomas: case-control study of subjects participating in the Nottingham fecal occult blood screening programme. Brit Med J 1993;307:285–289.

97. Schreinemachers, DM, Everson RB. Aspirin use and lung, colon and breast cancer incidence in a prospective study. Epidemiology 1994;5:138–146.

98. Luk GD. Prevention of gastrointestinal cancer—the potential role of NSAIDs in colorectal cancer. Schweiz Med Wochenschr 1996;126:801–812.

99. Narisawa T, Takahashi M, Niwa M, et al. Involvement of prostaglandin E2 in bile acid-caused promotion of colon carcinogenesis and anti-promotion by the cyclooxygenase inhibitor indomethacin. Jap J Cancer Res 1987;78:791–798.

100. Kargman S, O'Neill G, Vickers P, et al. Expression of prostaglandin G/H synthase-1 and -2 protein in human colon cancer. Cancer Res 1995;55:2556–2559.

101. Boland CR. Malignant tumors of the colon. In: Yamada T. ed. Textbook of gastroenterology. Philadelphia: JB Lippincott, 1995:1967–2027.

102. Lynch HT, Lanspa J, Bowman BM, et al. Hereditary nonpolyposis colorectal cancer—Lynch Syndrome I and II. Gastroenterol Clin North Am 1988;17:679–712.

103. Burt RW, Samowitz WS. The adenomatous polyp and the hereditary polyposis syndromes. Gastroenterol Clin North Am 1988;17:657–678.

104. Perzin KH, Bridge MF. Adenomatous and carcinomatous changes in hamartomatous polyps of the small intestine (Peutz-Jeghers Syndrome). Cancer 1982;49:971–983.

105. Haggitt RC, Reid BJ. Hereditary gastrointestinal polyposis syndromes. Am J Surg Pathol 1986;10:871–877.

106. Burt RW. Familial risk and colorectal cancer. Gastroenterol Clin North Am 1996;25:793–803.

107. Toribara NW, Sleisenger MH. Screening for colorectal cancer. New Engl J Med 1995;332:861–867.

108. Lynch HT, Smyrk TC, Watson P, et al. Genetics, natural history, tumor spectrum, and pathology of hereditary nonpolyposis colorectal cancer: an updated review. Gastroenterology 1993;104:1535–1549.

109. Jass JR, Smyrk TC, Stewart SM, et al. Pathology of hereditary nonpolyposis colorectal cancer. Anticancer Res 1994;114:1631–1634.

110. Burt RW, Bishop OT, Cannon ML, et al. Dominant inheritance of adenomatous colonic polyps and colorectal cancer. N Engl J Med 1985;312:1540–1544.

111. Cannon-Albright LA, Skolnick MH, Bishop T, et al. Common inheritance of susceptibility to colonic adenomatous polyps and associated colorectal cancers. N Engl J Med 1988;319:533–537.

112. Church JM, McGannon E, Hull-Boiner S, et al. Gastroduodenal polyps in patients with familial adenomatous polyposis. Dis Colon Rectum 192;35:1170–1173.

113. Spiro L, Olschwang S, Groden J, et al. Alleles of the APC gene: an attenuated form of familial polyposis. Cell 1993;75:951–957.

114. Hizawa K, Iida M, Matsumoto T, et al. Neoplastic transformation arising in Peutz-Jeghers polyposis. Dis Colon Rectum 1993;36: 953–957.

115. Desai DC, Neale KF, Talbot IC, et al. Juvenile polyposis. Br J Surg 1995;82:14–17.

116. Whitelaw SC, Murday VA, Tomlinson IPM, et al. Clinical and molecular features of the hereditary mixed polyposis syndrome. Gastroenterology 1997;112:327–334.

117. Lynch HT, Watson P, Lanspa SJ, et al. Natural history of colorectal cancer in hereditary nonpolyposis colorectal cancer (Lynch Syndromes I and II). Dis Colon Rectum 1988;31:439–444.

118. Mecklin JP. Frequency of hereditary colorectal carcinoma. Gastroenterology 1987;93:1021–1025.

119. Mecklin JP, Sipponen P, Jarvinen HJ. Histopathology of colorectal carcinoma in cancer family syndrome kindreds. Scand J Gastroenterol 1987;22:449.

120. Vasen HFA, Wijnen JT, Menko FH, et al. Cancer risk in families with hereditary nonpolyposis colorectal cancer diagnosed by mutation analysis. Gastroenterology 1996;110:1020–1027.

121. Lynch HT, Smyrk T, Landspa SJ. Natural history of colorectal cancer in hereditary nonpolyposis colorectal cancer (Lynch syndrome I and II). Dis Colon Rectum 1988;31:439–444.

122. Muto T, Kamiya J, Sawada T, et al. Small "flat adenomas" of the large bowel with special reference to its clinicopathologic features. Dis Colon Rectum 1985;28:847–851.

123. Faron ER, Vogelstein B. A genetic model for colorectal tumorigenesis. Cell 1990;61:759–767.

124. Hamilton SR. The molecular genetics of colorectal neoplasia. Gastroenterology 1993;105:3–7.

125. Fearon ER. Molecular genetic studies of the adenoma carcinoma sequence. Adv Intern Med 1994;39:123–147.

126. Wynder EL. The epidemiology of large bowel cancer. Cancer Res 1975;35:3388–3394.

127. Sandler RS. Epidemiology and risk factors for colorectal cancer. Gastroenterol Clin North Am 1996;25:717–735.

128. Hill MJ. Environmental and genetic factors in gastrointestinal cancer. In: Sherlock P, Morson BC, Barbara L, Veronesi U, eds. Precancerous lesions of the gastrointestinal tract. New York: Raven Press, 1983:1–22.

129. Phillips RL, Garfinkel L, Kuzma JW, et al. Mortality among California Seventh-Day Adventist for selected cancer sites. J Natl Cancer Inst 1980;65:1097–1107.

130. Reddy BS. Dietary fat and colon cancer: animal models. Prev Med 1987;16:460–467.

131. Giovannucci E, Rimm EB, Stampfer MJ, et al. Intake of fat, meat and fiber in relation to risk of colon cancer in men. Cancer Res 1994;54: 2390–2397.

132. Willett WC, Stampfer MJ, Colditz GA, et al. Relation of meat, fat and fiber intake to the risk of colon cancer in a prospective study among women. N Engl J Med 1990;323:1664–1672.

133. Nagengast FM. Grubben MJ. van Munster IP. Role of bile acids in colorectal carcinogenesis. Eur J Cancer 1995;31A:1067–1070.

134. Burnstein MJ. Dietary factors related to colorectal neoplasms. Surg Clin N Am 1993;73:13–29.

135. Sakaguchi M, Minoura T, Hiramatsu Y, et al. Effects of dietary saturated and unsaturated fatty acids on fecal bile acids and colon carcinogenesis induced by azoxymethane in rats. Cancer Res 1986; 46:61–65.

136. Minoura T, Takata T, Sakaguchi M, et al. Effect of dietary eicosapentaenoic acid on azoxymethane-induced colon carcinogenesis in rats. Cancer Res 1988;48:4790–4794.

137. Galloway DJ, Jarrett F, Boyle P, et al. Morphological and cell kinetic effects of dietary manipulation during colorectal carcinogenesis. Gut 1987;28:754–763.

138. Cummings JH, Hill MJ, Bone ES, et al. The effect of meat protein and dietary fiber on colonic function and metabolism II. Bacterial metabolites in feces and urine. Am J Clin Nutr 1979;32: 2094–2101.

139. Reddy BS, Wang CX, Maruyama H. Effect of restricted caloric intake on azoxymethane-induced colon tumor incidence in male f344 rats. Cancer Res 1987;46:1226–1228.

140. Tornberg SA, Holm LE, Carstensen JM, et al. Risks of cancer of the colon and rectum in relation to serum cholesterol and beta-lipoprotein. N Engl J Med 1986;315:1629–1633.

141. Hiramatsu Y, Takada H, Yamamura M, et al. Effect of dietary cholesterol on azoxymethane-induced colon carcinogenesis in rats. Carcinogenesis 1983;4:553–558.

142. Reddy BS, Cohen LA, McCoy GO, et al. Nutrition and its relationship to cancer. Adv Cancer Res 1980;32:237–245.

143. Wargovich MJ. New dietary anticarcinogens and prevention of gastrointestinal cancer. Dis Colon Rectum 1988;31:72–75.

144. Howe GR, Benito E, Castelleto R, et al. Dietary intake of fiber and decreased risk of cancers of the colon and rectum: evidence from the combined analysis of 13 case-control studies. J Natl Cancer Inst 1992;84:1887–1896.

145. Jacobs LR. Fiber and colon cancer. Gastroenterol Clin North Am 1988;17:747–760.

146. Jacobs JR. Modification of experimental colon carcinogenesis by dietary fibers. Adv Exp Med Biol 1986;266:105–118.

147. Smith-Barbaro P, Hanson D, Reddy BS. Carcinogen binding to various types of dietary fiber. J Natl Cancer Inst 1981;67: 495–497.

148. Thornton JR. High colonic pH promotes colorectal cancer. Lancet 1981;1:1081–1083.

149. Potter JD, Slattery ML, Bostick RM, et al. Colon cancer: a review of the epidemiology. Epidemiol Rev 1995;15:499–545.

150. Chen LH, Boissonneault GA, Glauert HP. Vitamin C, vitamin E and cancer. Anticancer Res 1988;8:739–748.

151. Willett WC: Selenium, vitamin E, fiber, and the incidence of human cancer: An epidemiologic perspective. Adv Exp Med Biol 1986;206: 27–34.

152. Vogel VG, McPherson RS. Dietary epidemiology of colon cancer. Hematol Oncol Clin North Am 1989;3:35–63.

153. Garland C, Skekelle RB, Barrett-Connor E, et al. Dietary vitamin D and calcium and risk of colorectal cancer: a 19-year prospective study in men. Lancet 1985;1:307–309.

154. Wargovich MJ, Baer AR, Hu PJ, et al. Dietary factors and colorectal cancer. Gastroenterol Clin North Am 1988;17:727–745.

155. Lipkin M, Friedman E, Winawer SJ, et al. Colonic epithelial cell proliferation in responders and nonresponders to supplemental dietary calcium. Cancer Res 1989;49:248–254.

156. Rozen P, Fireman Z, Fine N, et al. Oral calcium suppresses increased rectal epithelial proliferation of persons at risk of colorectal cancer. Gut 1989;30:650–655.

157. Carethers JM. The cellular and molecular pathogenesis of colorectal cancer. Gastroenterol Clin North Am 1996;25:737–754.

158. Giovannucci E, Stampfer MJ, Colditz GA, et al. Folate, methionine, and alcohol intake and risk of colorectal adenoma. J Natl Cancer Inst 1993;85:875–884.

159. Klatsky AL, Armstrong MA, Friedman GD, et al. The relationship of alcoholic beverage use to colon and rectal cancer. Am J Epidemiol 1988;128:1007–1015.

160. Giovannucci E, Rimm EB, Stampfer MJ, et al. A prospective study of cigarette smoking and risk of colorectal adenoma and colorectal cancer in U.S. men. J Natl Cancer Inst 1994;86:183–191.

161. Giovannucci E, Colditz GA, Stampfer MJ, et al. A prospective study of cigarette smoking and risk of colorectal adenoma and colorectal cancer in U.S. women. J Natl Cancer Inst 1994;86:192–199.

162. Kune S, Kune GG, Watson LF. Case-control study of alcoholic beverages as etiological factors: the Melbourne colorectal cancer study. Nutr Cancer 1987;9:43–56.

163. Karlin DA, McBath M, Jones RD, et al. Hypergastrinemia and colorectal carcinogenesis in the rat. Cancer Lett 1985;29:73–80.

164. Seitz J-F, Giovannini M, Gouvernet J, et al. Elevated serum gastrin levels in patients with colorectal neoplasia. J Clin Gastroenterol 1991;13:541–545.

165. Iishi H, Tatsuta M, Baba M, et al. Enhancement by vasoactive intestinal peptide of experimental carcinogenesis induced by azoxymethane in rat colon. Cancer Res 1987;46:4890–4893.

166. Hahn DL. Sex and race are risk factors for colorectal cancer within reach of the sigmoidoscope. J Fam Pract 1990;30:409–416.

167. Davis FG, Furner SE, Persky V, Koch M. The influence of parity and exogenous female hormones on the risk of colorectal cancer. Int J Cancer 1989;43:587–590.

168. Weiss NS, Darling JR, Chow WH. Incidence of cancer of the large bowel in women in relation to reproductive and hormonal factors. J Natl Cancer Inst 1981;57:57–60.

169. Kune GA, Kune S, Watson LF. Oral contraceptive use does not protect against large bowel cancer. Contraception 1990;41:19–25.

170. Francavilla A, DiLeo A, Polimeno L, et al. Nuclear and cytosolic estrogen receptors in human colon carcinoma and in surrounding noncancerous colonic tissue. Gastroenterology 1987;93:1301–1306.

171. Smironova IO, Turusov VS. 1,2-Dimethylhydrazine carcinogenesis in neonatally androgenized CBA mice. Carcinogenesis 1988;9:1927–1929.

172. Izbicki JR, Wambach G, Hamilton SR, et al. Androgen receptors in experimentally induced colon carcinogenesis. J Cancer Res Clin Oncol 1986;112:39–46.

173. Tutton PJ, Barkla DH. The influence of androgens, antiandrogens, and castration on cell proliferation in the jejunal and colonic crypt epithelia and in dimethylhydrazine- induced adenocarcinoma of rat colon. Virchows Arch (B) 1982;38:351–355.

174. Ituarte EM, Petrini J, Hershman JM, et al. Acromegaly and colon cancer. Ann Intern Med 1984;5:627–628.

175. Ron E, Gridley G, Hrusbec Z, et al. Acromegaly and gastrointestinal cancer. Cancer 1991;68:1673–1677.

176. Conteas CN, Desai TK, Arlow FA. Relationship of hormones and growth factors to colon cancer. Gastroenterol Clin North Am 1988;17:761–772.

177. Feig DS, Gottesman IS. Familial hyperparathyroidism in association with colonic carcinoma. Cancer 1987;60:429–432.

178. Bishop DT, Thomas HJW. The genetics of colorectal cancer. Cancer Survey 1990;9:585–604.

179. Stephenson BM, Finan PJ, Gascoyne J, et al. Frequency of familial colorectal cancer. Br J Surg 1991;78:1162–1166.

180. Winawer SJ, Schottenfeld D, Flehinger BJ. Colorectal cancer screening. J Natl Cancer Inst 1991;83:243–253.

181. Fuchs CS, Giovannucci EL, Colditz GA, et al. A prospective study of family history and the risk of colorectal cancer. N Engl J Med 1994;331:1669–1674.

182. St. John JB, McDermott FT, Hopper JL, et al. Cancer risk in relatives of patients with common colorectal cancer. Ann Intern Med 1993;118:785–790.

183. Slattery ML, Kerber RA. Family history of cancer and colon cancer risk: the Utah population database. J Natl Cancer Inst 1994;86:1618–1626.

184. Winawer SJ, Zauber AG, Gerdes H, et al. Risk of colorectal cancer in the families of patients with adenomatous polyps. N Engl J Med 1996;334:82–87.

185. Enblad P, Adami HO, Glimelius B, et al. The risk of subsequent primary malignant diseases after cancers of the colon and rectum. A nationwide cohort study. Cancer 1990;65:2091–2100.

186. Phipps RF, Perry PM. Familial breast cancer and the association with colonic carcinoma. Eur J Surg Oncol 1989;15:109–111.

187. Lyon JL, Gardner JW, West DW. Cancer risk and life-style cancer among Mormons from 1967-1975. Banbury Rep Ser 1980;4:3–30.

188. Garfinkel L, Stellman SD. Mortality by relative weight and exercise. Cancer 1988;62:1844–1850.

189. Sandler RS. Epidemiology and risk factors for colorectal cancer. Gastroenterol Clin North Am 1997;26:717–735.

190. Andrianopoulos G, Nelson RL, Bombeck CT, et al. The influence of physical activity in 1,2-dimethylhydrazine induced colon carcinogenesis in the rat. Anticancer Res 1987;7:849–852.

191. Giovannucci E, Ascherio A, Rimm EB, et al. Physical activity, obesity and risk for colon cancer and adenoma in men. Ann Intern Med 1995;122:327–334.

192. Vernick LJ, Kuller LH. A case-control study of cholecystectomy and right-side colon cancer: the influence of alternative data sources and differential interview participation proportions on odds ratio estimates. Am J Epidemiol 1982;116:86–101.

193. Mamianetti A, Cinto RO, Altolaguirre D, et al. Relative risk of colorectal cancer after cholecystectomy. A multicentre case-control study. Internat J Colorect Dis 1988;3:215–218.

194. Alley PG, Lee SP. The increased risk of proximal colonic cancer after cholecystectomy. Dis Colon Rectum 1983;26:522–524.

195. Giovannucci E, Colditz GA, Stampfer MJ. A meta-analysis of cholecystectomy and risk of colorectal cancer. Gastroenterology 1993;105:130–141.

196. Moorehead RJ, Mills JO, Wilson HK, et al. Cholecystectomy and the development of colorectal neoplasia: a prospective study. Ann R Coll Surg Engl 1989;71:37–39.

197. Sandler RS, Martin ZZ, Carlton NM, et al. Adenomas of the large bowel after cholecystectomy. A case-control study. Dig Dis Sci 1988;33:1178–1184.

198. Adami HO, Krusemo UB, Meirik O. Unaltered risk of colorectal cancer within 14–17 years of cholecystectomy: updating of a population-based cohort study. Br J Surg 1987;74:675–678.

199. Kune GA, Kune S, Watson LF. Large bowel cancer after cholecystectomy. Am J Surg 1988;156:359–362.

200. Rahman MI, Gibson-Shreve LD, Yuan Z, Morris HA. Selections from current literature: cholelithiasis, cholecystectomy and the risk of colorectal cancer. Fam Pract 1996;3:483–487.

201. Howden CE, Hornung CA. A systemic review of the association between Barrett's esophagus and colon neoplasms. Am J Gastroenterol 1995;90:1814–1819.

202. Post AB, Achkar E, Carey WD. Prevalence of colonic neoplasia in patients with Barrett's esophagus. Am J Gastroenterol 1993;88:877–880.

203. Tripp MR, Sampliner RE, Kogan FJ, Morgan TR. Colorectal neoplasms and Barrett's esophagus. Am J Gastroenterol 1996;81:1063–1064.

204. Mizusawa K, Kaibara N, Yonekawa M, et al. A prospective cohort study on the development of colorectal cancer after gastrectomy. Dis Colon Rectum 1990;33:298–301.

205. Offerhaus GJ, Tersmette AC, Tersmette KW, et al. Gastric, pancreatic, and colorectal carcinogenesis following remote peptic ulcer surgery. Review of the literature with the emphasis on risk assessment and underlying mechanism. Mod Pathol 1988;1:352–356.

206. Owen RW. Biotransformation of bile acids by clostridia. J Med Microbiol 1985;20;233–238.

207. Wargovich MJ, Eng VW, Newmark HL, et al. Calcium ameliorates the toxic effect of deoxycholic acid on colonic epithelium. Carcinogenesis 1983;4:1205–1207.

208. Ferguson LR, Parry JM. Mitotic aneuploidy as a possible mechanism for tumour promoting activity in bile acids. Carcinogenesis 1984;5:447–451.

209. Hill MJ. Bacterial metabolism and human carcinogenesis. Br Med Bull 1980;37:89–94.

210. Rogers AE, Nauss KM. Rodent models for carcinoma of the colon. Dig Dis Sci 1985;12:87S–102S.

211. Reddy BS, Narisawa T, Wright P, et al. Colon carcinogenesis with azoxymethane and dimethylhydrazine in germ-free rats. Cancer Res 1975;35:287–290.

212. Goldin BR, Gorbach SL. Effect of antibiotics on incidence of rat intestinal tumors induced by 1,2-dimethylhydrazine dihydrochloride. NJCI 1981;4:877–880.

213. Filipe MI, Scurr JH, Ellis H. Effects of fecal stream on experimental colorectal carcinogenesis morphologic and histochemical changes. Cancer 1982;50:2859–2865.

214. Oravec CT, Jones CA, Huberman E. Activation of the colon carcinogen 1,2-dimethylhydrazine in a rat colon cell-mediated mutagenesis assay. Cancer Res 1986;46:5068–5071.

215. Celik C, Mittleman A, Paolini NS, et al. Effects of 1,2-symmetrical dimethylhydrazine of jejunocolic transposition in Sprague-Dawley rats. Cancer Res 1981;41:2908–2911.

216. Rainey JB, Maeda M, Williamson RC. Distal transposition of rat caecum does not render it susceptible to carcinogenesis. Gut 1985;26:718–823.

217. Morson BC. Markers for increased risk of colorectal cancer. In: Sherlock P, Morson BC, Barbara L, Veronesi U, eds. Precancerous lesions of the gastrointestinal tract. New York: Raven Press, 1983:253–259.

218. Adachi M, Muto T, Moioka Y, et al. Flat adenoma and flat mucosal carcinoma (IIb type)—a new precursor of colorectal carcinoma? Report of two cases. Dis Colon Rectum 1988;31:236–243.

219. Ninto T, Bussey HJR, Morson BC. The evolution of cancer of the colon and rectum. Cancer. 1975;36:2251–2270.

220. O'Brien MJ, Winawer SJ, Zauber AG, et al. The National Polyp Study: patient and polyp characteristics associated with high-grade dysplasia in colorectal adenomas. Gastroenterology 1990;98:371–379.

221. Perzin KH, Bridge MF. Adenomas of the small intestine: a clinico-pathologic review of 51 cases and a study of their relationship to carcinoma. Cancer 1981;48:799–819.

222. Day DW. The adenoma-carcinoma sequence. Scand J Gastroenterol Suppl 1985;104:99–107.

223. Fenoglio CM, Pascal RR. Colorectal adenomas and cancer. Pathologic relationships. Cancer 1982;50:2601–2608.

224. Eide TJ. Remnants of adenomas in colorectal carcinomas. Cancer 1983;51:1866–1872.

225. Stryker SJ, Wolff BG, Culp CE, et al. Natural history of untreated colonic polyps. Gastroenterology 1987;93:1009–1013.

226. Willet W, MacMahon B. Diet and cancer: an overview. N Engl J Med 1984;310:633–638.

227. Winawer SJ, Zauber A, Ho MN, et al. Prevention of colorectal cancer by colonoscopic polypectomy. N Engl J Med 1993;329:1977–1981.

228. Enblad P, Busch C, Carlsson U, et al. The adenoma-carcinoma sequence in rectal adenomas. Support by the expression of blood group substances and carcinoma antigens. Am J Clin Pathol 1988;90:121–130.

229. Boland CR. Lectin histochemistry in colorectal polyps. Prog Clin Biol Res 1988;279:277–287.

230. Suzuki S, Mizuno M, Tomoda J, et al. Flow cytometric analysis of the DNA content in colorectal adenomas with focal cancers. Gastroenterology 1995;109:1098–1104.

231. Vogelstein B, Fearon ER, Hamilton SR, et al. Genetic alterations during colorectal-tumor development. N Engl J Med 1988;319:525–532.

232. Fearon ER. Molecular abnormalities in colon and rectal cancer. In: Mendelsohn J, Israel MA, Liotta LA. eds. The molecular basis of cancer. Philadelphia: WB Saunders, 1995:340–357.

233. Crawford BE, Stromeyer FW. Small nonpolypoid carcinomas of the large intestine. Cancer 1983;51:1760–1763.

234. Shimoda T, Ikegami M, Fujisaki J, et al. Early colorectal carcinoma with special reference to its development de novo. Cancer 1989;64:1138–1146.

235. Maskens AP, Dujardin-Loits RM. Experimental adenomas and carcinomas of the large intestine behave as distinct entities. Cancer 1981;47:81–89.

236. Ming SC, Yu PL. Histogenesis of experimental colonic carcinoma. Front Gastrointest Res 1991;18:200–224.

237. Goldman H, Ming SC, Hickok DF. Nature and significance of hyperplastic polyps of the human colon. Arch Pathol 1970;89:349–354.

238. Teoh HH, Delahunt B, Isbister WH. Dysplastic and malignant areas in hyperplastic polyps of the large intestine. Pathology 1989;21:138–142.

239. Jass JR, Filipe MI, Abbas S, et al. A morphologic and histochemical study of metaplastic polyps of the colorectum. Cancer 1984;53:510–515.

240. Longacre TA, Fenoglio-Preiser CM. Mixed hyperplastic adenomatous polyps/serrated adenomas. A distinct form of colorectal neoplasia. Am J Surg Pathol 1990;14:524–537.

241. Bentley E, Chandrasoma P, Radin R, Cohen H. Generalized juvenile polyposis with carcinoma. Am J Gastroenterol 1989;84:1456–1459.

242. Desaint B, Legender CI, Florent CH. Dysplasia and cancer in ulcerative colitis. Hepatogastroenterology 1989;36:219–226.

243. Broome U, Lindberg B, Lofberg R. Primary sclerosing cholangitis in ulcerative colitis—a risk factor for the development of dysplasia and DNA ploidy? Gastroenterology 1992;102:1877–1880.

244. MacDermott RP. Review of clinical aspects of cancer of the colon in patients with ulcerative colitis. Dig Dis Sci 1985;30:1145–1185.

245. Gilat T, Rozen P. Risk of colon cancer in ulcerative colitis in low incidence areas—a review. In: Winawer SJ, Schottenfeld D, Sherlock P, eds. Colorectal cancer: prevention, epidemiology and screening. New York: Raven Press, 1980:335–339.

246. Pascal RR. Dysplasia and early carcinoma in inflammatory bowel disease and colorectal adenomas. Hum Pathol 1994;25:1160–1171.

247. Bernstein C, Shanahan F, Weinstein WM. Are we telling the truth about surveillance colonoscopy in ulcerative colitis? Lancet 1994;343:71–74.

248. Riddell RH, Goldman H, Ransohoff DF, et al. Dysplasia in inflammatory bowel disease: standardized classification with provisional clinical applications. Hum Pathol 1983;14:931–968.

249. Korelitz BI. Carcinoma of the intestinal tract in Crohn's disease: results of a survey conducted by the National Foundation of Ileitis and Colitis. Am J Gastroenterol 1983;78:44–46.

250. Bernstein D. Rogers A. Malignancy in Crohn's disease. Am J Gastroenterol 1996;91:434–440.

251. Kvist N, Jacobsen O, Norgaard P, et al. Malignancy in Crohn's disease. Scand J Gastroenterol 1986;21:82–86.

252. Yardley JH. Comments on comparative pathology of colonic neoplasia in cotton-top marmoset (saguinus oedipus oedipus). Dig Dis Sci 1985;30:126S–133S.

253. Lushbaugh C, Humason G, Clapp N. Histology of colon cancer in saguinus oedipus oedipus. Dig Dis Sci 1985;30:119S–125S.

254. Xu Z, Su DL. Schistosoma japonicum and colorectal cancer: an epidemiological study in the People's Republic of China. Int J Cancer 1984;34:315–318.

255. Chen MC, Chuang CY, Chang PY, et al. Evolution of colorectal cancer in schistosomiasis. Transitional mucosal changes adjacent to large intestinal carcinoma in colectomy specimens. Cancer 1980;46:1661–1675.

256. Dimmette RM, Elwi AM, Sproat HF. Relationship of schistosomiasis to polyposis and adenocarcinoma of large intestine. Am J Clin Path 1956;26:266–276.

257. Williamson RCN, Rainey JB. The relationship between intestinal hyperplasia and carcinogenesis. Scand J Gastroenterol (Suppl) 1985;104:57–76.

258. Barthold SW, Beck D. Modification or early dimethylhydrazine carcinogenesis by colonic mucosal hyperplasia. Cancer Res 1980;40:4451–4455.

259. Jacobs R. Role of dietary factors in cell replication and colon cancer. Am J Clin Nutr 1988;48:775–779.

260. Spratt JS, Ackerman LV. Small primary adenocarcinomas of the colon and rectum. JAMA 1962;179:337–346.

261. Kjeldsberg CR, Altshuler JH. Carcinoma in situ of the colon. Dis Colon Rectum 1970;13:376–381.

262. Shimoda T, Ikegami M, Fujisaki J, et al. Early colorectal carcinoma with special reference to its development de novo. Cancer 1989;64:1138–1146.

263. Kudo S, Tamura S, Hirota S, et al. The problem of de novo colorectal carcinoma. Eur J Cancer 1995;31A:1118–1120.

264. Dawson PM, Habib NA, Rees HC, Wood CB. Mucosal field change in colorectal cancer. Am J Surg 1987;153:281–284.

265. Roby-Cafferty SS, Ro JY, Ordonez NG, Cleary KR. Transitional mucosa of colon. A morphological histochemical, and immunohistochemical study. Archives Pathol Lab Med 1990;114:72–75.

266. Schmidbauer G, Heilmann KL. Morphology and histochemistry of the mucosa surrounding small oligotubular adenomas of the large bowel. Pathol Res Pract 1985;180:45–48.

267. Dawson PA, Filipe MI. An ultrastructural and histochemical study of the mucous membrane adjacent to and remote from carcinoma of the colon. Cancer. 1976;37:2388–2398.

268. Mori M, Shimono R, Adachi Y, et al. Transitional mucosa in human colorectal lesions. Dis Colon Rectum 1990;33:498–501.

269. Caccamo D, Telenta M, Celener D. Concanavalin A binding sites in fetal, adult, transitional, and malignant rectosigmoid mucosa. Human Pathol 1989;20:1186–1192.

270. Ming S-C, Yu P-L. Histogenesis of experimental colonic carcinomas. In: Large bowel cancer: policy, prevention, research and treatment. Rozen P, Reich CB, Winawer SJ, eds. Front Gastrointest Res Basel: Karger, 1991;18:200–224.

271. Roncucci L, Medline A, Bruce WR. Classification of aberrant crypt foci and microadenomas in human colon. Cancer Epidemiol Biomarkers Prev 1991;1:57–60.

272. Pretlow TP, Barrow BJ, Ashton WS, et al. Aberrant crypts: putative preneoplastic foci in human colonic mucosa. Cancer Res 1991;51:1564–1567.

273. Otori K, Sugiyama K, Hasebe T, et al. Emergence of adenomatous

aberrant crypt foci (ACF) with concomitant increase in cell proliferation. Cancer Res 1995;55:4743–4746.

274. Roncucci L, Stamp D, Medline A, et al. Identification and quantification of aberrant crypt foci and microadenomas in the human colon. Hum Pathol 1991;22:287–294.

275. Yamashita N, Minamoto T, Ochiai A, et al. Frequent and characteristic K-ras activation in aberrant crypt foci of colon. Is there preference among K-ras mutants for malignant progression? Cancer 1995; 75(Suppl):1527–1533.

276. Yamashita N, Minamoto T, Ochiai A, et al. Frequent and characteristic K-ras activation and absence of $p53$ protein accumulation in aberrant crypt foci of the colon. Gastroenterology 1995;108: 434–440.

277. Pretlow TP, Roukhadze EV, O'Riordan MA, et al. Carcinoembryonic antigen in human colonic aberrant crypt foci. Gastroenterology 1994;107:1719–1725.

278. Smith AJ, Stern HS, Penner M, et al. Somatic APC and K-ras codon 12 mutations in aberrant crypt foci from human colons. Cancer Res 1994;54:5527–5530.

279. Bresalier RS, Kim YS. Malignant neoplasms of the large intestines. In: Sleisenger MH, Fordtran JS, eds. Gastrointestinal disease. Physiology, diagnosis, management. 5th ed. Philadelphia: WB Saunders, 1993:1449–1493.

280. Welin S, Youkers J, Spratt JS Jr. The rates and patterns of growth of 375 tumors of the large intestine and rectum observed serially by double contrast enema. (Malmo technique). Am J Roentgenol 1965;90:673–687.

281. Bolin S, Nilsson E, Sjodahl R. Carcinoma of the colon and rectum-growth rate. Ann Surg 1983;198:151–158.

282. Spratt JS Jr. Rates of growth of pulmonary metastases and host survival. Ann Surg 1964;159:161–171.

283. Havelaar I, Sugarbaker PH. Rate of growth of intraabdominal metastases from colon and rectal cancer followed by serial EOE CT. Cancer 1984;54:163–171.

284. Finlay IG, Brunton GF, Meed K, et al. Rate of growth of hepatic metastasis in colorectal carcinoma. Br J Surg 1982;69:689.

285. Peltomaki P, Aaltonen LA, Sistonen P, et al. Genetic mapping of a locus predisposing to human colorectal cancer. Science 1993;260: 810–819.

286. Marra G, Boland CR. DNA repair and colorectal cancer. Gastroenterol Clin N Am 1996;25:755–772.

287. Marra G, Boland CR. Hereditary nonpolyposis colorectal cancer: the syndrome, the genes and historical perspectives. J Natl Cancer Inst 1995;87:1114–1125.

288. Tanaka S, Imanishi K-I, Yoshihara M, et al. Immunoreactive transforming growth factor alpha is commonly present in colorectal neoplasia. Am J Pathol 1991;139:123–129.

289. Ohtani H, Nakamura S, Watanabe Y, et al. Immunocytochemical localization of basic fibroblast growth factor in carcinomas and inflammatory lesions of the human digestive tract. Lab Investigation 1993;68:520–527.

290. Van Laethem JL, Robberecht P. Growth factors in colorectal tumorigenesis. Acta Gastroenterol Belg 1995;58:274–279.

291. Hague A, Manning AM, van der Stappen JW, Paraskeva C. Escape from negative regulation of growth by transforming growth factor beta and from the induction of apoptosis by the dietary agent sodium butyrate may be important in colorectal carcinogenesis. Cancer Metastasis Rev 1993;12:227–237.

292. Cordon-Cardo C. Mutation of cell cycle regulators. Biological and clinical implications for human neoplasia. Am J Pathol 1995;147: 545–560.

293. Wang A, Yoshimi N, Ino N, et al. Overexpression of cyclin B1 in human colorectal cancers. J Cancer Res Clin Oncol 1997;123: 124–127.

294. Bresalier RS. The biology of colorectal cancer metastasis. Gastroenterol Clin North Am 1996;25:805–820.

295. Tsujitani S, Shirai H, Tatebe S, et al. Apoptotic cell death and its relationship to carcinogenesis in colorectal carcinoma. Cancer 1996; 77/78:1711–1716.

296. Wang L, Patel U, Ghosh L, et al. Mutation in the nm23 gene is associated with metastasis in colorectal cancer. J Cancer Res 1993; 53:717–720.

297. Campo E, Munoz J, Miquel R, et al. Cathepsin B expression in colorectal carcinomas correlates with tumor progression and shortened patient survival. Am J Pathol 1994;145:301–309.

298. Sinicrope FA, Ruan SB, Cleary KR, et al. Bcl-2 and $p53$ oncoprotein expression during colorectal tumorigenesis. Cancer Res 1995;55: 237–241.

299. Pedersen G, Brynskov J, Nielsen OH, Bendtzen K. Adhesion molecules in inflammatory and neoplastic intestinal diseases. Dig Dis 1995;13:322–336.

300. Arai T, Kino I. Role of apoptosis in modulation of the growth of human colorectal tubular and villous adenomas. J Pathol 1995;176: 37–44.

301. Agrez MV, Bates RC. Colorectal cancer and the integrin family of cell adhesion receptors: current status and future directions. Eur J Cancer 1994;30A:2166–2170.

302. Hamilton SR, Liu B, Parsons RE, et al. The molecular basis of Turcot's syndrome. N Engl J Med 1995;332:839–847.

303. Asltonen LA, Peltomaki P, Mecklin J-P, et al. Replication errors in benign and malignant tumors from hereditary nonpolyposis colorectal cancer. Cancer Res 1994;54:1645–1648.

304. Nicolaides NC, Papadopoulos N, Liu B, et al. Mutations of two PMS homologues in hereditary nonpolyposis colon cancer. Nature 1994; 371:75–80.

305. Bronner CE, Baker SM, Morrison PT, et al. Mutation in the DNA mismatch repair gene homologue hMLH1 is associated with hereditary non-polyposis colon cancer. Nature 1994;368:258–261.

306. Otori K, Sugiyama K, Hasebe T, et al. Emergence of adenomatous aberrant crypt foci (ACF) from hyperplastic ACF with concomitant increase in cell proliferation. Cancer Res 1995;55:4743–4746.

307. Heinen CD, Shivapurkar N, Tang Z, et al. Microsatellite instability in aberrant crypt foci from human colons. Cancer Res 1996;56:5339–5341.

308. Kern SE, Redston M, Seymour AB, et al. Molecular genetic profiles of colitis-associated neoplasms. Gastroenterology 1994;107: 420–428.

309. Benhattar J, Saraga E. Molecular genetics of dysplasia in ulcerative colitis. Eur J Cancer 1995;31A:1171–1173.

310. Greenwald BD, Harpaz N, Yin J, et al. Loss of heterozygosity affecting the $p53$, Rb, and mcc/apc tumor suppressor gene loci in dysplastic and cancerous ulcerative colitis. Cancer Res 1992;52; 741–745.

311. Cawkwell L, Lewis FA, Quirke P. Frequency of allele loss of DCC, $p53$, Rb1, WT1, NF1, NM23 and APC/MCC in colorectal cancer assayed by fluorescent multiplex polymerase chain reaction. Br J Cancer 1994;70:813–818.

312. Brentnall TA, Rubin CE, Crispin DA, et al. A germline substitution in the human MSH2 gene is associated with high-grade dysplasia and cancer in ulcerative colitis. Gastroenterology 1995;109: 151–155.

313. Suzuki H, Harpaz N, Tarmin L, et al. Microsatellite instability in ulcerative colitis-associated colorectal dysplasias and cancers. Cancer Res 1994;54:4841–4844.

314. Duckrey H. Production of colonic carcinomas by 1,2-dialkylhydrazines and azoxyalkanes. In: Burdette WJ, ed. Carcinoma of colon and antecedent epithelium. Springfield, Illinois: Charles C Thomas, 1970:267–279.

315. Fiala ES, Kulakis C, Bobotas G, Weisburger JH. Brief communication: detection and estimation of azomethane in expired air of 1,2-Dimethylhydrazine-treated rats. J Natl Cancer Inst 1976;56: 1271–1273.

316. Sumi Y, Miyakawa M. Gastrointestinal carcinogenesis in germ-free rats given N-methyl-N'-nitro-N-nitrosoguanidine in drinking water. Cancer Res 1979;39:2733–2736.

317. Sunter JP. Cell proliferation in gastrointestinal carcinogenesis. Scand J Gastroenterol 1985;104:45–55.

318. Rubio CA, Nylander G, Wahlin B, et al. Monitoring the histogenesis of colonic tumors in the Sprague-Dawley rat. J Surg Oncol 1986;31: 225–228.

319. Madara JL, Harte P, Deasy J, et al. Evidence for an adenoma-carcinoma sequence in dimethylhydrazine-induced neoplasms of rat intestinal epithelium. Am J Pathol 1983;110:230–235.

320. Inamori Y, Misumi A, Murakami A, Akagi M. The histogenesis of DMH-induced colonic carcinoma in rats. Gastroenterol Jap 1987; 22:7–17.

321. McGarrity TJ, Peiffer LP, Colony PC. Cellular proliferation in proximal and distal rat colon during 1,2-dimethylhydrazine-induced carcinogenesis. Gastroenterology 1988;95:343–348.

322. Moser AR, Luongo C, Gould KA, et al. ApcMin: a mouse model for intestinal and mammary tumorigenesis. Eur J Cancer 1995;31A:1061–1064.

323. Moser AR, Pitot HC, Dove WF. A dominant mutation that predisposes to multiple intestinal neoplasia in the mouse. Science 1990;247:322–324.

324. Dietrich WF, Lander ES, Smith JS, et al. Genetic identification of mom-1, a major modifier locus affecting min-induced intestinal neoplasia in the mouse. Cell 1993;75:631–639.

325. Dove WF, Gjould KA, Luongo C, et al. Emergent issues in the genetics of intestinal neoplasia. Cancer Surv 1995;25:335–355.

326. Kennedy AR, Beazer-Barclay Y, Kinzler KI, Newberne PM. Suppression of carcinogenesis of Min mice by the soybean derived Bowman-Birk inhibitor. Cancer Res 1996;56:679–682.

327. Sizer JS, Frederick PL, Osborne MP. Primary linitis plastica of the colon: report of a case and review of the literature. Dis Colon Rectum 1967;10:339–343.

328. Mathews JL, Cyle D Jr, Little WP. Primary linitis plastica of the rectum: report of a case. Dis Colon Rectum 1982;25:488–490.

329. Jackman RJ, Beahrs OH. Tumors of the large bowel. Philadelphia: WB Saunders, 1969.

330. Dionne L. The pattern of blood-borne metastasis from carcinoma of rectum. Cancer 1965;18:775–781.

331. Qizilbash AH. Pathologic studies in colorectal cancer: a guide to the surgical pathology examination of colorectal specimens and review of features of prognostic significance. Pathol Annu 1982;17(part 1):1–46.

332. Sarlin JG, Mori K. Morules in epithelial tumors of the colon and rectum. Am J Surg Pathol 1984;8:281–285.

333. Gibbs NM. Undifferentiated carcinoma of the large intestine. Histopathology 1977;1:77–84.

334. Iwafuchi M, Watanabe H, Ishihara N, Ito S. Neoplastic endocrine cells in carcinomas of the small intestine: histochemical and immunohistochemical studies of 24 tumors. Hum Pathol 1987;18:185–194.

335. Smith DM Jr, Haggitt RC. The prevalence and prognostic significance of argyrophil cells in colorectal carcinomas. Am J Surg Pathol 1984;8:123–128.

336. Jansson D, Gould VE, Gooch DT, et al. Immunohistochemical analysis of colon carcinomas applying exocrine and neuroendocrine markers. APMIS 1988;96:1129–1139.

337. Staren ED, Gould VE, Warren WH, et al. Neuroendocrine carcinomas of thee colon and rectum: a clinicopathologic evaluation. Surgery 1988;104:1080–1089.

338. Gould VE, Jao W, Chejfec G, et al. Neuroendocrine carcinomas of the gastrointestinal tract. Sem Diag Pathol 1984;1:13–18.

339. Lundqvist M, Wilander E. Exocrine and endocrine cell differentiation in small intestinal adenocarcinomas. Acta Pathol Microbiol Immunol Scand [A] 1983;91:469–474.

340. Shousha S. Paneth cell-rich papillary adenocarcinoma and a mucoid adenocarcinoma occurring synchronously in colon: a light and electron microscopic study. Histopathology 1979;3:489–501.

341. Kirkland SC. Clonal origin of columnar, mucous, and endocrine cell lineages in human colorectal epithelium. Cancer 1988;61:1359–1363.

342. Watson PH, Alguacil-Garcia A. Mixed crypt cell carcinoma. A clinicopathological study of the so-called 'goblet cell carcinoid.' Virchows Archiv (A) 1987;412:175–182.

343. Damjanov I, Amenta PS, Bosman FT. Undifferentiated carcinoma of the colon containing exocrine, neuroendocrine and squamous cells. Virchows Arch (A) 1983;401:57–66.

344. Palvio DH, Sorensen FB, Klove-Mogensen M. Stem cell carcinoma of the colon and rectum. Report of two cases and review of the literature. Dis Colon Rectum 1985;28:440–445.

345. Barkla DH, Whitehead RH, Foster H, Tutton PJ. Tuft (caveolated) cells in two human colon carcinoma cell lines. Am J Pathol 1988;132:521–525.

346. Seiler MW, Reilova-Velez J, Hickey W, et al. Ultrastructural markers of large bowel cancer. Prog Cancer Res Ther 1984;29:51–65.

347. Hickey WF, Seiler MW. Ultrastructural markers of colonic adenocarcinoma. Cancer 1981;47:140–145.

348. Elias H, Fong BB. Nuclear fragmentation in colon carcinoma cells. Hum Pathol 1978;9:679–684.

349. Hamilton PW, Allen DC, Watt PC, et al. Classification of normal colorectal mucosa and adenocarcinoma by morphometry. Histopathology 1987;11:901–911.

350. Graham AR, Paplanus SH, Bartels PH. Micromorphometry of colonic lesions. Laboratory Investigation 1988;59:397–402.

351. Watson PH, Carr I. A morphometric study of invasion and metastasis in human colorectal carcinoma. Clin Exp Metastasis 1987;5:311–319.

352. Jass JR, Sobin LH. Histological typing of intestinal tumours, 2nd ed. In: World Health Organization: International histological classification of tumours. Heidelberg: Springer-Verlag, 1989.

353. Umpleby HC, Ranson DL, Williamson RCN. Peculiarities of mucinous colorectal carcinoma. Br J Surg 1985;72:715–718.

354. Okuno M, Ikehara T, Nagayama M, et al. Mucinous colorectal carcinoma: clinical pathology and prognosis. Am Surgeon 1988;54:681–685.

355. Hanski C. Is mucinous carcinoma of the colorectum a distinct genetic entity? Br J Cancer 1995;72:1350–1356.

356. Minsky BD, Mies C, Recht A, Chaffey JT. Colloid carcinoma of the colon and rectum. Cancer 1987;60:3103–3112.

357. Spratt JS, Spjut HJ. Prevalence and prognosis of individual clinical and pathologic variables associated with colorectal carcinoma. Cancer 1967;20:1976–1985.

358. Sundblad AS, Paz RA. Mucinous carcinomas of the colon and rectum and their relationship to polyps. Cancer 1982;50:2504–2509.

359. Purtilo DT, Geelhoed GW, Li FP, et al. Mucinous colon carcinoma in a black family. Cancer Genet Cytogenet 1987;24:11–15.

360. Ojeda VJ, Mitchell KM, Wlaters MN, Gibson MJ. Primary colo-rectal linitis plastica type of carcinoma: report of two cases and review of the literature. Pathology 1982;14:181 189.

361. Giacchero A, Aste H, Baracchini P, et al. Primary signet-ring carcinoma of the large bowel. Report of nine cases. Cancer 1985;56:2723–2726.

362. Lui IOL, Kung ITM, Lee JMH, Boey JH. Primary colorectal signet-ring cell carcinoma in young patients: report of 3 cases. Pathology 1985;17:31–35.

363. Bonello JC, Sternberg SS, Quan SHQ. The significance of the signet-cell variety of adenocarcinoma of the rectum. Dis Colon Rectum 1980;23:180–183.

364. Almagro UA. Primary signet-ring carcinoma of the colon. Cancer 1983;52:1453–1457.

365. Fenoglio CM, Kaye GI, Lane N. Distribution of human colonic lymphatics in normal, hyperplastic and adenomatous tissue. Gastroenterology 1973;64:51–66.

366. Muto T, Kamiya J. Histological features of early cancer of the large intestine. Gan No Rinsho 1979;25:461–467.

367. Hermanek P, Gall FP. Early (microinvasive) colorectal carcinoma. Pathology, diagnosis, surgical treatment. Int J Colorectal Dis 1986;1:79–84.

368. Dukes CE. The classification of cancer of the rectum. J Pathol Bacteriol 1932;35:323–332.

369. Dukes CE. Cancer of the rectum: an analysis of 1000 cases. J Pathol Bacteriol 1940;50:527–539.

370. Kirklin JW, Dockerty MD, Waugh JM. The role of the peritoneal reflection in the prognosis of carcinoma of the rectum and sigmoid colon. Surg Gynecol Obstet 1949;88:326–331.

371. Astler VB, Coller FA. The prognostic significance of direct extension of the carcinoma of the colon and rectum. Ann Surg 1954;139:846–851.

372. Dukes CE. The surgical pathology of rectal cancer. J Clin Pathol 1949;2:95–98.

373. Dukes CE, Bussey HJR. The spread of rectal cancer and its effect on prognosis. Br J Cancer 1958;12:309–320.

374. Turnbull RB, Kyle K, Watson FR, et al. Cancer of the rectum: the influence of the no-touch isolation technic on survival rates. Ann Surg 1967;166:420–427.

375. Phillips RHS, Hittingger R, Blesovsky L, et al. Large bowel cancer: surgical pathology and its relationship to survival. Br J Surg 1984;71:604–610.

376. Gastrointestinal Tumor Study Group. Prolongation of the disease-free interval in surgically treated rectal carcinomas. N Engl J Med 1985;312:1465–1472.

377. Beahrs OH, Henson DE, Hutter RVP, Kennedy BJ, eds. Manual for staging of cancer. 4th ed. Philadelphia: JB Lippincott, 1992;69–73.

378. Jass JR, Love SB, Northover JM. A new prognostic classification of rectal cancer. Lancet 1987;1:1303–1306.

379. Jass JR, Morson BC. Reporting colorectal cancer. J Clin Pathol 1987;40:1016–1023.

380. Zarbo RJ. Interinstitutional assessment of colorectal carcinoma surgical pathology report adequacy: a College of American Pathologists Q-Probes study of practice patterns from 532 laboratories and 15,940 reports. Arch Pathol Lab Med 1992;116:1113–1119.

381. Association of Directors of Anatomic and Surgical Pathology. Recommendations for the reporting of resected large intestinal carcinomas. Modern Pathol 1996;9:73–76.

382. Barloon TJ, Lu CH, Honda H, et al. Primary adenocarcinoma of the duodenal bulb: radiographic and pathologic findings in two cases. Gastrointest Radiol 1989;14:223–225.

383. Perzin KH, Perterson M, Castiglione CL, et al. Intramucosal carcinoma of the small intestine arising in regional enteritis (Crohn's disease). Report of a case studied for carcinoembryonic antigen and review of the literature. Cancer 1984;54:151–162.

384. Meiselman MS, Ghahremani GG, Kaufman MW. Crohn's disease of the duodenum complicated by adenocarcinoma. Gastrointestinal Radiol 1987;12:333–336.

385. Cuvelier C, Bekaert E, De Potter C, et al. Crohn's disease with adenocarcinoma and dysplasia. Macroscopical, histological, and immunohistochemical aspects of two cases. Am J Surg Pathol 1989;13:187–196.

386. Spigelman AD, Williams CB, Talbot IC, et al. Upper gastrointestinal cancer in patients with familial adenomatous polyposis. Lancet 1989;2:783–785.

387. Jagelman DG, DeCosse JJ, Bussey HJ. Upper gastrointestinal cancer in familial adenomatous polyposis. Lancet 1988;1:1149–1151.

388. Dannenberg A, Godwin I, Rayburn J, et al. Multifocal adenocarcinoma of the proximal small intestine in a patient with celiac sprue. J Clin Gastroenterol 1989;11:73–76.

389. Levine ML, Dorf BS, Bank S. Adenocarcinoma of the duodenum in a patient with nontropical sprue. Am J Gastroenterol 1986;81:800–802.

390. Chen KTK, Workman RD, Kierkegaard DD. Adenocarcinoma of Meckel's diverticulum. J Surg Oncol 1983;23:41–42.

391. Persson GE, Bioesen PT. Cancer of aberrant pancreas in jejunum. Case report. Acta Chirurg Scand 1988;154:599–601.

392. Suarez V, Alexander-Williams J, O'Connor HJ, et al. Carcinoma developing in ileostomies after 25 or more years. Gastroenterology 1988;95:205–208.

393. Gadacz TR, McFadden DW, Gabrielson EW, et al. Adenocarcinoma of the ileostomy: the latent risk of cancer after colectomy for ulcerative colitis and familial polyposis. Surgery 1990;107:698–703.

394. Christie AC. Duodenal carcinoma with neoplastic transformation of the underlying Brunner's gland. Br J Cancer 1953;7:65–67.

395. Qizilbash AH. Epithelial neoplasms of the duodenum and periampullary region. In: Appelman HD. Pathology of the esophagus, stomach and duodenum. New York: Churchill Livingstone, 1984:145–173.

396. Bridge MF, Perzin KH. Primary adenocarcinoma of the jejunum and ileum. A clinicopathologic study. Cancer 1975;36:1876–1887.

397. Yamashina M. Primary adenocarcinoma of the small intestine with emphasis on microvillous differentiation. Acta Pathol Jap 1987;37:1061–1070.

398. Lien GS, Mori M, Enjoji M. Primary carcinoma of the small intestine. A clinicopathologic and immunohistochemical study. Cancer 1988;61:316–323.

399. Stern JB, Sobel HJ. Jejunal carcinoma with cells resembling Paneth cells. Arch Pathol 1961;72:47–50.

400. Yamaguchi K, Enjoji M. Carcinoma of the ampulla of Vater. A clinicopathologic study and pathologic staging of 109 cases of carcinoma and 5 cases of adenoma. Cancer 1987;59:506–515.

401. Lioe TF, Biggart JD. Primary adenocarcinoma of the jejunum and ileum: clinicopathological review of 25 cases. J Clin Pathol 1990;43:533–536.

402. Williamson RCN, Welch CE, Malt RA. Adenocarcinoma and lymphoma of the small intestine. Distribution and etiologic associations. Am Surg 1983;197:172–178.

403. Brophy C, Cahow CE. Primary small bowel malignant tumors. Unrecognized until emergent laparotomy. Am Surgeon 1989;55:408–412.

404. Yamaguchi K, Enjoji M, Kitamura K. Non-icteric ampullary carcinoma with a favorable prognosis. Am J Gastroenterol 1990;85:994–999.

405. Netscher DT, Larson GM. Colon cancer: the left to right shift and its implications. Surg Gastroenterol 1983;2:13–18.

406. Ghahremani GG, Dowlatshahi K. Colorectal carcinomas: diagnostic implications of their changing frequency and anatomic distribution. World J Surg 1989;13:321–324.

407. Kee F, Wilson RH, Gilliland R, et al. Changing site distribution of colorectal cancer. Br Med J 1992;305:158.

408. Cady B, Persson AV, Monson DO, Manuz DL. Changing patterns of colorectal carcinoma. Cancer 1974;33:422–426.

409. Slater GI, Haber RH, Aufses AH. Changing distribution of carcinoma of the colon and rectum. Surg Gynecol Obstet 1984;158:216–218.

410. Greene FL. Distribution of colorectal neoplasms. A left to right shift of polyps and cancer. Am Surg 1983;49:62–65.

411. Lockhart-Mummery HE, Morson BC. Crohn's disease of the large intestine. Gut 1964;5:493–509.

412. Thomas DM, Filipe MI, Smedley FH. Dysplasia and carcinoma in the rectal stump of total colitics who have undergone colectomy and ileo-rectal anastomosis. Histopathology 1989;14:289–298.

413. Hamilton SR. Colorectal carcinoma in patients with Crohn's disease. Gastroenterology 1985;89:398–407.

414. Teixeira CR, Tanaka S, Haruma K, et al. The clinical significance of the histologic subclassification of colorectal carcinoma. Oncology 1993;50:495–499.

415. Ponz de Leon M, Sacchetti C, Sassatelli R, et al. Evidence for the existence of different types of large bowel tumor: suggestions from the clinical data of a population-based registry. J Surg Oncol 1990;44:35–43.

416. Lazorthes F, Voigt JJ, Roques J, et al. Distal intramural spread of carcinoma of the rectum correlated with lymph nodal involvement. Surg Gynecol Obstet 1990;170:45–48.

417. Madsen PM, Christiansen J. Distal intramural spread of rectal carcinomas. Dis Colon Rectum 1986;29:279–282.

418. Kameda K, Furusawa M, Mori M, Sugimachi K. Proposed distal margin for resection of rectal cancer. Japanese J Cancer Res 1990;81:100–104.

419. Wood WQ, Wilkie DPD. Carcinoma of the rectum: an anatomico-pathologic study. Edinburgh Med J 1933;40:321–331.

420. Grinnell RS. Lymphatic block with atypical and retrograde lymphatic metastasis and spread in carcinoma of the colon and rectum. Ann Surg 1986;163:272–280.

421. Wolmark N, Cruz I, Redmond CK, et al. Tumor size and regional lymph node metastasis in colorectal cancer. A preliminary analysis from the NSABP clinical trials. Cancer 1983;51:1315–1322.

422. Jass JR, Atkin WS, Cuzick J, et al. The grading of rectal cancer: historical perspectives and a multivariate analysis of 447 cases. Histopathology 1986;10:437–459.

423. Watne AL, Moore GE, Burke E, et al. Cancer of the colon and rectum: a study of routes and metastases. Am J Surg 1961;101:7–10.

424. Kotanagi H, Fukuoka T, Shibata Y, et al. Blood vessel invasion in metastatic nodes for development of liver metastases in colorectal cancer. Hepatogastroenterology 1995;42:771–774.

425. Vider M, Maruyama Y, Narvaez R. Significance of the vertebral venous (Batson's) plexus in metastatic spread in colorectal carcinoma. Cancer 1977;40:67–71.

426. Berge T, Ekelund G, Mellner C, et al. Carcinoma of the colon and rectum in a defined population. An epidemiological, clinical and post mortem investigation of colorectal carcinoma and coexisting benign polyps in Malmo, Sweden. Acta Chirurg Scand Suppl 1973;438:1–86.

427. Gunn J, McCall JL, Yun K, Wright PA. Detection of micrometastases in colorectal cancer patients by K19 and K20 reverse-transcription polymerase chain reaction. Lab Invest 1996;75:611–616.

428. Braun S, Pantel K. Immunodiagnosis and immunotherapy of isolated

tumor cells disseminated to bone marrow of patients with colorectal cancer. Tumori 1995;81(Suppl):78–83.

429. Holtz F, Hart WR. Krukenberg tumors of the ovary: a clinicopathologic analysis of 27 cases. Cancer 1982;50:2438–2447.

430. Brennecke SP, McEvoy MI, Seymour AE, et al. Caecal adenocarcinoma metastatic to ovary inducing increased oestrogen production and postmenopausal bleeding. Austral N Z Obstet Gynaecol 1986; 26:158–161.

431. Blefari F, Risi O. Rare secondary carcinoma from colon to testis. Review of literature and report of a new case. Arch Ital Urol 1989;61:275–278.

432. Mast HL, Nissenblatt MJ. Metastatic colon carcinoma to the jaw: a case report and review of the literature. J Surg Oncol 1987;34:202–207.

433. McKay MJ, Carr PJ, Jawarski R, Kalnins I. Cancer of distant primary site relapsing in the nasopharynx: a report of two cases and review of the literature. Head Neck 1989;11:534–537.

434. Paling MR, Pope TL. Computed tomography of isolated osteoblastic colon metastases in the bony pelvis. J Comp Tomogr 1988; 2:203–207.

435. Hindley CJ, Metcalfe JW. A colonic metastatic tumor in the hand. J Hand Surg 1987;12:803–805.

436. Morris DC, Tomita T, Anderson HC. Heterotopic ossification: a case report and immunohistochemical observation. Hum Pathol 1989; 20:86–88.

437. Boreham P. Implantation metastases from cancer of the large bowel. Br J Surg 1958;46:103–108.

438. Slanetz CA, Herter FP, Grinnell RS. Anterior resection versus abdominoperineal resection for cancer of the rectum and rectosigmoid. Am J Surg 1972;123:110–117.

439. Mason AY. Cancer of the colon and rectum. Carcinoma of the lower two thirds of the rectum. Dis Colon Rectum 1976;19:11–14.

440. Guiss RL. The implantation of cancer cells with a fistula in ano: case report. Surgery 1954;36:136–139.

441. Schwartz D, Banner BF, Roseman DL, et al. Origin of Multiple "primary" colon carcinomas. A retrospective flow cytometric study. Cancer 1986;58:2082–2088.

442. August DA, Ottow RT, Sugarbaker PH. Clinical perspectives on human colorectal cancer metastasis. Cancer Metastasis Rev 1984;3: 303–324.

443. Gold P, Freeman SO. Specific carcinoembryonic antigens of the human digestive system. J Exp Med 1965;122:467–481.

444. Ho SB, Toribara NW, Bresalier RS, Kim YS. Biochemical and other markers of colon cancer. Gastroenterol Clin North Am 1988; 17:811–836.

445. Luk GD, Desai TK, Conteas CN, et al. Biochemical markers in colorectal cancer: diagnostic and therapeutic implications. Gastroenterol Clin North Am 1988;17:931–940.

446. Klavins JV. Gastrointestinal tumor markers, other than carcinoembryonic antigen, and alpha fetal protein. Cancer Detect Prev 1983; 6:131–136.

447. Mercer DW, Talamo TS. Multiple markers of malignancy in sera of patients with colorectal carcinoma. Preliminary clinical studies. Clin Chem 1985;31:1824–1828.

448. Nap M, Mollgard K, Burtin P, et al. Immunohistochemistry of carcinoembryonic antigen in the embryo, fetus and adult. Tumour Biol 1988;9:145–153.

449. Huitric E, Laumonier R, Burtin P, et al. An optical and ultrastructural study of the localization of carcinoembryonic antigen (CEA) in normal and cancerous human rectocolonic mucosa. Lab Invest 1976;34:97–108.

450. Fischbach W, Mossner J, Seyschab H, Hohn H. Tissue carcinoembryonic antigen and DNA aneuploidy in precancerous and cancerous colorectal lesions. Cancer 1990;65:1820–1824.

451. Guadagni F, Roselli M, Cosimelli M, et al. TAG-72 expression and its role in the biological evaluation of human colorectal cancer. Anticancer Res 1996;16:2141–2148.

452. Guadagni F, Roselli M, Cosimelli M, et al. Biologic evaluation of tumor-associated glycoprotein-72 and carcinoembryonic antigen expression in colorectal cancer, Part I. Dis Colon Rectum 1994; 37(Suppl):S16–S23.

453. Stamatiadis AP, St. Toumanidou M, Vyssoulis GP, et al. Value of serum acute-phase reactant proteins and carcinoembryonic antigen in

the preoperative staging of colorectal cancer. A multivariate analysis. Cancer 1990;65:2055–2057.

454. Sener SF, Imperato JP, Chmiel J, et al. The use of cancer registry data to study preoperative carcinoembryonic antigen level as an indicator of survival in colorectal cancer. CA 1989;39:50–57.

455. Angel CA, Pratt CB, Rao BN, et al. Carcinoembryonic antigen and carbohydrate 19-9 antigen as markers for colorectal carcinoma in children and adolescents. Cancer 1992;69:1487–1491.

456. Kuuselu P, Jalanko H, Roberts P, et al. Comparison of CA 19-9 and carcinoembryonic antigens (CEA) levels in the serum of patients with colorectal disease. Br J Cancer 1984;49:135–139.

457. Dahiya R, Itzkowitz SH, Byrd JC, et al. ABH blood group antigen expression, synthesis, and degradation in human colonic adenocarcinoma cell lines. Cancer Res 1989;49:4550–4556.

458. Kim YS, Yuan M, Itzkowitz SH, et al. Expression of ley and extended ley blood group-related antigens in human malignant, premalignant, and nonmalignant colonic tissues. Cancer Res 1986;46:5985–5992.

459. Cooper HS, Malecha MJ, Bass C, et al. Expression of blood group antigens H-2, Ley, and sialylated-Lea in human colorectal carcinoma: an immunohistochemical study using double-labeling techniques. Am J Pathol 1991;138:103–110.

460. Ota H, Nakayama J, Katsuyama T, Kanai M. Histochemical comparison of specificity of three bowel carcinoma-reactive lectins, Griffonia somplicifolia agglutinin-II, peanut agglutinin and Ulex europaeus agglutinin-I. Acta Pathol Jap 1988;38:1547–1559.

461. Pant KD, Shochat D, Nelson MO, Goldenberg DM. Colon-specific antigen-p (CSAp). I. Initial clinical evaluation as a marker for colorectal cancer. Cancer 1982;50:919–926.

462. Gold DV. Immunoperoxidase localization of colonic mucoprotein antigen in neoplastic tissues. Cancer Res 1981;41:767–772.

463. Bara J, Gautier R, Daher N, et al. Monoclonal antibodies against oncofetal mucin M1 antigens associated with precancerous colonic mucosae. Cancer Res 1986;46:3983–3989.

464. Pant KD, Fenoglio-Preiser CM, Berry CO, et al. COTA (colon-ovarian tumor antigen). An immunohistochemical study. Am J Clin Pathol 1986;86:1–9.

465. Birkje B, Histmark J, Skagen DW, et al. Flow cytometry of biopsy specimens from ulcerative colitis, colorectal adenomas, and carcinomas. Scand J Gastroenterol 1987;22:1231–1237.

466. Kouri M, Laasonen A, Mecklin JP, et al. Diploid predominance in hereditary nonpolyposis colorectal carcinoma evaluated by flow cytometry. Cancer 1990;65:1825–1829.

467. Hamada S, Itoh R, Nakanishi K, Fujita S. DNA distribution pattern of early adenocarcinomas of the colon and rectum and its possible meaning in the tumor progression. Cancer 1988;61:1555–1562.

468. Crissman JD, Zarbo RJ, Ma CK, Visscher DW. Histopathologic parameters and DNA analysis in colorectal adenocarcinomas. Pathol Annual 1989;24:103–147.

469. Visscher DW, Zarbo RJ, Ma CK, Crissman JD. Flow cytometric DNA and clinicopathologic analysis of Dukes' A&B colonic adenocarcinomas: a retrospective study. Mod Pathol 1990;3:709–712.

470. Hood DL, Petras RE, Edinger M, et al. Deoxyribonucleic acid ploidy and cell cycle analysis of colorectal carcinoma by flow cytometry. A prospective study of 137 cases using fresh whole cell suspensions. Am J Clin Pathol 1990;93:615–620.

471. Hoang C, Polivka M, Valleur P, et al. Immunohistochemical detection of proliferating cells in colorectal carcinomas and adenomas with the monoclonal antibody Ki-67. Preliminary data. Virchows Arch (A) 1989;414:423–428.

472. Lipkin M, Higgins P. Biological markers of cell proliferation and differentiation in human gastrointestinal diseases. Adv Cancer Res 1988;50:1–23.

473. Shepherd NA, Richman PI, England J. Ki-67 derived proliferative activity in colorectal adenocarcinoma with prognostic correlations. J Pathol 1988;155:213–219.

474. Fielding LP, Pettigrew N. College of American Pathologists Conference XXVI on clinical relevance of prognostic markers in solid tumors. Report of the Colorectal Cancer Working Group. Arch Pathol Lab Med 1995;119:45–51.

475. Chapman MAS, Hardcastle JD, Armitage NCM. Five-year prospective study of DNA tumor ploidy and colorectal cancer survival. Cancer 1995;76:383–387.

476. Cohn XH, Ornstein FL, Wang F, et al. The significance of allelic

deletions and aneuploidy in colorectal carcinoma. Results of a 5-year follow-up study. Cancer 1997;79:233–244.

477. Royds JA, Cross SS, Silcocks PB, et al. Nm23 'anti-metastatic' gene product expression in colorectal carcinoma. J Pathol 1994;172: 261–266.

478. Zeng ZS, Hsu S, Zhang AF, et al. High level of Nm23-H1 gene expression is associated with local colorectal cancer progression not with metastases. Br J Cancer 1994;70:1025–1030.

479. Ofner D, Riehemann K, Maier H, et al. Immunohistochemically detectable bcl-2 expression in colorectal carcinoma: correlation with tumor stage and patient survival. Br J Cancer 1995;72:981–985.

480. Lofberg R, Brostrom O, Karlen P, et al. DNA aneuploidy in ulcerative colitis: reproducibility, topographic distribution, and relation to dysplasia. Gastroenterology 1992;102:1149–1154.

481. Lanza G, Maestri IVA, Dubini A, et al. p53 expression in colorectal cancer. Relation to tumor type, DNA ploidy pattern and short term survival. Am J Clin Pathol 1996;105:604–612.

482. Poller DN, Baxter KJ, Shepherd NA. p53 and Rb1 protein expression: are they prognostically useful in colorectal cancer? Br J Cancer 1997;75:87–93.

483. Span M, Moerkerk PTM, DeGoeij AFPM, Arends JW. A detailed analysis of K-ras point mutations in relation to tumor progression and survival in colorectal cancer patients. Int J Cancer (Pred Oncol) 1996;69:241–245.

484. Shibata D, Reale MA, Lavin P, et al. The DCC protein and prognosis in colorectal cancer. N Engl J Med 1997;335:1727–1732.

485. Bockus HL, Kalser MH, Mouhran Y, et al. Early clinical manifestations of cancer of the colon and rectum. Dis Colon Rectum 1959;2:58–68.

486. Bloem Rm, Zwaveling A, Stijnene T. Adenocarcinoma of the colon and rectum: a report on 624 cases. Netherlands J Surg 1988;40: 121–126.

487. Kyllonen LE. Obstruction and perforation complicating colorectal carcinoma. An epidemiologic and clinical study with special reference to incidence and survival. Acta Chirurg Scand 1987;153: 607–614.

488. Kaufman Z, Eiltch E, Dinbar A. Completely obstructive colorectal cancer. J Surg Oncol 1989;41:230–235.

489. Nesbakken A, Haffner J. Colo-recto-anal intussusception. Case report. Acta Chirurg Scand 1989;155:201–204.

490. Bear HD, MacIntyre J, Burns HJ, et al. Colon and rectal carcinoma in the west of Scotland. Symptoms, histologic characteristics, and outcome. Am J Surg 1984;147:441–446.

491. Mandava N, Kumar S, Pizzi WF, Aprile IJ. Perforated colorectal carcinomas. Am J Surg 1996;172:236–238.

492. Panwalker AP. Unusual infections associated with colorectal cancer. Rev Infect Dis 1988;10:347–364.

493. Tabibian N, Clarridge JE. Streptococcus bovis septicemia and large bowel neoplasia. Am Fam Phys 1989;39:227–229.

494. Emiliani VJ, Chodos JE, Comer GM, et al. Streptococcus bovis brain abscess associated with an occult colonic villous adenoma. Am J Gastroenterol 1990;85:78–80.

495. Kornbluth AA, Danzig JB, Bernstein LH. Clostridium septicum infection and associated malignancy. Report of 2 cases and review of the literature. Medicine 1989;68:30–37.

496. Lee PH, Khauli RB, Baker S, Menon M. Prognostic and therapeutic observations of manifestations in the genitourinary tract of adenocarcinoma of the colon and rectum. Surg Gynecol Obstet 1989;169: 511–518.

497. Amico L, Caplan LR, Thomas C. Cerebrovascular complications of mucinous cancers. Neurology 1989;39:522–526.

498. Liel Y, Ariad S. Microangiopathic hemolytic anemia associated with metastatic carcinoma of the colon. South Med J 1988;81:1320–1321.

499. Macpherson A, Berth-Jones J, Graham-Brown RA. Carcinoma-associated dermatomyositis responding to plasmapheresis. Clin Ex Dermatol 1989;14:304–305.

500. Sung MW, Bruckner HW, Szabo S, Mitty HA. Extrahepatic obstructive jaundice due to colorectal cancer. Am J Gastroenterol 1988;83: 267–270.

501. Bak M. Nodular intra-abdominal panniculitis: an accompaniment of colorectal carcinoma and diverticular disease. Histopathology. 1996; 29:21–27.

502. McCallum A, Eastwood MA, Smith AN, Fulton PM. Colonic diverticulosis in patients with colorectal cancer and in controls. Scand J Gastroenterol 1988;23:284–286.

503. Morini S, de Angelis P, Manurita L, Colavolpe V. Association of colonic diverticula with adenomas and carcinomas. A colonoscopic experience. Dis Colon Rectum 1988;31:793–796.

504. Shemesh E, Czerniak A, Pines A, Bat L. Is there an association between gastric polyps and colonic neoplasms? Digestion 1989;42: 212–216.

505. Armstrong CP, Ahsan Z, Hinchley G, et al. Appendectomy and carcinoma of the caecum. Br J Surg 1989;76:1049–1053.

506. Yoshida J, Morisaki T, Yamaguchi K, et al. Carcinoma in adenoma of the ampulla of Vater synchronous with cancer of the sigmoid colon. Dig Dis Sci 1990;35:271–275.

507. Schmid KW, Galser K, Wykypiel H, Feichtinger H. Synchronous adenocarcinoma of the transverse colon, the gallbladder and the vermiform appendix. Klin Wochenschr 1988;66:1093–1096.

508. Klompje J, Petrelli NJ, Herrera L, Mittelman A. Synchronous and metachronous colon lesions in squamous cell carcinoma of the anal canal. J Surg Oncol 1987;35:86–88.

509. Takayama H, Nakagawa K, Onozuka S, et al. Nonfamilial Turcot syndrome presenting with astrocytoma—case report. Neurol Med Chir 1989;29:606–609.

510. el-Jabbour JN, Helm CW, McLaren KM, et al. Synchronous colonic adenocarcinoma and extragenital malignant mixed mesodermal tumour. Scot Med J 1989;34:567–568.

511. Kinn AC, Haggmark T, Willems JS. Aggressive mesenteric fibromatosis. Case report. Acta Chir Scand 1989;155:293–296.

512. Thomas WM, Pye G, Hardcastle JD, Mangham CM. Faecal occult blood screening for colorectal neoplasia: a randomized trial of three days or six days of tests. Br J Surg 1990;77:277–279.

513. McGarrity TJ, Long PA, Peiffer LP. Results of a repeat television-advertised mass screening program for colorectal cancer using fecal occult blood tests. Am J Gastroenterol 1990;85:266–270.

514. Hardcastle JD, Thomas WM, Chamberlain J, et al. Randomised, controlled trial of faecal occult blood screening for colorectal cancer. Results for first 107,349 subjects. Lancet 1989;1:1160–1164.

515. Ow CL, Lemar HJ, Weaver MJ. Does screening proctosigmoidoscopy result in reduced mortality from colorectal cancer? A critical review of the literature. J Gen Intern Med 1989;4:209–215.

516. Orrom WJ, Brzezinski WS, Wiens EW. Heredity and colorectal cancer. A prospective, community-based, endoscopic study. Dis Colon Rectum 1990;33:490–493.

517. Ahlquist DA. Fecal occult blood testing for colorectal cancer: can we afford to do this? Gastroenterol Clin North Am 1997;26:41–55.

518. Mandel JS, Bond JH, Church TR, et al. Reducing mortality from colorectal cancer by screening for fecal occult blood. N Engl J Med 1993;328:1365–1371.

519. Bond JH. Fecal occult blood testing for colorectal cancer: can we afford to do this? Gastroenterol Clin North Am 1997;26:57–70.

520. Dasmahapatra KS, Lopyan K. Rationale for aggressive colonoscopy in patients with colorectal neoplasia. Arch Surg 1989;124: 63–66.

521. Rex DK, Lehman GA, Hawes RH, et al. Screening colonoscopy in asymptomatic average-risk persons with negative fecal occult blood tests. Gastroenterology 1991;100:64–67.

522. Jarvinen HJ, Mecklin J-P, Sistonen P. Screening reduces colorectal cancer rate in families with hereditary nonpolyposis colorectal cancer. Gastroenterology 1995;108:1405–1411.

523. Rozen P, Baratz M, Fefer F, Gilat T. Low incidence of significant dysplasia in a successful endoscopic surveillance program of patients with ulcerative colitis. Gastroenterology 1995;108:1361–1370.

524. Stevenson G. Radiology in the detection and prevention of colorectal cancer. Eur J Cancer 1995;31A:1121–1126.

525. Hinder JM, Chu J, Bokey EL, et al. Use of transrectal ultrasound to evaluate direct tumour spread and lymph node status in patients with rectal cancer. Austral N Z J Surg 1990;60:19–23.

526. Thoeni RF, Rogalla P. Current CT/MRI examination of the lower intestinal tract. Baillieres Clin Gastroenterol 1994;8:765–796.

527. Kiefer PJ, Thorson AG, Christensen MA. Metachronous colorectal cancer. Time interval to presentation of a metachronous cancer. Dis Colon Rectum 1986;29:378–382.

528. Evers BM, Mullins RJ, Matthews TH, et al. Multiple adenocarcinomas of the colon and rectum. An analysis of incidences and current trends. Dis Colon Rectum 1988;31:518–522.

529. Kochhar R, Rajwanshi A, Wig JD. Fine needle aspiration cytology of rectal masses. Gut 1990;32:334–336.

530. Vobecky J, Leduc CP, Devroede G, Madarnas P. The reliability of routine pathologic diagnosis of colorectal adenocarcinoma. Cancer 1989;64:1261–1265.

531. Halvorsen TB. Tissue sampling and histological grading in colorectal cancer. Are routine sections representative? Acta Pathol Microbiol Immunol Scand 1989;97:261–266.

532. Eckharser FE, Knol JA. Surgery for primary and metastatic colorectal cancer. Gastroenterol Clin North Am 1997;26:103–127.

533. Beart RW. Colon, rectum, and anus. Cancer 1990;33:684–688.

534. Ottery FD, Bruskewitz RC, Weese JL. Endoscopic transrectal resection of rectal tumors. Cancer 1986;576:563–566.

535. Zauber AG, Winawer SJ. Initial management and follow-up surveillance of patients with colorectal adenomas. Gastroenterol Clin North Am 1997;26:85–101.

536. Shehata WM, Meyer RL, Jazy FK, et al. Regional adjuvant irradiation for adenocarcinoma of the cecum. Int J Radiat Oncol Biol Phys 1987;13:843–846.

537. Kopelson G. Adjuvant postoperative radiation therapy for colorectal carcinoma above the peritoneal reflection: I. Sigmoid colon. Cancer 1983;51:1593–1598.

538. Ernst CS, Shen JW, Litwin S, et al. Multiparameter evaluation of the expression in situ of normal and tumor-associated antigens in human colorectal carcinoma. J Natl Cancer Inst 1986;77:387–395.

539. Wadler S, Wiernik PH. Clinical update on the role of fluorouracil and recombinant interferon alpha-2a in the treatment of colorectal carcinoma. Sem Oncol 1990;17:16–21.

540. Moertel CG, Fleming TR, MacDonald JS, et al. Levamisole and fluorouracil for adjuvant therapy of resected colon carcinoma. New Engl J Med 1990;322:352–358.

541. Bismuth H, Castaing D, Traynor O. Surgery for synchronous hepatic metastases of colorectal cancer. Scan J Gastroenterol Suppl 1988;149:144–149.

542. Que FG. Nagorney DM. Resection of 'recurrent' colorectal metastases to the liver. Br J Surg 1994;81:255–258.

543. Schlag P, Hohenberger P, Holting T, et al. Hepatic arterial infusion (HAI) chemotherapy for liver metastasis of colorectal cancer using 5-FU. Eur J Surg Oncol 1990;16:99–104.

544. Cuncliffe WJ, Hasleton PS, Tweedle DE, Schofield PF. Incidence of synchronous and metachronous colorectal carcinoma. Br J Surg 1984;71:941–943.

545. Fenoglio CM, Pascal RR, Perzin KH. Tumors of the intestines. Atlas of tumor pathology, second series, fascicle 27. Washington, DC: Armed Forces Institute of Pathology, 1990.

546. Rex DK. Colonoscopy: a review of its yield for cancers and adenomas by indication. Am J Gastroenterol 1995;90:353–365.

547. Greenstein AJ, Slater G, Heimann TM, et al. A comparison of multiple synchronous colorectal cancer in ulcerative colitis, familial polyposis coli, and de novo cancer. Annals Surg 1986;203:123–128.

548. Gajraj H, Davies DR, Jackson BT. Synchronous small and large bowel cancer developing after pelvic irradiation. Gut 1988;29:126–128.

549. Johnson CD, Thomson H. Six synchronous colonic cancers in a pair of monozygotic twins. Dis Colon Rectum 1986;29:745–746.

550. Kaibara N, Koga S, Jinnai D. Synchronous and metachronous malignancies of the colon and rectum in Japan with special reference to a coexisting early cancer. Cancer 1984;54:1870–1874.

551. Langevin JM, Nivatvongs S. The true incidence of synchronous cancer of the large bowel. A prospective study. Am J Surg 1984;147:330–333.

552. Dasmahapatra KS, Lopyan K. Rationale for aggressive colonoscopy in patients with colorectal neoplasia. Arch Surg 1989;124:63–66.

553. Finan PJ, Ritchie JK, Hawley PR. Synchronous and 'early' metachronous carcinomas of the colon and rectum. Br J Surg 1987;74:945–947.

554. Yamagiwa H, Yoshimura H, Tomiyama H, et al. Squamous change of adenocarcinoma of the large intestine. Gan No Rinshoi 1984;30:233–238.

555. Comer TP, Beahrs OH, Docheertz MB. Primary squamous cell carcinoma and adenoacanthoma. Cancer 1971;28:1111–1117.

556. Schmidtmaun M. Zur kenntnis seltener krebsformen. Arch Pathol Anat 1919;226:100–118.

557. Michelassi F, Mishlove LA, Stipa F, Block GE. Squamous-cell carcinoma of the colon. Experience at the University of Chicago, review of the literature, report of two cases. Dis Colon Rectum 1988;31:228–235.

558. Lundquest DE, Marcus JN, Thorson AG, Massop D. Primary squamous cell carcinoma of the colon arising in a villous adenoma. Human Pathol 1988;19:362–364.

559. Burgers PA, Lupton EW, Talbot IC. Squamous-cell carcinoma of the proximal colon: report of a case and review of the literature. Dis Colon Rectum 1979;22:241–247.

560. Cerezo L, Alvarez M, Edwards O, Price G. Adenosquamous carcinoma of the colon. Dis Colon Rectum 1985;28:597–603.

561. Kontozoglou TE, Moyana TN. Adenosquamous carcinoma of the colon—an immunocytochemical and ultrastructural study. Report of two cases and review of the literature. Dis Colon Rectum 1989;32:719–721.

562. Berkelhammer CH, Baker AL, Block GE, et al. Humoral hypercalcemia complicating adenosquamous carcinoma of the proximal colon. Dig Dis Sci 1989;34:142–147.

563. Peonim V, Thakerngpol K, Pacharee P, Stitnimankarn T. Adenosquamous carcinoma and carcinoidal differentiation of the colon. Report of a case. Cancer 1983;52:1122–1125.

564. Vezeridis MP, Herrera LO, Lopez GE, et al. Squamous-cell carcinoma of the colon and rectum. Dis Colon Rectum 1983;26:188–191.

565. Michelassi F, Montag AG, Block GE. Adenosquamous-cell carcinoma in ulcerative colitis. Report of a case. Dis Colon Rectum 1988;31:323–326.

566. Pemberton M, Lendrum J. Squamous cell carcinoma of the caecum following ovarian adenocarcinoma. Br J Surg 1969;55:273–276.

567. Hickey WF, Corson JM. Squamous cell carcinoma arising in a duplication of the colon: case report and literature review of squamous cell carcinoma of the colon and of malignancy complicating colonic duplication. Cancer 1981;47:602–609.

568. Petrelli M, Tetangco E, Reid JD. Carcinoma of the colon with undifferentiated carcinoid and squamous cell features. Am J Clin Pathol 1981;75:581–584.

569. Knight BK, Hayes MM. Mixed adenocarcinoma and carcinoid tumour of the colon. A report of 4 cases with postulates on histogenesis. S African Med J 1987;72:708–710.

570. Moyana TN, Qizilbash AH, Murphy F. Composite glandular-carcinoid tumors of the colon and rectum. Report of two cases. Am J Surg Pathol 1988;12:607–611.

571. Jones MA, Griffith LM, West AB. Adenocarcinoid tumor of the periampullary region: a novel duodenal neoplasm presenting as biliary tract obstruction. Hum Pathol 1989;20:198–200.

572. Levendoglu H, Cox CA, Nadimpalli V. Composite (adenocarcinoid) tumors of the gastrointestinal tract. Dig Dis Sci 1990;35:519–525.

573. Mills SE, Allen MS, Cohen AR. Small-cell undifferentiated carcinoma of the colon. A clinicopathological study of five cases and their association with colonic adenomas. Am J Surg Path 1987;7:643–651.

574. Redman BG, Pazdur R. Colonic small cell undifferentiated carcinoma: a distinct pathological diagnosis with therapeutic implications. Am J Gastroenterol 1987;83:382–385.

575. Robidoux A, Monte M, Heppell J. Small-cell carcinoma of the rectum. Dis Colon Rectum 1984;28:594–596.

576. Wick MR, Weatherby RP, Weiland LH. Small cell neuroendocrine carcinoma of the colon and rectum: clinical, histologic, and ultrastructural study and immunohistochemical comparison with cloacogenic carcinoma. Hum Pathol 1987;18:9–21.

577. Bak M, Teglbjaerg PS. Pleomorphic (giant cell) carcinoma of the intestine, an immunohistochemical and electron microscopic study. Cancer 1989;64:2557–2564.

578. Jewell LD, Barr JR, McCaughey WT, et al. Clear-cell epithelial neoplasms of the large intestine. Arch Pathol Lab Med 1988;112:197–199.

579. Kubosawa H, Nagao K, Kondo Y, et al. Coexistence of adenocarcinoma and choriocarcinoma in the sigmoid colon. Cancer 1984;54:866–868.

580. Robey-Cafferty SS, Silva EG, Cleary KR. Anaplastic and sarcomatoid

carcinoma of the small intestine: a clinicopathologic study. Hum Pathol 1989;20:858–863.

581. Amano S, Yamada N. Endometrioid carcinoma arising from endometriosis of the sigmoid colon: a case report. Hum Pathol 1981;12:845–848.

582. Orr MM, Edwards AJ. Neoplastic change in duplication of the alimentary tract. Br J Surg 1975;62:269–274.

583. Wanebo HJ, Woodruff JM, Farr GH, Quan SH. Anorectal melanoma. Cancer 1981;47:1891–1900.

584. Hambrick E, Abacarian M, Smith D, Keller F. Malignant melanoma of the rectum in a Negro man: report of a case and review of the literature. Dis Colon Rectum 1974;17:360–364.

585. Sroujieh AS. Spontaneous regression of intestinal malignant melanoma from an occult primary site. Cancer 1988;62:1247–1250.

586. Raymond AR, Rorat E, Goldstein D, et al. An unusual case of malignant melanoma of the small intestine. Am J Gastroenterol 1984;79:689–692.

587. Beardmoir GL, Davies NC, McLeod R, et al. Malignant melanoma in Queensland: a study of 219 deaths. Aust J Dermatol 1969;10:158–168.

588. Wilson BG, Anderson JR. Malignant melanoma involving the small bowel. Postgrad Med J 1986;62:355–357.

589. Katon RM, Brendler SJ, Ireland K. Gastric linitis plastica with metastases to the colon: a mimic of Crohn's disease. J Clin Gastroenterol 1989;11:555–560.

590. Kanter MA, Isaacson NH, Knoll SM, Nochomovitz LE. The diagnostic challenge of metastatic linitis plastica. Two cases and a consideration of the problem. Am Surgeon 1986;52:510–513.

591. Levine MS, Drooz AT, Herlinger H. Annular malignancies of the small bowel. Gastrointest Radiol 1987;12:53–58.

592. Nyberg B, Sonnenfeld T. Metastatic breast carcinoma causing intestinal obstruction. Acta Chirurg Scand 1986;530:95–96.

593. Rabau MY, Alon RJ, Werbin N, Yossipov Y. Colonic metastases from lobular carcinoma of the breast. Report of a case. Dis Colon Rectum 1988;31:401–402.

594. Wegener M, Borsch G, Reitemeyer E, Schafer K. Metastasis to the colon from primary bronchogenic carcinoma presenting as occult gastrointestinal bleeding—report of a case. Zeitschr Gastroenterol 1988;26:358–362.

595. Pang JA, King WK. Bowel haemorrhage and perforation from metastatic lung cancer. Report of three cases and a review of the literature. Aust N Z J Surg 1987;57:779–783.

596. Fawaz F, Hill GJ 2d. Adult intussusception due to metastatic tumors. South Med J 1983;76:522–523.

PART VI

APPENDIX AND ANAL REGION

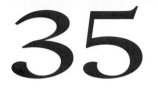

CHAPTER

35 | DISORDERS OF THE VERMIFORM APPENDIX

Chik-Kwun Tang

The human vermiform appendix can be involved by a wide range of diseases and its inflammatory condition, acute appendicitis, remains the most common acute abdominal condition (1). Other diseases, including congenital anomalies, various infectious conditions, and hyperplastic and neoplastic diseases, have also been observed in the appendix. Diseases other than acute appendicitis may produce symptoms and signs indistinguishable from those of acute appendicitis. Conversely, a complicated acute appendicitis may resemble other diseases, such as tumors. The accuracy of diagnosing acute appendicitis is high but far from perfect. When to operate thus continues to be one of the most common challenges to surgeons.

ANATOMY AND EMBRYOLOGY

The human vermiform appendix can be regarded developmentally as a part of the cecum. In the sixth week of gestational age, a blind-ended pouch, the cecal diverticulum, is formed on the antimesenteric border of the primitive midgut (2). The distal end of this pouch does not grow as rapidly as the proximal portion, thus becoming the appendix. The length of the appendix, however, increases during fetal development. Beginning at birth, the lateral wall of the cecum grows faster than the medial. This different growth rate results in the shift of the appendix from its end position to the side near the ileocecal valve.

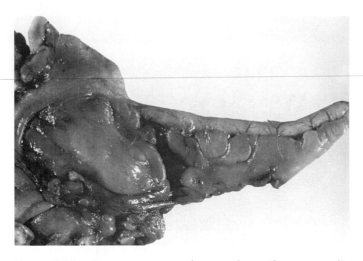

Figure 35.1 Gross appearance of a normal vermiform appendix showing smooth external surface attached to which is the extension of the mesentery. Blood vessels can be seen through the transparent peritoneum. The tenia coli end at the base of the appendix.

Approximately 70% of appendices are located behind the cecum (retrocecal), with its orifice opening into the cecum near the ileocecal valve (3). They may also be subcecal, pelvic, retrocolic, subhepatic, or buried in the cecal wall (2, 3). The appendiceal orifice varies in shape, from round to slit-like. The average length of the appendix ranges from 7 to 10 cm in normal adults (3, 4). Appendices are usually shorter in children. The external diameter ranges from 0.5 to 0.8 cm (3, 4). Because of its irregular shape, the diameter of the lumen is difficult to measure. The base of the appendix is anchored onto the posterior abdominal wall by the meso-appendix, which is an extension of the mesentery of the adjacent terminal ileum. The tip of the appendix is free. Although the three teniae coli meet at the base of the appendix, none is present in the appendix itself.

The appendicular artery, a branch of the ileocecal artery, provides the arterial blood supply. Its venous blood drains into the portal system via the superior mesenteric vein. The lymphatics of the appendix drain into the regional lymph nodes (3). Externally, the appendix is covered by the peritoneum through which small blood vessels are observed (3), and is pink, smooth, and glistening (Fig. 35.1). On cross sectioning, the appendiceal wall is a circular structure displaying pink-white color. The mucosa is soft, smooth, and pink and slightly protrudes into the lumen due to the prominent lymphoid tissue in the lamina propria.

The cells of the appendiceal mucosa are cytologically similar to those of the colon; different types of cells can be observed and are underlined by a basal lamina. They appear to differentiate towards columnar cells, including the goblet cells, early in fetal life (Fig. 35.2). The mucosa of the appendix does not form villi (Fig. 35.3). The columnar cells lining the surface function as absorptive elements, and the so-called M cells assist in luminal transport of antigens into the epithelium for appropriate immunologic processing (3). Nonbranching crypts (crypts of Lieberkuhn) are also lined by columnar cells. Here the goblet cells are more prominent than those in the surface. The goblet cells contain neutral

and acid sulfomucin, as demonstrated by periodic acid-Schiff (PAS) and alcian blue stains, respectively (3). At the bases of the crypts and mixed with the mucus-secreting cells are scattered enterochromaffin (Kultschitzky type) and Paneth's cells (3, 5). Also observed are the stem cells, mostly located at the base of the crypts (3).

The endocrine cells can be demonstrated by immunohistochemical techniques for chromogranin (3), neuron-specific-enolase (NSE), and serotonin, and are characterized by neurosecretory granules with electron microscopy (5). Enterochromaffin cells were found in the lamina propria as well, some of which appeared associated with the large cells resembling neurons in the submucosal Meissner's plexus, confirming Masson's original findings (5). These complexes have been termed "enterochromaffin-nerve-fibre" complexes, which may play a modulatory role between the epithelium and the deeper enteric nervous system medicated by serotonin neurotransmission under physiological conditions. Abnormal release of serotonin may cause acute inflammation and/or pain. It raises a question as to whether the pain in a case of clinical appendicitis with a histologically normal appendix is secondary to the abnormally secreted serotonin.

Like the intestine, the appendix is comprised of lamina propria, which itself is composed of loosely arranged fibrous connective tissue where histiocytes and lymphocytes are easily seen. The latter begin to appear as lymphoid nodules during fetal life. The percent-

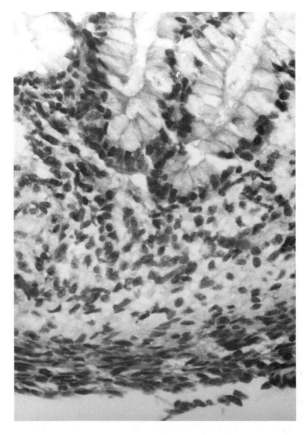

Figure 35.2 Normal vermiform appendix of a 13 week old fetus (gestational age) showing well developed goblet cells and thin muscular coat. Lymphoid follicles are absent.

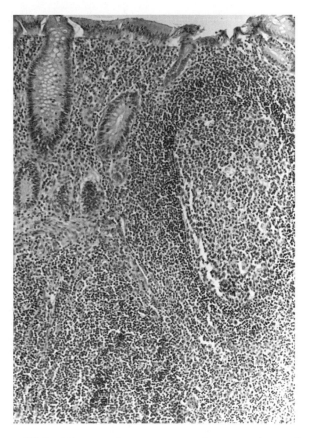

Figure 35.3 Microscopic appearance of a normal vermiform appendix of an adult. The epithelial lining the crypts of Lieberkuhn has prominent goblet cells. Lymphocytes and plasma cells are abundant in the lamina propria, with follicle and germinal center formation.

age of the lymphoid tissue of the appendix is the highest during the first decade of life and steadily decreases thereafter (6). The lymphoid follicles in a normal appendix typically show germinal centers, each of which is surrounded by a mantle of small lymphocytes (Fig. 35.3). Both the germinal center and the mantle zone are comprised of B cells with some admixed T cells, almost exclusively T helper cells. Immediately above the follicle is a zone of mixed cells (small and large lymphocytes) most of which are B cells. The overlying epithelium shows intraepithelial B and T suppressor lymphocytes. On either side of the follicle are diffuse small lymphocytes, macrophages, and plasma cells, the latter being the most prominent components. Beneath the follicle is the T-cell area where the helper to suppressor T cell ratio is approximately 8:1 (7).

The muscularis mucosae is poorly developed. The submucosa is composed of fibrous connective tissue in which blood vessels, nerves, and varying amounts of adipose tissue are present. The submucosa is surrounded by a circular and a longitudinal coat of smooth muscle, which are in turn covered by a serosa. Few ganglion cells are found in the submucosa. Other ganglion cells are haphazardly distributed in the muscle (8).

DEVELOPMENTAL ABNORMALITIES

CONGENITAL ABSENCE (AGENESIS)

Congenial absence (agenesis) of the appendix is rare, the frequency of which is 0.006% (9). It has been reported to be associated with other congenital anomalies caused by thalidomide (10). The diagnosis of congenital absence should be made only after other causes are excluded (11).

DUPLICATION

Duplication of the appendix is a rare condition and occurs commonly associated with other congenital anomalies (3), but may also occur with a normal cecum (12). Three different types may occur: Type A, a single cecum, a single appendiceal base and a bifurcated distal portion; Type B, a single cecum, two distinct appendiceal bases and two completely separate appendices; and Type C, two cecal structures, each with a single appendix (3).

DIVERTICULUM

Diverticula are found in 0.004 to 2.8% of surgical and autopsy material (13) and are more often acquired than congenital. The congenital diverticula are distinguished from their acquired counterparts by the presence of muscular coats and the absence of inflammation. Multiple congenital diverticula have also been described (14).

MALPOSITION

Malposition occurs occasionally associated with maldescent of the cecum, resulting in a sublhepatic cecum and appendix. Various types of malposition of appendix may also occur as consequences of different types of congenial malrotation of the intestine (2). Malposition may create diagnostic difficulty should acute appendicitis develop.

MISCELLANEOUS CONDITIONS

A unique case of appendix helicus was described in a 13 month old child. He was born with a lumbosacral meningomyelocele and a neurogenic bladder. The appendix helicus was found incidentally during cystectomy (15). Hirschsprung's disease (aganglionosis) may rarely involve the appendix with dilatation and even perforation (16). In neurofibromatosis (von Recklinghausen's disease), the appendix may rarely be involved, with associated appendicitis (17). Ectopic gastric and esophageal mucosa (18, 19), and aberrant pancreas (9) have been reported.

INFLAMMATORY DISORDERS

ACUTE APPENDICITIS

Acute appendicitis is acute inflammation of the vermiform appendix and the most common acute surgical condition of the abdomen (1). It has been generally accepted that Fitz was the first investigator to recognize acute appendicitis as a distinct clinicopathologic entity in 1886 (20, 21).

Acute appendicitis is far more common in Western than Eastern countries (22). The annual incidence is approximately 1.5 to 1.9 per 1,000 between the ages of 17 and 64 (23). The rate, however, has been noted to be declining after World War II (4). For instance, a current study showed a decrease in incidence from 100 per 100,000 down to 52 per 100,000 over a period of 15 years (24). It occurs in all ages but is rare before the age of two years. The peak incidence is in the second and third decades, teenagers being the most frequently affected. The incidence begins to decline after the age of 40 (23). The male to female ratio is 1:1 before puberty, 2:1 between 15 and 25 years, and after 25 returns to 1:1 again (1).

ETIOLOGY AND PATHOGENESIS

The etiology and pathogenesis of acute appendicitis are not entirely clear. However, observations and studies of the surgically removed appendices and experimental approaches have revealed contributory factors, among which obstruction, infection, and mucosal damage are the most important.

In their elegant study in dogs, Wangensteen and Bowers (25) demonstrated that complete obstruction of the cecal appendage (a canine equivalent to the human appendix) without prewashing the content resulted in acute appendicitis in six of eight dogs 6 to 24 hours after the ligation; the remaining two were normal. Complete obstruction of washed cecal appendage failed to produce appendicitis. If feces were introduced in the cecal appendage which had been ligated for five days, two of three animals developed appendicitis. In the same study, they carefully observed 91 human appendices surgically removed for acute appendicitis in order to correlate with their experimental results. Evidence of obstruction, usually by fecalith, was found in more than 70% of the specimens. The role of obstruction in the development of appendicitis was further confirmed in other experimental studies in rabbit (26), ape, and man (27).

In the study in humans (patients who had colonic cancer), their appendices were exteriorized and obstruction was created by ligating the base of the appendix. Seven to 49 hours after the initial obstruction, the intraluminal pressure was increased up to 126 cm of water in the majority of appendices. Histologic examination revealed a spectrum of changes, including mucosal appendicitis, diffuse appendicitis, and healing appendicitis. However, the appendix that served as a control (unobstructed) also demonstrated acute appendicitis.

Other factors may also be relevant and important in the development of appendicitis. Luminal pressure was increased after complete obstruction of the appendix was created (25–27). The increased pressure would then interfere with circulation, resulting in more accumulation of fluid in the lumen and further increasing the pressure, creating a vicious cycle. The deprivation of oxygen from the reduced blood flow would result in tissue damage thus favoring the invasion of bacteria (26).

Examination of the surgically removed appendices does not always reveal fecalith or other evidence of obstruction. The incidence of fecalith or other demonstrable obstruction in the surgically removed appendices ranges from 7 to 34% (28, 29). In a number of those that appear to be nonobstructive, lymphoid hyperplasia may play a role, especially in young patients in whom the lymphoid tissue is prominent and appendicitis common (4). Lymphoid hyperplasia of the appendix may be seen in measles (4), Coxsackie B virus infection (30, 31), and mononucleosis. However, the incidence of

appendicitis is not known to be increased in these conditions. Further complicating the interpretation is the fact that lymphoid hyperplasia may be secondary to inflammation of the appendix. The role of lymphoid hyperplasia in causing obstruction is therefore debatable, or at best, may only be a factor in a small number of appendicitis cases. Butler found no total obstruction of the appendiceal lumen by lymphoid hyperplasia nor distal dilatation in the specimens of acute appendicitis (29).

Mucosal ulceration is definitely an important pathogenic factor, which was found in 48 of 64 surgical specimens of acute appendicitis (32). Butler and Sisson et al. postulated that appendicitis begins as mucosal ulceration, followed by invasion of bacteria (29, 32). Because obstruction of their specimens was infrequent, these authors further suggested that obstruction was not fundamental in the development of appendicitis.

However, there are many specimens of acute appendicitis in which fecalith are found to be occupying the lumens. Experimentally, acute appendicitis does result from obstruction both in animals and men. Perhaps an attempt is in order to speculate on the possible role of obstruction in the development of mucosal ulcerations. The obstruction by a fecalith in humans may be similar to that created by ligature of the base of the appendix in that it would probably result in ischemia, which in turn would cause ischemic damage of the appendiceal mucosa. In some specimens, the ulcerated and inflamed mucosa appears to be similar to the ischemic changes of, for instance, the large intestine. The fecalith, which are hard and not entirely smooth (25), may mechanically damage the mucosa.

Butler raises another intriguing speculation that immune complex injury or delayed hypersensitivity may play a role in the pathogenesis based on the circumstantial evidence of lymphoid hyperplasia and inflammatory involvement of the lymphoid follicles in acute appendicitis (29). The role of diet in the pathogenesis of acute appendicitis is conflicting. Studies have shown that Europeans living in Africa who consume a low fiber diet have a higher incidence of appendicitis than do native Africans who eat a high fiber diet (22). Contrarily, a decreased incidence of appendicitis in Sweden occurred during a period in which there was a reduction in dietary fiber in the average diet (33). The relationship between dietary fiber and appendicitis remains uncertain.

From these studies, it is clear that the etiology and pathogenesis of appendicitis are multifactorial. Because the bacterial flora in the lumens of a normal appendix are essentially the same as those found in the inflamed appendices, their invasion into the appendiceal lymphoid tissue and other structures must be accomplished through the damaged mucosa, as advocated by Sisson et al. (32) and Butler (29), lest appendicitis be much more common than it is. The mucosal damage may be the result of virus infection (32), immune complex injury or delayed hypersensitivity (29), mechanical injury by fecalith, or ischemia due to obstruction. There remains a minority of cases in which the causative organism may itself be invasive without the assistance of pre-existing mucosal damage.

PATHOLOGY OF ACUTE APPENDICITIS

The morphologic appearance of acute appendicitis is basically that of acute inflammation with variations dependent on the severity and duration of the inflammatory process. The appendix is grossly congested and swollen with an increased diameter. The lumen is dilated in many specimens (Fig. 35.4A) and may contain pus and/or fecalith. The serosa is covered by fibrin or fibrinopurulent exudate

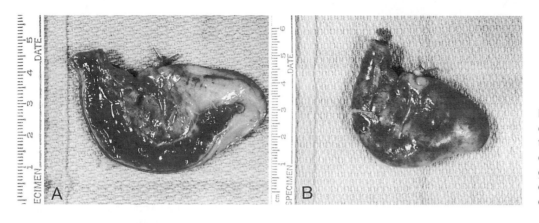

Figure 35.4 **(A)** Acute appendicitis showing hemorrhage in the dilated lumen. **(B)** The serosa of the same appendix is congested and hemorrhagic and covered by purulent exudate (See color plate).

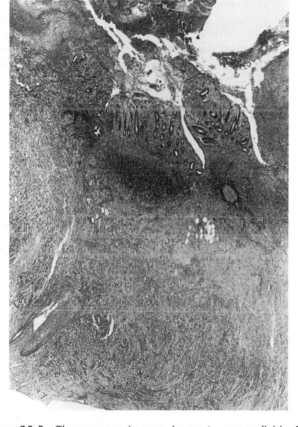

Figure 35.5 The mucosa is seen in acute appendicitis. The lymphoid follicles are distorted. The appendiceal wall is thickened.

(Fig. 35.4B). The presence of pus does not necessarily indicate perforation because suppuration may dissect the entire appendiceal wall into the periappendiceal tissue without a perforation (4). The mucosa is hyperemic (Fig. 35.4A) and may show mucosal necrosis or ulceration. In other instances, the lymphoid tissue may be so prominent that it forms soft-pink–tan, nodular protrusions into the appendiceal lumens. Microscopic examination shows characteristic features of acute appendicitis, including mucosal ulceration (Fig. 35.5) and infiltration by polymorphonuclear leukocytes,

eosinophils, plasm cells, and histiocytes throughout all appendiceal layers and frequently into the serosa. Many polymorphonuclear leukocytes may be found spilling out into the lumen. The appendiceal wall is edematous.

In the less severe cases, the gross appearance may reveal congestion on the serosa, and may even be normal. The inflammatory infiltrate of polymorphonuclear leukocytes is seen only in the mucosa, lamina propria, and submucosa. When this feature is associated with mucosal ulcerations, it is diagnostic of acute appendicitis. When it is not, it would be subject to controversial interpretation between an early acute appendicitis and the result of surgical manipulation, especially in patients with clinical presentations of acute appendicitis.

In the more advanced stage, the inflammatory process involves the full thickness of the appendiceal wall with partial necrosis or infarction of the wall where perforation may take place (Fig. 35.6). The tissue adjacent to the perforation is dull grey and covered by pus. Abscess may be formed in the periappendiceal tissue with some degree of organization characterized by granulation and fibrous tissue, resulting in a periappendiceal mass with adhesion to the adjacent structure, e.g. cecum, etc. This must be distinguished from a tumor or other conditions other than appendicitis, such as endometriosis or walled-off perforated diverticulitis of the adjacent bowel. Rarely, the pus may extend along the parabolic gutter, or spread to cause generalized peritonitis, subhepatic abscess, or pylephlebitis (4). Fistula may rarely be formed between the inflamed appendix and the adjacent organs (4, 9).

Occasionally, acute appendicitis occurs in the appendix with fibrosis of the lumen. Fibrous obliteration may have a protective mechanism (29).

Are histologically normal appendices removed from patients with clinical presentations always normal? Using in situ hybridization techniques, Wang et al. found that seven of 37 histologically normal appendices removed from symptomatic patients expressed tumor necrosis factor α (TNF-α) and interleukin-2 (IL-2) mRNA in germinal centers, submucosa, and lamina propria, both of which are molecular markers for inflammation (34). These findings were similar to those observed in the acutely inflamed appendices but not in the histologically normal appendices removed during elective surgery. At the molecular level, therefore, some of the histologically normal appendices removed from symptomatic patients are inflamed. The pain in these patients is considered to be due to leukotrienes, prostaglandins, serotonin, TNF-α, IL-1, and IL-8 (34).

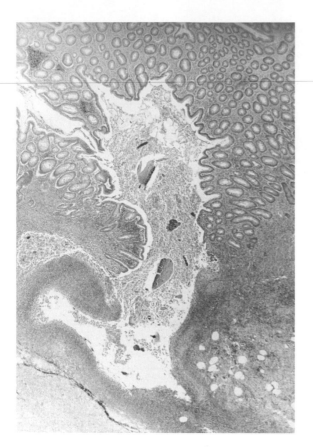

Figure 35.6 Acute gangrenous appendicitis displaying complete destruction of part of the appendiceal wall *(left)*, where only a layer of necrotic tissue is present (Courtesy of Dr. Si-Chun Ming, Temple University School of Medicine, Philadelphia, PA).

CLINICOPATHOLOGIC CORRELATION

In patients whose clinical manifestations are typical, i.e. anorexia, nausea, vomiting, fever, and right lower abdominal pain and tenderness, the diagnosis of acute appendicitis can be accurately made. However, disorders other than appendicitis may present symptoms and signs similar or identical to those of appendicitis (1). Needless to emphasize, the final diagnosis in most of these situations can only be made by pathologic examination. The removed appendices may even be histologically normal. It is well accepted that a certain percentage of appendices that are removed from patients with the clinical presentation of acute appendicitis would show no inflammation on microscopic examination, although the acceptable frequency of errors varies from institution to institution. This problem is probably best illustrated by the scenario created by King Edward VII's acute appendicitis.

In 1902, King Edward VII of England developed violent abdominal pain, nausea, vomiting, fast pulse, fever, and restlessness, which lasted for almost two weeks. That ended three days before his coronation, when his doctors decided that they should not wait any longer. They successfully removed a well-encapsulated abscess in which the appendix was totally destroyed (35). King Edward VII's appendicitis (perityphlitis) had made it a fashionable disease and triggered arguments as to when to operate. This decision remains a difficult one even today because an early and accurate diagnosis of an appendicitis is still a challenge to the surgeons. The highest perforation rate (29%) was associated with the best diagnostic accuracy (89%); the lowest perforation rate (14%) with the worst accuracy (67%) (21). Three percent (3%) of patients with perforated appendicitis died of peritonitis, intra-abdominal abscesses, or Gram-negative septicemia. The mortality rate in nonperforated appendicitis is about 0.1% (1). Morbidity in perforated appendicitis is also more common than in nonperforated appendicitis. To minimize the mortality and morbidity, it is inevitable that some of the appendices removed from patients with clinical symptoms and signs are histologically normal. What is a standard rate of error is not agreed upon. Malt considered that a 23% error rate might be reasonable (21). The diagnosis is difficult in the elderly and very young patients. In an analysis of 126,815 patients, Wen and Naylor found a perforation rate of 30 to 50% among patients over 45 years of age (36). The overall perforation rate was 50% in children under 5 years of age (37). In patients with HIV (human immunodeficiency virus), the clinical presentation is similar to that in those without HIV (38). However, the perforation rate was up to 40% due to diagnostic errors and delays in diagnosis (38, 39).

CHRONIC APPENDICITIS

The existence of chronic appendicitis still is a controversial subject (4). Conceptually, an acute stage of appendicitis may subside and become a chronic stage, among other possible consequences. The mere fibrosis obliterating the lumen may not necessarily result from an inflammatory process. Granulation tissue and fibrosis associated with chronic inflammatory infiltrate are regarded as manifestations of organizing acute appendicitis (4). The only acceptable cases of chronic appendicitis are those showing diffuse chronic inflammation with scarring and removed from patients with symptoms, in whom the symptoms can only be explained by inflammation of the appendix and are completely relieved after appendectomy (40).

ULCERATIVE COLITIS AND CROHN'S DISEASE

Approximately half of the appendices removed from patients with ulcerative colitis involving the right colon also have involvement of the appendix (41). A recent study showed that ulcerative appendicitis was observed in over 85% of the resected colons for ulcerative colitis (42). The involvement of the appendix is almost always part of a generalized colitis but in many specimens, the ulcerative colitis was distal to the appendix. The mucosa shows goblet cell depletion, crypt abscesses in some cases, and mucosal ulceration associated with inflammatory infiltrate, mostly of polymorphonuclear leukocytes. The submucosa may also be infiltrated by inflammatory cells. The lymphocytes and plasma cells are increased in the lamina propria. Some of these inflammatory features are essentially similar to those of ulcerative colitis, but may be difficult to distinguish from those of acute appendicitis (43). The histologic features may change depending on the phase of the disease (41).

Crohn's disease (transmural enteritis) can involve the appendix in approximately 25% of patients with Crohn's disease of the terminal ileum and in more than 50% of patients with colonic Crohn's disease (44). Controversy has been raised by some studies as to whether or not Crohn's disease limited to the appendix exists. Ariel et al. (45) and Dudley and Dean (46) found that none of their patients who had a histologic diagnosis of Crohn's disease of the appendix developed clinical symptoms of Crohn's diseases of other parts of the gastrointestinal tract 2 to 24 years after appendectomy. They concluded that primary Crohn's disease represents an idiopathic granulomatous appendicitis unrelated to Crohn's disease. The granulomas in these appendices were less frequent than those in the appendices involved as part of the generalized Crohn's disease. Huang and Appelman analyzed 20 cases of appendiceal Crohn's disease-like disease (ACLD), which histologically showed features similar to those of the typical Crohn's disease (47). Of the 15 patients with isolated ACLD, followed 5 weeks to 11.5 years, two developed Crohn's disease elsewhere in the bowel. The results of this study strongly suggest that isolated Crohn's disease of the appendix, or ACLD, dose exist. It is obviously a rare occurrence, however. The histologic features alone, including the density of the granulomas, do not always predict the clinical outcome (47). Patients presented with diffuse right lower abdominal pain, all of whom were diagnosed as appendicitis, clinically.

Grossly, the appendix is enlarged with a diameter of 1.5 cm or greater (Fig. 35.7). The microscopic features are basically similar to those of Crohn's disease elsewhere, including mucosal ulceration with polymorphonuclear leukocytic infiltration, transmural thickening by fibrosis, transmural chronic inflammation, noncaseating granulomas and giant cells, and superficial mucosal and submucosal fissures (Figs. 35.8A and 35.8B). However, granulomas are not a requirement for the diagnosis of ACLD (47). When granulomas are present and Crohn's disease is suspected, differential diagnosis of yersiniosis, sarcoidosis, tuberculosis, and other granulomatous diseases should be considered (47). Rarely, adenocarcinoma and carcinoid have been reported arising in the appendices involved by ulcerative colitis or Crohn's disease (48, 49).

ACQUIRED DIVERTICULUM AND DIVERTICULITIS

As previously mentioned in this chapter, acquired diverticula of the appendix are more common than the congenital type. Careful examination of the surgically removed appendix reveals an incidence of approximately 1% (50). They are usually small, 0.2 to 0.5 mm and found along both mesenteric and antimesenteric borders, as single or multiple beaded lesions (51, 52). The diverticula may be the site of inflammation, which may perforate or spread to cause appendicitis (4). Most of diverticula are incidental findings but they commonly show inflammation without involving the adjacent appendix. Their walls are composed of appendiceal mucosa and submucosa, including muscularis mucosa, but not muscularis propria (the congenital diverticula do), probably due to protrusion of these structures through the appendiceal wall resulting from increased luminal pressure (53). Gray Jr. and Wackym have identified diverticula in association with appendicitis, carcinoid and retention mucocele (4). When symptomatic, diverticular disease may clinically be similar to acute appendicitis (50).

INFECTIONS

BACTERIAL INFECTIONS

Most of the surgically removed, acutely inflamed appendices demonstrated, on culture, a variety of bacteria (54) without any particular responsible species. There remain small groups of inflammatory conditions for which a specific agent may be solely responsible. These conditions are presented in this section.

Campylobacter-*associated Appendicitis*

Recently, *Campylobacter* has been found to be responsible for a spectrum of disorders of the digestive system including the appendix (55). Patients with *Campylobacter* infection of the appendix are young, usually children, who often present with an appendicitis-like clinical picture. The appendices are grossly normal but the mesenteric lymph nodes are sometimes found to be swollen at operation.

The histologic abnormalities are similar to those of *Campylobacter* colitis. The mucosa is infiltrated by polymorphonuclear leukocytes and/or eosinophils, with degenerative changes or ulceration. Crypt abscesses may be present. There is subepithelial edema.

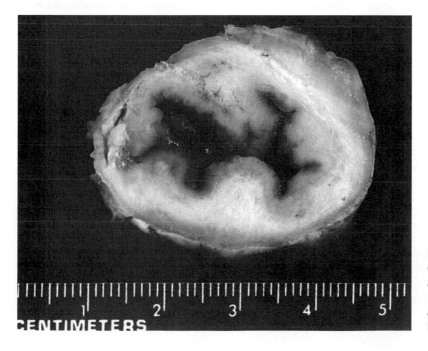

Figure 35.7 Cross section of an appendix involved by Crohn's disease. The entire organ is enlarged and the appendiceal wall is markedly thickened. The patient, a 35 year old woman, presented with symptoms of acute appendicitis. (Courtesy of Dr. Susan Yaron, Riddle Memorial Hospital, Granite Run, PA).

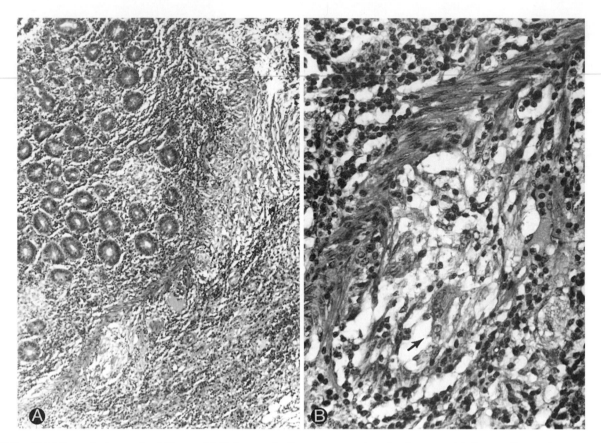

Figure 35.8 **(A)** Microphotograph of Figure 35.7 demonstrating a mucosal and submucosal inflammation, where a noncaseous granuloma is observed. **(B)** Scattered giant cells *(arrow)* are present in the granuloma. (Courtesy of Dr. Susan Yaron, Riddle Memorial Hospital, Granite Run, PA).

Sometimes the infiltration of histiocytes and lymphocytes in the mucosa acquires a granulomatous appearance. The submucosa, muscular layers, and serosa are not involved. Curved rod-shaped microorganisms can be found in the appendiceal lumen using Warthin-Starry indirect immunofluorescence and immunoperoxidase stains, and transmission electron microscopy (55). The offending microorganisms are *Campylobacter jejuni*, which is different from the *Helicobacter* genus (56).

Tuberculosis

Tuberculosis of the appendix more often presents as a part of the gastrointestinal or pulmonary infection than an isolated lesion (57). The rarity of the latter is reflected by the finding of only four cases out of 4,784 appendectomies (58). The patients usually present with symptoms of acute appendicitis. The tuberculous appendix is grossly thickened. The microscopic appearance is characterized by granulomas which usually contain a caseating center surrounded by epithelioid cells, lymphocytes, and histocytes. Despite characteristic features, the diagnosis of tuberculosis has to be confirmed by identifying the bacilli either by acid-fast stain and/or culture (59). In the isolated Tbc of the appendix, as in that of the gastrointestinal tract, the tuberculous bacilli are most likely the bovine type.

Yersinia *Infection*

Yersinia infection (yersiniosis) is caused by *Y. enterocolitica* in man. There have been reports of outbreaks of yersiniosis in the United States, and other countries (60). The patients are most commonly children and young adults who present with abdominal pain and fever. The organisms may be identified in culture and yield positive titers, both of which are important for confirming the diagnosis. Though systemic yersiniosis is usually fatal, enteric yersiniosis is a self-terminating illness (61). Because its clinical picture is often indistinguishable from that of acute appendicitis, many patients undergo an appendectomy.

Y. pseudotuberculosis and *Y. enterocolitica* are different but closely related, pleomorphic Gram-negative coccobacilli. The morphologic features produced by both organisms are similar (61). The mesenteric lymph nodes are almost always enlarged and frequently matted, and fleshy, reddish-grey with yellowish microabscesses. The appendices are either normal or congested. Microscopically, the appendiceal lymphoid follicles are enlarged with prominent reactive germinal centers in which granulomas may be present. The mucosa is infiltrated by eosinophils. The submucosal granulomas may be associated with ulcers of the overlying epithelium. Some of the granulomas have central necrosis, sometimes in the form of microabscess. Periappendiceal inflammation and fibrosis may be marked. Similar granulomas and lymphoid hyperplasia are found in the lymph nodes and other involved parts of the intestine. The differential diagnosis includes Crohn's disease, tuberculosis, sarcoidosis, tularemia, actinomycosis, amebiasis, and schistosomiasis (61).

Spirochetes

Spirochetes have been found in normal and inflamed appendices. Their colonization may account for the symptoms of appendicitis in patients with histologically normal appendices (62).

Actinomyces *Infection*

Actinomyces israelii may invade the appendiceal mucosa, causing mixed inflammation with symptoms indistinguishable from those of acute appendicitis. Colonies are formed by Gram-negative filamentous forms, which can be observed grossly as yellow, friable granules called "sulfur granules" (4). Polymorphonuclear leukocytes are found surrounding these granules and in the adjacent tissue, where granulation tissue and other types of inflammatory infiltrate are also present.

VIRAL INFECTIONS

Virus infection of the appendix is a difficult diagnosis to establish, and may be reflected by lymphoid hyperplasia.

Measles

Measles is a viral infection in which lymphoid hyperplasia of the appendix as well as multinucleated, Warthin-Finkeldey giant cells may be observed, changes that are similar to those of the tonsils and adenoids and may precede the clinical presentation of measles (63). The involvement of the appendix may produce a clinical picture indistinguishable from that of acute appendicitis.

Adenovirus

Adenovirus inclusions have been found in the appendices of young children presenting with ileal or ileocecal intussusception (64, 65). Grossly, the appendix is normal. By light microscopy, the epithelial cells display budlike proliferation and the adjacent surface epithelium is destroyed (65). Eosinophilic inclusions are found in the surface epithelial cells, usually intranuclear and surrounded by a halo (65), but they may also be intracytoplasmic as demonstrated by electron microscopy (64). The submucosal lymphoid follicles show hyperplastic changes.

Mononucleosis

Mononucleosis is caused by Epstein-Barr virus. All lymphoid tissues may be affected. Likewise, the appendix, when involved, shows lymphoid hyperplasia and marked infiltration of large immunoblasts, some of which resemble Reed-Sternberg cells, in the interfollicular zones, expanding the lamina propria (66).

Cytomegalovirus

Cytomegalovirus inclusions have been reported in the appendix of a homosexual man who was not immunosuppressed (67). The appendix was acutely inflamed and ruptured associated with a periappendiceal abscess. The inclusions were found in the histiocytes and endothelial cells but not in the epithelial cells.

PARASITIC INFECTIONS

Parasites are occasionally found in the appendices with or without accompanying inflammation. In their study, Dorfman et al. found parasites in 33 of 3,125 appendices with acute appendicitis; two of 49 with chronic appendicitis; and 15 of 253 normal appendices (68). It is not entirely clear why some parasites become invasive, causing tissue damage which is often complicated by bacterial infection.

Oxyuris vermicularis (pinworm) is the parasite most commonly found in the appendix, usually without associated tissue changes. However, Dorfman et al. found that *Trichuris trichiura* and *Ascaris lumbricoides* were the most common parasites in their series (68). Ashburn reported an incidence of 3% in the United States (69). Gray Jr. and Wackym observed a declining incidence (4). In their hospital, several instances were found annually in the 1950s, but not a single case in the last four years.

Both the worms (Figs. 35.9A and 35.9B) and eggs may be found in the appendiceal lumen. The appendix itself usually shows no tissue reaction. Less frequently, the parasite may be associated with an inflammatory picture indistinguishable from that of acute appendicitis or may be seen in the mucosa, surrounded by numerous eosinophils (70). There are many types of parasites that have been observed in the appendix (Table 35.1) (9, 71–76).

FUNGAL INFECTIONS

Histoplasma encapsulatum was found in 8.8% of 71,000 appendices (9). Rare fungal infections such as coccidioidomycosis, South American blastomycosis, sporotrichosis, cryptococcosis, and geotrichosis have also been reported (9).

SIMPLE OR RETENTION MUCOCELE

Simple or retention mucocele is dilatation of the appendix by accumulation of mucus with no evidence of hyperplasia or neoplasia (77). Patients with mucoceles range from 15 to 71 years of age.

Simple mucoceles are usually small and rarely exceed 5 cm in greatest diameter (Fig. 35.10). In addition to the content of mucin, simple mucoceles are lined by a layer of flattened appendiceal epithelium (Fig. 35.11), or devoid of epithelial lining. Obstruction may play a role in the formation of a mucocele. Experimentally, obstruction of the appendix has resulted in mucoceles in rabbits (78). Granulation tissue with chronic inflammation are observed around the mucus. In rabbits, intraperitoneal injection of chloroform-treated mucocele contents resulted in foreign body peritonitis (79). The mucin may become pearl-like lobules in or outside the mucocele, which has been termed myxoglobulosis (80).

Many authors have used the term "mucocele" to designate any lesions with cystic dilatation due to the accumulation of mucus, including simple mucocele, hyperplasia, or neoplasia. The author recommends that the term "mucocele" should be used for the simple mucocele as defined above and that lesions with mucus-containing cysts should be diagnosed specifically based on the features of which the lesions are composed, e.g. cystadenoma (not benign mucocele), cystadenocarcinoma (not malignant mucocele), etc.

EPITHELIAL HYPERPLASIA

Epithelial (or mucosal) hyperplasia is a benign proliferation of the appendiceal mucosa histologically and cytologically indistinguishable from those of hyperplastic polyps of the large intestine (77, 81, 82).

They occur in patients ranging from the teens to elderly but the majority of patients are over 40 years of age. Women are more often affected than men.

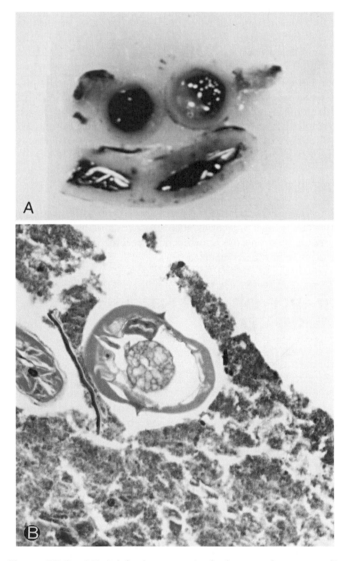

Figure 35.9   (A) Adult pin worms in the lumen of an appendix which is embedded in paraffin. (Courtesy of Dr. Theodore Krause, Episcopal Hospital, Philadelphia, PA). **(B)** Sections of the adult female worms showing ala on the sides, intestine, and uterus.

TABLE 35.1	Some Parasitic Infections of the Vermiform Appendix and Associated Pathologic Changes
Type of Parasite	**Associated Appendiceal Changes**
Oxyuris (Enterobius) vermicularis	No significant changes (majority); appendicitis, abscess
Ascaris lumbricoides[a]	No significant changes; acute appendicitis with or without perforation
Entameba histolytica[b]	Changes similar to those of intestine, mimicking those of appendicitis
Balantidium coli[c]	No significant changes; mucosal ulceration, appendicitis
Schistosoma mansoni[d]	Granulomatous inflammation
Trichuris trichiura[e]	Not mentioned
Trichuris vulpis[e]	Eosinophilic appendicitis
Strongyloides stercoralis[f]	Eosinophilic appendicitis with eosinophilic granuloma
Rictularia[g]	No significant changes

[a]Arean VM, Crandall CA. Ascariasis. In: Marcial-Rojas PA, ed. Pathology of protozoal and helminthic diseases with clinical correlation. Baltimore: Williams & Wilkins, 1971:784.

[b]Perez-Tamayo R, Brandt H. Amebiasis. In: Marcial-Rojas PA, ed. Pathology of protozoal and helminthic diseases with clinical correlation. Baltimore: Williams & Wilkins, 1971:159.

[c]Arean VM, Echevarria R. Balantidiasis. In: Marcial-Rojas PA, ed. Pathology of protozoal and helminthic diseases with clinical correlation. Baltimore: Williams & Wilkins, 1971:238.

[d]Gray GF Jr, Wackym PA. Surgical pathology of the vermiform appendix. In: Sommers SC, Rosen PP, Fechner RE, eds. Norwalk, Conn.: Appleton Century Crofts, Pathology Annual 1986;21(Part 2):111–144.

[e]Kenney M, Yermakov V. Infection of man with trichuris vulpis, the whipworm of dogs. Am J Trop Med Hyg 1980;29:1205–1208.

[f]Noodleman JS. Eosinophilic appendicitis demonstrating strongyloides stercoralis as a causative agent. Arch Pathol Lab Med 1981;105:148–149.

[g]Kenney M, Eveland LK, Yermakov V, et al. A case of riticularia infection of man in New York. Am J Trop Med Hyg 1975;24:596–599.

The gross appearance is often not described or described as normal. In a few cases, the appendices show a slightly dilated lumen with focal or diffuse thickening of the mucosa. Small papillary excrescences may be observed (81). On microscopic examination, the luminal surface of the hyperplastic focus is serrated or finely papillary. Cross sections of the glands show folded epithelium. The columnar cells and goblet cells interspace in an orderly fashion. Loss of lymphoid tissue is a common feature (77). Paneth cells are found in more than half of the cases and argentaffin cells, in all cases (82).

Epithelial hyperplasia of the appendix may be found alone or associated with acute inflammation, mucocele, villous papilloma of the appendix, adenomatous and hyperplastic polyps and adenocarcinoma of the colon, and mucinous cystadenoma of the ovary (81, 82). This lesion was regarded as nonneoplastic by Qizilbash, probably representing a response to mucosal injury (82).

NEOPLASIA

Though similar to the colonic epithelium, the appendiceal epithelium differs from it in that it rarely gives rise to neoplasms, either benign or malignant. Comparison between these two organs would inevitably raise a speculation that this difference is probably attributed to the smaller amount of appendiceal epithelium and the manner in which they are exposed to the environmental factor(s) within their lumens. The etiology and pathogenesis of appendiceal neoplasms are unknown. Table 35.2 shows the abbreviated classification of appendiceal neoplasms.

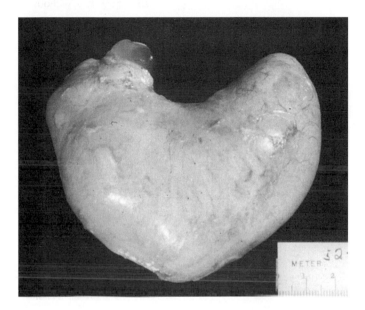

Figure 35.10 Simple mucocele of an appendix showing marked expansion of the organ, apparently as a result of accumulation of mucus. (Courtesy of Dr. Si-Chun Ming, Temple University School of Medicine, Philadelphia, PA).

EPITHELIAL NEOPLASMS

ADENOMA AND CYSTADENOMA

Adenomas of the appendix are benign epithelial tumors, which are usually diffuse lesions involving the entire circumference of the organ, and rarely polypoid. They are less common than their malignant counterparts. When adenomas are cystic, due to large mucus production by the neoplastic cells, they are regarded as cystadenomas.

Adenomas occur in patients ranging from 6 to 90 years of age with the mean age of 58.9 years (77). Clinically they are either asymptomatic, especially when the adenomas are small polypoid lesions measuring less than 1 cm (81), or present with symptoms and signs indistinguishable from those of acute appendicitis, or with a palpable abdominal mass (77, 81). Plain abdominal roentgenogram may demonstrate partial calcification of the wall of the cystadenoma (81).

Grossly, the appendix is either normal-appearing, or diffusely to cystically enlarged (81, 83, 84). The polypoid lesions are small. The diffuse adenomas display thickened mucosa, which is soft, pink, and protrudes into the lumen with many folds. The cystadenomas show a large amount of mucus content upon sectioning (Fig. 35.12), which is gelatinous and glistening. The inner surface may show solid areas. In others, there may be areas of fibrosis, disrupting the integrity of the wall, suggesting a rupture at this site. The mucus escapes from the ruptured site and into the adjacent tissue, creating a mass phenomenon regarding as pseudomyxoma peritonei.

Microscopically, appendiceal adenomas are divided into colonic type and mucinous type adenomas (77). The colonic type adenomas are characterized by increased immature columnar cells with reduction of goblet cells, hyperchromatism, and increased mitotic activities, similar to those of tubular adenomas of the colon. The mucinous type adenomas are more common than the colonic type. They show polypoid, diffuse or villous structures with long, slender, branching papillary projections composed of tall columnar

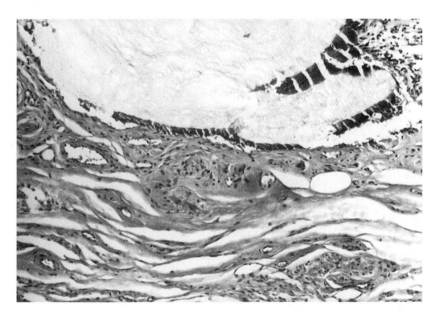

Figure 35.11 The simple mucocele is lined by a single layer of appendiceal epithelium.

cells and fibrovascular cores (Fig. 35.13). The columnar cells have basically located nuclei and often show eosinophilic or vacuolated cytoplasm. In the cross section of the diffuse villous adenoma, the entire circumference is lined by these villous structures. In cystad-

TABLE 35.2	Classification of Neoplasms of the Appendix

Epithelial Neoplasms
  Adenoma and cystadenoma
    Colonic type
    Mucinous type
  Mucinous tumor of unknown malignant potential (UMP).
  Adenocarcinoma and cystadenocarcinoma
    Colonic type
    Mucinous type
Neuroendocrine Neoplasms
  Carcinoids
    Insular
    Tubular
    Clear cell
  Adenocarcinoid (Goblet cell carcinoid)
Composite (chimeric) Neoplasms
  Cystadenoma-adenocarcinoid
  Mixed carcinoid-adenocarcinoma
Mesenchymal Neoplasms
Neural Neoplasms
Lymphoma
Metastatic Neoplasms

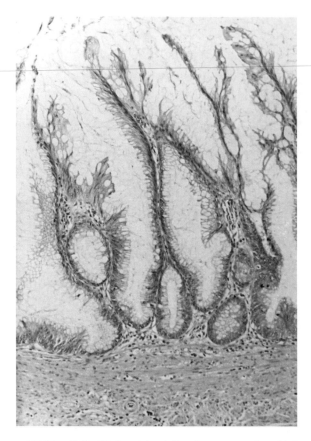

Figure 35.13   Tall villi lined by tall columnar and goblet cells with fibrovascular cores, characteristic of villous adenoma.

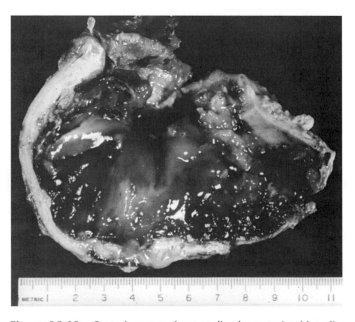

Figure 35.12   Cystadenoma of appendix characterized by glistening, nodular tumor tissue and gelatinous mucus admixed with blood in the cystic cavity. The wall is composed partly of the appendiceal muscular coat and partly by fibrous tissue. (Courtesy of Dr. Theodore Krause, Episcopal Hospital, Philadelphia, PA).

enomas, the neoplastic epithelium shows similar changes but these projections may be pushed toward the wall or even flattened to one cell thick. Mucosal ulceration is commonly present. Argentaffin cells have been found in 11 of 18 cystadenomas (83). Fragments of the neoplastic mucosa may or may not be observed in the pools of mucus in ruptured cystadenomas with fibrosis and acute and chronic inflammation. The neoplastic cells seen outside the appendix may cause difficulty in distinguishing a benign from a malignant tumor. Acellular mucin outside the appendix is usually not evidence of invasion (77).

Occasionally, small foci of well-differentiated adenocarcinoma may appear to arise from an otherwise benign adenoma (85). Some of the appendiceal cystadenomas are associated with ovarian cystadenomas or colonic adenocarcinoma.

Appendiceal cystadenomas have been treated both by simple appendectomy and right hemicolectomy. Follow-up has shown good prognosis even in patients who had mucus extension into the extraappendiceal spaces (81).

MUCINOUS TUMOR OF UNCERTAIN MALIGNANT POTENTIAL

In their recent study, Carr et al. found 20 mucinous appendiceal tumors, which were difficult to classify as either benign or malignant, and therefore, termed mucinous tumors of UMP (uncertain malignant potential) (77). The patients ranged from 24 to 93 years of age, with a mean age of 58.4 years. The most common clinical presentations were right lower quadrant or abdominal mass, followed by symptoms and signs indistinguishable from those of acute appendicitis. Some others were incidental findings at surgery.

Mucinous tumors UMP are composed of well-differentiated tall columnar, mucinous epithelial cells pushing deeply into the underlying tissue but without clear-cut invasion (77). Acellular mucin observed within or outside the appendiceal wall is usually not considered invasion. An irregular border of a well-differentiated mucinous tumor is equivocal in the interpretation of invasion, which may be the only evidence for diagnosing a malignant mucinous tumor. It was because of this difficulty that Carr et al. have separated these tumors from either benign or malignant mucinous tumors, and designated them as mucinous tumors UMP.

Patients with mucinous tumors UMP had a lower mortality rate than those with frank adenocarcinomas. Only two of 18 patients developed recurrence in a follow up period from 12 to 117 months (77). One of the two patients was treated by appendectomy alone.

ADENOCARCINOMA AND CYSTADENOCARCINOMA

Primary carcinomas of the appendix are rare, accounting for less than 0.5% of all gastrointestinal neoplasms (86). The rarity of appendiceal adenocarcinoma is also reflected by the finding of only 57 cases of 71,000 appendices (0.08%) (9). Adenocarcinoma and cystadenocarcinoma are two different forms of the same disease, namely, malignant epithelial tumor. They occur in patients from the second to the ninth decades, with the mean age around the mid-fifties (77, 86). Men are slightly more often affected than women.

Clinically the patients most commonly present with symptoms of acute appendicitis, followed by palpable masses, or other non-specific complaints. Some patients were operated for diseases of other organs, such as colonic carcinoma or ovarian tumor, and the appendiceal carcinomas were found incidentally. At operation, it is not unusual that the surgeon finds an inflammatory mass and requests an examination by a pathologist, who in turn diagnoses carcinoma on a frozen section. Occasionally, primary appendiceal adenocarcinoma presents as a uterine tumor (87) or bilateral

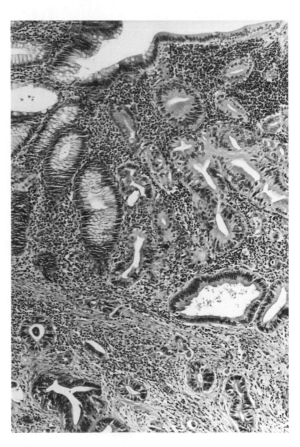

Figure 35.15   Noncystic well-differentiated adenocarcinoma of an appendix. The irregular, neoplastic glands invade the muscular wall. The tumor cells are pleomorphic and hyperchromatic. (Courtesy of Dr. Telesforo Reyes, North Arundel Hospital, Glen Burnie, MD).

Krukenberg tumors (81). It is extremely difficult to arrive at a precise clinical diagnosis of appendiceal adenocarcinoma. For instance, in one study none of the 94 patients was diagnosed to have appendiceal carcinomas preoperatively (86).

The gross appearance of a carcinomatous appendix may be indistinguishable from that of an acute appendicitis with walled-off perforation. The appendix is usually irregularly enlarged in the portion that is involved by the carcinoma and the accompanying fibrosis (Fig. 35.14). The latter may cause adhesion with the serosal surface of the adjacent cecum or other organ(s). The tumor is composed of creamy white or yellow-tan, hard tissue. In the cystic variant, the tumor is cystic due to the accumulation of varying amounts of mucus. The cystadenocarcinoma is grossly indistinguishable from its benign counterpart (81). When the mucus has accumulated in the tissue outside the cystic tumor, either through rupture or from production by infiltrating tumor cells, it is invariably accompanied with fibrosis and inflammation resulting in pseudomyxoma peritonei. Fibrous adhesion with the neighboring organ(s) may be extensive. A fistula tract may be formed (Fig. 35.15).

Microscopically, appendiceal adenocarcinomas are divided into mucinous and nonmucinous colonic types; the former are more common than the latter (77). The mucinous carcinomas consist of at least 50% of mucinous component and are composed of usually

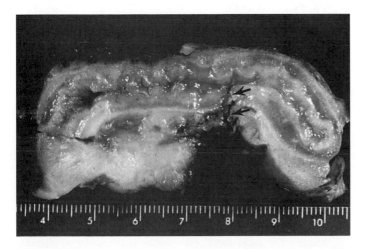

Figure 35.14   Noncystic adenocarcinoma of the appendix. The appendiceal mucosa and wall are markedly thickened by firm tumor and fibrous tissue, which is seen extending to the periappendiceal fat. A fistula tract is identified *(arrows)*.

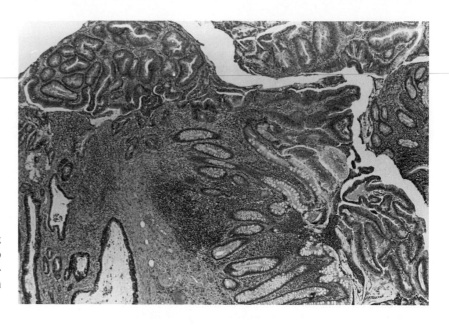

Figure 35.16   An epithelial tumor of the appendix showing transitional changes from the normal to adenomatous epithelium with focal adenocarcinoma. Foci of well differentiated adenocarcinoma are also seen invading the appendiceal wall.

well-differentiated, tall columnar epithelial cells. They may be noncystic, or cystic due to the accumulation of mucin. Because the clear differentiation of the tumor cells, mucinous adenocarcinomas may be difficult to distinguish from mucinous adenomas. Unless there is metastasis to lymph nodes(s) or organ(s), the only reliable criterion for diagnosing adenocarcinoma is invasion of the appendiceal wall or tissue outside the appendix (77, 81, 88, 89). Well-differentiated mucinous tumors displaying equivocal invasion have been classified as mucinous tumors UMP (77). The colonic type adenocarcinomas are composed of irregular glandular structures with focal clustering of tumor cells (Fig. 35.15). The tumor cells themselves are more atypical than those of appendiceal adenomas in that their nuclei are more pleomorphic and hyperchromatic. Approximately 38% of appendiceal adenocarcinomas were associated with lymph node metastasis (86). Other metastatic sites include liver, peritoneum, and lung (90). Occasionally, the neoplastic epithelium displays irregular microglandular patterns and markedly atypical columnar cells, which are indistinguishable from those of adenocarcinoma of the colonic type, thus allowing a carcinoma diagnosis even in the absence of invasion. Appendiceal adenocarcinomas can be graded into grades I, II, and III, representing well-differentiated, moderately-differentiated, and poorly-differentiated adenocarcinomas. Adenocarcinomas may be found arising in a background of adenocarcinoid (77), which were mucinous type and behaved similarly to appendiceal adenocarcinomas without such a background (77). Signet-ring cell carcinomas may rarely be observed in the appendix.

Adenomatous epithelium may be observed in continuity with the malignant component (Fig. 35.16). This association would naturally raise the possibility that there is an adenoma-carcinoma sequence. It is well accepted that this probably is the case in colonic neoplasms as it is supported by the remarkably common findings of carcinoma in colonic polyps, especially the villous type, and by follow-up study (91). Though a follow-up study of this type is impossible in appendiceal neoplasms, an endorsement of this concept is reasonable because of the close similarity between the two epithelia. In some other instances, the malignant epithelium may be seen in connection with the normal-appearing appendiceal epithe-

	TABLE 35.3 **Pathologic Staging of Appendiceal Carcinomas**	
	AJCC/UICC	Astler and Coller (Modified Dukes)
Stage 0	Carcinoma in situ; (Tis) no metastasis	
Stage I	Tumor invades the submucosa (T_1)	A
	No metastasis (N0; M0)	
	Tumor invades the muscularis propria (T_2)	B_1
	No metastasis (N0; M0)	
Stage II	Tumor invades through the muscularis propria and into the subserosa or mesentery (T_3)	B_2
	No metastasis (N0; M0)	
	Tumor directly invades other organs or structures and/or perforates the appendiceal peritoneum (T_4)	B_2
Stage III	Any T, metastasis to 1–3 regional lymph nodes (N_1), M0	C_1 or $_2$
	Any T, metastasis to 4 or more regional lymph nodes (N_2), M0	
Stage IV	Any T, any N and distant metastasis (M_1)	D

For Astler and Coller modification 1 = invasion of, but not through, muscularis propria; 2 = invasion through the subserosa or directly into adjacent organs.

Modified from Beahr OH, Henson DE, Hutter RVP, Kennedy BJ, eds. Manual for staging of cancer. 4th ed. Philadelphia: JB Lippincott, 1992.

lium. One must question then: Is the phenotypically normal epithelium undergoing a subtle, preneoplastic change?

Staging for appendiceal carcinomas is the same as that for colorectal carcinomas (92), the parameters are summarized in Table 35.3. Because mucin is observed frequently outside the appendix in adenocarcinoma and mucinous tumors UMP, the status of the primary tumor may be difficult to determine. Carr et al.

designate the tumor with acellular mucin as mucin-T, and mucin with neoplastic cells as cell-T (77). For instance, a tumor with neoplastic cells in the muscularis propria and acellular mucin in the serosa would be a cell-T2 and mucin-T3. A carcinoma with neoplastic cells in the serosa but acellular mucin beyond the visceral peritoneum would be a cell-T3 and mucin-T4.

The overall 5-year survival ranged from 55 to 65% (77, 86). The survival, however, may be affected by many parameters. According to their study, Nitcheki found that the grade of a tumor correlated with prognosis; the 5-year survival rates were 68%, 51%, and 7% for grades I, II, and III adenocarcinomas, respectively (86). Patients with mucinous carcinomas had a better 5-year survival than those with the colonic type (71% and 41%, respectively). When the Astler and Coller's modification of Dukes' staging was correlated with the outcome, the 5-year survival rates were 100%, 67%, 50%, and 6% for Astler and Coller's stages A, B, C, and D, respectively. The presence of acellular mucin outside the right lower quadrant of the abdomen and the presence of tumor cells outside the appendix reduced the survival (77). Acellular mucin outside the appendix and confined in the right lower quadrant did not significantly affect the survival.

The operative management is also a prognostic factor. Patients who underwent right hemicolectomy had a 5-year survival rate of 68% but those who underwent appendectomy alone, 20% (86).

No significant association was found between survival and age, sex, histologic patterns (for example, villous, undulating), or desmoplasia (77).

APPENDICEAL NEOPLASMS WITH SYNCHRONOUS AND METACHRONOUS NEOPLASMS OF OTHER ORGANS

Adenocarcinoma of the appendix may be present synchronously with adenomatous or villous adenomas or carcinoma of the colon. Eleven percent of patients with appendiceal adenocarcinomas had synchronous colorectal carcinomas (77), and less frequently,

metachronous colorectal carcinomas (77, 86). Other second malignant tumors reported included neoplasms of the ovary, pancreas, uterus, breast, kidney, prostate, hematopoietic, lung, thyroid, cartilage, esophagus, stomach, and bladder, and melanoma (77, 93).

Of particular interest are the synchronous appendiceal and ovarian mucinous tumors, either mucinous tumor of low malignant potential or mucinous adenocarcinomas. The association inevitably raises some questions: Are they two independent primaries? Is one the primary (either appendiceal or ovarian) and the other, a metastasis? A clinicopathologic study and comparative analysis of c-Ki-ras mutation showed that the pattern of the c-Ki-ras mutation was identical in the appendiceal and ovarian tumors in all six patients, suggesting that they are not independent tumors (94). In another study, Chuaqui et al. found that the genetic alteration occurred at 17q21.3-22 only in the ovarian tumors but not the appendiceal carcinomas in three cases, suggesting two independent primaries (95). In other cases, the loss of heterozygosity at the same loci was found in both the appendiceal and ovarian tumors, suggesting a single primary with metastasis to the other organ.

PSEUDOMYXOMA PERITONEI

Pseudomyxoma peritonei is characterized by implantation of mucus-producing epithelial cells on the peritoneal surface and accumulation of mucus in the peritoneal cavity (Figs. 35.17A and 35.17B) (4). Rupture of a cystadenoma or a cystadenocarcinoma of either appendiceal or ovarian origin, or invasion by a cystadenocarcinoma may result in pseudomyxoma peritonei. The accumulation of mucus in the peritoneum is invariably associated with polymorphonuclear leukocytic infiltration and granulation tissue in the adjacent areas, with fibrosis. The pseudomyxoma peritonei due to benign lesions may be self-limited whereas those resulting from a malignant lesion have a poor prognosis (81). Adhesions and intestinal obstruction are frequent complications (4). The presence

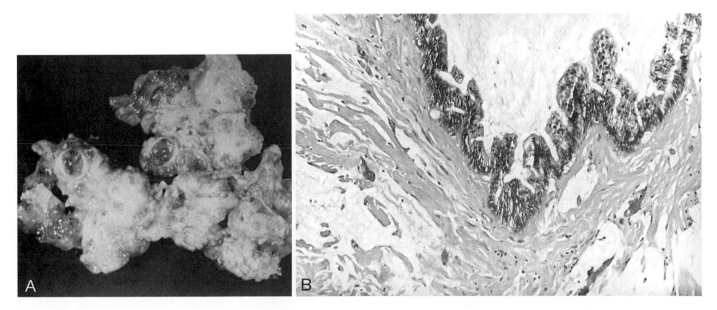

Figure 35.17   (A) Gross appearance of a pseudomyxoma peritonei. Lakes of the mucin are surrounded by firm, white tissue. **(B)** Microscopically, the firm areas are mostly fibrous connective tissue in which irregular, neoplastic glands are observed.

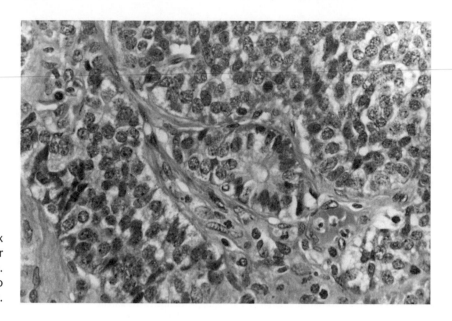

Figure 35.18 Carcinoid tumor of an appendix characterized by sheets of relatively uniform tumor cells with round to oval nuclei and scanty cytoplasm. A small gland is also seen (Courtesy of Dr. Telesforo Reyes, North Arundel Hospital, Glen Burnie, MD).

or absence of neoplastic cells in pseudomyxoma peritonei is an important prognostic factor. Therefore, the term should be limited to describing the gross appearance and should not be a pathologic diagnosis (77).

NEUROENDOCRINE NEOPLASMS

CARCINOID TUMOR

Carcinoid tumor of the appendix is an endocrine tumor histologically and cytologically similar to but biologically less aggressive than carcinoids arising from other parts of the gastrointestinal tract. The incidence of carcinoids is 0.32% (a 0.06 to 0.69% range) in surgically removed appendices; in an autopsy series, 0.054% (a 0.009 to 0.17% range) (96). They are the most common tumors of the appendix. Young adults ranging from 20 to 39 years of age are most often affected compared with other age groups. They are rare in children and adolescents but are still the most common gastrointestinal tract tumors in this age group (97). They occur more often in women than men. This has been attributed to the fact that women undergo appendectomy more often than men.

The majority of appendiceal carcinoids are less than 2 cm when discovered, and approximately 70% of carcinoids are located in the tip of the organ. The body of appendix is involved in 22% and the base 7%. Both the small size and the location probably explain why the majority of the patients are asymptomatic. The symptomatic patients most often present with symptoms and signs of appendicitis and only occasionally are their symptoms related to the obstruction of the lumen. Patients may rarely present with carcinoid syndrome (4) and Cushing's syndrome (98).

Appendiceal carcinoid tumors are oval or round, especially those arising in the tip, or appear to be a thickening of the wall. The tumors are usually firm, homogenous, and grey to yellow. Because of their small size, they are often overlooked grossly and only become evident microscopically. The appendiceal carcinoids are composed of uniform tumor cells with round to oval nuclei and relatively scanty amounts of cytoplasm. The majority of carcinoids are insular type, which are composed of sheets, nests or microglandular structures, or cords of tumor cells (Fig. 35.18). The periphery

of the sheets shows a palisading pattern characterized by parallel arrangement of their nuclei; inside, the tumor cells may form small, round structures, the microglandular pattern. The cytoplasm may show vacuolation. Mitoses are virtually absent. Other cases have been subclassified as tubular carcinoids, which are composed of tumor cells forming tubular structures and short trabeculae (99). They show different immunohistochemical characteristics when compared with the insular type. Particularly, the tubular carcinoids were positive for glucagon but the insular were negative (99). Using in situ hybridization, Shaw and Pringle detected proglucagon mRNA in all tubular carcinoids but none of the insular carcinoids (100). The appendiceal wall is often invaded by tumor. Lymphatic invasion is common. Both of these features are somewhat paradoxical to the excellent prognosis of the appendiceal carcinoids. Some carcinoids were positive for both Masson-Fontana (argentaffin) and Grimelius (argyrophil) (101, 102) whereas the tubular type was negative for argentaffinity (99). Immunohistochemical studies have showed that they were positive for many markers and some conflicting results came from different studies (Table 35.4). Electron microscopy demonstrates neurosecretory granules, similar to those of carcinoid tumor cells arising elsewhere.

While the histologic, immunohistochemical, and ultrastructural features have demonstrated the endocrine nature of appendiceal carcinoid, the histogenesis is somewhat controversial. The anatomic location and the histologic appearance and the similarity of the silver staining to that of the midgut carcinoids would support the concept that appendiceal carcinoids are midgut carcinoids, but some others have raised doubt primarily due to the much better behavior of appendiceal carcinoids than those of the jejunoileal carcinoids (101, 102). Based on the distribution of the nonneoplastic and neoplastic endocrine cells (101) and differential immunohistochemical staining between jejunoileal and appendiceal carcinoids, Moyana et al. and Wilander et al. suggest that appendiceal carcinoids arise from the subepithelial neuroendocrine complex (101, 102).

The prognosis of appendiceal carcinoids is excellent. None of the patients who had tumors less than 2 cm developed either recurrence or metastasis, or died of tumor 5 to 25 years after simple appendectomy (96, 103, 104). Patients with localized carcinoids larger than 2 cm also had an excellent prognosis. The appendiceal carcinoids invade the mesoappendix and metastasize to the regional lymph nodes in 1.4 to 8.8% of the cases (4). The metastasizing tumors are usually larger than 2 cm; the small tumors rarely metastasize (4). Extension into the periappendiceal fat alone is not a significant factor for metastasis or prognosis (97, 103). However, those who had carcinoids larger than 2 cm as well as unresectable metastasis at the time of operation may have a fatal outcome (103). Flow cytometric DNA analysis showed that two of seven carcinoids were aneuploid; one of the two carcinoids was associated with metastasis (105). Appendiceal carcinoids in patients less than 20 years of age are small tumors. Only five of 115 patients had carcinoids larger than 2 cm (97). They are rarely life threatening in this age group, even in patients with tumors larger than 2 cm and metastasis (97).

ADENOCARCINOID

Adenocarcinoid of the appendix is a tumor composed of both mucin-producing and endocrine cells. Since the first report in 1969, this appendiceal tumor has been termed adenocarcinoid, mucinous carcinoid, goblet cell carcinoid, and crypt cell carcinoma (106–110). The patients range in age from their 20s to 70s, with a mean age around 55 years. The symptomatic patients present with symptoms of appendicitis (108). Adenocarcinoids may

be an incidental finding, or rarely, present as bilateral ovarian tumors (111).

Similar to the conventional appendiceal carcinoid, adenocarcinoids are usually located in the distal portion of the appendix and less frequently, in the middle portion and the base. The tumor may sometimes be grossly inapparent, diffusely infiltrating the appendix without forming a discrete nodule. They usually involve an area of 1.0 to 1.8 cm (106). Grossly, adenocarcinoids are yellow to grey-white, soft or gelatinous. The microscopic appearance is characterized by microglandular formation and small nests composed of goblet cells (Fig. 35.19) filled with PAS-positive and Alcian blue-positive mucin (108). In some cases, the goblet cells may fuse and the tumor cells are identical to signet-ring cells. Focally, the tumor cells appear to arise from the crypt of Lieberkuhn (Fig. 35.19). Mitotic figures ranged from none to seven per ten high power fields, with an average of one per ten HPF (108). The submucosa, muscular wall, and the serosa are often infiltrated by tumor cells.

The histogenesis of adenocarcinoid is controversial. Supporting both the glandular and endocrine components are the findings of mucin content and neurosecretory granules in the tumor cells (108, 112). Recent studies have showed that adenocarcinoids were positive for serotonin, chromogranin, CEA, cytokeratin, HPP (108), and PYY in some cases (109). Table 35.4 shows the results of some immunohistologic studies (99, 102, 109, 113–115). Furthermore, the combination of adenocarcinoid and mucinous cystad-

TABLE 35.4	Immunohistochemical Markers in Appendiceal Neuroendocrine Tumors		
Markers	Insular Carcinoids	Tubular Carcinoids	Adenocarcinoids
Serotonin	D Pos[a,b,d]	Neg[a]	Pos[a]
Chromogranin	D Pos[a,b]	Variable; Weakly Pos[a]	Pos[a,c]
NSE	D Pos[a]	D Pos[a]	Neg[a,c]
CEA	Neg to F Pos[a]	D Pos[a]	D Pos[a]
Cytokeratin	F Pos[a]	D Pos[a]; Neg[b]	D Pos[a]
Glucagon	Neg[a]	D Pos[a]	Neg[a,c]
PYY	Pos[d]		
S-100	Pos in tumor[b,g] Pos around tumor[a,e]		
Calbindin-D	Pos[f]		
Protein gene product			Pos[c]
HPP			Pos[a,c]

D = Diffusely, Pos = Positive, Neg = Negative, F = Focal, PYY = Polypeptide YY, HPP = Human pancreatic polypeptide.

[a]Burke AP, Sobin LH, Federspiel BH, et al. Appendiceal carcinoids: correlation of histology and immunohistochemistry. Mod Pathol 1989;2:630–637.

[b]Wilander E, Scheibenpflug L. Cytokeratin expression in small intestinal and appendiceal carcinoids. A basis for classification. Acta Oncologica 1993;32:131–134.

[c]Anderson NH, Somerville JE, Johnston CF, et al. Appendiceal goblet cell carcinoids: a clinicopathological and immunohistochemical study. Histopathology 1991;18:61–65.

[d]Iwafuchi M, Watanbe H, Ajioka Y, et al. Immunohistochemical and ultrastructural studies of twelve argentaffin and six argyrophil carcinoid of the appendix vermiformis. Hum Pathol 1990;21:773–780.

[e]Goddard MJ, Lonsdale RN. The histogenesis of appendiceal carcinoid tumours. Histopathology 1992;20:345–349.

[f]Katsetos CD, Jami MM, Krishna L, et al. Novel immunohistochemical localization of 28000 molecular-weight (Mr) calcium binding protein (calbindin-D28k) in enterochromaffin cells of the human appendix and neuroendocrine tumors (carcinoids and small-cell carcinomas) of the midgut and foregut. Arch Pathol Lab Med 1994;118:633–639.

[g]Moyana TN, Satkunam N. A comparative immunohistochemical study of jejunoileal and appendiceal carcinoids. Implications for histogenesis and pathogenesis. Cancer 1992;70:1081–1088.

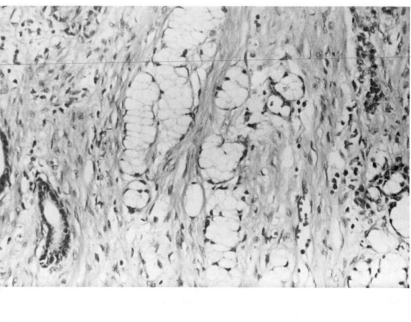

Figure 35.19 Adenocarcinoid of an appendix displaying prominent goblet cells. The tumor cells form small clusters of glandular structures infiltrating the lamina propria and appendiceal wall.

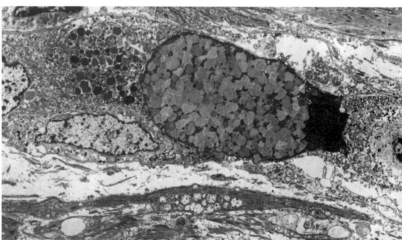

Figure 35.20 Electron micrograph of an adenocarcinoid showing prominent mucous granules in the cytoplasm of a neoplastic goblet cell and neurosecretory granules in two neighboring endocrine cells, one on the right and another, below the goblet cell. Apposing the left of the goblet cell is another cell containing both mucous and neurosecretory granules. (Courtesy of Dr. Bruce Elfenbein, Professor of Pathology, Temple University Hospital and School of Medicine, Philadelphia, PA).

enoma (116), and of adenocarcinoma and goblet cell carcinoid support the two different components (77, 108). The ultrastructural studies have shown few endocrine cells but no convincing evidence of mucin and secretory granules in the same cell (117, 118). An adenocarcinoid examined by us shows neoplastic mucin-containing and endocrine cells, and cells that contain both types of granules (Fig. 35.20). When both serotonin and mucosubstance are found in the same tumor cells, adenocarcinoid represents an amphicrine carcinoma (119). In Isaacson's study, however, the immunohistochemical stains demonstrated lysozyme, secretory component, and IgA, all of which are also present in the small intestine crypt cells but absent in the conventional carcinoids (117). Furthermore, only a few endocrine cells and scattered Paneth cells were mixed with the mucin-containing cells, prompting him to suggest that adenocarcinoids of the appendix are derived from the lysozyme-producing cells of the type normally present in the small intestinal crypts (117).

The behavior of adenocarcinoids is usually considered to be intermediate between that of conventional carcinoids and that of

adenocarcinomas of the appendix (106, 107, 112). When 23 of the original adenocarcinoids reported by Warkel were reviewed, seven were reclassified as mixed carcinoid-adenocarcinoma, without knowledge of the follow-up data (108). All seven patients developed metastases and died of disease in an average follow-up period of 71.3 months. The remaining 16 tumors were classified as goblet cell carcinoid; all 16 patients were alive in a mean follow-up period of 97 months. These observations raise a questions as to how many of the reported appendiceal adenocarcinoids represent mixed carcinoid-adenocarcinomas.

COMPOSITE (CHIMERIC) NEOPLASMS

Sporadic cases of combined mucinous cystadenoma and adenocarcinoid have been reported in the literature (116). As discussed in the section of adenocarcinoid, the glandular structures may show features of adenocarcinomas as prominent or major components in a background of adenocarcinoid. Appendiceal tumors comprising these diverse features have been regarded as mixed carcinoid-adenocarcinomas (108). The poor prognosis of patients with this type of tumor has prompted Burke et al. and Carr et al. to analyze these composite tumors as adenocarcinomas.

This chimeric phenomenon suggests that the different elements are either derived from a stem cell with divergent differentiation, or two different cells undergo neoplastic processes simultaneously.

Mesenchymal Neoplasms
LEIOMYOMA AND LEIOMYOSARCOMA

Both benign and malignant, smooth muscle tumors are rare. In a series of 8,699 appendices, two of the 101 appendiceal tumors were leiomyomas (120). Collins found an incidence of 1.7% in 71,000 appendices (9). In his series, leiomyomas were the most common benign tumors of the appendix. The leiomyomas are small and are usually incidental findings. The largest appendiceal leiomyoma recorded measured 15 × 11 × 12 cm and weighed 480 g (121).

The two reported appendiceal leiomyosarcomas were highly cellular and displayed marked cellular pleomorphism and high mitotic rate. Both patients died of advanced tumor within six months (122).

Neural Neoplasms
GRANULAR CELL TUMOR

Granular cell tumors of the appendix are rare. In a review of 74 granular cell tumors of the gastrointestinal tract, Johnston and Helwig found four cases of appendiceal origin (123). They should be distinguished from the degenerated smooth muscle cells (124).

NEUROMA

Neuromas are uncommon and usually located in the tip of the appendix. They can also be found in appendices with fibrous obliteration (125).

GANGLIONEUROMA

Ganglioneuromas of the appendix have been described in the literature (126). They range in size from a few millimeters to a pedunculated mass, causing obstruction of the lumen and appendicitis.

Lymphoma

Though the gastrointestinal tract is the most common extranodal site of primary lymphoma, the appendix is rarely affected (127, 128). Lymphoma of the appendix is more often an extension of the intestinal tumor than a solitary lesion. The overall incidence of primary appendiceal lymphoma is approximately 0.064% in 71,000 appendices (9). Pasquale et al. found 46 reported appendiceal lymphomas in the literature from 1898 to 1994 (128). They may occur both in adults and children, with the mean age of 25.7 years. Most patients presented with right lower quadrant pain and less frequently, a mass.

The pathologic features of the appendiceal lymphoma are those of non-Hodgkin's lymphomas, including the Burkitt's type

(127, 129). Follow-up information was available in 28 of the 46 primary reviewed by Pasquale et al.; only two patients died of primary lymphoma of the appendix (128).

Metastatic Neoplasms

Though only infrequently, carcinomas of the breast, stomach, bronchus, and prostate can metastasize to the appendix (130–132). Metastatic breast carcinoma and prostatic carcinoma may be difficult to distinguish from carcinoid tumors. Metastatic gastric signet-ring cell carcinoma may resemble adenocarcinoid (4). A Kaposi's sarcoma was found in the appendix as one of multiple foci in a patient afflicted with AIDS (133).

MISCELLANEOUS LESIONS
FIBROUS OBLITERATION

Fibrous obliteration is characterized by occlusion of a portion of the entire appendiceal lumen by bland fibrous tissue, replacing the normal mucosal and lymphoid components. It was found in 35% of 71,000 appendices (91% were surgical, the remaining autopsy specimens) (9). Most of these demonstrated obliteration of segments of the appendiceal lumens. In Butler's series, 14% of 276 surgically removed appendices showed fibrous obliteration (29). Kazzaz demonstrated argentaffin and argyrophil cells in the neuroma-like structures and suggested that the argentaffin and argyrophil cells migrate and cause hyperplasia of the nerve plexus leading to obstruction of the lumen (125). The lack of pre-existing appendicitis led to the belief that fibrous obliteration is a developmental event rather than the end stage of inflammation (134).

SARCOIDOSIS

The appendix may rarely be involved in sarcoidosis (135). The appendix shows noncaseating granulomas, with or without concomitant acute appendicitis. Since the granulomas are not diagnostic for sarcoidosis, infectious granulomas, Crohn's disease or other conditions which may cause granulomas must be considered in the differential diagnosis.

PERIAPPENDICITIS

Periappendicitis is a condition in which the inflammatory infiltrate is seen in the serosa and periappendiceal adipose tissue, usually secondary to an inflammatory process in the adjacent organs. The appendix proper is devoid of inflammation, although a severe case of periappendicitis may spread into the appendiceal wall. The common origins of periappendicitis is salpingitis, ileal Crohn's disease, Meckel's diverticulitis, etc. (4).

INTUSSUSCEPTION

Intussusception of the appendix occurs rarely; less than 200 cases have been reported in the medical literature (136). They occur more often in males than in females and in patients ranging from ten months to 75 years with the average age of 16 years. Clinically, intussusception may be asymptomatic or present with symptoms and signs of intussusception or those mimicking acute appendicitis. There are four types of intussusception of the appendix: the tip of the appendix is the intussusceptum and its proximal portion is the intussuscepien, the base of the appendix is the intussusceptum and the cecum is the intussuscepien, the proximal portion of the appendix is the intussusceptum and its distal part is the intussuscepien, and complete inversion of the appendix (inside out appendix) with accompanying ileocecal intussusception. All four types are well diagrammatically illustrated by Langsam et al. (136). Intussusception develops when the peristalsis of the appendix is increased or becomes irregular due to the foreign bodies, endometriosis, mucoceles, neoplasms, etc. (136).

ENDOMETRIOSIS

The appendix is an unusual site of endometriosis. However, when the intestinal tract is involved the appendix is often one of the affected sites, found in approximately one-third of the patients (137). Endometriosis is either an incidental finding or clinically present symptoms mimicking those of appendicitis. Foci of endometrial gland and stroma are found in the serosa or the appendiceal wall, which may or may not be associated with inflammation. There may be an associated muscular hyperplasia, forming a mass (138).

ARTERITIS

Arteritis may be found in up to 1% of appendices (4). Almost all of these cases are local and asymptomatic although the histologic features are indistinguishable from those of systemic arteritis nodosa. A case of polyarteritis nodosa, which presented as acute appendicitis, was reported recently (139). Necrotizing vasculitis was found in this surgically removed appendix without evidence of appendicitis.

CYSTIC FIBROSIS

Cystic fibrosis may clinically mimic "chronic appendicitis," resulting in appendectomy (140). The appendix showed increased activity of the mucus-secreting cells with mucus filling the distended crypts. Exceptionally, the appendiceal lumen may be markedly distended by the viscid mucus, resulting in the appearance of a mucocele.

SEPTA

Septa in the appendix has recently been described (141). By sectioning the appendix longitudinally, the septae are found to be complete and incomplete. All cases were found to be associated with acute appendicitis. Therefore, the question as to whether it is a congenital or an acquired lesion cannot be answered.

OTHER CONDITIONS

Melanosis (4), malakoplakia (142), Whipple's disease (143), and numerous other conditions (9) have been observed in the appendix.

APPENDICEAL DISORDERS IN PATIENTS WITH HIV

Acute appendicitis is not infrequent in HIV patients (38, 39). Other disorders that have been reported include metastatic Kaposi's sarcoma, cytomegalovirus, and streptococcus and mycobacterium

infections (133, 144, 145). The lymphoid tissue of the appendix may be affected. For instance, the author has observed that the lymphoid tissue was completely depleted in a patient who died of AIDS.

REFERENCES

1. Schwartz SI. Appendix. In: Schwartz SI, Shires GT, Spencer FC, Husser WC, eds. Principles of Surgery. New York: McGraw-Hill, 1994:1307–1318.
2. Moore KL, Persaud TVN. The developing human: clinically oriented embryology. 5th ed. Philadelphia: WB Saunders, 1993:251–254.
3. Segal GH, Petras RE. Vermiform appendix. In: Sternberg SS, ed. Histology for pathologists. New York: Raven Press, 1992:593–605.
4. Gray GF Jr, Wackym PA. Surgical pathology of the vermiform appendix. In: Sommers SC, Rosen PP, Fechner RE, eds. Norwalk, Conn.: Appleton Century Crofts, Pathology Annual 1986;21(Part 2):111–144.
5. Rode J, Dhillon AP, Papdaki L. Serotonin-immunoreactive cells in the lamina propria plexus of the appendix. Hum Pathol 1983;14:464–469.
6. Huang JMS, Krumbhaar EB. The amount of lymphoid tissue of the human appendix and its weight at different age periods. Am J Med Sci 1940;199:75–83.
7. Spencer J, Finn T, Isaacson PG. Gut associated lymphoid tissue: a morphological and immunocytochemical study of the human appendix. Gut 1985;26:672–679.
8. Emery JL, Underwood J. The neurological junction between the appendix and ascending colon. Gut 1970;11:118–120.
9. Collins DC. 71,000 human appendix specimens: a final report summarizing 40 years' study. Am J Protocol 1963;14:365–381.
10. Bremner DN, Mooney G. Agenesis of appendix: a further thalidomide anomaly [letter]. Lancet 1978;1:826e.
11. Rolff M, Jepsen LV, Hoffman J. The "absent" appendix. Arch Surg 1992;127:992.
12. Waugh TR. Appendix vermiform duplex. Arch Surg 1941;42:311–320.
13. George DH. Diverticulosis of the vermiform appendix in patients with cystic fibrosis. Hum Pathol 1987;18:75–79.
14. Favara BE. Multiple congenital diverticular of the vermiform appendix. Am J Clin Pathol 1968;49:60–64.
15. Mikat DM, Mikat KW. Appendix helicus: a unique anomaly of the vermiform appendix. Gastroenterology 1976;71:304–305.
16. Stone WD, Hendrix TR, Schuster MM. Aganglionosis of the entire colon in an adolescent. Gastroenterol 1965;48:636–641.
17. Merck C, Kindblom LG. Neurofibromatosis of the appendix in von Recklinghausen's disease. A report of a case. Acta Pathol Microbiol Scan Sect A 1975;83:623–627.
18. Aubrey DA. Gastric mucosa in the vermiform appendix. Arch Surg 1970;101:628–629.
19. Droga BW, Levine S, Baber JJ. Heterotopic gastric and esophageal tissue in the vermiform appendix. Am J Clin Pathol 1963;40:190–193.
20. Fitz RH. Perforating inflammation of the vermiform appendix: with special references to its early diagnosis and treatment. Am J Med Sci 1886;92:321–346.
21. Malt RA. The perforated appendix [Editorial]. N Engl J Med 1986;315:1546–1547.
22. Burkitt DP. The aetiology of appendicitis. Br J Surg 1971;58:695–699.
23. Sleisinger MH. Acute appendicitis (including the acute abdomen), In: Wyngaarden JB, Smith LH Jr, Bennett JC, eds. Cecil's textbook of medicine. Philadelphia: WB Saunders, 1992:746–749.
24. MaCahy P. Continuing fall in the incidence of acute appendicitis. Ann Roy Col Surg Engl 1994;76:282–283.
25. Wangansteen OH, Bowers WF. Significance of the obstructive factor in the genesis of acute appendicitis. An experimental study. Arch Surg 1937;34:496–526.
26. Pieper R, Kager L, Tidefeldt U. Obstruction of appendix vermiformis causing acute appendicitis. An experimental study in the rabbit. Acta Chir Scand 1982;148:63–72.

27. Buirge RE, Dennis C, Vardo RL, et al. Histology of experimental appendical obstruction (rabbit, ape and man). Arch Pathol 1940;30: 481–503.

28. Chang AR. An analysis of 3003 appendices. Aust N Z J Surg 1981;51:169–178.

29. Butler C. Surgical pathology of acute appendicitis. Hum Pathol 1981;12:870–878.

30. Tobe T, Horikoshi Y, Hamada C, et al. Virus infection as a trigger of appendicitis experimental investigation of Coxsackie B5 virus infection in monkey intestine. Surg 1967;62:927–934.

31. Tobe T. Inapparent virus infection as a trigger of appendicitis. Lancet 1965;1:1343–1346.

32. Sisson RG, Ahlvin RC, Hartlow MC. Superficial mucosal ulceration and the pathogenesis of acute appendicitis in childhood. Am J Surg 1971;122:378–380.

33. Arnbjornsson E, Asp NG, Westin SI. Decreasing incidence of acute appendicitis with special reference to the consumption of dietary fiber. Acta Chir Scand 1982;148:461–464.

34. Wang Y, Reen DJ, Puri P. Is a histologically normal appendix following emergency appendectomy always normal? Lancet 1996; 347:1076–1079.

35. Brooks SM. McBurney's point: the story of appendicitis. London: SC Barnes and Company, 1969:102.

36. Wen SW, Naylor D. Diagnostic accuracy and short term surgical outcomes in cases of suspected acute appendicitis. Can Med Assoc J 1995;152:1617–1626.

37. Williams N, Kapila L. Acute appendicitis in the under-5 year old. J Royal Coll Surg Edinburgh 1994;39:168–170.

38. Whitney TM, Macho JR, Russell TR, et al. Appendicitis in acquired immunodeficiency syndrome. Am J Surg 1992;164:467–471.

39. Binderow SR, Shaked AA. Acute appendicitis in patients with AIDS/HIV infection. Am J Surg 1991;162:9–12.

40. Mattei P, Sola JE, Yeo CJ. Chronic and recurrent appendicitis are uncommon entities often misdiagnosed. J Am Coll Surg 1994;178: 385–389.

41. Jahidi MR, Shaw ML. The pathology of the appendix in ulcerative colitis. Dis Colon Rectum 1976;19:345–349.

42. Croisman GM, George J, Harpaz N. Ulcerative appendicitis in universal and nonuniversal ulcerative colitis. Mod Pathol 1994;7: 322–325.

43. Larsen E, Axelsson C, Johansen A. The pathology of the appendix in morbus Crohn and ulcerative colitis. Acta Pathol Micro Scand 1970;212(Suppl):161–165.

44. Timmcke A. Granulomatous appendicitis: is it Crohn's disease. Report of a case and review of the literature. Am J Gastroenterol 1986;81:283–287.

45. Ariel I, Vinograd I, Hershlag A, et al. Crohn's disease isolated to the appendix: truth and fallacies. Hum Pathol 1986;17:1116–1121.

46. Dudley TH Jr, Dean PJ. Idiopathic granulomatous appendicitis, or Crohn's disease of the appendix revisited. Hum Pathol 1993;24: 595–601.

47. Huang JC, Appleman HD. Another look at chronic appendicitis resembling Crohn's disease. Mod Pathol 1996;9:975–981.

48. Odze RD, Medline P, Cohen Z. Adenocarcinoma arising in an appendix involved with chronic ulcerative colitis. Am J Gastroenterol 1994;89:1905–1907.

49. Le Marc'hadour F, Bost F, Peoc'h M, et al. Carcinoid tumours complicating inflammatory bowel disease. A study of two cases and review off the literature. Pathol Res Pract 1994;190:1185–1192.

50. Payan HM. Diverticular disease of the appendix. Dis Colon Rectum 1977;20:473–476.

51. Esparza AR, Pan CM, Diverticulosis of the appendix. Surgery 1970;67:922–928.

52. Rabinovitch J, Arden M, Barrett T, et al. Diverticulosis and diverticulitis of the vermiform appendix. Ann Surg 1962;155:434–440.

53. Deschenes L, Couture J, Garneau R. Diverticulitis of the appendix. Am J Surg 1971;121:706–709.

54. Leigh DA, Simmons K, Norman E. Bacterial flora of the appendix fossa in appendicitis and postoperative wound infection. J Clin Pathol 1974;27:997–1000.

55. Van Spreeuwel JP, Lindeman J, Bax R, et al. Campylobacter-associated appendicitis: prevalence and clinicopathologic features. In: Sommers SC, Rosen PP, Fechner RE, eds. Pathol Annual. Norwalk, Conn.: Appleton Century Crofts, 1987;22:55–65.

56. Jerris RC. Helicobactor. In: Murray PR, Baron EJ, Pfaller MA, Tenover FC, Yollen RH, eds. Manual of clinical microbiology. Washington DC: ASM Press 1995:483–491.

57. Mittal VK, Khanna SK, Gupta NM, et al. Isolated tuberculosis of appendix. Am Surgeon 1975;41:172–174.

58. Morrison H, Mixter CG, Schlesinger MJ, et al. Tuberculosis localized in the appendix. N Engl J Med 1952;246:329–331.

59. Parkin M, Robinson BL. Tuberculosis of the appendix. Br J Clin Pract 1964;18:741–742.

60. Black RE, Jackson RJ, Tsai T, et al. Epidemic yersinia enterocolotica infection due to contaminated chocolate milk. N Engl J Med 1978;298:76–79.

61. El-Maraghi NRH, Mair NS. The histopathology of enteric infection with yersinia pseudotuberculosis. Am J Clin Pathol 1979;71: 631–639.

62. Henrik-Nielson R, Lundbeck FA, Teglbjaerg PS, et al. Intestinal spirochetosis of the vermiform appendix. Gastroenterol 1985;88: 971–977.

63. Herzberg M. Giant cells in the lymphoid tissue of the appendix in the prodromal stage of measles. JAMA 1932;98:139–140.

64. Yunis EJ, Hashida Y. Electron microscopic demonstration of adenovirus in appendix vermiformis in a case of ileocecal intussusception. Pediatrics 1973;51:566–569.

65. Reif RM. Viral appendicitis. Hum Pathol 1981;12:193–196.

66. O'Brien A, O'Brien DS. Infectious mononucleosis: appendiceal lymphoid tissue involvement parallels characteristic lymph node changes. Arch Pathol Lab Med 1985;109:680–682.

67. Blackman E, Vimadalal S, Nash G. Significance of gastrointestinal cytomegalovirus infection in homosexual males. Am J Gastroenterol 1984;79:935–940.

68. Dorfman S, Talbot IC, Torres R, et al. Parasitic infection in acute appendicitis. Ann Trop Med Parasitol 1995;89:99–101.

69. Ashburn LL. Appendiceal oxyuris. Am J Pathol 1941;17:841–856.

70. Mogensen K, Pahle E, Kowalski K. Enterobius vermicularis and acute appendicitis. Acta Chir Scand 1985;151:705–707.

71. Arean VM, Crandall CA. Ascariasis. In: Marcial-Rojas PA, ed. Pathology of protozoal and helminthic diseases with clinical correlation. Baltimore: Williams & Wilkins, 1971:784.

72. Perez-Tamayo R, Brandt H. Amebiasis. In: Marcial-Rojas PA, ed. Pathology of protozoal and helminthic diseases with clinical correlation. Baltimore: Williams & Wilkins, 1971:159.

73. Arean VM, Echevarria R. Balantidiasis. In: Marcial-Rojas PA, ed. Pathology of protozoal and helminthic diseases with clinical correlation. Baltimore: Williams & Wilkins, 1971:238.

74. Kenney M, Yermakov V. Infection of man with trichuris vulpis, the whipworm of dogs. Am J Trop Med Hyg 1980;29:1205–1208.

75. Noodleman JS. Eosinophilic appendicitis demonstrating of strongyloides stercoralis as a causative agent. Arch Pathol Lab Med 1981; 105:148–149.

76. Kenney M, Eveland LK, Yermakov V, et al. A case of riticularia infection of man in New York. Am J Trop Med Hyg 1975;24: 596–599.

77. Carr NJ, McCarthy WF, Sobin LH. Epithelial noncarcinoid tumors and tumor-like lesions of the appendix. Cancer 1995;75:757–768.

78. Dachman AH, Nichols JB, Patrick DA, et al. Natural history of the obstructed rabbit appendix: observations with radiography, sonography and CT. AJR 1987;148:281–284.

79. Cheng KK. An experimental study of mucocele of the appendix and pseudomyxoma peritonei. J Pathol Bacteriol 1949;61:217–225.

80. Gonzaley JEG, Hann SE, et al. Myxoglobulosis of the appendix. Am J Surg Pathol 1988;12:962–966.

81. Higa E, Rosai J, Pizzimbono CA, et al. Mucosal hyperplasia, mucinous cystadenoma and mucinous cystadenocarcinoma of the appendix. A re-evaluation of the appendiceal "mucocele". Cancer 1973;32:1525–1544.

82. Qizilbash AH. Hyperplastic (metaplastic) polyps of the appendix. Report of 19 cases. Arch Pathol 1974;97:385–388.

83. Qizilbash AH. Mucoceles of the appendix. Their relationship to hyperplastic polyps, mucinous cystadenomas and cystadenocarcinomas. Arch Pathol 1975;99:548–555.

84. Wolfe M, Aimed N. Epithelial neoplasms of the vermiform appendix

(exclusive of carcinoid): II. Cystadenomas papillary adenomas, and adenomatous polyps of the appendix. Cancer 1976;37:2511–2522.

85. Mibu R, Itsh H, Iwashita A, et al. Carcinoma in situ of the vermiform appendix associated with adenomatosis of the colon. Dis Colon Rectum 1981;24:482–484.

86. Nitcheki SS, Wolf BG, Schlinkert R, et al. The natural history of surgically treated primary adenocarcinoma of the appendix. Ann Surg 1994;219:51–57.

87. Alenghat E, Talerman A. Adenocarcinoma of the vermiform appendix presenting as a uterine tumor. Gyn Oncol 1982;13:265–268.

88. Qizilbash AH. Primary adenocarcinoma of the appendix. A clinicopathologic study of 11 cases. Arch Pathol. 1975;99:556–562.

89. Wolfe M, Aimed N. Epithelial neoplasms of the vermiform appendix (exclusive of carcinoid): I. Adenocarcinomas of the appendix. Cancer 1976;37:2493–2510.

90. Cohen SE, Wolfman EF Jr. Primary adenocarcinoma of the vermiform appendix. Am J Surg 1974;127:704–707.

91. Lotfi AM, Spencer RJ, Ilstrup DM, et al. Colorectal polyps and the risk of subsequent carcinoma. Mayo Clinic Proc 1986;61:337–343.

92. Beahr OH, Henson DE, Hutter RVP, Kennedy BJ. eds. Manual for staging of cancer. 4th ed. Philadelphia: JB Lippincott, 1992.

93. Ferro M, Anthony PP. Adenocarcinoma of the appendix. Dis Colon Rectum 1985;28:457–459.

94. Cuatrecasas M, Matias-Guin X, Prat J. Synchronous mucinous tumors of the appendix and the ovary associated with pseudomyxoma peritonei. A clinicopathologic study of six cases with comparative analysis of c-Ki-ras mutations. Am J Surg Pathol. 1996;20:739–746.

95. Chuaqui RF, Zhuang Z, Emmert-Buck MR, et al. Genetic analysis of synchronous mucinous tumors of the ovary and appendix. Hum Pathol 1996;27:165–171.

96. Moertel CG, Dockerty MB, Judd ES. Carcinoid tumors of the vermiform appendix. Cancer 1968;21:270–278.

97. Corpron CA, Black CT, Herzog CE, et al. A half century of experience with carcinoid tumors in children. Am J Surg 1995;170:606–608.

98. Johnston WH, Waisman J. Carcinoid tumor of the vermiform appendix. Cancer 1968;21:270–278.

99. Burke AP, Sobin LH, Federspiel BH, et al. Appendiceal carcinoids: correlation of histology and immunohistochemistry. Mod Pathol 1989;2:630–637.

100. Shaw PA, Pringle JH. The demonstration of a subset of carcinoid tumors of the appendix by in situ hybridization using synthetic probes to proglucagon mRNA. L Pathol 1992;167:375–380.

101. Moyana TN, Satkunam N. A comparative immunohistochemical study of jejunoileal and appendiceal carcinoids. Implications for histogenesis and pathogenesis. Cancer 1992;70:1081–1088.

102. Wilander E, Scheibenpflug L. Cytokeratin expression in small intestinal and appendiceal carcinoids. A basis for classification. Acta Oncologica 1993;32:131–134.

103. Moertel CG, Weiland LH, Nagorney DM, et al. Carcinoid tumor of the appendix: treatment and prognosis. N Engl J Med 1987;317:1699–1701.

104. Roggo A, Wood WC, Ottinger LN. Carcinoid tumors of the appendix. Am J Surg 1993;217:385–390.

105. Goolsby CL, Punyarit P, Mehl PJ, et al. Flow cytometric DNA analysis of carcinoid tumors of the ileum and appendix. Hum Pathol 1992;23:1340–1343.

106. Warkel RL, Cooper PH, Helwig EB. Adenocarcinoid, a mucin-producing carcinoid tumor of the appendix. A study of 39 cases. Cancer 1978;42:2781–2793.

107. Edmonds P, Merino MJ, LiVolsi VA, et al. Adenocarcinoid (mucinous carcinoid) of the appendix. Gastroenterology 1984;86:302–309.

108. Burke AP, Sobin LH, Fedespiel BH, et al. Goblet cell carcinoids and related tumors of the vermiform appendix. Am J Clin Pathol 1990;94:27–35.

109. Anderson NH, Somerville JE, Johnston CF, et al. Appendiceal goblet cell carcinoids: a clinicopathological and immunohistochemical study. Histopathology 1991;18:61–65.

110. Butler JA, Houshiar A, Lin F, et al. Goblet cell carcinoid of the appendix. Am J Surg 1994;168:685–687.

111. Hood IC, Jones BA, Watts JC. Mucinous tumor of the appendix presenting as bilateral ovarian tumors. Arch Pathol Lab Med 1986;110:336–340.

112. Lewin KJ, Ulch T, Yang K, et al. The endocrine cells of the gastrointestinal tract tumors, Part II. Pathol Ann 1986;21:181–215.

113. Iwafuchi M, Watanbe H, Ajioka Y, et al. Immunohistochemical and ultrastructural studies of twelve argentaffin and six argyrophil carcinoid of the appendix vermiformis. Hum Pathol 1990;21:773–780.

114. Goddard MJ, Lonsdale RN. The histogenesis of appendiceal carcinoid tumours. Histopathology 1992;20:345–349.

115. Katsetos CD, Jami MM, Krishna L, et al. Novel immunohistochemical localization of 28000 molecular-weight (Mr) calcium binding protein (calbindin-D28k) in enterchromaffin cells of the human appendix and neuroendocrine tumors (carcinoids and small-cell carcinomas) of the midgut and foregut. Arch Pathol Lab Med 1994;118:633–639.

116. Al-Talib RK, Mason CH, Theaker JM. Combined goblet cell carcinoid and mucinous cystadenoma of the appendix. J Clin Pathol 1995;48:869–870.

117. Isaacson P. Crypt cell carcinoma of the appendix (so-called adenocarcinoid tumor). Am J Surg Pathol 1981;5:213–224.

118. Cooper PH, Warkel RL. Ultrastructure of the goblet cell type of adenocarcinoid of the appendix. Cancer 1978;42:2687–2695.

119. Chejfec G, Capella C, Solicia E, et al. Amphicrine cells, dysplasias, and neoplasias. Cancer 1985;56:2683–2690.

120. Schmutzer KJ, Bayer M, Zaki AE, et al. Tumors of the appendix. Dis Colon Rectum 1975;18:324–331.

121. Powell JL, Fuerst JF, Tapia RA. Leiomyoma of the appendix. South Med J 1980;73:1298–1299.

122. Jones PA. Leiomyosarcoma of the appendix: report of two cases. 1979;22:175–178.

123. Johnston J, Helwig EB. Granular cell tumors of the gastrointestinal tract and perianal region: a study of 74 cases. Dig Dis Sci 1981;26:807–816.

124. Sobel JH, Marquet E, Schwarz R. Granular degeneration of appendiceal smooth muscle. Arch Pathol 1971;92:427–432.

125. Kazzaz BA. Argentaffin and argyrophil cells in the appendix. J Pathol 1971;104:206–209.

126. Zarabi M, LaBach JP. Ganglioneuroma causing acute appendicitis. Hum Pathol 1982;13:1143–1146.

127. Lewin KJ, Ranchod M, Dorman RF. Lymphomas of the gastrointestinal tract. A study of 117 cases presenting with gastrointestinal disease. Cancer 1978;42:693–707.

128. Pasquale MD, Shabahang M, Bitterman P, et al. Primary lymphoma of the appendix. Case report and review of the literature. Surg Ankle 1994;3:243–248.

129. Sin IC, Ling ET, Prentice RA. Burkitt's lymphoma of the appendix: report of two cases. Hum Pathol 1980;11:465–470.

130. Latches KS, Canter J. Acute appendicitis secondary to metastatic carcinoma. Am J Surg 1966;111:220–223.

131. Dieter RA Jr. Carcinoma metastatic to the vermiform appendix report of three cases. Dis Colon Rectum 1970;13:336–340.

132. Answer MA, Pandas RLL, Chi YES, et al. Diagnosis of carcinoid-like metastatic prostatic carcinoma by an immunoperoxidase method. Am J Clin Pathol 1976;76:94–98.

133. Baker MS, Goldman H, Willie M, et al. Metastatic Kaposi's sarcoma presenting as acute appendicitis. Military Med 1986;151:45–47.

134. Howie JGR. The prussian blue reaction in the diagnosis of previous appendicitis. J Pathol Bacterial 1966;91:85–92.

135. Clarke H, Pollett W, Cattail S, et al. Sarcoidosis with involvement of the appendix. Arch Intern Med 1983;143:1603–1604.

136. Langsam LB, Raj PK, Galang CF. Intussuception of the appendix. Dis Colon Rectum 1984;27:387–392.

137. Mittal VK, Chondhury SP, Cortez JA. Endometriosis of the appendix presenting as acute appendicitis. Am J Surg 1981;142:519.

138. Panganiban W, Cornog JL. Endometriosis of the intestines and vermiform appendix. Dis Colon Rectum 1972;15:253–260.

139. Fayemi AO, Ali M, Braum EV. Necrotizing vasculitis of the gallbladder and the appendix. Similarity in the morphology of rheumatoid arthritis and polyarteritis nodosa. Am J Gastroenterol 1977;67:608–612.

140. Shwachman H, Holsclaw D. Examination of the appendix at laparotomy as a diagnostic clue in cystic fibrosis. N Engl J Med 1972;286:1300–1301.

141. Delafuente AA. Septa in the appendix, a previously undescribed condition. Histopathology 1985;9:1329–1337.

142. Blackshear W Jr. Malakoplakia of the appendix: a case reported. Am J Clin Pathol 1970;53:284–287.

143. Misra PS, Lebwohl P, Laufer H. Hepatic and appendiceal Whipple's disease with negative jejunal biopsies. Am J Gastroenterol 1981;75:302–306.

144. Domingo P, Ris J, Lopez-Contreras J, et al. Appendicitis due to mycobacterium avium complex in a patient with AIDS. Arch Intern Med 1996;156:1114.

145. Livingston RA, Sibery GK, Paidas CN, et al. Appendicitis due to mycobacterium avium complex in an adolescent infected with the human immunodeficiency virus. Clin Infect Dis 1995;20:1579–1580.

CHAPTER

36 | DISORDERS OF THE ANAL REGION

Robert R. Rickert

ANATOMY
DEVELOPMENTAL ABNORMALITIES
HEMORRHOIDS
PROLAPSE
INFLAMMATORY AND INFECTIOUS
  DISORDERS
  FISSURE
  FISTULA AND ABSCESS
  HIDRADENITIS SUPPURATIVA
  ANAL LESIONS IN INFLAMMATORY BOWEL DISEASE
    ULCERATIVE COLITIS
    CROHN'S DISEASE
  SEXUALLY TRANSMITTED DISEASES
    SYPHILIS
    GONORRHEA
    HERPES SIMPLEX
    CHLAMYDIA
    MOLLUSCUM CONTAGIOSUM
    LYMPHOGRANULOMA VENEREUM, CHANCROID,
      AND GRANULOMA INGUINALE
  TUBERCULOSIS
  OTHER CONDITIONS
BENIGN TUMORS AND
  TUMOR-LIKE LESIONS

CONDYLOMA ACUMINATUM
BOWENOID PAPULOSIS
ADNEXAL TUMORS
KERATOACANTHOMA
GRANULAR CELL TUMOR AND NEURILEMOMA
LEIOMYOMA
OLEOGRANULOMA
MALIGNANT TUMORS
  GENERAL CONSIDERATIONS
  CARCINOMA ARISING ABOVE THE DENTATE LINE
  CARCINOMA ARISING BELOW THE DENTATE LINE
  RISK FACTORS AND ETIOLOGY
  HISTOLOGIC FEATURES
  ANAL CANAL INTRAEPITHELIAL NEOPLASIA
  OTHER VARIANTS OF SQUAMOUS CELL
    CARCINOMA
    VERRUCOUS CARCINOMA
    GIANT CONDYLOMA ACUMINATUM
  ADENOCARCINOMA
  MALIGNANT MELANOMA
  EXTRAMAMMARY PAGET'S DISEASE
  BASAL CELL CARCINOMA
  OTHER MALIGNANT TUMORS

ANATOMY

Despite the frequency of many disorders of the anal region, their pathogenesis often is poorly understood. The confusion surrounding anal disorders relates largely to the rather complex gross and microscopic anatomy of the anal region, knowledge of which is essential to an understanding of its disease processes (1). Although uncommon, neoplasms arising in this area are also attended by considerable confusion with respect to classification and histogenesis.

As defined surgically, the anal canal measures 3 to 4 cm in length and extends from the upper to lower borders of the internal sphincter muscle (Fig. 36.1). It connects with the rectum superiorly and the true anal skin inferiorly. The so-called anatomic anal canal is defined as beginning at the dentate line and extending distally to the anal verge, which is that point where the walls of the anal canal come into contact in the resting state. This latter definition is unsatisfactory since the most typical anal neoplasms would arise outside of the anatomic anal canal (2). The most important and only reliably identifiable macroscopic landmark noted on inspection of the

mucosal surface is the dentate or pectinate line located at about the midline of the surgically defined canal. This line corresponds to the location of the anal valves, which are separated from each other by small papillae that represent the lower ends of six to ten vertical mucosal folds known as the anal columns of Morgagni. Above each of the crescentic anal valves lies a small recess or anal crypt. The dentate line marks the site of the fetal anal membrane corresponding to the junction of the endodermal part of the anal canal developed from the cloaca and the ectodermal portion derived from the anal pit (proctodeum).

Microscopically, the mucosal lining below the dentate line is of the stratified squamous type. Because its border with the dentate line grossly resembles a comb, it is also known as the pecten. The squamous mucous membrane of the anal canal is devoid of hair and other cutaneous appendages. The lower portion of the anal canal ends at the anal verge, where the squamous mucous membrane merges with true skin containing hair follicles, sweat glands, and apocrine glands.

The dentate line corresponds generally to the squamocolumnar junction. However, this is not an abrupt line of demarcation.

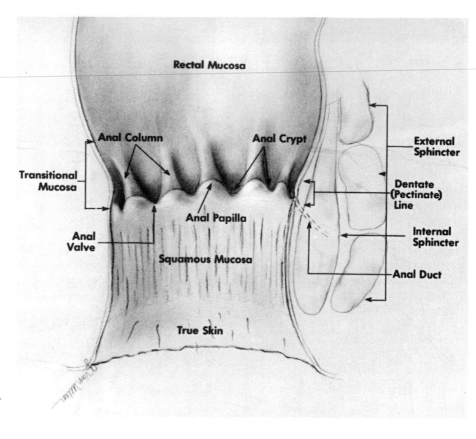

Figure 36.1 Diagram of the normal anatomy of anal region.

Instead, there is an intervening or anal transitional zone (ATZ) that measures from several millimeters to just over 1 cm in length. This narrow ring of transitional epithelium is of great interest and of presumed significance in the histogenesis of certain anal neoplasms (Fig. 36.2). Its microscopic appearance varies from an epithelium resembling lower urinary tract to one of stratified squamous, columnar, or cuboidal type (1–3). The most characteristic pattern is an epithelium containing cells of columnar to cuboidal shape arranged in four to nine rows (4). Small islands of colorectal type or of squamous epithelium, or both, may also be seen in this transitional zone. The upper border of the transitional zone merges with the normal mucosa of the rectum.

The above observations lend themselves to a zonal definition that recognizes three zones corresponding to the lining epithelium (2, 4). The upper zone is the *colorectal zone*, the middle zone is the *anal transitional zone* (ATZ) extending proximally from the dentate line to the junction with colorectal-type mucosa, and the distal zone is the *squamous zone* (pecten) lying between the dentate line and true perianal skin beginning at the anal verge. The squamous zone is lined by nonkeratinizing squamous epithelium. Another traditional, but I believe confusing, definition designates the squamous zone as the anal margin and the anal canal only as that portion from the dentate line proximally to its junction with rectal mucosa. The TNM staging system defines the anal canal as extending from the rectum to the perianal skin and lined by the mucous membrane overlying the internal sphincter (5). This definition includes the dentate line and the anal transitional zone epithelium as well as the non-hair–bearing and nonsweat-gland–bearing squamous mucosa

extending distally to its junction with skin. This definition, therefore, incorporates the histologic or zonal approach.

The anal ducts or glands open into the anal crypts. These long tubular structures usually extend distally for a short distance before penetrating into and occasionally through the internal sphincter muscle (Fig. 36.3). They may also extend proximally beneath the rectal mucosa. The ducts are lined by transitional or stratified columnar epithelium, and mucus-producing cells are commonly seen, especially in the terminal portion. Nodules of lymphoid tissue may surround the gland ducts.

Studies of the ATZ by scanning and transmission electron microscopy have suggested that the mucosa might be metaplastic squamous epithelium rather than urothelium, with which it is often compared (6). The anal canal epithelium has also been shown to contain endocrine cells and melanin-containing cells (7).

The hemorrhoidal plexus of veins surrounding the anal canal consists of an internal and an external portion. Above the dentate line the internal hemorrhoidal plexus drains into the portal venous system by means of the superior rectal and inferior mesenteric veins. The external hemorrhoidal plexus below the dentate line drains into the internal iliac veins of the systemic circulation by means of the internal pudendal veins, which receive blood from the inferior rectal veins.

The muscular wall of the anal canal consists of two portions. The internal sphincter is composed of smooth muscle and represents the expanded continuation of the circular layer of the muscularis propria of the rectum. The external sphincter is composed of skeletal (voluntary) muscle and is divided into a deep part, a superficial part,

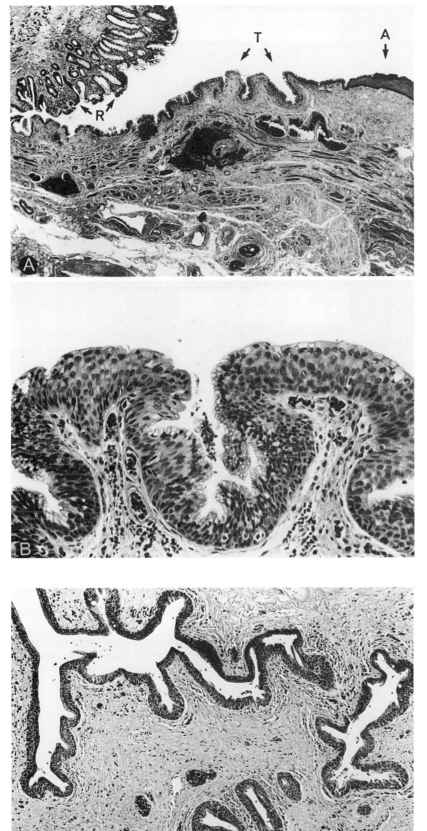

Figure 36.2   (A) Scanning photomicrograph of normal ATZ. Rectal mucosa is on the left *(R)*, transitional mucosa is in the broad central region *(T)*, and anal stratified squamous mucosa is on the right *(A)* (H & E, ×35). **(B)** Higher-power view of transitional mucosa, showing rows of cuboidal to columnar cells. Some mucus secreting cells are seen on the surface (H & E, ×330).

Figure 36.3 Anal ducts (glands) in the submucosal stroma, showing prominent branching. Ducts are lined by transitional epithelium (H & E, ×125).

and a subcutaneous part representing a downward extension of the puborectalis muscle.

The mucosa of the anal canal above the dentate line is supplied by autonomic nerves and is insensitive to pain. The squamous mucosa of the pecten, however, is supplied by inferior rectal nerves of somatic type, which render the lower canal sensitive to pain, touch, and temperature.

The lymphatic drainage of the anal canal, like the vascular supply, is in two directions. The drainage of the upper canal is into inferior mesenteric and internal iliac nodes, and that of the canal below the dentate line is into the inguinal nodes.

In this chapter the pathologic features of disorders of the anal region will be discussed. Several recent reviews elaborate more completely on the anatomic, clinical, and therapeutic aspects of diseases in this area (8, 9).

DEVELOPMENTAL ABNORMALITIES

Congenital abnormalities of the rectum and anus occur in about 1 out of every 5000 live births. Most have been somewhat loosely classified as examples of imperforate anus. After a period of extensive worldwide collaboration, a proposed "International Classification of Anorectal Anomalies" was presented in 1970 (10). This scheme is based on the relationships of the abnormality to the puborectalis muscle or levator sling and classifies lesions as low (translevator), intermediate, or high (supralevator).

The *low anomalies* comprise about 40% of lesions and may include anal stenosis, covered anus, anocutaneous fistula, anovulvar fistula, anovestibular fistula, anterior perineal anus, and vestibular anus. These tend to be the least severe types of defects. Pelvic innervation is normal. *Intermediate anomalies* are uncommon and account for about 15% of the total. They consist of anal agenesis or anorectal stenosis with or without the formation of fistula. The most significant lesions are the *high anomalies*, which make up 40% and are frequently associated with other sacral, neurologic, or urinary tract abnormalities. These are lesions of anorectal agenesis, and fistulas between the intestinal and urinary tracts occur only in this group (11). Rare additional anomalies that do not fit this classification include imperforate anal membrane. Further details on these anomalies are discussed elsewhere.

A report has suggested an increased risk of sacrococcygeal teratoma in patients with congenital anorectal malformations (12). Because the frequency of malignant change in sacrococcygeal teratomas increases proportionately with age, recognition of this apparent association and early treatment are important.

HEMORRHOIDS

Recognized since the time of Hippocrates, hemorrhoids have traditionally been regarded as varicosities of the submucosal plexus of the superior hemorrhoidal veins. More recent evidence suggests, however, that hemorrhoids are "cushions" of tissue normally present in the anal submucosa and are composed of blood vessels, smooth muscle, and connective tissue (13). They are located above the dentate line on the left lateral, right anterior, and right posterior aspects of the canal and are covered by transitional or rectal mucosa.

They are normally present at birth. It is suggested that their engorgement during defecation serves a protective role for the anal canal.

Additional evidence that hemorrhoids are not simply varicosities is their lack of relationship with portal hypertension. Surgeons also recognize that they are more than distended veins because much of the bleeding during surgery is arterial (14). Microscopically, hemorrhoids also contain more smooth muscle in their walls than do ordinary veins of similar size or in varicosities.

It has been suggested that with age these cushions bulge and then descend into the lumen of the anal canal (14). As they lose their support, the lining becomes more susceptible to the effects of straining, resulting in the common symptoms of bleeding and protrusion. Hereditary and environmental factors as well as individual habits may be responsible for the variations in size of hemorrhoids, presentation, or symptoms in different individuals.

Hemorrhoids are commonly defined by their anatomic location (8, 9). Those above the dentate line are internal hemorrhoids and are covered mostly by rectal mucosa. Those below the dentate line are external hemorrhoids and are covered by the squamous mucosa of the pecten or by perianal skin. If the communications between the internal and external venous plexuses enlarge, combined internal and external hemorrhoids result.

Clinical classification of internal hemorrhoids is based on the degree of prolapse (8, 9). First-degree hemorrhoids bleed but do not protrude. Second-degree hemorrhoids protrude during defecation but reduce spontaneously. Third-degree hemorrhoids protrude and must be reduced manually. Fourth-degree hemorrhoids cannot be reduced. Complications such as thrombosis, necrosis, and inflammation may occur. Organization of thrombosed hemorrhoids may result in the formation of fibrous polyps or tags. Since internal hemorrhoids are innervated by the autonomic system, they generally present without pain.

External hemorrhoids present usually because of thrombosis, which is often painful, or because of the appearance of tags or polyps, which may result from organization of previously thrombosed hemorrhoids. In my opinion, tissues submitted following hemorrhoid surgery should be routinely examined microscopically. Although rare, microscopic evidence of infections, Crohn's disease, or early neoplasms that were unsuspected clinically may be identified.

PROLAPSE

Rectal prolapse (procidentia) is defined as the circumferential descent of rectum through the anal sphincter (9). It is a condition seen most often in the very young or in the elderly. Prolapse of hemorrhoidal tissue also commonly occurs.

The reddened, protruding rectal mucosa in cases of procidentia and the surface of prolapsing hemorrhoids have a similar and very characteristic appearance. The histologic features include fibromuscular obliteration of the lamina propria, thickening and often fragmentation of the muscularis mucosae, hyperplasia of mucosal glands often with a villous configuration, and telangiectasia of the surface vessels (Fig. 36.4). Surface erosion may also occur.

These histologic features are entirely similar to the mucosal changes seen in the *solitary rectal ulcer syndrome* (15–17). It has been suggested that the solitary rectal ulcer syndrome results from ischemia due to internal prolapse of the rectal mucosa (15). In an effort to conceptually unify the similar nature of these processes the

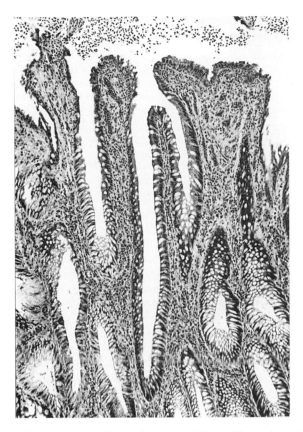

Figure 36.4 Prolapsed rectal mucosa. Note villous elongation and distortion of gland tubules, partial fibrous obliteration of lamina propria, and focal superficial erosion *(upper left)* (H & E, ×125).

term *mucosal prolapse syndrome* has been proposed (16). Recently added to this family of disorders has been *inflammatory cloacogenic polyp*, an unusual inflammatory polyp arising from the transitional zone of the anus (Fig. 36.5) (18). This lesion has many histologic features similar to prolapsed mucosa, suggesting that prolapse of transitional zone mucosa may be important in its pathogenesis. Further details on these disorders are discussed elsewhere.

INFLAMMATORY AND INFECTIOUS DISORDERS

FISSURE

An anal fissure is an elongated, triangular ulcer of the anal canal (8, 9). Fissures typically extend from the dentate line to the anal verge. The great majority are located in the posterior midline of the canal overlying the lower portion of the internal sphincter. Most of the rest are in the anterior midline.

The precise pathogenesis is not clear, but most believe the lesion is the result of traumatic tearing, especially during defecation with the passage of large, firm stools. Most fissures are superficial and may heal rapidly. They may, however, become chronic. Dysfunction of the internal sphincter may contribute to the chronicity of the lesion. Histologically, fissures are characterized by nonspecific inflammation. Large, deep chronic fissures are know as *anal ulcers*.

Frequently, chronic fissures are associated with hypertrophy of the anal papilla at the proximal end of the lesion to form a so-called *sentinel tag* or *pile*. Histologically, these are similar to other types of fibroepithelial papillomas and are covered by squamous mucosa. Occasionally, the stroma of large hypertrophied papillae may show cytologic atypia, which is regarded as a reactive phenomenon (19).

When fissures are located in atypical positions or when they fail to heal following appropriate treatment, other diagnostic possibilities should be considered. These include inflammatory bowel disease, especially Crohn's disease, specific infections such as tuberculosis or syphilis, and carcinoma.

FISTULA AND ABSCESS

An anal fistula (fistula in ano) is a passage one end of which opens into an anal crypt at the dentate line. The fistula may extend to the skin or may terminate in the perineal soft tissue. Because most do not have openings at both ends of the track, these lesions are more accurately regarded as sinuses rather than fistulae.

Knowledge of the normal muscular anatomy of the region is important to an understanding of anorectal suppurative disease. Structurally, the muscles are arranged as two funnels, one located within the other (20). The inner consists of the muscular wall of the

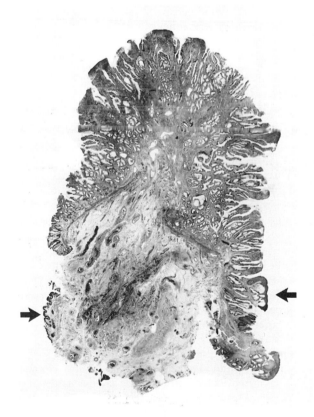

Figure 36.5. Scanning photomicrograph of inflammatory cloacogenic polyp. The mucosal surface has a microscopic appearance similar to that of the prolapsed mucosa in Figure 36.4. Remnants of transitional epithelium are present on the lower left *(arrow)* and of squamous epithelium on the lower right *(arrow)* (H & E, ×7).

rectum and anus including the terminal portion or internal sphincter. The outer funnel consists of the external sphincter and puborectalis muscles. Between the two is the intersphincteric space.

It is believed that the majority of suppurative processes in the area are the result of an initial infection of an anal duct, the anatomy of which provides a pathway between the anal canal and perianal soft tissues. The acute process in most cases is an abscess in the intersphincteric space. The formation of a fistula represents the chronic phase of this process. Anorectal abscess and fistula in ano are, therefore, different stages of the same basic condition (20, 21).

A detailed anatomic study has demonstrated that fistula in ano can be classified into four major groups based on the relationship of the track to the sphincteric muscles (20).

Intersphincteric, the most common type, in which the fistula extends only into the intersphincteric space.

Transsphincteric, the next most common, in which the fistula passes from the intersphincteric space through the external sphincter to the ischiorectal fossa.

Suprasphincteric, in which the fistula extends in the intersphincteric space over the top of the puborectalis muscle, then downward through the levator to the ischiorectal fossa.

Extrasphincteric, the least common type, in which the fistula passes from rectum to perianal skin completely external to the external sphincteric complex.

Histologically, the fistula is lined by granulation tissue and surrounded by a nonspecific acute and chronic inflammatory reaction. Giant cells of the foreign body type are frequently present and should not be confused with the granulomatous reaction seen in Crohn's disease. Fistulas do, however, occur in the course of inflammatory bowel disease, especially Crohn's disease, as well as in specific infections in the area. Carcinomas may also be associated with the formation of fistulas.

HIDRADENITIS SUPPURATIVA

Hidradenitis suppurativa is a chronic and acute inflammatory process involving the skin and subcutaneous tissues, especially where apocrine glands are found. The axilla is the most common site, but the anogenital area may also be affected. The term is actually a misnomer because involvement of the apocrine glands and adjacent deep structures is a secondary phenomenon. The primary event is probably related to follicular occlusion followed by a deep folliculitis, after which subcutaneous sinus tracts, abscesses, ulceration, and scarring may develop.

It is important to distinguish this inflammatory process from other disorders in the area that are associated with fistula formation. Several differential diagnostic observations have been offered using the internal sphincter as a point of reference (22). The sinus tract of hidradenitis is superficial to the sphincter muscle and involves the lower part of the canal distal to the dentate line. The fistula in ano penetrates and progresses deep to the sphincter muscle and originates in the crypt area of the dentate line. Finally, the fistula of Crohn's disease is often deep to all sphincter muscles and may involve rectal mucosa proximal to the dentate line.

ANAL LESIONS IN INFLAMMATORY BOWEL DISEASE

The pathologic features of idiopathic inflammatory bowel disease are covered in detail in a previous chapter. Involvement of the anal region, however, is sufficiently common and important to merit additional comment here.

ULCERATIVE COLITIS

In ulcerative colitis, anal involvement is usually nonspecific and not qualitatively different from that seen in patients without colitis. Superficial nonspecific inflammation is common, and acute lesions such as fissure, cryptitis, anorectal abscess, and fistula in ano may also occur.

CROHN'S DISEASE

Anal involvement in Crohn's disease is more frequent and important than in ulcerative colitis. Reports of the frequency of anal manifestations vary rather widely based mainly on what types of lesions are included as anal involvement (23–25). Generally, however, it is observed that 20 to 30% of patients with small bowel involvement and 50 to 80% of patients with large bowel involvement will develop anal lesions during the course of their disease. In some patients the anal manifestations may antedate by several years other clinical or radiographic evidence of disease in the more proximal intestinal tract (26).

The typical clinical features of anal Crohn's disease have been well described (23). Anal skin tags are common and tend to be larger, thicker, and firmer than tags in patients without Crohn's disease. Fissures are also common and are often large and deep with undermined edges. They also are more likely to occur in atypical positions than the non-Crohn's associated fissure. Fistula in ano may be similar to that in patients without Crohn's disease but is more frequently complex with multiple openings often at a considerable distance from the anus. The features most characteristic of Crohn's disease in anal inflammatory processes are absence of pain and presence of chronicity, induration, multiplicity, and cyanotic coloration.

The diagnosis of anal Crohn's disease may be confirmed by the histologic demonstration of a sarcoid-like granulomatous reaction in the tissue lesions described above (Fig. 36.6) (26). It is important to exclude anal tuberculosis with appropriate special stains. Care must also be taken not to confuse the giant-cell response to fecal debris commonly seen in fistula with the sarcoid-like reaction in Crohn's disease.

Recent attention has been given to a possible association between anal Crohn's disease and carcinoma of the anus. Several cases of anal squamous cell carcinoma and cloacogenic carcinoma in patients with anal Crohn's disease have been reported (27–29). Although a definite relationship between the two has yet to be established conclusively, careful clinical observation of patients with anal Crohn's disease with special attention to any new or unusual lesions is important.

SEXUALLY TRANSMITTED DISEASES

There has been a steady increase in the frequency of sexually transmitted diseases during recent decades (30). The increase has

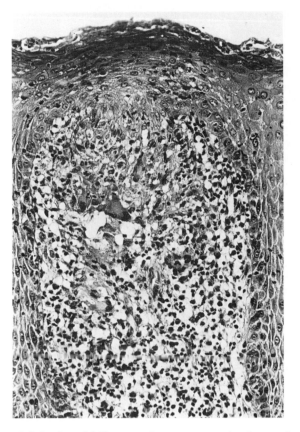

Figure 36.6 Sarcoid-like granulomatous reaction in an edematous anal tag from patient with advanced intestinal and anal Crohn's disease. Note the giant cell in the upper center of the field (H & E, ×330).

included not only such traditional venereal infections as syphilis, gonorrhea, lymphogranuloma venereum, chancroid, and granuloma inguinale but also, more dramatically, a host of other conditions including herpes, nonlymphogranulomatous chlamydial infections, candidiasis, condyloma acuminatum, and molluscum contagiosum. Anorectal venereal lesions are most commonly seen in male homosexuals who practice anorectal intercourse (31, 32). Patients may present with concurrent sexually transmitted infections of different types. In addition to the increased incidence of anorectal lesions in this population there is a risk of sexual transmission of enteric infections such as viral hepatitis, amebiasis, giardiasis, shigellosis, and *Campylobacter* enteritis.

During recent years there has been a dramatic increase in interest in sexually transmitted diseases. This is due to the noted increased frequency of these disorders as well as the enormous concern of both medical profession and general public with the acquired immunodeficiency syndrome (AIDS). Not only is AIDS most commonly transmitted sexually, but it is also often associated with other venereal disorders in the same patient. This section will review the common sexually transmitted diseases involving the anal region. Condyloma acuminatum will be considered later in a discussion of benign tumors.

SYPHILIS

Primary lesions of anogenital syphilis are frequently overlooked clinically. This is due both to the apparent trivial nature of the lesion as well as to its frequent similarity to other nonvenereal anal inflammatory disease, especially the common fissure. The typical lesion is an ulcer of the anal canal (30, 33). Unlike the primary ulcerated, indurated, and painless genital chancre, anal lesions of syphilis may be very painful (9). Histologically, the lesion is nonspecific. There is superficial ulceration with an underlying dense inflammatory infiltrate usually rich in plasma cells. Thick-walled blood vessels with prominent endothelial cells may be seen. Diagnosis may be accomplished by demonstration of spirochetes in fixed tissue by appropriate silver stains such as the Warthin-Starry stain, by darkfield microscopic examination of lesional scrapings, or by fluorescent treponemal antibody staining.

Secondary lesions of anogenital syphilis include the typical raised condylomata lata, which may be seen in association with a characteristic maculopapular rash (30). Other anorectal lesions seen in syphilis include polyps and smooth lobulated masses that may simulate neoplasms (34).

GONORRHEA

Anorectal gonorrhea is common in the male homosexual population (30, 32, 35). In women anorectal involvement is the result either of anorectal intercourse or of secondary spread from the vagina. The usual lesion is an acute or subacute proctitis, but the upper anal canal including anal crypts and ducts may also be affected.

HERPES SIMPLEX

Herpes of the anogenital region is usually due to infection of herpes simplex virus, type II (HSV-2) (9, 30, 34). It results in most cases from direct inoculation during anorectal intercourse. The patient first notes perianal itching and paresthesia several days to 2 weeks after exposure. This is followed by intense anal pain. Grossly the lesions are erythematous with small clustered vesicles that soon rupture and give rise to larger ulcers. The perianal skin and anal canal are most frequently involved, but the distal rectal mucosa may also be affected. Resolution usually occurs within 2 weeks, but recurrences are very common. Histologically, the lesions are similar to lesions of other cutaneous and mucosal surfaces caused by HSV-2. They are characterized by vesicle formation resulting from a reticular-type degeneration of the epithelium. Characteristic giant cells with prominent intranuclear inclusions are generally easily identified in early lesions.

CHLAMYDIA

Nonlymphogranulomatous chlamydial infection of the genitals is the most common sexually transmitted inflammatory disease (9, 30). The usual presentation is as a nonspecific urethritis in men or a nonspecific infection of the lower genital tract in women, but anorectal infection may occur in patients practicing anorectal intercourse.

MOLLUSCUM CONTAGIOSUM

Molluscum contagiosum is a contagious disorder characterized clinically by the appearance of multiple small, waxy papules with

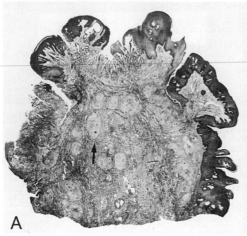

Figure 36.7   (A) Scanning power of a polypoid lesion of verrucous tuberculosis of the anus (H & E, ×7.5). **(B)** Higher-power view of the area marked by the arrow in A, showing a granuloma with early caseation. Acid-fast bacilli were easily identified (H & E, ×330).

umbilicated centers. Histologically, the lesions consist of epidermal lobules that extend into the dermis. Prominent inclusion bodies are characteristic. The disease, caused by a member of the poxvirus family, is spread by close body contact and, therefore, may be sexually transmissible. The most common sites of involvement are skin of abdomen, thigh, perineum, penis, scrotum, and vulva. The buttocks and perianal area, however, may occasionally be affected.

LYMPHOGRANULOMA VENEREUM, CHANCROID, AND GRANULOMA INGUINALE

These lesions are all rare venereal infections in industrialized countries (30). Each may occasionally be associated with anorectal lesions. There is a suspected though not proven relationship between lymphogranuloma venereum and carcinoma of the anus.

TUBERCULOSIS

Anorectal tuberculosis has steadily decreased in frequency in most parts of the world but remains quite common in those areas where pulmonary and intestinal tuberculosis are common. Involvement of the gastrointestinal tract results either exogenously from ingestion of contaminated milk or as endogenous spread from another site, especially the lung. Several types of anal and perianal tuberculosis have been described including ulcerative, hypertrophic, verrucous, lupoid, and miliary (36, 37). The ulcerative form is the most common. The verrucous form is the least common and presents as a warty mass in the anal canal (Fig. 36.7). All forms must be

distinguished from other types of anal inflammatory disease, especially Crohn's disease. The verrucous variant must also be distinguished from carcinoma.

OTHER CONDITIONS

A variety of other inflammatory, infectious, and nonneoplastic conditions are occasionally associated with anal involvement. Many dermatologic disorders may affect the anal region. Lichen sclerosus et atrophicus is rather common in the anogenital region of postmenopausal women but may also occur in children (38). Rare examples of malakoplakia have been reported in the anus (39). Eosinophilic colitis is usually seen in the proximal gastrointestinal tract, but anal involvement may occur (40). Another report presents a young patient with an anal abscess due to *Enterobius vermicularis* (41). A wide spectrum of anal inflammatory lesions including ulcers and abscesses have also been described in patients with hematologic disorders (42). A variety of microorganisms have been cultured from these lesions, the most frequent being *Escherichia coli* and *Pseudomonas aeruginosa*.

BENIGN TUMORS AND TUMOR-LIKE LESIONS

CONDYLOMA ACUMINATUM

Condyloma acuminatum, or common genital wart, is a sexually transmitted disease caused by members of the human papillomavirus family (HPV). The typical condyloma is a soft, fleshy, gray-tan to pink papillomatous growth that frequently occurs in multiples. In men genital warts are usually located on the penis, anus, or uncommonly the scrotum. In women the lesions are most frequent on the vulva, vaginal introitus, perineum, anus, and cervix.

Condyloma acuminatum is the most common tumor of the anal and perianal region. In this area the perianal skin is most frequently involved, but many patients have anal canal lesions as well. Condylomata of the anal region may be seen in association with penile warts in men or with vulvar warts in women, but they may also occur as the sole manifestation of infection in male homosexuals who practice anorectal intercourse (43). They frequently occur together with other sexually transmitted disorders.

Histologically the typical condyloma acuminatum is a papillomatous lesion characterized by pronounced acanthosis of the squamous epithelium (Fig. 36.8). At the base of the lesion the proliferating epithelium shows no evidence of invasion. There is orderly and progressive maturation of the epithelium, and the surface usually shows parakeratosis. Commonly present near the surface of the lesion are squamous cells with vacuolated cytoplasm surrounding variably enlarged and hyperchromatic nuclei. This feature, known as "koilocytotic" change or atypia, is a histologic hallmark of HPV infection.

Within the past decade there has been increasing interest in the relationship between HPV infection and neoplasia of the lower female genital tract, especially cervix and vulva (44–47). Of great significance in this area of active investigation is the observation that evidence of HPV infection of the cervix is usually in the subclinical form of a flat condyloma rather than the acuminate lesion described here. Several types of HPV have been implicated in anogenital lesions, including types 6, 11, 16, and 18. HPV-6 and HPV-11 are most likely to be associated with the grossly papillary benign condylomata acuminata, whereas HPV-16 and less commonly HPV-18 are associated with high-grade dysplastic lesions (45–47). Anal warts have been found to contain virus in low concentration, usually HPV-6 (43). The relationship between human papilloma viruses and anal squamous neoplasia will be further addressed later.

An important and as yet incompletely resolved issue concerns the premalignant potential of the anal condyloma. Several examples of carcinoma in situ associated with anal condylomata have been described (48, 49). Of particular interest in one of these reports is the observation that five of the nine patients had developed AIDS (49). Occasional cases of invasive squamous cell carcinoma arising in anal condylomata have also been described (50, 51). Care must be taken to distinguish malignant change in a condyloma from the bizarre atypia seen after topical treatment of these lesions with podophyllum resin (52). These changes may persist for several weeks after application.

BOWENOID PAPULOSIS

Bowenoid papulosis (dysplasia) was initially described as a lesion of the genitalia of young adults (53, 54). It is characterized clinically by multiple, small, pigmented papules. In addition to the common penile and vulvar involvement, anal lesions may also occur (55). Although clinically benign in appearance, these lesions have histologic features that are very similar to those of in situ squamous cell carcinoma (Bowen's disease). In contrast to classic Bowen's disease, however, bowenoid papulosis (dysplasia) usually presents a more

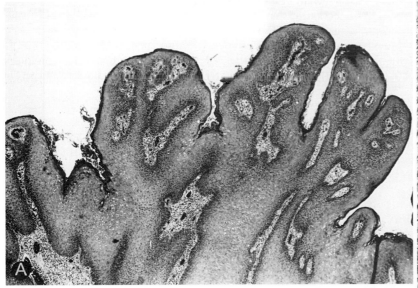
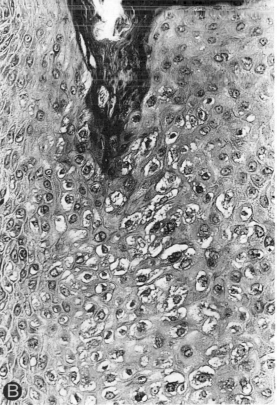

Figure 36.8 (A) Scanning photomicrograph of condyloma acuminatum showing typical papillary architecture (H & E, ×35). **(B)** Higher-power view of condyloma acuminatum showing vacuolated cytoplasm of koilocytotic cells (H & E, ×330).

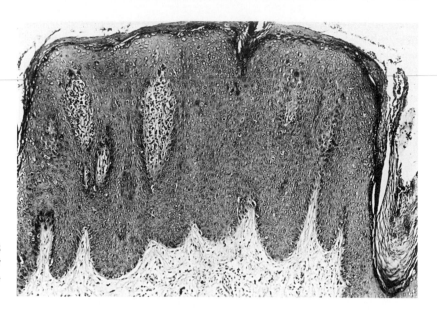

Figure 36.9 Perianal lesion of bowenoid papulosis (dysplasia) in a 31 year old woman. Note the markedly atypical but orderly squamous epithelium with nuclear uniformity (H & E, ×125).

orderly maturation of keratinocytes, greater nuclear uniformity, and milder cellular anaplasia (Fig. 36.9). Although clinical follow-up suggests that bowenoid papulosis (dysplasia) is a benign condition, it probably should be included with the spectrum of intraepithelial neoplasia (47). HPV-16 has been demonstrated in these lesions (56). In a study of vulvar lesions, many patients with these bowenoid lesions also had condylomata acuminata (54).

ADNEXAL TUMORS

Adnexal tumors of several varieties have been observed in the perianal skin. Most are of apocrine gland origin including such lesions as the apocrine gland adenoma and apocrine fibroadenoma (57, 58). Hidradenoma papilliferum, a benign sweat gland tumor usually found in the vulva, may also occur in the anal region.

KERATOACANTHOMA

Keratoacanthoma is a benign exophytic tumor of skin usually found on sun-exposed surfaces such as the dorsum of the hands and the face. Rare examples from the anal region have been described (59, 60). Just as in lesions of sun-exposed skin, it is important to distinguish this rapidly growing, "infiltrative" but clinically benign tumor from squamous cell carcinoma.

GRANULAR CELL TUMOR AND NEURILEMOMA

Granular cell tumors (myoblastomas) are common benign tumors that occur in a wide range of tissues and organs. The anal region is an infrequent site (61, 62). The lesions are composed of plump, granular cells that show diastase-resistant positivity with the periodic acid-Schiff (PAS) method. Although it was originally believed that the tumor was of muscle origin, it is now generally believed but not conclusively proved that the lesions are derived from Schwann's cells. A feature of special significance in granular cell tumors arising beneath mucosal surfaces is the frequent presence of pseudoepitheliomatous hyperplasia of the overlying epithelium (Fig. 36.10). Other benign neural tumors such as neurilemomas have also been described in the anal area (63).

LEIOMYOMA

Other benign lesions derived from mesenchymal tissue can also arise in this area. We have seen rare examples of leiomyoma arising from the internal sphincter, and a few others have been reported (64, 65).

OLEOGRANULOMA

Oleogranuloma is a benign reactive process that may grossly simulate a neoplasm. These lesions usually present as submucosal nodules in the lower rectum or anal canal, but ulcerated and annular lesions have also been described (66). The lesion is a foreign body reaction to oily substances most commonly employed in the injection of hemorrhoids. Histologically there are lipid granulomas with associated inflammation and fibrosis (Fig. 36.11).

MALIGNANT TUMORS

GENERAL CONSIDERATIONS

Before proceeding with a discussion of individual malignant neoplasms arising in the anal region, general considerations relating to the confusing subject of anal carcinoma will be addressed. The classification of malignant epithelial tumors of this region is complicated by an inadequate appreciation of the microscopic anatomy of the area as well as the related multiplicity of microscopic patterns expressed by these neoplasms.

The histologic junction between anus and rectum is not an abrupt interface between the squamous epithelium of the anal canal and the columnar, glandular mucosa of the lower rectum. Rather, there is an irregular, intervening "transitional" zone of presumed cloacogenic derivation. The existence of this special mucosa has been recognized for more than 100 years (67). However, it was not until more than 75 years had passed that it was suggested that neoplasms of a characteristic but varied histologic type arose from this epithelium (68). The term *transitional cloacogenic carcinoma* was proposed for these neoplasms. A host of descriptive terms has been used subsequently to designate members of this family of tumors including basaloid, transitional, nonkeratinizing squamous cell, cloacogenic, and mucoepidermoid carcinoma. It is appropriate to recognize this multiplicity of microscopic patterns of anal carcinoma as a reflection of the histologic variability of the transitional zone. The uncommon adenocarcinomas, the rare small cell anaplastic carcinoma, and other unusual malignant tumors of the region will be addressed later.

It is likely that the subject of anal carcinoma has been made unnecessarily complicated by focusing too much attention on the diverse histologic characteristics of these tumors. The vast majority of tumors in this region are variants of squamous carcinoma (69). They are uncommon tumors, representing only 2 to 4% of distal large bowel cancers. It should be emphasized that the most important issue is the site of origin of these tumors, that is, the distinction between tumors arising above or below the dentate line.

CARCINOMA ARISING ABOVE THE DENTATE LINE

These tumors are sometimes referred to as neoplasms of the anal canal proper and are nearly three times more common than tumors arising below the dentate line (squamous zone, pecten, or anal margin) (68). They arise grossly above or mainly above the dentate line. They arise from the mucous membrane of the upper anal canal (the ATZ) and include those neoplasms designated as cloacogenic carcinoma. They may be grossly indistinguishable from adenocarcinoma of the lower rectum. It may be difficult to ascertain the precise origin of the tumor grossly and endoscopically because these tumors may be large and obliterate normal anatomic landmarks. Tumors may extend proximally and/or distally and by biopsy may occasionally seem to arise from a site different from their true anatomic origin.

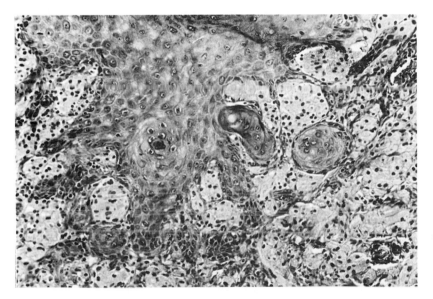

Figure 36.10 Granular cell tumor of the anal canal with pseudoepitheliomatous hyperplasia of the overlying squamous mucosa. The granular cells are noted between nests of proliferating squamous epithelium (H & E, ×320).

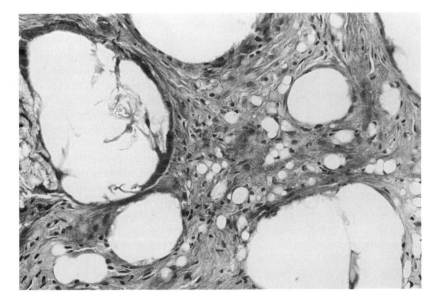

Figure 36.11 Oleogranuloma characterized by compressed empty spaces surrounded by flattened giant cells. Intervening tissue is fibrotic with smaller spaces that contained lipid droplets prior to processing (H & E ×330).

Anal canal carcinoma arising above the dentate line is two to three times more common in women than men, and the average age in most series is from 55 to 60 years (70–75). Common presenting symptoms are bleeding, anal pain, change in bowel habit, sensation of a mass, and pruritus ani. Treatment and survival data have been addressed in detail in several recent publications (71, 76–78). Of particular interest has been the change in therapeutic management of anal canal carcinoma during the past 20 years (79). This has also affected the ability of the pathologist to accurately assess the site of origin of anal carcinoma since most patients undergo combination chemoradiation therapy following biopsy diagnosis and clinical staging. Thus, the pathologist rarely has an opportunity to examine a resection specimen because of the rather impressive results of current combined chemoradiation therapy.

The most important prognostic indicators are depth of invasion and extent of spread of tumor. Various centers presenting series have developed their own staging schemes generally based on depth of invasion and extent of tumor (71–73). Anal canal carcinomas arising above the dentate line spread commonly into the lower one-third of the rectum and commonly involve the perirectal and later the inguinal lymph nodes. Specific histologic type has generally not been a significant predictor of survival, but differentiation has been useful and correlates with frequency of lymph nodes metastases (68, 80). The American Joint Committee on Cancer (AJCC) has developed universal staging systems for all anatomic sites including the anal canal (Tables 36.1 and 36.2) (5). This staging system recognizes the importance of clinical staging as well as the difficulty in pathologic assessment of extent of tumor due both to the frequent alteration of tumor appearance by radiation and chemotherapy as well as the infrequent opportunity for the pathologist to examine resection specimens. Assessment of the primary tumor (T) is based mainly on size, recognizing that for most histologic types the diameter of tumor correlates with the depth of invasion. It is hoped that widespread use of this common staging system will permit easier comparison of data concerning therapy and prognosis.

CARCINOMA ARISING BELOW THE DENTATE LINE

These carcinomas arise from the nonkeratinized squamous epithelium of the pecten (traditionally called anal margin) and the vast majority are typical squamous carcinoma. Tumors at this site are about four times more common in men than in women. Clinically, early lesions present as small, firm nodules, whereas more advanced tumors are often ulcerated. Verrucous forms of squamous cell carcinoma may also occur at this site. Coexisting conditions are more common in association with cancers of the distal canal and anal margin than of more proximal anal canal (81). These include condyloma, chronic fistulae, chronic pruritus, and a history of previous radiation treatment. Coexisting Bowen's disease may also occur. Carcinoma of the distal canal and anal margin grows more slowly than more proximal tumors, is more amenable to local treatment, and generally has a better prognosis. Anal margin tumors that arise from the most distal anal canal as defined in the AJCC TNM staging system—that is, the junction of the hair-bearing skin and the mucous membrane of the anal canal—are staged according to the system used for skin cancers (5). Metastases to inguinal lymph nodes may occur, but visceral metastases are uncommon.

TABLE 36.1	TNM Components in the American Joint Committee on Cancer (AJCC) for Staging Cancer of the Anal Canal

Primary Tumor (T)

TX	Primary tumor cannot be assessed
T0	No evidence of primary tumor
Tis	Carcinoma *in situ*
T1	Tumor 2 cm or less in greatest dimension
T2	Tumor more than 2 cm but not more than 5 cm in greatest dimension
T3	Tumor more than 5 cm in greatest dimension
T4	Tumor of any size invades adjacent organ(s), e.g., vagina, urethra, bladder (involvement of sphincter muscle(s) alone is not classified at T4)

Regional Lymph Nodes (N)

NX	Regional lymph nodes cannot be assessed
N0	No regional lymph node metastasis
N1	Metastasis in perirectal lymph node(s)
N2	Metastasis in unilateral internal iliac and/or inguinal lymph node(s)
N3	Metastasis in perirectal and inguinal lymph nodes and/or bilateral internal iliac and/or inguinal lymph nodes

Distant Metastasis (M)

MX	Presence of distant metastasis cannot be assessed
M0	No distant metastasis
M1	Distant metastasis

From Beahrs OH, Henson DE, Hutter RVP, Kennedy BJ. Manual for Staging of Cancer, 4th ed. Philadelphia: JB Lippincott, 1992:83–85.

RISK FACTORS AND ETIOLOGY

One of the most interesting topics for discussion concerning squamous neoplasia of the anal region is the rapidly evolving body of information related to risk factors and etiology. Studies investigating possible etiologic factors in anal carcinoma are somewhat confusing because of the failure of some reports to distinguish between anal canal carcinoma arising above and below the dentate line. Nonetheless, several interesting observations have been made (2, 82–89). A history of *genital warts* predisposes to the development of squamous cancer high in the anal canal, especially in homosexual men. A history of other *sexually transmitted diseases*, including lymphogranuloma venereum, syphilis, gonorrhea, genital herpes, chlamydia, and HIV, has long been known to be associated with an increased risk of anal cancer. A history of other *squamous genital neoplasms*, especially of cervix, vulva, and penis, increases risk of subsequent anal cancer. The *lifetime number of sexual partners* is correlated with risk of anal cancer. *Anal receptive intercourse* increases the risk of anal cancer by 33-fold in men but only 1.8-fold in women. Anal cancer has increased by 7-fold to 10-fold in homosexual men during the past two decades and also occurs at a younger age. *Immunosuppression* dramatically increases the risk of anal cancer not only in patients with AIDS but in transplant recipients in whom risk is estimated to be 100 times greater than in the immunocompetent population (90). *Cigarette smoking* in both females (relative risk 7.7) and men (relative risk 9.4) is associated with greater risk (91). Smoking is thought to have a late-stage or promotional effect in the etiology of anogenital cancer. *Geography*, especially related to areas of extreme poverty such as in parts of India and Brazil, has been related to an increase in squamous cancer of the anal margin (2). Finally, *Crohn's disease*, when fistulae are present, increases risk for both anal squamous carcinoma and adenocarcinoma (27–29, 92, 93).

What we have been witnessing, of course, is an evolving epidemiologic and risk factor profile that is remarkably similar to that of squamous neoplasia of the genital tract. Venereal transmission is clearly suspected and members of the HPV family are the main etiologic candidates. The increased risk for anal carcinoma among homosexual males has already been mentioned (82–88). Both in situ and invasive squamous cell carcinomas have been described and malignant change has been observed in condylomata from this patient population (49). A study that histologically examined all anal tissue submitted to a surgical pathology service identified 6.7% of 180 specimens from men with epithelial atypia as opposed to only 0.85% of 118 specimens from women (87). Some of these lesions contained koilocytotic changes suggestive of infection by HPV. Of 14 men with these atypical lesions whose sexual orientation was known, 11 (79%) were homosexual. Another study demonstrated HPV antigens by immunohistochemistry in both condylomata and squamous cell carcinomas of the areas in homosexual men (88). Subsequently, a study applying a more sensitive in situ hybridization technique detected HPV messenger RNA in 12 of 18 anal carcinomas (94).

A correlation exists between viral type isolated from a lesion and its malignant potential. HPV types 6 and 11 are found most frequently in anogenital warts and may be associated with low-grade dysplasia. In contrast, HPV types 16, 18, 31, 33, and 35 are found predominantly in association with high-grade dysplasia and in

TABLE	
36.2	**Stage Groupings in AJCC TNM Classification System for Staging Cancer of the Anal Canal**

Stage Grouping			
Stage 0	Tis	N0	M0
Stage I	T1	N0	M0
Stage II	T2	N0	M0
	T3	N0	M0
Stage IIIA	T1	N1	M0
	T2	N1	M0
	T3	N1	M0
	T4	N0	M0
Stage IIIB	T4	N1	M0
	Any T	N2	M0
	Any T	N3	M0
Stage IV	Any T	Any N	M1

From Beahrs OH, Henson DE, Hutter RVP, Kennedy BJ. Manual for Staging of Cancer, 4th ed. Philadelphia: JB Lippincott, 1992:83–85.

invasive carcinoma. The frequency of HPV detection in anal carcinoma has been shown to relate to the sensitivity of the detection system (94–99). For example, HPV-16 and HPV-18 can be detected by in situ hybridization in 17 to 50% of anal carcinoma. RNA probes increase the sensitivity to over 70% and polymerase chain reaction (PCR) detects HPV DNA in 78 to 85% of tumors. The majority of cases with detectable HPV have shown type 16. It has been suggested that HPV is not detectable in the basaloid (cloacogenic) variants of anal carcinoma by in situ hybridization (100). Other investigators, however, have found positive HPV expression by more sensitive techniques, and a recent study concludes that the prevalence of HPV in anorectal squamous cell carcinoma is unrelated to the presence or absence of a basaloid pattern (99). Another interesting observation has been that HPV-positive anal cancers tend to occur at a younger age than HPV-negative tumors (98).

HISTOLOGIC FEATURES

Carcinomas of anal canal arising above the dentate line are felt to develop from the mucosa of the ATZ and their microscopic patterns reflect the diverse histology of that epithelium. The majority of these tumors are nonkeratinizing squamous carcinomas similar to many lesions arising in the more distal anal canal pecten (Fig. 36.12). Others have a more widely varied histologic appearance that includes the basaloid (cloacogenic or transitional) variant. So-called "cloacogenic" carcinoma was defined as a tumor of the upper anal canal believed to arise from the transitional zone epithelium. Grinvalsky and Helwig were the first to suggest the potential of this special epithelium for giving rise to neoplasms histologically distinct from usual squamous cell (epidermoid) carcinoma (3). Others also have supported the contention that cloacogenic carcinoma is a distinct clinicopathologic entity (70, 100–102). Electron microscopic observations have suggested that both anal transitional epithelium and cloacogenic carcinoma are morphologically different from urothelium and squamous epithelium (102). A confusing profusion of descriptive terms has evolved, sometimes as synonyms for cloacogenic carcinoma and sometimes to define specific histologic subtypes. These include basaloid, transitional, nonkeratinizing squamous cell (epidermoid), and mucoepidermoid carcinoma (squamous carcinoma with mucinous microcysts). The most common designation for this "cloacogenic" histologic pattern currently is squamous carcinoma of basaloid type. Despite the fact that there may still be some controversy concerning the basaloid or cloacogenic histologic pattern as a specific subtype, the majority of observers support the position that they are variants of squamous carcinoma.

Low power view frequently shows an irregular, angulated, and trabeculated pattern (Fig. 36.13). Regardless of the dominant histologic pattern, foci of typical squamous differentiation are usually observed. One or more histologic subtypes may dominate the microscopic appearance, especially at higher power (Fig. 36.14). Basaloid or transitional patterns consist of nests and trabeculae of small cells without obvious intercellular bridges. Some observers reserve the term *basaloid* for tumors with recognizable palisading of cells at the periphery of the nests, a feature somewhat reminiscent of cutaneous basal cell carcinoma. Those without palisading have been morphologically compared with transitional cell tumors of urothelium. Many of these predominantly basaloid or transitional pattern

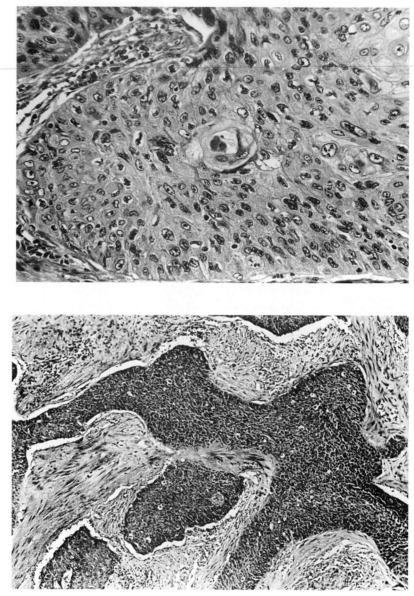

Figure 36.12 Moderately differentiated anal canal carcinoma arising from ATZ in a 65 year old woman. Tumor was a pure nonkeratinizing squamous cell carcinoma (H & E ×330).

Figure 36.13 Low-power view of invasive basaloid ("cloacogenic") carcinoma, showing a typical branching trabecular pattern (H & E, ×125).

tumors have small collections of squamoid cells or foci of indistinct pearl formation, often in the center of larger nests of tumor cells. Zones of central necrosis may also be a prominent feature. Still other tumors are characterized by the presence of small cystic or acinar foci lined by mucin-producing cells, formerly referred to as the mucoepidermoid pattern when this feature dominated. Since this pattern is usually only a minor component, many now prefer the designation of anal canal squamous or basaloid carcinoma with mucinous microcysts. Other areas may be histologically vaguely reminiscent of adenoid cystic carcinoma of salivary gland. Mitotic figures are not uncommon, but marked cellular pleomorphism is rare. It should be noted that any single tumor may show mixtures of all of these histologic patterns and should be emphasized again that most tumors will have at least some squamous differentiation. These tumors may extend proximally and/or distally. With proximal extension the tumor often undermines or ulcerates the columnar mucosa of the contiguous rectum further obscuring the precise site of origin. The adjacent mucosa frequently shows foci of high grade dysplasia or carcinoma in situ (anal canal intraepithelial neoplasia, ACIN) that may extend proximally across the surface of the rectal mucosa (Fig. 36.15). It is not rare to identify several patterns of associated intraepithelial neoplasia, with the more proximal component being basaloid and the more distal being typically squamous.

Neoplasms of this type may also occasionally arise from the anal duct epithelium, which shares a common embryologic origin with the ATZ. With large bulky tumors it may be difficult to identify the precise site of origin. Interestingly, some small lesions rarely may be associated with in situ carcinomatous changes of both anal duct and ATZ zone epithelium (55).

The significance of tumor grading and staging of anal canal carcinoma has been previously addressed. As noted, the degree of differentiation appears to be more significant than the specific subtype. It has also been observed that tumors with mucinous microcysts or pseudoadenoid cystic differentiation have a poorer prognosis (69, 77). Recent studies have also suggested that DNA ploidy may be an independent predictor of behavior (77).

Poorly differentiated basaloid carcinomas of the anal canal must also be distinguished from *small cell anaplastic neuroendocrine carcinoma* that may rarely arise in the distal rectum and extend into the contiguous anal canal (Fig. 36.16). These tumors resemble small cell carcinomas arising in other sites and tend to be highly aggressive neoplasms with early dissemination, especially to liver (103, 104). Distinction from the basaloid variant of anal squamous carcinoma often requires immunohistochemical or ultrastructural demonstration of neuroendocrine differentiation.

Carcinomas arising below the dentate line (pecten) are typically pure squamous carcinoma of ordinary type, although rare tumors with basaloid (cloacogenic) features may occur at this site. There is a tendency for the degree of differentiation and keratinization to be greater in tumors arising more distally (anal margin) (Fig. 36.17). Location is important because these pure squamous cell lesions, especially if small, are more amenable to local excision. As already noted, the AJCC TNM staging system classifies the distal (anal margin) tumors together with skin cancers.

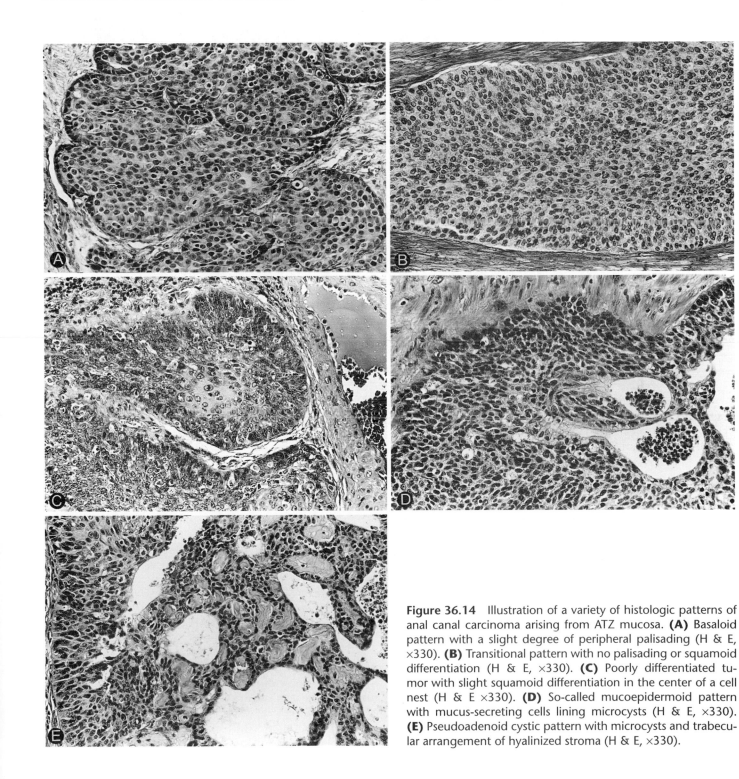

Figure 36.14 Illustration of a variety of histologic patterns of anal canal carcinoma arising from ATZ mucosa. **(A)** Basaloid pattern with a slight degree of peripheral palisading (H & E, ×330). **(B)** Transitional pattern with no palisading or squamoid differentiation (H & E, ×330). **(C)** Poorly differentiated tumor with slight squamoid differentiation in the center of a cell nest (H & E ×330). **(D)** So-called mucoepidermoid pattern with mucus-secreting cells lining microcysts (H & E, ×330). **(E)** Pseudoadenoid cystic pattern with microcysts and trabecular arrangement of hyalinized stroma (H & E, ×330).

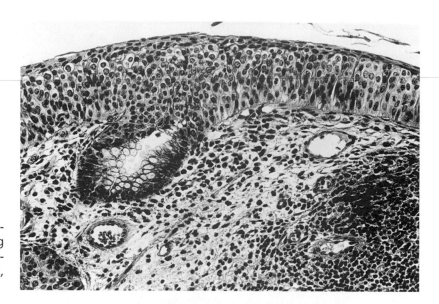

Figure 36.15 High-grade anal intraepithelial neoplasia (severe dysplasia/carcinoma in situ) extending into the lower rectum adjacent to invasive, predominantly basaloid, carcinoma of the anal canal (H & E, ×330).

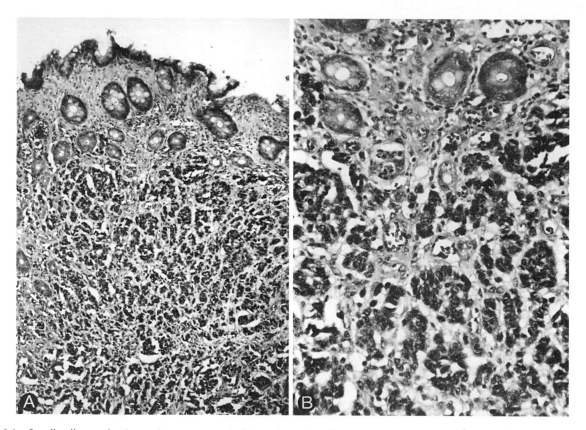

Figure 36.16 Small cell, anaplastic carcinoma extensively involving the distal rectum and anus of a 65 year old man. **(A)** Low power view showing tumor involving deep rectal mucosa (H & E, ×125). **(B)** Higher-power view showing poorly cohesive nests of anaplastic tumor cells, which were confirmed as neuroendocrine by immunohistochemistry and electron microscopy (H & E, ×330).

ANAL CANAL INTRAEPITHELIAL NEOPLASIA

Varying degrees of dysplasia including carcinoma in situ are frequently observed in mucosa adjacent to invasive carcinomas arising either above or below the dentate line (Fig. 36.15). The pattern of intraepithelial neoplasia often reflects the histologic appearance of the associated invasive lesion, that is, basaloid or typical squamous type. In keeping with terminology currently used in describing analogous lesions of other squamous epithelia, such as the lower female genital tract, the term anal canal intraepithelial neoplasia (ACIN) has been proposed (2, 105). These preinvasive changes may be seen also in the contiguous anal ducts. Similar changes also have been observed in condyloma acuminatum and in anal mucosa of homosexual men (49). Extension of perineal in situ carcinoma to the contiguous anal mucosa in women also has been reported (106).

Evidence supporting the precursor potential of this lesion is similar to that of the uterine cervix including a close histologic similarity, a younger average age than its invasive counterpart, and its extremely common occurrence adjacent to invasive cancers, especially those associated with HPV and in homosexual men. An interesting but not entirely unexpected observation is the occurrence of dysplastic mucosa in anal tissues removed for a variety of benign conditions (87, 107, 108). Its prevalence in the "general" population based on its incidental identification in minor anal surgical specimens is about 2 to 3 per 1000, but as high as 4.4% in a population that included a high proportion of young homosexual men (87). Another study describing unsuspected dysplastic changes in 2.3% of 306 surgical specimens removed for benign conditions noted no gender differences and did not comment in sexual orientation (107). In contrast to the well documented progression of HPV-associated premalignant lesions of the uterine cervix, the progression of anal intraepithelial neoplasia to invasive carcinoma appears to be rare (108). In fact, these authors conclude that incidentally discovered high-grade dysplasia in hemorrhoidal tissue is most often an innocuous, nonprogressive lesion usually cured by hemorrhoidectomy. Like its counterparts elsewhere in the anogenital region it is frequently associated with HPV infection. Another interesting but not surprising finding is the demonstration of only moderate agreement among experts in a study of interobserver variation in grading anal intraepithelial neoplasia (109).

Bowen's disease, a clinicopathologic variant of in situ squamous cell carcinoma, only rarely involves the anal region (110, 111). When anal involvement occurs, it is usually at the anal margin and adjacent perianal skin and may accompany more extensive perineal Bowen's disease. Clinically, Bowen's disease is manifested by discrete, red plaques with a scaly or fissured surface (112). Symptoms of itching and burning may occur. Histologically, the squamous epithelium exhibits striking disorganization with numerous large, atypical squamous cells and loss of normal polarity and orderly maturation (Fig. 36.18). Mitotic figures, often of markedly atypical type, may be seen at all levels of epithelium. In the perianal skin the process usually also extends for a variable distance into the epithelium of the cutaneous appendages. As noted earlier, Bowen's disease should be distinguished from the histologically similar but clinically benign bowenoid papulosis (Fig. 36.9).

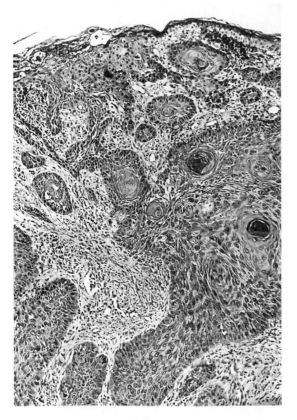

Figure 36.17 Moderately differentiated, focally keratinizing squamous cell carcinoma of the distal anal canal (anal margin) in a 64 year old man (H & E, ×125).

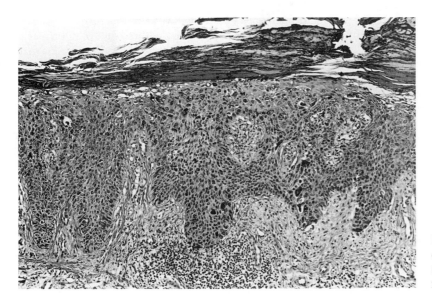

Figure 36.18 Bowen's disease (in situ squamous cell carcinoma). Note marked cellular anaplasia, disorderly maturation, and overlying parakeratotic scale (H & E, ×125).

Other Variants of Squamous Cell Carcinoma

As noted, many tumors that fit within the category of so-called cloacogenic (basaloid, transitional) carcinoma of the anal canal have variable degrees of squamous differentiation and are now generally regarded as variants of squamous cell carcinoma. The more distal lesions tend to have a greater degree of squamous differentiation. Carcinomas of the distal anal margin are typically pure squamous cell tumors, usually keratinizing, and of well-differentiated or moderately well-differentiated type (Fig. 36.17).

VERRUCOUS CARCINOMA

Verrucous carcinoma is an exceedingly well-differentiated variant of squamous cell carcinoma that occurs most commonly in the oral cavity (113). These tumors are characterized by a bulky, warty gross appearance and by a histologically benign appearance. They are locally invasive growths with pushing rather than infiltrating tumor margins. Only rare examples have been described involving the anal region (114).

GIANT CONDYLOMA ACUMINATUM

Giant condyloma acuminatum (Buschke-Loewenstein's tumor) was initially described as a tumor of the penis. Rare examples arising from the anorectal area have now been reported (115–118). These are large verrucous growths that tend to invade locally. It appears very likely that verrucous carcinoma and giant condyloma acuminatum are the same lesion (118). Furthermore, it appears that the tumor does not result from malignant transformation of a condyloma acuminatum but is a low-grade squamous cell carcinoma from its inception.

Adenocarcinoma

Adenocarcinomas of the anal region may arise from several available sources of glandular epithelium. These include the columnar mucosa of the lower rectum, the mucus-secreting cells of the ATZ epithelium, anal ducts (glands), and the apocrine glands of the perianal skin.

The most frequent type of adenocarcinoma to involve the anal region is simply a low-lying rectal cancer that extends downward into the upper anal canal. Differentiation from true anal adenocarcinoma is generally easy, as mucosal origin can usually be traced histologically to rectal columnar epithelium.

So-called cloacogenic carcinoma may show variable degrees of mucus secretion, a pattern sometimes referred to as mucoepidermoid carcinoma or anal squamous carcinoma with mucinous microcysts. These may arise from transitional epithelium of either the upper anal canal or the anal duct.

The most interesting type of primary adenocarcinoma of the anus is believed by most observers to arise from anal ducts (glands) and is known as perianal mucinous (colloid) adenocarcinoma (119–123). These are very rare neoplasms that have several clinical and pathologic features in common. They are slow-growing tumors and are frequently associated with long-standing perianal fistulae and abscesses. They arise in the deep perianal tissues without evidence of surface mucosal involvement. Presentation may be due to a painful mass in the buttock, occasionally accompanied by a gelatinous discharge. Anorectal bleeding or obstruction is not usually seen. Histologically, these are generally well-differentiated adenocarcinomas with abundant mucus production. Diagnosis requires a high degree of clinical suspicion. Multiple deep biopsies may be necessary to establish a diagnosis because the abundant mucus may make identification of tumor cells difficult. The clinical course is often followed by frequent recurrences when excision has been inadequate. Late metastases to inguinal lymph nodes may occur.

The relationship of this tumor to the commonly associated fistulae and abscesses continues to be controversial. Some believe that the perianal fistulae and abscesses antedate the carcinoma, but others believe that these typically slow-growing neoplasms undergo secondary fistulization. Most observers believe that these tumors arise from the mucous cells of anal ducts (glands). However, an alternative explanation suggests that they may arise from duplications of the lower end of the hindgut (123). Evidence offered in support of this theory is the occasional identification of normal rectal-type mucosa in anal fistulae, providing a possible epithelial source for this rare lesion. Histochemical studies of mucinous adenocarcinoma associated with chronic anal fistulae have been performed (124). In four of eight cases studied, the histochemical characteristics of the mucus were those of anal gland rather than rectal mucosa. Anal gland mucus has strong PAS reactivity, which is abolished by periodate borohydride saponification, indicating an absence or scarcity of O-acylated sialic acids.

Malignant Melanoma

Although rare, the anus is the third most common site after skin and eye of malignant melanoma, and the most common primary site in the gastrointestinal tract. Several excellent reviews of this tumor have been published (125–130). The median age (55 to 60 years) is similar to that of anal carcinoma. Reports of the largest numbers of cases suggest an approximately equal sex distribution. Bleeding is the most common presenting clinical symptom, followed by a mass, change in bowel habit, and pain.

Grossly, primary malignant melanoma of the anal canal usually appears as a polypoid mass that may be smooth or ulcerated. The average lesion measures 3 to 4 cm in diameter (129, 130). About two-thirds are grossly pigmented. The most common site of origin is at the dentate line and contiguous transitional zone. Pigment-producing cells have been identified at these sites in normal anal mucosa (7). Satellite nodules may be seen. Clinically the lesion may be confused with thrombosed hemorrhoids. Because extension of the growth into the lower rectum is common, a gross distinction between nonpigmented malignant melanoma and carcinoma of the anal canal or lower rectum is very difficult.

Histologically, malignant melanoma of the anal canal resembles its cutaneous counterpart (Fig. 36.19). Junctional involvement, either overlying or adjacent to extension is often of the acral-lentiginous type similar to other primary mucosal melanomas (128). In the absence of melanin pigment or identifiable lentiginous junctional change, differentiation from a poorly differentiated anal carcinoma may be very difficult. Adjunctive techniques such as electron microscopy or the immunohistochemical demonstration of S-100 protein or cytoplasmic melanoma antigen (HMB45) may also aid in establishing a correct diagnosis.

Anal malignant melanoma is a highly aggressive and usually lethal tumor. More than one-half of patients have evidence of

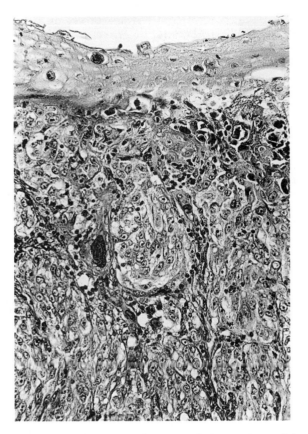

Figure 36.19 Malignant melanoma of the anal canal in an elderly woman. The lesion presented clinically as a prolapsing, pigmented mass (H & E, ×330).

metastasis at the time of diagnosis. The most common metastatic sites are the regional lymph nodes followed by liver and lung. The overall 5-year survival rate is 10 to 15% in most series.

EXTRAMAMMARY PAGET'S DISEASE

The most common site of involvement in extramammary Paget's disease is the vulva and contiguous perineal skin of postmenopausal white women. Much less commonly affected are sites such as the scrotum and axilla. Involvement of the contiguous perianal skin may also occur, but disease that is limited to perianal skin is rare. The clinical appearance of extramammary Paget's disease has been well described (131, 132). The typical lesions are erythematous patches or plaques, which may be scaly, crusted, eroded, or even ulcerated. Pruritus is common. The lesions vary greatly in size, and microscopic evidence of disease may extend beyond the grossly recognized limits of involvement.

Histologically, the disorder is characterized by the presence of large, cytologically malignant cells with pale, granular, and vacuolated cytoplasm scattered within the epidermis and sometimes the underlying cutaneous appendages (Fig. 36.20). The cells tend to be more numerous in the basal region, where they may form intraepidemal acinar structures. The involved epidermis may also show hyperkeratosis, parakeratosis, and acanthosis. The important differential diagnosis is distinction of extramammary Paget's disease from pagetoid malignant melanoma and Bowen's disease. An important

feature of the Paget's cell is the presence of cytoplasmic acid mucopolysaccharide, which may be demonstrated by a variety of special stains. Studies have also reported the immunohistochemical detection of carcinoembryonic antigen (CEA) in Paget's cells (133). The presence of melanin pigment within pagetoid cells does not establish a diagnosis of malignant melanoma, as melanin granules are occasionally seen both in Paget's cells and the neoplastic keratinocytes of Bowen's disease. Other differential diagnostic features of these disorders have been well described (132). The histologic appearance of mammary and extramammary Paget's disease is the same.

The histogenesis and pathogenesis of extramammary Paget's disease remain controversial topics. The area of greatest agreement is that the Paget's cell is a secretory (glandular) epithelial cell. It is well known that mammary Paget's disease is virtually always associated with an underlying ductal carcinoma of the breast. This constant association with an underlying carcinoma does not obtain in extramammary disease (131, 132). In fact, there appear to be variations in this association depending on the site of extramammary involvement. For example, in one series, 86% of 14 cases with perianal disease had underlying adnexal or visceral carcinomas, whereas a similar association was noted in only 33% of patients with nonperianal extramammary Paget's disease (131).

The most frequently espoused concepts of the nature of this disease suggest that (1) there is migration of Paget's cells into the epidermis from an underlying carcinoma or (2) the origin of the Paget's cells in the epidermis occurs independently or concomitantly with an underlying carcinoma (55). Most observers now regard extramammary Paget's disease as a form of intraepithelial adenocarcinoma that may progress to invasion of adjacent stroma. Another area of incompletely resolved controversy is the histogenetic source of the Paget's cells. Some favor an eccrine sweat gland origin, and others believe they arise from apocrine gland epithelium. Recent immunohistochemical demonstration of gross cystic disease fluid protein (GCDFP), a marker of apocrine epithelium, supports the most widely held view that extramammary Paget's disease is of apocrine cell derivation (134, 135). However, a recent report describes a patient with perianal Paget's disease occurring 8 months following resection of a low-lying rectal adenocarcinoma (136). There was virtually complete agreement between the immunohistochemical staining profile for both lesions suggesting that perianal Paget's disease may in some cases result from pagetoid spread from an underlying neoplasm.

BASAL CELL CARCINOMA

Basal cell carcinoma of the anus is a rare tumor that arises in the perianal skin. It is similar to cutaneous basal cell carcinoma arising in other sites and must be distinguished from a well-differentiated basaloid form of cloacogenic carcinoma of the anal canal (Fig. 36.21) (137, 138). The typical gross presentation is an ulcerated nodule with raised, pearly margins similar to that of other cutaneous basal cell carcinomas. The behavior is also similar to that of the usual basal cell carcinoma and distinctly different from that of carcinoma of the anal canal. Histologically, anal canal carcinoma of the basaloid type tends to have more cytologic atypia and greater numbers of mitoses than does basal cell carcinoma, but differential diagnosis may sometimes depend upon demonstration of the anal canal mucosal or perianal cutaneous origin of the particular neoplasm in question.

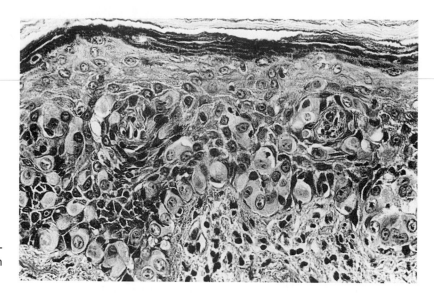

Figure 36.20 Perianal extramammary Paget's disease. Note the pale, granular cells singly and in nests in the basal portion of the epidermis (H & E, ×330).

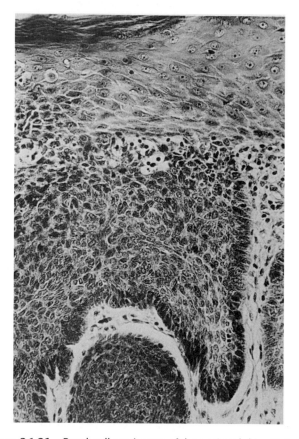

Figure 36.21 Basal-cell carcinoma of the perianal skin. Note the origin from the basal zone of the epidermis and the pronounced palisading of the cells at the periphery (H & E, ×330).

OTHER MALIGNANT TUMORS

Several other rare malignant tumors may arise in the anal region. A few cases of sarcomatoid carcinoma of the anus have been reported (139–141). Like their counterparts elsewhere, these tumors tend to be grossly polypoid and microscopically show carcinomatous areas in close approximation or admixed with the mesenchymal elements. Immunohistochemical and/or ultrastructural studies usually provide evidence of epithelial differentiation. The current general consensus is that most of these biphasic tumors are carcinomas with variable mesenchymal-like differentiation (142). However, a recent report describes an example of an aggressive anal tumor with documented neuroendocrine and rhabdomyoblastic features (141).

Leiomyosarcoma of the anorectal area has been described (65). It has been observed that not all stromal tumors of the anorectal region are malignant (143). It appears that while features such as location within muscularis propria, size, atypia, and tumor cell necrosis suggest malignancy, mitotic activity is the most important criterion indicative of aggressive behavior. Rare examples of embryonal rhabdomyosarcoma, usually of the botryoid type, have been seen in children (144). An anal mass has been reported as the presenting sign in a case of chronic lymphocytic leukemia (145).

Tumors from other sites may also secondarily involve the anus either as a result of metastasis or direct extension. The most common source of metastatic tumor of the anus is colorectal carcinoma. Extremely rare sources of metastatic disease such as the breast have also been reported (146). Direct extension of cancer to the anal and perianal tissue may occur from any site in the region including the lower urinary and genital tracts and the lower bowel.

REFERENCES

1. Fenger C. Histology of the anal canal. Am J Surg Pathol 1988;12:41–55.
2. Fenger C. Anal neoplasia and its precursors: facts and controversies. Sem Diag Pathol 1991;8:190–201.
3. Grinvalsky HT, Helwig EB. Carcinoma of the anorectal junction: histologic considerations. Cancer 1956;9:480–488.
4. Fenger C. The anal transitional zone: location and extent. Acta Pathol Microbiol Scand [A] 1979;87:379–386.
5. Beahrs OH, Henson DE, Hutter RVP, Kennedy BJ. Manual for staging of cancer. 4th ed. Philadelphia: JB Lippincott; 1992:83–85.
6. Fenger C, Knoth M. The anal transitional zone: a scanning and transmission electron microscopic investigation of the mucosal surface. Ultrastruct Pathol 1981;2:163–173.
7. Fenger C, Lyon H. Endocrine cells and melanin-containing cells in the anal canal epithelium. Histochem J 1982;14:631–639.

8. Lieberman D. Common anorectal disorders. Ann Intern Med 1984;101:837–846.
9. Fry RD, Kodner IJ. Anorectal disorders. Clin Symp 1985;37:2–32.
10. Santulli TV, Kiesewetter WB, Bill AH Jr. Anorectal anomalies: a suggested international classification. J Pediatr Surg 1970;5:281–287.
11. Parrott TS. Urologic implications of anorectal malformations. Urol Clin North Am 1985;12:13–21.
12. Moazam F, Talbert JL. Congenital anorectal malformations: harbingers of sacrococcygeal teratomas. Arch Surg 1985;120:856–859.
13. Thomson WH. The nature of hemorrhoids. Br J Surg 1975;62:542–552.
14. Haas PA, Fox TA Jr, Haas GP. The pathogenesis of hemorrhoids. Dis Colon Rectum 1984;27:442–450.
15. Rutter KRP, Riddell RH. The solitary ulcer of the rectum syndrome. Clin Gastroenterol 1975;4:505–530.
16. duBoulay CEH, Fairbrother J, Isaacson PG. Mucosal prolapse syndrome: a unifying concept for solitary ulcer syndrome and related disorders. J Clin Pathol 1983;36:1264–1268.
17. Saul SH, Sollenberger LC. Solitary rectal ulcer syndrome: its clinical and pathological underdiagnosis. Am J Surg Pathol 1985;9:411–421.
18. Lobert PF, Appelman HD. Inflammatory cloacogenic polyp: a unique inflammatory lesion of the anal transitional zone. Am J Surg Pathol 1981;5:761–766.
19. Schinella RA. Stromal atypia in anal papillae. Dis Colon Rectum 1976;19:611 613.
20. Parks AG, Gordon PH, Hardcastle JD. A classification of fistula-in ano. Br J Surg 1976;63:1–12.
21. Hanley PH. Anorectal abscess fistula. Surg Clin North Am 1978;58:487–503.
22. Culp CE. Chronic hidradenitis suppurativa of the anal canal: a surgical skin disease. Dis Colon Rectum 1983;26:669–676.
23. Alexander-Williams J, Buchmann P. Perianal Crohn's disease. World J Surg 1980;4:203–208.
24. Williams DR, Coller JA, Corman ML, et al. Anal complications in Crohn's disease. Dis Colon Rectum 1981;24:22–24.
25. Lockhart-Mummery HE. Anal lesions in Crohn's disease. Br J Surg 1985;72:S95–S96.
26. Gray BK, Lockhart-Mummery HE, Morson BC. Crohn's disease of the anal region. Gut 1965;6:515–524.
27. Daley JJ, Madrazo A. Anal Crohn's disease with carcinoma in situ. Dig Dis Sci 1980;25:464–466.
28. Preston DM, Fiona EF, Lennard Jones JE, Hawley PR. Carcinoma of the anus in Crohn's disease. Br J Surg 1983;70:346–347.
29. Slater G. Greenstein A, Aufses AH Jr. Anal carcinoma in patients with Crohn's disease. Ann Surg 1984;199:348–350.
30. Catterall RD. Sexually transmitted diseases of the anus and rectum. Clin Gastroenterol 1975;4:659–669.
31. Quinn TC, Corey L, Chaffer RG, et al. The etiology of anorectal infections in homosexual men. Am J Med 1981;71:395–406.
32. Rompalo AM, Stamm WE. Anorectal and enteric infections in homosexual men. West J Med 1985;142:647–652.
33. Samenius B. Primary syphilis of the anorectal region. Dis Colon Rectum 1968;11:462–466.
34. Quinn TC, Lukehart SA, Goodell S, et al. Rectal mass caused by Treponema pallidum: confirmation by immunofluorescent staining. Gastroenterology 1982;82:135–139.
35. Felman YM, Nikitas JA. Anorectal gonococcal infection. NY State J Med 1980;80:231–233.
36. Nepomuceno OR, O'Grady JF, Eisenberg SW, et al. Tuberculosis of the anal canal: report of a case. Dis Colon Rectum 1971;14:313–316.
37. Alankar K, Rickert RR, Sen P, Lazaro EJ. Verrucous tuberculosis of the anal canal: report of a case. Dis Colon Rectum 1974;17:254–257.
38. Laude TA, Narayanaswamy G, Rajkumar S. Lichen sclerosus et atrophicus in an eleven year old girl: report of a case. Cutis 1980;26:78–80.
39. Colby TV. Malakoplakia: two unusual cases which presented diagnostic problems. Am J Surg Pathol 1978;2:377–382.
40. Lee FI, Costello FT, Cowley DJ, et al. Eosinophilic colitis with perianal disease. Am J Gastroenterol 1983;78:164–166.
41. Mortensen NJ, Thomson JP. Perianal abscess due to Enterobius vermicularis: report of a case. Dis Colon Rectum 1984;27:677–678.
42. Vanheuverzwyn R, Delannoy A, Michaux JL, Dive C. Anal lesions in hematologic diseases. Dis Colon Rectum 1980;23:310–312.
43. Oriel JD. Epidemiology of human papilloma viruses. In: De Palo G, Rilke F, zur Hausen H, eds. Herpes and papilloma viruses. New York: Raven Press, 1986:55–61.
44. Meisels A, Morin C, Casas-Cordero M. Human papilloma-virus infection of the uterine cervix. Int J Gynecol Pathol 1982;1:75–94.
45. Crum CP, Ikenberg H, Richart RM, Gissman L. Human papilloma-virus type 16 and early cervical neoplasia. N Engl J Med 1984;310:880–883.
46. Kadish AS, Burk RD, Kress Y, et al. Human papillomaviruses of different types of precancerous lesions of the uterine cervix: histologic, immunocytochemical and ultrastructural studies. Hum Pathol 1986;17:384–392.
47. Gissman L, Schneider A. The role of human papilloma-viruses in genital cancer. In: De Palo G, Rilke F, zur Hausen H, eds. Herpes and papilloma viruses. New York: Raven Press, 1986:15–24.
48. Oriel JD, Whimster IW. Carcinoma-in situ associated with virus-containing anal warts. Br J Dermatol 1971;84:71–73.
49. Croxson T, Chabon AB, Rorat E, Barash IM. Intraepithelial carcinoma of the anus in homosexual men. Dis Colon Rectum 1984;27:325–330.
50. Kovi J, Tillman L, Lee SM. Malignant transformation of condyloma acuminatum: a light microscopic and ultrastructural study. Am J Clin Pathol 1974;61:702–710.
51. Ejeckman GC, Idikio HA, Nayak V, Gardiner JP. Malignant transformation in an anal condyloma acuminatum. Can J Surg 1983;26:170–173.
52. Connors RC, Ackerman AB. Histologic pseudomalignancies of the skin. Arch Dermatol 1976;112:167–180.
53. Wade TR, Kopf AW, Ackerman AB. Bowenoid papulosis of the penis. Cancer 1978;42:1890–1903.
54. Ulbright TM, Stehman FB, Roth LM, et al. Bowenoid dysplasia of the vulva. Cancer 1982;50:2910–2919.
55. Helwig EB. Neoplasms of the anus. In: Norris HT, ed. Pathology of the colon, small intestine and anus. New York: Churchill Livingstone, 1983:303–327.
56. Gross G, Hagedorn M, Ikenberg H, et al. Bowenoid papulosis: presence of human papillomavirus (HPV) structural antigens and HPV 16-related DNA sequences. Arch Dermatol 1985;121:858–863.
57. Weigand DA, Burgdorf WHC. Perianal apocrine gland adenoma. Arch Dermatol 1980;116:1051–1053.
58. Assor D, Davis JB. Multiple apocrine fibroadenomas of the anal skin. Am J Clin Pathol 1977;68:397–399.
59. Elliott GB, Fisher BK. Perianal keratoacanthoma. Arch Dermatol 1967;95:81–83.
60. Jensen SL, Sjolin K E. Keratoacanthoma of the anus: report of three cases. Dis Colon Rectum 1985;28:743–745.
61. Rickert RR, Larkcy IG, Kantor EB. Granular-cell tumors (myoblastomas) of the anal region. Dis Colon Rectum 1978;21:413–417.
62. Johnston J, Helwig EB. Granular cell tumors of the gastrointestinal tract and perianal region: a study of 74 cases. Dig Dis Sci 1981;26:807–816.
63. Abel ME, Kingsley AEN, Abcarian H, et al. Anorectal neurilemomas. Dis Colon Rectum 1985;28:960–961.
64. Kalima TV, Peltokallio P. Leiomyoma of the ischioanal region: report of a case. Dis Colon Rectum 1968;11:198–200.
65. Hishida Y, Ishida M. Smooth-muscle tumors of the rectum in Japanese. Dis Colon Rectum 1974;17:226–234.
66. Hernandez V, Hernandez IA, Berthrog M. Oleogranuloma simulating carcinoma of the rectum. Dis Colon Rectum 1967;10:205–210.
67. Herrmann G, Desfosses L. Sur la muqueuse de la region cloacale du rectum. Compt Rend Acad Sci 1880;90:1301–1302.
68. Morson BC, Pang LSC. Pathology of anal cancer. Proc R Soc Med 1968;61:623–624.
69. Williams GR, Talbott IC. Anal carcinoma—a histological review. Histopathology 1994;25:507–516.
70. Klotz RG Jr, Pamukcoglu T, Souilliard DH. Transitional cloacogenic carcinoma of the anal canal: clinicopathologic study of three hundred seventy-three cases. Cancer 1967;20:1727–1745.
71. Singh R, Nime F, Mittelman A. Malignant epithelial tumors of the anal canal. Cancer 1981;48:411–415.

72. Quan SHQ. Carcinoma of the anus. Int Adv Surg Oncol 1983;6: 323–335.

73. Boman BM, Moertel CG, O'Connell MJ, et al. Carcinoma of the anal canal: a clinical and pathologic study of 188 cases. Cancer 1984;54: 114–125.

74. Dougherty BG, Evans HL. Carcinoma of the anal canal: a study of 79 cases. Am J Clin Pathol 1985;83:159–164.

75. Greenall MJ, Quan SHQ, Decosse JJ. Epidermoid cancer of the anus. Br J Surg [Suppl] 1985;72:S97–S103.

76. Clark J, Petrelli N, Herrera L, Mittelman A. Epidermoid carcinoma of the anal canal. Cancer 1986;57:400–406.

77. Shepherd NA, Scholefield JH, Love SB, et al. Prognostic factors in anal squamous carcinoma: a multivariate analysis of clinical, pathologic and flow cytometric parameters in 235 cases. Histopathology 1990;16:545–555.

78. Beck DE, Karulf RE. Combination therapy for epidermoid carcinoma of the anal canal. Dis Colon Rectum 1994;37:1118–1125.

79. Nigro ND. The force of change in the management of squamous-cell cancer of the anal canal. Dis Colon Rectum 1991;34:482–486.

80. Hardcastle JD, Bussey HJR. Results of surgical treatment of squamous cell carcinoma of the anal canal and anal margin seen at St. Mark's Hospital, 1928-66. Proc R Soc Med 1968;61:629–630.

81. Greenall MJ, Quan SHQ, Stearns MW, et al. Epidermoid cancer of the anal margin: pathologic features, treatment, and clinical results. Am J Surg 1985;149:95–100.

82. Cooper HS, Patchefsky AS, Marks G. Cloacogenic carcinoma of the anorectum in homosexual men: an observation of four cases. Dis Colon Rectum 1979;22:557–558.

83. Daling JR, Weiss NS, Klopfenstein LL, et al. Correlates of homosexual behavior and the incidence of anal cancer. JAMA 1982;247: 1988–1990.

84. Peters RK, Mack TM. Patterns of anal carcinoma by gender and marital status in Los Angeles County. Br J Cancer 1983;48:629–636.

85. Daling JR, Weiss NS, Hislop TG, et al. Sexual practices, sexually transmitted diseases, and the incidence of anal cancer. N Engl J Med 1987;317:973–977.

86. Wexner SD, Milson JW, Dailey TH. The demographics of anal cancer are changing: identification of a high-risk population. Dis Colon Rectum 1987;30:942–946.

87. Nash G, Allen W, Nash S. Atypical lesions of the anal mucosa in homosexual men. JAMA 1986;256:873–876.

88. Gal AA, Meyer PR, Taylor CR. Papillomavirus antigens in anorectal condyloma and carcinoma in homosexual men. JAMA 1987;257: 337–340.

89. Dixon AR, Pringle JH, Holmes JT, Watkin DFL. Cervical intraepithelial neoplasia and squamous cell carcinoma of the anus in sexually active women. Postgrad Med J 1991;67:557–559.

90. Penn I. Cancers of the anogenital region in renal transplant recipients. Cancer 1986;58:611–616.

91. Daling JR, Sherman KJ, Hislop TG, et al. Cigarette smoking and the risk of anogenital cancer. Am J Epidemiol 1992;135:180–189.

92. Church JM, Weakley FL, Fazio VW, et al. The relationship between fistulas in Crohn's disease and associated carcinoma. Dis Colon Rectum 1985;28:361–366.

93. Chaikhouni A, Regueyra FI, Stevens JR. Adenocarcinoma in perianal fistulas of Crohn's disease. Dis Colon Rectum 1981;24:639–643.

94. Gal AA, Saul SH, Stoler MH. In situ hybridization analysis of human papillomavirus in anal squamous cell carcinoma. Mod Pathol 1989; 2:439–443.

95. Beckmann AM, Acker R, Christiansen AE, Sherman KJ. Human papillomavirus infection in women with multicentric squamous cell neoplasia. Am J Obstet Gynecol 1991;165:1431–1437.

96. Duggan MA, Boras VF, Inove M, McGregor SE. Human papillomavirus DNA in anal carcinomas: comparison of in situ and dot blot hybridization. Am J Clin Pathol 1991;96:318–325.

97. Zaki SR, Judd R, Coffield LM, et al. Human papillomavirus infection and anal carcinoma. Am J Pathol 1992;140:1345–1355.

98. Higgins GD, Uzelin DM, Philipps GE, et al. Differing characteristics of human papillomavirus, RNA-positive and RNA-negative anal carcinomas. Cancer 1991;68:561–567.

99. Shroyer KR, Brookes CG, Markham NE, Shroyer AL. Detection of human papillomavirus in anorectal squamous cell carcinoma: corre-

100. Wolber R, Dupuis B, Thiyagaratnam P, Owen D. Anal cloacogenic and squamous carcinomas: comparative histogenic analysis using in situ hybridization for human papillomavirus DNA. Am J Surg Pathol 1990;14:176–182.

101. Levin SE, Cooperman H, Freilich M, et al. Transitional cloacogenic carcinoma of the anus. Dis Colon Rectum 1977;20:17–23.

102. Gillespie JJ, MacKay B. Histogenesis of cloacogenic carcinoma: fine structure of anal transitional epithelium and cloacogenic carcinoma. Hum Pathol 1978;9:579–587.

103. Wick MR, Weatherby RP, Weiland LH. Small cell neuroendocrine carcinoma of the colon and rectum. Hum Pathol 1987;18:9–21.

104. Burke AB, Shekitka KM, Sobin LH. Small cell carcinomas of the large intestine Am J Clin Pathol 1991;95:315–321.

105. Fenger C, Nielsen VT. Intraepithelial neoplasia in the anal canal: the appearance and relation to genital neoplasia. Acta Pathol Microbiol Immunol Scand [A] 1986;94:343–349.

106. Schlaerth JB, Morrow CP, Nalick RH, Otis G Jr. Anal involvement by carcinoma in situ of the perineum in women. Obstet Gynecol 1984;64:406–411.

107. Fenger C, Nielsen VT. Dysplastic changes in the anal canal epithelium in minor surgical specimens. Acta Pathol Microbiol Scand 1981;89: 463–465.

108. Foust RL, Dean PJ, Stoler MH, Moinuddin SM. Intraepithelial neoplasia of the anal canal in hemorrhoidal tissue: a study of 19 cases. Hum Pathol 1991;22:528–534.

109. Carter PS, Sheffield JP, Shepherd N, et al. Interobserver variation in the reporting of the histopathological grading of anal intraepithelial neoplasia. J Clin Pathol 1994;47:1032–1034.

110. Scoma JA, Levy EI. Bowen's disease of the anus: report of two cases. Dis Colon Rectum 1975;18:137–140.

111. Strauss RJ, Fazio VW. Bowen's disease of the anal and perianal area: a report and analysis of twelve cases. Am J Surg 1979;137:231–234.

112. Rickert RR, Brodkin RH, Hutter RVP. Bowen's disease. CA 1977; 27:160–166.

113. Kraus FT, Perez-Mesa C. Verrucous carcinoma: clinical and pathologic study of 105 cases involving oral cavity, larynx and genitalia. Cancer 1966;19:26–38.

114. Gingrass PJ, Burbrick MP, Hitchcock CR, et al. Anorectal verrucose squamous carcinoma: report of two cases. Dis Colon Rectum 1978;21:120–122.

115. Knoblich R, Failing JF Jr. Giant condyloma acuminatum (Buschke-Loewenstein tumor) of the rectum. Am J Clin Pathol 1967;48: 389–395.

116. Elliot MS, Werner ID, Immelman EJ, Harrison AC. Giant condyloma (Buschke-Loewenstein tumor) of the anorectum. Dis Colon Rectum 1979;22:497–500.

117. Alexander RM, Kaminsky DB. Giant condyloma acuminatum (Buschke-Loewenstein tumor) of the anus: case report and review of the literature. Dis Colon Rectum 1979;22:561–565.

118. Prioleau PG, Santa Cruz DJ, Meyer JS, Bauer WC. Verrucous carcinoma: a light and electron microscopic, autoradiographic and immunofluorescence study. Cancer 1980;45:2849–2857.

119. Prioleau PG, Allen MS Jr, Roberts T. Perianal mucinous adenocarcinoma. Cancer 1977;39:1295–1299.

120. Askin FB, Muhlendorf K, Walz BJ. Mucinous carcinoma of anal duct origin presenting clinically as a vaginal cyst. Cancer 1978;42: 566–569.

121. Honore LH. Anal gland adenocarcinoma presenting as painless scrotal swelling in a 73 year old man: a case report. J Surg Oncol 1980;15:201–207.

122. Lee SH, Zucker M, Sato T. Primary adenocarcinoma of an anal gland with secondary perianal fistulas. Hum Pathol 1981;12:1034–1036.

123. Dukes CE, Galvin C. Colloid carcinoma arising within fistulae in the anorectal region. Ann R Coll Surg Engl 1956;18:246–261.

124. Fenger C, Filipe MI. Pathology of the anal glands with special reference to their mucinous histochemistry. Acta Path Microbiol Scand [A] 1977;85:273–285.

125. Morson BC, Volkstadt H. Malignant melanoma of the anal canal. J Clin Pathol 1963;16:126–132.

126. Mason JK, Helwig EB. Ano-rectal melanoma. Cancer 1966;19: 39–50.

127. Chiu YS, Unni KK, Beart RW Jr. Malignant melanoma of the anorectum. Dis Colon Rectum 1980;23:122–124.

128. Wanebo HJ, Woodruff JM, Farr GH, Quan SH. Anorectal melanoma. Cancer 1981;47:1891–1900.

129. Cooper, PH, Mills SE, Allen MS Jr. Malignant melanoma of the anus: report of 12 patients and analysis of 255 additional cases. Dis Colon Rectum 1982;25:693–703.

130. Brady M, Kavolius JP, Quan SHQ. Anorectal melanoma: a 64 year experience at Memorial Sloan-Kettering Cancer Center. Dis Colon Rectum 1995;38:146–151.

131. Helwig EB, Graham JH. Anogenital (extramammary) Paget's disease. Cancer 1963;16:387–403.

132. Jones RE Jr, Austin C, Ackerman AB. Extramammary Paget's disease: a critical reexamination. Am J Dermatopathol 1979;1:101–132.

133. Nadji M, Morales AR, Girtanner RE, et al. Paget's disease of the skin: a unifying concept of histogenesis. Cancer 1982;50:2203–2206.

134. Mazoujian G, Pinkus GS, Haagensen DE Jr. Extramammary Paget's disease: evidence for an apocrine origin: an immunoperoxidase study of gross cystic disease fluid protein-15, carcinoembryonic antigen, and keratin proteins. Am J Surg Pathol 1984;8:43–50.

135. Merot Y, Mazoujian G, Pinkus G, et al. Extramammary Paget's disease of the perianal and perineal regions: evidence of apocrine derivation. Arch Dermatol 1985;121:750–752.

136. Miller LR, McCunniff AJ, Randall ME. An immunohistochemical study of perianal Paget's disease: possible origins and clinical implications. Cancer 1992;69:2166–2171.

137. Nielsen OV, Jensen SL. Basal cell carcinoma of the anus: a clinical study of 34 cases. Br J Surg 1981;68:856–857.

138. White WB, Schneiderman H, Sayre JT. Basal cell carcinoma of the anus: clinical and pathological distinction from cloacogenic carcinoma. J Clin Gastroenterol 1984;6:441–446.

139. Kuwano H, Iwashita A, Enjoji M. Pseudosarcomatous carcinoma of the anal canal. Dis Colon Rectum 1983;26:123–128.

140. Kalogeropoulos NK, Antonakopoulos GN, Agapitos MB, et al. Spindle cell carcinoma (pseudosarcoma) of the anus: a light, electron microscopic and immunohistochemical study of a case. Histopathology 1985;9:987–994.

141. Roncaroli F, Montironi R, Feliciotti F, et al. Sarcomatoid carcinoma of the anorectal junction with neuroendocrine and rhabdomyoblastic features. Am J Surg Pathol 1995;19:217–223.

142. Iezzoni JC, Mills SE. Sarcomatoid carcinomas (carcinosarcomas) of the gastrointestinal tract: a review. Sem Diag Pathol 1993;10:176–187.

143. Haque S, Dean PJ. Stromal neoplasms of the rectum and anal canal. Hum Pathol 1992;23:762–767.

144. Srouji MN, Donaldson MH, Chatten J, Koblenzer CS. Perianal rhabdomyosarcoma in childhood. Cancer 1976;38:1008–1012.

145. Cresson DH, Siegal GP. Chronic lymphocytic leukemia presenting as an anal mass. J Clin Gastroenterol 1985;7:83–87.

146. Dawson PM, Hershman MJ, Wood CB. Metastatic carcinoma of the breast in the anal canal. Postgrad Med J 1985;61:1081.

INDEX

Page numbers in *italics* denote figures; those followed by "t" denote tables.